CAMPBELL'S UROLOGY

■

Edited by

Patrick C. Walsh, M.D.

David Hall McConnell Professor and Director
The Johns Hopkins University School of Medicine
Urologist-in-Chief
Brady Urological Institute
The Johns Hopkins Hospital
Baltimore, Maryland

Alan B. Retik, M.D.

Professor of Surgery (Urology)
Harvard Medical School
Chief, Department of Urology
Children's Hospital
Boston, Massachusetts

E. Darracott Vaughan, Jr., M.D.

James J. Colt Professor of Urology
Cornell University Medical College
Urologist-in-Chief
The New York Hospital–Cornell Medical Center
New York, New York

Alan J. Wein, M.D.

Professor and Chair, Division of Urology
University of Pennsylvania School of Medicine
Chief of Urology
University of Pennsylvania Medical Center
Philadelphia, Pennsylvania

■

CAMPBELL'S UROLOGY

Seventh Edition

VOLUME

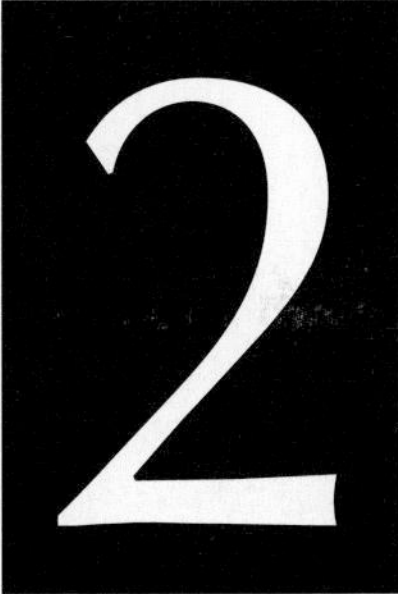

W.B. SAUNDERS COMPANY
A Division of Harcourt Brace & Company
Philadelphia London Toronto Montreal Sydney Tokyo

W.B. SAUNDERS COMPANY
A Division of Harcourt Brace & Company

The Curtis Center
Independence Square West
Philadelphia, Pennsylvania 19106

Library of Congress Cataloging-in-Publication Data

Campbell's Urology / [edited by] Patrick C. Walsh [et al.].—7th ed.

p. cm.

Includes bibliographical references and index.

ISBN 0-7216-4461-9

1. Urology. I. Campbell, Meredith F. (Meredith Fairfax). II. Walsh, Patrick C.
[DNLM: 1. Urogenital Diseases. 2. Urology—methods.
WJ 100 C192 1997]

RC871.C33 1998 616.6—dc21

DNLM/DLC 96-40836

Volume 1 ISBN 0-7216-4462-7
Volume 2 ISBN 0-7216-4463-5
Volume 3 ISBN 0-7216-4464-3
Set ISBN 0-7216-4461-9

Campbell's Urology

Printed in the United States of America

Last digit is the print number: 9 8 7 6 5 4 3 2 1

CONTRIBUTORS

Mark C. Adams, M.D.
Associate Professor of Urology and Pediatrics, Vanderbilt University School of Medicine, Vanderbilt University and The Vanderbilt University Children's Hospital, Nashville, Tennessee
AUGMENTATION CYSTOPLASTY

Ahmed Alkhunaizi, M.D.
Renal Fellow, University of Colorado School of Medicine, Denver, Colorado
ETIOLOGY, PATHOGENESIS, AND MANAGEMENT OF RENAL FAILURE

Rodney A. Appell, M.D.
Head, Section of Voiding Dysfunction and Female Urology, Department of Urology, The Cleveland Clinic Foundation, Cleveland, Ohio
PERIURETHRAL INJECTION THERAPY

Anthony Atala, M.D.
Assistant Professor, Harvard Medical School; Assistant in Surgery, Children's Hospital, Boston, Massachusetts
VESICOURETERAL REFLUX AND MEGAURETER

David M. Barrett, M.D.
Professor and Chair, Department of Urology, Mayo Clinic, Rochester, Minnesota
IMPLANTATION OF THE ARTIFICIAL GENITOURINARY SPHINCTER IN MEN AND WOMEN

John M. Barry, M.D.
Professor of Surgery and Chairman, Division of Urology and Renal Transplantation, The Oregon Health Sciences University; Staff Surgeon, University Hospital, Portland, Oregon
RENAL TRANSPLANTATION

Stuart B. Bauer, M.D.
Associate Professor of Urology, Harvard Medical School; Senior Associate in Surgery (Urology), The Children's Hospital, Boston, Massachusetts
ANOMALIES OF THE KIDNEY AND URETEROPELVIC JUNCTION
NEUROGENIC DYSFUNCTION OF THE LOWER URINARY TRACT IN CHILDREN

Arie Belldegrun, M.D.
Professor of Urology, Chief, Division of Urologic Oncology, and Director of Urological Research, Department of Urology, University of California, Los Angeles, School of Medicine, Los Angeles, California
RENAL TUMORS

Mitchell C. Benson, M.D.
Professor of Urology, Columbia University College of Physicians and Surgeons; Director, Urologic Oncology, Columbia-Presbyterian Medical Center, New York, New York
CONTINENT URINARY DIVERSION

Richard E. Berger, M.D.
Professor of Urology, University of Washington, Seattle, Washington
SEXUALLY TRANSMITTED DISEASES: THE CLASSIC DISEASES

Jerry G. Blaivas, M.D., FACS
Clinical Professor of Urology, Cornell University Medical College, The New York Hospital–Cornell Medical Center, New York, New York
URINARY INCONTINENCE: PATHOPHYSIOLOGY, EVALUATION, TREATMENT OVERVIEW, AND NONSURGICAL MANAGEMENT

David A. Bloom, M.D.
Professor of Surgery and Chief of Pediatric Urology, University of Michigan Medical School; Chief of Pediatric Urology, Mott Children's Hospital, Ann Arbor, Michigan
SURGERY OF THE SCROTUM AND TESTIS IN CHILDREN

Jon D. Blumenfeld, M.D.
Associate Professor of Medicine, Cornell University Medical College, New York, New York; Associate Attending in Medicine, Department of Medicine, The New York Hospital–Cornell Medical Center, New York, New York
RENAL PHYSIOLOGY
THE ADRENALS

Michael K. Brawer, M.D.
Professor, University of Washington; Chief, Urology Section, Seattle Veterans Administration Medical Center, Seattle, Washington
ULTRASONOGRAPHY OF THE PROSTATE AND BIOPSY

Charles B. Brendler, M.D.
Professor and Chief, Section of Urology, University of Chicago Hospitals and Pritzker School of Medicine, Chicago, Illinois
EVALUATION OF THE UROLOGIC PATIENT: HISTORY, PHYSICAL EXAMINATION, AND URINALYSIS

Gregory Broderick, M.D., FACS
Associate Professor of Surgery in Urology, University of Pennsylvania School of Medicine; Director of the Center for the Study of Male Sexual Dysfunction, University of Pennsylvania Health Systems, Philadelphia, Pennsylvania
EVALUATION AND NONSURGICAL MANAGEMENT OF ERECTILE DYSFUNCTION AND PRIAPISM

James D. Brooks, M.D.
Instructor of Urology, Department of Urology, Johns Hopkins Medical Institute, Baltimore, Maryland
ANATOMY OF THE LOWER URINARY TRACT AND MALE GENITALIA

H. Ballentine Carter, M.D.
Associate Professor of Urology and Oncology, The Johns Hopkins University School of Medicine; Department of Urology, The Johns Hopkins Hospital and Bayview Medical Center, Baltimore, Maryland
INSTRUMENTATION AND ENDOSCOPY
DIAGNOSIS AND STAGING OF PROSTATE CANCER

William Catalona, M.D.
Professor and Director, Division of Urology, Washington University School of Medicine, St. Louis, Missouri
UROTHELIAL TUMORS OF THE URINARY TRACT

Thomas S.K. Chang, Ph.D.
Associate Professor of Urology, Johns Hopkins School of Medicine, Baltimore, Maryland
PHYSIOLOGY OF MALE REPRODUCTION: THE TESTIS, EPIDIDYMIS, AND DUCTUS DEFERENS

Michael P. Chetner, M.D.
Associate Clinical Professor of Surgery and Oncology, University of Alberta; Director, Division of Urology, University of Alberta Hospital, Edmonton, Alberta, Canada
ULTRASONOGRAPHY OF THE PROSTATE AND BIOPSY

Robert L. Chevalier, M.D.
Genentech Professor of Pediatrics, University of Virginia School of Medicine; Director of Research, Children's Medical Center, University of Virginia, Health Sciences Center, Charlottesville, Virginia
RENAL FUNCTION IN THE FETUS, NEONATE, AND CHILD

Ashok Chopra, M.D.
Fellow of Reconstruction, Neurourology and Female Urology, Center for Health Sciences, University of California School of Medicine, Los Angeles, California
VAGINAL RECONSTRUCTIVE SURGERY FOR INCONTINENCE AND PROLAPSE

Ralph V. Clayman, M.D.
Professor of Urologic Surgery and Radiology, Washington University School of Medicine, St. Louis, Missouri
ENDOUROLOGY OF THE UPPER URINARY TRACT: PERCUTANEOUS RENAL AND URETERAL PROCEDURES

Donald S. Coffey, Ph.D.
Professor of Urology, Oncology, Pharmacology, and Experimental Therapeutics, Department of Urology, The Johns Hopkins Medical Institute, Baltimore, Maryland
THE MOLECULAR BIOLOGY, ENDOCRINOLOGY, AND PHYSIOLOGY OF THE PROSTATE AND SEMINAL VESICLES

Arnold Colodny, M.D.
Clinical Professor of Surgery, Harvard Medical School; Senior Surgeon and Associate Director of Urology, Boston Children's Hospital, Boston, Massachusetts
SURGERY OF THE SCROTUM AND TESTIS IN CHILDREN

Carlos Cordon-Cardo, M.D., Ph.D.
Associate Professor, Cornell University Medical Center; Director, Division of Molecular Pathology, Memorial Sloan-Kettering Cancer Center, New York, New York
AN OVERVIEW OF CANCER BIOLOGY

Jean B. deKernion, M.D.
Professor of Surgery/Urology, University of California, Los Angeles, School of Medicine; The Fran and Ray Stark Professor of Urology and Chairman, Department of Urology, UCLA Medical Center, Los Angeles, California
RENAL TUMORS

Charles J. Devine, M.D.
Professor of Urology, Eastern Virginia Medical School, Norfolk, Virginia
SURGERY OF THE PENIS AND URETHRA

William C. De Wolf, M.D.
Professor of Surgery, Harvard Medical School; Urologist-in-Chief, Division of Urology, Beth Israel Deaconess Medical Center, Boston, Massachusetts
PRINCIPLES OF MOLECULAR GENETICS

David A. Diamond, M.D.
Associate Professor of Surgery (Urology), Harvard Medical School; Associate in Surgery (Urology), Children's Hospital, Boston, Massachusetts
NEONATAL UROLOGIC EMERGENCIES

Giulio J. D'Angio, M.D.
Professor of Radiation Oncology Emeritus, University of Pennsylvania School of Medicine, Philadelphia, Pennsylvania
PEDIATRIC ONCOLOGY

George W. Drach, M.D.
Professor of Urology, University of Texas, Southwestern School of Medicine, Dallas, Texas
URINARY LITHIASIS: ETIOLOGY, DIAGNOSIS, AND MEDICAL MANAGEMENT

John W. Duckett, M.D.
Professor of Urology, University of Pennsylvania; Director of Pediatric Urology, Children's Hospital of Philadelphia, Philadelphia, Pennsylvania
HYPOSPADIAS

James A. Eastham, M.D.
Assistant Professor of Urology and Director of Urologic Oncology, Louisiana State University School of Medicine–Shreveport, Shreveport, Louisiana
RADICAL PROSTATECTOMY

Charles L. Edelstein, M.B., Ch.B., M.Med.
Renal Fellow, University of Colorado School of Medicine, Denver, Colorado; Senior Consultant Physician, Renal Unit, Department of Internal Medicine, University of Stellenbosch and The Tygerberg Hospital, Tygerberg, South Africa
ETIOLOGY, PATHOGENESIS, AND MANAGEMENT OF RENAL FAILURE

Mario A. Eisenberger, M.D.
Associate Professor of Oncology and Urology, Johns Hopkins Medical Institute, Baltimore, Maryland
CHEMOTHERAPY FOR HORMONE-RESISTANT PROSTATE CANCER

Jack S. Elder, M.D.
Professor of Urology and Pediatrics, Case Western Reserve University School of Medicine; Director of Pediatric Urology, Rainbow Babies and Children's Hospital, Cleveland, Ohio
CONGENITAL ANOMALIES OF THE GENITALIA

Jonathan I. Epstein, M.D.
Professor of Pathology, Urology, and Oncology, Johns Hopkins University School of Medicine; Associate Director of Surgical Pathology, The Johns Hopkins Hospital, Baltimore, Maryland
PATHOLOGY OF ADENOCARCINOMA OF THE PROSTATE

Audrey E. Evans, M.D.
Professor of Pediatrics, University of Pennsylvania School of Medicine, Philadelphia, Pennsylvania
PEDIATRIC ONCOLOGY

William R. Fair, M.D.
Professor of Urology, Cornell University Medical College; Chief of Urology and Vice-Chairman, Department of Surgery, Memorial Sloan-Kettering Cancer Center, New York, New York
AN OVERVIEW OF CANCER BIOLOGY

Diane Felsen, Ph.D.
Associate Research Professor of Pharmacology in Urology, Cornell University Medical College, The New York Hospital–Cornell Medical Center, New York, New York
PATHOPHYSIOLOGY OF URINARY TRACT OBSTRUCTION

Jeffrey Forman, M.D.
Professor of Radiation Oncology, Wayne State University School of Medicine, Detroit, Michigan
RADIOTHERAPY AND CRYOTHERAPY FOR PROSTATE CANCER

Jenny J. Franke, M.D.
Assistant Professor, Department of Urologic Surgery, Vanderbilt University, Nashville, Tennessee
SURGERY OF THE URETER

John P. Gearhart, M.D.
Professor of Pediatric Urology and Pediatrics, The Johns Hopkins University School of Medicine; Director of Pediatric Urology, The Johns Hopkins Hospital and Johns Hopkins Children's Center, Baltimore, Maryland
EXSTROPHY-EPISPADIAS COMPLEX AND BLADDER ANOMALIES

Robert P. Gibbons, M.D.
Chief of Staff, Section of Urology and Renal Transplantation, Virginia Mason Medical Center; Clinical Professor of Urology, University of Washington, Seattle, Washington
RADICAL PERINEAL PROSTATECTOMY

Kenneth I. Glassberg, M.D.
Professor of Urology, State University of New York, Health Science Center at Brooklyn; Director, Divisions of Pediatric Urology at University Hospital of Brooklyn, Kings County Hospital Center, Long Island College Hospital, Brooklyn; and Staten Island University Hospital, Staten Island, New York
RENAL DYSPLASIA AND CYSTIC DISEASE OF THE KIDNEY

Marc Goldstein, M.D.
Professor of Urology, Cornell University Medical College; Staff Scientist, Center for Biomedical Research, The Population Council; Attending Urologist and Director, Center for Male Reproductive Medicine and Microsurgery, Department of Urology, The New York Hospital–Cornell Medical Center, New York, New York
SURGICAL MANAGEMENT OF MALE INFERTILITY AND OTHER SCROTAL DISORDERS

Edmond T. Gonzales, Jr., M.D.
Professor of Urology, Scott Department of Urology, Baylor College of Medicine; Head, Department of Surgery, and Chief, Urology Service, Texas Children's Hospital, Houston, Texas
POSTERIOR URETHRAL VALVES AND OTHER URETHRAL ANOMALIES

Rafael Gosalbez, M.D.
Assistant Professor of Urology and Pediatrics and Chief of Pediatric Urology, Jackson Memorial Hospital, University of Miami, Miami, Florida
NEONATAL UROLOGIC EMERGENCIES

James E. Gow, M.D., Ch.M., FRCS
Late Clinical Lecturer, University of Liverpool, Liverpool, United Kingdom
GENITOURINARY TUBERCULOSIS

David Grignon, M.D.
Director of Anatomic Pathology, Harper Hospital; Associate Professor of Pathology, Detroit, Michigan
RADIOTHERAPY AND CRYOTHERAPY FOR PROSTATE CANCER

Frederick A. Gulmi, M.D.
Clinical Assistant Professor of Urology, State University of New York Health Sciences Center at Brooklyn; Associate Attending, Brookdale University Hospital and Medical Center, Brooklyn, New York
PATHOPHYSIOLOGY OF URINARY TRACT OBSTRUCTION

Philip Hanno, M.D.
Professor and Chairman, Department of Urology, Temple University School of Medicine, Philadelphia, Pennsylvania
INTERSTITIAL CYSTITIS AND RELATED DISEASES

W. Hardy Hendren, M.D., FACS, FAAP, FRCS(I)Hon.
Robert E. Gross Professor of Surgery, Harvard Medical School; Chief of Surgery, Massachusetts General Hospital; Visiting Surgeon, Children's Hospital, Boston, Massachusetts
CLOACAL MALFORMATIONS
URINARY UNDIVERSION: REFUNCTIONALIZATION OF THE PREVIOUSLY DIVERTED URINARY TRACT

Terry W. Hensle, M.D.
Professor of Urology, Columbia University, College of Physicians and Surgeons; Director of Pediatric Urology, Babies and Children's Hospital of New York, New York, New York
SURGICAL MANAGEMENT OF INTERSEXUALITY

Dianne M. Heritz, M.D., FRCSC
Lecturer, University of Toronto, Women's College Hospital, Toronto, Ontario, Canada
URINARY INCONTINENCE: PATHOPHYSIOLOGY, EVALUATION, TREATMENT OVERVIEW, AND NONSURGICAL MANAGEMENT

Harry W. Herr, M.D.
Associate Professor, Department of Urology, Cornell University Medical College; Associate Attending Surgeon, Urology Service, Department of Surgery, Memorial Sloan-Kettering Cancer Center, New York, New York
SURGERY OF PENILE AND URETHRAL CARCINOMA

Warren D. W. Heston, Ph.D.
Director, George M. O'Brien Urology Research for Prostate Cancer, Memorial Sloan-Kettering Cancer Center, New York, New York
AN OVERVIEW OF CANCER BIOLOGY

Stuart S. Howards, M.D.
Professor of Urology and Physiology, University of Virginia, Charlottesville, Virginia
MALE INFERTILITY
RENAL FUNCTION IN THE FETUS, NEONATE, AND CHILD

Jeffrey L. Huffman, M.D., M.H.A.
Professor of Urology, School of Medicine, and Associate Vice President for Health Affairs, University of Southern California, Los Angeles, California
URETEROSCOPY

Robert D. Jeffs, M.D.
Professor of Pediatric Urology and Pediatrics, The Johns Hopkins University School of Medicine, The Johns Hopkins Hospital, and Johns Hopkins Children's Center, Baltimore, Maryland
EXSTROPHY-EPISPADIAS COMPLEX AND BLADDER ANOMALIES

Gerald H. Jordan, M.D.
Professor of Urology, Eastern Virginia Medical School, Norfolk, Virginia
SURGERY OF THE PENIS AND URETHRA

John N. Kabalin, M.D.
Assistant Professor of Urology, Stanford University School of Medicine, Stanford, California
SURGICAL ANATOMY OF THE RETROPERITONEUM, KIDNEYS, AND URETERS

Louis R. Kavoussi, M.D.
Associate Professor and Director, Division of Endourology, Brady Urological Institute, The Johns Hopkins School of Medicine; Chief of Urology, Johns Hopkins Bayview Medical Center, Baltimore, Maryland
LAPAROSCOPY IN CHILDREN AND ADULTS

Michael A. Keating, M.D.
Private Practice, Orlando, Florida
VESICOURETERAL REFLUX AND MEGAURETER

William A. Kennedy II, M.D.
Fellow in Pediatric Urology, Children's Hospital of Philadelphia, Philadelphia, Pennsylvania
SURGICAL MANAGEMENT OF INTERSEXUALITY

Joseph M. Khoury, M.D.
Associate Professor of Surgery and Director, Urophysiology Division of Urology, Department of Surgery, University of North Carolina School of Medicine, Chapel Hill, North Carolina
RETROPUBIC SUSPENSION SURGERY FOR FEMALE SPHINCTERIC INCONTINENCE

Stephen A. Koff, M.D.
Professor of Surgery, The Ohio State University Medical Center; Chief, Section of Urology, Children's Hospital, Columbus, Ohio
ENURESIS

Karl J. Kreder, M.D.
Associate Professor of Urology, Department of Urology, University of Iowa Hospital and Clinics, Iowa City, Iowa
THE NEUROUROLOGIC EVALUATION

John N. Krieger, M.D.
Professor, Department of Urology, University of Washington School of Medicine; Attending Surgeon, University of Washington Medical Center, Seattle Veterans Administration Medical Center, Harborview Medical Center, and Children's Orthopedic Hospital, Seattle, Washington
ACQUIRED IMMUNODEFICIENCY SYNDROME AND RELATED CONDITIONS

Elroy D. Kursh, M.D.
Department of Urology, Cleveland Clinic, Cleveland, Ohio
EXTRINSIC OBSTRUCTION OF THE URETER

Gary E. Leach, M.D.
Associate Clinical Professor of Urology, University of California, Los Angeles; Chief of Urology, Kaiser-Permanente Medical Center, Los Angeles, California
SURGERY FOR CERVICOVAGINAL AND URETHROVAGINAL FISTULA AND URETHRAL DIVERTICULUM

Herbert Lepor, M.D.
Professor and Chairman, Department of Urology, and Professor, Department of Pharmacology, New York University School of Medicine; Urologist-in-Chief, New York University Medical Center, New York, New York
NATURAL HISTORY, EVALUATION, AND NONSURGICAL MANAGEMENT OF BENIGN PROSTATIC HYPERPLASIA

Ronald Lewis, M.D.
Professor of Surgery (Urology), Medical College of Georgia; Chief, Section of Urology, Medical College of Georgia Hospital, Augusta, Georgia
SURGERY FOR ERECTILE DYSFUNCTION

John A. Libertino, M.D.
Clinical Assistant Professor, Harvard Medical School, Boston; Chairman of Urology, Lahey Hitchcock Medical Center, Burlington, Massachusetts
RENOVASCULAR SURGERY

Mark R. Licht, M.D.
Head, Section of Sexual Dysfunction, and Staff, Department of Urology, Cleveland Clinic Florida, Ft. Lauderdale, Florida
IMPLANTATION OF THE ARTIFICIAL GENITOURINARY SPHINCTER IN MEN AND WOMEN

Peter Littrup, M.D.
Associate Professor of Radiology, Urology, and Radiation Oncology, Wayne State University School of Medicine, Detroit, Michigan
RADIOTHERAPY AND CRYOTHERAPY FOR PROSTATE CANCER

Tom F. Lue, M.D.
Professor of Urology, University of California School of Medicine, San Francisco, California
PHYSIOLOGY OF PENILE ERECTION AND PATHOPHYSIOLOGY OF ERECTILE DYSFUNCTION AND PRIAPISM
EVALUATION AND NONSURGICAL MANAGEMENT OF ERECTILE DYSFUNCTION AND PRIAPISM

Donald F. Lynch, Jr., M.D.
Associate Professor, Department of Urology, Eastern Virginia Medical School, Norfolk, Virginia
TUMORS OF THE PENIS

Max Maizels, M.D.
Professor of Urology, Northwestern University School of Medicine; Attending Pediatric Urologist, The Children's Memorial Hospital, Chicago, Illinois
NORMAL AND ANOMALOUS DEVELOPMENT OF THE URINARY TRACT

James Mandell, M.D.
Professor of Surgery and Pediatrics and Chief, Division of Urology, Albany Medical College, Albany, New York
PERINATAL UROLOGY
SEXUAL DIFFERENTIATION: NORMAL AND ABNORMAL

David J. Margolis, M.D.
Assistant Professor of Dermatology, University of Pennsylvania School of Medicine, Philadelphia, Pennsylvania
COLOR ATLAS OF GENITAL DERMATOLOGY
CUTANEOUS DISEASES OF THE MALE EXTERNAL GENITALIA

Fray F. Marshall, M.D.
Professor of Urology and Professor of Oncology, The Johns Hopkins University School of Medicine; Director, Division of Adult Urology, James Buchanan Brady Urological Institute, The Johns Hopkins Medical Institute, Baltimore, Maryland
SURGERY OF THE BLADDER

Thomas V. Martin, M.D.
Yale–New Haven Medical Center, New Haven, Connecticut
SHOCK-WAVE LITHOTRIPSY

John D. McConnell, M.D.
Professor and Chairman, Department of Urology, University of Texas Southwestern Medical Center, Dallas, Texas
EPIDEMIOLOGY, ETIOLOGY, PATHOPHYSIOLOGY, AND DIAGNOSIS OF BENIGN PROSTATIC HYPERPLASIA

David L. McCullough, M.D.
William H. Boyce Professor and Chairman of Department of Urology, Bowman Gray School of Medicine of Wake Forest University; Chief of Urology, North Carolina Baptist/Wake Forest University Medical Center, Winston-Salem, North Carolina
MINIMALLY INVASIVE TREATMENT OF BENIGN PROSTATIC HYPERPLASIA

W. Scott McDougal, M.D.
Walter S. Kerr, Jr., Professor of Urology, Harvard Medical School; Chief of Urology, Massachusetts General Hospital, Boston, Massachusetts
USE OF INTESTINAL SEGMENTS AND URINARY DIVERSION

Elspeth M. McDougall, M.D., FRCSC
Associate Professor of Urologic Surgery, Washington University School of Medicine, St. Louis, Missouri
ENDOUROLOGY OF THE UPPER URINARY TRACT: PERCUTANEOUS RENAL AND URETERAL PROCEDURES

Edward J. McGuire, M.D.
Professor and Director, Division of Urology, The University of Texas Health Science Center, Houston, Texas
PUBOVAGINAL SLINGS

Mani Menon, M.D.
Professor and Director, Division of Urology, University of Massachusetts, Worcester, Massachusetts
URINARY LITHIASIS: ETIOLOGY, DIAGNOSIS, AND MEDICAL MANAGEMENT

Edwin M. Meares, Jr., M.D.
Professor of Urology, Emeritus, Tufts University School of Medicine; Chairman, Department of Urology (Retired), New England Medical Center, Boston, Massachusetts
PROSTATITIS AND RELATED DISORDERS

Winston K. Mebust, M.D.
Valk Professor of Surgery/Urology and Chairman, Section of Urologic Surgery, University of Kansas Medical Center, Kansas City, Kansas
TRANSURETHRAL SURGERY

Edward M. Messing, M.D.
Winfield W. Scott Professor of Urology and Chairman, Department of Urology, University of Rochester Medical Center, Rochester, New York
UROTHELIAL TUMORS OF THE URINARY TRACT

James E. Montie, M.D.
Professor of Urology, University of Michigan, Ann Arbor, Michigan
RADIOTHERAPY AND CRYOTHERAPY FOR PROSTATE CANCER

Randall E. Morris, M.D.
Research Professor of Cardiothoracic Surgery and Director of Transplantation Immunology in the Department of Cardiothoracic Surgery, Stanford University School of Medicine, Stanford, California
TRANSPLANTATION IMMUNOBIOLOGY

Stephen Y. Nakada, M.D.
Assistant Professor of Surgery (Urology) and Head, Section of Endourology and Stone Disease, University of Wisconsin Medical School and University of Wisconsin Hospital and Clinics, Madison, Wisconsin

ENDOUROLOGY OF THE UPPER URINARY TRACT: PERCUTANEOUS RENAL AND URETERAL PROCEDURES

H. Norman Noe, M.D.
Professor of Urology and Chief of Pediatric Urology, University of Tennessee, Memphis; Chief of Pediatric Urology, LeBonheur Children's Medical Center, Memphis, Tennessee
RENAL DISEASE IN CHILDHOOD

Andrew C. Novick, M.D.
Professor of Surgery (Urology) Ohio State University School of Medicine; Chairman, Department of Urology, Cleveland Clinic Foundation, Cleveland, Ohio
SURGERY OF THE KIDNEY

Helen E. O'Connell, M.D.
Senior Lecturer, University of Melbourne, Department of Surgery; Attending Urologist, Royal Melbourne Hospital, Melbourne, Australia
PUBOVAGINAL SLINGS

Joseph E. Oesterling, M.D.
Professor and Urologist-in-Chief and Director, The Michigan Prostate Institute, University of Michigan, Ann Arbor, Michigan
RETROPUBIC AND SUPRAPUBIC PROSTATECTOMY

Carl A. Olsson, M.D.
John K. Lattimer Professor and Chairman, Department of Urology, College of Physicians and Surgeons of Columbia University; Director, Squier Urologic Clinic at The Columbia Presbyterian Hospital, New York, New York
CONTINENT URINARY DIVERSION

Nicholas Papanicolaou, M.D.
Professor of Clinical Radiology, Cornell University College of Medicine; Chief, Division of Abdominal Imaging, The New York Hospital–Cornell Medical Center, New York, New York
URINARY TRACT IMAGING AND INTERVENTION: BASIC PRINCIPLES

Alan W. Partin, M.D., Ph.D.
Associate Professor of Urology, Department of Urology, The Johns Hopkins Medical Institute, Baltimore, Maryland
THE MOLECULAR BIOLOGY, ENDOCRINOLOGY, AND PHYSIOLOGY OF THE PROSTATE AND SEMINAL VESICLES
DIAGNOSIS AND STAGING OF PROSTATE CANCER

Bhalchondra G. Parulkar, M.D.
Chief Resident, Division of Urological and Transplant Surgery, University of Massachusetts Medical Center, Worcester, Massachusetts
URINARY LITHIASIS: ETIOLOGY, DIAGNOSIS, AND MEDICAL MANAGEMENT

Craig A. Peters, M.D.
Assistant Professor of Surgery, Harvard Medical School; Assistant in Surgery, Children's Hospital, Boston, Massachusetts
PERINATAL UROLOGY
LAPAROSCOPY IN CHILDREN AND ADULTS

Paul C. Peters, M.D.
Professor Emeritus, University of Texas Southwestern Medical Center, Dallas, Texas
GENITOURINARY TRAUMA

Kenneth J. Pienta, M.D.
Associate Professor, University of Michigan School of Medicine, Ann Arbor, Michigan
ETIOLOGY, EPIDEMIOLOGY, AND PREVENTION OF CARCINOMA OF THE PROSTATE

Arthur T. Porter, M.D., FRCPC
Professor and Chairman, Wayne State University; Director of Clinical Care, Barbara Ann Karmanos Cancer Institute, Detroit, Michigan
RADIOTHERAPY AND CRYOTHERAPY FOR PROSTATE CANCER

Jacob Rajfer, M.D.
Professor of Surgery/Urology, University of California, Los Angeles, School of Medicine, Los Angeles; Chief, Division of Urology, Harbor–UCLA Medical Center, Torrance, California
CONGENITAL ANOMALIES OF THE TESTIS AND SCROTUM

R. Beverly Raney, M.D.
Professor of Pediatrics, University of Texas, M.D. Anderson Cancer Center, Houston, Texas
PEDIATRIC ONCOLOGY

Shlomo Raz, M.D.
Professor of Surgery/Urology, Center for Health Sciences, University of California School of Medicine, Los Angeles, Los Angeles, California
VAGINAL RECONSTRUCTIVE SURGERY FOR INCONTINENCE AND PROLAPSE

Martin I. Resnick, M.D.
Lester Persky Professor and Chairman, Department of Urology, Case Western Reserve University School of Medicine; Director, Department of Urology, University Hospitals of Cleveland, Cleveland, Ohio
EXTRINSIC OBSTRUCTION OF THE URETER

Neil M. Resnick, M.D.
Assistant Professor of Medicine, Harvard Medical School; Chief of Gerontology, Brigham and Women's Hospital, Boston, Massachusetts
GERIATRIC INCONTINENCE AND VOIDING DYSFUNCTION

Alan B. Retik, M.D.
Professor of Surgery/Urology, Harvard Medical School; Chief, Department of Urology, Children's Hospital, Boston, Massachusetts
PERINATAL UROLOGY
ANOMALIES OF THE URETER

Jerome P. Richie, M.D.
Elliott C. Cutler Professor of Surgery, Harvard Medical School; Chief of Urology, Brigham and Women's Hospital, and Chairman, Harvard Program in Urology (Longwood Area), Boston, Massachusetts
NEOPLASMS OF THE TESTIS

Richard C. Rink, M.D.
Associate Professor of Urology and Chief, Pediatric Urology, James Whitcomb Riley Hospital for Children, Indiana University School of Medicine, Indianapolis, Indiana
AUGMENTATION CYSTOPLASTY

Lauri J. Romanzi, M.D., FACOG
Assistant Professor, Cornell University Medical College; Director of Urogynecology, The New York Hospital–Cornell Medical Center, New York, New York
URINARY INCONTINENCE: PATHOPHYSIOLOGY, EVALUATION, TREATMENT OVERVIEW, AND NONSURGICAL MANAGEMENT

Shane Roy III, M.D.
Professor of Pediatrics, Section of Pediatric Nephrology, University of Tennessee, Memphis; Chief, Pediatric Nephrology, LeBonheur Children's Medical Center, Memphis, Tennessee
RENAL DISEASE IN CHILDHOOD

Thomas Rozanski, M.D.
Chief of Urology and Chief of Pediatric Urology, Brooke Army Medical Center, Ft. Sam Houston, Texas
SURGERY OF THE SCROTUM AND TESTIS IN CHILDREN

Daniel B. Rukstalis, M.D.
Chief of Urology, Allegheny University Hospital/Hahnemann, Philadelphia, Pennsylvania
PRINCIPLES OF MOLECULAR GENETICS

Arthur I. Sagalowsky, M.D.
Professor and Chief, Urologic Oncology, Department of Urology, The University of Texas Southwestern Medical Center; Attending, Zale Lipshy University Hospital, Dallas, Texas
GENITOURINARY TRAUMA

Jay I. Sandlow, M.D.
Assistant Professor, Department of Urology, The University of Iowa, Iowa City, Iowa
SURGERY OF THE SEMINAL VESICLES

Peter T. Scardino, M.D.
Russell and Mary Hugh Scott Professor and Chairman, Scott Department of Urology, Baylor College of Medicine; Chief, Urology Service, The Methodist Hospital, Houston, Texas
RADICAL PROSTATECTOMY

Anthony J. Schaeffer, M.D.
Professor and Chairman, Department of Urology, Northwestern University Medical School, Chicago, Illinois
INFECTIONS OF THE URINARY TRACT

Paul F. Schellhammer, M.D.
Professor and Chairman, Eastern Virginia Medical School, Norfolk; Active Staff, Sentara Health System: Norfolk General Hospital, Leigh Memorial Hospital, and Bayside, Norfolk and Virginia Beach, Virginia
TUMORS OF THE PENIS

Peter N. Schlegel, M.D.
Associate Professor of Urology, Cornell University Medical College; Staff Scientist, The Population Council; Associate Attending Urologist, The New York Hospital; Associate Visiting Physician, The Rockefeller University Hospital, New York, New York
PHYSIOLOGY OF MALE REPRODUCTION: THE TESTIS, EPIDIDYMIS, AND DUCTUS DEFERENS

Steven M. Schlossberg, M.D.
Professor of Urology, Eastern Virginia School of Medicine, Norfolk, Virginia
SURGERY OF THE PENIS AND URETHRA

Richard N. Schlussel, M.D.
Assistant Professor of Urology, Mount Sinai School of Medicine; Chief, Pediatric Urology, Mount Sinai Medical Center, New York, New York
ANOMALIES OF THE URETER

Robert W. Schrier, M.D.
Professor and Chairman, Department of Medicine, University of Colorado School of Medicine, Denver, Colorado
ETIOLOGY, PATHOGENESIS, AND MANAGEMENT OF RENAL FAILURE

Fritz H. Schröder, M.D.
Professor and Chairman, Department of Urology, Erasmus University, Rotterdam, The Netherlands
ENDOCRINE TREATMENT OF PROSTATE CANCER

Joseph I. Shapiro, M.D.
Associate Professor of Medicine and Radiology, University of Colorado School of Medicine, Denver, Colorado
ETIOLOGY, PATHOGENESIS, AND MANAGEMENT OF RENAL FAILURE

Linda M. Dairiki Shortliffe, M.D.
Professor and Chair of Urology, Stanford University School of Medicine; Chief of Pediatric Urology, Lucile Salter Packard Children's Hospital, Stanford, California
URINARY TRACT INFECTIONS IN INFANTS AND CHILDREN

Mark Sigman, M.D.
Assistant Professor of Urology, Brown University; Staff, Rhode Island Hospital, Veterans Administration Hospital, Providence, Rhode Island
MALE INFERTILITY

Donald G. Skinner, M.D.
Professor and Chairman, Department of Urology, University of Southern California School of Medicine, Los Angeles, California
SURGERY OF TESTICULAR NEOPLASMS

Eila C. Skinner, M.D.
Associate Professor of Clinical Urology, University of Southern California, Department of Urology, School of Medicine, Los Angeles, California
SURGERY OF TESTICULAR NEOPLASMS

Edwin A. Smith, M.D.
Assistant Clinical Professor of Surgery (Urology), Emory University School of Medicine; Attending, Egleston Children's Hospital and Scottish Rite Children's Medical Center, Atlanta, Georgia
PRUNE-BELLY SYNDROME

Jerome Hazen Smith, M.S.(Anat), M.Sc.Hyg., M.D.
Professor in Pathology, University of Texas Medical Branch; Pathologist, University of Texas Medical Branch Hospitals, Galveston, Texas
PARASITIC DISEASES OF THE GENITOURINARY SYSTEM

Joseph A. Smith, Jr., M.D.
William L. Bray Professor and Chairman, Department of Urologic Surgery, Vanderbilt University, Nashville, Tennessee
SURGERY OF THE URETER

Howard M. Snyder III, M.D.
Professor of Surgery in Urology, University of Pennsylvania School of Medicine, Philadelphia, Pennsylvania
PEDIATRIC ONCOLOGY
PRINCIPLES OF CONTINENT RECONSTRUCTION

R. Ernest Sosa, M.D.
Associate Professor of Urology, Cornell University Medical College; Associate Attending Urologist, The New York Hospital–Cornell Medical Center, New York, New York
RENOVASCULAR HYPERTENSION AND OTHER RENAL VASCULAR DISEASES
SHOCK-WAVE LITHOTRIPSY

William D. Steers, M.D.
Chairman and J.Y. Gillenwater Professor of Urology, University of Virginia School of Medicine, Charlottesville, Virginia
PHYSIOLOGY AND PHARMACOLOGY OF THE BLADDER AND URETHRA

Lynn Stothers, M.D., M.H.Sc.
Fellow of Reconstruction, Neurology, and Female Urology, Center for Health Sciences, University of California, Los Angeles, School of Medicine, Los Angeles, California
VAGINAL RECONSTRUCTIVE SURGERY FOR INCONTINENCE AND PROLAPSE

Stevan B. Streem, M.D.
Head, Section of Stone Disease and Endourology, Department of Urology, Cleveland Clinic Foundation, Cleveland, Ohio
SURGERY OF THE KIDNEY

Terry B. Strom, M.D.
Professor of Medicine, Harvard Medical School; Medical Director, Renal Transplant Service, and Director, Division of Immunology, Beth Israel Hospital; Physician, Brigham and Women's Hospital, Boston, Massachusetts
TRANSPLANTATION IMMUNOBIOLOGY

Manikkam Suthanthiran, M.D.
Professor of Medicine, Biochemistry, and Surgery, Cornell University Medical College; Chief, Division of Transplantation Medicine and Extracorporeal Therapy, and Chief, Division of Nephrology, Department of Medicine, The New York Hospital–Cornell Medical Center; Director, Immunogenetics and Transplantation Center, The Rogosin Institute, New York, New York
TRANSPLANTATION IMMUNOBIOLOGY

Ronald S. Swerdloff, M.D.
Professor of Medicine, University of California, Los Angeles, School of Medicine, Los Angeles; Chief, Division of Endocrinology, Harbor–UCLA Medical Center; Director, World Health Organization Collaborating Center of Reproduction, Torrance, California
PHYSIOLOGY OF HYPOTHALAMIC-PITUITARY FUNCTION

Brett A. Trockman, M.D.
Clinical Instructor, Department of Urology, Loyola University Medical Center, Maywood, Illinois
SURGERY FOR CERVICOVAGINAL AND URETHROVAGINAL FISTULA AND URETHRAL DIVERTICULUM

E. Darracott Vaughan, Jr., M.D.
James J. Colt Professor of Urology, Cornell University Medical College; Chairman, Department of Urology, and Attending Urologist-in-Chief, The New York Hospital–Cornell University Medical Center, New York, New York
RENAL PHYSIOLOGY
PATHOPHYSIOLOGY OF URINARY TRACT OBSTRUCTION
RENOVASCULAR HYPERTENSION AND OTHER RENAL VASCULAR DISEASES
THE ADRENALS

Franz von Lichtenberg, M.D.
Professor Emeritus of Pathology, Harvard Medical School; Senior Pathologist, Brigham and Women's Hospital, Boston, Massachusetts
PARASITIC DISEASES OF THE GENITOURINARY SYSTEM

R. Dixon Walker III, M.D.
Professor of Surgery and Pediatrics, University of Florida College of Medicine; Chief of Pediatric Urology, Shands Children's Hospital, Gainesville, Florida
EVALUATION OF THE PEDIATRIC UROLOGIC PATIENT

Patrick C. Walsh, M.D.
David Hall McConnell Professor and Director, Department of Urology, Johns Hopkins University School of Medicine; Urologist in Chief, James Buchanan Brady Urological Institute, Johns Hopkins Hospital, Baltimore, Maryland
THE NATURAL HISTORY OF LOCALIZED PROSTATE CANCER: A GUIDE TO THERAPY
ANATOMIC RADICAL RETROPUBIC PROSTATECTOMY

Christina Wang, M.D., FRACP, FRCP(Glas.)
Professor of Medicine, University of California, Los Angeles, School of Medicine, Los Angeles; Director, Clinical Study Center, Harbor–UCLA Medical Center, Torrance, California
PHYSIOLOGY OF HYPOTHALAMIC-PITUITARY FUNCTION

George D. Webster, M.B., Ch.B., FRCS
Professor of Surgery, Department of Surgery, Division of Urology, Duke University School of Medicine, Durham, North Carolina
THE NEUROUROLOGIC EVALUATION
RETROPUBIC SUSPENSION SURGERY FOR FEMALE SPHINCTERIC INCONTINENCE

Alan J. Wein, M.D.
Professor and Chair, Division of Urology, University of Pennsylvania School of Medicine; Chief of Urology, University of Pennsylvania Medical Center, Philadelphia, Pennsylvania
COLOR ATLAS OF GENITAL DERMATOLOGY
PATHOPHYSIOLOGY AND CHARACTERIZATION OF VOIDING DYSFUNCTION
NEUROMUSCULAR DYSFUNCTION OF THE LOWER URINARY TRACT AND ITS TREATMENT

Robert M. Weiss, M.D.
Professor and Chief, Section of Urology, Yale University School of Medicine, New Haven, Connecticut
PHYSIOLOGY AND PHARMACOLOGY OF THE RENAL PELVIS AND URETER

Richard D. Williams, M.D.
Professor and Head, Rubin H. Flocks Chair, Department of Urology, The University of Iowa, Iowa City, Iowa
SURGERY OF THE SEMINAL VESICLES

Gilbert J. Wise, M.D.
Professor of Urology, Health Science Center, State University of New York; Director of Urology, Maimonides Medical Center, Brooklyn, New York
FUNGAL INFECTIONS OF THE URINARY TRACT

John R. Woodard, M.D.
Clinical Professor of Surgery (Urology) and Director of Pediatric Urology, Emory University School of Medicine; Chief of Urology, Egleston Hospital for Children at Emory University, Atlanta, Georgia
PRUNE-BELLY SYNDROME

Subbarao V. Yalla, M.D.
Associate Professor of Surgery (Urology), Harvard Medical School, Boston, Massachusetts
GERIATRIC INCONTINENCE AND VOIDING DYSFUNCTION

Muhammad M. Yaqoob, M.D., Ph.D., MRCP
Consultant Nephrologist, The Royal London and St. Bartholomew's Hospitals, London, United Kingdom
ETIOLOGY, PATHOGENESIS, AND MANAGEMENT OF RENAL FAILURE

PREFACE
Seventh Edition of Campbell's Urology

The seventh edition of *Campbell's Urology* perpetuates over 70 years of association between the W.B. Saunders Company and the field of urology. In 1926, the classic textbook by Hugh Hampton Young, *Young's Practice of Urology* was first published. This was followed in 1935 by Frank Hinman Sr.'s *Textbook of Urology*. The first edition of *Campbell's Urology*, which was published in 1954, was edited by Meredith Campbell, Professor and Chairman of Urology at New York University. After his first and second editions he invited J. Hartwell Harrison to join him as a co-editor of the third edition. When Dr. Harrison expanded the editorial board for the fourth edition, the editors believed that Dr. Campbell's contribution to urology should be recognized in perpetuity by officially naming the textbook in his honor. This tradition continues today with the publication of the seventh edition.

With the field of urology undergoing rapid transformation, the editors believed that a major complete revision of *Campbell's Urology* was necessary within 5 years of publishing the last edition. This edition has been greatly expanded with the addition of 22 new chapters and 32 new authors. Dr. Alan Wein, Professor and Chairman of Urology at the University of Pennsylvania, has joined as a new editor and has added immeasurably to the sections on neuromuscular dysfunction of the urinary tract and incontinence.

In this edition we have used an organ systems orientation attempting wherever possible to aggregate physiology, pathophysiology, and medical and surgical management into individual sections, thereby providing a "mini" textbook for each subspecialty. We also believed that multidisciplinary authorship of some areas was very important, especially oncology. For this reason, you will note that prostate cancer is now subdivided into multiple chapters written by basic scientists, surgeons, medical oncologists, and radiation therapists. We have maintained an encyclopedic approach to each topic, but have encouraged the authors to use bold type to emphasize important concepts, thus making it easier to glean the essence from each chapter. Also, to make this edition more user friendly we have expanded the use of algorithms and decision trees wherever possible. Finally, this book will be accompanied by a study guide, which we have created to provide a structured approach to urologic education for residents, program directors, and certified urologists. At present, there is no structured curriculum for this purpose and it is the hope of the editors that this study guide will provide a systematic way to review many of the important areas in each field.

As we enter the 21st century it seemed appropriate to begin the book with the principles of molecular genetics, followed by the more traditional basic sciences such as anatomy. We have grouped renal physiology and pathophysiology together so that the reader can review the entire spectrum from normal physiology to the management of end-stage renal disease and hypertension. By building on a firm base of renal physiology, the reader can better understand the current thinking on acute renal failure, urinary tract obstruction, and renovascular disease.

Section V deals with the transport of urine to the lower urinary tract, normal and abnormal lower urinary tract storage and emptying, and the treatment of voiding dysfunction. Urinary incontinence is such an important topic that it and its treatment are considered in separate chapters in this section even though some overlap with other material is inevitable. Reconstructive and prosthetic surgery for sphincter incontinence are also considered separately here as well as other topics specifically related to female urology. Geriatric voiding dysfunction is likewise important enough to be accorded a separate chapter.

Sexual function and dysfunction, as well as reproductive function and dysfunction, follow in separate sections combining physiology, pathophysiology, and surgery. Benign prostatic hyperplasia represents one of the most common disorders managed by urologists. For this reason, it is now represented as a separate section with six chapters.

The entire section on pediatric urology has been reorganized, with new chapters "Evaluation of the Pediatric Urologic Patient" and "Renal Disease in Childhood." The chapter on "Normal and Anomalous Development of the Urinary Tract" has been expanded to include a section on molecular biology, and the chapter "Neonatal Urologic Emergencies" has been totally reorganized and stresses the most common conditions. In the chapter "Urinary Tract Infections in Infants and Children," there are now new sections discussing the management of girls with recurrent urinary tract infections without anatomic abnormalities and the incidence and detection of pyelonephritis in the absence of vesicoureteral reflux. Congenital disorders of the urinary tract have been subdivided into anomalies of the kidney and ureter, and the chapter "Vesicoureteral Reflux and Megaureter" has been totally rewritten with new authorship. Long-term results are now emphasized in the chapters on prune-belly syndrome, exstrophy of the bladder, cloacal malformations, and urinary undiversion.

The current approach to urinary stone disease as well as the use of emerging techniques in endourology and laparoscopy is now condensed. The chapter on the pathogenesis of urinary stone disease is immediately followed by alternatives for therapy including ESWL, ureteroscopy, and percutaneous approaches. These sections conclude with the chapter on percutaneous approaches for indications other than stone disease and an updated overview of the role of laparoscopy in both adults and children with urological problems. These chapters interface well with the following section, which is a compendium of the current status of urologic surgery, and includes open approaches to stone disease.

The editors are grateful for the support of the W.B. Saunders Company and especially to Richard Zorab, the editorial manager, who has facilitated our interactions. We also wish to express our thanks to Faith Voit, Hazel Hacker, Linda R. Garber, and the staff of the W.B. Saunders Company for their patience and help in bringing this ambitious undertaking to publication.

PATRICK C. WALSH, M.D.
For the Editors

CONTENTS

DRUG NOTICE

Medicine is an ever-changing field. Standard safety precautions must be followed, but as new research and clinical experience broaden our knowledge, changes in treatment and drug therapy become necessary or appropriate. Readers are advised to check the product information currently provided by the manufacturer of each drug to be administered to verify the recommended dose, the method and duration of administration, and contraindications. It is the responsibility of the treating physician, relying on experience and knowledge of the patient, to determine dosages and the best treatment for the patient. Neither the Publisher nor the editor assumes any responsibility for any injury and/or damage to persons or property.

The Publisher

VI
SEXUAL FUNCTION AND DYSFUNCTION

38
PHYSIOLOGY OF PENILE ERECTION AND PATHOPHYSIOLOGY OF ERECTILE DYSFUNCTION AND PRIAPISM

Tom F. Lue, M.D.

The penis does not obey the order of its master, who tries to erect or shrink it at will. Instead, the penis erects freely while its master is asleep. The penis must be said to have its own mind, by any stretch of the imagination.

LEONARDO DA VINCI

PHYSIOLOGY

Historical Aspects

The first description of erectile dysfunction dates from about 2000 B.C. and was set down on Egyptian papyrus. Two types were described: natural impotence ("the man is incapable of accomplishing the sex act"), and supernatural impotence (the result of evil charms and spells). Later, Hippocrates described many cases of male impotence among the rich inhabitants of Scythia and concluded that too much horseback riding was the cause. (The poor were not affected because they travelled on foot.) On penile erection, Aristotle stated that three branches of nerves carry spirit and energy to the penis and that erection is produced by the influx of air (Brenot, 1994). His theory was well accepted until Leonardo da Vinci (1504) noted a large amount of blood in the erect penis of hanged men and cast doubt on the concept of the air-filled penis. His writings, however, were kept secret until the beginning of this century (Brenot, 1994). Nevertheless, in 1585, in *Ten Books on Surgery* and the *Book of Reproduction*, Ambroise Pare gave an accurate description of penile anatomy and the concept of erection. He described the penis as being composed of concentric coats of nerves, veins, and arteries and of two ligaments (corpora cavernosa), a urinary tract, and four muscles. "When the man becomes inflamed with lust and desire, blood rushes into the male member and causes it to become erect." The importance of retaining blood in the penis was stressed by Dionis (1718, quoted by Brenot, 1994), who attributed this to the muscles cramping the veins at the proximal end of the penis, and by Hunter (1787), who thought that venous spasm prevented the exit of blood.

Many theories have since been added to explain the hemodynamic events that occur during erection and detumescence. In the 19th century, venous occlusion was thought to be the main factor involved in achieving and maintaining erection (Bochdalek, 1854; Waldeyer, 1899), but later investigators (Deysach, 1939; Christensen, 1954; Newman et al, 1964; Dorr and Brody, 1967) stressed the importance of increased arterial blood flow, and Newman and associates (1964), in human cadavers and volunteers, showed that erection could be induced by saline perfusion alone without venous constriction. However, radioactive xenon washout and cavernosography studies in human volunteers exposed to audiovisual sexual stimulation yielded conflicting results: Shirai and colleagues (1978) concluded that, although venous flow is increased, the markedly increased arterial flow overwhelms it; Wagner (1981) also showed increased arterial flow but concluded that venous drainage is decreased.

Even more controversial than the hemodynamics of erection is its anatomic mechanism. Various theories have been proposed to explain the erectile process: arterial polsters (Von Ebner, 1900; Kiss, 1921), arterial and venous polsters (Conti, 1952), the sluice theory (Deysach, 1939), an arteriovenous shunt (Newman et al, 1964; Newman and Northrup, 1981; Wagner et al, 1982), and contraction of the cavernous smooth muscles (Goldstein et al, 1982). Among these, Conti's hypothesis that arterial and venous polsters regulate penile blood flow is the most frequently quoted.

Since this volume's last edition, much progress has been made in the understanding of erectile function and dysfunction. In addition to the role of smooth muscle in regulating arterial and venous flow, the detailed structure of the tunica albuginea and its role in venous occlusion have been elucidated. An important breakthrough in the understanding of neural control of penile function is the identification of nitric oxide (NO) as the major neurotransmitter involved in erection. The role of endothelium in regulating smooth muscle tone and the intercellular link via gap junctions have also been clarified. In pathophysiology, the changes in the smooth muscle, endothelium, and fibroelastic framework that occur with diabetes, atherosclerosis, and aging have also been identified. These developments will be discussed in detail in this chapter.

Functional Anatomy of the Penis

The Tunica Albuginea

The tunica affords great flexibility, rigidity, and tissue strength to the penis (Hsu et al, 1992) (Fig. 38–1). **The tunical covering of the corpora cavernosa is a bilayered structure that has multiple sublayers:** (1) Inner layer bundles support and contain the cavernous tissue and are oriented circularly. Radiating from this inner layer are intracavernosal pillars (ICPs) acting as struts that augment the septum that provides essential support to the erectile tissue. (2) Outer layer bundles are oriented longitudinally, extending from the glans penis to the proximal crura; they insert into the inferior pubic ramus but are absent between the 5 and 7 o'clock positions. In contrast, the corpus spongiosum lacks an outer layer or intracorporeal struts, ensuring a low-pressure structure during erection.

The tunica is composed of elastic fibers that form an irregular, latticed network on which the collagen fibers rest. The detailed histologic composition of the tunica varies depending on anatomic location and function. Emissary veins run between the inner and outer layers for a short distance, often piercing the outer bundles in an oblique manner. Branches of the dorsal artery, however, take a more directly perpendicular route and are surrounded by a periarterial fibrous sheath.

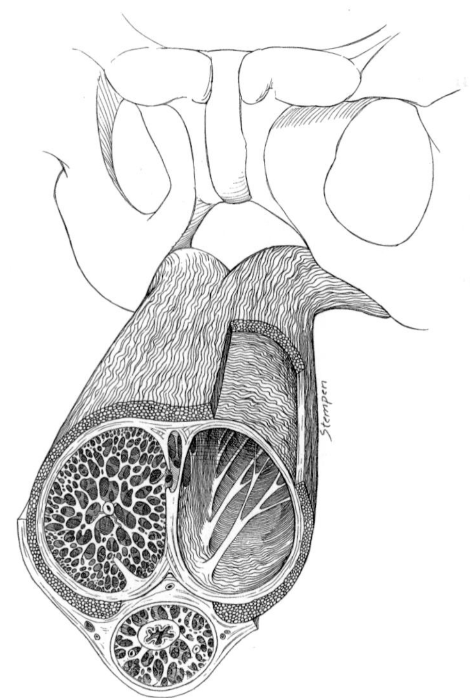

Figure 38–1. Cross section of the penis showing the intracavernous pillars supporting the erectile tissue and the inner circular and outer longitudinal layers of the tunica albuginea. The longitudinal layer is absent between the corpus cavernosum and the spongiosum. (From Lue TF, Akkus E, Kour NW: Physiology of erectile function and dysfunction. Campbell's Urology Update #12 1994; 1–10.)

The outer tunical layer appears to play an additional role in compression of the veins during erection. It also determines to a large extent variability in tunical thickness and strength (Hsu et al, 1992). At 7 o'clock the tunical thickness is 0.8 ± 0.1 mm, at 9 o'clock 1.2 ± 0.2 mm, and at 11 o'clock 2.2 ± 0.4 mm. At 3, 5, and 1 o'clock, the measurements are nearly identical in mirror-image fashion. (Differences at specific locations have been found to be statistically significant.)

The stress on the tunica before penetration has been measured as $1.6 \pm 0.2 \times 10^7$ newtons (N)/M^2 at the 7 o'clock position, $3.0 \pm 0.3 \times 10^7$ N/M^2 at 9 o'clock, and $4.5 \pm 0.5 \times 10^7$ N/M^2 at 11 o'clock.

The strength and thickness of the tunica correlate in a statistically significant way with location. The most vulnerable area is located on the ventral groove (between 5 and 7 o'clock), which lacks the longitudinally directed outer layer bundles; most prostheses tend to extrude here. Therefore, prosthesis extrusion often has an anatomic basis and is not merely a phenomenon caused by infection or compression.

Corpora Cavernosa, Corpus Spongiosum, and Glans Penis

The corpora cavernosa comprise two spongy paired cylinders contained in the thick envelope of the tunica albuginea. Their proximal ends, the crura, originate at the undersurface of the puboischial rami as two separate structures but merge under the pubic arch and remain attached up to the glans. **The septum between the two corpora cavernosa is incomplete in men** but is complete in some species, such as the dog.

The corpora cavernosa are supported by a fibrous skeleton that includes the tunica albuginea, intracavernous pillars, the intracavernous fibrous framework, and the periarterial and perineural fibrous sheath (Goldstein and Padma-Nathan, 1990; Hsu et al, 1992). Bitsch and associates (1990) believe that the intracavernous framework adds significant strength to the tunica albuginea. Within the tunica are the interconnected sinusoids separated by smooth muscle trabeculae surrounded by elastic fibers, collagen, and loose areolar tissue. The terminal cavernous nerves and helicine arteries are intimately associated with the smooth muscle. Each corpus cavernosum is a conglomeration of sinusoids, larger in the center and smaller in the periphery. In the flaccid state, the blood slowly diffuses from the central to the peripheral sinusoids, and the blood gas levels are similar to those of venous blood. During erection, the rapid entry of arterial blood into both the central and peripheral sinusoids changes the intracavernous blood gas levels to those of arterial blood. In a recent canine study, Azadzoi and associates (1995) demonstrated that subtunical oxygen tension in the penis is consistent with that of arterial blood, whereas the oxygen tension in the central portion of the corpus cavernosum is consistent with that of venous blood, suggesting that a shunting mechanism may exist.

The structure of the corpus spongiosum and glans is similar to that of the corpora cavernosa except that the sinusoids are larger; the tunica is thinner in the spongiosum (with only a circular layer [see earlier description]), and is absent in the glans.

Arterial Supply

The main source of blood supply to the penis is usually the internal pudendal artery, a branch of the internal iliac artery (Fig. 38–2). **In many instances, however, accessory arteries arising from the external iliac, obturator, vesical, and femoral arteries exist, and these may occasionally become the dominant or only arterial supply to the corpus cavernosum (Breza et al, 1989). Damage to these accessory arteries during radical prostatectomy or cystectomy may result in vasculogenic erectile dysfunction after surgery** (Aboseif et al, 1994; Kim et al, 1994). The internal pudendal artery becomes the common penile artery after giving off a branch to the perineum. The three branches of the penile artery are the dorsal, the bulbourethral, and the cavernous arteries. The cavernous artery is responsible for tumescence of the corpus cavernosum, and the dorsal artery controls engorgement of the glans penis during erection. The bulbourethral artery supplies the bulb and corpus spongiosum. The cavernous artery enters the corpus cavernosum at the hilum of the penis, where the two crura merge. Distally the three branches join to form a vascular ring near the glans. Along its course, the cavernous artery gives off many helicine arteries, which supply the trabecular erectile tissue and the sinusoids. These helicine arteries are contracted and tortuous in the flaccid state and become dilated and straight during erection. They help prevent backflow during the rigid erection phase (Tamaki, 1992).

Venous Drainage

The venous drainage from the three corpora originates in tiny venules leading from the peripheral sinusoids immediately beneath the tunica albuginea. **These venules travel in the trabeculae between the tunica and the peripheral sinusoids to form the subtunical venular plexus before exiting as the emissary veins.** Outside the tunica albuginea, the venous drainage is as follows:

1. The skin and subcutaneous tissue: Multiple superficial veins run subcutaneously and unite near the root of the penis to form a single (or paired) superficial dorsal vein, which in turn drains into the saphenous veins. Occasionally the superficial dorsal vein may also drain a portion of the corpora cavernosa.
2. The pendulous penis: The emissary veins from the corpus cavernosum and spongiosum drain dorsally to the deep dorsal, laterally to the circumflex, and ventrally to the periurethral veins. Beginning at the coronal sulcus, the prominent deep dorsal vein comprises the main venous drainage of the glans penis, corpus spongiosum, and distal two thirds of the corpora cavernosa. Usually one, but sometimes more than one, deep dorsal vein runs upward behind the symphysis pubis to join the periprostatic venous plexus.
3. The infrapubic penis: Emissary veins draining the proximal corpora cavernosa join to form cavernous and crural veins. These veins join the periurethral veins from the urethral bulb to form the internal pudendal veins.

The veins of the three systems communicate variably with each other. Variations in the number, distribution, and termination of the venous systems are common.

Hemodynamics and Mechanism of Erection and Detumescence

Corpora Cavernosa

The penile erectile tissue, specifically the cavernous smooth musculature and the smooth muscles of the arteriolar and arterial walls, plays a key role in the erectile process. **In the flaccid state, these smooth muscles are tonically contracted by the sympathetic discharge, allowing only a small amount of arterial flow for nutritional purposes.** The flaccid penis is in a moderate state of contraction, as evidenced by further shrinkage in cold weather and after phenylephrine injection.

Sexual stimulation triggers the release of neurotransmitters from the cavernous nerve terminals. This results in relaxation of these smooth muscles and the following events (Fig. 38–3): (1) dilation of the arterioles and arteries by increased blood flow in both the diastolic and systolic phases; (2) trapping of the incoming blood by the expanding sinusoids; (3) compression of the subtunical venular plexuses between the tunica albuginea and the peripheral sinusoids, reducing the venous outflow; (4) stretching of the tunica to its capacity, which encloses the

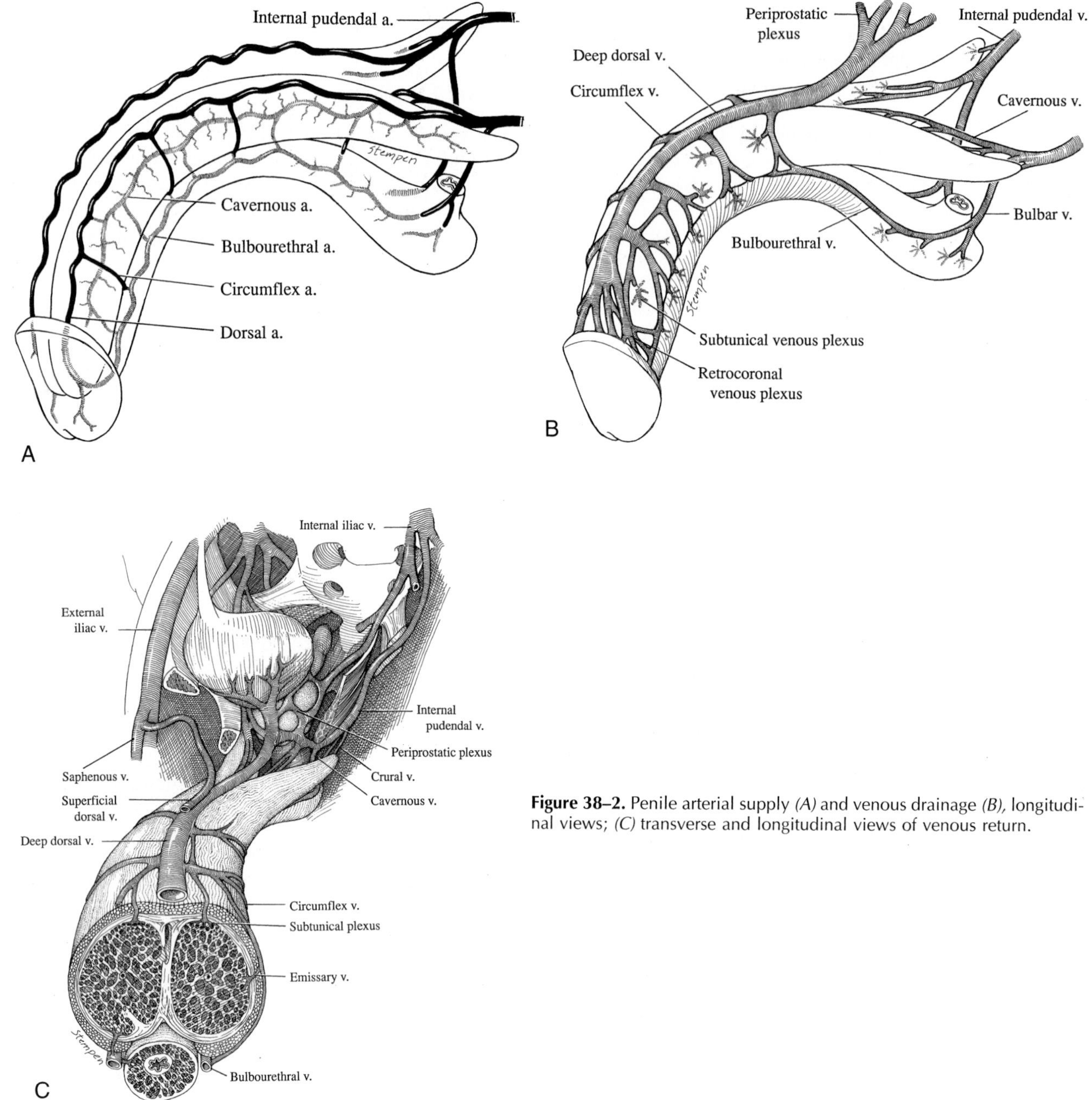

Figure 38–2. Penile arterial supply *(A)* and venous drainage *(B)*, longitudinal views; *(C)* transverse and longitudinal views of venous return.

emissary veins between the inner circular and the outer longitudinal layers and further decreases the venous outflow to a minimum; (5) an increase in intracavernous pressure (maintained at around 100 mm Hg), which raises the penis from the dependent position to the erect state (the full erection phase); and (6) a further pressure increase (to several hundred millimeters of mercury) with contraction of the ischiocavernosus muscles (rigid erection phase). The angle of the erect penis is determined by its size and its attachment to the puboischial rami (the crura) and the anterior surface of the pubic bone (the suspensory and funiform ligaments). In patients with a long heavy penis or a loose suspensory ligament, the angle usually is not greater than 90 degrees even with full rigidity.

Three phases of detumescence have been reported in an animal study (Bosch et al, 1991). The first entails a transient intracorporeal pressure increase, indicating the beginning of smooth muscle contraction against a closed venous system. The second phase involves a slow pressure decrease, suggesting a slow reopening of the venous channels with resumption of the basal level of arterial flow. In the third phase there is a fast pressure decrease and venous outflow capacity is fully restored.

Erection thus involves sinusoidal relaxation, arterial dilation, and venous compression (Lue et al, 1983). The importance of smooth muscle relaxation has been demonstrated in animal and human studies (Ignarro et al, 1990a; Saenz de Tejada et al, 1991b). To summarize the hemodynamic events of erection and detumescence, seven phases can be observed in animal experiments. The changes in and relationship be-

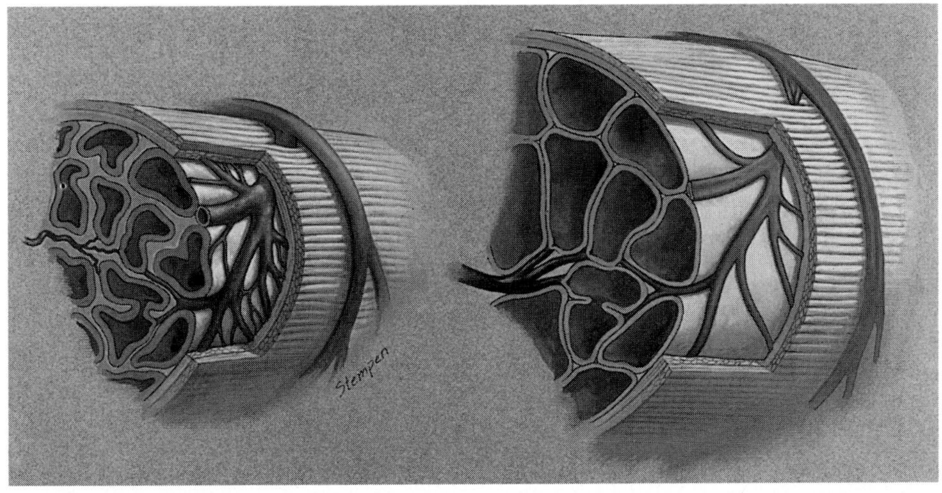

Figure 38–3. The mechanism of penile erection. In the flaccid state *(A),* the arteries, arterioles, and sinusoids are contracted. The intersinusoidal and subtunical venular plexuses are wide open, with free flow to the emissary veins. In the erect state *(B),* the muscles of the sinusoidal wall and the arterioles relax, allowing maximal flow to the compliant sinusoidal spaces. Most of the venules are compressed between the expanding sinusoids. Even the larger intermediary venules are sandwiched and flattened by distended sinusoids and the noncompliant tunica albuginea. This process effectively reduces the venous capacity to a minimum. (From Lue TF, Akkus E, Kour NW: Physiology of erectile function and dysfunction. Campbell's Urology Update #12 1994; 1–10.)

tween penile arterial flow and intracavernous pressure are shown in Figure 38–4.

Corpus Spongiosum and Glans Penis

The hemodynamics of the corpus spongiosum and glans penis are somewhat different from those of the corpora cavernosa. During erection, the arterial flow increases in a similar manner; however, the pressure in the corpus spongiosum and glans is only one-third to one-half that in the corpora cavernosa because the tunical covering (thin over the corpus spongiosum and virtually absent over the glans) ensures minimal venous occlusion. During the full erection phase, partial compression of the deep dorsal and circumflex veins between Buck's fascia and the engorged corpora cavernosa contribute to glanular tumescence, although the spongiosum and glans essentially function as a large arteriovenous shunt during this phase. In the rigid erection phase, the spongiosum and penile veins are forcefully compressed by the ischiocavernosus and bulbocavernosus muscles, resulting

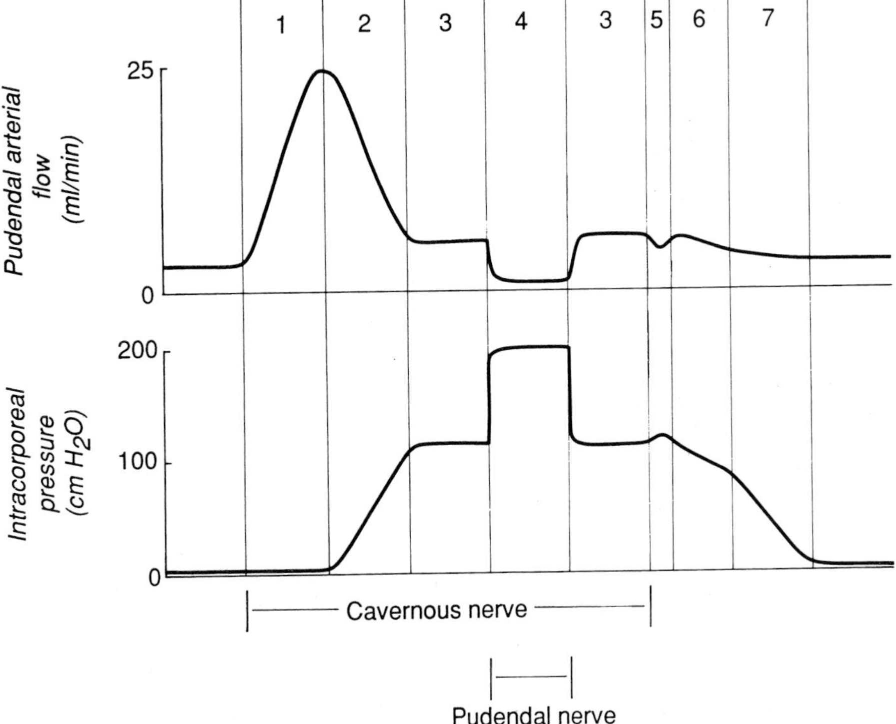

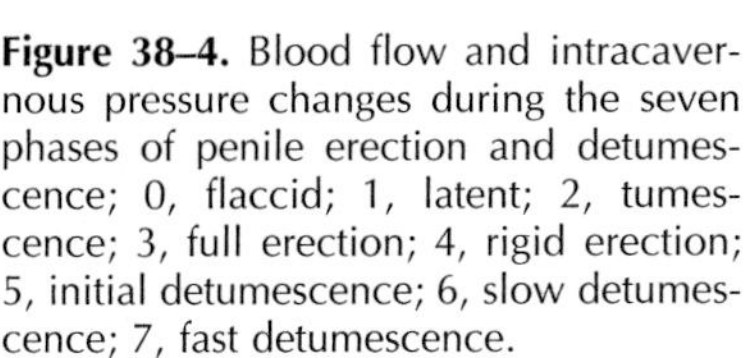

Figure 38–4. Blood flow and intracavernous pressure changes during the seven phases of penile erection and detumescence; 0, flaccid; 1, latent; 2, tumescence; 3, full erection; 4, rigid erection; 5, initial detumescence; 6, slow detumescence; 7, fast detumescence.

in further engorgement and increased pressure in the glans and spongiosum.

SMOOTH MUSCLE PHYSIOLOGY. Spontaneous contractile activity of cavernous smooth muscle has been recorded in in vitro and in vivo studies. In isolated strips of rabbit corpus cavernosum, Mandrek (1994) demonstrated spontaneous mechanical activity with a frequency of 6 to 30 contractions per minute accompanied by fluctuations in membrane potential. Stimulation of the tissue with tetraethylammonium chloride and noradrenaline produced strong tonic contractions with relative electrical silence. In a human study, Yarnitsky and associates (1995) found that two types of electrical activity were recorded from the corpus cavernosum: spontaneous and activity-induced. Levin and colleagues (1994) reported that in vitro spontaneous contractile activity is correlated with a phasic increase in intracellular calcium levels and a biphasic change in the NADH/NAD ratio, suggesting an initial increase and then a decrease in intracellular energy. Field stimulation results in a decrease in tension and intracellular calcium at low frequencies and an increase in tension with increased intracellular calcium at high frequencies. In general, the response to pharmacologic agents correlates with the change in intracellular calcium—for example, phenylephrine produces muscle contraction and an increase in intracellular calcium, while nitroprusside causes the opposite.

Neuroanatomy and Neurophysiology of Penile Erection

Peripheral Pathways

The innervation of the penis is both autonomic (sympathetic and parasympathetic) and somatic (sensory and motor) (Fig. 38–5). **From the neurons in the spinal cord and peripheral ganglia, the sympathetic and parasympathetic nerves merge to form the cavernous nerves, which enter the corpora cavernosa and corpus spongiosum to effect the neurovascular events during erection and detumescence.** The somatic nerves are primarily responsible for sensation and the contraction of the bulbocavernosus and ischiocavernosus muscles.

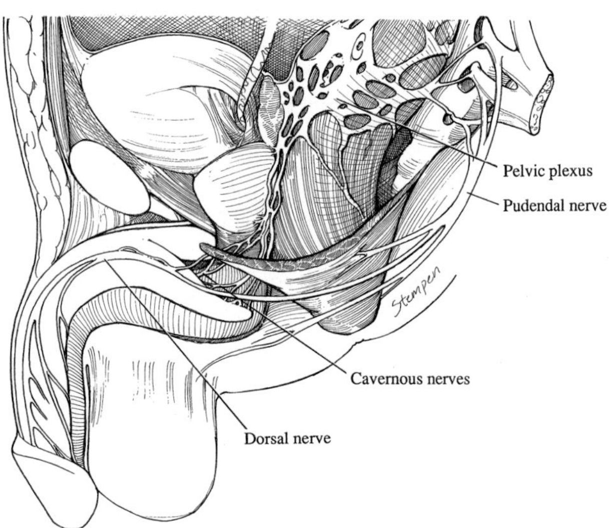

Figure 38–5. Penile neuroanatomy.

AUTONOMIC PATHWAYS. The sympathetic pathway originates from the eleventh thoracic to the second lumbar spinal segments and passes via the white rami to the sympathetic chain ganglia. Some fibers then travel via the lumbar splanchnic nerves to the inferior mesenteric and superior hypogastric plexuses, from which fibers travel in the hypogastric nerves to the pelvic plexus. In man, the T10–T12 segments are most often the origin of the sympathetic fibers, and the chain ganglia cells projecting to the penis are located in the sacral and caudal ganglia (DeGroat and Booth, 1993).

The parasympathetic pathway arises from neurons in the intermediolateral cell columns of the second, third, and fourth sacral spinal cord segments. The preganglionic fibers pass in the pelvic nerves to the pelvic plexus, where they are joined by the sympathetic nerves from the superior hypogastric plexus.

The cavernous nerves are branches of the pelvic plexus that innervate the penis. Other branches of the pelvic plexus innervate the rectum, bladder, prostate, and sphincters. The cavernous nerves are easily damaged during radical excision of the rectum, bladder, and prostate. A clear understanding of the course of these nerves is essential to prevent iatrogenic erectile dysfunction (Walsh et al, 1990). **Recent human cadaveric dissection has revealed medial and lateral branches of the cavernous nerves (the former accompany the urethra and the latter pierce the urogenital diaphragm 4 to 7 mm lateral to the sphincter) and multiple communications between the cavernous and dorsal nerves** (Fig. 38–6) (Paick et al, 1993).

Stimulation of the pelvic plexus and the cavernous nerves induces erection, whereas stimulation of the hypogastric nerve or the sympathetic trunk causes detumescence. This clearly implies that the sacral parasympathetic input is responsible for tumescence, and the thoracolumbar sympathetic pathway controls detumescence. In experiments with cats and rats, removal of the spinal cord below L4 or L5 reportedly eliminated the reflex erectile response, but placement with a female in heat or electrical stimulation of the medial preoptic area (MPOA) produced marked erection (Root and Bard, 1947; Courtois et al, 1993). Paick and Lee (1994) also reported that apomorphine-induced erection is similar to psychogenic erection in the rat and can be induced via the thoracolumbar sympathetic pathway if the sacral parasympathetic centers are injured. In man, many patients with sacral spinal cord injury retain psychogenic erectile ability even though reflexogenic erection is abolished. These cerebrally elicited erections are found more frequently in patients with lower motor neuron lesions below T12 (Bors and Comarr, 1960). No psychogenic erection occurs in patients with lesions above T9; the efferent sympathetic outflow is thus suggested to be at T11 and T12 (Chapelle et al, 1980). These authors have also reported that, in patients with psychogenic erections, lengthening and swelling of the penis are observed, but rigidity is insufficient.

It is therefore possible that cerebral impulses normally travel through sympathetic (inhibiting norepinephrine release), parasympathetic (releasing nitric oxide and acetylcholine), and somatic (releasing acetylcholine) pathways to produce a normal rigid erection. In patients with a sacral cord lesion, the cerebral impulse can still travel via the sympa-

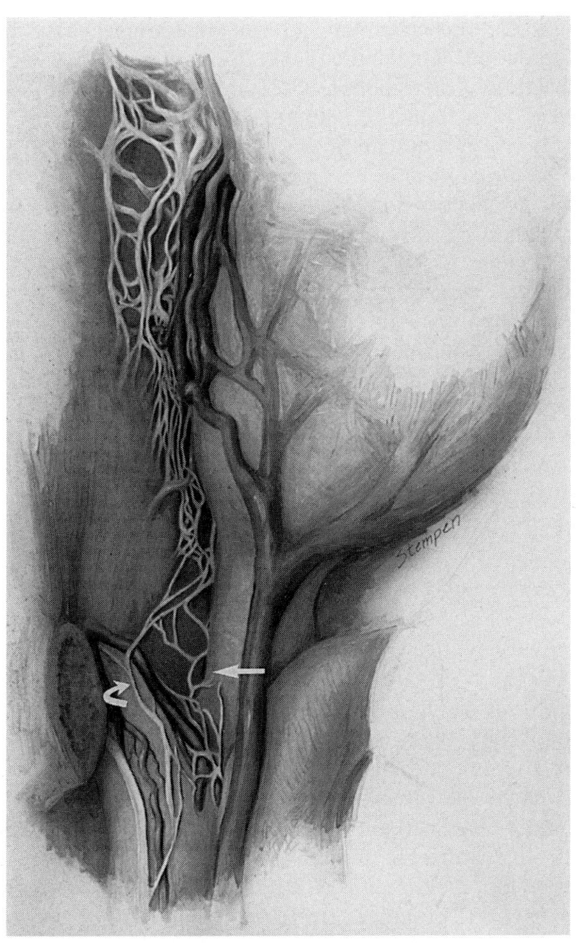

Figure 38–6. Drawing from human cadaveric dissection showing the medial *(straight arrow)* and lateral *(curved arrow)* bundles of the cavernous nerve distal to the prostate. (Reprinted by permission of the publisher from Paick JS, Donatucci CF, Lue TF: Anatomy of cavernous nerves distal to prostate: Microdissection study in adult male cadavers. Urology 1993; 42:145–149. Copyright 1993 by Elsevier Science Inc.)

thetic pathway to inhibit norepinephrine release, and nitric oxide and acetylcholine can still be released via synapse with postganglionic parasympathetic and somatic neurons. Because the number of synapses between the thoracolumbar outflow and postganglionic parasympathetic and somatic neurons is less than the sacral outflow, the resulting erection will not be as strong.

SOMATIC PATHWAYS. The somatosensory pathway originates at the sensory receptors in the penile skin, glans, urethra, and corpus cavernosum. In the human glans penis, there are numerous afferent terminations: free nerve endings and corpuscular receptors with a ratio of 10:1. The free nerve endings are derived from thin myelinated A-delta and unmyelinated C fibers and are unlike those in any other cutaneous area in the body (Halata and Munger, 1986). The nerve fibers from the receptors converge to form bundles of the dorsal nerve of the penis, which joins other nerves to become the pudendal nerve. Activation of these sensory receptors sends messages of pain, temperature, and touch via the dorsal and pudendal nerves, spinal cord, and spinothalamic tract to the thalamus and sensory cortex for sensory perception. The dorsal nerve of the penis used to be regarded as a purely somatic nerve; however, nerve bundles testing positively for nitric oxide synthase, which is parasympathetic in origin, have been demonstrated in the human by Burnett and colleagues (1993) and in rats by Carrier and co-workers (1995). Giuliano and associates (1993) have also shown that stimulation of the sympathetic chain at the L4–L5 level elicits an evoked discharge on the dorsal nerve of the penis, and stimulation of the dorsal nerve evokes a reflex discharge in the lumbosacral sympathetic chain in rats. These findings clearly demonstrate that the dorsal nerve is a mixed nerve with both somatic and autonomic components that enable it to regulate both erectile and ejaculatory function.

Onuf's nucleus in the second to fourth sacral spinal segments is the center of somatomotor penile innervation. These nerves travel in the sacral nerves to the pudendal nerve to innervate the ischiocavernosus and bulbocavernosus muscles. **Contraction of the ischiocavernosus muscles produces the rigid erection phase. Rhythmic contraction of the bulbocavernosus muscle is necessary for ejaculation.**

Supraspinal Pathways

Studies in animals have identified the MPOA and the paraventricular nucleus of the hypothalamus as important integration centers for sexual drive and penile erection (Sachs and Meisel, 1988; Marson et al, 1993): electrostimulation of this area induces erection, and lesions at this site limit copulation. Marson and colleagues (1993) injected pseudo-rabies virus into the rat corpus cavernosum and were able to trace labeled neurons from major pelvic ganglia to neurons in the spinal cord, brain stem, and hypothalamus. Mallick and associates (1994) also showed that stimulation of the dorsal nerve of the penis in the rat influenced the firing rate of about 80% of the neurons in the MPOA but not in other areas of the hypothalamus. Efferent pathways from the MPOA enter the medial forebrain bundle and the midbrain tegmental region (near the substantia nigra). Pathologic processes, such as Parkinson's disease or cerebrovascular accidents, in these regions are often associated with erectile dysfunction. A variety of neurotransmitters, including dopamine, norepinephrine, and serotonin, have been identified in the MPOA (Simerly and Swanson, 1988). **Recently, it has been suggested that dopaminergic and adrenergic receptors may promote sexual drive and that serotonin receptors inhibit it** (Foreman and Wernicke, 1990). Axonal tracing in monkeys, cats, and rats has shown direct projection from hypothalamic nuclei to the lumbosacral autonomic erection centers. The neurons in these hypothalamic nuclei contain peptidergic neurotransmitters, including oxytocin and vasopressin, which may be involved in penile erection (Sachs and Meisel, 1988).

In summary, the structures listed earlier are responsible for the three types of erection: psychogenic, reflexogenic, and nocturnal. Psychogenic erection is a result of audiovisual stimuli or fantasy. Impulses from the brain modulate the spinal erection centers (T11–L2 and S2–S4) to activate the erectile process. Reflexogenic erection is produced by tactile stimuli to the genital organs. The impulses reach the spinal erection centers; some then follow the ascending tract, resulting in sensory perception, and others activate the autonomic nuclei to send messages via the cavernous nerves to the penis to induce erection. This type of erection is preserved in patients with upper spinal cord injury. Nocturnal erection occurs mostly during rapid-eye-movement (REM) sleep. The mechanism is as yet unknown.

Neurotransmitters

PERIPHERAL NEUROTRANSMITTERS

Flaccidity and Detumescence (Fig. 38–7). Adrenergic nerve fibers and receptors have been demonstrated in the cavernous trabeculae and surrounding the cavernous arteries, and norepinephrine has generally been accepted as the principal neurotransmitter controlling penile flaccidity and detumescence (Hedlund and Andersson, 1985; Diederichs et al, 1990). Receptor-binding studies have shown that the number of alpha-adrenoceptors is ten times higher than the number of beta-adrenoceptors (Levin and Wein, 1980). It is also estimated that each human cavernous smooth muscle cell contains 65,000 alpha-adrenoceptor binding sites (Costa et al, 1993). **Currently, it is suggested that sympathetic contraction is mediated by activation of postsynaptic alpha$_{1a}$-, $_{1b}$-, and alpha$_{1c}$-adrenergic receptors** (Christ et al, 1990; Traish et al, 1995) **and is modulated by presynaptic alpha$_2$-adrenergic receptors** (Saenz de Tejada et al, 1989b).

Endothelin, a potent vasoconstrictor produced by the endothelial cells, has also been suggested as a neurotransmitter for detumescence (Holmquist et al, 1990; Saenz de Tejada et al, 1991a). Other vasoconstrictors such as thromboxane A$_2$, prostaglandin F$_{2\alpha}$, and leukotrienes have also been proposed (Hedlund et al, 1989; Azadzoi et al, 1992).

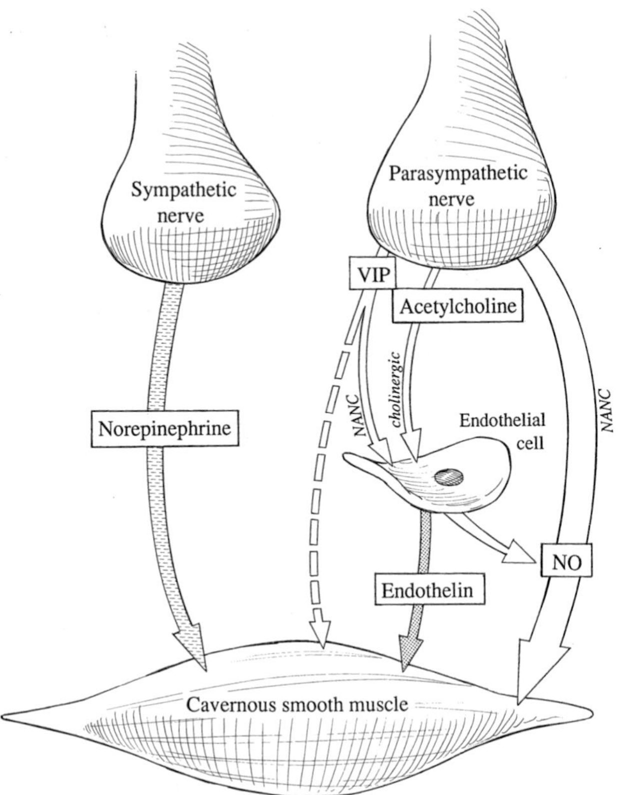

Figure 38–7. The interaction among cholinergic, adrenergic, non-adrenergic, and non-cholinergic (NANC) influences and their contribution to penile smooth muscle contraction and relaxation (*open arrows*, facilitation of smooth muscle relaxation; *patterned arrows*, smooth muscle contraction; *broken arrow* [VIP], = controversial effect; VIP, vasoactive intestinal polypeptide; NO, nitric oxide).

Erection. Acetylcholine is required for ganglionic transmission (by nicotinic receptors) and vascular smooth muscle relaxation (by muscarinic receptors). Cholinergic nerves have been demonstrated within the human cavernous smooth muscle and surrounding penile arteries, and ultrastructural examination has also identified terminals containing cholinergic vesicles in the same area (Steers et al, 1984). Acetylcholine has been shown to be released with electrical field stimulation of human erectile tissue (Blanco et al, 1989). Traish and colleagues (1990) report that the density of muscarinic receptors in cavernous tissue ranges from 35 to 65 fmol/mg protein; in endothelial cell membrane it ranges from 5 to 10 fmol/mg protein. Costa and associates (1993) estimate that the number of muscarinic receptor binding sites on isolated human cavernous muscle cells is 15 times less than the number of adrenoceptors. The muscarinic receptors of human corpus cavernosum are thought to be of the M$_2$ or M$_3$ subtype. However, intravenous or intracavernous injection of atropine has failed to abolish erection induced in animals by electrical neurostimulation (Stief et al, 1989) and in men by erotic stimuli (Wagner and Uhrenholdt, 1980). It has been suggested that acetylcholine stimulates the release of NO from endothelial cells and thus contributes directly to smooth muscle relaxation during erection (Saenz de Tejada et al, 1989a).

Recent observations strongly suggest that NO released from nonadrenergic-noncholinergic (NANC) neurons increases the production of cyclic guanosine monophosphate (cGMP), which in turn relaxes the cavernous smooth muscle (Ignarro et al, 1990a; Kim et al, 1991; Holmquist et al, 1991; Pickard et al, 1991; Burnett et al, 1992; Knispel et al, 1992; Rajfer et al, 1992; Trigo-Rocha et al, 1993a and b). **Kim and colleagues (1993) have also shown that the NO-mediated responses are progressively inhibited as a function of decreasing oxygen tension;** reversion to normal oxygen tension restores endothelium-dependent and neurogenic relaxation. **Currently, NO or an NO-like substance appears to be the most likely principal neurotransmitter causing penile erection.**

Nitric Oxide and cGMP in Relaxation of Smooth Muscle. NO was first described in 1979 as a potent relaxant of peripheral vascular smooth muscle, with an action mediated by cGMP (Gruetter et al, 1979). Subsequently, endothelium-derived relaxing factor was identified as NO or a chemically unstable nitroso precursor (Ignarro et al, 1987; Palmer et al, 1987). NO is synthesized from endogenous L-arginine by NO synthase (NOS) located in the vascular endothelium (Palmer et al, 1988). This enzyme can be inhibited by *N*-substituted analogues of L-arginine, such as *N*-methyl-L-arginine, *N*-nitro L-arginine, and *N*-amino-L-arginine. These compounds also inhibit endothelium-dependent relaxation (Fukuto et al, 1990; Buga et al, 1991; Rajfer et al, 1992). NO may be synthesized and released as a neurotransmitter by the NANC neurons after they are excited by either electrical or chemical stimulation. In this regard Ignarro and associates (1990b) suggest that NO is highly labile; therefore, it cannot be stored as a preformed neurotransmitter. Alternatively, another neurotransmitter such as vasoactive intestinal polypeptide (VIP) may interact with either endothelial or smooth muscle cells in the corpus cavernosum to trigger the local formation of NO.

There are at least three distinct forms of NOS (neuronal, endothelial, and macrophage [Table 38–1] [Lowenstein and Snyder, 1992]). In blood vessels and neurons, NOS is constitutive and is activated by calcium, which binds calmodulin as an enzyme cofactor (Bredt and Snyder, 1990). Bredt and colleagues (1991) have reported the cloning of NOS from rat brain. This neuronal NOS has multiple regulatory sites, including binding sites for nicotinamide adenine dinucleotide phosphate (NADPH), flavin adenine dinucleotide (FAD), and flavin mononucleotide (FMN). NOS also requires tetrahydrobiopterin. Neuronal NOS has a recognition site for calmodulin that is also present in endothelial NOS (Lamas et al, 1992; Janssens et al, 1992) and macrophage NOS (Lyons et al, 1992; Xie et al, 1992; Lowenstein et al, 1992). The three forms of NOS display about 50% identity in amino acid sequence. The constitutive isoforms are generally regulated by Ca^{2+}-calmodulin, whereas inducible forms are not. Most of the isoforms require NADPH, tetrahydrobiopterin, FAD, and FMN.

Previous studies have shown that cGMP induces the relaxation of numerous smooth muscle preparations including vascular, airway, and intestinal smooth muscle (Katsuki and Murad, 1977; Murad et al, 1978; Rapoport and Murad, 1983; Murad, 1986). The mechanism by which intracellular cGMP promotes smooth muscle relaxation is still unclear. Adams and colleagues (1989) report that cGMP maintains a very low intracellular concentration of free calcium, perhaps by promoting its intracellular binding to calcium-binding proteins, which in turn might cause relaxation of smooth muscle. Another possible mechanism is activation by cGMP-specific protein kinase, which results in the phosphorylation and inactivation of myosin light chain kinase, thereby causing light chain and smooth muscle relaxation (Draznin et al, 1986). Cyclic GMP may also alter calcium concentrations through other unknown mechanisms that are mediated independently of cGMP-dependent protein kinase activation. A considerable number of studies suggest that cGMP is a more potent relaxant of smooth muscle than cyclic adenosine monophosphate (cAMP).

The increased levels of cGMP in response to neurotransmitters are due to the activation of soluble or particulate forms of guanylyl cyclase in the cell. The soluble guanylyl cyclase is a heterodimer whose subunits have molecular weights of approximately 77.5 kD (a) and 70.5 kD (b) (Chinkers and Garbers, 1990). It is postulated that heterodimeric forms of guanylate cyclase may be associated with membranes and thus act through NO-sensitive membrane-mediated mechanisms (Murad et al, 1978; Garbers, 1992).

There are three mammalian forms of particulate guanylyl cyclase. Interestingly, the soluble guanylyl cyclase is clearly activated by the NO-releasing nitrovasodilator agents, but only some of the particulate isoforms of guanylyl cyclase can also be activated (Waldman et al, 1982).

Other investigators believe that VIP may be one of the neurotransmitters responsible for erection. VIP-immunoreactive nerve fibers have been identified within the cavernous trabeculae and surrounding penile arteries, and neurostimulation-induced cavernous smooth muscle relaxation has been shown to be blocked by a VIP antagonist or anti-VIP serum (Ottesen et al, 1984; Kim et al, 1995; Yeh et al, 1994). Interestingly, VIP-induced relaxation is reportedly inhibited by the NO synthesis blocker, N^{ω}-nitro L-arginine, which has led Kim and co-workers (1995) to suggest that NO generation is involved in VIP-stimulated smooth muscle relaxation. Both acetylcholine and VIP appear to be co-localized in parasympathetic pathways. Thus they may act synergistically to induce erection through inhibition of alpha$_1$-adrenergic activity by acetylcholine and release of NO by VIP, as suggested by Aoki and associates (1994). Other potential candidates include calcitonin gene–related peptide (CGRP) (Stief et al, 1990), peptide histidine methionine (Kirkeby et al, 1992), pituitary adenylate cyclase–activating polypeptide (Hedlund et al, 1994), and prostaglandins (Adaikan and Ratnam, 1988; Saenz de Tejada, 1989b). Prostaglandin E_1 receptor density is reported to be lower in impotent men (Aboseif et al, 1993). Although these neurotransmitters may participate in the erectile process, they are unlikely to play a major role. Nevertheless, because of the multiplicity of putative transmitters present in the corpus cavernosum and in perivascular nerves, further investigation is needed to elucidate the interactions between neurotransmitters and neuromodulators at the neuromuscular junction, and between the neural and endothelial control of vascular tone (Andersson and Holmquist, 1994).

Table 38–1. ISOFORMS OF NITRIC OXIDE SYNTHASE

Type	Co-Factors	Regulator	Molecular Weight (kD)	Source
Type Ia (soluble)	NADPH FAD/FMN	Ca^{2+}-calmodulin	155	Brain Cerebellum Neuroblastoma cells
Type Ib (soluble)	NADPH	Ca^{2+}-calmodulin	135	Endothelial cells
Type Ic (soluble)	NADPH FAD	Ca^{2+}	150	Neutrophils
Type II (soluble)	NADPH FAD/FMN	Unknown; induced by endotoxin/ cytokines	125	Macrophages
Type III (particulate)	NADPH FAD/FMN	Ca^{2+}-calmodulin	135	Endothelial cells
Type IV (particulate)	NADPH	Unknown; induced by endotoxin/ cytokines	?	Macrophages

NADPH, nicotinamide adenine dinucleotide phosphate; FAD, flavin adenine dinucleotide; FMN, flavin mononucleotide.

Intercellular Communication. During erection and detumescence, a communication should exist among cavernous smooth muscles to mediate synchronized relaxation and contraction (Christ et al, 1991). Although the electromyographic activity in the cavernous tissue of patients with normal erectile function is synchronous (Stief et al, 1991), the relatively sparse neuronal innervation of cavernous smooth muscle cannot explain this. **Several studies have demonstrated the presence of gap junctions in the membrane of adjacent muscle cells. These intercellular channels allow exchange of ions such as calcium and second-messenger molecules** (Christ et al, 1992). The major component of gap junctions is connexin 43, a membrane-sparing protein of less than 0.25 μm that has been identified between smooth muscle cells of human corpus cavernosum (Campos de Calvalho et al, 1993). Cell-to-cell communication through these gap junctions most likely explains the synchronized erectile response, although their pathophysiologic impact is still unclear.

CENTRAL NEUROTRANSMITTERS. A variety of neurotransmitters, including dopamine, norepinephrine, and serotonin, have been identified in the MPOA (Simerly and Swanson, 1988). **It is suggested that dopaminergic and adrenergic receptors may promote sexual drive, and that serotonin receptors inhibit it** (Foreman and Wernicke, 1990).

Dopamine. Clinical observations suggest that dopaminergic stimulation increases libido and produces erection. In men, apomorphine, which stimulates both D1 and D2 receptors, induces penile erection unaccompanied by sexual arousal (Danjou et al, 1988). In male rats, Hull and coworkers (1992) found that low levels of dopaminergic stimulation via the D1 receptor increase erection, but higher levels or prolonged stimulation produce seminal emission through D2 receptors. The erectile response induced by injection of apomorphine into the paraventricular area can be blocked by both dopamine receptor blockers and blockers of oxytocin receptors (Melis et al, 1989). Injection of oxytocin into the paraventricular area also induces erection, but this cannot be blocked by dopamine receptor blockers. These findings suggest that dopaminergic neurons activate oxytocinergic neurons in the paraventricular area and that the release of oxytocin produces erection (Melis et al, 1992).

Serotonin. General pharmacologic data indicate that serotonin (5-hydroxytryptophan [5-HT]) pathways inhibit copulation but that 5-HT may have both facilitory and inhibitory effects on sexual function depending on the receptor subtype and location and the species investigated (DeGroat and Booth, 1993). Andersson and Wagner (1995) summarized the results of administration of selective agonists and antagonists as follows: 5-HT-1A receptor agonists inhibit erectile activity but facilitate ejaculation; stimulation of 5-HT-1C receptors causes erection; and 5HT-2 agonists inhibit erection but facilitate seminal emission and ejaculation. It has also been reported that stimulation of both 5-HT-2 and 5-HT-1C receptors increases oxytocin secretion (Bagdy et al, 1992). In addition, 5-HT may also affect the spinal reflex because Marson and McKenna (1992) have reported that endogenous 5-HT may act in the lumbar cord to inhibit sexual reflexes, and Steers and DeGroat (1989) have shown that increased firing of the cavernous nerve and erection occur when *m*-chlorophenylpiperazine, a 5-HT-1C/1D receptor agonist, is given to rats.

Noradrenaline. Activation of alpha$_2$-adrenoceptors in the MPOA is associated with a decrease in sexual behavior in rats, and administration of clonidine, an alpha$_2$-adrenergic agonist, produces impotence and decreased libido in hypertensive patients. Yohimbine, an alpha$_2$-receptor antagonist, has been shown to increase sexual activity in castrated rats (Clark et al, 1985), but in impotent men the clinical effect is only marginal. Stimulation and blocking of alpha$_1$-adrenoceptors produce enhancement and inhibition, respectively, of sexual activity in rats.

Prolactin. Increased levels of prolactin suppress sexual function in men and experimental animals. In rats, high levels of prolactin decrease the genital reflex and disturb copulatory behavior. It is suggested that the mechanism of prolactin's action is through inhibition of dopaminergic activity in the MPOA.

Opioids. Endogenous opioids are known to affect sexual function, but the mechanism of action is far from clear. Injection of small amounts of morphine into the MPOA facilitates sexual behavior in rats. Larger doses, however, inhibit both penile erection and yawning induced by oxytocin or apomorphine. It is suggested that endogenous opioids may exert an inhibitory control on central oxytocinergic transmission (Argiolas, 1992).

Oxytocin. Oxytocin is known to be released into the circulation during sexual activity in humans and animals. It produces yawning and penile erection when injected into the paraventricular area in rats. It has been suggested that calcium is the second messenger mediating oxytocin-mediated penile erection. Because neurons in the paraventricular area have been shown to contain NOS, and NOS inhibitors prevent apomorphine- and oxytocin-induced erection, it is suggested that oxytocin acts on neurons whose activity is dependent on certain levels of NO (Vincent and Kimura, 1992; Melis and Argiolas, 1993).

Pharmacology of Penile Erection

Intracavernous and Topical Drugs

The introduction of intracavernous injection of vasoactive drugs has revolutionized the diagnosis and treatment of erectile dysfunction. Most researchers agree that erection results from relaxation of the smooth muscle of the arterioles and the cavernous trabeculae, whereas detumescence is the result of contraction of these smooth muscles. **Therefore, vasoactive drugs, injected intracavernously, can be used to induce erection (muscle relaxants) or detumescence (alpha-adrenergic agonists) through their effect on smooth muscle.** A number of newer agents have been reported recently, including the NO-releasing substances, nitroprusside (Brock et al, 1993a) and linsidomine chlorhydrate (SIN-1) (Stief et al, 1992).

The mechanism of smooth muscle relaxation in response to various vasodilators is complex and is not completely understood, especially when a combination of drugs such as papaverine, phentolamine, and prostaglandin E_1 is used. Fortunately, some recent reports have begun to shed light on this area. In a study of the effect of prostanoids on human erectile tissue, Kirkeby and colleagues (1993) found that prostaglandin E_1 does not affect resting tension but produces relaxation in tissue precontracted with noradrenaline. Prostaglandin E_2 increases the basal tone but is able to relax tissue precontracted by adrenaline. On the other hand, both prostaglandin $F_{2\alpha}$ and prostaglandin I_2 contract the cavernous muscles and may be involved in the detumescence mechanism. Derouet and associates (1994) examined the effect of prostaglandin E_1 on isolated human cavernous smooth muscle cells and found that it induced muscle relaxation by inhibiting voltage-dependent L-type Ca^{2+} current. In the case of calcium channel blockers, Kerfoot and colleagues (1993) showed that some are effective in relaxing cavernous smooth muscle; verapamil appears to be the best candidate for further testing.

Recently, several studies of the transdermal application of vasoactive drugs, including nitroglycerin cream or paste (Meyhoff et al, 1992), minoxidil (Cavallini, 1991), and stearyl-VIP (Gozes et al, 1994), have been reported. Transurethral application of vasoactive agents such as prostaglandin E_1 and E_2 has also shown promise (Wolfson et al, 1993). However, further studies must be done to evaluate their effectiveness and safety.

Inhibitors of phosphodiesterase, which normally degrades cGMP and cAMP, are an interesting group of compounds (Sparwasser et al, 1994). **They comprise five subtypes, and the specific cGMP inhibitor (type 5) (Sildenafil [Pfizer]) has been shown in preliminary human studies to enhance penile erection when given orally.** If it proves successful in clinical trials, this drug could be a major advance in the treatment of erectile dysfunction.

Centrally Acting Drugs

Drugs that activate central adrenergic receptors have been reported to increase the libido of patients who take L-dopa (a catecholamine precursor), amphetamines (catecholamine releaser), and L-deprenyl (a monoamine oxidase-B inhibitor that decreases the degradation of catecholamines). On the other hand, prazosin (an $alpha_1$ antagonist) and clonidine ($alpha_2$ agonist) suppress mating behavior, whereas yohimbine ($alpha_2$ antagonist) increases it (Clark et al, 1985).

Dopamine agonists (apomorphine and pergolide) and dopamine uptake inhibitors (nomifensine and bupropion) have been reported to enhance sexual drive in patients (Jeanty et al, 1984). In animal studies, selective activation of D_2-dopaminergic receptors by the systemic administration of agonists such as apomorphine and quinelorane increases sexual behavior, and this effect can be counteracted by centrally acting antagonists.

Serotonin (5-hydroxytryptamine [5-HT]) is believed to be an inhibitory transmitter in the control of sexual drive (Foreman et al, 1989). Suppressed libido in patients taking fenfluramine, a 5-HT–releasing agent, and elevated libido in patients taking buspirone, a 5-HT neuron suppressor, have been reported (Buffum, 1982). A metabolite of trazodone, *m*-chlorophenyl-piperazine, is a serotonergic agonist that induces erection in rats and rhesus monkeys and selectively increases the firing rate of the cavernous nerves in rats (Steers and DeGroat, 1989). Clinically, trazodone has been reported to enhance nocturnal penile erection and cause priapism in men (Saenz de Tejada et al, 1991c).

PATHOPHYSIOLOGY OF ERECTILE DYSFUNCTION

Incidence and Epidemiology

The increasing incidence of impotence with age was noted by Kinsey in 1948: only 1 of 50 men at age 40 but 1 in 4 by age 65 were impotent. In the United States alone, approximately 10 to 20 million men are affected (Furlow, 1985; Shabsigh et al, 1988), the majority of whom are over 65 years old. In 1990, Diokno and colleagues reported that 35% of married men aged 60 years and over suffer from erectile impotence. In older men, alterations in the vascular supply, hormonal changes, neurologic dysfunction, medication, and associated systemic diseases are the main causes.

A recent report from the Massachusetts Male Aging Study showed a combined prevalence of minimal, moderate, and complete impotence in 52% of noninstitutionalized men aged 40 to 70 years. The prevalence of complete impotence tripled from 5% to 15% between the ages of 40 and 70 years. Indeed, subject age was the variable most strongly associated with impotence. After adjustment for age, a higher probability of impotence was directly correlated with heart disease, hypertension, diabetes, associated medications, and index of anger and depression; it was inversely correlated with serum dehydroepiandrosterone, high-density lipoprotein, and an index of dominant personality. Cigarette smoking was associated with a greater probability of complete impotence in men with heart disease and hypertension (Feldman et al, 1994).

Classification

Many classifications have been proposed for erectile dysfunction. Some are based on the cause (diabetic, iatrogenic, traumatic, and so on), and some on the neurovascular mechanism of the erectile process (failure to initiate [neurogenic], failure to fill [arterial], and failure to store [venous] [Goldstein I, personal communication]). The following classification integrates the various causes of impotence with the modern understanding of erectile physiology and functional anatomy (Carrier et al, 1993) (Fig. 38–8).

Psychogenic

Previously, psychogenic impotence was believed to be the most common type, with 90% of impotent men thought to suffer from this condition (Masters and Johnson, 1970). This belief has given way to the realization that most men with erectile dysfunction have a condition that may be either predominantly functional or predominantly physical.

Sexual behavior and penile erection are controlled by the hypothalamus, the limbic system, and the cerebral cortex. Therefore, stimulatory or inhibitory messages can be relayed to the spinal erection centers to facilitate or inhibit erection.

Two possible mechanisms have been proposed to explain the inhibition of erection in psychogenic dysfunction: direct inhibition of the spinal erection center by the brain as an exaggeration of the normal suprasacral inhibition (Steers, 1990), and excessive sympathetic outflow or elevated peripheral catecholamine levels, which may increase penile smooth

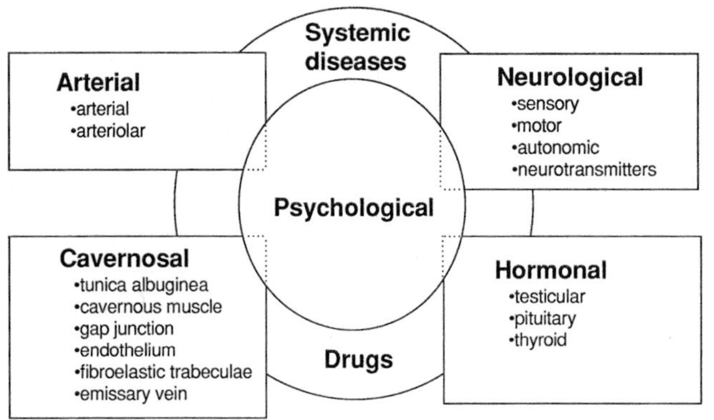

Figure 38–8. A functional classification of impotence. Note that it is unlikely for an individual patient's impotence to derive solely from one source. Most cases have a psychogenic component of varying degree, and systemic diseases and pharmacologic effects can be concomitant and causative. (Reprinted by permission of the publisher from Carrier S, Brock G, Kour NW, Lue TF: Pathophysiology of erectile dysfunction. Urology 1993; 42:468–481. Copyright 1993 by Elsevier Science Inc.)

muscle tone and thus prevent the relaxation necessary for erection. Recently, some results in animal studies demonstrated that activation of sympathetic nerves or systemic infusion of epinephrine causes detumescence of the erect penis (Diederichs et al, 1991a and b). Clinically, higher levels of serum norepinephrine have been reported in patients with psychogenic erectile dysfunction than in normal controls or patients with vasculogenic erectile dysfunction (Kim and Oh, 1992). Increased central sympathetic tone may be one of the causes of psychogenic erectile dysfunction and may explain why some patients respond poorly to injection therapy with no evidence of vascular or neurogenic disorders.

A subclassification of psychogenic erectile dysfunction has been proposed recently (Lue, 1994a): Type 1—anxiety, fear of failure (widower's syndrome, sexual phobia, performance anxiety, and so on); type 2—depression (including drug- or disease-induced depression); type 3—marital conflict, strained relationship; type 4—ignorance and misinformation (e.g., about normal anatomy, sexual function, or aging), religious scruples; type 5—obsessive-compulsive personality (anhedonia, sexual deviation, psychotic disorders).

It is hoped that this subclassification will serve as a catalyst for further work to improve the diagnosis and treatment of psychogenic erectile dysfunction.

Neurogenic

Because erection is a neurovascular event, any disease or dysfunction affecting the brain, spinal cord, cavernous and pudendal nerves, or receptors in the terminal arterioles and cavernous smooth muscles can induce dysfunction.

The MPOA with the paraventricular nucleus has been regarded as an important integration center for sexual drive and penile erection in animal studies (Sachs and Meisel, 1988). Pathologic processes affecting these regions, such as Parkinson's disease or stroke, are often associated with erectile dysfunction. Parkinsonism's effect may be caused by the imbalance of the dopaminergic pathways (Wermuth and Stenager, 1992). Other lesions in the brain noted to be associated with erectile dysfunction are tumors, Alzheimer's disease, and trauma.

In the patient with a spinal cord injury, the degree of erectile function that persists depends largely on the nature, location, and extent of the spinal lesion. Reflexogenic erection is preserved in 95% of patients with complete upper cord lesions, whereas only about 25% of those with complete lower cord lesions can achieve an erection (Eardley and Kirby, 1991). Sacral parasympathetic neurons are apparently important in the preservation of reflexogenic erection. However, the thoracolumbar pathway may compensate for loss of the sacral lesion through synaptic connections (Courtois et al, 1993). Other disorders at the spinal level (e.g., spina bifida, disc herniation, syringomyelia, tumor, and multiple sclerosis) may affect either the afferent or the efferent neural pathway in a similar manner.

Because of the close relationship between the cavernous nerves and the pelvic organs, surgery on these organs is a frequent cause of impotence. The incidence of iatrogenic impotence resulting from various procedures has been reported as follows: radical prostatectomy, 43% to 100% (Veenema et al, 1977; Finkle and Taylor, 1981; Walsh and Donker, 1982); perineal prostatectomy, 29% (Finkle and Taylor, 1981); abdominal perineal resection, 15% to 100% (Weinstein and Roberts, 1977; Yeager and Van Heerden, 1980); and external sphincterotomy at the 3 and 9 o'clock positions, 2% to 49% (McDermott et al, 1981). An improved understanding of the neuroanatomy of the pelvic and cavernous nerves (Walsh and Donker, 1982) has resulted in modifications of surgery for cancer of the rectum, bladder, and prostate, resulting in a lower incidence of iatrogenic impotence. For example, the introduction of nerve-sparing radical prostatectomy has reduced the incidence of impotence from nearly 100% to 30% to 50% (Catalona and Bigg, 1990; Quinlan et al, 1991). In patients with pelvic fracture, erectile dysfunction can be a result of cavernous nerve injury or vascular insufficiency or both. In a recent animal experiment in mature rats, Carrier and co-workers (1995), using NOS staining as a marker, showed that regeneration of the cavernous nerves after iatrogenic injury is more likely to be a result of sprouting from the remaining noninjured bundles than of reinnervation of the injured ones.

Alcoholism, vitamin deficiency, or diabetes may affect the cavernous nerve terminals, resulting in a deficiency of neurotransmitters. In diabetics, impairment of neurogenic and endothelium-dependent relaxation results in inadequate NO release (Saenz de Tejada, 1989a). Because there is no direct means of testing the autonomic innervation of the penis, clinicians should be cautious in making a diagnosis of neurogenic erectile dysfunction. Recently, NADPH diaphorase staining of the NANC nerve fibers in penile biopsy specimens has been proposed as an indicator of neurogenic status (Fig. 38–9) (Brock et al, 1993b). Stief and colleagues (1991) also proposed a single potential analysis of cavernous electrical activity to assess cavernous nerve function. Further studies are needed before these tests can be used routinely in clinical practice.

Bemelmans and associates (1991) performed somatosensory evoked potentials and sacral reflex latency measurements in impotent patients with no clinically overt neurologic disease and found that 47% of patients had at least one abnormal neurophysiologic measurement and that abnormal-

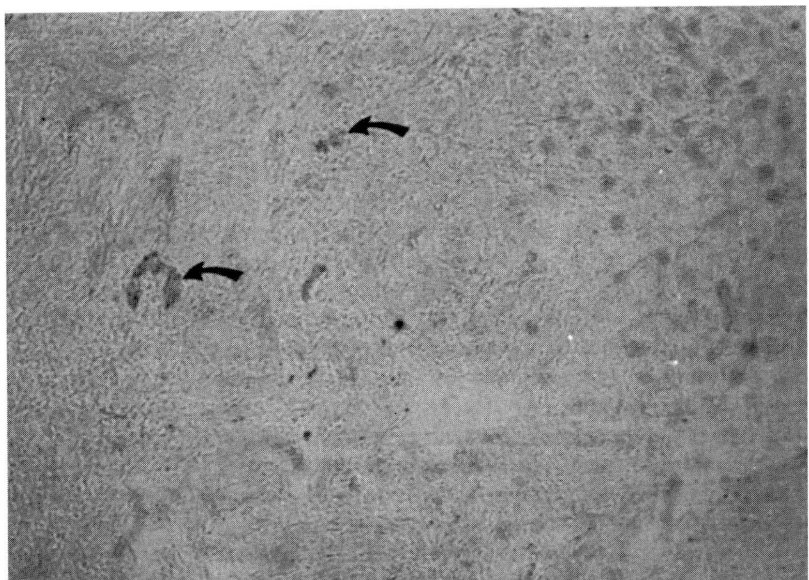

Figure 38–9. Photomicrograph of a biopsy specimen from a penis that has sustained no nerve injury. Several bundles staining positively for NADPH diaphorase are visible. (Reduced from ×40; reprinted with permission of the publisher from Brock G, Nunes L, Padma-Nathan H, et al: Nitric oxide synthase: A new diagnostic tool for neurogenic impotence. Urology 1993b; 42:412–417. Copyright 1993 by Elsevier Science Inc.)

ities were found more often in older patients. A decrease in penile tactile sensitivity with increasing age was also reported by Rowland and colleagues (1993). Sensory input from the genitalia is essential in achieving and maintaining reflexogenic erection, and the input becomes even more important when older people gradually lose the capability of psychogenic erection. Therefore, sensory evaluation should be an integral part of the evaluation for erectile dysfunction in all patients with or without an apparent neurologic disorder.

Endocrinologic

Endocrinopathy is a not infrequent finding in the impotent population. Androgens influence the growth and development of the male reproductive tract and secondary sex characteristics; their effects on libido and sexual behavior are well established. Androgen receptors have been found in the sacral parasympathetic cord and in the hypothalamus and limbic system, suggesting a possible role for central control and influence of erection (Rees and Michael, 1982). CGRP is thought to be a trophic factor produced by motor neurons to regulate expression of the acetylcholine receptor at the neuromuscular junction, and castration has been shown to reduce the number of CGRP-positive spinal motor neurons that innervate the bulbocavernosus muscle in mice (Wagner et al, 1994). Studies have shown that erection in response to visual sexual stimulation is not affected by androgen withdrawal in hypogonadal men, suggesting that androgen enhances but is not essential for erection (Bancroft and Wu, 1983). However, hypogonadal men have decreased nocturnal penile erectile activity that responds to androgen replacement (Cunningham et al, 1990). On the other hand, exogenous testosterone therapy in impotent men with borderline low testosterone levels reportedly has little effect on potency (Graham and Regan, 1992). The molecular mechanism of androgen's effect has been examined by several investigators. Matsumoto and colleagues (1994) found that the expression of beta-actin and beta-tubulin mRNA in androgen-sensitive motor neurons of the spinal nucleus of the bulbocavernosus muscle in adult male rats is regulated by androgen. Chamness and associates (1995) reported that nitrogen synthase activity and NOS decrease significantly in the penis but increase in the seminal vesicle after castration. Lugg and colleagues (1995) reported that dihydrotestosterone is the active androgen in the maintenance of NO-mediated penile erection in the rat. Beyer and Gonzales-Mariscal (1994) noted that testosterone and dihydrotestosterone are responsible for male pelvic thrusting and estradiol or testosterone for female pelvic thrusting during copulation.

Any dysfunction of the hypothalamic-pituitary axis can result in hypogonadism. Hypogonadotropic hypogonadism can be congenital or caused by a tumor or injury; hypergonadotropic hypogonadism may result from a tumor, injury, surgery, or mumps orchitis.

Hyperprolactinemia, whether resulting from a pituitary adenoma or drugs, leads to both reproductive and sexual dysfunction. Symptoms may include loss of libido, erectile dysfunction, galactorrhea, gynecomastia, and infertility. Hyperprolactinemia is associated with low circulating levels of testosterone, which appear to be secondary to inhibition of gonadotropin-releasing hormone secretion by the elevated prolactin levels (Leonard et al, 1989).

Erectile dysfunction may also be associated with both hyperthyroidism and hypothyroidism. Hyperthyroidism is commonly associated with diminished libido, which may be due to the increased circulating estrogen levels and less often with erectile dysfunction. In hypothyroidism, low testosterone secretion and elevated prolactin levels contribute to erectile dysfunction.

Diabetes mellitus, although the most common endocrinologic disorder, causes erectile dysfunction through its vascular, neurologic, endothelial, and psychogenic complications rather than through hormone deficiency per se. Changes in the cavernous arteries (Michal and Ruzbarsky, 1980) and in the cavernous erectile tissue (Saenz de Tejada et al, 1989a) have been reported. In a polysomnographic study, Hirshkowitz and colleagues (1990) reported that impotent men with diabetes have fewer sleep-related erections, less tumescence time, diminished penile rigidity, decreased heart rate response to deep breathing, and lower penile blood pressure than age-matched nondiabetic men. They concluded that neurologic and vascular factors are involved and diabetes may accelerate some age-related pathophysiologic processes.

Arteriogenic

Atherosclerotic or traumatic arterial occlusive disease of the hypogastric-cavernous-helicine arterial tree can decrease the perfusion pressure and arterial flow to the sinusoidal spaces, thus increasing the time needed to attain maximal erection and decreasing the rigidity of the erect penis. Michal and Ruzbarsky (1980) found that the incidence and age at onset of coronary disease and erectile dysfunction are parallel. In the majority of patients with arteriogenic erectile dysfunction, the impaired penile perfusion is a component of the generalized atherosclerotic process. Common risk factors associated with arterial insufficiency include hypertension, hyperlipidemia, cigarette smoking, diabetes mellitus, blunt perineal or pelvic trauma, and pelvic irradiation (Goldstein et al, 1984; Levine et al, 1990; Rosen et al, 1990). On arteriography, bilateral diffuse disease of the internal pudendal, common penile, and cavernous arteries has been found in impotent patients with atherosclerosis. **Focal stenosis of the common penile or cavernous artery is most often seen in young patients who have sustained blunt pelvic or perineal trauma** (Levine et al, 1990).

In one report, diabetic men and older men had a high incidence of fibrotic lesions of the cavernous artery, involving intimal proliferation, calcification, and luminal stenosis (Michal and Ruzbarsky, 1980). Hyperlipidemia is a well-known risk factor for arteriosclerosis. It enhances the deposition of lipid in the vascular lesions, causing atherosclerosis and eventual occlusion. Nicotine may adversely affect erectile function not only by decreasing arterial flow to the penis but also by blocking corporeal smooth muscle relaxation, thus preventing normal venous occlusion (Jünemann et al, 1987; Rosen et al, 1991).

Hypertension is another well-recognized risk factor for arteriosclerosis; a prevalence of about 45% has been noted in one series of impotent men (Rosen et al, 1991). However, in hypertension, the increased blood pressure itself does not impair erectile function; rather the associated arterial stenotic lesions are thought to be the cause (Hsieh et al, 1989).

Cavernosal (Venogenic)

Recently, failure of adequate venous occlusion has been proposed as one of the most common causes of vasculogenic impotence (Rajfer et al, 1988). **Veno-occlusive dysfunction may result from several possible pathophysiologic processes. (1) The presence or development of large venous channels draining the corpora cavernosa is frequently seen in patients with primary erectile dysfunction. (2) Degenerative changes (Peyronie's disease, old age, and diabetes) or traumatic injury to the tunica albuginea (penile fracture) results in inadequate compression of the subtunical and emissary veins.** In Peyronie's disease the inelastic tunica albuginea prevents the emissary veins from closing (Metz et al, 1983). Iacono and colleagues (1994) postulated that a decrease in elastic fibers in the tunica albuginea and an alteration in the microarchitecture (Iacono et al, 1993) may contribute to impotence in some men. Changes in the areolar layer associated with this disease may also disrupt the venous occlusion mechanism, and venous leakage can be seen in patients after surgery for Peyronie's disease (Dalkin and Carter, 1991). **(3) Structural alterations in the fibroelastic components of the trabeculae, cavernous smooth muscle, and endothelium may contribute. (4) Insufficient trabecular smooth muscle relaxation, causing inadequate sinusoidal expansion and insufficient compression of the subtunical venules, may occur in an anxious individual with excessive adrenergic tone or in a patient with inadequate neurotransmitter release from the parasympathetic nerves.** Alteration of alpha-adrenoceptors or other receptors may heighten the smooth muscle tone and impair its relaxation in response to endogenous muscle relaxant (Christ et al, 1990). **(5) Acquired venous shunts—the result of operative correction of priapism—can cause persistent glans-cavernosum or cavernosum-spongiosum shunting.**

FIBROELASTIC COMPONENT. Loss of compliance of the penile sinusoids may be the result of aging associated with increased deposition of collagen (Cerami et al, 1987). Hypercholesterolemia associated with altered collagen synthesis also may cause loss of compliance (Hayashi et al, 1987). Alterations in the fibroelastic structures can occur after penile trauma or priapism. Recently, Moreland and colleagues (1995) showed that prostaglandin E_1 suppresses collagen synthesis by transforming growth factor beta-1 ($TGF_{\beta 1}$) in human cavernous smooth muscle, which implies that intracavernous injection of prostaglandin E_1 may be beneficial in preventing intracavernous fibrosis.

SMOOTH MUSCLE. Wespes and co-workers (1991) demonstrated a decrease in the smooth muscle fiber in impotent men, primarily patients with arteriogenic and venogenic erectile dysfunction in whom the extent of dysfunction corresponded to the severity of vascular disease and the failure of erectile response to papaverine injection. In rabbits fed a high-cholesterol diet for 3 months, Jünemann and colleagues (1991) demonstrated significant smooth muscle degeneration with loss of cell-to-cell contact. Cavernous nerve injury seems also to affect cavernous smooth muscle relaxation, as demonstrated in neurotomized dogs (Paick et al, 1991). An in vitro biochemical study has shown impaired neurogenic and endothelium-related relaxation of penile smooth muscle in impotent diabetic men (Saenz de Tejada et al, 1989a). In vasculogenic and neurogenic erectile dysfunction, the damaged smooth muscle can be a key factor, aggravating the primary cause (Mersdorf et al, 1991). Pickard and associates (1994) showed that impairment of nerve-evoked relaxation and alpha-adrenergic–stimulated contraction of cavernous muscle and reduced muscle content occurred in men with venous or mixed venous-arterial impotence. In a study of three different potassium channel subtypes in cultured cavernous smooth muscle cells, Fan and co-workers (1995) reported an alteration of the maxi-K^+ channel in cells from impotent patients and suggested that impairment of the function or regulation of potassium channels may contribute to the decreased hyperpolarizing ability, altered calcium homeostasis, and impaired smooth muscle relaxation seen in impotence.

GAP JUNCTION. The intercellular communication

channels known as gap junctions can explain the synchronized and coordinated erectile response, although their pathophysiologic impact has yet to be clarified (Christ et al, 1991; Lerner et al, 1993). In patients with severe arterial disease, a loss or reduction of membrane contact occurs because of the presence of collagen fibers between cellular membranes (Persson et al, 1989). These findings imply that a malfunction or loss of gap junctions may alter the coordinated smooth muscle activity.

ENDOTHELIUM. By releasing vasoactive agents, the endothelium of the corpora can modify the tone of the adjacent smooth muscle and affect the development or inhibition of an erection. NO, prostaglandin, and the polypeptide endothelin (a strong vasoconstrictor) have been identified in the endothelial cell (Ignarro et al, 1990a and b; Saenz de Tejada et al, 1991a and b). Activation of cholinergic receptors on the endothelial cell by acetylcholine or stretching of the endothelial cells as a result of increased blood flow may elicit underlying smooth muscle relaxation through the release of NO (Saenz de Tejada et al, 1988; Rubanyi et al, 1989). Diabetes and hypercholesterolemia may also alter the function of endothelium-mediated relaxation of cavernous muscle (Azadzoi and Saenz de Tejada, 1991), impairing erection.

Drug-Induced

Various classes of therapeutic drugs can cause erectile dysfunction as an undesired side effect (Wein and Van Arsdalen, 1988). Slag and associates (1983) reported a 25% incidence of erectile dysfunction in a medical outpatient clinic population. For most drugs, the mechanism of action is unknown, and there are few well-controlled studies on the sexual effects of a particular drug.

In general, drugs that interfere with central neuroendocrine or local neurovascular control of penile smooth muscle have a potential for causing erectile dysfunction. Central neurotransmitter pathways, including 5-hydroxytryptaminergic, noradrenergic, and dopaminergic pathways involved in sexual function, may be disturbed by antipsychotics and antidepressants and some centrally acting antihypertensive drugs.

Centrally acting sympatholytics include methyldopa, clonidine (inhibition of the hypothalamic center via alpha$_2$-receptor stimulation), and reserpine (depletion of the stores of catecholamines and serotonin). Guanethidine, a peripheral sympatholytic, has been reported to cause erectile as well as ejaculatory dysfunction. Alpha-adrenergic blocking agents such as phenoxybenzamine and phentolamine also reportedly cause ejaculatory inhibition. Prazosin, a selective alpha$_1$-adrenergic blocking agent, may cause erectile dysfunction. Beta-adrenergic blockers have been reported to depress libido (Wein and van Arsdalen, 1988). Thiazide diuretics have been credited with widely differing effects on potency, and spironolactone produces erectile failure in 4% to 30% of patients and has been associated with decreased libido, gynecomastia, and mastodynia.

Major tranquilizers or antipsychotics can decrease libido, causing erectile failure and ejaculatory dysfunction. The mechanisms involved may include sedation, anticholinergic actions, a central antidopaminergic effect, alpha-adrenergic antagonist action, and release of prolactin. Among antidepressants, tricyclic antidepressants and monoamine oxidase (MAO) inhibitors reportedly cause erectile dysfunction through central or peripheral actions. The sexual side effects seen in patients taking minor tranquilizers may well be a result of the central sedative effects of these agents.

Cigarette smoking may induce vasoconstriction and penile venous leakage because of its contractile effect on the cavernous smooth muscle (Junemann et al, 1987). In a study of nocturnal penile tumescence in cigarette smokers, Hirshkowitz and colleagues (1992) reported an inverse correlation between nocturnal erection (both rigidity and duration) and the number of cigarettes smoked per day. Men who smoked more than 40 cigarettes a day had the weakest and shortest nocturnal erections. Alcohol in small amounts improves erection and sexual drive because of its vasodilatory effect and suppression of anxiety; however, large amounts can cause central sedation, decreased libido, and transient erectile dysfunction. Chronic alcoholism may result in liver dysfunction, decreased testosterone and increased estrogen levels, and alcoholic polyneuropathy, which also affects penile nerves (Miller and Gold, 1988). In an in vitro study of rabbits given 5% alcohol for 6 weeks, Saito and colleagues (1994) reported augmented smooth muscle contraction and relaxation in response to both electrical field stimulation and vasoconstrictors such as phenylephrine and potassium chloride but not to sodium nitroprusside, suggesting changes in neurovascular function. Cimetidine, a histamine H_2 receptor antagonist, has been reported to suppress the libido and produce erectile failure. It is thought to act as an antiandrogen and to increase prolactin levels (Wolfe, 1979).

Other drugs known to cause erectile dysfunction are estrogens and drugs with antiandrogenic action, such as ketoconazole and cyproterone acetate. Finally, many anticancer drugs may be associated with a progressive loss of libido and erectile failure.

Erectile Dysfunction Associated with Aging, Systemic Disease, and Other Causes

A number of studies have indicated a progressive decline in sexual function in "healthy" aging men. Masters and Johnson (1977) noted a number of changes in older men, including greater latency to erection, less turgid erection, loss of forceful ejaculation, decreased ejaculatory volume, and a longer refractory period. Decreased frequency and duration of nocturnal erection with increasing age was reported in a group of men who had regular intercourse (Schiavi and Schreiner-Engel, 1988). Other research has indicated a decrease in penile tactile sensitivity with age (Rowland et al, 1989). Recently, Garban and associates (1995) reported a decrease in NOS activity in the penile tissue of senescent rats. Heightened cavernous muscle tone was suggested to be the cause of decreased erectile response in older men by Christ and colleagues (1990). In one study, a decrease in testosterone levels in aging impotent men was associated with relatively normal gonadotropins, suggesting hypothalamic-pituitary dysfunction (Kaiser et al, 1988).

Chronic renal failure has frequently been associated with diminished erectile function, impaired libido, and infertility. In one study, by the time patients with uremia began maintenance dialysis, 50% were impotent (David and Koyle, 1990). In another study, 78% of the patients were found to have cavernous artery occlusive disease, and 90% had veno-occlusive dysfunction (Kaufman et al, 1994). The mechanism is probably multifactorial: depressed testosterone levels, diabetes mellitus, vascular insufficiency, multiple medications, autonomic and somatic neuropathy (Nogues et al, 1991), and psychological stress. After successful renal transplantation, 50% to 80% of patients return to their pre-illness potency (Salvatierra et al, 1975).

Patients with severe pulmonary disease often fear aggravating dyspnea during sexual intercourse. Patients with angina, heart failure, or myocardial infarction can become impotent from anxiety, depression, or arterial insufficiency. Other systemic diseases such as cirrhosis of the liver, scleroderma, chronic debilitation, and cachexia are also known to cause erectile dysfunction.

PRIAPISM

Priapism is the persistence of erection that does not result from sexual desire and fails to subside despite orgasm. Except in the high-flow type (nonischemic [see subsequent discussion]), priapism is often accompanied by pain and tenderness. It can occur in all age groups, including the newborn, but the peak incidence occurs between the ages of 5 and 10 and 20 to 50 years. In the younger group, priapism is most often associated with sickle-cell disease or neoplasm; in the older group, many cases are idiopathic (Hashmat and Rehman, 1993). Most incidents occur during nocturnal penile tumescence when the smooth muscle is relaxed and the venous channels are maximally compressed. Some occur after prolonged sexual activity, an insect bite, or drug use. Typically, priapism affects only the corpora cavernosa (very rarely the corpus spongiosum is also involved). Although no definitive distinction has been made between prolonged erection and priapism, the authors prefer to refer to erection of more than 6 hours' duration as priapism because, in the low-flow type, ischemia and acidosis occur at that time (Jünemann et al, 1986; Broderick et al, 1994).

Classification

Traditionally, priapism has been classified as primary or idiopathic and secondary. Hemodynamically, it can be separated into two distinct types: low-flow (ischemic) and high-flow (nonischemic). Because the low-flow state is caused by venous obstruction and the high-flow state by unregulated arterial flow, **Witt and colleagues (1990) have advanced a new classification: veno-occlusive and arterial priapism.** Priapism may also present as acute, intermittent (recurrent or stuttering), or chronic (usually as the high-flow type) (Hashmat and Rehman, 1993). Physiologically, the level of blood gases in the corpus cavernosum is similar to that of systemic venous blood in the flaccid state and reaches the arterial level during erection. It is to be remembered that every case of priapism begins with physiologic erection and well-oxygenated blood in the corpora. In high-flow priapism this condition persists, whereas in low-flow priapism the blood gases begin to show signs of ischemia and acidosis after 6 hours. However, in these patients well-oxygenated blood can also be aspirated during the resolution phase (whether this is spontaneous or is induced by medication or a shunting procedure). When in doubt, blood gas determination and duplex ultrasound scanning can be very helpful in the differential diagnosis.

Hauri and associates (1983) have demonstrated that in low-flow priapism venous drainage on cavernosography is delayed up to 15 minutes, and only the dorsal and bulbar arteries are opacified (not the cavernosal arteries) on arteriography. In high-flow priapism, cavernosography and arteriography show rapid venous drainage and pooling of blood in the corpus cavernosum from the ruptured cavernous artery.

Causes

In a review of the world literature, Pohl and colleagues (1986) reported the etiologic factors in 230 cases of priapism: one third were idiopathic, 21% involved alcohol abuse or drug therapy, 12% perineal trauma, and 11% sickle-cell anemia (Table 38–2). These factors are clearly affected by demographic factors. In one U.S. series (Nelson and Winter, 1977), sickle-cell disease accounted for 23% of adult cases and 63% of pediatric cases. Overall, 46% of cases were idiopathic, all with prior episodes.

Sickle-Cell Anemia

Sickle-cell disease affects 8% of black Americans. In a review of 321 pediatric patients, Tarry and colleagues (1987) found a 6.4% incidence of priapism among their sickle-cell clinic patients. Red cell sickling and later sludging of blood occur within the corpora cavernosa, perhaps as a result of abnormal endothelial adherence, the relatively acidic state of the corpora during erection, mild acidosis accompanying hypoventilation during sleep, or mild trauma with masturbation and intercourse. When the venous channels are maximally compressed during nocturnal penile tumescence, the sludged red blood cells can then block the microscopic subtunical venules and trigger diffuse veno-occlusion. In one study of adults with homozygous sickle-cell disease in a Jamaican clinic, stuttering nocturnal attacks of priapism lasting 2 to 6 hours reportedly affected 42% of patients (Serjeant et al, 1985). These attacks, which begin soon after puberty and are not related to other vaso-occlusive crises, may occur over weeks and culminate in a major episode lasting 3 to 5

Table 38–2. ETIOLOGY OF PRIAPISM

Idiopathic (primary)
Secondary
Thromboembolic (sickle-cell anemia and trait, leukemia, fat emboli, thalassemia, prolonged sexual activity?)
Neurogenic (spinal cord lesions, cauda equina compression, autonomic neuropathy, spinal stenosis, anesthesia)
Neoplastic (from metastatic cancer: prostate, bladder, lung, kidney)
Traumatic (perineal or genital; usually results in high-flow priapism)
Iatrogenic (intracavernous injection, arteriovenous or arteriocavernosum bypass surgery)
Infectious or toxic (malaria, rabies, scorpion sting)
Medications and chemicals (see Table 38–3)

days. Anecdotally, pediatric patients have been known to achieve erectile capability subsequently, but adults often do not recover it. The natural history of sickle-cell priapism is one of recurrence. Although almost all the cases are of the low-flow type, two cases of high-flow priapism in patients with sickle-cell disease have been reported (Ramos et al, 1995).

Intracavernous Injection

Injection of vasoactive substances into the corpora cavernosa is the cause most likely to confront urologists currently and in the future. The final common pathway for intracavernous drug therapy is smooth muscle relaxation. Although the venous channels are compressed temporarily during drug-induced erection, they should reopen when the smooth muscle regains its contractility. In cases of overdosage or heightened sensitivity to drugs, the smooth muscles do not regain contractility; thus priapism results.

In a literature review of cases worldwide in which intracavernous injection of papaverine was used in the diagnosis and treatment of impotence, Jünemann and Alken (1989) found that 5.3% of cases of priapism resulted from initial diagnostic testing and 0.4% resulted from home therapy. The majority of these prolonged erections occurred among patients with either neurogenic or psychogenic impotence.

Neurologic Disorders

For centuries, priapism has been noted in hanging victims. It has also been reported in patients with lumbar stenosis, cauda equina compression syndrome, spinal cord injury, and herniated disc. These conditions probably either enhance the release of erection-inducing neurotransmitters from the parasympathetic nerves or interfere with tonic discharge from the sympathetic nervous system. Persistent erection may occur during scrub preparation of patients under spinal or general anesthesia and can interfere with transurethral surgery (Van Arsdalen et al, 1983). This exaggerated response to genital stimulation (reflex erection) most likely results from blockage of the central inhibitory impulse by anesthesia. Nevertheless, this condition rarely persists after anesthesia is over (Van Arsdalen et al, 1983).

Malignancy

Although malignant infiltration itself does not result in priapism, it is conceivable that venous drainage may be obstructed or that the partial replacement of the sinusoids might promote stasis and thrombosis in the remaining tissue. This condition often presents as abnormal erection with pain (Wilson and Staff, 1982; Powell et al, 1985). The following conditions have been reported to metastasize to the penis and cause priapism: leukemia (Bhatia et al, 1992), prostate carcinoma (Schroeder-Printzen et al, 1994), renal carcinoma (Puppo et al, 1992), and melanoma (Sagar and Retsas, 1992).

Drug Therapy

Antihypertensive drugs such as hydralazine, guanethidine, and prazosin (Rubin, 1968), antipsychotic drugs of the phenothiazine group, especially chlorpromazine (Dorman and Schmidt, 1976), and antidepressants (notably trazodone [Priapism with trazodone, Med Lett, 1984]) have been associated with prolonged erection. A summary of drugs reported to induce priapism is listed in Table 38–3.

In a canine model, the intracavernous injection of trazodone and chlorpromazine resulted in increased arterial flow, venous resistance, and erection (Abber et al, 1987). Injection of a metabolite of trazodone, *m*-chlorophenylpiperazine, resulted in increased firing of the cavernous nerves in rat experiments, indicating possible central action (Steers and de Groat, 1989). In volunteers, trazodone was noted to prolong both nocturnal penile erection and detumescence (Saenz de Tejada et al, 1991).

The mechanism of priapism from these drugs is postulated to be related to alpha-adrenergic blockade or stimulation of serotonergic 1C/1D receptors. Nevertheless, priapism occurs in only a small percentage of patients taking these antipsychotic or antihypertensive medications and is not dosage-specific—a fact that highlights the importance of autonomic system dysregulation.

Total Parenteral Nutrition

Priapism associated with total parenteral nutrition has been reported by several authors (Klein et al, 1985; Ekstrom and Olsson, 1987), in each case after administration of 20% intravenous fat emulsion (Intralipid). Some patients describe recurrent episodes several hours later. These events resemble the stuttering priapism noted among sickle-cell patients. Dark venous blood is described on aspiration, suggesting the low-flow type. Several causative mechanisms have been proposed: (1) a direct increase in blood coagulability; (2) an

Table 38–3. DRUGS REPORTED TO CAUSE PRIAPISM

Antidepressants
Bupropion (Levenson, 1995)
Trazodone (Saenz de Tejada et al, 1991)
Fluoxetine (Murray and Hooberman, 1993)
Sertraline and lithium (Mendelson and Franko, 1994)
Antipsychotics
Clozapine (Rosen and Hanno, 1992; Seftel et al, 1992)
Tranquilizers
Mesoridazine (Starck et al, 1994)
Perphenazine (Tejera and Ramos-Lorenzi, 1992)
Antianxiety Agents
Hydroxyzine (Thavundayil et al, 1994)
Psychotropics
Chlorpromazine (Jackson and Walker, 1991)
Alpha-Adrenergic Blockers
Prazosin (Yaqoob et al, 1991)
Hormone
Gonadotropin-releasing hormone (in hypogonadal men) (Whalen et al, 1991)
Anticoagulants
Heparin
Coumadin
Recreational Drugs
Cocaine (intranasal—Fiorelli et al, 1990; topical—Rodrigues-Blaquez et al, 1990)
Alcohol

adverse effect on cellular elements of blood; and (3) fat emboli. To avoid priapism, the use of 10% fat emulsion, infused slowly and mixed with amino acid–dextrose solutions to prolong administration time, is recommended.

Trauma

Perineal or genital trauma can result in blockage of the penile venous drainage from thrombosis or severe hemorrhage or tissue edema at the base of the penis (low-flow priapism). Laceration of the cavernous artery within the corpora cavernosa due to trauma or intracavernous injection can also result in unregulated pooling of the blood into the sinusoidal spaces with consequent priapism (high-low priapism). High-flow priapism after blunt perineal trauma typically has a delayed onset (Ricciardi et al, 1993). Injury to the erectile tissue and the cavernous artery does not produce priapism until the patient has nocturnal erections, at which time vasodilation causes rupture of the damaged artery, resulting in unregulated high flow into the corpora cavernosa. However, the venous channels are able to compensate partially for the increased flow, and the result is a less than rigid erection without ischemia or pain. In some cases a ruptured arterial branch leading to a cavity is formed after the necrotic tissue is cleared away. This finding usually indicates more severe injury and less complete return of potency.

Pathophysiology

Early work with light microscopy revealed that, after days of idiopathic and secondary priapism, the corporeal tissue becomes thickened, edematous, and eventually fibrotic (Hinman, 1960). The natural sequela of prolonged priapism is impotence, with perhaps some erectile ability maintained in the proximal crura. Electron microscopic studies by Spycher and Hauri (1986) demonstrated trabecular interstitial edema after 12 hours of priapism, with destruction of sinusoidal endothelium, exposure of the basement membrane, and thrombocyte adherence at 24 hours. By 48 hours thrombi are noted in the sinusoidal spaces, and smooth muscle cell histopathologic findings vary from frank necrosis to fibroblast-like cell transformation.

Low-flow priapism is a failure of the detumescence mechanism from many causes, among which are excessive release of neurotransmitters, blockage of the draining venules, paralysis of the intrinsic detumescence mechanism, and prolonged relaxation of the intracavernous smooth muscles. The outcome is a persistently increased intracavernous pressure of 80 to 120 mm Hg and a gradually worsening ischemic state. Typically, pain does not ensue until 6 to 8 hours have passed. The degree of ischemia is a function of the number of emissary veins involved (roughly paralleling the rigidity) and the duration of venous occlusion. A recent study by Broderick and associates (1994) in rabbit cavernous muscle strips has uncovered several interesting findings that may partially explain the physiologic impairment seen in ischemic priapism: (1) anoxia eliminated spontaneous contractile activity and reduced tissue basal tension to a minimum; (2) under anoxic conditions, alpha-adrenergic agonists produced poorly sustained phasic contractile responses; anoxia eliminated the tonic contractile response to phenylephrine; (3) under anoxic conditions, field stimulation of cavernous smooth muscle that was precontracted with phenylephrine produced contraction rather than the relaxation seen in the normoxic state. The impaired contractile response seen in anoxia can be postulated to perpetuate erection with further worsening of the ischemic state.

One of the most intriguing aspects of penile blood is the lack of thrombosis, even after several days of low-flow priapism. In a study of the coagulative and fibrinolytic activities of blood in the cavernous body during pharmacologically induced erection, Rolle and colleagues (1991) reported that the cavernous fibrinolytic activity is three times higher than in peripheral blood. During prolonged erection, fibrinolysis is induced and results in local coagulopathy.

An interesting variant is recurrent priapism as a sequela of a priapic episode (Levine et al, 1991). The frequency of this condition can range from several times per day to once every several months, and it can be disabling. It is postulated that an initial episode of ischemic priapism results in a functional alteration of the adrenergic or endothelium-mediated mechanism that controls penile detumescence.

By definition, all priapism begins as high-flow priapism and the nonischemic state. In most cases priapism proceeds to a veno-occlusive disorder, acidosis, and anoxia and then to typical low-flow priapism. However, high arterial flow continues in some cases, with adequate venous outflow and well-oxygenated corpora cavernosa. **The most common cause of this condition is blunt perineal or genital trauma.** Because the venous channels are open, the erection is compressible and can vary from mild tumescence to slightly less than full rigidity. Pain is rare because the tissue is not ischemic. Some patients may be able to have an additional erection with sexual stimulation, but the majority actually present with the complaint of impotence. The erectile tissue usually appears normal even after as long as 3 years of persistent priapism (Brock et al, 1993). Most patients with high-flow priapism are able to regain adequate erection after embolization or surgical ligation of the ruptured artery, but it may take weeks to months (Bastuba et al, 1994) before full erection returns.

PERSPECTIVES

The past 5 years have seen a continuing explosion of new information on the physiology of penile erection and the pathophysiology of erectile dysfunction and priapism. These new discoveries have not only deepened our understanding of the disease process but also provided a solid basis for improving our methods of diagnosis and treatment. We can expect that the application of new research tools and information in molecular biology, signal transduction, and growth factors will raise the investigation of erectile function and dysfunction to an even higher level in the immediate future.

REFERENCES

Aboseif S, Riemer RK, Stackl W, et al: Quantification of prostaglandin E1 receptors in cavernous tissue of men, monkeys and dogs. Urol Int 1993; 50:148–152.

Aboseif S, Shinohara K, Breza J, et al: Role of penile vascular injury in erectile dysfunction after radical prostatectomy. Br J Urol 1994; 73:75–82.

Adaikan PG, Ratnam SS: Pharmacology of penile erection in humans. Cardiovasc Intervent Radiol 1988; 11:191–194.

Adams DJ, Barakeh J, Laskey R, Van Breemen C: Ion channels and regulation of intracellular calcium in vascular endothelial cells. FASEB J 1989; 3:2389–2400.

Andersson K-E, Holmquist F: Regulation of tone in penile cavernous smooth muscle. Established concepts and new findings. World J Urol 1994; 12:249–261.

Andersson K-E, Wagner G: Physiology of penile erection. Physiol Rev 1995; 75:191–236.

Aoki H, Matsuzaka J, Yeh KH, et al: Involvement of vasoactive intestinal peptide (VIP) as a humoral mediator of penile erectile function in the dog. J Androl 1994; 15:174–182.

Argiolas A: Oxytocin stimulation of penile erection. Pharmacology, site, and mechanism of action. Ann NY Acad Sci 1992; 652:194–203.

Azadzoi KM, Saenz de Tejada I: Hypercholesterolemia impairs endothelium-dependent relaxation of rabbit corpus cavernosum smooth muscle. J Urol 1991; 146:238–240.

Azadzoi KM, Kim N, Brown ML, et al: Endothelium-derived nitric oxide and cyclooxygenase products modulate corpus cavernosum smooth muscle tone. J Urol 1992; 147:220–225.

Azadzoi KM, Vlachiotis J, Pontari M, Siroky MB: Hemodynamics of penile erection: III. Measurement of deep intracavernosal and subtunical blood flow and oxygen tension. J Urol 1995; 153:521–526.

Bagdy G, Kalogeras KT, Szemeredi K: Effect of 5-HT1C and 5-HT2 receptor stimulation on excessive grooming, penile erection and plasma oxytocin concentrations. Eur J Pharmacol 1992; 229:9–14.

Bancroft J, Wu FC: Changes in erectile responsiveness during androgen replacement therapy. Arch Sex Behav 1983; 12:59–66.

Bemelmans BL, Meuleman EJ, Anten BW, et al: Penile sensory disorders in erectile dysfunction: Results of comprehensive neuro-urophysiological diagnostic evaluation in 123 patients. J Urol 1991; 146:777–782.

Beyer C, Gonzalez-Mariscal G: Effects of sex steroids on sensory and motor spinal mechanisms. Psychoneuroendocrinology 1994; 19:517–527.

Bitsch M, Kromann-Andersen B, Schou J, Sjontoft E: The elasticity and the tensile strength of tunica albuginea of the corpora cavernosa. J Urol 1990; 1943:642–644.

Blanco R, Saenz de Tejada I, Goldstein I, Krane RJ, et al: Cholinergic neurotransmission in human corpus cavernosum. II. Acetylcholine synthesis. Am J Physiol 1989; 254:H468–472.

Bochdalek V: Ergebnesse über einem bis getzt überschenen Teil des Erektion sapparates des Penis und der Clitoris. Vierteljahrschr Prakt Heilunde 1854; 43:115.

Bors E, Comarr AE: Neurological disturbances in sexual function with special reference to 529 patients with spinal cord injury. Urol Surv 1960; 10:191–222.

Bosch RJ, Benard F, Aboseif SR, et al: Penile detumescence: Characterization of three phases. J Urol 1991; 146:867–871.

Bredt DS, Hwang PH, Glatt C, et al: Cloned and expressed nitric oxide synthase structurally resemble cytochrome P-450 reductase. Nature 1991; 351:714–718.

Bredt DS, Snyder SH: Isolation of nitric oxide synthetase, a calmodulin-requiring enzyme (endothelium-derived relaxing factor/arginine/cGMP). Proc Natl Acad Sci USA 1990; 87:682–685.

Brenot PH: Male Impotence—A Historical Perspective. L'Esprit du Temps, France, 1994.

Breza J, Aboseif SR, Orvis BR, et al: Detailed anatomy of penile neurovascular structures: Surgical significance. J Urol 1989; 141:437–443.

Brock G, Breza J, Lue TF: Intracavernous sodium nitroprusside: Inappropriate impotence treatment. J Urol 1993a; 150:864–867.

Brock G, Nunes L, Padma-Nathan H, et al: Nitric oxide synthase: A new diagnostic tool for neurogenic impotence. Urology 1993b; 42:412–417.

Buffum J: Pharmacosexology: The effects of drugs on sexual function. A review. J Psychoactive Drugs 1982; 14:5–44.

Buga GM, Gold ME, Fukuto JM, Ignarro LJ: Shear stress-induced release of nitric oxide from endothelial cell growth on beads. Hypertension 1991; 17:187–193.

Burnett AL, Lowenstein CJ, Bredt DS, et al: Nitric oxide: A physiologic mediator of penile erection. Science 1992; 257:401–403.

Burnett AL, Tillman SL, Chang TS, et al: Immunohistochemical localization of nitric oxide synthase in the autonomic innervation of the human penis. J Urol 1993; 150:73–76.

Campos de Calvalho AC, Roy C, Moreno AP, et al: Gap junctions formed of connexin 43 are found between smooth muscle cells of human corpus cavernosum. J Urol 1993; 149:1568–1575.

Carrier S, Brock G, Kour NW, Lue TF: Pathophysiology of erectile dysfunction. Urology 1993; 42:468–481.

Carrier S, Zvara P, Nunes L, et al: Regeneration of nitric oxide synthase–containing nerves after cavernous nerve neurotomy in the rat. J Urol 1995; 153:1722–1727.

Catalona WJ, Bigg SW: Nerve-sparing radical prostatectomy: Evaluation of results after 250 patients. J Urol 1990; 143:538–543.

Cavallini G: Minoxidil versus nitroglycerin: A prospective double-blind controlled trial in a transcutaneous erection facilitation for organic impotence. J Urol 1991; 146:50–53.

Cerami A, Vlassara H, Brownlee M: Glucose and aging. Sci Am 1987; 256:90–96.

Chamness SL, Ricker DD, Crone JK, et al: The effect of androgen on nitric oxide synthase in the male reproductive tract of rat. Fertil Steril 1995; 63:1101–1107.

Chapelle PA, Durand J, Lacert P: Penile erection following complete spinal cord injury in man. Br J Urol 1980; 52:216–219.

Chinkers M, Garbers DL: Signal transduction by guanylyl cyclases. Ann Rev Biochem 1990; 60:553–575.

Christ GJ, Maayani S, Valcic M, Melman A: Pharmacologic studies of human erectile tissue: Characteristics of spontaneous contractions and alterations in alpha-adrenoceptor responsiveness with age and disease in isolated tissues. Br J Pharmacol 1990; 101:375–381.

Christ GJ, Moreno AP, Melman A, Spray DC: Gap junction–mediated intercellular diffusion of Ca^{2+} in cultured human corporal smooth muscle cells. Am J Physiol 1992; 263:C373–383.

Christ GJ, Moreno AP, Parker ME, et al: Intercellular communication through gap junctions: A potential role in pharmacomechanical coupling and syncytial tissue contraction in vascular smooth muscle isolated from the human corpus cavernosum. Life Sci 1991; 49:PL195–PL200.

Christensen GC: Angioarchitecture of the canine penis and the process of erection. Am J Anat 1954; 95:227–250.

Clark JT, Smith ER, Davidson JM: Evidence for modulation of sexual behavior by alpha-adrenoceptors in male rats. Neuroendocrinology 1985; 41:36–43.

Conti G: L'erection du penis humain et ses bases morphologico-vascularies. Acta Anat 1952; 14:217–262.

Costa P, Soulie-Vassal ML, Sarrazin B, et al: Adrenergic receptors on smooth muscle cells isolated from human penile corpus cavernosum. J Urol 1993; 150:859–863.

Courtois FJ, MacDougall JC, Sachs BD: Erectile mechanism in paraplegia. Physiol Behav 1993; 53:721–726.

Cunningham GR, Hirshkowitz M, Korenman SG, Karacan I: Testosterone replacement therapy and sleep-related erections in hypogonadal men. J Clin Endocrinol Metab 1990; 70:792–797.

Dalkin BL, Carter MF: Venogenic impotence following dermal graft repair for Peyronie's disease. J Urol 1991; 146:849–851.

Danjou P, Alexandre L, Warot D, et al: Assessment of erectogenic properties of apomorphine and yohimbine in man. Br J Clin Pharmacol 1988; 26:733–739.

David KRD, Koyle M: Impotence in chronic renal failure. *In* Rajfer Y, ed: Common Problems in Infertility and Impotence. Chicago, Year Book Medical Publishers, 1990, pp 368–375.

DeGroat WC, Booth AM: Neural control of penile erection. *In* Maggi CA, ed: The Autonomic Nervous System. Nervous Control of the Urogenital System. London, Harwood, 1993, pp 465–513.

Derouet H, Eckert R, Trautwein W, Ziegler M: Muscular cavernous single cell analysis in patients with venoocclusive dysfunction. Eur Urol 1994; 25:145–150.

Deysach LJ: Comparative morphology of erectile tissue of penis with especial emphasis on probable mechanism of erection. Am J Anat 1939; 64:111.

Diederichs W, Stief CG, Lue TF, Tanagho EA: Norepinephrine involvement in penile detumescence. J Urol 1990; 143:1264–1266.

Diederichs W, Stief CG, Benard F, et al: The sympathetic role as antagonist of erection. Urol Res 1991a; 19:123–126.

Diederichs W, Stief CG, Lue TF, Tanagho EA: Sympathetic inhibition of papaverine induced erection. J Urol 1991b; 146:195–198.

Diokno AC, Brown MB, Herzog AR: Sexual function in the elderly. Arch Int Med 1990; 150:197–200.

Dorr L, Brody M: Hemodynamic mechanisms of erection in the canine penis. Am J Physiol 1967; 213:1526.

Draznin MB, Rapoport RM, Murad F: Myosin light chain phosphorylation in contraction and relaxation of intact rat thoracic aorta. Int J Biochem 1986; 18:917–928.

Eardley I, Kirby RS: Neurogenic impotence. *In* Kirby RS, Carson CC, Webster GD, eds: Impotence: Diagnosis and Management of Male Erectile Dysfunction. Oxford, Butterworth-Heinemann, 1991, pp 227–231.

Fan SF, Brink PR, Melman A, Christ GJ: An analysis of the Maxi-K^+ (KCa) channel in cultured human corporal smooth muscle cells. J Urol 1995; 153:818–825.

Feldman HA, Goldstein I, Hatzichristou DG, et al: Impotence and its medical and psychosocial correlates: Results of the Massachusetts Male Aging Study. J Urol 1994; 151:54–61.

Finkle AL, Taylor SP: Sexual potency after radical prostatectomy. J Urol 1981; 125:350.

Foreman MM, Hall JL, Love RL: The role of the 5-HT_2 receptor in the regulation of sexual performance of male rats. Life Sci 1989; 45:1263–1270.

Foreman MM, Wernicke JF: Approaches for the development of oral drug therapies for erectile dysfunction. Semin Urol 1990; 8:107–112.

Fukuto JM, Wood KS, Byrns RE, Ignarro LJ: N^G-amino-L-arginine: A new potent antagonist of L-arginine-mediated endothelium-dependent relaxation. Biochem Biophys Res Commun 1990; 168:458–465.

Furlow WL: Prevalence of impotence in the United States. Med Aspects Human Sexuality 1985; 19:13–16.

Garban H, Vernet D, Freedman A, et al: Effect of aging on nitric oxide–mediated penile erection in rats. Am J Physiol 1995; 268:H467–475.

Garbers DL: Guanylyl cyclase receptors and their endocrine, paracrine and autocrine ligands. Cell 1992; 71:1–4.

Giuliano F, Rampin O, Jardin A, Rousseau JP: Electrophysiological study of relations between the dorsal nerve of the penis and the lumbar sympathetic chain in the rat. J Urol 1993; 150:1960–1964.

Goldstein AMB, Meehan JP, Zakhary R, et al: New observations on the microarchitecture of the corpora cavernosa in man and possible relationship to mechanism of erection. Urology 1982; 20:259–266.

Goldstein AMB, Padma-Nathan H: The microarchitecture of the intracavernosal smooth muscle and the cavernosal fibrous skeleton. J Urol 1990; 144:1145–1146.

Goldstein I, Feldman MI, Deckers PJ, et al: Radiation-associated impotence. A clinical study of its mechanism. JAMA 1984; 251:903–910.

Gozes I, Reshef A, Salah D, et al: Stearyl-norleucine–vasoactive intestinal peptide (VIP): A novel VIP analog for noninvasive impotence treatment. Endocrinology 1994; 134:2121–2125.

Graham CW, Regan JB: Blinded clinical trial of testosterone enanthate in impotent men with low or low-normal serum testosterone levels. Int J Impotence Res 1992; 4:P144.

Gruetter CA, Barry BK, McNamara DB, et al: Relaxation of bovine coronary artery and activation of coronary arterial guanylate cyclase by nitric oxide, nitroprusside and a carcinogenic nitrosoamine. J Cyclic Nucleotide Res 1979; 5:211–224.

Halata Z, Munger BL: The neuroanatomical basis for the protopathic sensibility of the human glans penis. Brain Res 1986; 371:205–230.

Hayashi K, Takamizawa K, Nakamura T, et al: Effects of elastase on the stiffness and elastic properties of arterial walls in cholesterol-fed rabbits. Atherosclerosis 1987; 66:259–267.

Hedlund H, Andersson K: Comparison of the responses to drugs acting on adrenoreceptors and muscarinic receptors in human isolated corpus cavernosum and cavernous artery. J Auton Pharmacol 1985; 5:81–88.

Hedlund H, Andersson K, Fovaeus M, et al: Characterization of contraction-mediating prostanoid receptors in human penile erectile tissues. J Urol 1989; 141:182–186.

Hedlund P, Alm P, Hedlund H, et al: Localization and effects of pituitary adenylate cyclase–activating polypeptide (PACAP) in human penile erectile tissue. Acta Physiol Scand 1994; 150:103–104.

Hirshkowitz M, Karacan I, Howell JW, et al: Nocturnal penile tumescence in cigarette smokers with erectile dysfunction. Urology 1992; 39:101–107.

Hirshkowitz M, Karacan I, Rando KC, et al: Diabetes, erectile dysfunction, and sleep-related erections. Sleep 1990; 13:53–68.

Holmquist F, Andersson K, Hedlund H: Actions of endothelin on isolated corpus cavernosum from rabbit and man. Acta Physiol Scand 1990; 139:113–122.

Holmquist F, Stief CG, Jonas U, Andersson KE: Effects of the nitric oxide synthase inhibitor NG-nitro-L-arginine on the erectile response to cavernous nerve stimulation in the rabbit. Acta Physiol Scand 1991; 143:299–304.

Hsieh JT, Muller SC, Lue TF: The influence of blood flow and blood pressure on penile erection. Int J Impotence Res 1989; 1:35–42.

Hsu GL, Brock G, Martinez-Pineiro L, et al: The three-dimensional structure of the human tunica albuginea: Anatomical and ultrastructural levels. Int J Impotence Res 1992; 4:117–129.

Hsu GL, Brock G, Martinez-Pineiro L, et al: Anatomy and strength of the tunica albuginea: Its relevance to penile prosthesis extrusion. J Urol 1994; 151:1205–1208.

Hull EM, Eaton RC, Markowski VP, et al: Opposite influence of medial preoptic D1 and D2 receptors on genital reflexes: Implications for copulation. Life Sci 1992; 51:1705–1713.

Hunter J: Treite des Maladies Veneriennes. Paris, Mequignon, 1787.

Iacono F, Barra S, DeRosa G, et al: Microstructural disorders of tunica albuginea in patients affected by Peyronie's disease with or without erection dysfunction. J Urol 1993; 150:1806–1809.

Iacono F, Barra S, DeRosa G, et al: Microstructural disorders of tunica albuginea in patients affected by impotence. Eur Urol 1994; 26:233–239.

Ignarro LJ, Buga GM, Wood KS, et al: Endothelium-derived relaxing factor produced and released from artery and vein is nitric oxide. Proc Natl Acad Sci USA 1987; 84:9265–9269.

Ignarro LJ, Bush PA, Buga GM, et al: Nitric oxide and cyclic GMP formation upon electrical field stimulation cause relaxation of corpus cavernosum smooth muscle. Biochem Biophys Res Comm 1990a; 170:843–850.

Ignarro LJ, Bush PS, Buga GM, Rajfer J: Neurotransmitter identity in doubt. Nature 1990b; 347:131–132.

Janssens SP, Shimouchi A, Quertermous T, et al: Cloning and expression of a cDNA encoding human endothelium-derived relaxing factor/nitric oxide synthase. J Biol Chem 1992; 267:14519–14522.

Jeanty P, Van den Kerchove M, Lowenthal A, De Bruyne H: Pergolide therapy in Parkinson's disease. J Neurol 1984; 231:148–152.

Jünemann K-P, Lue TF, Luo JA, et al: The effect of cigarette smoking on penile erection. J Urol 1987; 138:438–441.

Jünemann KP, Aufenanger J, Konrad T, et al: The effect of impaired lipid metabolism on the smooth muscle cells of rabbits. Urol Res 1991; 19:271–275.

Kaiser FE, Viosca SP, Morley JE, et al: Impotence and aging: Clinical and hormonal factors. J Am Geriatr Soc 1988; 36:511–519.

Katsuki S, Murad F: Regulation of cyclic 3′,5′-adenosine and cyclic 3′,5′-guanosine monophosphate levels and contractility in bovine tracheal smooth muscle. Mol Pharmacol 1977; 13:330–341.

Kaufman JM, Hatzichristou DG, Mulhall JP, et al: Impotence and chronic renal failure: A study of the hemodynamic pathophysiology. J Urol 1994; 151:612–618.

Kerfoot WW, Park HY, Schwartz LB, et al: Characterization of calcium channel blocker induced smooth muscle relaxation using a model of isolated corpus cavernosum. J Urol 1993; 150:249–252.

Kim ED, Blackburn D, McVary KT: Post-radical prostatectomy penile blood flow: Assessment with color flow Doppler ultrasound. J Urol 1994; 152:2276–2279.

Kim N, Azadzoi KM, Goldstein I, Saenz de Tejada I: A nitric oxide–like factor mediates nonadrenergic-noncholinergic neurogenic relaxation of penile corpus cavernosum smooth muscle. J Clin Invest 1991; 88:112–118.

Kim N, Vardi Y, Padma-Nathan H, et al: Oxygen tension regulates the nitric oxide pathway. Physiological role in penile erection. J Clin Invest 1993; 91:437–442.

Kim SC, Oh MM: Norepinephrine involvement in response to intracorporeal injection of papaverine in psychogenic impotence. J Urol 1992; 147:1530–1532.

Kim YC, Kim JH, Davies MG, et al: Modulation of vasoactive intestinal polypeptide (VIP)–mediated relaxation by nitric oxide and prostanoids in the rabbit corpus cavernosum. J Urol 1995; 153:807–810.

Kinsey AC, Pomeroy WB, Martin CE: Sexual Behavior in the Human Male. Philadelphia, W. B. Saunders Company, 1948, p 236.

Kirkeby HJ, Andersson KE, Forman A: Comparison of the effects of prostanoids on human penile circumflex veins and corpus cavernosum tissue. Br J Urol 1993; 72:220–225.

Kirkeby HJ, Fahrenkrug J, Holmquist F, Ottesen B: Vasoactive intestinal polypeptide (VIP) and peptide histidine methionine (PHM) in human penile corpus cavernosum tissue and circumflex veins: Localization and in vitro effects. Eur J Clin Invest 1992; 22:24–30.

Kiss F: Anatomisch-histologische Untersuchungen über die Erektion. Z Anat 1921; 61:455–521.

Knispel HH, Goessl C, Beckmann R: Nitric oxide mediates neurogenic relaxation induced in rabbit cavernous smooth muscle by electric field stimulation. Urology 1992; 40:471–476.

Lamas S, Marsden PA, Li GK, et al: Endothelial nitric oxide synthase: Molecular cloning and characterization of a distant constitutive enzyme isoform (signal transduction/gene family/endothelium-derived relaxing factor/cyclic GMP/guanylate cyclase). Proc Natl Acad Sci USA 1992; 89:6348–6352.

Leonard MP, Nickel CJ, Morales A: Hyperprolactinemia and impotence: Why, when and how to investigate. J Urol 1989; 142:992–994.

Lerner SE, Melman A, Christ GJ: A review of erectile dysfunction: New insights and more questions. J Urol 1993; 149:1246–1255.

Levin RM, Hypolite J, Broderick GA: Comparative studies on intracellular calcium and NADH fluorescence of the rabbit corpus cavernosum. Neurourol Urodynam 1994; 13:609–618.

Levin RM, Wein AJ: Adrenergic alpha receptors outnumber beta receptors in human penile corpus cavernosum. Invest Urol 1980; 18:225–226.

Levine FJ, Greenfield AJ, Goldstein I: Arteriographically determined occlusive disease within the hypogastric-cavernous bed in impotent patients following blunt perineal and pelvic trauma. J Urol 1990; 144:1147–1153.

Lowenstein CJ, Glatt CS, Bredt DS, Snyder SH: Cloned and expressed macrophage nitric oxide synthase contrasts with the brain enzyme. Proc Natl Acad Sci USA 1992; 89:6711–6715.

Lowenstein CJ, Snyder SH: Nitric oxide. A novel biological messenger. Cell 1992; 70:705–707.

Lue TF: Editorial comment. J Urol 1994a; 152:1661.

Lue TF: Erectile dysfunction associated with cavernous and neurological disorders. J Urol 1994b; 151:890–891.

Lue TF, Takamura T, Schmidt RA, et al: Hemodynamics of erection in the monkey. J Urol 1983; 130:1237–1241.

Lugg JA, Rajfer J, Gonzalez-Cadavid NF: Dihydrotestosterone is the active androgen in the maintenance of nitric oxide–mediated penile erection in the rat. Endocrinology 1995; 136:1495–1501.

Lyons CR, Orloff GJ, Cunningham JM: Molecular cloning and functional expression of an inducible nitric oxide synthase from a murine macrophage cell line. J Biol Chem 1992; 267:6370–6374.

Mallick HN, Manchanda SK, Kumar VM: Sensory modulation of the medial preoptic area neuronal activity by dorsal penile nerve stimulation in rats. J Urol 1994; 151:759–762.

Mandrek K: Electrophysiological methods in smooth-muscle physiology. Corpus cavernosum in vitro. World J Urol 1994; 12:262–265.

Marson L, McKenna ME: A role for 5-hydroxytryptamine in descending inhibition of spinal sexual reflexes. Exp Brain Res 1992; 88:313–320.

Marson L, Platt KB, McKenna KE: Central nervous system innervation of the penis as revealed by the transneuronal transport of pseudorabies virus. Neuroscience 1993; 55:280.

Masters WH, Johnson V: Human Sexual Response. Boston, Little, Brown, 1970.

Masters WH, Johnson VE: Sex after sixty-five. Reflections 1977; 12:31–43.

Matsumoto A, Arai Y, Urano A, Hyodo S: Androgen regulates gene expression of cytoskeletal proteins in adult rat motoneurons. Horm Behav 1994; 28:357–366.

McDermott DW, Bates RJ, Heney NM, Althausen A: Erectile impotence as complication of direct vision cold knife urethrotomy. Urology 1981; 18:467–469.

Melis MR, Argiolas A, Gessa GL: Evidence that apomorphine induces penile erection and yawning by releasing oxytocin in the central nervous system. Eur J Pharmacol 1989; 164:565–570.

Melis MR, Argiolas A: Nitric oxide synthase inhibitors prevent apomorphine- and oxytocin-induced penile erection and yawning in male rats. Brain Res Bull 1993; 32:71–74.

Melis MR, Stancampiano R, Gessa GL, Argiolas A: Prevention by morphine of apomorphine- and oxytocin-induced penile erection and yawning: Site of action in the brain. Neuropsychopharmacology 1992; 6:17–21.

Mersdorf A, Goldsmith PC, Diederichs W, et al: Ultrastructural changes in impotent penile tissue: A comparison of 65 patients. J Urol 1991; 145:749–758.

Metz P, Ebbehoj J, Uhrenholdt A, Wagner G: Peyronie's disease and erectile failure. J Urol 1983; 130:1103–1104.

Meyhoff HH, Rosenkilde P, Bodker A: Non-invasive management of impotence with transcutaneous nitroglycerin. Br J Urol 1992; 69:88–90.

Michal V, Ruzbarsky V: Histological changes in the penile arterial bed with aging and diabetes. *In* Zorgniotti AW, Rossi G, eds: Vasculogenic Impotence: Proceedings of the First International Conference on Corpus Cavernosum Revascularization. Springfield, IL, Charles C Thomas, 1980, pp 113–119.

Miller NS, Gold MS: The human sexual response and alcohol and drugs. J Subst Abuse Treat 1988; 5:171–177.

Moreland RB, Traish A, McMillin MA, et al: I. PGE1 suppresses the induction of collagen synthesis by transforming growth factor-beta 1 in human corpus cavernosum smooth muscle. J Urol 1995; 153:826–834.

Murad F, Mittal CK, Arnold WP, et al: Guanylate cyclase: Activation by azide nitro compounds, nitric oxide and hydroxyl radical and inhibition by hemoglobin and myoglobin. Adv Cyclic Nucl Res 1978; 9:145–158.

Murad F: Cyclic guanosine monophosphate as a mediator of vasodilation. J Clin Invest 1986; 78:1–5.

Newman HF, Northrup JD, Devlin J: Mechanism of human penile erection. Invest Urol 1964; 1:350–353.

Newman HF, Northrup JD: Mechanism of human penile erection: An overview. Urology 1981; 17:399–408.

Nogues MA, Starkstein S, Davalos M, et al: Cardiovascular reflexes and pudendal evoked responses in chronic haemodialysis patients. Funct Neurol 1991; 6:359–365.

Ottesen B, Wagner G, Virag R, Fahrenkrug J: Penile erection: Possible role for vasoactive intestinal polypeptide as a neurotransmitter. BMJ 1984; 288:9–11.

Paick JS, Donatucci CF, Lue TF: Anatomy of cavernous nerves distal to prostate: Microdissection study in adult male cadavers. Urology 1993; 42:145–149.

Paick JS, Goldsmith PC, Batra AK, et al: Relationship between venous incompetence and cavernous nerve injury: Ultrastructural alteration of cavernous smooth muscle in the neurotomized dog. Int J Impotence Res 1991; 3:185–195.

Paick JS, Lee SW: The neural mechanism of apomorphine-induced erection: An experimental study by comparison with electrostimulation-induced erection in the rat model. J Urol 1994; 152:2125–2128.

Palmer RMJ, Ashton DS, Moncada S: Vascular endothelial cells synthesize nitric oxide from L-arginine. Nature 1988; 333:664–666.

Palmer RMJ, Ferrige AG, Moncada S: Nitric oxide release accounts for the biological activity of endothelium-derived relaxing factor. Nature 1987; 327:524–526.

Pare A: Les Dix Livres de Chirurgie. Paris, 1585.

Persson C, Diederichs W, Lue TF, et al: Correlation of altered penile ultrastructure with clinical arterial evaluation. J Urol 1989; 142:1462–1468.

Pickard RS, King P, Zar MA, Powell PH: Corpus cavernosal relaxation in impotent men. Br J Urol 1994; 74:485–491.

Pickard RS, Powell PH, Zar MA: The effect of inhibitors of nitric oxide biosynthesis and cyclic GMP formation on nerve-evoked relaxation of human cavernosal smooth muscle. Br J Pharmacol 1991; 104:755–759.

Quinlan DM, Epstein JI, Carter BS, Walsh PC: Sexual function following radical prostatectomy: Influence of preservation of neurovascular bundles. J Urol 1991; 145:998–1002.

Rajfer J, Aronson WJ, Bush PA, et al: Nitric oxide as a mediator of relaxation of the corpus cavernosum in response to nonadrenergic, noncholinergic neurotransmission. N Engl J Med 1992; 326:90–94.

Rajfer J, Rosciszewski A, Mehringer M: Prevalence of corporal venous leakage in impotent men. J Urol 1988; 140:69–71.

Rapoport RM, Murad F: Endothelium-dependent and nitrovasodilator-induced relaxation of vascular smooth muscle: Role for cyclic GMP. J Cyclic Nucl Protein Phosphor Res 1983; 9:281–296.

Rees HD, Michael RP: Brain cells of the male rhesus monkey accumulate 3H-testosterone or its metabolites. J Comp Neurol 1982; 206:273–277.

Root WS, Bard P: The medication of feline erection through sympathetic pathways with some reference on sexual behavior after deafferentation of the genitalia. Am J Physiol 1947; 151:80–90.

Rosen MP, Greenfield AJ, Walker TG, et al: Arteriogenic impotence: Findings in 195 impotent men examined with selective internal pudendal angiography. Radiology 1990; 174:1043–1048.

Rosen MP, Greenfield AJ, Walker TG, et al: Cigarette smoking: An independent risk factor for atherosclerosis in the hypogastric-cavernous arterial bed of men with arteriogenic impotence. J Urol 1991; 145:759–763.

Rowland DL, Greenleaf W, Mas M, et al: Penile and finger sensory thresholds in young, aging, and diabetic males. Arch Sex Behav 1989; 18:1–12.

Rowland DL, Greenleaf WJ, Dorfman LJ, Davidson JM: Aging and sexual function in men. Arch Sex Behav 1993; 22:545–557.

Rubanyi GM, Romero JC, Vanhoutte PM: Flow-induced release of endothelium-derived relaxing factor. Am J Physiol 1989; 250:H1145–1149.

Sachs BD, Meisel RL: The physiology of male sexual behavior. *In* Knobil E, Neill JD, Ewing LL, eds: The Physiology of Reproduction. New York, Raven Press, 1988, pp 1393–1423.

Saenz de Tejada I, Blanco R, Goldstein I, et al: Cholinergic neurotransmission in human corpus cavernosum. I. Responses of isolated tissue. Am J Physiol 1988; 254:H459–467.

Saenz de Tejada I, Carson MP, de las Morenas A, et al: Endothelin: Localization, synthesis, activity, and receptor types in human penile corpus cavernosum. Am J Physiol 1991a; 261:H1078–1085.

Saenz de Tejada I, Goldstein I, Azadzoi K, et al: Impaired neurogenic and endothelium-mediated relaxation of penile smooth muscle from diabetic men with impotence. N Engl J Med 1989a; 320:1025–1030.

Saenz de Tejada I, Kim N, Lagan I, et al: Regulation of adrenergic activity in penile corpus cavernosum. J Urol 1989b; 142:1117–1121.

Saenz de Tejada I, Moroukian P, Tessier J, et al: Trabecular smooth muscle modulates the capacitor function of the penis. Studies on a rabbit model. Am J Physiol 1991b; 260:H1590–1595.

Saenz de Tejada I, Ware JC, Blanco R, et al: Pathophysiology of prolonged penile erection associated with trazodone use. J Urol 1991c; 145:60–64.

Saito M, Broderick GA, Wein AJ, Levin RM: Effect of chronic ethanol consumption on the pharmacological response of the rabbit corpus cavernosum. Pharmacology 1994; 49:386–391.

Salvatierra O, Fortmann JL, Belzer FO: Sexual function of males before and after renal transplantation. Urology 1975; 5:64–66.

Schiavi RC, Schreiner-Engel P: Nocturnal penile tumescence in healthy aging men. J Gerontology 1988; 43:M146–150.

Shabsigh R, Fishman IJ, Scott FB: Evaluation of erectile impotence. Urology 1988; 32:83–90.

Shirai M, Ishii N, Mitsukawa S, et al: Hemodynamic mechanism of erection in the human penis. Arch Androl 1978; 1:345–349.

Simerly RB, Swanson LW: Projections of the medial preoptic nucleus: A *Phaseolus vulgaris* leucoagglutinin anterograde tract-tracing in the rat. J Comp Neurol 1988; 270:209–242.

Slag MF, Morley JE, Elson MK, et al: Impotence in medical clinic outpatients. JAMA 1983; 249:1736–1740.

Sparwasser C, Drescher P, Will JA, Madsen PO: Smooth muscle tone regulation in rabbit cavernosal and spongiosal tissue by cyclic AMP– and cyclic GMP–dependent mechanisms. J Urol 1994; 152:2159–2163.

Steers WD, DeGroat WC: Effects of m-chlorophenylpiperazine on penile and bladder function in rats. Am J Physiol 1989; 257:R1441–1449.

Steers WD, McConnell J, Benson G: Anatomical localization and some pharmacological effects of vasoactive intestinal polypeptide in human and monkey corpus cavernosum. J Urol 1984; 132:1048–1053.

Steers WD: Neural control of penile erection. Semin Urol 1990; 8:66–70.

Stief C, Benard F, Bosch R, et al: Acetylcholine as a possible neurotransmitter in penile erection. J Urol 1989; 141:1444–1448.

Stief CG, Benard F, Bosch RJ, et al: A possible role of calcitonin-gene–related peptide in the regulation of the smooth muscle tone of the bladder and penis. J Urol 1990; 143:392–397.

Stief CG, Djamilian M, Anton P, et al: Single potential analysis of cavernous electrical activity in impotent patients: A possible diagnostic method for autonomic cavernous dysfunction and cavernous smooth muscle degeneration. J Urol 1991; 146:771–776.

Stief CG, Holmquist F, Djamilian M, et al: Preliminary results with the nitric oxide donor linsidomine chlorhydrate in the treatment of human erectile dysfunction. J Urol 1992; 148:1437–1440.

Tamaki M: Mechanism preventing backflow from the canine corpora cavernosa to arteries in the rigid phase of penile erection. Urol Int 1992; 48:64–70.

Traish AM, Carson MP, Kim N, et al: Characterization of muscarinic acetylcholine receptors in human penile corpus cavernosum: Studies on whole tissue and cultured endothelium. J Urol 1990; 144:1036–1040.

Traish AM, Netsuwan N, Daley J, et al: A heterogeneous population of alpha-1 adrenergic receptors mediates contraction of human corpus cavernosum smooth muscle to norepinephrine. J Urol 1995; 153:222–227.

Trigo-Rocha F, Aronson WJ, Hohenfellner M, et al: Nitric oxide and cGMP mediators of pelvic nerve–stimulated erection in dogs. Am J Physiol 1993a; 264:H419–H422.

Trigo-Rocha F, Hsu GL, Donatucci CF, Lue TF: The role of cyclic adenosine monophosphate, cyclic guanosine monophosphate, endothelium and nonadrenergic, noncholinergic neurotransmission in canine penile erection. J Urol 1993b; 149:872–877.

Veenema RJ, Gursel EO, Lattimer JK: Radical retropubic prostatectomy for cancer: A 20 year experience. J Urol 1977; 117:330.

Vincent SR, Kimura H: Histochemical mapping of nitric oxide synthase in the rat brain. Neuroscience 1992; 46:755–784.

von Ebner V: Uber Klappenartige Vorrichtungen in den Arterien der Schwellkorger. Anat Anz 1900; 18:79.

Wagner C, Bro-Rasmussen F, Willis EA, Neilsen MH: New theory on the mechanism of erection involving hitherto undescribed vessels. Lancet 1982; 1:416–418.

Wagner CK, Popper P, Ulibarri C, et al: Calcitonin gene–related peptide-like immunoreactivity in spinal motoneurons of the male mouse is affected by castration and genotype. Brain Res 1994; 647:37–43.

Wagner G, Uhrenholdt A: Blood flow measurement by the clearance method in the human corpus cavernosum in the flaccid and erect states. *In* Zorgniotti AW, Ross G, eds: Vasculogenic impotence. Proceedings of the First International Conference on Corpus Cavernosum Revascularization. Springfield, IL, Charles C Thomas, 1980, pp 41–46.

Wagner G: Erection, physiology and endocrinology. *In* Wagner G, Green R, eds: Impotence: Physiological, and Surgical Diagnosis and Treatment. New York, Plenum Press, 1981, pp 25–36.

Waldeyer W: Topographisch-anatomisch mit besonderes Beruchsichtigung der Chirurgie und gynakologie Dargestellt. *In* Das Decken, 1899, p 354.

Waldman SA, Lewicki JA, Brandwein HJ, Murad F: Partial purification and characterization of particulate guanylate cyclase from rat liver after solubilization with trypsin. J Cyclic Nucl Res 1982; 8:359–370.

Walsh PC, Brendler CB, Chang T, et al: Preservation of sexual function in men during radical pelvic surgery. Md Med J 1990; 39:389–393.

Walsh PC, Donker PJ: Impotence following radical prostatectomy: Insight into etiology and prevention. J Urol 1982; 128:492–497.

Wein AJ, Van Arsdalen K: Drug-induced male sexual dysfunction. Urol Clin North Am 1988; 15:23–31.

Weinstein MN, Roberts M: Sexual potency following surgery for rectal carcinoma. A follow-up of 44 patients. Ann Surg 1977; 185:295.

Wermuth L, Stenager E: Sexual aspects of Parkinson's disease. Semin Neurol 1992; 12:125–127.

Wespes E, Goes PM, Schiffmann S, et al: Computerized analysis of smooth muscle fibers in potent and impotent patients. J Urol 1991; 146:1015–1017.

Wolfe MM: Impotence of cimetidine treatment. N Engl J Med 1979; 300:94.

Wolfson B, Pickett S, Scott NE, et al: Intraurethral prostaglandin E-2 cream: A possible alternative treatment for erectile dysfunction. Urology 1993; 42:73–75.

Xie QW, Cho HJ, Calaycay J, et al: Cloning and characterization of inducible nitric oxide synthase from mouse macrophages. Science 1992; 256:225–228.

Yarnitsky D, Sprecher E, Barilan Y, Vardi Y: Corpus cavernosum electromyogram: Spontaneous and evoked electrical activities. J Urol 1995; 153:653–654.

Yeager ES, Van Heerden JA: Sexual dysfunction following proctocolectomy and abdominoperineal resection. Ann Surg 1980; 191:169.

Yeh KH, Aoki H, Matsuzaka J, et al: Participation of vasoactive intestinal polypeptide (VIP) as humoral mediator in the erectile response of canine corpus cavernosum penis. J Androl 1994; 15:187–193.

Priapism

Abber JC, Lue TF, Luo J, et al: Priapism induced by chlorpromazine and trazodone: Mechanism of action. J Urol 1987; 137:1039.

Bastuba MD, Saenz de Tejada I, Dinlenc CZ, et al: Arterial priapism: Diagnosis, treatment and long-term followup. J Urol 1994; 151:1231–1237.

Bhatia P, Arya LS, Chinnappan D, et al: Priapism in chronic myelogenous leukemia. Ind J Ped 1992; 59:130–132.

Brock G, Breza J, Lue TF, Tanagho EA: High flow priapism: A spectrum of disease. J Urol 1993; 150:968–971.

Broderick GA, Gordon D, Hypolite J, Levin RM: Anoxia and corporal smooth muscle dysfunction: A model for ischemic priapism. J Urol 1994; 151:259–262.

Dorman BW, Schmidt JD: Association of priapism in phenothiazine therapy. J Urol 1976; 116:51.

Ekstrom B, Olsson AM: Priapism in patients treated with total parenteral nutrition. Br J Urol 1987; 59:170.

Fiorelli RL, Manfrey SJ, Belkoff LH, Finkelstein LH: Priapism associated with intranasal cocaine abuse. J Urol 1990; 143:584–585.

Hashmat AI, Rehman J: Priapism. *In* Hashmat AI, Das S, eds: The Penis. Philadelphia, Lea & Febiger, 1993, pp 219–243.

Hauri D, Spycher M, Bruhlmann W: Erection and priapism: A new physiopathologic concept. Urol Int 1983; 38:138.

Hinman F Jr: Priapism reasons for failure of therapy. J Urol 1960; 83:420.

Jackson SC, Walker JS: Self-administered intraurethral chlorpromazine: An unusual cause of priapism. Am J Emerg Med 1991; 9:171–175.

Jünemann KP, Lue TF, Abozeid M, et al: Blood gas analysis in drug-induced penile erection. Urol Int 1986; 41:207–211.

Jünemann KP, Alken P: Pharmacotherapy of erectile dysfunction. Int J Impotence Res 1989; 1:71–93.

Klein EA, Montague DK, Steiger E: Priapism associated with the use of intravenous fat emulsion: Case reports and postulated pathogenesis. J Urol 1985; 133:857.

Levenson JL: Priapism associated with bupropion treatment [letter]. Am J Psychiatry 1995; 152:813.

Levine JF, Saenz de Tejada I, Payton TR, Goldstein I: Recurrent prolonged erections and priapism as a sequela of priapism: Pathophysiology and management. J Urol 1991; 145:764–767.

Mendelson WB, Franko T: Priapism with sertraline and lithium [letter]. J Clin Psychopharmacol 1994; 14:434–435.

Murray MJ, Hooberman D: Fluoxetine and prolonged erection [letter]. Am J Psychiatry 1993; 150:167–168.

Nelson JH, Winter CC: Priapism: Evolution of management in 48 patients in a 22-year series. J Urol 1977; 117:455.

Pohl J, Pott B, Kleinhans G: Priapism: A three phase concept of management according to etiology and prognosis. Br J Urol 1986; 58:113.

Powell BL, Craig JB, Muss HB: Secondary malignancies of the penis and epididymis: A case report and review of the literature. J Clin Oncol 1985; 3:110.

Priapism with trazodone (Desyrel): Med Lett 1984; 26:35.

Puppo P, Perachino M, Ricciotti G, Vitali A: Malignant priapism due to a huge renal carcinoma. Eur Urol 1992; 21:169–171.

Ramos CE, Park JS, Ritchey ML, Benson GS: High flow priapism associated with sickle cell disease. J Urol 1995; 153:1619–1621.

Ricciardi R Jr, Bhatt GM, Cynamon J, et al: Delayed high flow priapism: Pathophysiology and management. J Urol 1993; 149:119–121.

Rodriguez-Blaquez HM, Cardona PE, Rivera-Herrera JL: Priapism associated with the use of topical cocaine. J Urol 1990; 143:358.

Rolle L, Bazzan M, Bellina M, Fontana D: Coagulation and fibrinolytic activity of blood from corpus cavernosum. Arch Ital Urol Nefrol Androl 1991; 63:471–473.

Rosen SI, Hanno PM: Clozapine-induced priapism. J Urol 1992; 148:876–877.

Rubin SO: Priapism as a probable sequel to medication. Scand J Urol Nephrol 1968; 2:81.

Saenz de Tejada I, Ware JC, Blanco R, et al: Pathophysiology of prolonged penile erection associated with trazodone use. J Urol 1991; 145:60–64.

Sagar SM, Retsas S: Metastasis to the penis from malignant melanoma: A case report and review of the literature. Clin Oncol (R Coll Radiol) 1992; 4:130–131.

Schroeder-Printzen I, Vosshenrich R, Weidner W, Ringert RH: Malignant priapism in a patient with metastatic prostate adenocarcinoma. Urol Int 1994; 52:52–54.

Seftel AD, Saenz de Tejada I, Szetela B, et al: Clozapine-associated priapism: A case report. J Urol 1992; 147:146–148.

Serjeant GR, de Ceular K, Maude GH: Stilbestrol and stuttering priapism in homozygous sickle-cell disease. Lancet 1985; 2:1274.

Spycher MA, Hauri D: The ultrastructure of the erectile tissue in priapism. J Urol 1986; 135:142.

Starck LC, Talley BJ, Brannan SK: Mesoridazine use and priapism [letter]. Am J Psychiatry 1994; 151:946.

Steers WD, DeGroat WC: Effects of m-chlorophenylpiperazine on penile and bladder function in rats. Am J Physiol 1989; 257:1441–1449.

Tarry WF, Duckett JW Jr, Snyder H McC III: Urological complications of sickle cell disease in a pediatric population. J Urol 1987; 138:592.

Tejera CA, Ramos-Lorenzi JR: Priapism in a patient receiving perphenazine [letter]. J Clin Psychopharmacol 1992; 12:448–449.

Thavundayil JX, Hambalek R, Kin NM, et al: Prolonged penile erections induced by hydroxyzine: Possible mechanism of action. Neuropsychobiology 1994; 30:4–6.

Van Arsdalen K, Chen JW, Smith MJ: Vernon: Penile erection complications in transurethral surgery. J Urol 1983; 129:374.

Whalen RK, Whitcomb RW, Crowley WF Jr, McGovern FJ: Priapism in hypogonadal men receiving gonadotropin-releasing hormone. J Urol 1991; 145:1051–1052.

Wilson F, Staff WG: Malignant priapism: An unexpected response to local anesthetic infiltration of the dorsal nerves of the penis. Br J Surg 1982; 69:469.

Witt MA, Goldstein I, Saenz de Tejada I, et al: Traumatic laceration of intracavernosal arteries: The pathophysiology of nonischemic, high flow, arterial priapism. J Urol 1990; 143:129–132.

Yaqoob M, Parys B, Ahmad R: Prazosin-induced priapism in a patient on continuous ambulatory peritoneal dialysis (CAPD) [letter]. Periton Dial Int 1991; 11:363–364.

39
EVALUATION AND NONSURGICAL MANAGEMENT OF ERECTILE DYSFUNCTION AND PRIAPISM

Tom F. Lue, M.D.
Gregory Broderick, M.D.

Test of Congress

In France, the 16th and 17th centuries saw up to ten thousand legal judgements in cases of impotence as the basis for annulment of marriage. The lengthy procedure was divided into five stages. The first was the husband's confession. The second was a neighborhood inquiry. The third was a three-year trial period. The fourth was cross-examination by judges and genital examination of husband and wife by surgeons and matrons. The final stage was the Test of Congress—a public display of the consummation of the sexual act in the presence of doctors, surgeons, matrons, and judges.

BRENOT, 1994

DIAGNOSIS OF ERECTILE DYSFUNCTION

In the last decade, minimally invasive therapies such as the vacuum constriction device and intracavernous injection have replaced the penile prosthesis as the gold standard of treatment for erectile dysfunction. The introduction of these highly effective but nonspecific treatments has raised questions about the need for more sophisticated diagnostic tests. In these days of cost-consciousness and managed care competition, the diagnosis and treatment of erectile dysfunction will likely be dictated by insurance companies and government agencies rather than by the patient or his physician. This chapter attempts to formulate a commonsense approach to serve as a guide for urologists interested in treating erectile dysfunction.

We propose a two-level diagnostic approach, depending on the patient's and partner's goal and the patient's age, general health, and medical condition (Fig. 39–1). The first level consists of a detailed medical and psychosexual history, physical examination, and hormonal and laboratory testing followed by a discussion of treatment options and further diagnostic tests. This should be provided to everyone. The patient is then given a choice of either a therapeutic trial (with oral medication, a vacuum constriction device, or intracavernous injection) or a second level of evaluation. The latter is designed to elucidate the cause of the dysfunction and entails one or more of the following tests: psychologic consultation, nocturnal penile tumescence testing, advanced neurologic testing, and functional arterial and venous studies. The recommended diagnostic tests for each treatment option are described in Table 39–1.

The objectives of diagnostic evaluation are to (1) identify medical and psychosexual causes, (2) assess the degree and

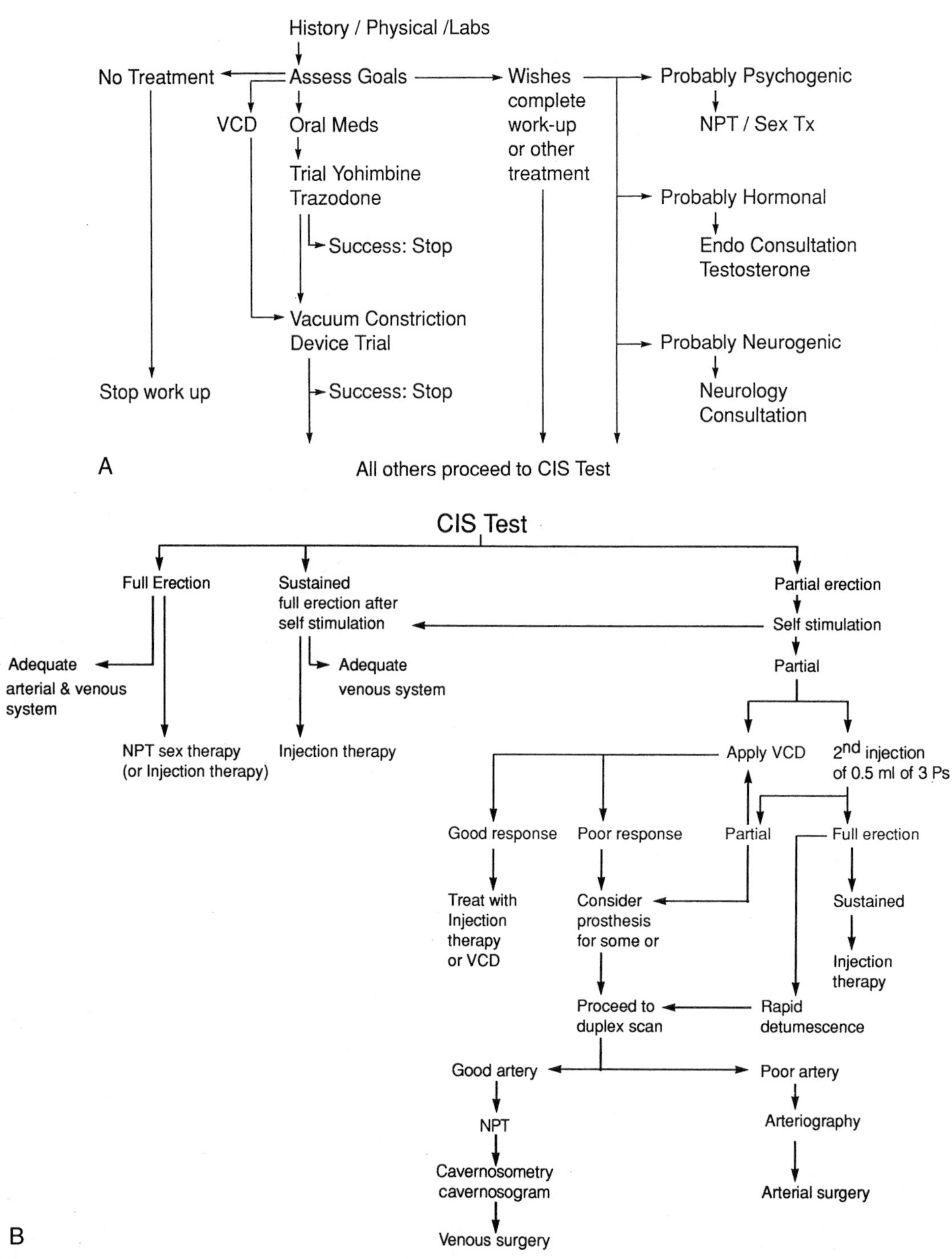

Figure 39–1. Patient's goal-directed approach for erectile dysfunction. 3Ps Solution, papaverine, phentolamine, and prostaglandin E_1. (Modified from Brock J, Lue TF: Impotence: A patient's goal-directed approach. Monographs In Urology 1992;13:99.)

junction with cognitive tasks (distraction and monitoring of erections). They found that about one third of the patients with purely psychogenic erectile dysfunction had an average increase in penile girth of more than 30 mm in response to combined vibration and film. None of the patients with organic involvement exceeded this 30-mm criterion. Rowland and associates (1994) also showed that vibratory stimulation, together with an erotic video, produced a greater penile response than the erotic video alone. Therefore, both groups of authors suggest that assessment of erection induced by vibrotactile and audiovisual stimulation can be an appropriate initial screening procedure. However, Rosso and colleagues (1994) analyzed the scientific community's attitude toward sexual stimulation video testing and warned that many factors may affect the outcome, such as the physician's fear of being accused of voyeurism, the physician's feelings about his or her own erotic fantasies and about pornography, and the castrating aspects of the hospital environment. Therefore, further studies are needed before visual or vibrotactile stimulation can be used as a screening test for the differential diagnosis of erectile disorders.

Psychometry and Psychologic Interview

Three groups of psychometric instruments are available for the evaluation of erectile dysfunction: (1) standardized personality questionnaires; (2) the depression inventory; and (3) questionnaires for sexual dysfunction and relationship factors. The Minnesota Multiphasic Personality Inventory (MMPI)–2 is a valuable tool for evaluating the patient's personality and its relevance to sexual dysfunction. The Beck Depression Inventory is a self-reported test for which a score exceeding 18 is considered indicative of significant clinical depression. For relationship assessment, the Short Marital Adjustment Test (for married couples) and the Dyadic Adjustment Inventory (for unmarried people) can be used to determine overall relationship quality. Specific factors examined include fidelity and level of commitment, as well as sexual relations, family finances, and relationships with friends. Although early reports of these tests claimed that they could differentiate psychogenic from physical causes, subsequent studies have been unable to substantiate these findings and consequently their use is limited.

A skillful diagnostic interview remains the mainstay of psychologic evaluation. Traditional psychoanalytic theory suggests that sexual disability is the symptomatic expression of an underlying neurotic conflict—in most cases related to unresolved oedipal problems. The newer concept popularized by Kaplan (1974, 1983) theorizes that the determinants of psychogenic impotence operate on different layers of causation, ranging from superficial and mild problems to those deeply rooted in early life. The immediate antecedents—particularly anxiety and fear of failure—are instrumental in all psychosexual dysfunction and are specific to the particular disorder. Deep intrapsychic conflicts and relationship problems can be operative in various degrees of severity and acuity but are unspecific for the particular dysfunction. Therefore, the diagnostic interview should focus more on the current sexual problem and its immediate causation and less on general personality traits. **Hartmann (1991) suggests that the interview should be focused on the following: (1) the current sexual problem and its history; (2) deeper causes of sexual dysfunction; (3) the relationship—dyadic causes; and (4) psychiatric symptoms.**

In obtaining the current sexual history, the interviewer should strive to determine whether the dysfunction is primary or secondary; constant, phasic, or situational; and partner specific. In determining immediate causes, the focus should be on sexual function, subjective experience, and emotional aspects. The information should cover the feeling during the course of sexual contact, the occurrence and timing of performance anxiety, interfering thoughts, the relationship between arousal and erection, the sexual excitement of the partner, and the partner's reaction to loss of erection. The interviewer should also obtain information on the degree of noncoital erections (masturbatory, nocturnal, or morning), knowing that the patient with psychogenic erectile dysfunction tends to underestimate his erections. If the patient complains of decreased sexual drive, one should attempt to determine if this occurs before or after the development of erectile dysfunction. The interviewer should also determine whether the patient has an appropriate concept of genital functioning and penile rigidity. Severely distorted demands for performance can be found not only in young and inexperienced men but also in older patients who cannot accept any age-related reduction of sexual functioning.

Identifying the deeper intrapsychic causes of sexual dysfunction is an important aspect of the diagnostic interview. The interviewer should solicit a history related to a traumatic experience, cultural or educational indoctrination, and neurotic processes in which the sexual symptoms serve as a defense against unconscious fear. In assessing a partner-related problem, the couple should be interviewed both together and apart, if possible. The history should include the partner's attitude and reaction to the dysfunction, the patient's erectile function with other partners, and other causes of marital discord such as failure of communication, lack of trust, and parental transference.

In soliciting psychiatric symptoms, the interviewer should determine whether psychopathologic symptoms such as alcoholism, depressive syndromes, anxiety disorder, and personality disorders have a dynamic connection to the erectile dysfunction. One should remember that psychiatric illness can be the cause of sexual dysfunction or it can be secondary or merely coincidental. In addition, although many psychiatric illnesses are associated with psychosexual problems, many patients with severe psychiatric disorders are capable of having normal sexual responses. A psychiatric illness often affects sexual desire more than erectile function, and many medications may affect both desire and erection (Hartmann, 1991).

Although psychologic consultation is not indicated for most patients with nonpsychogenic causes of erectile dysfunction, it is very useful in directing treatment in patients with deep-seated psychologic problems. For example, a patient with severe depression, a strained relationship, or unrealistic expectations will likely not enjoy a satisfactory outcome, even with a perfectly functioning penile prosthesis.

Neurologic Testing

Physiologically, there are three types of erections: nocturnal, psychogenic, and reflexogenic. In a broader sense, neurologic testing should assess peripheral, spinal, and supraspinal centers, and both somatic and autonomic pathways associated with all three types of erection and sexual arousal. However, although severe injury to the cavernous nerves (e.g., during radical prostatectomy) may completely eliminate spontaneous erection, a high percentage of patients with complete upper spinal cord injury are known to have adequate erections. In a recent report, Ghezzi and associates (1995) performed pudendal evoked potentials, motor evoked potentials of the bulbocavernosus muscle to magnetic stimulation, and bulbocavernosus reflex in 34 patients with multiple sclerosis and concluded that no relationship was found between neurophysiologic abnormalities and the presence or severity of erectile dysfunction, showing that these tests have little diagnostic usefulness in multiple sclerosis patients with impotence. In a study of men with Alzheimer's disease, Zeiss and co-workers (1990) found that 53% reported erectile dysfunction, although loss of erection was not related to degree of cognitive impairment, age, or depression. From the above-mentioned report, it is clear that the effect of neurologic deficit on penile erection is a complicated phenomenon and, with a few exceptions, neurologic testing will rarely change management. Moreover, there is no reliable test to assess neurotransmitter release, which leaves a major gap in the current assessment of overall neurologic function associated with penile erection. Therefore, for practical reasons, Carone and Bodo (1994) suggest that neurologic evaluation of impotence in patients with neurologic pathology should differ from that in other subjects; in particular, the aim is to identify or exclude a hidden or underestimated neurologic lesion. In our opinion, the aim of neurourologic testing is to (1) uncover reversible neurologic disease, such as dorsal nerve neuropathy secondary to long-distance bicycling; (2) assess the extent of neurologic deficit from a known neurologic disease, such as diabetes mellitus or pelvic injury; and (3) determine whether a referral to a neurologist is necessary (e.g., work-up for possible spinal cord tumor).

SOMATIC NERVOUS SYSTEM

Biothesiometry. This test is designed to measure the sensory perception threshold to various amplitudes of vibratory stimulation produced by a hand-held electromagnetic device (biothesiometer) placed on the pulp of the index fingers, both sides of the penile shaft, and the glans penis. Goldstein and Krane (1992) have developed a nomogram and have advocated using biothesiometry to select patients for further comprehensive testing (Table 39–5). In a recent study, Bemelmans and colleagues (1995) compared biothesiometry and neurourophysiologic investigations for the clinical evaluation of patients with erectile dysfunction and showed that penile glans biothesiometry yielded consistent results when measurements were repeated during one session. However, they found no relationship between results of penile glans biothesiometry and neurourophysiologic tests of the dorsal penile nerve, probably owing to the fact that vibration is not an adequate stimulus to the glanular skin, which contains free nerve endings only and hardly any vibration receptors. They argue that biothesiometric investigation of penile glans innervation is unsuited for the evaluation of penile innervation and cannot replace neurourophysiologic tests.

Table 39–5. PENILE BIOTHESIOMETRY*

Age Range (years)	Right Finger	Left Finger	Right Shaft	Left Shaft	Glans
17–29	5	5	5	5	6
30–39	5	5	6	6	7
40–49	5	5	6	6	7
50–59	6	6	8	8	9
60–69	6	6	9	9	10
>70	7	7	14	14	16

*Average vibration threshold to nearest whole number in potent control subjects with no neuropathology.

Modified from Goldstein I, Krane RJ: Diagnosis and therapy of erectile dysfunction. *In* Walsh PC, Retik AB, Stamey TA, Vaughan ED Jr, eds: Campbell's Urology. Philadelphia, W. B. Saunders Company, 1992, pp 3033–3072.

Sacral Evoked Response—Bulbocavernosus Reflex Latency. This test is performed by placing two stimulating ring electrodes around the penis, one near the corona, and the other 3 cm proximal. Concentric needle electrodes are placed in the right and left bulbocavernosus muscles to record the response. Square-wave impulses are delivered via a direct current stimulator. The latency period for each stimulus response is measured from the beginning of the stimulus to the beginning of the response. An abnormal bulbocavernosus reflex (BCR) latency time, defined as a value greater than three standard deviations above the mean (30–40 milliseconds), carries a high probability of neuropathology (Padma-Nathan, 1994). In a study of diabetic patients, Vodusek and associates (1993) showed a significant clinical and neurophysiologic correlation between the absence of the bulbocavernosus reflex on clinical examination and its prolonged latency on electrophysiologic measurement. However, the study also showed that the battery of electrophysiologic tests evaluating limb nerve function seems to be more sensitive in diagnosing neuropathy than electrophysiologic assessment of pudendal nerve function alone.

Dorsal Nerve Conduction Velocity. In patients with adequate penile length, it is possible to use two BCR latency measurements, one from the glans and one from the base of the penis, to determine the conduction velocity of the dorsal nerve (i.e., by dividing the distance between the two stimulating electrodes by the difference in latency between the base and the glans). Gerstenberg and Bradley (1983) have determined an average conduction velocity of 23.5 m/second with a range of 21.4 to 29.1 m/second in normal subjects.

Genitocerebral Evoked Potential Studies. This test involves electrical stimulation of the dorsal nerve of the penis, as described for the BCR latency test. Instead of recording EMG responses, this study records the evoked potential waveforms overlying the sacral spinal cord and cerebral cortex. The cerebral response to peripheral nerve stimulation is one of potentials of extremely low amplitude, and complex electronic equipment is used to store and average data of thousands of waveforms recurring as often as every tenth of a millisecond. The first latency recorded is the time of stimulation to the first replicated spinal response—the peripheral conduction time. The second is from the time of stimulation to the first replicated cerebral response—the total conduction time. The difference between the two is the central conduction time. Unlike BCR latency, this is a purely sensory evaluation. This study is not useful as a routine test, but it can provide an objective assessment of the presence, location, and nature of afferent penile sensory dysfunction in patients with subtle abnormalities on neurologic examination.

AUTONOMIC NERVOUS SYSTEM

Heart Rate Variability and Sympathetic Skin Response. Although autonomic neuropathy is an important cause of erectile dysfunction, direct testing is not available. However, many diseases that involve the autonomic nervous system affect innervation to multiple organ systems, and many tests have been developed to assess the integrity of the sympathetic and parasympathetic nervous systems. Several of these tests are discussed herein.

The test of heart rate control (mainly parasympathetic) consists of measuring heart rate variations during quiet breathing, during deep breathing, and in response to rising to one's feet. The normal parameters are (1) the heart rate variation coefficient of the mean RR variation during quiet breathing is less than 1.88 in the 41- to 60-year group and 2.52 for adults less than 40 years old; (2) the maximal average difference between the minimal heart rate of inspiration and maximal rate of expiration during three successive breathing cycles should be higher than 15 beats per minute in the younger group and 9 beats per minute in the older group; and (3) the ratio of the longest RR interval of the bradycardiac phase and the shortest RR interval of the tachycardiac phase should be greater than 1.11.

The test of blood pressure control (mainly sympathetic) measures the blood pressure response to standing up. The decrease in systolic blood pressure should be less than 13 mm Hg. Because heart rate and blood pressure responses can be affected by many external factors, these tests must be conducted under standardized conditions (Abicht, 1991).

Sympathetic skin response (SSR) measures the skin potential evoked by electric shock stimuli. For example, the electrical stimuli can be applied to the median or tibial nerve and the evoked potential recorded at the contralateral hand or foot or the penis. Daffertshofer and co-workers (1994) studied 50 men with erectile dysfunction with the SSR and other neurophysiologic tests and found that the SSR was absent in 11 of 30 cases but was normal in all patients with non-neurogenic erectile dysfunction. In three patients, the abnormal penile SSR was the only abnormality found. Dettmers and associates (1994) investigated 60 normal subjects and 30 patients with erectile dysfunction and found that the SSR was present in all normal subjects. The mean latency in the lower extremities was 2.16 ± 0.20 seconds. The SSR was compared with BCR and somatosensory evoked potentials (SSEP) of the pudendal nerve. Sensitivity for neurogenic dysfunction was 70% for the SSR and 60% for the BCR and SSEP. The SSR detects some patients with erectile dysfunction in whom other parameters are not indicative of pathology. Zgur and colleagues (1993) also studied 30 patients with moderate diabetic polyneuropathy and a control group of 30 normal subjects. In diabetics, two thirds reported autonomic symptoms and 60% of males reported erectile dysfunction. The SSR amplitudes were significantly lower (changed in 53%, absent in 20%) than in the controls. This abnormality correlated with some clinical and electroneurographic signs of neuropathy, suggesting similar impairment of sympathetic and somatic fibers. The Valsalva index was abnormal in 37% of patients, showing no correlation with clinical, electroneurographic or SSR changes. From these reports, SSR, especially if recorded from the penis, seems to be a useful method of testing penile autonomic innervation.

Smooth Muscle EMG and Single Potential Analysis of Cavernous Electrical Activity. Direct recording of cavernous electrical activity with a needle electrode during flaccidity and with visual sexual stimulation was first reported by Wagner and co-workers (1989). The normal resting flaccid electrical activity from the corpora cavernosa was a rhythmic slow wave with an intermittent burst of activity. These bursts virtually ceased during visual sexual stimulation or after intracavernous injection of a smooth muscle relaxant. The electrical activity returned during the detumescence phase. Patients with suspected autonomic neuropathy demonstrated a discoordination pattern with continuing electrical activity during visual sexual stimulation or after intracavernous injection of a smooth muscle relaxant.

Stief and associates (1991) used a different method of data processing by evaluating single potentials of the EMG. The following were analyzed: (1) first depolarization, (2) amplitude, (3) length, and (4) polyphasity. In a study of more than 500 patients with erectile dysfunction of various causes and 92 normal subjects, Djamilian and colleagues (1993) reported that, in normal subjects, single potential analysis of cavernous electrical activity (SPACE) shows a regular pattern of activity, with long phases of electrical silence at the usual amplification, interrupted by synchronous low-frequency, high-amplitude potentials. In patients with disruption of the peripheral autonomic supply, asynchronous potentials with higher frequencies and an irregular shape are typical. In those with complete spinal cord lesions, abnormal as well as normal electrical activity is found. In patients with a long history of insulin-dependent diabetes and (presumably) cavernous smooth muscle degeneration, SPACE recordings show irregular potentials with low amplitude and a slow depolarization speed; synchronization of electrical activity is usually absent.

Two international workshops on cavernous EMG have been convened and recording techniques standardized. It is now generally agreed that an analogue recording of cavernous EMG during flaccidity in normal subjects is reproducible (Fig. 39–3). **The cavernous EMG is characterized by highly reproducible waveforms (potentials) in the individual subject, mostly of comparable shape. Maximal peak-to-peak amplitude lies between 120 and 500 mV, and potentials have a mean duration of 12 seconds.* Obviously, more studies are needed to find the clinical utility and interpretation of the exact nature of cavernous EMG.**

Hormonal Testing

The value of routine endocrinologic testing in impotent men is controversial because the incidence of endocrinopathy has been reported to vary from 1.7% to 35%, with most large series closer to 1.7% (Johnson and Jarow, 1992). This large difference is likely due to differences in referral populations and the protocol used for screening. In a large series reported by Nickel and associates (1984), the overall incidence of endocrinopathy in impotent patients was 17.5%. However, in only 12% of cases did the endocrinopathy

*Gerstenberg T; Personal communication, 1995.

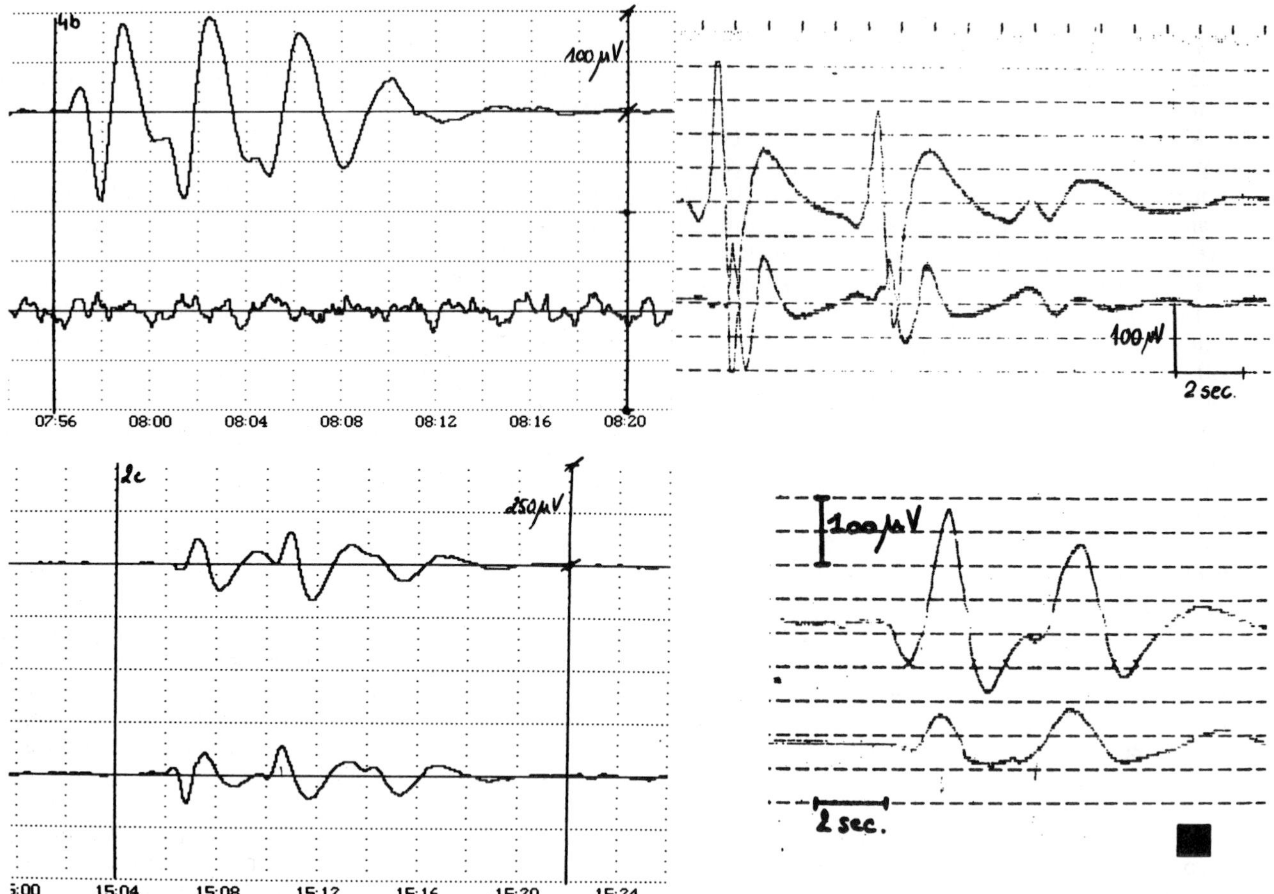

Figure 39–3. Electromyography of the corpus cavernosum in four men performed by different examiners shows the similarity of electrical activity recording. (From Merckx L, Gerstenberg TC, Pereira Da Silva J, et al: A consensus on the normal characteristics of corpus cavernosum EMG. Int J Impot Res. in press.)

clearly contribute to impotence. Indeed, it has been reported that up to 20% of elderly men who undergo estrogen therapy or surgical castration for prostate cancer can still maintain erections adequate for intercourse despite castrate levels of testosterone (Ellis and Grayhack, 1963). Thus, it has been suggested that routine endocrine screening of impotent men—with its high cost—may add little information beyond a complete history and physical examination. Therefore, some investigators have suggested that only men with clinical evidence of hypogonadism (i.e., bilateral testicular atrophy) or decreased libido need to be evaluated (Friedman et al, 1986; Johnson and Jarow, 1992; Akpunonu et al, 1994; Noldus and Huland, 1994).

Despite the above-mentioned arguments, it is well established that endocrinopathy leading to impotence may be a manifestation of a more serious, possibly life-threatening disease. In a small but significant number of patients, impotence may be the initial clinical manifestation of a serious disease such as a prolactin-secreting tumor (Carter et al, 1978; Maatman and Montague, 1986). In addition, most patients who are referred to a urologist for evaluation of erectile dysfunction have undergone little, if any, evaluation directed at identifying an underlying endocrinopathy. For these reasons, we still perform routine testosterone and prolactin measurements as part of our initial evaluation.

In serum, most of the testosterone is bound to albumin and testosterone-binding globulin (TeBG). Because TeBG is known to be decreased in hypothyroidism, obesity, and acromegaly, and increased in hyperthyroidism and estrogen therapy, it is necessary to measure the free biologically active hormone only in these conditions when total testosterone can be misleading. Testosterone is secreted episodically in response to luteinizing hormone (LH) pulses and has a diurnal pattern with an early morning peak. Some recommend three blood samples drawn at least 15 to 20 minutes apart in the morning, with an equal volume of serum from each pooled for a single determination (McClure and Marshall, 1994). For practical reasons, we usually obtain a single morning testosterone (normal 300–1000 ng/dl). If the result is abnormal, we repeat the test and obtain LH (normal, 1–15 mIU/ml) and follicle-stimulating hormone ([FSH]; normal, 1–15 mIU/ml) to differentiate primary from secondary hypogonadism. Only men with clearly documented hypogonadism are candidates for testosterone replacement therapy. We prefer to refer patients with secondary hypogonadism to an endocrinologist for further work-up of possible pituitary or hypothalamic dysfunction.

Abnormally elevated prolactin levels (>22 ng/ml) can lower testosterone secretion through inhibition of LH-releasing hormone (LHRH) secretion by the hypothalamus and result in impotence (Carter et al, 1978; Weideman and Northcutt, 1981; Maatman and Montague, 1986). Although the incidence of a prolactin-secreting tumor is extremely low in most large series of impotent patients, a large number of these patients (>90%) will have impotence and decreased libido as the presenting complaint (Carter et al, 1978; Maatman and Montague, 1986). Hyperprolactinemia may also be caused by certain drugs or medical conditions such as renal insufficiency and hypothyroidism, or it may be idiopathic (Weideman and Northcutt, 1981). Repeatedly elevated prolactin levels should, therefore, prompt a comprehensive evaluation to search for a treatable underlying cause.

Some men with gynecomastia or suspected androgen resistance (high serum testosterone and LH with undermasculinization) should undergo determination of serum estradiol and androgen receptors on the genital skin. Patients with a rapid loss of secondary sex characteristics may have both testicular and adrenal failure and should also be tested for adrenal function (McClure and Marshall, 1994). Other endocrine disorders such as hyperthyroidism and hypothyroidism and adrenocortical dysfunction or tumor may affect sexual function and should be investigated if suspected.

Vascular Evaluation

BIOCHEMICAL STUDY. It has been suggested that penile hypercoagulability predisposes the patient to penile vascular changes and impotence. Thromboxane A_2 is a potent vasoconstrictor and a stimulus of platelet aggregation, which may contribute to hypercoagulability. Contrarily, prostaglandin I_2 has exactly the opposite effect. Because the ratio of the prostacyclin concentration to the thromboxane A_2 concentration is constantly maintained in normal hemostatic responses, an imbalance between the two may be a factor in initiating vascular disease and decreasing blood flow. Kim and colleagues (1990) assessed the usefulness of the prostacyclin–to–thromboxane A_2 ratio in penile blood during erection for the diagnosis of arteriogenic impotence. The ratio in these patients was significantly lower than in patients with psychogenic and venogenic impotence. Measurement of the major urinary metabolites, 11-dehydro-thromboxane B_2 and 2,3-dinor-6-keto-prostaglandin F1-α (prostaglandin F1-α), by radioimmunoassay can accurately reflect in vivo the biosynthesis of thromboxane A_2 and prostaglandin I_2, respectively. Also, Lin and co-workers (1992) have reported that the mean urinary 11–dehydro-thromboxane B_2 level of patients with arteriogenic impotence is significantly greater than that of controls but that there is no significant difference in prostaglandin F1-α levels. Kohler and associates (1993) have also shown that the systemic prostacyclin–to–thromboxane A_2 ratio differs significantly between control rabbits and rabbits with hyperlipidemia. However, they could find no significant difference between patients suffering from organic and psychogenic erectile dysfunction.

PENILE BRACHIAL PRESSURE INDEX. The penile brachial index (PBI) represents the penile systolic blood pressure divided by the brachial systolic blood pressure. Use of the Doppler signal transducer to measure penile blood flow was introduced by Abelson in 1975. He reported that normal penile systolic blood pressure in the flaccid state was no more than 30 mm Hg below brachial systolic pressure. This test gained some initial popularity because of its low cost and noninvasiveness. The technique involves applying a small pediatric blood pressure cuff to the base of the flaccid penis and measuring the systolic blood pressure with a continuous-wave Doppler probe. A penile brachial index of 0.7 or less has been used to indicate arteriogenic impotence (Metz and Bengtsson, 1981).

Despite the initial enthusiasm, this test has many limitations. First, measurement in the flaccid state does not reveal the full functional capacity of the cavernous arteries in the erect state, and errors may also occur from improper fitting of the blood pressure cuff. Secondly, the continuous-wave Doppler probe does not discriminately select the arterial flow of the paired cavernous arteries, which are primarily involved in producing erection. In the flaccid state, the probe detects all pulsatile flow within its path and usually detects the higher blood flow of the dorsal penile artery, which is located superficially and supplies the glans penis, rather than the lower flow of the cavernous arteries. This error sometimes leads to the finding of a normal PBI in a patient with true arteriogenic impotence. **Therefore, a normal PBI cannot be relied upon to exclude arteriogenic impotence. Indeed, attempts to correlate PBI and other more established techniques have been disappointing:** For example, Mueller and associates (1990) found only a 39% correlation between PBI and pudendal arteriography. In another study, Aitchison and colleagues (1990) reported that up to 20% of patients deemed normal by one observer would be deemed abnormal by a second. They conclude that the PBI is inaccurate and poorly reproducible, and suggest no justification for its continued use.

PENILE PLETHYSMOGRAPHY (PENILE PULSE VOLUME RECORDING). This test is performed by connecting a 2.5- or 3-cm cuff to an air plethysmograph. The cuff is inflated to a pressure above brachial systolic pressure, which is then decreased by 10-mm Hg increments, and tracings are obtained at each level. The pressure demonstrating the best wave form is recorded. The normal wave form is similar to a normal arterial wave form obtained from a finger: a rapid upstroke, a sharp peak, a lower downstroke, and occasionally, a dicrotic notch. In patients with vasculogenic erectile dysfunction, the wave form shows a slow upstroke; a low, rounded peak; slow downstroke; and no dicrotic notch. Its height varies considerably; patients with vascular insufficiency usually have the lowest mean height (17.3 mm [deWolfe, 1988]). The proponents of this method argue that, because penile pulse volume recording measures the contributions of all the vessels at the root of the penis, it is more accurate than recording the pressure in an individual artery (as in PBI). However, this study is performed with the penis in the flaccid state and cannot distinguish whether the dorsal or the cavernous artery is impaired.

COMBINED INTRACAVERNOUS INJECTION AND STIMULATION TEST. Differentiation among psychogenic, neurogenic, and vascular causes is often difficult, even with a complete history, physical examination, and endocrine evaluation. Additional information regarding the vascular status of the penis is often helpful. Intracorporeal injection of papaverine, first introduced by Virag and associates (1984), was found to be a useful diagnostic tool, both inexpensive and minimally invasive, in patients with suspected vasculogenic impotence (Virag et al, 1984; Abber et al, 1986). The pharmacologic screening test allows the clinician to bypass neurogenic and hormonal influences and to evaluate the vascular status of the penis directly and objectively.

Pharmacologic evaluation of the impotent patient consists of testing the erectile response of the penis to an intracavernously administered vasodilating agent. This relaxes the penile vascular sinusoids and increases the blood flow in the cavernous arteries. The resultant engorgement of the corpora results in compression of the subtunical venules and decreases penile venous outflow. Therefore, to produce a normal erection, arterial vasodilation, sinusoidal relaxation, and decreased venous outflow must all occur in response to the vasodilating agent. In the past, a number of agents were used, including papaverine, a direct smooth muscle relaxant, and phentolamine, an alpha-adrenergic blocking agent. We use alprostadil (prostaglandin E_1), a potent vasodilating agent that is metabolized locally in the penis. The technique involves injecting 10 μg through a 28-gauge half-inch needle into the corpus cavernosum. The needle site is compressed manually for at least 5 minutes to prevent hematoma formation. The erectile response is periodically evaluated for both rigidity and duration. Normally, a full erection is achieved within 15 minutes (i.e., an erection > 90 degrees that is firm to palpation) and lasts longer than 15 minutes (Lue and Tanagho, 1987).

The pharmacologic test yields important information regarding penile vascular status. A normal finding rules out the possibility of venous leakage (although some patients [about 20%] with arterial insufficiency may achieve a rigid erection owing to an intact veno-occlusive mechanism [Pescatori et al, 1994]) and suggests that neurogenic, psychogenic, or hormonal factors may be primarily responsible, although it is unable to distinguish among them. Regardless, further evaluation for veno-occlusive dysfunction is rendered unnecessary.

An abnormal pharmacologic test result suggests penile vascular disease (arterial, venous, cavernous) and warrants further evaluation, although it may not always be indicative (Buvat et al, 1986; Lue and Tanagho, 1987; Steers, 1993). The patient's fear of injection often produces a heightened sympathetic response, which inhibits the response of the cavernous smooth muscle to the intracavernous agent. This problem may produce a false-positive result. To avoid this error, we have found it helpful to give patients as much privacy as possible during this study. They are also instructed to perform self-stimulation if a rigid erection does not result within 15 minutes. This technique is known as the combined injection and stimulation (CIS) test. In our experience, many patients (about 75%) who initially have a subnormal response to intracavernous injection have significant improvement in their erections after self-stimulation (Donatucci and Lue, 1992). Katlowitz and co-workers (1993), using audiovisual sexual stimulation after pharmacologically induced erection, also reported that 56.5% of patients experienced improved erection with their technique.

DOPPLER WAVE FORM ANALYSIS

Duplex Ultrasonography (Gray Scale and Color Coded). In 1985, Lue and associates introduced high-resolution sonography and pulsed Doppler blood flow analysis (duplex ultrasonography) with intracavernous injection of papaverine as a means of evaluating penile arterial insufficiency. The duplex ultrasound probe is composed of two piezoelectric transducers that allow simultaneous high-resolution imaging of the individual cavernous arteries in real time at a frequency of 7.5 to 10 MHz and pulsed range-gated Doppler analysis of blood flow at 4.5 MHz (Lue et al, 1985; Mueller and Lue, 1988). Duplex sonography provided clear advantages over previous techniques: First, in contrast to pudendal arteriography, duplex sonography is noninvasive and can be performed in the office setting; second, the high-resolution duplex ultrasound probe allows the ultrasonographer to image the individual cavernous arteries selectively and to perform Doppler blood flow analysis simultaneously within these vessels. The color-coded Doppler device provides an additional advantage of easier assessment of direction of blood flow and communication among the cavernous, dorsal, and spongiosal arteries, which are crucial in penile vascular and reconstructive surgeries (Fig. 39–4). It is the best tool available for the diagnosis of high-flow priapism and localization of arterial rupture (Fig. 39–5). It may also replace cavernosography in locating the sites of venous leakage.

The study is performed by first obtaining a baseline study of the flaccid penis. High-resolution ultrasonography is used to image the corpora cavernosa, the corpus spongiosum, and the tunica albuginea. The cavernous bodies should have a homogeneous, uniform echogenicity. The finding of echo-dense areas or calcification within the corporal bodies or the tunica albuginea may represent intrinsic sinusoidal disease, fibrosis, or Peyronie's disease (Aboseif et al, 1992). The cavernous arteries are usually identified near the septum at the base in the midshaft. The arterial diameter of the flaccid penis and the presence of any calcifications within the vessel wall are noted.

A pharmacologic erection is then induced by the intracavernous injection of a vasodilating agent such as papaverine (15 to 30 mg) or alprostadil (10 μg). Meuleman and colleagues (1992) have suggested 12.5 mg papaverine and 10 mcg alprostadil as the appropriate dosages for penile duplex ultrasonography for the optimal effect on cavernous arterial dilatation with a low risk of prolonged erection. (A low dose of papaverine or alprostadil has limited value, however, in the diagnosis of veno-occlusive dysfunction.) Sonographic assessment of the penis is then repeated 3 to 5 minutes after the injection. Each main cavernous and dorsal artery is individually assessed. Cavernous arterial diameter and pulsation are recorded. The presence of a communication between the paired cavernous arteries or between the dorsal and cavernous arteries should also be noted. An asymmetric appearance and response of the cavernous arteries or the lack of arterial pulsation may indicate a significant lesion (Benson et al, 1989).

In some patients, anxiety or fear of injection can lead to a sympathetic response that will inhibit erection. Therefore, we encourage all patients to perform manual self-stimulation in a private setting. Scanning is then repeated and, if necessary, a second injection and self-stimulation.

Pulsed Doppler analysis of the cavernous arteries provides a quantifiable functional assessment of the penile arterial flow during pharmacologic erection. In this respect, duplex sonography is superior to arteriography, which relies on radiographic criteria and provides mainly anatomic rather than functional information. Arteriography is most useful as a detailed roadmap of the penile arterial system and the recipient and donor arteries (usually the inferior epigastric) in patients who are candidates for penile revascularization. Duplex sonography, on the other hand, when

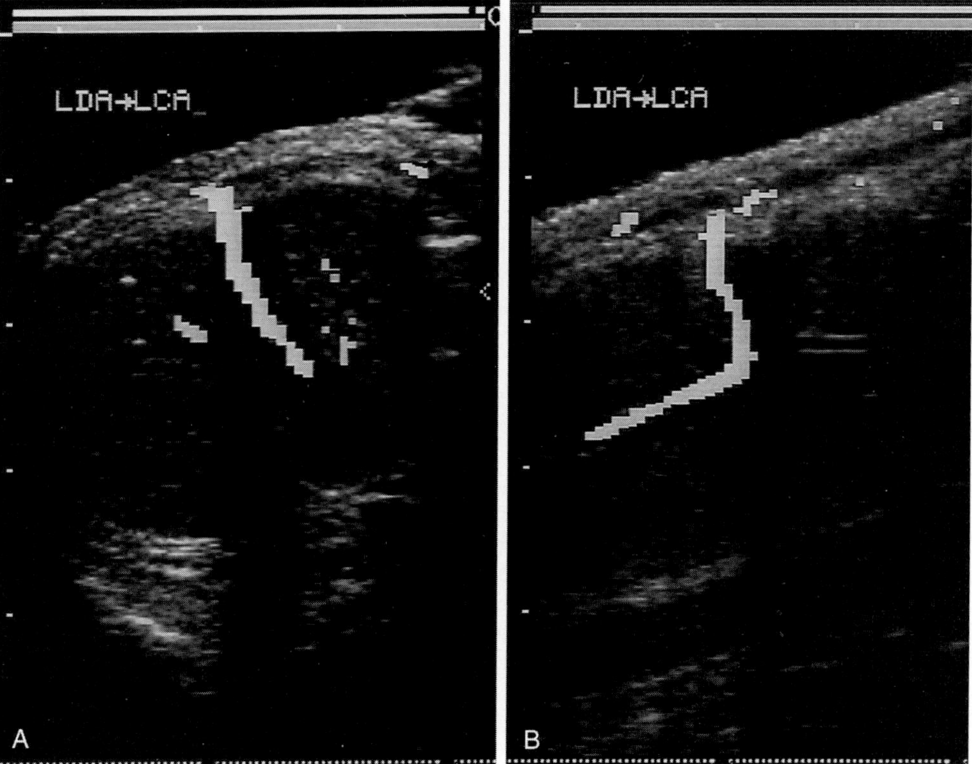

Figure 39–4. Collateral circulation between the cavernous and dorsal arteries shown by color-coded duplex ultrasound in transverse *(A)* and longitudinal *(B)* views.

properly employed provides the clinician with useful objective criteria with respect to blood flow velocity and arterial vasodilation, both of which have been demonstrated to correlate with arterial health.

Criteria for Normative Study. The criteria for a normal duplex sonogram in the evaluation of arteriogenic impotence have been the subject of some debate. Lue and associates reported several findings believed to be indicative of the normal penile arterial response to pharmacologic vasodilation (Lue et al, 1985). Intracavernous injection of a vasodilator produces arterial and arteriolar dilation, cavernous smooth muscle relaxation, and a drop of the peripheral vascular resistance of the penis. Together, these changes cause an increase in penile arterial inflow. This increase is then manifested as sonographically detectable increases in cavernous arterial diameter and blood flow velocity. The absence of these expected physiologic changes allows the experienced sonographer to detect and localize a significant arterial lesion.

Penile Blood Flow Velocity. An increase in penile arterial flow is necessary to penile erection. Total blood flow is a function of both arterial diameter and blood flow velocity.

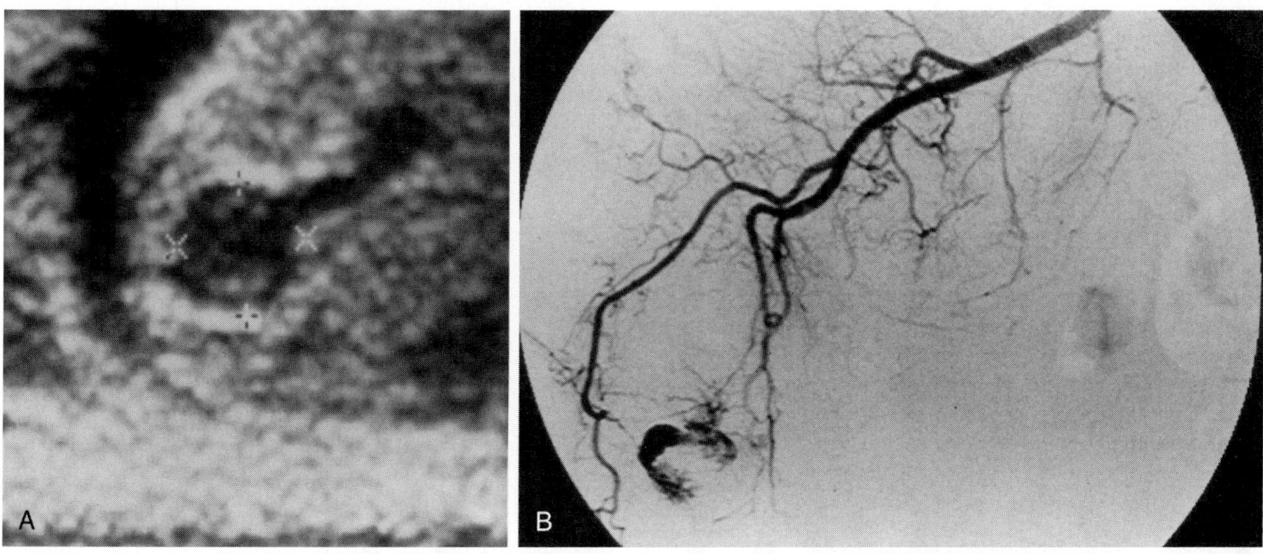

Figure 39–5. *A,* Ultrasonography in a patient with high-flow priapism shows a cavity in the corpus cavernosum. *B,* On selective penile arteriography, a ruptured branch of the cavernous artery is seen filling the cavity.

Not surprisingly, then, velocity has been shown to increase significantly during the early phase of erection. By evaluating a large number of patients with nonarteriogenic causes of impotence (e.g., neurogenic, pychogenic) Lue and associates established that the peak systolic velocity within the cavernous arteries should exceed 25 cm/second within 5 minutes of intracavernous injection of papaverine (Lue et al, 1985; Mueller and Lue, 1988) (see Fig. 39–2). These findings have been confirmed by other authors using similar sonographic techniques (Quam et al, 1989; Fitzgerald et al, 1991; Hwang et al, 1991; Jarow et al, 1993; Lee et al, 1993). Jarow and associates have suggested that a penile blood flow velocity index (defined as the sum of the right and left peak flow velocities) greater than 50 cm/second can be used to rule out arteriogenic impotence (Lopez et al, 1991; Jarow et al, 1993). Other researchers have suggested that a peak systolic velocity of at least 35 cm/second is indicative of normal arterial supply. At peak systolic velocities less than 35 cm/second, the likelihood and severity of arterial disease increase in proportion to the decrease, with a peak velocity less than 25 cm/second indicating a high likelihood of severe arterial disease (Benson et al, 1993). The above-mentioned investigators used different duplex ultrasound devices, which may account for their different standard.

Percent Arterial Dilation. An increase in penile arterial blood flow velocity after intracavernous injection is accompanied by an increase in cavernous arterial diameter. The finding of arterial vasodilation is an indication of adequate arterial wall compliance. Electronic caliper determinations of penile arterial diameter can be performed with high-resolution ultrasonography to within an accuracy of ± 0.1 mm (Lue et al, 1985). In the flaccid state, the cavernous arterial diameter is variable, ranging from 0.3 to 1.0 mm; with pharmacologic erection, Lue and associates determined that the mean increase should exceed 75% in patients without arteriogenic impotence (or a postinjection diameter of more than 0.7 mm) (Lue et al, 1985; Mueller and Lue, 1988). Patients with arterial insufficiency will show minimal or no vasodilation.

The accuracy of this particular criterion has been disputed by other investigators. Some have found a poor correlation between the percentage of arterial vasodilation and arteriographic evidence of arterial insufficiency (Benson et al, 1993; Rajfer et al, 1990; Jarow et al, 1993). Jarow and associates (1993) reported that, although peak systolic velocity correlated well with findings on arteriography, the percentage of arterial vasodilation did not. These findings may be related to the high number of patients in their study who had variant penile arterial anatomy. Moreover, the small size of the cavernous arteries may make the determination of diameter difficult by current ultrasound techniques and, therefore, less reproducible than peak systolic velocity. Nevertheless, a forceful pulsation with an appreciable change of arterial diameter between the systolic and diastolic phases indicates normal arterial compliance and function, and is seen only in patients who develop full erection after intracavernous injection. The relationship of diameter and velocity changes to the phases of erection is shown in Figure 39–6.

Blood Flow Acceleration. Blood flow acceleration is a function of peak systolic velocity. Cavernous blood flow acceleration is defined as the peak flow velocity divided by the pulse rise time. Because an increase in velocity can occasionally be seen in the absence of arterial vasodilation, some investigators have suggested that blood flow acceleration may be a useful parameter in the evaluation of arteriogenic impotence; Mellinger and associates (1990) have found it to correlate well with the subjective quality of erections. In a study comparing duplex ultrasound with arteriography, Valji and Bookstein (1993) reported significant differences in Doppler measurements (peak systolic velocity, acceleration, and resistance index) between patients with and without significant arterial disease. However, they suggested that duplex sonography of the cavernous arteries may be a useful screening tool in patients with suspected arteriogenic impotence only when acceleration is evaluated in combination with peak systolic velocity, which, unlike acceleration, has a well-defined lower limit of normal.

Comparison with Other Tests. Despite its significant limitations in applicability, pudendal arteriography with pharmacologic erection is still considered by many to be the gold standard for the evaluation of arteriogenic impotence. Attempts to correlate duplex sonography with pudendal arteriography have met with varying degrees of success (Quam et al, 1989; Mueller et al, 1990; Rajfer et al, 1990; Jarow et al, 1993). Nevertheless, most studies show a reasonable correlation. Shabsigh and colleagues (1990) compared duplex ultrasonography with NPT monitoring performed in a sleep laboratory and reported a good correlation, except in patients with neurogenic erectile dysfunction.

Knispel and Andresen (1993) studied patients with color-coded duplex sonography and penile blood gas measurements and reported a good correlation in 71%. In the remaining 29%, normal peak flow did not result in a cavernous oxygen tension of greater than 65 mm Hg, which prompted

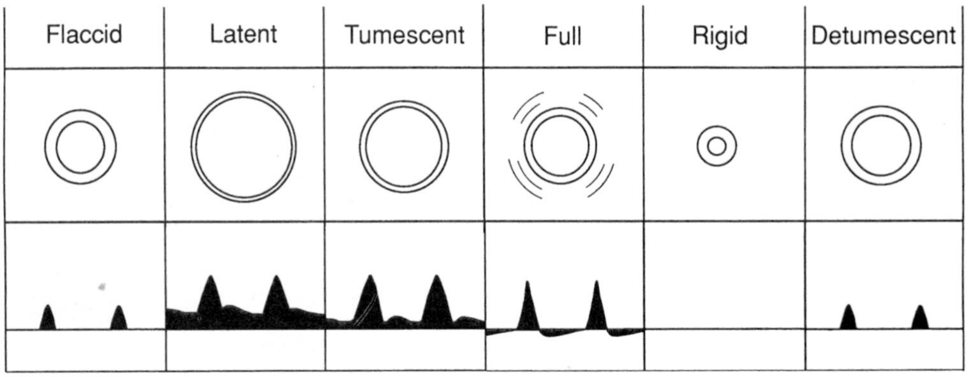

Figure 39–6. Artist's conception of the changes in diameter and flow wave form in the cavernous arteries induced by intracavernous injection of prostaglandin E_1 in a potent young man as demonstrated by duplex ultrasound. Forceful concentric pulsations are particularly noticeable during full erection.

them to suggest that cavernous perfusion defects may be responsible.

Variation in Penile Arterial Anatomy. Duplex ultrasonography relies on imaging the cavernous arteries at the base of the penis, where the anatomy is least variable and the blood flow is greatest. The variation in penile arterial anatomy can be a confounding factor. Jarow and associates (1993) found an excellent correlation between duplex sonography and pudendal arteriography in patients with classic penile arterial anatomy; however, the correlation was significantly lower in patients with variant anatomy. More significantly, both anatomic and radiographic studies show that a high percentage of patients have nonclassic penile arterial anatomy, which can potentially alter the interpretation of duplex sonography (Breza et al, 1989; Jarow et al, 1993). Significant variations include both the number and location of the cavernous arteries. Early branching or the presence of multiple vessels, for example, may make it difficult for the clinician to evaluate blood flow velocity through the main cavernous artery. The presence of distal arterial perforators from the dorsal or spongiosal arteries, if undetected, may lead the clinician to underestimate the total arterial blood flow and wrongly assign a diagnosis of arteriogenic impotence. Fortunately, with color-coded duplex ultrasonography, an experienced sonographer can now scan the entire penis from the crura to the tip and thus avoid underestimating penile blood flow.

Pitfalls of Ultrasonography. Although ultrasonography has been shown to be perhaps the most versatile technique for evaluating vasculogenic impotence, significant limitations have been pointed out. The fact that, like all radiologic tests, it is performed in a nonsexual setting with little privacy can increase the patient's anxiety level and cause a sympathetic response that will inhibit his response to injection (Diederichs et al, 1991; Donatucci and Lue, 1992). This may then reduce both the peak systolic blood flow velocity and arterial vasodilation, and lead the clinician to assign an incorrect diagnosis of arteriogenic impotence. We recommend that manual genital stimulation in a private setting after intracavernous injection be part of the test.

The result of the sonographic study may also be influenced by the temporal response to intracavernous injection. Arterial flow decreases significantly during the full erection phase, and ultrasonography performed during this period will yield a deceptively low peak velocity (Bongaerts et al, 1992). On the other hand, other investigators have found a small but significant number of patients who will show a delayed but eventually normal arterial response to intracavernous injection. Fitzgerald and colleagues (1991) have suggested that the sonographic examination be extended for up to 30 minutes after injection to detect these late responders. However, it is unclear if the delayed arterial response represents a normal variant or a mild form of arteriogenic impotence.

Relatively few studies have used normal volunteers and a standardized technique to establish a normal arterial response. Most criteria regarding peak systolic velocity and vasodilation have been established with patients with nonarteriogenic impotence (e.g., psychogenic, neurogenic) (Lue and Tanagho, 1987; Mueller and Lue, 1988; Fitzgerald et al, 1991), and the validity of using this particular patient population has been questioned. Lee and associates studied a group of potent volunteers and arrived at similar criteria for normal subjects (Lee et al, 1993). However, Mellinger and colleagues (1990) reported on a small number of potent volunteers studied by duplex sonography and found significantly higher values for both peak systolic velocity and percentage arterial vasodilation than are used by most investigators.

Last, ultrasonography is operator dependent. A thorough understanding of erectile physiology and anatomy is necessary to perform and interpret the examination properly. The experience of the clinician is critical to arriving at the correct diagnosis and avoiding the pitfalls outlined earlier.

Cavernous Arterial Occlusion Pressure. This variation of penile blood pressure determination was introduced by Padma-Nathan 1989 and Goldstein in 1990. It involves infusing saline solution into the corpora at a rate sufficient to raise the intracavernous pressure above the systolic blood pressure. A pencil Doppler transducer is then applied to the side of the penile base. The saline infusion is stopped, and the intracavernous pressure is allowed to fall. The pressure at which the cavernous arterial flow becomes detectable is defined as the cavernous artery systolic occlusion pressure (CASOP). A gradient between the cavernous and brachial artery pressures of less than 35 mm Hg and equal pressure between the right and left cavernous arteries have been defined as normal (Fig. 39–7). This technique offers several

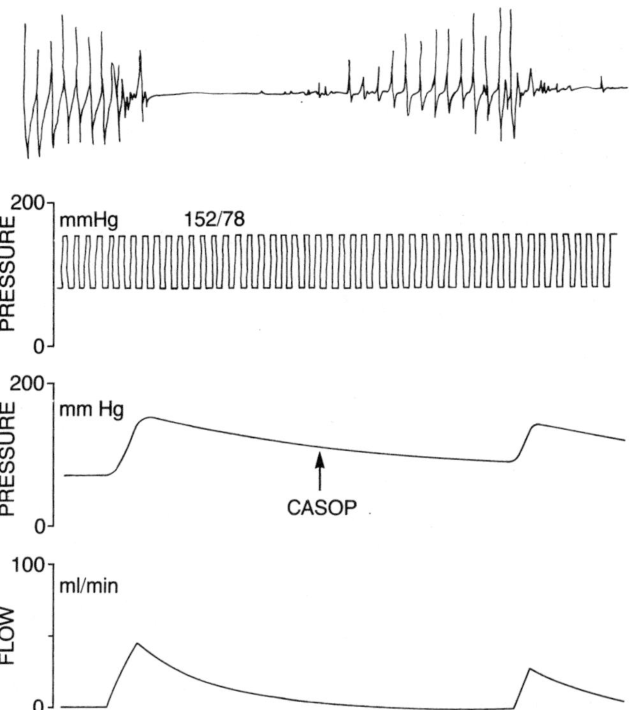

Figure 39–7. This tracing depicts four simultaneous variables obtained during the third phase of dynamic infusion cavernosometry and cavernosography. From top to bottom includes cavernosal artery flow recorded by utilizing a continuous wave Doppler ultrasound probe; systemic brachial systolic and diastolic arterial blood pressure (150/87 mm Hg); intracavernosal pressure, which varied from 70 to 160 mm Hg in this tracing; and intracavernosal heparinized saline inflow. The intracavernosal pressure at which the cavernosal artery pulsations returned, the effective cavernosal artery systolic occlusion pressure (CASOP), was 108 mm Hg. The gradient between the brachial and cavernosal artery systolic occlusion pressures was 150 to 108 or 42 mm Hg, which is abnormal.

advantages over the traditional PBI measurement. First, because a blood pressure cuff is not required, the Doppler probe can be directly applied to the base of the penis where the cavernous arteries are less likely to have branched. Second, continuous monitoring of the intracavernous pressure appears to be a more accurate way of determining the systolic arterial pressure of the cavernous arteries than the pressure cuff. **Last, unlike the PBI (which is performed on the flaccid penis), cavernous arterial systolic occlusion pressure after intracavernous injection of a vasodilating agent allows assessment of the functional capacity of the cavernous arteries in the erect state.** Results have been shown to correlate well with those of arteriography (Padma-Nathan et al, 1988) and peak systolic velocity obtained by high-resolution duplex Doppler ultrasound (Rhee et al, 1995). However, despite these advantages, dynamic infusion cavernosometry is nonetheless a more invasive procedure and more prone to psychologic inhibition, and is not feasible if the intracavernous pressure cannot be raised above the systolic blood pressure (e.g., in patients with severe venous leakage).

Radioisotopic Penography and Magnetic Resonance Imaging. Penile blood flow testing was first introduced by Shirai and co-workers (1978) and Wagner and Uhrenholdt (1980). Their original studies used a xenon 133 washout technique during visual sexual stimulation. Several investigators have modified the technique and use pharmacologic erection as well as different radioisotopes for the measurement of blood flow.

Chung and Choi (1990) examined 137 impotent patients with both nocturnal erections and audiovisual stimulation penography with technetium-99m. They reported a good correlation between the NPT study and penography in most patients, except in a group with unstable erection owing to severe fluctuations in blood flow. Grech and colleagues (1992) developed a method for measuring flow to the dependent portion of the penis with technetium-labeled red blood cells (^{99m}Tc-RBC). None of the subjects with arterial disease achieved flows greater than 20 ml/minute/100 mg tissue, whereas flow in patients without arterial disease exceeded this value. Hwang and associates (1990) reported a technique of combining penography with intracavernous injection. The skin test and corporeal xenon 133 penile washout test were conducted on each person before and 5 and 60 minutes after an intracavernous injection of alprostadil. The authors found the xenon 133 penile washout test helpful in assessing the hemodynamics of the cavernous and dorsal arteries.

Another technique of assessing penile function was reported by Kaneko and co-workers (1994), who used sequential contrast-enhanced magnetic resonance images of the penis in a flaccid state. They noted that subjects with normal erectile function showed gradual and centrifugal enhancement of the corpora cavernosa, whereas those with erectile dysfunction showed poor enhancement with abnormal progression.

Arteriography. Penile arteriography was introduced by the pioneering work of Michal and Pospichal (1978) and Ginestie and Romieu (1978). At present, selective pudendal arteriography performed with the aid of intracavernous injection is considered by many to be the gold standard for evaluating penile arterial anatomy (Struyven et al, 1979; Rajfer et al, 1990; Rosen et al, 1990). The study is performed by intracavernous injection of a vasodilating agent (papaverine, papaverine + phentolamine, or alprostadil), followed by selective cannulation of the internal pudendal artery and injection of a diluted contrast solution of low osmolarity. The anatomy and radiographic appearance of the cavernous arteries are then evaluated according to established criteria (Fig. 39–8).

Although angiography is most likely the most accurate single test for evaluating the anatomy of the cavernous arteries, significant limitations to its application have been pointed out. Like all invasive radiographic tests, the study is performed under artificial conditions, which may produce a significant sympathetic response and inhibit the erectile response. Inadequate vasodilation of the cavernous arteries,

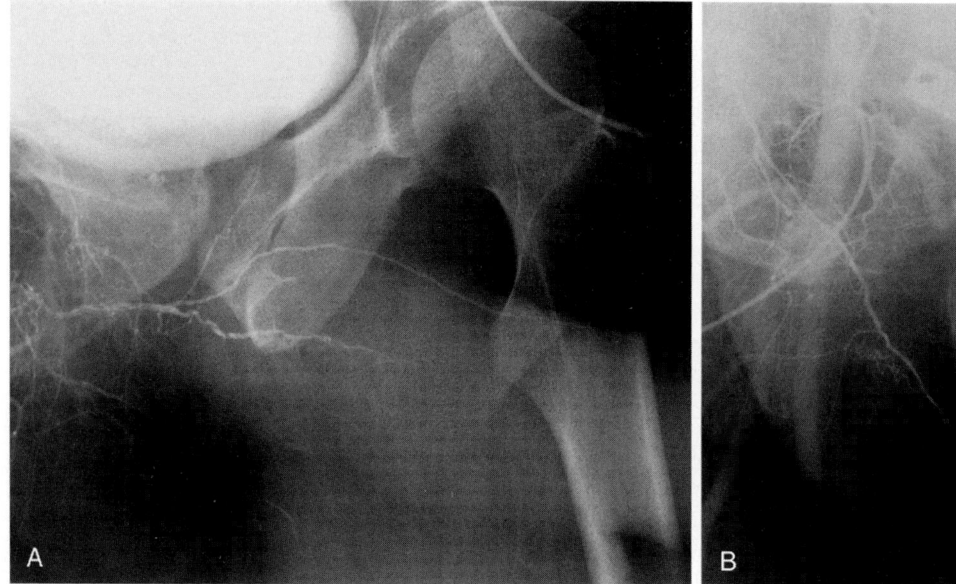

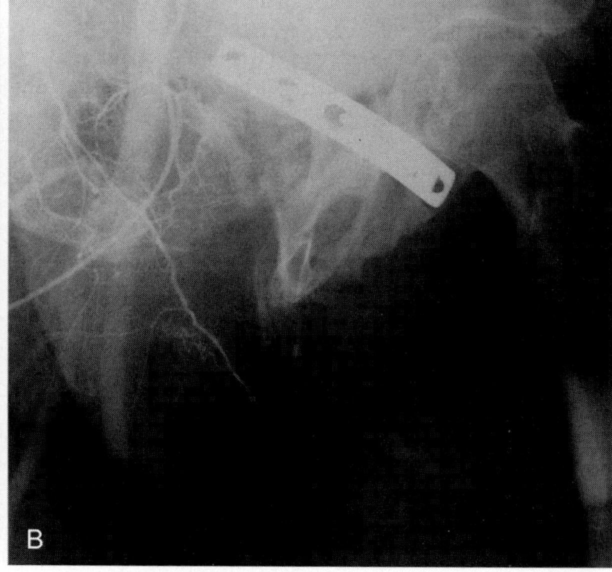

Figure 39–8. In this patient with a pelvic injury, pharmacologic penile arteriography (after intracavernous injection of 60 mg of papaverine) shows patent common penile, dorsal, and cavernous arteries *(A)* and nonvisualization of the common penile artery and its branches *(B)*.

vasospasm induced by cannulation, and injection of contrast solution may result in an abnormal radiographic appearance. To image the cavernous arteries optimally, contrast injection should be performed soon after intracavernous injection during the period of maximal vasodilation.

Arteriography is most useful in providing anatomic rather than functional information: It can detect vascular anomalies relatively easily, but it cannot provide information on blood flow velocity or acceleration within the cavernous arteries. Some investigators have also reported poor correlation between angiographic findings and those of other imaging studies, such as duplex ultrasonography, suggesting that one or both techniques may contain significant limitations (Montague, 1990; Rajfer et al, 1990). Last, owing to the relatively high cost and invasive nature of the study, only a small percentage of impotent patients are appropriate candidates (generally, only those who are candidates for arterial revascularization). Perhaps the strongest indication is in the young man with impotence secondary to a traumatic arterial disruption or in the rare patient with pelvic steal syndrome. In these very selected cases, a detailed roadmap of the arterial anatomy is essential to planning surgical reconstruction.

Veno-occlusive Dysfunction

The trapping of blood within the corpora cavernosa by decreased venous return is a necessary step to achieving and maintaining erection. Veno-occlusive incompetence is defined as the inability to achieve and maintain erection despite adequate arterial flow. Several diagnostic tests have been developed.

COMBINED INTRACAVERNOUS INJECTION AND STIMULATION TEST. As mentioned earlier, with CIS testing, rapid detumescence (within 5 min) after rigid erection has been achieved is indicative of veno-occlusive dysfunction. In one study, subsequent cavernosometry and cavernosography showed 84% of patients to have venous leakage (Donatucci and Lue, 1992). However, poor erection after the CIS test can result from arterial insufficiency or psychologic inhibition also. A repeat study with a stronger pharmacologic agent at another visit may rule out the latter. If indicated, arterial evaluation with the tests mentioned earlier will confirm the adequacy of arterial flow and the presence of venous leakage.

DUPLEX ULTRASOUND. Although Duplex sonography is most useful for evaluating arteriogenic erectile dysfunction, it can provide useful information regarding venogenic dysfunction as well. On occasion, color-coded duplex ultrasound can detect the presence of an abnormal communication between the corpus cavernosum and the corpus spongiosum or the glans penis (e.g., post-traumatic fistula, persistent corpora-to-glans shunt, or ectopic veins). More often than not, however, duplex sonography provides an indirect diagnosis of venogenic erectile dysfunction by ruling out arteriogenic dysfunction: For example, a poor erection in response to a vasodilating agent, despite a normal cavernous arterial response on duplex sonography, suggests veno-occlusive erectile dysfunction. For this reason, we believe that an evaluation for arteriogenic impotence by duplex sonography is always indicated before evaluating for veno-occlusive dysfunction (Lue et al, 1986).

Duplex sonography can also be used to detect venous leakage by directly imaging the most common leakage sites. Several investigators have reported that persistent flow in the dorsal vein during pharmacologically induced erection correlates well with the finding of venous leakage at that site during cavernosometry and cavernosography (Fitzgerald et al, 1991; Vickers et al, 1990). However, the presence of high flow in the deep dorsal vein is not indicative of venous leakage because this vein also drains the glans penis. Some investigators have similarly reported that transrectal ultrasonography after intracavernous injection of alprostadil can detect increased blood volume within the periprostatic venous plexus, signifying venous incompetence.

In addition to the above-mentioned findings, some investigators have shown good correlation between diastolic blood flow velocity within the cavernous arteries and the presence of venous leakage. In the normal erectile response, there should be little if any detectable flow within the cavernous arteries during the diastolic phase 15 to 20 minutes after intracavernous injection and self-stimulation. Montorsi and colleagues (1993) found that persistently elevated diastolic flow (>10 cm/second) in the cavernous arteries correlated positively with a diagnosis of venogenic erectile dysfunction obtained by dynamic infusion cavernosometry and cavernosography in almost 80% of cases. Others suggest that diastolic velocity greater than 5 cm/second is diagnostic of veno-occlusive dysfunction (Benson and Vickers, 1989; Fitzgerald et al, 1991).

Nisen and associates (1993) report that the resistance index is valuable in the diagnosis of venous leakage. Merckx and colleagues (1992) have found a good correlation between the results of duplex scanning and those of pharmacocavernosography and pharmacocavernosometry (93%) on the basis of clinical observation (inadequate erectile response to pharmacologic stimulation despite good arterial compliance), persistent diastolic flow, and the resistance index after 10 minutes.

CAVERNOSOMETRY AND CAVERNOSOGRAPHY. The standard diagnostic study for veno-occlusive dysfunction is pharmacologic cavernosometry and cavernosography. Cavernosography performed during visual sexual stimulation was introduced by Wagner (1981) and Shirai and Ishii (1981) to visualize veno-occlusive dysfunction. This technique was modified by Virag (1981) and Wespes and associates (1984), who introduced dynamic cavernosometry and cavernosography during artificial erection produced by saline infusion.

Cavernosometry involves simultaneous saline infusion and intracorporeal pressure monitoring. A more physiologic refinement is the addition of intracavernous injection of a vasodilating agent such as papaverine or alprostadil. The resultant vasodilation of the cavernous arteries produces an increase in penile arterial flow. The saline infusion rate necessary to maintain erection is thus directly related to the degree of venous leakage (Wespes et al, 1986). Kromann-Andersen and coworkers (1991) compared plain and pharmacologic cavernosometry, and reported that plain cavernosometry gave false-positive results in 6% and false-negative results in 16% and that pharmacologic cavernosometry was much more reproducible. Veno-occlusive dysfunction is indicated by either the inability to increase intracorporeal pressure to the level of the mean systolic blood pressure with saline infusion or a rapid drop of intracorporeal pressure after cessation of infusion (Puyau and Lewis, 1983; Rudnick et al, 1991; Shabsigh et al, 1991; Motiwala, 1993).

Puech-Leao and colleagues (1990) introduced a modification of the pump infusion cavernosometry technique by replacing the infusion pump mechanism with a gravity saline infusion set (gravity cavernosometry). The infusion source is placed approximately 160 cm above the penis (equivalent to 120 mm Hg pressure). With an intact veno-occlusive mechanism, the steady-state intracavernous pressure will closely approximate the pressure of the infusion source (above 110 cm H_2O); with a defective mechanism, it will remain significantly lower. Gravity infusion cavernosometry has been found to correlate well with pump infusion cavernosometry and may provide a simpler and more economical alternative (Puech-Leao et al, 1990; Meuleman et al, 1991).

Cavernosography involves the infusion of radiocontrast solution into the corpora cavernosa during an artificial erection to visualize the site of venous leakage. It should always be performed after activation of the veno-occlusive mechanism by intracavernous injection of a vasodilator (Fig. 39–9) (Lue et al, 1986); various leakage sites to the glans, corpus spongiosum, superficial and deep dorsal veins, and cavernous and crural veins can then be detected. In the majority of patients, more than one site can be visualized by cavernosography (Lue et al, 1986; Rajfer et al, 1988; Shabsigh et al, 1991). Although many impotent men studied with this technique are found to have venous leakage, the initial enthusiasm for venous ligation procedures has waned because of poor long-term results in many patients (Rossman et al, 1990; Yu et al, 1992; Kim and McVary, 1995). The development of collateral leakage sites is presumably one reason for the high failure rate (Yu et al, 1992). Also, it is becoming increasing clear that venous leakage is often the consequence of other abnormalities in the erectile mechanism such as intrinsic sinusoidal disease (Aboseif et al, 1992).

Technical factors may influence the findings on cavernosometry and cavernosography. The study is performed in a nonsexual setting with little privacy, leading to patient anxiety and an adverse effect on the erectile response. The phenomenon of incomplete trabecular smooth muscle relaxation will falsely suggest veno-occlusive dysfunction in some normal subjects (Montague and Lakin, 1992). In the clinical setting, this may lead a clinician to diagnose venous leakage in patients who may have another underlying cause of impotence (e.g., psychogenic, neurogenic). **Saenz de Tejada and colleagues have suggested that, to avoid overdiagnosis, cavernosometry should ideally be performed under the condition of complete trabecular smooth muscle relaxation (Saenz de Tejada et al, 1991; Hatzichristou et al, 1995), which their data indicate occurs in only 17% of patients with a single dose of vasoactive agent. Repeated dosages were required in the majority of patients** (Hatzichristou et al, 1995). The normal maintenance rate in patients with complete smooth muscle relaxation is reported to be less than 5 ml/minute, with a pressure decrease from 150 mm Hg of less than 45 mm Hg in 30 seconds.

Cavernous Assessment

CAVERNOUS SMOOTH MUSCLE. Wespes and coworkers have advocated corporal biopsies with light microscopy and computerized morphometric analysis as an adjunctive technique in the diagnosis of vascular impotence. In patients receiving penile implants and in cadaveric specimens, researchers have observed an age-related decrease in smooth muscle content within the corpora cavernosa (Wespes et al, 1992). When computerized morphometry was used to compare young patients with penile curvature but hemodynamically adequate erection with elderly patients with erectile dysfunction, the corpora cavernosa in the young were composed of 40% to 52% smooth muscle; in the elderly with corporal veno-occlusive dysfunction, 19% to 36% smooth muscle, and in those with arterial impotence, 10% to 25% smooth muscle (collagen was correspondingly increased) (Wespes et al, 1991). Malovrouvas and associates (1994) performed penile biopsies in 50 patients. They reported that the biopsy gun specimens were as representative as the open biopsy specimens. The most severe lesions were observed in the erectile tissue, in particular in the smooth muscle of the trabeculae and the helicine arteries, which had been reduced and replaced by connective tissue.

EXTRACELLULAR MATRIX. Changes in the extracellular matrix have similarly been disputed. Luangkhot and

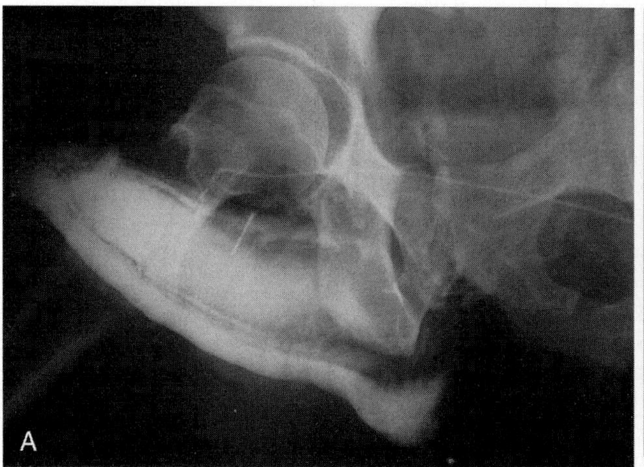

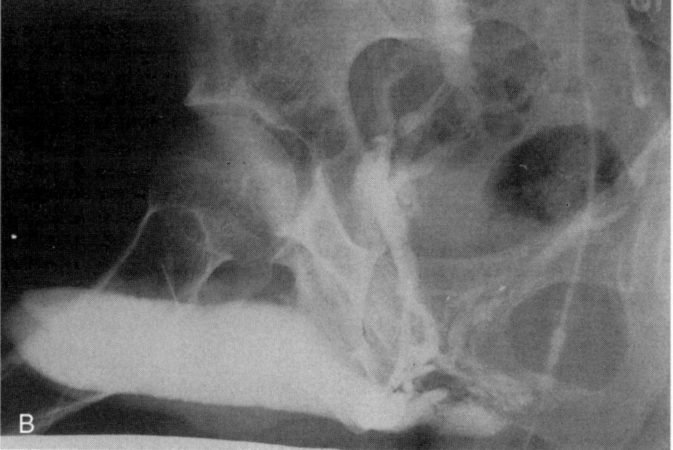

Figure 39–9. Pharmacologic cavernosography in *(A)* a patient 1 year after a penile fracture shows a communication between the corpus cavernosum and spongiosum; *(B)* in a 27-year-old man with primary impotence, it shows venous leakage from the crura.

colleagues (1992) found that the distribution pattern, quantity, and type of collagen within the corpora cavernosa did not vary with age or history of erectile dysfunction. These investigators found the mean collagen content in all patients to be 47%; collagen types I and IV predominate in the corpus cavernosum, with lesser amounts of type III. The tunica albuginea was noted to have equal proportions of types I and III. They and other investigators (Krane, 1985) have suggested that collagen type IV is a secretory product of basement membrane of blood vessels, concluding that its origin within the corpora is the endothelial cell lining of the sinusoids. Others have noted qualitative and quantitative differences in the collagenous architecture within the corpora of impotent patients receiving prostheses (Bornman et al, 1985; Jevtich et al, 1985; Goldstein and Padma-Nathan, 1990). Normal cavernous collagen content has been reported to range from 40% to 65%.

ULTRASTRUCTURAL STUDY. On electron microscopy, ultrastructural differences in the smooth muscle of the corpora cavernosa are found among patients with severe erectile dysfunction, but no single cause of dysfunction has been associated with a characteristic change in cavernous tissue, with the exception of diabetes, in which, as in other organ systems, a consistent alteration of the neural architecture is seen within the cavernous bodies (Saenz de Tejada et al, 1989: Mersdorf et al, 1991). Contrary to the above-mentioned studies, Vickers and co-workers (1990) examined the ultrastructure of cavernous smooth muscle and endothelium in patients with erectile dysfunction secondary to neural, arterial, venous, or fibrotic processes and found no pathognomonic changes.

NITRIC OXIDE SYNTHASE. In a study of biopsy specimens of cavernous tissue obtained from 25 men, Brock and colleagues (1993) determined the presence of nitric oxide synthase (NOS) (as shown by nicotinamide adenine dinucleotide phosphate [NADPH] diaphorase staining) in nerve fibers, smooth muscle, and sinusoidal endothelium. Positive staining for NOS correlated significantly ($P \leq .001$) with a clinical history of cavernous nerve integrity.

At present, cavernous biopsy remains a controversial issue. The proponents believe that it is essential for examining the cavernous tissue before arterial or venous surgery is contemplated. However, we believe that the less invasive tests, such as CIS and duplex ultrasonography, are adequate in predicting the integrity of the cavernous smooth muscle (Persson et al, 1989) and more studies are needed before the routine use of cavernous biopsy can be recommended.

NONSURGICAL TREATMENT OF ERECTILE DYSFUNCTION

Although the penile prosthesis remains one of the most effective treatments for all types of erectile dysfunction, nonsurgical management has replaced prosthetic surgery as the preferred choice in the last decade. Both specific and nonspecific treatments are available. Specific treatments include psychotherapy, replacement of offending medications, and hormone therapy; nonspecific treatments include the vacuum constriction device and intracavernous injection. Although nonspecific therapies appear to be more effective for most cases of erectile dysfunction, we believe that the patient should also be made aware of specific therapies to make an informed decision.

Lifestyle Change

Although it is difficult to prove its beneficial effect, a change of lifestyle should be encouraged (regular exercise, a healthy diet, smoking cessation, alcohol in moderation only). In rabbit experiments, the deleterious effect of a high-cholesterol diet on the cavernous smooth muscle was reversed several weeks after cholesterol was eliminated from the diet (Kim et al, 1994). We found that the best time to discuss this approach with the patient is at the time of vascular evaluation. If he is made aware that penile vascular disease is part of a generalized vascular disease that may involve other organs, he will more likely accept the advice.

Long-distance bicycle riding is another risk factor that should be discussed. Changing the bicycle seat or pursuing another form of exercise may be necessary if penile vascular compromise is found.

Change of Medication

When a patient complains of sexual dysfunction after taking a particular medication, it is important to determine whether the problem is related to loss of sexual drive or impaired erection or ejaculation. In many situations, changing the medication to a different class of agents is feasible. For example, older antihypertensive drugs such as methyldopa and reserpine have a high incidence of sexual dysfunction because of their central suppressive effect; newer drugs such as calcium channel blockers or angiotensin-converting enzyme inhibitors may reverse the dysfunction in some patients. Those who complain of sexual dysfunction after antidepressants may also benefit from substituting the drug with trazodone, which is known to improve erectile function.

Pelvic Floor Muscle Exercise

Claes and co-workers (1993) studied the anatomy of the ischiocavernosus muscle in cadavers and suggested that it influences venous leakage in the corpus cavernosum. They then gave 155 patients intensive physiotherapy consisting of electrical stimulation of the ischiocavernosus muscle, graded pelvic floor exercises with muscle training, and a home exercise program for lying, sitting, and standing positions. Intensive practice of increasing duration was encouraged. After 4 months, 69 patients were cured and 42 patients had improved. In another report, Claes and Baert (1993) studied a group of 150 consecutive male patients with erectile dysfunction and confirmed venous leakage, who were then assigned surgery or pelvic floor training on a random basis. The operative procedure consisted of dissection and removal of the deep dorsal vein and its tributaries or large veins draining into the internal or external pudendal system. The training program was given five times, in weekly sessions, and the patients were supervised by trained physiotherapists. Surgery was not superior to pelvic floor training either subjectively or objectively. Moreover, a significant improvement was found after the training program; 42% were satisfied with the outcome and refused surgery. The authors concluded that pelvic floor exercise is a realistic alternative to surgery in patients with mild venous leakage.

Psychosexual Therapy

Except in some clear-cut cases, the diagnosis of psychogenic erectile dysfunction is still one of exclusion. Sex therapy is certainly effective in a number of men with "organic" erectile dysfunction, and medical and surgical treatment is sometimes the choice for psychogenic erectile dysfunction (Hengeveld, 1991). Hengeveld (1991) has suggested contraindications for psychosexual therapy and medical and surgical therapy (Table 39–6); these contraindications may aid the decision when referral to a psychologist is considered. With our increased understanding of erectile physiology, some now argue that psychogenic erectile dysfunction is a subtype of neurogenic dysfunction and results from inadequate production or overinhibition of neurotransmitter release. Therefore, the choice of minimally invasive and highly effective therapies, such as a vacuum constriction device or intracavernous injection, may be better than a prolonged course of psychosexual therapy. **We believe, however, that in some cases psychosexual therapy should be the treatment of choice—if it can eliminate the specific underlying cause. Moreover, in some patients with mixed psychogenic and organic erectile dysfunction, psychosexual therapy may help relieve the anxiety and remove unrealistic expectations associated with medical or surgical therapy.**

Psychotherapy

There are two types of psychotherapy: psychoanalytic individual therapy and symptom-oriented counseling. Psychoanalytic individual therapy is based on the theory that the sexual dysfunction represents an underlying subconscious conflict, and psychoanalytic principles are used to treat the neurosis that has developed from the conflict. However, modern sexologists argue that psychoanalytic therapy is rarely indicated. Symptom-oriented treatment has been used by many physicians. The main elements are explanation of the cause, sexual information, reassurance, encouragement, and advice. The partner is often included in the therapy.

Table 39–6. PSYCHOSEXUAL CONTRAINDICATIONS

Relative Contraindications to Psychosexual Therapy
Uncooperative patient or sexual partner
Low sex drive
Homosexual orientation
Psychosis or major mood disorder
Major interpersonal problems with sexual partner
Failure of previous psychosexual treatment
Relative Psychosexual Contraindications to Treatment (Injection, Implant)
Unrealistic expectations
Psychosis or major mood disorder
Psychosomatic disorder (conversion disorder, chronic pain disorder, hypochondriasis)
Substance abuse
Crisis situation (divorce, grief, serious illness)
Major interpersonal problem with sexual partner
Sexual partner averse or psychiatrically disturbed

Sex Therapy

In the 1970s, Masters and Johnson (1970) developed a sensate focus exercise program for sex therapy and attracted many followers. Their aim was to detach sexuality from performance anxiety, inhibition, and guilt.

In the initial phase, the couple is advised to enjoy their bodies, using all senses in a relaxed and erotic way but to abstain completely from coitus. Subsequently, stimulation of sexual organs is encouraged, and when erection returns the couple can then progress to coitus. A major modification was made by Kaplan (1974, 1983), who emphasized the treatment of underlying personal or interpersonal conflicts. Others emphasize the importance of eliminating distorted beliefs, conflicts, and distractions and of enhancing the relationship.

Initially, Masters and Johnson (1970) reported a 70% success rate in restoring erectile function. Subsequent reports placed the success rate in the range of 35% to 80% with a significant recurrence rate (Hengeveld, 1983; LoPiccolo and Stock, 1986). Psychosexual therapy is reported to be less successful in patients with primary erectile dysfunction (Vickers et al, 1993).

Hormonal Therapy

We prefer to refer patients with thyroid, adrenal, pituitary, or hypothalamic dysfunction to endocrinologists for further work-up and treatment. Therefore, this discussion is limited to hypogonadism and hyperprolactinemia.

In a young hypogonadal man, testosterone replacement is clearly the treatment of choice. However, the risks may outweigh the benefits in older patients, in whom testosterone may speed up the growth of a hypertrophied prostate or occult prostate cancer. Nevertheless, there are a number of older hypogonadal patients whose libido and erectile function can be restored by testosterone therapy and who should not be denied the option. When a patient desires this, we routinely perform a digital rectal examination and obtain a serum prostate-specific antigen (PSA) level. When in doubt, ultrasound-guided biopsy is also performed before androgen therapy is given. Patients are followed every 6 months with a rectal examination and serum PSA as long as they are on therapy.

The androgen preparations commonly used are modifications by esterification of the 17-β-hydroxyl group or alkylation at the 17-α-group (McClure and Marshall, 1994) (Table 39–7). The alkylated testosterone preparations can be given orally, but absorption may be erratic with the risk of hepatotoxicity. The esterified preparation makes the testosterone more soluble in the fatty vehicles used for parenteral injection and slow release. The long-acting forms, testosterone cypionate and enanthate, are the drugs of choice for replacement therapy. In a study by Sokol and colleagues (1982), hypogonadal men receiving 200 mg of testosterone enanthate demonstrated a peak (supraphysiologic) level at 24 hours, which fell below eugonadal levels by day 9.

Table 39–7. ANDROGEN PREPARATIONS

Preparation	Dose (mg)	Route	Schedule
17-Alkylated androgens			
Methyltestosterone (Android, Metandren, Oreton)	25–50	Sublingual	Daily
Fluoxymesterone (Halotestin)	5–10	Oral	Daily
Methandrostenolone	5–10	Oral	Daily
Transdermal			
Testoderm	4–6	Scrotal skin	Daily
Androderm	5	Skin	Daily
Esterified testosterone			
Propionate	50	IM	3×/wk
Cypionate (Depo-Testosterone)	200	IM	Every 2–3 weeks
Enanthate (Delatestryl)	200	IM	Every 2–3 weeks

IM, Intramuscular.
Modified from McClure RD, Marshall G: Endocrinologic sexual dysfunction. *In* Singer C, Weiner WJ, (eds): Sexual Dysfunction: A Neuro-Medical Approach. Armonk, NY, Futura Publishing Company, 1994, pp 245–273.

Therefore, the recommend dose is 200 mg intramuscularly every 2 to 3 weeks.

Recently, two transdermal preparations, Testoderm (Alza Pharmaceuticals, Palo Alto, CA.) and Androderm (SmithKline Beecham Pharmaceuticals, Philadelphia, PA.) have been approved by the Food and Drug Administration. Testoderm is applied to the scrotal area and Androderm to any skin surface. In clinical trials, the transdermal system has been shown to increase serum testosterone concentrations to within the normal range in over 90% of patients. The most common adverse event has been dermal: itching (7%), chronic skin irritation (2%–5%), and allergic contact dermatitis (4%). In patients on long-term therapy, a periodic check of the hematocrit (to detect polythythemia), liver function, and PSA levels is recommended. The initial recommended dose of Androderm is two systems applied nightly for 24 hours, which will provide about 5 mg of testosterone per day. The initial therapeutic dose of Testoderm is 6 mg/day applied daily to the shaved scrotal skin. The morning serum testosterone concentration may be measured for titration of proper dosage. Both preparations are Schedule III controlled substances under the Anabolic Steroids Control Act.

Although endocrinopathy can certainly contribute to impotence, its role may result from its effects on central mechanisms (libido) rather than on the penile tissue itself; its overall contribution as a directly treatable cause of impotence is unclear. **The effectiveness of hormonal replacement in hypogonadal impotence has also been rather disappointing.** Morales and associates recently reported only a 9% response rate for patients treated with oral androgen replacement (Morales et al, 1994). The majority of older patients are more likely to suffer from concomitant neurovascular insufficiency than from androgen deficiency alone. If the aim of androgen replacement therapy is to restore erectile function, testosterone is a relatively poor choice when compared with others.

In patients with hyperprolactinemia with or without hypogonadism, testosterone therapy does not improve sexual function. Treatment should first be aimed at eliminating the offending drugs, such as estrogens, morphine, sedatives, or neuroleptics. Bromocriptine is a dopamine agonist that lowers the prolactin level and restores testosterone to normal. It is used to reduce tumor size in patients with a prolactin-secreting tumor. Surgery may occasionally be needed if the response is not satisfactory. In a study of 600 random patients, Netto Junior and Claro (1993) reported that moderate elevations of prolactin levels, without any associated disorder, occurred in 3.8% (23 of the 600 patients). In patients with prolactin levels ranging from 20 to 40 ng/ml, bromocriptine brought the values down to normal in all, but only one patient achieved full erection. In patients with levels higher than 40 ng/ml, nine of eleven achieved normal levels after treatment and 77.7% achieved full erection. These findings indicate that, in patients with a mild elevation of prolactin, other factors such as a vascular or neurologic deficit may be the underlying cause of erectile dysfunction. If a pituitary adenoma is identified (usually in patients with marked prolactin elevation), the treatment of choice is bromocriptine or surgical ablation.

Oral Agents

Centrally Acting Drugs

As discussed in Chapter 38, adrenergic, dopaminergic, and serotonergic receptors exist in the brain centers associated with libido, penile erection, and ejaculation. Therefore, a number of drugs are noted to affect sexual function, presumably through their action on these receptors.

ADRENOCEPTOR ANTAGONISTS. Phentolamine is an alpha$_1$-adrenergic antagonist and has been used in combination with papaverine for intracavernous injection. Oral phentolamine has been used in two clinical trials, with some reported improvement in erectile function (Gwinup, 1988; Zorgniotti, 1994).

Yohimbine, an alpha-adrenergic antagonist, is obtained from the bark of the yohim tree. In a controlled randomized study of patients with organic erectile dysfunction receiving 6 mg of yohimbine orally three times a day for 10 weeks, no statistically significant difference from those taking placebo was found (Morales et al, 1982). However, in a study in patients with psychogenic erectile dysfunction, a positive response rate of 62% was noted, whereas the placebo group only achieved a 16% response rate (Reid et al, 1987). **Clinically, although the response rate is marginal at best, yohimbine is widely prescribed—which attests to the public interest in an effective oral agent.**

DOPAMINERGIC AGONIST. Apomorphine is well known to cause yawning and erection in animals and humans. Lal and colleagues (1987) have shown that it induces erections when injected subcutaneously, and sublingual apomorphine is also reportedly successful and produces minimal side effects (occasional nausea and vomiting). Clinical trials are in progress (Heaton et al, 1995).

SEROTONERGIC DRUGS. Trazodone is a commonly prescribed mild antidepressant with a rare incidence of priapism. Its effect on penile erection is thought to be the result of serotonergic and alpha-adrenolytic activity. Several small clinical trials have shown a positive effect on nocturnal penile erection (Saenz de Tejada et al, 1991) and sexually stimulated erection (Lal et al, 1987). A combination of trazodone and yohimbine has also been reported to improve erectile function in some patients (Montorsi et al, 1994). Bondil (1992) investigated another drug combination, trazodone and moxisylyte, and reported that satisfactory sexual activity was restored in 28% of cases and an improvement in spontaneous erections was obtained in 42%. The major problem of trazodone is its marked sedative effect, which may render sexual activity more difficult. Some patients learn to take advantage of better nocturnal erections after trazodone and have sexual activity in the morning when the sedative effect is no longer a problem.

Peripherally Acting Drugs

Some oral vasoactive drugs have been reported to improve erectile function. Allenby and co-workers (1991) noted that patients who were given pentoxifylline for claudication of the lower extremities reported improved sexual function while taking the medication. In a double-blind randomized clinical trial conducted by Korenman and Viosca (1993), patients were given 12 weeks of treatment with placebo or 400 mg tid of pentoxifylline. Therapy was found to increase the PBI, and a significant number of men reported improved erectile function.

Recently, an oral type V phosphodiesterase inhibitor that inhibits the breakdown of cyclic guanosine monophosphate (cGMP) has been shown to be effective in several clinical trials.* If the efficacy of the drug is confirmed by further studies, this will represent another major breakthrough in the treatment of erectile dysfunction.

Transdermal and Intraurethral Medications

The high drop-out rate from intracavernous injection therapy has prompted researchers to seek alternate routes of delivering vasoactive drugs into the corpus cavernosum. Nitroglycerin, a smooth muscle relaxant, has been used in paste or cream form for angina for many years. Clinical trials of nitroglycerin paste have been conducted in the laboratory, and a better erectile response than to placebo has been demonstrated (Heaton et al, 1990). Cavallini (1991) conducted a double-blind study involving 33 patients, comparing minoxidil (1 ml of a 2% solution) with placebo and nitroglycerin (2.5 g of a 10% ointment). The application sites were the penile shaft (nitroglycerin) or glans penis (minoxidil and placebo). Increases in diameter and rigidity were measured with the Rigiscan device, and arterial flow was evaluated by conventional Doppler sonography. Minoxidil was shown to be more effective than nitroglycerin and placebo in increasing diameter, rigidity, and penile arterial flow.

Canale and co-workers (1992) also conducted a double-blind cross-over study with yohimbine ointment applied twice daily at the balanopreputial sulcus. In ten patients, the drug was also assayed by high-performance liquid chromatography in blood drawn from the corpora cavernosa. Rapid adsorption with a peak value of 58 ng/ml at 25 minutes was demonstrated. Treatment with yohimbine ointment was reported to be effective in patients with impotence of recent onset who had no major vascular alterations.

Intraurethral administration of prostaglandin E_2 was found to induce full tumescence in 30% and partial tumescence in 40% of patients (Wolfson et al, 1993). **Subsequently, alprostadil (prostaglandin E_1) was also found to be effective, and a large-scale clinical trial is now in progress.** Preliminary results show the most effective dose to be 500 mg, which is reported to induce adequate erection for sexual intercourse in about 50% of patients. Side effects include penile pain (10.9%), hypotension (2.8%), dizziness (3.8%), and urinary tract infection (0.2%).*

Intracavernous Injection

One of the most dramatic changes in urology has been the introduction of intracavernous injection of vasoactive drugs for the diagnosis and treatment of erectile dysfunction. De la Torre was the first to use intracavernous injection, with isoxsuprine,† and he obtained a U.S. patent in 1978. In 1982, Virag reported the incidental finding of erection induced by intracavernous injection of papaverine. The following year, at the annual meeting of the American Urological Association, Brindley personally demonstrated erection after injection of phenoxybenzamine. Subsequently, Zorgniotti and Lefleur (1985) reported their experience of instructing patients in the technique of autoinjection of a mixture of papaverine and phentolamine for home use. In the last decade, intracavernous injection therapy has gradually gained worldwide acceptance. A list of drugs that have been used clinically is presented in Table 39–8. Several of the most common drugs are discussed in more detail below.

Papaverine

Papaverine is an alkaloid isolated from the opium poppy. Its molecular mechanism of action is through its inhibitory effect on phosphodiesterase, leading to increased cyclic adenosine monophosphate (cAMP) and cGMP in penile erectile tissue.‡ Papaverine also blocks voltage-dependent calcium channels, thus impairing calcium influx, and it may also impair calcium-activated potassium and chloride currents (Brading et al, 1983). All of these actions relax cavernous smooth muscle and penile vessels. Papaverine is metab-

*Wicker P: Personal communication, 1995.

*Labasky R: Personal communication, 1995.
†Zorgniotti AW: Personal communication, 1993.
‡Dahiya R: Personal communication, 1995.

Table 39–8. COMMON INTRACAVERNOUS AGENTS

Drug	Dose Range	Advantages	Disadvantages/Side Effects
Papaverine	7.5–60 mg	Low cost Stable at room temperature	Fibrosis, priapism Elevation of liver enzymes
Papaverine + phentolamine	0.1–1 ml	More potent than papaverine alone	Fibrosis, priapism Requires refrigeration
Alprostadil	1–60 μg	Metabolized in penis Priapism rare	Painful erection Requires refrigeration Relatively expensive
Moxisylyte	10–30 mg	Priapism rare	Less potent
Papaverine + phentolamine + alprostadil	0.1–1 ml	Most potent	Requires refrigeration

olized in the liver, and the plasma half-life is about 1 to 2 hours.

Virag and colleagues (1984) originally used papaverine office injection followed by saline infusion to maintain a rigid erection for 15 minutes as a form of corporal dilation therapy. Some patients benefited after two or more treatments. However, the result was not as successful as expected. Home self-injection has since become popular, with the average dose ranging from 15 to 60 mg. Papaverine has been shown to be very effective in psychogenic and neurogenic erectile dysfunction. In paraplegic and tetraplegic patients, Kapoor and co-workers (1993) reported that satisfactory erection sufficient for coital penetration was possible in 98%. **The advantages are its low cost and stability at room temperature. The major disadvantages are the higher incidence of priapism (0%–35%) and corporal fibrosis (1%–33%), thought to be a result of low acidity (pH 3–4) (Barada and McKimmy, 1994), and occasional elevation of liver enzymes. The high incidence of priapism may partly be due to the investigators' learning curve in judging the right dose.** Younger men with better baseline erectile function and patients with psychogenic and neurogenic dysfunction are more likely to develop priapism (Lomas and Jarow, 1992). The fibrotic change appears to be dose dependent and cumulative, although significant fibrosis after only several injections has been reported (Corriere et al, 1988). The natural course of the fibrosis is not known. In our experience, some cases resolved several months after injection was discontinued, but others persisted. Systemic side effects include dizziness, pallor, and cold sweats, which may be the result of vasovagal reflex or hypotension from its vasodilatory effect in patients with veno-occlusive dysfunction. Tanaka (1990) measured systemic papaverine levels after intracavernous injection and found significantly higher peripheral blood levels in patients with poor erectile response suggestive of veno-occlusive dysfunction.

Alpha-Adrenergic Antagonists

PHENOXYBENZAMINE (DIBENZYLINE). In 1983, Brindley demonstrated that intracavernous injection of phenoxybenzamine (Dibenzyline) produces full erection. Phenoxybenzamine is a nonspecific alpha antagonist that binds covalently to alpha receptors and also blocks acetylcholine, histamine, and serotonin (Brindley, 1983; Wetterauer, 1991; Barada and McKimmy, 1994). It has prolonged vasoactive effects because of noncompetitive blockade, a long half-life (12 hours), and lipid solubility. Its systemic effects include hypotension, reflex tachycardia, nasal stuffiness, miosis, and retrograde ejaculation. Phenoxybenzamine crosses the blood-brain barrier and has central effects: hyperventilation, motor excitability, and nausea. It has a high incidence of priapism and pain at the injection site. Because peritoneal sarcomas have been noted after repeated intraperitoneal injection in rats and mice, clinical studies have ceased.

PHENTOLAMINE MESYLATE (REGITINE). Phentolamine mesylate (Regitine) is a competitive alpha-adrenoceptor antagonist with equal affinity for alpha$_1$- and alpha$_2$-receptors. It blocks receptors for 5-hydroxytryptamine (serotonin) and causes degranulation and histamine release from mast cells. Systemic hypotension, reflex tachycardia, nasal congestion, and gastrointestinal upset are the most common systemic side effects. It has a short plasma half-life (30 minutes). When injected intracorporally alone, it increases corporal blood flow but will not result in a significant rise in intracorporal pressure. It is hypothesized that, by blocking prejunctional alpha$_2$ receptors, phentolamine inadvertently increases intracorporal norepinephrine, preventing complete sinusoidal relaxation (Juenemann et al, 1986; Juenemann and Alken 1989).

MOXISYLYTE (THYMOXAMINE). Moxisylyte is a competitive blocker of alpha$_1$-adrenoceptors. It has a short duration of action (3–4 hours) and some antihistaminic properties. In vitro, it is less potent than phentolamine in relaxing cavernous smooth muscle precontracted by norepinephrine. Clinically, it is less effective as a single intracorporal agent than papaverine (Buvat et al, 1986, 1989). Because of its shorter duration of action, fewer systemic side effects, and low incidence of priapism, it is generally considered a safe intracorporal agent. Buvat and associates (1993) compared results in 72 patients receiving moxisylyte with those in 34 patients treated with papaverine during the same period of time. Complete and sustained erection was induced in 68% of patients treated with moxisylyte and 79% with papaverine. The rate of prolonged erection (1.3% versus 8.8%) and corporal fibrosis (1.3% versus 32%) was significantly less with moxisylyte.

Alprostadil (Prostaglandin E_1)

The discovery of prostaglandins goes back to the original observation by Kurzrok and Lieb (1930), who noticed that strips of human uterine muscle contract or relax when exposed to human semen. The substance was later identified as a lipid-soluble acid and was named prostaglandin. Alprostadil is the synthetic form of a naturally occurring unsaturated 20-carbon fatty acid (i.e., alprostadil is the exogenous form, and prostaglandin E_1 is the endogenous compound). It causes smooth muscle relaxation, vasodilation, and inhibition of platelet aggregation. Clinically, it was used for management of patent ductus arteriosus and peripheral vascular disease before being used for intracavernous injection. **Alprostadil is metabolized by the enzyme prostaglandin 15-hydroxydehydrogenase, which has been shown to be active in human corpus cavernosum (Roy et al, 1989). After intracavernous injection, 96% of alprostadil is locally metabolized within 60 minutes and no change in peripheral blood levels has been observed (van Ahlen et al, 1994).** In patients with veno-occlusive dysfunction, alprostadil may rise to ten times baseline, but up to 90% is metabolized on the first pass through the lungs.

Several formulations of alprostadil have been used for intracavernous injection (in alcohol, saline, and sterile water). It is not known whether different formulations vary in efficacy or tolerance. In the United States, the pediatric formulation (Prostin VR) was used first, followed by Caverject, a lyophilized powder specifically developed for intracavernous injection. In Caverject, every 20 μg of alprostadil also contains excipients of lactose (172 mg) and sodium citrate (47 mg). In a study comparing the efficacy of Caverject and Prostin VR in 120 patients, no significant difference was noted.

Consequent to the experimental report of Hedlund and Andersson (1985) of the relaxing effect of alprostadil on human penile tissue, Ishii and co-workers (1986) reported its use as an office diagnostic test. In 1988, Stackl and associates reported that alprostadil is safe and effective for home injection therapy. Since then, it has gained wide acceptance and has been the first drug approved by the Food and Drug Administration (FDA) for treating erectile dysfunction (Caverject). Several studies comparing the effect of alprostadil and papaverine have been reported. Alprostadil was shown to have a higher response rate and lower incidence of priapism and fibrosis, but the incidence of painful erection was much higher. Lee and co-workers (1989) compared it with papaverine and phentolamine and considered it superior for penile rigidity in 9 of 25 patients. The other 16 believed the two preparations were equivalent. No patient developed prolonged erection in either group, but painful erection was reported in 20 of the 25 treated with alprostadil. In another report, Lui and Lin (1990) also compared a papaverine and phentolamine mixture (7.5–60 mg papaverine plus 0.25–2.0 mg phentolamine) with alprostadil (10–20 μg). Adequate erection was seen in 67.1% of 51 patients given papaverine and phentolamine and in 79.1% of 76 patients given alprostadil. Four patients in the papaverine and phentolamine group developed prolonged erection.

In a review of the published literature, Linet and Neff (1994) found that, in doses of 10 to 20 μg, alprostadil produced full erections in 70% to 80% of patients with erectile dysfunction. The most frequent side effects were pain at the injection site or during erection (occurring in 16.8% of patients), hematoma and ecchymosis (1.5%), and prolonged erection and priapism (1.3%). Systemic side effects occurred rarely. To decrease the incidence and degree of painful erection, Schramek and colleagues (1994) used a combination of alprostadil (20 μg) and procaine (20 mg) and reported a significant decrease in local pain.

In summary, alprostadil is an effective agent for the diagnosis and treatment of erectile dysfunction. Its advantages are a lower incidence of prolonged erection, systemic side effects, and fibrosis (presumably because of its local metabolism by prostaglandin hydroxydehydrogenase present in the penile tissue). It is also the only FDA-approved agent for intracavernous injection in the United States at the present time. The disadvantages include a higher incidence of painful erection, higher cost, and shorter half-life if not refrigerated.

Vasoactive Intestinal Polypeptide

Vasoactive intestinal polypeptide (VIP), originally isolated from the small intestine, is a potent smooth-muscle relaxant. It is believed to be one of the nonadrenergic, noncholinergic (NANC) mediators of erection. Adaikan and associates (1986) proposed that VIP may be a neurotransmitter for penile erection. Recent evidence demonstrates that NANC relaxation results in the intracellular accumulation of cGMP, whereas VIP causes accumulation of cAMP.* Intracorporal injection of VIP does not produce rigid erection (Kiely et al, 1989).

Calcitonin Gene–Related Peptide

Calcitonin gene–related peptide (CGRP) is a potent vasodilator. Immunohistochemical techniques have localized CGRP in cavernous nerves, within the walls of cavernous arteries, and in cavernous smooth muscle (Stief et al, 1990). CGRP injection induces a dose-related increase in penile inflow. Clinically, the combination of CGRP and alprostadil has been reported to be effective in patients in whom other drugs were not (Djamilian et al, 1993). Systemic side effects include facial flushing and hypotension.

Nitric Oxide Donors

LINSIDOMINE. Linsidomine is an antianginal drug that releases nitric oxide to stimulate the production of cGMP and thus relax smooth muscle. When injected into the corpus cavernosum, it can produce penile erection with minimal side effects. Truss and co-workers (1994) studied the nitric oxide donor linsidomine chlorhydrate (SIN-1) as a treatment option. All normal control subjects had full rigid erections lasting 40 to 70 minutes. Of 113 patients, 78 (69%) had responses sufficient for intercourse with SIN-1, and no significant side effects were noted. However, Porst (1993) compared the effect of 1 mg linsidomine with 20 μg alprostadil in 40 patients with erectile dysfunction and reported that the erectile and hemodynamic response to linsidomine was more modest. Wegner and associates (1994) also performed a single-blind cross-over trial in 20 patients with erectile dysfunction of mixed etiology, comparing alprostadil with SIN-1 at two different dosages (1 and 2 mg). They reported that alprostadil always achieved the best response; the response to SIN-1 was significantly poorer regardless of the dosage

*Saenz de Tejada I: Personal communication, 1995.

used. They concluded that SIN-1 is not a useful alternative to alprostadil.

SODIUM NITROPRUSSIDE. Sodium nitroprusside, a nitric oxide donor, is an inorganic hypotensive agent whose main pharmacologic action is relaxation of vascular smooth muscle and consequent dilation of peripheral arteries and veins. The hypotensive effect is seen within a minute or two, and it dissipates almost as rapidly after infusion is stopped. The drug is cleared by intraerythrocytic reaction with hemoglobin and its half-life is about 2 minutes. Brock and associates (1993) reported that intracavernous injection of nitroprusside caused severe hypotension in their first three patients, which prompted discontinuation of a clinical trial. However, Martinez-Pineiro and colleagues (1995) performed a study comparing the effect of intracavernous administration of sodium nitroprusside (100 to 400 mg) with alprostadil (20 μg) in 105 patients and found that nitroprusside did induce penile erection in many patients with insignificant side effects. Nevertheless, they concluded that alprostadil was still a better choice.

Drug Combinations

Zorgniotti and Lefleur (1985) first reported the use of a combination of papaverine (30 mg) and phentolamine (0.5 mg) for self-injection. This was effective in 72% of 250 patients. Prolonged erection occurred in 1.6% during titration and in one patient on home therapy. Fibrosis developed in 4.1%. Goldstein and co-workers (1988) presented results of 300 patients using 0.1 to 1 ml of a solution containing 22.5 mg papaverine and 1.25 mg phentolamine/ml. Of patients who completed 3 months or more, 79% continued to do so. Seven patients (2.3%) developed prolonged erection and were treated with an injection of an alpha agonist. Stief and Wetterauer (1988) compared papaverine or phentolamine alone with a papaverine and phentolamine combination in men with organic erectile dysfunction and found that full erection occurred in 40% with papaverine alone, 7% with phentolamine alone, and in 87% with papaverine and phentolamine. The combination has been used successfully in patients with different types of erectile dysfunction: In general, those with neurogenic and psychogenic erectile dysfunction require a smaller amount to achieve erection; older patients and those with vasculogenic erectile dysfunction require more.

Kerfoot and Carson (1991) examined the effect of the papaverine and phentolamine combination in 65 patients 65 years or older (mean age 70 years) compared with a group of similar size but approximately 20 years younger (mean age 47 years). Treatment response rates were equal for the two age groups, although elderly patients required a higher dose to obtain an erection and used the medication less frequently. Complications were few, of minimal consequence, and occurred with equal frequency between the two age groups.

In a study by Armstrong and colleagues (1993), a total of 160 men with erectile failure received treatment with 13,030 intracavernous papaverine and phentolamine injections. An erection sufficient for sexual intercourse was achieved in 115 (72%). The response rates were as follows: vasculogenic (48%), psychogenic (93%), neurogenic (92%), diabetic (68%), idiopathic (63%), traumatic (60%), alcohol related (80%), and drug related (75%). After a mean follow-up period of 14.1 months, 55 (48%) were still successfully using intracavernous therapy. A total of 22 episodes of priapism occurred in 16 patients, and one patient developed corporeal fibrosis.

In summary, the combination of papaverine and phentolamine is an effective treatment and produces adequate erection in more than 70% of patients, with a greater than 75% satisfaction rate. Prolonged erection has been reported in 1% to 23% and fibrosis in 1.4% to 16%.

PAPAVERINE, PHENTOLAMINE, AND ALPROSTADIL. Virag and colleagues (1991) first used a combination of six drugs (Ceritine [which contains atropine], dipyridamole, ifenprodil, papaverine, piribedil, and yohimbine) in treating erectile dysfunction. In 1991, Bennett and associates introduced a three-drug mixture containing 2.5 ml of papaverine (30 mg/ml), 0.5 ml of phentolamine (5 mg/ml), and 0.05 ml of alprostadil (500 μg/ml) for intracavernous injection. Theoretically, because each of the three has a different mechanism of action, the combination should take advantage of the synergism among them and permit a much lower dose of each to be used, avoiding the side effects of high dosages. In the study by Bennett and co-workers (1991), 89% of the patients tested had adequate erection and went on to injection therapy at home. Overall, 74% of the 78 patients were maintained at a dose of less than 0.25 ml per injection, with a frequency averaging 3.1 uses per month. Two patients had a prolonged erection that required treatment. In another report from the same group, Barada and Bennett (1991) followed-up on 110 patients over 12 to 28 months: Sixty-five percent were continuing injection therapy, and of these, 89% were satisfied with the drug combination. Seven prolonged erections (5.6%) lasting more than 3 hours occurred. No patient developed fibrosis or nodules.

In another study (Goldstein et al, 1990), 32 patients in whom alprostadil alone or the dual combination of papaverine and phentolamine had failed had adequate erection when the triple combination was used. Eight patients reported painful erection. No prolonged erections or systemic side effects were noted. In a randomized cross-over study of 228 patients, McMahon (1991) likewise compared the triple drug combination with papaverine and phentolamine, and alprostadil alone. Statistically, the triple drug combination was more effective in patients with severe arteriogenic or mild veno-occlusive dysfunction. The incidence of prolonged erection was lower when compared with papaverine and phentolamine but not significantly different from alprostadil alone.

In summary, the triple drug combination has been shown to be as effective as alprostadil alone, but has a much lower incidence of painful erection. Further studies are needed to determine the long-term effects.

OTHER DRUG COMBINATIONS. Several other drug combinations have also been studied. Floth and Schramek (1991) reported that the combination of papaverine (7.5 mg) and alprostadil (5 μg) is more effective than alprostadil alone (10 μg) and might suitably replace papaverine and phentolamine or alprostadil alone in patients who do not respond well or who suffer side effects after high single doses. Montorsi and associates (1993b) used a mixture composed of 12.1 mg/ml of papaverine hydrochloride, 10.1 μg/ml of alprostadil, 1.01 mg/ml of phentolamine mesylate, and 0.15 mg/ml of atropine sulfate in a group of patients with veno-occlusive dysfunction; mean volume injected was 0.42 ± 0.09 ml (range 0.25 to 0.90 ml). They noted that 95% achieved sustained rigid erections. Four patients (7%) reported transient hypotension. Gerstenberg and co-workers (1992) reported a study of a combination of VIP (30 mg) and phentolamine (0.5–2.0 mg) in 52 men with erectile dysfunction. A total of 1380 self-injections were given. After sexual stimulation, all patients obtained adequate erection. None developed priapism, fibrosis, or systemic side effects. Although intracavernous VIP alone produced disappointing responses, in combination with papaverine it potentiated the response to this drug. Kiely and colleagues (1989) reported that a combination of papaverine and VIP produced penile rigidity similar to that with papaverine and phentolamine. Truss and co-workers (1994) reported the result of pharmacologic testing with a mixture of CGRP (5 mg) and alprostadil (10 μg) in 28 patients with erectile dysfunction and venous leakage in whom penile venous surgery had failed, 28 patients with erectile dysfunction and venous leakage who refused penile venous surgery, and 12 patients without venous leakage but a poor response to maximal doses of papaverine and phentolamine. Erections sufficient for intercourse were noted in 19 of the 28 patients in the first group (67.9%), 20 (71.4%) in the second, and 11 (91.7%) in the third.

Other Aspects of Intracavernous Injection Therapy

EFFICACY IN DIFFERENT TYPES OF ERECTILE DYSFUNCTION. It is obvious from the previous discussion that, **in patients with nonvascular causes (e.g., psychogenic, hormonal, neurogenic), the response rate to intracavernous injection is very high (80% to 100%). It is considerably lower in patients with vascular causes, and a higher dosage is required.** When the response is poor after repeated testing and sexual stimulation, the most likely diagnosis is severe vascular disease (arterial, venous, or both), although in rare cases, psychologic inhibition may be strong enough to impair the erectile response.

IMPROVEMENT IN SPONTANEOUS ERECTION. A number of patients experience improvement or recovery of spontaneous erections when practicing self-injection over the long term. Although reduction in performance anxiety may be involved in patients with a considerable psychogenic component, several blood flow studies have shown an improvement after long-term intracavernous injection (Porst et al, 1989; Marshall et al, 1994). In the study by Marshall and colleagues, 35 patients used either alprostadil or the triple drug mixture for 4 to 88 months. Cavernous arterial diameter and peak flow velocity were measured before and after self-injection (15 to 1296 injections). Significant improvement was noted in the peak flow velocity but not the diameter of the arteries. In ten matched controls who did not undergo self-injection over 15 to 77 months, none of the flow parameters changed significantly. During this study, 54% of the treated patients reported improvement in spontaneous erections. Although the improvement in blood flow and erection likely resulted from the vasodilatory effect of the injected drugs, an increase in sexual activity may also have contributed to the change because the control group was not sexually active.

Several other studies have examined improved spontaneous erection. Thiounn and associates (1993) reported that 85% of patients with psychogenic and 65% with organic erectile dysfunction experienced an improvement. In another study by Bucher and co-workers (1990), 9% of patients experienced complete recovery and 29% partial recovery (i.e., they required regular injections [every 2 to 3 weeks] to maintain the recovery of spontaneous erection).

PATIENT ACCEPTANCE AND DROPOUT RATE. In several studies, the percentage of patients accepting injection therapy when offered in the office ranges from 49% to 84% (Gerber and Levine, 1991; Chandeck Montesa et al, 1992; Hirsh et al, 1994). The reasons for declining include penile pain, inadequate response, fear of the needle, unnaturalness, and loss of sex drive. In long-term studies, 13% to 60% of patients drop out for a number of reasons. These include loss of interest, loss of the partner, poor erectile response, penile pain, concomitant illness, recovery of spontaneous erection, and ultimate choice of other therapy.

SERIOUS ADVERSE EFFECTS. Priapism and fibrosis are the two more serious side effects associated with intracavernous injection therapy. Linet and Neff calculated that priapism occurred in 1.3% of 8090 patients in 48 studies with alprostadil. The incidence was found to be about five times lower with alprostadil than with papaverine or the combination of papaverine and phentolamine (1.5% versus 10% versus 7%). Fibrosis can occur as a nodule, diffuse scarring, plaque, or curvature. The incidence is about ten times lower with alprostadil than with papaverine or papaverine and phentolamine (1% versus 12% versus 9% of patients) (Pastorini et al, 1993), although one study reported a 12% incidence with alprostadil.

DOSAGE AND ADMINISTRATION. Patients must have the first injection performed by medical personnel and receive appropriate training and education before performing self-injection at home. For alprostadil, an initial dose of 2.5 μg is recommended. If the response is inadequate, increases in 2.5-μg increments can be given until a full erection is achieved or a maximum of 60 μg is reached. There is no manufacturer's recommendation for other drugs used in intracavernous injection.

As a general rule, one should start with a small dose (such as 7.5 mg of papaverine, 0.1 ml of combination drugs), especially in patients with nonvascular erectile dysfunction. The goal is to achieve an erection that is adequate for sexual intercourse but that lasts for less than 1 hour. In patients who use excessive amounts to maintain erection for more than 1 hour, increasing doses may be required to achieve and maintain the same erection and eventually may fail to achieve erection at all.

CONTRAINDICATIONS. The use of intracavernous injection therapy is contraindicated in patients with sickle cell anemia, schizophrenia or a severe psychiatric disorder, severe venous incompetence, or severe systemic disease. In patients taking an anticoagulant or aspirin, compressing the injection site for 7 to 10 minutes after injection is recommended. In patients with poor manual dexterity, the sexual partner can be instructed to perform the injection.

Vacuum Constriction Device

The vacuum constriction device has become more popular in the last decade as an effective and safe treatment for erectile dysfunction. It consists of a plastic cylinder connected directly or by tubing to a vacuum-generating source (manual or battery-operated pump). After the penis is engorged by the negative pressure, a constricting ring is applied to the base to maintain the erection. To avoid injury, the ring should not be left in place for longer than 30 minutes.

The erection produced by a vacuum device is different from a physiologic erection or one produced by intracavernous injection. The blood oxygen level in the corpus cavernosum is less, and the portion of the penis proximal to the ring is not rigid, which may produce a pivoting effect. The penile skin may be cold and dusky, and ejaculation may be trapped by the constricting ring. The ring can be uncomfortable or even painful. However, in many patients, the device can produce an erection that is close to normal and rigidity sufficient for coitus. The device also engorges the glans and is useful for patients with glanular insufficiency.

In patients with severe proximal venous leakage or arterial insufficiency, fibrosis secondary to priapism, or an infection from a prosthesis, the device may not produce adequate erection. In these cases, combining intracavernous injection with the vacuum constriction device may enhance the erection (Marmar et al, 1988). The device can also be used successfully by men with a malfunctioning penile prosthesis in place (Sidi et al, 1990; Korenman and Viosca, 1992).

The majority of men using the device report satisfaction with penile rigidity, length, and circumference; partner satisfaction is likewise good (Sidi and Lewis, 1992). Patients also report an improvement in self-esteem and a sense of well-being. **Complications include penile pain and numbness, difficult ejaculation, ecchymosis, and petechiae. Patients taking aspirin or warfarin sodium (Coumadin) should exercise caution when using these devices.**

The patient's satisfaction rate has been reported to range from 68% to 83% (Cookson and Nadig, 1993). In a prospective study of the medical, sexual, and psychosocial outcome of vacuum devices in 29 men regularly using a device for 6 months, Turner and co-workers (1990) reported statistically significant improvement in erectile quality, frequency of intercourse attempts, frequency of orgasm, and sexual satisfaction, as well as decreased psychiatric symptoms, increased self-esteem, and a trend toward improved marital satisfaction. Of the partners, many reported improved sexual functioning, including increased frequency of orgasm, decreased masturbation, and greater sexual satisfaction, with no changes in psychosocial parameters.

The device is more acceptable to older men in a steady relationship than to young single men in search of a partner. It is very safe when used properly and is one of the least costly treatment options available. Although it can be used by any patient with erectile dysfunction, we still recommend that a reasonable work-up be conducted so that some easily correctable cause of the dysfunction is not overlooked.

For further reading relevant to both diagnosis and treatment, see the report of the NIH Consensus Development Panel on Impotence (NIH Consensus Conference, 1993).

Conclusion

Erection involves a complex series of psychologic, neurologic, and vascular events. Recent advances in the understanding of erectile physiology have made more accurate diagnosis of the different causes of erectile dysfunction possible. Technologic advances in imaging and diagnostic techniques have allowed physicians to counsel patients more effectively and to offer therapeutic options. It must be realized, however, that significant costs and limitations are associated with all these techniques and errors in diagnosis can occur. Therefore, the foundation of every patient evaluation remains a complete history and physical examination. A carefully directed approach to evaluating each patient and a thorough knowledge of available diagnostic modes is essential to producing a satisfactory therapeutic solution.

DIAGNOSIS OF PRIAPISM

Evaluation of Priapism

History and Physical Examination

The diagnosis of priapism is usually based on history and physical examination. Priapism associated with intracavernous pharmacotherapy occurs more often in patients with neurogenic and psychogenic impotence, and the diagnosis is evident. Sickle-cell priapism often occurs in teenagers, and recurrence is very common. **Acute low-flow (veno-occlusive) priapism, if lasting more than several hours, is usually painful because of changes associated with tissue ischemia. In contrast, most cases of high-flow (arterial) priapism are painless and usually follow perineal injury or direct injury to the penis. On physical examination, the corpora cavernosa are fully rigid in low-flow priapism and partial to fully rigid in high-flow priapism.** The glans and corpus spongiosum are not involved, except in very rare cases of tricorporal priapism (Sharpsteen et al, 1993). A thorough physical examination should include rectal, abdominal, and neurologic examinations. Chronic priapism and acute intermittent (stuttering) priapism may be more difficult to diagnose because of atypical physical findings. Our diagnostic approach is illustrated in Figure 39–10.

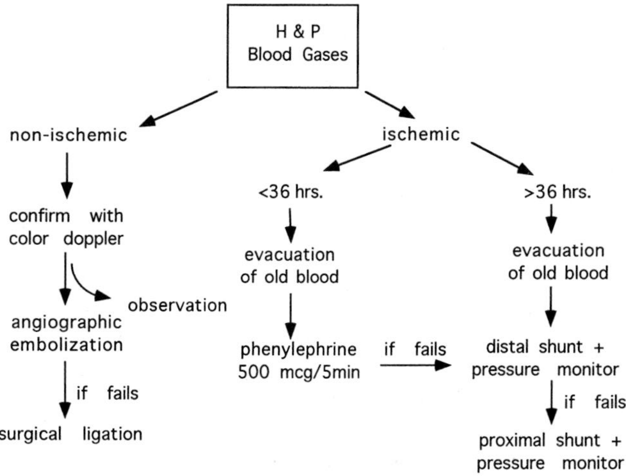

Figure 39–10. Medical management of priapism. (H & P, history and physical examination.)

Laboratory Testing

A blood sample should be obtained for hemoglobin S determination and to rule out leukemia. Urinalysis and urine culture should also be obtained to rule out urinary tract infection. Cavernous blood gas measurement is a very useful tool when the type of priapism needs to be determined: Blood gas values similar to those of venous blood are indicative of low-flow disease; values similar to arterial blood are suggestive of high-flow priapism (Lue et al, 1986). By definition, all cases of priapism begin as high flow; therefore, cavernous blood gas measurement, if performed early, may be misleading. The technetium-99m scan has been advocated as a means of differentiating between the two types: Uptake is high in arterial priapism and low in the veno-occlusive type (Hashmat, 1989). Cavernosography is another means of differentiating between the two (Bruhlmann et al, 1983; Hauri et al, 1983): Venous stasis is demonstrated in the veno-occlusive type and rapid drainage of the corpus cavernosum in the arterial type. **We prefer blood gas determination and, if doubt exists, a color-coded duplex ultrasound scan of the cavernous arteries and the corpora cavernosa. Minimal arterial flow with distended corpora cavernosa is seen in low-flow priapism, whereas a ruptured artery with unregulated blood pooling in the area of injury can often be seen in trauma-induced high-flow priapism** (Brock et al, 1993; Ilkay and Levine, 1995) (see Fig. 39–5).

NONSURGICAL TREATMENT OF PRIAPISM

Low-Flow Priapism

Treatment is aimed at the primary cause of priapism if it can be identified. The goal is to abort the erection, thereby preventing permanent damage to the corpora (which would lead to impotence), and to relieve pain. Medical management should always be tried before resorting to surgery. There is ample evidence that the risk of fibrosis and impotence increases with time. Generally, the incidence of impotence is less if erection is aborted in under 24 hours.

Medical Treatment

Medical treatment is aimed at decreasing arterial inflow and increasing venous outflow. **The first line of treatment involves aspiration of the corpora and intracavernous injection with an alpha-adrenergic agonist (Table 39–9). Epinephrine, norepinephrine, and phenylephrine all have similar effects. We recommend initial aspiration of the corpora via a 21-gauge butterfly needle, followed by injection of 250 to 500 μg phenylephrine, a pure alpha$_1$-adrenergic stimulant, every 5 minutes until detumescence takes place.** The phenylephrine solution is made by mixing 10 mg/ml of phenylephrine with 19 ml of normal saline. Irrigation with diluted alpha-adrenergic solution has also been described (Sidi, 1988; Molina et al, 1989). Alternatively, oral terbutaline has been shown to be effective in causing detumescence in some patients when priapism is related to intracavernous injection. A response rate of up to 36% has been reported in patients treated with either 5 or 10 mg of terbutaline, as compared with only 12% with placebo (Lowe and Jarow, 1993). However, in another study, terbutaline was found to have no benefit over placebo (Govier et al, 1994). Nevertheless, intracavernous injection of an alpha-adrenergic agonist remains the most effective treatment for low-flow priapism and is almost 100% effective if the priapism is treated within 12 hours of onset. Figure 39–10 shows the recommended algorithm for medical management.

Table 39–9. ALPHA-ADRENERGIC AGENTS FOR THE TREATMENT OF PRIAPISM*

Drug	Usual Dose
Epinephrine	10–20 μg
Phenylephrine	250–500 μg
Ephedrine	50–100 mg

*Intracavernous injection every 5 minutes until detumescence after aspiration of 10 to 20 ml of blood.

Sickle Cell Disease

Sickle cell disorder accounts for approximately 28% of all cases of priapism; 42% of adults and 64% of children with sickle cell disease eventually develop it. Although high-flow priapism in patients with sickle cell disease has been reported (Ramos et al, 1995), the majority of cases are of the low-flow type. Treatment should be prompt and conservative, because priapism often recurs in these patients. Having ruled out other causative factors, one should treat the patient by aggressive hydration, oxygenation, and metabolic alkalinization to reduce further sickling. Supertransfusion and erythrophoresis should be used as second-line therapy. Irrigation and injection, as noted earlier, should be performed as soon as possible.

Recurrent Priapism

Stuttering or recurrent priapism occurs often in patients with sickle cell trait or disease and in patients without sickle cell disease with prior episodes. The mechanism is unknown, although alteration of adrenoceptor or scarring of intracavernous venules might be partially responsible. **For sexually active patients, self-injection of an alpha-adrenergic agent such as phenylephrine (500 μg every 5 minutes until detumescence) can be used. If sexual function is not a concern, use of an antiandrogen or a gonadotropin-releasing hormone agonist** (Levine and Guss, 1993; Steinberg and Eyre, 1995), **which suppresses nocturnal penile erection, can be very helpful in preventing its recurrence.**

High-Flow Priapism

In the early stages, ice packing may cause vasospasm and spontaneous thrombosis of the ruptured artery. Three cases of spontaneous resolution have been observed by Ilkay and Levine (1995) and have prompted the authors to propose conservative treatment of high-flow priapism. **However,**

most of the cases with delayed cavernous arterial rupture (Ricciardi et al, 1993) **do not subside spontaneously, and arteriography with embolization of the internal pudendal artery is usually required** (Walker et al, 1990; Brock et al, 1993). Alternatively, injection of methylene blue to counteract the release of nitric oxide and embolization of the internal pudendal artery have been proposed by Steers and Selby (1991). A case of percutaneous autologous clot embolization of the arterial sinusoidal cavity has been reported by Ilkay and Levine (1995).

Complications

Untreated veno-occlusive priapism leads to corporeal fibrosis and impotence. Complications of treatment can be classified as early and late. Early complications include acute hypertension, headache, palpitation and cardiac arrhythmia from alpha-adrenergic agents, and bleeding, infection, and urethral injury from needle puncture. Two deaths and one case of skin necrosis have been reported after injection of undiluted metaraminol (2–4 mg) (Bondil and Guionie, 1988). Hematoma of the shaft after corporal aspiration and irrigation is also common. Infections are usually in the form of cellulitis. Therefore, strict asepsis in carrying out penile irrigation and use of antibiotics are both mandatory to avoid this potentially disastrous complication. If undiagnosed, it may lead to abscess formation. Urethral injury is a rare complication of treatment that may potentially lead to stricture or urethro-cutaneous fistula. Injury to the urethra can occur during needle aspiration and irrigation, when performing one of the distal shunts, or during the cavernoso-spongiosal shunt procedure.

The most important late complications of priapism are fibrosis and impotence. The incidence is directly related to the duration of priapism and the aggressiveness of treatment. Although the overall impotence rate in low-flow priapism has been reported to be as high as 50% in the literature, almost all patients will regain their previous potency if the priapism is aborted within 12 to 24 hours by medical therapy. In a study of intracavernous injection-induced priapism lasting 24 hours or longer, Kulmala and Tamella (1995) noted that most cases lasting less than 36 hours can be treated by aspiration and alpha-adrenergic drugs with no consequent fibrosis; after 36 hours, none of the patients responded to alpha-adrenergics, and all had some degree of intracavernous fibrosis. High-flow arterial priapism has a better prognosis, with a reported impotence rate of 20%.

Conclusion

Priapism is an uncommon condition, and low-flow priapism is a urologic emergency. Almost all cases can be successfully aborted with injection of a dilute alpha-adrenergic agonist, provided treatment begins within 12 hours of onset. Tissue damage can thus be prevented and potency preserved. High-flow priapism itself does not cause erectile tissue damage, but injury to the erectile tissue and nerves may be associated with delayed recovery of potency after treatment. The best diagnostic tool is a color-coded duplex ultrasonogram, and angiographic embolization is the treatment of choice.

REFERENCES

Diagnosis of Erectile Dysfunction

Abber JC, Lue TF, Orvis BR, et al: Diagnostic tests for impotence: A comparison of papaverine injection with the penile-brachial index and nocturnal penile tumescence monitoring. J Urol 1986;135:923.

Abelson D: Diagnostic value of the penile pulse and blood pressure: A Doppler study of impotence in diabetics. J Urol 1975;113:636.

Abicht JH: Testing the autonomic system. *In* Jonas U, Thon WF, Stief CG, (eds): Erectile Dysfunction. Berlin, Springer-Verlag, 1991; pp 187–193.

Aboseif SR, Baskin LS, Yen TS, Lue TF: Congenital defect in sinusoidal smooth muscles: A cause of organic impotence. J Urol 1992;148:58.

Ackerman MD, D'Attilio JP, Antoni MH, et al: The predictive significance of patient-reported sexual functioning in RigiScan sleep evaluations. J Urol 1991;146:1559.

Aitchison M, Aitchison J, Carter R: Is the penile brachial index a reproducible and useful measurement? Br J Urol 1990;66:202.

Aizenberg E, Zemishlany Z, Dorfman-Etrog P, Weizman A: Sexual dysfunction in male schizophrenic patients. J Clin Psychiatry 1995;56:137.

Akpunonu BE, Mutgi AB, Federman DJ, et al: Routine prolactin measurement is not necessary in the initial evaluation of male impotence. J Gen Intern Med 1994;9:336.

Allen R, Brendler CB: Snap-gauge compared to a full nocturnal penile tumescence study for evaluation of patients with erectile impotence. J Urol 1990;143:51.

Allen RP, Engel RM, Smolev JK, Brendler CB: Comparison of duplex ultrasonography and nocturnal penile tumescence in evaluation of impotence. J Urol 1994;151:1525.

Allen RP, Smolev JK, Engel RM, Brendler CB: Comparison of RigiScan and formal nocturnal penile tumescence testing in the evaluation of erectile rigidity. J Urol 1993;149:1265.

Armenakas NA, McAninch JW, Lue TF, et al: Posttraumatic impotence: Magnetic resonance imaging and duplex ultrasound in diagnosis and management. J Urol 1993;149:1272.

Barry JM, Blank B, Boileau M: Nocturnal penile tumescence monitoring with stamps. Urology 1980;15:171.

Bemelmans BL, Hendrick LB, Koldewijn EL, et al: Comparison of biothesiometry and neuro-urophysiological investigations for the clinical evaluation of patients with erectile dysfunction. J Urol 1995;153:1483.

Benson CB, Vickers MA: Sexual impotence caused by vascular disease: Diagnosis with duplex sonography. AJR Am J Roentgenol 1989;153:1149.

Benson CB, Aruny JE, Vickers MA, Jr: Correlation of duplex sonography with arteriography in patients with erectile dysfunction. AJR Am J Roentgenol 1993;160:71.

Bondil P, Louis JF, Daures JP, et al: Penile extensibility and erectile function. Preliminary results. Ann Urol 1990;24:373.

Bongaerts AH, deKorte PJ, Delaere KP, van Thillo EL: Erectile dysfunction: Timing of spectral wave-form analysis in the assessment of the function of the cavernosal arteries. Europ J Radiol 1992;15:140.

Bornman MS, du Plessis DJ, Ligthelm AJ, van Tonder HJ: Histological changes in the penis of the Chacma baboon—a model to study aging penile vascular impotence. J Med Primatol 1985;14:13.

Bradley WE, Timm GW, Gallagher JM, Johnson BK: New method for continuous measurement of nocturnal penile tumescence and rigidity. Urology 1985;26:4.

Breza J, Aboseif SR, Orvis BR, et al: Detailed anatomy of penile neurovascular structures: Surgical significance. J Urol 1989;141:437.

Brock G, Nunes L, Padma-Nathan H, et al: Nitric oxide synthase: A new diagnostic tool for neurogenic impotence. Urology 1993;42:412.

Brock G, Lue TF: Impotence: A patient's goal-directed approach. Monogr Urol 1992;13:99.

Buvat J, Lemaire A, Marcolin G, et al: Intracavernous injections on vasoactive drugs. J Urol 1986;92:111.

Carone R, Bodo G: Neurological evaluation of erectile impotence. Arch Ital Urol Nefrol Androl 1994;66:207.

Carroll JL, Baltish MH, Bagley DH: The use of PotenTest in the multidisciplinary evaluation of impotence: Is it a reliable measure? Jefferson Sexual Function Center. Urology 1992;39:226.

Carter JN, Tyson JE, Tolis G, et al: Prolactin-screening tumors and hypogonadism in 22 men. N Engl J Med 1978;299:847.

Chung WS, Choi HK: Erection versus nocturnal erection. J Urol 1990;143:294.

Cilurzo P, Canale D, Turchi P, et al: The RigiScan system in the diagnosis of male sexual impotence. Arch Ital Urol Nefrol Androl 1992;64:2.

Colombo F, Fenice O, Austoni E: NPT: Nocturnal penile tumescence test. Arch Ital Urol Androl 1994;66:159.

Condra M, Morales A, Surridge DH, et al: The unreliability of nocturnal penile tumescence recording as an outcome measurement in the treatment of organic impotence. J Urol 1986;135:280.

Daffertshofer M, Linden D, Syren M, et al: Assessment of local sympathetic function in patients with erectile dysfunction. Int J Impotence Res 1994;6:213.

Davis-Joseph B, Tiefer L, Melman A: Accuracy of the initial history and physical examination to establish the etiology of erectile dysfunction. Urology 1995;45:498.

Dettmers C, van Ahlen H, Faust H. Evaluation of erectile dysfunction with the sympathetic skin response in comparison to bulbocavernosus reflex and somatosensory evoked potentials of the pudendal nerve. Electromyogr Clin Neurophysiol 1994;34:437.

deWolfe VG: Non-invasive vascular evaluation. *In* Montague DK, ed. Disorders of Male Sexual Function. Chicago, Year Book Publishers, 1988, pp 44–59.

Diedrich GK, Stock W, LoPiccolo J: A study on the mechanical reliability of the Dacomed snap gauge: Implications for the differentiation between organic and psychogenic impotence. Arch Sex Behav 1992;21:509.

Diederichs W, Stief CG, Lue TF, Tanagho EA: Sympathetic inhibition of papaverine induced erection. J Urol 1991;146:195.

Djamilian M, Stief CG, Hartmann U, Jonas U: Predictive value of real-time RigiScan monitoring for the etiology of organogenic impotence. J Urol 1993;149:1269.

Donatucci CF, Lue TF: The combined intracavernous injection and stimulation test: Diagnostic accuracy. J Urol 1992;148:61.

Ek A, Bradley WE, Krane RJ: Nocturnal penile rigidity measured by the snap-gauge band. J Urol 1983;129:964.

Ellis WJ, Grayhack JT: Sexual function in aging males after orchiectomy and estrogen therapy. J Urol 1963;89:895.

Fineman KR, Rettinger HI: Development of the male function profile/impotence questionnaire. Psychol Rep 1991;68:1151.

Fischer C: Cycle of penile erection synchronous with dreaming sleep. Arch Gen Psychiatry 1965;12:29.

Fitzgerald SW, Erickson SJ, Foley WD, et al: Color Doppler sonography in the evaluation of erectile dysfunction: Patterns of temporal response to papaverine. AJR Am J Roentgenol 1991;157:331.

Friedman DE, Clare AW, Rees LH, Grossman A: Should impotent males who have no clinical evidence of hypogonadism have routine endocrine screening? (Letter.) Lancet 1986;1(8488):1041.

Geisser ME, Murray FT, Cohen MS: Use of the Florida Sexual History Questionnaire to differentiate primary organic from primary psychogenic impotence. J Androl 1993;14:298.

Gerstenberg TC, Bradley W: Nerve conduction velocity measurements of dorsal nerve of the penis in normal and impotent males. Urology 1983;21:90.

Ghezzi A, Malvestiti GM, Baldini S, et al: Erectile impotence in multiple sclerosis: A neurophysiological study. J Neurol 1995;242:123.

Ginestie JF, Romieu A: Radiologic exploration of impotence. The Hague, Martinus Nijhoff, 1978.

Goldstein AM, Padma-Nathan H: The microarchitecture of the intracavernosal smooth muscle and the cavernosal fibrous skeleton. J Urol 1990;144:1144.

Goldstein I, Krane RJ: Diagnosis and therapy of erectile dysfunction. *In* Walsh PC, Retik AB, Stamey TA, Vaughan ED Jr, eds: Campbell's Urology. Philadelphia, W. B. Saunders Company, 1992, pp 3033–3072.

Grech P, Dave S, Cunningham DA, Witherow RO: Combined papaverine test and radionuclide penile blood flow in impotence: Method and preliminary results. Br J Urol 1992;69:408.

Halverson HM: Genital and sphincter behavior of the male infant. J Gen Psychol 1940;56:95.

Hartmann U: Psychological evaluation and psychometry. *In* Jonas U, Thon WF, Stief CG, eds: Erectile Dysfunction. Berlin, Springer-Verlag, 1991, pp 93–103.

Hatzichristou DG, Saenz de Tejada I, Kupferman S, et al: In vivo assessment of trabecular smooth muscle tone, its application in pharmacocavernosometry and analysis of intracavernous pressure determinants. J Urol 1995;153:1126.

Hauri D, Spycher M, Bruhlmann W: Erection and priapism: A new physiopathological concept. Urol Int 1983;38:138.

Hirshkowitz M, Ware JC: Studies of nocturnal penile tumescence and rigidity. *In* Singer C, Weiner WJ, eds: Sexual Dysfunction: A Neuro-Medical Approach. Armonk, NY, Futura Publishing Company, Inc. 1994, pp 77–99.

Hwang, TI, Lin MS, Yang CR: Evaluation of vasculogenic impotence using dynamic penile washout test. J Formos Med Assoc 1990;89:992.

Hwang TI, Liu PZ, Yang CR: Evaluation of penile dorsal arteries and deep arteries in arteriogenic impotence. J Urol 1991;146:46.

Janssen E, Everaerd W, Van Lunsen RH, Oerlemans S: Validation of a psychophysiological waking erectile assessment (WEA) for the diagnosis of male erectile disorder. Urology 1994;43:686, discussion 695.

Jarow JP, Pugh VW, Routh WD, Dyer RB: Comparison of penile duplex ultrasonography to pudendal arteriography. Variant penile arterial anatomy affects interpretation of duplex ultrasonography. Invest Radiol 1993;28:806.

Jevtich MJ, Kass M, Khawand N: Changes in the corpora cavernosa of impotent diabetics: comparing histological with clinical findings. J Urol 1985;91:281.

Johnson AR, Jarow JP: Is routine endocrine testing of impotent men necessary? J Urol 1992;147:1542.

Kaneko K, De Mouy EH, Lee BE: Sequential contrast-enhanced MR imaging of the penis. Radiology 1994;191:75.

Kaneko S, Mizunaga M, Miyata M, et al: Analysis of nocturnal penile tumescence with continuous monitoring of penile rigidity. Nippon Hinyokika Gakkai Zasshi 1990;81:1889.

Kaneko S, Yachiku S, Miyata M, et al: Continuous monitoring of penile rigidity and tumescence in Japanese without erectile dysfunction. Nippon Hinyokika Gakkai Zasshi 1991;82:955.

Kaplan HS: The Evaluation of Sexual Disorders. New York, Brunner/Mazel, 1983.

Kaplan HS: The New Sex Therapy. New York, Brunner/Mazel, 1974.

Karacan I: Clinical value of nocturnal penile erection in the prognosis of impotence. Med Aspects Hum Sexuality 1970;4:27.

Katlowitz NM, Albano GJ, Morales P, Golimbu M: Potentiation of drug-induced erection with audiovisual sexual stimulation. Urology 1993; 41:431.

Kessler WO: Nocturnal penile tumescence. Urol Clin North Am 1988;15:81.

Kim SC, Choi IG, Oh CH, Cha YJ: Prostacyclin-to-thromboxane A2 ratio in arteriogenic impotence. J Urol 1990;144:1373.

Kim ED, McVary KT: Long-term results with penile vein ligation for venogenic impotence. J Urol 1995;153:655.

Knispel HH, Anderson R: Evaluation of vasculogenic impotence by monitoring of cavernous oxygen tension. J Urol 1993;149:1276.

Kohler H, Sohn M, Klein CL, et al: Intracavernosal kinetics of eicosanoids and endothelin during erection. Data from human and animal studies on intrapenile and systemic prostaglandins. Int J Impotence Res 1993;5:3.

Krane SM: The turnover and degration for collagen. Ciba Found Symp 1985;114:97.

Kromann-Andersen, B, Nielsen KK, Nordling J: Cavernosometry: Methodology and reproducibility with and without pharmacological agents in the evaluation of venous impotence. Br J Urol 1991;67:517.

Lee B, Sikka SC, Randrup ER, et al: Standardization of penile blood flow parameters in normal men using intracavernous prostaglandin E1 and visual sexual stimulation. J Urol 1993;149:49.

Lin JS, Lui SM, Chen CM, and Chang WC: The change of urinary 11-dehydro-thromboxane B2 and 2, 3-dinor6-keto-prostaglandin F_1 alpha in arteriogenic impotence. J Urol 1992;148:311.

Lopez JA, Espeland MA, Jarow JP: Interpretation and quantification of penile blood flow studies using duplex ultrasonography. J Urol 1991;146:1271.

Luangkhot R, Rutchik S, Agarwal V: Collagen alterations in the corpus cavernosum of men with sexual dysfunction. J Urol 1992;148:467.

Lue TF, Tanagho EA: Physiology of erection and pharmacological management of impotence. J Urol 1987;137:829.

Lue TF, Hricak H, Marich KW, Tanagho EA: Vasculogenic impotence evaluated by high-resolution ultrasonography and pulsed Doppler spectrum analysis. Radiology 1985;155:777.

Lue TF, Hricak H, Schmidt RA, Tanagho EA: Functional evaluation of penile veins by cavernosography in papaverine-induced erection. J Urol 1986;135:479.

Lue TF: Impotence: A patient's goal-directed approach to treatment. World J Urol 1990;8:67.

Maatman TJ, Montague DK: Routine endocrine screening in impotence. Urology 1986;27:499.

40 SURGERY FOR ERECTILE DYSFUNCTION

Ronald Lewis, M.D.

Surgery similar to what is practiced today for the relief of erectile dysfunction was first reported at the turn of the 20th century (Gee, 1975; Lewis, 1990; Das, 1994). Lowsley and Reuda (1953) reported results in 273 impotent patients treated with multiple corporeal and venous plication procedures as an update to a previous report in 1936. Kim and Carson (1993) reviewed the history of placement of prostheses for impotence. Beheri in 1966 (in over 700 patients) and Pearman in 1972 reported intracavernous placement of polyethylene and silicone prostheses, respectively, with dilation of the corporeal space with Hegar dilators. In 1973, Scott and co-workers reported on the first five patients who underwent implant surgery to receive an inflatable penile prosthesis. The first use of the Small-Carrion prosthesis was reported in 1975 (Small et al, 1975).

Ebbehoj and Wagner (1979) can be given credit for the first modern surgical approach to correction of abnormal drainage of the cavernous tissue based on diagnostic dynamic cavernosography techniques. Vaclav Mikal (1980) should be considered the father of modern vascular surgery for impotence with his presentation of various arterial vascular procedures to treat the disorder in the 1970s. Another pioneer in the revascularization procedures for treating impotence is Ronald Virag (1982), who first introduced deep dorsal vein arterialization.

Today, surgical treatment for erectile dysfunction consists of placement of a penile prosthesis or, in very carefully selected patients, vascular surgery. In addition, in this chapter, a discussion of surgery for treatment of priapism is included, which is less often needed since the introduction of pharmacologic reversal.

PATIENT COUNSELING FOR ERECTILE DYSFUNCTION SURGERY

It is imperative that **alternative nonsurgical treatment modalities be fully explained** to the potential patient. Decisions for management of impotence should be in the context of **patient** (and, when at all possible, the partner) **goal-directed therapy,** as presented by Lue in Chapter 39. Patients who have first failed more conservative treatment for their erectile problem will tend to be more satisfied with a later choice of surgical intervention. There are individual patients, however, who will benefit from surgical intervention as a primary choice. Table 40–1 provides the elements of informed consent that are necessary for prosthetic surgery.

The **choice of incision** for erectile surgery varies markedly, and this should also be explained to the patient in the preoperative counseling sessions. For placement of semirigid devices or self-contained cylinder inflatable devices, or for performance of a corpus cavernosal-glans shunt in priapism, a subcoronal partial or complete circumferential incision is adequate, but circumcision, if foreskin is present, is necessary to avoid a edematous inner tube deformity of the subglanular skin. However, if balanitis or posthitis is present, a first-stage circumcision is necessary before placement of a penile prosthesis, because the risk of infection would be too

Table 40–1. WHAT THE POTENTIAL PROSTHETIC PATIENT NEEDS TO KNOW

- Any other possible conservative treatment options
- What the prosthesis will do for him, and what change in body status will result
- Explanation in lay terms where device is to be placed
- What options are available to solve the problem
- Expected functional and cosmetic result
- Possible involvement of others who will be involved with the patient in prosthetic care and/or use
- Explanation of possible complications
  - stress what disease process in patient may affect complication rate
  - stress major complications and incidence
  - stress the possibility of revision surgery
- Encourage the patient to ask questions about prosthesis and surgery
- When possible, give the patient an idea of the longevity of prosthesis

great with simultaneous placement. For placement of a two- or three-piece inflatable penile prosthesis, a penile scrotal or infrapubic incision (in either case vertical or horizontal) is optimal, depending on the preference of the surgeon. It is easier to place the suprapubic reservoir, and the tubing from the cylinders is in a more protected position in the infrapubic incision, but dilation of the corpora is slightly more difficult. On the other hand, dilation and access to the intracavernous space with clearer vision of the urethra, a definite advantage in the presence of intracavernosal fibrosis, is easier with the penile-scrotal incision, but placement of a suprapubic reservoir is more difficult and is performed blindly. Tubing from one of the penile cylinders to the pump crosses over the urethra with this incision, and the tubing is covered by less overlying tissue. A semicircular incision on one side of the scrotal skin around the base of the penis, through which the entire penile shaft and access to the infrapubic region can be obtained, is the incision of choice for penile vein dissection and ligation surgery. Although some authors believe that a paramedian incision is the best way to expose the inferior epigastric vessel complex in penile revascularization, I prefer a midline abdominal incision from umbilicus to base of penis, which will provide access to bilateral inferior epigastric vessel complexes, if this becomes necessary, without having to make a second paramedian incision. The more preferable incision for more extensive cavernosal to spongiosal shunts in the management of persistent priapism is the midline perineal incision, which is also the best way to approach a crural erosion of a cylinder.

PENILE PROSTHESES

Penile prostheses are basically of **two broad categories: the malleable or semirigid, and the inflatable devices** (Table 40–2, and Figs. 40–1 to 40–4). The malleable or semi-rigid devices are of pure silicone rubber, or contain an intertwined central or spiral metallic core or polytetrafluoroethylene (PFTE)–coated interlocking polysulfone rings connected by a spring loaded cable, which locks the rings in a rod column with activation of the device and unlocks them for the flaccid state. The inflatable devices are either self-contained cylinders or so-called two- or three-piece devices. The former holds fluid in the crural base part of the cylinder

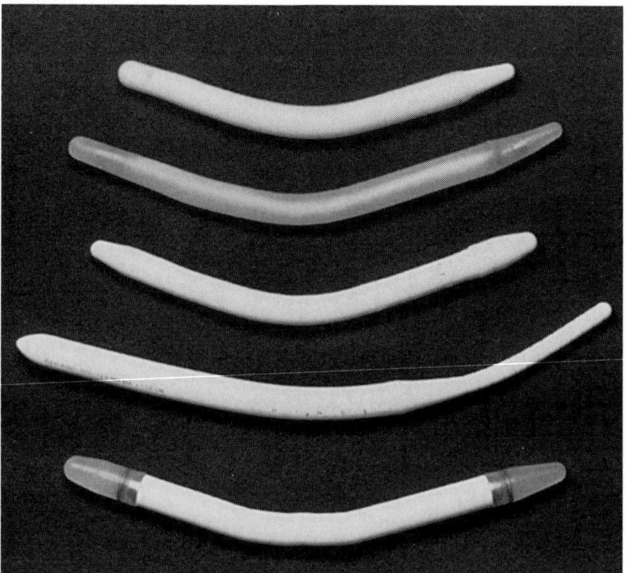

Figure 40–1. Varieties of semirigid and malleable penile prostheses. From top to bottom, the American Medical Systems (AMS) malleable prosthesis, the Bard Jonas prothesis, the Mentor malleable prosthesis, the Surgitech Flexirod (no longer produced), and the Dacomed Duraphase.

and the space between the outer silicone layer and the reinforcing central Dacron sleeve in the flaccid state. This is transferred to the central cylinder during rigidity activation via a pump mechanism in the glanular end of the cylinder; release for flaccidity is accomplished by overcoming a valve with bending of the device. In the United States, there are two companies who make these more sophisticated two- or three-piece devices. The first, the originator of inflatable devices, continues to make the device entirely of silicone polymers except for Dacron reinforcement sleeves in the cylinders. The second company constructs the cylinders and reservoirs of a proprietary polyurethane-containing compound but uses silicone polymer tubing and some silicone polymers for tubing connection sites and the pump. **No penile prostheses contain silicone gel.** Several of the two- and three-piece device pumps and cylinders are preconnected by tubing, and some are prefilled with saline. One available model has length expansion. The two-piece devices contain a combination scrotal reservoir/pump, and the three-piece devices have a scrotal pump and a reservoir, which is placed suprapubically, usually in the space between the rectus muscle and the peritoneum or intraperitoneally.

Selection of the appropriate device for the individual

Table 40–2. CURRENTLY AVAILABLE PENILE IMPLANTS

Rods	Self-contained
AMS 600 (AMS)	Dynaflex (AMS)
Jonas (Bard)	Inflatable (multiple components)
Small-Carrion (Mentor)	700 CX and Ultrex (AMS)
Malleable (Mentor)	Ambicor (AMS)
Mechanical	Alpha I (Mentor)
Duraphase (Dacomed)	GFS Mark II (Mentor)

AMS, American Medical Systems, Minnetonka, MN; Bard, C.R. Bard, Covington, GA; Dacomed, Dacomed Corporation, Minneapolis, MN; Mentor, Mentor Urology, Inc., Santa Barbara, CA.

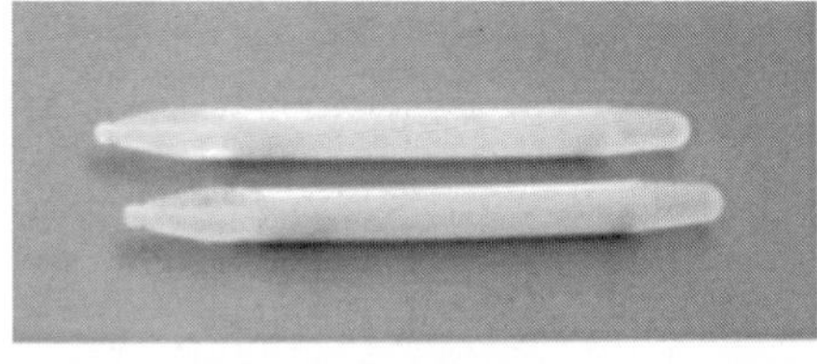

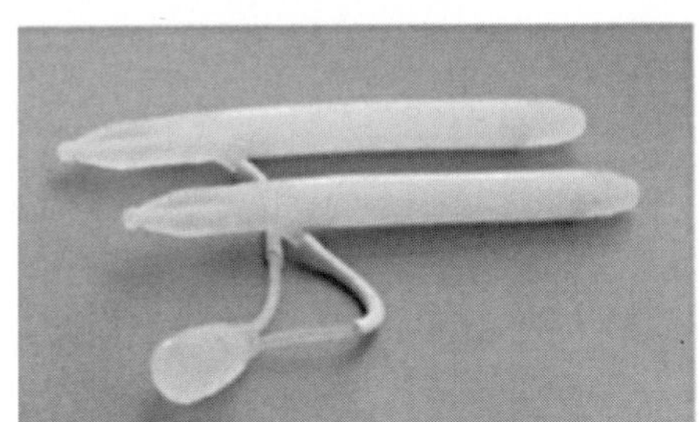

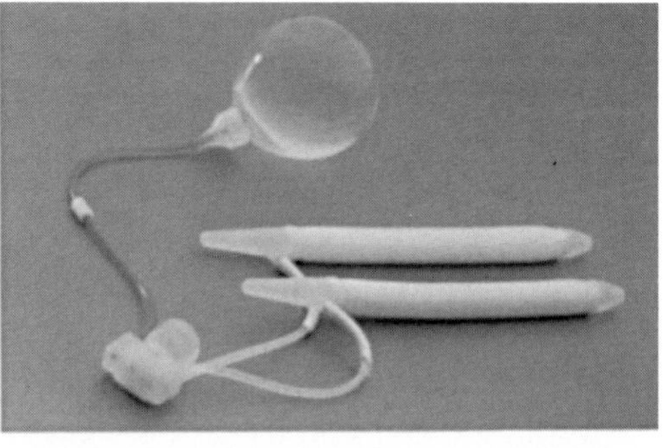

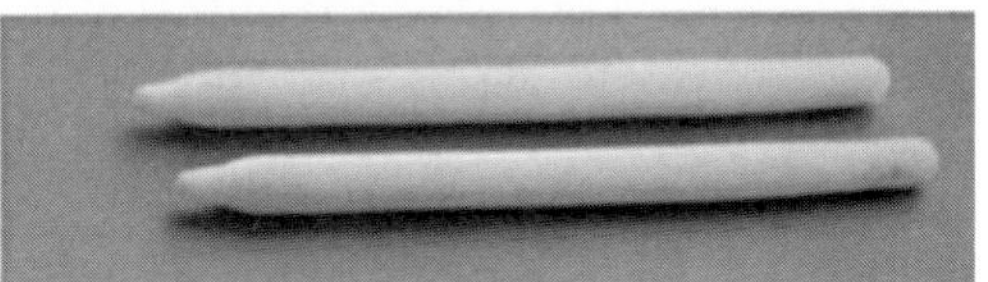

Figure 40–2. Penile prostheses produced by AMS. Clockwise from top left, the Dynaflex self-contained inflatable penile prosthesis, the Ultrex Plus three-piece inflatable prosthesis, the Malleable 600 penile prosthesis, and the two-piece Ambicor.

patient is largely based on **three considerations: the patient's preference, the cost of the device, and the surgeon's preference.** The advantages of the various devices should be explained in order for the patient to make a more informed choice. The advantages of the semirigid device are easier placement, less chance of failure due to wear, and lower cost. The more rigid cylinder will be a greater aid in holding a condom collection device in place, but the self-contained inflatable device is also a good choice for this particular circumstance, because of the more rigid and developed glanular pump end of the cylinder. Patients who use condom catheters are more likely to have neurologic disease and lack of penile sensation, and are, therefore, more prone to cylinder erosion with the semirigid or malleable devices. Besides this drawback of the semirigid devices, other disadvantages include less concealability and inability of change in girth. An advantage of the two-piece device includes easier surgical placement, because of lack of need for suprapubic reservoir placement, but because less fluid is transferred in and out of the cylinders with the erect and flaccid states, the degree of rigidity and change in girth and length is not as good as with the three-piece inflatable device. In one of the two-piece devices, which retains many features of the self-contained device, the flaccidity is not as good as with the three-piece device. The three-piece devices provide a flaccid and erect state that more closely mimics natural erection, but one mandatory caution to be made to the prospective recipient is that **no penile prosthesis will restore the full length previously achieved by the patient with his natural erection.** Also, because the inflatable prostheses contain multiple mechanical parts, the chance of me-

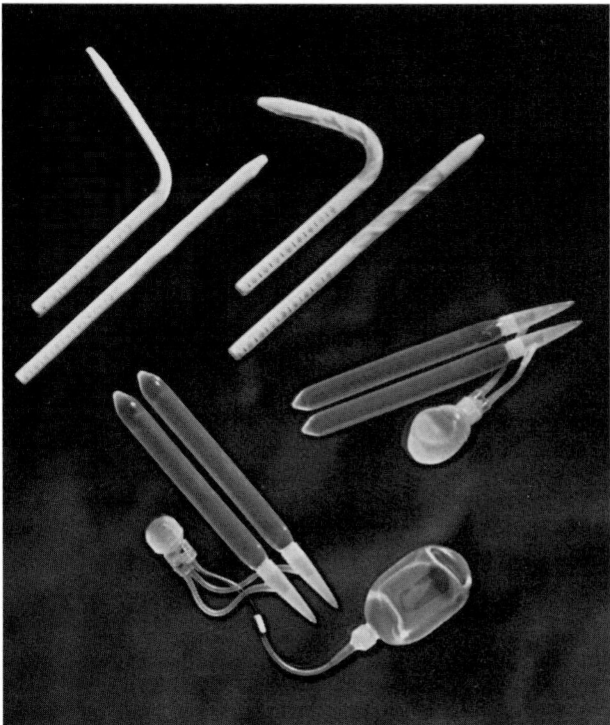

Figure 40–3. Penile prostheses produced by Mentor Urology, Inc. Two varieties of malleable devices *(top),* the two-piece GFS Mark II inflatable penile prosthesis *(middle right),* and the three-piece Alpha 1 inflatable penile prosthesis.

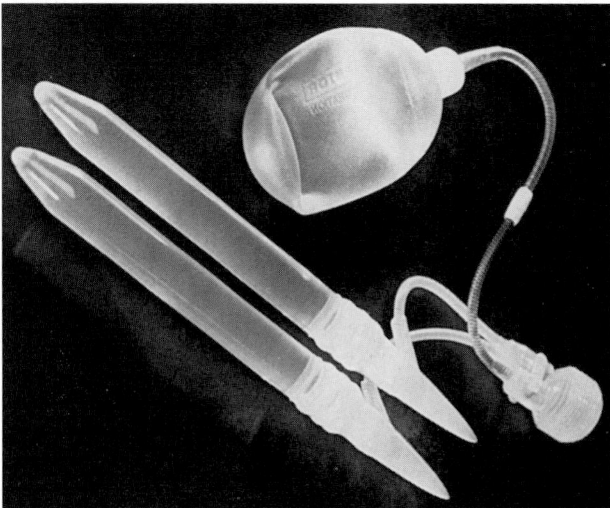

Figure 40–4. A proposed penile prosthesis by Mentor Urology, Inc., which will have the ability to expand in length based on an accordion base. This has not been released and does not have approval of the Food and Drug Administration.

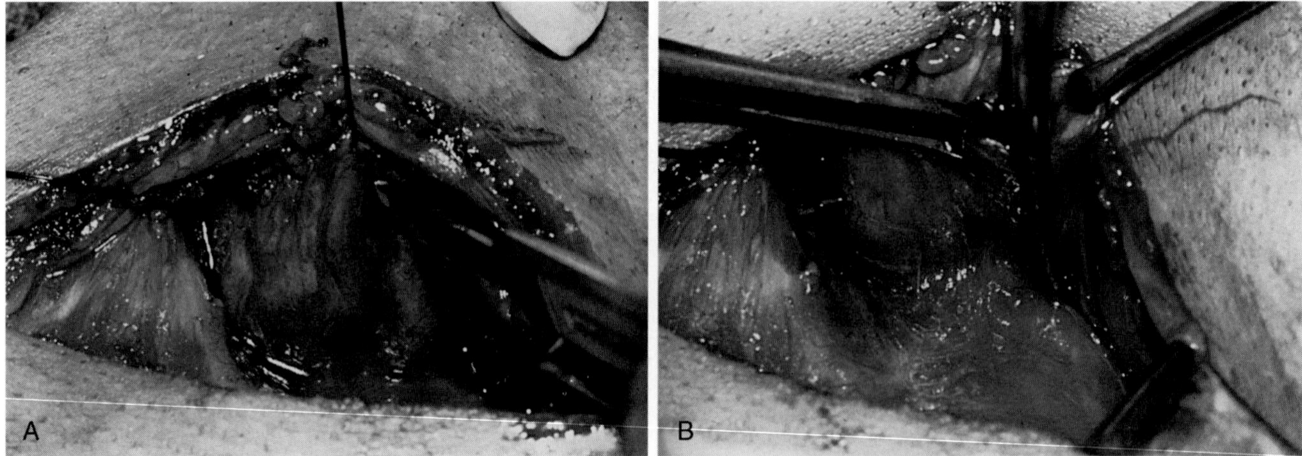

Figure 40–5. *A,* Using a No. 15 blade, the beginning corporotomy incision is made just below a traction suture on the lateral surface of the right corpora cavernosum. *B,* The corporotomy incision is extended for a distance of 2 to 4 cm with Mayo scissors.

chanical wear is higher than that experienced with the more simple devices. Some surgeons prefer the more permanently rigid devices for impotence surgery associated with Peyronie's disease, but, others prefer the three-piece device inflatable device for this type of patient. Patients with severe arthritis or restrictive hand problems may have difficulty working a scrotal pump and may want to avoid such a device unless a willing partner is available to assist.

Techniques of Implant Surgery

A large part of the **preparation of the patient** is ensuring that he does have realistic expectations for the device and an understanding that any present erectile ability may be lost, particularly if the entire device ever has to be removed, and that future revision surgery may be necessary. Infection prophylaxis is discussed later in this chapter.

Most experienced implant surgeons prefer to place the patient in the **supine position. Placement of a Foley urinary catheter is recommended,** especially in patients with corporal fibrosis and in patients who will have placement of a suprapubic reservoir, because an empty bladder facilitates creation of the reservoir pouch and avoids injury to the bladder. It is not absolutely required for primary placement of other devices. Special tools are limited but consist of tools to dilate the corpora cavernosa tissue for placement of the cylinders (a set of Hegar dilators [No. 7/8 to No. 13/14], a dilamezinsert, or Brooks dilators), a cylinder-measuring device, cylinder protection devices for placement of tunica albuginea corporal sutures once the cylinders are in place, a long-nosed nasal forceps for assistance in placement of the suprapubic reservoir via a penile scrotal incision, shodded hemostatic clamps for safe temporary clamping of device tubing, special connector pliers for those devices requiring this type of connector placement, special blunt-tipped needles for filling of components of the inflatable devices, and a cylinder placement tool. Suture used to close the corporotomy can be permanent but absorbable monofilament suture (polydioxanone, Ethicon, Inc/Johnson & Johnson, Somerville, NJ) of 2-0 size is my preference.

Once the appropriate incision (see discussion above) is made and the **tunica albuginea surface is exposed on the lateral surface of the corpus cavernosum, a corporotomy incision** is started with a No. 15 blade and then extended with a straight Mayo scissors for a distance of 2.5 to 4 cm (Fig. 40–5*A* and *B*). If the device is placed via a circumcision-like incision the corporotomy is started distally 2 to 3 cm from the glanular edge and carried proximally toward the crural portion of the corpora until the appropriate length is achieved. If the incision in the corporal bodies is more proximal, such as that achieved with a penile scrotal or infrapubic incision, the most proximal incision is best placed 6 to 7 cm from the crural end of the corpora. This allows minimal extender use and ensures exit of the cylinder tubing in a more direct manner, which will eliminate later cylinder wear from tubing lying against cylinder under the tunica albuginea (Fig. 40–6).

The next step is **dilation of the corporal space.** This should be carefully done by placement of the dilation tool of choice toward the crura or the glans, taking care to abut against the ischial tuberosity in the crural direction, because

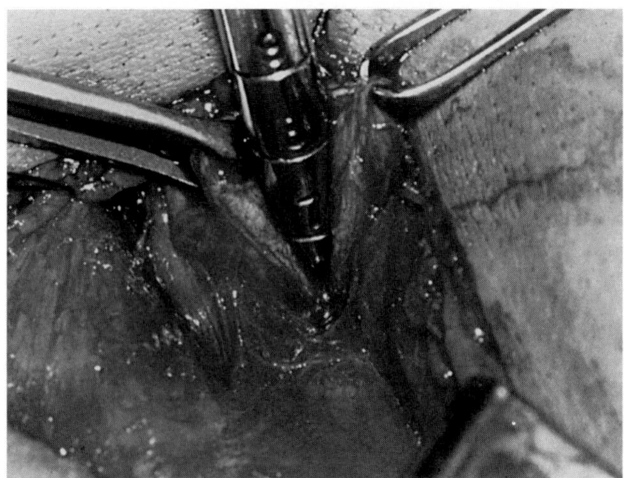

Figure 40–6. The incision is planned so that the lower part of the corporotomy opening is approximately 6 to 7 cm from the crural end of the corpora as shown in this figure. The most proximal depth of the incision is at 6.5 cm.

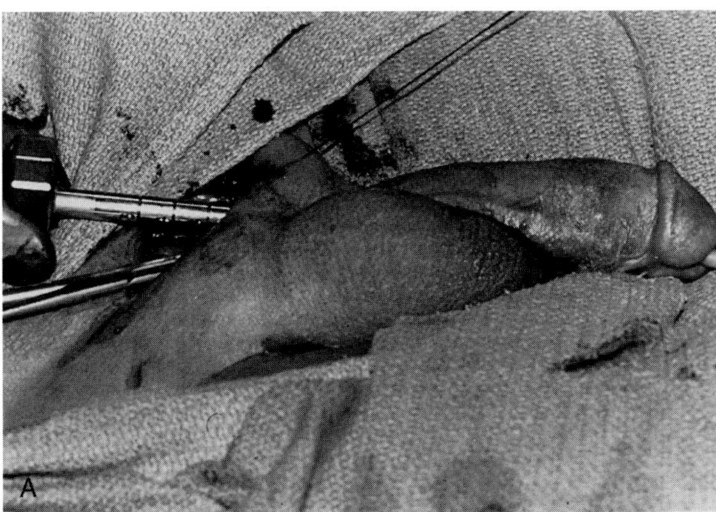

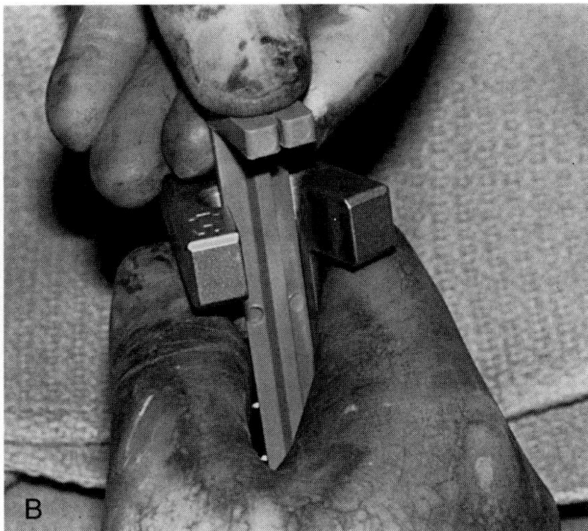

Figure 40–7. *A,* Dilation of the right corpora. Notice that the penis is twisted so that the end of the dilation tool can be followed along the lateral surfaces of the corpora as it is introduced. This shows introduction through an infrapubic incision. *B,* Using the central dilation core, the corpora is dilated in a single maneuver. This picture shows dilation of the crural portion of the corpora. Notice that the base of the insert is rested on the hand in order to lessen the chance of perforation.

this is where intraoperative perforation is most likely to occur, and to advance under the glans distally to ensure proper placement of the cylinder in order to avoid a floppy SST deformity of the glans. This distal dilation is safely performed by keeping the tip of dilator lateral as it is advanced under the glans. Perforation into the urethra may also result if too vigorous distal dilation is performed or in patients with some distal corporal fibrosis. Corporal dilation should be easily performed, and any difficulty should suggest to the surgeon an improper plane, cross-over into the opposite corpora through the midline septum, or perforation (Fig. 40–7*A* and *B*).

Once dilation of a corporal body has been accomplished proximally and distally, the **corporal closure sutures** can be placed on either side of the corporotomy, which makes closure of the corporotomy incision much easier and less risky for an inflatable cylinder perforation (Fig. 40–8*A* and *B*). Montague (1993) suggested a novel way of tying horizontally placed sutures in two stages, tying the distal strands of opposite sutures first followed by a second knot of the proximal strands, so that two knots are made with each oppositely placed suture. This is a excellent closure for primary device placement, but double-strand tying of opposite preplaced vertical sutures is recommended for replacement or revision surgery. Preplacement of the corporotomy sutures is not necessary for noninflatable cylinders, because this closure can be interrupted or running and be made over the cylinder. A protective tool is used for placement of suture over a previously placed inflatable cylinder.

Most surgeons make the corporotomy incision and perform corporal dilation bilaterally **before placement of either cylinder.** If there is a question of not being able to place the maximum diameter device of the model selected for the patient, placement of a Hegar dilator into both of the corporal spaces will indicate a tightness that will require selection of a smaller diameter. Careful measurement of the length of

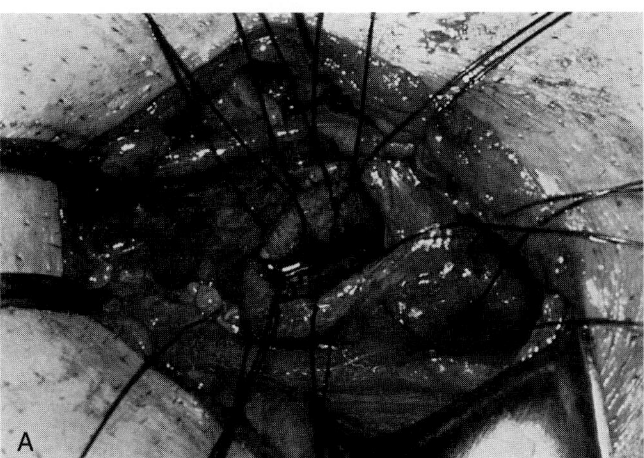

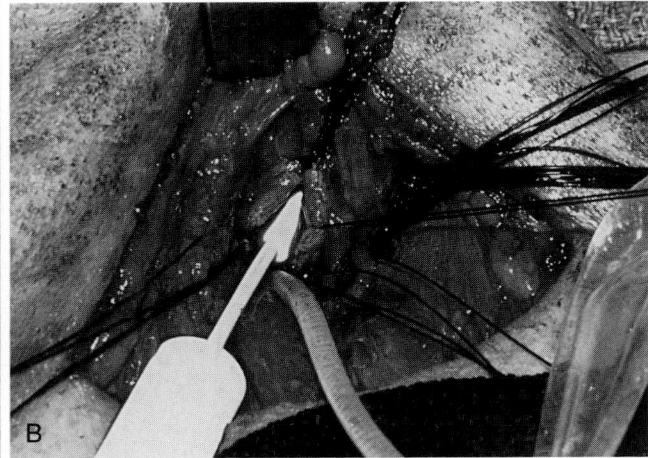

Figure 40–8. *A,* Preplacement of 2-0 PDS sutures into either side of the corporotomy incision. Note that there are four sutures on either side of the corporotomy. To the far right, there is also a traction suture that is still in place. *B,* Illustration of several points. Notice that the exit tubing comes straight out because of the proximal extension of the corporotomy incision. For placement of other sutures, a protector should be used for placement of suture over an inflatable cylinder. Shown here is the Mentor Urology, Inc., tool. A Furlow protective tool can also be used.

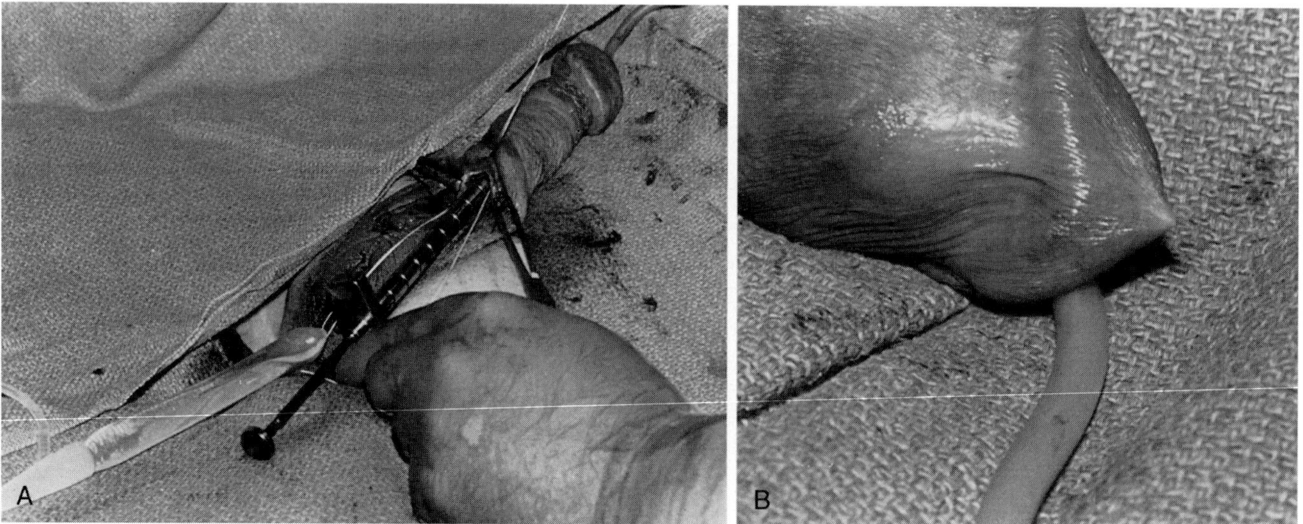

Figure 40–9. *A,* Demonstration of placement of the Furlow introducer that has been preloaded with a threaded Keith needle into the distal corpora through a penile scrotal incision. *B,* Demonstration of the proper exit site for the Keith needle as it is pushed through the distal end of the corpora through the glans. Note the relationship to the indwelling Foley catheter.

the corporal space is made using the special cylinder-measuring device. The appropriate length individual cylinders with or without rear-tip extenders (total length 1 cm less with the AMS Ultrex cylinder) are then placed into their respective intracorporal spaces directly for the semirigid devices and with a cylinder placement tool for inflatable devices. The tool incorporates a cylinder suture attached to a Keith needle, which is inserted through the glans (Fig. 40–9*A* and *B*). Immediately before placement of the cylinders, the corporal spaces are irrigated with an antibiotic solution, as are all subsequent spaces for the pump and the reservoir at the time of exposure. For placement of semirigid devices, it is usually easier to place the crural end of the device first. For the Duraphase (Dacomed Corp) device, due to its lesser flexibility, the subcoronal approach is the easiest with placement of the crural end first. Then, using a small hooked retractor, such as an eyelid retractor, to elevate the more distal end of the corporotomy incision, the glanular end can be flipped into the dilated corporal space. Length selection with this device is somewhat different, and the manufacturer's instructions for measurement should be followed. With inflatable cylinders that have attached tubing, direct exit at the tubing connection site is preferable, and care is taken in tying the previous placed coporotomy suture on either side of the tubing to ensure this (Fig. 40–10). For the semirigid devices, once the cylinders are placed and the corporotomies are closed, skin closure using chromic catgut or other absorbable braided suture completes the surgery.

For the two- and three-piece devices, a space is created in the sub-Dartos scrotum for **placement of the reservoir/pump or the pump** with the index and middle finger or sometimes with a large Hegar dilator or Kelly clamp (Fig. 40–11). Preattached pump devices are placed in this space, after antibiotic irrigation, and the tubing from each of the cylinders is sometimes separated with sutured tissue to keep them separated to prevent tubing to tubing wear. I have not found this to be a common cause of mechanical failure in patients who have not routinely had this compartmentaliza-

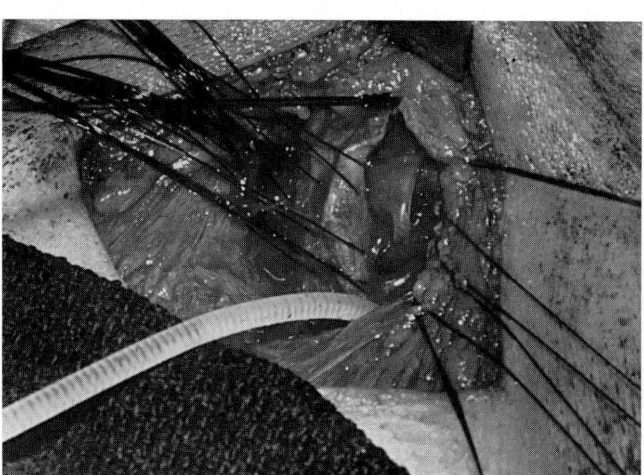

Figure 40–10. A cylinder is in place in the right corpora. The first set of sutures has been tied. Notice the proper exit of the tubing from the cylinder.

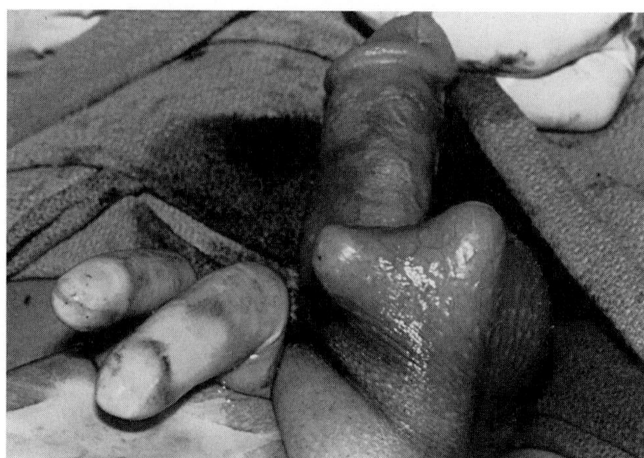

Figure 40–11. Development of a subcutaneous scrotal space for placement of a pump.

tion. If the pump is not preconnected to the cylinders, the order of reservoir or pump placement is not important.

For **placement of the suprapubic reservoir** in three-piece devices, a space is created behind the rectus muscle by making a midline vertical incision in the rectus fascia first and, under direct vision, creating a space behind the rectus muscle preperitoneally. Some surgeons make the reservoir space through the external inguinal ring, puncturing the inguinal floor and subsequently dilating the space behind the rectus muscle. This can be facilitated by a long-nosed nasal speculum or a special dilation tool. Placing the pump into the peritoneum has been advocated by some surgeons to eliminate risk of entrapment of the reservoir, which might lead to autoinflation. This can be avoided by carefully creating an adequate space initially, which can be ascertained when filling the reservoir after placement. I add 5 mL more than the size of the capacity of the reservoir and leave the tubing connected to the syringe, expecting to see spontaneous filling of the syringe to 5 mL once pressure is taken off the barrel of the syringe. If more than 5 mL returns, I check the position of the reservoir and expand the space until this no longer occurs. If the reservoir continues to fill the syringe passively with more than the 5 mL, it is left filled with this zero pressure volume (which may be less than the recommended volume) to avoid autoinflation. Once the reservoir is placed and filled, the tubing is shod clamped and the opening in the rectus fascia, if made for placement of the reservoir, is closed with No. 1 braided absorbable suture. Once the reservoir and pump are in place, appropriate connections are made between the tubing of the various components, and the tubing is separated from other tubing. The device is inflated and deflated several times to ensure proper position and function. It is left in the deflated state. The wound is closed in a couple of layers, and appropriate dressings are put in place. A surgical drain is not usually required, although some implant surgeons prefer a fenestrated tubular suction drain for 24 to 48 hours postoperatively, specifically when there is a large amount of intraoperative bleeding. If an indwelling Foley catheter was placed, it is removed the morning following surgery. The patient is most comfortable with the penis taped to the lower abdomen. An attempt is made to inflate the device 4 to 6 weeks after surgery. For noninflatable devices, intercourse trials can begin, if all wounds are healed, at this same time. Individual surgeons who have described operative techniques that may be more variable than that described above are included in the reference section (Small, 1991; Montague and Lakin, 1993; Mulcahy, 1993).

Complications of Penile Prosthesis Surgery

These will be divided for the sake of discussion into the following four categories: intraoperative technical problems, infection, other postoperative surgical problems, and mechanical failure.

A common **intraoperative problem** is crural perforation. This can be managed with a separate perineal direct closure of the tear after placement of the device or, as suggested by Mulcahy, an artificial windsock repair (Mulcahy, 1987; Fishman, 1993) (Fig. 40–12*A* and *B*). With the two- or three-piece inflatable devices with attached tubing, I have found that placing a tunica albuginea closure suture on either side of the exit tubing keeps the cylinder in place, provided the ischial tuberosity can be sounded with the dilation or measuring device and the ipsilateral cylinder can be placed similar to the opposite cylinder, so that repair of a simple tear is not necessary. If this approach is followed, the device should remain in the deflated state for 6 weeks. If a distal corporal perforation occurs on the first side of dilation in primary implant procedures, the procedure should be abandoned and rescheduled at a later time. However, if this occurs in patients with severe intracorporeal scarring or a previous history of such an injury and the surgeon has prepared the patient for urinary diversion, a catheterized diverting perineal urethrostomy can be performed, if the perforation can be directly repaired via a circumcision-like incision. The patient should be kept on broad-spectrum antibiotics for 2 to 3 weeks postoperatively, and a retrograde urethrogram at that time should be normal before removing the diverting catheter. The perineal catheter is preferred over the suprapubic route because bladder spasm around the catheter usually results in leakage in the perineum and not into the penile urethra. Also, bladder spasms are less often seen with the urethral catheter. The placement of a penile catheter is not recommended because of friction at the site of the repair and greater chance of infection ascending into the urethra along the catheter. There is less agreement on a recommendation for management of distal perforation at the time of dilation of the second corpora after an atraumatic dilation of the opposite side. Again, the distal injury must be identified and repaired. No cylinder is placed on the side of the perforation, but urinary diversion can make the placement of the contralateral cylinder and the remainder of the device possible. The reasoning for such placement is that stopping the operation and returning at another time, which is an option, will result in bilateral corporal fibrosis. If the procedure is abandoned, the placement of fenestrated tubular drains into the corporal spaces for around the clock irrigation with an antibiotic solution every 4 hours for 2 to 3 postoperative days will decrease subsequent fibrosis (Maatman and Montague, 1984).

One of the most dreaded complications associated with penile prostheses is **infection.** In excellent reviews by Carson (1989, 1993), the incidence is 0.6% to 8.9%. Infection is more common in patients with spinal cord injuries, those with diabetes mellitus (particularly those who are under poor control; implantation should not be performed in patients with glycosylated hemoglobin greater than 11.5%), those with a history of urinary tract infections, and those having a replacement device operation (Rossier and Fam, 1984; Kabalin and Kessler, 1988; Bishop et al, 1992; Radomski and Herschorn, 1992; Quesada and Light, 1993; Lewis, 1995). Most infection associated with penile prostheses occurs in the first 3 months following surgery, but delayed infection or infection from hematogenous sources have been reported in the literature (Carson and Robertson, 1988; Kabalin and Kessler, 1988). It is probably wise to advise patients with penile prostheses, who are going to have dental work or other surgery where there is a high risk of infection, to have prophylactic antibiotic coverage.

Table 40–3 presents preventive measures, which are probably the most important elements in the management of

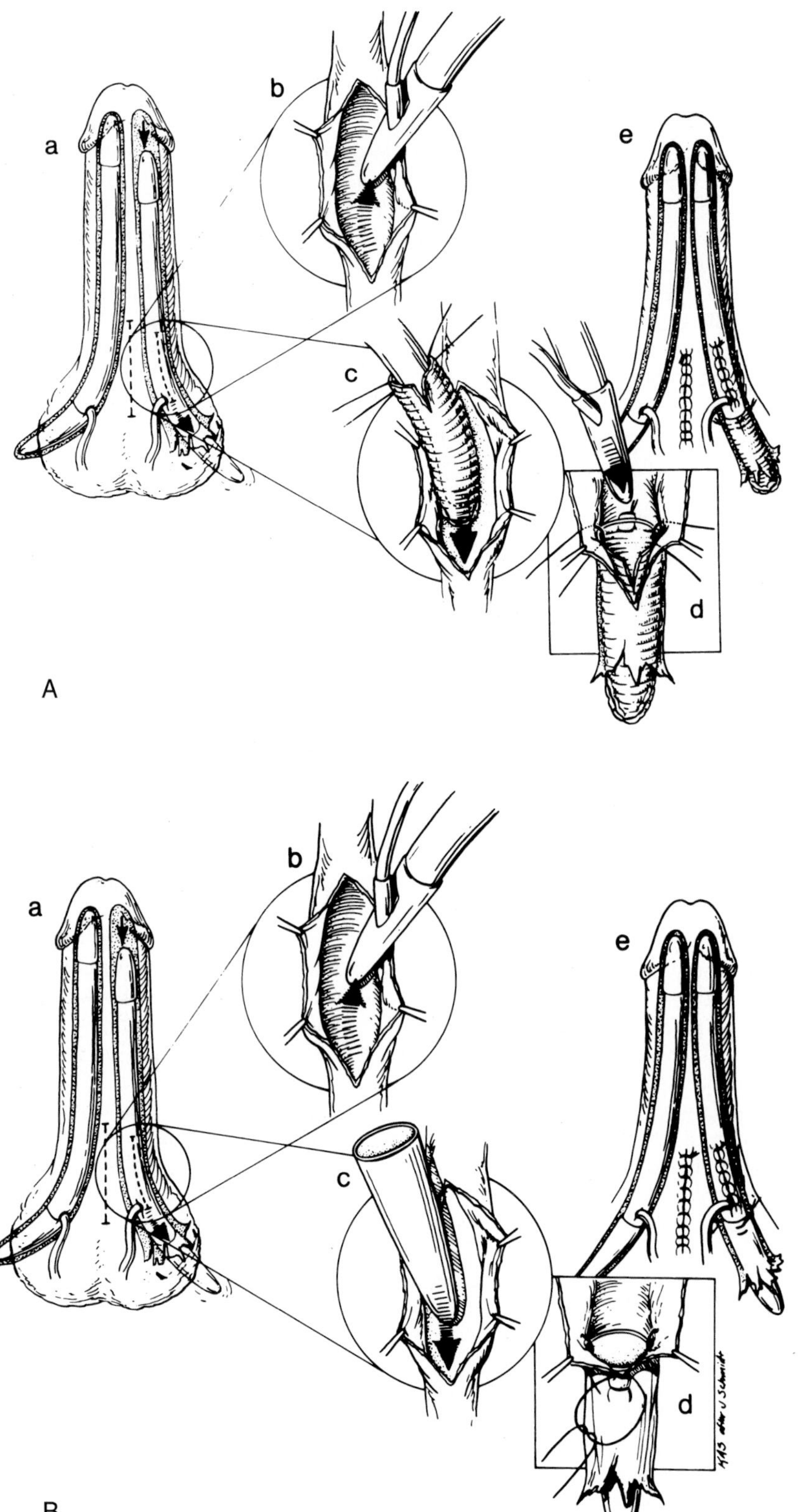

Figure 40–12. *A,* Example of the technique of neocorpus cavernosum windsock from synthetic material. *B,* Use of a fixed cylinder extender as a sutured fixed site for the cylinder introduction in the case of crural corpora perforation. (From Fishman I. Perforation and erosion of penile prostheses. Contemporary Urology 1991; 3:55–56. Reproduced by permission of Contemporary Urology/Medical Economics.)

Table 40–3. PROSTHETIC INFECTION PREVENTION

- Short hospital stay preoperatively and postoperatively
- Elimination of other sites of infection preoperatively
- Discontinuation of chronic indwelling catheters 2 weeks before surgery and diversion of urine drainage
- Antiseptic soap shower or bath night before and morning of surgery
- Prophylactic perioperative antibiotics
- Shaving immediately before surgery (in holding area or operating room)
- 10- to 15-minute skin preparation
- Strict intraoperative sterile technique (curtail operating room traffic)
- Intraoperative antibiotic wound irrigation and prosthesis soaking

infection. In those patients who have no previous history of genitourinary or prosthetic infection, a first-generation cephalosporin given as surgical prophylaxis is adequate. For others, a combination of an aminoglycoside and vancomycin surgical prophylaxis is recommended. The use of oral postoperative antibiotics is variable (Rossier and Fam, 1984; Kabalin and Kessler, 1988; Bishop et al, 1992; Radomski and Herschorn, 1992; Quesada and Light, 1993; Lewis 1995) but certainly should be considered in those patients who have had previous penile prosthetic infection or surgery.

Salvage surgery for infection in penile prostheses is debatable, but in carefully selected patients, such an approach is not unreasonable (Lewis and McLaren, 1993; Wilson and Delk, 1995). It is advisable that in the face of frank purulent material, the entire device be removed. If the device is removed, intracorporal drainage with intermittent antibiotic irrigation is recommended to help decrease subsequent fibrosis (Maatman and Montague, 1984). Table 40–4 outlines principles of prosthesis salvage technique (Fig. 40–13).

Other surgical complications include problems with position, pain, cosmetics and size, encapsulation, and pressure erosion. The three most common position problems are inadequate cylinder length, resulting in an SST deformity, a high-riding pump or pump/reservoir combination, and a kinked reservoir neck. The SST deformity is corrected by the Ball procedure (Ball, 1980) (Fig. 40–14) and the other disorders

Table 40–4. SALVAGE TECHNIQUES FOR PENILE PROSTHESIS

- Options
  - New components in same space (drains are always used) or a new site
  - Retention of some components of the device
  - Perineal urethrostomy diversion with immediate repair of urethral perforation
  - Early replacement after local and systemic antibiotics over 3 weeks
- Tubular fenestrated drains (irrigation with antibiotics)
  - Old infected sites
  - Same site with immediate replacement
  - Corpora spaces without devices to decrease future fibrosis
  - 1 to 5 drains may be used in a patient
  - Majority are irrigated around the clock with 2 to 7 mL every 4 to 8 hours for 5 to 7 days
- Dabs antibiotic solution for irrigation consists of:

500 mg of neomycin 80 mg of gentamicin 100 mg of polymyxin	1000 mL isotonic saline

- Long course of postoperative oral antibiotics

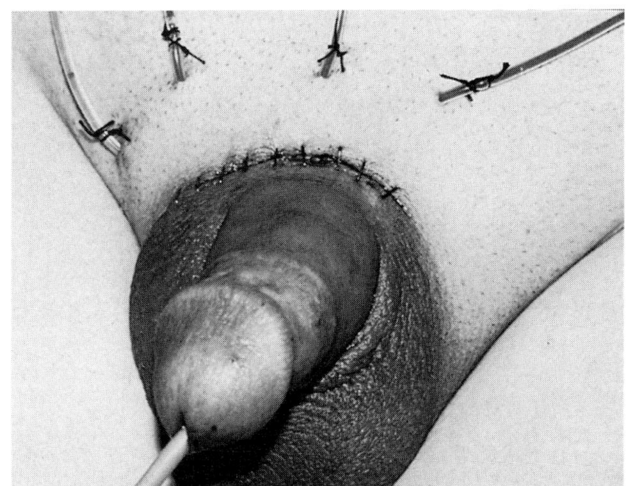

Figure 40–13. Example of a salvage procedure in which four tubular fenestrated drains have been placed in various sites. This patient had an infected pump removed on the right side. One of the drains is for this space. One of the cylinders had been replaced, and the second is a drain from this site. The third is a drain around the connector sites, and the fourth is from the opposite scrotum, where a new pump was placed. This patient was successfully salvaged without removal of the entire device. Notice the main incision, a curvilinear incision just above the penile base.

by open surgical repair if the position problem is interfering with the function of the device. It is not unusual for the patient to experience some degree of discomfort or minor penile pain 4 to 6 weeks postoperatively. Severe pain or that associated with an elevated white blood cell count or temperature elevations should alert the physician to the possibility of infection during this early postoperative period. Persistence of pain beyond this time also suggests a smoldering infection. The use of oversized cylinders can also produce pain. Encapsulation of a reservoir or a pump/reservoir can lead to the inability to fully deflate the cylinders of an inflatable device and also autoinflation, both of which necessitate open surgery to repair. Exposure is usually limited to connection sites where tubing can be hydraulically dilated to rupture the encapsulation. Pressure erosion does not necessarily indicate the need to remove the entire device, especially in the absence of frank pus (Furlow and Goldwasser, 1987).

Mechanical complications of the penile prostheses have decreased over time because devices have been modified in response to the identification of problem areas. There have been numerous peer-reviewed articles in the urologic literature describing mechanical problems with and reliability of the various prostheses, but the value of many are limited because of subsequent change in the devices and lack of long term follow-up. A recent review article attempts to clarify for the surgeon what to present to the patient as to the mechanical reliability of the various devices still presently used. Table 40–5 is a modification of one presented in this review and tabulates this data in useful form for physician and patient discussion (Lewis, 1995). There are certain clarifications that should be discussed regarding the data presented in Table 40–5. The American Medical System (AMS; Minnetonka, MN) 700 series were performed before Dacron sleeve reinforcement of the cylinders and the double-

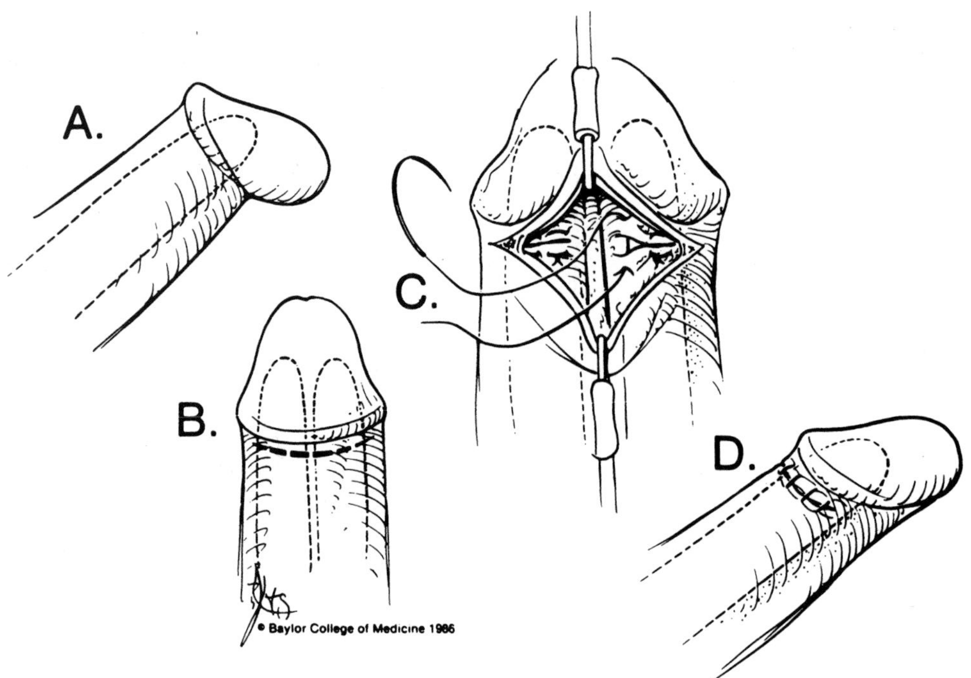

Figure 40–14. Technique for closure of the corpora for an SST deformity by plication suture. (From Fishman IJ: Complicated implantation of an inflatable penile prosthesis. Urol Clin North Am 1987; 14:217.)

wall layer of silicone, which is present in the 700 CX and Ultrex Plus. The AMS-PPT was an investigational device. Many of the mechanical failures reported by Wilson for the Mentor Corporation (Santa Barbara, CA) device were metallic connector problems; these connectors were subsequently discontinued. Although the follow-up data for the AMS-700 was from the same institution in the reports by Furlow and colleagues and Lewis and McLaren, the increased mechanical failure in the latter report was the result not only of longer follow-up but also the fact that the latter report included patients who had had the device placed at other institutions as well. The earlier report and the later 1995 report by Lewis included only patients who had the device placed at the Mayo Clinic. The unusually low mechanical failure rate of the AMS-700 CX reported by Quesada and Light has not been the experience of many other implanters; silicone polymer cylinders do have significant wear reported in other series. However, series with higher rates of secondary placement usually result in higher subsequent mechanical failure, perhaps suggesting a difference in wear owing to patient variability in handling the device. The reports by Woodworth and colleagues (1991) and Wilson and associates (1988) center on primary placement patients only. Merrill (1988), along with Steinkohl and Leach (1991), report decreasing mechanical failure rates over time with the Mentor inflatable penile prostheses, with improvement in the device design. The follow-up in the Goldstein (1993) report of the connectorless Mentor device is short term, because the device is relatively new; the report of the two-piece Mentor device by Fein (1992) is similar. In our report of mechanical failures of the Mentor two-piece device, we found most of these were due to a design problem of the reservoir/pump, leading to encapsulation; this problem dramatically decreased once this part of the device was changed. The newer AMS two-piece device and the recently modified AMS self-contained inflatable device are either too new, or there are no reports in the literature of significantly followed populations, to include longevity data. The Lewis 1995 data cannot be used to compare the three-piece device of two different companies because there were many more secondary placements of the AMS devices and the period of follow-up was much shorter for the Mentor device. However, the superior resistance to wear of the polyurethane cylinder appears to be real. Actual long-term results for semirigid devices in large series of patients is lacking in the literature, but two of the best are included in the table.

In summary, what can be said about mechanical reliability of the modern penile prosthesis based on analysis of the reported literature? We must try to base our knowledge of **long-term reliability** of a particular device only after it has been **followed for at least 5 years,** which has been difficult in the past because of the many design changes in response to attempts to deliver an improved device to the patient. Real-time follow-up, preferably in a prospective manner, versus life table statistics is a better way of determining actual mechanical reliability of a given prosthetic. It is preferable to have large populations followed by single institutions or a combination of institutions with significant numbers from each participant. Some multigroup reports indicate that two or three implants were used per participant. **For patients who have primary placement of a modern penile prosthesis, reoperation for mechanical failure can be expected in 5% of the cases when the device has been in place for 5 to 10 years. The chance of mechanical failure is greater in patients who have experienced previous prosthetic problems. These patients requiring secondary placement also have a more significant risk for infection, as well as those with other predisposing infection risk factors.**

Reoperation for Penile Prostheses

Reoperation may be necessary for one of the complications that have been discussed above. Such surgery can be difficult, particularly owing to intracorporal scarring, more likely if the device had to be removed previously for infection. Reoperation guidelines have been reviewed extensively, and the reader is referred to these references for details (Fishman, 1989, 1993; Lewis and McLaren, 1993). In patients who have intracorporal fibrosis from previous infection, **selection of smaller cylinders than those previously in place** will often be necessary. Tunical tears are more apt to occur in this type of patient, and the possibility of intraoperative repair of these should be part of the informed consent regimen for these patients. Some of these **repairs may include urinary diversion,** as mentioned in the discussion of intraoperative complications above. **Penile numbness is more commonly seen** in patients requiring cylinder revision surgery because more dissection is required over the tunica albuginea of the corpora cavernosa, with the possibility of injury to the penile sensory nerves. If there is concern about penile arterial injury because of the necessity of extensive corporeal surgery, a hand-held intraoperative Doppler probe will help identify the penile arterial branches.

In operating for **leakage of fluid** from an inflatable penile prosthesis with tubing connectors, **exploration of the connector sites first is recommended, because this is the area most frequently associated with pressure-induced failure.** This complication, of course, is less likely to occur in those devices in which connectors between the cylinders and the pump have been eliminated. If only a connector has to be replaced in the AMS device, a tie-on connector has to be used instead of the quick connector. **The second most likely source of fluid leak after tubing and tubing connectors is the cylinders, and the site of wear is most often near the input tubing attachment.** It is rare to find reservoir problems or leakage in the three-piece inflatable devices. Hydraulic rupture of encapsulation of a reservoir, when a problem, can usually be accomplished at the tubing connector site, and exposure of the reservoir is rarely needed. **When replacing a failed part of a multicomponent device, it is recommended that, if the device has been present for 5 years or longer, all of the device be replaced.**

The **most difficult problem** in reoperation is **intracorporal fibrosis.** It is **often necessary to make more than one corporal incision** to prepare a space for placement of a

Table 40–5. LONG-TERM RESULTS OF PENILE PROSTHESES

Study (Year Reported)	Year Implant Performed	Follow-up (Months)	Total Number of Patients	Type of Prosthesis	Product Failure (%)	Reoperation Other Than Mechanical Failure (%)
Fishman et al (1984)	1983	12	113	AMS-700*	2 (1.8)	5 (4.45)
Furlow et al (1988)	Unknown	6–20	120	AMS-700	10 (8.3)	11 (9.2)
Knoll et al (1990)	1983–1988	3–46 (avg 24)	94	AMS-700 CX	6 (6.4)	14 (15)
Woodworth et al (1991)§	1979–1988	22–70 ?–21 (mean 14)	99 43	AMS-700 AMS-700 CX	10 (10) 2 (5)	3 (3.33) 1 (1)
Hackler (1986)	1982–1985	6–46 (avg 21)	46	Mentor 3 piece†	0	6 (13)
Merrill (1988)	1982–1987	2–60 (mean 32)	301	Mentor 3 piece	18 (6)	12 (4)
Steinkohl and Leach (1991)	1982–1987	Unknown	46	Mentor 3 piece	13 (28)	Not reported
Fein (1992)	1988–1991	6–27	80	Mentor GFS Mark II (2 piece)	0	0
Wilson et al (1988)§	1976–1984 1986–1987 1984–1987	30–132 6–18 6–48	120 29 67	AMS-PPT AMS-700 CX Mentor 3 piece	56 (46) 4 (14) 13 (19)	Not reported
Lewis and McLaren (1993)	1983–1990 1986–1991 1983–1991 1987–1991	24–108 12–72 12–84 12–60	Unknown 275 64 61	AMS-700 AMS-700 CX Mentor 3 piece Mentor 2 piece	95 13 (4.7) 12 (18.8) 13 (21)	105 20 (73) 9 (14) 11 (18)
Lewis (1995)	1984–1993	67 37 (mean)	164 56	AMS-700 CX Mentor Alpha 1	44 (26.8) 1 (1.8)	31 (18.9) 3 (5.6)
Goldstein et al (1993)	1989–1991	4–26 (mean 8 ± 5)	112	Mentor Alpha 1 3 piece	4 (3.6)	5 (4.5)
Quesada and Light (1993)	1984–1991	8–86	214	AMS-700 CX	4 (1.9)	5 (4.5)
Benson et al (1985)	?–1982	20–38 (mean 30)	97	Jonas‡	2 (2)	6 (6)
Dorflinger and Bruskewitz (1986)	1983–1985	2–24 (median 11)	57	AMS Malleable*	0	5 (8.8)

*American Medical Systems (Minnetonka, MN)
†Mentor Corporation (Santa Barbara, CA)
‡Bard Urological (Naperville, IN)
§Included primary placement only

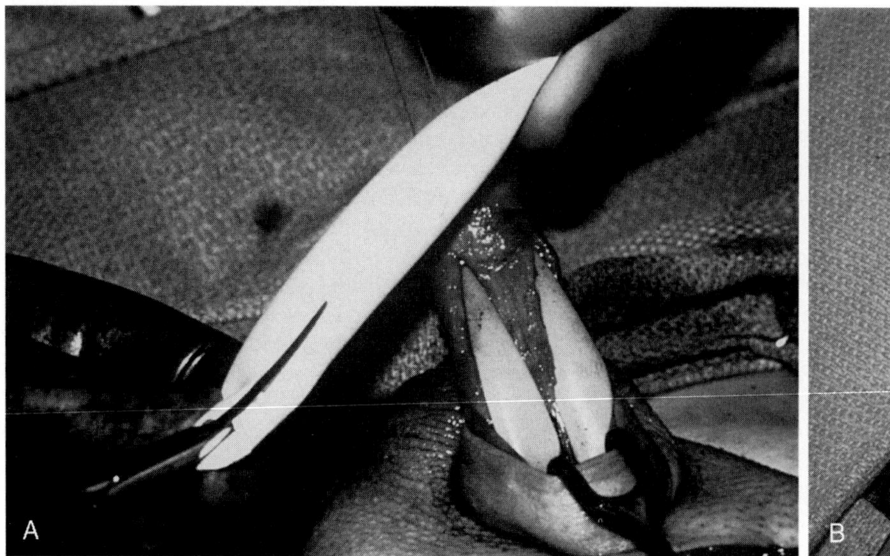
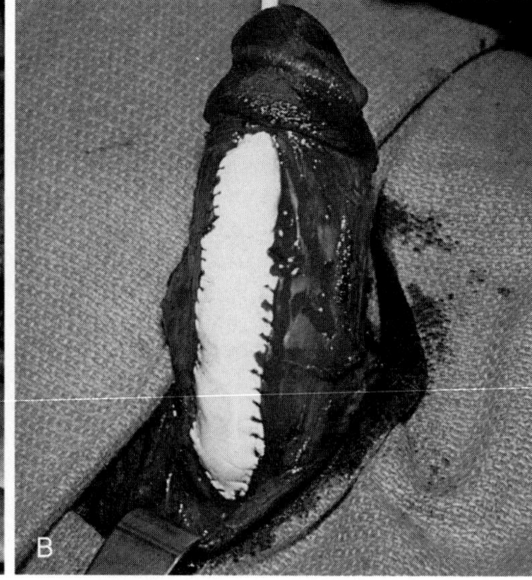

Figure 40–15. *A,* Placement of bilateral cylinders into severely fibrosed corpora cavernosa shows a defect in the corporeal wall. Appropriate graft of Gore-Tex material is being fashioned. *B,* One of the grafts has been sewn in place to the normal wall of the tunica albuginea of the left corpora cavernosa.

new cylinder. A penile scrotal incision may be the best for total corporal exposure. Sometimes, it is necessary to develop a plane between the dense fibrotic tissue and the internal surface of the tunica albuginea sharply under direct vision. Special tools such as the Carrion-Rossello dilator may be helpful. If there is a paucity of tunica albuginea for coverage after removal of the fibrous tissue, it may be necessary to cover the cylinder with a patch of Dacron or PFTE (Fig. 40–15).

Patient and Partner Outcome After Penile Prostheses

Six articles in the urologic literature have presented detailed data on patient and partner satisfaction with the penile prosthesis. Tables 40–6 and 40–7 summarize these data. **No major large prospective studies have been performed to determine actual patient and partner satisfaction.** Most have relied on questionnaires sent to the patient after the device has been in place for a while, and **response rate has varied from 56% to 85%.** Many of the partner satisfaction series were recorded by the patient, as opposed to the actual response of the partner. A small population has shown improvement in satisfaction over time. An enhancement of sexual and nonsexual relationships between the partners has been consistently reported. **A common dissatisfaction expressed is inadequate length. In general, patient and partner satisfaction with penile prostheses ranges from 60% to 80%.**

Penile Prostheses in Peyronie's Disease

A discussion of the surgical management of Peyronie's disease is given in Chapter 107. An excellent review of this

Table 40–6. PENILE PROSTHESES PATIENT AND PARTNER OUTCOME

Study	Device	Method of Patient Follow-up	Patient Follow-up			Patient Results	
			No.	*%*		*% Satisfied*	*% Dissatisfied*
Gerstenberger, Osborne, and Furlow (1979)	AMS inflatable	Mailed questionnaire	61/96	63.5		74	
Pedersen, Tiefer, Ruiz, and Melman (1988)	Mentor inflatable (54) and semirigid (18)	Telephone interview	52/72	72		64	
Krauss et al (1989)	Rigid device	Prospective study and 6–12 month postoperative structured telephone interview	19	100	6 mo 12 mo	66.7* 75	8.3† 8.3† 8.3‡
Fallon and Ghanen (1990)	AMS inflatable (80) and semirigid (62)	Mailed questionnaire	142/252	56		83	6
McLaren and Barrett (1992)	AMS-700 inflatable	Mailed questionnaire and telephone interview	272/387	70		83.5	11.7
Goldstein et al (1993)	Mentor Alpha I	Mailed questionnaire	96/112	85		85	15

*0 (Completely dissatisfied) to 100 (completely satisfied)—to be considered satisfied score of 80 or above.
†Score of 60 to 69 out of 100.
‡Score of <50 out of 100.

Table 40–7. PENILE PROSTHESES PATIENT AND PARTNER OUTCOME

Study	Method of Partner Assessment	Partner Follow-up		Partner Results		Comments
		No.	*%*	*Satisfied*	*Dissatisfied*	
Gerstenberger, Osborne, and Furlow (1979)	Questionnaire completed by patient	59/96	60	74.5		30% equal erections achieved with implant 35% penis shorter 61% improvement in nonsexual relationship with partner
Pedersen, Tiefer, Ruiz, and Melman (1989)	Interview	22/41	54	75		88% satisfied with erection 50% penis smaller and orgasm unchanged 19% penis larger 33% longer orgasm 15% unable to deflate/inflate device properly
Krauss et al (1989)	Structured interview same as patient and separate	19	100	41.7	25	92% patients would repeat operation (90% partners) At 1 yr, >50% couples increased frequency of intercourse Significant adjustment to device occurred from 6–12 month follow-up 50% would have liked larger prosthesis
Fallon and Ghanen (1990)	Questionnaire completed by patient	133/252	54	80	13	25% delayed orgasm and/or ejaculation 11% believed they chose wrong prosthesis (6% of inflatable and 18% semirigid) 25% prosthesis did meet their expectations 92% were glad they had surgery 91% felt this "best solution" 11% thought prosthesis source of conflict with partner
McLaren and Barrett (1992)	Mailed questionnare and telephone interview	265/387	68.5	69.8	9.4	87% increased or no change in sexual desire (72% partners) 10% decrease in sexual desire 29% orgasm better (26% partners) 19% orgasm worse (8% partners) Only 67% with previous implants satisfied
Goldstein et al (1993)	Questionnaire completed by patient	Unknown		85	15	80% patients able to have intercourse 92% able to achieve orgasm & ejaculation 82% implant fulfilled expectations 76% improved self-confidence 87% pleased with ease of concealment 89% pleased with ease of deflation/inflation 81% satisfied with rigidity and width 88% would recommend implant to a friend

subject has been prepared by Benson and colleagues (1993). **Office injection of smooth muscle relaxants often demonstrates the degree of deformity and the extent of the erection that the patient is able to obtain. In patients with significant erectile failure associated with the disease, the most prudent treatment course may be placement of a penile prosthesis with or without incision or excision of the penile plaque.** Some experts have preferred semirigid devices, and others have preferred the inflatable three-piece devices, which I believe are preferable. After penile lengthening procedures, a synthetic patch coverage is usually necessary if the resultant tunical defect is larger than 1.5 cm.

VASCULAR SURGERY FOR ERECTILE DYSFUNCTION

Vascular surgery for impotence can be divided into **two major areas: penile revascularization and surgery for a veno-occlusive disorder.** Although this type of surgery has been reported only in the last 15 years, a number of review and technique articles exist and are recommended for further details that are not presented in these pages (Metz, 1986; Lewis, 1990a and b, 1993; Sohn et al, 1992; Hatzichristou and Goldstein, 1993; Goldstein et al, 1994; Sharlip, 1994).

Selection Criteria for Erectile Dysfunction Vascular Surgery

This area is discussed to some extent in the previous chapter by Tom Lue. **It is a rare patient with erectile dysfunction who should be offered the choice of vascular surgery. Those patients with discrete focal arterial lesions found on pudendal arteriography, particularly younger patients who have a history of trauma, who do not have**

insulin-dependent diabetes, who are not currently users of tobacco, and who do not have neurologic disease are the best candidates for penile revascularization procedures. They should not have systemic arteriosclerosis or major veno-occlusive dysfunction. These patients should have demonstrated functional arterial disease, based on findings on the second phase of the dynamic infusion cavernosometry and cavernosography (DICC) of Goldstein (a gradient of greater than 30 mm Hg between the penile occlusion pressure and the mean brachial pressure), or have poor peak systolic velocities (<25 cm/sec) in the penile arteries on color duplex Doppler sonographic studies, before considering pudendal arteriography. Patients with arterial disease or a combination of arterial and veno-occlusive disease should be offered an in-depth discussion of alternative therapeutic choices such as vacuum constriction devices and penile prostheses. Many patients with mild to moderate vascular disease will also respond to vasoactive agent injection with improved erections that are suitable for vaginal intercourse.

Criteria for recommending surgery for a veno-occlusive disorder consist of the following: (1) a patient complaint of short duration erections or tumescence only with sexual stimulation, (2) failure to obtain or maintain an erection from the use of intracavernous injection on multiple trials with different agents with sexual stimulation, (3) normal cavernous arteries on color duplex Doppler studies or second phase of DICC, (4) determination of a faulty veno-occlusive mechanism as determined by infusion pump or gravity cavernosometry, (5) location of the site of venous leakage from the corpora cavernosa on pharmacocavernosography, (6) no medical contraindication to surgery, (7) complete elimination of tobacco use, (8) selection after presentation of alternative therapeutic choices in the face of a long-term success rate of 40% to 50%. It is a rare patient who should be offered venous surgery for the treatment of erectile dysfunction.

Techniques of Vascular Surgery for Erectile Dysfunction

Penile vascular surgery is performed with the patient under general intubated or spinal anesthesia. The patient is placed in a supine position with the legs in a slightly abducted position. Some surgeons prefer a dorsal lithotomy position for venous dissection and ligation surgery, and if crural banding or ligation is planned as part of the procedure, this is also the position of choice. Some surgeons prefer the use of loupes for the early dissection in the arterial cases and for all of the venous surgery cases. A hand-held Doppler probe is an excellent accessory tool for monitoring of the dorsal artery and checking for runoff into revascularized arteries or arterialized veins. A lighted suction instrument is also useful, particularly in the infrapubic dissection of the penile veins. Placement of an indwelling penile urethral catheter is recommended, particularly for the arterial cases; it is also helpful for any venous dissection near the urethra. The choice of incision for the venous surgery is the anterior scrotal peripenile incision, first introduced by Lue (1988) (see Fig. 40–19). The choice of incision for arterial surgery is the lower abdominal midline, because both inferior epigastric artery vessel bundles can be dissected from the lower surface of the rectus muscle, if necessary. Others prefer a paramedian incision for dissecting the inferior epigastric artery complex.

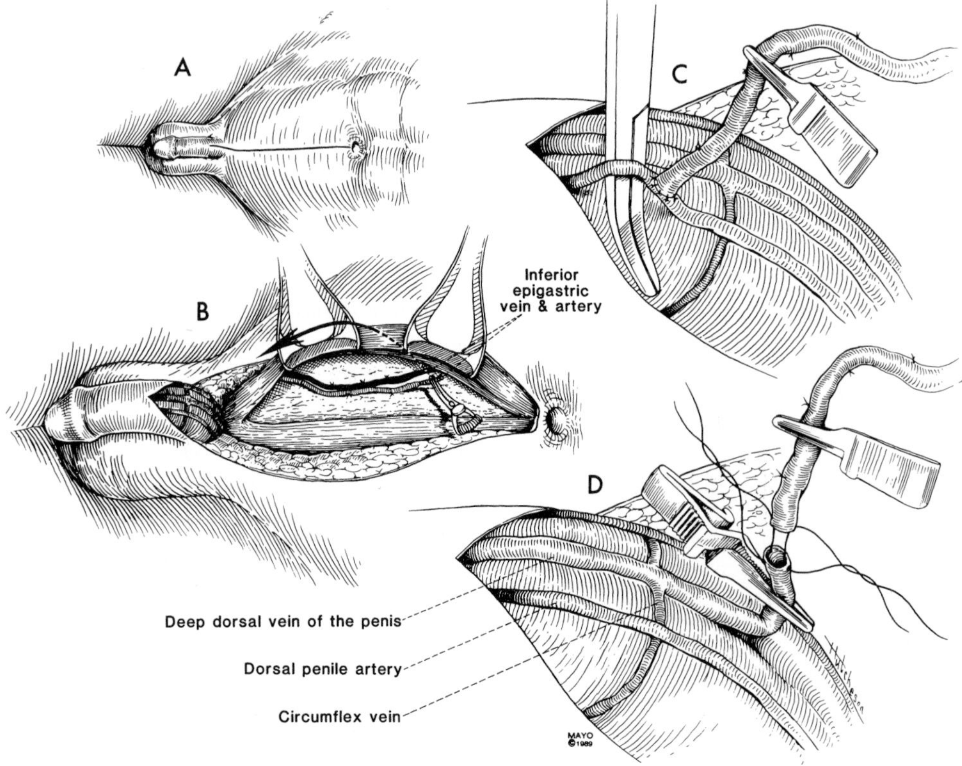

Figure 40–16. Steps in revascularization procedures of the penis using the inferior epigastric artery. *A,* Midline incision. *B,* Dissection of the inferior epigastric vessels from the lower surface of the rectus muscle. *C,* Anastomosis of the inferior epigastric artery in an end-to-side fashion to the left dorsal artery. *D,* Anastomosis of the inferior epigastric artery to the deep dorsal vein in an end-to-end configuration. Details are described in the text. (Reproduced by permission of Mayo Clinic Foundation.)

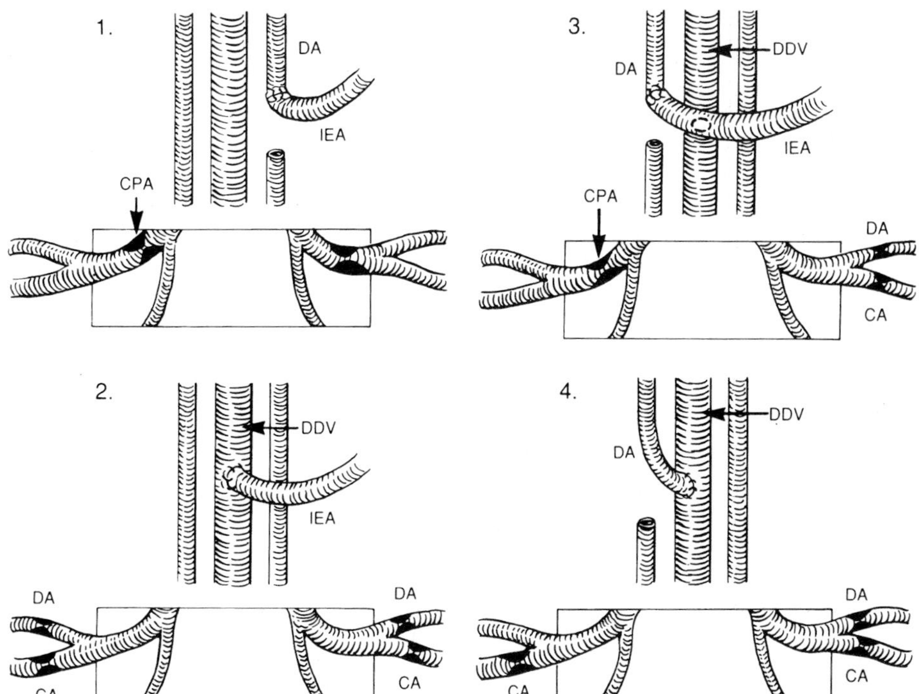

Figure 40–17. Types of arteriographic patterns and the associated types of bypass procedures. DDV, Deep dorsal vein; DA, doral artery; IEA, inferior epigastric artery; CA, cavernosa artery; CPA, common penile artery. (From Hatzichristou D, Goldstein I: Penile microvascular arterial bypass surgery. Urol Clin North Am 1993; 1:42.)

Hatzichristou and Goldstein (1993) have presented an excellent description of penile revascularization surgery stressing microvascular arterial surgery principles. Surgical technique is illustrated in Figures 40–16 to 40–18, and the general nature of this type of vascular surgery is presented in Table 40–8. Certain points of technique need to be stressed. **There is no single type of revascularization surgery that fits every case** (see Fig. 40–17). The preoperative arteriogram is necessary for selection of the preferable recipient vessel. It is preferable to connect the donor arterial vessel, usually the inferior epigastric artery (occasionally in the absence of a suitable epigastric artery, a saphenous vein connected to the femoral artery may serve as the input arterial supply) to a branch of the dorsal penile artery in an end-to-side fashion, or when able, with an end-to-end anastomosis, which allows the most efficient run-off. This is possible if the dorsal artery has demonstrated good connections to the intracavernosal deep penile artery on the preoperative arteriogram. When there is no such connection nor suitable dorsal arteries, revascularization of an isolated segment of deep dorsal vein with good communicators to the intracavernous tissue is the choice for recipient vessel. Another possibility is the use of a Y-branch of the inferior epigastric artery or two inferior epigastric arteries for anastomosis to the dorsal artery and an isolated segment of deep dorsal vein.

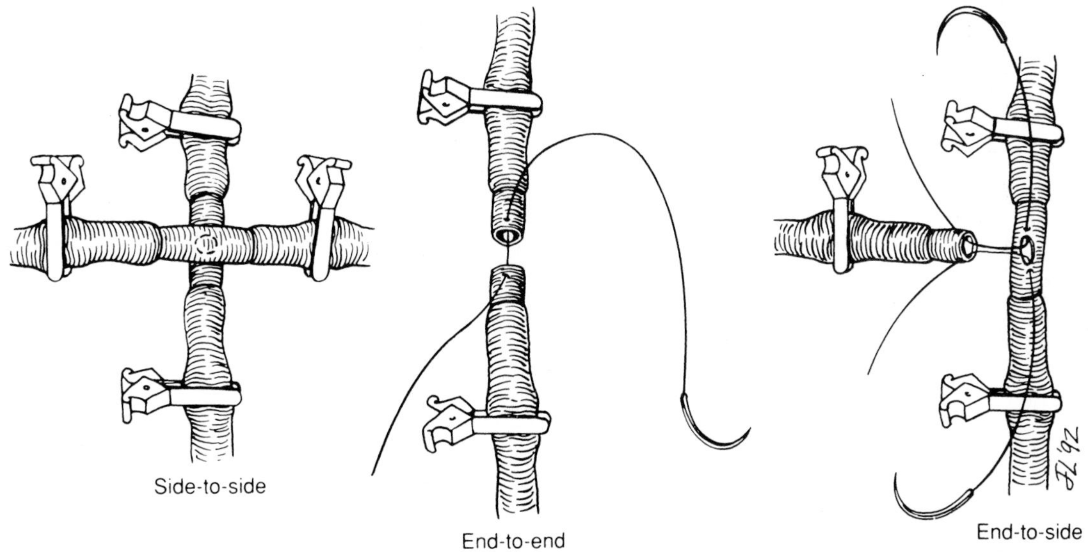

Figure 40–18. The different types of microvascular anastomoses. Notice the adventitial tissue is removed from the vessel only at the site of the anastomosis. (From Hatzichristou D, Goldstein I: Penile microvascular arterial bypass surgery. Urol Clin North Am 1993; 1:42.)

Table 40–8. CURRENT MAJOR PENILE REVASCULARIZATION PROCEDURES

- Use of inferior epigastric artery or saphenous vein bypass from femoral vein as input source
- Microvascular surgery (endothelium preserving)
- Modification of Michal procedure—distal or proximal end-to-end to dorsal artery or end-to-side to dorsal artery
- Arterialization (modification of Virag procedure) of isolated segment of deep dorsal vein
- Direct anastomosis to deep penile cavernous artery

The dissection of the epigastric artery incorporates the accompanying veins, because separation is almost impossible or would be too time consuming in order to control bleeding venous branches. Usually, branches isolated during the dissection are both artery and vein, which can be commonly ligated or clipped using small vascular clips. The inferior epigastric artery is dissected as far distally as possible, usually to the level or slightly above the level of the umbilicus. Small branches near its origin are also ligated or clipped so that once divided, the full arterial length can be used as the artery is brought to the base of the penis for microscopic anastomosis in gentle curving nontension fashion. **The recipient vessel should be prepared before the inferior epigastric artery is divided.**

Hatzichristou and Goldstein recommend preservation of the fundiform and suspensory ligament of the penis. I prefer an end-to-end anastomosis to the deep dorsal vein if this is the vessel to be used and thus take down these structures to prepare a good free vein for anastomosis. I do reanastomose the base of the penis back to the infrapubic periosteum after such vein preparation with a silk suture. When anastomosing to the deep dorsal artery in either an end-to-side or end-to-end fashion, the two ligaments can be preserved. The initial multiple branches of the deep dorsal vein near the glans are ligated with a nonpermanent suture, as well as large trunks of the deep dorsal vein that anastomose to the spongiosum laterally along the shaft of the penis. Valves in the deep dorsal vein are removed with a 2-mm LeMaitre valvulotome or a similarly sized Fogarty balloon catheter. Adventitia is removed only at the sites of anastomosis of the two vessels. **The anastomosis is accomplished microscopically using 8 to 10-0 monofilament vascular suture.** I prefer the 10-0 suture. The vessels are clamped with low-tension vascular bulldog clamps. The inferior epigastric artery is usually flushed with a dilute heparin and/or papaverine solution just prior to the anastomosis.

For **venous dissection and ligation surgery,** the entire penis can be inverted into the wound for access to all-important venous channels along the shaft of the penis using a combination of sharp and blunt dissection. See Figure

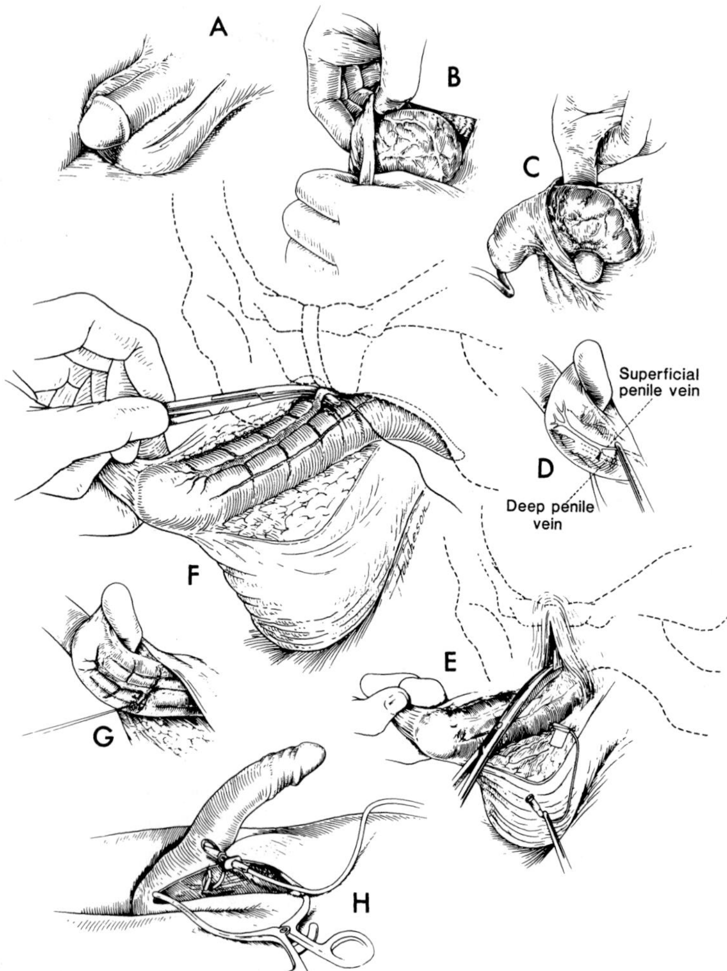

Figure 40–19. Steps in the performance of deep penile vein ligation and dissection surgery. *A,* The peri-penile anterior scrotal incision. *B* and *C,* Eversion of the penile deep tissues through the wound. *D,* Ligation of communicators identified between the superficial and deep penile venous system. *E,* Release of the suspensory ligament in the infrapubic region. *F,* Ligation of the vein on the penile shaft. Once this ligation is accomplished, the vein is dissected proximately and distally. *G,* Distal dissection of the penile vein in the mid penile shaft. Direct communicators and communicators from the circumflex vessels are ligated and exposed. *H,* An operative cavernosometry to produce an erection and show that adequate veno-occlusion has been obtained from the surgery. (Reproduced by permission of Mayo Clinic Foundation.)

Table 40–9. RESULTS OF SURGERY FOR VENO-OCCLUSIVE SEXUAL DYSFUNCTION

Study (Years of Study)	No. of Patients	Excellent	Improved	Immediate Success/Later Failure	Failures	Average Follow-up (Months)
Lewis-Tulane series (1981–1987)	49	12 (24%)	12 (24%)	8 (16%)	17 (35%)	15
Wespes et al (1982–1986)	67*	31 (46%)	16 (24%)		20 (30%)	24
Donatucci and Lue (1986–1988)	100	44 (44%)	24 (24%)		32 (32%)	(12–50)
Bondil et al (1981–1988)	60	25 (42%)†			35 (58%)	22
Lunglmayr et al (1984–1986)	29	9 (31%)†		10 (34.5%)	10 (34.5%)	to 24
Weidner et al						
(1985–1987)	51	28 (55%)		8 (16%)‡	15 (29%)‡	12
(1988–1989)	40	24 (60%)		11 (27.5%)‡	5 (12.5%)‡	12
Gilbert et al (1985–1990)	134	26 (19.4%)	47 (35.1%)		61 (45.5%)	12.9
Lewis-Mayo series						
(1987–1988)	28	7 (25%)	4 (14%)	8 (29%)	9 (32%)	48
(1988–1989)	32	9 (28%)	13 (41%)	5 (15.5%)	5 (15.5%)	24
Knoll et al (1987–1989)	41	19 (46%)	Unknown	Unknown	22 (54%)	28
Kropman et al (1987–1989)	20	6 (30%)	4 (20%)	8 (40%)	2 (10%)	15
Rossman et al (1985–1988)	16	2 (12.5%)	2 (12.5%)	10 (62.5%)	2 (12.5%)	Unknown
Claes and Baert (1987–1989)	72	30 (41.7%)	23 (31.9%)		19 (26.4%)	>12
Montague et al (1988–1990)	18	11 (61%)		6 (33%)	1 (6%)	24
Freedman et al (1986–1991)	46	11 (24%)	8 (17%)	23 (50%)	4 (9%)	31–33

*Sixty-seven patient questionnaire responses to 105 letters sent.
†Series reported as excellent or improved as a group, not in each individual category.
‡Seventeen of 39 are now able to achieve erection with pharmacologic agent injection.

40–19 for a general outline of the steps of venous dissection surgery. Communicating veins between the deep and superficial system are ligated as exposed with absorbable suture because the patient will be able to palpate permanent ligatures, and these can often be a nuisance. After the penile shaft eversion is accomplished a butterfly needle can be placed into one of the corpora cavernosa, fixing this in place with a purse-string ligature in the tunica albuginea, for introduction of indigo carmine for greater demarcation of draining cavernosal veins or intraoperative or postdissection pharmacocavernosometry.

As the penis is dissected more proximally and as the fundiform and suspensory ligaments are dissected and divided, communicating veins to the perineal side wall and the pubic region are usually isolated and divided so that exposure of the deeper venous drainage system is facilitated. The suspensory ligament must be taken down in its entirety for proper exposure to the more distal deep dorsal penile vein and the cavernosal veins, when present. Once the penis is fully mobilized, an incision in Buck's fascia directly over the deep dorsal penile vein is made in the midshaft, the vein divided between ligatures, and then distal or proximal dissection is begun, ligating communicating tributaries encountered in this dissection of the deep dorsal vein or veins. Care is taken to stay in the midline over the deep dorsal vein to avoid injury to the slightly more laterally positioned dorsal penile arteries and penile sensory nerves. Distally along the penile shaft, the dissection of the deep dorsal vein is taken to 1 to 1½ cm from the glanular sulcus where the multitrunk origins of this vein are dissected and individually ligated. Along the penile shaft, communicating circumflex veins near the corpora cavernosa and the spongiosum are identified, exposed under Buck's fascia, and ligated. Any use of electrocoagulation along the penile shaft should be performed with a bipolar unit to prevent transmission of possible coagulation to arteries or nerves of the penile shaft. The deep dorsal vein is dissected proximally to under the pubis, where it is ligated with a heavy permanent suture. It is in this area that the cavernosal veins can be found for dissection and ligation. Some expert surgeons also recommend crural plication sutures along the lateral surface of the tunical albuginea of each of the corpora cavernosa. An attempt is made after the venous dissection to reapproximate the suspensory ligament attachment of the base of the penis, using a permanent suture from the pubis to the midline tunica albuginea of the corpora in the midline sulcus, where the deep dorsal vein had been. A fenestrated tubular drain is placed in the infrapubic region and exits out a separate stab wound where it is affixed to the skin. This stays usually for 24 to 48 hours and is removed at the time of minimal drainage. The skin closure is done carefully to match the various layers of depth and equal side-to-side approximation; failure to do so will result in dense fixation of this scrotal or infrapubic skin to the penile shaft. A loose elastic dressing is applied to the penile shaft, and the catheter is usually removed the following morning. This dressing is used to avoid glanular edema. Some authors recommend perineal plication procedures or spongiosolysis, which I have described in a previous publication, but these procedures are rarely indicated (Lewis, 1993).

Complications of Vascular Surgery for Erectile Dysfunction

Penile edema is common after vascular surgery of the penis. A lightly applied elastic wrapping dressing of the penis for 24 hours after surgery greatly aids in controlling this postoperative minor complication, and any mild to moderate edema after the removal of the dressing usually resolves without sequelae 2 to 3 weeks after surgery. Superficial ecchymosis and bruising of the penile shaft and scrotum is not unusual nor debilitating; serious wound hematomas

Table 40–10. SUCCESS RATE OF ARTERIAL SURGERY FOR IMPOTENCE

Study, Year	Procedure	Patients (No.)	Result
Virag, 1982	V4-V6	36	41.6% good, 33.3% fair
Michal et al, 1986	Michals	73	60% success
Balko et al, 1986	V6	11	73% significantly improved
U. S. Society for Study of Impotence, 1988*	V-5 or modified V-5	56	46% success, 14% improved
Lizza and Zorgniotti, 1988	V-5 or modified V-5	13	77% success
Sharlip, 1988/1990	Mixed/V-5	30/7	50% success, 40% success
Virag and Bennett, 1991	V-5	100	38% good, 30% improved
Furlow et al, 1990	Modified V-5	95	78% success
Sohn, 1992	Mixed	65	54% good or improved
Bock and Lewis, 1992	Mixed	36	53% success, 28% improved

*Reported by Belker and Bennett, 1988.

can be avoided by the use of the tubular fenestrated drain postoperatively for 24 to 48 hours.

Two significant complications of penile vascular surgery are penile numbness or hypoesthesia and penile shortening due to scar entrapment, which is experienced in as many of 20% of patients. Penile sensation usually returns 12 to 18 months after surgery if no major penile sensory nerve has been significantly severed. The **penile shortening** due to severe scar entrapment **may require subsequent scar release surgery** and the use of relaxing Z-plasty incisions or scrotal flap coverage.

Mechanical disruption of the microvascular anastomosis has been reported by Hatzichritou and Goldstein (1993). Resumption of sexual activity should begin 6 weeks after this surgery. **Another complication of deep dorsal penile vein arterialization is glans hyperemia, which occurs when a communicating vein from the revascularized deep dorsal vein to the glans in the distal dissection is missed.** Surgical exploration and ligation of the arterialized communicator resolves the problem.

Results of Vascular Surgery for Erectile Dysfunction

Tables 40–9 and 40–10 list reported results of venous and arterial surgery for erectile dysfunction. **In summary, long-term success rates of 50% to 60%** are less than optimal and have led some to question the possible benefits from this type of surgery (Donatucci and Lue, 1992; Lewis, 1992, 1994; Sohn et al, 1992; Wespes and Schulman, 1993; Sharlip, 1994). Sohn's report of lack of correlation of results as reported by the patient to preoperative and postoperative objective testing in the arterial surgical treatment of erectile dysfunction would suggest that much scientific understanding is lacking for this treatment modality. **Although a crucial part of the erectile cycle is veno-occlusion, it is not agreed that veno-occlusive surgery (which generally removes veins outside of the corpora cavernosa) is an effective or even reasonable therapy.** There are three reasons for this: (1) Veno-occlusion is dependent on arterial inflow and relaxation of the sinus smooth muscle; thus, poor veno-occlusion may be a reflection of sinus smooth muscle disease for the most part, and there is no current way to diagnose this possible damage. (2) There is controversy as to the type of test and the criteria of particular tests used to diagnose veno-occlusive disorder. (3) The surgical approach to veno-occlusive disease has been variable, and comparison between different surgical reports is difficult.

SURGERY FOR PRIAPISM

Surgery for priapism is rarely indicated today. Nonischemic priapism can usually be treated nonoperatively and often certain cases of early ischemic priapism can, with vigorous penile irrigation, be converted into nonischemic

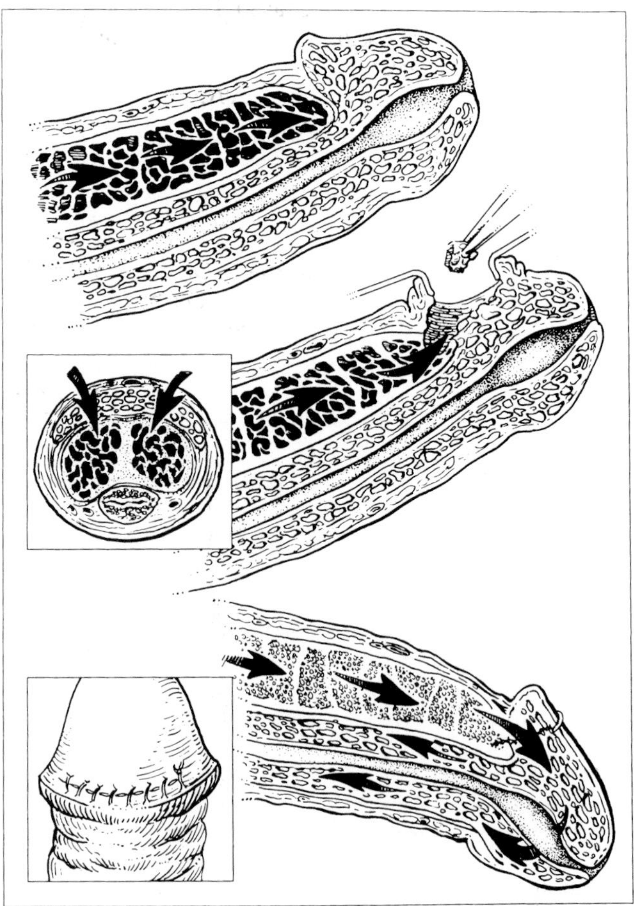

Figure 40–20. Steps in the formation of the more radical cavernosal shunt of the El-Ghoreb procedure. (From Lewis RW: How to evaluate and treat priapism. Contemporary Urology 1995; 7:33. Reproduced by permission of Contemporary Urology/Medical Economics.)

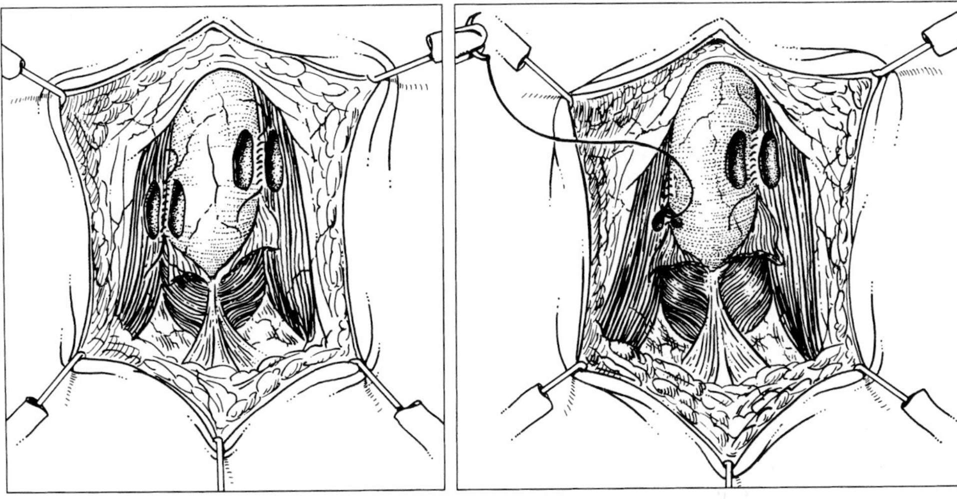

Figure 40–21. The Sacher procedure, in which bilateral cavernosum and spongiosum shunts are created. This illustration shows the staggered placement of the shunts so that they are not placed exactly opposite from each other; such placement could lead to urethral compression. (From Lewis RW: How to evaluate and treat priapism. Contemporary Urology 1995; 7:33. Reproduced by permission of Contemporary Urology/Medical Economics.)

priapism and managed with the same nonsurgical approach. Infiltrative priapism and thromboembolic priapism should have specific medical therapy. The diagnosis and management of priapism has recently been extensively reviewed (Padma-Nathan, 1993; Lewis, 1995) and is covered in Chapter 39. High-flow arterial priapism after penile trauma is established by penile arteriography and can usually be successfully treated at the time of the diagnostic study by embolization by the interventional radiologist. However, in rare cases, this is not possible, and principles of this type of surgery are outlined below.

When a shunting procedure is indicated, the use of a transglanular to corpus cavernosal scalpel or needle core biopsy technique of Ebbehoj or Winter is the first reasonable approach (Ebbehoj, 1974; Winter, 1976). The El-Ghorab procedure, illustrated in Figure 40–20, is a more aggressive open surgical modification of this type of shunting maneuver (Ercole et al, 1981). On the rare occasion that more involved surgery is needed, the best is that described by Sacher via a perineal approach, as seen in Figure 40–21 (Sacher, 1972). One caution should be stated about this approach: The anastomotic windows should be placed at different levels so that a urethral stricture can be avoided. The suture used for this procedure is 2-0 chromic catgut.

In those patients who have postarterial traumatic high-flow priapism and have fistulous flow into the cavernous tissue that the interventional radiologist has been unable to embolize, careful surgical approach to ligate the feeding arterial vessel is needed. I have performed this procedure in three individuals using intraoperative color duplex ultrasonography to help localize the site of entry into the corpus cavernosum, in order to localize the feeding vessel above the tear for ligation. Surgery was successful, and after 6 months, all had regained potency, presumably by collateral circulation because permanent suture material was used for ligation. All of the patients were young individuals who had sustained some perineal trauma.

In summary, the patient who suffers from erectile dysfunction does have several surgical therapeutic options, depending on the cause of the impotence and the general health and age of the individual. All conservative nonoperative choices should be carefully explained to the patient, and he should be encouraged to try these first. However, the young patient with a specific focal arterial lesion who is not a smoker and otherwise is generally healthy can be successfully rearterialized in about 50% to 70% of the time using careful microscopic procedures. In general, it is a rare patient who will be helped with venous dissection and ligation surgery, and the long-term success rates are between 40% and 50%. On the other hand, a penile prosthesis usually results in an acceptable solution for 70% to 80% of patients who undergo this surgery. The modern devices are mechanically reliable, and with the complicated inflatable devices, the failure rate after use for 5 to 10 years is 5%. The infection rate is 1% to 9%, and if this occurs, it usually results in total removal of the device.

REFERENCES

History of Erectile Dysfunction Surgery

Beheri GE: Surgical treatment of impotence. Plast Reconstr Surg 1966; 38:92–97.

Das S: Early history of venogenic impotence. Int J Impotence Res 1994; 4:183–189.

Ebbehoj J, Wagner G: Insufficient penile erection due to abnormal drainage of cavernous bodies. Urology 1979; 13:507–509.

Gee WF: A history of surgical treatment of impotence. Urology 1975; 5:401–405.

Kim JH, Carson CC: History of urologic prostheses for impotence. Probl Urol 1993; 7:283–288.

Lewis RW: Venous ligation surgery for venous leakage. Int J Impotence Res 1990; 2:1–19.

Lowsley OS, Reuda EA: Further experience with an operation for the cure of certain types of impotence. J Int Coll Surg 1953; 19:69–77.

Mikal V: Revascularization procedures of the cavernous bodies in vasculogenic impotence. *In* Zorgniotti A, Rossi G, eds: Proceedings of the First International Conference of Corpus Cavernosum Revascularization. Springfield, IL, Charles C Thomas, 1980, pp 239–255.

Pearman RO: Insertion of a Silastic penile prosthesis for the treatment of organic sexual impotence. J Urol 1972; 107:802–806.

Scott FB, Bradley WE, Timm GW: Management of erectile impotence—use of implantable inflatable prosthesis. Urology 1973; 2:80–82.

Small MP, Carrion HM, Gordon JA: Small Carrion penile prosthesis: A new implant for the management of impotence. Urology 1975; 5:479–486.

Virag R: Revascularization of the penis. *In* Bennett AH, ed: Management of Male Impotence. Baltimore, Williams & Wilkins, 1982, pp 219–233.

Penile Prostheses

Ball TP: Surgical repair of "SST" deformity. Urol 1980; 15:603–604.

Benson RC Jr, Knoll LD, Furlow WL: Penile prostheses and Peyronie's disease. Probl Urol 1993; 7:342–349.

Benson RC Jr, Patterson DE, Barrett DM: Long term results with the Jonas Malleable penile prosthesis. J Urol 1985; 134:899–901.

Bishop JR, Moul JW, Sihelnik SA, et al: Use of glycosylated hemoglobin to identify diabetics at high risk for penile periprosthetic infections. J Urol 1992; 147:386–388.

Carson CC: Infections in genitourinary prostheses. Urol Clin North Am 1989; 16:139–147.

Carson CC: Management of penile prosthesis infection. Probl Urol 1993; 7:368–380.

Carson CC, Robertson CN: Late hematogenous infection of penile prostheses. J Urol 1988; 139:50–52.

Dorflinger T, Bruskewitz R: AMS malleable penile prosthesis. Urology 1986; 38:480–485.

Fallon B, Ghanem H: Sexual performance and satisfaction with penile prostheses in impotence of various etiologies. Int J Impotence Res 1990; 2:35–42.

Fein RL: The G.F.S. Mark II inflatable penile prosthesis. J Urol 1992; 147:66–68.

Fishman IJ: Corporeal reconstruction procedures for complicated penile implants. Urol Clin North Am 1989; 16:73–90.

Fishman IJ: Corporeal reconstruction of penile prosthesis implantation. Probl Urol 1993; 7:350–367.

Fishman IJ, Scott FB, Light JK: Experience with inflatable penile prosthesis. Urology 1984; 23(Suppl 5):86–92.

Furlow WL, Goldwasser B: Salvage of the eroded inflatable penile prosthesis: New concept. J Urol 1987; 138:312–314.

Furlow WL, Goldwasser B, Gundian JC: Implantation of Model AMS 700 penile prosthesis: Long-term results. J Urol 1988; 139:741–742.

Gerstenberger DL, Osborne D, Furlow WL: Inflatable penile prosthesis: Followup study of patient-partner satisfaction. Urology 1979; 14:583–587.

Goldstein I, Bertero EB, Kaufman JM, et al: Early experience with the first pre-connected 3-piece inflatable penile prosthesis: The Mentor Alpha 1. J Urol 1993; 150:1814–1818.

Hackler RH: Mentor inflatable penile prosthesis: A reliable mechanical device. Urology 1986; 28:489–491.

Kabalin JM, Kessler R: Infectious complications of penile prosthesis surgery. J Urol 1988; 139:953–955.

Knoll LD, Furlow WI, Motley RC: Clinical experience implanting an inflatable penile prosthesis with controlled-expansion cylinder. Urology 1990; 36:502–504.

Krauss DJ, Lantinga LJ, Carey MP, et al: Use of the malleable penile prosthesis in the treatment of erectile dysfunction: A prospective study of postoperative adjustment. J Urol 1989; 142:988–991.

Lewis RW: Long term results of penile prosthetic implantations. Urol Clin North Am 1995; 22:847–863.

Lewis RW, McLaren R: Reoperation for penile prosthesis implantation. Probl Urol 1993; 7:381–401.

Maatman TJ, Montague DK: Intracorporal drainage after removal of infected penile prosthesis. Urol 1984; 23:184–185.

McLaren RH, Barrett DM: Patient and partner satisfaction with the AMS 700 penile prosthesis. J Urol 1992; 147:62–65.

Merrill DC: Clinical experience with the Mentor inflatable penile prostheses in 301 patients. J Urol 1988; 140:1424–1427.

Montague DK: Penile prosthesis corporotomy closure: A new technique. J Urol 1993; 150:924–925.

Montague DK, Lakin MM: Inflatable penile prostheses: The AMS experience. Probl Urol 1993; 7:328–333.

Mulcahy JJ: A technique of maintaining penile prosthesis position to prevent proximal migration. J Urol 1987; 137:294–296.

Mulcahy JJ: Implantation of hydraulic penile prostheses. Urol Clinics North Am 1993; 1:71–92.

Pedersen B, Tiefer L, Ruiz M, Melman A: Evaluation of patients and partners 1 to 4 years after penile prosthesis surgery. J Urol 1988; 139:956–958.

Quesada ET, Light JK: The AMS 700 inflatable penile prosthesis: Long-term experience with the controlled expansion cylinder. J Urol 1993; 149:46–48.

Radomski SB, Herschorn S: Risk factors associated with penile prosthesis infection. J Urol 1992; 147:383–385.

Rossier AB, Fam BA: Indicators and results of semirigid penile prosthesis in spinal cord injury patients: Long term follow-up. J Urol 1984; 131:59–61.

Small MP: Penile prostheses. *In* Glenn J, ed: Urologic Surgery, 4th ed. Philadelphia, J. B. Lippincott, 1991, pp 877–899.

Steinkohl WB, Leach GE: Mechanical complications associated with Mentor inflatable penile prosthesis. Urology 1991; 38:32–34.

Wilson SK, Delk JR: Inflatable penile implant infection: Predisposing factors and treatment suggestions. J Urol 1995; 153:659–661.

Wilson SK, Wahman GE, Lange JL: Eleven years of experience with inflatable penile prostheses. J Urol 1988; 139:951–952.

Woodworth BE, Carson CC, Webster GD: Inflatable penile prosthesis: Effect of device modification on functional longevity. Urology 1991; 38:533–536.

Vascular Surgery for Erectile Dysfunction

Balko A, Malhotra CM, Winize JP, et al: Deep penile vein arterialization for arterial and venous impotence. Arch Surg 1986; 121:774–777.

Barada JH, Bennett AH: Penile revascularization: Where do we stand? Int J Impotence Res 1990; 2:79–86.

Belker AM, Bennett AH: Applications of microsurgery in urology. Surg Clin North Am 1988; 68:1177–1178.

Bock D, Lewis RW: Treatment of vasculogenic impotence: Penile revascularization. Int J Impotence Res 1992; 4:223–230.

Bondil P, Schauvliege T, Nguyen Qui JL: Venocavernous leakage: Considerations in 60 operated cases. *In* Proceedings of Sixth Biennial Corpora Cavernosum Revascularization and Third Biennial World Meeting on Impotence. Boston, International Society of Impotence Research (ISIR), 1988, p 189.

Claes H, Baert L: Cavernosometry and penile vein resection in corporeal incompetence: An evaluation of short-term and long-term results. J Impotence Res 1991; 3:129.

Donatucci CF, Lue TF: Venous surgery: Are we kidding ourselves? *In* Lue TF, ed: World Book of Impotence. London, Smith-Gordon and Company, 1992, pp 221–227.

Freedman AL, Neto FC, Rajfer J: Long-term results of penile vein ligation for impotence from venous leakage. J Urol 1993; 149:1301–1303.

Furlow WL, Fisher J, Knoll LD, Benson Jr RC: Current status of penile revascularization with deep dorsal vein arterialization: Experience with 95 patients. Int J Impotence Res 1990; 2(Suppl 2):348–349.

Gilbert P, Sparwasser C, Beckert R, et al: Venous surgery in erectile dysfunction. The role of dorsal penile-vein ligators and spongiosolysis for impotence. Urol Int 1992; 49:40–47.

Goldstein I, Hatzichristou DG, Pescatori EG: Pelvic, perineal, and penile trauma-associated arteriogenic impotence: Pathophysiologic mechanisms and the role of microvascular arterial bypass surgery. *In* Bennett AH, ed: Impotence—Diagnosis and Management of Erectile Dysfunction. Philadelphia, W. B. Saunders Company, 1994, pp 213–228.

Hatzichristou D, Goldstein I: Penile microvascular and arterial bypass surgery. Urol Clin North Am 1993; 1:39–60.

Knoll LD, Furlow WL, Benson RC: Penile venous ligation surgery for the management of cavernosal venous leakage. Urol Int 1992; 49:33–39.

Kropman RF, Nijeholt AABL, Giespers AGM, Swarten J: Results of deep penile vein resection in impotence caused by venous leakage. Int J Impotence Res 1990; 2:29–34.

Lewis RW: Venous surgery for impotence. Urol Clin North Am 1988; 15:115–121.

Lewis RW: Vascular surgery in the management of erectile dysfunction. *In* Rous SN, ed: A Urology Annual. East Norwalk, CT, Appleton and Lange, 1990a, pp 1–25.

Lewis RW: Venous ligation surgery for venous leakage. Int J Impotence Res 1990b; 2:1–19.

Lewis RW: Arteriovenous surgeries: Do they make any sense? *In* Lue TF, ed: World Book of Impotence. London, Smith-Gordon and Company, 1992, pp 199–220.

Lewis RW: Venous surgery in the patient with erectile dysfunction. Urol Clin North Am 1993; 1:21–38.

Lewis RW: Venogenic impotence: Is there a future? Curr Opin Urol 1994; 6:340–342.

Lizza E, Zorgniotti A: Penile revascularization for impotence: Comparison of the V-S and the Furlow operations. J Urol 1988; 139:298A (Abstract 544).

Lue TF: Treatment of venogenic impotence. *In* Tanagho EA, Lue TF, McClure RD, eds: Contemporary Management of Impotence and Infertility. Baltimore, Williams & Wilkins, 1988, pp 175–177.

Lunglmayr G, Nachtigall M, Gindl K: Long-term results of deep dorsal penile vein transection in venous impotence. Eur Urol 1988; 15:209–212.

Metz P: Arteriogenic erectile impotence. Dan Med Bull 1986; 33:134–150.

Michal V, Krysl I, Klika T, Fará P: Revascularization of the cavernous bodies. Presented at Biennial Meeting of the International Society for Impotence Research, Prague, June 1986.

Montague DK, Angermeier KW, Lakin M, Ignaut CA: Penile venous ligation in 18 patients with 1 to 3 years of follow-up. J Urol 1993; 149:306–307.

Rossman B, Mieza M, Melman A: Penile vein ligation for corporeal incompetence: An evaluation of short-term and long-term results. J Urol 1990; 144:679–682.

Sharlip ID: Vasculogenic impotence secondary to atherosclerosis/dysplasia. *In* Bennett AH, ed: Impotence—Diagnosis and Management of Erectile Dysfunction. Philadelphia, W. B. Saunders Company, 1994, pp 205–212.

Sharlip ID: The role of vascular surgery in arteriographic and combined arteriographic and venous impotence. Semin Urol 1990: 8:129–137.

Sohn MH, Sikora RR, Bohndorf KK, et al: Objective follow-up after penile revascularization. Int J Impotence Res 1992; 4:73–84.

Virag R: Revascularization of the penis. *In* Bennett AH, ed: Management of male impotence. Baltimore, Williams & Wilkins, 1982:219–233.

Virag R, Bennett AH: Arterial and venous surgery for vasculogenic impotence: A combined French and American experience. Arch Ital Urol Nefrol Androl 1991: 63:95–100.

Weidner W, Weiske WH, Rudnick J, et al: Venous surgery in veno-occlusive dysfunction: Long-time results after deep dorsal vein resection. Urol Int 1992: 49:24–28.

Wespes E, Delcour L, Prejzerowixc L, et al: Long-term follow-up of operations for venous leakage. *In* Proceedings of Sixth Biennial International Symposium for Corpora Cavernosum Revascularization and Third Biennial World Meeting on Impotence. Boston, International Society of Impotence Research (ISIR), 1988, p 193.

Wespes E, Schulman C: Venous impotence: Pathophysiology, diagnosis and treatment. J Urol 1993; 149:1238–1245.

Surgery for Priapism

Ebbehoj J: A new operation for priapism. Scand J Plast Reconstr Surg. 1974; 8:241–242.

Ercole CJ, Pontes JE, Pierce JM Jr: Changing surgical concepts in the treatment for priapism. J Urol 1981; 125:210–211.

Lewis RW: How to evaluate and treat priapism. Contemp Urol 1995; 7:29–42.

Padma-Nathan H: Surgical management of priapism. Urol Clin North Am 1993; 1:109–115.

Sacher EC, Sayegh E, Frensilli F, et al: Cavernospongiosum shunt in the treatment of priapism. J Urol 1972; 108:97–100.

Winter CC: Cure of idiopathic priapism: New procedure for creating fistula between glans penis and corpora cavernosa. Urol 1976; 8:389–391.

VII
REPRODUCTIVE FUNCTION AND DYSFUNCTION

41
PHYSIOLOGY OF HYPOTHALAMIC-PITUITARY FUNCTION

Ronald S. Swerdloff, M.D.
Christina Wang, M.D.

THE HYPOTHALAMIC-PITUITARY-GONADAL AXIS

The reproductive hormonal axis in men consists of five main components: (1) the extrahypothalamic central nervous system, (2) the hypothalamus, (3) the pituitary gland, (4) the testis, and (5) the gonadal steroid-sensitive end organs (Fig. 41–1). The components of this system function in a closely regulated manner to produce the concentrations of circulating gonadal steroids required for normal male sexual development and maintenance of sexual behavior. The reproductive axis also regulates the maturation of sperm necessary for normal fertility.

The hypothalamus is the site of production of the peptide hormone gonadotropin-releasing hormone (GnRH), which is transported to the pituitary gland by a short portal venous system connecting the two areas. **GnRH stimulates the synthesis and release of two gonadotropic hormones: luteinizing hormone (LH) and follicle-stimulating hormone (FSH).** These two hormones, named after their function in females but produced in both sexes, are secreted into the general circulation and transported to the testis. In the testis, they stimulate gonadal steroid secretion and are important in the initiation and maintenance of spermatogenesis. **The secreted testicular androgens testosterone and dihydrotestosterone (DHT) act on numerous end organs to cause development of male secondary sexual characteristics and to control (or inhibit) the secretion of gonadotropins.** Nonsteroid secretory products of the testis, such as inhibin, activin, and follistatin, may also have regulatory effects on gonadotropins. In addition to inhibin, the testes produce a large number of proteins and growth factors that may have local paracrine or autocrine effects on the testes. These Sertoli cell products may serve as the mediators of interaction between germ cells, Leydig cells, peritubular myoid cells, and Sertoli cells of the testis (see the section on the testis).

The pituitary also secretes the lactotropic hormone prolactin (PRL). The physiologic inhibitor of PRL release is the hypothalamic neurotransmitter dopamine. The hypothalamic peptides thyrotropin-releasing hormone and vasoactive intestinal peptide stimulate the release of PRL from the pituitary and may be the putative PRL-releasing hormones in men. PRL affects testicular function in men by inhibiting GnRH release from the hypothalamus and gonadotropin secretion from the pituitary (Fig. 41–2). Additional inhibitory effects of PRL on the gonadotroph cells of the pituitary and Leydig cells and the testes may exist, although they are of secondary importance.

An understanding of the reproductive axis is critical for the assessment of hypogonadism, infertility, gynecomastia, abnormal sex organ development (pseudohermaphroditism), and delayed and precocious puberty, and it is important in the assessment and management of patients with benign hypertrophy and carcinoma of the prostate. The function and control of each of the components of the reproductive axis are considered in detail in this chapter.

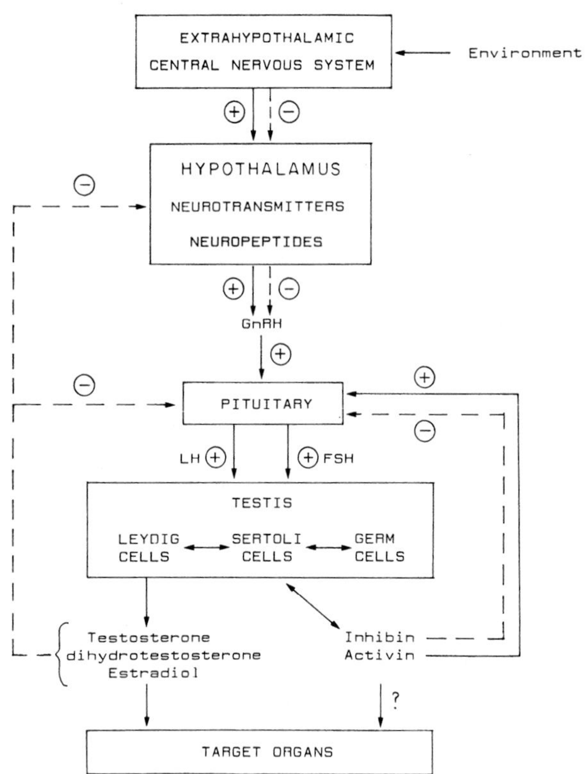

Figure 41–1. Diagram of the hypothalamic-pituitary-testicular axis. LH, luteinizing hormone; FSH, follicle-stimulating hormone.

The Extrahypothalamic Central Nervous System

There is ample evidence in experimental animals that the extrahypothalamic brain, such as the amygdala, the hippocampus, and mesencephalon tissue, has both augmentary and inhibitory influences on reproductive function (Sawyer, 1972). The amygdala, a portion of the limbic system, sends signals that affect neuroendocrine function of both the anterior hypothalamic area and the ventromedial hypothalamus. The hippocampus, another portion of the limbic system, also sends projections to the ventromedial hypothalamus but through a different pathway. The midbrain connections to many areas of the hypothalamus, including the preoptic, anterior, arcuate, and medial basal hypothalamus, have been long established and include neurons containing the neurotransmitters norepinephrine and serotonin (Fig. 41–3). Although there is considerable controversy concerning the roles that the amygdala and hippocampus play in influencing gonadotropin secretion (Ellendorff and Parvizi, 1980), it is clear that they are involved in conveying information from sensory systems to the hypothalamus. The sensory systems of olfaction and vision are known to have important influences on reproductive function in lower animals (Bronson, 1968; Michael, 1975; Reppert and Klein, 1980), but not all of these effects have been demonstrated in humans.

Evidence that higher cortical function may influence reproductive function in humans includes the frequent occurrence of menstrual abnormalities in emotionally stressed women and the demonstration of depressed serum testosterone levels in mentally stressed (Kreutz et al, 1972) and severely ill men (Handelsman, 1994).

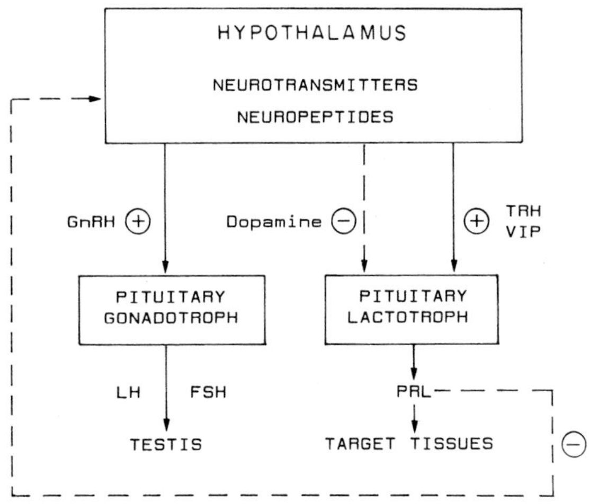

Figure 41–2. Relationship of prolactin to the hypothalamic-pituitary-testicular axis. VIP, vasoactive intestinal peptide; TRH, thyrotropin-releasing hormone; GnRH, gonadotropin-releasing hormone.

The Pineal Gland and Melatonin

In rats, the diurnal rhythm of gonadotropins appears to be related to the light-dark cycle and the effects seem to be mediated through a visual-pineal pathway, influencing melatonin production. Data to support this concept include the identification of the neural pathway by which light-induced neural signals pass through the suprachiasmatic nucleus in the hypothalamus and extend to the pineal gland through noradrenergic pathways from the superior cervical ganglia (Moore, 1973). These noradrenergic signals stimulate the synthesis and activity of enzymes required for melatonin synthesis (Klein and Moore, 1979); melatonin, in turn, modulates gonadotropin secretion. Thus, light inhibits noradren-

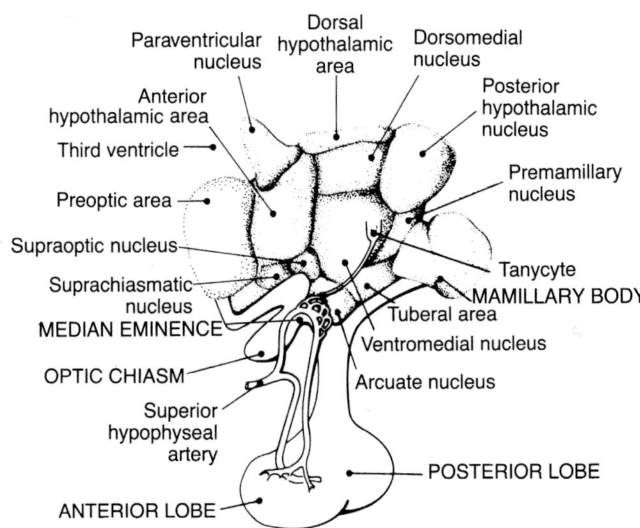

Figure 41–3. Nuclear organization of the hypothalamus. (Modified from Moore RY: Neuroendocrine mechanisms: Cells and systems. *In* Yen SSC, Jaffe RB, eds: Reproductive Endocrinology, 2nd ed. Philadelphia, W. B. Saunders Company, 1986, pp 3–31.)

ergic activity and lowers melatonin levels during the day; in the absence of light exposure, melatonin increases at night (Wilkinson et al, 1977). Levels of melatonin in the blood and urine respond rapidly to changes in photic stimulation in mammals, including nonhuman primates, producing a circadian rhythm. The role of melatonin is especially important in mammals exhibiting seasonal changes in reproduction (Reiter, 1980). Data in the human are less clear. However, the circadian rhythm in humans, unlike that in other mammals, is not abolished by constant light nor does constant exposure to light at night cause a marked decrease in melatonin levels. Melatonin exhibits a circadian pattern in the human, with low daytime and high nighttime levels (Attanasio et al, 1985), and has been suggested to have potential functions in sexual maturation, circadian rhythmicity, and so on (Vaughan, 1984; Wurtman and Waldhauser, 1986). Circumstantial evidence linking visual stimuli and the reproductive system includes the observations of Zacharias and Wurtman (1964), who demonstrated that menarche occurs earlier in blind girls. Melatonin has been implicated in the prepubertal suppression of gonadotropin secretion. This is supported by the negative correlation between melatonin and gonadotropin levels in children (Waldhauser et al, 1984), increased melatonin levels in patients with delayed puberty (Cohen et al, 1982), and decreased levels with precocious puberty (Attanasio et al, 1983). However, these findings were not confirmed in prepubertal primates, in which an increase in gonadotropins was not demonstrated after pinealectomy (Plant and Zorub, 1986).

The Hypothalamus

The hypothalamus is the integrating center of the reproductive hormonal axis. It is at this level that both neural messages from the central nervous system and at least part of the humoral messages from the testis act to modulate the secretion of GnRH, which is released into the hypophyseal-portal vessels that connect the median eminence with the adenohypophysis. Anatomically, the hypothalamus (see Fig. 41–3) is bounded anteriorly by the optic chiasm, posteriorly by the mamillary bodies, laterally by the sulci formed with the temporal lobes, and superiorly by the thalamus. The most inferior portion of the hypothalamus is the medial eminence, from which descends the pituitary stalk. The hypothalamus contains a large number of nuclei that are responsible for homeostatic control of many endocrine and nonendocrine systems. The medial basal hypothalamus is particularly involved in control of gonadotropin secretion.

Neurotransmitter Regulation of GnRH Secretion

The role of neurotransmitter regulation of GnRH synthesis and release by the hypothalamus is well established. The detailed modulations of these processes are complex and subject to large species differences. In monkey and human brains, the GnRH nerve cells are localized in the medial basal hypothalamus and the neurons project both to the median eminence and on other neurosecretory neuronal elements (Halasz et al, 1989). These neurons are influenced by input from other hypothalamic structures and extrahypothalamic pathways and, in particular, are modulated by gonadal steroids. Immunocytochemical studies indicate catecholaminergic, serotoninergic, gamma-aminobutyric acid (GABA)–ergic, opioid peptidergic, immunoreactive substance P, and corticotropin-releasing hormone axons synapse on GnRH neurons. Other putative regulators, such as the excitatory amino acids (aspartate and glutamate), vasoactive intestinal peptide, oxytocin, cholecystokinin, angiotensin 11, and neuropeptide Y, may also be effectors of GnRH release (Fig. 41–4). The effects of excitatory amino on GnRH release may be mediated in part through nitric oxide release. Several peptides provided in the paraventricular and arcuate nuclei (e.g., corticotropin-releasing hormone, oxytocin, beta-endorphin) are inhibitory to release of GnRH, as are substance P, neuropeptide K, and gamma, alpha, and beta interleukin. It appears likely that the primary stimulation of the GnRH pulse generator is norepinephrine (Barraclough and Wise, 1982; Kalra and Kalra, 1983; Nowak and Swerdloff, 1985; Gitler and Barraclough, 1987). Dopamine stimulates in vitro GnRH release from human hypothalamus (Jarjour et al, 1986; Rasmussen, 1986), but in vivo studies showed that dopamine administration is predominantly inhibitory in the human (Sawyer, 1975; Leblanc et al, 1976; Lachelin et al, 1977; Kalra, 1983). Some of the inhibition may be mediated through reduced PRL secretion (Yen, 1986).

Opioid peptides are consistently inhibitory to GnRH secretion. Male opiate addicts have low LH and testosterone levels and are sometimes sexually impotent (Wang et al, 1978). Administration of naloxone, a specific opiate receptor

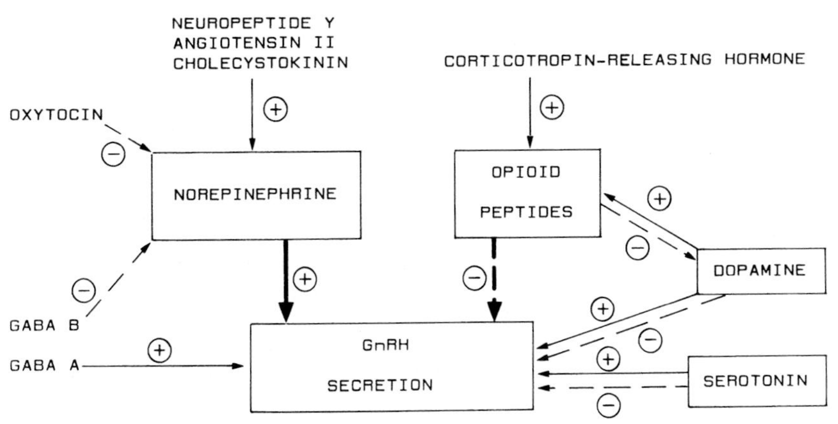

Figure 41–4. Schematic diagram of the major components of the neurotransmitter regulation of gonadotropin-releasing hormone (GnRH) secretion.

antagonist, elicits a rise in LH levels and an increase in frequency and amplitude of pulsatile LH secretion in both men and women (Delitala et al, 1981; Ropert et al, 1981). Subsequent administration of beta-endorphin, an endogenous opiate, promptly suppresses the elevated, circulating LH levels (Reid et al, 1981). In addition, dopaminergic and opioid peptidergic activity may interact in the regulation of GnRH secretion (Rasmussen, 1986). Dopamine stimulates in vitro release of beta-endorphin from the human hypothalamus, and beta-endorphin inhibits hypothalamic dopaminergic activity.

Serotoninergic influence may be stimulatory or inhibitory on GnRH release, depending on the endocrine milieu (Weiner and Ganong, 1978). GABA may stimulate GnRH secretion through GABA-A type receptors directly but can interact with norepinephrinergic or opioid peptidergic terminals through GABA-B type receptors to inhibit GnRH secretion. Other neurotransmitters, such as neuropeptide Y (stimulatory) or oxytocin (inhibitory), may influence GnRH secretion via the norepinephrinergic system (Masotto et al, 1989).

It is well recognized that stress can produce gonadal dysfunction of varying duration. Corticotropin-releasing hormone has been implicated in stress-mediated decrease in gonadotropin secretion. It is most likely that the suppressive effect of corticotropin-releasing hormone on GnRH release and the consequent pulsatile LH secretion are mediated primarily by endogenous opioid peptides, independent of the effect of corticotropin-releasing hormone on glucocorticoid levels (Gindoff and Ferin, 1987).

Gonadotropin-Releasing Hormone

A single hypothalamic decapeptide GnRH (Schally et al, 1971) has stimulatory effects on the pituitary gland that result in enhanced synthesis and release of both gonadotropic hormones LH and FSH.

Although GnRH has been identified in many areas of the central nervous system, it is most concentrated in the medial basal region of the hypothalamus, extending caudally and ventrally from the suprachiasmatic region to the arcuate nucleus and median eminence. GnRH is synthesized in the neurosecretory neurons and is transported by axoplasmic flow to the axon terminals in the median eminence (McCann and Moss, 1975).

GnRH is released into the portal circulation in pulses, occurring at a frequency averaging one pulse every 70 to 90 minutes (Carmel et al, 1976; Knobil, 1980). GnRH has a very short half-life in the blood (approximately 2 to 5 minutes). The pituitary gland is, therefore, exposed to high levels of GnRH in hypophyseal-portal blood for brief periods of time. This pulsatile pattern of GnRH release appears to be essential for stimulatory effects on LH and FSH release (Belchetz et al, 1978; Wildt et al, 1981), whereas constant exposure of the gonadotropins to GnRH results in paradoxical inhibitory effects on LH and FSH release (Belchetz et al, 1978). The latter observation has been exploited by the development of long-acting GnRH analogues that suppress LH and testosterone secretion (Labrie et al, 1978; Swerdloff et al, 1983) for use as a medical treatment of metastatic prostate cancer (Tolis et al, 1982). More recently, GnRH antagonists have been developed for the same purpose (Vickery, 1986).

Variations in the pulse frequency of GnRH release may be important in determining the relative ratio of LH and FSH secreted into the peripheral circulation. Data now accumulating indicate that shortening the pulse frequency of GnRH release increases the LH to FSH ratio; lengthening the interval between GnRH pulses decreases the ratio of LH to FSH (Wildt et al, 1981). Neurotransmitters, pituitary gonadotropins, and gonadal steroids may all modulate the pulse frequency and amplitude of GnRH secretion.

Although systems have been developed to assay GnRH in body fluids, attempts to measure this substance in the peripheral blood of animals or humans have been fraught with problems. Bioassays using large amounts of peripheral blood have been performed (Malacara et al, 1972), but these do not lend themselves well to dynamic testing; the radioimmunoassays currently available appear to be of borderline sensitivity and are adversely affected by nonspecific substances in the serum or plasma of humans (Keye et al, 1973; Arimura et al, 1974; Ben-Jonathan et al, 1974; Nett et al, 1974). Clinically useful measurements of GnRH in systemic blood are not available at the present time.

GnRH has been synthesized and is available for administration in research and diagnostic studies in both experimental animals and humans. When administered intravenously, it acts rapidly, resulting in prompt release of LH and, to a much lesser extent, of FSH into the blood stream (Fig. 41–5) (Wollesen et al, 1976). The response of the pituitary to GnRH is influenced by the presence of gonadal steroids (see later discussion of feedback). Testosterone deficiency in patients with testicular disorders results in an augmented response (Marshall, 1975).

Because administered GnRH should have a direct effect on the pituitary gland, it was hoped that GnRH testing would distinguish patients with hypogonadotropic hypogonadism of pituitary origin from those with hypothalamic disease. It was reasoned that those with pituitary disease would not respond to GnRH, whereas those with hypothalamic disorders would secrete LH and FSH normally after administration of GnRH. Unfortunately, a single pulse dose of GnRH is inadequate to distinguish between these two varieties of hypogonadotropic hypogonadism reliably (Marshall et al, 1972). One probable reason for the decreased pituitary response to GnRH in some patients with hypothalamic disorders causing hypogonadotropic hypogonadism is that the

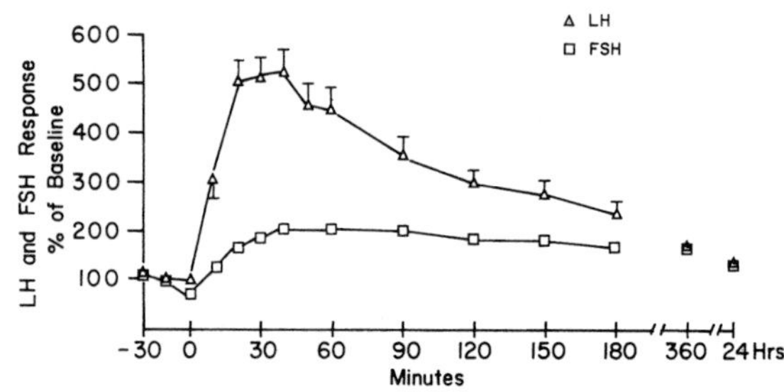

Figure 41–5. Serum luteinizing hormone (LH) and follicle-stimulating hormone (FSH) response to a 300-μg bolus dose of gonadotropin-releasing hormone (GnRH) in normal men. A peak response of LH is seen at 20 to 40 minutes after injection. (Modified from Wollesen F, et al: Metabolism, 1976; 25:1275.)

pituitary gland is chronically understimulated and has developed neither the stored reserves nor the biosynthetic machinery to respond normally to a single bolus dose of the hypothalamic hormone. This concept has been supported by evidence that repeated GnRH administration to patients with hypothalamic GnRH deficiency results in a greater response to each individual bolus dose of GnRH (Besser and Mortimer, 1974; Yoshimoto et al, 1975). This approach with repeated pulsatile administration of GnRH has been used with success in the induction of puberty, maintenance of secondary sex characteristics, and initiation of fertility in patients with hypothalamic GnRH deficiency (Crowley et al, 1985).

The Pituitary

Secretion and Measurements of Gonadotropins (Luteinizing Hormone and Follicle-Stimulating Hormone)

The bulk of immunocytologic evidence indicates that a single cell type secretes both LH and FSH (Bhasin and Swerdloff, 1995). Some gonadotrophins, however, may stain only for FSH or LH, and it is not clear if these monohormonal cells represent separate cell types or similar cell types in different secretory phases. LH and FSH are glycopeptides consisting of two peptide chains (alpha and beta) (Papkoff et al, 1973; Ward et al, 1973; Reichert and Ward, 1974; Shome and Parlow, 1974). LH and FSH share a common alpha peptide chain (alpha chain) with thyroid-stimulating hormone (TSH) and human chorionic gonadotropin (hCG), and differ from each other by the presence of a specific beta chain, the latter providing specificity of biologic action (Pierce, 1971). The genes for both subunits have been cloned for a number of species (for a review of this topic, see Bhasin and Swerdloff, 1995). Individual subunits are not biologically active; formation of the heterodimer is essential for biologic activity. The subunits are linked internally by disulfide bonds. The location of the cystines helps confer the three-dimensional structure of the glycoprotein by determining folding (Pierce and Parsons, 1981; Gharib et al, 1990). The role of the carbohydrate side chains was reviewed by Bhasin and Swerdloff in 1995. The function of the carbohydrate portions of the molecules has been investigated. One important role of glycosylation is protection from biologic degradation (Van Hall et al, 1971). There is evidence suggesting that alteration of glycosylation of these hormones leads to changes in biologic activity (Dahl et al, 1988).

LH and FSH are synthesized in the pituitary gland, released into the systemic blood circulation, and carried to the gonad, where they exert their effects. Both hormones are usually measured in the blood by immunoassay techniques. These techniques have replaced older bioassay methods (e.g., mouse uterine weight bioassay for total urinary gonadotropin) (Swerdloff and Odell, 1968), which were more cumbersome and often less specific in their ability to separate LH, FSH, and TSH. Until recently, the LH radioimmunoassay that was generally available did not distinguish between LH and hCG. Although the latter substance is found only in pregnant women (normal and abnormal), a closely related substance is usually found in high concentrations in the blood of subjects with choriocarcinoma of the testis and may also be produced by a large number of other neoplasms (Odell, 1974). Neoplastic production of gonadotropin was best assessed by a beta hCG assay, which does not detect the normal LH levels in men. In the past few years, commercial two-site–directed immunoradiometric or non-isotope methods (e.g., immunofluorometric or immunochemiluminescent) have been available. These assays have a high degree of specificity and much greater sensitivity (Hammila, 1984; Jaakkola, 1990). Under certain circumstances, the biologic activity of LH or FSH may differ from its immunologic measurement. In general, the immunofluorometric assay correlates well with biologic activity; however, in vitro bioassays (stimulation of testosterone release from Leydig cells for LH and stimulation of aromatase activity from granulosa cells for FSH) have also been developed (Dufau et al, 1974; Wang, 1988). Bioassays for LH and FSH are usually reserved for special research problems. Free alpha subunit of the glycopeptides can be measured in the serum (Whitcomb, 1990). Alpha-subunit levels may be elevated in patients with glycopeptide-secreting pituitary adenomas (Snyder, 1985).

Because the metabolic clearance rate of LH is considerably greater than that of FSH, there is a more rapid disappearance of the former hormone from the circulation. **Both hormones are secreted in an episodic fashion by the pituitary gland, but the longer survival time of FSH in the circulation is reflected by a more constant serum level of that hormone than of the more rapidly metabolized LH (Kohler et al, 1968; Coble et al, 1969; Marshall et al, 1973).** The episodic secretion of LH and FSH results in considerable short-term variation in the serum concentrations of the two hormones. The peak-and-trough pattern of blood levels of gonadotropins is of practical clinical importance in that single measurements of circulating LH may be as much as 50% above or below mean integrated hormone concentrations (Fig. 41–6) (Santen and Bardin, 1973). The amplitude of the swings in serum values produced by episodic secretion of gonadotropins is least in prepubertal children and greatest in hypogonadal patients with testicular failure. **Episodic secretion of LH and FSH begins to appear before puberty, at which time it is related to sleep, but the greatest sleep-related changes in LH pulse occur after the onset of puberty (Boyar et al, 1972; Wu et al, 1990).** As sexual maturation progresses, the periodic secretion of LH becomes generalized throughout the sleep-wake cycle and specific sleep-related elevations become less apparent. Other than these pubertal sleep-related elevations, diurnal variations of LH and FSH do not appear to be significant in the evaluation of adult humans.

Interrelationship Between Prolactin and Gonadotropins

Hyperprolactinemia is associated with disturbed reproductive functions, as reflected by lowered serum testosterone levels and symptoms of hypogonadism (Carter et al, 1978). The mechanisms by which hyperprolactinemia induces testosterone deficiency are complex, but serum LH levels are suppressed or inappropriately low (relative to serum testosterone) in most cases, indicating that the hypothalamic-pituitary axis fails to respond to reduced testicular testosterone production. It appears that PRL may inhibit

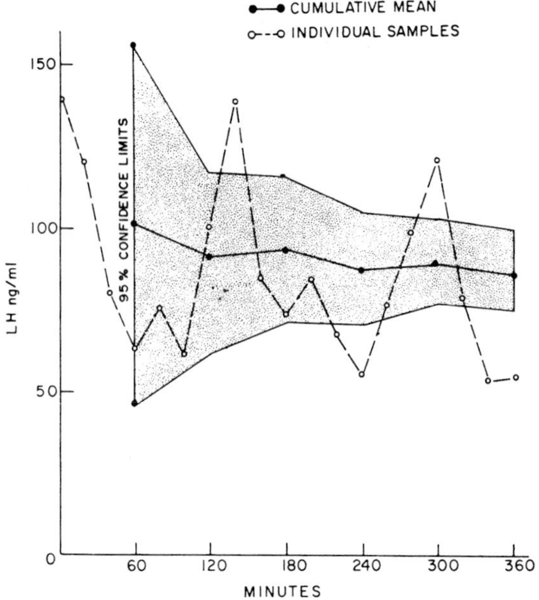

Figure 41–6. The solid line and shaded area represent the cumulative mean lutenizing hormone (LH) level and the 95% confidence limits of that mean at hourly intervals for 6 hours in a single patient. For comparison, the dotted lines and open circles represent the actual estimates of serum LH in samples obtained at 20-minute intervals. (From Santen RJ, Bardin CW: J Clin Invest, 1973; 52:2617. By copyright permission of the American Society for Clinical Investigation.)

GnRH secretion either directly or through modulation of the tuberoinfundibular dopaminergic pathway. The pituitary responds normally to GnRH administration, and the pulse frequency of LH secretion is impaired in hyperprolactinemic patients. Prompt and dramatic improvement in sexual function occurs in many hyperprolactinemic men treated with bromocriptine (dopamine agonist with PRL-lowering activity) (Carter et al, 1978; Spark et al, 1980; Thorner et al, 1980). There is evidence thay suggests that hyperprolactinemia may impair sexual function in men both by its direct effect on the central nervous system and by inhibition of androgen secretion. The direct central nervous system effect is supported by clinical data demonstrating that androgen replacement therapy of hyperprolactinemic hypoandrogenized men did not return libido to normal as long as PRL levels remained elevated (Carter et al, 1978). **Finally, it must be recognized that some patients with macroadenomas including prolactinomas have hypogonadotropic hypogonadism produced by the mass lesion itself.**

Feedback Control of Gonadotropins

As depicted in Figure 41–1, the hypothalamic-pituitary-gonadal system consists of a closed-loop feedback control mechanism directed at maintaining normal reproductive function. In this system, gonadal hormones have inhibitory effects on the secretion of LH and FSH. This is easily demonstrated by the rise in serum LH and FSH that occurs after orchiectomy (Fig. 41–7) (Walsh et al, 1973). As seen in Figure 41–7, LH and FSH levels continue to rise for a long period after castration, reaching maximum levels as late as 25 to 50 days after surgery. In studies in experimental animals, changes in serum levels of LH and FSH are preceded by elevations of pituitary mRNA for αβ, and FSH-β subunits, although the changes in FSH-β are more modest (Gharib, 1987).

Although it is generally held that testosterone, the major secretory product of the testis, is the primary inhibitor of LH secretion in men, a number of testis products, including estrogens and other androgens, have the ability to inhibit LH secretion (Swerdloff and Walsh, 1973). Finkelstein has reexamined the issue of whether testosterone suppresses gonadotropins at the pituitary or indirectly at the hypothalamic level and concluded that the effects occur at both functional levels (Finkelstein, 1991).

Estradiol, a potent estrogen, is produced both from the testis and from peripheral conversion of androgens and androgen precursors (Longcope et al, 1969). Although the concentration of estradiol in the blood of men is relatively low compared with that of testosterone, it is a much more potent inhibitor of LH and FSH secretion (approximately 1000-fold) (Swerdloff and Walsh, 1973). In addition to the potential direct role of estradiol in inhibition of the hypothalamic-pituitary axis, local metabolic conversion (aromatization) of testosterone or other androgen precursors to estradiol may occur in the hypothalamus, where estradiol inhibits GnRH production (Naftolin et al, 1971). However, androgens that cannot be converted to estradiol are very potent inhibitors of LH and FSH (Swerdloff et al, 1972; Naftolin and Feder, 1973; Stewart-Bentley et al, 1974). In order to better define the relative role of androgens and estrogens in the control of LH secretions in intact men, attempts have been made to infuse steroids in amounts that would produce physiologic concentrations of the hormones in the blood (Sherins and Loriaux, 1973; Stewart-Bentley et al, 1974). These studies demonstrate suppression of LH levels by physiologic concentrations of both testosterone and estradiol, suggesting that both hormones may be important in LH regulation. Although it is possible that a synergistic effect of the two hormones may be responsible for physiologic control of LH, data from experimental animals fail to demonstrate such synergism (Gay and Dever, 1971; Swerdloff and Walsh, 1973). Testolactone, an aromatase inhibitor, attenuates the testosterone-induced inhibition of LH secretion in both normal and GnRH-deficient men (Finkelstein et al, 1991). Testosterone alone decreased mean LH levels, the decrease being greater in men that received testosterone alone than testolactone plus testosterone. These data suggest that the inhibitory effects of testosterone are mediated both directly by testosterone itself and indirectly through aromatization to estradiol (Finkelstein, 1991). Despite this factor, DHT, which is non-aromatizable, also inhibits LH secretion, confirming the concept that aromatization is not obligatory for LH feedback (Santen, 1975). Conversion of testosterone to DHT is not required for feedback effects of testosterone either, because the potent 5α-reductase inhibitor finasteride, given short term (days) to normal men, does not elevate either LH or FSH levels (Rittmaster, 1992). It is notable that patients with congenital end-organ resistance to testosterone (testicular feminization) may have a female phenotypic appearance associated with normal or above-normal serum estradiol levels and high blood LH concentrations (Judd et al, 1972; Faiman and Winter, 1974). **These findings in their totality may suggest that both testosterone and estradiol are important physiologic controllers of LH secretion.**

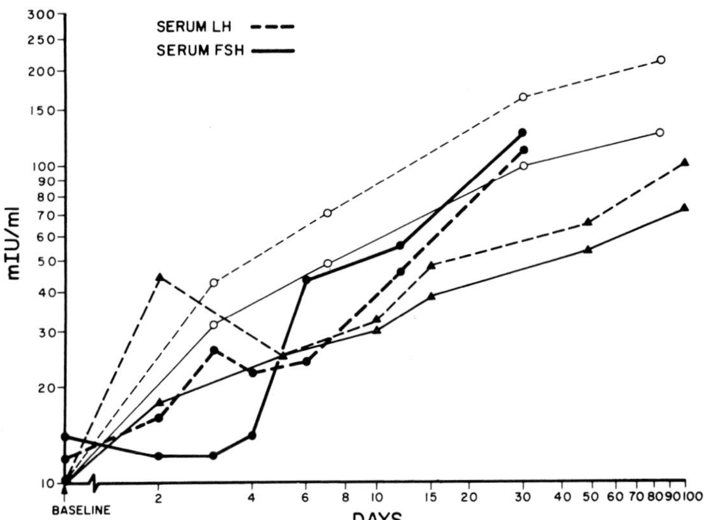

Figure 41–7. Effect of bilateral orchiectomy on serum luteinizing hormone (LH) and follicle-stimulating hormone (FSH) concentrations in three men. (From Walsh PC, Swerdloff RS, Odell WD: Acta Endocrinol, 1973; 74:449.)

The mechanism of feedback control of FSH secretion is even more controversial than that of LH. The rise in serum FSH after castration (see Fig. 41–7) demonstrates the important role of the testis in the feedback control of FSH secretion. As for LH, both testosterone and estradiol are capable of suppressing FSH serum levels, although the relative importance of these two gonadal steroids remains undefined. In one study, Stewart-Bentley and associates (1974) infused near-physiologic amounts of testosterone and estradiol and reported suppression of LH but not FSH. In other studies in men, Sherins and Loriaux (1973), using higher doses of steroids, reported suppression of both LH and FSH. Testosterone suppression of LH and FSH occurs even when aromatization to estradiol is blocked (Marynick et al, 1979).

There is considerable evidence that a nonsteroidal tubular factor may also be important in the feedback regulation of FSH. This concept dates back to the work of McCullagh and Walsh (1935), who suggested that a substance originating in the germinal epithelium inhibits pituitary FSH production. They named this substance inhibin. Elevations of serum FSH concentrations are found in men with azoospermia in whom the germinal epithelium is selectively injured, as shown by normal serum or urinary LH and testosterone levels. Circumstances in which this group of findings are seen include irradiation of the testis (Paulsen, 1968), use of antispermatogenic agents (Van Thiel et al, 1972), and early cryptorchidism (Swerdloff et al, 1971), as well as some cases of oligospermia or azoospermia (Rosen and Weintraub 1971; deKretser and Burger, 1972; Leonard et al, 1972).

Inhibin has been isolated and characterized in follicular fluid. It is produced by the Sertoli cells of the testis and the granulosa cells of the ovary. Inhibin has two subunits, alpha and beta. Two forms of inhibin have been isolated. They have the same alpha subunit, and their beta subunits are different. Both inhibin A (α, β A subunits) and inhibin B (α, β B subunits) have been shown to cause selective suppression of FSH release in vitro (Ling et al, 1985; Miyamoto et al, 1985; Rivier et al, 1985; Robertson et al, 1985). Combinations of the two beta subunits (heterodimers and homodimers) led to the formation of activins. Activins increase the secretion of FSH in vitro. In addition to inhibin, a number of gonadal peptides and growth factors, such as follistatin and transforming growth factor-β are also modulators of FSH secretion. All of these gonadal peptides have been shown to have a paracrine or autocrine role in regulation of the function of gonadal cells (Ying, 1988).

In male rats, testicular inhibin is regulated by pituitary hormones, because testicular inhibin concentrations decline after hypophysectomy. FSH increases testicular inhibin content and stimulates inhibin release from cultured Sertoli cells (Au et al, 1985). Nevertheless, immunoneutralization studies in rats reveal that infusion of anti-inhibin sera leads to an increase in serum FSH only in the female and prepubertal male animal but not in the adult male (Rivier, 1986; Ying, 1987). When Leydig cells in adult male rats are destroyed by a Leydig cell-specific toxin, EDS, administration of anti-inhibin sera leads to an increase in serum FSH (Culler and Negro-Vilar, 1990). In women, an inverse relationship between inhibin and FSH has been demonstrated (McLachlan et al, 1987). In men, immunoreactive α inhibin increases in parallel with LH and FSH during puberty, rises after GnRH stimulation in patients with idiopathic hypogonadotropic hypogonadism, and declines during gonadotropin suppression by testosterone (McLachlan et al, 1988; Sheckter et al, 1988; Burger et al, 1988). However, not only purified FSH but also LH and hCG increase inhibin levels in gonadotropin-suppressed men (McLachlan et al, 1988). Moreover, inhibin is released into human spermatic veins in well-defined pulses that coincide with episodes of testosterone release, suggesting the involvement of LH in the regulation of inhibin release from the testis (Winters, 1990). Surprisingly, studies in men with primary testicular insufficiency showed no significant changes in serum α inhibin levels measured by radioimmunoassay (deKretser et al, 1989). The interrelationship between inhibin and gonadotropins in the human male was clarified when β inhibin was shown to have a negative correlation with serum FSH levels (Illingworth, 1996).

It must be emphasized that even in pathologic states in which marked damage to the germinal tissue occurs, serum FSH is not elevated to castration levels unless Leydig cell function is also impaired. **Although the relative roles need to be better understood, both gonadal steroids and pep-**

tides appear to be important in maintaining normal serum FSH concentrations.

The Testis

Hormonal Control of Spermatogenesis

Spermatogenesis is a complex process whereby a primitive stem cell, the type A spermatogonium, passes through a complex series of transformations to give rise to spermatozoa. In humans, this takes 73 days. The development of the male germ cells in the seminiferous tubule essentially consists of three phases: spermatogonial multiplication, meiosis, and spermatogenesis. In the seminiferous epithelium, cells in these developmental phases are arranged in defined associations or stages. Along the seminiferous tubules, in most mammals, these stages follow one another in a regular fashion, giving rise to the wave of the seminiferous epithelium. The time interval between the appearance of the same cell association at a given point of the tubule is called the cycle of the seminiferous epithelium (Parvinen, 1982).

Although the dependence of spermatogenesis on pituitary FSH and on intratesticular testosterone has been emphasized, the precise nature of interaction between these hormones and germ cells remains poorly understood. FSH and androgens seem to have different preferential sites of action during the cycle of the seminiferous epithelium. Stages VII and VIII appear to be androgen dependent, whereas maximal binding of FSH and activation of FSH-dependent enzymes occurs in stages XIII to XV of the spermatogenic cycle (Ritzen et al, 1981; Gordeladze et al, 1982).

Recent studies, using the transillumination-assisted microdissection technique, further demonstrate a small but significant peak of FSH-stimulated cAMP production late in stage VII, suggesting a stimulatory effect of FSH on stage VII (Parvinen, 1993). This notion is further supported by in vivo studies showing that recombinant preparation of human FSH can, in a significant manner, prevent the regressive changes in spermatogenesis at stage VII in the adult rat 1 week after hypophysectomy (Russell et al, 1993) or GnRH antagonist treatment (Sinha-Hikim and Swerdloff, 1995).

The hormonal control of spermatogenesis has been the subject of numerous studies over many years. However, despite this intensive study, the specific role and relative contribution of FSH and LH in regulation of spermatogenesis in adult mammals remain far from settled. Earlier studies have shown that quantitatively normal spermatogenesis (assessed by measurements of homogenization-resistant advanced [steps 17 to 19] spermatids) can be restored by exogenous administration of testosterone alone in adult rats made azoospermic by treating them with implants of testosterone and estradiol (Awoniyi et al, 1989a) or by active immunization against either LH or GnRH (Awoniyi et al, 1989b). In a separate study, these authors have also reported that testosterone alone is capable of maintaining advanced spermatid numbers in adult rats actively immunized against GnRH (Awoniyi et al, 1992). These results of qualitative maintenance or restoration of spermatogenesis by testosterone alone in rats in the absence of both radioimmunoassayable LH and FSH suggest that FSH has no effect on the regulation of spermatogenesis in the adult rat. Quantitative maintenance of spermatogenesis has also been achieved in adult rats in which LH and FSH had been suppressed pharmacologically by a GnRH antagonist with testosterone alone, when administered at higher doses (Rea et al, 1986; Bhasin et al, 1988). However, because testosterone supplementation increases both the serum concentrations and pituitary content of FSH in GnRH-antagonist–treated rats, the observed quantitative maintenance of spermatogenesis in these rats (Rea et al, 1986; Bhasin et al, 1988) cannot be attributed with certainty to testosterone alone. In a recent study, McLachlan and colleagues (1994) have shown that spermatogenesis is not quantitatively restored in the GnRH-immunized rat that received pharmacologic amounts of testosterone as used in the earlier studies and further emphasizes the need for both FSH and testosterone in the restoration of spermatogenesis. Similarly, in most studies of hypophysectomized rats, spermatogenesis is not quantitatively maintained (Sun et al, 1989; Santuli et al, 1990) or restored (Roberts et al, 1991) by exogenous administration of testosterone, suggesting that FSH and other pituitary hormones might be required for complete regulation of spermatogenesis in this species.

A definitive role of FSH on the maintenance of spermatogenesis in adult rats under various experimental situations has been suggested previously by a number of investigators (Bartlett et al, 1989; Chandolia et al, 1991; Kerr et al, 1992; Russell et al, 1993; Vaishnav et al, 1994). These studies were, however, of limited duration. Thus, stimulatory effects of FSH on spermatogenesis that are obvious after 1 or 2 weeks of gonadotropin and testosterone deprivation might not become so obvious after long-term treatment. The most definitive evidence, however, comes from a recent study (Sinha-Hikim and Swerdloff, 1995) that shows that recombinant human FSH replacement to GnRH-A treated rats fully attenuated the early (1 week) GnRH-A–induced reduction in germ cell numbers at stage VII as well as the number of advanced (steps 17–19) spermatids. In addition, FSH treatment effectively prevented GnRH-A–induced reduction in the number of pachytene spermatocytes and step-7 spermatids for 2 weeks. It is also noted in that study that FSH replacement to GnRH-A treated rats for 4 weeks generated an increase in the number of B spermatogonia available for entry into meiosis and maintained the number of preleptotene spermatocytes.

Unlike in the rat, exogenous administration of testosterone to hypogonadotropic men does not induce spermatogenesis, probably because of the practical limits of the dose of testosterone that can be administered. In humans, when the onset of hypogonadotropic hypogonadism occurs before puberty, the initiation of sperm production generally requires both LH and FSH (Sherins, 1977). LH affects spermatogenesis by increasing intratesticular testosterone levels. The levels of FSH required to initiate spermatogenesis in these patients are variable but are probably very low. Thus, in both humans and rats, both FSH and LH are required for the initiation of a complete cycle of spermatogenesis. However, in patients with gonadotropin deficiency that is acquired after puberty, sperm production can be stimulated with LH alone, suggesting that the reinitiation and maintenance of spermatogenesis in adults can be achieved only by LH. Studies of selective gonadotropin replacement in normal men, in whom hypogonadotropic hypogonadism was induced with exogenous testosterone administration, show that qualitatively normal sperm production can be achieved by replacement of either FSH or LH alone. **Both FSH and LH are necessary to maintain quantitatively normal spermatogenesis in humans (Matsumoto et al, 1983, 1986; Schaison et al, 1993).**

In addition to LH (androgens) and FSH, many peptides and growth factors (e.g., inhibin, activin, insulin-like growth factor-1, transforming growth factor-β are secreted locally in the seminiferous tubules. The role of these proteins as mediators of cell-to-cell interactions involved in the local control of spermatogenesis remains to be characterized.

Hormonal Control of Testicular Steroidogenesis

Acting on its specific LH receptor in the Leydig cells, LH stimulates testicular steroidogenesis. The response of Leydig cells to trophic hormones such as LH involves the mobilization of cholesterol from the cellular stores to the outer mitochondrial inner membrane. The transfer of cholesterol to the mitochondrial membrane is dependent on the synthesis of a novel protein, steroidogenic acute regulatory protein (STAR). This protein stimulates steroidogenesis in the absence of trophic hormone (Clark et al, 1995). Mutations of the gene for STAR led to cessation of adrenal and gonadal steroidogenesis, resulting in the clinical disorder of congenital lipid adrenal hyperplasia (Lin et al, 1995). In addition to LH, FSH may indirectly affect Leydig cell function by an action on Sertoli cells and spermatogenesis. In experiments in which disruption of spermatogenesis is induced, functional changes occur in the Leydig cells. In addition, a number of testicular peptides (e.g., GnRH-like peptide, insulin growth factor-1, transforming growth factor-β) may have a role in the local control of testicular steroidogenesis (Bhasin et al, 1983; Risbridger and deKretser, 1989).

Changes in the Reproductive Axis with Age

Changes During Sexual Maturation

The human fetal pituitary gland has the capacity not only to synthesize and store FSH and LH but also to secrete these hormones in high concentrations during early gestation. Fetal serum FSH and LH levels seem to peak at midgestation (Kaplan et al, 1976). The decline during late gestation may be the result of maturation of the capacity of the hypothalamic-pituitary-gonadal axis to respond to negative feedback by gonadal steroids. The same authors have noted a sex difference in fetal gonadotropins, in that females have higher peak levels (particularly of FSH) than do males.

During the first years of life, serum LH and FSH levels are detectable in the blood; the concentrations of both hormones are low at birth but rise for several months after birth and then decline to very low levels by 9 to 12 months (Faiman and Winter, 1974). Figure 41–8 presents serum LH, FSH, and testosterone concentrations in boys aged 2 to 21 years (Swerdloff and Odell, 1975).

There is a progressive rise in LH and FSH from approximately age 6 to 8 years through the completion of puberty, with the increase in FSH slightly preceding the increase in LH concentrations. Earlier studies using radioimmunoassay for LH and FSH showed a slow progressive rise in gonadotropins during the prepubertal years. Later studies using more sensitive immunofluorometric assays described a 116-fold increase in serum LH between age 7 years and adulthood (Apter, 1989). In early puberty, the mean LH level increased much more than that of FSH. For LH, the increase in mean levels was due to an increase in both pulse amplitude and frequency; for FSH, the increase was progressive from prepuberty to midpuberty (Dunkel et al, 1992). There is a much steeper increase in blood testosterone, beginning at approximately 10 to 12 years of age. Figure 41–9 shows the sleep-related development of the episodic secretion of LH and FSH seen in children at mid-

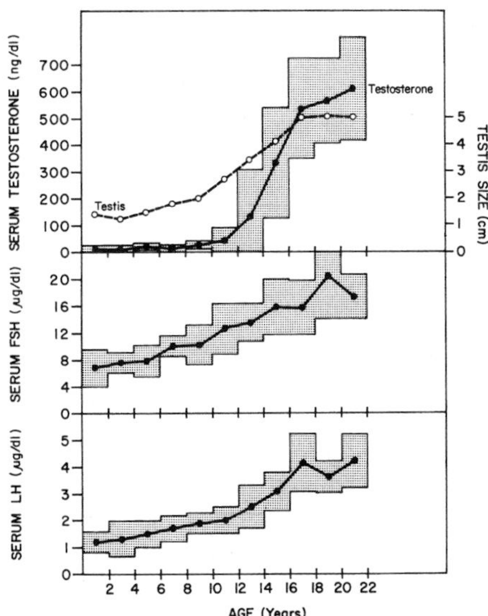

Figure 41–8. Cross-sectional data demonstrating the changes in testis size and serum luteinizing hormone (LH), follicle-stimulating hormone (FSH), and testosterone levels during sexual maturation in boys. Not shown are the relatively higher LH and FSH levels seen in the first year of life. (From Swerdloff RS, Odell WD: Postgrad Med J, 1975; 51:200. Used by permission.)

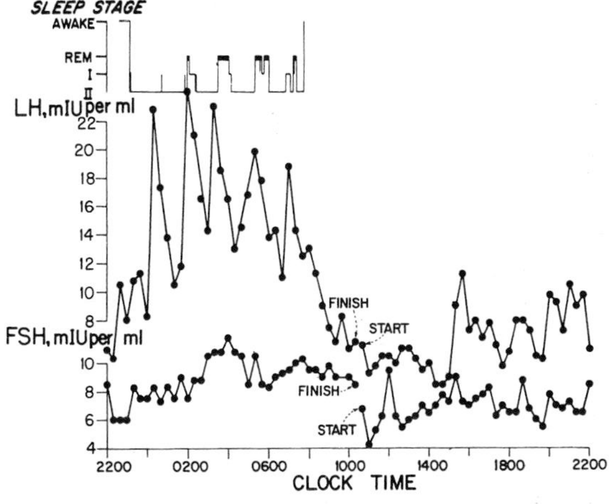

Figure 41–9. Plasma luteinizing hormone (LH) and follicle-stimulating hormone (FSH) concentration samples every 20 minutes for 24 hours in a normal pubertal child. Gonadotropin levels are elevated during sleep. (From Boyar RM, et al: Reprinted with permission of the New England Journal of Medicine, 1973; 289:283.)

puberty (Boyar et al, 1972). More recent studies have confirmed the nocturnal hypersecretion of LH at midpuberty but failed to show a dermal variation in FSH (Dunkel et al, 1992). As described in previous and subsequent sections, LH is the primary stimulus for testosterone secretion, whereas both LH and FSH are important determinants of the induction and maintenance of the spermatogenic process.

Changes in Old Age

Decreased testicular function is frequently seen in elderly men (Vermeulen et al, 1972; Swerdloff and Heber, 1982). Although associated ill health may depress testicular function, lower serum total and especially free testosterone concentrations are common in healthy elderly men (Fig. 41–10) (Rubens et al, 1974; Baker et al, 1976; Harman and Tsitouras, 1980; Sparrow et al, 1980). Other androgens such as 5α-DHT, androstanediol, and androstanediol glucuronide also decrease with aging (Lewis et al, 1976). In contrast, serum estradiol and estrone levels increase with age due in part to increased peripheral aromatization of androgen to estrogen (Greenblatt, 1976).

Circulating levels of both LH and FSH are increased with aging (Christiansen, 1972; Haug et al, 1974; Rubens et al, 1974; Snyder et al, 1975; Baker et al, 1976; Greenblatt et al, 1976), providing further evidence for a primary defect at a testicular level (Fig. 41–11). Despite the wide individual variations shown in Figure 41–11, there is a consistent increase in gonadotropin levels in men over the age of 40. It has been reported that the ratio of bioactive to immunoreactive LH and FSH levels is lower in older than in younger men (Warner et al, 1985; Tenover et al, 1987). This suggests that the LH and FSH secreted in the elderly male may have lower biologic activity. A relatively greater increase in FSH compared with LH has been reported (Christiansen, 1972), suggesting that seminiferous tubule degeneration with decreased inhibin production occurs to a greater extent than do decreases in Leydig cell function. Walsh and co-workers (1973) found that those elderly men with the highest FSH elevations showed significant changes in seminiferous tubule morphology.

Although the evidence for primary testicular abnormalities in older men has been clearly established, an additional or secondary hypothalamic-pituitary defect has been suggested, based on the observation that serum testosterone concentrations remain below normal, whereas the testes retain the ability to respond to exogenous gonadotropin with increased testosterone secretion. The increases in blood gonadotropin levels in androgen-deficient elderly men may be blunted in contrast to those in younger men with similar degrees of androgen deficiency. This concept is supported by the observation that the responses of the gonadotropins following standard GnRH testing are lower and delayed in older than younger men (Haug et al, 1974; Snyder et al, 1975; Winters and Troen, 1982). Further evidence of altered hypothalamic function in the elderly man is the loss of the diurnal rhythm of testosterone present in younger men (Bremner et al, 1983).

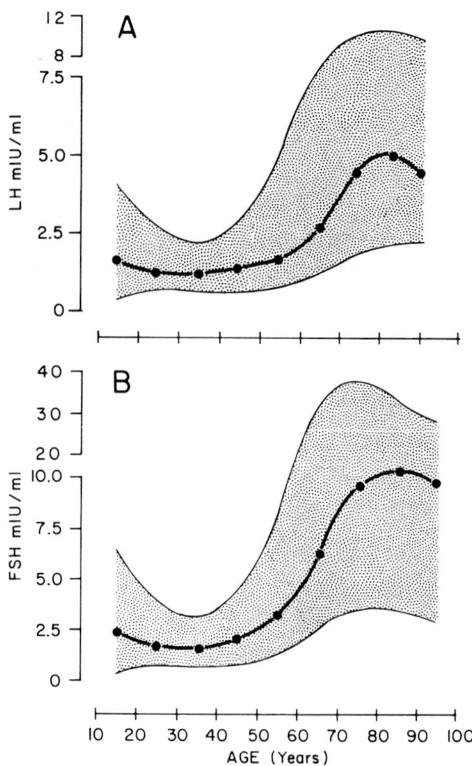

Figure 41–11. *A,* Rise in serum luteinizing hormone (LH) with aging. *B,* Rise in serum follicle-stimulating hormone (FSH) with aging. The shaded area represents range of individual values. (From Baker HWG, Burger HG, deKretser DM, et al: Endocrinology of aging: Pituitary testicular axis. Proc. 5th Intl. Congress of Endocrinology, 1976, pp 479–483.)

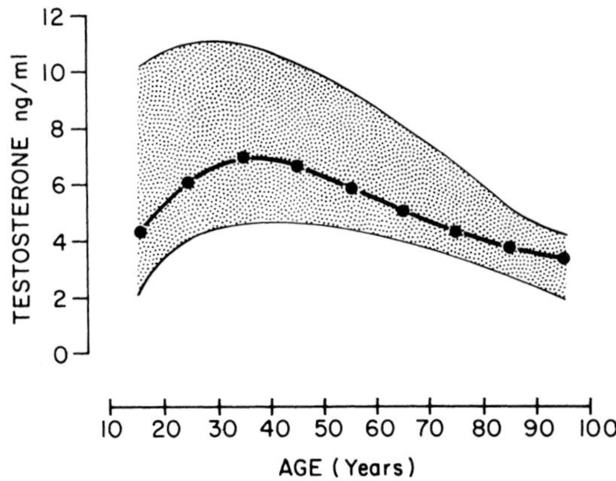

Figure 41–10. Decline with age of total testosterone. The shaded area represents the range of individual values. (From Baker HWG, Burger HG, deKretser DM, et al: Endocrinology of aging: Pituitary testicular axis. Proc. 5th Intl. Congress of Endocrinology, 1976, pp 479–483.)

Several explanations for decreased pituitary function with aging have been proposed. Kley and associates (1974) suggested that increased levels of estrogen and other circulating steroids tend to inhibit gonadotropin secretion despite lowered levels of testosterone. Alternatively, centers mediating hypothalamic sensitivity to steroid feedback (the "gonadostat") might be altered to respond to lowered levels of testosterone in aged men with inhibition of pituitary function. Such increased sensitivity to steroidal feedback occurs in prepubertal boys and may also occur in elderly men (Muta et al, 1981; Winters and Troen 1982). Finally, there may be an age-related decrease in pituitary gonadotroph cellular responsiveness secondary to changes in pituitary GnRH receptor number or steps beyond receptor binding or other events mediating gonadotropin secretion.

In summary, a primary defect in the reproductive hormonal axis with aging occurs at a gonadal level as a result of decreased numbers of Leydig cells and degenerative seminiferous tubule changes. These changes at a testicular level result in elevations of circulating gonadotropins, but there is evidence of decreased pituitary gonadotropin secretory responses, at least to exogenous GnRH. The normal range for testosterone varies according to laboratory. In general, levels below 300 ng/dl are considered abnormal for a healthy young male population. About 20% of men between 60 and 80 years of age have serum testosterone levels below 300 ng/dl. Serum LH and FSH levels were highly variable in this 20% of the older male population with low testosterone levels. It remains unclear to what extent relatively low serum testosterone levels reflect clinically important pathology. Because hypogonadal men have an increased incidence of sexual dysfunction, osteoporosis, decreased muscle mass and strength, lowered vigor, and increased depressive symptoms, the implication of a low testosterone level is of great relevance. Treatment may reduce fractures, increase strength and vigor, and lead to an improved quality of life. Balanced against this are the potential risks of lowered HDL cholesterol (possibly increased atherosclerosis) and aggravation of benign prostatic hyperplasia and prostate cancer. Prospective studies are under way to clarify the risk or reward of such treatment (Swerdloff and Wang, 1993; Tenover, 1994).

THE HYPOTHALAMIC-PITUITARY-GONADAL AXIS AND THE ASSESSMENT OF HYPOGONADAL PATIENTS

Patients with under-androgenization and lowered serum testosterone levels usually fall into one of two pathophysiologic classes: those with a primary testicular disease or those with a hypothalamic-pituitary disorder. These two general categories (hypergonadotropic and hypogonadotropic hypogonadism) can be differentiated by the measurement of serum levels of LH and FSH.

Patients with primary Leydig cell damage exhibit diminished feedback inhibition of gonadotropin secretion, resulting in high serum LH and FSH concentrations; this is, therefore, classified as hypergonadotropic hypogonadism. Such patients would be expected to have a diminished Leydig cell reserve and a blunted testosterone response to administered LH or to the LH-like effects of hCG (Paulsen et al, 1968). Patients with hypogonadotropic hypogonadism (see later) respond to hCG with increases in testosterone. However, this test adds little new information to the diagnosis. The major use of the hCG stimulation test is to exclude anorchia in cryptorchid boys with impalpable testes (Handelsman and Swerdloff, 1985).

Patients with low serum testosterone and low or inappropriately low-normal serum LH levels are classified as having hypogonadotropic hypogonadism. Such patients have an abnormality involving either the hypothalamus or the pituitary gland. This defect can be structural, such as a hypothalamic or pituitary tumor. More frequently, it is due to one of the following: (1) administration of drugs that inhibit the hypothalamic axis, such as tranquilizers or estrogens; (2) congenital inability to synthesize or release GnRH or LH and FSH, as in congenital hypogonadotropic hypogonadism (such patients can have isolated LH or FSH deficiency or multiple tropic hormone defects); or (3) altered hypothalamic control mechanisms, as in starvation or anorexia nervosa. The most common form of congenital hypogonadotropic hypogonadism is part of Kallmann's syndrome, characterized by delayed or arrested sexual development and anosmia. Other, less common somatic manifestations include color blindness, cleft lip and palate, and cranial nerve defects (Santen, 1973).

The site of the hypothalamic or pituitary lesion should be localized, if possible, by computed tomography scan or magnetic resonance imaging. A serum PRL must be measured to exclude the presence of hyperprolactinemia. A single test dose of GnRH (usually 100 g intravenously) does not distinguish hypothalamic from pituitary disease. A GnRH test preceded by a period of "priming" the pituitary gonadotrophs by repeated low-dose stimulation has been used to diagnose hypothalamic disorders. The GnRH test with prior priming can demonstrate that low or absent LH responses to a single dose of GnRH in hypothalamic disorders can be augmented to give normal LH levels, whereas priming has no effect in pituitary disorders (Snyder et al, 1979). Difficulty also exists in distinguishing delayed sexual maturation from incomplete hypogonadotropic hypogonadism because basal LH and FSH levels may be similarly low in both circumstances (Boyar et al, 1973). GnRH testing may be of potential value but is limited by the smaller LH response in normal prepubertal children that can overlap with the response of patients with incomplete hypogonadotropic hypogonadism. Newborns with hypogonadotropic hypogonadism may be identified by measuring the testicular volume sequentially during the first 3 months of life. Normal children apparently double the testicular volume during this period (Cassorla et al, 1981). The GnRH test, however, is very useful in distinguishing precocious puberty that is due to central hypothalamic causes from that due to testicular or adrenal disorders in both boys and girls.

The clomiphene test is based on the observation that an increase in FSH and LH occurs after clomiphene administration. Although the mechanism of action of clomiphene is not absolutely clear, most evidence indicates that it interferes at a hypothalamic level with steroid feedback inhibition of gonadotropin secretion (Marshall, 1975). Because an intact pituitary is required for normal LH and FSH secretion, adult patients with either hypothalamic or pituitary defects demonstrate an impaired response to clomiphene. This test is of little value with the advent of the GnRH priming stimulation test (Handelsman and Swerdloff, 1985).

Patients with severe germinal epithelial damage without concomitant loss of androgen function may show modest isolated elevation of serum FSH levels. Such a monotropic increase in FSH in patients with azoospermia or severe oligospermia is believed to be due to a decrease in the production of inhibin from the germinal epithelium.

In rare instances, phenotypic male patients with clinical evidence of under-androgenization may have normal, high-normal, or elevated serum testosterone levels (Walsh et al, 1974; Wilson et al, 1974). Such patients have a partial peripheral defect in testosterone responsiveness. (Classification of these disorders is presented in Chapter 37.) Serum LH levels in such patients may be either elevated or normal, depending on whether hypothalamic response to testosterone is also impaired.

REFERENCES

Apter D, Cacciatore B, Alfthan H, Stenmain U-H: Serum LH concentrations increase 100-fold in females from 7 years of age to adulthood, as measured by time-resolved immunofluorometric assay. J Clin Endocrinol Metab 1989; 68:53–57.

Arimura A, Kastin AJ, Schally AV, et al: Immunoreactive LH-releasing hormone in plasma: Midcycle elevation in women. J Clin Endocrinol Metab 1974; 38:510.

Attanasio A, Borrelli P, Gupta D: Circadian rhythms in serum melatonin from infancy to adolescence. J Clin Endocrinol Metab 1985; 61:388–390.

Attanasio A, Borelli P, Marini R, et al: Serum melatonin in children with early and delayed puberty. Neuroendocrinol Lett 1983; 5:387.

Au CL, Robertson DM, deKretser DM: Effects of hypophysectomy and subsequent FSH and testosterone treatment on inhibin production by adult rat testes. J Endocrinol 1985; 105(1):1–6.

Awoniyi CA, Santulli R, Sprando RL, et al: Restoration of advanced spermatogenic cells in the experimentally regressed rat testis: Quantitative relationship to testosterone concentration within the testis. Endocrinology 1989a; 124:1217–1223.

Awoniyi CA, Santulli R, Chandrashekar V, et al: Quantitative restoration of advanced spermatogenic cells in adult male rats made azoospermic by active immunization against luteinizing hormone or gonadotropin-releasing hormone. Endocrinology 1989b; 125:1303–1309.

Awoniyi CA, Zirkin BR, Chandrashekar V, Schlaff WD: Exogenously administered testosterone maintains spermatogenesis quantitatively in adult rats actively immunized against gonadotropin-releasing hormone. Endocrinology 1992; 130:3283–3288.

Baker HWG, Burger HG, deKretser DM, Hudson B: Endocrinology of aging: Pituitary testicular axis. Proceedings of the 5th International Congress of Endocrinology, Hamburg, FRG, 1976, pp 479–483.

Barraclough CA, Wise PM: Thc role of catecholamines in the regulation of pituitary luteinizing hormone and follicle-stimulating hormone secretion. Endocr Rev 1982; 3(1):91–119.

Bartlett JMS, Weinbauer GF, Nieschlag E: Differential effects of FSH and testosterone on the maintenance of spermatogenesis in the adult hypophysectomized rat. J Endocrinol 1989; 121:49–58.

Belchetz PE, Plant TM, Nakai Y, et al: Hypophysial responses to continuous and intermittent delivery of hypothalamic gonadotropin releasing hormone. Science 1978; 202:631.

Ben-Jonathan N, Mical RS, Porter JC: Transport of LRF from CSF to hypophysial portal and systemic blood and the release of LH. Endocrinology 1974; 95:18.

Besser GM, Mortimer CH: Effects of the gonadotropin releasing hormone in patients with hypothalamic-pituitary-gonadal diseases. Acta Fertil Eur 1974; 5:65.

Bhasin S, Heber D, Peterson M, et al: Partial isolation and characterization of testicular GnRH-like factors. Endocrinology 1983; 112:1144.

Bhasin S, Fielder T, Peacock N, et al: Dissociating antifertility effects of GnRH-antagonist from its adverse effects on mating behavior in male rats. Am J Physiol 1988; 254:E84–E91.

Bhasin S, Swerdloff RS: Follicle-stimulating hormone and luteinizing hormone. *In* Melmed S, ed: The Pituitary. Cambridge, MA, Blackwell Scientific Publications, 1995, pp 230–276.

Boyar R, Finkelstein J, Roffwarg H, et al: Synchronization of augmented luteinizing hormone secretion with sleep during puberty. N Engl J Med 1972; 287:582.

Boyar RM, Finkelstein JW, Witkin M, et al: Studies of endocrine function in "isolated" gonadotropin deficiency. J Clin Endocrinol Metab 1973; 36(1):64–72.

Bremner WJ, Vitiello MV, Prinz PN: Loss of circadian rhythmicity in blood testosterone levels with aging in normal men. J Clin Endocrinol Metab 1983; 56:1278.

Bronson FH: Pheromonal influences on mammalian reproduction. *In* Diamond M, ed: Perspectives in Reproduction and Sexual Behavior. Bloomington, Indiana University Press, 1968, pp 341–361.

Burger HG, McLachlan RI, Banyah M, et al: Serum inhibin concentrations rise throughout normal male and female puberty. J Clin Endocrinol Metab 1988; 67(4):689–694.

Carmel PW, Arani S, Ferin M: Pituitary stalk portal blood collection in rhesus monkeys: Evidence of pulsatile release of gonadotropin releasing hormone (GnRH). Endocrinology 1976; 99:243.

Carter JN, Tyson JE, Tolis G, et al: Prolactin-secreting tumors and hypogonadism in 22 men. N Engl J Med 1978; 299(16):847–852.

Cassorla FG, Golden SM., Johnsonbaugh RE, et al: Testicular volume during early infancy. J Pediatr 1981; 99:742.

Chandolia RK, Weinbauer GF, Fingscheidt U, et al: Effects of flutamide on testicular involution induced by an antagonist of gonadotropin-releasing hormone and on stimulation of spermatogenesis by follicle-stimulating hormone in rats. J Reprod Fertil 1991; 93:313–323.

Christiansen P: Urinary follicle-stimulating hormone and luteinizing hormone in normal adult men. Acta Endocrinol (Copenh) 1972; 71:1.

Clark BJ, Wells J, King SR, Stocco DM: The purification, cloning and expression of a novel luteinizing hormone–induced mitochondrial protein in MA-10 mouse Leydig tumor cells. Characterization of the steroidogenic acute regulatory protein (StAR). J Biol Chem 1994; 269:28314.

Coble YD Jr, Kohler PO, Cargille CM, Ross GT: Production rates and metabolic clearance rates of human follicle-stimulating hormone in premenopausal and postmenopausal women. J Clin Invest 1969; 48:359.

Cohen HN, Hay LD, Annesley TM, et al: Serum immunoreactive melatonin in boys with delayed puberty. Clin Endocrinol (Oxf) 1982; 17(5):517–521.

Crowley WF Jr, Filicori M, Spratt DI, Santoro NF: The physiology of gonadotropin releasing hormone (GnRH) secretion in men and women. Rec Prog Horm Res 1985; 41:473–531.

Culler MD, Negro-Vilar : Destruction of testicular Leydig cells reveals a role of endogenous inhibin in regulating follicle-stimulating hormone secretion in the adult male rat. Mol Cell Endocrinol 1990; 70:89–98.

Dahl KD, Bicsak TA, Hsueh AJ: Naturally occurring antihormones: Secretion of FSH antagonists by women treated with a GnRH analog. Science 1988; 239:72.

deKretser DM, Burger HG, Fortune D, et al: Hormonal, histological and chromosomal studies in adult males with testicular disorders. J Clin Endocrinol Metab 1972; 35(3):392–401.

deKretser DM, McLachlan RI, Robertson DM, Burger HG: Serum inhibin levels in normal men and men with testicular disorders. J Endocrinol 1989; 12:517.

Delitala G, Devilla L, Arata L: Opiate receptors and anterior pituitary hormone secretion in man: Effects of naloxone infusion. Acta Endocrinol (Copenh) 1981; 97(2):150–156.

Dufau ML, Mendelson CR, Catt KJ: A highly sensitive in vitro bioassay for LH and hCG: Testosterone production by dispersed Leydig cells. J Clin Endocrinol Metab 1974; 39:610.

Dunkel L, Alfthan H, Stenman U, et al: Developmental changes in (24 hour profiles) of luteinizing hormone and follicle-stimulating hormone from prepuberty to midstages of puberty in boys. J Clin Endocrinol Metab 1992; 74:890–897.

Ellendorff F, Parvizi N: Role of extrahypothalamic centers in neuroendocrine integration. *In* Motta M, ed: The Endocrine Functions of the Brain. New York, Raven Press, 1980, pp 297–325.

Faiman C, Winter JS: The control of gonadotropin secretion in complete testicular feminization. J Clin Endocrinol Metab 1974; 39:631.

Finkelstein JS, Whitcomb RW, O'Dea St L, et al: Sex steroid control of gonadotropin secretion in the human male I. Effects of testosterone administration in normal and GnRH deficient men. J Clin Endocrinol Metab 1991; 73:609–620.

Gay VL, Dever NW: Effects of testosterone propionate and estradiol benzoate alone or in combination on serum LH and FSH in orchidectomized rats. Endocrinology 1971; 89(1):161–168.

Gharib SD, Wierman ME, Badger TM, Chin WW: Sex steroid hormone regulation of FSH subunit mRNAs levels in the rat. J Clin Invest 1987; 80:294–299.

Gharib SD, Wierman ME, Shupnik MA, Chin WW: Molecular biology of the pituitary gonadotropins. Endocr Rev 1990; 11:177–199.

Gindoff PR, Ferin M: Endogenous opioid peptides modulate the effect of corticotropin-releasing factor on gonadotropin release in the primate. Endocrinology 1987; 121(3):837–842.

Gitler MS, Barraclough CA: Locus coeruleus (LC) stimulation augments LHRH release induced by medial preoptic stimulation: Evidence that the major LC stimulatory component enters contralaterally into the hypothalamus. Brain Res 1987; 422(1):1–10.

Gordeladze JO, Parvinen M, Clausen OPF, Hansson V: Stage dependent variation in Mn^{++}-sensitive adenyl cyclase (AC) activity in spermatid and FSH sensitive Sertoli cells. Arch Androl 1982; 8:43.

Gormley G, Ridgmaster R: Effect of finasteride, a 5-alpha reductase inhibitor, on serum gonadotropins in normal men. Endocrinology 1991; 73:145A.

Greenblatt RB, Oettinger M, Bohler CS: Estrogen-androgen levels in aging men and women: Therapeutic considerations. J Am Geriatr Soc 1976; 24:173.

Halasz B, Kiss J, Molnar J: Regulation of the gonadotropin-releasing hormone (GnRH) neuronal system: Morphological aspects. J Steroid Biochem 1989; 33(4B):663–668.

Handelsman, DJ: Testicular dysfunction in systemic disease. Endocrinol Metab Clin North Am 1994; 23:839–856.

Handelsman DJ, Swerdloff RS: Male gonadal dysfunction. J Clin Endocrinol Metab 1985; 14(1):89–124.

Harman SM, Tsitouras PD: Reproductive hormones in aging men. I. Measurement of sex steroids, basal luteinizing hormone and Leydig cell response to human chorionic gonadotropin. J Clin Endocrinol Metab 1980; 51:35.

Haug EA, Aakvaag A, Sand T, Torjesen PA: The gonadotropin response to synthetic GnRH in males in relation to age, dose and basal serum Ievels of testosterone, estradiol-17 beta and gonadotrophins. Acta Endocrinol (Copenh) 1974; 77:625.

Hemmila I, Dakubu S, Mukkala VM, et al: Europium as a label in time-resolved immunofluormetric assays. Anal Biochem 1984; 137:335–343.

Illingsworth PJ, Groome NP, Byrd W, et al: Inhibin-B: A likely candidate for the physiologically important form of inhibin in men. J Clin Endocrinol Metab 1996; 81:1321–1325.

Jaakkola T, Ding YQ, Kellokumpu-Lehtinen P, et al: The ratios of serum bioactive/immunoactive LH and FSH in various clinical conditions with increased and decreased gonadotropin secretion: Reevaluation by a highly sensitive immunometric assay. J Clin Endocrinol Metab 1990; 70:1496–1505.

Jarjour LT, Handelsman DJ, Raum WJ, Swerdloff RS: Mechanism of action of dopamine in the in vitro release of gonadotropin-releasing hormone. Endocrinology 1986; 119(4):1726–1732.

Judd HL, Hamilton CR, Barlow JJ, Yen SSC, Kliman B: Androgen and gonadotropin dynamics in testicular feminization syndrome. J Clin Endocrinol Metab 1972; 34(1):229–234.

Kallmann F, Schoenfeld W, Barrera S: The genetic aspects of primary eunuchoidism. Am J Ment Defi 1944; 48:203–236.

Kalra SP: Opioid peptides—inhibitory neuronal systems in regulation of gonadotropin secretion. *In* McCann SM, Dhindsa D, eds: Role of Peptides and Proteins in Control of Reproduction. New York, Elsevier Biomedical, 1983, pp 63–87.

Kalra SP, Kalra PS: Neural regulation of luteinizing hormone secretion in the rat. Endocr Rev 1983; 4(4):311–351.

Kaplan SL, Grumbach MM, Aubert ML: The ontogenesis of pituitary hormones and hypothalamic factors in the human fetus: Maturation of central nervous system regulation of anterior pituitary function. Rec Prog Horm Res 1976; 32:161.

Kerr JB, Maddocks S, Sharpe RM: Testosterone and FSH have independent, synergistic and stage-dependent effects upon spermatogenesis in the rat testis. Cell Tissue Res 1992; 268:179–189.

Keye WR Jr, Kelch RP, Niswender GD, Jaffe RB: Quantitation of endogenous and exogenous gonadotropin releasing hormone by radioimmunoassay. J Clin Endocrinol Metab 1973; 36:1263.

Klein DC, Moore RY: Pineal *N*-acetyltransferase and hydroxyindole-O-methyltransferase: Control by the retina hypothalamic tract and the suprachiasmatic nucleus. Brain Res 1979; 174(2):245–262.

Kley HK, Nieschlag E, Bidlingmaier F, Kruskemper HL: Possible age dependent influence of estrogens on the binding of testosterone in plasma of adult men. Horm Metab Res 1974; 6(3):213–216.

Knobil E: The neuroendocrine control of menstrual cycle. Rec Prog Horm Res 1980; 36:53.

Kohler PO, Ross GT, Odell WD: Metabolic clearance and production rates of human luteinizing hormone in pre- and postmenopausal women. J Clin Invest 1968; 47:38.

Kreutz LE, Rose RM, Jennings R: Suppression of plasma testosterone levels and psychologic stress. Arch Gen Psychiatry 1972; 26(5):479–482.

Labrie F, Auclair C, Cusan L, et al: Inhibitory effects of LHRH and its agonists on testicular gonadotropin receptors and spermatogenesis in the rat. Int J Androl 1978; 2(Suppl):303.

Lachelin GCL, Leblanc H, Yen SSC: The inhibitory effect of dopamine agonists in LH in women. J Clin Endocrinol Metab 1977; 44(4):728–732.

Leblanc H, Lachelin GC, Abu-Fadil S, Yen SSC: Effects of dopamine infusion on pituitary hormone secretion in humans. J Clin Endocrinol Metab 1976; 43(3):668–674.

Leonard JM, Leach RB, Couture M, Paulsen CA: Plasma and urinary follicle-stimulating hormone levels in oligospermia: J Clin Endocrinol Metab 1972; 34(1):209–214.

Lewis JG, Ghanadian R, Chisholm GD: Serum 5 alphadihydrotestosterone and testosterone: Changes with age in men. Acta Endocrinol 1976; 82:444.

Lin D, Sugawara T, Strauss JF, et al: Role of steroidogenic acute regulatory protein in adrenal and gonadal steroidogenesis. Science 1995; 267:1828.

Ling N, Ying SY, Ueno N, et al: Isolation and partial characterization of a Mr32,000 protein with inhibin activity from porcine follicular fluid. Proc Natl Acad Sci USA 1985; 82(21):7217–7221.

Longcope C, Kato T, Horton R: The conversion of blood androgens to estrogens in normal adult men and women. J Clin Invest 1969; 48(12):2191–2201.

Malacara JM, Seyler LE Jr, Reichlin S: Luteinizing hormone releasing factor activity in peripheral blood from women during the midcycle luteinizing hormone ovulatory surge. J Clin Endocrinol Metab 1972; 34:271.

Marshall JC: Clinics in endocrinology and metabolism. Investigative procedures. Clin Endocrinol Metab 1975; 4:545.

Marshall JC, Anderson DC, Fraser TR, Harsoulis P: Human luteinizing hormone in man: Studies of metabolism and biological action. Endocrinology 1973; 56:431.

Marshall JC, Harsoulis P, Anderson DC, et al: Isolated pituitary gonadotropin deficiency: Gonadotrophin secretion after synthetic luteinizing hormone and follicle stimulating hormone-releasing hormone. BMJ 1972; 4:643.

Marynick SP, Loriaux DL, Sherins RJ, et al: Evidence that testosterone can suppress pituitary gonadotropin secretion independently of peripheral aromatization. J Clin Endocrinol Metab 1979; 49(3):396–398.

Masotto C, Wisniewski G, Negro-Vilar A: Different γ-aminobutyric acid receptor subtypes are involved in the regulation of opiate-dependent and -independent luteinizing hormone-releasing hormone secretion. Endocrinology 1989; 125(1):548–553.

Matsumoto AM, Karpas AE, Bremner WJ: Chronic human chorionic gonadotropin administration in normal men: Evidence that follicle stimulating hormone is necessary for the maintenance of quantitatively normal spermatogenesis in man. J Clin Endocrinol Metab 1986; 62:1186.

Matsumoto AM, Karpas AE, Paulsen CA, Bremner WJ: Reinitiation of sperm production in gonadotropin-suppressed normal men by administration of follicle-stimulating hormone. J Clin Invest 1983; 72:1005.

McCann SM, Moss RL: Putative neurotransmitter involved in discharging gonadotropin-releasing neuro-hormones and the action of LH releasing hormone on the CNS. Life Sci 1975; 16:833.

McCullagh DR, Walsh EL: Experimental hypertrophy and atrophy of thc prostate gland. Endocrinology 1935; 19:466–470.

McLachlan RI, Matsumoto AM, Burger HG, et al: Relative roles of follicle-stimulating hormone and luteinizing hormone in the control of inhibin secretion in normal men. J Clin Invest 1988; 82:880–884.

McLachlan RI, Robertson DM, deKretser DM, Burger HG: Inhibin, a nonsteroidal regulation of pituitary follicle stimulating hormone. Baillieres Clin Endocrinol Metab 1987; 1(1):89–112.

McLachlan RI, Wreford ND, Tsonis C, DeKretser D, Robertson DM: Testosterone effects on spermatogenesis in the gonadotropin-releasing hormone-immunized rat. Biol Reprod 1994; 50:271–280.

Michael RP: Hormonal steroids and sexual communication in primates. J Steroid Biochem 1975; 6(3–4):161–170.

Miyamoto K, Hasegawa Y, Fukuda M, et al: Isolation of porcine follicular fluid inhibin of 32K daltons. Biochem Biophys Res Comm 1985; 129(2):396–403.

Moore RY: Retinohypothalamic projection in mammals: A comparative study. Brain Res 1973; 49(2):403–409.

Muta K, Kato K-I, Akamine Y, Ibayashi H: Age related changes in the feedback regulation of gonadotropin secretion by sex steroids in men. Acta Endocrinol 1981; 96(2):154–162.

Naftolin F, Feder HH: Suppression of luteinizing hormone secretion in male rats by 5 alpha-androstan-17 beta-ol-3-one (dihydrotestosterone) propionate. J Endocrinol 1973; 56(1):155–156.

Naftolin F, Ryan KJ, Petro Z: Aromatization of androstenedione by the diencephalon. J Clin Endocrinol Metab 1971; 33(2):368–370.

Nett TM, Akbar AM, Niswender GD: Serum levels of luteinizing hormone and gonadotropin-releasing hormone in cycling, castrated and anestrous ewes. Endocrinology 1974; 94:713.

Nowak FV, Swerdloff RS: Gonadotropin-releasing hormone (GnRH) release by superfused hypothalami in response to norepinephrine. Biol Reprod 1985; 33(4):790–796.

Odell WD: Humoral manifestations of nonendocrine neoplasms—ectopic hormone production. *In* Williams RH, ed: Textbook of Endocrinology, 5th ed. Philadelphia, W. B. Saunders Company, 1974, p 1105.

Papkoff H, Sairam MR, Farmer SW, Li CH: Studies on the structure and function of interstitial-cell stimulating hormone. Recent Prog Horm Res 1973; 29:563.

Parvinen M: Regulation of the seminiferous epithelium. Endocr Rev 1982; 3:404.

Parvinen M: Cyclic function of Sertoli cells. *In* Russell LD, Griswold MD, eds: The Sertoli Cell. Clearwater, FL, Cache River Press, 1993, pp 331–347.

Paulsen CA: Discussion. *In* Rosenberg E, ed: Gonadotropins. Los Altos, Geron-X, 1968, pp 163–166.

Paulsen CA, Gordon DL, Carpenter RW, et al: Klinefelter's syndrome and its variants: A hormonal and chromosomal study. Recent Prog Horm Res 1968; 24:321–363.

Pierce JG: The subunits of pituitary thyrotropin—their relationship to other glycoprotein hormones. Endocrinology 1971; 89:1331.

Pierce JG, Parsons TF: Glycoprotein hormones structure and function. Annu Rev Biochem 1981; 50:465–496.

Plant TM, Zorub DS: Pinealectomy in agonadal infantile male rhesus monkeys (Macaca mulatta) does not interrupt initiation of the prepubertal hiatus in gonadotropin secretion. Endocrinology 1986; 118(1):227–232.

Rasmussen DD: New concepts in the regulation of hypothalamic gonadotropin releasing hormone (GnRH) secretion. J Endocrinol Invest 1986; 9(5):427–437.

Reichert LE, Ward DN: On the isolation and characterization of thc alpha and beta subunits of human pituitary follicle-stimulating hormone. Endocrinology 1974; 94:655.

Reid RL, Hoff JD, Yen SSC, Li CH: Effects of exogenous beta h-endorphin on its disappearance rate in normal human subjects. J Clin Endocrinol Metab 1981; 52(6):1179–1184.

Reiter RJ: Thc pineal and its hormones in the control of reproduction in mammals. Endocr Rev 1980; 1(2):109–131.

Reppert SM, Klein DC: Mammalian pineal gland: Basic and clinical aspects. *In* Motta M, ed: The Endocrine Functions of thc Brain. New York, Raven Press, 1980, pp 327–371.

Rea MA, Marshall GR, Weinbauer GF, Nieschlag E: Testosterone maintains pituitary and serum FSH and spermatogenesis in GnRH-antagonist suppressed rats. J Endocrinol 1986; 108:101–107.

Risbridger GP, deKretser DM: Paracrine regulation of the testis. *In* Burger H, deKretser D, eds: The Testis. New York, Raven Press, 1989, pp 255–268.

Rittmaster RS, Lemay A, Zwicker H, et al: Effect of finasteride, a 5α-reductase inhibitor, on serum gonadotropins in normal men. J Clin Endocrinol Metab 1992; 75:484–488.

Ritzen EM, Hansson V, French FS: The Sertoli cell. *In* Burger H, deKretser D, eds: The Testis. New York, Raven Press, 1981, pp 171-194.

Rivier J, Spiess J, McClintock R, et al: Purification and partial characterization of inhibin from porcine follicular fluid. Biochem Biophys Res Comm 1985; 133(1):120–127.

Rivier C, Rivier J, Vale W: Inhibin mediated feedback control of FSH secretion in the female rat. Science 1986; 234:205–208.

Roberts KP, Awoniyi CA, Santulli R, Zirkin BR: Regulation of Sertoli cell transferrin and sulfated glycoprotein-2 messenger ribonucleic acid levels during the restoration of spermatogenesis in the adult hypophysectomized rat. Endocrinology 1991; 129:3417–3423.

Robertson DM, Foulds LM, Levershar L, et al: Isolation of inhibin from bovine follicular fluid. Biochem Biophys Res Comm 1985; 126(1):220–226.

Ropert JF, Quigley ME, Yen SSC: Endogenous opiates modulate pulsate luteinizing hormone release in humans. J Clin Endocrinol Metab 1981; 52(3):583–585.

Rosen SW, Weintraub BD: Monotropic increase of serum FSH correlated with low sperm count in young men with idiopathic oligospermia and aspermia. J Clin Endocrinol Metab 1971; 32(3):410–416.

Rubens R, Dhont M, Vermeulen A: Further studies on Leydig cell function in old age. J Clin Endocrinol Metab 1974; 39:40.

Russell LD, Corbin TJ, Borg KE, et al: Recombinant human follicle-stimulating hormone is capable of exerting a biological effect in the adult hypophysectomized rat by reducing the number of degenerating germ cells. Endocrinology 1993; 133:2062–2070.

Santen RJ, Paulsen CA: Hypogonadotropic eunuchoidism I. Clinical study of the mode of inheritance. J Clin Endocrinol Metab 1973; 36:47–54.

Santen RJ, Bardin CW: Episodic luteinizing hormone secretion in man: Pulse analysis, clinical interpretation, physiologic mechanisms. J Clin Invest 1973; 52:2617.

Santen RJ: Is aromatization of testosterone to estradiol required for inhibition of LH secretion in men? J Clin Invest 1975; 56:1555–1563.

Santulli R, Sprando RL, Awoniyi CA, et al: To what extent can spermatogenesis be maintained in the hypophysectomized adult rat testis with exogenously administered testosterone? Endocrinology 1990; 126:95–101.

Sawyer CH: Functions of the amygdala related to feedback actions of gonadal steroid hormones. In Eleftheriou BE, ed: Neurobiology of the Amygdala. New York, Plenum Press, 1972, pp 745–752.

Sawyer CH: Some recent developments in brain-pituitary ovarian physiology. Neuroendocrinology 1975; 17(2):97–124.

Schaison G, Young J, Pholsena M, et al: Failure of combined follicle-stimulating hormone–testosterone administration to initiate and/or maintain spermatogenesis in men with hypogonadotropic hypogonadism. J Clin Endocrinol Metab 1993; 77:1545–1549.

Schally AV, Nair RM, Redding A, Arimura TW: Isolation of the luteinizing hormone and follicle-stimulating hormone–releasing hormone from porcine hypothalami. J Biol Chem 1971; 246:7230.

Sheckter CB, McLachlan RI, Tenover JS, et al: Stimulation of serum inhibin concentrations by gonadotropin-releasing hormone in men with idiopathic hypogonadotropic hypogonadism. J Clin Endocrinol Metab 1988; 67 (6):1221–1224.

Sherins RJ, Loriaux DL: Studies of the role of sex steroids in the feedback control of FSH concentrations in men. J Clin Endocrinol Metab 1973; 36(5):886–893.

Sherins RJ, Winters SJ, Wachslicht H: Studies of the role of hCG and low dose FSH in initiating spermatogenesis in hypogonadotropic men. (Abstract.) Chicago, Annual Meeting of The Endocrine Society, June, 1977.

Shome B, Parlow AF: Human follicle stimulating hormone: First proposal for the amino acid sequence of the hormone-specific, beta subunit (hFSH)b. J Clin Endocrinol Metab 1974; 39:203.

Sinha-Hikim AP, Swerdloff RS: Temporal and stage-specific effects of recombinant human follicle-stimulating hormone on the maintenance of spermatogenesis in gonadotropin-releasing hormone antagonist-treated rat. Endocrinology 1995; 136:253–261.

Snyder PJ. Reitano JF, Utiger RD: Serum LH and FSH responses to synthetic gonadotrophin releasing hormone in normal men. J Clin Endocrinol Metab 1975; 41:938.

Snyder PJ, Rudenstein RS, Garder DF, Rothman JA: Repetitive infusion of gonadotropin-releasing hormone distinguishes hypothalamic from pituitary hypogonadism. J Clin Endocrinol Metab 1979; 48:864.

Snyder PJ: Gonadotroph cell adenomas of the pituitary. Endocr Rev 1985; 6:552–563.

Spark RF, White RA, Connolly PB: Impotence is not always psychogenic: Newer insights into hypothalamic-pituitary-gonadal dysfunction. JAMA 1980; 243:750–755.

Sparrow D, Bossc R, Rowe JW: The influence of age, alcohol consumption and body build on gonadal function in men. J Clin Endocrinol Metab 1980; 51:5S.

Steinberger E: Hormonal control of mammalian spermatogenesis. Physiol Rev 1971; 51(1):1–22.

Stewart-Bentley M, Odell WD, Horton R: The feedback control of luteinizing hormone. J Clin Endocrinol Metab 1974; 38(4):545–553.

Sun YT, Wreford NG, Roberston DM, deKretser DM: Quantitative cytological studies of spermatogenesis in intact and hypophysectomized rats: Identification of androgen-dependent stages. Endocrinology 1990; 127:1215–1223.

Swerdloff RS, Bhasin S, Heber D: Effect of GnRH superactive analogs (alone and combined with androgen) on testicular function in man and experimental animals. J Steroid Biochem 19:491, 1983.

Swerdloff RS, Heber D: Effects of aging on male reproductive function. *In* Korenman S, ed: The Endocrinology of Aging. New York, Elsevier, 1982, pp 119–135.

Swerdloff RS, Jacobs HS, Odell WD: Hypothalamic-pituitary-gonadal interrelationships in the rat during sexual maturation. *In* Saxena BB, Beling CG, Gandy HM, et al, eds: Gonadotropins. New York, John Wiley & Sons, 1972, pp 546–566.

Swerdloff RS, Odell WD: Gonadotropins: Present concepts in the human. Calif Med 1968; 109:467.

Swerdloff RS, Odell WD: Hormonal mechanisms in the onset of puberty. Postgrad Med 1975; J 51:200.

Swerdloff RS, Walsh PC: Testosterone and estradiol suppression of LH and FSH in adult male rats: Duration of castration, duration of treatment and combined treatment. Acta Endocrinol 1973; 73(1):11–21.

Swerdloff RS, Walsh PC, Jacobs HS, Odell WD: Serum LH and FSH during sexual maturation in thc male rat: Effect of castration and cryptorchidism. Endocrinology 1971; 88(1):120–128.

Swerdloff RS, Walsh PC, Odell WD: Control of LH and FSH secretion in the male: Evidence that aromatization of androgens to estradiol is not required by inhibition of gonadotropin secretion. Steroids 1972; 20(1):13–22.

Swerdloff RS, Wang C: Androgen deficiency and aging in men. West J Med 1993; 159:579–585.

Tenover JS: Androgen administration to aging men. Endocrinol Metab Clin North Am 1994; 23:877–892.

Tenover JS, Dahl KD, Hsueh AJW, et al: Serum bioactive and immunoreactive follicle-stimulating hormone in levels and the response to clemiphere in healthy young and elderly men. J Clin Endocrinol Metab 1987; 64:1103.

Tenover JS, Matsumoto AM, Clifton DK, Bremner WJ: Age-related alterations in the circadian rhythms of pulsatile luteinizing hormone and testosterone secretion in healthy men. J Gerontol 1988; 43(6):M163–169.

Thorner MO, Evans WS, MacLeod RM, et al: Hypoprolactinemia: Current concepts of management including medical therapy with bromocriptine. *In* Goldstein M, Lieberman A, Cahre DB, Thorner MO, eds: Advances in Biochemical Psychopharmacology, Vol. 23. Ergot Compounds and Brain Function. Neuroendocrine and Neuropsychiatric Aspects. New York, Raven Press, 1980, pp 165–189.

Tolis G, Ackman D, Stellos A, et al: Tumor growth inhibition in patients with prostatic carcinoma treated with LHRH agonists. Proc Natl Acad Sci USA 1982; 79:1658.

Vaishnav M, Moudgal NR: Role of FSH in regulating testicular germ cell transformation in the rat: A study using DNA flow cytometry. Andrologia 1994; 26:111–117.

Van Hall EV, Vaitukaitis JL, Ross GT,et al: Immunological and biological activity of HCG following progressive desialylation. Endocrinology 1971; 88:456–464.

Van Thiel DH, Sherins RJ, Myers GH Jr, DeVita VT Jr: Evidence for a specific seminiferous tubular factor affecting follicle-stimulating hormone secretion in man. J Clin Invest 1972; 51(4):1009–1019.

Vaughan GM: Melatonin in humans. *In* Reiter RJ ed: Pineal Research Reviews, Vol. 2. New York, Alan R. Liss, 1984, pp 141–201.

Vermeulen A, Rubens R, Verdonck L: Testosterone secretion and metabolism in male senescence. J Clin Endocrinol Metab 1972; 34:730.

Vickery BH: Comparison of the potential for therapeutic utilities with gonadotropin-releasing hormone agonists and antagonists. Endocr Rev 1986; 7:115.

Waldhauser F, Weiszenbacher G, Frisch H, et al: Fall in nocturnal serum melatonin during pre-puberty in pubescence. Lancet 1984; 1(8373):362–365.

Walsh PC, Madden JD, Harrod MJ, et al: Familial incomplete male pseudohermaphroditism: Type II. Decrease dihydrotestosterone formation in pseudovaginal perineoscrotal hypospadias. N Engl J Med 1974; 291:944.

Walsh PC, Swerdloff RS, Odell WD: Feedback control of FSH in the male: Role of estrogen. Acta Endocrinol 1973; 74:449.

Wang C: Bioassays of follicle-stimulating hormone. Endocr Rev 1988; 9:374.

Wang C, Chan V, Yeung RTT: The effect of heroin addiction on pituitary-testicular function. Clin Endocrinol 1978; 9(5):455–461.

Ward DN, Reichert LE Jr, Liu WK, et al: Chemical studies of luteinizing hormone from human and ovine pituitaries. Recent Prog Horm Res 1973; 29:533.

Warner BA, Dufau ML, Santen RJ: Effects of aging and illness on the pituitary testicular axis in men: Qualitative as well as quantitative changes in luteinizing hormone. J Clin Endocrinol Metab 1985; 60:263.

Weiner RI, Ganong WF: Role of brain monoamines and histamine in regulation of anterior pituitary secretion. Physiol Rev 1978; 58(4):905–976.

Whitcomb RW, O'Dea L St, Finkelstein JS, et al: Utility of free alpha-subunit as an alternative neuroendocrine marker of GnRH stimulation of the gonadotroph in the human: Evidence from normal and GnRH-deficient men. J Clin Endocrinol Metab 1990; 70:1654–1661.

Wildt L, Hansler A, Marshall G, et al: Frequency and amplitude of gonadotropin-releasing hormone stimulation and gonadotropin secretion in the Rhesus monkey. Endocrinology 1981; 109:376.

Wilkinson M, Arendt J, Bradtke J, de Ziegler D: Determination of a dark-induced increase in pineal *N*-acetyl-transferase activity and simultaneous radioimmunoassay of melatonin in pineal, serum, and pituitary tissue of the male rat. Endocrinology 1977; 72(2):243–244.

Wilson JD, Harrod MJ, Goldstein JL, et al: Familial incomplete male pseudohermaphroditism: Type I. N Engl J Med 1974; 290:1097.

Winters SJ: Inhibin is released together with testosterone by the human testis. J Clin Endocrinol Metab 1990; 70:548–550.

Winters SJ, Troen P: Episodic luteinizing hormone (LH) secretion and the response of LH and follicle-stimulating hormone to LH-releasing hormone in aged men: Evidence for coexistent primary testicular insufficiency and an impairment in gonadotropin secretion. J Clin Endocrinol Metab 1982; 55:560.

Wollesen F, Swerdloff RS, Odell WD: LH and FSH responses to luteinizing releasing hormones in normal adult human males. Metabolism 1976; 25:1275.

Wollesen F, Swerdloff RS, Peterson M, Odell WD: Testosterone (T) modulation of pituitary response to LRH: Differential effects on luteinizing hormone (LH) and follicle-stimulating hormone (FSH). J Clin Invest 1974; 53:85a.

Wu FCW, Butler GE, Kelnar CJ, Sellar RE: Patterns of pulsatile luteinizing hormone secretion before and during the onset of puberty in boys: a study using an immunoradiometric assay. J Clin Endocrinol Metab 1990; 70:629.

Wurtman RJ: Fall in nocturnal serum melatonin during prepuberty and pubescence. Lancet 1984; 1:362.

Wurtman RJ, Waldhauser F: Melatonin in humans. J Neurol Transm 1986; 21(Suppl):1–8.

Yen SSC: Prolactin in human reproduction. *In* Yen SSC, Jaffe RB eds: Reproductive Endocrinology: Physiology, Pathophysiology and Clinical Management. Philadelphia, W. B. Saunders Company, 1986, pp 237–263.

Ying SY, Czvik J, Becker A, et al: Secretion of FSH and production of inhibin are reciprocally related. Proc Natl Acad Sci USA 1987; 84:4631–4635.

Ying SY: Inhibins, activins and follistatins: Gonadal proteins modulating the secretion of follicle-stimulating hormone. Endocr Rev 1988; 9:267–293.

Yoshimoto Y, Moridera K, Imura H: Restoration of normal pituitary gonadotropin reserve by administration of luteinizing hormone–releasing hormone in patients with hypogonadotropic hypogonadism. N Engl J Med 1975; 292:242.

Zacharias L, Wurtman R: Blindness: Its relation to age of menarche. Science 1964; 144:1154–1155.

42

PHYSIOLOGY OF MALE REPRODUCTION: THE TESTIS, EPIDIDYMIS, AND DUCTUS DEFERENS

Peter N. Schlegel, M.D.
Thomas S. K. Chang, Ph.D.*

Testis
- Gross Structures and Vascularization
- Cytoarchitecture and Functions of the Testis
- Sertoli Cell–to–Germ Cell Associations
- The Germinal Epithelium
- Hormonal Regulation of Spermatogenesis
- Age-Related Changes in the Testis and in Spermatogenesis

Epididymis
- Gross Structures
- Contractile Tissue
- Innervation
- Vascularization
- Epididymal Epithelium
- Functions of the Epididymis
- Control of Epididymal Function

Spermatozoa

Ductus Deferens
- Vascularization and Innervation
- Cytoarchitecture of the Ductus Deferens
- Functions of the Ductus Deferens

Regnier de Graaf's treatise of 1668 asserting that the fertilizing portion of semen was produced in the testis was followed by van Leuwenhoek's initial description of spermatozoa in 1677 and von Kolliker's demonstration in 1841 that spermatozoa were produced through cellular division within the seminiferous tubules. Subsequently, Leydig presented the first critical study of the intertubular tissue of the testis in 1850 and Sertoli described the nongerminal cells of the seminiferous tubules in 1865. In this century, reports by Young in 1930 and Belonoshkin in 1942 established that spermatozoa undergo fertility and motility maturation, respectively, in the epididymis.

These early investigations prompted an exponential increase in the number of studies of male reproductive physiology over the past 50 years; studies that show that the production of spermatozoa is a complex process that requires many weeks from the initial mitotic divisions through the myriad changes readying it for ejaculation and fertilization. Highlights of this intricate process within the testis include (1) the initial mitotic divisions that produce either a set of stem cells relatively resistant to external injury or a population of rapidly proliferating germ cells destined to become spermatozoa; (2) meiosis, within a unique intratesticular environment created in part by Sertoli and interstitial cells, that results in the formation of the haploid gamete; and (3) the dramatic differentiation of the prospective gamete into a specialized cell ideally suited for transit through the female reproductive tract and, ultimately, fertilization. Epididymal maturation processes involving spermatozoa include the acquisition of the capacity for progressive motility and the ability to fertilize.

New laboratory procedures involving assisted reproductive technologies have permitted spermatozoa and their precursors to fertilize under circumstances that would otherwise preclude fertilization (Kimura and Yanagimachi, 1995; Palermo et al, 1995; Tesarik et al, 1995). These laboratory procedures, in combination with molecular studies of male reproductive function, have underscored the importance of understanding the role of the male reproductive tract in the normal production and development of spermatozoa and

*Published posthumously.

the unique contributions of spermatozoa to the fertilization process and embryo development (Cummins and Jequier, 1994; Schatten, 1994). The objective of this chapter is to summarize earlier and more recent studies describing the structure and function of the human testis, epididymis, ductus deferens, and spermatozoon. Where there is a paucity of information about the human systems, we will provide knowledge obtained from the study of experimental animals.

TESTIS

Gross Structures and Vascularization

In healthy young men, the ovoid testis measures 15 to 25 ml in volume (Prader, 1966) and has a length of approximately 4.5 to 5.1 cm (Tishler, 1971; Winter and Faiman, 1972). The testicular parenchyma is surrounded by a capsule made up of three layers—the outer visceral layer of the tunica vaginalis, the tunica albuginea, and the innermost layer of the tunica vasculosa. The tunica albuginea contains large numbers of branching smooth muscle cells that course through the predominantly collagenous tissue (Langford and Heller, 1973). These smooth muscle cells may impart a contractile capability to the human testicular capsule because contractions have been elicited in the isolated testicular capsule from humans (Rikimaru and Shirai, 1972) and other species (Davis and Langford, 1969, 1970; Rikimaru and Suzuki, 1972) by electrical stimulation and specific autonomic drugs. In humans and several other species, capsular smooth muscle tone or contractions may affect blood flow into the testis (Schweitzer, 1929), because the testicular artery traverses the capsule at an oblique angle. Whether capsular smooth muscle contraction plays a significant role in promoting the flow of seminiferous tubule fluid out of the testis (Davis and Horowitz, 1978) is uncertain because some fluid flow from the rat rete testis is maintained after removal of the capsule (Free et al, 1980).

Within the capsule, the testis is divided into compartments separated by the septum of the testis. Within each septum are the seminiferous tubules, which contain the developing germ cells, as well as interstitial tissue. **Interstitial tissue is comprised of Leydig cells, mast cells, and macrophages, as well as nerves and blood and lymph vessels. In humans, interstitial tissue takes up 20% to 30% of the total testicular volume** (Setchell and Brooks, 1988). The relationship between seminiferous tubules and interstitial tissue is demonstrated in Figure 42–1.

The seminiferous tubules are long U-shaped tubules. The combined length of the 600 to 1200 tubules in the human testis is approximately 250 meters (Lennox and Ahmad, 1970) (Fig. 42–2). The two ends of each seminiferous tubule are connected to short, straight segments, the tubuli recti, which open into the rete testis. Roosen-Runge and Holstein (1978) suggested that the rete testis topography acts as a valve with a built-in mechanism for activating the flow of fluid and spermatozoa toward the epididymis. The rete testis coalesces to form the ductuli efferentes, which act as conduits to carry testicular fluid and spermatozoa into the caput epididymis (see Fig. 42–2). Readers are referred to publications by Ilio and Hess (1994) and Setchell and coworkers (1994) for detailed descriptions of the anatomy and

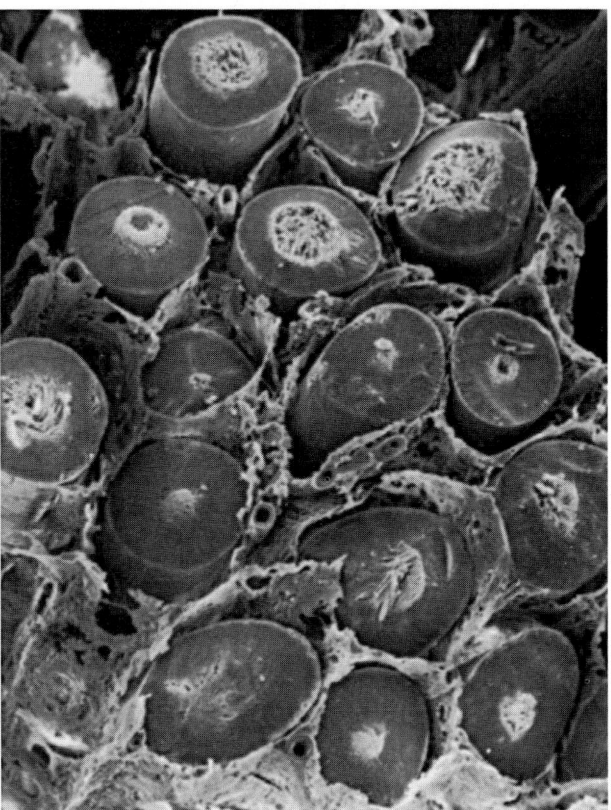

Figure 42–1. Scanning electron micrograph of the cut surface of the human testis. Note the relationship of interstitial tissue to seminiferous tubules. (From Christensen AK: *In* Greep RO, Astwood WB, eds: Handbook of Physiology, Section 7. Male Reproductive System. Baltimore, The Williams & Wilkins Company, 1975, pp 339–351. Copyright 1975, The American Physiological Society, Bethesda, Md.)

histology of the rete testis in animals and humans. **In humans, 6 to 15 ductuli efferentes lead from the rete testis to the epididymis** (Jonte and Holstein, 1987; Saithoh et al, 1990; Ilio and Hess, 1994). In an excellent study, Yeung and colleagues (1991) reported that the ductuli efferentes leave the testis as straight tubules, then, traveling distally, in succession become highly coiled lobules, branch into thin tubules, and join a network of coiled dark tubules that ultimately connect with the epididymis proper in both end-to-end and end-to-side junctions.

The testis has no somatic innervation but receives autonomic innervation primarily from the intermesenteric nerves and renal plexus (Mitchell, 1935). These nerves run along the testicular artery to the testis. Baumgarten and associates (1968) found that the testicular adrenergic innervation is restricted primarily to small blood vessels supplying clusters of Leydig cells. These authors concluded that the sympathetic-adrenergic innervation is of little importance for the functional integrity of the testis in humans. Other studies, however, suggest that vascular tone in the testis appears to be at least partially under nervous control (Linzell and Setchell, 1969). (See Hodson [1970] for a complete discussion of testicular and epididymal innervation.)

The human testicular parenchyma is provided with approximately 9 ml of blood/100 g of tissue/minute (Petterson et al, 1973). Fritjofsson and co-workers (1969) claimed that in humans, blood flow to the left testis varies from 1.6 to

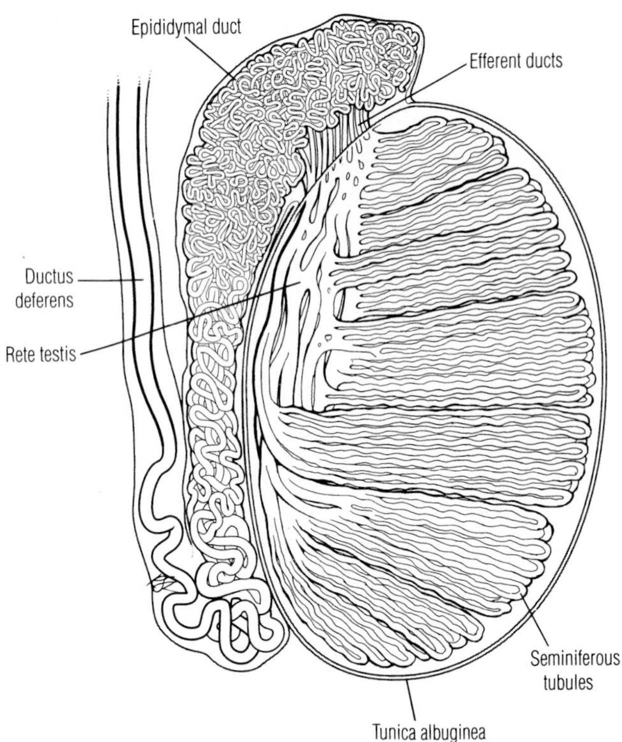

Figure 42–2. The human testis showing the seminiferous tubules, epididymis, and ductus deferens. (Illustration based on dissections in Hirsh AV: The anatomical preparations of the human testis and epididymis in the Glasgow Hunterian Collection. Human Reproduction Update 1995, 1995; 1:515–521.)

12.4 ml/100 mg/minute, whereas that to the right testis ranges from 3.2 to 38.5 ml/100 g/minute. The significance of this variation in testicular blood flow is unknown.

The vasculature of the mammalian testis has been thoroughly discussed in excellent reviews (Gunn and Gould, 1975; Free, 1977; Setchell and Brooks, 1988). **The arterial supply to the human testis and epididymis is derived from three sources: the internal spermatic artery, the deferential artery, and the external spermatic or cremasteric artery** (Harrison and Barclay, 1948). The internal spermatic artery arises from the abdominal aorta just below the renal artery and becomes a component of the spermatic cord above the internal inguinal ring. From a practical standpoint, it is important to consider the number of testicular arteries that are present in the spermatic cord at the inguinal level. **Jarow and colleagues (1992) found an average of two arteries during intraoperative dissection with loupes, but 2.4 arteries in the inguinal region could be identified in cadaveric dissections. Another intraoperative dissection study of over 100 spermatic cords identified a single artery at 10 to 15 × magnification in 50% of cases, two arteries in 30%, and three arteries in 20%** (Beck et al, 1992). Within the spermatic cord, the arteries are intimately associated with a network of anastomotic veins that eventually form the pampiniform plexus. **The vascular arrangement in the pampiniform plexus, with the counterflowing artery and veins separated only by the thickness of their vascular walls in some areas (Harrison, 1949a), facilitates the exchange of heat and small molecules.** For example, testosterone is transported from the vein to the artery via a concentration-limited, passive diffusion process in men (Bayard et al, 1975). The countercurrent exchange of heat in the spermatic cord provides blood to the testis that is 2 to 4°C lower than rectal temperature in the normal individual (Agger, 1971). A loss of the temperature differential is associated with testicular dysfunction in humans with idiopathic infertility, as well as those with varicocele (Mieussett et al, 1987) and cryptorchidism (Marshall and Elder, 1982).

Leaving the pampiniform plexus and extending to the mediastinal area of the testis, the spermatic artery becomes highly coiled and branches before entering the testis. Kormano and Suoranta (1971) completed an angiographic study of the arterial pattern of 78 human autopsy testes and observed that **a single artery enters the testis in 56% of cases, two branches enter in 31% of cases, and three or more branches enter in 13% of cases.** Within the testis, the artery divides into a series of centrifugal arteries that penetrate the testicular parenchyma. Subsequent branches give rise to a dual set of arterioles that supply blood to individual intertubular and peritubular capillaries (Muller, 1957). The capillaries inside the columns of interstitial tissue are called the intertubular capillaries, whereas the rope ladder–like capillaries running near the seminiferous tubules are called the peritubular capillaries. In their study of testicular microvasculature, Takayama and Tomoyoshi (1981) have questioned whether this distinct intertubular and peritubular capillary arrangement is present throughout the human testis.

Testicular blood flow appears to be regulated at several levels. Autoregulation of flow through the testicular artery may involve myogenic mechanisms in the subcapsular region of the artery, at least in the rat (Davis, 1990). In addition, although total testicular blood flow is relatively constant, the regional distribution of flow within the testis is thought to vary significantly based on local metabolic needs. For example, local peptide effectors such as luteinizing hormone (LH) appear to be transported relatively rapidly across the continuous endothelium of testicular capillaries, while testosterone, produced in the interstitium, emerges from the testis predominantly in testicular venous effluent, not in lymph (Desjardins, 1989). Finally, differential dilation and constriction of terminal arterioles allow capillary units to be perfused selectively. Taken together, these observations suggest a highly specialized function for the microvasculature of the testis. (See Desjardins [1989] for an excellent discussion of testicular microcirculation.) The exact mechanisms by which the microvasculature may facilitate or affect local testicular function remains to be elucidated.

The veins within the testis are unusual in that they do not run with the corresponding intratesticular arteries. The small veins in the parenchyma empty into either the veins on the surface of the testis or into one of a group of veins near the mediastinum that travel toward the region of the rete (Setchell and Brooks, 1988). These two sets of veins join together with deferential veins to form the pampiniform plexus. Ishigami and colleagues (1970) stated that blood in this venous system tends to stagnate because the spermatic vein is thin-walled, poorly muscularized, and lacks effective valves except at the inflow points into the inferior vena cava or the renal vein. This issue remains controversial.

There are prominent lymphatic ducts in the spermatic cord of the human testis (Wenzel and Kellerman, 1966; Hundeiker, 1971). **The lymph capillaries that give rise to these**

lymph ducts originate within the intertubular spaces and do not penetrate the seminiferous tubules. Obstruction of the lymphatic ducts in the spermatic cord invariably is followed by dilatation of the interstitium but not the seminiferous tubules, suggesting that although the extracellular space of the interstitium is drained via the lymphatics, the seminiferous tubules are not. In some species, testicular lymph is transported to the ipsilateral epididymis (Setchell and Brooks, 1988), suggesting an effect of testicular lymph on epididymal function. Whether there is a testis-epididymis lymphatic system in humans is not known.

The extracellular fluid bathing the Sertoli cells and germinal cells flows from the seminiferous tubules into the rete to form rete testis fluid, which is transported into the caput epididymidis. It was previously thought that the fluid probably originates both from primary secretions within the seminiferous tubules and from epithelial secretions directly into the rete (Tuck et al, 1970; Kormano et al, 1971; Levine and Marsh, 1971). However, Setchell and Waites (1975) suggested that "the majority of the fluid leaving the rete, originates in the tubules." Whatever its origin, rete testis fluid is a dilute suspension of spermatozoa in a fluid isosmotic with plasma.

Setchell and Waites (1975) reported that in the ram, the ion composition and the carbohydrate, amino acid, and protein content of rete testis fluid are markedly different from those in blood plasma or lymphatics. They correctly pointed out that "differences in composition between the fluid inside the seminiferous tubules and excurrent ducts of the testis and blood plasma or testicular lymph make it clear that substances do not diffuse freely into and out of tubules." Extrapolation of this idea led to the concept of a blood-testis barrier, which exists to a greater or lesser extent in numerous species (Setchell and Waites, 1975) including humans (Koskimies et al, 1973). This topic is discussed in detail later in this chapter.

Cytoarchitecture and Functions of the Testis

Interstitium

The interstitium of the testis contains blood vessels, lymph vessels, fibroblastic supporting cells, macrophages, mast cells, and Leydig cells (Fig. 42–3). Macrophages within the testis have been shown to be involved in the regulation of testicular parenchymal cells, including Leydig cells (Hutson, 1994). Stereologic analysis (Kaler and Neaves, 1978) showed that **a testis from a 20-year-old man contained approximately 700 million Leydig cells. Leydig cells alone account for about 5% to 12% of the total volume of the human testis** (Christensen, 1975; Kaler and Neaves, 1978). The mechanisms by which Leydig cells develop and mature are reviewed by Huhtaniemi and Pelliniemi (1992) and Hardy and associates (1991). Evidence obtained after ablation of Leydig cells from mature rat testes with ethane dimethyl sulfonate suggests that paracrine factors within the testis and pituitary luteinizing hormone (LH) influence the differentiation of Leydig cells from precursor cells (Teerds et al, 1988; Keeney and Ewing, 1990). Hardy and co-workers (1991) demonstrated that insulin-like growth factor-I (IGF-I) enhances the production of androgen by purified immature rat Leydig cells and suggested that IGF-I may have a role in the differentiation of Leydig cells during puberty.

The Leydig cell is responsible for the bulk of testicular steroid production. Testosterone, synthesized from the steroid precursor cholesterol, is the principal steroid produced by the human testis (Lipsett, 1974), **although numerous C_{18}, C_{19}, and C_{21} steroids are also produced** (Lipsett, 1974; Ewing and Brown, 1977). It is unclear at present whether the bulk of cholesterol used for testosterone biosynthesis is derived from blood plasma (Andersen and Dietschy, 1977) or from de novo biosynthesis (Charreau et al, 1981). In either event, Figure 42–4 shows that cholesterol from the metabolically active pool must be transported into the mitochondria where a cholesterol side-chain cleavage enzyme converts it to pregnenolone and the C6 fragment, isocaproaldehyde. Pregnenolone must then be transported out of the mitochondrial membrane into the smooth endoplasmic reticulum, where it is converted to testosterone. Testosterone probably then diffuses across the cell membrane and is trapped in the extracellular fluid and blood plasma by steroid-binding macromolecules. This biosynthetic process is schematically demonstrated in Figure 42–4.

The control of Leydig cell steroidogenesis has been reviewed exhaustively (Rommerts et al, 1974; Christensen, 1975; Eik-Nes, 1975; Catt and Dufau, 1976; Dufau and Catt, 1978; Ewing, 1983; Dufau, 1988; Payne and Youngblood, 1995). Suffice it to say that **the primary, acute regulation of testosterone production is dependent on LH.** Facilitated transport of LH (human chorionic gonadotropin) to Leydig cells appears to be mediated by endothelial cells via receptor-mediated transport of LH through the endothelial cells (Ghinea et al, 1994.) **Within Leydig cells, LH probably results in the transport of cholesterol into mitochondria or in the binding of cholesterol to the cholesterol side-chain cleavage enzyme.** Pituitary peptides other than LH (e.g., follicle-stimulating hormone and prolactin) have also been shown to modify LH-stimulated Leydig cell steroidogenesis (see Ewing, 1983). Nonpituitary factors capable of altering the production of steroids by Leydig cells include luteinizing hormone–releasing hormone (Sharpe, 1984); inhibin and activin (Bardin et al, 1989); epidermal growth factor, IGF-I, and transforming growth factor-β (Ascoli and Segaloff, 1989; Saez et al, 1991); prostaglandins (Eik-Nes, 1975); and adrenergic stimulation (Eik-Nes, 1975). Most of this information, however, is derived from in vitro experiments using laboratory animals, and the role of these factors in normal testicular function in humans is uncertain. Other poorly understood autocrine and paracrine effectors of Leydig cell function also have been proposed (for a review of this literature see Skinner et al, 1991). Finally, direct inhibition of Leydig cell steroidogenesis via estrogens and androgens may exist (Ewing, 1983).

Testosterone concentrations in the peripheral blood of men change dramatically during the life cycle. Figure 42–5 shows that a testosterone peak occurs in the blood of the human fetus between 12 and 18 weeks of gestation. Another testosterone peak occurs at approximately 2 months of age (see Fig. 42–5). Testosterone reaches a maximum concentration during the second or third decade of life, then reaches a plateau, and declines thereafter (see Fig. 42–5). Additionally, annual and daily rhythms (see Fig. 42–5, insets

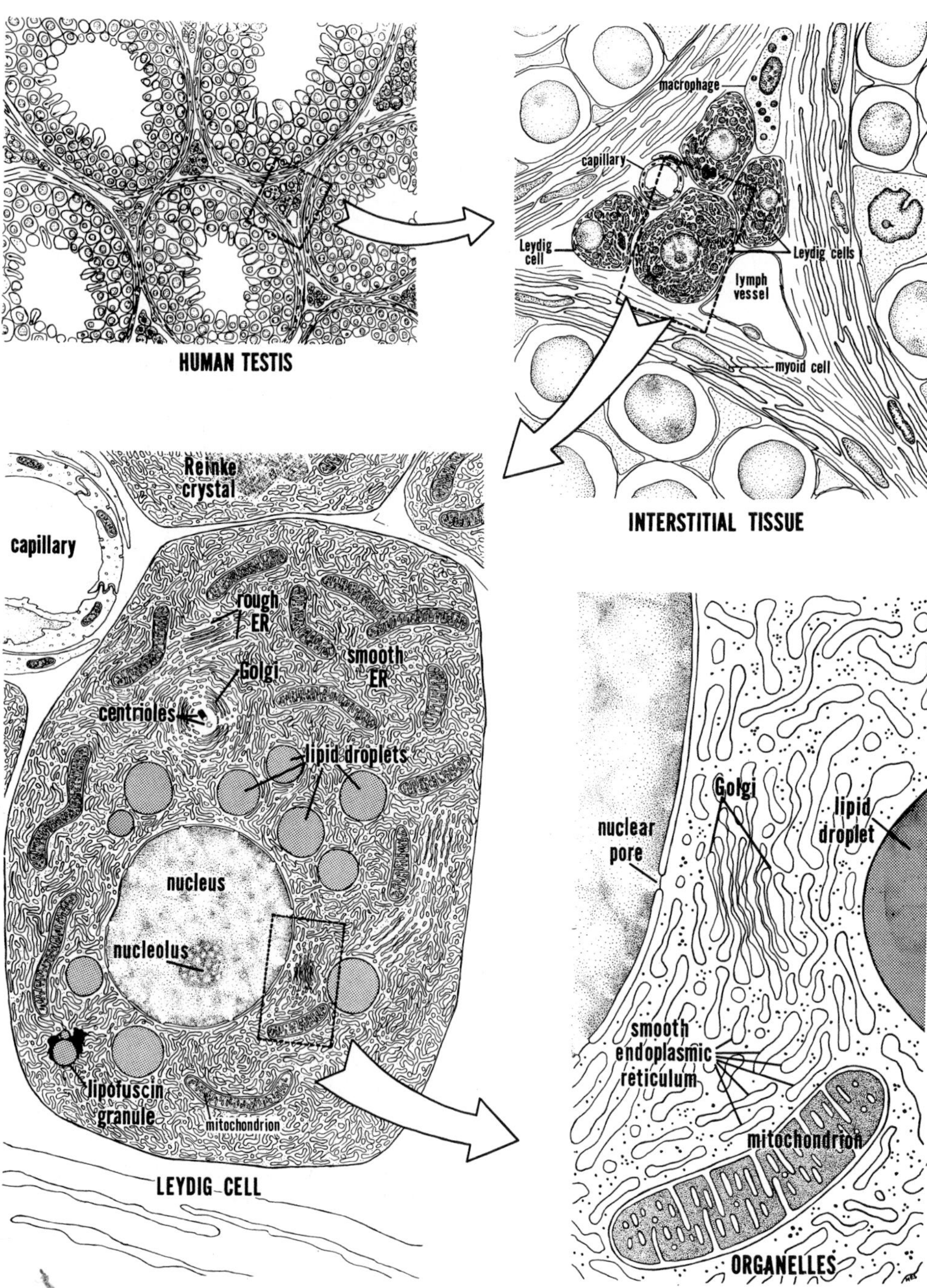

Figure 42–3. Location and fine structure of human Leydig cells. Leydig cells occur in clusters in the interstitial tissue between the seminiferous tubules *(upper left)*. Interstitial tissue *(upper right)* contains macrophages and fibroblasts as well as capillaries and lymph vessels. Seminiferous tubules are surrounded by a boundary layer of myoid cells. The most abundant organelle within the cytoplasm of the Leydig cell is the smooth endoplasmic reticulum *(lower left)*. Some of the organelles are seen in greater detail in a selected area of cytoplasm *(lower right)*. (From Christensen AK. *In* Greep RO, Astwood WB, eds: Handbook of Physiology, Section 7. Male Reproductive System. Baltimore, The Williams & Wilkins Company, 1975; pp 339–351. Copyright 1975, The American Physiological Society, Bethesda, Md.)

A and B) in testosterone concentration occur. Superimposed on these rhythms are irregular fluctuations in testosterone concentration in peripheral blood (see Fig. 42–5, inset C). (See the review by Ewing and colleagues [1980] for a thorough discussion of this subject.)

In those species that have been studied thoroughly, **the major epochs in testosterone production represent an orderly sequence of temporal signals that cause the following: first, the differentiation and development of the fetal reproductive tract; second, the neonatal organization or imprinting of androgen-dependent target tissues, ensuring their appropriate response later in puberty and adulthood; third, the masculinization of the male at puberty; and fourth, the maintenance of growth and function of androgen-dependent organs in the adult.** In part, these temporal changes in testosterone production reflect a complex interaction between the pituitary gland and the testis. For a thorough discussion of this topic, see Reyes and colleagues (1989), Swerdloff and Heber (1981), DiZerga and Sherins (1981), and Santen (1981).

Seminiferous Tubules

The seminiferous tubules, with their germinal elements and supporting cells, provide a unique environment for the production of germ cells. The supporting cells include the sustentacular cells of the basement membrane and the Sertoli cells. The germinal elements comprise a population

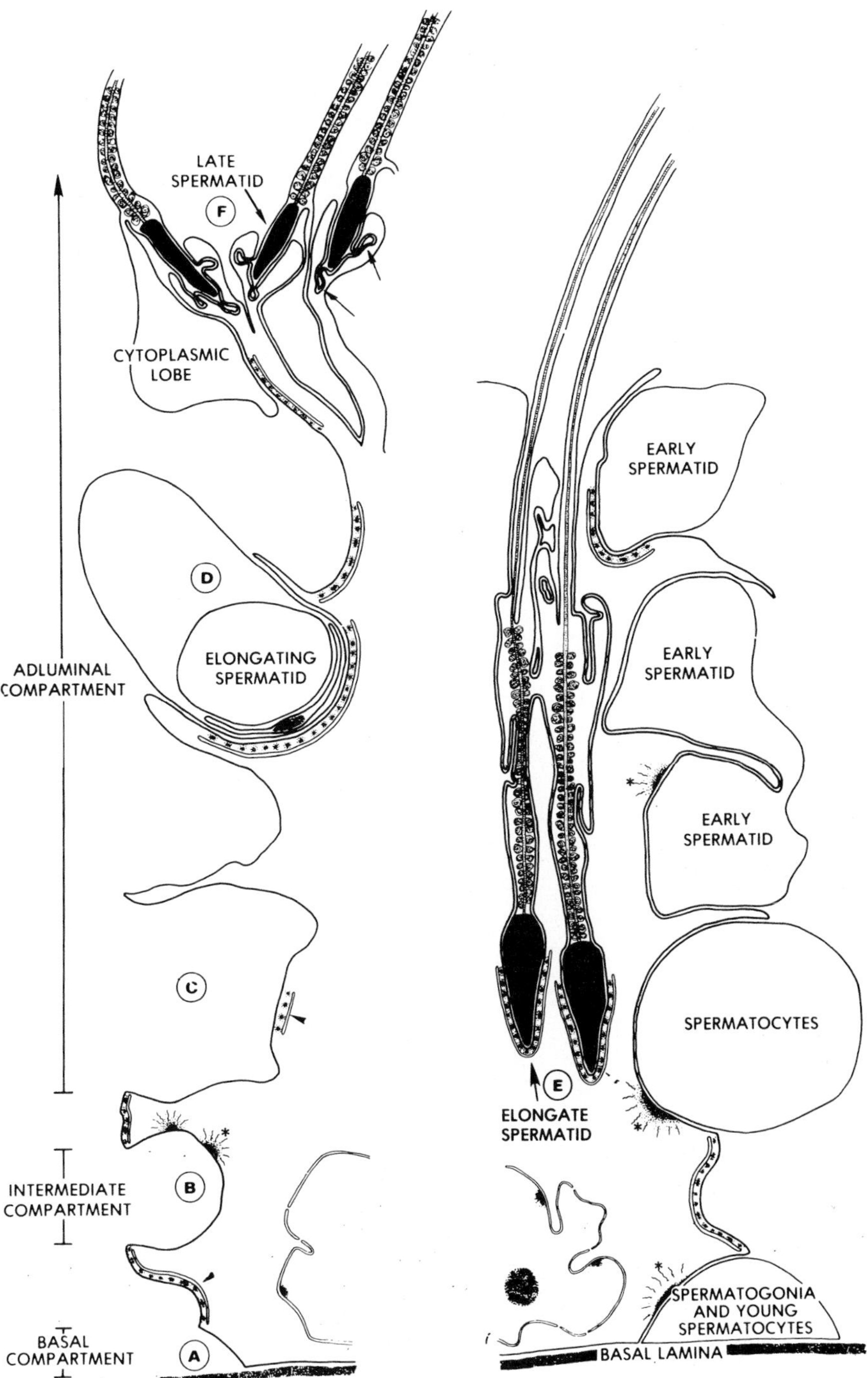

Figure 42–9. The tree-shaped Sertoli cell with a thickened central portion, or "trunk," and more delicate processes, or "limbs." The diagram is split vertically to allow the presentation of major configurational changes that occur during the spermatogenic cycle. Note the basal, intermediate, and adluminal compartments of the seminiferous epithelium. *A,* Spermatogonia and early spermatocytes share a position on the basal lamina and are overreached by one surface of adjacent Sertoli cells that join to form occluding junctions (site of blood-testis barrier). *B,* Sertoli cells form junctional complexes both above and below leptotene-zygotene spermatocytes in the process of being translocated from the basal to the adluminal compartment. *C,* The spermatocytes enter the adluminal compartment of the seminiferous epithelium when the higher Sertoli junctions dissociate. *D,* The elongating spermatid becomes situated within a narrow recess of the trunk of the Sertoli cell. *E,* As the spermatid elongates further, the cell becomes lodged within the body of the Sertoli cell. *F,* The advanced spermatid moves toward the lumen of the seminiferous epithelium in preparation for spermiation. Only the head region remains in intimate contact with the Sertoli cell. Specialized cell-to-cell contacts: Asterisks represent desmosome–gap junction complex; arrowheads represent ectoplasmic specializations; isolated arrows represent tubulobulbar complexes. (From Russell LD., Gamete Res 1980; 3:179–202.)

cytoplasm is lost from condensing spermatids by Sertoli cell phagocytosis of tubulobulbar complexes.

In summary, physical contact between the Sertoli cell and the germ cell may play some role in propelling the germ cell upward toward the lumen of the seminiferous tubule. Moreover, the intimate association between the condensing spermatid and the apical portion of the Sertoli cell during spermiogenesis is associated with the casting off of the residual cytoplasm from the developing spermatid. Lastly, the junctional complexes between adjacent Sertoli cells clearly form an important component of the blood-testis barrier with all its consequences.

The Germinal Epithelium

The epithelium of the seminiferous tubule is populated by cells that give rise to approximately 123 × 10⁶ (range 21 to 374 × 10⁶) spermatozoa daily in the human male (Amann and Howards, 1980). This process of sperm production is called spermatogenesis. It involves a proliferative phase during which spermatogonia divide either to replace their number (stem cell renewal) or to produce daughter cells committed to become spermatocytes; a meiotic phase when spermatocytes undergo reduction division, resulting in haploid spermatids; and a spermiogenic phase, when spermatids undergo a dramatic metamorphosis in size and shape to form mature spermatozoa. Because of the complexity of the topic, lack of complete information regarding humans, and space limitations in this chapter, the following discussion of spermatogenesis is general in nature and references are not always made to original research. Instead, the discussion rests heavily on excellent reviews by Heller and Clermont (1964), Ewing and colleagues (1980), DiZerga and Sherins (1981), Kerr (1991), deKretser and Kerr (1994), and Sharpe (1994).

Histologic examination of the human testis with the aid of a light microscope reveals large numbers of germ cells arrayed among Sertoli cells and extending from the basement membrane to the lumen of the seminiferous tubule. **Morphologic analysis (Clermont, 1963; Heller and Clermont, 1964) reveals the presence of at least 13 recognizable germ types in the human testis (Fig. 42–10). These cells represent different steps in the developmental process.** Proceeding from the least to the most differentiated, they are dark type A spermatogonia (Ad); pale type A spermatogonia (Ap); type B spermatogonia (B); preleptotene primary spermatocytes (R); leptotene primary spermatocytes (L); zygotene primary spermatocytes (Z); pachytene primary spermatocytes (P); secondary spermatocytes (II); and Sa, Sb_1, Sb_2, Sc, Sd_1, and Sd_2 spermatids (see Fig. 42–10).

Testis Development

Prenatal development of the testis involves migration of primordial germ cells to the gonadal ridge and association of these precursors with Sertoli cells to form primitive testicular cords (Witschi, 1948; Fritz, 1994; George and Wilson, 1994). The primitive germ cells of the undifferentiated gonad are referred to as gonocytes after the gonad differentiates into a testis by forming seminiferous cords. **The gonocytes are located in a central position within the seminiferous cords and are classified subsequently as spermatogonia only after they migrate to the periphery of the tubule** (Gondos, 1971).

The numbers of gonocytes change in fetal and prepubertal testes. Prior to birth, from the 8th to the 22nd week of pregnancy, a steep increase in the number of germ cells per tubule (from 1.1 to 3.5) occurs. Thereafter, there is a slight

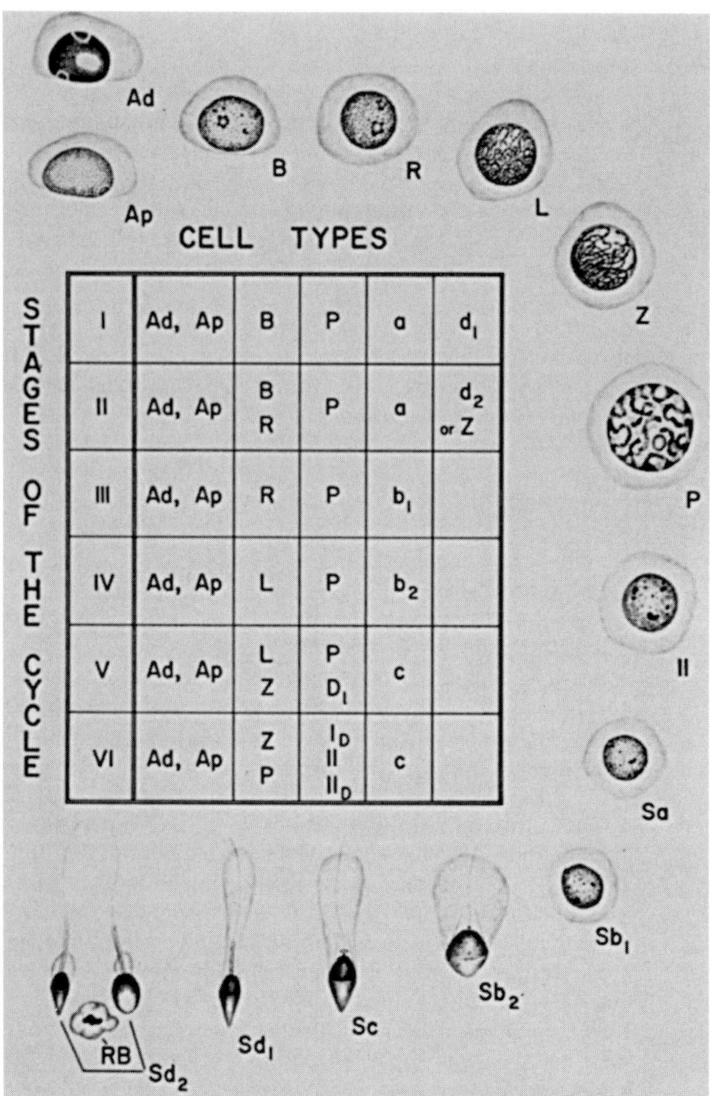

I	Ad, Ap	B	P	a	d_1
II	Ad, Ap	B R	P	a	d_2 or Z
III	Ad, Ap	R	P	b_1	
IV	Ad, Ap	L	P	b_2	
V	Ad, Ap	L Z	P D_1	c	
VI	Ad, Ap	Z P	I_D II II_D	c	

Figure 42–10. The steps of spermatogenesis in humans. The table shows the cells that make up the six stages of the cycle of the seminiferous epithelium (I to VI): D_1, diakinesis; I_D and II_D, first and second maturation divisions of spermatocytes. Ad, dark type A spermatogonium; AP, pale type A spermatogonium; B, type B spermatogonium; R, resting or preleptotene primary spermatocyte; L, leptotene spermatocyte; Z, zygotene spermatocyte; P, pachytene spermatocyte; II, secondary spermatocyte; Sa(a), $Sb_1(b_1)$, $Sb_2(b_2)$, Sc(c), $Sd_1(d_1)$, $Sd_2(d_2)$, spermatids; Rb, residual body. (Modified from Clermont Y: Am J Anat 1966; 118:509–524.)

decrease in the number of germ cells per Sertoli cell until 4 months after birth. This relative decrease in germ cells is due to proliferative activity of immature Sertoli cells during this period of time (Hilscher and Engemann, 1992). Until approximately 7 years of life, there appears to be very little morphologic change of the human testis. From 7 to 9 years of life, mitotic activity of gonocytes is detectable, with spermatogonia populating the base of the seminiferous tubule in numbers equal to those of the Sertoli cells (Muller and Skakkebaek, 1983). There appears to be little further morphologic change in spermatogonia until spermatogenesis begins at the time of puberty. Further observations regarding the maturation of gonocytes and their migration to the base of the seminiferous tubule, including the factors that may be responsible for these changes, may provide greater insight into clinical problems affecting the testis, including cryptorchidism.

Spermatogonial Proliferation and Stem Cell Renewal in Adult Testes

Pale type A spermatogonia are located in the basal compartment of the seminiferous tubule that is formed by overreaching Sertoli-to-Sertoli tight junctions. These **Ap spermatogonia divide at 16-day intervals in the human (Clermont, 1972) to form B spermatogonia, which are committed to becoming spermatocytes.** Interestingly, the spermatogonial cytoplasm generally does not separate completely when the nucleus divides following mitosis. Therefore, cytoplasmic bridges are formed between adjacent spermatogonia. Evidently, this process continues during meiosis, because cytoplasmic bridges have been observed between all classes of germ cells (Ewing et al, 1980). Although the functional significance of cytoplasmic bridges remains unknown, their presence could be important for the synchronization of cellular proliferation, differentiation, and possibly the control of gene expression in haploid cells.

Periodically, the population of undifferentiated spermatogonia must be replenished. This process of stem cell renewal has been reviewed recently by deKretser and Kerr (1994) and Sharpe (1994). **In humans, the best evidence is that by division, type Ad spermatogonia give rise, in a renewal process, to other type Ad spermatogonia as well as type Ap spermatogonia, the cells that differentiate into type B spermatogonia and ultimately into spermatozoa** (Heller and Clermont, 1964). The mechanisms by which spermatogonia both replenish their population and generate precursors for spermatogenesis are not completely clear. Recent studies in rodents have suggested that the c-kit transmembrane tyrosine kinase receptor and its Steel factor ligand may be involved in spermatogonial stem cell self-renewal. The c-kit receptor is a marker for type A spermatogonia in rats (reviewed by Dym, 1994). The result of this process is that in the rat, some stem cells differentiate into intermediate and then type B spermatogonia that proceed through spermatogenesis, in a c-kit dependent process, whereas other stem cells renew the stem cell population of spermatogonia (Yoshinaga et al, 1991).

MEIOSIS. Type B spermatogonia interconnected by cytoplasmic bridges divide mitotically to form preleptotene primary spermatocytes that will undergo meiosis. This process has been described in general (Ewing et al, 1980; Sharpe, 1994) and for the human by Kerr and deKretser (1981) and by Kerr (1991). **In the meiotic phase of spermatogenesis, a reductional division is followed by an equatorial division, resulting in the production of daughter cells with the haploid chromosome number and, as a consequence of recombination, with different genetic information.** Specifically, in the first meiotic division, primary spermatocytes, which are 2N in DNA content and contain the diploid number of chromosomes, are transformed by reduction division into secondary spermatocytes, which are 2N in DNA content and haploid in chromosomal number. The secondary spermatocytes then undergo a second meiotic division, which results in the formation of round Sa spermatids, which are 1N in DNA and haploid in chromosomal content (see Fig. 42–10). Accordingly, each primary spermatocyte gives rise to four round spermatids. **The meiotic and all subsequent phases of spermatogenesis occur behind the blood-testis barrier created by the Sertoli-to-Sertoli cell tight junctions.** Interestingly, a significant number of germ cells undergo degeneration as they differentiate from primary spermatocytes to late spermatids; approximately 40% of germ cells degenerate in humans (Barr et al, 1971; Johnson et al, 1984b) and about 66% of germ cells in the rat undergo programmed cell death (Allan et al, 1992).

SPERMIOGENESIS. During spermiogenesis, the products of meiosis, the round Sa spermatids, metamorphose into mature spermatids (see Fig. 42–10). During this metamorphosis, extensive changes occur in both the spermatid cytoplasm and the nucleus. These changes have been described in detail by Kerr and deKretser (1981) and include loss of cytoplasm, formation of the acrosome, formation of the flagellum, and migration of cytoplasmic organelles to positions characteristic of the mature spermatozoon. If the human is similar to the rat, then the clone of spermatids are connected to each other via cytoplasmic bridges and to Sertoli cells via ectoplasmic specializations.

In humans, the entire spermatogenic process, from its onset with the appearance of Ap spermatogonia in stage V through four complete cycles and to its completion when spermatozoa are released from the seminiferous epithelium in stage II of the fifth cycle (see Fig. 42–10), requires approximately 74 days (Heller and Clermont, 1964; reviewed by Sharpe, 1994). **If spermatogenesis is viewed from a fixed point in a seminiferous tubule, six recognizable cellular associations (stages of the cycle of the seminiferous epithelium) occur one after another in a predictable and constant fashion during this 74-day interval (Heller and Clermont, 1964; Fig. 42–11). Each complete cycle of the seminiferous epithelium requires about 16 days**. Accordingly, the proliferative phase of spermatogenesis (differentiation of Ap to B spermatogonia) is initiated four times during the period required for an Ap spermatogonium to differentiate into a spermatozoon. The result is that the adult human testis is populated by one or two cohorts of spermatogonia, one or two cohorts of spermatocytes, and one or two cohorts of spermatids. This stage-specific production of spermatogonia allows the efficient production of millions of spermatozoa a day.

In rodents, the stages of spermatogenesis occur more or less consecutively from the first to the last stage along a given segment of the tubule in repeating sequences. **One complete series of segments representing the recognized**

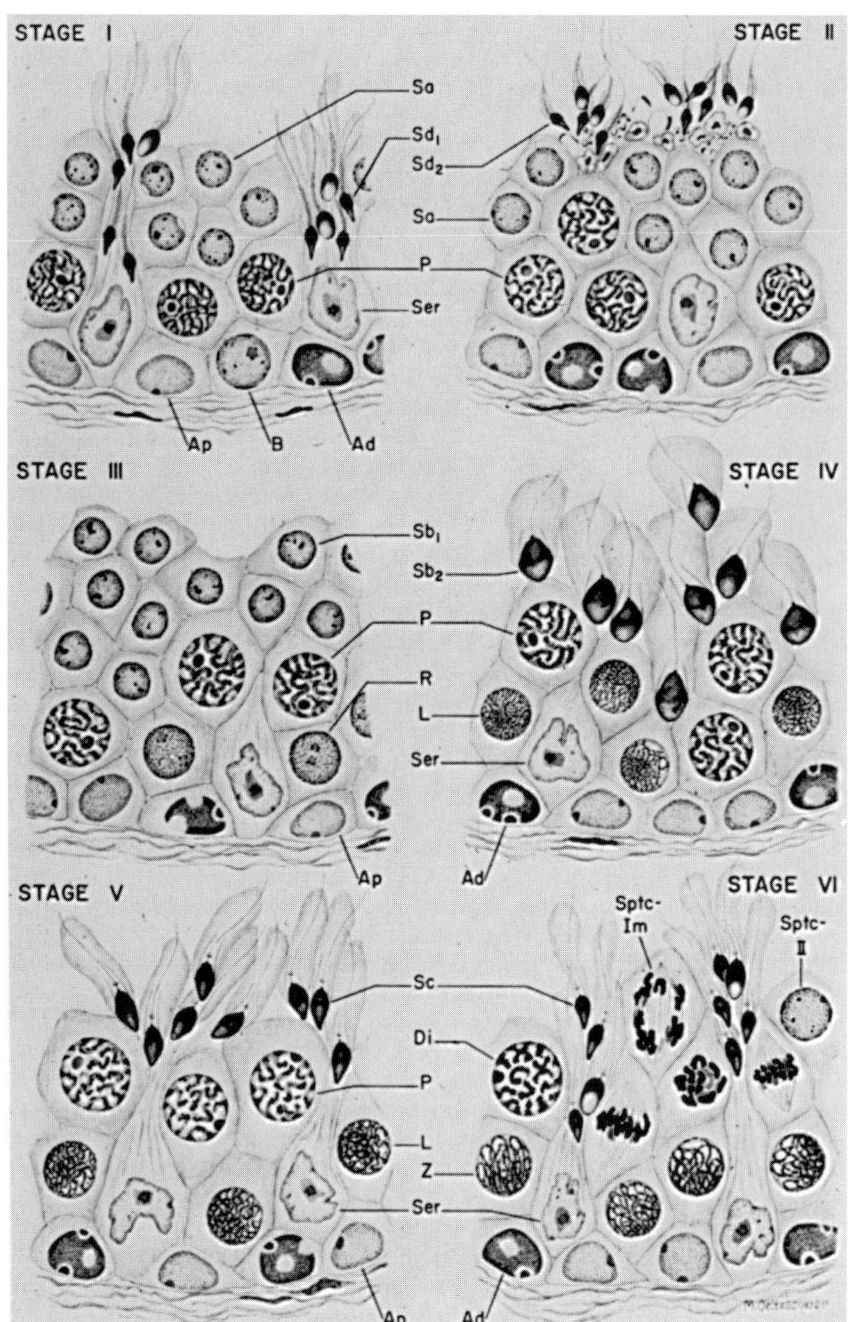

Figure 42–11. Cellular composition of the six cellular associations (stages I to VI) found in human seminiferous tubules. Ser, Sertoli nuclei; Ad and Ap, dark and pale type A spermatogonia; B, Type B spermatogonia; R, resting (preleptotene) primary spermatocytes; L, leptotene-spermatocytes; Z, zygotene spermatocytes; P, pachytene spermatocytes; Di, diplotene spermatocytes; Sptc-Im, primary spermatocytes in division; Sptc-II, secondary spermatocytes in interphase; Sa, Sb_1, Sb_2, Sc, Sd_1, Sd_2, spermatids at various steps of spermatogenesis. (Modified from Heller CG, Clermont Y: Rec Prog Horm Res 1964; 20:545–575.)

cellular associations (stages) is called the wave of the seminiferous epithelium. It has long been claimed (Roosen-Runge and Barlow, 1953; Heller and Clermont, 1964; Leidl and Waschke, 1970) that humans do not exhibit a wave of the seminiferous epithelium. Instead, the stages occupy only a portion of the circumference of the tubule, thus forming a mosaic rather than a well-defined linear array of succeeding stages of spermatogenesis. This concept has been challenged by Schulze (1989) who, using computer-aided three-dimensional imaging, reported **an orderly sequence of stages in oblique orientation that implies a helical arrangement of stages of the seminiferous tubule in humans (Fig. 42–12).** The exact configuration of the spermatogenic wave in the human testis remains to be confirmed.

Hormonal Regulation of Spermatogenesis

The role of hormones in the initiation of spermatogenesis at puberty, the maintenance of spermatogenesis during adulthood, and the reinitiation of spermatogenesis following pathologic or chemically induced hypogonadism is summarized in excellent reviews by McLachlan and colleagues (1995), Sharpe (1994), and Weinbauer and Nieschlag (1991). **There is general agreement that FSH and to a lesser extent LH, through the stimulation of testosterone production, are normally involved in the initiation of spermatogenesis at puberty.** In animals, FSH has been shown to stimulate the maturation of Sertoli and perhaps Leydig

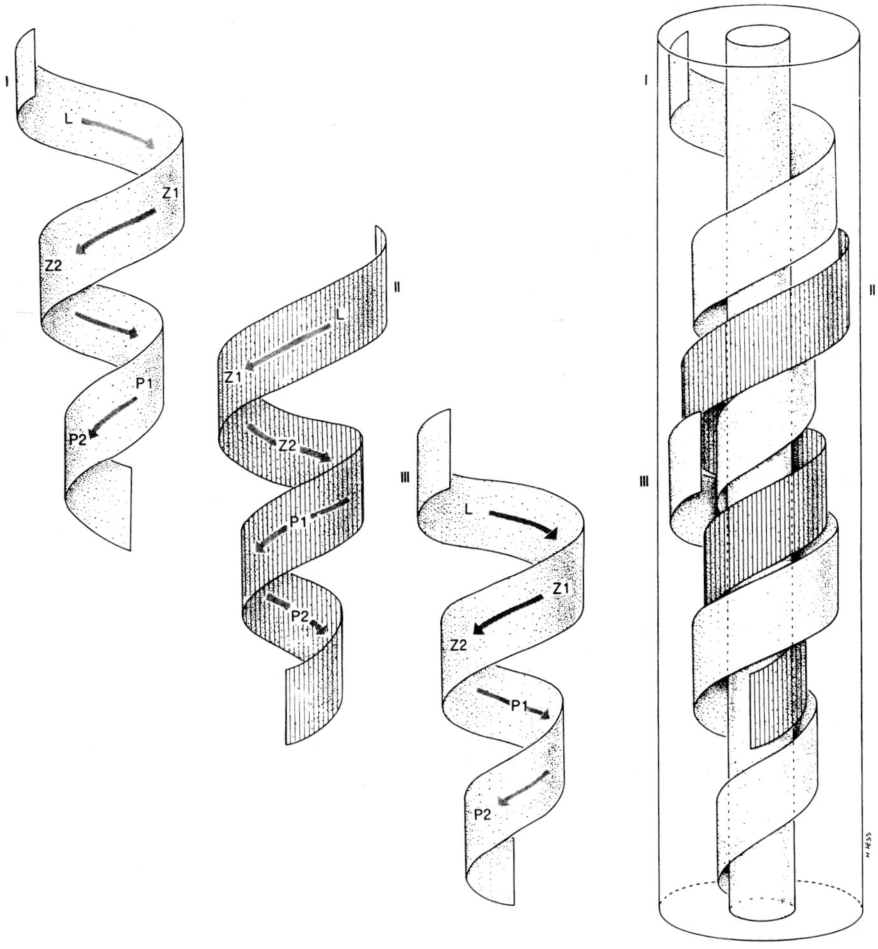

Figure 42–12. Three-dimensional model for the arrangement of primary spermatocytes in the human seminiferous tubule. The helices on the left (I, II and III) represent three cohorts of developing spermatocytes. L, leptotene; Z1, early zygotene; Z2, late zygotene; P1, early/midpachytene; P2, late pachytene. In the cylindrical representation of the seminiferous tubule on the right, each cohort of spermatocytes occupies a distinct helical region in the epithelium, with the more advanced cells closer to the lumen of the tubule. (From Schulze W, Rehder U: Cell Tissue Res 1984; 237:395–407. Courtesy of Springer-Verlag, Heidelberg.)

cells (Gondos and Berndison, 1993; Sharpe, 1994). Although definitive studies have not been conducted, FSH likely plays similar roles in the initiation of spermatogenesis in humans (Sharpe, 1994). It has also been reported that in humans, testosterone alone can induce spermatogenesis in prepubertal boys with Leydig cell tumors (Steinberger et al, 1973; Chemes et al, 1982) or familial testotoxicosis (Rosenthal et al, 1983; Reiter et al, 1986), although only qualitative spermatogenesis was achieved.

In adults, testosterone produced as a consequence of LH stimulation is the major factor responsible for the maintenance of spermatogenesis (see reviews by McLachlan et al, 1995; Sharpe, 1994). As stated by Zirkin and associates (1994) (p 276) "In nearly all animals, including man and most other primates, testosterone alone is able to maintain qualitatively complete spermatogenesis; the role of FSH may be to influence the quantity of spermatozoa produced, and this may be effected at pre-meiotic and/or post-meiotic levels, depending on the species." Testosterone regulates spermatogenesis, probably via an effect on the Sertoli cell (Lyon et al, 1975). In rats, the effect of testosterone on Sertoli cells is mediated through the testosterone-induced stimulation of P-Mod-S production in peritubular cells (Skinner and Fritz, 1985; Skinner, 1995); whether this also occurs in humans remains to be proved.

The effect of pituitary gonadotropins on spermatogenesis has been reviewed (DiZerga and Sherins, 1981; Sharpe, 1994; Zirkin et al, 1994). Hypophysectomy results in testicular atrophy in numerous species (Steinberger, 1971), including humans (Mancini et al, 1969, 1972). **Testes of hypophysectomized men are characterized by Leydig cell atrophy, peritubular hyalinization, and germinal depletion that varies from tubules containing only spermatogonia to those with scattered spermatocytes** (Mancini et al, 1969). There is little evidence at present to suggest that LH acts other than by stimulating endogenous testosterone production. It is likely that FSH is important for the maintenance of spermatogenesis in humans (Matsumoto et al, 1986), although additional studies are required in order to fully understand the role of hormones in maintaining spermatogenesis in humans.

The hormonal regimen required to restore spermatogenesis after testicular regression such as that following hypophysectomy depends on whether spermatogenesis is to be maintained immediately after hypophysectomy or reinitiated after the germinal epithelium has been allowed to regress completely. Moreover, the amount of hormone required depends on the desired end point—production of a few advanced spermatids (qualitative) or complete restoration of spermatid numbers (quantitative). **In men with suppressed levels of FSH, qualitative spermatogenesis can be achieved by treatment with testosterone alone (Matsumoto and Bremner, 1985); normal quantitative spermatogenesis requires treatment with FSH in combination with testoster-**

one (Matsumoto et al, 1986). Quantitative maintenance of spermatogenesis in the human male by testosterone alone has not been achieved to date, probably because of the difficulty in achieving a high enough blood level of testosterone. Using an alternative approach, Turner and co-workers (1990b) maintained quantitative spermatogenesis in gonadotropin-releasing hormone antagonist–treated rats by injection of testosterone-laden microspheres directly into the testis. Subsequent studies by Sawchuk and Turner (1993) demonstrated that spermatozoa produced in gonadotropin-releasing hormone antagonist–treated animals following treatment with testosterone-laden microspheres were fertile.

The localization of specific genes that are critical for spermatogenesis are being investigated. The detection of microdeletions of a region of the Y chromosome, referred to as interval 6, in 5% to 10% of azoospermic men has focused attention on this area as the site for a critical gene that is important for spermatogenesis (Chandley and Cooke, 1994). One gene that has been localized on the long arm of the Y chromosome is DAZ (deleted in azoospermia). One study of 89 men with nonobstructive azoospermia indicated that 12 (13%) had deletions of DAZ (Reijo et al, 1995). Other testicular autocrine and paracrine factors are probably involved, directly or indirectly, in the regulation of spermatogenesis: seminiferous growth factor, basic fibroblast growth factor, IGF-I, Sertoli cell–secreted growth factor, transforming growth factor-α, interleukin-1 (IL-1), chalones, meiosis-inhibiting substances, and meiosis-preventing substances. The reader is referred to excellent reviews on these topics by Bellve and Zheng (1989), Saez and associates (1991), Lamb (1993), and Skinner (1995).

Age-Related Changes in the Testis and in Spermatogenesis

Johnson and colleagues (1984a, 1984b) reported that **the testes of young men contain a total of approximately 500 million Sertoli cells, but at ages greater than 50 years, the number of Sertoli cells is reduced by about half. The number of Leydig cells is also reduced significantly with age; approximately 50% of Leydig cells are lost after the age of 60 (Neaves et al, 1984, 1985). These changes in the testes with increasing age are accompanied by a decrease in spermatogenesis.** Paniagua and co-workers (1991) reported that in men aged 27 to 42 years, approximately 85% of seminiferous tubules exhibit normal spermatogenesis, whereas men 70 to 79 and 80 to 89 years of age have normal spermatogenesis in only 31% and 16% of seminiferous tubules, respectively. The decline in spermatogenesis is accompanied by increasing numbers of tubules with moderate to marked hypospermatogenesis, maturation arrest, Sertoli cell only, and sclerosis. The mechanisms by which testes change with age are not fully understood.

EPIDIDYMIS

Recent advances in assisted reproductive technology such as microsurgical epididymal sperm aspiration and intracytoplasmic sperm injection have made possible the fertilization of eggs using spermatozoa recovered from proximal regions of the epididymis and even from the testis. As a result, previously accepted principles concerning the necessity for the maturation of spermatozoa within the epididymis have been challenged (Schoysman, 1993; Schoysman et al, 1993; Silber et al, 1995; Schlegel et al, 1995). Although the success of assisted reproductive technology should be acknowledged, one must not overlook the fact that by circumventing the normal barriers to fertilization presented by the female reproductive tract and by the egg itself, these new technologies allow fertilization by spermatozoa that otherwise would have very little chance of fertilizing. **Under normal circumstances following coitus, fertilization requires that spermatozoa survive within the female tract, migrate to the site of fertilization, bind to the egg, and undergo the processes of capacitation and acrosome reaction. Numerous studies in animals and men have established that in order to perform these functions and ultimately fertilize eggs in the absence of assisted reproductive technology, spermatozoa must undergo a maturation process while passing through some portion of the epididymis** (for reviews see Cooper, 1990; Bedford, 1994; and Turner, 1995). Unfortunately, the mechanisms by which the epididymis supports the maturation of spermatozoa (and the impact of ductal obstruction on epididymal physiology) remain largely unknown. The following sections describe the structure and functions of the epididymis and discuss the physiologic and biochemical events associated with sperm epididymal maturation.

Gross Structures

In men, the epididymal tubule is 3 to 4 meters in length (Jenkins et al, 1978). The entire length of the epididymal tubule is coiled and encapsulated within the sheath of connective tissue of the tunica vaginalis (Lanz and Neuhäuser, 1964). Extensions from this connective tissue sheath enter the interductal spaces, forming septa that divide the duct into histologically similar regions (Kormano and Reijonen, 1976). A loose network of tissue arises from the septa, supporting the ducts and their associated vascular supply and innervation.

Anatomically, the epididymis is divided into three regions: the caput, the corpus, and the cauda epididymidis (Fig. 42–13). On the basis of histologic criteria, each of these regions can be subdivided into distinct zones separated by transition segments (Baumgarten et al, 1971). **Most of the human caput epididymidis consists of ductuli efferentes that, on leaving the testis, form a network of ducts that join into a common tubule that ultimately gives rise to the epididymal tubule proper** (Fig. 42–14). As described in an elegant study by Yeung and associates (1991), this complex of tubules contains seven types of ducts characterized by unique epithelia and eight types of junctions. The epididymal tubule emerges posterior to the junction of the last joining cranial efferent ducts. At this point, the epididymal lumen is oval in shape and its diameter remains relatively constant throughout the corpus, or body, of the epididymis. In the bulky cauda epididymidis, the diameter of the duct enlarges substantially, and the lumen acquires an irregular shape. Progressing distally, the duct gradually assumes the characteristic appearance of the ductus deferens.

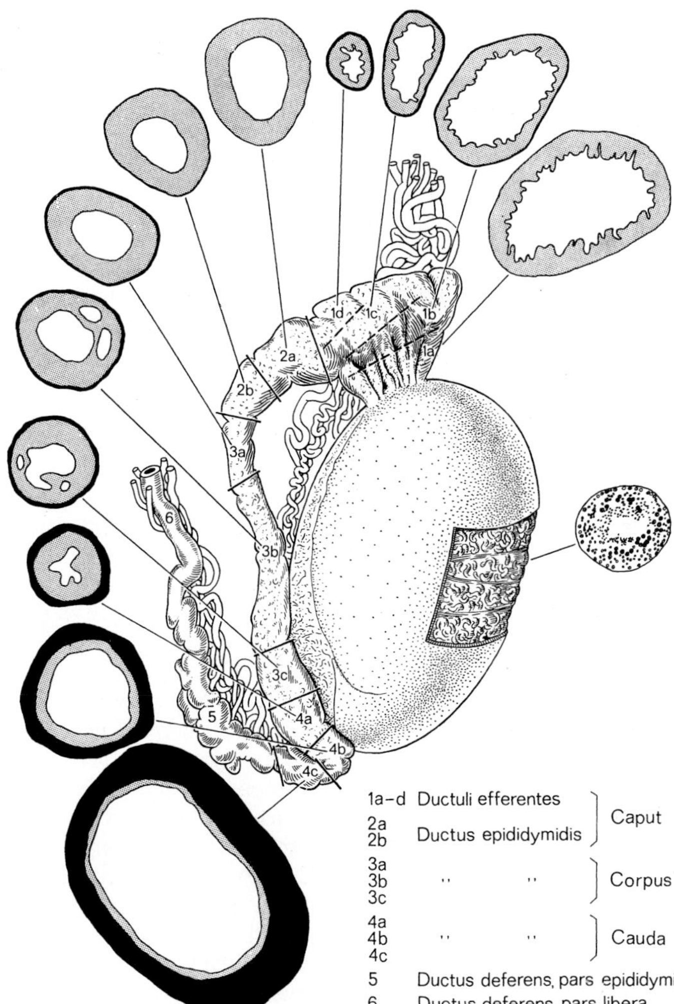

Figure 42–13. The human epididymis showing regionalization of the ductal epithelium and muscle layer. (From Baumgarten HG, Holstein AF, Rosengren E: Z Zellforsch Mikrosk Anat 1971; 120:37–79. Courtesy of Springer-Verlag, Heidelberg.)

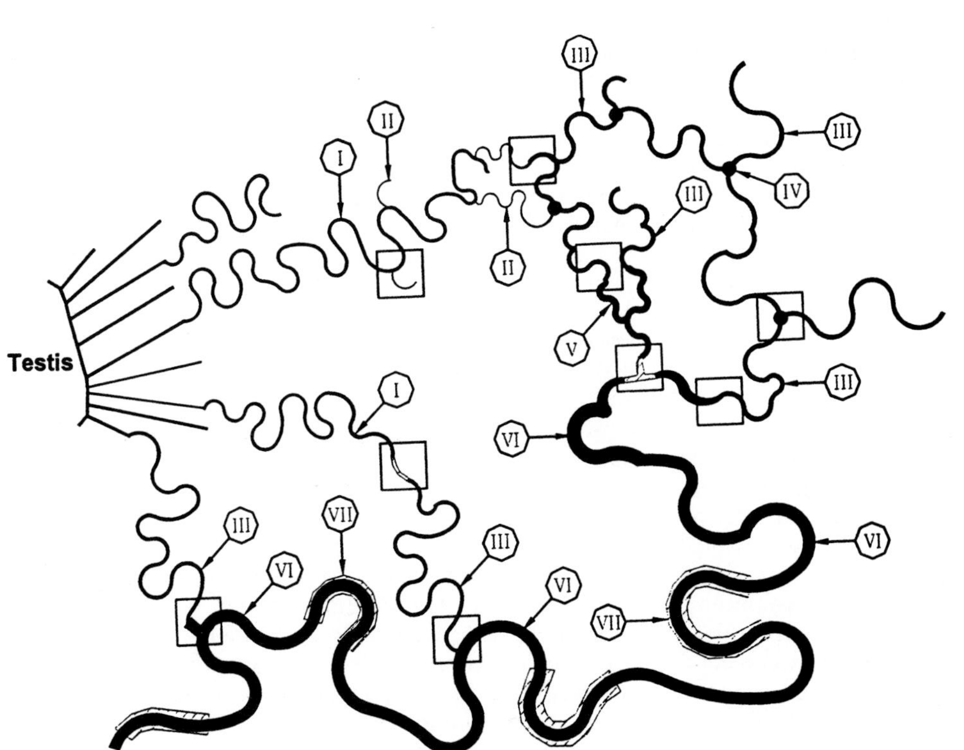

Figure 42–14. The complex tubular network within the human caput epididymidis. Note that, as depicted by different line thicknesses and Roman numerals (I–VII), there are seven types of tubules each characterized by a unique epithelium. The tubules join through eight distinctive types of junctions shown in boxes. (Modified from Yeung CH, Cooper TG, Bergmann M, Schulze H: Am J Anat 1991; 191:261–279. Copyright © John Wiley & Sons, Inc. Reprinted by permission of Wiley-Liss, Inc., a division of John Wiley & Sons, Inc.)

Contractile Tissue

External to the basal lamina of the ductuli efferentes and the epididymal tubule are contractile cells of varying architecture and quantity (Baumgarten et al, 1971). In the ductuli efferentes, the distal regions of the caput epididymidis, and the proximal segments of the corpus epididymidis, the contractile cells form a loose layer two to four cells deep around the tubule. These cells contain myofilaments and are connected by numerous nexus-like junctions. In the distal regions of the corpus epididymidis, other contractile cells are present. These cells are much larger than the contractile cells in the more proximal regions, have fewer nexus-like intracellular junctions, and resemble thin smooth muscle cells. In the cauda epididymidis, the thin contractile cells decrease in number and are replaced by thick smooth muscle cells that form three layers—the outer two layers oriented longitudinally and the central layer circularly. This contractile layer increases in thickness distally and ultimately joins the ductus deferens.

Innervation

The innervation of the human epididymis is derived primarily from the intermediate and inferior spermatic nerves, which, in turn, arise from the superior portion of the hypogastric plexus and from the pelvic plexus, respectively (Mitchell, 1935). The ductuli efferentes and the proximal segments of the ductus epididymidis are sparsely innervated by sympathetic fibers (Baumgarten and Holstein, 1967; Baumgarten et al, 1968). In these regions, the fibers are present in a peritubular plexus and are principally associated with blood vessels. The number of nerve fibers rises significantly at the level of the midcorpus epididymidis and progressively increases distally along the epididymis, coincident with the appearance and proliferation of smooth muscle cells (Baumgarten et al, 1971). **The differential distribution of the contractile cells and the sympathetic nerves within the epididymis may be responsible for the rhythmic peristaltic movements of the ductuli efferentes and the initial segments of the epididymis, as well as the intermittent contractile activity of the normally quiescent cauda epididymidis and the ductus deferens during emission and ejaculation** (Risley, 1963). The significance of these physiologic events to the movement of spermatozoa through the epididymis is discussed in a later section.

Vascularization

In humans, the caput and the corpus epididymidis receive arterial blood via a single branch from the testicular artery, which divides into the superior and inferior epididymal branches (MacMillan, 1954). The cauda epididymidis is supplied by branches from the deferential artery (artery of the vas deferens), which also communicates with the arteries of the caput and corpus epididymidis. The vasal and cremasteric arteries serve as collateral sources to the epididymis in the event that the main testicular artery is obstructed or ligated.

The arterial branches leading to the epididymis enter along the septa formed by the connective tissue sheath. Once they enter the epididymis, these vessels become extensively coiled before transforming into the straight vessels of the microvascular bed (Kormano and Reijonen, 1976). The microvascularization varies significantly along the length of the ductus epididymidis, the proximal segments of the caput epididymidis containing a dense subepithelial capillary network and the degree of vascularization decreasing distally along the epididymal duct.

According to MacMillan (1954), venous drainage from the corpus and cauda epididymidis join to form the vena marginalis epididymis of Haberer. The capital veins communicate with the pampiniform plexus or the vena marginalis, the latter then joining the vena marginalis testis, the pampiniform plexus, the cremasteric vein, or the deferential vein.

Lymphatic drainage of the epididymis occurs through two routes (Wenzel and Kellermann, 1966). Lymph from the caput and corpus epididymidis is removed via the same vessels draining the testis. These vessels follow the internal spermatic vein through the inguinal canal and ultimately terminate in the preaortic nodes. Lymph vessels from the cauda epididymidis join those draining the ductus deferens and terminate in the external iliac nodes.

Epididymal Epithelium

The histology of the human ductus epididymidis has been reviewed by Holstein (1969), Vendrely (1981), and Yeung and associates (1991). **The epithelium consists of two major cells types, principal cells and basal cells, which vary in composition along the length of the duct** (Fig. 42–15). Principal cells change in height and length of stereocilia, generally being tall (120 μm), with long stereocilia in the proximal regions of the epididymis, and small (50 μm), with short stereocilia in the more distal regions. The nuclei in these cells are elongated and often possess large clefts and one or two nucleoli. The presence of numerous coated pits, micropinocytotic vesicles, multivesicular bodies, and irregularly shaped membranous vesicles near the apex of these cells, in addition to an extensive Golgi apparatus, suggests that principal cells carry out both absorptive and secretive processes. In humans, the number of coated pits and vesicles, multivesicular bodies, and Golgi apparatus in principal cells vary quantitatively along the epididymis, suggesting that these cells possess a differential ability for absorption and secretion along the length of the duct (Vendrely and Dadoune, 1988).

Basal cells are dispersed among the more numerous principal cells within the epithelium. These tear-shaped cells rest on the basal lamina and extend approximately 25 μm toward the lumen, their apices forming threads between adjacent principal cells. The morphology of basal cells remains relatively constant throughout the epididymal duct. **Recent ultrastructural and immunohistochemical studies by Yeung and co-workers (1994) characterized basal cells in the human corpus epididymidis as tissue-fixed macrophages.** These authors proposed that epididymal basal cells may be involved in a local immune defense mechanism and that "macrophages are the progenitors of basal cells and replenish a slowly turning over population of basal cells that

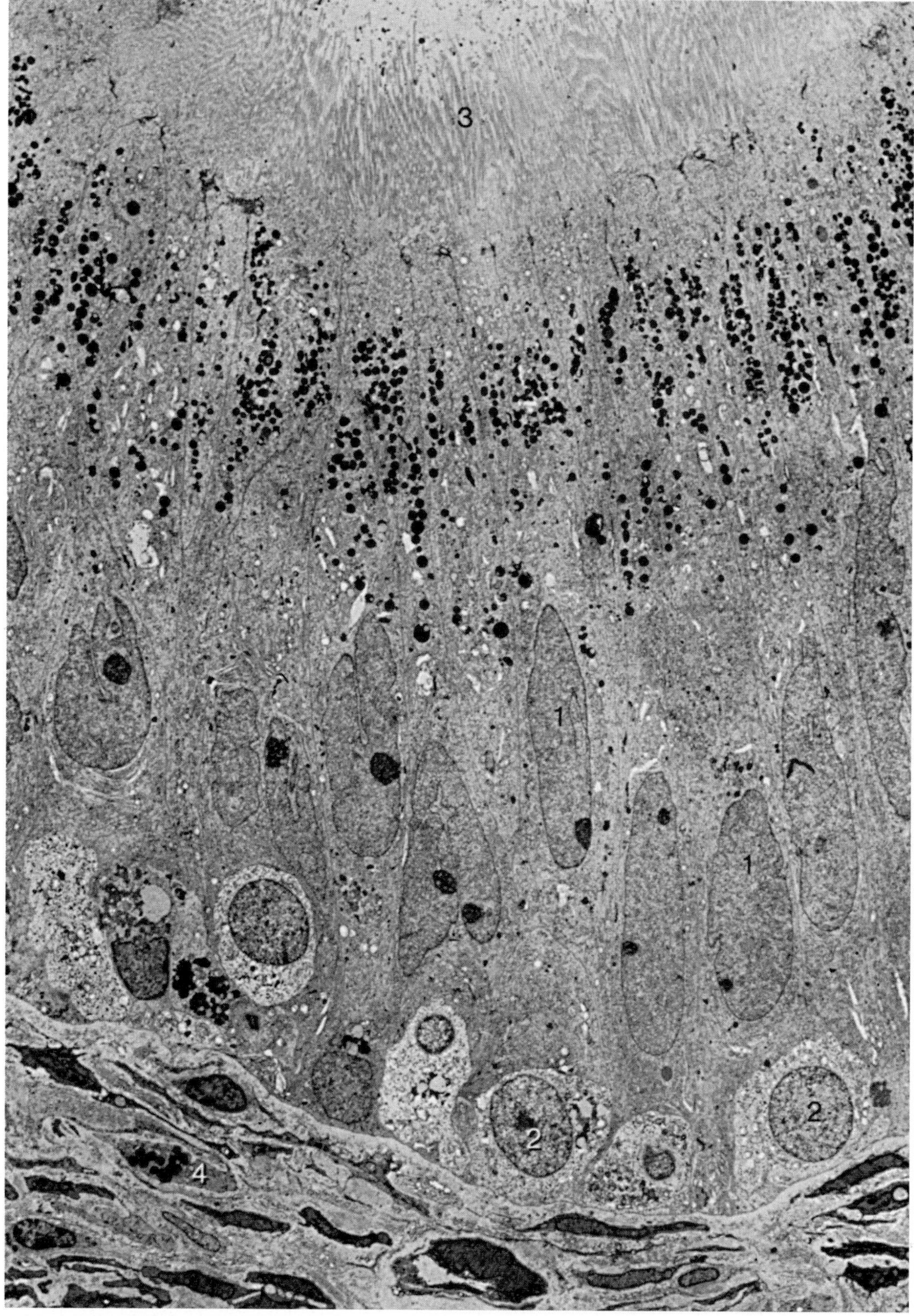

Figure 42–15. Electron micrograph of a cross-section through the human ductus epididymidis. Major components of the luminal epithelium are principal cells (1), basal cells (2), stereocilia (3), and myofilaments (4). Magnification approximately × 1800. (From Holstein AF: *In* Hafez ESE, ed: Human Semen and Fertility Regulation in Men. St. Louis, The C. V. Mosby Company, 1976, pp 23–30. Copyright 1976, The C. V. Mosby Company, St. Louis.)

become overloaded with detritus (sperm degradation products) removed from the epithelium."

Intraepithelial lymphocytes present in the epididymis also have been suggested to play a role in immune defense. Using lymphocyte cell surface–specific monoclonal antibodies, Ritchie and colleagues (1984) identified epithelial lymphocytes as T cells. These authors further characterized most of the intraepithelial lymphocytes as belonging to the suppressor and cytotoxic T-cell subset and suggested that these cells may participate in a mechanism for tolerance to sperm autoantigens.

Another potential immune defense system within the epididymis is formed by intercellular tight junctions. In laboratory animals, tight junctions between epithelial cells within the ductuli efferentes and the caput epididymidis are thought to form a blood-epididymis barrier analogous to the blood-testis barrier (Suzuki and Nagano, 1978; Hoffer and Hinton, 1984). **The blood-epididymis barrier probably extends from the caput into the cauda epididymidis.** Howards and associates (1976) demonstrated that the barrier in the hamster cauda epididymidis is permeable to low-molecular-weight substances, such as water and urea, but is impermeable to inulin, a compound with a molecular weight of 5000. The function of the blood-epididymis barrier as well as the involvement of epithelial lymphocytes and basal cells in an epididymal immune defense system deserve additional study. As is discussed later, the blood-epididymis barrier may also play an important role in influencing the composition of fluid present within different segments of the epididymal lumen (Turner, 1991; Hinton and Palladino, 1995).

Functions of the Epididymis

Regional differences in (1) the anatomic structures of the epididymal tubule, (2) the innervation and vascularization of the duct, and (3) the histology of the epithelium suggest that the epididymis is actually a succession of different tissues (Vendrely, 1981). The following sections describe the functions of this complex system—specifically, sperm transit and storage, and sperm fertility and motility maturation. Additional information concerning epididymal function can be obtained from reviews by Robaire and Hermo (1988), Moore and Smith (1988), Bedford, (1994), and Hinton and Palladino (1995).

Sperm Transport

Depending on the measurements employed, **sperm transport through the human epididymis has been observed to require anywhere from an average of about 1 day to 11 to 12 days** (Rowley et al, 1970; Amann, 1981; Johnson and Varner, 1988). Sperm transit time through the caput-corpus portion of the epididymis is roughly similar to the transit time through the cauda epididymidis. Amann (1981) suggested that sperm epididymal transit time is influenced by daily testicular sperm production rather than by a direct influence of age. This hypothesis was confirmed by Johnson and Varner (1988), who found no difference in sperm epididymal transit time between groups of men aged 20 to 49 and 50 to 79 years. Moreover, Johnson and Varner (1988) observed that sperm epididymal transit time averaged only 2 days in men with a high daily sperm production rate (137 million per testis), compared with an average of 6 days in men with a low daily sperm production rate (34 million per testis). With respect to sexual activity, Amann (1981) reported that whereas sperm transit time through the caput and corpus epididymidis is not affected, **recent emissions reduce transit time through the cauda epididymidis by 68%.**

Because it is generally accepted that human spermatozoa are immotile within the epididymal lumen, other mechanisms must be involved in the movement of the spermatozoa through the epididymis. These mechanisms may be inferred from the results of animal studies (Bedford, 1975; Hamilton, 1977; Courot, 1981; Jaakkola and Talo, 1982; Jaakkola, 1983). Initially, spermatozoa are carried into the ductuli efferentes by rete testis fluid; the flow of the fluid is facilitated by the resorption of water by ductal epithelial cells. Motile cilia and the contraction of the myoid cells surrounding the ductuli efferentes may also assist the movement of spermatozoa into the epididymis. The principal mechanism responsible for moving spermatozoa through the epididymis is probably the spontaneous rhythmic contractions of the contractile cells surrounding the epididymal duct. The regionalization of the smooth muscle cells, and the adrenergic innervation within the epididymis described earlier, serve to optimize the ability of the epididymal duct to transport spermatozoa to the ductus deferens.

Sperm Storage

After migrating through the caput and corpus epididymidis, spermatozoa are retained in the cauda epididymidis for varying lengths of time, depending on the degree of sexual activity. Amann (1981) observed that **in a group of men 21 to 55 years of age, an average of about 155 to 209 million spermatozoa were present in each epididymis.** Similar observations concerning epididymal sperm storage in men were made by Johnson and Varner (1988). **In humans, approximately half of the total number of epididymal spermatozoa are stored in the caudal region.**

As discussed in the following sections, spermatozoa stored in the cauda epididymidis are capable of undergoing progressive motility and have the capacity to fertilize eggs. The length of time that spermatozoa can be stored within the epididymis in a potentially fertile state is uncertain. Early studies using experimental animals demonstrated that spermatozoa can be maintained in a viable state for several weeks within the cauda epididymidis following ligation of the ductus deferens (Hammond and Asdell, 1926; Young, 1929). Other studies, however, showed that rabbit (Cooper and Orgebin-Crist, 1977) and rat (Cuasnicu and Bedford, 1989) sperm fertility, measured in vivo, diminished when spermatozoa were retained in the epididymis for longer than normal times. Johnson and Varner (1988) speculated, without presenting data, that in humans, the aging of sperm as a result of extended epididymal transit time (prolonged storage) "may contribute to reduced fertility." This hypothesis was supported recently by studies that suggested that long-term storage of spermatozoa resulted in decreased motility (Yeung et al, 1993) and decreased ability of retained spermatozoa to fuse with zona pellucida–free hamster eggs (Zeuzes et al, 1992). The influence of epididymal storage on sperm motility, fertility, and viability clearly requires further study.

The fate of unejaculated epididymal spermatozoa in humans is unknown. Studies using experimental animals suggest a variety of sperm-removal mechanisms. In the rat and guinea pig, spermatozoa are lost via spontaneous seminal discharge and oral self-cleaning (Martan and Risley,

1963; Martan, 1969). Rams lose approximately 90% of their daily production of 7 billion spermatozoa into urine (Lino et al, 1967), whereas bulls may lose about 50% of the spermatozoa produced by the testis owing to resorption in the epididymis (Amann and Almquist, 1961). In humans, phagocytosis of spermatozoa by macrophages within the lumen of the epididymis is observed following ligation of the ductus deferens (Phadke, 1964). However, removal of large numbers of spermatozoa from the epididymis of unvasectomized men by spermiophages, spontaneous emission, or epididymal resorption has not been reported. Spermiophagy in the ampullary region of the vas deferens is discussed in a later section.

Maturation of Spermatozoa

Studies in laboratory and domestic animals established that beyond serving as a mere conduit and storage depot for spermatozoa, the epididymis sustains maturation processes that support the acquisition of progressive motility and fertility by spermatozoa. Several reports suggest that similar processes also occur in humans. The following sections discuss sperm epididymal maturation, with reference to human studies where appropriate. The possible effects of reproductive tract obstruction on sperm epididymal maturation are also discussed.

SPERM MOTILITY MATURATION. Human spermatozoa develop an increased capacity for motility as they migrate through the epididymis. This process of motility maturation is expressed as a change in the pattern of sperm motility, as well as in an increase in the percentage of spermatozoa exhibiting more mature motility patterns. Bedford and colleagues (1973) observed that the majority of spermatozoa taken from the ductuli efferentes and resuspended in culture medium are immotile or exhibit only weak tail movements. A few spermatozoa from these samples have immature tail movements characterized by wide-arced, thrashing beats that result in little forward progression (Fig. 42–16*A*). The number of spermatozoa possessing this immature motility pattern increases in the initial segment of the epididymis. More distally, in the midcorpus region, the proportion of spermatozoa exhibiting the immature motility decreases, with a corresponding increase in the number of spermatozoa possessing a mature motility pattern characterized by high-frequency, low-amplitude beats that result in progressive motility (Fig. 42–16*B*). In the cauda epididymidis, more than 50% of spermatozoa possess the mature motility pattern when diluted in culture medium, the remainder of the spermatozoa being immotile or having the immature motility forms observed in the proximal regions of the epididymis. Moore and associates (1983) confirmed the observations regarding the increased capacity of human spermatozoa for progressive motility during epididymal transit. Using more precise techniques involving computer-aided sperm analysis following suspension in physiologic diluent, Yeung and co-workers (1993) observed increases in straight-line and curvilinear sperm swimming velocities from the ductuli efferentes to the cauda epididymidis. However, they found that although the percentage of motile sperm increased from the ductuli efferentes to the corpus epididymidis, there was a decrease in the percentage of motile spermatozoa from the distal corpus to the cauda epididymidis. The authors attributed the decrease in sperm motility within the cauda to prolonged storage.

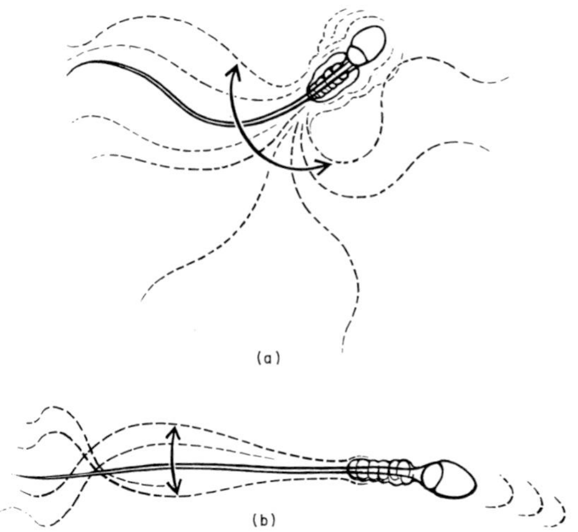

Figure 42–16. Patterns of tail movement in human epididymal spermatozoa. *A,* The pattern shown by spermatozoa taken from proximal regions of the epididymis is characterized by a high-amplitude, low-frequency beat, producing little forward movement. *B,* In contrast, tail movement in a large proportion of spermatozoa from the cauda epididymidis is characterized by low-amplitude, rapid beats that result in forward progression. (From Bedford JM, Calvin HI, Cooper GW: J Reprod Fertil [Suppl] 1973; 18:199–213.)

Studies involving experimental animals indicate that motility maturation may be, in part, an intrinsic sperm process that occurs independent of specific interactions with the epididymis. Although hamster and rabbit spermatozoa are generally immotile in the caput epididymidis, motile spermatozoa were found in this region following ligation of the duct at the level of the corpus epididymidis (Horan and Bedford, 1972; Orgebin-Crist, 1969). However, the time required for the development of motility in the spermatozoa entrapped proximally by the ligature was much longer than that required for the maturation of motility when spermatozoa were allowed to migrate through the epididymal duct. In addition, the motility observed in sperm of the caput epididymidis following ligation of the corpus did not persist for more than a very brief period (see Bedford, 1975). These data suggest that **spermatozoa are inherently able to develop some degree of motility, but that normally, the maturation of sperm motility is potentiated through interaction with the epididymis during migration into more distal regions of the duct.**

Whether, and to what degree, epididymal sperm motility maturation in humans is dependent on specific epididymal regions is not clear. Studies of patients with congenital absence of the vas deferens or with epididymal obstruction frequently report poor motility in spermatozoa aspirated from the caput epididymidis (Schoysman and Bedford, 1986; Jardin et al, 1988; Silber, 1989; Schlegel et al, 1994). However, these observations may reflect an alteration or decrement in epididymal function in these patients rather than in intrinsic sperm processes. Unquestionably, the process of sperm motility maturation in the human epididymis requires additional investigation.

SPERM FERTILITY MATURATION. Convincing evidence from experimental studies demonstrated that testicular spermatozoa are intrinsically incapable of fertilizing eggs (Orgebin-Crist, 1969; Bedford, 1974). **In most animals, the ability to fertilize eggs is gradually acquired as the spermatozoa migrate into the distal regions of the epididymis.** For example, Orgebin-Crist (1969) showed that spermatozoa from the caput, corpus, and cauda epididymidis of the rabbit are able to fertilize 1%, 63%, and 92% of exposed rabbit eggs, respectively (Fig. 42–17).

Evidence has also been presented for epididymal sperm fertility maturation in humans. Using zona pellucida–free hamster eggs to assess the fertilizing capacity of human epididymal spermatozoa, Hinrichsen and Blaquier (1980) demonstrated that although spermatozoa from the proximal regions of the epididymis are able to bind to the zona pellucida–free eggs, only spermatozoa from the cauda epididymidis are able to both bind and penetrate the eggs. Essentially, the same observations were made by Moore and colleagues (1983). **Taken together, these studies suggest that sperm fertility maturation in humans is, for the most part, achieved at the level of the distal corpus or proximal cauda epididymidis** (Fig. 42–18).

More recent studies, however, have questioned whether sperm fertility maturation in humans requires sperm migration into the distal regions of the epididymis. In these studies, patients with ductal obstruction or with congenital absence of the vas deferens were able to achieve pregnancies following vasoepididymostomy up to the level of the ductuli efferentes (Schoysman and Bedford, 1986; Silber, 1989). The pregnancy rate was higher when the anastomosis was performed lower in the epididymis. Additional studies using assisted reproductive techniques with spermatozoa aspirated from men with congenital absence of the vas deferens or secondary genital duct obstruction confirmed that the fertilizing capacity of spermatozoa is improved when a greater length of epididymis is present (Schlegel et al, 1994; Chen et al, 1995). **Taken together, these studies demonstrate that in patients with ductal obstruction or with congenital absence of the vas deferens, some degree of sperm fertility maturation occurs in the caput epididymidis but that sperm fertilizing capacity is enhanced with further migration through the epididymis.** The most distal region of the obstructed epididymis contains only senescent, dead, and degenerating spermatozoa (Schlegel et al, 1994).

The apparent discrepancy between the studies using zona pellucida–free hamster eggs and those on patients with ductal obstruction in localizing the site of fertility maturation in the human epididymis may be explained by earlier studies on laboratory animals. These studies showed that following ductal obstruction by surgical ligation of the epididymis or vas deferens, the normal location of fertility maturation along the epididymal duct is skewed proximally (see Bedford, 1967; Orgebin-Crist, 1969; Bedford, 1988). Moreover, postobstruction change in the epididymis may be irreversible. Turner and co-workers (1990a) reported that the flow of fluid through the lumen of the epididymis is reduced significantly, even after the restoration of ductal patency. Viewing these results collectively, Bedford (1994) and Yeung (1993) suggested that, as in laboratory animals, ductal obstruction in humans also may result in a shift, or skewing, of the normal pattern of sperm fertility maturation in the epididymis. Clearly, additional studies are required to determine the site and process of sperm fertility maturation in the normal human epididymis and in the epididymis following ductal obstruction or congenital absence of the vas deferens.

Controversy exists concerning the outcome of fertilization by spermatozoa that have just acquired fertilizing capacity in the proximal regions of the epididymis. Overstreet and Bedford (1976) reported that embryonic mortality in the rabbit is not increased after fertilization with spermatozoa taken from the distal corpus epididymidis. However, other studies using rabbits (Orgebin-Crist, 1981; Orgebin-Crist and Jahad, 1977; Brackett et al, 1978), sheep (Fournier-Delpech et al, 1979), and rats (Paz et al, 1978) indicated that fertilization using immature or young spermatozoa from proximal regions of the epididymis results in a higher rate of embryonic mortality compared with fertiliza-

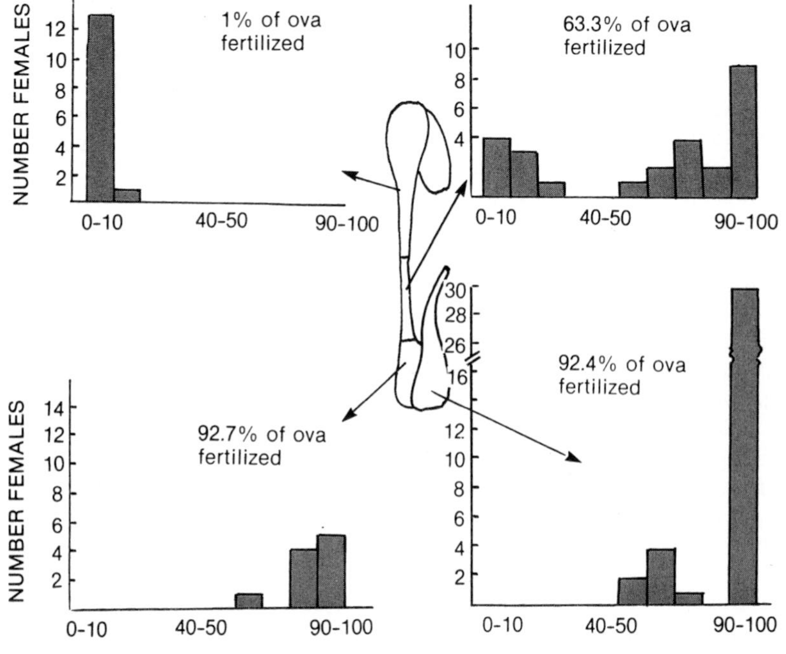

Figure 42–17. Sperm fertility maturation in the rabbit epididymis. Spermatozoa taken from distal regions of the epididymis possess higher fertilizing ability than do spermatozoa from proximal epididymal regions. (From Orgebin-Crist MC: Biol Reprod [Suppl] 1969; 155:1–15.)

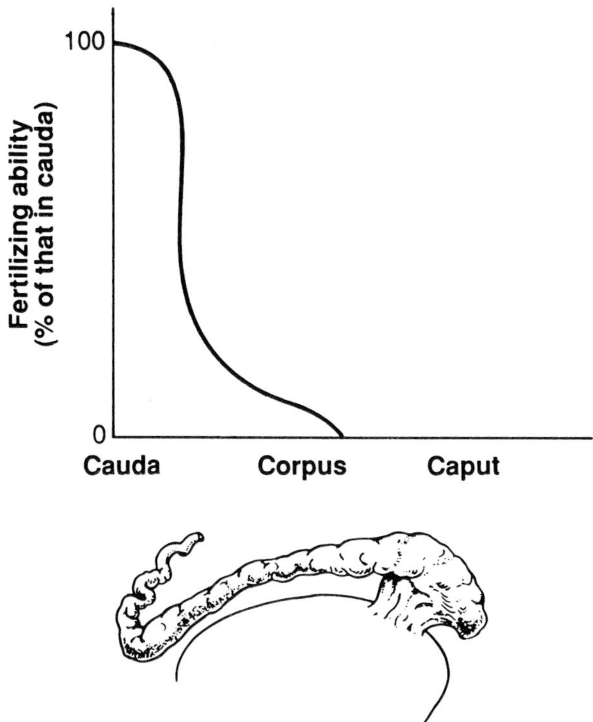

Figure 42–18. Sperm fertility maturation in the human epididymis. Sperm-fertilizing ability is assessed using zona pellucida–free hamster eggs and by changes in motility, which increases in the distal regions of the human epididymis. (Based on Hinrichsen MJ, Blaquier JA. J Reprod Fertil 1980; 60:291–294; Moore HD, Hartman TD, Pryor JP. Int J Androl 1983; 6:310–318). (From Bedford JM: Ann NY Acad Sci 1988; 541:284–291.)

tion using ejaculated spermatozoa or mature spermatozoa from the distal epididymis. Because of the increasing occurrence of high vasoepididymostomies, the use of spermatozoa of the caput epididymidis for in vitro fertilization, and especially with the increasing application of intracytoplasmic sperm injection using epididymal or testicular spermatozoa, this controversy and its relevance to humans must be resolved by future studies.

BIOCHEMICAL CHANGES IN SPERMATOZOA DURING EPIDIDYMAL MATURATION. Spermatozoa undergo a myriad of biochemical and molecular changes as they pass through the epididymis. The topic of sperm modification in the epididymis has been reviewed extensively (see Jones, 1989; Robaire and Hermo, 1988; Hinton and Palladino, 1995; and Yanagimachi, 1994). Although information from human studies is sparse, it is apparent that sperm surface membranes assume an increasingly negative net charge during epididymal transit (Bedford et al, 1973). This alteration in surface charge is probably the result of deletions, additions, and modifications of the sperm surface and integral membrane components that are in part also reflected as changes in sperm surface antigenicity (Tezon et al, 1985; Ross et al, 1990). Other modifications in human spermatozoa during epididymal maturation include the oxidation of sulfhydryl groups to disulfides in the sperm membrane (Reyes et al, 1976), as well as in the sperm head and sperm tail structures (Bedford et al, 1973). Bedford and coworkers (1973) suggested that the formation of intracellular disulfide bonds may provide the sperm tail and head with the structural rigidity necessary for progressive motility and successful penetration of eggs.

Studies on laboratory animals have described yet other sperm membrane changes that may occur in human spermatozoa during epididymal migration. These modifications include alterations in sperm lectin-binding properties (Nicolson et al, 1977; Courtens and Fournier-Delpech, 1979; Olson and Danzo, 1981; Hermo et al, 1992), phospholipid and lipid content (Nikolopoulou et al, 1985), glycoprotein composition (Fournier-Delpech et al, 1977; Olson and Danzo, 1981; Brown et al, 1983), immunoreactivity (Killian and Amann, 1973; Brooks and Tiver, 1984), and iodination characteristics (Nicolson et al, 1979; Olson and Danzo, 1981). Orgebin-Crist and Fournier-Delpech (1982) demonstrated that in the rat, sperm membrane modifications during epididymal passage result in an increased ability to adhere to the zona pellucida of the egg. Blobel and colleagues (1990) described a guinea pig sperm integral membrane glycoprotein (PH-30) that is modified during epididymal transit. Although it is controversial whether this protein is involved in sperm-egg fusion or in reorganizing the egg's cytoskeleton at the site of sperm attachment (Green, 1993), this protein likely plays a key role in fertilization. Another integral sperm membrane glycoprotein (PH-20) that is modified during epididymal transit was found to have hyaluronidase activity and, accordingly, was suggested to enable spermatozoa to penetrate the cumulus cell mass surrounding the egg (Lathrop et al, 1990; Lin et al, 1994). These observations provide important insight into the maturation of sperm fertility in the epididymis.

Spermatozoa also undergo numerous metabolic changes during epididymal transit (see reviews by Voglmayr [1975] and Dacheux and Paquignon [1980]). Studies using experimental animals describe the acquisition of an increased capacity for glycolysis (Hoskins et al, 1975), changes in intracellular pH and calcium content, modification of adenylate cyclase activity (Casillas et al, 1980), and alterations in cellular phospholipid and phospholipid-like fatty acid content (Voglmayr, 1975). Whether similar modifications occur in human spermatozoa during epididymal migration is unknown. However, such changes are likely because human spermatozoa exhibit an increased ability for motility and fertility as they traverse the epididymis (see the previous discussion on sperm motility maturation in the epididymis).

Factors Involved in Epididymal Function

Although the mechanisms by which the epididymis carries out its functions of sperm transport, sperm maturation, and sperm storage are unclear, the consensus is that these processes are influenced by the fluids and secretions within the epididymal lumen. The constituents of this fluid have been reviewed by Hinton and Palladino (1995), Turner (1991, 1995), Robaire and Hermo (1988), and Hermo and colleagues (1994). Studies using laboratory animals demonstrated that the biochemical composition of epididymal fluid not only differs from that of blood serum but also undergoes regional changes within the epididymis. For a thorough discussion of the regionalization of epididymal fluid, the reader is referred to excellent reviews by Turner (1991) and Robaire and Hermo (1988). Suffice it to say that the osmolarity, electrolyte content, and protein composition of luminal fluid varies significantly from region to region in the epididymis. This fluid compartmentalization may reflect the multifunctional nature of the epididymis and is probably the consequence of the differential vascularization along the epididymal tubule, the semipermeability of the blood-epididymis barrier, and the selective absorption and differential secretion of fluid constituents along the length of the duct. In this regard, several studies have described regionalized protein synthesis (Junera et al, 1988) and differential gene expression within specific regions of the epididymis in laboratory animals (Brooks et al, 1986; Ghyselinck et al, 1989; Douglass et al, 1991; Garrett et al, 1990; Cornwall and Hann, 1995a) and in humans (Kirchhoff et al, 1990). Two human epididymal-specific genes have been cloned and sequenced, and their corresponding gene products have been characterized. The HE2 gene is expressed in the caput and proximal corpus epididymidis and encodes a 10 kD secretory glycopeptide that is localized within the epididymal epithelium and in the subacrosomal equatorial region of the sperm head (Osterhoff et al, 1994). A 10-kD HE4 gene product is present in the corpus and cauda epididymidis, and is homologous to extracellular proteinase inhibitors (Kirchhoff et al, 1991). Further characterization of these human epididymal-specific gene products is needed in order to understand their roles in the epididymal maturation of spermatozoa.

Specific constituents of epididymal fluid identified in laboratory studies include glycerylphosphorylcholine, carnitine, and sialic acid. In addition, **epididymal fluid contains proteins that have physiologic effects on spermatozoa—proteins that are believed to have a sperm-protective role, and other proteins that may be important for sperm-egg interactions.** Examples of proteins that affect sperm function are forward motility protein (Brandt et al, 1978), sperm survival factor (Morton et al, 1978), progressive motility–sustaining factor (Sheth et al, 1981), sperm motility–inhibiting factor (Turner and Giles, 1982), acidic epididymal glycoprotein (Pholpramool et al, 1983), and the EP2-EP3 proteins that induce sperm binding to the zona pellucida (Cuasnicu et al, 1984b; Blaquier et al, 1988). Epididymal proteins suggested to protect spermatozoa against proteolytic degradation or oxidative damage during epididymal transit include proteinase inhibitors (Kirchhoff et al, 1991; Cornwall et al, 1992; Cornwall and Hann, 1995b), glutathione peroxidase (Ghyselinck et al, 1991), and gamma-glutamyl transpeptidase (Hinton et al, 1991). Two types of epididymal proteins are believed to influence sperm-egg interaction: proteins that may directly participate in sperm-egg binding, and epididymal enzymes that modify sperm membrane glycoproteins. Examples of proteins involved in sperm-egg binding include PH-30 (Kirchhoff et al, 1990), protein D/E (Cuasnicu et al, 1984a), and α-D-mannosidase (Cornwall et al, 1991). Glycosyltransferase enzymes and β-D-glactosidase are reported to modify sperm membrane carbohydrates and thereby facilitate sperm-egg binding (Skudlarek et al, 1992; Tulsiani et al, 1993). In summary, the inorganic, organic, and macromolecular constituents of epididymal fluid provide a unique and optimal environment capable of supporting maturation processes whereby spermatozoa acquire the ability to carry out the steps necessary for normal fertilization in the female tract.

Control of Epididymal Function

From animal studies, it is clear that **the functions of the epididymis are androgen dependent** (see reviews by Orgebin-Crist et al [1975], Brooks [1983], and Robaire and Hermo [1988]). Clearly, the synthesis of some, but not all, epididymal proteins is regulated by androgen (Jones et al, 1980; Brooks, 1983; Charest et al, 1989; Toney and Danzo, 1989). Bilateral castration results not only in the loss of androgen-dependent epididymal proteins but also in the loss of epididymal weight, the perturbation of luminal histology, and changes in the synthesis and secretion of epididymal fluid components including glycerylphosphorylcholine, carnitine, and sialic acid. Ultimately, the epididymis loses the ability to sustain the processes of sperm motility and fertility maturation and sperm storage. Most of these degenerative processes can be reversed by androgen replacement therapy. However, the effects of androgen on the initial segments of the epididymis are thought to be mediated by ABP and possibly other testicular factors. Thus, the consequences of androgen deprivation on the initial epididymal regions cannot be reversed following castration or ligation of the ductuli efferentes, treatments that prevent the entrance of ABP and testicular factors into the epididymis (Fawcett and Hoffer, 1979).

Studies using laboratory animals indicated that, **compared with the accessory sex glands, the epididymis requires higher levels of androgen for maintenance of its structure and functions** (Rajalakshmi et al, 1976). **The regulatory effects of androgen on the epididymis appear to be mediated through dihydrotestosterone, the primary androgen in epididymal tissue extracts (Vreeburg, 1975; Pujol et al, 1976), and 5α-androstane-3αβ-diol (3A-diol)** (Lubicz-Nawrocki, 1973; Orgebin-Crist et al, 1975). The enzymes {+grk}D{-grk}^{4}-5α-reductase, which catalyzes the formation of dihydrotestosterone from testosterone, and 3α-hydroxysteroid dehydrogenase, which converts dihydrotestosterone to 3α-diol, are present in the epididymis and have been localized within the subcellular fractions of epididymal homogenates from humans (Kinoshita et al, 1980; Larminat et al, 1980) and experimental animals (Robaire et al, 1977; Scheer and Robaire, 1983).

Studies in the rat demonstrated that epididymal functions are also influenced by temperature (Foldesy and Bedford, 1982; Wong et al, 1982). Abdominal placement of the epididymis, resulting in exposure to body temperature, causes the loss of sperm storage and electrolyte transport functions. Whether the functions of the human epididymis are similarly affected by body temperature is unknown. The potential influence of temperature on epididymal function in humans may be an important consideration in investigating the relationships between varicocele or cryptorchidism and male fertility.

Evidence from studies in the rat has also suggested that the ability of the epididymis to store spermatozoa may be influenced by the sympathetic nervous system. Surgical partial denervation of the epididymis resulted in an abnormal accumulation of spermatozoa within the cauda epididymidis and a decrease in the curvilinear and straight-line swimming speed of the retained spermatozoa (Billups et al, 1990a, 1990b). These results suggest that chemical or surgical sympathetic denervation or nerve trauma may have an adverse effect on subsequent fertility.

SPERMATOZOA

Because of its highly specialized morphology and physiology, the spermatozoon is marvelously suited for its single purpose—reproduction. For reviews of sperm structure and function, the reader is referred to Fawcett and Bedford (1979), Tash and Means (1988), Fouquet and Kann (1994), Lindemann and Kanous (1989), and Majumder and colleagues (1990). Mature spermatozoa stored within the cauda epididymidis and the ductus deferens are highly differentiated cells (Fig. 42–19). **The human spermatozoon is approximately 60 μm in length** (Fléchon and Hafez, 1976). The oval sperm head, which is about 4.5 μm long and 3 μm wide, consists principally of a nucleus that contains the highly compact chromatin material. In hamster (Ward and Coffey, 1990) and human (Barone et al, 1994) spermatozoa, **nuclear DNA is highly organized into loop domains attached at their bases to a nuclear matrix** (for a review of DNA organization in human spermatozoa see Ward and Coffey [1991]). Surrounding the anterior portion of the sperm head is the acrosome, a membrane-bound organelle that contains the enzymes required for penetration of the outer vestments of the egg prior to fertilization (Chang and Hunter, 1975; Yanagimachi, 1994).

The middle piece of the spermatozoon is a highly organized segment consisting of helically arranged mitochondria surrounding a set of outer dense fibers and the characteristic 9 + 2 microtubular structure of the sperm axoneme. The outer dense fibers, which are rich in disulfide bonds, are thought to provide the sperm tail with the rigidity necessary for progressive motility (Bedford et al, 1973). The sperm mitochondria contain the enzymes required for oxidative metabolism and for the production of adenosine triphosphate, the primary energy source for the cell. **The sperm axoneme contains the enzymes and structural proteins necessary for transduction of the chemical energy of adenosine**

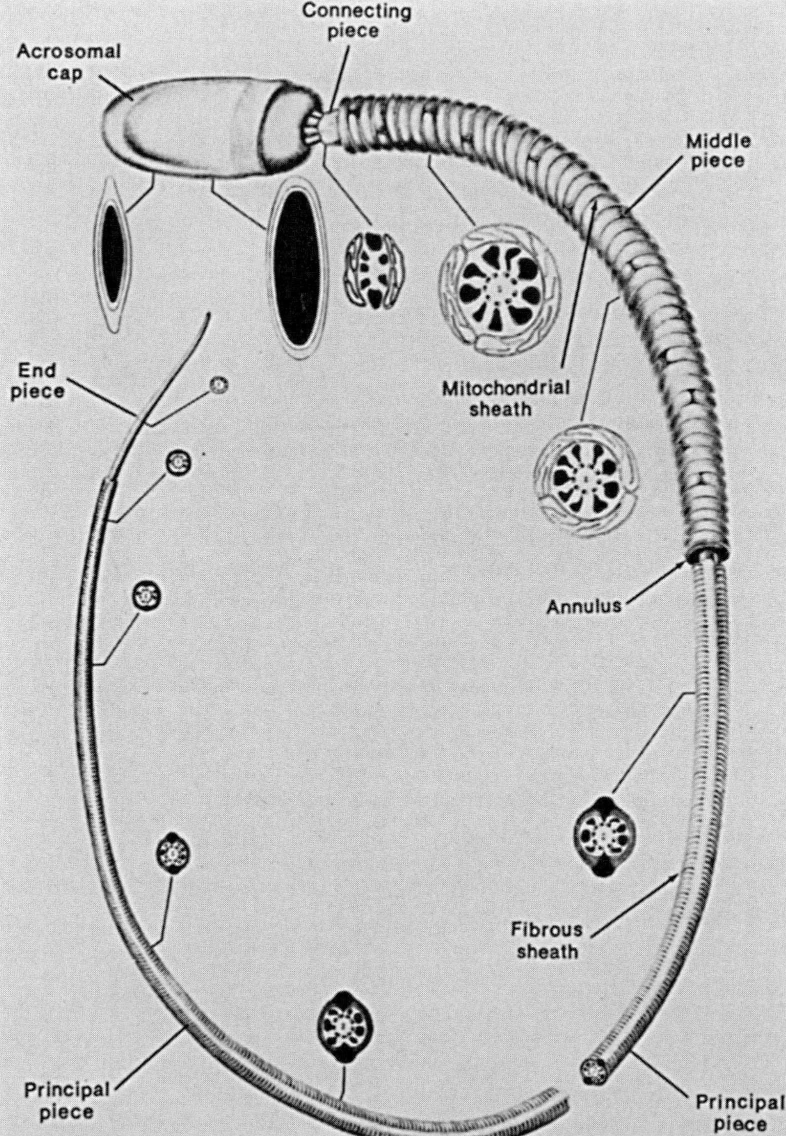

Figure 42–19. A typical mammalian spermatozoon. The plasma membrane is omitted in order to illustrate the major components of the spermatozoon. Cross-sectional insets show the orientation of the internal cell structures. (From Fawcett DW: The mammalian spermatozoon. Dev Biol 1975a; 44:394–436.)

triphosphate into mechanical movement, resulting in motility. The outer dense fibers and axonemal structures present in the middle piece continue, with slight modification, through the principal piece of the spermatozoon, which is surrounded by a fibrous sheath. At the distal end of the principal piece, the outer dense fibers terminate, leaving the axonemes as the primary structure in the end-piece region. Except for the end piece, the spermatozoon is enveloped by a highly specialized plasma membrane that regulates the transmembrane movement of ions and other molecules (Friend, 1989). Moreover, as shown in studies with laboratory animals, **the plasma membrane covering the sperm head region contains specialized proteins that participate in sperm-egg interactions during the early stages of fertilization** (for reviews see Dietl and Rauth [1989], Saling [1989], and Myles [1993]). In particular, carbohydrate-binding proteins on the sperm membrane interact with the species-specific ZP3 protein in the egg zona pellucida, which results in sperm binding to the zona and subsequently in the induction of the acrosome reaction (O'Rand, 1988; Wassarman, 1988; Dietl and Rauth, 1989; Shabanowitz, 1990). As described earlier, other sperm membrane proteins, such as PH-30 and D/E, are present on spermatozoa and function as fusion proteins between the sperm and egg plasma membranes during fertilization (Cuasnicu et al, 1984b; Blobel et al, 1990).

In addition to the obvious role of spermatozoa in providing genetic material during fertilization, recent work has suggested that **other components of the male gamete may have significant importance for embryonic development** (see reviews by Barton et al [1991] and Wyrobek [1993]). Normally in humans the mitotic activity of embryos appears to be organized by the paternally derived centrosome (Schatten, 1994; Simerly et al, 1995). **In the absence of this contribution from a male gamete, mitotic activity of the human embryo is chaotic and a viable embryo is not produced** (Palermo et al, 1994). Emphasizing the importance of spermatozoa in postfertilization embryonic development, Chan and associates (1993) stated that "we should drastically change our attitude from one of the spermatozoon as a robust, simple initiator of embryonic development, and embrace the idea of the vulnerability of such germ cells both during and after their production, and how detrimental influences on this might profoundly affect embryogenesis after successful fertilization." Further observations and experiments are required to delineate exactly what components of the male gamete are necessary to facilitate embryo development.

The functionally competent spermatozoon is a result of the complex processes of spermatogenesis and epididymal maturation. For excellent reviews of sperm function during fertilization (e.g., capacitation, egg binding, and the acrosome reaction), see Yanagimachi (1994), Garbers (1989), Dietl and Rauth (1989), and Myles (1993).

DUCTUS DEFERENS

The ductus deferens is a tubular structure derived embryologically from the mesonephric (wolffian) duct. **In humans, the ductus deferens is approximately 30 to 35 cm in length;** it begins at the cauda epididymidis and terminates in the ejaculatory duct near the prostate gland. Lich and colleagues (1978) stated that the ductus deferens may be divided into five portions: (1) the convoluted region of the ductus deferens within the tunica vaginalis, (2) the scrotal portion, (3) the inguinal division, (4) the retroperitoneal or pelvic portion, and (5) the ampulla. In cross section, the ductus deferens consists of an outer adventitial connective tissue sheet that contains blood vessels and small nerves, a muscular coat that is made up of a middle circular layer surrounded by inner and outer longitudinal muscle layers, and a mucosal inner layer made up of an epithelial lining (Neaves, 1975). The lumen of the tubule is approximately 0.05 cm in diameter.

Vascularization and Innervation

The ductus deferens receives its blood supply from the deferential artery via the inferior vesicle artery (Harrison, 1949b). Kormano and Reijonen (1976) discovered that **the microvascularization of the sheathless portion of the human ductus deferens is divided into an outer network within the adventitial layer and an inner subepithelial capillary network.**

The ductus deferens of the human receives nerve fibers from both the sympathetic and the parasympathetic nervous system (Sjöstrand, 1965). The cholinergic supply is of minor importance in the motor activity of the ductus deferens (Baumgarten et al, 1975). In contrast, **the human ductus deferens has a rich supply of sympathetic adrenergic nerves (Sjöstrand, 1965; Alm, 1982; McConnell et al, 1982) derived from the hypogastric nerves via the presacral nerve** (Batra and Lardner, 1976). Interestingly, the ductus deferens receives a special type of short adrenergic nerve (Sjöstrand, 1965). McConnell and co-workers (1982) reported that adrenergic nerve fibers were observed in all three layers of the tunica muscularis, with the greatest concentration in the outer longitudinal layer. Recently, Amobi and associates (1995) reported that the action of noradrenaline on the vas deferens is mediated through alpha$_1$-adrenoceptors and that selected alpha$_1$-adrenoceptor agonists evoked differential responses in the longitudinal and circular muscles of the ductus deferens. Neurons containing other neurotransmitter substances, such as neuropeptide Y, tyrosine hydroxylase, and vasoactive intestinal polypeptide, have also been identified (Alm, 1982; McConnell et al, 1982; Tainio, 1995). It remains to be shown how the actions of these neurotransmitters are coordinated in support of the physiologic functions of the ductus deferens.

Cytoarchitecture of the Ductus Deferens

There have been numerous studies in experimental animals describing the cytoarchitecture of the ductus deferens (for a review, see Hamilton [1975]). Similar detailed descriptions of the human ductus deferens at the light and electron microscopic level have been presented (Popovic et al, 1973; Friend et al, 1976; Hoffer, 1976; Paniagua et al, 1981; Riva et al, 1982; Nistal et al, 1992). Paniagua and co-workers (1981) observed that the ductus deferens was lined by pseudostratified epithelium, that the epithelial height decreased along the length of the ductus; that the longitudinal folds of the epithelium were simple in the proximal region and became more complex toward the distal segments; and that the thickness of the entire muscle layer gradually decreased along the length of the ductus deferens. Hoffer (1976) and Paniagua and colleagues (1981) reported that the pseudostratified epithelium lining the lumen of the ductus deferens is composed of basal cells and three types of tall thin columnar cells. The latter, which extend from the base of the epithelium to the lumen, include principal cells, pencil cells, and mitochondrion-rich cells. All of these cells show stereocilia and irregular convoluted nuclei. According to Paniagua and associates (1981), principal cells are the most frequent cell type in the proximal portion of the ductus deferens. In contrast, the portion of both pencil cells and mitochondrion-rich cells increases toward the distal end of the ductus deferens.

The complexity of the muscular layers, the specialized and rich adrenergic innervation, the variety of epithelial cells in the mucosal layer, and the changing structural characteristics from the proximal to the distal end strongly suggest that the ductus deferens in humans is more than a passive conduit for the transport of sperm from the cauda epididymidis to the urethra.

Functions of the Ductus Deferens

Spermatozoa Transport

There are numerous theories to explain the transport of spermatozoa through the ductus deferens in humans (Gunha et al, 1975; Neaves, 1975; Batra and Lardner, 1976). Unfortunately, data supporting these theories are fragmentary and the issue remains unresolved. However, several pertinent observations have been made. Apparently, **the human ductus deferens exhibits spontaneous motility (Ventura et al, 1973). Also, the human ductus deferens has the capacity to respond when stretched (Bruschini et al, 1977). Finally, the contents of the ductus deferens can be propelled into the urethra by strong peristaltic contractions that are elicited either by electrical stimulation of the hypogastric nerve (Bruschini et al, 1977) or by adrenergic neurotransmitters** (Ventura et al, 1973; Bruschini et al, 1977; Lipshultz et al, 1981).

Prins and Zaneveld (1979, 1980a, 1980b) have obtained interesting results regarding the transport of spermatozoa through the ductus deferens at sexual rest, after sexual stimulation, and after ejaculation. Using the rabbit as a model, Prins and Zaneveld (1979) showed that during the sexual rest, epididymal contents were transported distally through the vas deferens into the urethra in small amounts and at irregular intervals, supporting the idea that urethral disposal is a mechanism for ridding the epididymis of excess spermatozoa. Further, they showed that when rabbits were sexually stimulated, spermatozoa were transported from the cauda epididymidis and proximal ductus deferens toward the distal ductus deferens. If ejaculation occurred, spermatozoa were propelled into the urethra.

After sexual stimulation and ejaculation, an interesting phenomenon occurred. The contents of the ductus deferens were propelled proximally and even into the cauda epididymidis because the distal portion of the ductus deferens contracted with greater amplitude, frequency, and duration than did the proximal portion of the ductus deferens (Prins and Zaneveld, 1980b). Importantly, this process was reversed on prolonged sexual rest, and the excess cauda epididymal spermatozoa that derived from daily spermatozoa production were once again transported distally. These results were interpreted to mean that the ductus deferens of the rabbit played an important role not only in sperm transport during sexual activity but also in the maintenance of epididymal sperm reserves. It remains to be seen whether similar mechanisms are at work in sperm transport through the human ductus deferens.

Absorption and Secretion

Based on morphologic criteria, it has been suggested that the human ductus deferens may have both absorptive and secretory functions. **The stereocilia, apical blebbing, and primary and secondary lysosomes of principal cells in the human ductus deferens are characteristic of cells involved in absorptive functions** (Hoffer, 1976; Paniagua et al, 1981, Murakami and Yokoyama, 1989). However, although protein absorption from the tubular lumen of the rat ductus deferens has been observed (Friend and Farquhar, 1967), direct evidence of fluid or protein absorption by the epithelium in the human vas deferens has not been reported.

Cooper and Hamilton (1977) have shown that the terminal region and gland of the rat ductus deferens have the capacity to phagocytose and absorb spermatozoa. Using scanning electron microscopy, Murakami and colleagues (1982) reported spermiophagy by epithelial cells in the ampullary region of the ductus deferens in men and monkeys. Whether the amount of spermiophagy in the ampulla and in other regions of the excurrent duct is sufficient for the removal of excess spermatozoa in men remains to be seen.

Hoffer (1976), Paniagua and associates (1981), and Nistal and co-workers (1992) reported that **the principal cells of the human ductus deferens have characteristics typical of cells that are capable of synthesizing and secreting glycoproteins.** This is in keeping with reports by Gupta and colleagues (1974) and Bennett and associates (1974) that the rat ductus deferens synthesizes and secretes glycoproteins into the tubular lumen. In an attempt to explain successful pregnancies achieved after high epididymovasostomy or efferentiovasostomy, Bedford (1994) suggested that the absorptive and secretory functions of the vas deferens may create a luminal environment capable of supporting the maturation of sperm fertility. Unfortunately, we were unable to find experimental results in the human that would confirm a secretory function in the vas deferens or support the idea of sperm maturation within the vas deferens.

The structure and function of the ductus deferens probably depends on androgen stimulation because (1) the human ductus deferens converts testosterone to dihydrotestosterone (Dupuy et al, 1979), (2) castration causes atrophy of—and testosterone treatment causes restoration of—monkey vas deferens function (Dinaker et al, 1977), and (3) spontaneous as well as alpha- and beta-adrenergic stimulated contractions of the rat ductus deferens are altered by castration and testosterone treatment (Borda et al, 1981).

REFERENCES

Agger P: Scrotal and testicular temperature: Its relation to sperm count before and after operation for varicocele. Fertil Steril 1971; 22:286–291.

Allan DJ, Harmon BV, Roberts SA: Spermatogonial apoptosis has three morphologically recognizable phases and shows no circadian rhythm during normal spermatogenesis in the rat. Cell Prolif 1992; 25:241–250.

Allenby G, Foster PM, Sharpe RM: Evidence that secretion of immunoactive inhibin by seminiferous tubules from the adult rat testis is regulated by specific germ cell types: Correlation between in vivo and in vitro studies. Endocrinology 1991; 128:467–476.

Alm P: On the autonomic innervation of the human vas deferens. Brain Res Bull 1982; 9:673–681.

Amann RP: A critical review of methods for evaluation of spermatogenesis from seminal characteristics. J Androl 1981; 2:37–45.

Amann RP, Almquist JO: Reproductive capacity of dairy bulls. VI. Effect of unilateral vasectomy and ejaculation frequency on sperm reserves: Aspects of epididymal physiology. J Reprod Fertil 1962; 3:260–268.

Amann RP, Howards SS: Daily spermatozoal production and epididymal spermatozoal reserves of the human male. J Urol 1980; 124:211–215.

Amobi N, Smith CH: The human vas deferens: Correlation of response pattern to noradrenaline and histological structure. Eur J Pharmacol 1995; 273:25–34.

Andersen JM, Dietschy JM: Regulation of sterol synthesis in 15 tissues of rat. II. Role of rat and human high and low density plasma lipoproteins and of rat chylomicron remnants. J Biol Chem 1977; 252:3652–3659.

Ascoli M, Segaloff DL: Regulation of the differentiated functions of Leydig tumor cells by epidermal growth factor. Ann NY Acad Sci 1989; 564:99–115.

Bardin CW, Cheng CY, Musto NA, Gunsalus GL: The Sertoli cell. *In* Knobil E, Neill JD, eds: The Physiology of Reproduction, 2nd ed. New York, Raven Press, 1994, pp 1291–1333.

Bardin CW, Morris PL, Shaha C, et al: Inhibin structure and function in the testis. Ann NY Acad Sci 1989; 564:10–23.

Barone JG, De Lara J, Cummings KB, Ward WS: DNA organization in human spermatozoa. J Androl 1994; 15:139–144.

Barr AE, Moore DJ, Paulsen CA: Germinal cell loss during human spermatogenesis. J Reprod Fertil 1971; 25:75–80.

Barton SC, Ferguson-Smith AC, Fundele R, Surani MA: Influence of paternally imprinted genes on development. Development 1991; 113:679–687.

Batra SK, Lardner TJ: Sperm transport in the vas deferens. *In* Hafez ESE, ed: Human Semen and Fertility Regulation in Men. St. Louis, The CV Mosby Company, 1976, pp 100–106.

Baumgarten HG, Falck B, Holstein AF, et al: Adrenergic innervation of the human testis, epididymis, ductus deferens and prostate: A fluorescence microscopic and fluorimetric study. Z Zellforsch Mikrosk Anat 1968; 90:81–95.

Baumgarten HG, Holstein AF: Catecholaminehaltige nervenfasern im hoden des menschen. Z Zellforsch Mirosk Anat 1967; 79:389–395.

Baumgarten HG, Holstein AF, Rosengren E: Arrangement, ultrastructure, and adrenergic innervation of smooth musculature of the ductuli efferentes, ductus epididymidis and ductus deferens of man. Z Zellforsch Mikrosk Anat 1971; 120:37–79.

Baumgarten HG, Owan C, Sjoberg NO: Neural mechanisms in male fertility. *In* Sciarra JJ, Markland C, Speidel JI, eds: Control of Male Fertility. Hagerstown, Harper & Row, 1975, pp 26–40.

Bayard F, Boulard PY, Huc A, Pontonnier F: Arterio-venous transfer of testosterone in the spermatic cord of man. J Clin Endocrinol Metab 1975; 40:345–346.

Beck EM, Schlegel PN, Goldstein M: Intraoperative varicocele anatomy: A macroscopic and microscopic study. J Urol 1992; 148:1190–1194.

Bedford JM: Effect of duct ligation on the fertilizing ability of spermatozoa from different regions of the rabbit epididymis. J Exp Zool 1967; 166:271–281.

Bedford JM: Report of a workshop: Maturation of the fertilizing ability of mammalian spermatozoa in the male and female reproductive tract. Biol Reprod 1974; 11:346–362.

Bedford JM; Maturation, transport and fate of spermatozoa in the epididymis. *In* Greep RO, Astman EB, eds: Handbook of Physiology. Section 7, Male Reproductive System. Baltimore, The Williams & Wilkins Company, 1975, pp 303–317.

Bedford JM: The bearing of epididymal function in strategies for *in vitro* fertilization and gamete intrafallopian transfer. Ann NY Acad Sci 1988; 541:284–291.

Bedford JM: The status and the state of the human epididymis. Hum Reprod Update 1994; 9:2187–2199.

Bedford JM, Calvin HI, Cooper GW: The maturation of spermatozoa in the human epididymis. J Reprod Fertil (Suppl)1973; 18:199–213.

Bellvé AR, Zheng W: Growth factors as autocrine and paracrine modulators of male gonadal functions. J Reprod Fertil 1989; 85:771–793.

Belonoschkin B. Biologie der spermatozoen in menschlichen hoden und nebenhoden. Arch Gynaek 1942; 174:357–362.

Bennett G, Leblond CP, Haddad A: Migration of glycoprotein from the Golgi apparatus to the surface of various cell types as shown by autoradiography after labelled fucose injection into rats. J Cell Biol 1974; 60:258–284.

Billups KL, Tillman S, Chang TSK: Ablation of the inferior mesenteric plexus in the rat: Alteration of sperm storage in the epididymis and vas deferens. J Urology 1990a; 143:625–629.

Billups KL, Tillman S, Chang TSK: Reduction of epididymal sperm motility after ablation of the inferior mesenteric plexus in the rat. Fert Steril 1990b; 53:1076–1082.

Blaquier J, Cameo MS, Cuasnicu PS, et al: On the role of epididymal factors in sperm fertility. Reprod Nutr Dev 1988; 28:1209–1216.

Blobel CP, Myles DG, Primakoff P, White JM: Proteolytic processing of a protein involved in sperm-egg fusion correlates with acquisition of fertilization competence. J Cell Biol 1990; 111:69–78.

Borda E, Agostini M del C, Gimeno, MF, Gimeno AL: Castration alters the stimulatory and inhibitory adrenergic influences on isolated rat vas deferens. Pharmacol Res Comm 1981; 13:981–996.

Brackett BJ, Hall JL, Oh YK: In vitro fertilizing ability of testicular, epididymal, and ejaculated rabbit spermatozoa. Fertil Steril 1978; 29:571–582.

Brandt H, Acott TS, Johnson DJ, Hoskins DD: Evidence for an epididymal origin of bovine sperm forward motility protein. Biol Reprod 1978; 19:830–835.

Brooks DE: Epididymal functions and their hormonal regulation. Aust J Biol Sci 1983; 36:205–221.

Brooks DE, Tiver K: Analysis of surface proteins of rat spermatozoa during epididymal transit and identification of antigens common to spermatozoa, rete testis fluid and cauda epididymal plasma. J Reprod Fertil 1984; 71:249–257.

Brooks DE, Means AR, Wright EJ, et al: Molecular cloning of the cDNA for two major androgen-dependent secretory proteins of 18.5 kilodaltons synthesized by the rat epididymis. J Biol Chem 1986; 26:4956–4961.

Brown CR, von Glos KI, Jones R: Changes in plasma membrane glycoproteins of rat spermatozoa during maturation in the epididymis. J Cell Biol 1983; 96:256–264

Bruschini H, Schmidt RA, Tanagho EA: Studies on the neurophysiology of the vas deferens. Invest Urol 1977; 15:112–116.

Casillas ER, Elder CM, Hoskins DD: Adenylate cyclase activity of bovine spermatozoa during maturation in the epididymis and the activation of sperm particulate adenylate cyclase by GTP and polyamines. J Reprod Fertil 1980; 59:297–302.

Catt KJ, Dufau ML: Basic concepts of the mechanism of action of peptide hormones. Biol Reprod 1976; 14:1–15.

Chan SY, Tucker MJ, Leung CK, Leong MK: Association between human in vitro fertilization rate and pregnancy outcome: A possible involvement of spermatozoal quality in subsequent embryonic viability. Asia Oceania J Obstet Gyneacol 1993; 19:357–373.

Chan SYW, Loh TT, Wang C, Tang LC: Seminal plasma transferrin and seminiferous tubular dysfunction. Fertil Steril 1986; 45:687–691.

Chandley AC, Cooke HJ: Human male fertility: Y-linked genes and spermatogenesis. Hum Molec Genet 1994; 3:1449–1452.

Chang MC, Hunter RHF: Capacitation of mammalian sperm: Biological and experimental aspects. *In* Greep RO, Astman EB, eds: Handbook of Physiology. Section 7, Male Reproductive System. Baltimore, The Williams & Wilkins Company, 1975, pp 339–351.

Charest NJ, Petrusz P, Ordronneau P, et al: Developmental expression of an androgen-regulated epididymal protein. Endocrinol 1989; 125:942–947.

Charreau EH, Calvo JC, Nozu K, et al: Hormonal modulation of 3-hydroxy-3-methylglutaryl coenzyme A reductase activity in gonadotropin stimulated and desensitized testicular Leydig cells. J Biol Chem 1981; 256:12719–12724.

Chemes H, Dym M, Fawcett DW, et al: Pathophysiological observations of Sertoli cells in patients with germinal aplasia or severe germ cell depletion. Ultrastructural findings and hormone levels. Biol Reprod 1977; 17:108–123.

Chemes HF, Pasqualini T, Rivarola MA, Bergada C: Is testosterone involved in the initiation of spermatogenesis in humans? A clinicopathological presentation and physiological consideration in four patients with Leydig cell tumors of the testis or secondary Leydig cell hyperplasia. Int J Androl 1982; 5:229–245.

Chen CS, Chu SH, Soong YK, Lai YM: Epididymal sperm aspiration with assisted reproductive techniques—difference between congenital and acquired obstructive azoospermia. Hum Reprod 1995; 10:1104–1108.

Christensen AK: Leydig cells. *In* Greep RO, Hamilton DW, eds: Handbook of Physiology. Section 7, Male Reproductive System. Baltimore, The Williams & Wilkins Company, 1975, pp 339–351.

Cigorraga SB, Chemes H, Pellizzari E: Steroidogenic and morphogenic characteristics of human peritubular cells in culture. Biol Reprod 1994; 51:1193–205.

Clermont Y: The cycle of the seminiferous epithelium in man. Am J Anat 1963; 112:35–51.

Clermont Y: Kinetics of spermatogenesis in mammals: Seminiferous epithelium cycle and spermatogonial renewal. Physiol Rev 1972; 52:198–236.

Connell CJ: The Sertoli cell of the sexually mature dog. Anat Rec 1974; 178:333.

Cooper TG: In defense of a function for the human epididymis. Fertil Steril 1990; 54:965–975.

Cooper TG, Hamilton DW: Phagocytosis of spermatozoa in the terminal region and gland of the vas deferens of the rat. Am J Anat 1977; 150:247–267.

Cooper TG, Orgebin-Crist MC: Effect of aging on the fertilizing capacity of testicular spermatozoa from the rabbit. Biol Reprod 1977; 16:258–266.

Cornwall GA, Hann SR: Specialized gene expression in the epididymis. J Androl 1995a; 16:379–383.

Cornwall GA, Hann SR: Transient appearance of CRES protein during spermatogenesis and caput epididymal sperm maturation. Mol Reprod Dev 1995b; 41:37–46.

Cornwall GA, Orgebin-Crist MC, Hann SR: The CRES gene: A unique testis-regulated gene related to the cystatin family is highly restricted in its expression to the proximal region of the mouse epididymis. Molec Endocrinol 1992; 6:1653–1664.

Cornwall GA, Tulsiani DRP, Orgebin-Crist: Inhibition of mouse, sperm-D-mannosidase inhibits sperm-egg binding in vitro. Biol Reprod 1991; 44:913–921.

Courot M: Transport and maturation of spermatozoa in the epididymis of mammals. *In* Bollack C, Clavert A, eds: Progress in Reproductive Biology. Vol 8, Epididymis and Fertility: Biology and Pathology. Basel, S. Karger, 1981, pp 67–79.

Courtens JL, Fournier-Delpech S: Modifications in the plasma membranes of epididymal ram spermatozoa during maturation and incubation in utero. J Ultrastruct Res 1979; 68:136–148.

Cuasnicu PS, Bedford JM: The effect of moderate epididymal aging on the kinetics of the acrosome reaction and fertilizing ability of hamster spermatozoa. Biol Reprod 1989; 40:1067–1073.

Cuasnicu PS, Echeverri FG, Piazza AD, et al: Antibodies against epididymal glycoproteins block fertilizing ability in rat. J Reprod Fert 1984a; 72:467–471.

Cuasnicu PS, Gonzales-Echeverria F, Piazza A, et al: Epididymal proteins mimic the androgenic effect of zona pellucida recognition by immature hamster spermatozoa. J Reprod Fertil 1984b; 71:427–431.

Cummins JM, Jequier AM: Treating male infertility needs more clinical andrology, not less. Hum Reprod 1994; 9:1214–1219.

Dacheux JL, Paquignon M: Relations between the fertilizing ability, motility and metabolism of epididymal spermatozoa. Reprod Nutr Dev 1980; 20:1085–1099.

Davis AG: Role of FSH in the control of testicular function. Arch Androl 1981; 7:97–108.

Davis JR: Myogenic tone of the rat testicular subcapsular artery has a role in autoregulation of testicular blood supply. Biol Reprod 1990; 42:727–735.

Davis AG, Horowitz AM: Age-related differences in the response of the isolated testicular capsule of the rat to norepinephrine, acetylcholine and prostaglandins. J Reprod Fertil 1978; 54:269–274.

Davis JR, Langford GA: Response of the testicular capsule to acetyl choline and noradrenaline. Nature 1969; 222:386–387.

Davis JR, Langford GA: Response of the isolated testicular capsule of the rat to autonomic drugs. J Reprod Fertil 1969; 19:595–598.

deKretser DW, Burger HG: Ultrastructural studies of the human Sertoli cell in normal men and males with hypogonadotropic hypogonadism before and after gonadotropic treatment. *In* Saxena BB, Beling CG, Gandy HM, eds: Gonadotropins. New York, Wiley Interscience, 1972, pp 640–656.

deKretser DM, Kerr JB: Cytology of the testis. *In* Knobil E, Neill JD, eds: The Physiology of Reproduction, 2nd ed. New York, Raven Press, 1994, pp 1177–1290.

Desjardins C: The microcirculation of the testis. Ann NY Acad Sci 1989; 564:243–249.

Dietl JA, Rauth G: Molecular aspects of mammalian fertilization. Hum Reprod 1989; 4:869–875.

Dinakar RA, Dinaker N, Prasad MRN: Response of the epididymis, ductus deferens and accessory glands of the castrated prepubertal rhesus monkey to exogenous administration of testosterone 5-dihydrotestosterone. Indian J Exp Biol 1977; 15:829–836.

DiZerga GS, Sherins RJ: Endocrine control of adult testicular function. *In* Burger H, DeKretser D, eds: The Testis. New York, Raven Press, 1981; pp 127–140.

Douglass J, Garrett SH, Garret JE: Differential patterns of regulated gene expression in the adult rat epididymis. *In* Robaire B, ed: The Male Germ Cell: Spermatogonium to Fertilization. New York, The New York Academy of Sciences, 1991, pp 384–398.

Dufau ML: Endocrine regulation and communicating functions of the Leydig cell. Ann Rev Physiol 1988; 50:483–508.

Dufau ML, Catt KJ: Gonadotrophin receptors and regulation of steroidogenesis in the testis and ovary. Vitam Horm 1978; 36:461–592.

Dupuy GM, Boulanger KD, Roberts KD, et al: Metabolism of sex steroids in the human and canine vas deferens. Endocrinol 1979; 104:1553–1558.

Dym M: The fine structure of the monkey Sertoli cell and its role in maintaining the blood-testis barrier. Anat Rec 1973; 175:639–656.

Dym M: Spermatogonial stem cells of the testis. Proc Natl Acad Sci USA 1994; 91:11287–11289.

Dym M, Fawcett DW: The blood-testis barrier in the rat and the physiological compartmentation of the seminiferous epithelium. Biol Reprod 1970; 3:308–318.

Dym M, Raj HGM, Chemes HE: Response of the testis to selective withdrawal of LH or FSH using antigonadotropic sera. *In* Troen P, Nankin HR, eds: The Testis in Normal and Infertile Man. New York, Raven Press, 1977, pp 97–117.

Eik-Nes KB: Biosynthesis and secretion of testicular steroids. *In* Greep RO, Astwood EB, eds: Handbook of Physiology> Section 7, Male Reproductive System. Baltimore, The Williams & Wilkins Company, 1975, pp 95–115.

Ewing LL: Leydig cell. *In* Lipshultz LI, Howards S, eds: Infertility in the Male. New York, Churchill Livingstone, 1983, pp 43–69.

Ewing LL, Brown B: Testicular steroidogenesis. *In* Johnson AD, Gomes WR, eds: The Testis, Vol 4. New York, Academic Press, 1977, pp 239–287.

Ewing LL, Davis JC, Zirkin BR: Regulation of testicular function. A spatial and temporal view. *In* Greep RO, ed: International Review of Physiology, Vol. 22. Baltimore, University Park Press, 1980, pp 41–115.

Fawcett DW: Interactions between Sertoli cells and germ cells. *In* Mancini RE, Mancini L, eds: Male Fertility and Sterility. New York, Academic Press, 1974, pp 13–36.

Fawcett DW: Ultrastructure and function of the Sertoli cell. *In* Greep RO, Hamilton DW, eds: Handbook of Physiology. Section 7, Male Reproductive System. Baltimore, The Williams & Wilkins Company, 1975b, pp 21–55.

Fawcett DW: The cell biology of gametogenesis in the male. Perspect Biol Med 1979; 22:S56–S73.

Fawcett DW, Bedford JM, eds: The Spermatozoon. Maturation, Motility, Surface Properties and Comparative Aspects. Baltimore, Urban & Schwarzenberg, 1979, pp 23–35.

Fawcett DW, Hoffer AP: Failure of exogenous androgen to prevent regression of the initial segments of the rat epididymis after efferent duct ligation or orchiectomy. Biol Reprod 1979; 20: 162–181.

Fléchon JE, Hafez ESE: Scanning electron microscopy of human spermatozoa. *In* Hafez ESE, ed: Human Semen and Fertility Regulation in Men. St. Louis, The C.V. Mosby Company, 1976, pp 76–82.

Flickinger C, Fawcett DW: The junctional specializations of Sertoli cells in the seminiferous epithelium. Anat Rec 1967; 158:207–221.

Foldesy RG, Bedford JM: Biology of the scrotum. I. Temperature and androgen as determinants of the sperm storage capacity of the rat cauda epididymis. Biol Reprod 1982; 26:673–682.

Fouquet J-P, Kann M-L: The cytoskeleton of mammalian spermatozoa. Biol Cell 1994; 81:89–93.

Fournier-Delpech S, Colas G, Courot M, et al: Epididymal sperm maturation in the ram: Motility, fertilizing ability, and embryonic survival after uterine artificial insemination in the ewe. Ann Biol Anim Biochim Biophys 1979; 19:579–586.

Fournier-Delpech S, Danzo RJ, Orgebin-Crist MC: Extraction of concanavalin A affinity material from rat testicular and epididymal spermatozoa. Ann Biol Anim Biochim Biophys 1977; 17:207–215.

Free MJ: Blood supply to the testis and its role in local exchange and transport of hormones. *In* Johnson AD, Gomes WR, eds: The Testis, Vol 4. New York, Academic Press, 1977, pp 39–90.

Free MJ, Jaffe RA, Morford DE: Sperm transport through the rete testis in anaesthetized rats: Role of the testicular capsule and effect of gonadotropins and prostaglandins. Biol Reprod 1980; 22:1073–1078.

Friend DS: Sperm maturation: membrane domain boundaries. Ann NY Acad Sci 1989; 567:208–221.

Friend DS, Farquhar MG: Functions of coated vesicles during protein absorption in the rat vas deferens. J Cell Biol 1967; 35:357–376.

Friend DS, Galle J, Silber S: Fine structure of human sperm, vas deferens epithelium, and testicular biopsy specimens at the time of vasectomy reversal. Anat Rec 1976; 184:584.

Fritjofsson A, Persson JE, Petterson S: Testicular blood flow in man measured with xenon-133. Scand J Urol Nephrol 1969; 3:276–280.

Fritz IB: Somatic cell-germ cell relationships in mammalian testes during development and spermatogenesis. Ciba Found Symp 1994; 182:271–274.

Garrett JE, Garrett SH, Douglas J: A spermatozoa-associated factor regulates proenkephalin gene expression in the rat epididymis. Mol Endocrinol 1990; 4:108–118.

George FW, Wilson JD: Sex determination and differentiation. *In* Knobil E, Neill JD, eds: The Physiology of Reproduction, 2nd ed. New York, Raven Press, 1994, pp 3– 28.

Ghinea N, Mai TV, Groyer-Picard MT, Milgrom E: How protein hormones reach their target cells: Receptor-mediated transcytosis of hCG through endothelial cells. J Cell Biol 1994; 125:87–97.

Ghyselinck NB, Jimenez C, Courty Y, Dufaure JP: Androgen-dependent messenger RNA(s) related to secretory proteins in the mouse epididymis. J Reprod Fertil 1989; 85:631–639.

Ghyselinck NB, Jimenez C, Dufaure JP: Sequence homology of androgen-regulated epididymal proteins with glutathione peroxidase in mice. J Reprod Fert 1991; 93:461–466.

Gondos B, Berndison WE: Postnatal and pubertal development. *In* Russell LD, Griswold MD, eds: The Sertoli Cell. Clearwater, Florida, Cache River Press, 1993, pp 115–153.

Gondos B, Hobel CJ: Ultrastructure of germ cell development in the human fetal testis. Z Zellforsch 1971; 119:1–20.

Green DP: Mammalian fertilization as a biological machine: A working model for adhesion and fusion of sperm and oocyte. Hum Reprod 1993; 8:91–96.

Griswold MD: Interactions between germ cells and Sertoli cells in the testis. Biol Reprod 1995; 52:211–216.

Griswold MD: Protein secretion by Sertoli cells: General considerations. *In* Russel LD, Griswold MD, eds: The Sertoli Cell. Clearwater, Florida, Cache River Press, 1993; pp 195–200.

Griswold MD, Morales C, Sylvester SR: Molecular biology of the Sertoli cell. Oxf Rev Reprod Biol 1988; 10:53–123.

Gunha SK, Kaur H, Ahmed AM: Mechanics of spermatic fluid transport in the vas deferens. Med Biol Eng 1975; 13:518–522.

Gunn SA, Gould TC: Vasculature of the testes and adnexa. *In* Greep RO, Astwood EB, eds: Handbook of Physiology. Section 7, Male Reproductive System. Baltimore, The Williams & Wilkins Company, 1975, pp 117–142.

Gupta G, Rajalakshmi N, Prasad MRN, Moudgal NR: Alteration of epididymal function and its relation to maturation of spermatozoa. Andrologia 1974; 6:35–44.

Hadley MA, Byers SW, Suarez-Quian CA, et al: Extracellular matrix regulates Sertoli cell differentiation, testicular cord formation and germ cell development *in vitro*. J Cell Biol 1985; 101:1511–1522.

Hamilton DW: Structure and function of the epithelium lining the ductuli efferentes, ductus epididymides, and ductus deferens in the rat. *In* Greep RO, Astwood EB, eds: Handbook of Physiology. Section 7, Male Reproductive System. Baltimore, The Williams & Wilkins Company, 1975, pp 259–301.

Hamilton DW: The epididymis. *In* Greep RO, Kablinsky T, eds: Frontiers in Reproduction and Fertility Control. Part 2. Cambridge, MIT Press, 1977, pp 411–426.

Hammond, J, Asdell SA: The vitality of the spermatozoa in the male and female reproductive tract. J Exp Biol 1926; 4:155–162.

Hansson V, Djoseland O: Preliminary characterization of the 5-dihydrotestosterone binding protein in the epididymal cytosol fraction: In vivo studies. Acta Endocrinol 1972; 71:614–624.

Hardy MP, Gelber SJ, Zhou Z, et al: Hormonal control of Leydig cell differentiation. *In* Robaire B, ed: The male Germ Cell: Spermatogonium to Fertilization. New York, The New York Academy of Sciences, 1991, pp 152–163.

Harrison RG. The comparative anatomy of the blood supply of the mammalian testis. Proc Zool Soc London 1949a; 119:325–344.

Harrison RG: The distribution of the vasal and cremasteric arteries to the testis and their functional importance. J Anat 1949b; 83:267–282.

Harrison RG, Barclay AE: The distribution of the testicular artery (internal spermatic artery) to the human testis. Br J Urol 1948; 20:57–66.

Heller CG, Clermont Y: Kinetics of the germinal epithelium in man. Rec Prog Horm Res 1964; 20:545–575.

Hermo L, Lalli M, Clermont Y: Arrangement of connective tissue elements in the walls of seminiferous tubules of man and monkey. Am J Anat 1977; 148:433–446.

Hermo L, Oko R, Morales CR: Secretion and endocytosis in the male reproductive tract: A role in sperm maturation. Int Rev Cytol 1994; 154:106–189.

Hermo L, Winikoff R, Kan FW: Quantitative changes in *Ricinus communis* agglutinin I and *Helix promatia* lectin binding sites in the acrosome of rat spermatozoa during epididymal transit. Histochemistry 1992; 98:93–103.

Hilscher B, Engemann A: Histological and morphometric studies on the kinetics of germ cells and immature Sertoli cells during human prespermatogenesis. Andrologia 1992; 24:7–10.

Hinrichsen MJ, Blaquier JA: Evidence supporting the existence of sperm maturation in the human epididymis. J Reprod Fertil 1980; 60:291–294.

Hinton BT, Palladino MA: Epididymal epithelium: its contribution to the formation of a luminal fluid microenvironment. Microsc Res Tech 1995; 30:67–81.

Hinton BT, Palladino MA, Mattmeuller DR, et al: Expression and activity of gamma-glutamyl transpeptidase in the rat epididymis. Molec Reprod Dev 1991; 28:40–46.

Hodson N: The nerves of the testis, epididymis and scrotum. *In* Johnson AD, Gomes WR, Vandemark NL, eds: The Testis, Vol 1. New York, Academic Press, 1970, pp 47–99.

Hoffer AP: The ultrastructure of the ductus deferens in man. Biol Reprod 1976; 14:425–445.

Hoffer AP, Hinton BT: Morphological evidence for a blood-epididymis barrier and the effects of gossypol on its integrity. Biol Reprod 1984; 30:991–1004.

Holstein AF: Morphologische studien am nebenhoden des menschen. *In* Bargmann W, Doerr W, eds: Zwanglose Abhandlungen aus dem Gebeit der normalen und pathologischen Anatomie. Stuttgart, Georg Thiem Verlag, 1969, pp 1–17.

Horan AH, Bedford JM: Development of the fertilizing ability of spermatozoa in the epididymis of the Syrian Hamster. J Reprod Fertil 1972; 30:417–423.

Hoskins DD, Munsterman D, Hall ML: The control of bovine sperm glycolysis during epididymal transit. Biol Reprod 1975; 12:566–572.

Howards SS, Jessee SJ, Johnson A: Micropuncture studies of the blood-seminiferous barrier. Biol Reprod 1976; 14:264–269.

Huhtaniemi I, Pelliniemi LJ: Fetal Leydig cells: Cellular origin, morphology, life span, and special functional features. Proc Soc Exp Biol Med 1992; 201:125–140.

Hundeiker M: Lymphgefasse in parenchym des menschlichen hodens. Versuch einer Darstellung durch injektion. Arch Klin Exp Dermatol 1969; 235:271–276.

Hutson JC: Testicular macrophages. Int Rev Cytol 1994; 149:99–143.

Ilio KY, Hess RA: Structure and function of the ductuli efferentes: A review. Microsc Res Tech 1994; 29:432–467.

Ishigami K, Yoshida Y, Hirooka M, Mohri K: A new operation for varicocele: Use of microvascular anastomosis. Surgery 1970; 67:620–623.

Jaakkola UM: Regional variations in transport of the luminal contents of the rat epididymis *in vivo*. J Reprod Fertil 1983; 68:465–470.

Jaakkola UM, Talo A: Relation of electrical activity to luminal transport in the cauda epididymis of the rat *in vitro*. J Reprod Fertil 1982; 64:121–126.

Jardin A, Izard V, Benoit G, et al: *In vivo* and *in vitro* fertilizing ability of immature human epididymal spermatozoa. Reprod Nutr Dev 1988; 28:1375–1385.

Jarow JP, Ogle A, Kaspar J, Hopkins M: Testicular artery ramification within the inguinal canal. J Urol 1992; 147:1290–1292.

Jegou B: Spermatids are regulators of sertoli cell function. *In* Robaire B, ed: The Male Germ Cell: Spermatogonium to Fertilization. New York, The New York Academy of Sciences, 1991, pp 340–353.

Jenkins AD, Turner TT, Howards SS: Physiology of the male reproductive system. Urol Clin North Am 1978; 5:437–450.

Johnson L, Petty CS, Neaves WB: Influence of age on sperm production and testicular weights in men. J Reprod Fertil 1984a; 70:211–218.

Johnson L, Petty CS, Porter JC, Neaves WB: Germ cell degeneration during postprophase of meiosis and serum concentrations of gonadotropins in young adult and older adult men. Biol Reprod 1984b; 31:770–784.

Johnson L, Varner DD: Effect of daily spermatozoon production but not age on transit time of spermatozoa through the human epididymis. Biol Reprod 1988; 39:812–817.

Jones R: Membrane remodelling during sperm maturation in the epididymis. Oxf Rev Reprod Biol 1989; 11:285–337.

Jones R, Brown CR, Von Glos IK, Parker MG: Hormonal regulation of protein synthesis in the rat epididymis. Biochem J 1980; 188:667–676.

Jonte G, Holstein AF: On the morphology of the transitional zones from the rete testis into the ductuli efferentes and from the ductuli efferentes into the ductus epididymidis. Andrologia 1987; 41:398–412.

Junera HR, Alfonsi M-F, Fain-Maurel M-A, Dadoune JP: Characterization of regional proteins in tissues and fluid in the human epididymis. Reprod Nutr Dev 1988; 28:1267–1273.

Kaler LW, Neaves WB: Attrition of human Leydig cell population with advancing age. Anat Rec 1978; 192:513–518.

Kaya M, Harrison RG: The ultrastructural relationship between Sertoli cells and spermatogenic cells in the rat. J Anat 1976; 121:279–290.

Keeney DS, Ewing LL: Effects of hypophysectomy and alterations in the spermatogenic function on Leydig cell volume, number, and proliferation in adult rats. J Androl 1990; 11:367–378.

Kerr JB: The cytology of the human testis. *In* Burger H, deKretser D, eds: The Testis, 2nd ed. New York, Raven Press, 1989, pp 197–229.

Kerr JB: Ultrastructure of the seminiferous epithelium and intertubular tissue of the testis. J Elec Microsc Tech 1991; 19:215–240.

Killian GJ, Amann RP: Immunophoretic characterization of fluid and sperm entering and leaving the bovine epididymis. Biol Reprod 1973; 9:489–499.

Kimura Y, Yanagimachi R: Development of normal mice from oocytes injected with secondary spermatocyte nuclei. Biol Reprod 1995; 53:855–862.

Kinoshita Y, Hosaka M, Nishimura R, Takai S: Partial characterization of 5α-reductase in the human epididymis. Endocrinol Jpn 1980; 27:277–284.

Kirchhoff C, Habben I, Ivell R, Krull N: A major human epididymis-specific cDNA encodes a protein with sequence homology to extracellular proteinase inhibitors. Biol Reprod 1991; 45:350–357.

Kirchhoff C, Osterhoff C, Habben I, Ivell R: Cloning and analysis of mRNAs expressed specifically in the human epididymis. Int J Androl 1990; 13:155–167.

Kormano M: Dye permeability and alkaline phosphatase activity of testicular capillaries in the postnatal rat. Histochemie 1967; 9:327–338.

Kormano M, Koskimies AI, Hunter RL: The presence of specific proteins, in the absence of many serum proteins, in the rat seminiferous tubule fluid. Experientia 1971; 27:1461–1463.

Kormano M, Reijonen K: Microvascular structure of the human epididymis. Am J Anat 1976; 145:23–27.

Kormano M, Suoranta H: An angiographic study of the arterial pattern of the human testis. Anat Anz 1971; 128:69–76.

Koskimies AI, Kormano M, Alfthan O: Proteins of the seminiferous tubule fluid in man—evidence for a blood-testis barrier. J Reprod Fertil 1973; 32:79–86.

Lamb DJ: Growth factors and testicular development. J Urol 1993; 150:583–592.

Langford GA, Heller CG: Fine structure of muscle cells of the human testicular capsule: Basis of testicular contractions. Science 1973; 179:573–575.

Lanz T von, Neuhäuser G: Morphometrische analyse des menschlichen nebenhodens. Z Anat Entwicklungsgesch 1964; 124:126–133.

Larminat MA de, Hinrichsen MJ, Scroticati C, et al: Uptake and metabolism of androgen by the human epididymis in vitro. J Reprod Fertil 1980; 59:397–402.

Lathrop WF, Carmichael EP, Myles DG, Primikoff P: cDNA cloning reveals molecular structure of a sperm surface protein, PH-20 involved in sperm-egg adhesion and the wide distribution of its gene among mammals. J Cell Biol 1990; 111:2939–2949.

Leidl W, Waschke B: Comparative aspects of the kinetics of the spermiogenesis, *In* Holstein AF, Hortmann E, eds: Morphological Aspects of Andrology. Berlin, Grosse, 1970, pp 21–38.

Lennox B, Ahmad KN: The total length of tubules in the human testis. J Anat 1970; 107:191.

Levine N, Marsh DJ: Micropuncture studies of the electrochemical aspects of fluid and electrolyte transport in individual seminiferous tubules, the epididymis and the vas deferens in rats. J Physiol 1971; 213:557–570.

Lich Jr R, Howerton LW, Amin M: Anatomy and surgical approach to the urogenital tract in the male. *In* Harrison JH, et al, eds: Campbell's Urology, Vol 1. Philadelphia, W. B. Saunders Company, 1978, pp 3–33.

Lin Y, Mahan K, Lathrop WF, et al: A hyaluronidase activity of the sperm plasma membrane protein PH-20 enables sperm to penetrate the cumulus cell layer surrounding the egg. J Cell Biol 1994; 125:1157–1163.

Lindemann CB, Kanous KS: Regulation of mammalian sperm motility. Arch Androl 1989; 23:1–22.

Lino BF, Braden AWH, Turnbull KE: Fate of unejaculated spermatozoa. Nature 1967; 213:594–595.

Linzell JL, Setchell BP: Metabolism, sperm and fluid production of the isolated perfused testis of the sheep and goat. J Physiol 1969; 201:129–143.

Lipsett MB: Steroid secretion by the testis in man. *In* James VHT, Serio M, Martini L, eds: The Endocrine Function of the Human Testis, Vol II. New York, Academic Press, 1974, pp 1–12.

Lipshultz LI, McConnell J, Benson GS: Current concepts of the mechanism of ejaculation. J Reprod Med 1981; 26:499–507.

Lubahn DB, Golding TS, Couse JF, et al: Alteration of reproductive function but not prenatal sexual development after insertional deletion of the mouse estrogen receptor gene. Proc Natl Acad Sci USA 1993; 90:11162–11166.

Lubicz-Nawrocki CM: The effect of metabolites of testosterone on the viability of hamster epididymal spermatozoa. J Endocrinol 1973; 58:193–198.

Lyon MF, Glenister PH, Lamoreux ML: Normal spermatozoa from androgen-resistant germ cells of chimeric mice and the role of androgen in spermatogenesis. Nature 1975; 258:620–622.

MacMillan EW: The blood supply of the epididymis in man. Br J Urol 1954; 26:60–71.

Maddocks S, Setchell BP: The physiology of the endocrine testis. Oxf Rev Reprod Biol 1988; 10:53–123.

Majumder GC, Dey CS, Haldar S, Barua M: Biochemical parameters of initiation and regulation of sperm motility. Arch Androl 1990; 24:287–303.

Mancini RE, Loret AP, Guitelman A, Ghirlanda J: Effect of testosterone in the recovery of spermatogenesis in hypophysectomized patients. Hormone antagonists. Gynecol Invest 1971; 2:98–115.

Mancini RE, Seigner AC, Loret AP: Effect of gonadotropins on the recovery of spermatogenesis in hypophysectomized patients. J Clin Endocrinol Metab 1969; 29:467–478.

Marshall FF, Edler JS: Cryptorchidism and Related Anomalies. New York, Praeger Publishers, 1982, pp 27–46.

Martan J: Epididymal histochemistry and physiology. Biol Reprod (Suppl 1) 1969; 1:34–54.

Martan J, Risley PL: The epididymis of mated and unmated rats. J Morphol 1963; 113:1–15.

Mather JP, Gunsalus GL, Musto NA, et al: The hormonal and cellular control of Sertoli cell secretion. J Steroid Biochem 1983; 19:41–51.

Matsumoto AM, Bremner WJ: Stimulation of sperm production by human chorionic gonadotropin after prolonged gonadotropin suppression in normal men. J Androl 1985; 6:137–143.

Matsumoto AM, Karpas AE, Bremner WJ: Chronic hCG administration in normal men: Evidence that FSH is necessary for the maintenance of quantitatively normal spermatogenesis in man. J Clin Endocrinol Metab 1986; 62:1184–1192.

McConnell J, Benson GS, Wood JG: Autonomic innervation of the urogenital system: Adrenergic and cholinergic elements. Brain Res Bull 1982; 9:679–694.

McLachlan RI, Wreford NG, Robertson DM, de Kretser DM: Hormonal control of spermatogenesis. Trends Endocrinol Metab 1995; 6:95–101.

Mieusset R, Bujan L, Mondinat C, et al: Association of scrotal hyperthermia with impaired spermatogenesis in infertile men. Fertil Steril 1987; 48:1006–1011.

Mitchell GAG: The innervation of the kidney, ureter, testicle and epididymis. J Anat 1935; 70:10–32.

Moore HD, Hartman TD, Pryor JP: Development of the oocyte-penetrating capacity of spermatozoa in the human epididymis. Int J Androl 1983; 6:310–318.

Moore HD, Smith CA: The role of the epididymis during maturation of mammalian spermatozoa *in vivo* and *in vitro*. Reprod Nutr Dev 1988; 28:1217–1224.

Morton BE, Fraser C, Sagdraca R: Inhibition of sperm dilution damage by purified factors from hamster cauda epididymidis and by defined diluents. Fertil Steril 1978; 32:107–114.

Muller I: Kanalchen und Capillararchitektonik des ratten Hodens. Z Zellforsch 1957; 45:522–537.

Muller J, Skakkebaek NE: Quantification of germ cells and seminiferous tubules by stereological examination of testicles from 50 boys who suffered from sudden death. Int J Androl 1983; 6:143–156.

Murakami M, Sugita A, Hamasaki M: Scanning electron microscopic observations of the vas deferens in man and monkey with special reference to spermiophagy in its ampullary region. Scand Electron Microsc 1982; 3:1333–1339.

Murakami M, Yokoyama R: SEM observations of the male reproductive tract with special reference to epithelial phagocytosis. Prog Clin Biol Res 1989; 296:207–214.

Myles DG: Molecular mechanisms of sperm-egg membrane binding and fusion in mammals. Dev Biol 1993; 158:35–45.

Neaves WB: Biological aspects of vasectomy. *In* Greep RO, Astwood EB, eds: Handbook of Physiology. Section 7, Male Reproductive System. Baltimore, The Williams & Wilkins Company, 1975, pp 383–404.

Neaves WB, Johnson L, Petty CS: Age-related change in numbers of other interstitial cells in testes of adult men: Evidence bearing on the fate of Leydig cells lost with increasing age. Biol Reprod 1985; 33:259–269.

Neaves WB, Johnson L, Porter JC, et al: Leydig cell numbers, daily sperm production and serum gonadotropin levels in aging men. J Clin Endocrinol Metab 1984; 55:756–763.

Nicolson GL, Brodginski AB, Beattie G, Yanagimachi R: Cell surface changes in the proteins of rabbit spermatozoa during epididymal passage. Gamete Res 1979; 2:153–162.

Nicolson GL, Usui N, Yanagimachi R, et al: Lectin-binding sites on the plasma membranes of rabbit spermatozoa. Changes in surface receptors during epididymal maturation and after ejaculation. J Cell Biol 1977; 74:950–962.

Nikolopoulou M, Soucek DA, Vary JC: Changes in the lipid content of board sperm plasma membranes during epididymal maturation. Biochim Biophys Acta 1985; 815:486–498.

Nistal M, Abaurrea MA, Panaigua R: Morphological and histometric study on the human Sertoli cell from birth to the onset of puberty. J Anat 1982; 14:351–363.

Nistal M, Santamaria L, Paniagua R: The ampulla of the ductus deferens in man: Morphological and ultrastructural aspects. J Anat 1992; 180:97–104.

Olson GE, Danzo BJ: Surface changes in rat spermatozoa during epididymal transit. Biol Reprod 1981; 24:431–443.

O'Rand MG: Sperm-egg recognition and barriers to interspecies fertilization. Gam Res 1988; 19:315–328.

Orgebin-Crist MC: Studies on the function of the epididymis. Biol Reprod 1969; 1(Suppl)155.

Orgebin-Crist MC: Epididymal physiology and sperm maturation. *In* Bollack C, Clavert A, eds: Progress in Reproductive Biology, Vol 8. Epididymis and Fertility: Biology and Pathology. Basel, S. Karger, 1981, pp 80–89.

Orgebin-Crist MC, Danzo BJ, Davies J: Endocrine control of the development and maintenance of sperm fertilizing ability in the epididymis. *In* Greep RO, Astman EB, eds: Handbook of Physiology. Section 7, Male Reproductive System. Baltimore, The Williams & Wilkins Company, 1975, pp 319–338.

Orgebin-Crist MC, Fournier-Delpech S: Sperm-egg interaction. Evidence for maturational changes during epididymal transit. J Androl 1982; 3:429–433.

Orgebin-Crist MC, Jahad N: Delayed cleavage of rabbit ova after fertilization by young epididymal spermatozoa. Biol Reprod 1977; 16:358–362.

Osterhoff C, Kirchhoff C, Krull N, Ivell R: Molecular cloning and characterization of a novel human sperm antigen (HE2) specifically expressed in the proximal epididymis. Biol Reprod 1994; 50:516–525.

Overstreet JW, Bedford JM: Embryonic mortality in the rabbit is not increased after fertilization of young epididymal spermatozoa. Biol Reprod 1976; 15:54–57.

Palermo G, Munne S, Cohen J: The human zygote inherits its mitotic potential from the male gamete. Hum Reprod 1994; 9:1220–1225.

Palermo GD, Cohen J, Alikani M, et al: Intracytoplasmic sperm injection: a novel treatment for all forms of male factor infertility. Fertil Steril 1995; 63:1231–1240.

Paniagua R, Nistal M, Saez FJ, Fraile B: Ultrastructure of the aging human testis. J Electron Microsc Tech 1991; 19:241–260.

Paniagua R, Regader J, Nistal M, Abaurrea MA: Histological, histochemical an ultrastructural variations along the length of the human vas deferens before and after puberty. Acta Anat 1981; 111:190–203.

Parvinen M, Vihko KK, Toppari J: Cell interactions during the seminiferous epithelial cycle. Int Rev Cytol 1986; 104:115–151.

Payne AH, Youngblood GL: Regulation of steroidogenic enzymes in Leydig cells. Biol Reprod 1995; 52:217–225.

Paz GF, Kaplan R, Yedwab G, et al: The effect of caffeine on rat epididymal spermatozoa: Motility, metabolism and fertilizing capacity. Int J Androl 1978; 1:145–152.

Petterson S, Soderholm B, Persson JE, et al: Testicular blood flow in man measured with venous occlusion plethysmography and xenon-133. Scan J Urol Nephrol 1973; 7:115–119.

Phadke AM: Fate of spermatozoa in cases of obstructive azoospermia and after ligation of vas deferens in man. J Reprod Fertil 1964; 7:1–12.

Pholpramool C, Lea OA, Burrow PV, et al: The effects of acidic epididymal glycoprotein (AEG) and some other proteins on the motility of rat epididymal spermatozoa. Int J Androl 1983; 6:240–248.

Pineau C, de la Calle JFV, Pinon-Lataillade G, Jegou B: Assessment of testicular function after acute and chronic irradiation: Further evidence for an influence of late spermatids on Sertoli cell function in the adult rat. Endocrinology 1989; 124:2720–2728.

Pinon-Lataillade G, de la Calle JFV, Viguier-Martinez MC: Influence of germ cells upon Sertoli cells during continuous low-dose rate γ-irradiation of adult rats. Mol Cell Endocrinol 1988; 58:51–63.

Popovic NA, McLeod DG, Borski AA: Ultrastructure of the human vas deferens. Invest Urol 1973; 10:266–277.

Prader A: Testicular size: Assessment and clinical importance. Triangle 1966; 7:240–243.

Prins GS, Zaneveld LJD: Distribution of spermatozoa in the rabbit vas deferens. Biol Reprod 1979; 21:181–185.

Prins GS, Zaneveld LJD: Contractions of the rabbit vas deferens following sexual activity: A mechanism for proximal transport of spermatozoa. Biol Reprod 1980a; 23:904–909.

Prins GS, Zaneveld LJD: Radiographic study of fluid transport in the rabbit vas deferens during sexual rest and after sexual activity. J Reprod Fertil 1980b; 58:311–319.

Pujol A, Bayard F, Louvet JP, Boulard C: Testosterone and dihydrotestosterone concentrations in plasma, epididymal tissues and seminal fluid of adult rats. Endocrinol 1976; 98:111–113.

Rajalakshmi M, Arora R, Bose TK, et al: Physiology of the epididymis and induction of functional sterility in the male. J Reprod Fertil (Suppl)1976; 24:71–94.

Reijo R, Lee T-Y, Salo P, et al: Diverse spermatogenic defects in humans caused by Y chromosome deletions encompassing a novel RNA-binding protein gene. Nature Genet 1995; 10:383–393.

Reiter EO, Brown SR, Longcope C Beitins IZ: Male-limited familial precocious puberty in three generations; apparent Leydig cell autonomy and elevated glycoprotein hormone alpha subunit. N Engl J Med 1986; 311:515–519.

Reyes A, Mercado E, Goicoechea B, Rosado A: Participation of membrane sulfhydryl groups in the epididymal maturation of human and rabbit spermatozoa. Fertil Steril 1976; 27:1452–1458.

Reyes FI, Winter JSD, Faiman C: Endocrinology of the fetal testis. *In* Burger H, deKretser D, eds: The Testis, 2nd ed. New York, Raven Press, 1989, pp 119–142.

Richardson LL, Kleinman HK, Dym M: Basement membrane gene expression by Sertoli and peritubular myoid cells in vitro in the rat. Biol Reprod 1995; 52:320–330.

Rikimaru A, Shirai M: Responses of the human testicular capsule to electrical stimulation and to autonomic drugs. Tohoku J Exp Med 1972; 108:303–304.

Rikimaru A, Suzuki T: Mechanical response of the isolated rabbit testis to electrical stimulation and to autonomic drugs. Tohoku J Exp Med 1972; 108:283–289.

Risley PL: Physiology of the male accessory organs. *In* Hartman CG, ed: Mechanisms Concerned with Conception. New York, Pergamon Press, 1963, pp 73–133.

Ritchie AWS, Hargreave TB, James K, Chisholm GD: Intra-epithelial lymphocytes in the normal epididymis. A mechanism for tolerance to sperm auto-antigens? Br J Urol 1984; 56:79–83.

Ritzen EM, Hansson V, French FS: The Sertoli cell. *In* Burger H, deKretser D, eds: The Testis. New York, Raven Press, 1981, p 171.

Ritzen EM, Hansson V, French FS: The Sertoli cell. *In* Burger H, deKretser DM, eds: The Testis, 2nd ed. New York, Raven Press, 1989, pp 269–302.

Ritzen EM, Nayfeh SN, French FS, Dobbins MC: Demonstration of androgen binding components in rat epididymis cytosol and comparison with binding components in prostate and other tissues. Endocrinol 1971; 89:143–151.

Riva A, Testa-Riva F, Usai E, Cossu M: The ampulla ductus deferentis in man, as viewed by SEM and TEM. Arch Androl 1982; 8:157–164.

Robaire B, Ewing LL, Zirkin BR, Irby DC: Steroid {+grk}Da{-grk} reductase and 3α-reductase dehydrogenase in the rat epididymis. Endocrinol 1977; 101:1379–1390.

Robaire B, Hermo L: Efferent ducts, epididymis, and vas deferens: Structure, functions and their regulation. *In* Knobil E, Neill J, eds: The Physiology of Reproduction. New York, Raven Press, 1988, pp 999–1080.

Rommerts FFG, Cooke BA, van der Molen HJ: The role of cyclic AMP in the regulation of steroid biosynthesis in testis tissue. A review. J Steroid Biochem 1974; 5:279–285.

Romrell LJ, Ross MH: Characterization of Sertoli cell-germ junctional specializations in disassociated testicular cells. Anat Rec 1979; 193:23–41.

Roosen-Runge EC, Barlow FD: Quantitative studies in human spermatogenesis. I. Spermatogonia. Am J Anat 1953; 93:143–120.

Roosen-Runge EC, Holstein AF: The human rete testis. Cell Tissue Res 1978; 189:409–433.

Rosenthal SM, Grumbach MM, Kaplan SL: Gonadotrophin-independent familial sexual precocity with premature Leydig and germinal cell maturation (familial Testoxicosis): Effects of a potent LHRH agonist and medroxyprogesterone acetate therapy in four cases. J Clin Endocrinol Metab 1983; 57:571–579.

Ross P, Kan FW, Antaki P, et al: Protein synthesis and secretion in the human epididymis and immunoreactivity with sperm antibodies. Mol Reprod Dev 1990; 26:12–23.

Rowley MJ, Teshima F, Heller CG: Duration of transit of spermatozoa through the human male ductular system. Fertil Steril 1970; 21:390–396.

Russell L: Desmosome-like junctions between Sertoli cells and germ cells in the rat testis. Am J Anat 1977; 148:301–312.

Russell LD: Sertoli-germ cell interactions: A review. Gamete Res 1980; 3:179–202.

Russell LD, Clermont Y: Anchoring device between Sertoli cells and late spermatids in rat seminiferous tubules. Anat Rec 1976; 185:259–278.

Saez JM, Avallet O, Lejeune H, Chatelain PG: Cell-cell communication in the testis. Horm Res 1991; 36:104–115.

Saithoh K, Terada T, Hatakeyama S: A morphological study of the efferent ducts of the human epididymis. Int J Androl 1990; 13:369–376.

Saling PM: Mammalian sperm interaction with extracellular matrices of the egg. Oxf Rev Reprod Biol 1989; 11:339–388.

Santen RJ: Feedback control of luteinizing hormone and follicle stimulating hormone secretion by testosterone and estradiol in men: Physiologic and clinical implications. Clin Biochem 1981; 14:243–251.

Sawchuk TJ, Turner TT: Restoration of spermatogenesis and subsequent fertility by direct intratesticular hormonal therapy. J Urol 1993:1997–2001.

Schatten G: The centrosome and its mode of inheritance—the reduction of the centrosome during gametogenesis and its restoration during fertilization. Dev Biol 1994; 165:299–335.

Scheer H, Robaire B: Subcellular distribution of steroid {+grk}D{-grk}^{4}-5α-reductase and 3α-hydroxysteroid dehydrogenase in the rat epididymis during sexual maturation. Biol Reprod 1983; 29:1–10.

Schlegel PN, Berkeley AS, Goldstein M, et al: Epididymal micropuncture with in vitro fertilization and oocyte micromanipulation for the treatment of unreconstructable obstructive azoospermia. Fertil Steril 1994; 61:895–901

Schlegel PN, Palermo GD, Alikani M, et al: Micropuncture retrieval of epididymal sperm with IVF: Importance of in vitro micromanipulation techniques. Urol 1995; 46:238–241.

Schoysman R: Clinical situations challenging the established concept of epididymal physiology in the human. Acta Eur Fertil 1993; 24:55–60.

Schoysman R, Vanderzwalmen P, Nijs M, et al: Successful fertilization by testicular spermatozoa in an in-vitro fertilization programme. Hum Reprod 1993; 8:1339–1440.

Schoysman RJ, Bedford JM: The role of the human epididymis in sperm maturation and sperm storage as reflected in the consequences of epididymovasostomy. Fertil Steril 1986; 46:293–299.

Schweitzer R: Uber die bedeutung der vascularisation, der binnendruckes und der zwischenzellen fur die biologie des hodens. Z Anat Entwickl 1929; 89:775–796.

Schulze W: Structural principles underlying the spermatogenic process in man and a non-human primate (Macaca Cynomolgus). Diesbach Verlag, Reproductive Biology and Medicine, 1989, pp 58–65.

Setchell BP, Brooks DE: Anatomy, vasculature, innervation and fluids of the male reproductive tract. *In* Knobil E, Neill JD, eds: The Physiology of Reproduction. New York, Raven Press, 1988, pp 753–836.

Setchel BP, Maddocks S, Brooks DE: Anatomy, vasculature, innervation, and fluids of the male reproductive tract. *In* Knobil E, Neill JD, eds: The Physiology of Reproduction, 2nd ed. New York, Raven Press, 1994, pp 1063–1175.

Setchell BP, Waites GMH: The blood-testis barrier. *In* Greep RO, Astwood EB, eds: Handbook of Physiology. Section 7, Male Reproductive System. Baltimore, The Williams & Wilkins Company, 1975, pp 143–172.

Shabanowitz RB: Mouse antibodies to human zona pellucida: Evidence that human ZP3 is strongly immunogenic and contains two distinct isomer chains. Biol Reprod 1990; 43:260–270.

Sharpe RM: Intratesticular factors controlling testicular function. Biol Reprod 1984; 30:29–49.

Sharpe RM: Regulation of spermatogenesis. *In* Knobil E, Neill JD, eds: The Physiology of Reproduction, 2nd ed. New York, Raven Press, 1994, pp 1364–1434.

Sheth AR, Gunjikar AN, Shah GV: The presence of progressive motility sustaining factor (PMSF) in human epididymis. Andrologia 1981; 13:142–146.

Silber SJ: Role of the epididymis in sperm maturation. Urology 1989; 33:47–51.

Silber SJ, Devroey P, Tournaye H, Vansteirteghem AC: Fertilizing capacity of epididymal and testicular sperm using intracytoplasmic sperm injection (ICSI). Reprod Fertil Dev 1995; 7:281–293.

Simerly C, Wu G-J, Zoran S, et al: The paternal inheritance of the centrosome, the cell's microtubule-organizing center, in humans, and the implications for infertility. Nature Med 1995; 1:47–51.

Sjöstrand NO: The adrenergic innervation of the vas deferens and the accessory male genital glands. Acta Physiol Scand 257(Suppl) 1965; 65:5–22.

Skinner MK: Interactions between germ cells and Sertoli cells in the testis. Biol Reprod 1995; 52:211–216.

Skinner MK, Fritz IB: Testicular peritubular cells secrete a protein under androgen control that modulates Sertoli cell functions. Proc Nat Acad Sci, USA 1985; 82:114–118.

Skinner MK, Norton JN, Mullaney BP, et al: Cell-cell interactions and the regulation of testis function. Ann NY Acad Sci 1991; 637:354–363.

Skudlarek MD, Tulsiani DRP, Orgebin-Crist M: Rat epididymal luminal fluid acid β-D-galactosidase optimally hydrolyzes glycoprotein substrate at neutral pH. Biochem J 1992; 286:907–914.

Steinberger E. Hormonal control of mammalian spermatogenesis. Physiol Rev 1971; 51:1–22.

Steinberger E, Root A, Fischer M, Smith KO: The role of androgens in the initiation of spermatogenesis is man. J Clin Endocrinol Metabol 1973; 37:746–751.

Suvanto O, Kormano M. The relation between *in vitro* contractions of the rat seminiferous tubules and the cyclic stage of the seminiferous epithelium. J Reprod Fertil 1970; 21:227–232.

Suzuki F, Nagano T: Development of tight junctions in caput epididymal epithelium of mouse. Dev Biol 1978; 63:321–334.

Swerdloff RS, Heber D: Endocrine control of testicular function from birth to puberty. *In* Burger H, deKretser D, eds: The Testis. New York, Raven Press, 1981, pp 107–126.

Tainio H: Peptidergic innervation of the human prostate, seminal vesicle and vas deferens. Acta Histochem 1995; 97:113–119.

Takayama H, Tomoyoshi T: Microvascular architecture of rat and human testes. Invest Urol 1981; 18:341–344.

Tash JS, Means AR: cAMP-dependent regulatory processes in the acquisition and control of sperm flagellar movement. Prog Clin Biol Res 1988; 267:335–355.

Teerds KJ, DeRooij DG, Rommerts FF, Wensing CJ: The regulation of the proliferation and differentiation of rat Leydig cell precursor cells after EDS administration or daily HCG treatment. J Androl 1988; 9:343–351.

Tesarik J, Mendoza C, Testart J: Viable embryos from injection of round spermatids into oocytes. (Letter.) New Engl J Med 1995; 333:525.

Tezon JC, Ramella E, Cameo MS, et al: Immunochemical localization of secretory antigens in the human epididymis and their association with spermatozoa. Biol Reprod 1985; 32:591–597.

Tishler PV: Diameter of testicles. N Engl J Med 1971; 285:1489.

Toney TW, Danzo BJ: Androgen and estrogen effects on protein synthesis by the adult rabbit epididymis. Endocrinol 1989; 125:243–249.

Toyama Y: Actin-like filaments in the myoid cell of the testis. Cell Tis Res 1977; 177:221–226.

Tuck RR, Setchell BP, Waites GMH, Young JA: The composition of fluid collected by micropuncture and catheterization from the seminiferous tubules and rete testes of rats. Eur J Physiol 1970; 318:225–243.

Tulsiani DRP, Skudlarek MD, Holland MK, Orgebin-Crist M: Glycosylation of rat sperm plasma membrane during epididymal maturation. Biol Reprod 1993; 48:417–428.

Tung PS, Skinner MK, Fritz IB: Fibronectin synthesis is a marker for peritubular contaminants in Sertoli cell-enriched cultures. Biol Reprod 1984; 30:199–211.

Turner TT: Spermatozoa are exposed to a complex microenvironment as they traverse the epididymis. *In* Robaire B, ed: The Male Germ Cell: Spermatogonium to Fertilization. New York, The New York Academy of Sciences, 1991, pp 364–383.

Turner TT: On the epididymis and its role in the development of the fertile ejaculate. J Androl 1995; 16:292–298.

Turner TT, Giles RD: Sperm motility-inhibiting factor in rat epididymis. Am J Physiol 1982; 242:R199–R203.

Turner TT, Gleavy JL, Harris JM: Fluid movement in the lumen of the rat epididymis: Effect of vasectomy and subsequent vasovasostomy. J Androl 1990a; 11:422–428.

Turner TT, Howards SS, Gleavy JL: On the maintenance of male fertility in the absence of native testosterone secretion: Site-directed hormonal therapy in the rat. Fertil Steril 1990b; 54:149–160.

Vendrely E: Histology of the epididymis in the human adult. *In* Bollack C, Clavert A, eds: Progress in Reproductive Biology, Vol 8. Epididymis and Fertility: Biology and Pathology. Basel, S. Karger, 1981; pp 21–33.

Vendrely E, Dadoune JP: Quantitative ultrastructural analysis of the principal cells in the human epididymis. Reprod Nutr Develop 1988; 28:1225–1235.

Ventura WP, Freund M, Davis J, Pannuti MS: Influence of norepinephrine on the motility of the human vas deferens: A new hypothesis of sperm transport by the vas deferens. Fertil Steril 1973; 24:68–77.

Vitale R: The development of the blood-testis barrier in Sertoli-cell-only rats. Anat Rec 1975; 181:501.

Voglmayr JK: Metabolic changes in spermatozoa during epididymal transit. *In* Greep RO, Astman EB, eds: Handbook of Physiology. Section 7, Male Reproductive System. Baltimore, The William & Wilkins Company, 1975, pp 437–451.

Vreeburg JTM: Distribution of testosterone and 5α-dihydrotestosterone in rat epididymis and their concentration in efferent duct fluid. J Endocrinol 1975; 67:203–210.

Ward WS, Coffey DS: Specific organization of genes in relation to the sperm nuclear matrix. Biochem Biophys Res Comm 1990; 173:20–25.

Ward WS, Coffey DS: DNA packaging and organization in mammalian spermatozoa: Comparison with somatic cells. Biol Reprod 1991; 44:569–574.

Wassarman PM: Zona pellucida glycoproteins. Ann Rev Biochem 1988; 57:415–442.

Weinbauer GF, Nieschlag E: Peptide and steroid regulation of spermatogenesis in primates. *In* Robaire B, ed: The Male Germ Cell: Spermatogonium to Fertilization. New York, New York Academy of Sciences, 1991, pp 107–121.

Wenzel J, Kellerman P: Vergleichende untersuchungen uber das lymphgefasssytem des nebenhodens und hodens von mensch, hund unk kaninchen. Z Mikrosk Anat Forsch 1966; 75:368–375.

Winter JSD, Faiman C: Pituitary-gonadal relations in male children and adolescents. Pediatr Res 1972; 6:126–131.

Witschi E: Migration of the germ cells of human embryos from the yolk sac to the primitive gonadal fold. Carnegie Institute Wash Contrib Embryol 1948; 209:67–80.

Wong PYD, Au CL, Bedford, JM: Biology of the scrotum. II. Suppression by abdominal temperature of transepithelial ion and water transport in the cauda epididymis. Biol Reprod 1982; 26:683–689.

Wyrobek AJ: Methods and concepts in detecting abnormal reproductive outcomes of paternal origin. Reprod Toxicol (Suppl 1) 1993; 7:3–16.

Yanagimachi R: Mammalian fertilization. *In* Knobil E, Neill JD, eds: The Physiology of Reproduction, 2nd ed. New York, Raven Press, 1994, pp 189–317.

Yeung CH, Cooper TG, Oberpenning F, et al: Changes in movement characteristics of human spermatozoa along the length of the epididymis. Biol Reprod 1993; 49:274–280.

Yeung CH, Cooper TG, Bergmann M, Schulze H: Organization of tubules in the human caput epididymidis and the ultrastructure of their epithelia. Am J Anat 1991; 191:261–279.

Yeung CH, Nashan D, Sorg C, et al: Basal cells of the human epididymis—antigenic and ultrastructural similarities to tissue-fixed macrophages. Biol Reprod 1994; 50:917–926.

Yoshinaga K, Nishikawa S, Ogawa M, et al: Role of c-kit in mouse spermatogenesis: Identification of spermatogonia as a specific site of c-kit expression and function. Development 1991; 113:689–699.

Young WC: A study of the function of the epididymis. II. The importance of an aging process in sperm for the length of the period during which fertilizing capacity is retained by sperm isolated in the epididymis of the guinea pig. J Morphol 1929; 48:475–489.

Young WC: A study of the function of the epididymis. III. Functional changes undergone by spermatozoa during their passage through the epididymis and vas deferens in the guinea pig. J Expl Biol 1930; 8:151–166.

Zeuzes MT, Reed TE, Nieschlag E: Non-Poisson distribution of sperm from grandfathers in zona-free hamster ova. Urol Res 1992; 20:275–280.

Zirkin BR, Awoniyi C, Griswold MD, et al: Is FSH required for adult spermatogenesis? J Androl 1994; 15:273–276.

43
MALE INFERTILITY

Mark Sigman, M.D.
Stuart S. Howards, M.D.

OVERVIEW

The field of infertility has undergone and continues to undergo rapid changes. In the 1950s, 1960s, and 1970s, the management of the infertile couple focused on the female, with evaluation of the male being an often neglected component. The 1980s witnessed an awareness of the frequency of male factor infertility, leading to increased emphasis on the evaluation of the male partner. At the same time, the development of in vitro fertilization (IVF) led to an explosive rise in the use of this technology for the treatment of both male and female factor infertility. This led to a shift in emphasis from treatment designed to improve fertility toward treatment designed to achieve conception by bypassing fertility problems. In the 1990s, we are witnessing the refinement of micromanipulation procedures such as intracytoplasmic sperm injection, assisted hatching, embryo biopsy, and the potential for embryo cloning. With the success of these high-technology, high-cost procedures, the evaluation of the male is often bypassed, because it is thought of as a tedious and ineffective evaluation. This approach ignores the fact that many causes of male infertility such as varicocele, ductal obstruction, and infections are easily and effectively treated. In addition, without a full evaluation, significant diseases such as testicular cancer, pituitary tumors, and neurologic disease may be overlooked (Jarow, 1994). Several factors have led to a re-examination of the use of assisted reproductive techniques (ARTs) as primary therapy. The recent debate on health care reform has emphasized the high cost of ARTs. The recently proposed and defeated Clinton Health Care Plan specifically excluded IVF treatment. The reports of an increased incidence of ovarian cancer in women who had been treated with fertility drugs in the past has led many couples to re-examine this approach.

The chance of a normal couple conceiving is estimated to be approximately 25% per month, 75% by 6 months, and 90% by 1 year (Spira, 1986). In addition, fertility rates are at their peak in men and women at age 24. Beyond that age, fertility rates begin to decline with age (van Noord–Zaadstra et al, 1991). Thus, although most couples achieve conception within 1 year, approximately 10% to 15% of couples are unable to do so (Greenhall et al, 1990). **Approximately 20% of cases of infertility are due entirely to a male factor, with an additional 30% of cases involving both male and female factors** (Mosher, 1991). Therefore, roughly one half of infertile unions involve male factor infertility. Of infertile couples without treatment, 25% to 35% will conceive at some time by intercourse alone (Collins et al, 1983). Within the first 2 years, 23% will conceive, whereas an additional 10% will do so within 2 more years (Aafjes et al, 1978). This baseline pregnancy rate must be understood when evaluating the results of therapy for these couples. **With the advancing age of infertile couples, we do not recommend deferring an initial evaluation until 12 months of attempted conception have been completed. A basic, simple, cost-effective evaluation of both the male and female should be initiated at the time of presentation.**

The approach to the evaluation of the infertile male should be similar to that used to evaluate other medical problems. A thorough history should be taken, with particular attention to those areas that may affect fertility. This should be followed by a physical examination. An initial series of laboratory tests completes the basic evaluation. The results of the history, physical examination, and initial laboratory testing is used to formulate a differential diagnosis that may lead to more specific testing. Many tests are available to evaluate different aspects of male infertility, but not all patients need all tests.

Ideally, the evaluation of the infertile man should result in the identification of the specific abnormality responsible for infertility. Although this is possible in some instances, many men demonstrate abnormal semen analyses for which no etiology can be identified. When possible, specific treatment is directed toward a specific etiology. However, both empirical therapies and ARTs may be of value in the absence of known etiologic factors. It is important to remember that therapeutic donor insemination and adoption are treatment alternatives. The infertile couple should be made aware of these options, with the physician playing a counseling role to avoid excessively prolonged, futile treatments.

Table 43–1. COMPONENTS OF THE HISTORY IMPORTANT FOR THE EVALUATION OF THE INFERTILE MALE

I. Sexual History
- Duration of sexual relations with and without birth control
- Methods of birth control
- Sexual technique: Potency, use of lubricants (some are spermatocidal)
- Frequency and timing of coitus

II. Past History
- Developmental: History of cryptorchidism, age of puberty, gynecomastia, congenital abnormalities of urinary tract or central nervous system
- Surgical: Orchiopexy, pelvic or retroperitoneal surgery, herniorrhaphy, sympathectomy, vasectomy, injury to genitals, spinal cord injury, testicular torsion
- Medical: Urinary infections, sexually transmitted diseases, mumps, renal disease, diabetes mellitus, radiotherapy, recent febrile illness, epididymitis, tuberculosis, smallpox (causes obstructive azoospermia) or other chronic diseases, anosmia, midline defects
- Drugs: Complete list of all past and present medications. Many drugs interfere with spermatogenesis, erection, and ejaculation.
- Occupation and habits: Exposure to chemicals and heat, hot baths, steam baths, radiation, cigarettes, alcohol
- Past marital history of both partners, including pregnancies and miscarriages; any offspring with other partners
- Previous infertility evaluations and treatments

III. Family History
- Testicular atrophy
- Hypogonadotropism
- Cryptorchidism
- Congenital midline defects

IV. Female Reproductive History

HISTORY

The evaluation of the infertile male should include a thorough history exploring all aspects related to fertility (Table 43–1). The duration of infertility, details of prior pregnancies, methods of birth control used in the past, and the couple's frequency of sexual intercourse as well as the time of coitus should be recorded. It should be determined whether the couple realizes that the ovulatory period occurs during the midmenstrual cycle. Sperm remain viable within the cervical mucus and crypts for approximately 48 hours. **Although there is some controversy, most experts advise intercourse every 2 days, which ensures that viable sperm are present during the 12- to 24-hour period in which the oocyte is within the fallopian tube and is capable of being fertilized.** Intercourse that is too frequent may result in inadequate numbers of sperm being deposited in the vaginal vault, and similarly, if sexual activity is too infrequent, the ovulatory period may be missed.

Both potency and ejaculatory function should be addressed. In addition, the lubricants used for intercourse should be noted. Most of the commonly used lubricants, such as Lubafax, K-Y Jelly, Keri Lotion, Surgilube, and saliva, adversely affect sperm motility (Tagatz et al, 1972; Goldenberg and White, 1975; Tulandi et al, 1982; Boyers et al, 1987). Lubricants that do not impair in vitro sperm motility include peanut oil, safflower oil, vegetable oil, and raw egg white. In general, a couple should be advised to use a lubricant only if necessary and to use a minimal amount of one that does not impair sperm function.

The developmental history of the patient should be explored. **Unilateral cryptorchidism slightly decreases fertility, and bilateral cryptorchidism results in a significant reduction in fertility** (Cendron et al, 1989). There is considerable recent experimental and clinical evidence that as long as the onset is prepubertal, the timing of orchidopexy does not affect the findings of spermatogenic abnormalities in these testes (Lipshultz et al, 1976; Cendron et al, 1989; Pryor et al, 1989). A history of delayed or absent puberty may be associated with an endocrinopathy or androgen receptor abnormality. A history of gynecomastia may be associated with prolactin or estrogen abnormalities.

The patient's past surgical history may be of particular importance. Pelvic or retroperitoneal surgery may affect erectile and ejaculatory function. Bladder neck surgery may result in retrograde ejaculation. Retroperitoneal node dissections may injure the sympathetic nerves, resulting in anejaculation or retrograde ejaculation. Some modifications have resulted in a preservation of the sympathetic nerves, allowing the retention of ejaculatory function in most patients (Jewett, 1990; Donohue et al, 1993). The vas deferens may be inadvertently injured or stripped of its blood supply during a herniorrhaphy. Testicular trauma or torsion may result in testicular atrophy; such patients may also be predisposed to the development of antisperm antibodies.

The patient should be questioned for a history of urinary tract infections or sexually transmitted diseases. A history of prostatitis or pyospermia, or both, should be noted, although there is no convincing evidence that these conditions actually cause infertility (McConnell, 1991). Prepubertal mumps does not affect the testes; however, mumps orchitis may develop if the disease occurs postpubertally. Approximately 30% of patients affected after the ages of 11 to 12 develop unilateral mumps orchitis, whereas 10% may be affected bilaterally (Werner, 1950). A history of an absent or low-volume ejaculate suggests the possibility of retrograde ejaculation, ejaculatory duct obstruction, or congenital hypoplasia or absence of the vas deferens and seminal vesicles. Ejaculatory dysfunction or erectile abnormalities may develop in patients with diabetes mellitus or multiple sclerosis. Infertility is common in patients with renal failure. **Oligospermia is identified in approximately 60% or more of patients with testicular cancer or lymphoma at the time of diagnosis** (Carrol et al, 1987; Nijman et al, 1987; Rustin, 1987). Chemotherapy or radiotherapy may further impair testicular function. Spermatogenesis may take up to 4 to 5 years to return following radiation therapy or chemotherapy (Orecklin et al, 1973; Rustin et al, 1987). The initial depression in spermatogenesis following chemotherapy is due to direct cytotoxicity to rapidly dividing germ cells. Various agents effect different steps in spermatogenesis. If the stem cells are irreversibly damaged, permanent azoospermia results. The prognosis can be predicted if the details of the chemotherapeutic regimen, including the specific agents, the doses, and the duration of treatment, are known (Oates, 1992). **Following a febrile illness, spermatogenesis may be impaired for 1 to 3 months. In patients with abnormal semen analyses and a history of a systemic illness within 3 months of the evaluation, semen analysis should be continued over a 3- to 6-month period to adequately assess the patient's baseline fertility status.** Azoospermia in a patient with a history of epididymitis suggests epididymal obstruction. Immotile cilia syndrome or *Kartagener's syndrome* should be suspected in patients with immotile sperm, a history of frequent respiratory infections, and situs inversus. If the vas deferens is absent bilaterally in an azoospermic patient, he may have a mild form of cystic fibrosis, which is an autosomal recessive disorder. Most of these men have no other manifestations of cystic fibrosis. They should undergo genetic screening, and possibly pulmonary and gastrointestinal evaluation, and be advised that brothers have a 50% chance of having the disease. Children born using the patient's sperm (with ART) will most likely be carriers of the gene and may have the disease depending on the carrier status of the partner. Azoospermia associated with a history of frequent respiratory infections also suggests the possibility of Young's syndrome. In patients with this condition, epididymal obstruction due to inspissation of secretions accounts for azoospermia. A history of severe headaches, galactorrhea, or impaired visual fields should raise the possibility of a central nervous system tumor. *Kallmann's syndrome* is hypogonadotropic hypogonadism associated with anosmia. Many medications and drugs, including nitrofurantoin, cimetidine sulfasalazine, cocaine, nicotine, marijuana, and caffeine, have been implicated as impairing spermatogenesis (Kolodny et al, 1974; Van Thiel et al, 1975; Abel et al, 1989; Berul and Harclerode, 1989; Marshburn et al, 1989; Schlegel et al, 1991). Spermatogenesis may return to normal after cessation of these agents.

Anabolic steroids have been used increasingly by athletes. Hypogonadotropic hypogonadism may result from the androgenic component of the steroids. Normal hormonal function usually returns after these agents are discontinued, but this is not always the case (Holma, 1977). Exposure to other agents such as pesticides should be noted, because these may be gonadotoxic. Testicular temperatures are normally 1 to 2.5°F below body temperature. Impaired semen quality and spermatogenesis have resulted from experimental hyperthermia (MacLeod and Hotchkiss, 1941). Similarly, the frequent use of hot tubs has been found to result in a 10% decrease in sperm motility (Procope, 1965). Therefore, the use of saunas and hot tubs should be discontinued in those patients with suboptimal semen analyses. There is no scientific evidence that wearing jockey shorts affects spermatogenesis.

Vine and colleagues (1994) performed a meta-analysis of 21 studies on the effect of cigarette smoking on semen quality. They concluded that smoking lowered sperm density by 13% to 17%, although 14 of the studies did not document an effect. Androgen receptor abnormalities should be suspected in patients with a family history of intersex disorders. In utero exposure to diethylstilbestrol causes an increased incidence of epididymal cysts, a slightly increased frequency of cryptorchidism, but little or no effect on semen quality in those men who do not have an undescended testis. Finally, the physician should be aware of the results of the wife's fertility evaluation.

EVALUATION OF THE FEMALE

Female factors are involved in a large percentage of infertility cases. The urologist must have a general understanding of the causes of female infertility, as well as the diagnostic and treatment approaches to these problems. Fallopian tube pathology is present in 30% to 40% of infertile couples, often involving endometriosis or pelvic adhesions. Fifteen to twenty percent of cases of infertility are related to ovulatory dysfunction, and cervical factors are present in approximately 5% of cases.

Evaluation of Ovulation

The evaluation of the female is similar to that in the male, consisting of a thorough history and physical examination, followed by appropriate laboratory testing. The adequacy of ovulation is examined by several methods. Irregularity of the menstrual cycle suggests ovulatory dysfunction. Basal body temperature charting is often an initial and easy method of evaluation. Additional information may be obtained by urinary LH testing, midluteal progesterone levels, and endometrial biopsy. Also, ultrasonic monitoring of the development and disappearance of ovarian follicles may be useful.

Generally, combinations of the above-mentioned methods are used over several cycles to determine the adequacy and consistency of ovulation. A normal biphasic basal body temperature chart demonstrates an increased temperature of at least 0.4°F for 12 to 15 days following ovulation. A temperature drop prior to the rise correlates with the time of ovulation. Luteal phase defects are characterized by a sustained increase in temperature lasting less than 11 days. Serum progesterone levels are obtained during the midluteal phase. Adequate progesterone levels require ovulation and corpus luteum function. The endometrial biopsy is usually performed several days before the time of expected menstruation. It is used to diagnose a luteal phase defect and to confirm ovulation. Ovarian ultrasound is used prior to ovulation to evaluate follicular development and oocyte release. It is often used in combination with urinary LH testing to predict the time of ovulation.

Evaluation of the Fallopian Tubes

The hysterosalpingogram is performed by injecting dye through the cervix to outline the uterus and fallopian tubes. It determines the patency of the fallopian tubes as well as the shape of the uterus. It is generally performed in the early follicular phase of the cycle following cessation of menstrual bleeding. Both oil-based and water-based dyes are used. There are limited data suggesting higher pregnancy rates with intercourse following oil-based hysterosalpingogram studies. Laparoscopy may be performed if prior tests have suggested pelvic pathology, such as uterine leiomyomas, pelvic adhesions, or endometriosis. It may also be performed when all prior tests have been normal to identify previously unsuspected pathologies. Because the above-mentioned tests and procedures are usually performed during particular periods of the menstrual cycle, the evaluation of the female takes longer than that of the male. It is important to take the age of the female into consideration when recommending therapy. Conception rates drop in the 35- to 39-year-old age group. Thus, it is common to recommend more aggressive therapy in couples in which the woman is approaching 40 years old and to take a slower stepwise approach in younger couples. With a basic understanding of the evaluation of the female, the urologist is better able to counsel the couple as to which treatments are most appropriate given both the female and male infertility factors.

PHYSICAL EXAMINATION

The physical examination should be geared toward identifying any abnormalities that may be associated with infertility. The patient's habitus as well as the pattern of virilization should be noted. Situs inversus raises the possibility of Kartagener's syndrome associated with immotile cilia.

Genital Examination

Specific attention should be directed toward the genital examination. The penis should be examined for evidence of hypospadias, which may interfere with the cervical deposition of semen. Similarly, severe chordee may interfere with intercourse. **With the patient standing in a warm room to allow relaxation of the cremaster muscle, the scrotal contents should be evaluated.** The testes should be palpated for consistency and size. **Because the majority of the testicular volume consists of seminiferous tubules and germinal elements, a reduction in the number of these cells is manifested as testicular atrophy.**

The dimensions of the testes should be measured. This may be performed using calipers, an orchidometer, or sonography. **The normal fertile adult testis is greater than 4 cm in length** and greater than 20 ml in volume (Table 43–2) (Carney and Tuttle, 1960). Decreased testicular size, whether unilateral or bilateral, correlates with impaired spermatogenesis (Lipshultz, 1977). **Careful palpation of the epididymis should determine the presence of the head, body, and tail.** The possibility of epididymal obstruction is suggested by the presence of induration or cystic change of the epididymis. **Palpation of the vas deferens is performed** to ensure its presence as well as to rule out areas of atrophy.

Examination of the spermatic cords should be performed to identify the presence of a varicocele. **Small varicoceles (grade I) are palpable only during the Valsalva maneuver. Moderate-sized varicoceles (grade II) are palpable with the patient in the standing position, whereas large varicoceles (grade III) are visible through the scrotal skin and are palpable when the patient is in the standing position.** Asymmetry of the spermatic cords, accentuated by the Valsalva maneuver, suggests the presence of a varicocele. In patients with strong cremasteric reflexes, or in those with high-riding testicles, slight traction on the testes during the Valsalva maneuver allows for a more accurate examination of the spermatic cords. Thickening and asymmetry of the spermatic cords that persist in the supine position suggest the possibility of a lipoma of the cord or caval obstruction due to a renal tumor. Varicoceles decrease in size when the patient is in the supine position. Similarly, bilateral thickening of the cords, resolving with the patient in the supine position, suggests the presence of bilateral varicoceles.

Many diagnostic methods have been employed to identify subclinical varicoceles, those that are not palpable by physi-

Table 43–2. COMPARISONS OF TESTICULAR DIMENSIONS (LENGTH × WIDTH) AND VOLUME FOR PREPUBERTAL AND PUBERTAL BOYS AND NORMAL ADULT MEN

Clinical Status	Volume (ml)	Length × Width (cm) (cm)
Prepubertal	1	1.6 × 1.0
	2	2.0 × 1.2
	3	2.3 × 1.4
	4	2.5 × 1.5
	5	2.7 × 1.6
	6	2.9 × 1.8
Pubertal	8	3.1 × 2.0
	10	3.4 × 2.1
	12	3.7 × 2.3
	15	4.0 × 2.5
Adult*	20	4.5 × 2.7
	25	5.0 × 3.0
	30	5.5 × 3.2

*Normal adult testicular size 24±4 (SD) ml (n = 44).

cal examination. Venography has been used for many years; however, this procedure is invasive and the results are affected by the pressure of injection, the position of the catheter, and the judgment of the examiner. In addition, venography is not without complications (Seyferth et al, 1981). The presence of a venous rushing sound, which is increased with the Valsalva maneuver, is used to identify the presence of a varicocele with the Doppler stethoscope (Perrin et al, 1980; Gonzalez et al, 1983; Ponchietti et al, 1983; Netto et al, 1984; World Health Organization, 1985). Both real-time scrotal ultrasonography and duplex scrotal ultrasonography have been used to visualize dilated spermatic veins in the scrotum. The presence of more than three veins that enlarge in the upright position, with at least one larger than 3 mm, is believed by some authorities to be indicative of a varicocele (McClure and Hriacac, 1986). Higher temperatures in the scrotum or testicle that are identified with contact scrotal thermography are believed to correlate with the presence of a varicocele (Lewis and Harrison, 1980; Yamaguchi et al, 1989). With the use of these techniques, up to 91% of patients with idiopathic infertility have been identified as having subclinical varicoceles (Perrin et al, 1980; Naryan et al, 1981; Gonzalez et al, 1983). Bilateral varicoceles have been demonstrated in up to 58% of patients (Perrin et al, 1980; Gonzalez et al, 1983), whereas only 10% of patients are identified as having bilateral varicoceles by clinical examination alone. **There have been no controlled studies demonstrating improved pregnancy rates following the diagnosis and treatment of subclinical varicoceles. Therefore, we do not recommend evaluating patients for the presence of subclinical varicoceles.**

Finally, many experts recommend that a careful rectal examination should be performed to evaluate the prostate as well as the areas above the prostate for evidence of cystic dilatation of the seminal vesicles. Significant prostatic tenderness raises the possibility of a prostatic infection.

INITIAL BASIC LABORATORY EVALUATION

The next step in the evaluation of the male partner in an infertile marriage, after a history and physical examination, is appropriate laboratory testing. First, all patients need a semen analysis.

Semen Analysis

The semen analysis remains the cornerstone of the laboratory evaluation of the infertile man. Despite this, it is important to realize that the measurement of semen parameters does not constitute a measure of fertility. **Except in cases of azoospermia, the semen analysis does not allow for the separation of patients into sterile and fertile groups. Because semen parameters decrease in quality, the statistical chance of conception decreases but does not reach zero.** Nevertheless, an accurately performed semen analysis remains an important tool for the evaluation of the infertile man.

Collection

To compare different semen samples from the same patient with accuracy, it is important to maintain consistency in the length of sexual abstinence prior to collection of the specimen. Changes in the intervals between ejaculations often result in an increased variability of the results of the semen analyses. Even with this precaution, the results of semen analyses are often inconsistent, and therefore, multiple analyses are indicated in equivocal or difficult situations. Clean, wide-mouth containers should be used for specimen collection. These containers should be obtained from the physician because residual chemicals in other containers may injure the sperm. The specimen may be collected in the physician's office or at home and brought to the office by placing the container in a shirt pocket next to the body to keep it warm during transit.

Most specimens are obtained by masturbation. In those cases in which the patient objects to collecting the specimen through masturbation, special condoms without spermotoxic agents designed for semen collection may be used, allowing the couple to have intercourse. Coitus interruptus may also be used as an alternative method for obtaining the specimens if care is taken to ensure complete collection.

The specimen should be examined in the laboratory within 2 hours of collection. A label on the container should state the patient's name, the date, the time of collection, and the abstinence period. **In most cases, two to three specimens examined over a period of several weeks will give an adequate assessment of baseline spermatogenesis.** In those occasional cases in which parameters differ markedly in the initial semen specimens, additional specimens, collected over a 2- to 3-month period, may be obtained.

Physical Characteristics

Freshly ejaculated semen is a coagulum that liquefies over a 5- to 25-minute period. The seminal vesicles secrete the substance responsible for coagulation. Patients with **congenital bilateral absence of the vas** usually have absent or hypoplastic seminal vesicles. **Semen in these patients does not coagulate and has a low volume.** Secretions from the testis, epididymis, bulbourethral glans (Cowper's glands), glands of Littre (periurethral glans), prostate, and seminal vesicles compose the normal seminal fluid. The fluid is released from the glands in a specific sequence during ejaculation. Prior to the ejaculation of the major portion of the ejaculate, a small amount of fluid from the glands of Littre and the bulbourethral glands is secreted. This is followed by a low-viscosity opalescent fluid from the prostate containing a few sperm. The principal portion of the ejaculate contains the highest concentration of sperm, along with secretions from the testis, epididymis, and vas deferens, as well as some prostatic and seminal vesicle fluids. The last fraction of the ejaculate consists of seminal vesicle secretions. **The secretions from Cowper's glands account for 0.1 to 0.2 ml, prostatic secretions account for 0.5 ml, and the secretions from the seminal vesicles account for 1.5 to 2.0 ml. The majority of ejaculated sperm come from the distal epididymis, with a small contribution from the ampulla of the vas. The unobstructed seminal vesicle is not a reservoir for sperm.**

Although the seminal vesicles are responsible for the formation of a coagulum, proteinase secreted by the prostate is responsible for semen liquefaction. Several proteases, including prostate-specific antigen and plasminogen activators, play a role in semen liquefaction. Tissue plasminogen activator levels have been shown to be lower in the semen of patients with nonliquefaction than in normal semen (Arnaud et al, 1994). It is unclear whether or not male infertility may be due to failure of semen liquefaction. Some patients with nonliquefying semen have normal postcoital test (PCT) results. In addition, sperm may be found in the cervical mucus prior to semen liquefaction (Santomauro, 1972). Failure of liquefaction should be differentiated from semen that remains hyperviscous after liquefaction. Nonliquefying semen remains a coagulum and does not change consistency following ejaculation. Hyperviscous liquefied semen becomes less of a coagulum following ejaculation; however, its consistency remains thicker than normal. Liquefaction of semen may be induced by the addition of seminin, a seminal proteinase, or alpha-amylase. However, there is no evidence that this procedure increases the fertility of these samples (Syner et al, 1975; Wilson and Bunge, 1975). Normally, liquefied semen should be able to be poured drop by drop. Hyperviscous semen forms thick strands instead of drops. The viscosity of hyperviscous specimens may be reduced by passing the specimen through an 18-gauge needle with a syringe three to five times (Amelar, 1962). In those cases in which the semen demonstrates nonliquefaction or hyperviscosity, a PCT should be performed. If results are normal, demonstrating adequate numbers of motile sperm in the cervical mucus, the consistency of the semen may be disregarded. The consistency of the seminal fluid may be of significance if the PCT demonstrates few sperm with good-quality mucus. In these cases, a cross-mucus hostility test or an in vitro cervical mucus–sperm interaction test may be employed (see later). If these tests suggest that either nonliquefaction or hyperviscosity are contributing to the infertility, the best treatment is semen processing and intrauterine insemination (IUI) of the husband's sperm.

The volume of the ejaculate should be measured to the nearest milliliter. In our laboratory, with an abstinence period of 2 to 3 days, most normal men have seminal volumes between 1.5 and 5.0 ml.

Small-volume ejaculates may be produced in patients with partial retrograde ejaculation, absence of the vas deferens and seminal vesicles, obstruction of the ejaculatory ducts, androgen deficiency, sympathetic denervation, calcification of the vas deferens and seminal vesicles, bladder neck surgery, or drug therapy. The significance of high-volume ejaculates remains unclear. Dilution may result in oligospermic sperm concentrations with normal total numbers of sperm. Therapeutic insemination of the female partner has been recommended for these cases. However, not all investigators agree on this point. A normal PCT result strongly suggests that a high-volume ejaculation is not a factor in infertility. If high seminal volume is believed to be the etiologic factor, semen processing with concentration of sperm and IUI may be employed.

Concentration

The semen specimen should be well mixed prior to determination of sperm concentration. Standard methods for determining sperm concentration have been outlined by several groups. A Newbauer standard blood cell counting chamber is commonly employed. The specimen is diluted at a 1:20 ratio in a test tube. The diluent may consist of distilled water or sodium bicarbonate with 1% phenol in order to immobilize the spermatozoa. A drop of this specimen is placed on a counting chamber, and a coverslip is applied. Spermatozoa are counted within five blocks containing 16 squares each. All spermatozoa within this area and touching the lower and right-hand sides of each block are included. This number, multiplied by 10^6, represents the count per milliliter. Two sets of five blocks should be counted and an average calculated. A dilution of 1:10 should be used in those specimens with low sperm densities. The number of sperm within five blocks should be divided by 2 and then multiplied by 10^6 to obtain the sperm concentration. Counting chambers have been developed that allow for the examination of undiluted semen. In these chambers, a drop of undiluted sperm is placed on the slide, and the number of sperm with the grid are counted. The number of sperm within ten blocks represents the number of sperm in millions per milliliter. The sperm may be immobilized by cooling the specimen in ice water or by heating it to 50 degrees. Dilution of the specimen is still required with high sperm densities. Hyperviscous semen may elevate the coverslip, increasing the volume of semen counted. These specimens may be passed through an 18-gauge syringe, as previously noted. In the past, a white blood cell pipette has been used to perform dilutions of semen. Hand-held, variable-volume pipettors with disposable tips allow for quicker and easier dilutions. With this technique, the margin of error is at least 10%. If no sperm are identified, the specimen should be centrifuged and the pellet examined for the presence of sperm.

Computer-Aided Semen Analysis

Computer-aided semen analysis (CASA) refers to a semi-automated technique used to visualize and digitize static and dynamic sperm images using computer-assisted image analysis. Most systems employ video with multiple frames, which when played back, creates moving images. These techniques correlate, albeit imperfectly, with standard methods.

The computerized systems are able to determine parameters not measurable manually. Curvilinear velocity is the average distance per unit time between successive positions of an individual sperm. Straight-line velocity is the speed of a sperm in a forward direction. This is a measure of forward progression. Linearity is determined by dividing straight-line velocity by curvilinear velocity. Additional measurements include lateral head displacement, flagellar beat frequency, and circular movement analysis. Hyperactivation is a state of motility that sperm attain after capacitation in which large-amplitude movements of the head and tail of the sperm are coupled with a slow or nonprogressive motility (Yanagimachi, 1970). It has been found that prior to capacitation, about 0.4% of spermatozoa demonstrate a hyperactivated pattern. Following capacitation, 22% of fertile samples demonstrate hyperactivation, whereas only 8.5% of sperm from oligospermic patients demonstrate these patterns (Burkman, 1984). There are insufficient data to determine which, if any, of these reportable parameters may prove useful by distinguishing fertile from infertile patients above and beyond what is presently obtained with a manual semen analysis. Many factors, including the frequency of sampling, dilution of the sample, number of cells imaged, sensitivity of the imaging, and temperature of the sample, affect the results. **The advantages of CASA are that one gets quantitative data. It can be standardized, and it may be useful in marketing. The disadvantages include the following: the equipment is expensive, the method is labor intensive, the variables mentioned above can affect the results, the method is not yet standardized, and thus far, it has not been documented to give a more accurate prognosis or to affect treatment** (Davis and Katz, 1993).

Motility

Motility refers to the number (in percent) of sperm that have flagellar motion. The evaluation should be performed within 2 hours of ejaculation, and the sample should be kept at 37°C. A drop of fresh semen is placed on a clean, standard microscopic slide, and a coverslip is positioned over the drop. The specimen may be examined at 250 × to 400 × magnification. Although a phase-contrast microscope facilitates the observation of sperm, a standard bright-field microscope may be used. Ten random fields are examined, and the percentage of sperm that are moving is calculated. In specimens with counts of fewer than 40 to 60 million sperm per milliliter, exact numbers of motile and nonmotile sperm may be counted. In specimens of higher concentrations, motility is most often estimated, although some investigators recommend diluting the specimen prior to motility determination. Estimates performed by skilled technicians are consistent. An assessment of the quality of forward movement of the sperm should be noted. This is graded on an arbitrary scale of forward progression. A rating of 0 signifies no motility; 1 denotes sluggish or nonprogressive movement; 2 refers to sperm moving with a slow, meandering forward progression; 3 signifies sperm moving in a reasonably straight line with moderate speed; and 4 indicates sperm moving in a straight line with high speed (Amelar et al, 1973). It is unnecessary and of no proven value to determine motility parameters at repeated time points after seminal collection. This is a nonphysiologic measurement because sperm leave the semen and enter the cervical mucus within minutes of deposition within the vaginal vault (MacLeod, 1965). The motility may be depressed if the abstinence period has been prolonged.

Occasional clumps of agglutinated sperm are of no consequence. However, frequent sperm agglutination is abnormal and suggests the presence of antisperm antibodies. Notation should be made of the presence of other cell types. In the unstained, wet mount semen specimen, white blood cells and immature germ cells are similar in appearance and are known as *round cells*. An estimate of the number of these cells per high-power field should be made. Special stains are used to differentiate white blood cells from immature germ cells (see the section on white blood cell staining). The concentration of white blood cells in the infertile and fertile populations overlaps considerably. However, excessive numbers of white blood cells may be associated with the presence of an infection or inflammation. The concentration of immature germ cells is proportional to the concentration of sperm, although many men with poor semen quality have a higher percentage of immature cells than do fertile men. However, the patient-to-patient variation is considerable and is of unclear significance (Wolff et al, 1990). Although necrospermia is used to refer to those cases in which no motile sperm are identified, this terminology is inaccurate. In many cases, these sperm are alive with ultrastructural defects in the axonemal component of the flagella. Although immotile, these sperm may appear morphologically normal.

Morphology

The morphologic examination of spermatozoa is a sensitive indicator of the quality of spermatogenesis and of fertility (Talbot and Chacon, 1981; Kruger et al, 1988). Whereas some gross morphologic abnormalities can be identified with bright-field examination of unstained semen, this is a very insensitive determination. A more detailed morphologic examination of a wet mount may be obtained with the use of phase-contrast microscopy. However, the most accurate assessments involve the use of a stained specimen. A drop of semen may be placed on a glass slide and a second slide used to smear the specimen over the slide's surface. The smear may be allowed to air dry; however, the use of a spray cytologic fixative, such as that used for Papanicolaou (Pap) smears, will result in better preservation of morphology. The specimen may then be stained using a routine Pap stain (MacLeod, 1964) or Diff Quik (Baxter Healthcare Corporation, Miami FL). There is no consensus as to the classification of sperm morphology, and more than 70 variations have been described. However, a practical classification divides the cells into normal (oval head), amorphous (irregular head), tapered head, large- and small-headed, and immature (Fig. 43–1) (MacLeod, 1965). The human spermatozoal head is normally 3.0 to 5.0 microns long and 2.0 to 3.0 microns wide. Immature spermatozoa contain retained cytoplasmic droplets surrounding the midpiece. Specimens from individual patients maintain remarkable consistency in morphology from sample to sample (MacLeod, 1964). Testicular stresses, due to infection, heat, radiation, or varicoceles, may result in more than 2% to 3% of immature forms being demonstrated in specimens. These cells may appear in the ejaculate within 2 to 3 weeks of the onset of an illness. Increased numbers of amorphous and tapering forms commonly accompany an increase in immature cells in the semen (MacLeod, 1964). Although many variations in methodologies exist using the above-mentioned classification system, normal specimens contain 60% or more normal forms with less than 3% immature forms.

Strict Criteria Morphology

Van Zyl first described a system of strict criteria for normal sperm morphology (SCM) in 1972 (Van Zyl, 1972) and found that men who had more than 40% normal morphology by his criteria had a higher rate of impregnation than those who did not meet this standard. He also noted that SCM was a better predictor of fertility than any of the standard semen analysis parameters. He emphasized that with this technique, the thickness of the smear must be well controlled so that each cell can be well visualized and stained. He gave special attention to the characteristics of

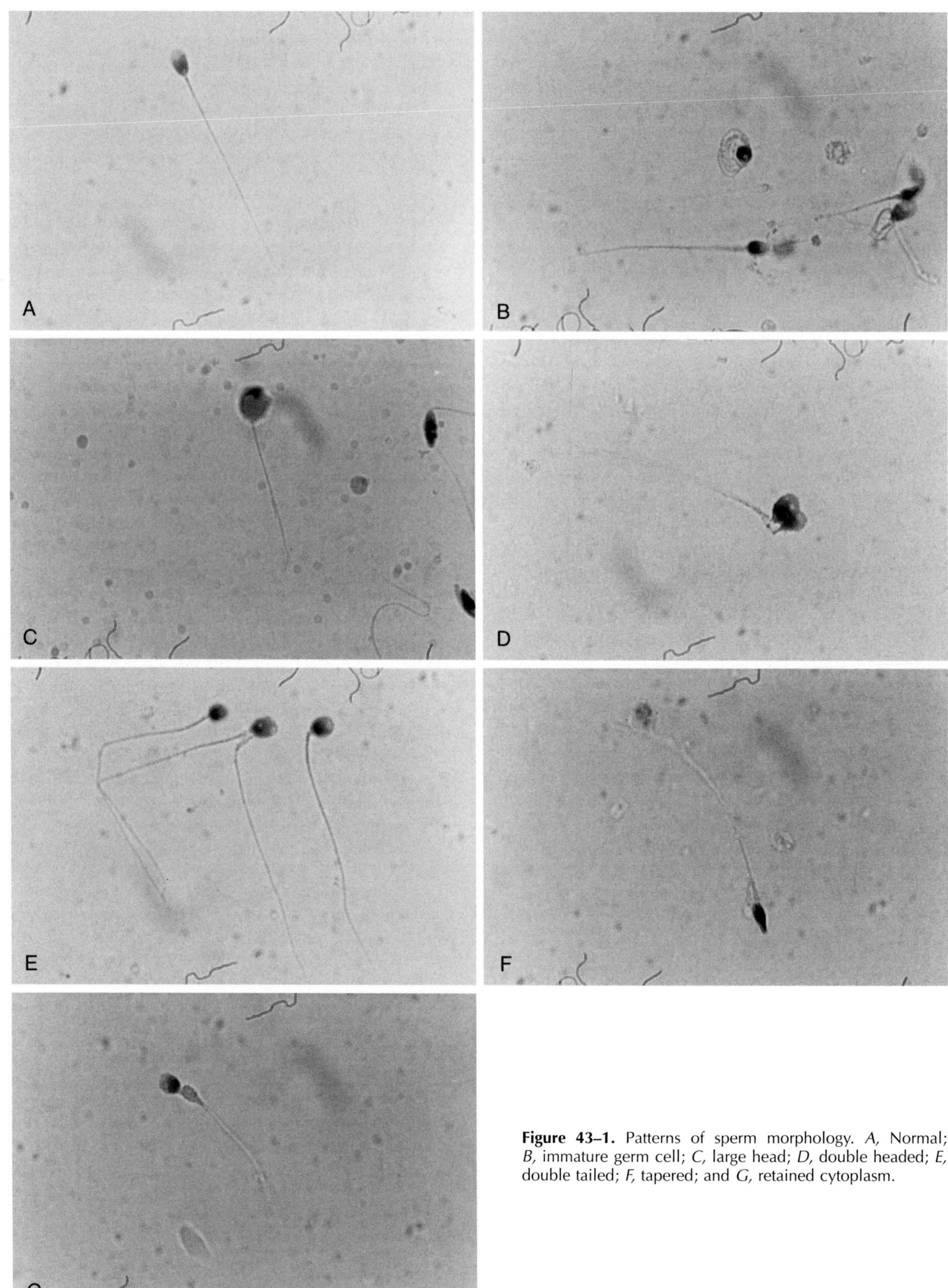

Figure 43–1. Patterns of sperm morphology. *A,* Normal; *B,* immature germ cell; *C,* large head; *D,* double headed; *E,* double tailed; *F,* tapered; and *G,* retained cytoplasm.

the acrosome and emphasized that each part of the sperm cell must be measured and compared with a standard (Van Zyl, 1980). These standards, as modified by Kruger, are depicted in Figure 43–2. In 1986, Kruger and associates found that in a group of men with sperm densities greater than 20 million per milliliter and motility greater than 30%, IVF rates were 37% for those with less than 14% normal sperm by SCM and 91% for those with greater than 14% normal sperm. Furthermore he noted that men with less than 4% normal SCM had an IVF rate of 7.6%, whereas those with 4% to 14% normal forms had a 63.9% fertilization rate. Subsequent studies have confirmed the correlation between SCM and IVF rate. However, several recent investigations have not shown a convincing correlation between SCM and fertility (Comhaire et al, 1994; Grow et al, 1994). Also, most of the recent work in this area has examined the relationship between SCM and IVF, not the fertility of men practicing normal sexual intercourse.

Additional Semen Parameters

Measurements have been made of many semen components. For the most part, however, these have not proved to be of clinical value. The pH of semen varies between 7.05 and 7.80 (Raboch and Skachova, 1965). The seminal vesicles produce fructose in an androgen-dependent process. Normal semen fructose concentrations range from 120 to 450 mg/dl. Conditions such as inflammation of the seminal vesicles resulting in dysfunction, androgen deficiency, partial obstruction of the ejaculatory ducts, or incomplete ejaculation may result in concentrations below 120 mg/dl. **In cases of absent seminal vesicles, fructose is usually absent from the semen. Patients with obstructed seminal vesicles and congenital absence of the seminal vesicles, which are usually associated with bilateral absence of the vas deferens, demonstrate acidic, fructose-negative semen and small-volume ejaculates that do not coagulate.** Transrectal ultrasonography (TRUS) is more commonly used to diagnose absence or anatomic abnormalities of the seminal vesicles and ejaculatory ducts. Measurements of other components of seminal fluids, such as citric acid phosphatase, spermine, aminotransferases, zinc concentrations, magnesium, and other ions, have not yielded clinically useful information.

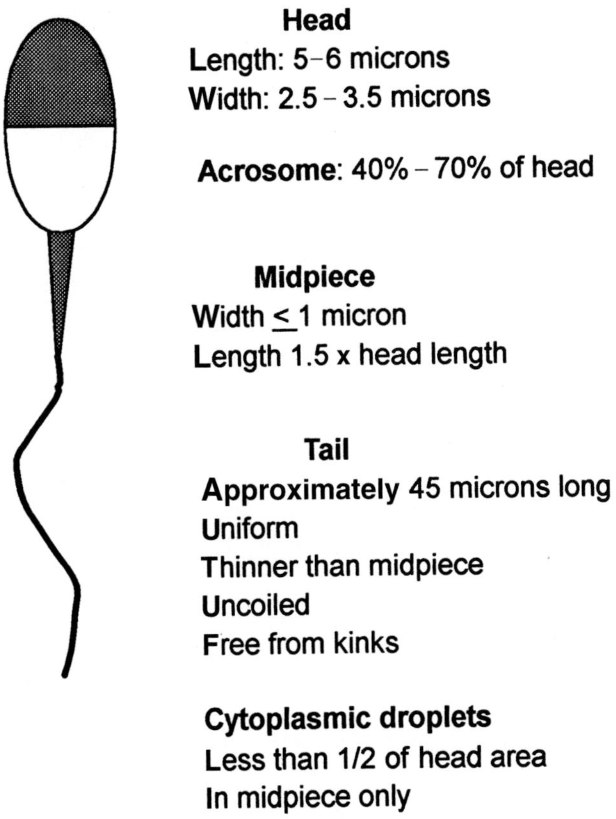

Figure 43–2. Criteria for normal sperm by rigid criteria.

Normal Values

Patients and physicians are often confused as to the difference between an *average* semen analysis and the *minimal* semen parameters required for normal fertility. Mean sperm densities between 70 and 80 million per milliliter have been found in fertile populations (Naghma-E-Rehan et al, 1975; Greenberg, 1977). Although this measurement represents the mean of fertile populations, this is not indicative of the minimal parameters required for conception. There is some evidence that semen quality has declined over the last several decades (Carlsen, 1992; Auger, 1995) Statistics from infertile populations demonstrate that the chances of initiating pregnancy decrease as semen quality decreases. **An ideal diagnostic test completely distinguishes normal from abnormal populations with no overlap (i.e., there are no false-positive or false-negative results). Most tests we deal with in medicine have overlap between two groups at approximately 2 standard deviations from the mean of the normal group. Unfortunately, in the case of semen analysis data, there is almost complete overlap between fertile and infertile men. Of course, all azoospermic men are infertile, and men with very high sperm densities and percent motilities are very likely to be fertile. Nevertheless, the vast majority of patients have semen quality that does not allow one to state unequivocally whether or not the patient is fertile.** Smith and co-workers (1977) reported a 25% pregnancy rate in couples whose husbands demonstrated counts of fewer than 12.5 million sperm per milliliter, whereas 44% of couples conceived when the count was between 12.5 and 25 million sperm per milliliter. Other investigators have found similar results (Schoysman and Gerris, 1983).

Thus, one must differentiate *subfertility* from *sterility*. Each laboratory defines its own set of standard values. **We define a minimally adequate specimen as one with the following criteria:**

- **A seminal volume of 1.5 to 5.0 ml**
- **A total sperm count of greater than 50 million**
- **Motility greater than or equal to 50%**
- **Forward progression greater than 2.0**
- **Fifty percent or more of sperm having normal morphology by standard criteria. Although by strict criteria abnormal samples are defined as having less than 14% normal forms, we have not found significant fertilization defects in most samples with greater than 1% normal forms using strict criteria.**

In addition, there should be minimal agglutination, and viscosity should be normal. As mentioned earlier, this provides a basis for making an educated estimate, not a definite diagnosis, of fertility. Although semen contains millions of sperm, IVF studies have determined that 50,000 to 500,000 sperm may be required to fertilize an ovum (Wolf et al, 1984). Clinical studies in women who have undergone hysterectomy have determined that only one of every 5000 sperm placed in the vagina reaches the cervical mucus and one out of every 14 million sperm in the vagina reaches the oviduct (Settladge, 1973). Further, it should be realized that levels that may constitute requirements for natural conception do not apply to ARTs, wherein fertilization may occur with suboptimal semen specimens. Lastly, it has become clear, from IVF, that the standard semen parameters are inadequate to measure the fertility potential of individual sperm.

Hormonal Evaluation

Fewer than 3% of cases of male infertility are due to a primary hormonal abnormality. Such abnormalities are rare in patients with sperm concentrations greater than 5 million sperm per milliliter (Baker et al, 1986). In the presence of normal spermatogenesis, follicle-stimulating hormone (FSH) secretion is regulated by negative feedback by inhibin. With primary testicular failure, inadequate Leydig and Sertoli cell function result in elevated gonadotropin levels with normal or low testosterone levels (Table 43–3). Hypothalamic or pituitary dysfunction resulting in inadequate levels of gonadotropins causes low peripheral levels of testosterone and an absence of spermatogenesis. As a result of the pulsatile secretion of gonadotropin-releasing hormone (GnRH), gonadotropins are secreted episodically, resulting in variation in the serum concentrations of these hormones, particularly luteinizing hormone (LH). Some investigators believe that for proper hormonal determination, measurements should be made on a pooled sample consisting of individual samples taken at 15-minute intervals. **Despite the inaccuracies of single determinations, it is rare for a patient's clinical endocrine status to be inaccurately determined with a single measurement. We recommend a pooled blood sample only when the results of one hormonal determination do not fit the clinical situation** (Bain et al, 1988).

Throughout early childhood, gonadotropin and testosterone levels remain low. LH and FSH levels begin increasing from approximately 6 to 8 years of age. Testosterone levels begin increasing at 10 to 12 years of age (Rifkind et al, 1967). During the reproductive years, gonadotropin and testosterone levels remain relatively constant. Later in life, testosterone levels, particularly free testosterone levels, decrease and gonadotropin concentrations rise (Albert, 1956). Degeneration of seminiferous tubules and decreased numbers of Leydig cells are thought to be responsible for these changes.

Table 43–3. HORMONAL STATUS AS A FUNCTION OF CLINICAL DIAGNOSIS

Clinical Status	FSH (mIU/ml)	LH (mIU/ml)	Testosterone (ng/100 ml)
Normal men	Normal	Normal	Normal
Germinal aplasia	↑	Normal	Normal
Testicular failure	↑	↑	Normal or ↓
Hypogonadotropic hypogonadism	↓	↓	↓

FSH, Follicle-stimulating hormone; LH, luteinizing hormone.

There is no agreement as to what should constitute an initial endocrine evaluation. **We recommend that all men with an indication in the history, physical examination, or a sperm density less than 5 to 10 million per milliliter have measurements taken of LH, FSH, and testosterone.** However, many experts believe that all infertile men should undergo these tests. If an isolated serum testosterone level is low or borderline and the LH is not elevated, we recommend that testosterone and free testosterone measurements be taken in the morning, because levels of testosterone are higher in the morning and free testosterone levels are useful in equivocal cases. If the testosterone level remains low, a serum prolactin measurement and a pituitary magnetic resonance imaging (MRI) study or computed tomography (CT) scan should be obtained (see later).

Impaired visual fields or severe headaches suggest the presence of a central nervous system tumor. Prolactin determination should be performed in these patients. However, in men with pituitary tumors, serum prolactin concentration may be normal. Most men with prolactin-secreting tumors present with macroadenomas (greater than 1 cm). Prolactin levels in these patients are usually higher than 200 ng/ml. Hypogonadotropism, coupled with low androgen levels, is commonly found in these patients. However, mild prolactin elevation is more frequent in infertile patients. Evaluation of the central nervous system often fails to identify a tumor. These patients with idiopathic hyperprolactinemia have normal gonadotropin and testosterone levels. We do not recommend treatment of isolated mild hyperprolactinemia because, in our experience this has not resulted in improved spermatogenesis. However these patients should be evaluated to rule out a pituitary tumor. The GnRH stimulation test is often abnormal in men with suboptimal semen quality; however, at this time, the finding of an abnormal GnRH test does alter treatment. Therefore, we do not advocate routine GnRH stimulation testing.

Male infertility secondary to congenital adrenal hyperplasia (CAH) is very rare. Patients with this condition may have a history of precocious puberty, a family history of CAH, short stature due to premature closure of the epiphyseal plates, and testicular enlargement that may be indicative of adrenal rest tumors of the testis. Measurement of the plasma 17-hydroxyprogesterone reveals elevated levels in these patients. Partial, late-onset CAH has been found in some cases of male infertility; however, this is uncommon (Augarten et al, 1991). We do not advocate routine screening for CAH. Estrogen excess may be endogenous or exogenous. Patients with estrogen excess may present with bilateral gynecomastia, impotence, and atrophic testes. Normal levels of plasma FSH, LH, and testosterone are usually found in cases of elevated levels of plasma estrogens. Thyroid function studies do not need to be determined unless there is clinical evidence of thyroid abnormalities.

INTERPRETATION OF THE INITIAL EVALUATION

Based on the initial history, physical examination, and laboratory studies, a differential diagnosis may be developed

Table 43–4. CLASSIFICATION OF MALE INFERTILITY STATUS BY CRITERIA OF SEMEN ANALYSIS

I. Absent Ejaculation

1. Drugs
2. Surgery
3. Vascular occlusion
4. Diabetes mellitus
5. Psychologic disturbances

II. Azoospermia

1. Seminiferous tubular sclerosis
   a. Klinefelter's syndrome
   b. Chromatin-negative Klinefelter's syndrome
2. Germinal aplasia
   a. Idiopathic
   b. Drug/radiation exposure
   c. Klinefelter's syndrome with mosaicism
   d. XYY syndrome
3. Maturation arrest
   a. Idiopathic
   b. XYY syndrome
   c. Varicocele
4. Ductal obstruction
5. Endocrinopathy

III. Oligospermia

1. Idiopathic
2. Cryptorchidism
3. Varicocele
4. Drugs
5. Systemic infection
6. Endocrinopathy

IV. Normal But Infertile

1. Gynecologic abnormality
2. Abnormal coital habits
3. Acrosomal defects
4. Immunologic
5. Unexplained

V. Asthenospermia

1. Spermatozoal structural defects
2. Prolonged abstinence
3. Idiopathic
4. Genital tract infection
5. Antisperm antibodies

(Table 43–4). Further, more specific testing allows the physician to place the patient into an etiologic category. The frequency of semen abnormalities and etiologic categories in a group of our patients are listed in Tables 43–5 and 43–6.

Absent or Low-Volume Ejaculate

Absent ejaculation may be due either to retrograde ejaculation or lack of emission (no expulsion of semen through the vas deferens into the posterior urethra) (Fig. 43–3). **Neurologic abnormalities, bladder neck surgery, drug therapy, androgen deficiency, or retroperitoneal surgery may account for absent or retrograde ejaculation. In addition, psychologic disturbances associated with an inability to obtain orgasm present with similar findings.** A combination of antegrade and retrograde ejaculation presents with a low-volume ejaculate. Because the majority of seminal fluid is contributed by the seminal vesicles, **in the absence of retrograde ejaculation, a low-volume ejaculate suggests the lack of seminal vesicle contribution. The patient should be examined for the presence of the vas deferens because it may be absent when there is agenesis of the seminal vesicles. Partial or**

Table 43–5. DISTRIBUTION OF PATIENTS PRESENTING WITH INFERTILITY BY FINDINGS ON SEMEN ANALYSIS

Semen Pattern	Number of Patients	Percent
Multiple Parameters, Abnormal	664	38.67
Asthenospermia	413	24.05
Normal	409	23.82
Teratazoospermia	172	10.02
Oligospermia	31	1.81
Low Volume	28	1.63

Table 43–6. DISTRIBUTION OF PATIENTS BY DIAGNOSTIC CATEGORY AFTER FULL EVALUATION

Category	Number	Percent
Varicocele	650	38.17
Idiopathic	422	24.78
Obstruction	224	13.15
Normal	168	9.86
Cryptorchidism	61	3.58
Antisperm antibodies	43	2.52
Ejaculatory dysfunction	22	1.29
Drug use	17	1
Endocrinopathy	17	1
WBC	17	1
Sexual dysfunction	10	0.59
Testicular failure	5	1.47
Genetic	4	0.23
Ultrastructural	4	0.23
Sertoli cell–only	4	0.23
Cancer	3	0.18
Heat	1	0.06
Radiation exposure	1	0.06
Systemic illness	1	0.06
Testicular cancer	1	0.06

complete ejaculatory duct obstruction also causes a low-volume ejaculate. Some men produce low-volume ejaculates when masturbating into a container but produce normal volumes when ejaculation is accomplished by intercourse. Collection of a specimen with intercourse using a seminal collection condom will identify these cases. Finally, incomplete specimen collection should be ruled out, as well as a decreased abstinence period. All cases of absent ejaculation and low-volume ejaculation should be evaluated with a postejaculate urine specimen. This is performed by centrifuging the specimen for 10 minutes at 300 g or more. The pellet should then be inspected and interpreted in relationship to the patient's clinical findings. In patients with absent ejaculation, the finding of more than 5 to 10 sperm per high-power field indicates retrograde ejaculation. In patients with low-volume ejaculates, the finding of more sperm in the urine than in the antegrade specimen suggests a significant component of retrograde ejaculation. Finally, in patients with azoospermia, the finding of any sperm in the postejaculate urine rules out complete bilateral ductal obstruction. In the absence of sperm in the postejaculate urine, ejaculatory duct obstruction should be suspected. **Although traditionally fructose determination was used to evaluate the presence of seminal vesicle contributions to the ejaculate, presently TRUS is most commonly employed. If the TRUS is normal, further evaluation depends on whether the patient is azoospermic or not.** In the azoospermic patient, a testis biopsy with touch prep should be performed to determine whether or not spermatogenesis is present. If spermatogenesis is present, then the genital ducts do not carry sperm either due to a physical obstruction or malfunction of the ejaculatory duct apparatus (such as from neurologic injury or calcification of the vas deferens as found in diabetics). To identify a physical obstruction, a scrotal exploration with vasogram and sampling of vasal fluid is indicated (see Chapter 44). In low-volume oligospermic patients, there is generally very little reason to perform a testis biopsy because spermatogenesis must be present. In some of these cases, evidence of ejaculatory duct obstruction

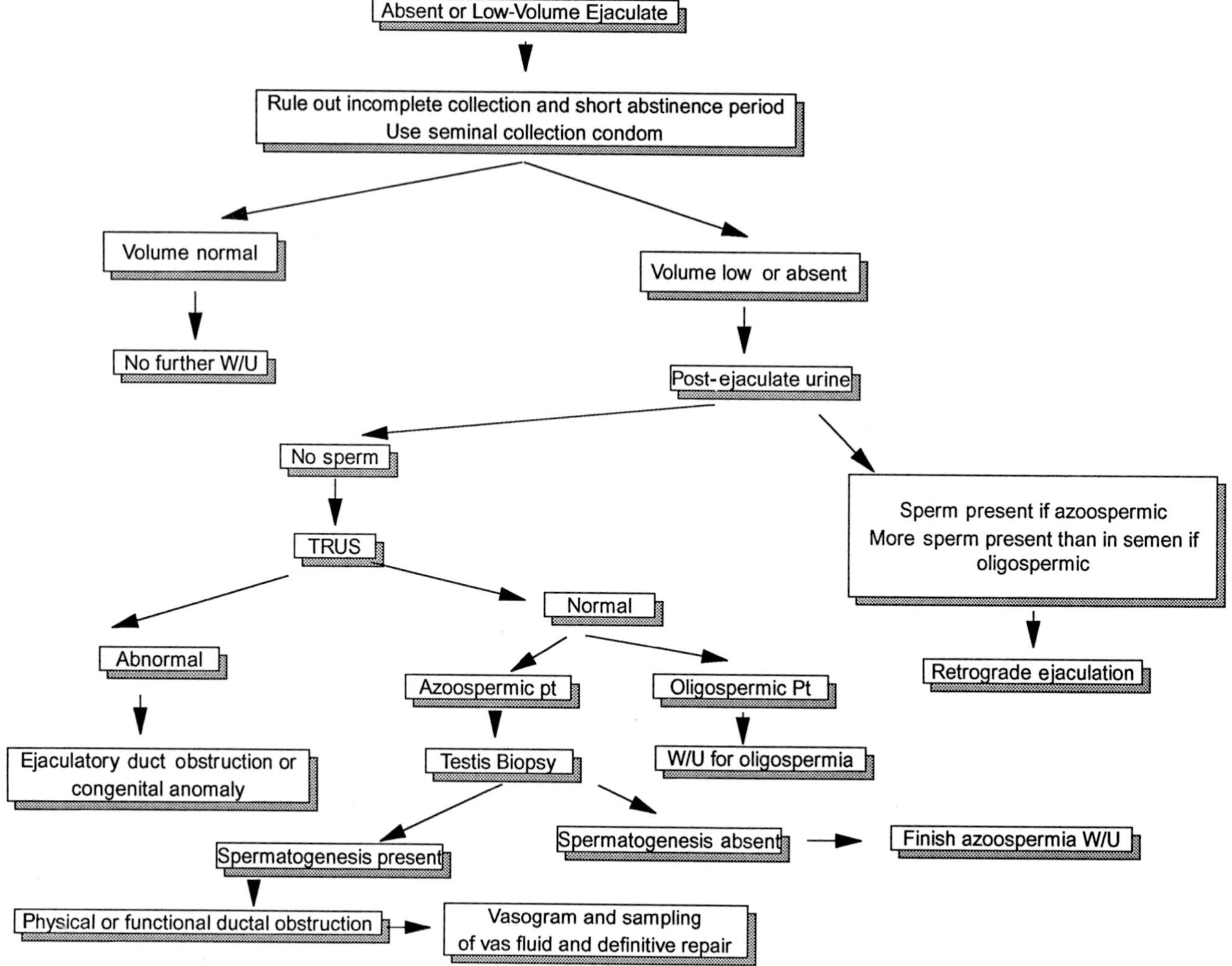

Figure 43–3. Algorithm for evaluation of the patient with a low-volume ejaculate. TRUS, Transrectal ultrasonography; W/U, work-up.

may be suggested by the TRUS. These cases of partial ejaculatory duct obstruction are uncommon.

Azoospermia

Ductal obstruction, chromosomal abnormalities, varicoceles, endocrinopathies, gonadotoxins, and idiopathic causes account for azoospermia (Fig. 43–4). **The evaluation of the azoospermic patient should be geared toward determining whether azoospermia is due to a lack of spermatogenesis or to physical or functional ductal obstruction.** The initial step should be to centrifuge the semen specimen. The presence of any sperm in the pellet rules out bilateral ductal obstruction, and the patient should be evaluated for oligospermia. Ductal obstruction may occur at any level from the ejaculatory duct to the vas deferens and the epididymis, as well as the efferent ductules. This may be congenital (e.g., congenital absence of the vas deferens [CBAVD]) or acquired (e.g., vasectomy). CBAVD is identified by physical examination and should be worked up as described below. In azoospermic patients with palpable vas deferens, the results of endocrine studies guide further evaluation. In patients with normal hormonal studies (see Fig. 43–4), a testis biopsy and touch preparation should be performed. The presence of spermatogenesis on the biopsy suggests a ductal obstruction. A scrotal exploration with vasogram and sampling of intraoperative vasal fluid should be performed (see Chapter 44). In patients with no spermatogenesis on biopsy, any correctable abnormality accounting for the spermatogenic defect should be corrected. Vasography is not indicated in these cases. **In patients with small testes and FSH concentrations greater than 2 to 3 times normal, severe germ cell failure is present, and the ultimate outlook is poor. A testis biopsy usually does not change therapy; therefore, further evaluation in these cases should be performed with a guarded prognosis.** It should be kept in mind that in some of these cases, occasional mature sperm may be found in the seminiferous tubules. Thus, testicular biopsies may be indicated for therapy and not diagnosis in these cases. Patients with azoospermia and small testes may have karyotyping performed to identify chromosomal abnormalities. Patients with a normal-sized testis on one side and an atrophic or absent testis on the contralateral side should undergo a testis biopsy even if the FSH is elevated because they may have obstruction associated with normal spermatogenesis in the healthy testis.

The finding of a low FSH and LH or an inappropriate LH

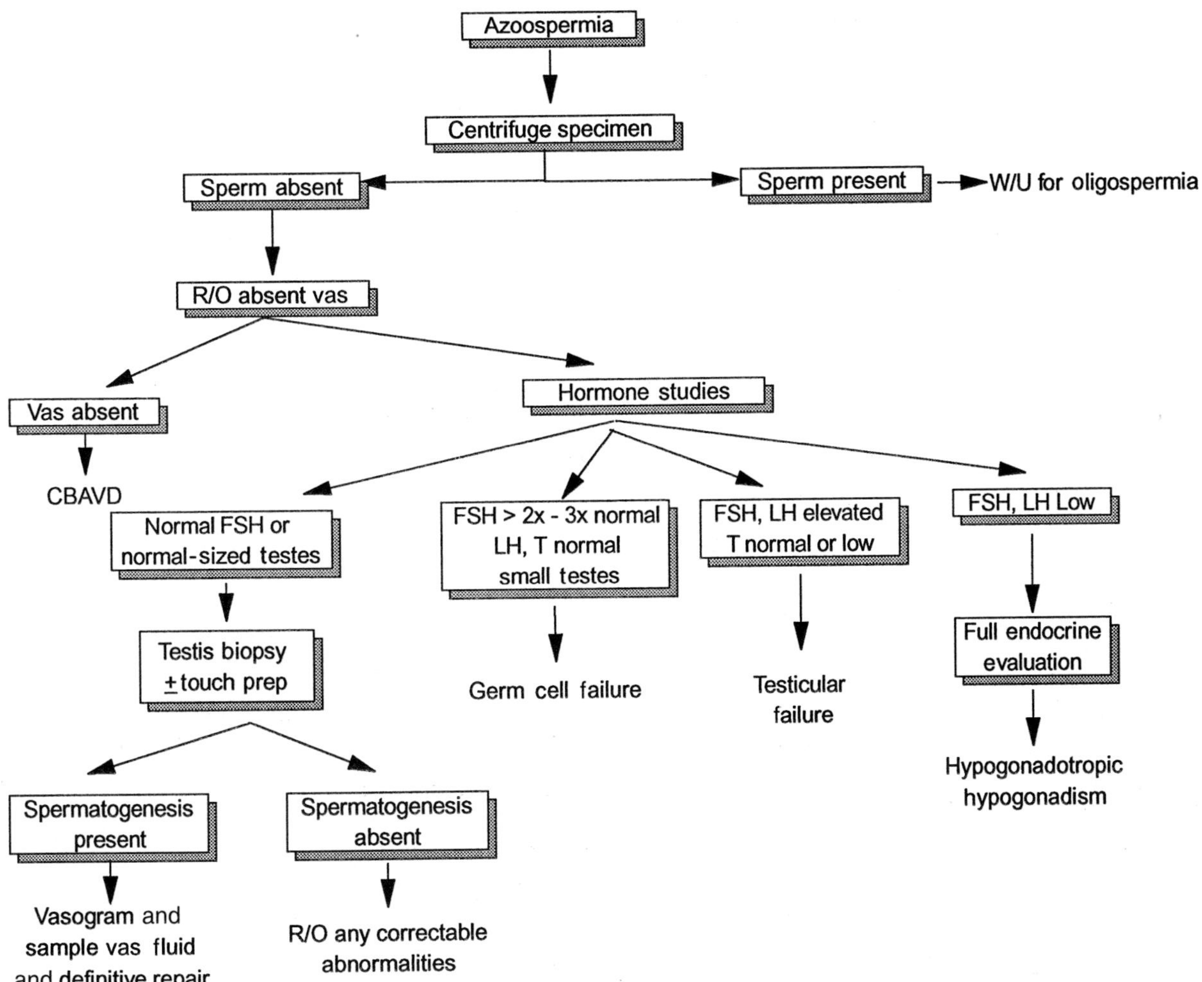

Figure 43–4. Algorithm for evaluation of the patient with azoospermia. CBAVD, Congenital absence of the vas; FSH, follicle-stimulating hormone; LH, luteinizing hormone; R/O, rule out; T, testosterone; W/U, work-up.

level in the presence of a low testosterone level suggests hypogonadotropic hypogonadism. These patients should undergo a complete endocrine evaluation to rule out a pituitary tumor or panhypopituitarism.

In the patient with CBAVD, a serum FSH should be determined. In the presence of a normal serum FSH and normal-sized testes, there is no indication for a testis biopsy because these patients almost uniformly have normal spermatogenesis. If the history or physical examination suggests an abnormality of spermatogenesis, a biopsy may be performed. Because CBAVD is associated with unilateral renal agenesis, a renal ultrasound should also be obtained in these patients. Although a TRUS is often performed in these patients to identify abnormalities of the seminal vesicles, this is not a necessary component of the evaluation and will not affect treatment.

The evaluation of a group of azoospermic patients determined that 41% had normal spermatogenesis. Sertoli cell–only syndrome was identified in 38% of patients, maturation arrest in 20%, and focal scarring in 2% (Jarow et al, 1989).

Oligospermia

Oligospermia refers to sperm densities of less than 20 million sperm per milliliter or a total count of less than 50 million sperm. Isolated oligospermia with normal movement and morphology parameters is uncommon. In severe oligospermia (less than 5–10 million per milliliter), hormone studies, specifically LH, FSH and testosterone levels, should be evaluated. If these levels are abnormal, a complete hormonal evaluation should be obtained, as outlined in the hormonal evaluation section. Hormone deficiency should be treated appropriately, as described later in this chapter. Patients with normal results on hormonal studies and isolated oligospermia are candidates for empiric medical therapy and ARTs.

Asthenospermia

Defects in sperm movement (asthenospermia) refer to low levels of motility or forward progression, or both. Spermatozoal structural defects, prolonged abstinence periods, genital tract infection, antisperm antibodies, partial ductal obstruction, and idiopathic causes may be responsible for these cases (Fig. 43–5). The finding of asthenospermia or significant sperm agglutination raises the possibility of immunologic infertility. An antisperm antibody assay, preferably a direct assay, should be performed. Patients with antisperm antibodies are candidates for immunosuppression or

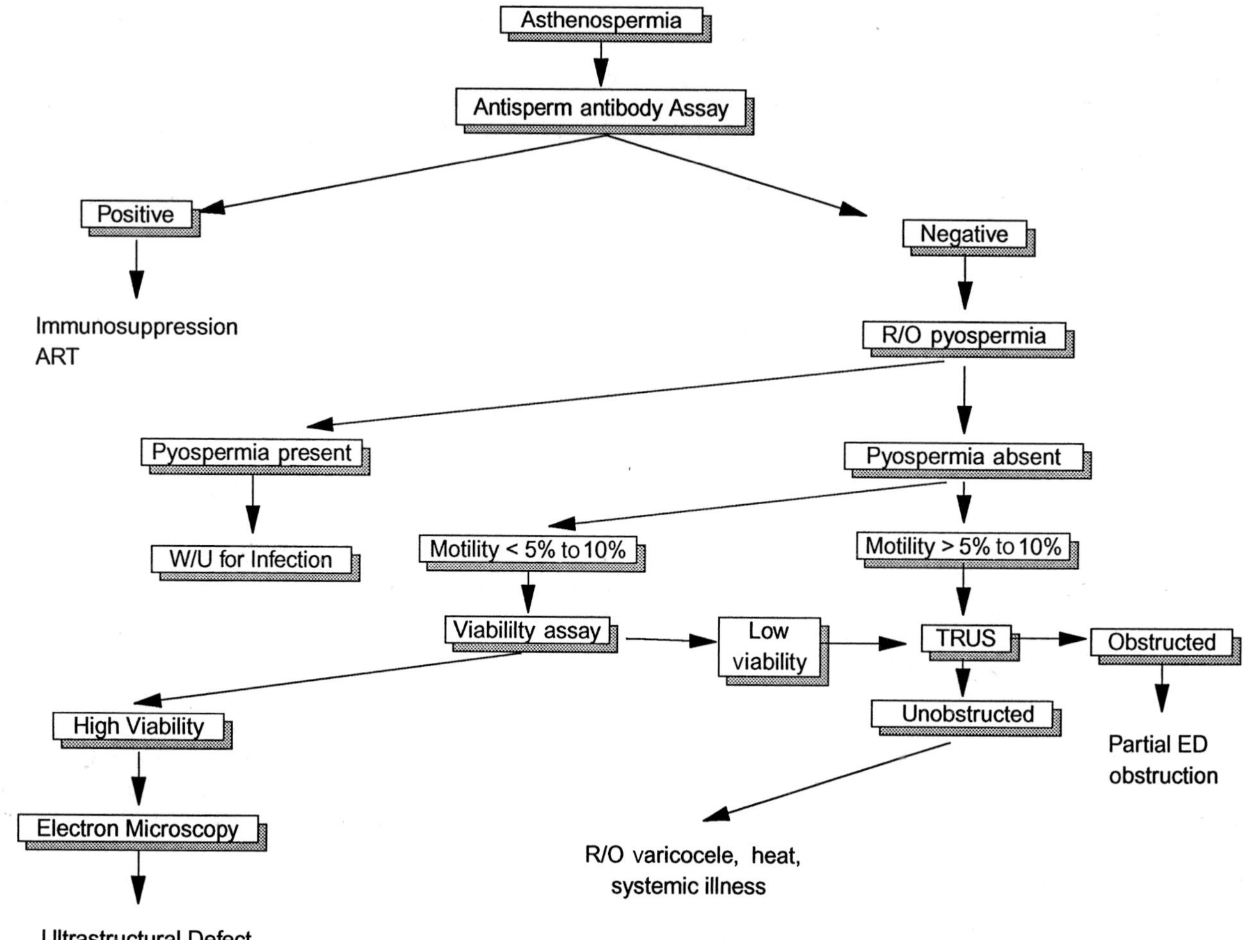

Figure 43–5. Algorithm for evaluation of the patient with asthenospermia. ART, Assisted reproductive techniques; ED, ejaculatory duct; R/U rule out; TRUS, transrectal ultrasonography; W/U, work-up.

ARTs. Hormonal studies rule out an endocrine deficiency; however, this type of deficiency is uncommon in the presence of normal sperm densities. Infection should be suspected if increased numbers of round cells have been reported in the semen analysis. In these instances, a study to differentiate immature germ cells from white blood cells, such as the Endtz test or immunohistochemical staining, may be considered. True pyospermia may be evaluated further by cultures or swabs to detect the presence of *Mycoplasma* and *Chlamydia*. In addition, a urinalysis should be performed to rule out the presence of a urinary tract infection. Semen cultures may be performed but are often contaminated by distal urethral organisms.

A varicocele is the most common surgically correctable abnormality found in infertile men and may be responsible for sperm motility defects as well as defects in sperm count and shape. Partial ejaculatory duct obstruction may be suspected in asthenospermic patients, particularly in the presence of borderline low volume and very poor forward progression. TRUS may be performed in these instances. Complete absence of sperm motility or cases with motilities with less than 5% should be evaluated by a sperm viability assay. The finding of a high fraction of viable sperm in the presence of low or absent sperm motility suggests an ultrastructural abnormality, such as that found in the immotile cilia syndrome and Kartagener's syndrome (immotile cilia syndrome associated with situs inversus). Patients with classic immotile cilia syndrome present with a history of chronic respiratory tract infections. This is due to a lack of dynein arms in the axoneme of the cilia of the respiratory tract and in the flagella of the spermatozoa. Situs inversus is present in approximately 50% of these patients (see section on structural abnormalities of spermatozoa). Electron microscopic evaluation of spermatozoa identifies these cases. Occasionally, excessively prolonged abstinence periods may result in severely depressed motility.

Teratospermia

Defects in morphology are termed teratospermia and have become more common with the utilization of rigid criteria for the evaluation of sperm morphology. Temporary insults to spermatogenesis and varicoceles may exist in these cases. Rarely, specimens consisting of round-headed sperm missing the acrosome may be found.

Multiple Defects in Seminal Parameters

Defects in sperm density, motility, and morphology are frequently due to a varicocele effect. This lesion should have been discovered on the physical examination (Fig. 43–6). In patients without clinical evidence of a varicocele, we do not advocate studies to detect subclinical varicoceles. Partial ejaculatory duct obstruction may also cause similar findings. This condition should be suspected in the patient with borderline seminal volumes with pronounced defects in forward progression. This possibility may be evaluated with TRUS. Other causes of multiple sperm defects include cryptorchidism; temporary insults to spermatogenesis such as heat, either environmental or endogenous due to a fever; or environmental toxins. If a temporary insult is suspected, several semen analyses should be performed over 1 to 2 spermatogenic cycles (3 to 6 months) once the inciting agent is removed.

Normal Semen Parameters

Normal semen analyses in infertile couples suggest the possibility of a female factor as well as immunologic infertility or incorrect coital habits. A PCT should be obtained in these instances. If no sperm are identified, the couple must be questioned about their coital technique. Both partners in couples with unexplained infertility should be evaluated for the presence of antisperm antibodies. A direct assay is preferred in the male, whereas an indirect one is performed in the female. The female should also be carefully evaluated to rule out significant female factors. If no abnormalities are found, sperm function testing should be performed in the male. Tests such as the sperm penetration assay (SPA) or the inducibility of the acrosome reaction should be considered. If the PCT is consistently abnormal, in the absence of antisperm antibodies, then an in vitro sperm cervical mucus assay should be performed. A normal result suggests a cervical mucus abnormality, whereas an abnormal result suggests a sperm migration problem. Abnormal sperm function testing results should instigate a re-evaluation of the male in a search for correctable abnormalities. If no abnormalities are detected, ARTs should be considered. If sperm function testing is normal, re-evaluation of the female should be undertaken.

SECOND-LEVEL TESTING

Based on the initial evaluation and the differential diagnoses suggested by this evaluation, additional, more specific testing may be indicated. The purpose of second-level testing is to rule in or rule out specific etiologies. It must be remembered that there are specific indications for obtaining these tests and not all patients need all tests.

Antisperm Antibodies

In the postpubertal male, the blood-testis and blood-epididymal barrier prevents exposure of sperm to the immune system. The basis of this barrier is the tight junctions that develop between cells. In addition, there may be active immunosuppression by T-suppressor cells (El-Demry and James, 1988), as well as immunosuppressive factors such as prostaglandin E_2 in the seminal plasma (Quayle et al, 1989). Antisperm antibodies develop if these barriers are disrupted.

There is clear evidence that ductal obstruction leads to the development of antisperm antibodies. Other possible etiologies include epididymal or testicular infection, torsion of the testicle, cryptorchidism, genital trauma, and varicoceles (Iqbal et al, 1989; Jarow and Sanzone, 1992; Knudson et al, 1994; Urry et al, 1994). Antisperm antibodies have been identified in approximately 60% of men following vasectomy (Ansbacher, 1971; Fuchs and Alexander, 1983). Surface-bound antisperm antibodies were found on sperm retrieved from the epididymis in 35% of men with CBAVD (Patrizio et al, 1992). Testicular torsion or trauma may lead to the development of antisperm antibodies.

Immunoglobulins may enter the genital tract through the seminiferous tubules, epididymis, or prostate. Immunoglobu-

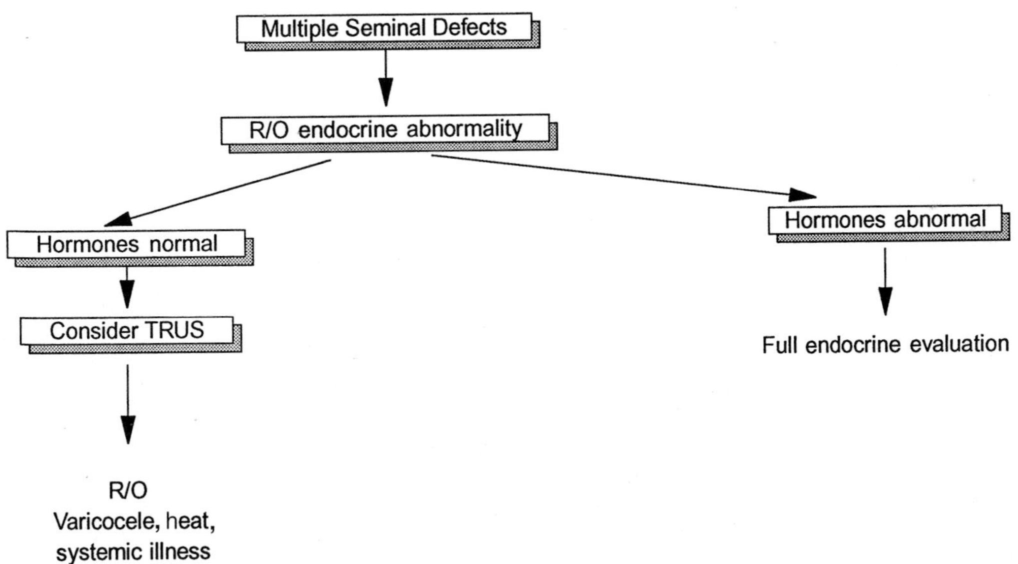

Figure 43–6. Algorithm for evaluation of the patient with multiple seminal defects. R/O, Rule out; TRUS, transrectal ultrasonography.

lin A (IgA) and immunoglobulin G (IgG) may both passively diffuse into the genital tract; however, IgA is also actively secreted. **Because immunoglobulins may be secreted locally in the genital tract, it is not surprising that there may be antisperm antibodies present on the sperm surface that are not found in the serum.**

Antisperm antibodies can affect sperm function at several different levels. Cervical mucus penetration may be impaired in sperm coated with antibodies. There appears to be some reaction between the cervical mucus and the Fc region of the antibody (Aitken et al, 1988). Some antibodies have been found to cause premature induction of the acrosome reaction, whereas in other cases, impairment of zona binding or fertilization of ova have been identified (Clarke et al, 1985b; DeAlmeida et al, 1989; Mahoney et al, 1991). In addition, there is recent evidence that some surface-bound antibodies may not interfere with fertilization but with subsequent embryo cleavage of fertilized ova (Naz, 1992).

An association between the presence of antisperm antibodies and infertility has been known for many years. Pregnancy rates are significantly lower in couples in whom the male has demonstrated the presence of antisperm antibodies (Ayvaliotis et al, 1985). There is considerable disagreement as to which are the most valid antibody assays and even what levels of antibodies in a specific assay constitute clinically significant levels. This has resulted in a plethora of antisperm antibody assays. In the past, the presence of antisperm antibodies was most commonly determined from a serum sample. The presence of antisperm antibodies in the serum is not always associated with the presence of these antibodies on the sperm (Hellstrom et al, 1988; Sigman et al, 1989). In general, the higher the titer of antibodies in the serum, the more likely there will be antibodies in the semen. **Most investigators believe that only antibodies present on the spermatozoal surface are clinically significant.** Thus, most recent investigations have been aimed at direct assays determining the presence of sperm-bound antibodies instead of the indirect detection of serum antisperm antibodies.

In enzyme-linked immunosorbent assays, sperm or sperm antigens are bound to a plastic well. An antihuman antibody to which an enzyme is bound is then added to the well. Commonly, sperm are fixed or disrupted prior to their plating in the well, which may expose intracellular antigens. These intracellular antigens are probably of no clinical significance.

We recommend the direct Immunobead Assay, which has become increasingly used for the detection of antisperm antibodies. This assay employs micron-sized polyacrylamide beads, to which rabbit antihuman antibodies have been linked. The beads are mixed with washed spermatozoa and bind to the portion of the sperm containing the antisperm antibodies. Immunobead binding is determined by examination under a phase-contrast microscope. Beads containing anti-IgG or anti-IgA are commonly used and allow for the determination of the class of antibody as well as the site of antibody binding. Scoring is based on the percentage of motile sperm with bead binding (Ayvaliotis et al, 1985; Clarke et al, 1985a). Ayvaliotis and associates (1985) found a 43% pregnancy rate when fewer than 50% of sperm demonstrated to Immunobead Assay binding, whereas there was 21% pregnancy rate in those couples in whom the sperm demonstrated greater than 50% Immunobead Assay binding. An indirect Immunobead Assay may be performed by using patient serum with donor sperm. The indirect assay is associated with a high false-positive rate and, therefore, is not an ideal test. The Sperm Mar test (Ortho Diagnostic Systems, Beerse, Belgium) creates a mixed agglutination reaction between IgG-coated polystyrene microspheres, sperm, and anti-IgG antiserum. The Immunobead Assay must be performed on washed sperm, whereas the Sperm Mar assay is performed on unwashed semen; it is therefore easier to perform. Comparison studies between the Sperm Mar assay and the Immunobead Assay have yielded conflicting results (Hellstrom et al, 1989; Sedor and Hirsch, 1994). Most patterns of bead binding to sperm appear to have comparable detrimental effects on fertility (Ayvaliotis et al, 1985).

Fertility may also be impaired in the presence of antisperm antibodies in the female. Of necessity, indirect assays must be used on females and therefore are subject to the same problems as indirect assays in the male. Although serum is easier to work with, antisperm antibodies in the cervical mucus are more clinically significant; however, this substance is technically difficult to work with.

We believe that patients with the previously mentioned risk factors, those demonstrating impaired sperm motility, sperm agglutination, abnormal PCT findings, and couples with unexplained infertility should be tested for the presence of antisperm antibodies. Because the presence of serum antisperm antibodies does not affect the decision to proceed with vasectomy reversals, we do not recommend preoperative testing in these patients. Testing may be performed in patients with patent anastomoses after reversal who are not able to impregnate their spouses.

White Blood Cell Staining of Semen

Under wet mount microscopy, immature germ cells and leukocytes appear similar and are known as round cells. The presence of greater than 1 to 3 million white blood cells per milliliter suggests a genital tract infection or inflammation. Both infection and infertility have been associated with pyospermia (Caldamone et al, 1980; Berger et al, 1982; Maruyama et al, 1985). Most studies suggest detrimental effects of leukocytes on sperm function. However, many patients with pyospermia do not have genital tract infections. Approximately one third of the cases demonstrating increased numbers of round cells will be found to have true pyospermia, with the remainder of cases having increased numbers of immature germ cells (Sigman and Lopes, 1993). In addition, not all studies of patients with increased numbers of leukocytes in the semen report decreased fertility rates (Tomlinson et al, 1993). Infertile couples have been found to have greater concentrations of white blood cells than did fertile populations (Wolff and Anderson, 1988). The morphologic differentiation of round cells may be made using traditional staining techniques, such as the Pap stain. However, these methods necessitate a highly trained observer. Monoclonal antibodies directed against white blood cell surface antigens have been combined with immunohistochemical techniques to aid in the differentiation of round cells (Homyk et al, 1990). The red-brown staining pattern of leukocytes allows their easy differentiation from immature germ cells (Wolff and Anderson, 1988). A technique relying on the presence of peroxidase in white blood cells identifies granulocytes but may miss samples that consist primarily of macrophages. Peroxidase-positive white blood cells stain dark brown with this simple procedure (Endtz, 1974).

We recommend some type of white blood cell staining of semen in patients with more than 10 to 15 round cells per high-power field or more than 1 to 3 million round cells per milliliter. If the majority of cells are white blood cells and the concentration is greater than 1 to 3 million blood cells per milliliter, the patient should be evaluated for a genital tract infection. The treatment of true pyospermia in the absence of symptomatic infection remains problematic (Yanushpolky et al, 1995).

Cultures of the Genital Tract

Genital tract infections very infrequently contribute to male infertility. Many organisms, including aerobic and anaerobic organisms, as well as *Mycoplasma*, have been cultured from human semen (Swenson et al, 1980; Lewis et al, 1981; Busolo et al, 1984; Upadhyaya et al, 1984; Naessens et al, 1986). Although studies have found that bacteria may be spermicidal (Paulson and Polakowski, 1977), others have found no consistent effect on fertility (Makler et al, 1981; Berger et al, 1982). **In the presence of a clear genital tract infection, such as cystitis, urethritis, or prostatitis, appropriate treatment should be instituted. However, routine genital tract bacterial culturing is not indicated in the absence of evidence of infection or pyospermia.**

Mycoplasmas are aerobic bacteria that bind to cell membranes and do not stain with Gram's stain. Both *Mycoplasma hominis* and *Ureaplasma urealyticum* have been associated with nongonococcal urethritis in humans (Bowie et al, 1977). Increased pregnancy rates have been reported in uncontrolled studies of patients treated for these organisms (Kundsin, 1986). However, controlled studies have not confirmed these findings (Indress et al, 1978). Similarly, there have been conflicting studies on the relationship between the presence of *Mycoplasma* in the genital tract and seminal parameters. Upadhyaya and co-workers (1984) found normal sperm motility, viability, and morphology but a decrease in sperm concentration in patients whose genital tracts were colonized with this organism. Other studies have found no effect on semen parameters (Soffer et al, 1990). Some investigators have found evidence of adherence of *Mycoplasma* to sperm (Busolo et al, 1982; Lewis et al, 1981; Upadhyaya et al, 1984). Cultures from *Mycoplasma* have been difficult to obtain in the past. Office-based systems based on culture of seminal plasma have increased the availability and ease of these cultures (Wood et al, 1985).

Chlamydia infections have become the most prevalent sexually transmitted disease in the United States (Thompson and Washington, 1983). This obligate intracellular bacterium is a common cause of epididymitis and nongonococcal urethritis. Cultures of semen, prostatic secretions, and urine have documented the presence of *Chlamydia* (Thompson et al, 1983). Traditional culturing methods require monolayered cultures of McCoy cells. Fluorescent monoclonal antibody techniques have been developed to detect *Chlamydial* antigens in direct smears of semen or urethral swabs without the need for culturing.

Our approach is to take a culture in patients with clinical evidence of an inflammatory or infectious process and to test it for *Mycoplasma* and *Chlamydia*. In addition, semen may be cultured for bacterial organisms; however, these frequently yield low concentrations of multiple organisms from distal urethral contamination. At present, we do not advise routine cultures in patients without evidence of disease. Urine cultures should also be obtained in those patients with evidence of cystitis or urethritis.

Testicular Biopsy

The testicular biopsy is performed primarily on azoospermic patients. In cases of symmetric testes, unilateral biopsies should be performed. However, in patients with asymmetric testes in which the physician suspects different lesions (such as primary testicular failure on one side and ductal obstruction on the other), bilateral biopsies or biopsy of the more normal testis may be performed. In cases of bilaterally atrophic testes associated with markedly elevated FSH values, testicular specimens usually demonstrate an absence of germ cells. Biopsies in these cases are usually unnecessary but at times may be performed to give the couple a definitive diagnosis and avoid unnecessary treatments. Mature spermatozoa have been extracted from testicular tissue of nonobstructed azoospermic patients. These sperm may then be used for in vitro fertilization with intracytoplasmic sperm injection. Similarly, a biopsy is not indicated in most cases of oligospermia, because the results will not alter therapy. A biopsy very occasionally is performed to rule out partial ductal obstruction in patients with severe oligospermia, normal-sized testes, and normal FSH values. Partial ductal obstruction is suggested in these cases if the biopsy specimen demonstrates normal spermatogenesis. The details of the technique of testicular biopsy are discussed in Chapter 44. The interpretation of testicular biopsies is subjective and suffers from a lack of uniformity of the systems of classification. The examination should evaluate the size and number of seminiferous tubules, the thickness of the tubule basement membrane, the relative number and types of germ cells within the seminiferous tubules, the degree of fibrosis in the interstitium, and the presence and condition of Leydig cells. Very commonly, more than one pattern is identified in a single biopsy specimen. This has contributed to inconsistencies in classification systems. The following classification scheme is commonly used and clinically practical.

Normal Testes

The majority of normal testes are made up of seminiferous tubules that are separated by a thin layer of loose interstitium containing Leydig cells, blood vessels, lymphatics, and connective tissue (Fig. 43–7). Leydig cells are acidophilic, round to polygonal cells found in groups, and may contain crystalloids of Reinke. The basement membrane of the seminiferous tubule is lined by Sertoli cells and spermatogonia. Germ cells in all stages of spermatogenesis should be seen within the seminiferous tubules. However, not all tubules necessarily contain all stages of spermatogenesis. Normal testicular biopsy specimens are usually found in azoospermic patients with ductal obstruction.

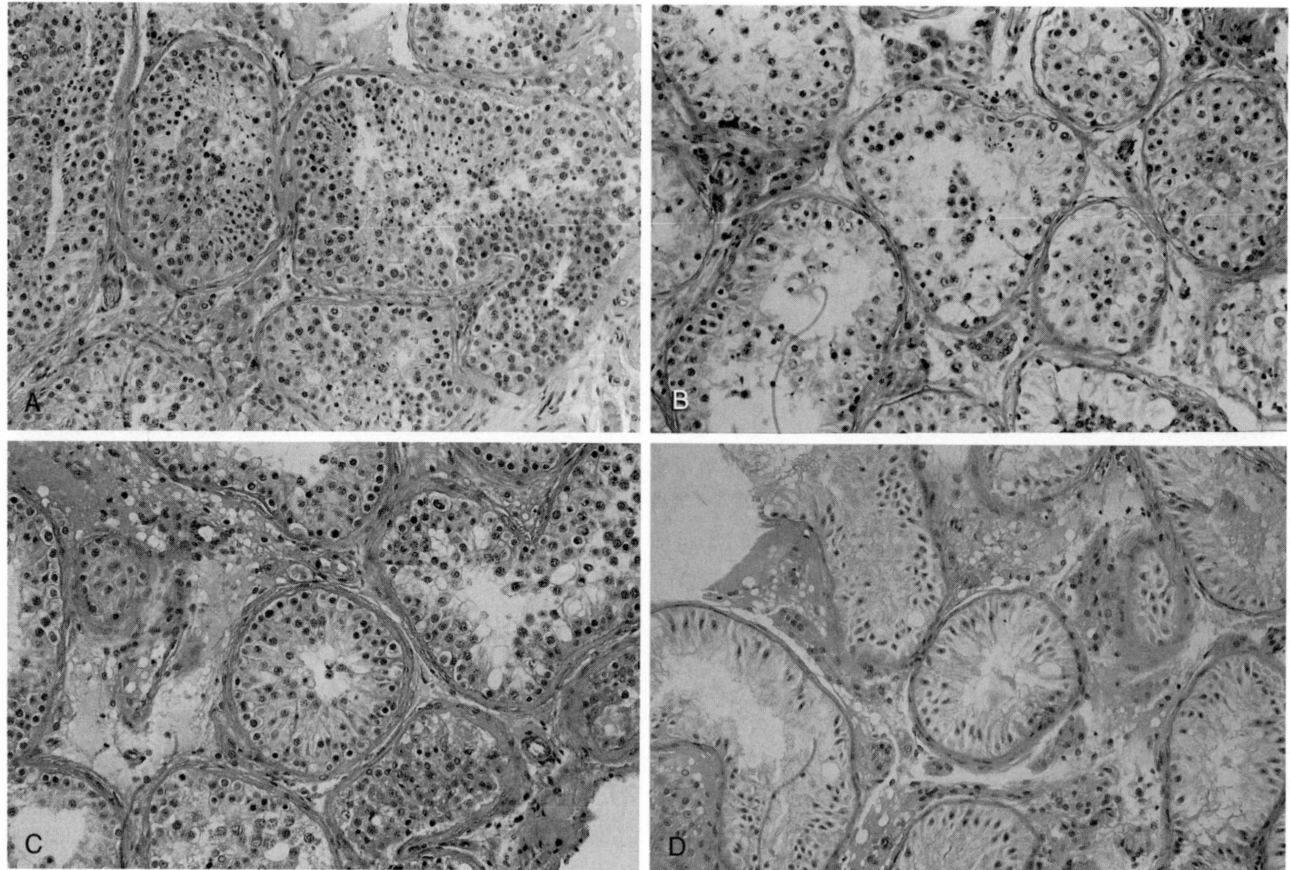

Figure 43–7. Patterns of spermatogenesis on testis biopsy. *A,* Normal; *B,* hypospermatogenesis; *C,* complete early maturation arrest; and *D,* Sertoli cell only.

Hypospermatogenesis

A reduction in the number of all germinal elements within the seminiferous tubule is present in cases of hypospermatogenesis. Thus, histologic examination reveals thinner layers of germ cells within the seminiferous tubules. The organization of the germinal epithelium may be disrupted, and immature germ cells may be found in the lumen in some instances. The interstitium and Leydig cells are normal. Clinically, these patients demonstrate oligospermia.

Maturation Arrest

Histologic examination of these testes reveals spermatogenesis proceeding normally through a specific stage, at which point no further maturation of germ cells is identified. The arrest may occur at the primary spermatocyte, secondary spermatocyte, or spermatid stage. In a given patient, the block is at a consistent stage. Some cases of late maturation arrest may be difficult to differentiate from normal spermatogenesis. A testicular touch preparation does not reveal mature sperm in cases of late maturation arrest. In other cases, the arrest appears to be partial such that the relative number of maturing germ cells after the point of arrest is decreased. Thus, mature sperm may be produced but in decreased numbers. These patients demonstrate oligospermia, and in many cases, biopsy specimens may reveal sections of partial maturation arrest as well as hypospermatogenesis.

Germinal Aplasia

This condition is also known as Sertoli cell–only syndrome. Testicular histology reveals seminiferous tubules containing Sertoli cells with a complete absence of all germ cells. The diameter of the seminiferous tubules is reduced, and the interstitium is usually minimally altered. **Patients with this condition clinically exhibit small to normal-sized testes associated with normal or elevated levels of FSH.** Although there is no therapy to induce spermatogenesis, mature sperm have been found in testicular tissue in some of these cases. These patients may be candidates for in vitro fertilization with intracytoplasmic sperm injection. This condition should be differentiated from end-stage testes, which commonly contain sclerosis, with some tubules containing only Sertoli cells.

End-Stage Testes

Tubular and peritubular sclerosis is characteristic of end-stage testes. Germ cells are absent from the sclerotic seminiferous tubules. Sertoli cells may or may not be present. Leydig cells may be absent or decreased in number within the sclerotic interstitium. Clinically, these testes are bilaterally atrophic and firm. A gradual decrease in spermatogenic activity leads to a reduction and disappearance of all germ and Sertoli cells in the testes of patients with Klinefelter's syndrome. Tubular sclerosis and hyalinization usually result. Clumping of Leydig cells may be apparent.

Other Patterns

In cases of hypogonadotropic hypogonadism, seminiferous tubules remain very small, demonstrating an absence of germ cells and Leydig cells. This is the pattern of a 7-month-old fetus. In cases of isolated LH deficiency (fertile eunuchs), normal spermatogenesis or hypospermatogenesis may be present. However, Leydig cell numbers may be reduced. Testicular atrophy, exhibited as normal-sized seminiferous tubules with a depletion of germ cells, is found in hypophysectomized adult males who were sexually mature at the time of gonadotropin depletion. Leydig cells may be depleted or absent in these specimens.

The testicular biopsy is rarely pathognomonic of a single etiology. The most common abnormalities in infertile men are hypospermatogenesis and maturation arrest. In addition, several patterns may be present in an individual biopsy specimen. Thus, in most cases, a testicular biopsy does not result in the identification of a specific etiologic factor of a patient's infertility. As mentioned above, testicular biopsies may be performed for therapy to retrieve sperm for ARTs rather than for diagnosis.

Percutaneous fine needle aspiration cytology has been used to determine the presence of spermatogenesis (Cohen et al, 1984). This technique may be performed in the office without anesthesia but requires a highly skilled cytologist. The interpretation is similar to that of a testicular touch preparation. Flow cytometry may be combined with fine needle aspiration and the ploidy patterns correlated with the state of spermatogenesis (Chan et al, 1984). Finally, some investigators have promoted quantitative methods of scoring testicular biopsies in attempts to correlate the histologic pattern with the results of the semen analysis. These techniques have been difficult to reproduce and have not gained widespread use.

Transrectal Ultrasonography

The purpose of radiologic evaluation of the genital system is to identify evidence of ductal obstruction, either complete or partial. TRUS allows for the anatomic visualization of the prostate, seminal vesicles, and distal vas deferens (Fig. 43–8). **This study is clearly indicated in azoospermic patients with acidic small seminal volumes in whom the semen does not coagulate.** Obstruction of the ejaculatory ducts is suggested by dilatation of the seminal vesicles to greater than 1.0 to 1.5 cm in anteroposterior diameter. Hypoplasia or absence of the seminal vesicles is easily diagnosed. Shinohara and associates (1985) studied a group of infertile patients with low ejaculate volumes or nonpalpable vas deferens and identified seminal vesicle abnormalities in 75% of patients. Of significance, some fructose was found in the semen of two thirds of those patients with bilateral absence of the seminal vesicles. Some investigators have interpreted ultrasound findings as demonstrating partial ejaculatory duct obstruction. Seminal findings in these cases have included normal or low-normal seminal volumes with low motility and particularly poor forward progression. This study should be performed on patients with normal hormonal profiles and normal-sized testes. Although dilated seminal vesicles greater than 1 to 1.5 cm and a dilated ejaculatory duct leading up to the verumontanum are clearly suggestive of ejaculatory duct obstruction, other findings remain controversial. It has been suggested that the finding of cystic areas seen within the seminal vesicles as well as hyperechoic lesions in the region of the ejaculatory ducts at the level of the verumontanum indicate evidence of partial ejaculatory duct obstruction. It has also been suggested that the finding of a large number of motile sperm in a seminal vesicle aspirate is consistent with a partial or complete ejaculatory duct obstruction. Although this assumption remains unproven, the procedure may be performed using a 22-gauge needle at the time of TRUS. At present, the indications for obtaining TRUS in the search for partial ejaculatory duct obstruction as well as the ultrasonic criteria to diagnose this condition remain controversial (Jarow, 1994). Ejaculatory duct obstruction should be suspected in a patient who describes pain with ejaculation; a decrease in ejaculate volume, particularly following an episode of prostatitis; or hematospermia.

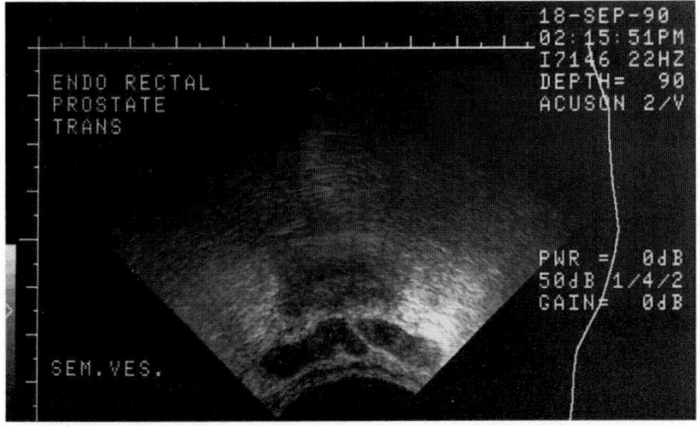

Figure 43–8. Normal transrectal ultrasonograph of seminal vesicles.

Vasography

The evaluation of the vas deferens requires vasography. This procedure is most commonly performed in the operating room and is discussed in detail in Chapter 44. In the past, retrograde vasography was performed to visualize the proximal vas deferens and epididymis; however, this approach is contraindicated, because it may result in a rupture of the epididymal tubule and subsequent epididymal obstruction. **This test is most commonly indicated in the azoospermic patient with normal-sized testes, normal FSH levels, and spermatogenesis present on testis biopsy.** In this situation, ductal obstruction is ruled out as the cause of azoospermia if a unilaterally patent vas is identified. If sterile saline injected into the vas toward the bladder flows freely, the vas is not obstructed and there is no need to inject contrast media and perform an x-ray study. At the time of vasography, the vas fluid may be inspected under 400 × microscopy to determine the presence of sperm. Presence of sperm in the vas fluid suggests an obstruction distal (toward the bladder) to the vasotomy site, whereas the absence of sperm in the vas fluid suggests a more proximal obstruction. Vasography may also be indicated in the severely oligospermic patient in whom there is reason to suspect a unilateral vasal obstruction (such as from a hernia repair) with an abnormal contralateral testis. In the oligospermic patient with no evidence of vasal obstruction by history or physical examination and symmetric testes, there is generally no indication for vasography. In an unobstructed system, the vas deferens, seminal vesicle, and ejaculatory duct should be visualized, and dye should enter the prostatic urethra and bladder. If an obstruction is identified on vasography, we recommend surgical correction at the time of the vasography.

Functional Evaluation of Spermatozoa

Sperm–Cervical Mucus Interaction Assays

For conception to occur following intercourse, sperm must travel through the cervical mucus. The PCT assesses this interaction. The examination should be performed just prior to ovulation, at which point the cervical mucus becomes clear and thin. A drop of cervical mucus is examined under a microscope (Moghissi, 1976). Although the test has been used for more than 60 years, there is no agreement as to how the test should be performed, the timing of the test, or the grading system.

A normal test result is usually defined as one in which more than 10 to 20 sperm are identified per high-power field (400 ×). Progressive motility should be present in the majority of the sperm. **The PCT should be performed in cases of hyperviscous semen, unexplained infertility, and low-volume or high-volume semen specimens with good sperm density.** Most investigators agree that in the face of normal postcoital findings, a cervical factor or semen deposition abnormality is not involved in the couple's infertility. However, abnormal PCT may result from many causes. Inappropriate timing of the PCT is the most common cause for an abnormal result. Other causes include anatomic abnormalities, semen or cervical mucus antisperm antibodies, inappropriately performed intercourse, and abnormal semen.

In an attempt to standardize the cervical mucus interaction, in vitro cervical mucus tests have been developed. In the slide test, a drop of sperm is placed adjacent to cervical mucus under a coverslip. The ability of the sperm to penetrate the mucus is then examined microscopically. This test is simple; however, it may be difficult to reproduce and is not quantifiable. To quantitate this cervical mucus sperm interaction more easily, cervical mucus may be placed in a capillary tube, which is then placed in contact with a semen specimen. The migration distance, penetration density, and quality of progressive movement can then be determined.

Finally, to localize the etiology of an abnormal PCT to either partner, cross-mucus hostility testing may be performed. In this procedure, the woman's mucus is placed in contact with donor sperm as well as with the partner's sperm. Similarly, the partner's sperm, as well as the donor's sperm, is placed in contact with the woman's mucus (Morgan et al, 1977). To completely remove the female factor from the assay, bovine cervical mucus has been used for in vitro testing. The migration of sperm into human and bovine cervical mucus appears to be similar (Gaddum-Rosse et al, 1980; Alexander, 1981; Mangione et al, 1981; Moghissi et al, 1982). Bovine cervical mucus interaction assays allow for the use of mucus with consistent quality, thereby eliminating the effect of the female factor.

The quality of the semen specimen (particularly motility parameters) correlates with the quality of the cervical mucus penetration tests. However, poor cervical mucus interaction tests have been found in some patients with normal semen parameters (Takemoto et al, 1985; Keel et al, 1987). Much confusion remains as to the precise role cervical mucus penetration tests should play in the evaluation of the infertile male. Poor reproducibility caused by the many factors affecting outcome limit the utility of the PCT despite its simplicity and physiologic basis. Although some of the drawbacks of the PCT are eliminated with in vitro cervical mucus assays, the results remain dependent on the quality of the female cervical mucus.

We believe that in most cases, the standard PCT should constitute the initial assessment of cervical mucus sperm interaction. This should be performed in couples in whom the semen analysis is of reasonably good quality. Because patients with very-poor-quality semen invariably have a poor PCT, it is not necessary to perform a PCT in this group of patients. A persistently abnormal PCT in the face of reasonably good semen parameters should lead the physician to question the quality of the cervical mucus. The quality of the mucus is rated by inspecting its ferning and spinnbarkeit. This is usually performed by the gynecologist at the time of the PCT. If mucus quality is reported to be good, then poor timing relative to the time of ovulation is not likely to be involved. If no sperm are seen in good quality cervical mucus, the couple should be questioned about their coital technique, and the physician should be sure the patient does not have severe hypospadias, which would lead to a sperm deposition problem. The finding of good-quality mucus and few or nonmotile sperm or immobilized sperm demonstrating a shaking motion should lead to the evaluation of both the male and female partner for the presence of antisperm antibodies. Following an abnormal PCT, in vitro cervical mucus interaction tests may then be performed. The particular in vitro test chosen depends on the availability of the individual test as well as the couple's specific circumstances.

Acrosome Reaction

Fertilization requires sperm to undergo capacitation and the acrosome reaction. Visualization of the human acrosome requires specific staining to differentiate acrosome-reacted sperm from nonacrosome-reacted sperm. Transmission electron microscopy clearly defines the status of the acrosome, but it is an expensive and labor-intensive procedure and is not suitable for routine clinical use. Traditional tissue-staining techniques have been developed to examine the acrosome. Trypan blue stains nonviable sperm, and rose bengal stains intact acrosomes pink (Talbot and Chacon, 1981). Other techniques, including indirect immunofluorescence and labeled lectins have been used to examine the sperm acrosome (Talbot and Chacon, 1980; Cross et al, 1986; Kallajoki et al, 1986; Lee et al, 1987; Mortimer et al, 1987). Sperm must undergo capacitation prior to the acrosome reaction. In vitro, capacitation generally takes about 3 hours. Following capacitation, sperm may be induced to undergo the acrosome reaction by exposing them to acrosome-inducing agents. Acrosome reaction studies may determine the percent of cells in the semen sample that have spontaneously undergone the acrosome reaction as well as the percent of cells that may be induced to undergo the acrosome reaction following capacitation and exposure to an inducing agent. In general, normal semen samples demonstrate a spontaneous acrosome reaction rate of less than 5% and an induced acrosome reaction rate of 15% to 40%. Samples from infertile populations have demonstrated high spontaneous rates of acrosome-reacted sperm and low inducibility of the acrosome reaction (Fenichel et al, 1991). This assay is indicated in patients with unexplained poor fertilization rates obtained in IVF. If an acrosome reaction defect is identified, in vitro treatment of sperm may improve the inducibility of the acrosome reaction, or micromanipulation may be used with IVF (Tesarik and Mendoza, 1993; Yovich et al, 1994). Acrosome reaction assays are not widely available but have begun to be offered in some clinical laboratories. Because normal penetration in an SPA requires the sperm to undergo the acrosome reaction, an SPA may be performed if an acrosome reaction assay is not available.

Sperm Penetration Assay

Cross-species fertilization is prevented by the zona pellucida. This glycoprotein layer surrounds the ovum of most species. In 1976, Yanagimachi demonstrated that following the removal of the zona pellucida, human sperm could fuse with hamster oocytes. For penetration to occur, the sperm must be capacitated in vitro. Scoring is performed by determining the percentage of ova that have been penetrated or by calculating the number of sperm that have penetrated each ovum. Thus, this assay requires (1) sperm to be able to undergo capacitation, (2) the acrosome reaction, (3) fusion with the oolemma, and (4) incorporation into the ooplasm. Samples are commonly believed to be normal if the sperm penetrate between 10% and 30% of ova. Unfortunately, the assay is a bioassay with variable results and is not standardized. Therefore, there are conflicting results and significant controversies as to its interpretation. Some investigators have found no correlation of the SPA with semen parameters, whereas others have found some correlation (Aitken et al, 1982). In most instances, motility correlated most closely with the results of the SPA. In a study of 27 patients with abnormalities of count, motility, and morphology, Aitken and co-workers (1985) found an average of 3% of ova penetrated in the male factor group compared with 44% of ova penetrated in the control group. IVF of human oocytes remains the gold standard for validation of the SPA. Again, contrasting findings have been reported when IVF is correlated with the SPA. In 15 couples in whom the male had normal semen parameters, all patients with a normal SPA fertilized human ova in vitro, whereas no patient with a negative SPA fertilized human ova in vitro (Swanson et al, 1983). Other investigators have found conflicting results. Of 42 couples in whom the semen analysis was normal, Auzmanas and associates (1985) found that 96% of those couples in whom the male had a normal SPA fertilized human ova, whereas 100% of 11 couples in whom the husband had a negative SPA fertilized human ova. When the male partner demonstrated an abnormal semen analysis, similar results were obtained. The fertilization of most hamster oocytes can be obtained by alteration of laboratory conditions, according to Smith and associates (1987), who believed that the number of penetrations per egg represented a more sensitive indicator of the fertilizing capacity of sperm. With this technique, couples with a normal SPA demonstrated a 95% chance of fertilizing human ova in vitro in contrast to a 50% chance in those couples with an abnormal SPA. These inconsistencies make it clear that for proper interpretation of the SPA, the physician must be familiar with the laboratory that is performing this assay and should be aware of what correlations have been documented between the results of the assay and actual human fertilization. The correlation between the results of the SPA and natural in vivo pregnancy also has been examined. No relation between pregnancy and the results of the SPA was found in a study by Aitken and colleagues (1985) of 27 oligospermic patients followed for a mean of 4.2 years.

Another study (Corson et al, 1988) correlated the results of the SPA with conception in 227 infertile couples followed for a mean of 17.9 months. Those couples with an SPA of greater than 11% of ova penetrated demonstrated pregnancy rates twice as high as those couples with an SPA of less than 11%. Similar results have been found by other investigators (Kretzer et al, 1988).

There remains little agreement on the utility and interpretation of the SPA. Despite these controversies, we believe the SPA should be obtained in couples with unexplained infertility. In addition, it is helpful in couples who are proceeding with ARTs. We encourage couples with an abnormal SPA to consider IVF in lieu of IUI to document whether or not a fertilization defect exists.

Hemizona Assay

In the Hemizona Assay, the human zona pellucida is microscopically divided in half. Each half is then incubated with either patient sperm or sperm from a fertile donor. A Hemizona Index is then calculated by counting the number of sperm bound to each zona half and dividing the number of sperm bound from the patient by the number of sperm bound from the donor. Most male patients who do not fertilize human ova in vitro demonstrate a Hemizona Index of less than 0.60 (Burkman et al, 1988). Because this assay requires a source of human ova and significant micromanipulation skills, it has not gained widespread use. This test is indicated in cases in which IVF has not resulted in fertilization in the presence of a normal SPA. The SPA is performed on zona-free ova, therefore sperm that have a defect limited to zona binding but retain the capacity to fuse with the oolemma will demonstrate a normal SPA but an abnormal Hemizona Index. This is not a common finding because the majority of cases with abnormal fertilization also have broad defects in sperm function that would be detected by both assays (Oehlinger et al, 1991). Patients demonstrating defects in the Hemizona Assay are appropriately treated with micromanipulation combined with IVF.

TREATMENT OVERVIEW

Based on the results of the history, physical examination, and laboratory studies, the physician should place the patient into an etiologic category. The clinician is then faced with two treatment options. The male patient may be treated in an attempt to improve spermatogenesis and subsequent fertility potential through intercourse. The alternate management approach is to bypass the problem of the male by using either his spermatozoa with ARTs or proceeding with donor insemination or adoption. **We believe that as a general rule, it is preferable to treat the male to improve spermatogenesis rather than ignore the male factor and use high-cost, high-technology ARTs.** On the other hand, often it is not possible to improve spermatogenesis, or attempted treatment may fail. In these instances, it is very appropriate to proceed with ART. These two management approaches are not mutually exclusive, and in some couples, attempts may be made to treat the male at the same time the couple proceeds with ARTs. This more aggressive approach may be used in the older couple in which the female's reproductive potential is diminishing because of age. Finally, both donor insemination and adoption need to be suggested as alternatives in appropriate cases.

DIAGNOSTIC CATEGORIES

The results of the history, physical examination, and laboratory testing allow the clinician to place the patient into a diagnostic classification. These categories may imply a cause for the patient's subfertility, although no cause can be determined for the infertility for a large percent of patients, which places them in the category of idiopathic infertility.

Endocrine, or Pretesticular, Causes

Endocrine causes of male infertility are often referred to as *pretesticular.* Impairment of fertility in these cases is secondary to a hormone imbalance.

Pituitary Disease

Pituitary function may be affected in cases of pituitary surgery, infarction, tumors, radiation, or infectious diseases. Patients with prepubertal onset of pituitary disease are usually diagnosed prior to a fertility evaluation as a result of growth retardation or adrenal or thyroid deficiency. Infertility, impotence, visual field abnormalities, and severe headaches may be presenting symptoms in the adult male with pituitary dysfunction. Normal male secondary sexual characteristics are usually present unless adrenal insufficiency exists. Small, soft testes may be demonstrated on physical examination. This is in contrast to cases of primary testicular failure with tubular and peritubular sclerosis, in which case the testes are small and firm to palpation. Plasma testosterone levels are low, and gonadotropin levels are low or normal. Thus, a normal LH value associated with a low serum testosterone value is abnormal and further evaluation is required. Evaluation of other pituitary hormones and endocrine functions should be performed in appropriate cases.

Isolated Hypogonadotropic Hypogonadism

Gonadotropin deficiency may occur in the presence of otherwise normal pituitary function. **This condition may be due to *Kallmann's syndrome* (hypogonadotropic hypogonadism associated with anosmia), which occurs in sporadic and familial forms (Biben and Gordon, 1955) or idiopathic hypogonadotropic hypogonadism.** In Kallmann's syndrome, a failure of GnRH secretion by the hypothalamus appears to be responsible for the gonadotropin deficiency leading to secondary testicular failure (Hoffman and Crowley, 1982). Anosmia may be complete or partial. Autosomal dominant inheritance from male to male with variable penetrance is the most common pattern. However, X-linked transmission and autosomal recessive inheritance have been suggested (Ewer, 1968). Del Castillo (1992) reported that the gene for X-linked Kallman's syndrome maps to Xp 22.3 and has a homologous locus, Kalp, on Yq11. Genetic studies suggest that idiopathic hypogonadism is not due to an abnormality of the GnRH gene (Weiss 1991) but may involve the genes responsible for development and migration of GnRH neurons (Dacou-Voutetakis, 1992).

Several other congenital anomalies such as craniofacial asymmetry, cleft palate, harelip, color blindness, congenital deafness, cryptorchidism, and renal anomalies may be associated with this syndrome (Danish et al, 1980). A delay in pubertal development is the hallmark of the syndrome and most commonly causes the patient to present for medical evaluation. The diagnosis may occasionally be made in childhood because of the presence of cryptorchidism or micropenis. As a result of a delay in the androgen-dependent closure of the epiphyseal plates, the length of the arms and legs may be greater than that of the trunk. In addition, the testes are prepubertal in appearance, usually being smaller than 2 cm in diameter. In the prepubertal male, differentiating between Kallmann's syndrome and delayed sexual maturation may be very difficult. The diagnostic evaluation has been reviewed by Whitcomb and Crowley (1993). A family history of Kallmann's syndrome or the presence of somatic midline defects or anosmia may help in the prepubertal diagnosis.

The first sign of puberty is testicular growth. Thus, if the testes are enlarged, the patient is experiencing delayed puberty rather than hypogonadotropic hypogonadism. Normal males experiencing early puberty demonstrate LH pulses if frequent blood samples are obtained. These pulses are not present in patients with Kallmann's syndrome (Boyar et al, 1972). GnRH stimulation testing results in an absent or blunted rise in gonadotropins. However, repeated GnRH injections prime the pituitary, resulting in rises of both gonadotropins. This pattern of response is also found in prepubertal boys (Snyder et al, 1979). Finally, following doses of 5000 IU of human chorionic gonadotropin (hCG), prepubertal and pubertal boys demonstrate larger rises in testosterone levels than do patients with Kallmann's syndrome. **Androgen replacement with testosterone or hCG is adequate treatment for the teenager and results in virilization. However, it must be remembered that treatment with exogenous androgens results in suppression of intratesticular testosterone production. Thus, spermatogenesis and testicular growth are not stimulated in these patients.** Prior treatment with androgens does not impair subsequent testicular response to gonadotropin therapy (Martin, 1967). Androgen therapy should be given in parenteral form as testosterone enanthate or cypionate. Intramuscular injections of 200 mg every other week are usually sufficient to induce full virilization in most patients. Although oral androgens are available as fluoxymesterone and 17-methyltestosterone, they are less potent and may result in a higher incidence of hepatic abnormalities. Reversible intrahepatic cholestasis resulting in elevations of plasma transaminase, lactate dehydrogenase, and bilirubin may be noted. Transdermal testosterone skin patch treatment has not been extensively evaluated in this group of patients.

Gonadotropin therapy is required for the initiation of spermatogenesis. Given as 2000 IU IM three times per week, hCG initiates spermatogenesis in most patients. **However, the completion of spermiogenesis occurs in only 20% of patients with hCG therapy alone. The addition of FSH is required in most patients and is commonly given after 6 months of hCG therapy.** FSH is usually given in the form of human menopausal gonadotropin (hMg [Pergonal]), which contains 75 IU of FSH and 75 IU of LH per vial. The intramuscular administration of one-half vial three times per week usually results in the completion of spermatogenesis (Finkel et al, 1985). Stimulation of the testes with FSH and LH results in testicular growth, although the final testis volume may remain below normal. Whereas the semen motility parameters are usually good, oligospermia with counts below 10 million sperm per milliliter are common (Paulsen et al, 1970). However, in contrast to patients with idiopathic oligospermia who are often infertile with these sperm densities, many patients with hypogonadotropic hypogonadism are able to conceive despite these low sperm densities.

GnRH supplied via intermittent subcutaneous injections or via an infusion pump with 90-minute pulses may be used in these patients. In one study, Shargil (1987) compared twice-daily injections of GnRH with treatment given by means of a pulsatile infusion pump. Pulsatile infusion resulted in superior endocrine responses as well as improved spermatogenesis and fertility compared with subcutaneous injections. Eight of 18 patients treated with subcutaneous injections achieved pregnancy in contrast to 10 of 12 patients treated with the pulsatile infusion pump. Kliesch and associates (1994) have also reported such results with this method. The authors usually use hCG followed by hMG as the initial treatment and reserve infusion pump therapy for those patients who respond poorly.

Fertile Eunuch Syndrome

Isolated LH deficiency occurs rarely in patients with normal FSH levels. Men with this condition demonstrate a variably eunuchoid habitus, large testes, and small-volume ejaculates that may contain a few spermatozoa (Faiman et al, 1968). Plasma testosterone and LH levels are low, but FSH levels are in the normal range. Testicular biopsy specimens demonstrate maturation of the germinal epithelium. However, Leydig cells may not be apparent because of insufficient LH stimulation. A rise in serum testosterone following hCG therapy documents normal Leydig cell function in these patients. Sufficient intratesticular testosterone is produced to support some spermatogenesis. However, inadequate peripheral androgen levels result in a lack of virilization.

Isolated Follicle-Stimulating Hormone Deficiency

Patients with this rare disorder demonstrate normal virilization, normal LH and testosterone levels, and normal-sized testes. Owing to a lack of FSH, oligospermia or azoospermia is present. Administration of hMG improves spermatogenesis (Al-Ansari et al, 1984). More specific treatment may be given in the form of pure FSH (Metrodin).

Other Congenital Syndromes

The Prader-Willi syndrome consists of obesity, hypotonic musculature, mental retardation, small hands and feet, short stature, and hypogonadism. There is a familial tendency. The locus for Prader-Willi syndrome has been mapped to chromosome 15q11–q13. The cause of the syndrome is a deletion or uniparental disomy. The DNA probe PW71 can be used to make the diagnosis (Lerer et al, 1994). Patients demonstrate LH and FSH deficiencies because of a lack of GnRH. Treatment is identical to that for Kallmann's syndrome. As a result of the multiple anomalies in these patients, however, infertility is often not a clinical problem (Bray et al, 1983). A similar picture is found in Laurence-Moon-Bardet-Biedl syndrome, which consists of hypogonadotropic hypogonadism, retinitis pigmentosa, polydactyly, and hypomnesia.

Androgen Excess

Gonadotropin production is inhibited by negative feedback from estrogens and androgens at the hypothalamus and pituitary. A hypogonadal state, therefore, may be induced by androgen excess whether it is due to exogenous sources, such as anabolic steroids used by athletes, or to endogenous production, such as a metabolic abnormality or an androgen-producing tumor. The seminiferous tubules are exposed to very high levels of testosterone when synthesis takes place in the Leydig cells because it diffuses into the tubules. Thus, exogenous androgens will cause a decrease in LH production. This, in turn, results in decreased stimulation of Leydig cells and decreased intratesticular androgen production. Nontesticular androgens do not result in the same high androgen concentrations in the seminiferous tubules creating a relative hypogonadal state. In addition, the peripheral androgens suppress FSH production, which may impair spermatogenesis. CAH is the most common cause of endogenous androgen excess. A congenital deficiency of 21-hydroxylase is the most common of the five enzyme defects responsible for this syndrome. Defects in the encoding gene have been documented to cause the endocrine disease in the case of all but one of the steroidogenic enzyme deficiencies (including 21-hydroxylase). The diagnosis can be made in the first trimester of pregnancy by DNA analysis of biopsies of the chorionic villi (New, 1994). A deficiency of 21-hydroxylase results in a decrease in cortisone synthesis, which leads to increased pituitary production of adrenocorticotropic hormone. Elevated levels of adrenocorticotropic hormone result in hyperstimulation of the adrenal gland and in increased production of adrenal androgens. Excess androgens feed back to the pituitary, inhibiting the production of gonadotropins and leading to a hypogonadal state. Short stature and precocious puberty develop in these patients. As a result of androgen stimulation, premature enlargement of the penis may occur; however, because of a lack of gonadotropin stimulation, the testes remain underdeveloped. Basal plasma 17-hydroxyprogesterone levels are often elevated 50 to 200 times above normal levels. In addition, elevated urinary 17-ketosteroid and pregnanetriol levels may occur. Not all patients with this syndrome demonstrate fertility abnormalities. Urban and co-workers (1978) studied 20 patients with CAH. Almost all patients demonstrated normal serum gonadotropin and testosterone levels. Two patients were untreated, and three had been poorly treated; however, four of these patients had children. Of the 15 treated patients, eight had conceived. In some patients, the adrenal androgen levels appear to be sufficient to stimulate complete maturation of germ cells. Glucocorticoid therapy results in a reduction of adrenocorticotropic hormone levels, which induces a decrease in peripheral testosterone, thus stimulating endogenous gonadotropin secretion. This approach can be used to render men with infertility secondary to CAH fertile (Augarten et al, 1991). Bilateral testicular adrenal rest tumors may develop in occasional patients. These tumors may resolve with hormonal therapy (Cutfield et al, 1983). Patients with 21-hydroxylase deficiency, complicated by adrenal rest tumors, may present with infertility that may be permanent because of fibrosis, whereas patients without these tumors may be fertile. Partial 21-hydroxylase deficiency may be present in some patients. These cases may remain cryptic because mild androgen elevations may not be evident in men. Occasional case reports have found cryptic 21-hydroxylase deficiency in infertile men.

Excess androgen production may also be due to adrenal or testicular tumors. This results in the failure of testicular development in prepubertal patients. Tubular and peritubular sclerosis may occur in the postpubertal patient secondary to a state of hypogonadotropism caused by excess androgens. This condition may be irreversible.

Estrogen Excess

Pituitary gonadotropin secretion is suppressed by peripheral estrogens. A state of secondary testicular failure may be induced by estrogen-secreting tumors in the adrenal cortex or in the testis. Testicular Sertoli cell tumors or interstitial cell tumors may produce estrogen. Excess peripheral estrogens may also result from hepatic dysfunction. Peripheral adipose tissue converts androgen into estrogen. Elevated estrogen levels have been identified in morbidly obese patients; however, not all investigators have confirmed this finding (Schneider et al, 1979; Hargreave et al, 1988). Impotence, gynecomastia, and testicular atrophy may be present in the face of estrogen excess. Hormonal studies demonstrate low levels of FSH, LH, and testosterone in the presence of elevated estrogens. Urinary 17-ketosteroid levels may also be elevated. Treatment is directed at the underlying condition.

Prolactin Excess

Both impotence and infertility have been associated with hyperprolactinemia. Routine screening of infertile men for hyperprolactinemia is not useful (Eggert-Kruse, 1991). In patients with pituitary adenomas, gonadotropin as well as testosterone levels are depressed, whereas prolactin levels are markedly elevated. However, some patients with hyperprolactinemia demonstrate mild elevations, and investigation reveals small microadenomas or no evidence of pituitary tumors. Levels of serum gonadotropins and testosterone may be normal. Although most women present with microadenomas, most men presenting with prolactinomas have macroadenomas ($\geq$1.0 cm). A persistent elevation of prolactin should be investigated with a CT scan or a MRI study of the head. Bromocriptine, surgery, and radiotherapy have been used for the treatment of macroadenomas. Bromocriptine therapy alone is often used for the treatment of microadenomas. New, long-acting oral and intramuscular preparations of bromocriptine are effective in treating microadenomas and macroadenomas, and are useful to increase patient compliance (Zgliczynski 1992; Haase et al 1993). Cases of idiopathic hyperprolactinemia are treated with bromocriptine, which may be withdrawn yearly to determine whether hyperprolactinemia persists (Dollar and Blackwell, 1986; Wang et al, 1987).

Thyroid Abnormalities

Although hyperthyroidism has been associated with infertility, patients present with symptoms of thyroid dysfunction and do not present primarily with infertility (Clyde et al, 1976; Kidd et al, 1979). Testicular and pituitary abnormalities as well as elevated levels of circulatory estradiol have been identified in patients with hyperthyroidism. In addition, maturation arrest patterns have been identified on testicular biopsy specimens.

Glucocorticoid Excess

Glucocorticoid excess may suppress LH secretion, resulting in androgen deficiency and testicular dysfunction. Glucocorticoid excess may be secondary to endogenous production as in Cushing's syndrome or secondary to exogenous intake from medical therapy. Hypospermatogenesis or maturation arrest patterns are found on testicular biopsy specimens (Gabrilove et al, 1974). Therapy is directed at correction of the underlying glucocorticoid abnormality.

Testicular Causes

Genetic Abnormalities

Approximately 6% of infertile men are found to have chromosomal abnormalities, with the incidence increasing as the sperm count decreases. The highest incidence is found in azoospermic patients, with 10% to 15% of patients demonstrating abnormalities of the karyotype (Bourrouillou et al, 1992). The incidence falls to 4% to 5% in oligospermic patients and 1% in normospermic patients (Mastuda et al, 1992). Karyotype analysis of white blood cells detects only gross alterations in the genetic material. Recent techniques, such as the polymerase chain reaction and fluorescent in situ hybridization allow for the detection of mutations that do not alter the karyotypic appearance of chromosomes. Using these techniques, more subtle genetic mutations have been identified in infertile patients considered to have otherwise normal karyotypes. The majority of fertility related karyotypic abnormalities are associated with Klinefelter's syndrome or XYY syndrome. Some authors recommend routine karyotypes in this patient population. Others argue that this procedure is unnecessary because the condition is not treatable and may result in the development of significant psychologic stress to the patient and the couple. With the recent ability to perform intracytoplasmic sperm injection and the possible use of round spermatid nuclear injection combined with IVF in patients with severe oligospermia or maturation arrest, there may be new emphasis on genetic screening of couples prior to these procedures.

KLINEFELTER'S SYNDROME

The presence of an extra X chromosome is the genetic hallmark of Klinefelter's syndrome. This is due to nondysjunction of the meiotic chromosomes of the gametes from either parent. **This results in a hypogonadal man demonstrating the classic triad of small, firm testes; gynecomastia; and elevated urinary gonadotropins** (Klinefelter et al, 1942). This syndrome is identified in one of every 600 male births (MacLean et al, 1964; Paulsen et al, 1968). Although secondary sexual characteristics begin developing at the appropriate time, the completion of puberty is usually delayed, at which point eunuchoidism, gynecomastia, or impotence may be noted. Virilization may be complete in some patients and the diagnosis delayed until adulthood, at which point the patient may present with infertility with associated gynecomastia and small, firm testes. Mental retardation and various psychiatric disturbances have been identified in some of these patients (Becker et al, 1966; Theilgaard et al, 1984). Azoospermia is typically present. Seminiferous tubular sclerosis is commonly identified on testicular biopsy. However, occasional Sertoli cells or spermatozoa may be found. Plasma FSH levels are usually markedly elevated as a result of the severe seminiferous tubular injury, whereas LH levels are elevated or normal. Total plasma testosterone levels are decreased in 60% of patients and normal in 40% (Paulson et al, 1968). The physiologically active free testosterone concentrations are usually decreased. In addition, plasma estradiol levels are usually increased, stimulating increased levels of testosterone-binding globulin and resulting in a decreased testosterone-to-estrogen ratio, which is believed to be responsible for gynecomastia (Chopra et al, 1973; Wang et al, 1975). The diagnosis may be made with a chromatin-positive buccal smear, indicating the presence of an extra X chromosome. Karyotypes usually demonstrate 47,XXY or, less commonly, a mosaic pattern of 46,XY/47XXY. Less severe abnormalities are present in patients with the mosaic form of Klinefelter's syndrome, and occasional patients are fertile (Foss and Lewis, 1971).

There is no therapy to improve spermatogenesis in Klinefelter's syndrome. For the patient with mosaic Klinefelter's syndrome and severe oligospermia, intracytoplasmic injection combined with IVF is a technical possibility. Recently, intracytoplasmic sperm injection (ICSI) has been used in this situation with fertilization and embryo transfer; however, no pregnancy was obtained (Harari et al, 1995). Although the authors argued that ICSI should be a safe procedure in mosaic cases because only the normal 46XY cell line (not the 47XXY cell line) would proceed through spermatogenesis, this has not been proved. Of concern, recent studies examining the chromosomal complement of sperm cells from patients with mosaic Klinefelter's syndrome have revealed an increased incidence of abnormal chromosomal complements in sperm from these patients. This finding indicates that 47XXY cells are able to undergo meiosis and form spermatozoa (Cozzi et al, 1994).

XYY SYNDROME

This karyotype has been linked to aggressive and criminal behavior (Jacobs et al, 1965; Walzer and Gerald, 1976; Freyne and O'Connor, 1992). Not all investigators agree that this behavior is secondary to the karyotype but believe that it may be secondary to tall stature, which may predispose individuals to this behavior (Hook, 1973). This karyotype occurs in 0.1% to 0.4% of newborn infants (Balodimos et al, 1966; Price et al, 1966; Walzer and Gerald, 1976). Patients are characteristically tall, and semen analyses typically reveal severe oligospermia or azoospermia. Recent fluorescent in situ hybridization studies of spermatozoa from a 47XYY male revealed an increased incidence of diploid and tetraploid cells in the raw semen sample. However, when only motile sperm were examined, no increased incidence of abnormal genotypes were identified, suggesting that the functional sperm do not carry the extra Y chromosome (Han et al, 1994). Testicular biopsy specimens reveal patterns ranging from maturation arrest to complete germinal aplasia, as well as occasional cases demonstrating seminiferous tubular sclerosis (Santen et al, 1970; Skakkebaek et al, 1973; Baghdassarian et al, 1975). In addition, occasional patients have been fertile (Stenchever and MacIntyre, 1969). Plasma gonadotropins and testosterone levels are most often within the normal range in these patients (Lundberg and Helstrom, 1970). However, elevations of plasma FSH levels may be found in association with more severe patterns of testicular dysfunction. The testicular abnormalities in this syndrome are not amenable to current treatment modalities.

XX MALE

Findings similar to those of Klinefelter's syndrome are found in patients with the XX male syndrome (sex reversal syndrome). These patients demonstrate small, firm testes; frequent gynecomastia; small to normal-sized penises; and azoospermia. Testicular biopsy may demonstrate seminiferous tubule sclerosis, resulting in elevated gonadotropins and decreased testosterone levels (Perez-Palacios et al, 1981). Unlike typical patients with Klinefelter's syndrome, these individuals have shorter than normal average heights, show no higher incidence of mental deficiency, and have an increased incidence of hypospadias (de la Chapelle, 1981). Although karyotypes demonstrate 46XX chromosomal complements, molecular biologic mapping has suggested that portions of the Y chromosomes are present (Page et al, 1987; Burgoyne, 1989). Studies of males with XX sex reversal have revealed various genetic scenarios. Translocation of portions of the Y chromosome onto the X chromosome have been identified. It is hypothesized that in these patients, the portion of the Y chromosome containing the testes determining factor (SRY gene) has been translocated, whereas the azoospermia factor gene is not present in these patients, resulting in azoospermia. Mutation of an autosomal or X chromosome gene, which results in testis determination, has also been proposed to occur in patients without evidence of Y chromosomal material (Fechner et al, 1993; Boucekkine et al, 1994).

ANDROGEN ABNORMALITIES

Androgens act by binding to cytoplasmic receptors that travel to the cell nucleus and interact with the nuclear matrix, stimulating messenger RNA synthesis. Androgen abnormalities may involve a deficiency in androgen synthesis, a deficiency in conversion of testosterone to dihydrotestosterone (5α-reductase deficiency) or androgen receptor abnormalities. Both defects in androgen synthesis and 5α-reductase deficiency commonly result in ambiguous genitalia and are therefore discussed in Chapter 70. Defects in androgen receptors result in androgen-resistant syndromes. Karyotypically, these patients are 46,XY males, with phenotypes ranging from pseudohermaphroditism to a normal male phenotype with infertility. Aimann and colleagues (1979) reported that in a group of phenotypically normal men with azoospermia and severe oligospermia, fibroblasts cultured from genital skin demonstrated androgen-resistant deficiencies. These patients had elevated serum levels of LH and testosterone. These authors calculated an androgen insensitivity index (serum testosterone x serum LH) to identify those men. It was found that 11.6% of patients with azoospermia or severe oligospermia showed abnormally high androgen insensitivity indices, indicating the presence of an androgen receptor defect (Schulster et al, 1983.) Other investigators have found that few patients were identified with the use of this index (Griffin and Wilson, 1980). Recent molecular studies of the androgen receptor gene have not found a high incidence of mutations in infertile men (Puscheck et al, 1994). Because the androgen receptor gene is located on the X chromosome, this syndrome is inherited as an X-linked recessive trait. The phenotypic abnormalities are the result of abnormal receptor function or decreased receptor number.

NOONAN'S SYNDROME

The phenotypic appearance of patients with this syndrome is similar to that found in Turner's syndrome (X0). Thus, these patients have short stature and demonstrate hypertelorism, webbed neck, low-set ears, cubitus valgus, ptosis, and cardiovascular abnormalities (Collins and Turner, 1973). Chromosomal analysis reveals a 46XY karyotype. Cryptorchidism and testicular atrophy are commonly present with associated elevations of gonadotropins. Although androgens may be given to complete virilization, there is no treatment for the fertility abnormality in these patients.

OTHER CHROMOSOMAL ABNORMALITIES

Chromosomal abnormalities have been found in infertile patients without Klinefelter's or the XYY syndrome. Various patterns of translocations involving the somatic chromosomes have been associated with some cases of oligospermia (Plymate et al, 1976; Sarto and Therman, 1976). In addition, testicular biopsy specimens of oligospermic men have demonstrated meiotic abnormalities of the germ cells but with normal peripheral karyotypes (Hulten et al, 1970; Pearson et al, 1970; Skakkebaek et al, 1973; Koulischez and Schoysman, 1974). Biopsy specimens of subjects with Down syndrome have demonstrated patterns ranging from maturation arrest to complete germinal aplasia (Shroder et al, 1971). Elevations of both FSH and LH levels have also been found in these patients (Campbell et al, 1982).

Karyotypic abnormalities have been identified in the male partners of women who have undergone recurrent abortions. Both meiotic and mitotic abnormalities have been found in peripheral blood cells as well as in testicular tissue (Blumberg et al, 1982; Fortuny et al, 1988).

Several syndromes with a genetic component are associated with male infertility. Prune-belly syndrome is associated with absence of the abdominal wall musculature, cryptorchidism, and urogenital tract abnormalities. An autosomal dominant inheritance pattern is suggested (Riccardi and Grum, 1977). The Prader-Willi and Laurence-Moon-Biedl syndromes have genetic basis and are discussed earlier (see the section on endocrine causes).

Other Causes of Testicular Impairment

BILATERAL ANORCHIA

Also known as vanishing testes syndrome, bilateral anorchia is found in genetic XY males with nonpalpable testes. Patients demonstrate prepubertal male phenotypes, indicating that testicular tissue, secreting androgens, must have been present in utero. It is thought that the testes may have been lost in utero secondary to infection, vascular injury, or testicular torsion. Molecular analysis of DNA from these patients have shown no abnormalities in the testis determining regions (SRY gene) (Lobaccaro et al, 1993). Low plasma testosterone and elevated gonadotropin levels are present in these males (Aynsley-Green et al, 1976). Virilization may be induced with testosterone administration; however, the infertility associated with the condition is not treatable.

CRYPTORCHIDISM

Cryptorchidism is present in about 3% to 4% of full-term boys (Scorer and Farrington, 1971; John Radcliffe Hospital, 1992). By 1 year of age, 1% to 1.6% (Scorer and Farrington, 1971; John Radcliffe Hospital, 1992) of boys demonstrate undescended testes. After 6 months of age, the undescended testis is unlikely to descend on its own. Two thirds of cases are unilateral, whereas one third of cases are bilateral. **Sperm concentrations below 12 to 20 million per milliliter are found in 50% of patients with bilateral cryptorchidism and in 25% to 30% of patients with unilateral cryptorchidism** (Lipshultz, 1976; Lipshultz et al, 1976; Okuyama et al, 1989). Testicular biopsy of the cryptorchid testis reveals decreased numbers of Leydig cells. Within the first 6 months of life, the number of germ cells in the cryptorchid testis is within the normal range; however, the normal increase in germ cell numbers does not occur. By 2 years of age, 38% of unilateral and bilaterally cryptorchid testes have lost germ cells. The descended testis, in cases of unilateral cryptorchidism, also may demonstrate abnormalities with lower numbers of germ cells. **In general, the higher the cryptorchid testis, the more severe the testicular dysfunction. Absence of germ cells is found in 20% to 40% of inguinal or prescrotal testes in contrast to 90% of intra-abdominal testes** (Hadziselimovic, 1983). Both mechanical and hormonal etiologic factors have been suggested to explain the mechanism of cryptorchidism. Increasing evidence points to a defect in the hypothalamic-pituitary-gonadal axis in these patients (Canlorbe et al, 1974). It is important to differentiate the *cryptorchid testis* from the *retractile testis*, which is caused by a hyperactive cremasteric reflex, and from an ectopic testis. The latter two cases are not associated with testicular dysfunction. The finding of histologic changes in cryptorchid testis within the first year of life has led to therapy directed at correction of cryptorchidism by 1 to 2 years of age. Retrospective studies report fertility rates from 78% to 92% in patients with surgically corrected unilateral cryptorchidism (Kumar et al, 1987; Cendron et al, 1989; Puri and O'Donnell, 1990).

VARICOCELE

A varicocele is an abnormal tortuosity and dilation of the testicular veins within the spermatic cord. **Varicoceles are found in approximately 30% of infertile males (Dubin and Amelar, 1971; Cockett et al, 1979; Aafjes and vander Vijver, 1985; Marks et al, 1986).** The varicocele is the most common surgically correctable cause of male infertility.

Varicoceles do not occur with equal frequency on the left and right sides, because approximately 90% are left sided, although some clinicians report a high incidence of bilateral varicoceles. Differences in the venous drainage patterns of the right and left testicular veins may account for this left-sided predominance. The left testicular vein drains into the left renal vein, whereas the right testicular vein drains into the inferior vena cava. In addition, there is a higher incidence of absent venous valves in the left side than in the right (Ahlberg et al, 1966). Lastly, the left renal vein may be compressed between the superior mesenteric artery and the aorta. This "nutcracker phenomenon" may result in increased pressure in the left testicular venous system (Coolsaet, 1980). The finding of unilateral right-sided varicoceles is uncommon and raises the possibility of thrombosis or occlusion of the vena cava or situs inversus (Grillo-Lopez, 1971). Various mechanisms have been suggested to account for the testicular dysfunction associated with varicoceles (Howards, 1995). Intrascrotal temperatures have been demonstrated to be 0.6°C higher in oligospermic varicocele patients compared with patients without varicoceles (Zorgniotti and MacLeod, 1973). Intratesticular temperatures have also been found to be increased by 0.78°C in the testis of patients with a varicocele; in contrast, a decrease of 0.5°C is seen in the testis in patients without varicoceles when they rise from a supine to a standing position (Yamaguchi et al, 1989). Other studies have found that elevated intratesticular temperatures are common in oligospermic patients regardless of the cause of the spermatogenic defect (Mieusset et al, 1989). Not all investigators have found an association between higher intratesticular temperatures and varicoceles (Tessler and Krahan, 1966; Stephenson and O'Shaughnessy, 1968).

Reflux of renal and adrenal metabolites from the renal vein (Comhaire and Vermeulen, 1974), decreased blood flow (Saypol et al, 1981), and hypoxia (Chakraborty et al, 1985) have also been postulated to account for the varicocele effect. Infertility in varicocele patients may be multifactorial. There is evidence that smoking in the presence of a varicocele has a greater adverse effect than either factor alone (Klaiber et al, 1987; Peng et al, 1990). Experimental animal models have demonstrated that following production of unilateral varicocele, bilateral increases in testicular blood flow and temperature occur. Thus, it may be that an increase in blood flow leads to a secondary increase in testicular temperature, resulting in an impairment of spermatogenesis (Saypol et al, 1981). Subsequent repair of these experimental varicoceles has resulted in a normalization of blood flow and temperature (Green et al, 1984). These data may explain the bilateral effect of unilateral varicoceles. An elegant description of the seminal abnormalities of patients with varicoceles was presented by MacLeod (1965). **Decreased motility was the most common finding, being present in 90% of patients. Sperm concentrations of fewer than 20 million sperm per milliliter were demonstrated in 65% of patients. In addition, morphologic abnormalities were common. MacLeod (1965) described the so-called stress pattern of sperm morphology. This pattern consists of increased numbers of amorphous cells and immature germ cells, as well as more than 15% tapered forms.** Similar patterns were found associated with viral illnesses and the ingestion of antispermatogenic compounds. Rodriguez-Rigau and colleagues (1981) found no difference in the incidence of the stress patterns between infertile patients with and without varicoceles. Other investigators have confirmed these findings (Portuondo et al, 1981; Ayodeiji and Baker, 1986). However, these questions have been reopened by Naftulin and colleagues (1991), who found more tapered forms in varicocele patients than they did in controls. On the other hand, even these authors did not believe that the presence of significant numbers of tapered forms was adequate to make a diagnosis of varicocele.

As mentioned previously, the authors believe that the diagnosis of varicoceles rests on a thorough physical examination and that there is insufficient evidence to warrant investigations for subclinical varicoceles.

Varicoceles become clinically manifest at the time of puberty. Increasing incidences are reported at different stages of pubertal development, with an incidence of 15% by age 13 (Oster, 1971; Steeno et al, 1976; Berger, 1980). Many investigators have reported that varicoceles retard the growth of the testis and inhibit spermatogenesis in adolescent boys and young men (Steeno et al, 1976; Sayfan et al, 1988; Laven et al, 1992). The effect of varicocele repair on the adolescent was studied by Cass and Belman (1987). These investigators treated 20 adolescents with grade II or III varicoceles and ipsilateral loss of testicular volume. A significant increase in testicular volume was demonstrated in 16 of these patients following varicocele repair. Subsequently, a favorable effect on testis growth and semen quality of repair of a varicocele in adolescent boys has been confirmed by several investigators (Okuyama et al, 1988; Hoesli, 1990). **It is recommended that varicocele repair be performed in adolescents with grade II or III varicoceles associated with ipsilateral testicular growth retardation.** Because not all adults with varicoceles are infertile, present efforts are being directed at determining which patients will develop testicular dysfunction.

There is abundant evidence that varicoceles decrease semen quality in men. However, the majority of men with varicoceles remain fertile because the effect is modest or they were blessed with excellent reserve fertility potential. Normal gonadotropin and testosterone levels are usually found on hormonal studies, whereas elevations of FSH may be found in some patients (Swerdloff and Walsh, 1975). However, abnormal GnRH stimulation tests are often present in both adolescents and subfertile men with varicoceles.

Treatment of varicoceles is directed at ligation or occlusion of the dilated testicular veins. Surgical, radiographic, and laparoscopic techniques have been used toward this end and are discussed in depth in Chapter 44. Medical therapy has been suggested to be efficacious in the treatment of varicoceles. However, there are no well-designed studies to support this contention (Netto et al, 1984). **Improvement in seminal parameters is demonstrated in approximately 70% of patients following surgical varicocele repair. Improvements in motility are most common, occurring in 70% of patients, with improved sperm densities in 51% and improved morphology in 44% of patients. However, conception rates are less, averaging 40% to 50%** (Tulloch, 1955; Brown, 1976; Glezerman et al, 1976; Dubin and Amelar, 1977; Cockett et al, 1979; Marks, 1986).

There are very few controlled studies of the effect of varicocele repair on fertility. A controlled study by Nilsson (1979) demonstrated no effect of varicocele repair on semen quality or fertility. Other studies, including those of Baker and colleagues (1986) and Vermeulen and associates (1986) show no beneficial effect of varicocele repair. However, none of these studies have large enough numbers or are controlled well enough to be definitive. Indeed, similar controlled, but not randomized, studies have shown a definite beneficial effect of correction of varicocele over medical treatment or no treatment (Aafjes and van der Vijver, 1985; Gerris, 1988).* A recently published controlled randomized study is particularly convincing. Forty-five men who were partners in infertile marriages and who had clinical varicocele, suboptimal semen quality, normal endocrine parameters, and normal wives were divided into a control group and an operative group. The pregnancy rate in the control group at 1 year was 10%, whereas the rate in the operated group was 60% at 1 year and 72% at 2 years. The control group was treated after 1 year. Pregnancy rates 1 and 2 years after surgery were then 44% and 66%, respectively (Madgar et al, 1995).

In one study, Steckel and co-workers (1993) found that men with large varicoceles demonstrated poorer preoperative semen quality than did patients with smaller varicoceles. Following surgical repair, patients with larger varicoceles demonstrated greater improvement in semen parameters than did patients with small or medium-sized varicoceles. In contrast, other investigators have found that the size of the varicocele was not a significant factor (Dubin and Amelar, 1977).

It must be remembered that many varicoceles are not associated with infertility; therefore, not all varicoceles necessitate correction. The presence of a clinically detectable varicocele associated with an abnormal semen analysis in an infertile couple is an appropriate indication for treatment after the female partner has been evaluated. Although azoospermia in the presence of a varicocele portends a poor prognosis for fertility, occasional patients have responded to varicocele repair (Mehan, 1976).

Sertoli Cell–Only Syndrome

The etiology of Sertoli cell–only syndrome is unknown and is probably multifactorial. Patients usually present with small to normal testes and azoospermic semen specimens. Phenotypically, these patients are normally virilized males. Seminiferous tubules are lined by Sertoli cells with a complete absence of germ cells and a normal interstitium (Rothmon et al, 1982). Plasma FSH levels are often but not invariably elevated because of the absence of germ cells, whereas plasma testosterone and LH levels are normal.

Myotonic Dystrophy

Myotonic dystrophy consists of myotonia, which is a condition of delayed muscle relaxation after contraction. In addition, patients demonstrate premature frontal baldness, posterior subcapsular cataracts, and cardiac conduction defects. Significantly, testicular atrophy develops in up to 80% of patients (Drucker et al, 1963) during adulthood. Leydig cells typically are uninvolved, with biopsy specimens demonstrating severe tubular sclerosis. Serum FSH levels are elevated (Mahler and Parizel, 1982). The disease is transmitted as an autosomal dominant trait with variable penetrance. The abnormality is due to an unstable CTG sequence in a protein kinase gene (Jansen et al, 1994). There is no therapy for the testicular dysfunction in these patients.

Gonadotoxic Agents

Many physical and chemical agents may injure the germinal epithelium. Because the seminiferous epithelium consists of rapidly dividing cells, it is susceptible to agents that interfere with cell division. In addition, because spermatogenesis is an androgen-dependent process, drugs that interfere with androgen production or action may adversely affect fertility. Lastly, although many chemicals and drugs are known to affect spermatogenesis, there remain many environmental exposures for which there are no data regarding their antifertility effects.

Chemotherapy

Spermatogenesis is adversely affected by most chemotherapeutic agents (Parvinen et al, 1984). **The most susceptible cells are those most actively dividing and consist of spermatogonia and spermatocytes up to the preleptotene stage.** The specific combination of drugs used for therapy, the dose administered, and the age of the patient at the time of treatment are determinants of the specific effect on the gonads. Studies of large groups of patients who survived cancers in childhood have demonstrated that fertility rates of patients treated with alkylating agents were 60% lower than in nontreated controls. As single drugs, alkylating agents and procarbazine seem to result in the greatest amount

*Lipshultz, LI: Personal communication, 1991.

ductules to the ejaculatory duct may be involved. Obstructions may be congenital, because of malformation or absence of ductal structures, or acquired, secondary to infection, stricture, or vasectomy.

Congenital hypoplasia or absence of the vas is an uncommon cause of male infertility, representing 11% to 50% of cases of congenital ductal obstruction (El-Itreby and Girgis, 1961; Charny and Gillenwater, 1965; Amelar and Hotchkiss, 1963). Careful physical examination reveals a range of epididymal findings, from the presence of a full epididymis to the presence of only portions of the epididymis. There is usually associated hypoplasia or absence of the seminal vesicles and ampulla. Unilateral renal agenesis has also been noted in some patients. As noted previously, low-volume azoospermic ejaculates are characteristic of patients with this condition. Testicular biopsies generally demonstrate the presence of spermatogenesis. Surgical treatment with alloplastic spermatoceles has resulted in pregnancy rates between 0% and 4% and is not recommended. The advent of IVF has allowed a new avenue of treatment for this condition. Temple-Smith and colleagues (1985) reported a pregnancy following epididymal sperm aspiration from a patient with secondarily obstructed azoospermia. This technique has been used to treat patients with CBAVD. **At present, the most useful form of treatment for these men is epididymal sperm aspiration with intracytoplasmic sperm injection (see later).** If there is no epididymis or epididymal sperm are not available, testicular biopsy with sperm harvesting and intracytoplasmic sperm injection may be used. Men with epididymal or vasal obstruction can be rendered fertile with microsurgical repair (see Chapter 44) or the abovementioned methods. Failure of emission and retrograde ejaculation are functional forms of ductal obstruction and can be treated as described later. Obstruction of the ejaculatory ducts can be evaluated with TRUS. If there is hypoplasia or absence of the seminal vesicles, the diagnosis can be easily confirmed with TRUS. If partial or unilateral obstruction is suspected because of a low-volume ejaculate or, as some would suggest, because of a normal volume ejaculate with low motility and poor forward progression, TRUS can be used to identify dilated seminal vesicles. If present, this condition can be treated with transurethral resection of the ejaculatory ducts. We recommend that consideration be given to performing this procedure with ultrasound guidance. Some authors believe that partial obstruction of the seminal vesicles can cause poor motility and a decreased sperm count. They recommend aspiration of the seminal vesicles and transurethral resection of the ducts if significant numbers of sperm are present in the seminal vesicles. This approach is unproven and requires more investigation.

Ejaculatory Problems

Any process that interferes with the innervation of the vas deferens and bladder neck may result in lack of emission or retrograde ejaculation. This problem should be suspected in any patient who reports a low-volume or absent ejaculate; the finding of greater than 10 to 15 sperm per high-power field in a postejaculate urine specimen confirms the presence of retrograde ejaculation. This condition may follow transurethral resection of the prostate, bladder neck surgery, retroperitoneal lymph node dissections, and extensive pelvic surgery involving the colon and rectum. Medical illnesses, such as diabetes mellitus, multiple sclerosis, and pharmacologic therapy involving interference with sympathetic tone, may also affect ejaculation. **When retrograde ejaculation is not due to surgical changes of the bladder neck or in cases of lack of emission, pharmacologic therapy may be employed.** Phenylpropanolamine hydrochloride (75 mg bid), ephedrine sulfate (25 to 50 mg four times per day), pseudoephedrine hydrochloride (60 mg four times per day), and imipramine hydrochloride (25 mg bid) may induce ejaculation secondary to an increase in the tone of the internal sphincter and vas deferens. In addition, some cases of lack of emission may be converted to retrograde ejaculation by this therapy. These drugs are more effective if given for 4 days than if given in only one or two doses. If no effect is found within 2 weeks, success is unlikely. **Cases of retrograde ejaculation that are unresponsive to medical therapy or due to ablation of the bladder neck may be treated by recovery of sperm from the bladder combined with IUI (Shargold et al, 1990).** Fluid intake should be adjusted so that the urine is in the isotonic range to limit its gonadotoxic effect on sperm. The addition of sodium bicarbonate (650 mg four times per day for 48 hours prior to collection) may also improve the viability of recovered sperm. Sperm that are recovered are then washed in media, such as Hamms F10 with albumin, prior to insemination. If poor sperm viability persists, sperm-washing media may be instilled into the patient's bladder prior to ejaculation, lessening the toxic effect of urine. In cases of postoperative bladder neck changes, surgical techniques have been applied in attempts to treat this dysfunction (Abrahams et al, 1975). With the advancement in semen processing techniques, this surgery is rarely indicated today.

Penile vibratory stimulation results in ejaculation in approximately 70% of spinal cord–injured men (Oates et al, 1990; Ohl and Menge, 1995). Although specially designed equipment with specific vibration frequency and amplitudes are available, many practitioners have found good results using vibrators intended for general muscle relaxation available at routine department stores. **This approach should be used in patients with upper motor neuron lesions such as spinal cord injury. Patients with lesions below T12 usually do not respond to vibratory ejaculation. Patients with distal motor neuron lesions do not respond to this form of therapy. Electroejaculation involves the application of pulsed electrical current applied to the periprostatic plexus with the use of a rectal probe or needle electrodes.** Ejaculation has been successfully induced in patients following spinal cord injury and retroperitoneal lymph node dissections, and in multiple sclerosis, transverse myelitis, and diabetes mellitus. **Ejaculation occurs in approximately 75% of patients** (Brindley, 1981; Shaban et al, 1988; Ohl et al, 1989). In spinal cord–injured patients with complete cord lesions, the procedure may be performed in an office setting without anesthesia. However, in patients with incomplete cord lesions or intact pelvic sensation, general anesthesia is required (Bennett et al, 1987). **Electroejaculation should be attempted in patients not responsive to vibratory stimulation or those who are not candidates for vibratory stimulation.** Autonomic dysreflexia may occur in patients during vibratory or electroejaculation. This problem occurs primarily in patients with lesions above the T4 level. Pretreatment of these patients with 20 mg of nifedipine given subinguinally, 15 minutes before the procedure, usually allows the procedure to be performed safely (Steinberger et al, 1990).

The presence of indwelling urethral catheters or urinary tract infection has been associated with poor sperm quality as compared with patients with sterile urine managed by clean intermittent catheterization. Following semen processing of the obtained specimens, IUI, IVF, or IVF with ICSI may be performed.

ASSISTED REPRODUCTIVE TECHNIQUES

ARTs involve the manipulation of sperm or ova, or both, in an attempt to improve conception and live birth rates. The methodology and variety of techniques has continued to advance at a rapid pace. The simplest techniques involve only manipulation of sperm, whereas more sophisticated procedures involve manipulation of sperm and ova. Fertilization may occur in vivo or in vitro. These techniques are indicated in idiopathic male infertility, unexplained infertility, or in cases in which no therapy has been effective in resulting in conception. With the reported high success rates of IVF combined with intracytoplasmic sperm injection, some practitioners believe that it is best to proceed directly to these techniques rather than evaluate the basis of the male's infertility. In a recent cost-benefit analysis, Schlegel (1995) reported that the cost of delivery following a varicocele repair was $10,626 as compared with $62,898 for the same couple undergoing IVF. Thus, it is important that ARTs be used in appropriate settings and not as broad cure-all techniques. **For many couples in whom infertility is due to a mild-to-moderate male factor, IUI or IVF is an appropriate therapy. Owing to the significantly lower cost of IUI, this is often the initial treatment, and couples failing to conceive may proceed to IVF. If there is reason to believe the sperm may not fertilize ova without assistance, then IVF with ICSI may be the initial treatment.** Such cases include severe male factor infertility in which inadequate numbers of motile sperm are available for regular IVF or IUI. In addition, cases with abnormal sperm function testing, such as a zero score on the SPA, may proceed with IVF rather than IUI. If a regular IVF cycle demonstrated fertilization, the couple may then proceed with IUI in lieu of further IVF cycles.

Semen Processing

Semen must be processed prior to use for ARTs. A variety of procedures are used, including simple sperm washing, swim-ups (allowing pelleted sperm to swim up into a supernatant), sedimentations, and Percoll gradient centrifugations (Pousette et al, 1986; Adeghe, 1987; Pardo et al, 1988; Tanphaichitr et al, 1988; McClure et al, 1989). Seminal plasma is removed in all of these procedures, whereas others also select only motile sperm, removing nonmotile sperm and leukocytes. It is generally believed that the removal of seminal plasma is necessary. There is no agreement as to the value of selecting only motile sperm for these procedures. Increased fertilizing capacity of suboptimal semen specimens has been demonstrated following the in vitro addition of compounds such as pentoxifylline (Yovich, et al, 1988) or TEST-yolk buffer incubation of spermatozoa (Barak et al, 1992; Paulson et al, 1992). Larger studies have not demonstrated consistent increases in most couples treated with these techniques (Sigman et al, 1995).

Intrauterine Insemination

Intrauterine insemination has been used for many years for the treatment of male factor as well as female factor infertility. However, considerable controversy exists as to the efficacy of this procedure in increasing the chances of conception in male factor cases. A small catheter is used to inject processed sperm through the cervix into the uterine cavity in this procedure. It is hoped that by bypassing the cervical mucus, higher numbers of motile sperm will be able to progress to the fallopian tubes, thus increasing the chances of conception. **Male factor infertility, unexplained infertility, cervical mucus abnormalities, and anatomic abnormalities interfering with the deposition of sperm at the cervical os (severe hypospadias, retrograde ejaculation) are all indications for intrauterine insemination.** There is considerable variation in reported pregnancy rates using intrauterine insemination for male factor infertility. Belker and Cook (1987) found pregnancy rates ranging from 0% to 66% in a review of 17 published series. Kerin and colleagues (1984) reported a 21% pregnancy rate per cycle in 35 patients undergoing washed sperm IUI in women with nonstimulated menstrual cycles. This was compared with zero pregnancies occurring during intercourse cycles. Other studies have found little significant difference (Kirby et al, 1991) or no significant difference between IUI cycles and intercourse cycles (Ho et al, 1989; te Velde et al, 1989). The injection of raw semen is contraindicated because seminal prostaglandins may cause severe uterine cramping, and pelvic infection may be induced by bacterial contamination of the seminal fluid. A recent study demonstrated higher pregnancy rates with washed versus unwashed sperm IUI (Goldenberg et al, 1992). Ovarian hyperstimulation protocols, similar to those used for IVF, have been combined with IUI for male factor infertility. **Controlled studies have reported pregnancy rates of 7% to 19% per cycle compared with 0% to 2.2% in nonstimulated cycles** (Cruz et al, 1986; Kemmann et al, 1987; Melis et al, 1987; Nulsen et al, 1993; Ho et al, 1992; Nan et al, 1994).

In Vitro Fertilization

Following the report of a successful human pregnancy using IVF of human ova by Edwards and co-workers in 1980, this technique has been widely employed for the treatment of infertility. Initial attempts had been limited to female infertility secondary to blockage of fallopian tubes; however, because of the advances in IVF technology, a significant portion of IVF cycles now involve male factor infertility. Most centers employ some type of ovarian hyperstimulation to induce maturation of more than one oocyte in a given cycle. Oocyte development is monitored ultrasonically, and ova are harvested prior to ovulation with the use of ultrasound-guided needle aspiration. In vitro insemination is accomplished by mixing processed sperm with recovered oocytes. If fertilization takes place, the developing embryos are placed into the uterus transcervically. Only 20% to 30% of transferred embryos will implant and result in clinical pregnancies. Increased implantation rates have been reported following placement of zygotes or embryos into the fallopian tube instead of the uterus or by weakening the zona pellucida (assisted hatching) to improve the ability of the embryo to hatch through the zona. **In couples in whom infertility is not due to a male factor, 90% of inseminated oocytes are fertilized. However, in couples in whom infertility is due to a male factor, fertilization rates are significantly less.** Fertilization rates following insemination with higher numbers of sperm in the male factor couples do not compare with fertilization rates of non–male factor couples, emphasizing the fact that even motile sperm from male factor couples do not fertilize as well as equal numbers of motile sperm from non–male factor couples. Up to 40% of couples failed to fertilize any oocytes in vitro in contrast to only 10% of non–male factor couples (Cohen et al, 1985; Ben-Chetrit et al, 1995). Many centers find that couples who fail to fertilize on the first IVF attempt also fail to fertilize in subsequent attempts (Cohen et al, 1985). However, some centers report no association between the failure to fertilize on the first cycle and the results on a subsequent cycle (Ben-Schlomo et al, 1992). With the increasing availability of intracytoplasmic sperm injection, **most centers recommend that the couple proceed to an IVF cycle with micromanipulation if an initial cycle resulted in very poor fertilization.** The suboptimal fertilization rates of male factor couples in standard IVF result in lower pregnancy rates for these couples as compared with non–male factor couples. Pregnancy rates per egg retrieval cycle for severe male factor couples have been in the range of 7.8% as compared to 22.4% in less severe male factor couples (Ben-Chetrit et al, 1995). It should be realized that pregnancy rates are not live birth rates because approximately 30% of pregnancies miscarry and not all cycles in which women begin ovarian stimulation result in retrieval of oocytes. Live birth rates average 16.6% per egg retrieval cycle for male factor couples undergoing standard IVF (without micromanipulation) as compared with 21.5% for non–male factor couples (American Society for Reproductive Medicine, Society for Assisted Reproductive Technology in the United States and Canada, 1995).

Tubal Gamete Placement

Traditional in vitro fertilization-embryo transfer (IVF-ET) involves intrauterine placement of embryos. As mentioned previously, only 20% to 30% replaced embryos implant, resulting in pregnancy. Following intercourse, in vivo fertilization occurs in the fallopian tubes, followed by transport of the embryo down the fallopian tube into the uterus. Intrafallopian placement of gametes has been performed in the hope that this more physiologic placement will result in higher pregnancy rates. In GIFT, retrieved oocytes and sperm are placed in the fallopian tube prior to fertilization. If pregnancy is not achieved by this technique, it is not possible to determine whether it is due to a lack of implantation or a lack of fertilization. Because of this problem, some investigators believe that GIFT is not an optimal treatment for male factor infertility. Pregnancy rates in male factor and non–male factor couples are similar or higher than those for IVF. Because this procedure does not specifically attempt to improve the fertilizing capacity of sperm from male factor couples, pregnancy rates in these couples remain lower than pregnancies in GIFT cycles from non–male factor couples (Assisted Reproductive Technology in the United States and Canada, 1995). By replacing zygotes or embryos into the fallopian tube following IVF, tubal transfer techniques combine the benefits of GIFT with those of IVF. Fertilized eggs may be transferred at the zygote stage, as in pronuclear stage tubal transfer and zygote intrafallopian transfer, or at early embryo stage, as in tubal embryo transfer and tubal embryo stage transfer. There is no consensus as to whether tubal gamete placement yields better pregnancy rates than intrauterine embryo placement as with IVF when performed on comparable patients. **Results published by the American Fertility Society and the Society for Assisted Reproductive Technology (1995) report IVF yielding an 18.6% delivery rate per retrieval cycle as compared with rates of 28.1% with GIFT and 24.4% with zygote intrafallopian transfer. Although the GIFT and zygote intrafallopian transfer rates are higher than the IVF rates in this survey, the procedures are not necessarily performed on comparable patients. In addition, there are many IVF programs that achieve IVF pregnancy rates equal to GIFT pregnancy rates.** The recent development of assisted hatching (a micromanipulation technique that thins or tears the zona pellucida to allow easier hatching and implantation of the embryo) has resulted in improved implantation and pregnancy rates in appropriate IVF patients (Liu et al, 1993; Stein et al, 1995).

Micromanipulation

Although implantation rates may be increased by the use of intrafallopian transfer techniques and the more recent assisted hatching procedure, micromanipulation procedures have developed to address the poor fertilizing capacity of sperm from male factor couples. Sperm must traverse the zona pellucida prior to fertilization. Various procedures have been developed to alter the zona pellucida in attempts to allow sperm to reach the oolemma. A hole or tear is made in the zona pellucida with zona drilling and partial zona dissection. Subzonal insertion of sperm involves the use of a sharp micropipette to inject sperm into the perivitelline space between the plasma membrane and the zona pellucida. Although initial studies with these techniques yielded promising results (Malter and Cohen, 1989), as the procedures became more widely available, it became clear that results were suboptimal in the majority of patients. Recently, direct ICSI has been successfully used in cases of severe male factor infertility. In this procedure, one individual sperm is injected directly into the cytoplasm of a human ova (VanSteirteghem et al, 1993a). Pregnancy rates of 25% to 35% per egg retrieval cycle have been reported (VanSteirteghem et al, 1993b; Payne et al, 1994). This technique also appears to be efficacious with sperm obtained through microsurgical epididymal sperm aspiration using either fresh or frozen epididymal sperm as well as sperm retrieved from testicular biopsy specimens (Nagy et al, 1995). Follow-up of children born via micromanipulation procedures have revealed no increased incidence of major congenital abnormalities (Bonduelle et al, 1994). Of significance, this procedure can be performed in men with just a few viable sperm in their semen specimens as well as in patients with spermatogenesis but unreconstructible ductal obstruction. This procedure has also been successfully used in nonobstructed azoospermic patients with almost complete spermatogenic arrest on testicular biopsy by using spermatozoa retrieved from testicular tissue (Yemini et al, 1995). Finally, a few human pregnancies have been achieved following the injection of isolated nuclei from round spermatid into human ova in patients with complete maturation arrest (Sofikitis et al, 1995). Although this technology clearly has made pregnancy possible in many situations, the safety of these procedures in the most severe male factor cases has not been proved. It is not clear that genetic defects may not be passed on to offspring in these types of cases.

REFERENCES

Overview

Aafjes JH, Vijver JCM, Schenck PE: The duration of infertility: An important datum for the fertility prognosis of men with semen abnormalities. Fertil Steril 1978; 30:423–425.

Collins JA, Wrixon W, Janes LB, Wilson EH: Treatment-independent pregnancy among infertile couples. N Engl J Med 1983; 309:1201–1206.

Greenhall E, Vessey M: The prevalence of subfertility: A review of the current confusion and a report of two new studies. Fertil Steril 1990; 54:978–983.

Jarow JP: Life-threatening conditions associated with male infertility. Urol Clin North Am 1994; 21:409–415.

Mosher WD, Pratt WF: Fecundity and infertility in the United States: Incidence and trends. Fertil Steril 1991; 56:192–193.

Spira A: Epidemiology of human reproduction. Human Reprod 1986; 1:111–115.

van Noord-Zaadstra BM, Looman CW, Alsbach H, et al: Delaying childbearing: Effect of age on fecundity and outcome of pregnancy. BMJ 1991; 302:1361–1365.

History

Abel EL, Moore C, Waselewsky D, et al: Effects of cocaine hydrochloride on reproductive function and sexual behavior of male rats on the behavior of their offspring. J Androl 1989; 10:17–27.

Berul CI, Harclerode JE: Effects of cocaine hydrochloride on the male reproductive system. Life Sci 1989; 45:91–95.

Boyers SP, Corrales MB, Huszar G, DeCherney AH: The effects of lubrin on sperm motility in vitro. Fertil Steril 1987; 47:882–884.

Carrol PR, Whitmore WF, Herr HW, et al: Endocrine and exocrine profiles of men with testicular tumors before orchiectomy. J Urol 1987; 137:420–423.

Cendron M, Keating MA, Huff DS, et al: Cryptorchidism, orchidopexy and infertility: A critical long-term retrospective analysis. J Urol 1989; 142:559–562.

Donohue JP, Thornhill JA, Foster RS: Retroperitoneal lymphadenectomy for clinical stage A testis cancer (1965–1989): Modifications of technique and impact on ejaculation. J Urol 1993; 149:237–243.

Goldenberg RL, White R: The effect of vaginal lubricants on sperm motility in vitro. Fertil Steril 1975; 26:872–873.

Holma PK: Effects of an anabolic steroid (metandienone) on spermatogenesis. Contraception 1977; 15:151–162.

Jewett MAS: Nerve sparing technique for retroperitoneal lymphatinectomy in testis cancer. Urol Clin North Am 17:449–456, 1990.

Kolodny RC, Masters WH, Kolodny RM, Toro G: Depression of plasma testosterone levels after chronic intensive marijuana use. N Engl J Med 1974; 290:872–874.

Lipshultz LI, Caminos-Torres R, Greenspan CS, Snyder PJ: Testicular function after orchiopexy for unilaterally undescended testes. N Engl J Med 1976; 295:15–18.

MacLeod J, Hotchkiss RS: The effect of hyperpyrexia upon spermatozoa counts in men. Endocrinology 1941; 28:760.

Marshburn PB, Sloan CS, Hammond MG: Semen quality in association with coffee drinking, cigarette smoking and ethanol consumption. Fertil Steril 1989; 52:162–165.

McConnell JD: Abnormalities in sperm motility; techniques of evaluation and treatment. *In* Lipshultz LF, Howards S, eds: Infertility in the Male, 2nd ed. St. Louis, Mosby–Year Book, 1991, pp 266–267.

Nijman JM, Koops H, Kremer J, et al: Gonadal function after surgery and chemotherapy in men with stage II and III non-seminimonous testicular tumors. J Clin Oncol 1987; 5:651–656.

Oates RD: Nonsurgical treatment of infertility: Specific therapy. *In* Lipshultz L, Howards SS, eds: Infertility in the Male, 2nd ed. St. Louis, Mosby–Year Book, 1992, pp 376–394.

Orecklin JR, Koffman JT, Thompson RW: Fertility in patients treated for malignant testicular tumors. J Urol 1973; 109:293–295.

Procope BJ: Effect of repeated increase of body temperature on human sperm cells. Int J Fertil 1965; 10:333–339.

Pryor JL, Hurt GS, Caloras D, et al: Histologic analysis of orchiopexy in a cryptorchid rabbit model. J Urol 1989; 142:413–417.

Rustin GJ, Pektasides D, Bagshawe KD, et al: Fertility and chemotherapy for male and female germ cell tumors. Int J Androl 1987; 10:389–392.

Schlegel PN, Chang TS, Marshall FF: Antibiotics: potential hazards to male fertility. Fertil Steril 1991; 55:235–242.

Tagatz GE, Okagaki T, Sciarra JJ: The effect of vaginal lubricants on sperm motility and viability in vitro. Am J Obstet Gynecol 1972; 113:88–90.

Tulandi T, Plouffe L Jr, McInnes RA: Effect of saliva on sperm motility and activity. Fertil Steril 1982; 38:721–723.

Van Thiel DH, Gavaler JS, Lester R, Goodman MD: Alcohol induced testicular atrophy. An experimental model for hypogonadism occurring in chronic alcoholic men. Gastroenterology 1975; 69:326–332.

Vine MF, Margolin BH, Morrison HI, Hulka BS: Cigarette smoking and sperm density: A meta-analysis. Fertil Steril 1994; 61:35–43.

Werner CA: Mumps orchitis and testicular atrophy. Ann Intern Med 1950; 32:1066.

Physical Examination

Carney SW, Tuttle W: The spermatogenic potential of the undescended testis before and after treatment. J Urol 1960; 83:697–705.

Gonzalez R, Reddy P, Kaye KW, Marayan P: Comparison of Doppler examination and retrograde spermatic venography in the diagnosis of varicocele. Fertil Steril 1983; 40:96–99.

Lewis RW, Harrison RN: Contact scrotal thermography: II. Use in the infertile male. Fertil Steril 1980; 34:259–263.

Lipshultz LI, Corriere JN Jr: Progressive testicular atrophy in the varicocele patient. J Urol 1977; 117:175–176.

McClure RD, Hriacac H: Scrotal ultrasound in infertile man: Detection of subclinical unilateral and bilateral varicoceles. J Urol 1986; 135:711–715.

Naryan P, Amplatz K, Gonzalez R: Varicocele in male subfertility. Fertil Steril 1981; 36:92–97.

Netto NR Jr, Lemos GC, Barbosa EN: The value of thermography and of the Doppler ultrasound in varicocele diagnosis. Int J Fertil 1984; 29:176.

Perrin P, Rollet J, Durand L: The Doppler stethoscope in the diagnosis of subclinical varicocele. Br J Urol 1980; 52:390–391.

Ponchietti R, Crarselli GF, Noci I, et al: Telethermography and echo-Doppler. Evaluation of the subclinical varicocele in infertile men. Acta Eur Fertil 1983; 14:283–284.

Seyferth W, Jecht E, Zeitler E: Percutaneous sclerotherapy of varicocele. Radiology 1981; 139:335–340.

World Health Organization: Comparison among different methods for the diagnosis of varicocele. Fertil Steril 1985; 43:575–581.

Yamaguchi M, Sakatoku J, Takihara H: The application of intrascrotal deep temperature measurement for the non-invasive diagnosis of varicoceles. Fertil Steril 1989; 52:295–301.

Initial Basic Laboratory Evaluation

Semen Analysis

Amelar RD: Coagulation, liquefaction and viscosity of human semen. J Urol 1962; 87:187–190.

Amelar RD, Dubin L, Schoenfild C: Semen analysis. Urology 1973; 2:605–611.

Arnaud A, Schved JF, Gris JC, et al: Tissue-type plasminogen activator level is decreased in human seminal plasma with abnormal liquefaction. Fertil Steril 1994; 61:741–745.

Auger J, Kunstmann JM, Czyglik F, Jouannet P: Decline in semen quality among fertile men in Paris during the past 20 years. N Engl J Med 1995; 332(5):281–281.

Burkman LJ: Characterization of hyperactivated motility by human spermatozoa during capacitation: Comparison of fertile and oligo-zoospermic sperm populations. Arch Androl 1984; 13:153–165.

Carlsen E, Giwercman A, Keiding N, Skakkebaek NE: Evidence for decreasing quality of semen during past 50 years. BMJ 1992; 305:609–613.

Comhaire F, Schoonjans F, Vermeulen L, DeClercq N: Methodological aspects of sperm morphology evaluation: Comparison between strict and liberal criteria. Fertil Steril 1994; 62:857–861.

Davis RO, Katz DF: Computer-aided sperm analysis: Technology at a crossroads. Fertil Steril 1993; 59:953–955.

Greenburg SH: Varicocele and male infertility. Fertil Steril 1977; 28:699–706.

Grow DR, Oehninger S, Seltman HJ, et al: Sperm morphology as diagnosed by strict criteria: Probing the impact of teratozoospermia on fertilization rate and pregnancy outcome in a large in vitro fertilization population. Fertil Steril 1994; 62:559–567.

Kruger TF, Acosta AA, Simons KF, et al: Predictive value of abnormal sperm morphology in in vitro fertilization. Fertil Steril 1988; 49:112–117.

Kruger TF, Menkveld R, Stander FS, et al: Sperm morphologic features as a prognostic factor in in vitro fertilization. Fertil Steril 1986; 46(6):1118–1123.

MacLeod J: Human seminal cytology as a sensitive indicator of the germinal epithelium. Int J Fertil 1964; 9:1281–1285.

MacLeod J: The semen examination. Clin Obstet Gynecol 1965; 8:115–121.

Naghma-E-Rehan, Sobrero AJ, Fertig JW: The semen of fertile men: Statistical analysis of 1300 men. Fertil Steril 1975; 26:492–502.

Raboch J, Skachova J: The pH of human ejaculate. Fertil Steril 1965; 16:252.

Santomauro AG, Sciarra JJ, Varma AO: A clinical investigation of the role of the semen analysis and postcoital test in the evaluation of male infertility. Fertil Steril 1972; 23:245–251.

Schoysman R, Gerris J: 12-year follow-up study of pregnancy rates in 1291 couples with idiopathically impathically impaired male fertility. Acta Eur Fertil 1983; 14:51–56.

Settladge DSF, Motoshima M, Tredway DR: Sperm transport from the external cervical os to the fallopian tubes in women: A time and quantitation study. Fertil Steril 1973; 24:655–661.

Smith KD, Rodriguez-Rigau LJ, Steinberger E: Relation between indices of semen analysis and pregnancy rate in infertile couples. Fertil Steril 1977; 28:1314–1319.

Syner FN, Moghisi KS, Yanez J: Isolation of a factor from normal human semen that accelerates dissolution of abnormally liquefying semen. Fertil Steril 1975; 26:1064–1069.

Talbot P, Chacon RS: A triple stain technique for evaluating normal acrosome reactions of human sperm. J Exp Zool 1981; 215:201–208.

Van Zyl JA: Review of the male factor in 231 infertile couples. S Afr J Obstet Gynecol 1972; 10:17–24.

Van Zyl JA: The infertile couple. Part II. Examination and evaluation of semen. S Afr Med J 1980; 485–491.

Wilson VG, Bunge RG: Infertility and semen non-liquefication. J Urol 1975; 113:509–510.

Wolf DP, Byrd W, Dandekar P, Quigley MN: Sperm concentration in the fertilization of human eggs in vitro. Biol Reprod 1984; 31:837–848.

Wolff H, Politch JA, Martinez A, et al: Leukocytospermia is associated with poor semen quality. Fertil Steril 1990; 53:528–536.

Yanagimachi R: The movement of golden hamster spermatozoa before and after capacitation. J Reprod Fertil 1970; 23:193–196.

Hormonal Evaluation

Albert A: Human urinary gonadotropins. Recent Prog Horm Res 1956; 12:266.

Augarten A, Weissenberg R, Pariente C, Sack J: Reversible male infertility in late onset congenital adrenal hyperplasia. J Endocrinol Invest 1991; 14:237–240.

Bain J, Langevin R, D'Costa M, et al: Serum pituitary and steroid hormone levels in the adult male: One value is as good as three. Fertil Steril 1988; 49:123–126.

Baker HWG, Burger HG, de Krester DM, et al: Relative incidence of etiologic disorders in male infertility. *In* Stanten RJ, Swerdloff RS, eds: Male Reproductive Dysfunction. Diagnosis and Management of Hypogonadism, Infertility and Impotence. New York, Marcel Dekker, Inc., 1986, pp 247–250.

Rifkind AB, Kulin HE, Ross GT: Follicle-stimulating hormone (FSH) and luteinizing hormone (LH) in the urine of prepubertal children. J Clin Invest 1967; 46:1925–1931.

Azoospermia

Jarow JP, Espeland M, Lipshultz LI: Evaluation of the azoospermic patient. J Urol 1989; 142:62–65.

Second-Level Testing

Antisperm Antibodies

Aitken RJ, Parslow JM, Hargreave JB, Hendrey WF: Influence of antisperm antibodies on human sperm function. Br J Urol 1988; 62:367–373.

Ansbacher R: Sperm-agglutinating and sperm-immobilizing antibodies in vasectomized men. Fertil Steril 1971; 22:629–632.

Ayvaliotis B, Bronson R, Rosenfield D, Cooper G: Conception rates in couples where autoimmunity to sperm is detected. Fertil Steril 1985; 43:739–742.

Clarke GN, Elliot PM, Smaila C: Detection of sperm antibodies in semen using the Immunobead test: A survey of 813 consecutive patients. Am J Reprod Immunol Microbiol 1985a; 7:118–123.

Clarke GN, Lopata A, McBain JC, et al: Effect of sperm antibodies in males in human in vitro fertilization (IVF). Am J Reprod Immunol 1985b; 8:62–66.

De Almeida M, Gazagne I, Jeulin C, et al: In vitro processing of sperm with autoantibodies and in vitro fertilization results. Hum Reprod 1989; 4:49–53.

El-Demry M, James K: Lymphocytes, subjects, and macrophages in the male genital tract in health and disease. Eur J Urol 1988; 14:226–245.

Fuchs EF, Alexander NJ: Immunologic considerations before and after vasovasostomy. Fertil Steril 1983; 40:497–499.

Hellstrom JG, Samuels SJ, Waits AB, Overstreet JW: A comparison of the usefulness of the Sperm Mar and Immunobead tests for the detection of antisperm antibodies. Fertil Steril 1989; 52:1027–1031.

Hellstrom WJ, Overstreet JW, Samuels SJ, Lewis EL: The relationship of circulating antisperm antibodies to sperm surface antibodies in infertile men. J Urol 1988; 140:1039–1044.

Iqbal PK, Adeghe AJ, Hughes Y, et al: Clinical characteristics of subfertile men with antisperm antibodies. Br J Obstet Gynaecol 1989; 96:107–110.

Jarow JP, Sanzone JJ: Risk factors for male partner antisperm antibodies. J Urol 1992; 148:1805–1807.

Knudson G, Ross L, Stuhldreher D, et al: Prevalence of sperm bound antibodies in infertile men with varicocele: The effect of varicocele ligation on antibody levels and semen response. J Urol 1994; 151:1260–1262.

Mahoney MC, Blackmore PF, Bronson RA, Alexander NJ: Inhibition of human sperm–zona pellucida tight binding in the presence of antisperm antibody positive polyclonal patient sera. J Reprod Immunol 1991; 19:287–301.

Naz RK: Effects of antisperm antibodies on early cleavage of fertilized ova. Biol Reprod 1992; 46:130–139.

Patrizio P, Silber SJ, Ord T, et al: Relationship of epididymal sperm antibodies to their in vitro fertilization capacity in men with congenital absence of the vas deferens. Fertil Steril 1992; 58:1006–1010.

Quayle AJ, Kelly RW, Hargreave TB, James K: Immunosuppression by seminal prostaglandin. Clin Exp Immunol 1989; 75:387–391.

Sedor J, Hirsch IH: Office based screening of sperm autoimmunity. J Urol 1994; 152:2017–2019.

Sigman M, Basshum B, Lipshultz LI, et al: Predictive value of the indirect Immunobead assay in the male. Presented at the 45th Annual Meeting of the American Fertility Society. San Francisco, Nov. 13–16, 1989.

Urry RL, Carrell DT, Starr NT, et al: The incidence of antisperm antibodies in infertility patients with a history of cryptorchidism. J Urol 1994; 151:381–383.

White Blood Cell Straining of Semen

Berger RE, Karp LE, Williamson RA, et al: The relationship of pyospermia and seminal fluid bacteriology to sperm function as reflected in the Sperm Penetration Assay. Fertil Steril 1982; 37:557–564.

Caldamone AA, Emilson LBV, Al-Juburi A, Cockett ATK: Prostatitis: Prostatic secretory dysfunction affecting fertility. Fertil Steril 1980; 34:602–606.

Endtz AW.: A rapid staining method for differentiating granulocytes from germinal cells in Papanicolaou stained semen. Acta Cytol 1974; 18:2–7.

Homyk M, Anderson DJ, Wolff H: Differential diagnosis of immature germ cells in semen utilizing monoclonal antibodies MHS-10. Fertil Steril 1990; 53:323–330.

Maruyama DK, Hale RW, Rogers BJ: Effects of white blood cells on the in vitro penetration of zona free hamster eggs by human spermatozoa. J Androl 1985; 6:127–135.

Sigman M, Lopes L: The correlation between round cells and white blood cells in semen. J Urol 1993; 149(5 part 2):1338–1340.

Tomlinson MJ, Barrett CL, Cook ID: Prospective study of leukocytes and leukocyte subpopulations in semen suggest they are not a cause of male infertility. Fertil Steril 1993; 60:1069–1075.

Wolff H, Anderson DJ: Immunohistologic characterization and quantitation of leukocyte subpopulations in human semen. Fertil Steril 1988; 49:497–504.

Yanushpolky IH, Politch JA, Hill JA, Anderson DJ: Antibiotic therapy and leukocytospermia: A prospective, randomized, controlled study. Fertil Steril 1995; 63:142–147.

Cultures of the Genital Tract

Berger RE, Karp LE, Williamson RA, et al: The relationship of pyospermia in seminal fluid bacteriology to sperm function as reflected in the sperm penetration assay. Fertil Steril 1982; 37:557–564.

Bowie WR, Wang SP, Alexander ER, et al: Etiology of nongonococcal urethritis: Evidence for *Chlamydia trachomatis* and *Ureaplasma urealyticum*. J Clin Invest 1977; 59:735–742.

Busolo F, Zanchetta R, Lanzone E, Cusianato R: Microbial flora in semen of asymptomatic men. Andrologia 1984; 16:269–275.

Indress W, Patton WC, Taymor ML: On the etiologic role of *Ureaplasma urealyticum* (T-mycoplasma): Infection in infertility. Fertil Steril 1978; 30:293–296.

Kundsin RB, Falk L, Hertig AT: *Mycoplasma, Chlamydia,* Epstein-Barr, herpes I and II, and AIDS infections among 100 consecutive infertile female patients and husbands: Diagnosis, treatment, and results. Int J Fertil 1986; 31:356–359.

Lewis RH, Harrison RM, Domonique GJ: Culture of seminal fluid in a fertility clinic. Fertil Steril 1981; 35:194–198.

Makler A, Urbach Y, Lefler E, Merzbach D: Factors affecting sperm motility: VI. Sperm viability under the influence of bacterial growth in human ejaculates. Fertil Steril 1981; 35:666–670.

Naessens A, Foulon W, Debrucker P, et al: Recovery of micro-organisms in semen and relationship to semen evaluation. Fertil Steril 1986; 45:101–105.

Paulson JD, Polakowski KL: Isolation of a spermatozoal immobilization factor from *Escherichia coli* filtrates. Fertil Steril 1977; 28:182–185.

Soffer Y, Ron-El R, Golan A, et al: Male genital *Mycoplasma* and *Chlamydia trachomatis* culture: Its relationship with accessory gland functions, sperm quality, and autoimmunity. Fertil Steril 1990; 53:331–336.

Swenson CE, Toth A, Toth C, et al: Asymptomatic bacteriospermia in infertile men. Andrologia 1980; 12:7–11.

Thompson SE, Washington AE: Epidemiology of sexually transmitted *Chlamydia trachomatis* infections. Epidemiol Rev 1983; 5:96–123.

Upadhyaya M, Hibbard BM, Walker SM: The effect of *Ureaplasma urealyticum* on semen characteristics. Fertil Steril 1984; 41:304–308.

Wood JC, Lu RN, Peterson EN, delaMaza LM: Evaluation of Mycotrim-GU for isolation of *Mycoplasma* species and *Ureaplasma urealyticum*. J Clin Microbiol 1985; 22:789–792.

Radiologic Procedures and Testicular Biopsy

Chan SL, Lipshultz LI, Schwartzendruber D: Deoxyribonucleic acid (DNA) flow cytometry: A new modality for quantitative analysis of testicular biopsies. Fertil Steril 1984; 41:485–487.

Cohen MD, Frye S, Warner RS, Leiter E: Testicular needle biopsy in diagnosis of infertility. Urology 1984; 24:439–442.

Jarow JP: Seminal vesicle aspiration in the management of patients with ejaculatory duct obstruction. J Urol 1994; 152:899–901.

Shinohara K, Lipshultz LI, Scardino PT: Transrectal ultrasonography of the seminal vesicles in the azoospermic patient. Presented to the South Central Section Meeting of the American Urologic Association. Guadalajara, Mexico, November 1985.

Functional Evaluation of Spermatozoa

Aitken RJ: Diagnostic value of the zona-free hamster oocyte penetration test and sperm movement characteristics in oligospermia. Int J Androl 1985; 8:348–356.

Aitken JR, Best FSM, Richardson DW, et al: An analysis of semen quality and sperm function in cases of oligozoospermia. Fertil Steril 1982; 38:705–711.

Alexander MF: Evaluation of male infertility with an in vitro cervical mucus penetration test. Fertil Steril 1981; 36:201–208.

Auzmanas M, Tureck RW, Blasco L, et al: The zona-free hamster egg penetration assay as a prognostic indicator in a human in vitro fertilization program. Fertil Steril 1985; 43:433–437.

Burkman LJ, Coddington CC, Fraken DR, et al: The Hemizona Assay (HZA): Development of a diagnostic test for the binding of human spermatozoa to the human hemizona pellucida to predict fertilization potential. Fertil Steril 1988; 49:688–697.

Corson SL, Batzer FR, Marmar J, Maislin G: The human sperm–hamster egg penetration assay: Prognostic value. Fertil Steril 1988; 49:328–334.

Cross NL, Morales P, Overstreet JW, Hanson FW: Two simple methods for detecting acrosome-reacted human sperm. Gamete Res 1986; 15:213–226.

Fenichel P, Donzeau M, Farahifar D, et al: Dynamics of human sperm acrosome reaction: Relation with in vitro fertilization. Fertil Steril 1991; 55(5):994–999.

Gaddum-Rosse P, Blandau RJ, Lee,WI: Sperm migration into cervical mucus in vitro: II. Human spermatozoa in bovine mucus. Fertil Steril 1980; 33:644–648.

Kallajoki M, Virtanen I, Suominen J: The fate of acrosomal straining during the acrosome reaction of human spermatozoa as revealed by a monoclonal antibody and PNA-lectin. Int J Androl 1986; 9:181–194.

Keel BA, Kelly RW, Webster BW, et al: Application of a bovine cervical mucus penetration test. Arch Androl 1987; 19:33–41.

Kretzer P, Pope E, Younger J, Blackwell R: Long-term follow-up of patients with zero hamster tests. Presented at the 44th Annual Meeting of the American Fertility Society, Atlanta. October 8–13, 1988.

Lee MA, Trucco GS, Bechtol KB, et al: Capacitation and acrosome reactions in human spermatozoa monitored by a chlortetracycline fluorescence assay. Fertil Steril 1987; 48:649–658.

Mangione CM, Medley NE, Menge AC: Studies on the use of estrous bovine cervical mucus in the human sperm cervical mucus penetration technique. Int J Fertil 1981; 26:20–24.

Moghissi KS: Post-coital test: Physiologic basis, technique, and interpretation. Fertil Steril 1976; 27:117–129.

Moghissi KS, Siegel S, Meinhold D, Agronow SJ: In vitro sperm cervical mucus penetration: Studies in human and bovine cervical mucus. Fertil Steril 1982; 37:823–827.

Morgan H, Hendry WF, Stedronski J, et al: Sperm/cervical mucus crossed hostility testing and antisperm antibodies in the husband. Lancet 1977; 1:1228–1230.

Mortimer D, Curtis EF, Miller RG: Specific labeling by peanut agglutinin of the outer acrosomal membrane of the human spermatozoon. J Reprod Fertil 1987; 81:127–135.

Oehlinger S, Acosta AA, Veeck LL, et al: Recurrent failure of in vitro fertilization: Role of the Hemizona assay in the sequential diagnosis of specific sperm-oocyte defects. Am J Obstet Gynecol 1991; 164:1210–1215.

Smith RG, Johnson A, Lamb DJ, Lipshultz LI: Functional tests of spermatozoa: Sperm Penetration Assay. Urol Clin North Am 1987; 14:451–458.

Swanson RJ, Mayer JF, Jones KH, et al: Hamster ova/human sperm penetration: Correlation with count, motility and morphology for in vitro fertilization. Arch Androl Suppl 1984; 12:69–77.

Takemoto FS, Rogers BJ, Wiltbank MC, et al: Comparison of the penetration ability of human spermatozoa into bovine cervical mucus and zona free hamster eggs. J Androl 1985; 6:162–170.

Talbot P, Chacon RS: A new procedure for rapidly scarring acrosome reactions of human sperm. Gamete Res 1980; 3:211–216.

Talbot P, Chacon RS: A triple stain technique for evaluating normal acrosome reactions of human sperm. J Exp Zool 1981; 215:201–208.

Tesarik J, Mendoza C: Sperm treatment with pentoxifylline improves the fertilizing ability in patients with acrosome reaction insufficiency. Fertil Steril 1993; 60:141–148.

Yanagimachi R, Yanagimachi H, Rogers BJ: The use of zona-free animal ova as a test system for the assessment of the fertilizing capacity of human spermatozoa. Biol Reprod 1976; 15:471–476.

Yovich JM, Edirisinghe WR, Yovich JL: Use of the acrosome reaction to ionophore challenge test in managing patients in an assisted reproduction program: A prospective, double-blind, randomized controlled study. Fertil Steril 1994; 61:902–910.

Diagnostic Categories

Endocrine Causes

Al-Ansari AA, Khalil TH, Kelani Y, et al: Isolated follicle-stimulating hormone deficiency in men: Successful long term gonadotropin therapy. Fertil Steril 1984; 42:618–626.

Augarten A, Weissenberg R, Pariente C, Sack J: Reversible male infertility in late onset congenital adrenal hyperplasia. J Endocrinol Investigation 1991; 14(3):237–240.

Biben RL, Gordon GS: Familial hypogonadotropic eunuchoidism. J Clin Endocrinol 1955; 15:931.

Boyar R, Finkelstein J, Roffwarg H, et al: Synchronization of augmented luteinizing hormone secretion with sleep during puberty. N Engl J Med 1972; 287:562–586.

Bray GA, Dahms WT, Swerdloff RS, et al: The Prader-Willi syndrome: A study of 40 patients and a review of the literature. Medicine 1983; 62:59–80.

Clyde HR, Walsh PC, English RW: Elevated plasma testosterone and gonadotropin levels in infertile males with hyperthyroidism. Fertil Steril 1976; 27:662–666.

Cutfield RG, Bateman JM, Odell WD: Infertility caused by bilateral testicular masses secondary to congenital adrenal hyperplasia (21-hydroxylase deficiency). Fertil Steril 1983; 40:809–814.

Dacou-Voutetakis C: Hypogonadotropic hypogonadism: The genetic defect. A hypothesis based on human and animal prototypes. Horm Res 1992; 37(Suppl 3):62–64.

Danish RK, Lee PA, Mazur T, et al: Micropenis: II. Hypogonadotropic hypogonadism. Johns Hopkins Med J 1980; 146:177–184.

del Castillo I, Cohen-Salmon M, Blanchard S, et al: Structure of the X-linked Kallmann syndrome gene and its homologous pseudogene on the Y chromosome. Nat Genet 1992; 2(4):305–310.

Dollar JR, Blackwell RE: Diagnosis in management of prolactinomas. Cancer Metastasis Rev 1986; 5:125–138.

Eggert-Kruse W, Schwalbach B, Gerhard I, et al: Influence of serum prolactin on semen characteristics and sperm function. Int J Fertil 1991; 36(4):243–251.

Ewer RW: Familial monotropic pituitary gonadotropin insufficiency. J Clin Endocrinol Metab 1968; 28:783–788.

Faiman C, Hoffman DL, Ryan RJ, Albert A: The "fertile eunuch" syndrome: Demonstration of isolated luteinizing hormone deficiency by radioimmunoassay technique. Mayo Clin Proc 1968; 43:661–667.

Finkel DM, Phillips JL, Snyder PJ: Stimulation of spermatogenesis by gonadotropins in men with hypogonadotropic hypergonadism. N Engl J Med 1985; 313:651–655.

Gabrilove JL, Nicols GL, Sohval AR: The testis in Cushings's syndrome. J Urol 1974; 112:95–99.

Haase R, Jaspers C, Schulte HM, et al: Control of prolactin-secreting macroadenomas with parenteral, long-acting bromocriptine in 30 patients treated for up to 3 years. Clin Endocrinol 1993; 38(2)165–176.

Hargreave TB, Elton RA, Sweeting VM, Basreliam K: Estradiol and male fertility. Fertil Steril 1988; 49:871–875.

Hoffman AR, Crowley WF: Induction of puberty in men by long-term pulsatile administration of low-dose gonadotropin releasing hormone. N Engl J Med 1982; 307:1237–1241.

Kidd GS, Glass AR, Vigersky RA: The hypothalamic-pituitary testicular excess in thyrotoxicosis. J Clin Endocrinol Metab 1979; 48:798–802.

Kliesch S, Behre HM, Nieschlag E: High efficacy of gonadotropin or pulsatile gonadotropin-releasing hormone treatment in hypogonadotropic hypogonadal men. European Journal of Endocrinology 1994; 131(4):347–354.

Lerer I, Meiner V, Pashut-Lavon I, Abeliovich D: Molecular diagnosis of Prader-Willi syndrome: Parent-or-origin dependent methylation sites and non-isotopic detection of (CA)n dinucleotide repeat polymorphisms. Am J Med Genet 1994; 52(1):79–84.

Martin FIR: The stimulation and prolonged maintenance of spermatogenesis by human pituitary gonadotropins in a patient with hypogonadotropic hypogonadism. J Endocrinol 1967; 38:431–437.

New MI: 21-Hydroxylase deficiency congenital adrenal hyperplasia. J Steroid Biochem Mol Biol 1994; 48(1):15–22.

Paulsen CA, Espeland DH, Michaels EL: Effects of HCG, HMG, HLH and HGH administration on testicular function. *In* Rosenberg E, Paulsen CA, eds: The Human Testis. New York, Plenum Press, 1970, pp 547–551.

Schneider G, Kirschner MA, Berkowitz R, Ertel NH: Increased estrogen production in obese men. J Clin Endocrinol Metab 1979; 48:633–638.

Shargil AA: Treatment of idiopathic hypogonadotropic hypogonadism in men with luteinizing hormone–releasing hormone: A comparison of treatment with daily injections and with the pulsatile infusion pump. Fertil Steril 1987; 47:492–501.

Snyder PJ, Rudenstein RS, Gardner DF, Rothman JG: Repetitive infusion of gonadotropin-releasing hormone distinguishes hypothalamic from pituitary hypogonadism. J Clin Endocrinol Metab 1979; 48:864–868.

Urban MD, Lee PA, Migeon CJ: Adult weight and fertility in men with congenital adrenal hyperplasia. N Engl J Med 1978; 299:1392–1396.

Wang C, Lam KSL, May JTC, et al: Long-term treatment of hyperprolactinemia with bromocriptine: Effect of drug withdrawal. Clin Endocrinol 1987; 27:363–371.

Weiss J, Adams E, Whitcomb RW, et al: Normal sequence of the gonadotropin-releasing hormone gene in patients with idiopathic hypogonadotropic hypogonadism. Biol Reprod 1991; 45(5):743–747.

Whitcomb RW, Crowley WF Jr: Male hypogonadotropic hypogonadism. [Review.] Endocrinol Metabol Clin North Am 1993; 22(1):125–143.

Zgliczynski W, Zgliczynski S, Makowska A, et al: New long-acting bromocriptine (Parlodel MR and Parlodel LAR) in the treatment of pituitary tumors with hyperprolactinemia. Endocrynol Pol 1992; 43(3):234–241.

Testicular Causes

Klinefelter's Syndrome

Becker KL, Hoffman DL, Albert A, et al: Klinefelter's syndrome. Arch Intern Med 1966; 118:314–321.

Chopra IJ, Tulchinsky D, Greenway FL: Estrogen-androgen imbalance in men with hepatic cirrhosis. Ann Intern Med 1973; 79:198–203.

Cozzi J, Chevret E, Rousseaux S, et al: Achievement of meiosis in XXY germ cells: Study of 543 sperm karyotypes from an XY/XXY mosaic patient. Hum Genet 1994; 93:32–34.

Foss GL, Lewis FJW: A study of 4 cases with Klinefelter's syndrome, showing motile spermatozoa in their ejaculates. J Reprod Fertil 1971; 25:401–408.

Harari O, Bourne H, Baker G, et al: High fertilization rate with intracytoplasmic sperm injection in mosaic Klinefelter's syndrome. Fertil Steril 1995; 63:182–184.

Klinefelter HG Jr, Reifenstein EC Jr, Albright F: Syndrome characterized by gynecomastia, aspermatogenesis without a-Leydigism and increased secretion of follicle-stimulating hormone. J Clin Endocrinol 1942; 2:615.

MacLean N, Harnden DJ, Bond J, et al: Sex-chromosome abnormalities in new born babies. Lancet 1964; 1:286.

Matsuda T, Horii Y, Ogura K, et al: Chromosomal survey of 1001 subfertile males: Incidence and clinical features of males with chromosomal anomalies. Hinyokika Kiyo 1992; 38:803–809.

Paulsen CA, Gordon DL, Carpenter RW, et al: Klinefelter's syndrome and its variants: A hormonal and chromosomal study. Recent Prog Horm Res 1968; 24:321–363.

Theilgaard A: A psychologized study of the personalities of XYY and XXY men. Acta Psychiatr Scand Suppl 1984; 315:1–133.

Wang C, Baker HWG, Burger HG, et al: Hormonal studies in Klinefelter's syndrome. Clin Endocrinol 1975; 4:399–411.

XYY Syndrome

Baghdassarian A, Bayard F, Borganakar S, et al: Testicular function in XYY men. Johns Hopkins Med J 1975; 136:15–24.

Balodimos MC, Lisco H, Berwin I, et al: XYY karyotype in a case of familial hypogonadism. J Clin Endocrinol 1966; 26:443–452.

Freyne A, O'Connor A: XYY genotype and crime: 2 cases. Med Sci Law 1992; 32:201–203.

Han TH, Ford JH, Flaherty SP, et al: A fluorescent in situ hybridization analysis of the chromosome constitution of ejaculated sperm in a 47 XYY male. Clin Genet 1994; 45:67–70.

Hook EB: Behavioral implications of the human XYY genotype. Science 1973; 179:139–150.

Jacobs PA, Brunton M, Melville MM, et al: Aggressive behavior, mental subnormality and the XYY male. Nature 1965; 208:1351.

Lundberg PO, Helstrom J: Hormone levels in men with extra Y chromosomes. Lancet 1970; 2:1133.

Price WH, Strong JA, Whatmore PB, McClemont WF: Criminal patients with XYY sex chromosome complement. Lancet 1966; 1:565–506.

Santen RJ, de Kretser DM, Paulson CA, Vorhees J: Gonadotropins and testosterone in XYY syndrome. Lancet 1970; 2:371.

Skakkebaek NE, Zeuthen E, Neilsen J, Yde H: Abnormal spermatogenesis in XYY males: A report on 4 cases ascertained through a population study. Fertil Steril 1973; 24:390–395.

Stenchever MC, MacIntyre MN: A normal XYY man. Lancet 1969; 1:680.

Walzer S, Gerald PS: Social class and frequency of XYY and XXY. Science 1976; 190:1228–1229.

Other Chromosomal Abnormalities

Aiman J, Griffin JE, Gazak JM, et al: Androgen insensitivity as a cause of infertility in otherwise normal men. N Engl J Med 1979; 300:223–227.

Blumberg BD, Khulkin JD, Rotter JI, et al: Minor chromosomal variants and major chromosomal anomalies in couples with recurrent abortion. Am J Hum Genet 1982; 34:948–960.

Boucekkine C, Toublanc JE, Abbas N, et al: Clinical and anatomical spectrum in the XX sex-reversed patients. Relationship to the presence of Y specific DNA sequences. Clin Endocrinol 1994; 40:733–742.

Bourrouillou G, Bujan L, Calvas P, et al: Role and contribution of karyotyping in male infertility. Prog Urol 1992; 2:189–195.

Burgoyne PS: Mammalian sex determination: Thumbs down for zinc finger. Nature 1989; 342:860–862.

Campbell WA, Lowther J, McKenzie I, Price WH: Serum gonadotropins in Down's syndrome. J Med Genet 1982; 19:98–99.

Collins E, Turner G: The Noonan syndrome: A review of the clinical and genetic features of 27 cases. J Pediatr 1973; 83:941–950.

de la Chapelle A: The etiology of maleness in XX men. Hum Genet 1981; 58:105–116.

Fechner PY, Marcantonio SM, Jaswaney V, et al: The role of the sex-determining region Y gene in the etiology of 46,XX maleness. J Clin Endocrinol Metab 1993; 76:690–695.

Fortuny A, Carrio A, Soler A, et al: Detection of balanced chromosome rearrangements in 445 couples with repeated abortion and cytogenetic prenatal testing in carriers. Fertil Steril 1988; 49:774–779.

Griffin JE, Wilson JD: The syndromes of androgen resistance. N Engl J Med 1980; 302:198–209.

Hulten M, Eliasson R, Tillinger KG: Low chiasma count and other meiotic irregularities in 2 infertile 46,XXY men with spermatogenic arrest. Hereditas 1970; 65:285–290.

Koulischez L, Schoysman R: Chromosomes and human infertility. Clin Genet 1974; 5:116–126.

Page DC, Brown LG, de la Chapelle A: Exchange of terminal portions of X- and Y-chromosomal short arms in human XX males. Nature 1987; 328(6129):437–440.

Pearson PL, Ellis JD, Evans HJ: A gross reduction in chiasma formation during meiotic prophase and a defective DNA repair mechanism associated with a case of human male infertility. Cytogenetics 1970; 9:460–467.

Perez-Palacios G, Medina M, Ullao-Aguirre A, et al: Gonadotropin dynamics in XX males. J Clin Endocrinol Metab 1981; 53:254–257.

Plymate SR, Bremner WF, Paulsen CA: The association of D-group chromosomal translocations and defective spermatogenesis. Fertil Steril 1976; 27:139–144.

Puscheck EE, Behzadian MA, McDonough PG: The first analysis of exon 1 (the transactivation domain) of the androgen receptor gene in infertile men with oligospermia or azoospermia. Fertil Steril 1994; 62:1035–1038.

Riccardi VM, Grum CM: The prune belly anomaly: Heterogeneity and superficial X-link mimicry. J Med Genet 1977; 14:266–272.

Sarto GE, Therman E: Large translocation t(3q−;4p+) as probable cause of semisterility. Fertil Steril 1976; 27:784–788.

Schroder J, Lydecken K, De la Chapelle A: Meiosis and spermatogenesis in G-trisomic males. Humangenetik 1971; 13:15–24.

Schulster A, Ross L, Scommegna A: Frequency of androgen insensitivity in infertile phenotypically normal men. J Urol 1983; 130:699–701.

Skakkebaek NE, Bryant JI, Phillips J: Studies on meiotic chromosomes in infertile men and controls with normal karyotypes. J Reprod Fertil 1973; 35:23–36.

Other Causes of Testicular Impairment

Anorchia and Cryptorchidism

Aynsley-Green A, Zachmann M, Illig R, et al: Congenital bilateral anorchia in childhood: A clinical, endocrine and therapeutic evaluation of 21 cases. Clin Endocrinol 1976; 5:381–391.

Canlorbe P, Toublanc JE, Roger M, et al: Etude de la fonction endocrine dans 125 cas de cryptorchidies. Ann Med Interne (Paris) 1974; 125:365–369.

Cendron M, Keating MA, Hoff DS: Cryptorchidism, orchiopexy and infertility. J Urol 1989; 142:559–562.

Hadzielimovic F: Cryptorchidism: Management and Implications. New York, Springer-Verlag, 1983.

John Radcliffe Hospital Cryptorchidism Study Group: Cryptorchidism: A prospective study of 7500 consecutive male births, 1984–1988. Arch Dis Child 1992; 67:892–899.

Kumar D, Bremner N, Brown PW: Fertility after orchiopexy for cryptorchidism: A new approach to assessment. Br J Urol 1987; 64(5):516–520.

Lipshultz LI: Cryptorchidism in the subfertile male. Fertil Steril 1976; 27:609–620.

Lipshultz LI, Caminos-Torres R, Greenspan C, Snyder PJ: Testicular function after unilateral orchiopexy. N Engl J Med 1976; 295:15–18.

Lobaccaro JM, Medlej R, Berta P, et al: TCR analysis and sequencing of the SRY sex determining gene in 4 patients with bilateral congenital anorchia. Clin Endocrinol 1993; 38:197–201.

Okuyama A, Nonomura N, Nakamura M, et al: Surgical management of undescended testis: Retrospective study of potential fertility in 274 cases. J Urol 1989; 142:749–751.

Puri P, O'Donnell B: Semen analysis of patients who had orchiopexy at or after seven years of age. Lancet 1988; 2:1051–1052.

Scorer CG, Farrington HG: Congenital Deformities of the Testis and Epididymis. London, Butterworth's, 1971.

Varicocele

Aafjes JH, vander Vijver JCM: Fertility of men with and without a varicocele. Fertil Steril 1985; 43:901–904.

Ahlberg NE, Bartley O, Chidekel N: Right and left gonadal veins: An anatomical and statistical study. Acta Radiol Diagn 1966; 4:593–601.

Ayodeiji O, Baker HWG: Is there a specific abnormality of sperm morphology in men with varicoceles? Fertil Steril 1986; 45:839–842.

Baker HWG, Burger HG, de Kretser DM, et al: Relative incidence of etiologic disorders in male infertility. *In* Stante RJ, Swerdloff RS eds: Male Reproductive Dysfunction. Diagnosis and Management of Hypogonadism, Infertility and Impotence. New York, Marcel Dekker, Inc., 1986, pp 247–250.

Berger OG: Varicocele in adolescents. Clin Pediatr 1980; 19:810–811.

Brown JS: Varicocelectomy in the subfertile male: A 10 year experience in 295 cases. Fertil Steril 1976; 27:1046–1053.

Cass EJ, Belman AB: Reversal of testicular growth value by varicocele ligation. J Urol 1987; 137:475–476.

Chakraborty J, Sinha Hikim AP, Jhunjhunwala JS: Stagnation of blood in the microcirculatory vessels in the testes of men with varicocele. J Androl 1985; 6:117–126.

Cockett ATK, Urry RL, Dougherty KA: The varicocele and semen characteristics. J Urol 1979; 121:435–436.

Comhaire F, Vermeulen A: Varicocele sterility: Cortisol and catecholamines. Fertil Steril 1974; 25:88–95,

Coolsaet BLRA: The varicocele syndrome: Venography determining the optimal level for surgical management. J Urol 1980; 124:833–839.

Dubin L, Amelar RD: 986 cases of varicocelectomy: A 12 year study. Urology 1977; 10:446–449.

Dubin L, Amelar RD: Etiologic factors in 1,294 consecutive cases of male infertility. Fertil Steril 1971; 22:469–474.

Gerris J, Van Neuten J, Van Camp C, et al: Clinical aspects in the surgical treatment of varicocele in subfertile men. I. Comparison of observed and expected pregnancy rates. Eur J Obstet Gynecol Reprod Biol 1988; 27(1):33–41.

Glezerman M, Rakowszczyk M, Lunenfeld B, et al: Varicocele in oligospermic patients: Pathophysiology and results after ligation and division of the internal spermatic vein. J Urol 1976; 115:562–565.

Green KF, Turner TT, Howards SS: Varicocele: Reversal of the testicular blood flow and temperature effects by varicocele repair. J Urol 1984; 131:1208–1211.

Grillo-Lopez AJ: Primary right varicocele. J Urol 1971; 105:540–541.

Hoesli Z: Follow-up studies after operation of varicocele in adolescence. Dialogues in Pediatric Urology 1990; 13(4):4–5.

Howards SS: Treatment of male infertility. N Engl J Med 1995; 332(5):312–317.

Klaiber EL, Broverman DM, Pokoly TB: Interrelationships of smoking, testicular varicoceles and seminal fluid indexes. Fertil Steril 1987; 47:481–486.

Laven JES, Haans LCF, Mali WPTM, et al: Effects of varicocele treatment in adolescents: A randomized study. Fertil Steril 1992; 58:756–762.

MacLeod J: Seminal cytology in the presence of varicocele. Fertil Steril 1965; 16:735–757.

Madgar I, Weissenberg R, Lunefeld B, et al: Controlled trial of high spermatic vein ligation for varicocele in infertile men. Fertil Steril 1995; 63:120–124.

Marks JL, McMahon R, Lipshultz LI: Predictive parameters of successful varicocele repair. J Urol 1986; 136:609–612.

Mehan DJ: Results of ligation of internal spermatic vein in the treatment of infertility in azoospermic patients. Fertil Steril 1976; 27:110–114.

Mieusset R, Bujan L, Plantavid M, Grandjean H: Increased levels of FSH and LH associated with intrinsic testicular hyperthermia in oligospermic infertile men. J Clin Endocrinol Med 1989; 68:419–425.

Naftulin BN, Samuels SF, Hellstrom WJG, et al: Semen quality in varicocele patients is characterized by tapered sperm cells. Fertil Steril 1991; 56:149–151.

Netto JNA, Fakiani EP, Lemos GC: Varicocele: Clinical or surgical treatment. Int J Fertil 1984; 29:164–167.

Nilsson S, Edvinsson A, Nilsson B: Improvement of semen and pregnancy rate after ligation and division of the internal spermatic vein: Fact or fiction? Br J Urol 1979; 51:591–596.

Okuyama A, Nakamura M, Vamiki M, et al: Surgical repair of varicocele at puberty: Preventive treatment for fertility improvement. J Urol 1988; 139:562–564.

Oster J: Varicocele in children and adolescents. An investigation of the incidence among Danish school children. Scand J Urol Nephrol 1971; 5:27–32.

Peng BCH, Tomashefsky P, Nagler HM: The cofactor effect: Varicocele and infertility. Fertil Steril 1990; 54:143–148.

Portuondo JA, Calabozo M, Echanojareigui AD: Morphology of spermatozoa in infertile men with and without varicocele. J Androl 1981; 4:312–315.

Rodriguez-Rigau LJ, Smith KD, Steinberger E: Varicocele and the morphology of spermatozoa. Fertil Steril 1981; 35:54–57.

Sayfan J, Soffer Y, Manor H, et al: Varicocele in youth. A therapeutic dilemma. Ann Surg 1988; 207(2):223–227.

Saypol DC, Howards SS, Turner TT, et al: Influences of surgically induced varicocele on testicular blood flow temperature and histology in adult rats and dogs. J Clin Invest 1981; 68:39–45.

Steckel J, Dicker AP, Goldstein M: The influence of varicocele size on response to varicocelectomy. J Urol 1993; 149:769–771.

Steeno O, Knops J, DeClerck L, et al: Prevention of fertility disorders by detection and treatment of varicocele at school and college age. Andrologia 1976; 8:47–53.

Stephenson JD, O'Shaughnessy EJ: Hypospermia and its relationship to varicoceles and intrascrotal temperature. Fertil Steril 1968; 19:110–117.

Swerdloff RS, Walsh PC: Pituitary and gonadal hormones in patients with varicocele. Fertil Steril 1975; 26:1006–1012.

Tessler AN, Krahan HP: Varicocele and testicular temperature. Fertil Steril 1966; 17:201–203.

Tulloch WS: Varicocele in subfertility: Results of treatment. Br Med J 1955; 2:356.

Vermeulen A, Vandeweghe M, Deslypere JP: Prognosis of subfertility in men with corrected or uncorrected varicocele. J Androl 1986; 7(3):147–155.

Yamaguchi M, Sakatoku J, Takahara H: The application of intrascrotal deep body temperature measurement for the noninvasive diagnosis of varicoceles. Fertil Steril 1989; 52:295–301.

Zorgniotti A, MacLeod J: Studies in temperature, human sperm quality and varicoceles. Fertil Steril 1973; 24:854–863.

Sertoli Cell–Only Syndrome and Myotonic Dystrophy

Drucker WD, Blanc WA, Rowland MM, et al: The testis in myotonic muscular dystrophy: A clinical and pathologic study with a comparison with Klinefelter's syndrome. J Clin Endocrinol Metab 1963; 23:59.

Jansen G, Willems P, Coerwinkel M, et al: Gonasomal mosaicism in myotonic dystrophy patients: Involvement of myotatic events in (CTG) in repeat variation and selection against extreme expansion in sperm. Am J Hum Genet 1994; 54:575–585.

Mahler C, Parizel G: Hypothalamic-pituitary function in myotonic dystrophy. J Neurol 1982; 226:233–242.

Rothmon CM, Sims CA, Stotts CL: Sertoli only syndrome. Fertil Steril 1982; 38:388–390.

Chemotherapy

Anselmo AP, Cartoni C, Bellantuono P, et al: Risk of infertility in patients with Hodgkin's disease treated with ABVD versus MOPP versus ABVD/MOPP: Hematologica 1990; 75:155–158.

Berthelsen JG, Skakkebaek NE: Gonadal function in men with testis cancer. Fertil Steril 1983; 39:68–75.

Bokemeyer C, Schmoll HJ, Van Rhee J, et al: Long-term gonadal toxicity after therapy for Hodgkin's and non-Hodgkin's lymphoma. Ann Hematol 1994; 68:105–110.

Drasga RE, Eihorn LH, William SD, et al: Fertility after chemotherapy for testicular cancer. J Clin Oncol 1983; 1:179.

Fossa SD, Ous S, Abyholm T, et al: Post-treatment fertility in combination chemotherapy and retroperitoneal surgery on hormone and sperm production. Br J Urol 1985; 57:210–214.

Hendry WF, Stedronska J, Jones CR, et al: Semen analysis in testicular cancer and Hodgkin's disease: Pre- and post-treatment findings and implications for cryopreservation. Br J Urol 1983; 55(6):769–773.

Kader HA, Rostom AY: Follicle stimulating hormone levels as a predictor of recovery of spermatogenesis following cancer therapy. Clin Oncol 1991; 3:27–40.

Kreuser ED, Xiros N, Hetzel WD, et al: Reproductive endocrine gonadal capacity in patients treated with COPP chemotherapy for Hodgkin's disease. J Cancer Res Clin Oncol 1987; 113:260–266.

Nijman JM, Schraffordt Koops H, Kremer J, Sleijfer DT: Gonadal function after surgery and chemotherapy in men with stage II and III nonseminomatous testicular tumors. J Clin Oncol 1987; 5(4):651–656.

Parvinen M, Lahdetie J, Parvinen LM: Toxic and mutogenic influences on spermatogenesis. Arch Toxicol 1984; 7(Suppl):128–139.

Roeser HP, Stocks AE, Smith AJ: Testicular damage due to cytotoxic drugs and recovery after cessation of therapy. Aust N J Med 1978; 8:250–254.

Rustin GJS, Pektasides D, Bagshawe KD, et al: Fertility and chemotherapy for male and female germ cell tumors. Int J Androl 1987; 10:389–392.

Waxman J: Chemotherapy and the adult gonad: A review. J R Soc Med 1983; 76:144–148.

Radiation Exposure

Byrne J, Hulvihill JJ, Myers MH, et al: Effects of treatment on fertility in long-term survivors of childhood or adolescent cancer. N Engl J Med 1987; 317:1315–1321.

Clifton DK, Bremner WJ: The effect of testicular x-irradiation on spermatogenesis in man: A comparison with the mouse. J Androl 1983; 4:387–392.

Delic JI, Bush C, Peckham MJ: Protection from procarbazine-induced damage of spermatogenesis in the rat by androgen. Cancer Res 1986; 46:1909–1914.

Nygaard R, Clausen N, Siimes MA, et al: Reproduction following treatment for childhood leukemia: A population-based prospective cohort study of infertility and offspring. Med Pediatr Oncol 1991; 19:459–466.

Rowley MJ, Leach DR, Warner GA, Heller CG: Effect of greater doses of ionizing radiation on the human testis. Radiat Res 1974; 59:665–678.

Schlappack OK, Delic JI, Harwood JR, Stanley JA: Attempted protection of spermatogenesis from single doses of gamma-irradiation in the androgen pre-treated rat. Arch Androl 1987; 19:269–274.

Senturia VD, Peckham CS, Peckham MJ: Children fathered by men treated for testicular cancer. Lancet 1985; 2:766–769.

Commonly Prescribed Drugs and Ingested Compounds

Bracken MB, Eskenazi D, Sachse K, et al: Association of cocaine use with sperm concentration, motility, and morphology. Fertil Steril 1990; 53:315–322.

Close CE, Roberts PL, Berger RE: Cigarettes, alcohol and marijuana are related to pyospermia in infertile men. J Urol 1990; 144:900–903.

Cosgrove MD, Benton B, Henderson BE: Male genital urinary/abnormalities and maternal diethylstilbestrol. J Urol 1977; 117:220–222.

Dikshit RK, Buch JG, Mansuri SM: Effect of tobacco consumption on semen quality of a population of hypofertile males. Fertil Steril 1987; 48:334–336.

Dunphy BC, Barratt CL, Cooke ID: Male alcohol consumption and fecundity in couples attending an infertility clinic. Andrologia 1991; 23:219–221.

Evans HJ, Fletcher J, Torrance M, and Hargreave TB: Sperm abnormalities in cigarette smoking. Lancet 1981; 1:627–629.

Fraser L: Mechanisms controlling mammalian fertilization. Oxf Rev Reprod Biol 1984; 6:174–225.

Gordon CG, Altman K, Southern AL, et al: Effect of alcohol (ethanol) administration on sex-hormone metabolism in normal men. N Engl J Med 1976; 295:793–797.
Harmon J, Aliapoulios MA: Gynecomastia in marijuana users. N Engl J Med 1972; 287:936.
Hembree WC, Zeidenbert P, Nahas G: Marijuana effects on human gonadal function. *In* Nahas G, Poton WDM, Indanpaan-Heittila J, eds: Marijuana: Chemistry. Biochemistry and Cellular Effects. New York, Springer-Verlag, Inc., 1976, pp 521–527.
Lancranjan I, Popescu HI, Gavanescu O, Gavanescu O, Klepsch I, Serbanescu M: Reproductive ability of workmen occupationally exposed to lead. Arch Environ Health 1975; 30:396–401.
Lipshultz LI, Ross CE, Whorton D, et al: Dibromochloropropane and its effect on testicular function in man. J Urol 1980; 124:464–468.
Marshburn PB, Sloan CS, Hammond MG: Semen quality and association with coffee drinking, cigarette smoking and ethanol consumption. Fertil Steril 1989; 52:162–165.
Mendelson JH, Mello NK, Ellingboe J: Effects of acute alcohol intake on pituitary-gonadal hormones in normal human males. J Pharmacol Exp Ther 1977; 202:676–682.
Nelson WO, Steinburger E: The effect of Furadroxyl upon the testis of the rat. Anat Rec 1952; 112:367.
Nelson WO, Bunge RB: The effect of therapeutic dosages of nitrofurantoin upon spermatogenesis in man. J Urol 1957; 77:275–282.
Osser S, Beckman-Ramirez A, Liedholm P: Semen quality of smoking and nonsmoking men in infertile couples in a Swedish population. Acta Obstet Gynecol Scand 1992; 71:215–218.
Rodriguez-Rigau LJ, Smith KD, Steinburger E: Cigarette smoking and semen quality. Fertil Steril 1982; 38:115–116.
Toth A: Reversible toxic effect of salicylazosulfapyridine on semen quality. Fertil Steril 1979; 31:538–540.
Van Thiel DH, Gavaler JS, Smith WF, et al: Hypothalamic-pituitary-gonadal dysfunction in men using cimetidine. N Engl J Med 1979; 300:1012–1015.

Ultrastructural Abnormalities of Sperm

Baccetti B, Selmi MG, Soldani P: Morphogenesis of "decapacitated" spermatozoa in a man. J Reprod Fertil 1984; 70:395–397.
Bianchi E, Savasta S, Calligara A, et al: HLA haplotype segregation and ultrastructural study in familial immotile cilia syndrome. Hum Genet 1992; 89:270–274.
Chemes HE, Carizza C, Scarinci F, et al: Lack of a head in human spermatozoa from sterile patients: A syndrome associated with impaired fertilization. Fertil Steril 1987; 47:310–316.
Eliasson R, Mossberg B, Camner P, Afzelius BA: The immotile cilia syndrome: A congenital ciliary abnormality as an etiologic factor in chronic airway infections and male sterility. N Engl J Med 1977; 297:1–6.
Feneux D, Serres C, Jouannet P: Sliding spermatozoa: A dyskinesia responsible for human infertility? Fertil Steril 1985; 44:508–511.
Florke-Gerloff S, Topfer-Petersen E, Muller-Esterl W, et al: Biochemical and genetic investigation of round-headed spermatozoa in infertile men including two brothers and their father. Andrologia 1984; 16:187–202.
Jouannet PS, Escalier D, Serres C, David G: Motility of human sperm without outer dynein arms. J Submicrosc Cytol Pathol 1983; 15:67–71.
Kullander S, Rousing A: On round-headed human spermatozoa. Int J Fertil 1975; 20:33–40.
Rossman CM, Forrest JB, Less RNKW, et al: The dyskinetic cilia syndrome: Abnormal ciliary motility in association with abnormal ciliary ultrastructure. Chest 1981; 80:860–865.
Sturgess JM, Chao J, Wong J, et al: Cilia with defective radial spokes: A cause of human respiratory disease. N Engl J Med 1979; 300:53–56.
Zanboni L: The ultrastructural pathology of the spermatozoan as a cause for infertility: The role of electron microscopy in the evaluation of semen quality. Fertil Steril 1987; 48:711–734.

Orchitis

Beard CM, Benson RC, Kelalis PP, et al: The incidence of mumps orchitis in Rochester, Minnesota, 1935–1974. Mayo Clinic Proc 1977; 52:3–7.
McKendrick GDW, Nishtar T: Mumps orchitis and sterility. Public Health 1976; 80:277–278.

Immunologic Infertility

Bollendorf A, Check JH, Katsoff D, Fedele A: The use of chymotrypsin/galactose to treat spermatozoa bound with anti-sperm antibodies prior to intra-uterine insemination. Hum Reprod 1994; 9:484–488.
Confino E, Friberg J, Dudkiewicz AB, et al: Intrauterine inseminations with washed human spermatozoa. Fertil Steril 1986; 46–60:55.
Hendry WF, Hughes L, Scammell G, et al: Comparison of prednisolone and placebo in subfertile men with antibodies to spermatozoa. Lancet 1990; 335:85–88.
Kremer J, Jager S, Kuiken J: Treatment of infertility caused by antisperm antibodies. Int J Fertil 1978; 23:270–276.
Lenzi A, Gandini L, Claroni F, et al: Immunological usefulness of semen manipulation for artificial insemination homologous (AIH) in subjects with antisperm antibodies bound to sperm surface. Andrologia 1988; 20:314–321.
Medical Research International, Society for Assisted Reproductive Technology, The American Fertility Society: In vitro fertilization—embryo transfer (IVF-ET) in the United States: 1989 results from the IVF-ET Registry. Fertil Steril 1991; 55:14–23.
Shulman S: Treatment of immune male infertility with methylprednisolone. Lancet 1976; 2:1243.

Idiopathic Infertility

Abel BJ, Carswell G, Elton R, et al: Randomised trial of clomiphene citrate treatment and vitamin C for male infertility. Br J Urol 1982; 54:780–784.
Aulitzky W, Frick J, Hadziselimovic F: Pulsatile LHRH therapy in patients with oligozoospermia and disturbed LH pulsatility. Int J Androl 1989; 12:265–272.
Brigante C, Motta G, Fusi F, et al: Treatment of idiopathic oligozoospermia with tamoxifen. Acta Eur Fertil 1985; 16:361–364.
Buvat J, Ardaens K, Lemaire A, et al: Increased sperm count in 25 cases of idiopathic normogonadotropic oligospermia following treatment with tamoxifen. Fertil Steril 1983; 39:700–703.
Charny CW: The use of androgens for human spermatogenesis. Fertil Steril 1959; 10:557–570.
Charny CW, Gordon JA: Testosterone rebound therapy: A neglected modality. Fertil Steril 1978; 29:64–68.
Charny CW: Clomiphene therapy in male infertility: A negative report. Fertil Steril 1979; 32:551–555.
Chehval MF, Mehan DJ: Chorionic gonadotropins in the treatment of the subfertile male. Fertil Steril 1979; 31:666–668.
Clark RV, Sherins RJ: Treatment of men with idiopathic oligozoospermic infertility using the aromatase inhibitor, testolactone: Results of a double-blinded randomized, placebo-controlled trial with crossover. J Androl 1989; 10:240–247.
Dony JMJ, Smals AGH, Rolland R, et al: Effect of chronic aromatase inhibition by C^{1}-testolactone on pituitary-gonadal function and sperm indexes in oligozoospermic men. Andrologia 1986; 18:69–78.
Fauser BCJM, Rolland R, Dony JMJ, Corbey RS: Long-term, pulsatile, low dose, subcutaneous luteinizing hormone-releasing hormone administration in men with idiopathic oligozoospermia: failure of therapeutic and hormonal response. Andrologia 1985; 17:143–149.
Foss GL, Tindal VR, Birkett JP: The treatment of subfertile men with clomiphene citrate. J Reprod Fertil 1973; 32:167–170.
Homonnai ZT, Peled M, Paz GF: Changes in semen quality and fertility in response to endocrine treatment of subfertile men. Gynecol Obstet Invest 1978; 9:244–255.
Howards SS: Treatment of male infertility. N Engl J Med 1995; 332(5):312–317.
Jungck EC, Roy S, Greenblatt RB, Mahesh VB: Effect of clomiphene citrate on spermatogenesis in the human. Fertil Steril 1964; 15:40–43.
Keough EJ, Burger HG, de Kresterc DM, Hudson B: Nonsurgical management of male infertility. *In* Hafez ESE, ed: Human semen and fertility regulation in men. St. Louis, C.V. Mosby, 1976, pp 452–463.
Lamensdorf H, Compere D, Begley G: Testosterone rebound therapy in the treatment of male infertility. Fertil Steril 1975; 26:469–472.
Margalioth EJ, Laufer N, Persistz E, et al: Treatment of oligoasthenospermia with human chorionic gonadotropin: Hormonal profiles and results. Fertil Steril 1983; 39:841–844.
Micic S, Dotlic R: Evaluation of sperm parameters in clinical trial with clomiphen citrate of oligospermic men. J Urol 1985; 133:221–222.
Newton R, Schinfield JS, Schiff I: Clomiphene treatment of infertile men: Failure of response with idiopathic oligospermia. Fertil Steril 1980; 34:399–400.
Noci I, Chelo E, Saltarelli O, et al: Tamoxifen and oligospermia. Arch Androl 1985; 15:83–88.
Palti Z: Clomiphene therapy in defective spermatogenesis. Fertil Steril 1970; 21:838–843.
Paulson DF, Hammond CB, deVere White R, Wiebe RH: Clomiphene

citrate: Pharmacologic treatment of hypofertile male. Urology 1977; 9:419–421.

Pusch HH, Purstner P, Haas J: Treatment of asthenozoospermia with HCG. Andrologia 1986; 18:201–207.

Ronnberg L: The effect of clomiphene treatment on different sperm parameters in men with idiopathic oligozoospermia. Andrologia 1980; 12:261–265.

Rowley MJ, Heller CG: The testosterone rebound phenomenon in the treatment of male infertility. Fertil Steril 1972; 23:498–504.

Ross LS, Kandel GL, Prinz LM, Auletta F: Clomiphene treatment of the idiopathic hypofertile male: High-dose, alternate-day therapy. Fertil Steril 1980; 33:618–623.

Schellen TM, Beck JM: The influence of high doses of mesterolone on the spermiogram. Fertil Steril 1972; 23:712–714.

Schellen TM, Beck JJ: The use of clomiphene treatment for male sterility. Fertil Steril 1974; 25:407–410.

Schwarzstein L, Aparicio NJ, Turner D, et al: Use of synthetic luteinizing hormone–releasing hormone in treatment of oligospermic men: A preliminary report. Fertil Steril 1975; 26:331.

Sokol RZ, Steiner BS, Bustillo M, et al: A controlled comparison of the efficacy of clomiphene citrate in male infertility. Fertil Steril 1988; 49:865–870.

Torok L: Treatment of oligozoospermia with tamoxifen (open and controlled studies). Andrologia 1985; 17:497–501.

Vermeulen A, Comhaire F: Hormonal effects of an antiestrogen, tamoxifen, in normal and oligospermic men. Fertil Steril 1978; 29:320–327.

Vigersky RA, Glass AR: Effect of delta 1 testolactone on the pituitary-testicular axis in oligospermic men. J Clin Endocrinol Metab 1981; 52:897–902.

Wang C, Chan CW, Wong KK, Yeung KK: Comparison of the effectiveness of placebo, clomiphene citrate, mesterolone, pentoxfylline, and testosterone rebound therapy for the treatment of idiopathic oligospermia. Fertil Steril 1983; 40:358–365.

World Health Organization: A double-blind trial of clomiphene citrate for the treatment of idiopathic male infertility. Int J Androl 1992; 15:299–302.

World Health Organization Task Force on the Diagnosis and Treatment of Infertility: Mesterolone and idiopathic male infertility: A double-blind study. Int J Androl 1989; 12:254–264.

Zarate A, Valdes-Vallina F, Gonzales A, et al: Therapeutic effect of synthetic luteinizing hormone–releasing hormone (LH-RH) in male infertility due to idiopathic azoospermia and oligospermia. Fertil Steril 1973; 24:485–486.

Ductal Obstruction

Amelar RD, Hotchkiss RS: Congenital aplasia of the epididymides and vasa deferentia: Effects on semen. Fertil Steril 1963; 14:44.

Charny CW, Gillenwater JY: Congenital absence of the vas deferens. J Urol 1965; 93:399–401.

Dubin L, Amelar RD: Etiologic factors in 1,294 consecutive cases of male infertility. Fertil Steril 1971; 22:469–474.

El-Itreby AA, Girgis S.: Congenital absence of vas deferens in male sterility. Int J Fertil 1961; 6:409.

Greenburg SH, Lipshultz LI, Wein AJ: Experience with 425 subfertile male patients. J Urol 1978; 119:507–510.

Temple-Smith PD, Southwick GJ, Yates CA, et al: Human pregnancy by in vitro fertilization (IVF) using sperm aspirated from the epididymis. J In Vitro Fert Embryo Transfer 1985; 2:119–122.

Ejaculatory Problems

Abrahams JI, Solish GI, Boorjan P, et al: The surgical correction of retrograde ejaculation. J Urol 1975; 114:888–890.

Bennett CJ, Seager SWF, McGuire EJ: Electroejaculation for recovery of sperm after retroperitoneal lymph node dissection: Case report. J Urol 1987; 137:513–515.

Brindley GS: Electroejaculation: Its technique, neurologic implications and uses. J Neurol Neurosurg Psychiatry 1981; 44:9–18.

Oates RD, Stakin DR, Krane RJ: Penile laboratory stimulation in the spinal cord injured male to induce ejaculation. J Urol 1990; 143:344a–346a.

Ohl DA, Bennett CJ, McCabe M, et al: Predictors of success in electroejaculation of spinal cord injured men. J Urol 1989; 142:1483–1486.

Ohl DA, Menge AC: Penile vibratory stimulation in SCI males—does a penile prosthesis impair results? Presented at the 90th annual meeting of the American Urological Association, April 23–28, 1995, Las Vegas, Nevada.

Shaban SF, Seager SW, Lipshultz LI: Electroejaculation. Med Instrum 1988; 22:77–81.

Shargold GA, Cantor B, Schreiber JR: Treatment of infertility due to retrograde ejaculates: A simple cost effective method. Fertil Steril 1990; 34:175–176.

Steinberger REO, Ohl BA, Bennett CJ, et al: Nifedipine pretreatment for autonomic dysreflexia during electroejaculation. Urology 1990; 36:228–231.

Assisted Reproductive Techniques

Adeghe AJ: Effect of washing on sperm surface autoantibodies. Br J Urol 1987; 60:360–363.

American Society for Reproductive Medicine, Society for Assisted Reproductive Technology in the United States and Canada: 1993: Results generated from the American Society for Reproductive Medicine. Fertil Steril 1995; 64:13–21.

Barak Y, Ammit A, Lessing JB, et al: Improved fertilization rate in an in vitro fertilization program by egg yolk treated sperm. Fertil Steril 1992; 58:197–198.

Belker AM, Cook CL: Sperm processing and intrauterine insemination for oligospermia. Urol Clin North Am 1987; 14:597–607.

Ben-Chetrit A, Senoz S, Greenblatt EM, Casper RF: In vitro fertilization outcome in the presence of severe male factor infertility. Fertil Steril 1995; 63:1932–1037.

Ben-Schlomo I, Bider D, Dor J, et al: Failure to fertilize in vitro in couples with male factor infertility: What next? Fertil Steril 1992; 58:187–189.

Bonduelle M, Desmyttere S, Buysse A, et al: Prospective follow-up study of 55 children born after subzonal insemination and intracytoplasmic sperm injection. Hum Reprod 1994; 9:1765–1769.

Cohen J, Edwards R, Fehilly C, et al: In vitro fertilization: A treatment for male infertility. Fertil Steril 1985; 43:422–432.

Cruz RI, Kemmann E, Brandeis VT, et al: A perspective study of intrauterine insemination of processed sperm from men with oligoasthenospermia in superovulated women. Fertil Steril 1986; 6:673–677.

Edwards RG, Steptoe PC, Purdy JM: Establishing full-term human pregnancies using cleaved embryos grown in vitro. Br J Obstet Gynaecol 1980; 87:737–756.

Goldenberg M, Rabinovici J, Bider D, et al: Intra-uterine insemination with prepared sperm vs unprepared first split ejaculates. A randomized study. Andrologia 1992; 24:135–140.

Ho PC, Poon ENL, Chan SYW, Wang C: Intrauterine insemination is not useful in oligoasthenospermia. Fertil Steril 1989; 51:682–684.

Ho PC, So WK, Chan YF, Yeung WS: Intrauterine insemination after ovarian stimulation as a treatment for subfertility because of subnormal semen: A prospective randomized controlled trial. Fertil Steril 1992; 58:995–999.

Kemmann E, Bohrer M, Sheldon R, et al: Active ovulation management increases the monthly probability of pregnancy occurrence in ovulatory women who receive intrauterine insemination. Fertil Steril 1987; 48:916–920.

Kerin JF, Kirby C, Peek J, et al: Improved conception rate after intrauterine insemination of washed spermatozoa from men with poor quality semen. Lancet 1984; 1:533–535.

Kirby CA, Flaherty SP, Godfrey BM, et al: A prospective trial of intrauterine insemination of motile spermatozoa versus timed intercourse. Fertil Steril 1991; 45:102–107.

Liu HC, Cohen J, Alikani M, et al: Assisted hatching facilitates earlier implantation. Fertil Steril 1993; 60:871–875.

Malter HE, Cohen J: Partial zona dissection of the human oocyte: A non-traumatic method using micromanipulation to assist zona pellucida penetration. Fertil Steril 1989; 51:139–148.

McClure RD, Nunes L, Tom R: Semen manipulation: Improved sperm recovery and function with a 2-layer Percoll gradient. Fertil Steril 1989; 51:874–877.

Melis GB, Poaletti AN, Stringini F, et al: Pharmacologic induction of multiple follicular development improves the success rate of artificial insemination with husband's semen in couples with male related or unexplained infertility. Fertil Steril 1987; 47:441–445.

Nagy Z, Liu J, Cecile J, et al: Using ejaculated, fresh, and frozen-thawed epididymal and testicular spermatozoa gives rise to comparable results after intracytoplasmic sperm injection. Fertil Steril 1995; 63:808–815.

Nan PM, Kohlen BJ, TeVelde ER, et al: Intra-uterine insemination or timed intercourse after ovarian stimulation for male subfertility? A controlled study. Hum Reprod 1994; 9:2022–2026.

Nulsen JC, Walsh S, Dumoz S, Metzger DA: A randomized and longitudinal study of human menopausal gonadotropin with intrauterine insemination in the treatment of infertility. Obstet Gynecol 1993; 82:780–786.

Pardo M, Barri PN, Bancells N, et al: Spermatozoa selection in discontinuous Percoll gradients for use in artificial insemination. Fertil Steril 1988; 49:505–509.

Paulson RJ, Sauer MV, Francis MM, et al: A prospective controlled evaluation of TEST-yolk buffer in the preparation of sperm for human in vitro fertilization in suspected cases of male infertility. Fertil Steril 1992; 58:551–555.

Payne D, Flaherty SP, Geffrey R, et al: Successful treatment of severe male factor infertility in 100 consecutive cycles using intracytoplasmic sperm injection. Hum Reprod 1994; 9:2051–2057.

Pousette A, Akerlof E, Rosenborg L, Fredricsson B: Increase in progressive motility and improved morphology of human spermatozoa following their migration through Percoll gradients. Int J Androl 1986; 9:1–13.

Schlegel PN: Is varicocelectomy a cost effective treatment for male infertility in the ICSI era? Presented at the 51st Meeting of the American Society for Reproductive Medicine. Seattle, WA, October 7–12, 1995.

Sigman M, Frishman G, Hanning R, et al: Test yolk buffer treatment of sperm for male factor IVF. Presented at the 90th Annual Meeting of the American Urological Association, Las Vegas, Nevada, April 23–28, 1995. J Urol 1995; 153:65.

Sofikitis N, Miyagawa I, Sharlip I, et al: Human pregnancies achieved by intra-ooplasmic injections of round spermatid (RS) nuclei isolated from testicular tissue of azoospermic men. Presented at the 90th Annual Meeting of the American Urological Association, Las Vegas, Nevada, April 23 to 28, 1995. Abstract #368.

Stein A, Rufas O, Amit S, et al: Assisted hatching by partial zona dissection of human pre-embryos in patients with recurrent implantation failure after in vitro fertilization. Fertil Steril 1995; 63:838–841.

Tanphaichitr N, Agulnick A, Seibel N, Taymor M: Comparison of the in vitro fertilization rate by human sperm capacitated by multiple-tube swim-up and Percoll gradient centrifugation. J In Vitro Fert Embryo Transfer 1988; 5:119–122.

te Velde ER, van Kooy RJ, Waterreus JJH: Intrauterine insemination of washed husband's spermatozoa: A controlled study. Fertil Steril 1989; 51:182–185.

VanSteirteghem AC, Liu J, Joris H, et al: Higher success rate by intracytoplasmic sperm injection than by a subzonal insemination. Report of a second series of 300 consecutive treatment cycles. Hum Reprod 1993a; 8:1955–1060.

VanSteirteghem AC, Nagy Z, Joris H, et al: High fertilization and implantation rates after intracytoplasmic sperm injection. Hum Reprod 1993b; 8:1961–1066.

Yemini M, Vanderzwalmen P, Mukaida T, et al: Intracytoplasmic sperm injection, fertilization, and embryo transfer after retrieval of spermatozoa by testicular biopsy from an azoospermic male with testicular tubal atrophy. Fertil Steril 1995; 63:1118–1120.

Yovich JL, Edirisinghe WR, Cummins JM, Yovich JM: Preliminary result using pentoxifylline in a pronuclear stage tubal transfer (PROST) program for severe male factor infertility. Fertil Steril 1988; 50:179–181.

44
SURGICAL MANAGEMENT OF MALE INFERTILITY AND OTHER SCROTAL DISORDERS

Marc Goldstein, M.D.

OVERVIEW

Advances have been made in reproductive biology that were unthinkable at the time the previous edition of Campbell's Urology was published. The widespread use and success of in vitro fertilization (IVF) with intracytoplasmic injection of a single sperm into a mature oocyte (ICSI) has expanded our ability to treat all but the most severe cases of testicular failure. Immature haploid germ cells (round spermatids) have been injected into oocytes and achieved fertilization, pregnancy, and live healthy births in humans (Tesarik et al, 1995). Diploid germ cell nuclei obtained from secondary spermatocytes undergo meiosis after injection into mouse oocytes to produce live young (Kimura and Yanagimachi, 1995).

These techniques, initially feared by urologists as a replacement for male infertility treatment, have instead pushed back the frontiers of male reproductive surgery. Pregnancy rates with micropuncture epididymal sperm aspiration in men with unreconstructable obstructions now approach 50% (Schlegel and Goldstein, 1993a; Schlegel et al, 1995). Testicular sperm has been used to achieve pregnancy as well. Microsurgical varicocelectomy has resulted in return of sperm to the ejaculate in 60% of azoospermic men with testicular failure making pregnancy possible using IVF with ICSI in 38% of men (Matthews and Goldstein, 1996a).

Varicocele, long known to be associated with male infertility, has now clearly been shown to result in progressive, duration-dependent testicular injury (Russell, 1957; Lipshultz and Corriere, 1977; Nagler et al, 1985; Harrison et al, 1986; Kass et al, 1987; Hadziselimovic et al, 1989; Gorelick and Goldstein, 1993). Whereas surgical repair of varicocele has previously been reserved for the already infertile male, early repair of varicocele, using safer and more effective surgical techniques, is expanding the urologist's role from that of salvaging remaining testicular function to that of preventing future infertility.

When surgery for male infertility and scrotal disorders is undertaken, only rarely is the life of the patient at stake. What is at stake when the surgery described in this chapter is undertaken is new life, with the potential for altering not only the quality of a couple's life but the future of our species. The responsibilities assumed by the surgeon in these circumstances demands the utmost in judgment and skill. **Many of the procedures described in this chapter are among the most technically demanding in all of urology.** Acquisition of the skills required to perform them demands intensive laboratory training in microsurgery and a thorough knowledge of the anatomy and physiology of the male reproductive system. **Attempting such surgery only occasionally and without proper training is a terrible disservice to the patient, the couple, and future humanity.**

SURGICAL ANATOMY

The scrotal contents are unique in their accessibility for physical examination, imaging modalities, and surgical intervention. The success of surgery for male infertility and scrotal disorders is predicated on selection of the correct operation and most appropriate surgical approach. The details of the history and careful physical examination, followed by confirmatory, judiciously selected laboratory and imaging procedures, are presented in Chapter 43. When surgical intervention for diagnostic or therapeutic purposes is indicated, a thorough understanding of the anatomy and physiology of the male reproductive system (see Chapter 42) is requisite for planning and carrying out a surgical procedure with the highest probability of success and lowest morbidity.

TESTIS BIOPSY

Indications

The indications for testis biopsy are detailed in Chapter 43. Briefly, **testis biopsy is indicated in azoospermic men with testis of normal size and consistency, palpable vasa deferentia, and normal serum follicle-stimulating hormone (FSH) levels.** Under these circumstances, **a biopsy distinguishes obstructive azoospermia from primary seminiferous tubular failure.** In the testes of men with absent vasa, a biopsy always reveals at least some spermatogenesis (Goldstein and Schlossberg, 1988), and a biopsy is not necessary before sperm aspiration and in vitro procedures.

The ability to achieve pregnancy with only a single testicular sperm or a haploid germ cell nucleus has broadened the indications for testis biopsy to virtually all azoospermic men, and has turned biopsy into a potentially therapeutic as well as a diagnostic procedure. Even men with markedly elevated serum FSH levels and small soft testes, in whom testicular failure is certain, often harbor rare mature sperm in their testes. A biopsy is indicated in those men if the couple is willing to undergo costly ($12,500–$15,000 per attempt) IVF with ICSI.

The recently discovered heterogeneity of the testes, coupled with the ability of testicular sperm to acquire motility (Jow et al, 1993), has resulted in changes in the techniques of testis biopsy. **Examination of fresh unfixed tissue for the presence of sperm with tails** and possible motility, **and examination of multiple biopsy sites if sperm are not found, is now mandatory.**

The biopsy should usually be performed bilaterally. Good spermatogenesis is sometimes found in small firm testes, whereas biopsies of large healthy testes may reveal maturation arrest.

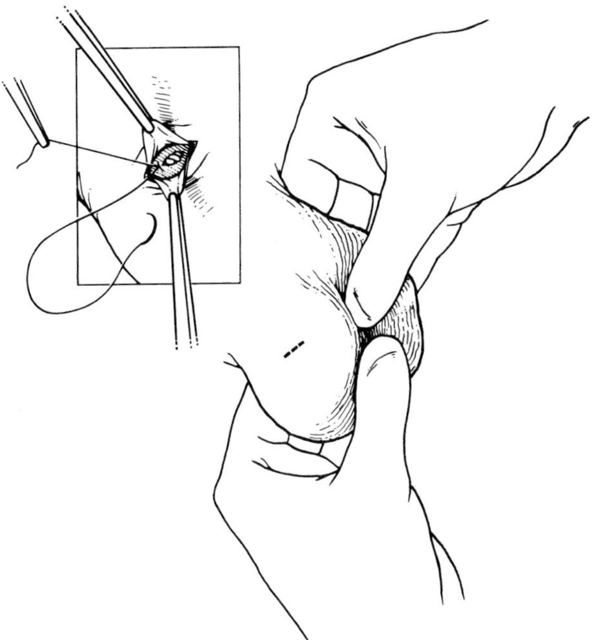

Figure 44–1. Testis biopsy. Transverse incision of 0.5 cm over upper lateral or medial aspect of testis. Transfixing suture in tunica albuginea maintains control and is used for closure. Hemostats hold open edges of tunica vaginalis.

Open Testis Biopsy

Open testis biopsy may be performed using either general, spinal, or local anesthetic. Some advocate local anesthesia with spermatic cord block; however, in rats, the incidence of accidental damage to the testicular artery during blind cord block is 5% (Goldstein et al, 1983). Local anesthesia of just the skin and tunics without a cord block is uncomfortable. General or spinal anesthetic is essential if there has been previous scrotal surgery with scar or adhesions.

When performing testis biopsy, the surgeon must provide an adequate tissue sample, use a technique that avoids trauma to the specimen, and avoid injury to the epididymis and testicular blood supply. Open biopsy under direct vision satisfies these requirements.

An assistant stretches the scrotal skin tightly over the anterior surface of the testis and confirms that the epididymis is posterior. Bilateral 1-cm transverse scrotal incisions provide good exposure with a minimum of scrotal skin bleeding. Alternatively, a single vertical incision in the median raphe may be employed. The incision is carried through the skin and dartos muscle, and the tunica vaginalis is opened. **If the anatomy is distorted from previous surgery or the epididymis cannot be clearly palpated posteriorly, or if the tunica albuginea cannot be clearly identified, the incision should be enlarged and the testis delivered. Testis biopsy material for permanent fixation should not be handled or traumatized in any way because this may distort the testicular architecture.** The edges of the tunica vaginalis are held open with hemostats, and any bleeding vessels are cauterized. Use of loupes or the operating microscope allows ready identification of a spot relatively free of visible surface vessels. The tunica albuginea of the testis is transfixed with a 5-0 polypropylene suture armed with a small, tapered needle (cutting needles are more likely to cause bleeding). The wound should be dry prior to incising the tunic to prevent saturation of the biopsy with blood. A 3- to 4-mm incision is made in the tunic with a 15-degree microknife. Small crossing vessels can be cauterized with a bipolar cautery and divided before excising a pea-sized sample of seminiferous tubules with a pair of razor-sharp iris scissors (Fig. 44–1). The specimen is then deposited directly into either Bouins, Zenkers, or collidine buffered glutaraldehyde solution. Formalin fixation results in distortion of testicular histology and should not be used for testis biopsy. **A so-called touch-prep is made by blotting the cut surface of the testis several times with a glass slide and adding a drop of saline or lactated Ringer's and a coverslip. Examination under high power using a light microscope with or without phase contrast reveals the presence of sperm with tails and allows assessment of motility (Fig. 44–2). If no sperm are found on the touch-prep, a second specimen may be cut for a wet squash-prep.** In this case, the specimen is placed on a slide, a drop of saline is added,

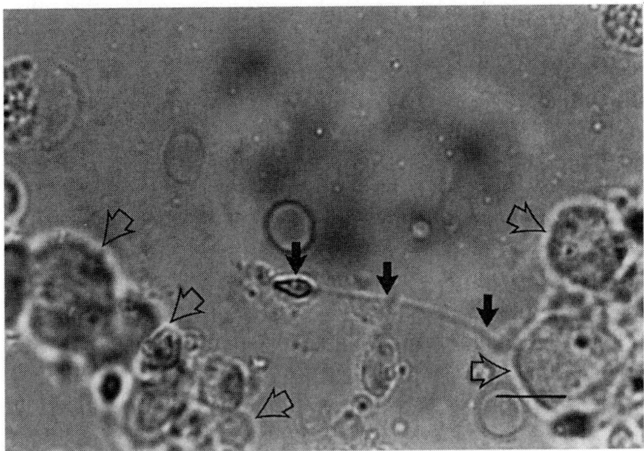

Figure 44–2. Intraoperative wet prep reveals sperm with tails *(solid arrows)*. Immature germ cells are seen as well *(open arrows)*.

and the specimen is crushed under a coverslip (Jow et al, 1993). If no sperm are found, the tunic is closed with the previously placed transfixing suture and another area is biopsied through the same skin incision.

The tunica vaginalis is closed with a running 5-0 polypropylene suture for hemostasis. **Polypropylene is less reactive than absorbable suture or nylon and prevents the formation of adhesions. This approach facilitates any future scrotal explorations such as epididymal reconstruction, aspiration, or therapeutic rebiopsy for testicular sperm retrieval** at the time of IVF with ICSI. The skin may be closed with a subcuticular 5-0 Monocryl suture or left open because these small wounds heal quickly. The wounds are covered with bacitracin ointment, and a fluff-type dressing is secured with snug scrotal support. Antibiotics are unnecessary.

Percutaneous Testis Biopsy

Percutaneous testis biopsy using the same 16- to 18-gauge biopsy gun employed for prostatic biopsy **is a blind procedure and could result in unintentional injury to either the epididymis or testicular artery.** This technique should not be used when previous surgery has resulted in scarring and obliteration of normal anatomy. Specimens obtained in this way often contain few tubules with poorly preserved architecture. When it is performed under local anesthesia without blind cord block, the procedure can be painful. Re-exploration of men who have undergone this type of biopsy has uniformly revealed adhesions and obliteration of the tunica vaginalis space, making exploration for vasoepididymostomy, epididymal aspiration, or rebiopsy more difficult.

Percutaneous Testicular Aspiration

Testicular aspiration performed with a 23-gauge needle is probably less risky and painful than percutaneous biopsy. Although flow cytometric evaluation of this material can distinguish haploid from diploid cells and, therefore, confirm the presence or absence of late stages of spermatogenesis (Chan et al, 1984), direct wet examination of the aspirate for sperm and assessment of motility provides the most useful information. Three or four aspirations can be performed until sperm are identified. These sperm can be used for IVF with ICSI (Craft and Tsirigotis, 1995) in cases in which sperm could not be retrieved from the epididymis.

Complications of Testis Biopsy

When it is carefully performed, testis biopsy is associated with few complications. **The most serious complication associated with testis biopsy is inadvertent biopsy of the epididymis.** If histologic evaluation of the biopsy material reveals epididymis with sperm within the epididymal tubule, obstruction of the epididymis at the site of the biopsy is certain. If, however, there are no sperm within the epididymal tubules, the patient is either obstructed above the level of the biopsy or has primary seminiferous tubular failure and no harm has been done.

The most common complication of testis biopsy is hematoma. Hematomas can be large and may require drainage. Placement of a transfixing suture in the tunica albuginea prior to incising it will avoid loss of exposure of the biopsy site and will help prevent this complication. If the biopsy site is lost before closure, the incision should be enlarged and the testis delivered. The tunica vaginalis also has a good blood supply and its edges should be carefully oversewn.

Because of the rich blood supply of the scrotum and its contents, wound infection is rare in the absence of hematoma, and antibiotics are unnecessary.

VASOGRAPHY

Indications

The absolute indications for vasography are

1. Azoospermia, plus
2. Complete spermatogenesis with many mature spermatids on testis biopsy, plus
3. At least one palpable vas.

Relative indications for vasography are

1. Severe oligospermia with normal testis biopsy.
2. Highly positive sperm-bound antibodies.
3. Low semen volume and very poor sperm motility (partial ejaculatory duct obstruction).

Vasography should answer the following questions:

1. Are there sperm in the vasal fluid?
2. Is the vas obstructed?

If the testis biopsy reveals many sperm, then

1. Absence of sperm in vasal fluid indicates an epididymal obstruction. Vasography is performed in this case with saline or methylene blue to confirm patency prior to vasoepididymostomy.
2. Copious vasal fluid containing many sperm indicates vasal or ejaculatory duct obstruction, and formal contrast vasography is performed as described later.
3. Copious thick white fluid in a dilated vas without sperm indicates both vasal or ejaculatory duct obstruction and secondary epididymal obstruction.

Vasography with radiographic contrast media and intraoperative x-ray study is rarely indicated. There is no need to perform vasography at the time of testis biopsy unless touch- or wet-prep biopsy reveals sperm with tails, and in this case, immediate reconstruction is undertaken. If performed carelessly, vasography can cause stricture or even obstruction at the vasography site, which can complicate subsequent reconstruction. In addition, because the majority of nonvasectomy-related obstructions are epididymal, vasography is of no value in making the diagnosis.

If testis biopsy reveals normal spermatogenesis and the vasa are palpable, vasography, if necessary, should be performed at the time of scrotal exploration and definitive repair of obstruction.

General anesthesia provides the most flexibility for scrotal exploration, vasography, and repair of obstruction. Although local anesthesia can provide adequate analgesia, patients are often unable to lie still through several hours of microsurgery. Long-acting hypobaric spinal or continuous epidural anesthesia can be satisfactory.

Technique of Vasography and Interpretation of Findings

If the site of obstruction is unknown and there is no previous inguinal incision, the testis is delivered through a high vertical scrotal incision. The vas deferens is identified and isolated at the junction of the straight and convoluted portions of the vas deferens. Using an operating microscope and 10-power magnification, the vasal sheath is vertically incised and the vasal vessels carefully preserved.

A clean segment of bare vas is delivered and surrounded with a vessel loop. A straight clamp is placed beneath the vas to act as a platform. Under 15-power magnification, a 15-degree microknife is used to transect the vas until the lumen is revealed (Fig. 44–3). **Any fluid exuding from the lumen is placed on a slide, mixed with a drop of saline, and sealed with a coverslip for microscopic examination. If the vasal fluid is devoid of sperm, after milking the epididymis and convoluted vas and repeated sampling, epididymal obstruction is present.** The seminal vesicle end of the vas is then cannulated with a 24-gauge angiocatheter sheath and is injected with saline to confirm its patency (Fig. 44–4). If the saline passes easily, formal vasography is not necessary. If further proof of patency of the vas deferens is desired, dilute methylene blue or indigo carmine may be injected and the bladder catheterized. The presence of blue dye in the urine confirms patency of the vas.

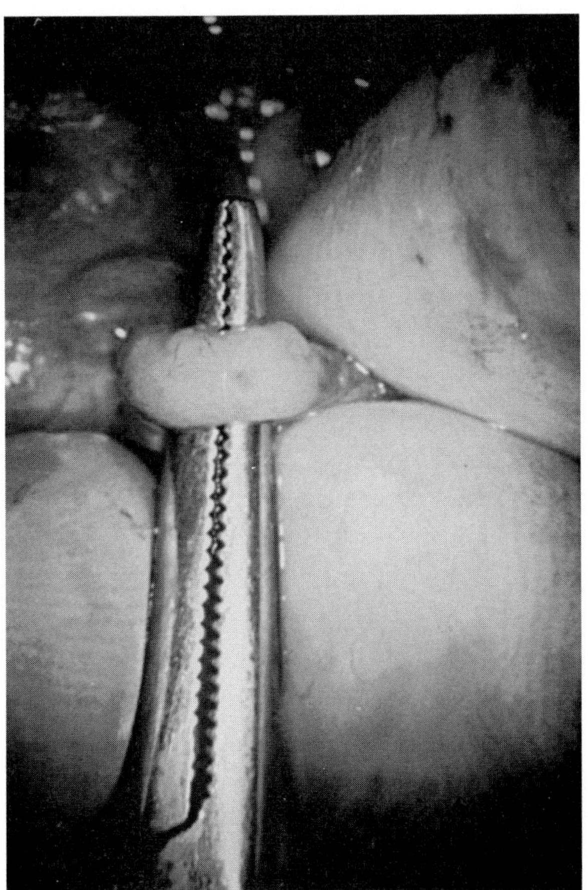

Figure 44–3. Hemitransected vas. Vasal vessels are excluded and preserved.

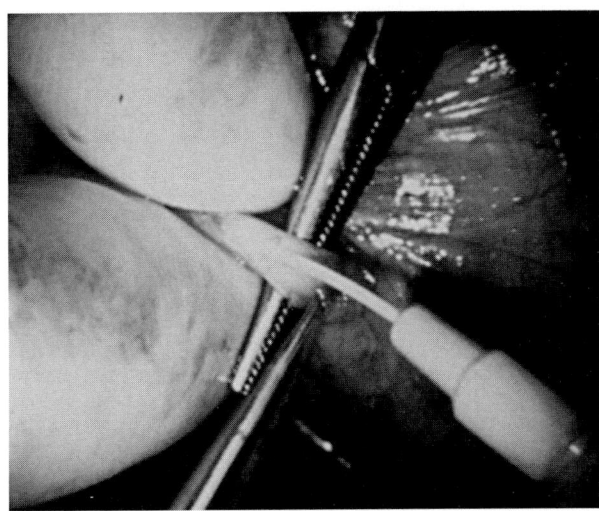

Figure 44–4. Cannulation of vasal lumen with a 24-gauge angiocath sheath. (From Goldstein M: Vasography and technique of testis biopsy. *In* Rajfer J, ed: Common Problems in Infertility and Impotence. New York, Mosby–Year Book, 1990.)

If a large amount of fluid is found in the vasal lumen and microscopic examination reveals the presence of sperm, the obstruction is toward the seminal vesicle end of the vas. In these cases, the vas is usually markedly dilated and a No. 3 whistle-tip ureteral catheter can be gently passed toward the seminal vesicle end of the vas. A No. 16 Fr Foley catheter is placed in the bladder, and the balloon is filled with 5 ml of air. Placing the balloon on gentle traction prior to vasography prevents reflux of contrast into the bladder, which can obscure detail (Fig. 44–5). The balloon also identifies the location of the bladder neck relative to any obstruction. After the vasa have been cannulated, vasograms are performed with the injection of 50% water-soluble contrast media (Fig. 44–6). **If vasography reveals obstruction at the site of the ejaculatory ducts (Fig. 44–7), methylene blue is injected in both vasa to facilitate a transurethral resection (TUR) of the ejaculatory ducts.** If both vasa are visualized after injection of contrast into only one vas (Fig. 44–8), it indicates that both vasa empty into a single cavity, usually a midline cyst.

Vasography may reveal the vas deferens ending blindly far from the ejaculatory ducts (Fig. 44–9). This finding indicates congenital partial absence of the vas deferens, and patients with this abnormality should be tested for cystic fibrosis. If this abnormality is found bilaterally (Fig. 44–10), reconstruction is impossible but vasal or epididymal sperm can be aspirated into fine glass pipettes (see the section entitled Sperm Retrieval Techniques) and cryopreserved for future IVF with ICSI. If vasography reveals obstruction in the inguinal region (Fig. 44–11), either inguinal vasovasostomy or crossed transseptal vasovasostomy may be performed. **Vasography sites are carefully closed microsurgically** using two or three interrupted 10-0 monofilament

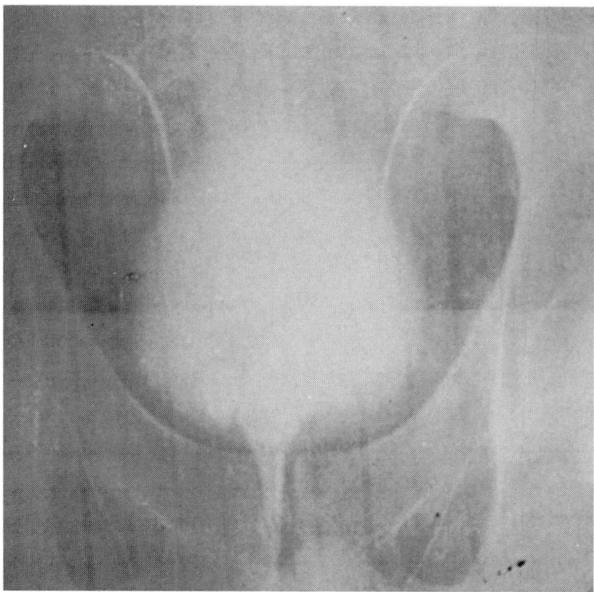

Figure 44–5. Vasogram without occlusion of bladder neck. Contrast material refluxing into the bladder obscures detail. (From Goldstein M: Vasography and technique of testis biopsy. *In* Rajfer J, ed: Common Problems in Infertility and Impotence. New York, Mosby–Year Book, 1990.)

polypropylene for the mucosa and 9-0 for the muscularis and adventitia (as described in Vasovasostomy in this chapter).

If the vasal fluid reveals no sperm and vasography confirms patency of the abdominal end of the vas, the vas is completely transected and the seminal vesicle end is prepared for vasoepididymostomy (see the section entitled Surgery of the Epididymis). If the vasal fluid reveals many sperm and vasography is normal, either retrograde ejaculation, lack of emission, or aperistalsis of the vas is the cause of the azoospermia.

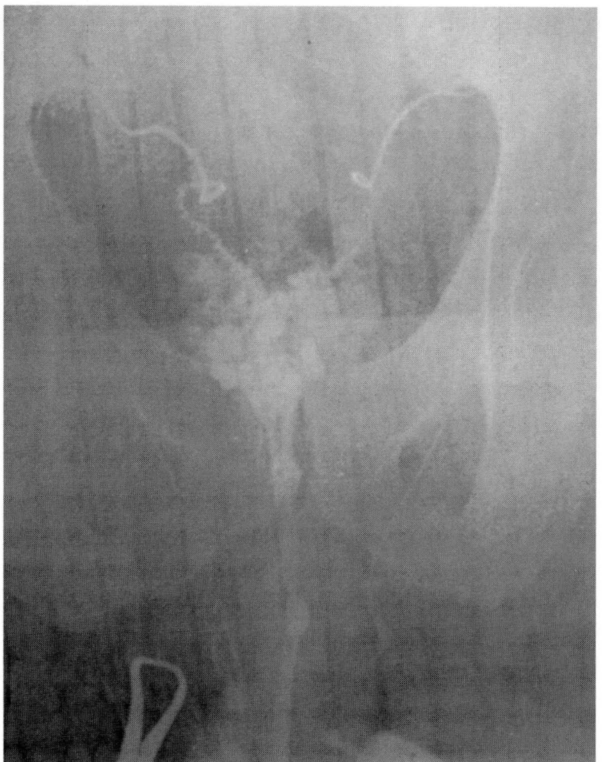

Figure 44–6. Normal vasogram with Foley catheter occluding bladder neck. (From Goldstein M: Vasography and technique of testis biopsy. *In* Rajfer J, ed: Common Problems in Infertility and Impotence. New York, Mosby–Year Book, 1990.)

Fine Needle Vasography

Exposure of the vas in its straight portion may allow vasography to be performed with a fine needle, obviating the need for hemitransection of the vas. Dewire and Thomas (1995) employ a 30-gauge lymphangiogram needle attached to Silastic tubing. When the sensation of puncture of the lumen is detected, 50% water-soluble contrast is injected to confirm patency radiographically. This has proved to be a difficult technique for even experienced microsurgeons to master. Accurate evaluation of vasal fluid for sperm is diffi-

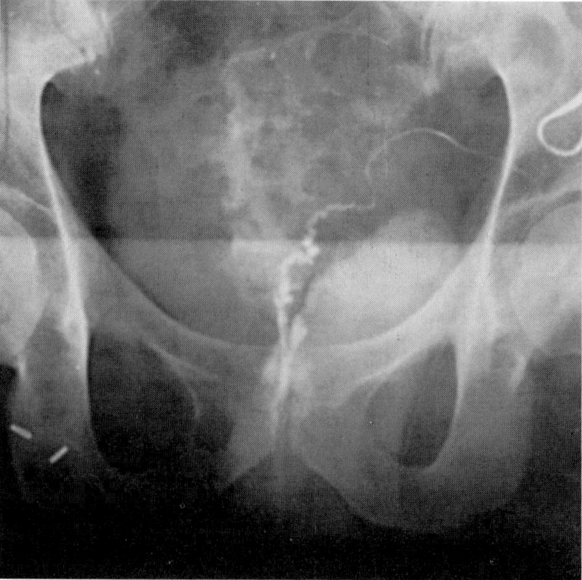

Figure 44–7. Ejaculatory duct obstruction. (From Goldstein M: Vasography and technique of testis biopsy. *In* Rajfer J, ed: Common Problems in Infertility and Impotence. New York, Mosby–Year Book, 1990.)

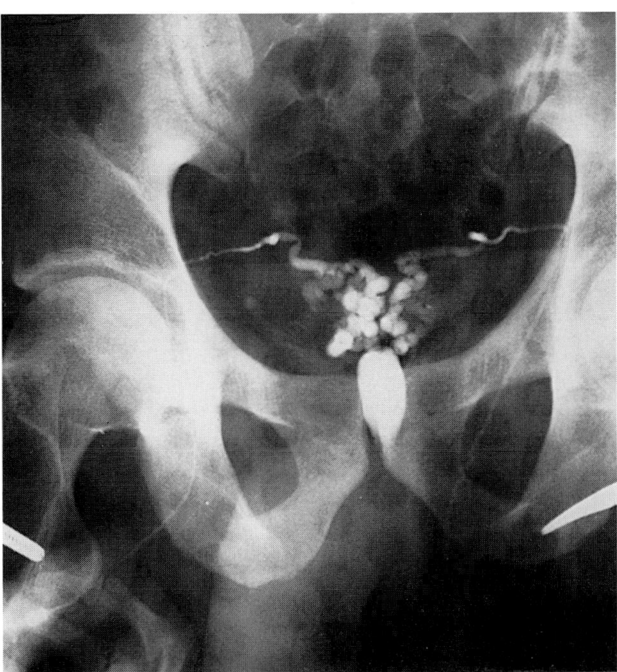

Figure 44–8. Both vasa are visualized after injection of contrast into only the right side. The vasa empty into a common cavity.

cult because it is so scant. If barbotage with 0.1 ml of saline or lactated Ringer's reveals the presence of sperm, then epididymal obstruction has been excluded and contrast can be injected. Collection of vasal sperm for cryopreservation is difficult with this technique.

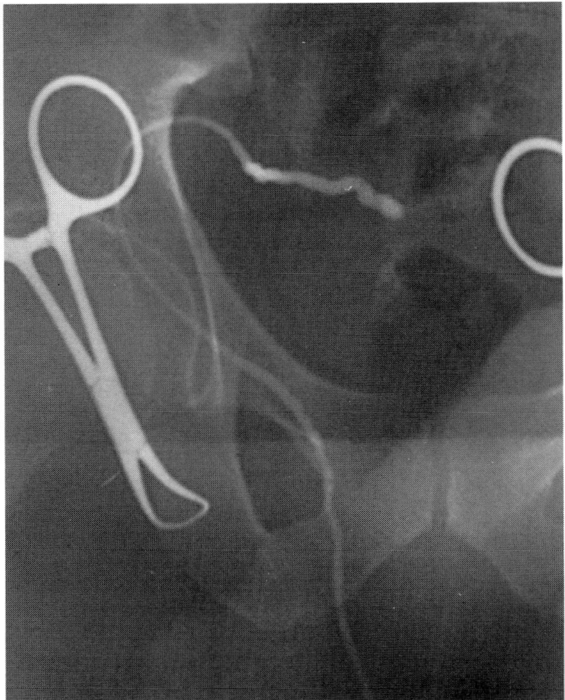

Figure 44–9. Unilateral partial agenesis of the vas deferens. (From Goldstein M: Vasography and technique of testis biopsy. *In* Rajfer J, ed: Common Problems in Infertility and Impotence. New York, Mosby–Year Book, 1990.)

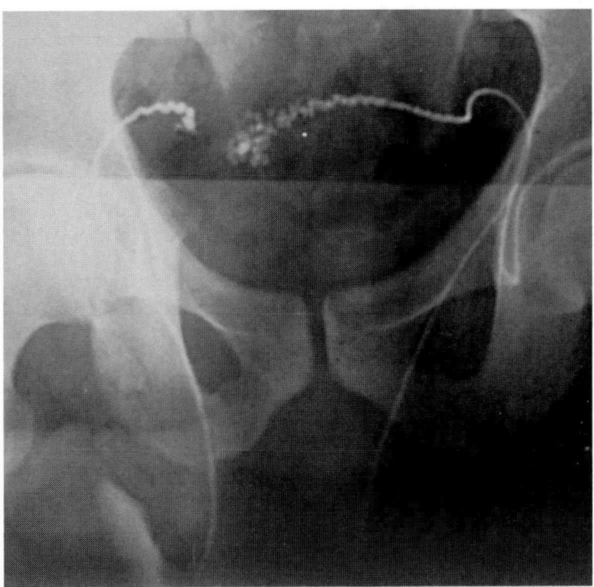

Figure 44–10. Bilateral partial agenesis of vas deferens. (From Goldstein M: Vasography and technique of testis biopsy. *In* Rajfer J, ed: Common Problems in Infertility and Impotence. New York, Mosby–Year Book, 1990.)

Percutaneous vasography through the scrotal skin has been successfully performed in China using the same ringed percutaneous fixation clamp employed for the no-scalpel vasectomy (see the section entitled No-Scalpel Vasectomy). After fixation of the vas beneath the scrotal skin, the vas lumen is punctured with a 22-gauge sharp needle and cannulated with a 24-gauge blunt needle through which vasography is performed. This technique is even more difficult than the

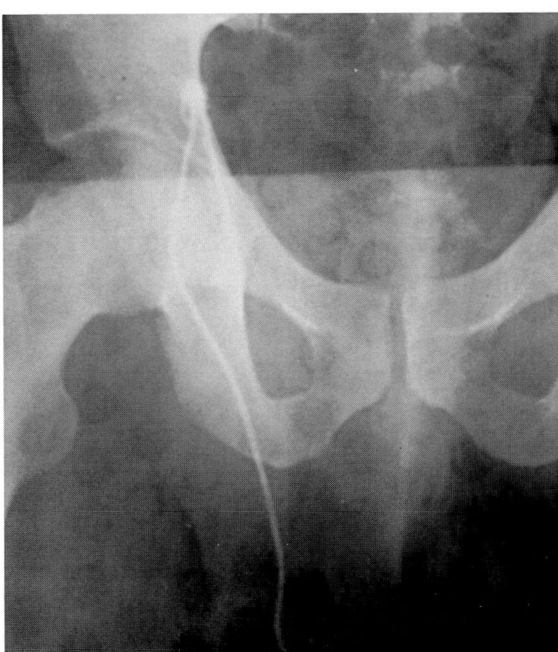

Figure 44–11. Inguinal obstruction of vas deferens. (From Goldstein M: Vasography and technique of testis biopsy. *In* Rajfer J, ed: Common Problems in Infertility and Impotence. New York, Mosby–Year Book, 1990.)

direct vision technique described by Dewire and Thomas (1995).

Contrast Agents for Vasography

When performing vasography, Ringer's lactate or normal saline should be used first. **If the fluid injects easily toward the seminal vesicle end of the vas, contrast vasography is unnecessary. For confirmation of patency,** or if injection of saline requires undue pressure, **methylene blue can be injected and the bladder catheterized.** The presence of dye in the bladder indicates patency. Inability to inject requires formal vasography with 50% diluted water-soluble contrast material. If vasography reveals ejaculatory duct obstruction, methylene blue is instilled to assist in TUR of the ejaculatory ducts. A 2-0 nylon or polypropylene suture may be threaded into the vas lumen to localize an inguinal obstruction. When groin scars are present, however, exploration is best performed directly through the old scar. This approach will lead to the inguinal obstruction and obviate the need for a separate vasotomy or vasogram.

Complications of Vasography

Stricture

Multiple attempts at percutaneous vasography using sharp needles can result in stricture or obstruction at the vasography site. Careless or crude closure of a vasostomy can also result in stricture and obstruction. Nonwater-soluble contrast agents may also result in stricture and should not be employed for vasography.

Injury to the Vasal Blood Supply

If the vasal blood supply is injured at the site of vasography, vasovasostomy proximal to the vasography site may result in ischemia, necrosis, and obstruction of the intervening segment of vas.

Hematoma

A bipolar cautery should be used for meticulous hemostasis at the time of vasostomy to prevent hematoma in the perivasal sheath.

Sperm Granuloma

Leaky closure of a vasography site may lead to the development of a sperm granuloma, which can result in stricture or obstruction of the vas. The microsurgical technique for closure of vasography sites is identical to that employed for vasovasostomy described later in this chapter.

Transrectal Vasography and Seminal Vesiculography

If transrectal ultrasound reveals markedly dilated seminal vesicles or a midline müllerian duct cyst, or both, in a man with obstructive azoospermia, transrectal aspiration followed by instillation of methylene blue mixed with radiographic contrast is a useful diagnostic and potentially therapeutic maneuver (Jarrow, 1994; Katz et al, 1994).

The same bowel prep and antibiotic coverage used for transrectal prostate biopsy is employed. The fine needle aspirate is examined for sperm. If sperm are present, it means at least one vas and epididymis are patent. One-half milliliter of methylene blue is diluted with 1.5 ml of 50% water-soluble contrast and is instilled. If a flat plate reveals a potentially resectable lesion, a TUR of the ejaculatory ducts is performed (see the section entitled Transurethral Resection of the Ejaculatory Ducts). Visualization of methylene blue effluxing from the ejaculatory ducts or unroofed cyst aids in determining the adequacy of the resection.

The aspirated sperm are analyzed and then frozen for possible future IVF with ICSI in the event that surgery fails.

If no sperm are found in the aspirated fluid, it suggests that secondary epididymal obstruction exists. At the time of surgery, the tunica vaginalis is opened and the epididymis is inspected under the operating microscope. If there is clear evidence of epididymal obstruction, that is, an epididymal sperm granuloma or a clear line of demarcation in the epididymis with dilated and indurated tubules above and soft and collapsed tubules below, vasoepididymostomy is performed (see the section entitled Surgery of the Epididymis). This should only be performed if a TUR has been successfully accomplished.

This technique obviates the need for formal open scrotal vasography in men with transrectally or transperineally accessible lesions. If sperm are found in the aspirate, a TUR may immediately be undertaken without violating the scrotum. Sperm-laden aspirates may be frozen for future IVF with ICSI (see the section entitled Oocyte Micromanipulation Techniques for Facilitated Fertilization) if surgery fails.

Summary

1. Perform vasography only if biopsy confirms obstruction.

2. Perform vasography only at the time of planned reconstruction.

3. Always sample vasal fluid first.

4. Formal vasography with x-ray contrast is needed only to locate obstructions proximal to the internal inguinal ring.

5. If transrectal ultrasound reveals dilated seminal vesicles or a midline (müllerian duct) cyst, or both, transrectal fine needle aspiration followed by instillation of contrast and methylene blue should be performed.

VASECTOMY

Vasectomy is a safe and effective method of permanent contraception employed by nearly 7% of all married couples and performed on approximately one-half million men per year in the United States (more than any other urologic surgical procedure). Impressive as these numbers may seem,

tive hematomas and lessen the possibility of future vasectomy reversal. Most urologists insist on removing a segment of vas for pathologic verification, primarily for medicolegal reasons. Even from the legal point of view, a pathologist's report confirming the presence of vas in the vasectomy specimen offers little or no protection from litigation. **Documented counseling, diligent follow-up to obtain at least two azoospermic semen specimens postoperatively, and careful selection of appropriate candidates for vasectomy in the first place provide the best protection from malpractice suits.**

Preferred Methods of Occlusion

Occlusion techniques that result in very low rates of recanalization without destruction of excessively long segments of vas or complicated, time-consuming strategies include the following:

1. Removal of a 1-cm segment followed by intraluminal thermal cautery with a battery-driven device for a distance of 1 cm in each direction, plus application of a medium hemoclip on each end distal to the cauterized segment (this is the author's preferred technique).

2. Intraluminal cautery, as described earlier, plus separation of the vasal ends into different tissue planes with or without removal of a segment.

3. Double medium hemoclips on each end placed 1 cm apart after removal of a 1-cm segment with or without separation into different tissue planes.

Postoperative Semen Analysis

No technique of vasal occlusion, short of removing the entire scrotal vas, is 100% effective. **Follow-up semen analysis with the goal of obtaining two absolutely azoospermic specimens 4 to 6 weeks apart is essential. If any motile sperm are found in the ejaculate 3 months after vasectomy, the procedure should be repeated.** If rare nonmotile sperm are found, contraception may be cautiously discontinued and repeat semen analysis performed every 3 months. Rare complete sperm in a spun semen analysis pellet are found in 10% of semen specimens at a mean of 10 years after vasectomy (Lemack and Goldstein, 1996).

Open-Ended Vasectomy

For over 20 years, attempts have been made to develop reversible methods of vasectomy. Until recently, most of these efforts focused on the use of mechanical valves that could be opened and closed. Unfortunately, these attempts have not been successful because of the damage to the epididymis that occurs after long-term obstruction. There is now some evidence that leakage of sperm at the vasectomy site prevents this pressure-induced damage and may increase the chances of successful reversal when accurate microsurgical vasovasostomy is performed (Silber, 1977). If the testicular end of the vas deferens is not sealed (open-ended technique), a sperm granuloma forms at the vasectomy site and damage to the epididymis is reduced. Early experience with this technique resulted in an unacceptably high incidence of vasectomy failure, varying from 7% to 50% (Shapiro and Silber, 1979; Goldstein, 1983). Better methods of sealing and burying the abdominal end of the vas reduce the failure rate of open-ended vasectomy to about 4%. This is still a substantially higher incidence of failure than that obtained with the closed occlusion techniques described earlier. Because recanalization after vasectomy is invariably associated with sperm granuloma formation, it is likely that open-ended vasectomy will always be associated with higher failure rates unless extraordinary efforts are made to separate widely the vasal ends or very long lengths of vas are destroyed on the seminal vesicle side. These measures, however, would either unduly complicate the performance of vasectomy or, paradoxically, make it less reversible.

Complications of Vasectomy

Hematoma and Infection

Hematoma is the most common complication of vasectomy, with an average incidence of 2% but a range of 0.09% to 29% (Kendrick et al, 1987). Infection is surprisingly common, with an average rate of 3.4%, but several series report rates from 12% to 38% (Appell and Evans, 1980; Randall et al, 1983; Randall et al, 1985). **The experience of the vasectomist is the single most important factor relating to complications** (Kendrick et al, 1987). **The hematoma rate was significantly higher among physicians performing 1 to 10 vasectomies (4.6%) than among those performing 11 to 50 vasectomies (2.4%) or greater than 50 vasectomies per year (1.6%).** A similar relationship was seen for the hospitalization rate.

Sperm Granuloma

Sperm granulomas form when sperm leak from the testicular end of the vas. Sperm are highly antigenic, and an intense inflammatory reaction occurs when sperm escape outside the reproductive epithelium. Sperm granuloma are rarely symptomatic. The presence or absence of a sperm granuloma at the vasectomy site seems to be of importance in modulating the local effects of chronic obstruction on the male reproductive tract. The sperm granuloma's complex network of epithelialized channels provides an additional absorptive surface that helps vent the high intraluminal pressure in the obstructed excurrent ducts. Numerous animal studies have correlated the presence or absence of sperm granuloma at the vasectomy site with the degree of epididymal and testicular damage. Species that always develop granulomas after vasectomy have minimal damage to the seminiferous tubules. Some studies of men undergoing vasectomy reversal have revealed somewhat higher success rates in men who have a sperm granuloma at the vasectomy site (Silber, 1977), whereas another large study has not (Belker et al, 1991).

Although sperm granulomas at the vasectomy site are present microscopically in 10% to 30% of men undergoing reversal, it is likely that, given enough time, virtually all men develop sperm granulomas at the vasectomy site, the epididymis, or the rete testis.

When chronic postvasectomy pain is localized to the granuloma, excision and occlusion of the vasa with intraluminal cautery usually relieve the pain and prevent recurrence (Schmidt, 1979). On the other hand, men with postvasectomy congestive epididymitis may be relieved of their pain by open-ended vasectomy designed to purposefully produce a pressure-relieving sperm granuloma.

Long-Term Effects of Vasectomy

Long-term effects of vasectomy in humans include vasitis nodosa, chronic testicular or epididymal pain, alterations in testicular function, chronic epididymal obstruction, postulated systemic effects of vasectomy, and possibly, an increased incidence of prostate cancer. Although vasitis nodosa has been reported in up to 66% of vasectomy specimens in men undergoing vasectomy reversal (Freund et al, 1989), this entity does not appear to be associated with pain or significant medical sequelae.

In humans, micropuncture studies have revealed that the markedly increased pressures that occur on the testicular side of the vas as well as the epididymis after vasectomy are not transmitted to the seminiferous tubules (Johnson and Howards, 1975). Therefore, little disruption of spermatogenesis is expected in humans. Biopsies up to 15 years after vasectomy show the testes to be essentially normal on light microscopy. Electron microscopic studies, however, have revealed thickening of the basal lamina and scattered areas of disrupted spermatogenesis in portions of the biopsy specimens (Jarow et al, 1985). Chronic orchialgia or epididymal pain, or both, after vasectomy occurs in approximately 1 in 2000 patients. In some cases, vasectomy reversal might be considered or, alternatively, an open-ended vasectomy may be used, as described previously. **The brunt of pressure-induced damage after vasectomy falls on the epididymis and efferent ductules.** These structures become markedly distended and then adapt to reabsorb large volumes of testicular fluid and sperm products. When pain and tenderness are localized in the epididymis, total epididymovasectomy, including removal of the testicular vasal remnant, relieves pain in 95% of men (Selikowitz and Schned, 1985) (see the section entitled Epididymectomy).

Systemic effects of vasectomy have been postulated. **Vasectomy disrupts the blood-testis barrier, resulting in detectable levels of serum antisperm antibodies in 60% to 80% of men** (Lepow and Crozier, 1979; Fuchs and Alexander, 1983). Some studies suggest that the antibody titers diminish 2 or more years after vasectomy. Others suggest that these antibody titers persist. However, neither circulating immune complexes nor deposits are increased after vasectomy in humans (Witkin et al, 1982). **Studies in animals and humans have failed to find any association between antisperm antibodies and immune complex–mediated diseases such as lupus erythematosus, scleroderma, rheumatoid arthritis, or myasthenia gravis** (Massey, 1984). Although one study in cynomolgus monkeys found more frequent and extensive atherosclerosis of the major vessels in previously vasectomized monkeys fed a high-cholesterol diet (Alexander and Clarkson, 1978), **no evidence of excess cardiovascular disease (Walker et al, 1981a), illness requiring hospitalization (Walker et al, 1981b; Petitti et al, 1982), or biochemical alterations (Smith and Paulson, 1980) have been found in more than 15 reports (12 employing matched controls) examining thousands of men** (Schuman et al, 1993).

One of the controversies is the possible link between vasectomy and prostate cancer. **Studies have found an increased risk of prostate cancer in men who had a vasectomy 20 years previously. But two large-scale cohort studies evaluated men from a wide range of socioeconomic strata and did not find a link between vasectomy and prostate cancer.** Another study of vasectomy sequelae found no increased incidence of cancer or other diseases (Schuman et al, 1993).

The most likely explanation for the increased diagnosis of prostate cancer in vasectomized men is detection bias. Vasectomized men are more likely to visit a urologist and, therefore, are more likely to have cancer diagnosed earlier. Further, men who choose to undergo vasectomy may be more likely to seek health care, increasing their opportunity for prostate cancer detection. **A recent multidisciplinary National Institutes of Health panel concluded that the epidemiologic associations between vasectomy and prostate cancer are weak. It recommended no change in clinical or public health practice and said that screening for prostate cancer should not be any different for vasectomized men** (Healy, 1993).

Nevertheless, men seeking vasectomy should be informed of these and other related studies and be counseled about the controversies. The American Urological Association now recommends annual digital rectal examination and serum prostate-specific antigen assay for men who had a vasectomy more than 20 years ago or who were older than 40 at the time of vasectomy.

VASOVASOSTOMY

The number of American men who undergo vasectomy has remained stable at about 500,000 per year, as has the divorce rate of 50%. Surveys suggest that 2% to 6% of vasectomized men will ultimately seek reversal. Furthermore, obstructive azoospermia is the result of iatrogenic injuries to the vas deferens (usually from hernia repair) in 6% of azoospermic men (Hendin et al, 1992).

Preoperative Evaluation

Physical Examination

1. Testis: Small or soft testes suggest impaired spermatogenesis and predict a poor outcome.
2. Epididymis: An indurated irregular epididymis often predicts secondary epididymal obstruction, necessitating vasoepididymostomy.
3. Sperm granuloma: **A sperm granuloma at the testicular end of the vas means sperm have been leaking at the vasectomy site. This vents the high pressures away from the epididymis and probably improves the prognosis for restored fertility** regardless of the time interval since vasectomy.
4. Vasal gap: When a very destructive vasectomy has

been performed, most of the scrotal straight vas may be absent or fibrotic and the patient should be advised that inguinal extension of the scrotal incision is necessary to enable a tension-free anastomosis.

5. Scars from previous surgery: Operative scars in the inguinal or scrotal region should alert one to the possibility of iatrogenic vasal or epididymal obstruction.

Laboratory Tests

1. **Semen analysis with centrifugation and examination of the pellet for sperm should be performed preoperatively. Complete sperm with tails are found in 10% of preoperative pellets a mean of 10 years after vasectomy (Lemack and Goldstein, 1996). Under these circumstances, sperm are certain to be found in the vas on at least one side, improving the prognosis for restored fertility.** Men with a low semen volume should have a transrectal ultrasound to alert one to the possibility of ejaculatory duct obstruction.

2. Serum and antisperm antibody studies: The presence of serum antisperm antibodies corroborates the diagnosis of obstruction and the presence of active spermatogenesis.

3. Serum FSH: Men with small soft testes should have serum FSH measured. An elevated FSH predicts impaired spermatogenesis and a poorer prognosis.

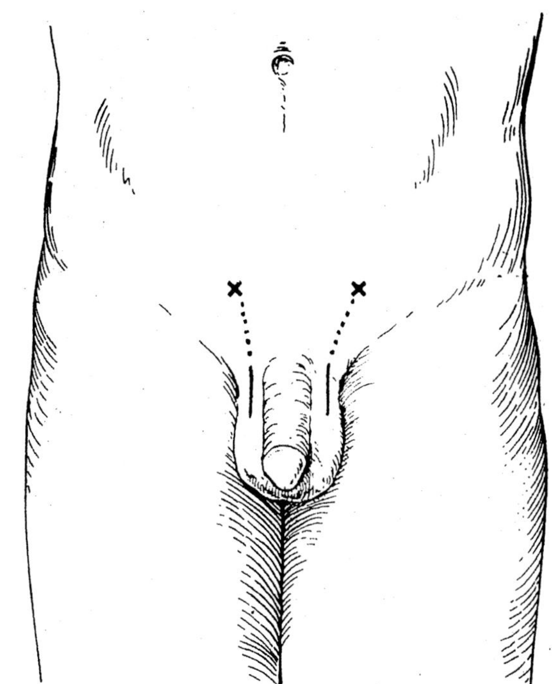

Figure 44–23. Preferred incisions for vasectomy reversal allow extension to external inguinal ring (marked by *X*) when abdominal vas is short.

Anesthesia

Light general anesthesia is preferred. In cooperative patients, regional or even local anesthesia with sedation can be employed if the time interval since vasectomy is short, the vasal ends are easily palpable, or a sperm granuloma is present, decreasing the likelihood of secondary epididymal obstruction. Slight movements are greatly magnified by the operating microscope and disturb performance of the anastomosis. When large vasal gaps are present, extensions of the incisions into the inguinal canal may be necessary. Furthermore, if vasoepididymostomy is necessary, the operating time could exceed 4 or 5 hours. **Local anesthesia limits the options available to the surgeon.** Hypobaric spinal anesthesia with long-acting agents such as bupivacaine (Marcaine) can provide 4 to 5 hours of anesthesia time and has the advantage of eliminating lower body motion. Epidural anesthesia with an indwelling catheter can be equally effective.

Surgical Approaches

Scrotal

Bilateral high vertical scrotal incisions provide the most direct access to the obstructed site in cases of vasectomy reversal. Length is usually a problem on the abdominal end but not the testicular end. Mark the location of the external inguinal ring (Fig. 44–23). **If the vasal gap is large or the vasectomy site is high, this incision can easily be extended inguinally toward the external ring.** If the vasectomy site is low, it is easy to pull up the testicular end. This incision should be made at least 1 cm lateral to the base of the penis. **The testis should be delivered with the tunica vaginalis left intact.** This method provides excellent exposure of the entire scrotal vas deferens and, if necessary, the epididymis.

Infrapubic Incision

An infrapubic incision provides excellent exposure when the abdominal end of the vas is short but is awkward when vasoepididymostomy is necessary. It also may give the false impression that there is no tension on the anastomosis when vasal gaps are large. There is no advantage over inguinal extension of a high scrotal incision.

Inguinal Incision

An inguinal incision is the preferred approach in men with suspected obstruction of the inguinal vas deferens from prior herniorrhaphy or orchiopexy. Incision through the previous scar usually leads directly to the site of obstruction. If the obstruction turns out to be scrotal or epididymal, it is a simple matter to deliver the testis through the inguinal incision or through a separate scrotal incision.

Preparation of the Vasa

The vas is grasped above and below the site of obstruction with two Babcock clamps. Penrose drains replace the Babcock clamps and facilitate the dissection. The vasal vessels and periadventitial sheath are included. The vas is mobilized enough to allow a tension-free anastomosis. In order to preserve good blood supply, **the vas should not be stripped of its sheath.** The obstructed segment and, if present, sperm granuloma at the vasectomy site should be dissected out and excised. By staying right on the vas or sperm granuloma, or both, during this dissection, the risk of injuring the testicular artery is reduced. **Injury to adjacent cord structures, especially the testicular artery, is likely to result in testicular atrophy because the vasal artery has usually been interrupted at the vasectomy site.**

When large vasal gaps are present, a gauze-wrapped index finger is used to separate the cord structures from the vas. Blunt finger dissection through the external ring will free the vas to the internal inguinal ring if additional abdominal length is necessary. These maneuvers will leave all the vasal vessels intact. **When the vasal gap is extremely large, additional length can be achieved by dissecting the entire convoluted vas free of its attachments to the epididymal tunic** (Fig. 44–24), allowing the testis to drop upside down. These maneuvers can provide an additional 4 to 6 cm of length. In order to maintain the integrity of the vasal vessels, this dissection is best performed using magnifying loupes or the operating microscope under low power. If the amount of vas removed is so large that even these measures fail to allow a tension-free anastomosis, the incision can be extended to the internal inguinal ring, the floor of the inguinal canal cut, and the vas rerouted under the floor, as in a difficult orchiopexy. An additional 4 to 6 cm of length can be obtained by dissecting the epididymis off of the testis from the vasoepididymal (VE) junction to the caput epididymis (Fig. 44–25). The superior epididymal vessels are left intact and provide adequate blood supply to the testicular end of the vas. With this combination of maneuvers, 15-cm gaps can be bridged.

After the vasa have been freed, the testicular end of the vas is cut tranversely. An ultrasharp knife drawn through a slotted 2- to 3-mm diameter nerve clamp (Accurate Surgical and Scientific Instrument Corp., Westbury, NY) yields a perfect 90-degree cut (Fig. 44–26). The cut surface of the testicular end of the vas deferens is inspected using 8- to 15-power magnification. **A healthy white mucosal ring that springs back immediately after gentle dilation should be seen. The muscularis should be smooth and soft, not gritty.** The cut surface should look like a bull's eye, with the three vasal layers distinctly visible. Healthy bleeding should be noted from both the cut edge of the mucosa as well as the surface of the muscularis. If the blood supply is poor or the muscularis is gritty, the vas is recut until healthy

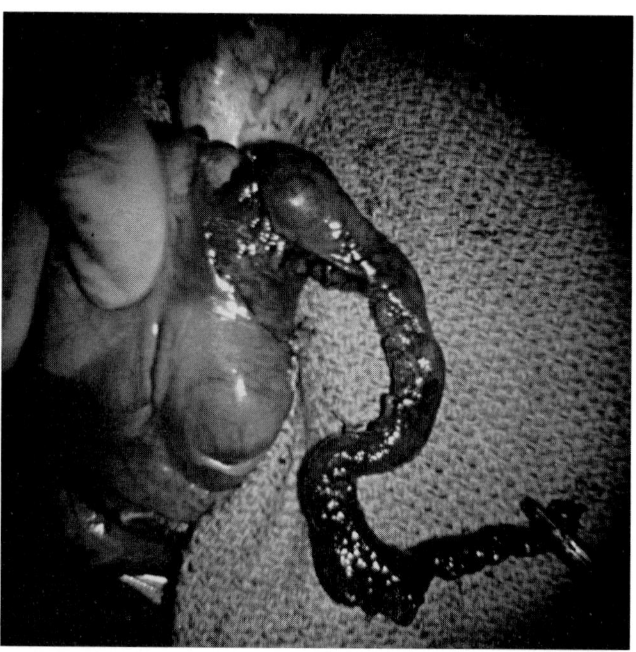

Figure 44–25. Entire vasoepididymal complex dissected to caput epididymis to bridge massive vasal gaps.

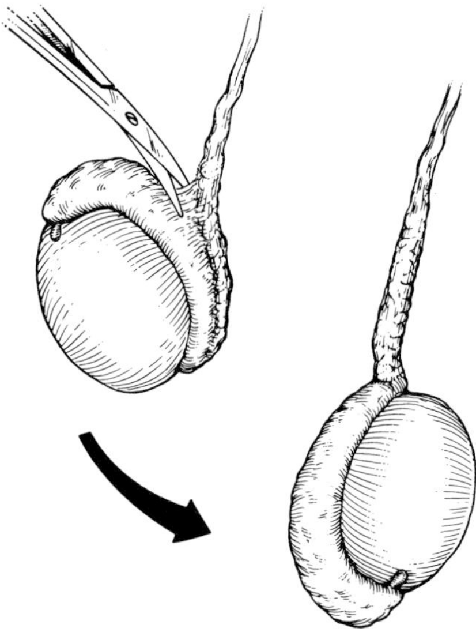

Figure 44–24. Convoluted vas dissected off of epididymal tunic provides additional length on testicular side.

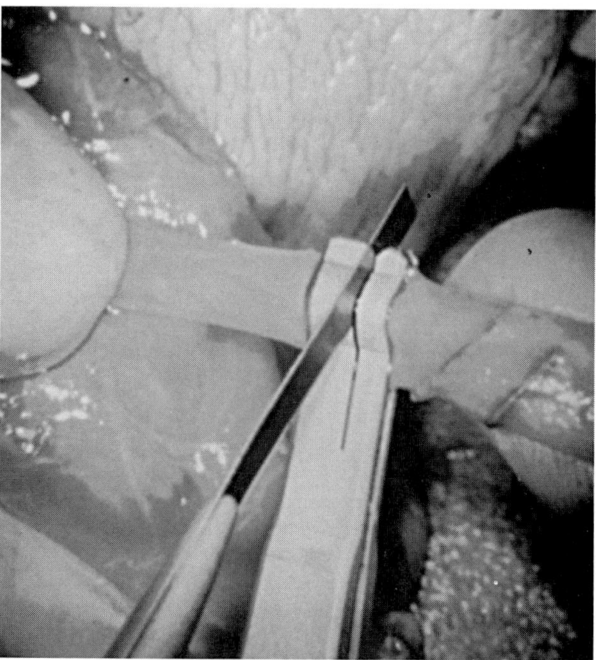

Figure 44–26. Ultrasharp knife drawn through a 2- to 3-mm slotted nerve holding clamp (from Accurate Surgical and Scientific Instrument Corporation, Westbury, NY) produces a perfect 90-degree cut.

tissue is found. The vasal artery and vein are then clamped and ligated with 6-0 polypropylene. Small bleeders are controlled with a microbipolar forcep set at low power. Once a patent lumen has been established on the testicular end, the vas is milked and a clean glass slide is touched to its surface. The vasal fluid is immediately mixed with a drop or two of saline or Ringer's lactate and preserved under a coverslip for microscopic examination. The abdominal end of the vas deferens is prepared in a similar manner, and the lumen is gently dilated with a microvessel dilator and is cannulated with a 24-gauge angiocatheter sheath. Injection of saline or Ringer's lactate confirms its patency. **A minimum of instrumentation of the mucosa should be performed.**

After preparation, the ends of the vasa are stabilized with a Microspike approximating clamp (Goldstein, 1985) to remove all tension prior to performing the anastomosis. Isolating the field through a slit in a rubber dam prevents microsutures from sticking to the surrounding tissue. A sterile tongue blade covered with a large Penrose drain is placed beneath the ends of the vasa to provide a platform on which to perform the anastomosis.

When to Perform Vasoepididymostomy

The gross appearance of fluid expressed from the testicular end of the vas is usually predictive of findings on microscopic examination (Table 44–1). If microscopic examination of the vasal fluid reveals the presence of sperm with tails, vasovasostomy is performed. If no fluid is found, a 24-gauge angiocatheter sheath is inserted into the lumen of the testicular end of the vas and barbotaged with 0.1 ml of saline while the convoluted vas is vigorously milked. The barbotage fluid is expressed onto a slide and examined. **Men with large sperm granulomas often have virtually no dilation of the testicular end of the vas and little or no fluid initially; however, with barbotage and vigorous milking, invariably sperm can be found in this scant fluid.** If there is no sperm granuloma, and the vas is absolutely dry and spermless after multiple samples are examined, vasoepididymostomy is indicated. If the fluid expressed from the vas is found to be thick, white, water insoluble, and toothpaste like in quality, microscope examination rarely reveals sperm. Under these circumstances, the tunica vaginalis is opened and the epididymis inspected. If clear evidence of obstruction is found, that is, an epididymal sperm granuloma with dilated tubules above and collapsed tubules below, vasoepididymostomy is performed. **When the surgeon is in doubt or if he or she not experienced with vasoepididymostomy, vasovasostomy should be performed.** In about 30% of men with bilateral absence of sperm in the vasal fluid, sperm returns to the ejaculate after vasovasostomy.

When copious, crystal clear, water-like fluid squirts out from the vas and no sperm are found in this fluid, a vasovasostomy is performed because the likelihood is that sperm will return to the ejaculate after vasovasotomy is performed.

Multiple Vasal Obstructions

If saline injection reveals that the abdominal end of the vas deferens is not patent, a 2-0 nylon or polypropylene suture is gently threaded into the vas lumen to determine the site of obstruction. If the obstruction is within 5 cm of the original vasectomy site, the abdominal end of the vas deferens may be dissected to this site and excised. The incision should then be extended inguinally to free the vas up extensively toward the internal inguinal ring. The testicular end then should also be freed up to the VE junction. If the site of the second obstruction is so far from the vasectomy site that two vasovasostomies are necessary, a single crossed vasovasostomy should be performed to yield one good system. If this is not possible, vasal or epididymal sperm is aspirated into micropipettes and cryopreserved for future IVF with ICSI (see the section entitled Sperm Retrieval Techniques). **Simultaneous vasovasostomies at two separate sites may lead to devascularization of the intervening segment with fibrosis and necrosis.**

Varicocelectomy and Vasovasostomy

When men presenting for vasovasostomy or vasoepididymostomy are found to have significant varicoceles on physical examination, it is tempting to repair the varicoceles at the same time. The surgeon should resist this temptation. **When varicocelectomy is properly performed, all spermatic veins are ligated and the only remaining avenues for testicular venous return are the vasal veins.** In men who have had vasectomy and are presenting for reversal, the vasal veins are likely to be compromised from either the original vasectomy or the reversal itself. Furthermore,

Table 44–1. RELATIONSHIP BETWEEN GROSS APPEARANCE OF VASAL FLUID AND MICROSCOPIC FINDINGS

Vasal Fluid Appearance	Most Common Findings on Microscopic Examination	Surgical Procedure Indicated
Copious, crystal clear, watery	No sperm in fluid	Vasovasostomy
Copious, cloudy thin, water soluble	Usually sperm with tails	Vasovasostomy
Copious, creamy yellow, water soluble	Usually many sperm heads, occasional sperm with short tails	Vasovasostomy
Copious, thick white toothpaste-like, water insoluble	No sperm	Vasoepididymostomy
Scant, white thin fluid	No sperm	Vasoepididymostomy
Dry spermless vas—no granuloma at vasectomy site	No sperm	Vasoepididymostomy
Scant fluid, granuloma present at vasectomy site	Barbotage fluid reveals sperm	Vasovasostomy

the integrity of the vasal artery in those men is also likely to be compromised. Varicocelectomy in such men requires preservation of the testicular artery as the primary remaining testicular blood supply, as well as preservation of some avenue for venous return.

Microscopic varicocelectomy can ensure preservation of the testicular artery in most cases. Deliberate preservation of the cremasteric veins provides venous return. Of 570 men presenting for vasectomy reversal, 19 had large varicoceles (19 left, 7 bilateral). Microsurgical varicocelectomy was performed at the same time as vasovasostomy. The cremasteric veins and the fine network of veins adherent to the testicular artery were left intact for venous return and to minimize the chances of injury to the testicular artery. Postoperatively, 5 of 26 varicoceles recurred (22%) and two testes atrophied (8%) (Goldstein, 1995). This compares to a recurrence rate of 1% and no cases of atrophy in 640 varicocelectomies performed by the author in nonvasectomized men in whom the vasal vessels were intact and the cremasteric veins and periarterial venous network were ligated.

Because of the significantly increased risk of testicular atrophy and varicocele recurrence, **varicocelectomy should usually not be performed at the same time as vasovasostomy or vasoepididymostomy**. The vasovasostomy or vasoepidymostomy should be performed first. The semen quality should then be assessed postoperatively. If necessary, varicocelectomy can be safely performed 6 months or more later, when venous and arterial channels have formed across the anastomotic line. This two-stage delayed approach has been completed a dozen times with no atrophy or recurrence. The varicocelectomy should be performed microscopically to preserve the testicular artery, because atrophy can occur after testicular artery ligation, even when the vasal blood supply to the testis is intact.

Interestingly, the marked increase in recurrences when the cremasteric veins and periarterial venous network were left intact suggest that these veins contribute to a significant proportion of recurrences of varicoceles.

Anastomotic Techniques: Keys to Success

All successful vasovasostomy techniques depend on adherence to surgical principles that are universally applicable to anastomoses of all tubular structures. These principles include accurate mucosa-to-mucosa approximation, creation of an anastomosis that is leakproof and tension free, provision of a good blood supply, use of healthy mucosa and muscularis, and use of good atraumatic anastomotic technique.

Accurate Mucosa-to-Mucosa Approximation

In human vasovasostomy, the lumen on the testicular side is usually dilated, often to diameters 3 to 6 times that of the abdominal side. Techniques that work well with lumina of equal diameters may be less successful when applied to lumina of markedly discrepant diameters.

Leakproof Anastomosis

Sperm are highly antigenic and provoke an inflammatory reaction when they escape from the normally intact lining of the excurrent ducts of the male reproductive tract. Extravasated sperm adversely influence the success of vasovasostomy (Hagan and Coffey, 1977). **Unlike blood vessel anastomoses, in which platelets and clotting factors seal the gaps between sutures, vasal and epididymal fluid contains no platelets or clotting factors, so the watertightness of the anastomosis is entirely dependent on the mucosal sutures.**

Tension-Free Anastomosis

When an anastomosis is performed under tension, sperm may appear in the ejaculate for several months after surgery. Ultimately, sperm counts and motility will decrease and azoospermia may ensue. At re-exploration, only a thin fibrotic band is found at the anastomotic site. This can be prevented by adequately freeing up of the end of the vasa and placement of reinforcing sutures in the sheath of the vas.

Good Blood Supply

If the cut vas exhibits poor blood supply, it should be recut until healthy bleeding is encountered. If extensive resection is necessary, additional length should be obtained using the techniques previously described.

Healthy Mucosa and Muscularis

If the mucosa or cut surface of the vas exhibits poor distensibility after dilation, peels away from the underlying muscularis, or shreds easily, then the vas should be cut back until healthy mucosa is found. If the muscularis is found to be fibrotic or gritty, the vas must be recut until healthy tissue is found.

Good Atraumatic Anastomotic Technique

If multiple surgical errors occur during the procedure, such as cutting of the mucosa with the needles, tearing through of sutures, or backwalling of the mucosa, the anastomosis should be resected and redone immediately.

Set-Up

An operating microscope providing variable magnification from 6 to 32 power is employed. A diploscope providing identical fields for both surgeon and assistant is preferred. Foot pedal controls for a motorized zoom and focus leave the surgeon's hands free.

Both surgeon and assistant should be comfortably seated on well-padded stools to stabilize the lower body. The author prefers a simple rolling stool with a round bean bag (meditation pillow) taped on top for padding. **Two arm boards, placed on either side of the surgeon and built up to the appropriate height with folded blankets taped to the board, provide excellent arm support and dramati-**

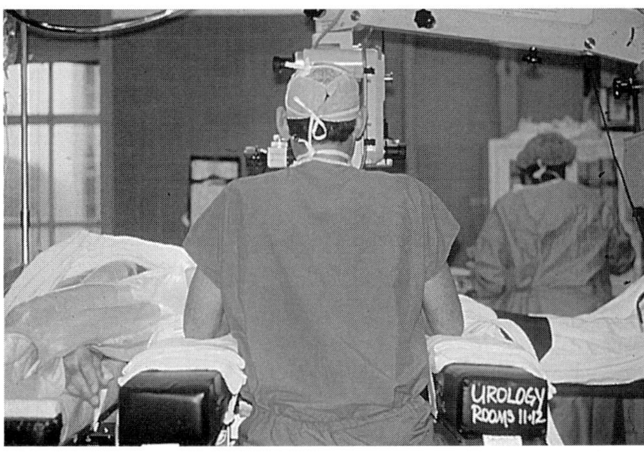

Figure 44–27. Two arm boards, placed on either side of the surgeon and assistant, and built up to the right height with folded blankets taped to the board, provide excellent arm support and dramatically improve stability and accuracy.

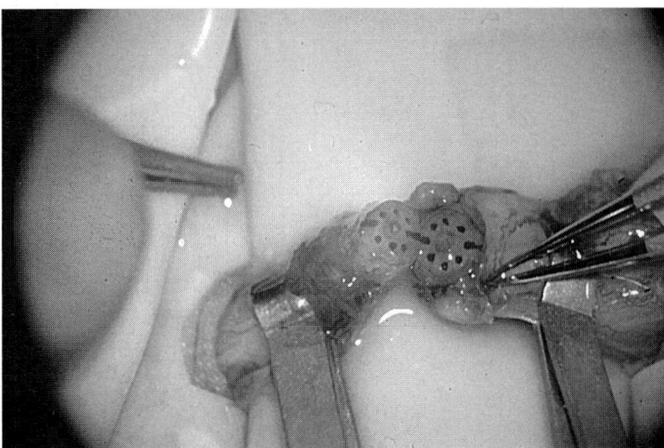

Figure 44–29. Precision placement of sutures is facilitated by drying the cut surface of the vas with a Weck cell and using a microtip marking pen to map out planned needle exit points. Lines are drawn on the most anterior and posterior dots to help match them up. This mapping prevents dog ears and leaks when the lumen diameters are discrepant.

cally improve stability and accuracy (Fig. 44–27). This set-up is flexible and maneuverable and is a fraction of the cost of cumbersome electric microsurgery chairs. **If you are a right-handed surgeon, sit on the patient's right side,** so your forehand stitch is always on the smaller, more difficult abdominal side lumen.

Microsurgical Multilayer Microdot Method

This method of vasovasostomy can handle lumina of markedly discrepant diameters in the straight or convoluted vas. **The microdot technique ensures precise suture placement by exact mapping of each planned suture. The microdot method separates the planning from the placement.** This approach allows focus on only one task at a time and results in dramatically improved accuracy.

A microtip marking pen (Devon Skin Marker Extra Fine #151; 1-800-DEVON PO) is used to map out planned needle exit points. **Exactly eight mucosal sutures are used for every anastomosis** (Fig. 44–28) because it is easy to map out and always results in a leakproof closure, even when the lumen diameters are discrepant.

Immediately after drying, the cut surface of the testicular end of vas with a Weck cell, a dot is made at 3 o'clock, halfway between the mucosal ring and the outer edge of the muscle layer. A line is extended out from this dot to serve as a reference point. The second dot is made at 9 o'clock, and a line is extended from this dot as well. Additional dots are at 12 o'clock and 6 o'clock. Finally, four more dots are evenly spaced between each of these. The abdominal end of the vas is marked in the same way to exactly match the testicular end (Fig. 44–29). Monofilament 10-0 polypropylene sutures, double-armed with 70-μ diameter taper-point needles bent into a fishhook configuration (available from Sharpoint and Ethicon) are used. **Double-armed sutures allow inside-out placement (Fig. 44–30), eliminating the need for manipulation or dilation of the mucosa and the possibility of backwalling.** If the mucosal rings are not sharply defined, stain the cut surfaces of the vasal ends with indigo carmine to highlight the mucosa. The anastomosis is begun with the placement of four 10-0 mucosal sutures anteriorly (Fig. 44–31). If the mucosal edges of the small abdominal side lumen are not clearly visualized, gently and momentarily dilate the lumen with a microvessel dilator just prior to placement of the sutures. For accurate mucosal approximation, include only a small amount of mucosa but half the muscle wall thickness. **Include exactly the same amount of tissue in the bites on each side. The needle**

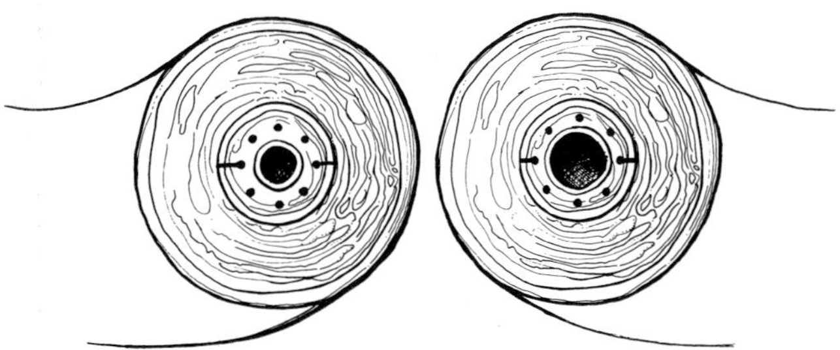

Figure 44–28. Location of eight mucosal sutures is indicated.

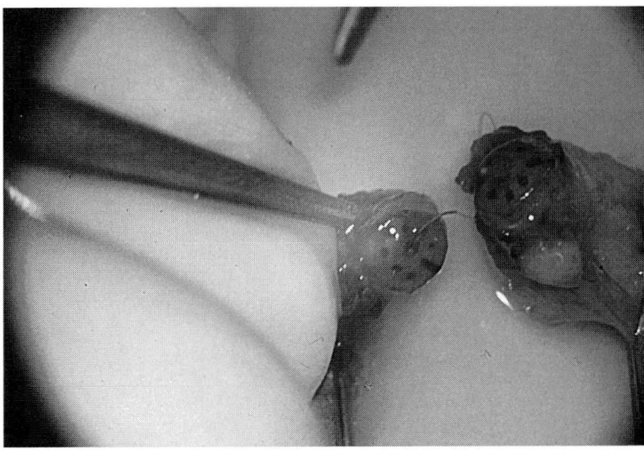

Figure 44–30. Inside-out placement of mucosal sutures using double-armed fishhook-shaped needles.

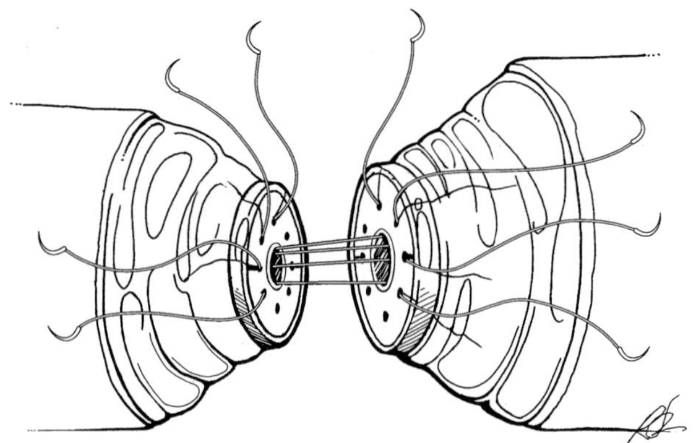

Figure 44–31. Placement of first four mucosal sutures. Sutures exit through microdots.

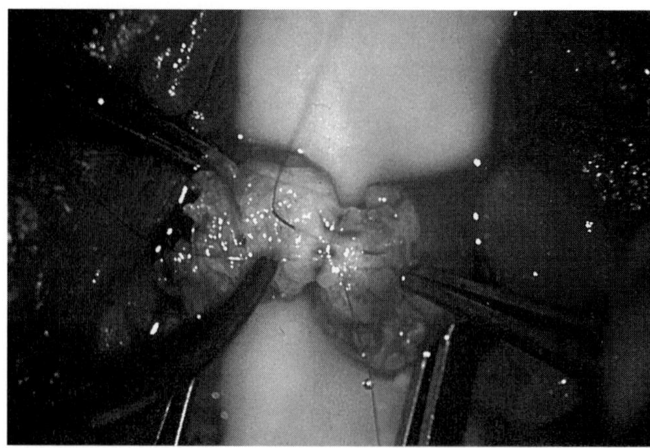

Figure 44–33. Placement of 9-0 sutures just above but not through the mucosa to seal gaps between mucosal sutures.

should exit through the center of each dot. After placement, tie the four mucosal sutures. Place three 9-0 monofilament polypropylene deep muscularis sutures exactly in between the previously placed mucosal sutures just above but not through the mucosa (Fig. 44–32) and then tie them. These sutures seal the gaps between the mucosal sutures (Fig. 44–33) without trauma to the mucosa from the larger 100-μ diameter cutting needle required to penetrate the tough vas muscularis and adventitia. Rotate the vas 180 degrees (Fig. 44–34) and place four additional 10-0 sutures through each microdot and then tie them to complete the mucosal portion of the anastomosis (Figs. 44–35 and 44–36). Just prior to tying the last mucosal suture (Fig. 44–37), irrigate the lumen with heparinized Ringer's lactate to prevent the formation of clot in the lumen. After completion of the mucosal layer, place five more 9-0 deep muscularis sutures exactly in between each mucosal suture just above but not penetrating the mucosa. **Place each 9-0 suture, cut it long, place the next one, cut it long, then tie the previously placed suture.** Leave the previously placed 9-0 untied until the next 9-0 suture is placed. This facilitates more accurate placement (Fig. 44–38). Finish the anastomosis by approximating the vasal sheath with six to eight interrupted sutures of 6-0 polypropylene (Fig. 44–39*A*). This layer completely covers the anastomosis, relieving it of all tension (see Fig. 44–39*B*).

Anastomosis in the Convoluted Vas

Vasovasostomy performed in the convoluted portion of the vas deferens is technically more demanding than anastomoses in the straight portion. Fear of cutting back into the convoluted vas in order to obtain healthy tissue may lead surgeons to complete an anastomosis in the straight portion when the testicular end of the vas has poor blood supply, unhealthy or friable mucosa, or gritty fibrotic muscularis. Adherence to the following principles will enable anastomosis in the convoluted vas to succeed as often as those in the straight portion:

1. A perfect transverse cut yielding a round ring of mucosa and a lumen directed straight down is essential (Fig. 44–40*A*). A very oblique lumen with a thin flap of muscle and mucosa on one side is not acceptable (see Fig. 44–40*B*). The vas should be recut at 0.5-mm intervals until a perfect cut with good blood supply and healthy tissue is obtained. A slotted nerve clamp 2.5 or 3 mm in diameter and ultrasharp knife facilitates this part of the procedure (see Fig. 44–26). Often, the vas must be recut two or three times until a satisfactory or proper cut is obtained.

2. The convoluted vas should not be unraveled. This disturbs the blood supply at the anastomotic line.

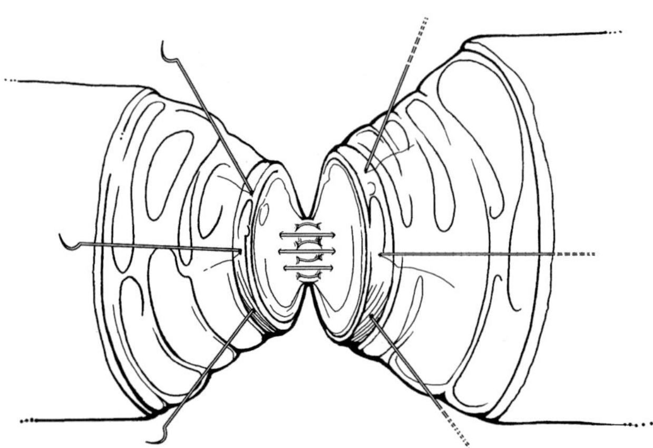

Figure 44–32. Deep mucularis sutures placed between mucosal sutures.

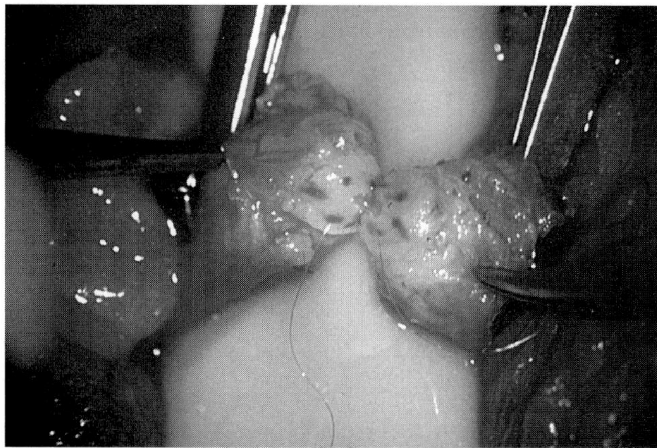

Figure 44–34. Appearance of anastomosis after vas is rotated 180 degrees.

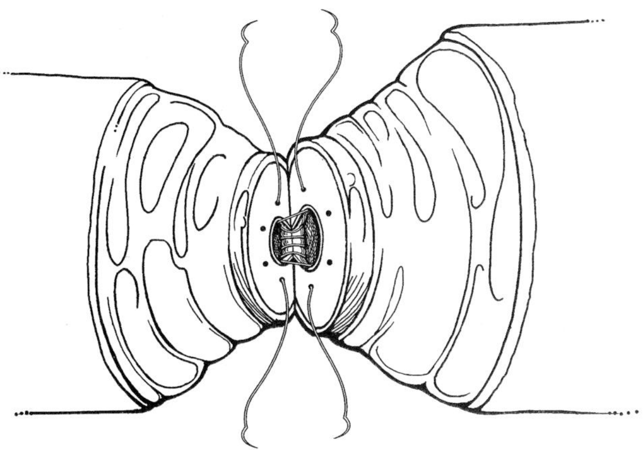

Figure 44–35. Scheme for placement of four additional mucosal sutures.

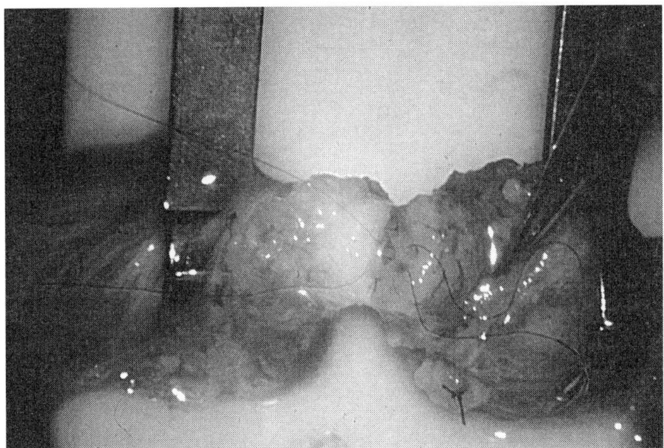

Figure 44–37. Mucosal layer nearing completion. Note absence of dog ears.

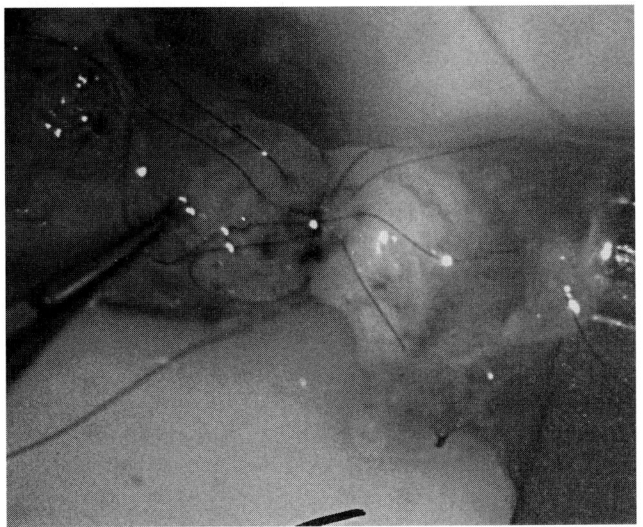

Figure 44–36. Placement of four additional 10-0 mucosal sutures. Note sutures exit through microdots.

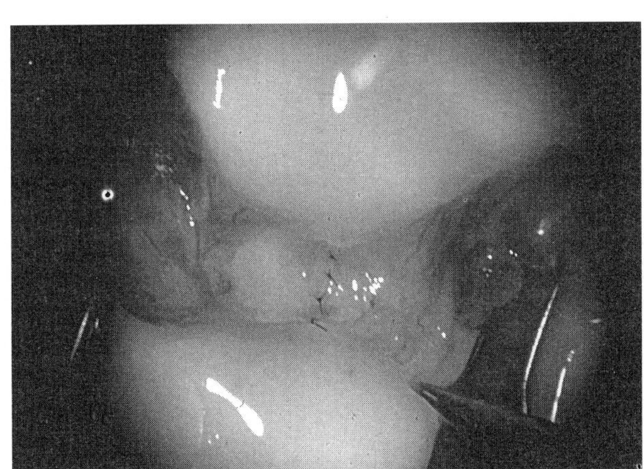

Figure 44–38. Completed 9-0 layer.

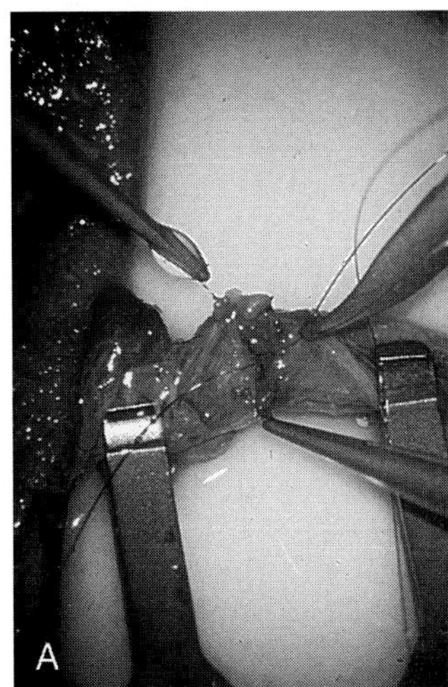

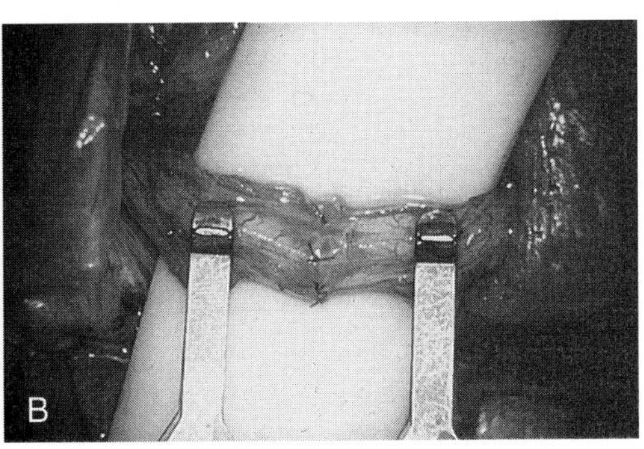

Figure 44–39. *A* and *B*, Approximation of vasal sheath with 6-0 polypropylene sutures.

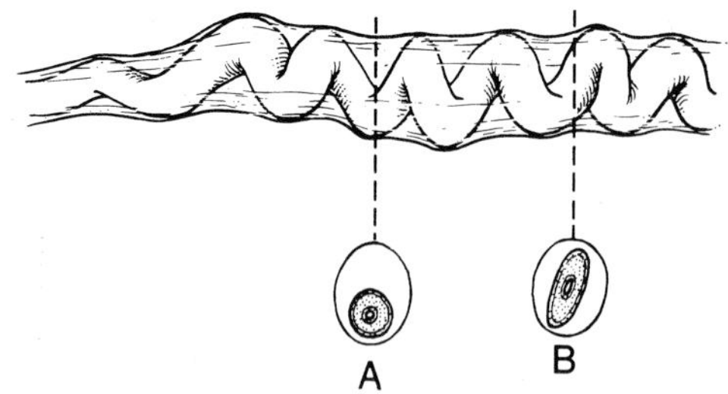

Figure 44–40. *A*, Round lumen essential for success in convoluted anastomoses. *B*, Oblique cut is not acceptable.

3. The sheath of the convoluted vas may be carefully dissected free of its attachments to the epididymal tunic (see Fig. 44–24). This will minimize disturbance of its blood supply and provide the necessary length to perform a tension-free anastomosis.
4. Care must be taken to avoid taking large bites of the muscularis and adventitial layers on the convoluted side to prevent inadvertent perforation of adjacent convolutions.
5. Reinforce the anastomosis by approximating the vasal sheath of the straight portion to the sheath of the convoluted portion with six to eight polypropylene sutures. This will remove all tension from the anastomosis.

Crossed Vasovasostomy

This is a useful procedure that often provides an easy solution for otherwise difficult problems (Lizza et al, 1985, Hamidinia, 1988). Crossover vasovasostomy is indicated in the following circumstances:

1. Unilateral inguinal obstruction of the vas deferens associated with an atrophic testis on the contralateral side.
2. Unilateral obstruction or aplasia of the inguinal vas or ejaculatory duct and contralateral obstruction of the epididymis.

It is preferable to perform one anastomosis with a high probability of success (vasovasostomy) than two operations with a much lower chance of success, such as unilateral vasovasoepididymostomy and contralateral TUR of the ejaculatory ducts.

3. In general, opt for one good anastomosis instead of two mediocre ones. Opt for one good vasovasostomy rather than a unilateral vasoepididymostomy and contralateral mediocre vasovasostomy.

Technique

Transect the vas attached to the atrophic testis at the junction of its straight and convoluted portion, and confirm its patency with a saline or methylene blue vasogram (Fig. 44–41). Dissect the contralateral vas toward the inguinal obstruction. Clamp it as high up as possible with a right angle clamp. Transect it and cross it through a capacious opening made in the scrotal septum and proceed with vasovasostomy, as described above. This procedure is much easier than trying to find both ends of the vas within the dense scar of a previous inguinal operation.

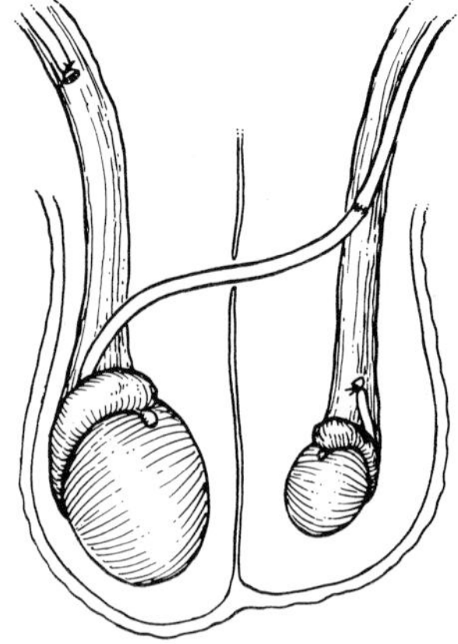

Figure 44–41. Transseptal crossed vasovasostomy.

Transposition of the Testis

Occasionally, when vasal length is critically short, a tension-free crossed anastomosis can best be accomplished by testicular transposition (Fig. 44–42).

Wound Closure

If the vasal dissection was extensive, Penrose drains are brought out through the dependent portion of the right and left hemiscrota and fixed in place with sutures and safety pins prior to beginning the anastomosis. Placement of drains at the end of the procedure may potentially disturb the anastomosis. The dartos muscle is loosely approximated with interrupted absorbable sutures and the skin with subcuticular sutures of 5-0 Monocryl. The wound heals with a fine scar and none of the railroad tracks associated with through-and-through skin closures. **Virtually all of our procedures are performed on an ambulatory basis.** If drains were placed, the patients are given detailed instructions (with explicit drawings) on how to remove the drains the next morning.

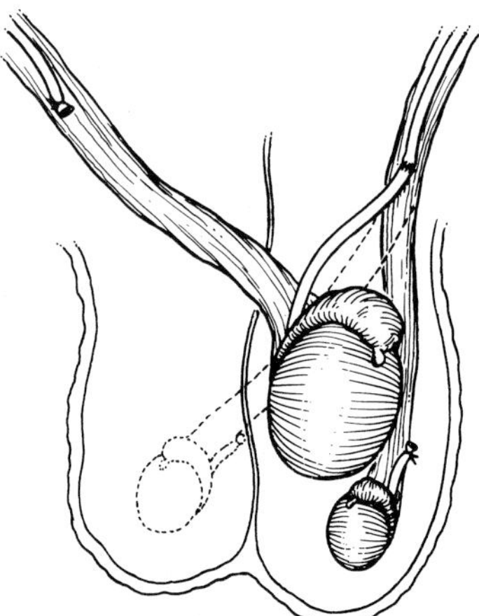

Figure 44–42. Testicular transposition.

Postoperative Management

Sterile fluffs are held in place with a snug-fitting scrotal supporter. Only perioperative antibiotics are used. Patients are discharged with a prescription for Tylenol with codeine. They shower 48 hours after surgery. **They wear a scrotal supporter at all times (except in the shower), even when sleeping, for 6 weeks postoperatively. Thereafter, a comfortable scrotal supporter is worn whenever the patient is upright, until pregnancy is achieved.** Desk work is resumed in 3 days. No heavy work or sports are allowed for 3 weeks. **No intercourse or ejaculation is allowed for 4 weeks postoperatively.** Semen analyses are obtained at 1, 3, and 6 months postoperatively and every 6 months thereafter. If azoospermia persists at 6 months, the procedure will have to be redone or a vasoepididymostomy will be necessary.

Postoperative Complications

The most common complication is hematoma. In 1300 operations, seven small hematomas occurred. None required surgical drainage. Most were walnut sized and perivasal. They take 6 to 12 weeks to resolve if wound infection has not occurred. Late complications include sperm granuloma at the anastomotic site (~5%). This usually is a harbinger of eventual obstruction. Late stricture and obstruction are disappointingly common (see later). **Progressive loss of motility followed by decreasing counts indicates stricture.** The author's recent switch to **polypropylene sutures** (shown in rat studies to be less reactive than nylon) (Chen et al, 1993), **use of the microdot system to prevent leaks, minimizing disturbance of the vasal blood supply, and use of scrotal support until pregnancy is established may reduce this incidence. Because of the significant rate of late stricture and obstruction, the author strongly encourages cryopreservation of semen specimens as soon as motile sperm appear in the ejaculate.**

Long-Term Follow-Up Evaluation After Vasovasostomy

When sperm are found in the vasal fluid on at least one side at the time of surgery, the anastomotic technique described results in appearance of sperm in the ejaculate in 99% of men (Matthews et al, 1995). **Late obstruction, after initial patency, will occur in 12% of men by 14 months postoperatively** (Matthews et al, 1995). Pregnancy has occurred in 63% of couples followed for at least 2 years when female factors are excluded and sperm were found in the vas on at least one side at the time of vasovasostomy.

SURGERY OF THE EPIDIDYMIS

Detailed knowledge of epididymal anatomy and physiology (presented in Chapter 42) is essential before undertaking surgery of this delicate but important structure. Sperm motility and fertilizing capacity progressively increase during passage through the 200-μ diameter, 12- to 15-foot-long, tightly coiled, single tubule. When the epididymis is obstructed and functionally shortened after vasoepididymostomy, even very short lengths of epididymis are able to adapt and allow some sperm to acquire motility and fertilizing capacity (Silber, 1989; Jow et al, 1993). Adaptation may gradually continue for up to 2 years after surgical reconstruction, with progressive improvement in the fertility and motility of sperm. Nevertheless, preservation of the greatest possible length of functional epididymis is most likely to result in the best sperm quality after vasoepididymostomy (Schoysman and Bedford, 1986). Furthermore, because the wall of the epididymis is thinnest in the caput region and gradually thickens, owing to the increasing numbers of smooth muscle cells in its more distal (inferior) end, anastomoses are technically easier to perform and more likely to succeed in its distal regions. **Because the epididymis is a single tubule with a very small diameter, injury or occlusion of a tubule anywhere along its length will lead to total obstruction of output from that epididymis.** For these reasons, **magnification, with loupes for macrodissection and with the operating microscope for anastomosis, is essential for performing all epididymal surgery.**

Fortunately, the epididymis is blessed with a rich blood supply derived from the testicular vessels superiorly and the deferential vessels inferiorly (see Chapter 42). Because of the extensive interconnections between these branches, either the testicular or deferential branches (but not both) to the epididymis may be divided without compromising epididymal viability.

Conversely, because the epididymal branches of the testicular artery are medial to and separate from the main testicular artery and veins, surgical procedures may be performed on the epididymis without compromise to testicular blood supply.

Epididymectomy

Epididymectomy may be indicated in men with chronic infection or abscess of the epididymis unresponsive to antibiotic therapy. Men with acquired immunodeficiency syndrome (AIDS) may develop cytomegalovirus infection of the epididymis requiring epididymectomy (Randazzo et al, 1986). **Chronic unremitting epididymal pain after vasectomy may be relieved by total epididymectomy** (Selikowitz and Schmed, 1985). All patients should be counseled preoperatively that the procedure may impair their fertility, or render them sterile if bilateral epididymectomy is performed.

Surgical Technique

The testis is delivered through a vertical median raphe or transverse scrotal incision, and the vas deferens isolated at the junction of its straight and convoluted regions, and is doubly ligated and divided, including the deferential vessels. The convoluted vas is then dissected free of its attachments to the epididymal tunic and traced to the VE junction (see Fig. 44–24). The tunica vaginalis is opened, and the dissection is continued in the plane between the epididymis and the testis (see Fig. 44–25). Optical loupe magnification

(2.5 ×) and elevation of the epididymis with an encircling Penrose drain, with transillumination of the mesentery between the testis and epididymis, allows for better visualization of the epididymal blood supply and avoids injury to the spermatic cord vessels that are encountered at the junction of the middle and upper thirds of the testis, entering medial to the epididymis. The efferent ducts, located superior to the testicular vascular pedicle, are ligated with an absorbable suture, and the epididymectomy specimen is removed. The edges of the tunica vaginalis along the base of the resected epididymis should be oversewn with a continuous absorbable suture for hemostasis. The dartos muscle is loosely closed with absorbable sutures, and the skin is closed with a subcuticular 5-0 monofilament absorbable suture.

Spermatocelectomy

A spermatocele is the epididymal equivalent of a berry aneurysm; the lesion may occur anywhere in the epididymis but is more common in the caput region. They are exceedingly common, increasing in frequency with age, and identified incidentally in up to 30% of men undergoing high-resolution scrotal ultrasonography. Intervention for spermatocele is rarely indicated. Spermatoceles are usually painless and do not obstruct the epididymal tubule from which they arise. **Resection of the spermatocele may cause epididymal obstruction.** Spermatocelectomy is indicated when the spermatocele is associated with unremitting pain or when it has grown to a an uncomfortably large size. By definition, spermatoceles contain sperm. Puncture with a 30-g needle and identification of sperm in the aspirated fluid confirm the diagnosis. Stagnant sperm within a spermatocele occasionally leads to antisperm antibody formation, and excision may eliminate these antibodies.

Surgical Technique

The testis is delivered through a median raphe or transverse scrotal incision, and the tunica vaginalis opened. The spermatocele is dissected free of the epididymis using the operating microscope to avoid inadvertent injury to epididymal tubules. The attachment of the spermatocele to the epididymis is ligated with 6-0 polypropylene or monofilament absorbable suture to prevent extravasation of sperm and granuloma formation. The tunica vaginalis is reapproximated with a continuous 5-0 polypropylene suture, and the dartos muscle and skin are closed in two layers.

Excision of Epididymal Tumors and Cysts

Most nontransilluminable epididymal masses are benign adenomatoid tumors. Malignant epididymal tumors are exceedingly rare. Like any potentially malignant testicular mass, they should be managed by inguinal exploration, clamping of the cord, and delivery of the testis. If the diagnosis of malignancy is uncertain, the field should be isolated and cooled with ice prior to opening the tunica vaginalis for direct inspection and biopsy. This modification of Chevassu's maneuver (Goldstein and Waterhouse, 1983) is particularly useful for exploration of epididymal tumors, which are usually benign, and prevents needless orchiectomy. If the diagnosis of malignancy has been excluded, the epididymal tumor or cyst is excised in an identical fashion to that employed for a spermatocele.

Vasoepididymostomy

Before the development of microsurgical techniques, accurate approximation of the vasal lumen to that of a specific epididymal tubule was not possible. Vasoepididymostomy was performed by aligning the vas deferens adjacent to a slash made in multiple epididymal tubules and hoping a fistula would form. Results with this primitive technique were poor. Microsurgical approaches allow accurate approximation of the vasal mucosa to that of a single epididymal tubule (Silber, 1978), resulting in marked improvement in patency and pregnancy rates (Schlegel and Goldstein, 1993). **Microsurgical vasoepididymostomy, however, is the most technically demanding procedure in all of microsurgery.** In virtually no other operation are results so dependent on technical perfection. **Microsurgical vasoepididymostomy should be attempted only by experienced microsurgeons who perform the procedure frequently.**

Indications

The indications for vasoepididymostomy at the time of vasectomy reversal are reviewed in the section entitled Vasovasostomy. For obstructive azoospermia that is not a result of vasectomy, vasoepididymostomy is indicated when the testis biospy reveals complete spermatogenesis and scrotal exploration reveals the absence of sperm in the vasal lumen and no obstruction of the vasa or ejaculatory ducts. The preoperative evaluation is identical to that described in the section entitled Preoperative Evaluation under the heading Vasovasostomy.

Microsurgical End-to-Side Vasoepididymostomy

This is the preferred technique for proximal epididymal obstruction and when vasal length is not compromised.

End-to-side vasoepididymostomy has the advantage of being minimally traumatic to the epididymis and relatively bloodless (Wagenknecht et al, 1980; Krylov and Borovikov, 1984; Fogdestam et al, 1986; Thomas, 1987). **The end-to-side technique does not disturb the epididymal blood supply.** When the level of epididymal obstruction is clearly demarcated by the presence of markedly dilated tubules proximally and collapsed tubules distally, the site at which the anastomosis should be performed is readily apparent. This method obviates the necessity for identifying the single tubule effluxing sperm among the many tubules cut when the epididymis is sectioned transversely. **The end-to-side approach has the advantage of allowing accurate approximation of the muscularis and adventitia of the vas deferens to a precisely tailored opening in the tunic of the epididymis.** This is the preferred technique when vasoepididymostomy is performed simultaneously with inguinal vasovasostomy because it is possible to preserve the vasal blood supply deriving from epididymal branches of the testicular artery (Fig. 44–43). This provides blood supply to the segment of vas intervening between the two anastomoses. Maintenance of the deferential artery's contribution to the testicular blood supply is also important in situations in which the integrity of testicular artery is in doubt owing to previous surgery such as orchiopexy, nonmicroscopic varicocelectomy, or hernia repair.

The testis is delivered through a 3- to 4-cm high vertical scrotal incision. The vas deferens is identified, isolated with a Babcock clamp, and then surrounded with a Penrose drain at the junction of the straight and convoluted portions of the vas deferens. Using 8- to 15-power magnification provided by the operating microscope, the vasal sheath is vertically incised with a microknife and a bare segment of vas stripped of its carefully preserved vessels is delivered. The vas is hemitransected with the ultrasharp knife until the lumen is entered (see Fig. 44–3). **The vasal fluid is sampled. If microscopic examination of this fluid reveals the absence of sperm, the diagnosis of epididymal obstruction is confirmed.** Saline vasography is performed by cannulating the abdominal end of the vas with a 24-g angiocatheter sheath to confirm patency of the vas and ejaculatory ducts (see Fig. 44–4). The vas is then completely transected using a 2.5-mm slotted nerve clamp (see Fig. 44–26), and the vas is prepared for vasovasostomy, as described earlier (see the section entitled Preparation of the Vasa).

After opening the tunica vaginalis, the epididymis is inspected under the operating microscope. An anastomotic site is selected above the area of suspected obstruction, proximal to any visible sperm granulomas, where dilated epididymal tubules are clearly seen beneath the epididymal tunic. A relatively avascular area is grasped with sharp jeweler's forceps, and the epididymal tunic tented upward. **A 3- to 4-**

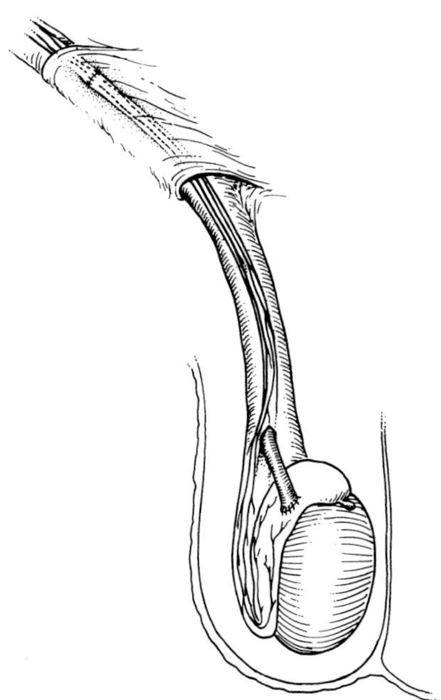

Figure 44–43. Simultaneous inguinal vasovasostomy and scrotal vasoepididymostomy with preservation of the vasal branches of the epididymal artery.

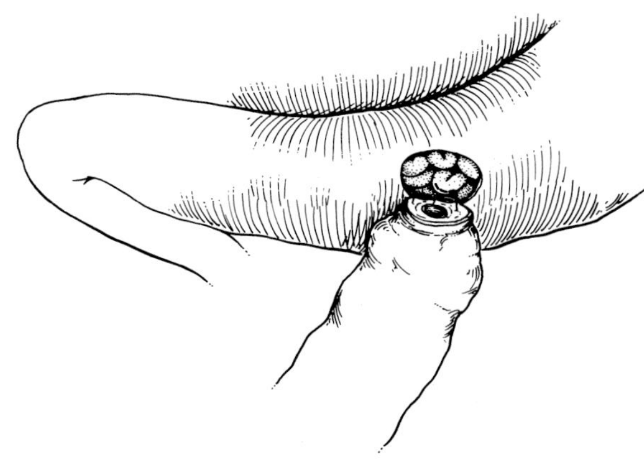

Figure 44–44. Preparation for end-to-side vasoepididymostomy. The 9-0 sutures approximate the posterior lip of the vasal adventitia to the lower edge of the opening tailored in the epididymal tunic.

mm buttonhole is made in the tunic with microscissors to create a round opening that matches the outer diameter of the previously prepared vas deferens. The tubules are then gently dissected with a combination of sharp and blunt dissection until dilated loops of tubule are clearly exposed.

The vas deferens is drawn through an opening in the tunica vaginalis and secured in proximity to the anastomotic site with two to four interrupted sutures of 6-0 polypropylene placed through the vasal adventitia and the tunica vaginalis. **The vasal lumen should reach the opening in the epididymal tunic easily with length to spare.** The posterior edge of the epididymal tunic is then approximated to the posterior edge of the vas muscularis and adventitia with three interrupted sutures of double-armed 9-0 nylon (Fig. 44–44). This is done in such a way as to bring the vasal lumen in close approximation to the epididymal tubule selected for anastomosis. Under 25 to 32 power magnification, using small curved microscissors, an opening about 0.3 to 0.5 mm in diameter is made in the selected tubule by buttonholing a tiny window. Epididymal fluid is touched to a slide, diluted with saline or Ringer's lactate, and inspected under the microsope for sperm. If no sperm are found, the opening in the tubule is closed with 10-0 sutures, the vas detached, and the tunic incision closed with 9-0 nylon. The procedure is then repeated more proximally in the epididymis.

Once sperm are identified, they are aspirated with glass capillary tubes and flushed into media for cryopreservation (see Fig. 44–51, in the section entitled Open Tubule Technique) (Matthews et al, 1995). **Methylene blue solution is dripped on the cut tubule to outline the mucosa.** The posterior mucosal edge of the epididymal tubule is approximated to the posterior edge of the vasal mucosa with two interrupted sutures of 10-0 monofilament polypropylene sutures double armed with fishhook 70-μ diameter tapered needles (Fig. 44–45). The lumen is irrigated with Ringer's solution just prior to placement of each suture to keep the epididymal lumen open. After these mucosal sutures are tied, the anterior mucosal anastomosis is completed with three to four additional 10-0 sutures. Use the system shown in Figure 44–48 to prevent a confusing tangle of untied sutures. The outer muscularis and adventitia of the vas are then approximated to the cut edge of the epididymal tunic

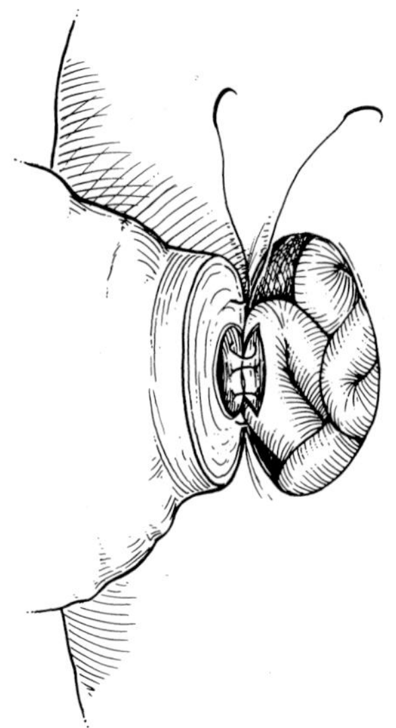

Figure 44–45. Posterior row of 10-0 mucosal sutures placed inside out.

with 8 to 12 additional interrupted sutures of 9-0 nylon double armed with 100-μ diameter needles (Fig. 44–46). The vasal sheath is secured to the epididymal tunic with three to five sutures of 9-0 or 6-0 polypropylene. The testis and epididymis are gently returned to the tunica vaginalis, which is closed with 5-0 polypropylene. Penrose drains are usually not necessary. The scrotum is closed as previously described.

Microsurgical Vasoepididymostomy: End-to-End Anastomosis

An end-to-end operation is the preferred technique for obstructions in the cauda epididymis and at or near the VE junction. At this point, the outer diameter of the epididymis is narrower and more closely matches that of the vas deferens. In addition, there is more muscle around the epididymis distally and the anastomosis resembles a vasovasostomy in the convoluted vas. Furthermore, it is possible to perform a more distal anastomosis when the epididymis is dissected completely to the VE junction and transversely sectioned. An end-to-side operation cannot be performed easily in the distal cauda of the epididymis, near the VE junction, especially if the vas is short as in vasectomy reversal.

An end-to-end anastomosis is also useful when vasal length is compromised and the epididymis is obstructed distally, a situation commonly encountered during vasectomy reversal. If the epididymis is obstructed distally, it can be dissected off of the testis right up to the efferent ductules, if necessary, and flipped up to provide 3 to 5 cm of additional length (see Fig. 44–25). The superior epididymal branches of the epididymal artery are preserved and provide excellent blood supply to the distal epididymis.

The correct level in the epididymis at which the anastomosis should be performed can be more rapidly and accurately assessed with an end-to-end technique. The epididymis is rapidly, serially transected at 1- to 2-mm intervals until a tubule with high flow and good quality fluid containing abundant sperm is found. In contrast, with end-to-side operations, the opening in the tunic must first be prepared and the tubule dissected out before opening the tubule.

Surgical Technique for Microsurgical End-to-End Vasoepididymostomy

When end-to-end vasoepididymostomy is performed, it is particularly important to avoid stripping the vas of its sheath. The vas should be sectioned with as much sheath and periadventitial tissue left attached to the vas as possible. This is critical for completing the outer layer of the anastomosis, especially in the more proximal epididymis, where the diameter of the epididymal tunic is much larger than that of the stripped vas.

After the vas has been prepared, the tunica vaginalis is opened and the testis delivered. Inspection of the epididymis under the operating microscope may reveal a clearly delineated site of obstruction. Often, a discrete yellow sperm granuloma is noted, above which the epididymis is indurated and the tubules dilated, and below which the epididymis is soft and the tubules collapsed. Under these circumstances, the epididymis is encircled with a small Penrose drain at the level of obstruction and, using 2.5-power loupe magnifica-

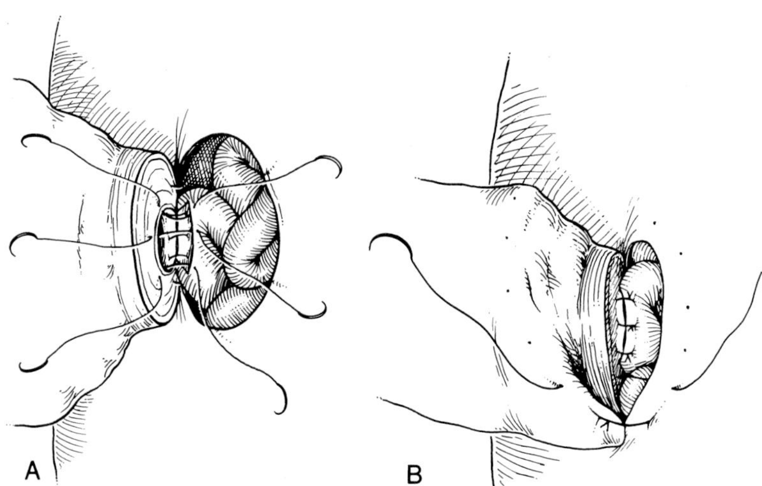

Figure 44–46. After completion of the anterior mucosal portion of the anastomosis *(A),* the second layer of 9-0 nylon sutures is placed to provide a watertight seal *(B).*

tion, is dissected proximally 3 to 5 cm off of the testis, yielding sufficient length to perform the anastomosis. Usually, a nice plane can be found between the epididymis and testis, and injury to the epididymal blood supply can be avoided by staying right on the tunica albuginea of the testis. The inferior and, if necessary, middle epididymal branches of the testicular artery are doubly ligated and divided to free up an adequate length of epididymis. The superior epididymal branches entering the epididymis at the caput are always preserved and can provide adequate blood supply to the entire epididymis. The tunica vaginalis is then closed over the testis with 5-0 polypropylene. This method prevents drying of the testis and thrombosis of the surface testicular vessels during the anastomosis. The dissected epididymis remains outside of the tunica vaginalis.

When the site of obstruction is not obvious or the epididymis is indurated and dilated throughout its length, the epididymis is dissected to the VE junction. This dissection is often facilitated by first dissecting the convoluted vas to the VE junction from below, and then, after encircling the epididymis with a Penrose drain, dissecting the epididymis to the VE junction from above. In this way, the entire VE junction can be freed up. This approach will allow preservation of maximal epididymal length in cases of distal obstruction near the VE junction.

When the dissection has been completed, the operating microscope is brought into the field. At the VE junction, or if clearly delineated, at the site of obstruction, the epididymis is encircled with a slotted nerve clamp of appropriate diameter (3–7 mm) and transversely sectioned using an ultrasharp knife (Fig. 44–47). The distal epididymal stump is ligated, and the proximal cut surface of the epididymis inspected under high-power magnification.

The epididymis is serially sectioned until a gush of cloudy fluid is seen effluxing from a single epididymal tubule. After hemostasis has been obtained with a bipolar cautery, a touch prep of epididymal fluid is made, a drop of saline or Ringer's solution is added, and careful microscopic examination of the slide performed. If many sperm are present, the single tubule continually effluxing fluid is identified. **A drop of methylene blue placed on the cut surface of the epididymis helps clearly outline the cut edges of the epididymal tubules.** Defunctionalized tubules empty in seconds and no longer efflux fluid. The tubule effluxing fluid is gently probed with a microvessel dilator to identify the direction of its lumen. **If no sperm are found or if the cut tubule is obliquely sectioned, the epididymis is recut until sperm-bearing fluid is found continually effluxing from a round clearly visualized tubule.** If fluid continuously effluxes from more than one site, a tubule or tubules may have been tangentially cut. The epididymis is sectioned again a few millimeters proximally until efflux is noted from only one round tubule. In the proximal caput, where the six to seven efferent ducts enter the epididymis, fluid may continually efflux from more than one tubule. Pick the tubule with the best flow and most clearly visualized edges. Cauterize the others with the bipolar cautery. **Painstakingly meticulous attention must paid to the attainment of absolutely perfect hemostasis with a very fine-tipped bipolar coagulation forcep.** Major epididymal vessels at the edge of the tunic are ligated with 6-0 polypropylene. **Sperm are aspirated into micropippettes and cryopreserved,** as described later in the section entitled Open Tubule Technique (Matthews and Goldstein, 1996b).

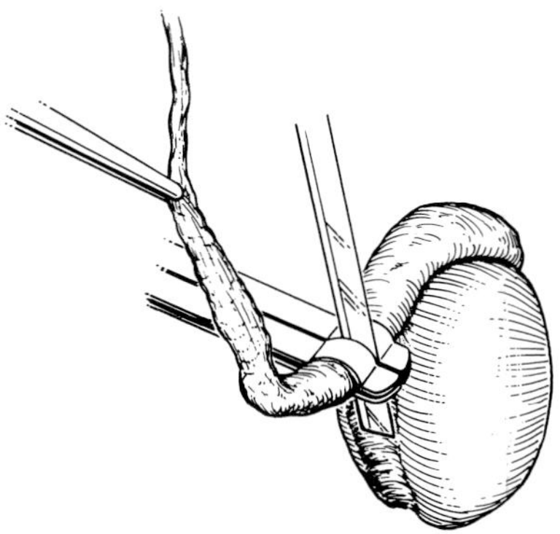

Figure 44–47. Preparation for end-to-end vasoepididymostomy.

The epididymis and vas deferens are stabilized with a Microspike approximating clamp so that the mucosa of the vas and single epididymal tubule are immediately adjacent to each other, kissing. The anastomosis is begun with the placement of two to three posterior mucosal sutures of 10-0 monofilament polypropylene double armed with 70-μ fish-hook–shaped taper-point needles. Inside-out placement of these sutures helps prevent backwalling of the mucosa. Two to four additional anterior mucosal sutures are placed, and all sutures are tied.

To avoid a spaghetti-like tangle of untied sutures, use the following system to identify which end belongs to which: (Fig. 44–48)

Suture 1—Place posteriorly and away, then remove needles from both ends (no needles).
Suture 2—Place posteriorly and near. Leave both needles intact.
Suture 3—Place anterior and away. Straighten both needles.
Suture 4—Place anteriorly and near. Hyperbend both needles.

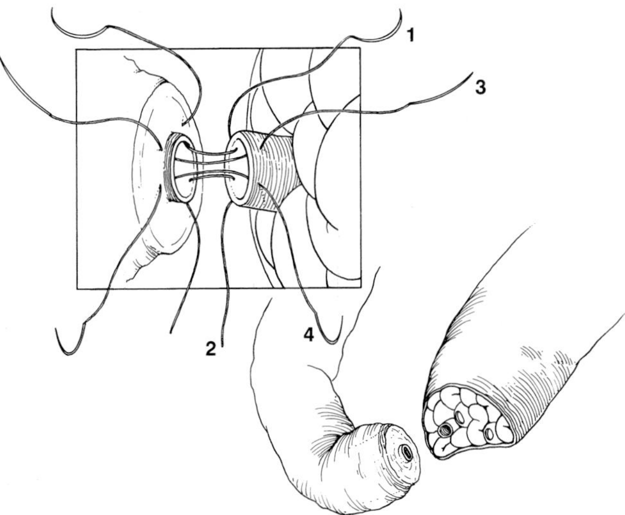

Figure 44–48. The scheme for the placement of 10-0 mucosal sutures for end-to-end vasoepididymostomy.

Tie the sutures according to the order in which they were placed. Fill in any gaps anteriorly with additional sutures. Thin bites are taken of the vasal mucosa to match the amount of tissue included on the epididymal side.

It is important to **avoid taking overly wide bites during placement of epididymal mucosal sutures to prevent inadvertent occlusion of an adjacent convolution of the epididymal tubule.** After completion of the mucosal anastomosis, interrupted 9-0 polypropylene sutures are used to approximate the sheath of the vas deferens to the epididymal tunic (Fig. 44–49). These sutures are placed in such a way as to keep the mucosal anastomosis exactly aligned. Creativity is often required, and 15 to 25 sutures may be necessary to secure a watertight anastomosis. This design will create a situation in which the path of least resistance for epididymal fluid is through the vasal lumen. As during vasovasostomy, persistent leakage of sperm with subsequent granuloma formation is likely to compromise the results of vasoepididymostomy. **Avoid deep bites on the epididymal tunic side to prevent occlusion of a proximal epididymal tubule.**

The anastomosis is now turned over, and additional 9-0 sutures are placed to complete the second layer of the anastomosis. Hemostasis is obtained, and if necessary, Penrose drains are brought out through a dependent location of the hemiscrotum and fixed in place with 2-0 silk and safety pins before the anastomosis is performed. This prevents inadvertent disturbance of the anastomosis from drain placement. The testis is replaced in the scrotum in a natural position, without torsion, to allow a tension-free anastomosis. The scrotum is closed as described for vasovasostomy. The drains are removed the day after surgery.

Long-Term Follow-Up Evaluation and Results

In the hands of experienced and skilled microsurgeons, microsurgical vasoepididymostomy results in the appearance of sperm in the ejaculate in 50% to 80% of men. In the author's hands, the patency rate is 70%, and 43% of men with sperm will impregnate their wives after a minimum follow-up of 2 years (Schelegal and Goldstein, 1993). Pregnancy rates are higher the more distal the anastomosis is performed. **At 14 months after surgery, 25% of initially patent anastomoses have shut down** (Matthews et al, 1995a). **For this reason, we recommend banking sperm both intraoperatively** (Matthews and Goldstein, 1996b) **and as soon as they appear in the ejaculate postoperatively.** In men with very low counts or poor sperm quality postoperatively and in men who remain azoospermic but have sperm that was cryopreserved intraoperatively, IVF with ICSI (described later in the section entitled Oocyte Micromanipulation Techniques for Facilitated Ferilization) yields a 38.5% delivery rate at Cornell. Persistently azoospermic men without cryopreserved sperm can opt for either a redo vasoepidymostomy and/or microscopic epididymal sperm aspiration combined with IVF and ICSI (see the section entitled Sperm Retrieval Techniques).

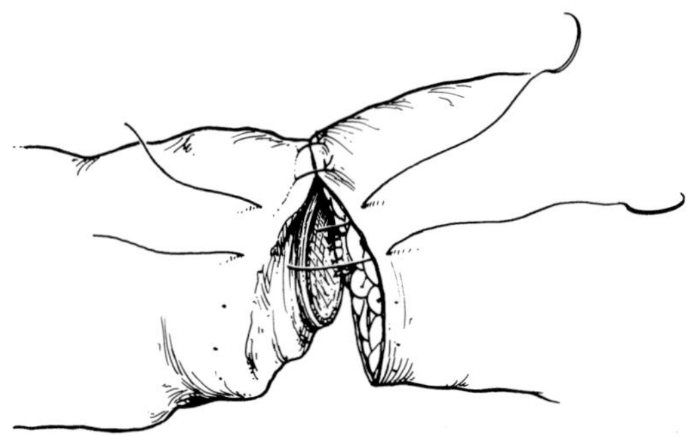

Figure 44–49. Second layer of 9-0 polypropylene approximating vasal adventitia and perivasal sheath to cut edge of the epididymal tunic.

TRANSURETHRAL RESECTION OF THE EJACULATORY DUCTS

Ejaculatory duct obstruction is usually a congenital anomaly that represents the opposite end of the spectrum of vasal and epididymal anomalies that begin with congenital complete absence of the vas deferens and most of the epididymis. When the aplastic segment occurs at the terminal end of the vas, where the ejaculatory duct enters the urethra, it is potentially correctable by TUR. Occasionally, ejaculatory duct obstruction results from chronic prostatitis or extrinsic compression of the ejaculatory ducts by prostate or seminal vesical duct cysts.

Diagnosis

The work-up leading to the diagnosis of probable ejaculatory duct obstruction is covered in Chapter 43. Briefly, **ejaculatory duct obstruction is suspected in azoospermic or severely oligospermic or asthenospermic men with at least one palpable vas deferens, a low semen volume and negative, or low semen fructose levels.** If these men have normal serum levels of FSH and testis biopsy reveals normal spermatogenesis, the diagnosis of ejaculatory duct obstruction is entertained.

Digital rectal examination may reveal a midline cystic structure. **Transrectal sonography has revolutionized the diagnosis and treatment of ejaculatory duct obstruction.** A midline cystic lesion or dilated ejaculatory ducts and seminal vesicles can be visualized sonographically. As described in the section entitled Transrectal Vasography and Seminal Vesiculography earlier in this chapter, **transrectal ultrasound–guided aspiration of the cystic or dilated ejaculatory duct or seminal vesicles is performed** (Jarow, 1994). **The aspirate is examined microscopically, and if sperm are found, they are cryopreserved and 2 to 3 ml of methylene blue diluted with water-soluble radiographic contrast is instilled. If an x-ray study confirms a potentially resectable lesion, TUR of the ejaculatory ducts is performed without the need for prior vasography** because the presence of sperm indicates that at least one epididymis is patent and that the cyst or dilated ejaculatory duct communicates with a nonobstructed vas. The instillation of methylene blue assists in localizing the opening of the ejaculatory duct and confirms when resection has entered the system. **Transrectal sonography with aspiration should be performed immediately before anticipated surgery and employs the same bowel prep and antibiotic prophylaxis used for transrectal prostate biopsy.**

If no sperm are found in the aspirate, vasography, as described earlier, is necessary. If no sperm are found in the vas when the vasotomy is made but vasography reveals a resectable lesion, a TUR is performed as described below. Vasoepididymostomy may be performed at the same time if (1) repeat sampling of the vasal fluid at the completion of the TUR still fails to reveal sperm, (2) the fluid quality and appearance of the epididymis clearly indicate epididymal obstruction (see the section entitled When To Perform Vasoepididymostomy), or (3) the surgeon is very experienced at vasoepididymostomy. If ejaculatory duct obstruction is confirmed by vasography employing a 50% water-soluble contrast medium, the No. 3 Fr whistle-tip ureteral vasography stents are left in place so that a dilute methylene blue solution can be injected by the assistant to aid resection.

Technique

Cold knife incision alone almost always leads to reobstruction. The resectoscope, with the No. 24 Fr cutting loop, is engaged with a finger placed in the rectum providing anterior displacement of the posterior lobe of the prostate. The ejaculatory ducts course between the bladder neck and the verumontanum, and exit at the level of and along the lateral aspect of the verumontanum (Fig. 44–50). **Resection of the veru often reveals the dilated ejaculatory duct orifice or cyst cavity. Resection should be carried out in this region with great care in order to preserve the bladder neck proximally, the striated sphincter distally, and the rectal mucosa posteriorly.** Efflux of methylene blue from dilated orifices confirms adequate resection. **Avoid excessive coagulation.** If formal vasography was performed, the hemivasotomies are closed employing microsurgical technique. A Foley catheter is left overnight, and the patient receives an additional 7 days of oral antibiotics.

Complications

Reflux

Reflux of urine into the ejaculatory ducts, vas, and seminal vesicles occurs after a majority of resections. This can be documented by voiding cystourethography or measuring semen creatinine levels (Malkevich et al, 1994). Contamination of semen by urine impairs sperm quality.

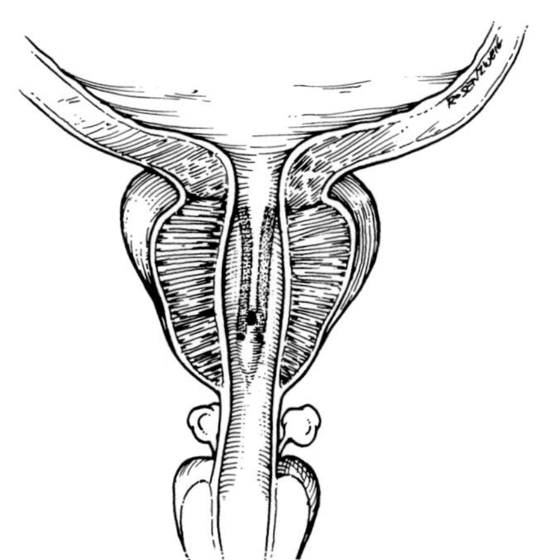

Figure 44–50. Transurethral resection of the ejaculatory ducts showing the location of resection.

Epididymitis

Reflux can lead to acute and chronic epididymitis. Recurrent epididymitis often results in epididymal obstruction. The incidence of epididymitis after TUR is probably underestimated. Symptomatic chemical epididymitis may occur from refluxing urine. **Chronic low-dose antibacterial suppression, such as that employed for vesicoureteral reflux, may be necessary until pregnancy is achieved.** If epididymitis is chronic and recurrent, vasectomy or even epididymectomy may be necessary.

Retrograde Ejaculation

Even when care has been taken to spare the bladder neck, retrograde ejaculation is common after TUR. Pseudoephedrine (Sudafed), 120 mg orally, given 90 minutes before ejaculation, or phenylpropanolamine and chlorpheniramine (Ornade spansules), given twice a day for a week, may prevent this. If this is not successful, sperm can be retrieved from alkalinized urine and used for either intrauterine insemination or IVF with ICSI.

Results

TUR of the ejaculatory ducts results in increased semen volume about two thirds of the time and the appearance of sperm in the ejaculate in about 50% of previously azoospermic men. Pregnancy rates are based on case reports and small series (Goldwasser et al, 1985). If viable sperm appear in the ejaculate but the quality is poor, IVF with ICSI is recommended, which currently yields delivery rates of up to 38.5% per attempt. Because of the potential for serious complications, TUR should only be performed in azoospermic men or severely oligoasthenospermic men and only after the couple has stated they are unwilling to undergo IVF and have been fully apprised of the risks of TUR.

ELECTROEJACULATION

Men with neurologic impairments in sympathetic outflow, such as is seen in traumatic spinal cord injury, demyelinating neuropathies (multiple sclerosis), and diabetes following retroperitoneal lymph node dissection, frequently have abnormalities in or absence of seminal emission. **Ejaculation can be induced in many of these men, especially those with high spinal cord injury, with vibratory stimulation** (Schellan, 1968; Brindley, 1981). **For those men that do not respond to vibratory stimulation, electroejaculation has proved to be a safe and effective means of obtaining motile sperm suitable for assisted reproduction techniques (intrauterine insemination [IUI], IVF).**

The procedure is performed under general anesthesia, except in men with a complete spinal cord injury, who do not require anesthesia. In men with a high thoracic spinal cord lesion (above T6) or in those men with prior history of autonomic dysreflexia, pretreatment (15 minutes prior to the procedure) with 20 mg of sublingual nifedipine is employed. An intravenous access should be created in these men, and their blood pressure and pulse monitored every 2 minutes before, during, and for 20 minutes following electroejaculation. In the event of a sympathetic outflow (autonomic dysreflexia), termination of the procedure should be sufficient to break the response; however, intravenous access allows for delivery of sympatheticolytic agents should they become necessary.

Prior to placing the patient in the lateral decubitus position, the bladder is catheterized and emptied. An unlubricated No. 12 or 14 Fr Silastic catheter is used because commonly employed lubricants are spermicidal. The urine pH is tested, and if it is under 6.5, 10 ml of buffer (*N*-2-hydroxyethylpiperazine-*N'*-2-ethane sulfonic acid–bovine serum albumin [HEPES-BSA]) is instilled into the bladder and urethra. Before the electroejaculation sequence, a digital rectal examination and anoscopy are performed. The rectal probe is well lubricated, inserted with the electrodes facing anteriorly, and applied against the posterior aspect of the prostate and seminal vesicles. The probe is connected to a variable output power source, which simultaneously records probe temperature through a thermistor in the rectal probe. Electrostimulation is started at 3 to 5 volts and increased in 1-volt increments with each stimulation. An assistant records probe temperatures and number of stimulations to full erection and ejaculation, and collects the ejaculate in a sterile wide-mouth plastic container. The number of stimulations and maximum voltage required are variable, and the ejaculate may be retrograde. If probe temperature rises rapidly or above 40°C, stimulation is suspended until the temperature falls below 38°C or probes are changed. At the completion of stimulation, anoscopy is again performed to check for rectal injury. The bladder is recatheterized to obtain any retrograde-ejaculated sperm. The specimens are then delivered to the laboratory for processing.

By employing this technique, sperm can be recovered in greater than 90% of men. Overall pregnancy rates of up to 40% can be achieved after multiple cycles with insemination (Bennett et al, 1987). Use of IVF with ICSI yields close to 40% live delivery rates for a single (albeit costly) procedure if motile sperm are obtained.

SPERM RETRIEVAL TECHNIQUES

Men with congenital absence or bilateral partial aplasia of vas deferens, or those with failed or surgically unreconstructable obstructions can now be treated by using sperm retrieval techniques in conjunction with IVF (Silber et al, 1990; Schlegel, et al, 1994). These techniques are also useful for intraoperative retrieval of sperm during reconstructive procedures such as vasoepididymostomy, which have significant failure rates. The intraoperatively retrieved sperm may be used immediately if the wife has been prepared for IVF, or the sperm may be cryopreserved for a future IVF with ICSI cycle in the event the reconstructive surgery is unsuccessful. Sperm obtained from chronically obstructed systems usually have poor motility and decreased fertilizing capacity. **The use of ICSI combined with IVF is essential to achieve optimal results.**

Microsurgical Epididymal Sperm Aspiration Techniques

Open Tubule Technique

The technique described here can be employed for either intraoperative sperm retrieval at the time of vasoepididymostomy or in men with congenital absence of the vas or unreconstructable obstructions (Matthews and Goldstein, 1996b). A median raphe approach allows delivery of both testes through a single incision in men undergoing sperm retrieval only. The tunica vaginalis is opened, and the epididymis is inspected under 16 to 25 power magnification using the operating microscope. The epididymal tunic is incised over a diluted tubule, as described previously for vasoepididymostomy. Meticulous hemostasis is obtained using the bipolar cautery. A dilated tubule is isolated and incised with a 15-degree microknife or buttonholed with a curved microscissors, if preparing for an end-to-side vasoepididymostomy. The fluid is touched to a slide, a drop of saline or Ringer's lactate is added, a coverslip is placed, and the fluid is examined. If no sperm are obtained, the epididymal tubule and tunic are closed with 10-0 and 9-0 monofilament polypropylene sutures, respectively, and an incision is made more proximally in the epididymis or even at the level of the efferent ductules until motile sperm are obtained.

As soon as motile sperm are found, a dry micropipette (5 μl; Drummond Scientific Company, Broomall, PA) is placed adjacent to the effluxing epididymal tubule (Fig. 44–51*A*). A standard hematocrit pipette is less satisfactory but can be used if micropipettes are not available. **Sperm are drawn into the micropipette by simple capillary action.** Negative pressure, as is generated by action of an in-line syringe, should not be applied during sperm recovery because this may potentially disrupt the delicate epididymal mucosa. Multiple micropipettes may be employed simultaneously to increase speed of sperm recovery.

The highest rate of flow is observed immediately following incision of the tubule. Progressively better quality sperm are often found following the initial washout. **Gentle compression of the testis and epididymis enhances flow from the incised tubule.** With patience, 10 to 20 L of epididymal fluid can be recovered.

The micropipette is connected to a short (3- to 5-cm) segment of medical grade silicone tubing (American Scientific Products, McGaw Park, IL). Alternatively, the tubing attached to a 22-g butterfly needle may be employed. A 20-gauge needle fitted to a Luer-tip syringe is then placed in line (see Fig. 44–51*B*). The fluid is flushed with IVF media (0.5–1.0 ml) into a sterile container. Once a micropipette has been used, it is discarded. Residual fluid in the pipette will disrupt capillary action. A typical procedure requires 4 to 12 micropipettes. The sperm bank should be instructed to cyropreserve the aspirate in multiple vials (aliquots) so that several IVF cycles may be attempted, if required.

Experience with the technique has revealed that, **paradoxically, in obstructed systems, sperm motility is better as one moves more proximally in the epididymis, with the**

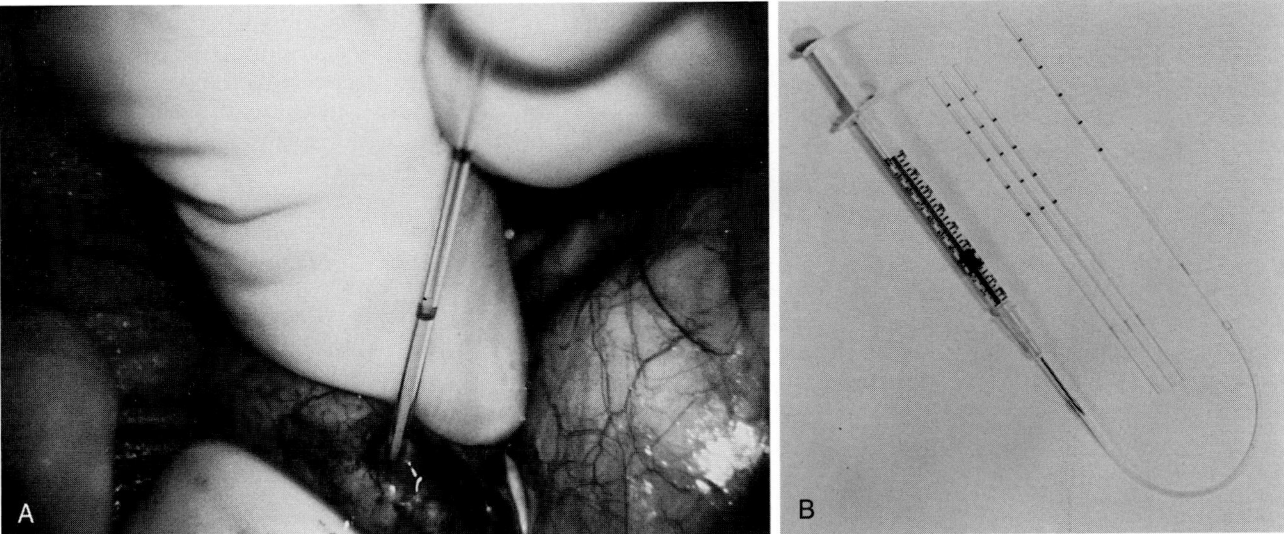

Figure 44–51. *A*, Sperm drawn into micropipette by capillary action. *B*, System employed to flush sperm-laden micropipettes.

most motile sperm often found in the efferent ductules. The environment in the obstructed epididymis appears to promote a natural swim-up. Initial motility and, consequently, fertilization rates are highest in men who have the longest length of epididymal tubule available. Even when obstructed with debris distally, the epididymal tubule may be capable of secreting substances that can diffuse proximally and benefit sperm motility and fertilizing capacity.

Micropuncture Techniques

Micropuncture of the epididymal tubule in laboratory animals has been employed for studies of epididymal function (Howards et al, 1975). When epididymal sperm is collected by incision into an epididymal tubule and aspiration of the effluxing fluid, contamination with some blood and tissue fluid is inevitable, regardless of meticulous attempts at hemostasis with a microbiopolar cautery. Even microscopic quantities of such contaminants have an adverse effect on sperm motility and fertilizing capacity. Although ICSI has overcome these problems, **specimens that are free of contamination are more easily processed for IVF and cryopreservation.** To circumvent the contamination problem, the micropuncture technique perfected in animals has been adapted for aspiration of human epididymal sperm (Schlegel et al, 1994). **This is the ideal technique for primary epididymal sperm retrieval in men with congenital absence of the vas deferens or unreconstructable reproductive tract obstructions. It should not be employed at the time of vasovasostomy or vasoepididymostomy because tubule puncture proximal to an anastomosis may result in obstruction.**

Glass capillary tubes, 0.9 mm (o.d.) × 0.6 mm (i.d.) are washed and pulled to a tip width of 250 to 350 μ, and the tips are sharpened on a fine grinding wheel. The micropuncture pipettes are again washed, siliconized, and attached to medical grade silicone tubing. A collecting system, similar to that used for epididymal micropuncture in animals, is employed (Fig. 44–52).

The epididymis is exposed and prepared as described previously using an operating microscope. Under 15 to 32 power magnification, with an assistant stabilizing the epididymis and gently squeezing the testis and epididymis, the epididymal tubule is punctured in an area devoid of blood vessels. Successful puncture is heralded by free flow of epididymal sperm and fluid up the pipette (Fig. 44–53). The pipette tip is gently advanced 0.5 to 1.0 mm into the lumen and adjusted for maximum flow. When no further fluid can

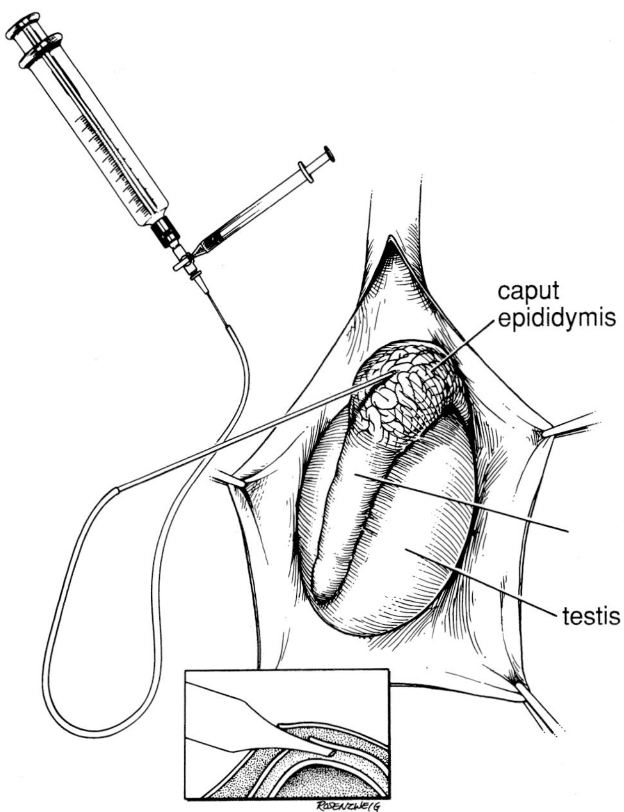

Figure 44–52. Micropuncture of the human epididymal tubule. Collection system.

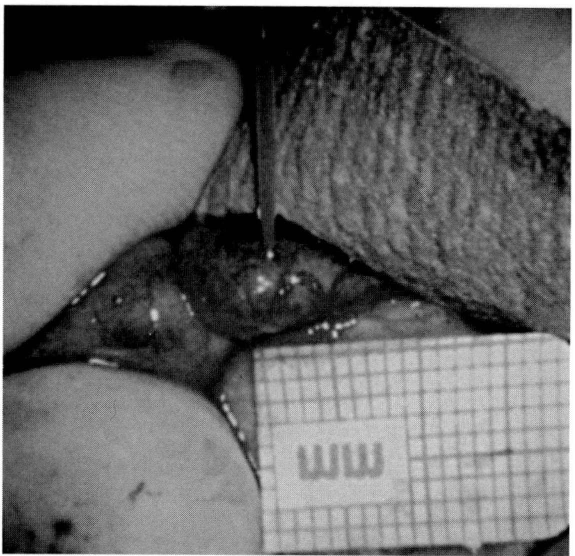

Figure 44–53. Successful micropuncture of the epididymal tubule.

be collected, the pipette is removed from the tubule and the collected fluid flushed out with media for examination and processing. The puncture hole is sealed with a single stitch of 10-0 monofilament polypropylene. Repetitive punctures can be made progessively more proximal until motile sperm are retrieved. The efferent ductules can be punctured with equal success. **Enough sperm can be retrieved for immediate use as well as cryopreservation into multiple vials for future IVF.**

Through the employment of standard ICSI, 13 of 24 (54%) ongoing pregnancies or deliveries have been achieved with this technique (Schlegel et al, 1995) as compared with a 25% pregnancy rate prior to ICSI (Schlegel et al, 1994). **Using a new ICSI technique of aggressive sperm immobilization, the pregnancy rate has been boosted to 82% of 17 cycles** (Palermo et al, 1996). At present, **pregnancies have been achieved in 65% of cases using cryopreserved epididymal sperm.** If these results with cryopreserved sperm are maintained, sperm aspiration can be performed electively in selected ideal cases, with the cryopreserved sperm used for future IVF cycles.

Percutaneous Epididymal Sperm Aspiration

Percutaneous puncture of the epididymis with a fine needle has been successfully employed to obtain sperm and achieve pregnancies (Shrivastav et al, 1994; Craft and Tsirigotis, 1995). The technique is not reliable and the small quantities of sperm obtained are inadequate for cryopreservation. In view of the enormous costs and effort involved in IVF, epididymal sperm retrieval under direct vision is the preferred technique.

Autogenous Spermatocele

Although epididymal aspiration has proved to be very successful in men with unreconstructable tracts, costly IVF with ICSI is necessary and repeat procedures, each with their own anesthetic, may be required. Creation of an autogenous sperm reservoir was described by Moni and Lalitha (1992a). Using sperm percutaneously aspirated from the reservoir, they reported a pregnancy in one out of four couples using simple intrauterine insemination. The procedure can only be performed in patients with an intact tunica vaginalis and no adhesions from prior surgery. Because men with congenital absence of the vas have normal spermatogenesis, biopsy in men with normal testis volume and serum FSH is unnecessary. We have attempted to refine the method by using microsurgical techniques (Matthews and Goldstein, 1996).

Following exposure through a median raphe incision, the tunica vaginalis is sharply opened with a 15-degree microknife away from the epididymis. A dilated epididymal tubule is identified, and **a 1-mm buttonhole is made sharply in the overlying visceral tunic. This opening is much smaller then the 3- to 4-mm opening made for vasoepididymostomy.** Too large an opening in the tunic will result in tearing of the epididymal tubule when marsupialization is attempted. The dilated tubule is sharply incised for 1 mm with a microknife or is buttonholed with microscissors. If sperm are found in the fluid, the mucosa of the incised epididymal tubule is marsupialized to the edge of the buttonholed visceral tunica vaginalis with six to eight interrupted sutures of 10-0 polypropylene (Fig. 44–54). **Constant irrigation of the epididymal surface with Ringer's solution is mandatory to prevent drying out of the epididymal surface, resulting in subsequent adhesions and failure. Abundant sperm are aspirated for either immediate IVF or cryopreservation, or both,** as described previously in the section entitled Open Tubule Technique. One-half milliliter of triamcinolone (Kenalog) mixed with 10 ml of lactated Ringer's is instilled in the tunica vaginalis before closure of the parietal tunic with a 6-0 polypropylene continuous suture.

Beginning 6 weeks postoperatively and timed to their partner's cycle, patients undergo ultrasonographic imaging of the reservoirs with percutaneous aspiration of any fluid collections. To date, with a mean follow-up of 5 months in 19 men, 75% of patients imaged have demonstrated fluid collections sonographically and 44% of those aspirated have

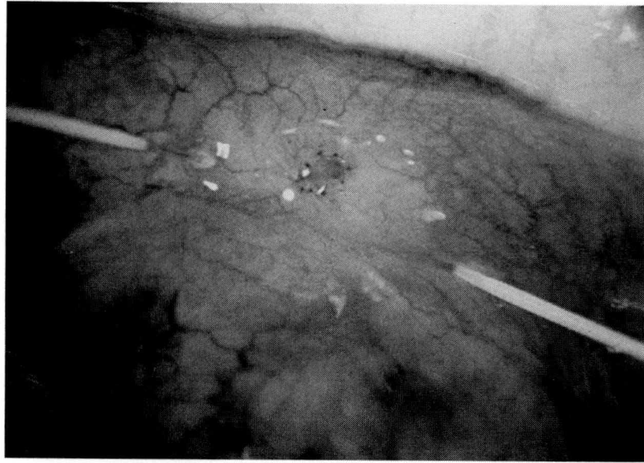

Figure 44–54. Marsupialized epididymal tubule for creation of autogenous spermatocele.

yielded viable sperm. IUI has not yet yielded a pregnancy, but frozen sperm obtained at the time of the surgery or postoperatively from the reservoir has resulted in four ongoing pregnancies using IVF with ICSI (Matthews and Goldstein, 1996c).

Alloplastic Spermatocele

Before the development of IVF techniques, attempts to treat men with surgically unreconstructable obstructive azoospermia involved the creation or implantation of an artificial silicone sperm reservoir, or alloplastic spermatocele. The reservoir would be percutaneously aspirated to obtain spermatozoa for artificial insemination. These attempts have been largely unsuccessful. A review of over 200 attempted implantations of alloplastic spermatoceles in humans by different authors revealed only three term pregnancies (Turner, 1988). However, these results were reported before the use of IVF with ICSI. The remarkable success of IVF with ICSI using relatively simple sperm retrieval techniques has resulted in a halt to any further attempts at development of an improved alloplastic spermatocele.

Testicular Sperm Retrieval

Pregnancies have now been achieved using sperm retrieved directly from the testis (Craft et al, 1995; Schlegel et al, 1997). All of these pregnancies have employed IVF with ICSI. **The indications for testicular sperm retrieval are**

1. **Failure to find sperm in the epididymis** in the presence of the spermatogenesis or complete absence of the epididymis.
2. **Severe hypospermatogenesis in which no sperm are found in the ejaculate or in the epididymis but some sperm are found in the testis.**

Testicular sperm retrieval should be used as a procedure of last resort because (1) testicular sperm numbers, motility, and viability are low; (2) dissection of sperm out of testicular tissue requires extraordinary technical expertise; (3) cryopreservation is difficult; (4) epididymal sperm retrieval has been successfully employed on hundreds of men and is the gold standard.

Testicular sperm have been retrieved employing one of three techniques:

1. **Open biopsy** allows retrieval of the largest number of sperm with potential for cryopreservation; this **is the best technique to use in men with severe hypospermatogenesis** (Schlegel et al, 1997).
2. Percutaneous core biopsy uses the same equipment as for prostate biopsy.
3. Percutaneous aspiration with a high-suction glass syringe and a 23-gauge needle is the least invasive method, but it requires several passes to obtain an adequate yield.

The percutaneous methods are most appropriate in men with normal spermatogenesis and obstructive azoospermia in whom adequate numbers of sperm can be retrieved in a small amount of tissue (Craft et al, 1995b). The pros and cons of these three methods are discussed in the section entitled Testis Biopsy.

Postmortem Sperm Retrieval

Postmortem sperm retrieval and cryopreservation (but no pregnancies) was initially reported by Rothman in 1980, and the procedure employed removal and mincing of the epididymis. The retrieved sperm can be frozen and subsequently used to achieve pregnancy. Pregnancy has now been achieved with sperm retrieved postmortem using IVF with ICSI.

Retrieval of sperm from the vas can be performed using the technique described for the no-scalpel vasectomy (see the section entitled Vasectomy). Once the vas has been delivered, a hemivasotomy is made with a number 15 microknife. The testicular end of the vas is cannulated with a 22-gauge angiocatheter, and the vas is irrigated with 0.2 ml of human tubal fluid medium while the convoluted vas and epididymis are massaged.

Twenty-four million sperm, with 70% considered grade I motile, were retrieved 13 hours after death with this technique.* The ethical appropriateness of such retrieval is the most important issue surrounding its use.

OOCYTE MICROMANIPULATION TECHNIQUES FOR FACILITATED FERTILIZATION

In vitro fertilization combined with the assisted fertilization technique of ICSI has enabled the highly successful treatment of severe male factor infertility (Palermo et al, 1992; Van Steirteghem et al, 1993). **These techniques** do not replace treatment of the male but instead **offer the opportunity for the urologist to treat men that would not have been candidates for any therapeutic interventions just 5 years ago.** Examples of those who could not be helped include

1. **Men with surgically unreconstructable obstruction such as congenital absence of the vas deferens.**
2. **Men with less than 100 viable sperm in the total ejaculate.**
3. **Azoospermic men with varicoceles. Sixty percent of these men respond to varicocelectomy with the return of enough sperm to achieve pregnancy using IVF with ICSI** (Matthews and Goldstein, 1996a).

Intracytoplasmic Sperm Injection

Earlier techniques of oocyte micromanipulation such as partial zona dissection or subzonal insertion have been supplanted by (ICSI) (Palermo et al, 1992). With ICSI, a viable sperm is injected directly into the oocyte (Fig. 44–55) after the sperm tail is immobilized to prevent oocyte destruction. Only one viable sperm is needed for each oocyte retrieved. In experienced hands (Van Steirteghem et al, 1993), fertiliza-

*Schlegel, personal communication, 1995.

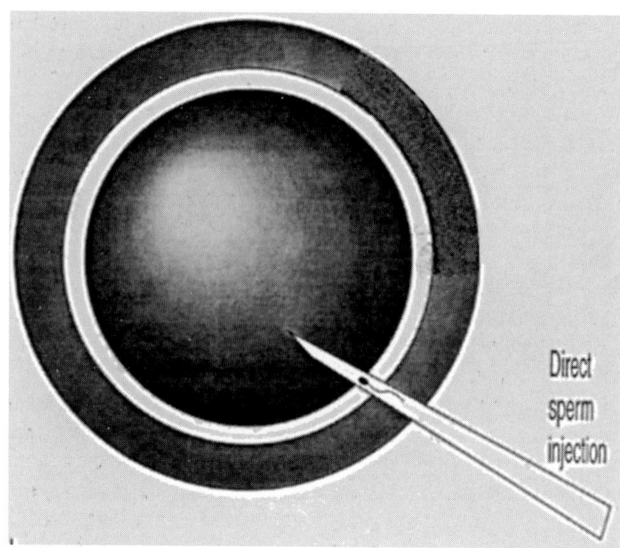

Figure 44–55. Intracytoplasmic sperm injection (ICSI).

tion rates are in the range of 60% to 70% and delivery rates per retrieval are 38.5% in the first 560 couples at the author's institution. The rate of oocyte damage is less than 10%. The incidence of major fetal abnormalities is 3.2% compared with 1.6% in natural conception. **IVF with ICSI is now the treatment of choice for severe uncorrectable male factor infertility.** ICSI is costly ($12,000–$15,000 for a single attempt) and usually is not covered by most forms of health insurance. It also involves putting the female partner through a month of intramuscular injections, frequent sonographic monitoring, and measurement of blood hormone levels, culminating in the transvaginal retrieval of multiple oocytes under sedation or general anesthesia. If embryos develop, they are transferred to the uterus transvaginally 3 days later. Aside from the cost and discomfort, each attempt is an emotional roller coaster for the couple. **These procedures should not be applied indiscriminately. Every attempt should be made to treat the male and enable the couple to conceive as naturally as possible. Most couples prefer natural conception.** Microsurgical vasovasotomy, with a better than 50% natural pregnancy rate, and varicocelectomy with a natural pregnancy rate of 40% to 70% should be the first level of therapy.

Frontiers in Fertilization

Until now, pregnancy was not possible without sperm. Work in animals (Sofikitis et al, 1994) and humans (Tesarik et al, 1995) has resulted in pregnancy and live births after the injection of haploid germ cells (round spermatids) into the oocyte. Fertilization rates with this technique are low, but further research is likely to result in improved results. The germ cells are retrieved from testis biopsy tissue. Because immature germ cells can often be identified in the semen, eventually biopsy may not be necessary. In the mouse diploid germ cell, nuclei have been injected into oocytes and found to undergo meiosis in the oocyte, form an embryo, and produce live young (Kimura and Yanagimachi, 1995).

The last frontier is the induction of meiosis in nongerm cells enabling even men with Sertoli-cell only or anorchia to father children.

VARICOCELECTOMY

Varicocelectomy is by far the most commonly performed operation for the treatment of male infertility. **Varicocele is found in approximately 15% of the general population, in 35% of men with primary infertility, and in 75% to 81% of men with secondary infertility.** Animal and human studies have demonstrated that **varicocele is associated with a progressive and duration-dependent decline in testicular function** (Russell, 1957; Lipshultz and Corriere, 1977; Nagler et al, 1985; Harrison et al, 1986; Kass and Belman, 1987a; Hadziselimovic et al, 1989; Chehval and Purcell, 1992; Gorelick and Goldstein, 1993; Witt and Lipshultz, 1993).

Repair of varicocele will halt any further damage to testicular function (Kass et al, 1987b) and, in a large percentage of men, result in improved spermatogenesis (Dubin and Amelar, 1977; Goldstein et al, 1992) as well as enhanced Leydig cell function (Su et al, 1995). The potentially important role of urologists in preventing future infertility underscores the importance of using a varicocelectomy technique that minimizes the risk of complications and recurrence. Table 44–2 summarizes the pros and cons of various methods of varicocele repair.

Scrotal Operations

A variety of surgical approaches have been advocated for varicocelectomy. The earliest recorded attempts at repair of varicocele date to antiquity and involved external clamping of the scrotal skin, including the enlarged veins. In the early 1900s, an open scrotal approach was employed, involving the mass ligation and excision of the varicosed plexus of veins. At the level of the scrotum, however, the pampiniform plexus of veins is intimately entwined with the coiled testicular artery. Therefore, **scrotal operations are to be avoided because damage to the arterial supply of the testis frequently results in testicular atrophy and further impairment of spermatogenesis and fertility.**

Retroperitoneal Operations

Retroperitoneal repair of varicocele involves incision at the level of the internal inguinal ring (Fig. 44–56*A*), splitting

Table 44–2. TECHNIQUES OF VARICOCELECTOMY

Technique	Artery Preserved	Hydrocele (%)	Failure (%)	Potential for Serious Morbidity
Retroperitoneal	No	7	15–25	No
Conventional inguinal	No	3–30	5–15	No
Laparoscopic	Yes	12	?5–15	Yes
Radiographic	Yes	0	15–25	Yes
Microscopic inguinal or subinguinal	Yes	0	1.0	No

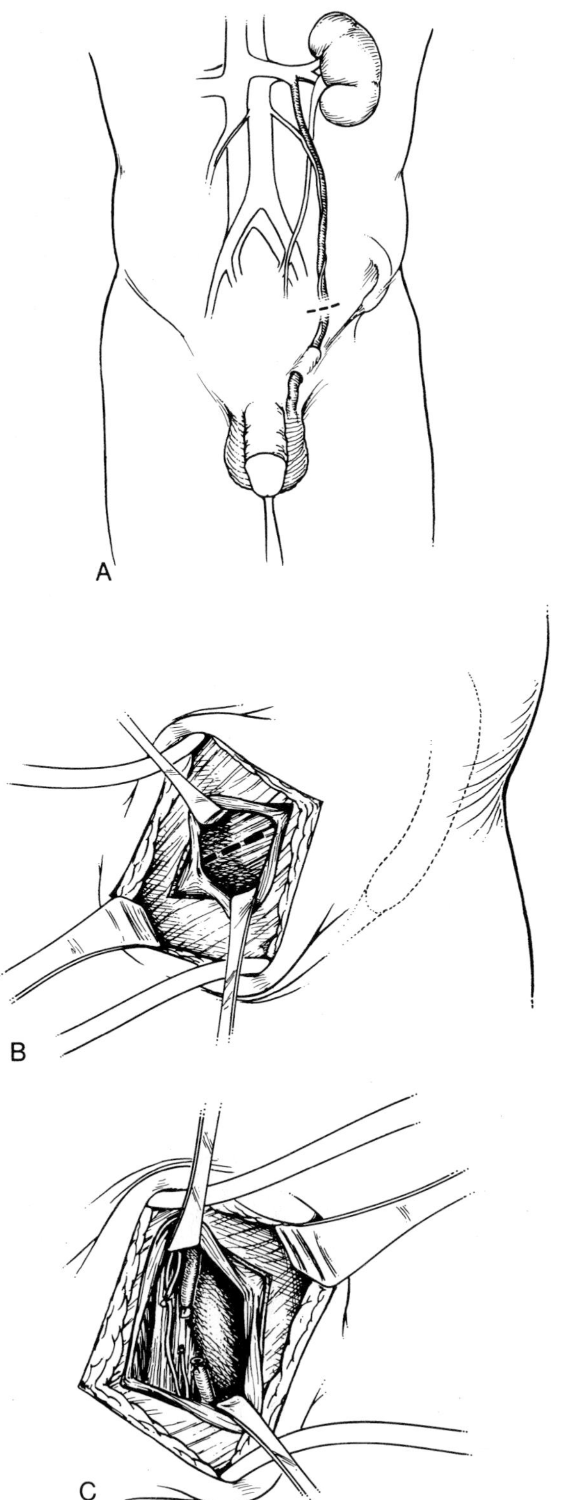

Figure 44–56. *A* to *C,* Retroperitoneal varicocelectomy.

of the external and internal oblique muscles (see Fig. 44–56*B*), and exposure of the internal spermatic artery and vein retroperitoneally near the ureter (see Fig. 44–56*C*). This approach has the advantage of isolating the internal spermatic veins proximally, near the point of drainage into the left renal vein. At this level, only one or two large veins are present and, in addition, the testicular artery has not yet branched and is often distinctly separate from the internal spermatic veins. Retroperitoneal approaches involve ligation of the fewest number of veins. This approach is still a commonly employed method for the repair of varicocele, especially in children.

A disadvantage of a retroperitoneal approach is the high incidence of recurrence of varicocele, especially in children and adolescents, when the testicular artery is intentionally preserved. Recurrence rates after retroperitoneal varicocelectomy are approximately 15% (Homonnai et al, 1980; Rothman et al, 1981). Failure is usually due to preservation of the periarterial plexus of fine veins (venae comitantes) along with the artery. These veins have been shown to communicate with larger internal spermatic veins (Beck et al, 1992). If they are left intact, they may dilate and cause recurrence. Less commonly, failure is due to the presence of parallel inguinal or retroperitoneal collaterals, which may exit the testis and bypass the ligated retroperitoneal veins rejoining the internal spermatic vein proximal to the site of ligation (Sayfan et al, 1981; Murray et al, 1986). Dilated cremasteric veins, another cause of varicocele recurrence (Sayfan et al, 1980), cannot be identified with a retroperitoneal approach. Positive identification and preservation of the 0.5- to 1.5-mm testicular artery via the retroperitoneal approach is difficult, especially in children, in whom the artery is small. The operation involves working in a deep hole, and because at this level the internal spermatic vessels cannot be delivered into the wound, they must be dissected and ligated in situ in the retroperitoneum. In addition, the difficulty in positively identifying and preserving lymphatics using this approach results in postoperative hydrocele formation after 7% to 33% of retroperitoneal operations (Szabo and Kessler, 1984). The incidence of recurrence appears to be higher in children, with rates reported between 15% and 45% in adolescents (Gorenstein et al, 1986; Levitt et al, 1987; Reitelman et al, 1987). Kass (1992) reports that **recurrence can be markedly reduced in children and adolescents by intentional ligation of the testicular artery.** This approach ensures ligation of the periarterial network of fine veins. Although reversal of testicular growth failure has been documented with intentional testicular artery ligation at the time of retroperitoneal repair in children, **the effect of artery ligation on subsequent spermatogenesis is uncertain.** In adults, bilateral artery ligation has been documented to cause azoospermia and testicular atrophy occasionally. At least, **it is inarguable that testicular artery ligation does not enhance testicular function.**

Laparoscopic Varicocelectomy

In essence, laparoscopic repair is a retroperitoneal approach and many of the advantages and disadvantages are similar to those of the open retroperitoneal approach.

Using the laparoscope, the internal spermatic vessels and vas deferens can be clearly visualized through the laparoscope as they course through the internal inguinal ring. **The magnification provided by the laparoscope allows visualization of the testicular artery. With experience, the lymphatics may be visualized and preserved as well.** With laparoscopic varicocelectomy, the internal spermatic veins are ligated at the same level as the retroperitoneal (Palomo) approach described earlier in the section entitled Retroperitoneal Operations. Laparoscopic varicocelectomy allows preservation of the testicular artery in a majority of cases, as well as preservation of lymphatics. The incidence of varicocele recurrence would be expected to be similar to that associated with open retroperitoneal operations. These recurrences are due to collaterals joining the internal spermatic vein near its entrance to the renal vein or entering the renal vein separately.

Reported series of laparoscopic varicocelectomy are too small and the follow-up interval too short to determine the incidence of recurrence and complications. The potential complications of laparoscopic varicocelectomy (injury to bowel, vessels or viscera, air embolism, peritonitis) are significantly more serious than those associated with open techniques. Furthermore, laparoscopic varicocelectomy requires a general anesthetic. The microsurgical techniques described next can be performed using local or regional anesthesia and employ a 2.5- to 3.0-cm incision for unilateral repair. This is equal to or less than the sum of incisions employed for a laparoscopic approach. Furthermore, laparoscopic varicocelectomy takes at least twice as long to perform and is less cost effective than open varicocelectomy. Finally, postoperative pain and recovery from the laparoscopic technique are the same as those associated with subinguinal varicocelectomy.

In the hands of an experienced laparoscopist, the approach is a reasonable alternative for the repair of bilateral varicoceles (Donovan and Winfield, 1992).

Microsurgical Inguinal and Subinguinal Operations: The Preferred Approaches

Inguinal and subinguinal varicocelectomy are the most popular approaches. They have the advantage of allowing the spermatic cord structures to be pulled up and out of the wound so that the testicular artery, lymphatics, and small periarterial veins may be more easily identified. In addition, **an inguinal or subinguinal approach allows access to external spermatic and even gubernacular veins,** which may bypass the spermatic cord and result in recurrence if they are not ligated. Last, an inguinal or subinguinal approach allows access to the testis for biopsy or examination of the epididymis for obstruction.

Traditional approaches to inguinal varicocelectomy involve a 5- to 10-cm incision made over the inguinal canal, opening of the external oblique aponeurosis, and encirclement and delivery of the spermatic cord. The cord is then dissected, and all the internal spermatic veins are ligated (Dubin and Amelar, 1977). The vas deferens and its vessels are preserved. An attempt is made to identify and preserve the testicular artery and, if possible, the lymphatics. In addition, the cord is elevated, and any external spermatic veins that are running parallel to the spermatic cord or perforating the floor of the inguinal canal are identified and ligated. Compared with retroperitoneal operations, conventional nonmagnified inguinal approaches lower the incidence of varicocele recurrence but do not alter the incidence of either hydrocele formation or testicular artery injury. **Conventional inguinal operations are associated with an incidence of postoperative hydrocele formation varying from 3% to 15% with an average incidence of 7%** (Szabo and Kessler, 1984). Analysis of the hydrocele fluid has clearly indicated that hydrocele formation following varicocelectomy is due to ligation of the lymphatics (Szabo and Kessler, 1984). The incidence of testicular artery injury during nonmagnified inguinal varicocelectomy is unknown. Case reports, however, suggest that this complication may be more common than is now realized. It can result in testicular atrophy, and if the operation is performed bilaterally, azoospermia may ensue in a previously oligospermic man. Furthermore, Starzl and his transplant group (Penn et al, 1972) reported a 14% incidence of testicular atrophy and a 70% incidence of hydrocele formation when the spermatic cord was divided and only the vas and vasal vessels preserved.

The introduction of **microsurgical technique** to varicocelectomy **has resulted in a substantial reduction in the incidence of hydrocele formation.** This is **because the lymphatics can be more easily identified and preserved.** Furthermore, the use of **magnification enhances the ability to identify and preserve the 0.5- to 1.5-mm testicular artery, thus avoiding the complications of atrophy or azoospermia.**

Anesthesia

If the testis is delivered, as described later, regional or light general anesthesia is preferred. If only the cord is delivered, local anesthesia with a combination of equal amounts of 0.25% bupivacaine and 1% lidocaine is satisfactory with adjunctive intravenous heavy sedation. After infiltration of the skin and subcutaneous tissues, the cord is infiltrated prior to delivery. Blind cord block carries with it a small risk of inadvertent testicular artery injury (Goldstein et al, 1983). Therefore, a 30-gauge needle should be employed for cord block to minimize the risk of injury and hematoma.

Inguinal and Subinguinal Approaches

The introduction of the subinguinal approach, just below the external inguinal ring (Marmar et al, 1985a), obviates the necessity for opening any fascial layer and is associated with less pain and a rapid recovery comparable to laparoscopic procedures. At the subinguinal level, however, significantly more veins are encountered, the artery is more often surrounded by a network of tiny veins that must be ligated, and the testicular artery is often divided into two or three branches, making arterial identification and preservation more difficult.

Subinguinally, the arterial pulsations are often dampened by compression on the edge of the external ring, making its identification somewhat more difficult than when the external oblique is opened. Table 44–3 summarizes the criteria for performing the operation inguinally (external oblique opened) versus subinguinally (fascia intact). **In general, it is best to use a subinguinal approach in men with a history of inguinal surgery.** Under these circumstances, the cord is usually stuck to the undersurface of the external oblique, and opening the fascia risks injury to the cord. A subinguinal approach is easier in obese men in whom opening and closing the fascia is difficult through a small incision. A subinguinal approach is easier in men with high,

Table 44–3. INDICATIONS FOR INGUINAL (EXTERNAL OBLIQUE OPENED) VERSUS SUBINGUINAL (FASCIA INTACT) VARICOCELECTOMY

Inguinal	Subinguinal
Children or prepubertal adolescents	Prior inguinal surgery
Solitary testis	Obesity
Tight, low external ring	Lax, capacious external ring
Thin men	High external ring
	Long cord with low-lying testis
Less experienced with microsurgical repair	Very experienced with microsurgical repair

lax, capacious external rings and in men with long cords and low-lying testes. In these men, the level of the external ring is fairly proximal to the testis and opening the fascia will not result in a significant diminution in the number of veins to be ligated or in the branching of the testicular artery.

Always open the external oblique in children or prepubertal adolescents who have not undergone inguinal surgery previously. In children, the testicular artery is very small and systemic blood pressure is low, making identification of the artery very difficult in a subinguinal approach. The fascia should also be opened in men with a solitary testis in whom preservation of the artery is critical. Exposure of the cord more proximally (at the inguinal level), allows identification of the artery before it has branched, where clear pulsations are more readily observed.

Open the fascia in thin men with tight, low external rings; high-riding testes; and short cords. The microdissection will be quicker and easier, and it is easy to open and close the fascia in thin men.

A subinguinal operation is significantly more difficult than a high inguinal operation, and the procedure should only be used by surgeons who perform the operation frequently.

Before making the incision, the location of the external inguinal ring is determined by invagination of the scrotal skin and is marked. The size of the incision is determined by the size of the testis when delivery of the testis (see later) is planned. Atrophic testes can be delivered through a 2- to 2.5-cm incision. Large testes require a 3- to 3.5-cm incision.

If the decision is made to perform an inguinal operation and thus to open the fascia, the incision is begun at the external ring and extended laterally 2 to 3.5 cm along Langer's lines (Fig. 44–57). If the operation is to be performed subinguinally, the incision is placed in the skin lines just below the external ring (see Fig. 44–57). Camper's fascia and Scarpa's fascia are divided with the electrocautery between the blades of a Crile clamp. The superficial epigastric artery and vein, if encountered, are retracted or, alternately, may be clamped, divided, and ligated (or clipped).

If the decision was made to use the inguinal approach, the external oblique aponeurosis is cleaned and opened the length of the incision to the external inguinal ring in the direction of its fibers. A 3-0 absorbable suture placed at the apex of the external oblique incision facilitates later closure.

The spermatic cord is grasped with a Babcock clamp and delivered through the wound. The ilioinguinal and genital branches of the genitofemoral nerve are excluded from the cord, which is then surrounded with a large Penrose drain.

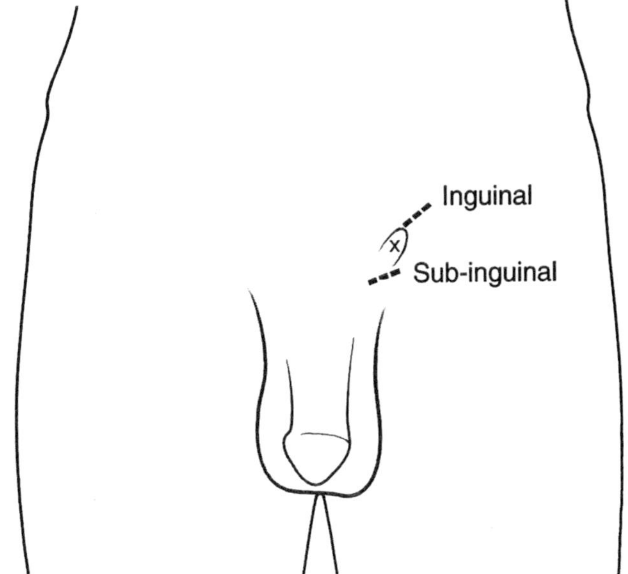

Figure 44–57. Inguinal incision beginning at the external inguinal ring (X) and extending 3 cm laterally along the skin lines. Subinguinal incision just below the ring.

If a subinguinal incision was made, Camper's and Scarpa's fascia are incised, as described earlier. The surgeon's index finger is introduced into the wound and along the cord into the scrotum. The index finger is then hooked under the external inguinal ring, retracting it cephalad. A small Richardson retractor is slid along the back of the index finger and retracted caudad over the cord toward the scrotum (Fig. 44–58). The spermatic cord is revealed between the index finger and retractor. The assistant grasps the cord with a Babcock clamp and delivers it through the wound. The cord is surrounded with a large Penrose drain.

Delivery of the Testis

Delivery of the testis through a small inguinal or subinguinal incision guarantees direct visual access to all possi-

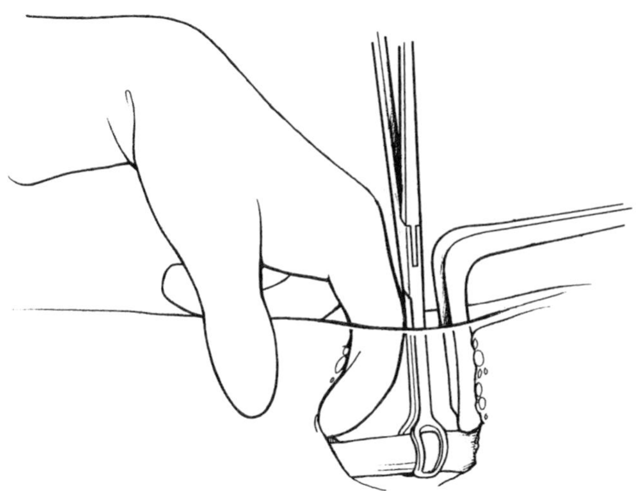

Figure 44–58. Index finger hooked under external ring and retraction caudad to expose cord.

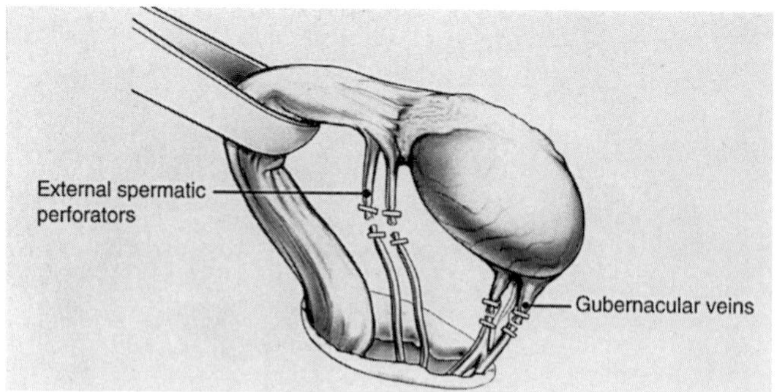

Figure 44–59. Delivery of the testis, providing exposure of external spermatic and gubernacular venous collaterals.

ble avenues of testicular venous drainage. Delivery of only the cord allows access to most external spermatic collaterals but may miss those close to the testis and will not allow access to scrotal or gubernacular collaterals, which have been demonstrated radiographically to be the cause of 10% of recurrent varicoceles (Kaufman et al, 1983). With gentle upward traction on the cord and upward pressure on the testis through the invaginated scrotum, the testis is easily delivered through the wound. All external spermatic veins are identified and doubly ligated with hemoclips and divided (Fig. 44–59). The gubernaculum is inspected for the presence of veins exiting from the tunica vaginalis. These are either cauterized or doubly clipped and divided. **When this step is completed, all testicular venous return must be within the cord surrounded by the Penrose drain.** The testis is then returned to the scrotum, and the Penrose drain is left beneath the cord structures (Fig. 44–60).

Dissection of the Cord

The operating microscope is then brought into the field. Under 4 to 6 power magnification the external and internal spermatic fascias are opened (Fig. 44–61). The magnification is increased to 8 to 15 power, and after irrigation with 1% papaverine solution, the cord is inspected for the presence of pulsations revealing the location of the testicular artery. **If the testicular artery is identified, it is dissected free of all surrounding tissue, tiny veins, and lymphatics, using a fine-tipped nonlocking microneedleholder and microforceps.** The artery is encircled with a 0 silk for positive identification and gentle retraction (Fig. 44–62). The suspected artery is tested by elevating the artery with the tips of the microneedleholder until it is completely occluded, and then it is slowly lowered until a pulsating blush of blood appears just over the needleholder. If the artery is not immediately identified, the cord is carefully dissected beginning with the largest veins. The veins are stripped clean of adherent lymphatics, and the undersides of the largest veins are inspected for an adherent artery. **In approximately 40% of cases, the testicular artery is adherent to the undersurface of a large vein** (Beck et al, 1992). All veins within the cord, with the exception of the vasal veins, are doubly ligated with either hemoclips (Fig. 44–63*A*) or by passing two 4-0 silk ligatures, one black and one white, beneath the vein (see Fig. 44–63*B*). These ligatures are then tied and the vein divided. Medium hemoclips are used for veins 5 mm or larger, small hemoclips are used for veins 1 to 5 mm, and 4-0 silk is used for veins smaller than 2 mm. **The use of an automatic clip applier** (Ligaclip small size, Ethicon,

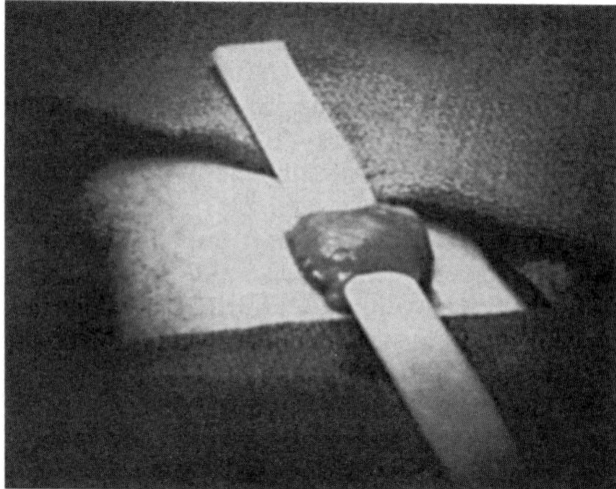

Figure 44–60. The testis has been returned to the scrotum, and the spermatic cord has been elevated over a large Penrose drain.

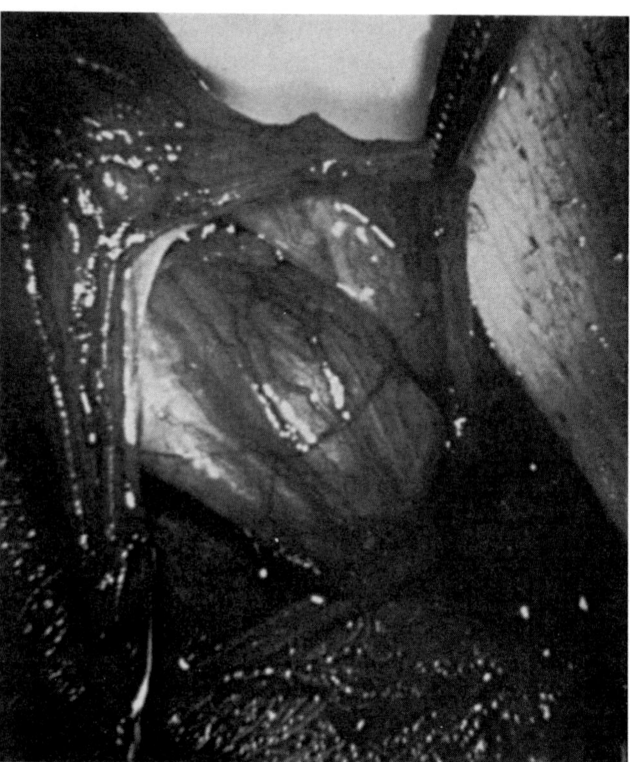

Figure 44–61. The external and internal spermatic fascias are opened. (From Gilbert BR, and Goldstein M: Microsurgery 1988;9:281–285.)

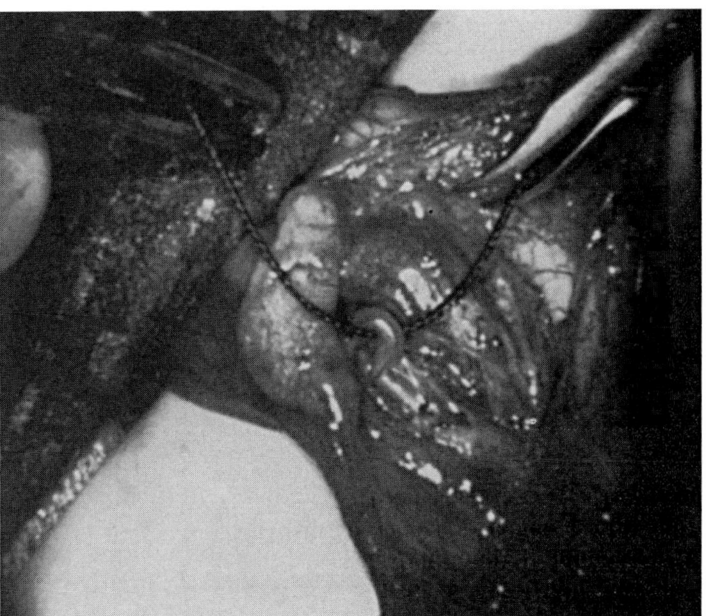

Figure 44–62. The testicular artery is identified and tagged with a 0 silk suture. (From Gilbert BR, Goldstein M: Microsurgery 1988;9:281–285.)

Somerville, NJ) **significantly reduces operating time.** The bipolar cautery can be used for veins smaller than 0.5 mm. The vasal veins are preserved providing venous return. If the vas deferens is accompanied by dilated veins larger than 3 mm in diameter, they are dissected free of the vasal artery and ligated. The vas deferens is always accompanied by two sets of vessels. **As long as at least one set of vasal veins remains intact, venous return will be adequate.** At the completion of the dissection, the cord is run over the index finger and inspected to verify that all veins have been identified and ligated. Small veins adherent to the testicular artery are dissected free and ligated or, if they are smaller than 1 mm, cauterized using a bipolar unit with a jeweler's forceps tip and divided. **At the completion of the dissection, only the testicular artery, cremasteric artery and cremasteric muscle, lymphatics (Fig. 44–64), and vas deferens with its vessels remain.** After adequate hemostasis is achieved, the cord is returned to its bed. The external oblique aponeurosis, if opened, is reapproximated with continuous suturing using the previously placed 3-0 suture. Scarpa's and Camper's fascia are reapproximated with a single or continuous 3-0 plain catgut suture, and the skin is approximated with a 5-0 monofilament absorbable subcuticular suture reinforced by 2 Steri-Strips (Fig. 44–65). A scrotal supporter is applied and stuffed with fluff-type dressings. The patient is discharged on the day of surgery with a prescription for Tylenol with codeine. Light work may be resumed in 2 or 3 days.

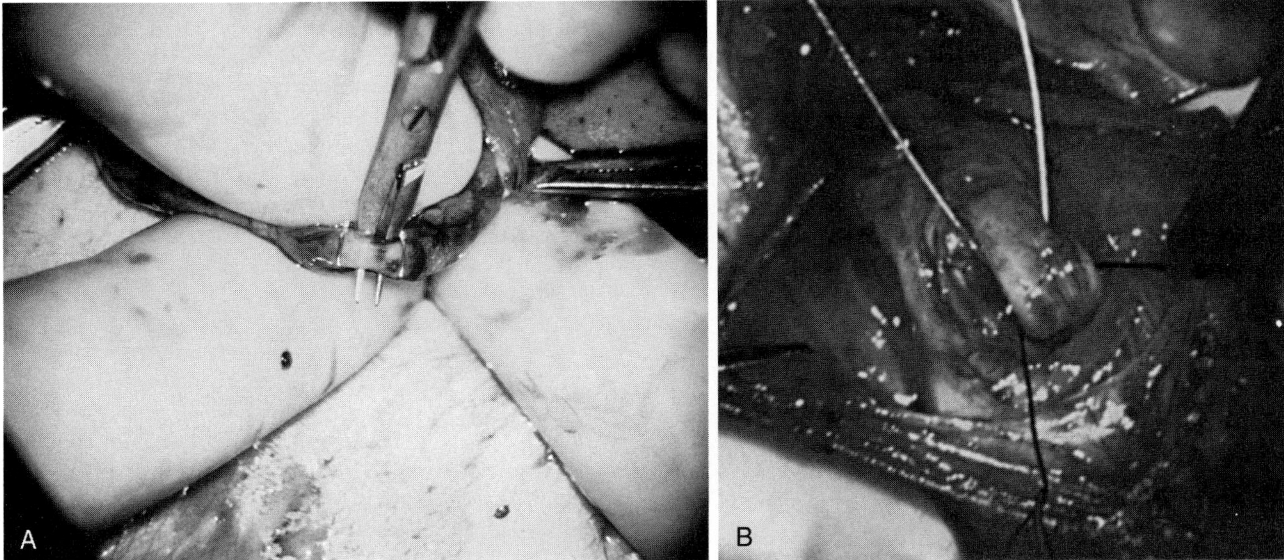

Figure 44–63. Internal spermatic veins are cleaned and ligated with either hemoclips *(A)* or double 4-0 silks, one black and one white, passed beneath them prior to ligation and division *(B)*. (From Gilbert BR, Goldstein M: Microsurgery 1988;9:281–285.)

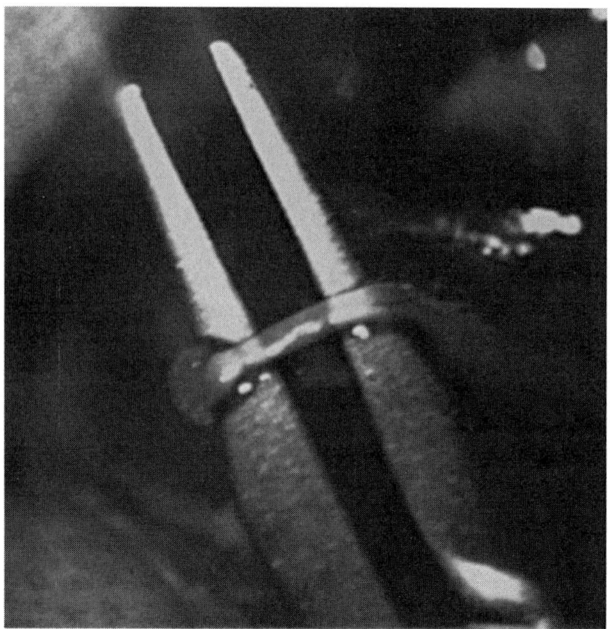

Figure 44–64. Lymphatics are clearly identified and preserved.

Radiographic Occlusion Techniques

Intraoperative venography has been employed to visualize the venous collaterals, that if left unligated, may result in varicocele recurrence (Sayfan et al, 1981; Belgrano et al, 1984; Levitt et al, 1987; Zaontz and Firlit, 1987). Intraoperative venography does reduce the incidence of varicocele recurrence, but the two-dimensional view afforded often does not enable the surgeon to identify the location of all collaterals.

Radiographic balloon or coil occlusion of the internal spermatic veins has been successfully employed for varicoceles (Lima et al, 1978; Walsh and White, 1981; Weissbach et al, 1981). These techniques are performed under a local anesthetic through a small cut-down incision over the femoral vein. The recurrence rate after balloon occlusion was originally 11%, and more recently, it is reportedly as low as 4% (Kaufman et al, 1983; Mitchell et al, 1985; Murray et al, 1986; Matthews et al, 1992). Failure to successfully cannulate small collaterals and external spermatic veins results in recurrence. **Venographic placement of a balloon or coil in the internal spermatic vein is successfully accomplished in 75% to 90% of attempts** (White et al, 1981; Morag et al, 1984); **therefore, a significant number of men undergoing attempted radiographic occlusion will ultimately require a surgical approach.** In addition, radiographic techniques take between 1 and 3 hours to perform compared with 25 to 45 minutes required for surgical repair. Although rare, serious complications of radiographic balloon or coil occlusion have included migration of the balloon or coil into the renal vein, resulting in loss of a kidney, pulmonary embolization of the coil or balloon (Matthews, et al, 1992), femoral vein perforation or thrombosis, and anaphylactic reaction to radiographic contrast medium. Antegrade scrotal sclerotherapy via cannulation of a scrotal vein has been employed in Europe (Tauber and Johsen, 1994). The recurrence rate is similar to that of balloon or coil techniques. Long-term follow-up is not available, and the consequence of escape of the sclerosing agent into the renal vein and vena cava is unknown.

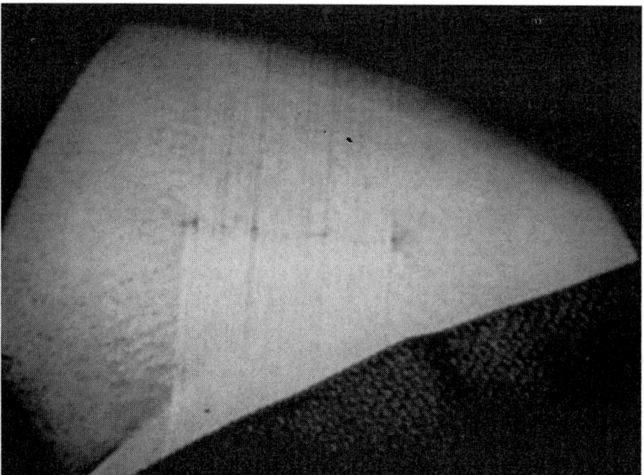

Figure 44–65. Steri-Strip closure of the skin.

Complications of Varicocelectomy

Hydrocele

Hydrocele formation is the most common complication reported after nonmicroscopic varicocelectomy. The incidence of this complication varies from 3% to 33%, with an average incidence of about 7%. Analysis of the protein concentration of hydrocele fluid indicates that **hydrocele formation after varicocelectomy is due to lymphatic obstruction** (Szabo and Kessler, 1984). At least half of postvaricocelectomy hydroceles grow to a size large enough to warrant surgical excision due to the discomfort. The effect of hydrocele formation on sperm function and fertility is uncertain. It is known that men with varicocele have significantly elevated intratesticular temperatures (Zorgniotti and MacLeod, 1979; Goldstein and Eid, 1989), and this factor appears to be an important pathophysiologic phenomenon mediating the adverse effects of varicocele on fertility (Saypol et al, 1981). The development of a large hydrocele creates an abnormal insulating layer that surrounds the testis. This insulating layer may impair the efficiency of the countercurrent heat exchange mechanism and, therefore, obviate some of the benefits of varicocelectomy.

Use of magnification to identify and preserve lymphatics can virtually eliminate the risk of hydrocele formation after varicocelectomy (Goldstein et al, 1992; Marmar and Kim, 1994). Also, radiographic balloon or coil occlusion techniques eliminate the risk of hydrocele formation.

Testicular Artery Injury

The diameter of the testicular artery in humans is 0.5 to 1.5 mm. Microdissections of the human spermatic cord have revealed that the testicular artery is closely adherent to a large internal spermatic vein in 40% of men. In another 20% of men, the testicular artery is surrounded by a network of tiny veins (Beck et al, 1992). During the course of cord dissection for varicocelectomy, the artery may develop a spasm and, even in its unconstricted state, is often difficult to positively identify and preserve. **Injury or ligation of the testicular artery carries with it the risk of testicular atrophy or impaired spermatogenesis, or both.** Starzl's transplant group (Penn et al, 1972) reported a 14% incidence of frank testicular atrophy when the testicular artery was purposely ligated. The actual incidence of testicular artery ligation during varicocelectomy is unknown, but some studies suggest that it is common (Wosnitzer and Roth, 1983). Animal studies indicate that the risk of testicular atrophy after testicular artery ligation varies from 20% to 100% (MacMahon et al, 1976; Goldstein et al, 1983). In humans, atrophy after artery ligation is probably less likely owing to the contribution of the cremasteric as well as vasal arterial supply. **In children, the potential for neovascularization and compensatory hypertrophy of the vasal and cremasteric vessels is probably greater than that in adults, making atrophy after testicular artery ligation less likely.** Use of magnifying loupes, or preferably an operating microscope or a fine-tipped Doppler probe, facilitates identification and preservation of the testicular artery and, therefore, minimizes the risk of testicular injury. Radiographic balloon or coil occlusion techniques also eliminate this risk.

Varicocele Recurrence

The incidence of varicocele recurrence following surgical repair varies from 0.6% to 45%. Recurrence is more common after repair of pediatric varicoceles. Radiographic studies of recurrent varicoceles visualize periarterial, parallel inguinal, or midretroperitoneal collaterals or, more rarely, transscrotal collaterals (Kaufman et al, 1983). **Retroperitoneal operations miss parallel inguinal collaterals.** Nonmagnified inguinal operations have a lower incidence of varicocele recurrence but fail to address the issue of scrotal collaterals or small veins surrounding the testicular artery. The microsurgical approach with delivery of the testis lowers the incidence of varicocele recurrence to less than 1% compared with 9% using conventional inguinal techniques (Goldstein et al, 1992; Marmar and Kim, 1994).

Results

Varicocelectomy results in significant improvement in semen analysis in 60% to 80% of men. Reported pregnancy rates after varicocelectomy vary from 20% to 60%. A randomized controlled trial of surgery versus no surgery in infertile men with varicoceles revealed a pregnancy rate of 44% at one year in the surgery group versus 10% in the control group (Madgar et al, 1995). In our series of 1500 microsurgical operations, 43% of couples were pregnant at 1 year (Goldstein et al, 1992) and 69% at 2 years when couples with female factors were excluded. **Microsurgical varicocelectomy results in return of sperm to the ejaculate in 60% of azoospermic men with palpable varicoceles** (Matthews and Goldstein, 1996a).

The results of varicocelectomy are also related to the size of the varicocele. **Repair of large varicoceles results in a significantly greater improvement in semen quality than repair of small varicoceles** (Steckel et al, 1993; Jarow et al, 1996) (Fig. 44–66). In addition, large varicoceles are associated with greater preoperative impairment in semen quality than small varicoceles, and consequently, overall pregnancy rates are similar regardless of varicocele size. Some evidence suggests that the younger the patient is at the time of varicocele repair, the greater the improvement after repair and the more likely the testis is to recover from varicocele-induced injury (Kass et al, 1987b). Varicocele recurrence, testicular artery ligation, and postvaricocelectomy hydrocele formation are often associated with poor postoperative results. **In infertile men with low serum testosterone levels, microsurgical varicocelectomy alone results in substantial improvement in serum testosterone levels** (Su et al, 1995).

Summary

Varicocele is an extremely common entity and is found in 15% of the male population. Varicoceles are found in approximately 35% of men with primary infertility and 75% to 81% of men with secondary infertility. Mounting evidence clearly demonstrates that varicocele causes progressive duration-dependent injury to the testis. Larger varicoceles appear to cause more damage than small varicoceles, and conversely, repair of large varicoceles results in greater improvement of semen quality. **Varicocelectomy can halt the progressive duration-dependent decline in semen quality found in men with varicoceles.** The earlier the age at which varicocele is repaired, the more likely is recovery of spermatogenic function. **Variococelectomy can also improve Leydig cell function, resulting in increased testosterone levels.**

The most common complications after varicocelectomy are hydrocele formation, testicular artery injury, and varicocele persistence or recurrence. **The incidence of** these **complications can be reduced by employing microsurgical techniques, inguinal or subinguinal operations, and exposure of the external spermatic and scrotal veins.** Employment of these advanced techniques of varicocelectomy provides a safe, effective approach to elimination of varicocele, preservation of testicular function, and in a substantial number of men, an increase in semen quality and likelihood of pregnancy.

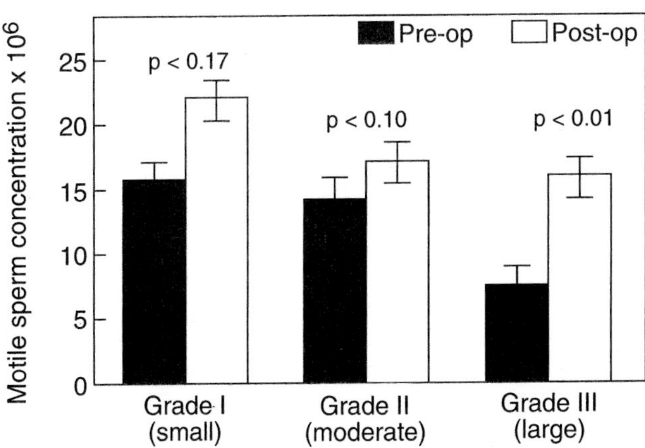

Figure 44–66. Relationship between varicocele size and response to repair.

HYDROCELECTOMY

Inguinal Approach

High-resolution scrotal ultrasound should be performed in all men with hydrocele. An inguinal approach to hydrocelectomy is indicated when sonography or palpation reveals any indication of an intratesticular mass. The surgical approach is identical to that employed for radical orchiectomy. A modification of the Chevassu's maneuver is employed (Goldstein and Waterhouse, 1983). The cord is doubly occluded with rubber-shod clamps, the hydrocele delivered, and the gubernaculum ligated and divided prior to opening the sac. The field is isolated and the testis cooled after the sac is opened. This technique allows inspection of the testis and epididymis and biopsy of suspicious areas without risk of seeding malignant cells. If no malignancy is found, needless orchiectomy is avoided. Hydrocelectomy is then performed using one of the techniques described later.

Scrotal Approach

Scrotal hydrocelectomy may be safely performed when sonographic examination is normal, especially in men with a clear etiology for hydrocele, such as after varicocelectomy or epididymitis. Under these circumstances, either a transverse incision within the scrotal folds and between the scrotal vessels or a median raphe incision results in minimal bleeding and a virtually invisible postoperative scar.

Methods of Repair

If excision techniques of repair are employed, the hydrocele sac is exposed, dissected, and delivered intact. It is opened in an avascular area anteriorly, away from the testis, epididymis, vas deferens, and cord structures. If indicated, samples of hydrocele fluid are collected for cultures and cytology. **Large hydroceles can severely distort the normal anatomic relationships.** The internal spermatic vessels and vas deferens are encircled with Penrose drains for positive identification, and their courses are traced to avoid injury to these structures. The opening in the sac is enlarged using a Bovie cautery in a direction away from the testis, epididymis, vessels, and vas. The testis and epididymis are inspected for masses, evidence of epididymitis, or dilated epididymal tubules suggestive of obstruction. **The margins of the epididymis may be difficult to clearly identify.** In large long-standing hydroceles, the epididymis may be splayed out far from the testis. The convoluted portion of the vas deferens may be distorted and splayed out within the layers of the hydrocele sac. **Loupe magnification is sometimes useful in positively identifying the margins of the epididymis.**

After inspection and identification of all the key structures within and adjacent to the hydrocele sac, repair is accomplished using one of the techniques described later.

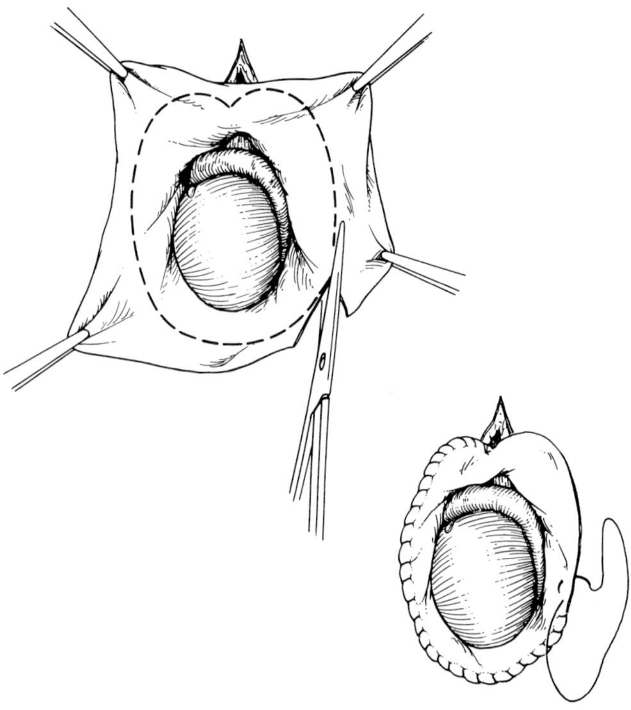

Figure 44–67. Simple excision of thick-walled hydrocele sac with oversewn edges.

Excisional Techniques

Excisional techniques are most certain to result in permanent elimination of the hydrocele. Excision is performed for long-standing hydroceles with thick-walled sacs and multiloculated hydroceles. After simple excision, leaving a one finger-breadth margin to avoid injury to the epididymis, the edges are oversewn with a 4-0 chromic catgut baseball stitch (Fig. 44–67). When large, thin, floppy sacs are excised, the bottleneck operation, in which the sac edges are sewn together behind the cord (Fig. 44–68), reduces the chance of recurrence caused by reapposition of the edges of the hydrocele sac. When the bottleneck operation is employed, the sac margins should be left 1 cm wider to prevent

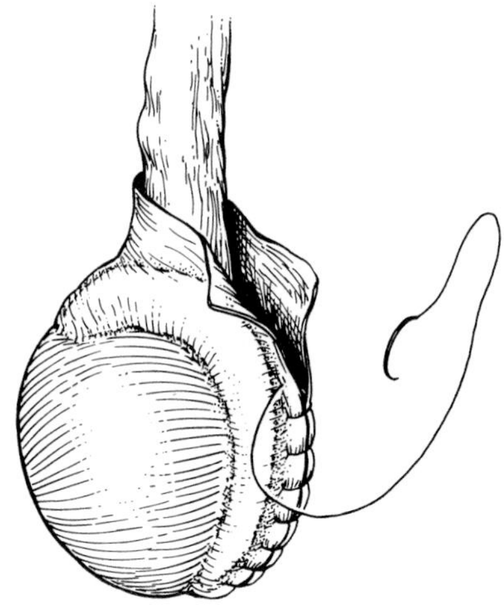

Figure 44–68. Bottleneck technique for excision of thin, floppy sacs.

constriction of the cord. If necessary, a Penrose drain is brought out through the dependent portion of the hemiscrotum and fixed in place with a 2-0 silk suture and a safety pin. The dartos muscle is closed with a continuous catgut suture and the skin with a subcuticular absorbable suture. Fluff dressings are stuffed inside a snug-fitting scrotal supporter.

Plication Techniques

Plication operations (Lord, 1964) can be employed for thin sacs but are not suitable for multiloculated hydroceles or long-standing thick-walled hydroceles because plication will leave a large bundle of residual tissue within the scrotum. Because the sac is not dissected, plication is quick and relatively bloodless.

The sac is opened, and the cut edges are cauterized or oversewn for hemostasis. The testis is delivered, and the sac is inverted. Beginning one finger breadth away from the testis and epididymis, 8 to 12 catgut sutures are placed radially to plicate the sac (Fig. 44–69). Drains are not necessary. Closure is performed as described earlier.

Window Operations

Window operations offer a quick, bloodless method of repair but are associated with a high recurrence rate if they are used for large hydroceles. It is useful for small hydroceles, especially those discovered at the time of varicocelectomy. After the sac is exposed, a 1- to 2-cm buttonhole is removed in an avascular area. The sac edge is oversewn using a continuous everting stitch of 5-0 polypropylene, grasping first the inner epithialialized edge and then tacking it to the outer parietal layer of the tunic with each stitch. The suture line is interrupted halfway one half of the way around (Fig. 44–70).

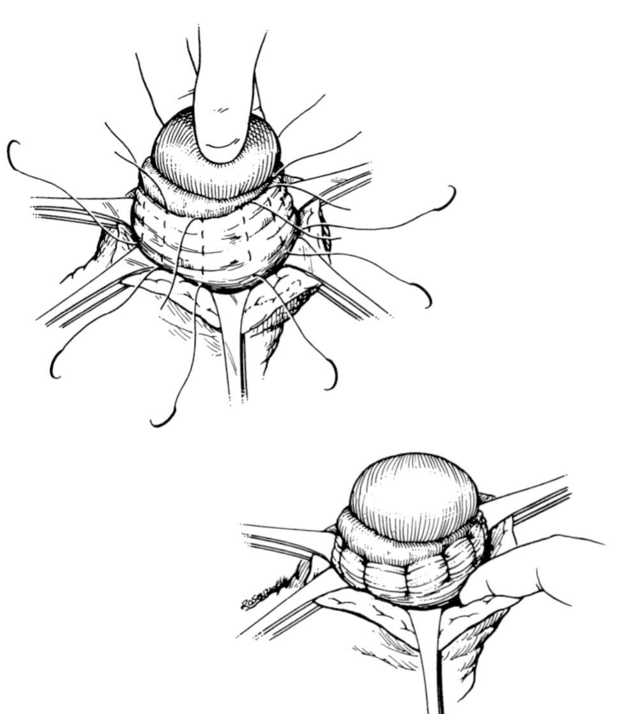

Figure 44–69. Lord's plication technique.

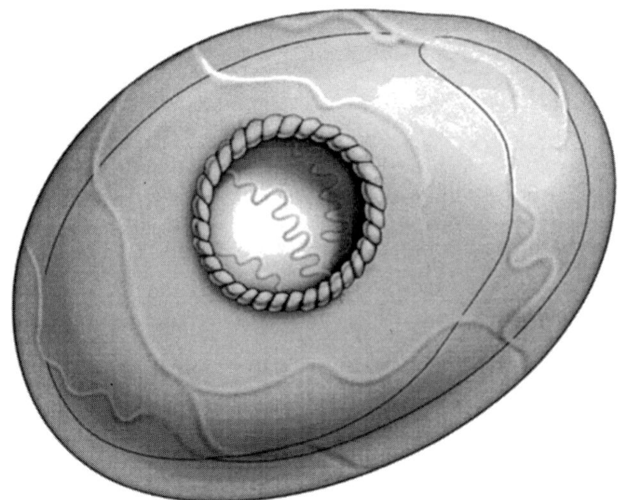

Figure 44–70. Window operation.

Dartos Pouch Technique

The dartos pouch technique is suitable for thin-walled sacs. As in the plication and window techniques, sac dissection is not required and bleeding is minimal. After delivery of the testis, the cut edges of the sac opening are cauterized or oversewn with catgut for hemostasis, and a Dartos pouch is created exactly as for adult scrotal orchiopexy (see the section entitled Scrotal Orchiopexy for Adult Retractile Testis and to Prevent Torsion).

Sclerotherapy

Sclerotherapy has also been used with some success in the treatment of hydrocele. **Sclerotherapy with tetracycline derivatives or other irritating agents may result in epididymal obstruction** (Osegbe, 1991; Ross and Flom, 1991), sometimes is associated with substantial postoperative pain, and is often followed by hydrocele recurrence (Odell, 1979; Osegbe, 1991). When a recurrent hydrocele forms after sclerotherapy, it is usually multiloculated and more difficult to repair. **Sclerotherapy is most useful in older men in whom fertility is no longer an issue** (Sigurdsson et al, 1994).

Complications

Hematoma is the most common complication of hydrocelectomy. When excision techniques are employed, the incidence of hematoma can be minimized by meticulously oversewing all raw edges of the sac and draining the scrotum, when necessary.

In men desiring to maintain their fertility for the future, the primary dangers associated with hydrocelec-

tomy operations are injury to the epididymis or the vas deferens. In some large hydroceles, the anatomy can be extremely distorted. The epididymis may not be identifiable. The vas deferens, especially in its convoluted portion, may be splayed out within the hydrocele layers. Regardless of the approach to hydrocelectomy, the vas deferens and the epididymis should be positively identified and care taken to avoid injury to these structures. The internal spermatic vessels should also be positively identified and encircled with a Penrose drain to prevent injury during excision of the hydrocele sac.

SCROTAL ORCHIOPEXY FOR ADULT RETRACTILE TESTES AND TO PREVENT TORSION

Spermatogenesis is exquisitely temperature sensitive. It is well known that varicocele is associated with elevated testicular temperature, and this factor is believed to be the primary pathophysiologic feature of that disorder (Zorgniotti and MacLeod, 1979; Saypol et al, 1981; Goldstein and Eid, 1989). It is also well known that cryptorchidism is associated with a high incidence of infertility, even when it is unilateral. Both animal and human studies have shown that artificial elevation of testicular temperature results in impaired spermatogenesis. In pigs, testes that are pushed into the abdomen and secured there will stop producing sperm (Wensing, 1986). Orchiopexy restores spermatogenesis. In pigs with surgically created cryptorchid testes, cooling of the testes with an intra-abdominal cooling device restores spermatogenesis (Frankenhui, 1979). Long hot baths and saunas in humans, on a regular basis, have been shown to impair spermatogenesis.

Retractile testes in boys are usually not surgically repaired if the testes can be manually manipulated down into the scrotum either in the office or under anesthesia. The fate of persistently retractile testis in adults is unknown. A subset of infertile men have retractile testis. The semen analyses of these men are similar to those of men with varicoceles. These men, however, do not have palpable varicoceles. They all have at least one testis and frequently both that retract out of the scrotum and into the abdomen and remain there for an hour or more a day. In some men, these testes remain in the abdomen virtually all of the time, except when in a warm shower or under anesthesia. It is likely that these testes will suffer from impaired temperature regulation and impaired spermatogenesis. Scrotal orchiopexy can improve the semen quality and fertility of some of these men.

When scrotal orchiopexy is performed for retractile testis, a dartos pouch operation should be performed. Simple suture orchiopexy of the tunica albuginea of the testis to the dartos, such as is performed sometimes to prevent torsion, will not prevent retraction of these testes into the groin. Creation of a dartos pouch will keep the testis well down into the scrotum and permanently prevent retraction. **This is also the most reliable and safest technique for the prevention of testicular torsion** (Redman 1995a).

A 3- to 4-cm transverse incision is made in the low scrotal skin folds overlying the testis. **The incision is kept very superficial, just through the dermis and not into the dartos. A large pouch must be created to accommodate the adult testis.** The dissection is above the dartos and just below the skin, which is kept thin.

After a capacious pouch is created, the dartos and underlying tunica vaginalis are vertically incised and the testis delivered. The cremasteric fibers are divided and ligated to minimize the tendency of the testis to retract. The opening in the dartos muscle is closed around the cord (but not too tightly) to prevent the testis from falling out of the pouch. The cut edge of the everted tunic is approximated to the opening in the dartos muscle with interrupted synthetic monofilament absorbable sutures. This method allows placement of the testis in the pouch without the need for fixation sutures in the tunica albuginea (Redman 1995). The skin is closed over the testis with interrupted sutures of 4-0 chromic catgut. This technique obviates the risk of inadvertent injury to and bleeding from the testicular artery, which courses just under the tunica albuginea (Jarow, 1990).

ACKNOWLEDGMENT

I thank Jean Schweis and Linda McKeiver of the Population Council, who provided invaluable assistance in the preparation of this manuscript. Thanks to Sarah Girardi, M.D., and Armand Zini, M.D., for their critical review of this manuscript.

REFERENCES

Overview

Gorelick J, Goldstein M: Loss of fertility in men with varicocele. Fertil Steril 1993; 59:613–616.

Hadziselimovic F, Herzog B, Liebundgut B, et al: Testicular and vascular changes in children and adults with varicocele. J Urol 1989; 142:583–585.

Harrison RM, Lewis RW, Roberts JA: Pathophysiology of varicocele in nonhuman primates: Long-term seminal and testicular changes. Fertil Steril 1986; 46:500–510.

Kass EJ, Chandra RS, Belman AB: Testicular histology in the adolescent with a varicocele. Pediatrics 1987; 79:996–998.

Kimura Y, Yanagimachi R: Mouse oocytes injected with testicular spermatozoa or round spermatids can develop into normal offspring. Development 1995; 121:2397–2405.

Lipshultz LI, Corriere JN: Progressive testicular atrophy in the varicocele patient. J Urol 1977; 117:175–176.

Matthews GJ, Goldstein M: Induction of spermatogenesis and pregnancy after microsurgical varicocelectomy in azoospermic men. Presented at the Annual Meeting of American Urological Association, May 4–9, Orlando 1996a; 154:abstract.

Nagler HM, Li X-Z, Lizza EF, et al: Varicocele: Temporal considerations. J Urol 1985; 134:411–413.

Russell JK: Varicocele, age, and fertility. Lancet 1957; II:222.

Schlegel PN, Goldstein M: Microsurgical vasoepididymostomy: Refinements and results. J Urol 1993; 150:1165–1168.

Schlegel PN, Palermo GD, Alikani M, et al: Micropuncture retrieval of epididymal sperm with in vitro fertilization: Importance of in vitro micromanipulation techniques. Urology 1995; 46:238–241.

Tesarik J, Mendoza C, Testart J: Viable embryos from injection of round spermatids into oocytes. N Engl J Med 1995; 333(8):525.

Testis Biopsy

Chan SL, Lipshultz LI, Schwartzendruber D: Deoxyribonucleic acid (DNA) flow cytometry: A new modality for quantitative analysis of testicular biopsies. Fertil Steril 1984; 41:485–487.

Craft I, Tsirigotis M: Simplified recovery, preparation and cryopreservation of testicular spermatozoa. Hum Reprod 1995; 10:1623–1627.

Goldstein M, Young GPH, Einer-Jensen N: Testicular artery damage due to infiltration with a fine gauge needle: Experimental evidence suggesting that blind cord block should be abandoned. Surgical Forum 1983; 24:653–656.

Goldstein M, Schlossberg S: Men with congenital absence of the vas deferens often have seminal vesicles. J Urol 1988; 140:85–86.

Jow WW, Steckel J, Schlegel PN, et al: Motile sperm in human testis biopsy specimens. J Androl 1993; 14:194–198.

Vasography

Dewire DM, Thomas AV: Microsurgical end-to-side vasoepididymostomy. *In* Goldstein M, ed: Surgery of Male Infertility. Philadelphia, W. B. Saunders, 1995, pp 128–134.

Jarrow JP: Seminal vesicle aspiration in the management of patients with ejaculatory duct obstruction. J Urol 1994; 152:899–901.

Katz D, Mieza M, Nagler HM: Ultrasound guided transrectal seminal vesiculaography; a new approach to the diagnosis of male reproductive tract abnormalities. Annual Meeting of the American Urological Association, San Francisco, 1994.

Vasectomy

Alexander NJ, Clarkson TB: Vasectomy increases the severity of diet-induced atherosclerosis in *Macaca fasciculoris*. Science 1978; 201:538.

Appell R, Evans P: Vasectomy: Etiology of infectious complications. Fertil Steril 1980; 33:52–53.

Ban SL: Sterility by vas injection method. Hu Nan Med J 1980; 5:49–50.

Belker AM, Thomas AV, Fuchs EEF: Results of 1469 microsurgical vasectomy reversals by vasovasostary study group. J Urol 1991; 145:505.

Bennett AH: Vasectomy without complication. Urology 1976; 7:184.

Esho JO, Cass AS: Recanalization rate following methods of vasectomy using interposition of fascial sheath of vas deferens. J Urol 1978; 120:178–179.

Freund MJ, Weidmann JE, Goldstein M, et al: Microrencanalization after vasectomy in man. J Androl 1989; 10:120–132.

Fuchs EF, Alexander N: Immunologic considerations before and after vasovasostomy. Fertil Steril 1983; 40:497–499.

Goldstein M: Vasectomy failure using an open ended technique. Fertil Steril 1983; 40:699–700.

Healy B: From the National Institutes of Health. Does vasectomy cause prostate cancer? JAMA 1993; 269:2620.

Jarow JP, Budin RE, Dym M, et al: Quantitative pathological changes in the human testis after vasectomy. N Engl J Med 1985; 313:1252–1255.

Johnson AL, Howards SS: Intratubular hydrostatic pressure in testis and epididymis before and after vasectomy. Am J Physiol 1975; 228:556.

Kendrick J, Gonzales B, Huber D, et al: Complications of vasectomies in the United States. J Fam Prac 1987; 25:245–248.

Lemack GE, Goldstein M: Presence of sperm in the pre-vasectomy reversal semen analysis: Incidence and implications. J Urol 1996; 155:167–169.

Lepow IH, Crozier R: Vasectomy: Immunologic and Pathophysiologic Effects in Animal and Man. New York, Academic Press, 1979.

Li S: Ligation of vas deferens by clamping method under direct vision. Chin Med J 1976; 4:213–214.

Li S: Percutaneous injection of vas deferens. Chin. J. Urol. 1980; 1(4): 193–198.

Li S, Goldstein M, Zhu J, Huber D: The no-scalpel vasectomy. J Urol 1991; 145:341–344.

Massey FJ: Vasectomy and health: Results from a large cohort study. JAMA 1984; 252:1023.

Moss WM: Sutureless vasectomy, an improved technique; 1300 cases performed without failure. Fertil Steril 1974; 27:1040–1045.

Nirapathpongporn A, Huber DH, Krieger JN: No-scalpel vasectomy at the King's birthday vasectomy festival. Lancet 1990; 335:894–895.

Petitti DB, Klein R, Kipp H, Friedman GD: Vasectomy and the incidence of hospitalized illness. J Urol 1982; 129:760–762.

Randall PE, Ganguli L, Marcuson RW: Wound infection following vasectomy. Br J Urol 1983; 55:564–567.

Randall PE, Ganguli LA, Keaney MGL, Marcuson RW: Prevention of wound infection following vasectomy. Br J Urol 1985; 57:227–229.

Schmidt SS: Spermatic granuloma: An often painful lesion. Fertil Steril 1979; 31:178–181.

Schmidt SS: Vasectomy. Urol Clin North Am 1987; 14:149–166.

Schuman LM, Coulson AH, Mandel JS, et al: Health status of American men: A study of post-vasectomy sequelae. J Clin Epidemiol 1993; 46:697–958.

Selikowitz AM, Schned AR: A late post-vasectomy syndrome. J Urol 1985; 134:494–497.

Shapiro EI, Silber SJ: Open-ended vasectomy, sperm granuloma, and post-vasectomy orchialgia. Fertil Steril 1979; 32:546–550.

Silber SJ: Sperm granulomas and reversibility of vasectomy. Lancet 1977; 2:588–589.

Smith MS, Paulson DF: The physiologic consequences of vas ligation. Urological Survey 1980; 30:31–33.

Tao T: Vas deferens sterility by injection method. Qeng Dao Med J 1980; 5:65–68.

Walker AM, Hunter JR, Watkins RN, et al: Vasectomy and non-fatal myocardial infarction. Lancet 1981a; 1:13–15.

Walker AM, Jick H, Hunter JR, et al: Hospitalization rates in vasectomized men. JAMA 1981b; 245:2315–2317.

Witkin SS, Zelikovsky G, Bongiovanni AM: Sperm-related antigens, antibodies, and circulating immune complexes in sera of recently vasectomized men. J Clin Invest 1982; 70:33–40.

Vasovasostomy

Chen L-E, Seaber AV, Urbaniak JR: Comparison of 10-0 polypropylene and 10-0 nylon sutures in rat arterial anastomosis. Microsurgery 1993; 14:328–333.

Goldstein M: Microspike approximator for vaso-vasostomy. J Urol 1985; 134:74.

Goldstein M: Simultaneous microsurgical vasovasostomy and varicocelectomy: Caveat emptor. American Society of Reproductive Medicine, 51st Annual Meeting, 1995.

Hagan KF, Coffey DS: The adverse effects of sperm during vasovasostomy. J Urol 1977; 118:269–273.

Hamidinia A: Transvasovasostomy—an alternative operation for obstructive azoospermia. J Urol 1988; 140:1545–1548.

Hendin BN, Schlegel PN, Goldstein M: Microsurgical reconstruction of iatrogenic injury to the vas deferens. American Fertility Society, 48th Annual Meeting, 1992; 140:1545–1548.

Lemack GE, Goldstein M: Presence of sperm in the pre-vasectomy reversal semen analysis: Incidence and implications. J. Urol. 1996; 155: 167–169.

Lizza EF, Marmar JL, Schmidt SS, et al: Transseptal crossed vasovasostomy. J Urol 1985; 134:1131–1132.

Matthews GJ, Schlegel PN, Goldstein M: Patency following microsurgical vasoepididymostomy and vasovasostomy: Temporal considerations. J Urol 1995; 154:2070–2073.

Surgery of the Epididymis

Fogdestam I, Fall M, Nilsson S: Microsurgical epididymovasotomy in the treatment of occlusive azoospermia. Fertil Steril 1986; 46:925.

Goldstein M, Waterhouse K: When to use the Chevassu maneuver during exploration of intrascrotal masses. J Urol 1983; 130:1199–1200.

Jow WW, Steckel J, Schlegel PN, et al: Motile sperm in human testis biopsy specimens. J Androl 1993; 14:194–198.

Krylov VS, Borovikov AM: Microsurgical method of reuniting ductus epididymis (sic). Fertil Steril 1984; 41:418–423.

Matthews GJ, Schlegel PN, Goldstein M: Patency following microsurgical vasoepididymostomy and vasovasostomy: Temporal considerations. J. Urol 1995a; 154: 2070–2073.

Matthews GJ, Goldstein M: A simplified technique of epididymal sperm aspiration. Urology 1996b; 47:123–125.

Randazzo RF, Hulette CM, Gottlieb MS, Rajfer J: Cytomegalovirus epididymitis in a patient with the acquired immune deficiency syndrome. J Urol 1986; 136:1095–1096.

Schlegel PN, Goldstein M: Microsurgical vasoepididymostomy: Refinements and results. J Urol 1993; 150:1165–1168.

Schoysman RJ, Bedford JM: The role of the human epididymis in sperm maturation and sperm storage as reflected in the consequences of epididymovasostomy. Fertil Steril 1986; 46:292–299.

Selikowitz AM, Schned AR: A late post-vasectomy syndrome. J Urol 1985; 134:494–497.

Silber SJ: Microscopic vasoepididymostomy. Specific microanastomosis to the epididymal tubule. Fertil Steril 1978; 30:565.

Silber SJ: Role of epididymis in sperm maturation. Fertil Steril 1989; 33:47–51.

Thomas AJ Jr: Vasoepididymostomy. Urol Clin North Am 1987; 14:527.

Wagenknecht LV, Klosterhalfen H, Schirren C: Microsurgery in andrologic urology. J Microsurg 1980; 1:370.

Transurethral Resection of the Ejaculatory Ducts

Goldwasser BZ, Weinerth JL, Carson CF: Ejaculatory duct obstruction: The case for aggressive diagnosis and treatment. J Urol 1985; 134:964–966.

Jarow JP: Seminal vesicle aspiration in the management of patients with ejaculatory duct obstruction. J Urol 1994; 152:899–901.

Malkevich DA, Mieza M, Nagler HM: Patency of ejaculatory ducts after transurethral resection of ejaculatory ducts verified by reflux seen on voiding cystourethrogram. J Urol 1994; 151:301A.

Electroejaculation

Bennett CJ, Ayers JWT, Randolph JF Jr, et al: Electroejaculation of paraplegic males followed by pregnancies. Fertil Steril 1987; 48:1070–1072.

Brindley GS: Reflex ejaculation under vibratory stimulation in paraplegic men. Paraplegia 1981; 19:299.

Schellan TM: Induction of ejaculation by electrovibration. Fertil Steril 1968; 19:566.

Sperm Retrieval Techniques

Craft I, Tsirigotis M: Simplified recovery, preparation and cryopreservation of testicular spermatozoa. Hum Reprod 1995; 10:1623–1627.

Craft IL, Tsirigotis M, Bennet V, et al: Percutaneous epididymal sperm aspiration (PESA) and intracytoplasmic sperm injection (ICSI) in the management of infertility due to obstructive azoospermia. Fertil Steril 1995; 63:1038–1042.

Howards SS, Jesse S, Johnson A: Micropuncture and microanalytic studies of the effect of vasectomy on the rat testis and epididymis. Fertil Steril 1975; 26:20.

Matthews GJ, Goldstein M: Microsurgical autogenous sperm reservoir with simultaneous epididymal sperm aspiration: A novel approach for the man with surgically unreconstructable obstruction. Techniques in Urology 1995; 1:120–125.

Matthews GJ, Goldstein M: Simplified method of epididymal sperm aspiration. Urology 1996; 47:123–125.

Moni VN, Lalitha PA: Moni's window operation: A new surgical technique to create a sperm reservoir in congenital vasal agenesis. J Urol 1992; 148:843.

Palermo GD, Schlegel PN, Colombero LT, et al: Aggressive sperm immobilization prior to intractoplasmic sperm injection with immature spermatozoa improves fertilization and pregnancy rates. Hum Reprod 1996; 11:1023–1029.

Rothman CM: A method for obtaining viable sperm in the post-mortem state. Fertil Steril 1980; 34:512.

Schlegel PN, Berkeley AS, Goldstein M, et al: Epididymal micropuncture with IVF for treatment of surgically unreconstructable vasal obstruction. Fertil Steril 1994; 61:895–901.

Schlegel PN, Palermo GD, Alikani M, et al: Micropuncture retrieval of epididymal sperm with in vitro fertilization: Importance of in vitro micromanipulation techniques. Urology 1995; 46:238–241.

Schlegel PN, Palermo GD, Goldstein M, et al: Testicular sperm extraction with ICSI for non-obstructive azoospermia. Urology 1997. In press.

Shrivastav P, Nadkarni P, Wensvoort S, Craft I: Percutaneous epididymal sperm aspiration for obstructive azoospermia. Hum Reprod 1994; 9:2058–2061.

Silber SJ, Ord T, Balmaceda J, et al: Congenital absence of the vas deferens: The fertilization capacity of human epididymal sperm. N Engl J Med 1990; 323:1788–1792.

Turner TT: On the development and use of alloplastic spermatoceles. Fertil Steril 1988; 49:387–394.

Oocyte Micromanipulation Techniques for Facilitated Fertilization

Kimura Y, Yanagimachi R: Mouse oocytes injected with testicular spermatozoa or round spermatids can develop into normal offspring. Development 1995; 121:2397–2405.

Matthews GJ, Goldstein M: Induction of spermatogenesis and pregnancy after microsurgical varicocelectomy in azoospermic men. Presented at the Annual Meeting of American Urological Association, May 4–9, Orlando, 1996a (abstract).

Palermo G, Joris H, Devroey P: Pregnancies after intracytoplasmic injection of single spermatozoon into an oocyte. Lancet 1992; 340:17.

Sofikitis NV, Miyagawa I, Agapitos E, et al: Reproductive capacity of the nucleus of the male gamete after completion of meiosis. J Asstd Reprod Genet 1994; 11:335–341.

Tesarik J, Mendoza C, Testart J: Viable embryos from injection of round spermatids into oocytes. Lancet 1995; 333:525.

Van Steirteghem AC, Nagy Z, Joris H, Liu J: High fertilization and implantation rates after intracytoplasmic sperm injection. Hum Reprod 1993; 8:1061–1066.

Varicocelectomy

Beck EM, Schlegel PN, Goldstein M: Intraoperative varicocele anatomy: A macro and microscopic study. J Urol 1992; 148:1190–1194.

Belgrano E, Puppo P, Quattrini S, et al: The role of venography and sclerotherapy in the management of varicocele. Eur Urol 1984; 10:124–129.

Chehval MJ, and Purcell MH: Deterioration of semen parameters over time in men with untreated varicocele: Evidence of progressive testicular damage. Fertil Steril 1992; 57:174–177.

Donovan JF, Winfield HN: Laparoscopic varix ligation. J Urol 1992; 147:77.

Dubin L, Amelar R: Varicocelectomy: 986 cases in a 12 year study. Urology 1977; 10:446–449.

Goldstein M, Young GPH, Einer-Jensen N: Testicular artery damage due to infiltration with a fine gauge needle: Experimental evidence suggesting that blind cord block should be abandoned. Surgical Forum 1983; 24:653–656.

Goldstein M, Eid JF: Elevation of intratesticular and scrotal skin surface temperature in men with varicocele. J Urol 1989; 142:743–745.

Goldstein M, Gilbert BR, Dicker AP, et al: Microsurgical inguinal varicocelectomy with delivery of the testis: An artery and lymphatic sparing technique. J Urol 1992; 148:1808–1811.

Gorelick J, Goldstein M: Loss of fertility in men with varicocele. Fertil Steril 1993; 59:613–616.

Gorenstein A, Katz S, Schiller M: Varicocele in children: "To treat or not to treat"—venographic and manometric studies. J Pediatr Surg 1986; 21:1046–1050.

Hadziselimovic F, Herzog B, Liebundgut B, et al: Testicular and vascular changes in children and adults with varicocele. J Urol 1989; 142:583–585.

Harrison RM, Lewis RW, Roberts JA: Pathophysiology of varicocele in nonhuman primates: Long-term seminal and testicular changes. Fertil Steril 1986; 46:500–510.

Homonnai ZT, Fainman N, Engelhard Y, et al: Varicocelectomy and male fertility: Comparison of semen quality and recurrence of varicocele following varicocelectomy by two techniques. Int J Androl 1980; 3:447–456.

Jarow JP, Ogle SR, Eskew LA: Seminal improvement following repair of ultrasound detected subclinical varicoceles. J Urol 1996; 155:1287–1290.

Kass EJ, Belman AB: Reversal of testicular growth failure by varicocele ligation. J Urol 1987a; 137:475.

Kass EJ, Chandra RS, Belman AB: Testicular histology in the adolescent with a varicocele. Pediatrics 1987b; 79:996–998.

Kass EJ, Marcol B: Results of varicocele surgery in adolescents: A comparison of techniques. J Urol 1992; 148:694–696.

Kaufman SL, Kadir S, Barth KH, et al: Mechanisms of recurrent varicocele after balloon occlusion or surgical ligation of the internal spermatic vein. Radiology 1983; 147:435.

Levitt S, Gill B, Katlowitz N, Kogan SJ, Reda E: Routine intraoperative post-ligation venography in the treatment of the pediatric varicocele. J Urol 1987; 137:716–718.

Lima SS, Castro MP, Costa OF: A new method for the treatment of varicocele. Andrologia 1978; 10:103.

Lipshultz LI, Corriere JN: Progressive testicular atrophy in the varicocele patient. J Urol 1977; 117:175.

MacMahon RA, O'Brien B McG, Cussen LJ: The use of microsurgery in the treatment of the undescended testis. J Pediatr Surg 1976; 11:521.

Madgar I, Weissenberg R, Lunenfeld B, et al: Controlled trial of high spermatic vein ligation for varicocele in infertile men. Fertil Steril 1995; 63:120–124.

Marmar JL, DeBenedictis TJ, Praiss D: The management of varicoceles by microdissection of the spermatic cord at the external inguinal ring. Fertil Steril 1985; 43:583–588.

Marmar JL, Kim Y: Subinguinal microsurgical varicocelectomy: A technical critique and statistical analysis of semen and pregnancy data. J Urol 1994; 152:1127–1132.

Matthews GJ, Goldstein M: Induction of spermatogenesis and pregnancy after microsurgical varicocelectomy in azoospermic men. Presented at the Annual Meeting of American Urological Association, May 4–9, Orlando 1996a (abstract).

Matthews RD, Roberts J, Walke, WA, Sands JP: Migration of intravascular balloon after percutaneous embolotherapy of varicocele. Urology 1992; 39:373–375.

Mitchell SE, White RI, Chang R, et al: Long-term results of outpatient balloon embolotherapy in 300 varicoceles. Radiology 1985; 157:90.

Morag B, Rubinstein ZJ, Goldwasser B, et al: Percutaneous venography and occlusion in the management of spermatic varicoceles. Am J Roentgenol 1984; 143:635–640.

Murray RR, Mitchell SE, Kadir S, et al: Comparison of recurrent varicocele anatomy following surgery and percutaneous balloon occlusion. J. Urol. 1986; 135: 286–289.

Nagler HM, Li X-Z, Lizza EF, et al: Varicocele: Temporal considerations. J Urol 1985; 134:411–413.

Penn I, Mackie G, Halgrimson CG, Starzl TE: Testicular complications following renal transplantion. Ann Surg 1972; 176:697.

Reitelman C, Burbige KA, Sawczuk IS, Hensle TW: Diagnosis and surgical correction of the pediatric varicocele. J Urol 1987; 138:1038–1040.

Rothman LP, Newmark M, Karson R: The recurrent varicocele. A poorly recognized problem. Fertil Steril 1981; 35:552.

Russell JK: Varicocele, age, and fertility. Lancet 1957; ii:222.

Sayfan J, Adam YG, Soffer Y: A new entity in varicocele subfertility: The "cremasteric reflux." Fertil Steril 1980; 33:88.

Sayfan J, Adam YG, Soffer Y: A natural "venous bypass" causing postoperative recurrence of a varicocele. J Androl 1981; 2:108–110.

Saypol DC, Howards SS, Turner TT: Influence of surgically induced varicocele on testicular blood flow, temperature, and histology in adult rats and dogs. J Clin Invest 1981; 68:39.

Steckel J, Dicker AP, Goldstein M: Influence of varicocele size on response to microsurgical ligation of the spermatic veins. J Urol 1993; 149:769–771.

Su L-M, Goldstein M, Schlegel PN: The effect of varicocelectomy on serum testosterone levels in infertile men with varicoceles. J Urol 1995; 154:1752–1755.

Szabo R, Kessler R: Hydrocele following internal spermatic vein ligation: A retrospective study and review of the literature. J Urol 1984; 132:924–925.

Tauber R, Johsen N: Antegrade scrotal sclerotherapy for the treatment of varicocele: Technique and late results. J Urol 1994; 151:386–390.

Walsh PC, White RI: Balloon occlusion of the internal spermatic vein for the treatment of varicoceles. JAMA 1981; 246:1701.

Weissbach L, Thelen M, Adolphs H-D: Treatment of idiopathic varicoceles by transfemoral testicular vein occlusion. J Urol 1981; 126:354–356.

White RI, Kaufman SL, Barth KH, et al: Occlusion of varicoceles with detachable balloons. Radiology 1981; 139:327.

Witt MA, Lipshultz LI: Varicocele: A progressive or static lesion? Urology 1993; 42:541–543.

Wosnitzer M, Roth JA: Optical magnification and Doppler ultrasound probe for varicocelectomy. Urology 1983; 22:24–26.

Zaontz MR, Firlit CF: Use of venography as an aid in varicocelectomy. J Urol 1987; 138:1041–1042.

Zorgniotti AW, MacLeod J: Studies in temperature, human semen quality, and varicocele. Fertil Steril 1979; 24:40.

Hydrocelectomy

Goldstein M, Waterhouse K: When to use the Chevassu maneuver during exploration of intrascrotal masses. J Urol 1983; 130:1199–1200.

Lord PH: A bloodless operation for the radical cure of idiopathic hydrocele. Br J Surg 1964; 51:914.

Odell TH: Sclerosant treatment for hydroceles and epididymal cysts. Br Med J 1979; 2:704.

Osegbe DN: Fertility after sclerotherapy for hydrocele. Lancet 1991; 337:172.

Ross LS, Flom LS: Azoospermia: A complication of hydrocele repair in fertile population. J Urol 1991; 146:1991.

Sigurdsson T, Johansson JE, Jahnson S, et al: Polidocanol sclerotheraphy for hydroceles and epididymal cysts. J Urol 1994; 151:898–901.

Scrotal Orchiopexy for Adult Retractile Testes and to Prevent Torsion

Frankenhui MT, Wensing CJG: Induction of spermatogenesis in the naturally cryptorchid pig. Fertil Steril 1979; 31:428.

Goldstein M, Eid JF: Elevation of intratesticular and scrotal skin surface temperature in men with variocele. J Urol 1989; 142:743–745.

Jarow JP: Intratesticular arterial anatomy. J Androl 1990; 11:255–259.

Redman JF, Barthold JS: A technique for atraumatic scrotal pouch orchiopexy in the management of testicular torsion. J Urol 1995; 154:1511–1512.

Saypol DC, Howards SS, Turner TT: Influence of surgically induced varicocele on testicular blood flow, temperature, and histology in adult rats and dogs. J Clin Invest 1981; 68:39.

Wensing CJG: Testicular descent in the rat and a comparison of this process with that in the pig. Anat Rec 1986; 214:154.

Zorgniotti AW, MacLeod J: Studies in temperature, human semen quality, and varicocele. Fertil Steril 1979; 24:40.

VIII
BENIGN PROSTATIC HYPERPLASIA

45
THE MOLECULAR BIOLOGY, ENDOCRINOLOGY, AND PHYSIOLOGY OF THE PROSTATE AND SEMINAL VESICLES

Alan W. Partin, M.D., Ph.D.
Donald S. Coffey, Ph.D.

The sex accessory tissues include the prostate, seminal vesicles, and bulbourethral glands. At present, there is a lack of firm insight into the specific biologic functions of the male sex accessory tissues. They require the continued function of the testes for their development, growth, and maintenance of the secretions that form the major components of the ejaculate. The tremendous variation in the evolution of these sex accessory glands is expressed by marked species differences of anatomy, biology, and function. For example, the seminal vesicles are large and prominent in the human and rat but are absent in both the cat and dog.

The presence of the prostate is *universal* in mammals. However, it is marked by considerable variation in anatomy, biochemistry, and pathology. This species variation is reflected in the comparative volume of ejaculate: 250 ml in the boar, 70 ml in the stallion, 9 ml in the dog, 4 ml in the bull, 3 ml in the human, and only 1 ml in the ram. Whereas the human ejaculate forms a clot and subsequently lyses, in rodents, a solid copulatory plug is formed. In the human ejaculate, the major anion is citrate, whereas in the dog ejaculate, it is chloride ion.

The human sex accessory tissues produce very high concentrations of many potent biologic substances that appear in the seminal plasma, such as fructose (2 mg/ml), citric acid (4 mg/ml), spermine (3 mg/ml), prostaglandins (200 μg/ml), zinc (150 μg/ml), proteins (40 mg/ml), and enzymes such as immunoglobulins, proteases, esterases, and phosphatases. With the exception of specific enzyme activities in the clotting and lysing process occurring with seminal plasma proteins, there is limited knowledge of the physiologic function of many of the other potent secretory products within the seminal plasma. The seminal plasma may not contain factors that are absolutely essential for fertilization. Nevertheless, the secretions may optimize conditions for fertilization by providing a buffered effect, increasing sperm motility, or enhancing sperm survival or sperm transport in both the male and female reproductive tracts. These sex accessory glands are uniquely positioned to block the entrance of pathogens by secreting potent biologic protective substances into the urethra. These substances include high concentrations of metal ions (zinc) or highly charged organic molecules (spermine) or potent proteases (lysozymes and prostatic-specific antigen). The mechanical washing of the urethra by these secretions, as well as the establishment of a hostile milieu to invading pathogens, may be one of the primary functions of the sex accessory tissues and may account for the large variability in structure and composition of these glands between species.

Abnormal growth of the sex accessory tissues is primarily limited to the prostate of the human and dog. Why all other mammals such as the horse, bull, and cat are completely devoid of prostate tumors is still a mystery. It is also unknown why only the prostate gland in the human has such a high incidence of benign and malignant tumors, whereas the bulbourethral glands and the seminal vesicles are essentially devoid of tumors. Approximately 50% of men develop symptoms from benign prostatic hyperplasia (BPH), and 10% develop clinically detectable cancer within their lifetime. In contrast, tumors have never been reported in the bulbourethral gland. This is difficult to explain because both of these glands arise from the same developmental anlagen, the urogenital sinus, and the same hormonal stimulus by dihydrotestosterone (DHT). Both glands have similar vascular and neuronal stimulation, as well as the same exposure to urine. It is unknown whether or not the differences in the pathology between these two glands are caused by intrinsic or extrinsic environmental factors. The answer to these questions may provide an important insight into BPH, carcinogenesis, and the prevention of prostate cancer. For detailed reviews of prostate physiology, see Small and Prins (1995), Luke and Coffey (1994a), Lepor and Lawson (1993), and the early classics of Mann and Mann (1981) and Aumuller (1979).

DEVELOPMENT AND CELL BIOLOGY

Embryonic Development

The sex accessory glands differ in their embryonic origin and in the type of steroid that induces their developmental growth. Aumuller (1979) has provided the most detailed classic review of the embryologic, histologic, and endocrinologic aspects of both the prostate and seminal vesicle development (Cunha, 1994; Randall, 1994; Small and Prins, 1995). **Under the influence of testosterone, the wolffian ducts develop into the seminal vesicles, epididymis, vas deferens, and ejaculatory ducts.** The growth of these wolffian-derived sex accessory glands is primarily completed by the 13th week of gestation. **The prostate develops from the urogenital sinus during the third fetal month under the influence of DHT produced from fetal testosterone through the action of the enzyme 5α-reductase. The five paired epithelial buds arise on the posterior side of the urogenital sinus on both sides of the verumontanum and invade the mesenchyme to form the prostate.** The top pairs of buds form the inner zone of the prostate and appear to be of mesoderm origin, whereas the lower buds form the outer zone of the prostate and appear to be of endoderm origin. **This is of potential importance because BPH arises from the inner zone, whereas the outer zone contains the primary origin of cancer.** The inner and outer zones of the prostate develop as concentric circles around the urethra. The long-branched ducts along the outer zone form the thick peripheral layer of the true prostate gland. The central portion of the prostate contains the mucosal and submucosal glands, a remnant of the müllerian duct (the utriculus prostaticus, which forms the prostatic utricle), and the ejaculatory ducts, which traverse both zones. The prostate is histologically well differentiated by the fourth fetal month. There has been much debate, and several divergent views on the development of the zones of the prostate have been offered (see Chapter 3). This debate has been reviewed earlier in detail by McNeal (1980) and by Aumuller (1979). The full embryology of the prostate in relation to its zones still requires modern biologic and molecular techniques for a precise definition.

The prostate forms acini and collecting ducts by arborization that branches from the urethra and may be compared to a small tree, with growth occurring primarily at the tips of the ducts as they extend and branch during development. The belief that these dynamic growth processes occur along a budding and branching system was developed from studies on the mouse and rat prostate (Sugimura et al, 1986; Banerjee et al, 1993a, 1993b; Cunha, 1994).

At 3 1/2 months (14 weeks) of gestation, the prostate is composed of 70 ducts surrounded by stromal components that arise from the mesonephric and paramesonephric mesenchyme. In response to high maternal levels of estradiol, at 5 months of development, an extensive squamous cell metaplasia appears, peaks at 36 weeks, and then starts to subside. The decrease in squamous cell growth following birth results in a diminution in the size of the prostate at 3 months. **The male fetus is dependent on androgens synthesized by the Leydig cells, which become activated during the second month of gestation and reach a peak secretory activity by the fourth month.**

During development of the prostate from the urogenital sinus, there is a close reciprocal interaction between the stromal and epithelial tissue components (Verhoeven et al, 1992; Cunha, 1994). DHT is produced from testosterone by 5α-reductase within the mesenchymal elements (stroma) of the prostate. Although the theory has not been proved, one can hypothesize that DHT is formed in the stromal cells and has an autocrine effect within the stromal cell and a paracrine effect on DHT receptors in nearby secretory epithelial nuclei. This process, in turn, stimulates the morphogenesis of the epithelial cells. This process is thought to occur by induction of DHT by specific soluble growth factors such as epidermal growth factor (EGF), keratinocyte growth factor (KGF, fibroblast growth factor-7 [FGF-7]), insulin-like growth factor (IGF), and transforming growth factor-β). In addition, DHT induces alterations in the insoluble extracellular matrix components interfacing the stromal and epithelial cells. Identifying the exact growth factors and extracellular matrix changes related to these temporal events will be an important basic research frontier in andrology and urology.

In the development of other organs, it is apparent that growth factors have several functions: they can either stimulate or inhibit growth depending on concentrations, combination, and sequence of presentation to target cells. For example, EGF interacts with TGF-β, IGF, and gonadotropins to affect the differentiation of the other types of reproductive cells. It is expected that similar roles will be further elucidated for various types of prostate cells as well (Bendell and Dorrington, 1990; Cohen et al, 1991; Martinoli and Pelletier, 1991; Yan et al, 1992; Cohen et al, 1993; Steiner, 1993; Sikes et al, 1995). **Growth factors are discussed later, but it is important to note that müllerian inhibiting substance (MIS) is expressed early in gonadal differentiation of the male and causes the regression of the müllerian duct**. The requirement for MIS in human male development is well established; the human gene has been isolated, the primary amino acid sequence of MIS has been determined. It now appears that MIS is closely related to a family of proteins that include TGF-β, a very potent inhibitor of normal epithelial growth, and has functions in a wide variety of cell types.

The temporal events that are involved in the development of the male reproductive tract, as well as the involvement of both steroids and growth hormones, are of fundamental importance in developmental biology but also may be of great interest in the study of the development of pathology in the prostate. It has been proposed by McNeal (1978) that BPH may be caused by reactivation of dormant embryonic growth in the adult stroma: The proliferation of the stromal elements can stimulate the ingrowth of epithelial cells to produce a benign growth. Animal models using sandwiches of chimeric tissues composed of embryonic urogenital mesenchyme and adult prostate tissues have demonstrated that the fetal mesenchyme can drive both the differentiation and growth of adult urogenital cells (Cunha et al, 1983b; Chung and Cunha, 1983, 1984, 1987; Thompson and Chung, 1986; Cunha, 1994; Sikes et al, 1995).

Postnatal Development and Hormone Imprinting of Growth

At birth, the majority of the prostatic acini are lined with squamous and metaplastic epithelial cells, which have scattered secretory activity and lead to the formation of lumen of varying sizes and shapes (Andrews, 1951; Aumuller, 1979). The stimulation of this development is believed to be controlled by residual maternal steroids such as estrogens. With the withdrawal of maternal estrogens, a prostatic involutional phase occurs during the first 5 months following birth. Large transient surges of serum androgen, estrogen, and progesterone levels normally occur very early in postnatal life in both rats and in humans. **In the human male, neonatal surges in testosterone are observed to peak between 2 and 3 months of age. During this period, serum testosterone levels rise to 60 times that of normal prepubertal levels and often reach the adult serum testosterone range of about 400 ng/dl (Forest, 1979; Pang et al, 1979).** Serum estradiol levels are very high at birth in both humans and rats but quickly fall to near undetectable levels in the first few days after birth. There is a subsequent transient prepubertal surge in serum estradiol levels in the rat but not in humans. Human progesterone levels are high at birth and are believed to be elevated from placental progesterone production. There is a second transient progesterone surge that occurs in humans at approximately 2 months of age (Forest, 1979).

Studies in the rat have shown that neonatal and prepubertal steroids are of critical importance in determining the long-term growth regulation of the prostate that occurs later in life when the organ is subjected to testosterone stimulation (Kincl et al, 1963; Swanson et al, 1963; Morrison and Johnson, 1966; Bronson et al, 1972; Rajfer and Coffey, 1979a, 1979b; Chung and McFadden, 1980; Naslund and Coffey, 1986, 1987; Prins and Birch, 1995). **The ability of neonatal and prepubertal steroids to imprint the prostate has been established as a critical factor in animal studies but has not been fully defined for the human prostate.** It is important to note that there are differences in the postnatal development of the male reproductive tract between human and rodents, but the correlation of these prepubertal surges of steroid blood levels in both the rat and human may indicate that a similar imprinting process may be expected in the human. Naslund and Coffey (1986, 1987) have proposed that neonatal imprinting may be an important factor in setting the response of the prostate in later adult life and could have implications for BPH as well. Higgins and associates (1982) have shown that differentiation in the rat prostate may be determined, in part, by DNA methylation of specific genes in the seminal vesicles and ventral prostate. Recent work has demonstrated that in utero exposure to lactational toxins (e.g., 2,3,7,8-tetrachlorodibenzo-*p*-dioxin) can inhibit rat ventral prostate imprinting for size and protein expression but does not inhibit imprinting of testosterone response (Bjerke et al, 1994). Prins (1992) demonstrated that neonatal estrogen exposure can alter prostatic growth in the rat and produces lobe-specific changes in the androgen receptor expression in the adult gland (Prins and Birch, 1995). **Testosterone, DHT, and estrogen can vary in their effect on the prostate at various times during development, postnatal imprinting, puberty, adulthood, and aging.** These changes are often associated with a redistribution of steroid receptors and the response to stimulation of specific patterns of growth factors with their concomitant receptors.

Overview of the Gross Anatomy of the Sex Accessory Glands

The prostate contains a number of individual glands composed of 30 to 50 lobules leading to 15 to 30 secretory ducts that open into the urethra lateral to the colliculus seminalis (Narbaitz, 1974; Aumuller, 1979). In the discussion of prostate organization, the term lobes has been replaced by zones (McNeal, 1988, 1990). The shape of the prostate has been compared to a horse chestnut, with the length of the anterior aspect being between 3 and 4 cm and its width between 3.5 to 5 cm. **The normal adult human prostate weighs approximately 20 g, plus or minus 6 g (Berry et al, 1984) and lies immediately below the base of the bladder surrounding the proximal portion of the urethra.** The gland is located posterior to the inferior part of the symphysis pubis, superior to the urogenital diaphragm and anterior to the rectum. The gland is composed of alveoli lined by tall columnar secretory epithelial cells. The acini of these alveoli drain, by a system of branching ducts and tubules, into the floor and lateral surfaces of the posterior urethra. The alveoli and ducts are embedded within a stroma of fibromuscular tissue.

The seminal vesicles weigh 8 to 9 g in the human and develop as paired pouches (capacity, 4.5 ml each) from the vas deferens. The glands are 4 to 5 cm in length and are located directly posterior to the bladder adjacent to the rectum. The glands are composed of tubular alveoli containing viscous secretions. The ducts can be highly variable from a simple tube to the more common short main ducts with clusters of large side ducts. **Their secretions contribute to semen but are not stored. The ampulla at the distal end of the vas deferens does store sperm, and the seminal vesicles join the ampulla to form the beginning of the ejaculatory ducts**. The ejaculatory ducts pass through the prostate and finally terminate below the utricle within the prostate urethra at the verumontanum.

The bulbourethral, or Cowper's, gland is a paired, pea-sized, typically mucous, compound tubular gland located directly below the prostate within the urogenital sinus. This gland was named after its founder, William Cowper, who first described it in 1698. It is variable in evolution, being a very large gland in the squirrel and boar but absent in the dog. The glands empty into the urethra, and the function and composition of their secretions are poorly understood, except that they contain high concentrations of sialic acid. **Very small periurethral glands, termed glands of Littre, line the penile urethra. It is believed that the Cowper's and Littre glands function to lubricate the urethra, thus facilitating intromission. All of these sex accessory tissues depend on androgens for development, growth, and maintenance of their size and secretory products, and contribute to the composition of the seminal plasma of the ejaculate.**

Prostate Anatomy

For many years, the prostate was believed to have a lobular structure. Prior to 1906, when Home described the middle lobe, the prostate was considered to be composed of only two lateral lobes (LeDuc, 1939). For the next century, the importance of the two or three lobes of the prostate was widely debated. However, in 1912, Lowsley proposed the existence of five prostatic lobes based on embryologic findings: two lateral lobes, an anterior lobe, a posterior lobe, and the middle lobe. The anterior lobe, which was present in fetal material, atrophied and disappeared by the time of birth. This concept was adopted widely for the next 50 years. Franks (1954) has emphasized that these divisions were only identifiable in the embryo; from the last months of gestation into postnatal life, no divisions into separate glands were possible. Furthermore, LeDuc (1939) was unable to demonstrate a posterior row of prostatic ducts, challenging the existence of the posterior lobe of the prostate given such anatomic prominence by Lowsley. **Urologic surgeons frequently refer to midline and laterally projecting nodules of BPH as middle and lateral lobes, respectively. However, these so-called lobes are not reference points of normal anatomy but exist only as lobular enlargement of hyperplastic tissue in men with BPH.**

Today, the concept of a lobular structure has been replaced by a concept based on concentric zones. Many authors have suggested that the prostate could be separated into at least two independent structures, an inner and an outer zone (Young, 1926; Huggins and Webster, 1948; Franks, 1954). In more recent years, the morphology of the prostate has come under intense study by several talented investigators (McNeal, 1968, 1976, 1980, 1981, 1988, 1990; Tissell and Salander, 1975; Blacklock and Bouskill, 1977). Of these, McNeal's work appears to be the most widely accepted. A historical and comparative analysis of McNeal's terminology to the contributions of others has been made (McNeal, 1980). Rather than dividing the prostate into arbitrary lobes, McNeal has identified zones that appear to have morphologic, functional, and pathologic significance. To understand his descriptions of the prostate, it is important to recognize that the prostatic urethra is not a straight tube. Rather, at the midpoint of the prostatic urethra between the apex of the prostate and the bladder neck (i.e., at the upper end of the verumontanum) the posterior wall of the urethral is angled anteriorly in such a way that the entire proximal urethra is angled 35 degrees anterior to the course of the distal urethral segment. Previously, many investigators used transverse sections of the prostate taken at the level of the verumontanum for their studies. However, McNeal (1968) has emphasized the need for planes other than conventional transverse sections to demonstrate differences between one part of the prostate and the other. Using sagittal, coronal, and oblique sections, he has divided the prostate into four distinct zones. Each zone makes contact with a specific portion of the prostatic urethra, which can be taken as the primary anatomic landmark for defining them. The subsequent descriptions of these zones are taken directly from McNeal's many contributions (McNeal, 1968, 1976, 1980, 1981, 1988, 1990).

The *anterior fibromuscular stroma* is a thick sheet of connective tissue that covers the entire anterior surface of the prostate. It is a continuous sheet of smooth muscle that surrounds the urethra proximally at the bladder neck, where it emerges with the internal sphincter and detrusor muscle. Near the apex, the smooth muscle merges with transverse loops of striated muscle, which represent a proximal extension of the external sphincter, thus forming an incomplete sphincter along the anterior aspect of the distal urethral segment. **The anterior fibromuscular stroma comprises up to one third of the total bulk of the prostate**. It is entirely lacking in glandular elements.

***The peripheral zone* is the largest anatomic subdivision of the prostate**. It is a flat disk of secretory tissue whose ducts branch out laterally from either side of the distal urethra. Laterally, some of the terminal ducts curve anteriorly to form a shallow cup around the striated sphincter and then anchor into the lateral extent of the anterior fibromuscular stroma. **This zone contains 75% of the total glandular tissue of the prostate. In this region, a majority of carcinomas arise. Furthermore, this is the tissue sampled in most random biopsies of the prostate.**

The *central zone* is the smaller of the two subdivisions of functioning glandular prostate, making up about 25% of its mass. It contacts the urethra only at the upper end of the verumontanum, where its ductal orifices open in a tight circle immediately around the ejaculatory duct orifices. The ducts branch laterally to form a flat wedge of glandular tissue with its apex at the verumontanum and its base at the base of the prostate posterior to the bladder neck. The central zone surrounds the ejaculatory ducts, completing the proximal quadrant of glandular tissue above and behind the verumontanum. McNeal distinguishes the central from the peripheral zone based on differences in architecture of the glands and cytologic detail. He believes that the architecture and histologic features of the central zone closely resemble those of the seminal vesicle, suggesting that the central zone could be of wolffian duct origin. This possibility correlates with the uncommon occurrence of carcinoma in both the seminal vesicle and central zone.

The *preprostatic tissue*, which surrounds the anteriorly displaced urethra proximal to the upper end of the verumontanum, is the smallest of the four regions and most complex in its arrangement of glandular and nonglandular elements. This term has been applied to this zone because of its sphincteric function at the time of ejaculation to prevent reflux of seminal fluid into the bladder. Its main component is a cylindrical smooth muscle sphincter surrounding the entire preprostatic urethra. Inside this cylinder of smooth muscle are the tiny periurethral glands, which constitute less than 1% of the mass of the glandular prostate. They do not possess their own periglandular musculature and are confined in their extent to the immediate periurethral stroma. Because the smooth muscle cylinder limits the expansion of the glands laterally away from the urethra, these glands grow proximally toward the bladder neck. However, at the distal margin of the smooth muscle sphincter, some ducts escape below the most distal rings of the smooth muscle sleeve, thus enabling them to develop outside its confines.

The *transition zone* is a small group of ducts, arising at a single point at the junction of the proximal and distal urethral segments. The ducts in this region, which comprise less than 5% of the mass of the normal glandular prostate, demonstrate more branching and acinar proliferation than the other periurethral ducts. Although they are insignificant in size and functional importance, the transition zone and the other periurethral glands are the origin of BPH.

Seminal Vesicle Anatomy

The seminal vesicles (glands) consist of hollow tubes approximately 15 cm long, which are coiled into two vesicle-like glands located near the base of the bladder in close approximation to the prostate. For years, after the initial anatomic description of the seminal vesicles, it was incorrectly assumed that these organs stored seminal fluid because sperm were found within the fluid that was expressed from them. **It is now widely accepted that the seminal vesicles do not store sperm. A more appropriate term would be seminal glands because their major function is secretory in nature and not to serve as a reservoir or vesicle. Although it has not been proven, it is assumed that the fluid secreted from the seminal vesicles is involved in supporting the function of the sperm.**

The seminal vesicles are paired in the human, horse, rat, and guinea pig. The size of the seminal vesicles varies from species to species; they are comparatively large in the rat, guinea pig, and hamster, and are enormous in the boar which has an ejaculate volume of nearly 300 ml. Seminal vesicles are absent in marsupials, carnivores, and interestingly, in some primates (present in baboons and humans). Variation also exists within certain subgroups (e.g., some species of rabbit have seminal vesicles and others do not). It has been speculated that the presence of the seminal vesicles in some species is primarily to provide seminal volume and proteins, which can assist in the lysis of the seminal coagulum. This theory has been challenged because the rat and mouse, which have relatively large seminal vesicles, produce abundant secretions and a so-called ejaculatory plug, which represents a very concentrated thick lump of spermatozoa. This small-volume plug is not lysed. A second theory has speculated that the seminal vesicles, which are usually present in higher species, have supplanted the accessory reproductive function played by the kidney in lower species such as reptiles, amphibians, and fish (Price and Williams-Ashman, 1973).

The epithelium lining the intricately folded tubes is generally pseudostratified, consisting of a row of round basal cells under a single row of low columnar cells. The remainder of the gland is composed of loose connective tissue and a layer of smooth muscle. The lumen of the seminal vesicle, being wide at the proximal portion, gradually narrows as it passes distally toward the prostate, where it meets the vas deferens to become the ejaculatory duct. **The seminal vesicles are composed of three layers: (1) an inner mucosal epithelial layer, (2) an intermediate smooth muscular layer and (3) an outer layer of loose areolar tissue surrounded by a peritoneal covering. The muscular layer contracts just prior to ejaculation to expel the seminal secretions. The secretory epithelium (columnar epithelium) and the goblet cells secrete the principal volume of the ejaculate, which is high in fructose and provides nutritional support to the sperm.**

Prostate Cell Types

Epithelial Cells

A summary of the tissue and cellular elements and the organization of the prostate are listed in Table 45–1. **The prostatic epithelium in the human is composed of three major cell types: secretory epithelial cells, basal cells, and neuroendocrine cells.** In most glands with renewing cell populations, there is a steady state flow of cells from quiescent reserve stem cells to a more rapidly dividing pool of transient proliferating cells. This proliferating population finally proceeds to the formation of the fully mature nondividing, terminally differentiated secretory cells then, via programmed apoptosis, to senesce and death (Tenniswood et al, 1992; Isaacs, 1993; Kyprianou, 1994). It has been carefully investigated how this generalized scheme of apoptotic cell death functions in the normal, hyperplastic, and cancerous prostate (reviewed by Isaacs, 1993).

In the prostate, the most common tall (12–10 μm) columnar secretory epithelial cells are terminally differentiated and are easily distinguished by their morphology, abundant secretory granules. These cells stain for prostate-specific antigen (PSA), acid phosphatase, and other enzymes, such as leucine amino peptidase. These tall columnar secretory cells look like rows of a picket fence resting next to each other. They are connected by cell adhesion molecules (CAMs), and their bases are attached to a basement membrane through integrin receptors. The nucleus is at the base just below a clear zone (2–8 μm) of abundant Golgi apparati, and the upper cellular periphery is rich in secretory granules and enzymes. The apical plasma membrane facing the lumen possesses microvilli, and secretions move out into the open collecting spaces of the acinus. These epithelial cells ring the periphery of the acinus and produce secretions into the acini that drain into the ducts that connect to the urethra. With androgen ablation, the typical secretory cells decrease by 90% in number, become cuboidal, and shrink by 80% in volume and 60% in height (DeKlerk et al, 1976). **Kastendieck (1977) identified five different prostatic epithelial cell types; type I, the basal cell; type II, the immature nonsecretory glandular cell; type III, the mature secretory glandular cell; type IV, the nonsecreting predegenerative glandular cell; and type V, the degenerating glandular cell.**

Table 45–1. SUMMARY OF THE ANATOMY AND CELL BIOLOGY OF THE PROSTATE GLAND

Components	Properties
Development	
Seminal vesicles	From wolffian ducts via testosterone stimulation
Prostate	From urogenital sinus via DHT stimulation
Prostate Zones	
Anterior fibromuscular	30% of prostate mass, no glandular elements, smooth muscle
Peripheral	Largest zone, 75% of prostate glandular elements, site of carcinomas
Central	25% of prostate glandular elements, surrounds ejaculatory ducts, may be of wolffian duct origin, seminal vesicle like
Preprostatic transition	Smallest, surround upper urethra, complex, sphincter 5% of prostate glandular elements, site of BPH 15% to 30% of prostate volume
Epithelial Cells	
Basal	Small undifferentiated, keratin-rich (type 4, 5, 6) pluripotent cells, less than 10% of epithelial cell number
Transient proliferating	Incorporate thymidine
Columnar secretory	Terminal differentiated, nondividing, rich in acid phosphatase and PSA. 20 μ tall, most abundant cell, keratin type 8, 18, 19.
Neuroendocrine cells	Serotonin rich, APUD type
Stroma Cells	
Smooth muscle	Actin-rich, myosin
Fibroblast	Vimentin-rich and associated with fibronectin
Endothelial	Associated with fibronectin, alkaline phosphatase positive
Tissue Matrix	
Extracellular	
Basement membrane	Type IV collagen meshwork, laminin rich, fibronectin
Connective tissue	Type I and Type III fibrillar collagen, elastin
Glycosaminoglycans	Sulfates of dermatan, chondroitin, and heparin; hyaluronic acid
Cytomatrix	Tubulin, actin, and intermediate filaments of keratin
Nuclear matrix	DNA tight-binding proteins, RNA and residual nuclear proteins

BPH, Benign prostatic hyperplasia; DHT, dehydrotestosterone.

Basal and Stem Cells

In comparison to the secretory epithelial cells, the basal cells are much smaller and less abundant, comprising less than 10% of the secretory epithelial cells. These small cells are round with little cytoplasm and large irregularly shaped nuclei. They are less differentiated and almost devoid of secretory products such as acid phosphatase. Basal cells always rest on the basement membrane and appear wedged between the bases of adjacent tall columnar epithelial cells (reviewed by Bonkhoff et al, 1996). The plasma membrane is rich in ATPase, suggesting that these cells may be involved in active transport, are rich in 5-nm tonofilaments, and stain brightly with fluorescent antibodies to keratin (Isaacs, 1984). **Clinical work by Wojno and Epstein (1995) has demonstrated that immunohistochemical identification of basal cells with basal cell–specific anticytokeratin monoclonal antibodies (34-beta-E12) markedly improves the histologic diagnosis of prostate cancer.** Although normal and hyperplastic prostatic acini are lined with 34-beta-E12 positive–staining basal cells, the acini of prostatic adenocarcinoma lack these basal cells and are devoid of staining, thus making it a useful tool in confirming or establishing the diagnosis of prostate cancer.

It was originally believed that these basal cells were myoepithelial (Franks, 1954), but this may not be the case because they are not rich in actin or myosin. Presently, it is believed that these undifferentiated basal cells give rise to secretory epithelial cells and, as such, function as a type of stem cell (Merk et al, 1982). Evans and Chandler (1987) used pulse chase DNA labeling experiments to confirm the concept of the basal cell as a stem cell for secretory epithelial cells. Basal cell proliferation has been measured in relation to BPH (Dermer, 1978). The importance of understanding the biology of these basal cells is realized because of the growing evidence that many neoplasms, both benign and malignant, may represent stem cell diseases. The stem cell concept of normal and abnormal growth has been reviewed by Isaacs and Coffey (1989) and Bonkhoff and Remberger (1996).

The precise identification of stem cells and the transient proliferating cells within the prostate has not been realized. Indeed, there may be several types of stem cells as well as several types of secretory cells. Lectins as cell markers have been used to identify some types of basal and secretory cells (Sinowatz et al, 1990). Merk and colleagues (1986) have presented evidence that canine prostatic basal cells have a pluripotentiality response and can change their keratin pattern following treatment with estrogens or androgens, or both. Bonkhoff and co-workers (1996) studied the immunoprofile of three well-characterized proliferating antigens (Ki-67, proliferating cell nuclear antigen [PCNA], and MIB-1, which is a specific clone of Ki-67) in normal and hyperplastic prostate and demonstrated that basal cells may serve a proliferative role in epithelial cell renewal within the prostate. Finally, Walensky and associates (1993) reported on a novel M_r-32,000 (pp32) nuclear phosphoprotein that was expressed by prostate cells and seminal vesicle basal cells that were competent for self-renewal (stem cells). This protein, and its RNA, were present in the stem cell population within the rat prostate; the mRNA, but not the protein, was present within the dividing population of cells, and neither the message nor the product of pp32 was present in the terminally differentiated transient population of cells. Meeker and Coffey (1996) have reported that telomerase activity may reside within the rat stem cell, producing its immortalization characteristics.

Neuroendocrine Cells

There are significant populations of neuroendocrine cells residing among the abundant secretory epithelium in the normal prostate gland (reviewed by diSant-Agnese and Cockett, 1994). These cells are found in the epithelium of the acini and in ducts of all parts of the gland, as well as in the urothelium of the prostatic urethral mucosa (Abrahamason et al, 1987, 1989; Davis, 1987; diSant Agnese and Cockett; 1994). The distribution, morphology, and secretory products of these cells have been studied in both normal and BPH tissues (diSant-Agnese et al, 1984, 1985). **There are three types of prostate neuroendocrine cells, with the major type containing both serotonin and thyroid-stimulating hormone. The two minor cell types contain calcitonin and somatostatin (Abrahamsson and Lilja, 1989). Neuroendocrine cells are also termed APUD, for amine precursor uptake decarboxylase cells, and regulate cellular activity through secretion of hormonal polypeptides or biogenic amines such as serotonin (5-hydroxytryptamine), which are a common markers for these cells.** High-pressure liquid chromatography measurements have shown that normal human prostate tissue contains approximately 1400 ng of serotonin per gram of tissue, and this would certainly emphasize the importance of these cells (Davis, 1987). It is most probable that these neuroendocrine cells may be involved in the regulation of prostatic secretory activity and cell growth. Chung and his co-workers (1984) have shown that rat ventral prostate growth can be uncoupled from secretory function by transplanting the ventral prostate subcutaneously. In this model, synthesis of prostatin, a secretory protein, can be restored by beta-agonist treatment using L-isoproterenol, thus suggesting beta-adrenergic receptors in the regulation of prostatic epithelial cells (Guthrie et al, 1990). They also demonstrated that norepinephrine has a direct mitogenic effect on cultured prostatic stromal cells. Guthrie and colleagues (1990) also demonstrated that norepinephrine and 5-hydroxytryptamine were greatly increased in the prostate of castrated animals and that the level of a biogenic amine was regulated reversibly by androgens (Chung et al, 1987; Thompson et al, 1987; Guthrie et al, 1990).

Higgins and Gosling (1989) have studied the structure and intrinsic innervation of the normal human prostate and have observed acetylcholine esterase nerves associated with smooth muscle in both the peripheral and central parts of the prostate. In addition, they have shown that the majority of the acini in the peripheral and central regions possess a rich plexus of autonomic nerves and that vasoactive intestinal peptide (VIP)–positive nerve fibers were found in relation to the epithelial lining acini in the central and peripheral regions of the gland. They concluded that autonomic innervation in the peripheral and central regions of the gland was indistinguishable, and they were unable to find a distinct transitional zone morphologically. In contrast, Reese and associates (1988) have found plasminogen activator as a marker of the functional zones within the human prostate gland.

Lepor and Kuhar (1984) characterized and studied the location of the muscarinic cholinergic receptor in human prostate tissue and localized it to the epithelial cells. Their findings are consistent with the observation that a muscarinic cholinergic agonist has a marked positive effect on the volume of prostatic secretions. In addition, the alpha$_1$-adrenergic receptor has also been studied in the human prostate. This is of clinical importance because of the use of selective alpha$_1$-adrenergic antagonists to alleviate bladder outlet obstruction symptoms secondary to BPH (Lepor and Shapiro, 1984; Lepor et al, 1988; Lepor, 1990; Lepor, 1993). **Recent work has demonstrated three subtypes of the alpha$_1$-adrenergic receptor (alpha$_{1A}$, alpha$_{1B}$, and alpha$_{1D}$), of which the alpha$_{1A}$ receptor appears to be the most abundant in the prostate (70%).** In both laboratory as well as preliminary clinical trials, pharmacologic agents (tamsulosin) directed against the alpha-$_{1A}$ receptor have demonstrated effectiveness against BPH (Lepor, 1995).

The Stroma and Tissue Matrix

A tissue matrix system is defined as a biologic scaffolding or residual skeleton structure that organizes and locates cells and their polarity and interactions within the organ (Getzenberg et al, 1990). The tissue matrix system forms an interacting three-dimensional framework and is one of the most active areas of modern cell biology involving the interaction of the matrix components, including the extracellular matrix, cytoskeleton, and nuclear matrix. **It is believed that structural phase shifts and communication through these matrix elements may play a central role in controlling prostatic development and function. The transmission of structural signals from the cell periphery to the DNA may play a central role in regulating chromatin structure and gene expression (Getzenberg et al, 1990).** The epithelial cells rest on the basement lamina or membrane, which is about 100-nm thick and surrounds the acini. The basement membrane is not a membrane but a complex structure containing, in part, collagen types IV and V, glycosoaminoglycans, complex polysaccharides and glycolipids. This layer forms an interface to the stromal compartment that consists of a structural extracellular matrix, ground substance, and a variety of stromal cells, including the fibroblasts, capillary and lymphatic endothelial cells, smooth muscle cells, neuroendocrine cells, and axons (Aumuller, 1983; Mawhinney, 1989). The smooth muscle cells are clustered around the acinar structure and are believed to be mechanically involved in the secretion of ejaculate under neural stimulation. In BPH, these smooth muscle cells change their morphology (Rohr and Bartsch, 1980). The authors hypothesize that under hormonal stimulation, the smooth muscle produces collagen, which forms part of the extracellular matrix and enhances epithelial growth by stromal-epithelial interactions (see later discussion). All mammalian cells are composed of a cytomatrix or cytoskeleton network that is formed from a network of microtubules of 20 nm (tubulins), microfilaments of 6 nm (actins), and intermediate filaments of 10 nm (keratin, desmin, or vimentin). **Tubulin is ubiquitous in all cells as a microtubular structure that appears to anchor many cellular structures and is a critical factor in determining the shape of the cell.** The microfilaments are composed primarily of actin, which has the ability to polymerize and depolymerize, and as such, forms one of the important structural chemomechanical systems when it interacts with myosin within the cell. There are several types of intermediate filaments of the cytomatrix that are extremely important because they vary in type and composition with differentiation and appear to define the various cell or tissue types within the body. For example, **one of the intermediate filaments called desmin is a central component of all muscle cells, while the intermediate filament vimentin is found in all fibroblasts.** The keratin intermediate filaments are universal to the cytomatrix of all epithelial cells. There is usually just one type of vimentin and desmin in the fibroblast or muscle cells. In contrast, within the epithelial cells, the keratins occur in over 20 different molecular types that vary with the state of cellular differentiation and the types of epithelial cells. Keratins can change in prostate epithelial cells with disease (BPH or cancer) or hormonal stimulation (Ellis et al, 1984; Isaacs, 1984; Purnell et al, 1984; Achtstatter et al, 1985; Brawer et al, 1985; Merk et al, 1986).

The cytomatrix (cytoplasmic skeleton) just described terminates in the center of the cell by direct attachment to the nuclear matrix (Fig. 45–1). Therefore, the prostatic epithelial cell has direct structural linkage via the cytoskeletal-nuclear matrix systems from the DNA to the plasma membrane. The cytomatrix then makes direct contact with the basement membrane and extracellular matrix and ground substance of the stroma. This entire interlocking tissue scaffolding or superstructure is termed the *tissue matrix* (Getzenberg et al, 1990), and it may have dynamic properties in ordering biologic processes and the transport of secretion from the sex accessory tissues.

Understanding the biologic components of the tissue matrix system within sex accessory tissues is of paramount importance (see review by Getzenberg et al, 1990). The epithelial cell is anchored to the basement membrane or basement lamina by an extracellular matrix protein called laminin. **The laminin proteins are glycoproteins of the extracellular matrix that mediate attachment of cells to the type IV collagen of the basement membrane. *Laminin is produced by epithelial cells but not by fibroblasts*, and is a large molecule with molecular domains that interact with type IV collagen of the basement membrane and integrin type of receptors within the cell surface glycocalyx of the epithelial cell.** Laminin surrounds the basement membrane of prostate acinar epithelial cells, capillaries, smooth muscle, and nerve fibers but not the lymphatics, lymphocytes, or fibroblasts, and the laminin distribution becomes disrupted in high-grade prostate neoplasms (Sinha et al, 1989).

A second type of prostatic glycoprotein involved in cell adherence to the extracellular matrix is fibronectin, which binds to the integrin family of receptors. **Fibronectin is secreted primarily by prostatic fibroblasts and forms an adhesive material that makes a binding interface of mesenchymal and epithelial cells to various types of collagen and proteoglycans of the extracellular matrix. There are several types of fibronectin, and they have been proposed**

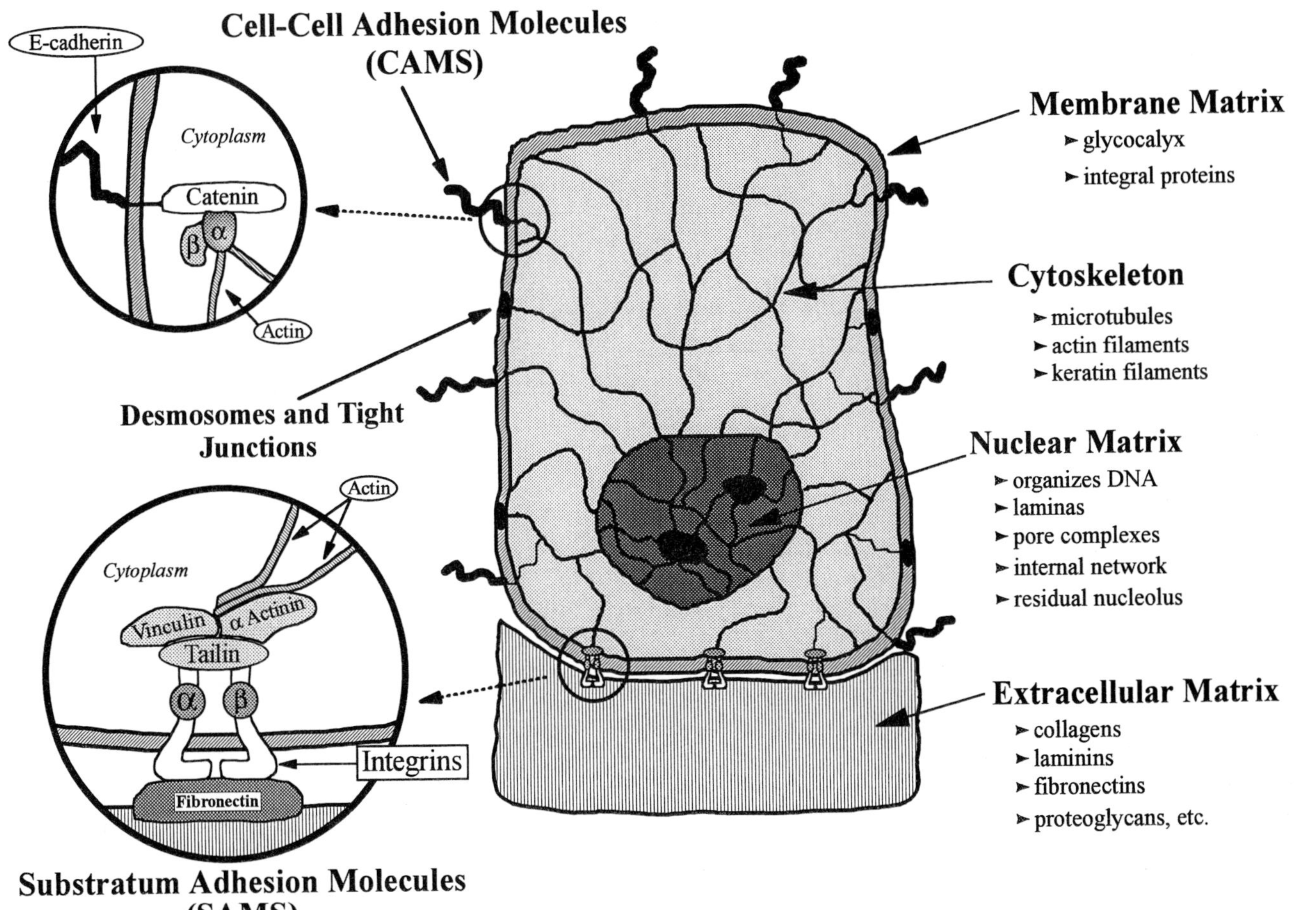

Figure 45–1. The tissue matrix system, a superstructure scaffold network that connects the extracellular matrix components to the integrin receptors that extend through the plasma membrane and connect directly to the cytomatrix structures. The cytomatrix directly couples to the nuclear matrix that attaches and organizes the DNA. The cell adhesion molecules (CAMs) and desmosome connect neighboring cells. (From Getzenberg RH, Pienta KJ, Coffey DS: The tissue matrix: Cell dynamics and hormone action. Endocr Rev 1990; 11:399–416.)

to play a key role in morphogenesis and control of cell growth.

The connective tissue of the prostate is primarily collagen of type I and III, which form the interstitial collagen (Bartsch et al, 1984), while type IV and type V are found primarily in the basement membrane, woven through the stroma and connective tissue of the extracellular matrix in a complex network of glycosaminoglycans (GAGs) and complex polysaccharides. **GAGs are large, negatively charged polymers (polyanions) that have proved to be critical factors in the signaling of extracellular matrix events in many different tissues (Hay, 1981). These large polysaccharide polymers have long been proposed to play an important role in prostate growth (Arcadi, 1954). DeKlerk (1983) has isolated and quantitated these important GAGs from normal and benign human prostates and report that dermatan sulfate is the predominant (40%) GAG followed by heparin (20%), chondroitin (16%), and hyaluronic acid (20%).** Fetal prostates are devoid of dermatan sulfate, and chondroitin sulfate increases with development of BPH. Chan and Wong (1989a, 1989b) have studied the histochemical distribution in the guinea pig lateral prostate and have identified three different types of proteoglycan fibers in different tissue compartments. It will be of interest to determine the role of GAGs in sex accessory tissue function. It has been shown that synthesis of proteoglycans can be regulated in the rat prostate by androgens (Hiler, 1987; Kofoed et al, 1990).

In the near future, one of the more active areas of unraveling the control of sex accessory tissue function will revolve around a clearer understanding of the interactions of these complex tissue matrix components. At present, there have been several important studies (Cunha et al, 1983b; DeKlerk, 1983; Chung et al, 1984) that all point to the importance of these structural elements. Of particular importance are the studies that have shown the localization of keratins (Wojno and Epstein, 1995), laminin, fibronectin, and actin within the various cell types of the prostate, with other studies (Bartsch et al, 1984; Thornton et al, 1984) focusing on the collagen distribution and subtypes within the prostate (Mawhinney, 1989).

In summary, the shape of a cell determines the func-

tion of the cell. This shape, in turn, is determined by the formation of a tissue matrix system that hardwires the cell to the DNA so that the DNA can receive and respond to its environment in an appropriate manner. This is analogous to the floppy disk of a computer, in that the DNA is the software that contains all of the potential information, and the cell's structural elements are analogous to the computer hardware, which reads or processes the DNA information. They work in concert to produce the final output (Getzenberg et al, 1990; Pienta et al, 1993a; Sommerfield et al, 1995). This system allows a histologist to determine a cell type by observing its structure, and a pathologist to detect a disease by visual changes in cell structure. Also, this system may have self-organizing principles referred to as the *interphase between chaos and order*, which forms a new field called complexity that attempts to explain such complex emergent properties (Sommerfeld et al, 1995). In prostate cancer, there is a dramatic change in the composition of the tissue matrix system (Pienta et al, 1993a).

In summary, each cell type has a specific three-dimensional organization of its genome in relation to different cell type–specific compositions of the nuclear matrix (Getzenberg et al, 1990; Sommerfeld et al, 1995). Whether this tissue-specific organization accounts for why the bulbourethral gland in the human is impervious to the formation of cancer whereas the prostate gland is highly susceptible to carcinogenesis remains to be elucidated.

SEX ACCESSORY GLAND SECRETIONS

The seminal plasma is formed primarily from the secretions of the sex accessory tissues. **Normal human ejaculate is approximately 3 ml and is composed of two components—spermatozoa and the seminal plasma. The spermatozoa, which represent less than 1% of the total ejaculate, are present in the range of 100 million/ml. The major contribution to the volume of the seminal plasma derives from the seminal vesicles (3 ml), from the prostate (1.5–2 ml), and from Cowper's gland (0.5 ml) and glands of Littre (0.1 to 0.2 ml).** During ejaculation, the secretions of these glands are released in a sequential manner (Amelar and Hotchkiss, 1965; Tauber et al, 1975). **The first fraction of the human ejaculate is rich in sperm and prostatic secretions. Fructose, which represents a major secretory product of the seminal vesicles, is elevated in the later fraction of the ejaculate.** The overall chemical composition of prostatic secretions and the normal human and rodent seminal plasma have been studied by many laboratories, and the results have been summarized (Mann and Mann, 1981; Zaneveld and Tauber, 1981; Aumuller and Seitz, 1990; Daniels and Grayhack, 1990; Chow et al, 1993; Gonzales et al, 1993).

In relation to other body fluids, the seminal plasma is unusual because of its very high concentrations of potassium, zinc, citric acid, fructose, phosphorylcholine, spermine, free amino acids, prostaglandins, and enzymes, most notably acid phosphatase, diamine oxidase, beta-glucuronidase, lactic dehydrogenase (LDH), alpha-amylase, prostatic-specific antigen, and seminal proteinase (Table 45–2).

Table 45–2. COMPOSITION OF PROSTATIC FLUID

pH	6.6–7.2
Specific gravity	1.027 ± 0.002
Protein	25 mg/ml
Lipid	3 mg/ml
Sodium	153 mM
Potassium	48 mM
Calcium	30 mM
Magnesium	20 mM
Chloride	38 mM
Bicarbonate	20 mM
Citrate	98 mM
Zinc	488 μg/ml
Spermine	2.4 mg/ml
Cholesterol	0.9 mg/ml

Data from Daniels and Grayhack, 1990; Zaneveld and Chatterton, 1982; Mann and Mann, 1981.

Citric Acid

Citric acid is formed in the prostate at 100 times higher concentrations than that seen in other soft tissues (e.g., prostate tissue has 30,000 nmoles/g, and other tissues have a range of 150–450 nmoles/g). **The concentration of citrate in the ejaculate is 500 to 1000 times higher than in the plasma. Prostate secretory epithelial cells form citrate from aspartic acid and glucose. The high concentrations seen within the prostate results partly from the inability of the mitochondria of the prostate cells to readily oxidize citrate once it is formed; therefore, the rate of citrate synthesis far exceeds the rate of citrate oxidation (Costello and Franklin, 1989, 1994).** Kavanagh (1994) measured citrate and isocitrate levels in the prostate, which are catalyzed by aconitase, and demonstrated ratios of 33:1 in the prostate while other tissues demonstrate ratios of 10:1. This decreased activity of aconitase might explain the high levels of citrate within the prostate.

Diamine oxidase, an enzyme that degrades polyamines within the prostate, has been linked to citric acid concentrations and indirectly to sperm motility and fertility (Le Calve et al, 1995; Gonzales, 1994). Yacoe and associates (1991) used nuclear magnetic resonance (NMR) spectroscopy to investigate the relationship between citrate metabolism and prostate cancer, and demonstrated statistically insignificant differences between normal epithelium and prostate cancer cell lines. The relationship between prostatic inflammatory disease and citric acid has also been investigated (Wolff et al, 1991a, 1991b).

One of the major anions in the human seminal plasma is citrate (mean, 376 mg/100 ml) in the range of 20 mM or 60 mEq/L. This is compared with the chloride ion concentration (155 mg/100 ml) at 40 mM. Citrate is a potent binder of metal ions, and the seminal plasma concentration of citrate, 20 mM, is comparable to that of the total divalent metals at 13.6 mM (calcium, 7 mM; magnesium, 4.5 mM; zinc, 2.1 mM). Prostatic citrate levels are approximately 15.8 mg/ml (Zaneveld and Tauber, 1981), and the values for seminal vesicle citric acid secretions are almost 100-fold less, being only 0.2 mg/ml.

Fructose

The source of fructose in human seminal plasma is the seminal vesicles (Mann and Mann, 1981). Patients with

tissue in the human prostate than in the rat prostate. The clinical aspects of PAP were reviewed by Romas and Kwan (1993) and Lowe and Trauzzi (1993).

Prostate-Specific Membrane Antigen

Although it is not a secretory protein, prostate-specific membrane antigen (PSMA) is a very important membrane-bound protein of the prostatic epithelial cell. This transmembrane glycoprotein (PSMA) is found on the surface of prostatic epithelial cells and has a molecular weight of 100,000 (Wright et al, 1995). The cDNA for PSMA has been cloned and the deduced amino acid sequence determined (Israeli et al, 1993). Based on the amino acid sequence, there are many glycosylation sites available, which suggest that the extracellular domain of this transmembrane peptide is heavily glycosylated (Wright et al, 1995). A monoclonal murine IgG1 antibody (7E11-C5) was prepared against purified PSMA (Horoszweicz et al, 1987), which recognizes the antigen on prostatic epithelial cells. 7E11-C5 immunoreacts weakly with normal and BPH prostatic epithelium and strongly with malignant epithelium from the prostate. 7E11-C5 does not react with most other tumors and other normal tissues (Horoszweicz et al, 1987). PSMA expression in prostate tumors appears to correlate with the degree of differentiation of the tumor and not with tumor stage (Wright et al, 1995). The monoclonal antibody to PSMA, 7E11-C5, has been covalently linked to Indium^{111} (^{111}In-CYT-356) and is under investigation as an imaging tool to localize prostate cancer metastases and disease recurrence following radical surgery. Evidence has demonstrated that the cDNA sequence for PSMA and the cDNA sequence for *N*-acetylated alpha-linked acidic dipeptidase (NAALADase), an enzyme localized to the brain (Stauch-Slusher et al 1992) that catalyzes the cleavage of glutamate from *N*-acetyl-L-aspartyl-L-glutamate (NAAG), are similar (Carter et al, 1996). The clinical usefulness of PSMA for diagnosis, monitoring, and imaging of men with prostatic disease is under investigation.

Prostate-Specific Protein–94, Beta-Microseminoprotein, and Beta-Inhibin

A major 16-kD MW protein has been found in prostatic secretions that contain 94 amino acids and has been termed PSP-94. This protein had previously been designated as beta-inhibin and also as beta-microseminoprotein (Dube et al, 1987; Ulvsback et al, 1989). Transcripts of messenger RNA for this protein have also been identified in nongenital tissues (Ulvsback et al, 1989). **It remains to be determined how useful PSP-94 will be in diagnosing or monitoring prostate cancer.**

Zn-α2-Glycoprotein

Lin and Clinton (1986) identified a 40-kD glycoprotein that they had purified from seminal plasma that is similar to Zn-α_2-glycoprotein isolated from blood plasma. It receives its name from its ability to be precipitated by zinc acetate. It is present in the kidney and other biologic fluids, and its function is unknown.

Leucine Aminopeptidase

Aminopeptidases hydrolyze the *N*-terminal amino acid from small polypeptides (reviewed by Pretlow et al, 1994). Leucine aminopeptidases are particularly active against the substrate L-leucyl-glycine, and some of these enzymes are referred to as arylamidases because the optimal substrate is L-leucyl-β-naphthylamine. The human prostate is rich in the latter arylamidase type of leucine aminopeptidase with an activity in prostatic fluid of 30,000 units/ml. Mattila (1969) demonstrated two forms of the enzyme in human prostatic tissue (107,000 and 305,000 MW), only one of which was similar to that of the kidney. The kidney is one of the richest sources of leucine aminopeptidases, but at present, the tissue-specific nature of any of these isoenzymes has not been established.

Leucine aminopeptidase is a product of the epithelial cells of the prostate (Niemi et al, 1963) and is secreted into the lumen of the acini (Kirchheim et al, 1964; Vafa et al, 1993). Rackley and associates (1991) demonstrated that extracts from areas affected by prostatic carcinoma contained less leucine aminopeptidase activity than tissue obtained from areas affected by BPH.

Lactic Dehydrogenase

The isoenzyme ratios of LDHs in human semen may be altered in a patient with prostatic cancer (Oliver et al, 1970; Grayhack et al, 1977). LDH (150,000 MW) is composed of four subunits (each of 35,000 MW) of only two different types of proteins, denoted M and H. The LDH of muscle has four M units and that of heart has four H units. Five isoenzymes of LDH can be found in tissues with a four subunit composition as follows: LDH I, MMMM; LDH II, MMMH; LDH III, MMHH; LDH IV, MHHH; and LDH V, HHHH. The M and H subunits appear to be the same in all tissues, but the amounts of LDH I to V can vary. Denis and Prout (1963) observed increased levels of LDH IV and V in prostatic cancer tissue. Several investigators have observed elevated ratios of LDH V and LDH I in human prostatic cancer (Elhilali et al, 1967; Oliver et al, 1970; Flocks and Schmidt, 1972).

Immunoglobulins, C3 Complement, and Transferrin

There are many reports establishing the presence of immunoglobulins in human seminal plasma (reviewed by Liang et al, 1991; Gahankari and Golhar, 1993). It is possible to measure levels of IgG from 7 to 22 mg/100 ml and IgA from 0 to 6 mg/100 ml; IgM is, however, very low and often not detected (Friberg and Tilly-Friberg, 1976). The complete source of these antibodies is not known, although they are found in expressed prostatic fluid (Grayhack et al, 1979) and may be related to infections (Fowler and Mariano, 1982). They are usually found at lower levels in seminal plasma than in blood, but the possibility of diffusion across the so-called blood-seminal plasma barrier has not been eliminated (see discussion by Friberg and Tilly-Friberg, 1976). Expressed prostatic fluid contains considerable amounts of the C_3 component of complement, being present at 1.82 mg/100 ml, and this increases almost 10-fold in fluid collected from patients with prostatic adenocarcinoma to levels of 16.9 mg/100 ml (Grayhack and Lee, 1981). Prostatitis also has been shown to be related to C_3 among men with chronic prostatitis (Blenk and Hofstettet, 1991). Prostatitis and BPH only increase the level approximately twofold. In the same manner, a protein-carrying iron, termed transferrin, is increased in a similar manner, going from normal levels of prostatic fluid of 5.3 mg/dl to 42.4 mg/dl in prostatic carcinoma (Grayhack and Lee, 1981). The function of these serum proteins in the secretion of prostatic fluid remains to be determined.

Seminal Vesicle Secretory Proteins

Williams-Ashman presented a classic review (1983) on the regulatory features of the seminal vesicles' development and function (reviewed by Cunha et al, 1992). The secretory proteins of the seminal vesicles are major proteins and enzymes involved in the rapid clotting of the ejaculate. **The major clotting protein has been termed seminogelin (Lilja et al, 1985) which has been shown to be the seminal vesicle–specific antigen**. These proteins from the seminal vesicle serve as substrates for PSA from the prostate, which enzymatically lyses the seminal clot through its protease activity (Lilja, 1985; Aumuller et al, 1990). Beyond this coagulation reaction, it is uncertain what role these seminal vesicle proteins play, but their effect on fertility and uterine sperm motility have been studied in the mouse. Many of the proteins secreted by the seminal vesicle are under androgen regulation (Higgins and Hemingway, 1991; Hagstrom et al, 1992). Recent work (Harvey et al, 1995) has identified an androgen-regulated protease with elastase-like activity within seminal vesicle secretions.

Coagulation and Liquefaction of Semen

Within 5 minutes following ejaculation, human semen coagulates into a semisolid gel, and on further standing for a 5- to 20-minute period, the clot spontaneously liquefies to form a viscous liquid (Huggins and Neal, 1942; Tauber and Zaneveld, 1976; Mann and Mann, 1981). Calcium-binding substances such as sodium citrate and heparin do not inhibit the coagulation process, nor are prothrombin, fibrinogen, or factor XII required, because they are absent in seminal plasma (for review, see Mann and Mann, 1981). The seminal clot is formed of fibers 0.15 to 10 nm in width, and its morphology differs from that of a blood fibrin clot (Huggins and Neal, 1941; Tauber and Zaneveld, 1976; Mann and Mann, 1981). Factors affecting blood coagulation do not regulate semen viscosity (Amelar, 1962). From these observations and others, it appears that the coagulation of human semen is different from that of blood.

Examination of split human ejaculates indicates that the first fraction, originating primarily from Cowper's gland and the prostate, contains the liquefaction factors, and the final fraction of the ejaculate is enriched in seminal vesicle secretions and is responsible for the coagulation of the ejaculate (Lilja et al, 1987).

It has long been known that prostatic fluid has a dramatic fibrinolytic-like activity and that 2 ml of this secretion can liquefy 100 ml of clotted blood in 18 hours at 37°C (Huggins and Neal, 1942; Mann and Mann, 1981). The factors involved in such proteolytic activity in semen have been resolved (Huggins and Neal, 1942; Syner et al, 1975; Tauber and Zaneveld, 1976; Tauber et al, 1976b; Mann and Mann, 1981; Zaneveld and Chatterton, 1982; Lilja et al, 1987). **Two types of seminal plasma proteolytic enzymes appear to be major factors in the liquefaction process—plasminogen activators and PSA. Two plasminogen activators have been isolated from seminal plasma; they have molecular weights of 70,000 and 74,000 and appear to be related to urokinase (Propping et al, 1974).** It is believed that the plasminogen activators originate from prostatic secretions.

The seminal plasma contains a variety of other proteolytic enzymes, including pepsinogen, lysozyme, alpha-amylase, and hyaluronidase. **In addition, human semen inhibits the activity of the proteolytic enzyme trypsin, and this is due to the presence in the seminal plasma of such proteinase inhibitors as alpha$_1$-antitrypsin and alpha$_1$-antichymotrypsin.** Coagulation and liquefaction vary in different species. For example, the semen of the bull or dog does not coagulate, whereas the semen of rodents such as the rat and guinea pig ejaculate a firm pellet that does not appear to liquify (Tauber et al, 1975; Tauber and Zaneveld, 1976). In rodents, the plugs form through the action of an enzyme called vesiculase, which comes from the anterior lobe of the prostate and reacts with seminal vesicle secretions. Because of this action, the anterior lobe of the rodent prostate is also called the coagulating gland. Vesiculase is not identical with thrombin because it does not coagulate fibrinogen and thrombin does not clot the secretions of the seminal vesicles. Williams-Ashman and co-workers (1977) have established that vesiculase has transamidase activity, catalyzing the formation of gamma-glutamyl-ϵ-lysine crosslinks in the seminal vesicles. This seminal vesicle protein, which serves as a substrate for vesiculase, is a very basic substance with a molecular weight of 17,900; it has been characterized by Notides and Williams-Ashman (1967) in regard to its physical properties.

In summary, it appears that seminal plasma coagulation and liquefaction are under enzymatic control, but the biologic purpose of this process has not been determined. Enzymes and proteins of the seminal vesicles and prostate glands are involved in this system. There have been reports that some infertile men may have impairment of the liquefaction process (Bunge and Sherman, 1954; Bunge, 1970; Eliasson, 1973; Amelar and Dubin; 1977).

Prostatic Secretions and Drug Transport

Aumuller and Seitz (1990) have reviewed the secretory mechanism for the sex accessory tissues. Isaacs (1983) has also reviewed the concepts related to the fluid and drug transport properties of the prostate and seminal vesicles. Isaacs has compared the composition and volume of prostatic secretion under basal stimulation and under neurologic stimulation during ejaculation or pilocarpine stimulation. This work reveals that under neurologic stimulation an increase of 205-fold in the total potassium, chloride, and sodium output over the basal secretory rate, and has shown that the prostate is capable of secreting five times its total content of sodium and chloride during this active secretion. This demonstrates the tremendous transport powers of this system. Smith and his colleagues (1985) have studied the transepithelial voltage changes during prostatic secretion in the dog and have concluded that sodium may move passively through the plasma in the prostatic fluid during ejaculation but that the movement of potassium and chloride ions involves active transcellular transport. Isaacs and associates (1981) have shown that the androgen-induced secretions can be blocked in the presence of estrogen, although the growth properties and biologic properties of the androgen on the prostate are not markedly altered. This factor suggests a direct effect of estrogen in blocking a major transport system in the prostate.

Only a few compounds are capable of entering the semen by simple diffusion, including ethanol, iodine, and a few antibiotics (see review of Reeves, 1982). Drugs entering prostatic secretions have been of interest because of the prevalence of prostatitis and the need for new modalities of chemotherapy. Stamey and colleagues have made extensive studies of the ability of chemotherapeutic agents to concentrate in the prostatic fluid of humans and dogs (Hessl and Stamey, 1971; Stamey et al, 1973), and many other laboratories have also contributed to this knowledge (Madsen et al, 1968, 1976, 1978; Fowle and Bye, 1972). **Few drugs reach concentrations in the prostatic secretion that approach or surpass their concentrations in blood, but some exceptions are the basic macrolides, erythromycin, and oleandomycin; sulfonamides; chloramphenicol; tetracycline; and clindamycin, trimethoprim, and fluoroquinolones (see review of Reeves, 1982)**. In general, these drugs are assumed to pass across the membrane by nonionic diffusion, possibly by lipid solubility through the membrane. When they reach the more acidic prostatic fluid, they are protonated and acquire a more positive charge; thus, the charged drugs become relatively trapped within the prostatic secretions. Several factors are critical, including the pK' of the drug and the pH of the prostatic secretions, as well as the drug binding to proteins in each compartment. Basic drugs would be more positively charged in acidic prostatic fluid than in blood. Slight changes in pH can have significant effects on this nonionic diffusion. Samples of prostatic secretions from humans varied widely in pH from 6 to 8, with a mean value of 6.6; however, **with prostatic inflammation, the pH tended to be 7** or greater (White, 1975). It should be realized that although prostatic secretions are slightly acidic, the pH of freshly ejaculated human semen is slightly alkaline (pH 7.3 to 7.7); on standing, semen first becomes more alkaline with the loss of carbon dioxide and then acidic owing to accumulation of lactic acid.

Drugs may be developed in the future that are transported into the prostate as therapeutic agents or chemoprotectors, or as a route to the semen to regulate fertility; however, more must be learned about the fundamental transport system into and out of the male reproductive tract before such an approach is feasible.

THE ENDOCRINE CONTROL OF PROSTATE GROWTH

Endocrine Overview

The prostate, like other sex accessory tissues, is stimulated to grow and is maintained in size and secretory function by the continued presence of serum testosterone; it is converted by metabolism within the prostate into the more active androgen DHT. It is important to realize that testosterone is synthesized in the testes from the precursor of progesterone by a series of reversible reactions. When testosterone is reduced by 5α-reductase action to form DHT, or to estrogens by aromatase action, it is irreversible. **In other words, although testosterone can be converted into DHT and into estrogens, estrogens and DHT cannot be converted into testosterone**. Androgens, estrogens, and adrenal steroids are believed to have strong effects on different cells and tissues in the body that can vary with development and age. This varies from embryonic development and differentiation into neonatal imprinting, through to puberty, and on into adult maintenance and later senescence. Therefore, androgen ablation or androgen treatment have a wide variety of physiologic effects that must be taken into consideration.

The generalized effect of the endocrine glands on the prostate is depicted in Figure 45–2. The hypothalamus releases a small protein with only 10 amino acids (decapeptide) referred to as luteinizing hormone–releasing hormone (LHRH) or gonadotropin-releasing hormone. Under the stimulation of LHRH, the pituitary releases luteinizing hormone, which is transported to the testes and acts directly on the Leydig cells to stimulate steroid synthesis. The release of testosterone becomes the major serum androgen, with the potential for stimulating prostatic growth. **Most of the estrogen in the male is also derived from peripheral conversion of testosterone to estrogens through an enzymatic aromatization reaction**.

Other androgens capable of stimulating prostate growth include adrenal androgens such as androstenedione. However this is not a major pathway because, in both animals and humans, castration leads to almost complete involution of the prostate, implying that insufficient adrenal androgens are present to stimulate any meaningful growth of the normal prostate (Oesterling et al, 1986). Only when the adrenals are stimulated by excess adrenocorticotropic hormone or are overactive do they have any significant effect in stimulating prostatic growth (e.g., the adrenogenital syndrome). The role of adrenal androgens is minor, but this is a very controversial issue and has led to the concept of total androgen blockade, which some investigators claim provides control of prostate cancer by eliminating adrenal androgens or their function. This is the basis of the therapeutic concept of using LHRH analogues to block testicular androgen production in combination with antiandrogens, such as flutamide, theoretically to block any residual androgen stimulation of the prostate from the adrenal gland.

Prolactin has often been postulated to enhance androgen-induced growth; however, several decades of study have failed to indicate the mechanism of this action, but it does not appear at present to be a major means of regulating normal prostatic growth. **Prolactin is believed to enhance the uptake of androgens into the prostate and to affect the synthesis of citric acid**. Estrogen treatment induces prolactin release from the pituitary. The following section reviews endocrine factors released by other organs, and their synthesis, serum levels, and transport to the prostate.

Androgen Production by the Testes

Because the testes produce the major serum androgen supporting prostate and sex accessory tissue growth, it is

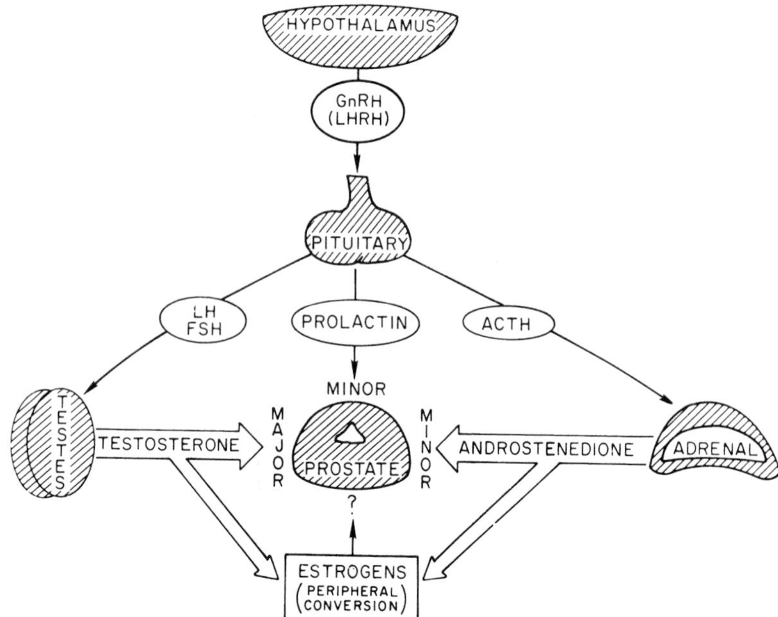

Figure 45–2. Simplified endocrinology of the prostate. Luteinizing hormone–releasing hormone (LHRH), also termed gonadotropin-releasing hormone (GnRH), stimulates the pituitary to release the gonadotropins LH and FSH, which stimulate the Leydig cells of the testes to synthesize testosterone. Testosterone is the major serum androgen stimulating prostatic growth. Peripheral conversion of testosterone by aromatization forms the estrogens in the male. The adrenal gland is under ACTH stimulation and releases the minor androgens, such as androstenedione, which is also converted peripherally to estrogens. Prolactin has also been shown to have a minor effect in stimulating androgen-induced prostatic growth. The prostate can produce its own growth factors (autocrine or paracrine) or respond to circulating growth factors.

important to briefly review this function. **In the normal human male, the major circulating serum androgen is testosterone, which is almost exclusively (more than 95%) of testicular origin. Under normal physiologic conditions, the Leydig cells of the testis are the major source of the testicular androgens**. The Leydig cells are stimulated by the gonadotropins (primarily luteinizing hormone) to synthesize testosterone from acetate and cholesterol. The spermatic vein concentration of testosterone is 40 to 50 μg/100 ml and is approximately 75 times more concentrated than the level detected in the peripheral venous serum (Hammond et al, 1978), which is approximately 600 ng of testosterone per 100 ml. Other androgens also leave the testes by the spermatic vein, and these include androstenediol, androstenedione (3 μg/100 ml), dehydroepiandrosterone (7 μg/100 ml), and DHT (0.4 μg/100 ml). Therefore, concentrations of these other androgens are much lower in the spermatic vein than those of testosterone (15%). The testosterone that enters the plasma is referred to as the testosterone blood production rate and is 6 to 7 mg/day in the human (Fig. 45–3). **Although other steroids, such as androstenedione from the adrenals, can be converted by peripheral metabolism to testosterone, they probably account for less than 5% of the overall production of plasma testosterone. The mean metabolic clearance rate for testosterone is around 1000 L per 24 hours and results in a plasma half-life of only 10 to 20 minutes. The average testosterone concentration in adult human male plasma is approximately 611 ± 186 ng/100 ml, with a normal range of 300 to 1000; this is equal to 10.4 to 34.7 nmol/L in SI units** (Table 45–4). Serum testosterone levels are not remarkably related to age between 25 and 70 years, although they do decline gradually to approximately 500 ng/100 ml after age 70 years. It is recognized that plasma concentrations of testosterone can vary widely in an individual in any one day and may reflect both episodic and diurnal variations in the production rate. Testosterone levels are higher in the morning than at any other time of the day.

Only 2% of the total serum testosterone is not protein bound. This is termed the free testosterone in the plasma and exists at a concentration of approximately 15 ng/100 ml, or less than 1 nM. It is only this free testosterone that is available to the prostate for uptake and metabolism to DHT or for uptake by the liver and intestine to primarily form 17-ketosteroids. Metabolic androgens, such as the 17-ketosteroids, are then secreted into the urine as water-soluble steroid conjugates with either sulfuric acid or glucuronic acid. **The total 17-ketosteroids in the urine in adult males is from 4 to 25 mg/24 hours and is not an accurate index of testosterone production, because other steroids from the adrenals as well as nonandrogenic steroids can be metabolized to 17-ketosteroids**. Only small (25 to 160 μg/day) amounts of testosterone enter the urine without metabolism, and this urinary testosterone represents less than 2% of the daily testosterone production.

Although testosterone is the primary plasma androgen inducing growth of the prostate gland and other sex accessory tissues, it appears to function as a prohormone. The active form of the androgen in the prostate is not testosterone but a more androgenic metabolite, DHT (Farnsworth and Brown, 1963; Shimazaki et al, 1965a; Anderson and Liao, 1968; Bruchovsky and Wilson, 1968a, 1968b) (see Fig. 45–3). The formation of DHT involves the reduction of the double bond in the A ring of testosterone through the enzymatic action of the enzyme 5α-reductase (Fig. 45–4). This conversion can take place directly in the prostate and seminal vesicles or in peripheral tissues such as the liver. **DHT concentration in the plasma of normal men is very low, 56 ± 20 ng/100 ml, in comparison to testosterone, which is 11-fold higher at approximately 611 ng/100 ml** (see Table 45–4).

In summary, although DHT is a potent androgen (1.5–2.5 times as potent as testosterone in most bioassay systems), its low plasma concentration and tight binding to plasma proteins diminishes its direct importance as a circulating androgen affecting prostate and seminal vesicle growth. **In**

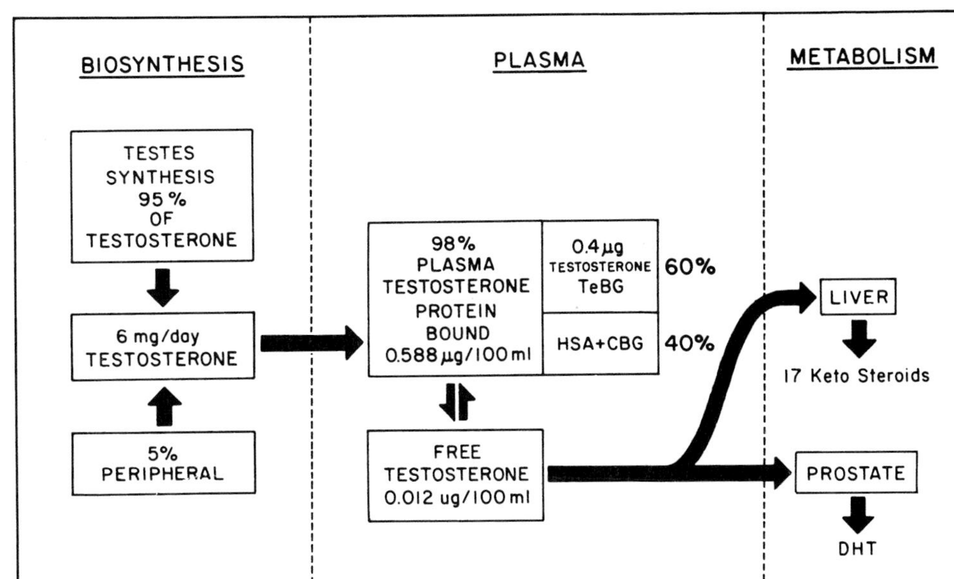

Figure 45–3. A quantitative assessment of the testicular biosynthesis, plasma transport, and metabolism of testosterone. Plasma testosterone is bound to testosterone-binding globulin (TeBG), human serum albumin (HSA), and cortisol-binding globulin (CBG). All numbers are average values for the normal adult male.

contrast, DHT is of paramount importance within the prostate, where it is formed from testosterone. DHT is the major form of androgen found within the prostate gland (5 ng/g tissue wet weight) and is fivefold higher than testosterone, that is only at approximately 1 ng/g. In the prostate, DHT binds to specific androgen receptors within the nucleus of the epithelial cells, where approximately 100,000 DHT molecules reside per nucleus. DHT becomes the major androgen regulating the cellular events of growth, differentiation, and function in the prostate. Normal adult male plasma levels of some important steroids are summarized in Table 45–4, and these values are derived as averages from numerous studies and the individual values can fluctuate with age, time of day, stress, hospitalization, and environmental changes.

Adrenal Androgens

There is evidence that hyperstimulation of the adrenal cortex can cause an overproduction of adrenal steroids, which may then stimulate the growth of the prostate gland. For example, in humans, abnormal virilism has been observed in immature males with hyperfunction of the adrenal cortex resulting from neoplasia or hyperplasia of the adrenal gland (e.g., adrenogenital syndrome). In rodents, overstimulation of the adrenals can also induce limited prostate growth, even in the absence of testicular androgens. For example, administration of exogenous adrenocorticotropic hormone to castrated animals significantly increases the growth of sex accessory tissue (Tullner, 1963; Tisell, 1970; Walsh and Gittes, 1970).

The effect of normal levels of adrenal androgens on the prostate in noncastrated humans and adult male rats may not be significant because adrenalectomy has very little effect on prostate size, DNA, or morphology of the sex accessory tissue (Mobbs et al, 1973; Oesterling et al, 1986). Furthermore, following castration in animals, with the adrenals intact, the prostate will finally diminish to a very small size (90% reduction in total cell mass). Finally, the small involuted ventral prostate in the castrated rat cannot be significantly reduced further by performing additional adrenalec-

Table 45–4. AVERAGE PLASMA LEVELS OF SEX STEROIDS IN HEALTHY HUMAN MALES

	Plasma Concentration		Daily Blood	
Steroid (common name)	***ng/100 ml***	***Relative Molarity***	**Production Rate (mg/day)**	**Relative Androgenicity Rat VP assay**[1]
Testosterone	611 ± 186	100	6.6 ± 0.5	100
Dihydrotestosterone (DHT)	56 ± 20	9	0.3 ± 0.06	181
5α-androstane-3α,17β-diol (3α-androstanediol)	14 ± 4	2	0.2 ± 0.03	126
5α-androstane-3β,17β-diol (3β-androstanediol)	<2	<0.3		18
Androstenediol	161 ± 52	26		0.21
Androsterone	54 ± 32	9	0.28	53
Androstenedione	150 ± 54	25	1.4	39
Dehydroepiandrosterone (DHEA)	501 ± 98	81	29	15
Dehydroepiandrosterone sulfate (DHEAS)	135,925 ± 48,000	17,619		<1
Progesterone	30	4.5		
17β-Estradiol (E_2)	2.5 ± 08	0.4	0.75	
Estrone	4.6	0.8	0.045	

[1]VP assay, Ventral prostate growth in castrate rat.

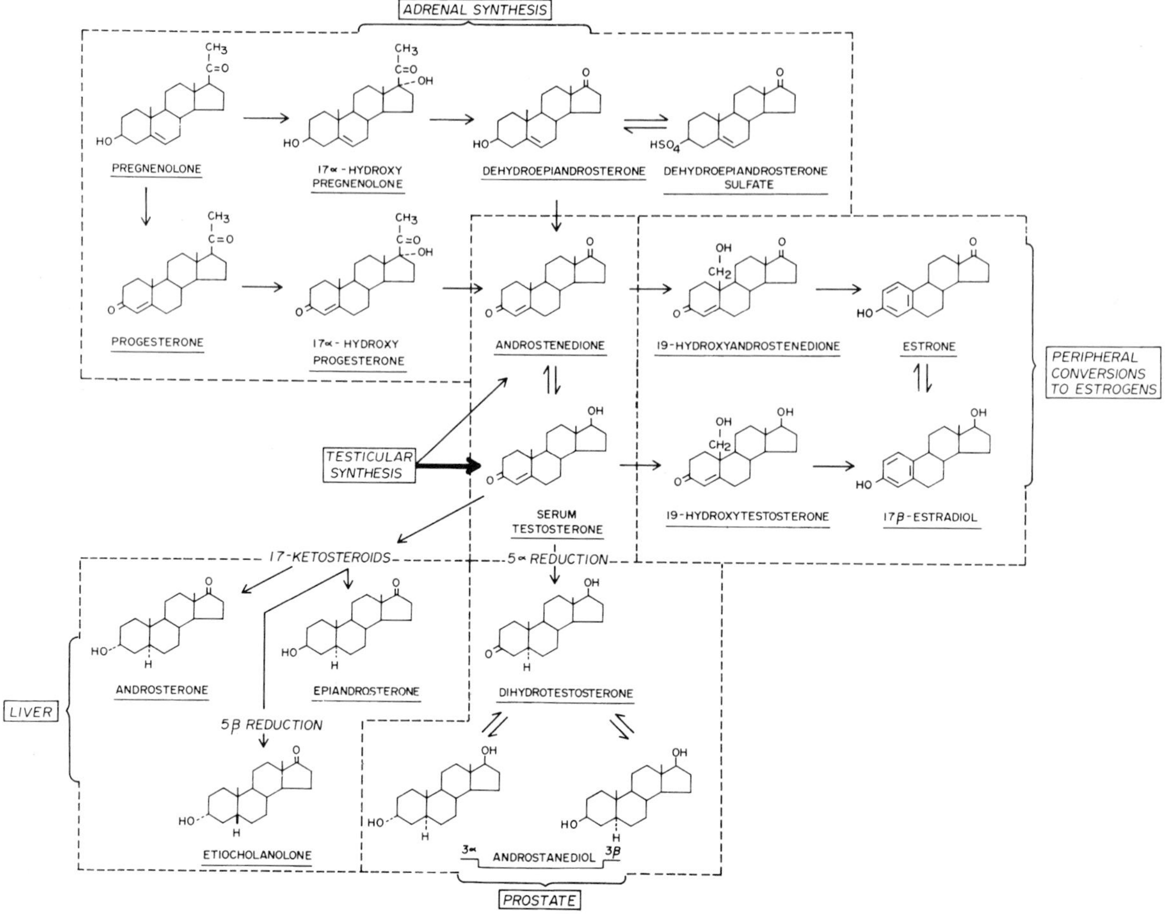

Figure 45–4. Overview of the synthesis and metabolism of testosterone in four main body compartments: (1) adrenal synthesis of androstenedione; (2) peripheral conversion of androgens (androstenedione and testosterone) to estrogen; (3) formation of active dihydrotestosterone within the prostate; and (4) inactivation in the liver of testosterone to three types of 17-ketosteroids.

tomy or hypophysectomy (Kyprianou and Isaacs, 1987). In rats that are castrated, the DHT level in the prostatic tissue is approximately 20% of that in normal intact animals. Adrenalectomy lowers the DHT to nondetectable levels without further diminution in prostate growth. This indicates that a threshold level of DHT is required in the prostate to stimulate growth and that the castrate level is below this threshold. It has also been concluded similarly that, in humans, the prostate does not restore itself following castration, indicating that adrenal androgens are insufficient to compensate for the loss of testicular function. Quantitative morphometry of the human prostate (Oesterling et al, 1986) also confirms that the adrenal gland has little effect on the normal prostate epithelial cell size.

The adrenal steroids, dehydroepiandrosterone, and the conjugate dehydroepiandrosterone sulfate, as well as androstenedione, are androgens synthesized from acetate and cholesterol (see Fig. 45–4), which are secreted by the normal human adrenal glands. **Essentially, all of the dehydroepiandrosterone in male plasma originates from the adrenal cortex, and the production rate in humans is 10 to 30 mg/day. Less than 1% of the total testosterone in the plasma is derived from dehydroepiandrosterone (Horton, 1976; MacDonald, 1976).**

The prostate and seminal vesicles of the rat and the human prostate can slowly hydrolyze dehydroepiandrosterone sulfate to free steroids through prostate sulfatase enzymatic activity, but the degree of conversion is low, thereby explaining why dehydroepiandrosterone sulfate is not a very potent androgen.

A second adrenal androgen is androstenedione, and the plasma concentration in adult males is approximately 150 ± 54 ng/100 ml (see Table 45–4). The blood production rate of androstenedione in human males is about 2 to 6 mg/day, with approximately 20% of the androstenedione being generated by peripheral metabolism of other steroids. **Androstenedione cannot be converted directly to DHT and, therefore, is a weak androgen.** An important role for androstenedione in the male may be its peripheral conversion to estrogens through the aromatase reaction (see Fig. 45–4).

The adrenal gland also produces C 21 steroids (e.g., progesterone). The plasma production rate at 0.75 mg/day is low, producing a low plasma progesterone concentration of 30 ng/100 ml. **Although progesterone is weakly androgenic, it does not exert a significant effect on the prostate at the low concentrations present in normal male plasma. In summary, under normal conditions, the adrenals do not support significant growth of prostatic tissue.**

Estrogens in the Male

Only small amounts of estrogen are produced directly by the testes. Approximately 75% to 90% of the estro-

gens in the plasma of young healthy human males is derived from the peripheral conversion of androstenedione and testosterone to estrone and estradiol via the aromatase reaction (see Fig. 45–4) (Horton, 1976; MacDonald, 1976). The androgenic C19 steroids (testosterone and androstenedione) are converted to the estrogenic C18 steroids first by removing the 19-methyl group and subsequently by formatting an aromatic or phenolic steroid ring (aromatase reaction), present in both estradiol and estrone. Estradiol is formed from testosterone and estrone from androstenedione; these two estrogens are then interconvertible (see Fig. 45–4). **The daily production of estradiol in the human male is about 40 to 50 μg, and only 5 to 10 μg (10% to 25%) can be accounted for by direct testicular secretion**. The dynamics of the synthesis of estrogens in human males have been quantitated by Siiteri and MacDonald (1973), who showed that of the 7.0 mg of testosterone produced in the human male each day, only 0.35% is converted directly to estradiol, forming 24 μg/day. Of the 2.5 mg of androstenedione produced per day, 1.7% is converted to estrone, producing 42 μg/day. The interconversion of estrone and estradiol yields a final total peripheral production of approximately 40 μg of estradiol per day. **The exact location in the periphery where estrogen production occurs has not been elucidated on a quantitative basis, but it is believed that most of the daily production may involve adipose tissue.** The small amount of estrogens secreted directly from the testes may originate in part from the Sertoli cells, because in culture, these cells respond to follicle-stimulating hormone by producing small amounts of estradiol (Dorrington and Armstrong, 1975); in the adult rat, the Leydig cell may be the source of estradiol.

Men older than 50 years of age may have an increase in total plasma estradiol levels of approximately 50%, with minimal change (less than 10%) in the free estradiol levels because of increases in binding of the estradiol by elevated serum testosterone-estradiol–binding globulin (TeBG) levels, which are also age related (Vermeulen, 1976). **The age-related decrease in the plasma-free testosterone level while the free estradiol level is maintained produces a 40% increase in the ratio of free estradiol and free testosterone (Vermeulen et al, 1969; Vermeulen, 1976). It is apparent that the availability of estrogens and androgens in the serum is regulated not only by their total level but by the free (i.e., unbound) level as well. Because the steroid-binding proteins in the serum can regulate the free levels, it is important to understand how they function.**

Androgen-Binding Proteins in the Plasma

The great bulk of serum steroids do not circulate freely in males but are reversibly bound to a variety of serum proteins. Less than 2% of the total testosterone in human plasma is free or unbound, and the remaining 98% is bound to several different types of plasma proteins (see Fig. 45–3). The plasma proteins that bind steroids include human serum albumin, TeBG (also called steroid-binding globulin [SBG]), corticosteroid-binding globulin (also termed transcortin), progesterone-binding globulin, and to a lesser extent, the alpha-acid glycoprotein. The total amount of testosterone bound to progesterone-binding globulin and alpha-acid glycoprotein is not large and is usually ignored.

The regulation of the amount of androgen that is free is an important physiologic factor that varies among different species. **The total amount of steroid-bound androgen receptor depends on two factors: (1) the *affinity* of the steroid to bind to a specific protein, and (2) the *capacity* (maximal potential binding when all of a binding protein is saturated), which is governed by the amount of binding protein in the plasma**. Serum albumin has a relatively low affinity for testosterone, but because albumin is at high concentration in the plasma, it can bind appreciable quantities of testosterone. Therefore, albumin is termed a low-affinity, high-capacity binding protein. In contrast, TeBG, which has been isolated from plasma, has a high affinity for binding steroids, but the protein is present in relatively low concentrations; however, the plasma molarity of each binding protein exceeds the plasma molarity for total testosterone concentration. **The majority of testosterone bound to plasma protein is associated with TeBG**. For example, Vermeulen (1973) has calculated that in the normal human male, 57% of testosterone in the plasma is bound to TeBG and 40% is bound to human serum albumin. Less than 1% is bound to corticosteroid-binding globulin, and only 2% of the total testosterone is free (see Fig. 45–3). The normal plasma free testosterone level is therefore 12.1 ± 3.7 ng/100 ml or 0.42 nM; this nonprotein-bound free testosterone is available to diffuse into the sex accessory tissue and into liver cells for metabolism. In addition, a large percentage of the TeBG is saturated, whereas only a small fraction of the total capacity of corticosteroid-binding globulin and albumin is used under normal conditions. As testosterone levels increase in the plasma, the order of increasing saturation of the plasma proteins proceeds from TeBG to corticosteroid-binding globulin to albumin. Therefore, the binding of androgen is a dynamic equilibrium between various serum proteins.

The total plasma levels of TeBG can be altered by hormone therapy. **Administration of testosterone decreases TeBG levels in the plasma, while estrogen therapy stimulates the production of TeBG (Forest et al, 1968; Vermeulen et al, 1969; Burton and Westphal, 1972)**. Estrogen also competes with testosterone to bind to TeBG, but estrogen has only one third of the binding affinity of testosterone. **Therefore, administration of small amounts of estrogen increases the total concentration of TeBG, and this effectively increases the binding of testosterone and thus lowers the free testosterone plasma concentration**.

Therefore, because free testosterone enters sex accessory tissue, the binding of testosterone to plasma proteins inhibits the uptake into the prostate (Lasnitzki and Franklin, 1972). It is apparent that androgenic activity is regulated in part by the extent of binding of an androgen to the steroid-binding proteins in the plasma. Indeed, Anderson and colleagues (1972) have postulated that altered testosterone binding to plasma proteins might produce amplified changes in free estrogen and androgen levels, and this could be an important factor in inducing gynecomastia and impotence.

Prolactin

Exogenous androgens can restore the normal adult prostate to 80% of its original size in hypophysectomized rats.

To obtain full restoration with androgens in these hypophysectomized rats, supplements of exogenous prolactin are required (Grayhack et al, 1955). This early observation has been confirmed in numerous animal experiments, in which prolactin was shown to be synergistic with androgens on prostate growth (Assimos et al, 1984). In addition, prolactin increases zinc uptake in the tissue (Moger and Geschwind, 1972), alters androgen uptake and metabolism (Lloyd et al, 1973), and regulates citric acid and fructose levels. Prolactin receptors have been identified in prostatic tissue (Aragona and Friesen, 1975). Prolactin has a permissive effect on the growth of the lateral prostate of the rat, and this effect may be associated with increased nuclear androgen levels (Manandhar and Thomas, 1976; Assimos et al, 1984). The direct action of prolactin on prostate epithelial cells has also been suggested through tissue and organ culture experiments (McKeehan et al, 1984). The aforementioned evidence that prolactin affects prostatic growth in animals has led to much speculation about a similar role in humans. Prolactin levels in human blood are elevated by treatment with estrogens or some tranquilizing drugs and stress, and can be decreased by L-dopa and ergot derivatives. With improved assays, the levels have been monitored in patients of advanced age and in those with BPH, but no clear correlation between prolactin effect and a cause of prostate pathology is yet apparent (Birkoff et al, 1974).

REGULATION OF PROSTATIC GROWTH AT THE CELLULAR LEVEL BY STEROIDS AND PROTEIN GROWTH FACTORS

Overview

It now appears that there are multiple levels of cell regulation that include steroid hormone action, growth factors, direct cell-to-cell communication, and interactions with the extracellular matrix. These interactive types of growth control are usually accomplished by several generalized systems, as depicted in the schematic in Figure 45–5. The types include (1) *endocrine factors,* or long-range signals arriving at the prostate by serum transport of hormone originating from the secretions of distant organs (this includes serum hormone–like steroids such as testosterone and estrogens, and serum endocrine polypeptide hormones like prolactin and gonadotropins); (2) *neuroendocrine* signals originating from neural stimulation such as 5-hydroxytryptamine, acetylcholine, and norepinephrine; (3) *paracrine factors* or soluble tissue growth factors that stimulate or inhibit growth that are elaborated over short ranges between neighboring cells within the prostate tissue compartment such as FGF and EGF; (4) *autocrine factors*, which are growth factors that are produced and released by a cell and then fed back on the same cell's external membrane receptors to regulate its own growth or function such as autocrine motility factor; (5) *intracrine factors*, which are autocrine factors that are not released outside but work inside the cell; (6) *extracellular matrix factors*, which are insoluble tissue matrix systems that make direct and coupled contact by being attached through integrins and adhesion molecules of the basal membrane and couple cytoskeleton organization with the extracellular matrix components that include the GAGs, such as heparan sulfate (Getzenberg et al, 1990); (7) *cell-to-cell interactions* of the epithelial or stromal cells occurring through tight membrane junctions on intramembrane proteins such as the CAMs, like E-cadherin, that couple neighboring cells.

Of these seven growth control systems, the first extensively studied in the regulation of prostate growth was the endocrine effect of androgenic steroid involving changes in serum testosterone levels, conversion to DHT, and steroid receptor interactions. Androgens are permissive or required for full prostate growth, but in the last decade, rapid progress has been made in the understanding of the other systems, particularly the interactive role of growth factors and their receptors. At present, how these receptors use cell signaling in the nucleus and how structural elements are used in cellular control involving the tissue matrix is being studied. These mechanisms are reviewed starting with androgen action at the prostate cell level, beginning with the arrival of testosterone in the serum.

Androgen Action at the Cellular Level

Testosterone in the serum arrives at the prostate bound to albumin or SBGs as depicted in the schematic in Figure 45–6. Only the free testosterone enters the prostate cell, where it is then subjected to a variety of steroid metabolic steps that appear to regulate the activity, and finally, the inactivation of this steroid hormone. The temporal sequence of intracellular events is depicted in Figure 45–6. The sequence includes (1) cellular diffusion of testosterone; (2) conversion of testosterone to DHT by metabolism of 5α-reductase; (3) the binding of DHT or testosterone to specific androgen receptors in the nucleus; (4) activation of the steroid receptor in the nucleus by conformational change, phosphorylation, and binding of the receptor to androgen receptor elements (ARE), by binding of the receptor to tissue-specific proteins of the nuclear matrix; (5) production of receptor-induced changes in DNA loop topology and chromatin structure; (6) the receptor's acting as a transcription factor and, when bound to the DNA and matrix in proximity to androgen target genes, increasing the RNA polymerase transcription of the DNA into messenger RNA (mRNA), (7) transcription of the message (mRNA), which is very large and contains introns, exons, and a poly-A tail section (only the exon portion of the mRNA will be retained in the final message; the trimming and processing of the mRNA is accomplished on the nuclear matrix as it is transported through the nucleus and out through the nuclear pore complex); (8) transportion of stabilized mRNA into the cytoplasmic compartment to be translated at the ribosome into protein, (9) transportation of the proteins to specific cellular sites and its subsequent post-translational modification, and finally, (10) the storage of the protein in secretory granules poised for secretion into the lumen on neurologic command during the physiologic process of ejaculation.

The epithelial cell is the primary unit in secretion, but specific genes are also activated in the stromal cells; these events are also regulated by testosterone, estrogens, and growth factors in a similar chain of events, as discussed

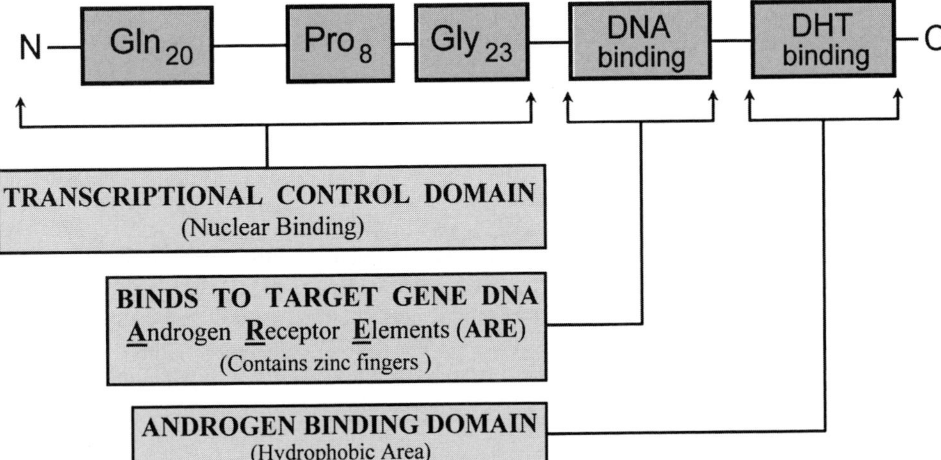

Figure 45–8. Structure of the human androgen receptor protein showing the repetitive amino acid components that make up the three domains that regulate transcription, DNA binding, and steroid specificity.

cell line of prostate cancer render it able to be activated by inappropriate steroids such as estrogens or even antiandrogens. This factor may have profound implications on how prostate cancer may become androgen insensitive and continue to grow in the absence of androgens by producing a steroid receptor that functions without a steroid, or how antiandrogens can paradoxically maintain growth of the cancer.

The hormone-responsive elements to which the normal androgen receptors have been shown to belong to the glucocorticoid-responsive element (GRE)/progesterone-responsive element (PRE) subgroup (French et al, 1990). A consensus sequence for the ARE has been determined to be GG(A/T)ACAnnnTGTTCT (Roche et al, 1992). Some degree of sequence variation exists among the identified AREs (Luke and Coffey, 1994b). Androgen binding to the receptor is required to transport the androgen receptor into the nucleus, but once there, androgen is not required for the receptor to bind to the AREs of DNA (Luke and Coffey, 1994b). AREs have been identified within the last few years for various genes that are responsive to androgen action (Luke and Coffey, 1994b). The androgen-regulated rat secretory protein C3 of prostatein has an ARE within its first intronic element, which has been shown to function as an androgen-responsive promoter (Claessens et al, 1989). PSA is a major protein in the human male ejaculate that is androgen regulated. An androgen regulatory element has been found upstream of the PSA gene's first exon in the promoter region (Reigman et al, 1992).

The transcription domain of the androgen receptor codes for important information involved in nuclear binding. Much of this interaction may be defined by the repetitive amino acids sequences that are unique and fall in three domains of approximately 20 repeating glutamine, followed by a space containing eight repetitive proline, and following 23 repetitive glycine units (see Fig. 45–8). The glutamine repeats form a beta sheet, which helps form protein-protein interactions. Barrack and colleagues (Schoenberg et al, 1994) have reported that these glutamine repeat sequences, which are coded by a CAG repeat in the gene, vary in prostate cancer. In the normal population, this sequences varies over a length of 11 to 31 CAG repeats, and this configuration is called polymorphism. This means that different people have alleles of variant polyglutamine repeat units. This variation is racially defined, and it has been suggested that this may be related to the differences in the incidence of rates of prostate cancer in different ethnic groups. Barrack and colleagues (unpublished data) have observed that there is a relation between the aggressiveness of prostate cancer and the CAG repeat, with the smaller units being more associated with tumor-positive lymph nodes. In this regard, it has also been reported that patients with X-linked spinal and bulbar muscular atrophy, termed Kennedy's disease, possess a larger glutamine repeat in the range of 40 to 60 copies (LaSpada, 1991). **It is obvious that the genetic studies of inherited diseases of both androgen insensitivity and overvirilization, as well as changes in the androgen receptor mutation associated with prostate cancer and its biologic properties, will be of great help in unraveling the role of the human androgen receptor in relation to its structure.**

The development of the androgen receptor during embryonic development appears first in the mesenchyme of both the rat ventral prostate and seminal vesicle and, a few days later, appears in the epithelial cells; it is unknown what regulates this timing. In the development of the seminal vesicles and the wolffian duct, testosterone appears to be the primary androgen in the glandular development, and in the ventral prostate, which forms from the urogenital sinus, the androgen is primarily DHT. Both testosterone and DHT can bind to the androgen receptor; however, on a molar basis, the DHT is 3 to 10 times more potent. This decrease in potency of testosterone is believed to be due to the rapid off rates of the testosterone once bound so that equilibrium results in less receptor occupancy when compared with DHT at similar levels. It now appears that a series of modulator proteins can interact with the androgen receptor that can modify its tissue specificity, DNA binding properties, and transport to the nucleus. The androgen receptors can form dimers with themselves, which are referred to an homodimers, and they can also form heterodimers to these cytoplasmic and nuclear modulator proteins that can regulate their biologic properties.

What produces the tissue specificity in receptor action? Two cell types in different tissues from the same animal can contain the same androgen receptors present in their nuclei, but a cell in one tissue type will respond to the receptor by making one type of androgen-induced protein, whereas another cell in a different tissue will produce a second type of androgen-induced protein. For example, in the rat, the ventral prostate and the seminal vesicles both have androgen receptors, and in the presence of DHT, they bind to the same genome (DNA) in their nuclei; however, the prostate makes a different pattern of androgen-controlled gene expression of secretory proteins from the secretory proteins induced by androgen in the seminal vesicles. How two cells with the same DNA respond to the same receptor in a totally different manner remains a mystery. Is it because the receptors are different in these two tissues in some subtle way or that certain DNA sequences have been slightly modified by methylation or changes in topology or chromatin structure? This is one of the major frontiers of endocrine molecular biology.

The Role of the Nuclear Matrix in Androgen Action

The nuclear matrix is an important structural modulator of nuclear regulation and is an ideal target for hormonal regulation. Indeed, the nuclear matrix is a major site of steroid hormone receptor binding (Barrack and Coffey, 1982; Wilson and Colvard 1984; Alexander et al, 1987; Barrack, 1987; Donnelly et al, 1983; Metzger and Korach, 1990; Luke and Coffey, 1994a). In the prostate, over 60% of all nuclear androgen receptors are associated with the nuclear matrix (Barrack and Coffey, 1982). The matrix is also a target for many other types of regulatory interactions, including the nuclear products of oncogenes and viral proteins that can also induce growth regulation similar to that of hormone-induced growth. For example, the nuclear matrix is reported to be a cellular target for the retrovirus myc oncogene protein, the adenovirus E1A transforming protein, as well as the polyoma large T antigen. All of these transformation proteins that bind to the nucleus are believed to be early molecular events in carcinogenesis or transformation. For a more detailed review of the matrix in hormone action, see the review of Luke and Coffey (1994b) and Getzenberg and colleagues (1990), and for the role of the nuclear matrix in cancer, see Pienta and associates (1989).

Stromal-Epithelial Interactions

It is now apparent that there is a dynamic and reciprocal interaction between the functions of the epithelial cells and the function of the stromal cells (Cunha, 1994; Sikes et al, 1995; Steiner, 1993). These cross-talk interactions are interfaced as well as mediated by and through the spatial organization of the extracellular matrix elements that form the basement membrane linkage that presents, filters, and organizes the two-way paracrine signals and the flow of information between those two cellular compartments (Fig. 45–9). For example, fluids, gases, nutrients, hormones, and many growth factors arriving in the prostate via the circulation must first pass through the stroma ground substance, the extracellular matrix, and the membrane basement to finally reach the base of the secretory epithelial cells.

Therefore, it is important to define stromal-epithelial interactions. The noncellular stroma and connective tissue of the prostate comprise what is termed the ground substance and the extracellular matrix in what was first suggested by Arcadi (1954) to play an important role in prostate function and pathology. Later, an interactive tissue matrix system was proposed that extended from the extracellular matrix to the nucleus and linked all cells (Getzenberg et al, 1990; Isaacs et al, 1981). The extracellular matrix has long been recognized as one of the important inductive components during normal development of many different types of cells (Grobstine, 1975; Cunha, 1976; Hay, 1981; Bissell et al, 1982). The extracellular matrix is far more than just a supporting scaffolding for cells because it has been shown to play a central role in the development and control of cellular function (Hay, 1981; Getzenberg et al, 1990). Cell-to-cell interactions can also modify the type of response that a cell makes to hormones and growth factors. **In summary, what a cell touches determines how a cell develops and how it responds to its environment and extracellular signals.**

There has been increasing interest in the role of stromal tissue elements in inducing the growth of the sex accessory tissue since the early suggestions of Franks in 1970 that epithelial cells require stroma for their growth. In addition, the classic tissue reconstruction experiments of Cunha and colleagues (1983), Chung and Cunha (1983), Biller and coworkers (1985), and Cunha (1994) have clearly shown the direct importance of the isolated embryonic mesenchyme on the induction of differentiation of normal prostatic epithelial cells (see earlier discussion). McNeal (1978) proposed that in BPH, the stroma may be reactivated in adult life to return to an embryonic state, thus stimulating abnormal growth; this concept has generated a great deal of interest and effort to understand these tissue components of the prostate. To test whether adult prostate cells could be stimulated by embryonic factors, Chung and colleagues (1984a, 1984b, 1992) transplanted a fetal urogenital sinus into an adult rat prostate and induced a large hyperplastic overgrowth of adult prostatic tissue that was apparently stimulated by the presence of the factors from the fetal tissue. It is unknown whether direct contact with an insoluble embryonic extracellular matrix or soluble diffusible growth factor(s), or both, and steroids are responsible for these observations (see review of Sikes et al, 1995). Figure 45–9 illustrates the pathways of coupling stromal-epithelial interactions involving both soluble (growth factors and steroids) and insoluble (extracellular matrix, cell-to-cell, and integrin) interactions.

Cell-matrix interactions can also serve as a brake or negative factor to suppress or limit growth. Muntzing (1980) proposed that collagen of the prostate might suppress pros-

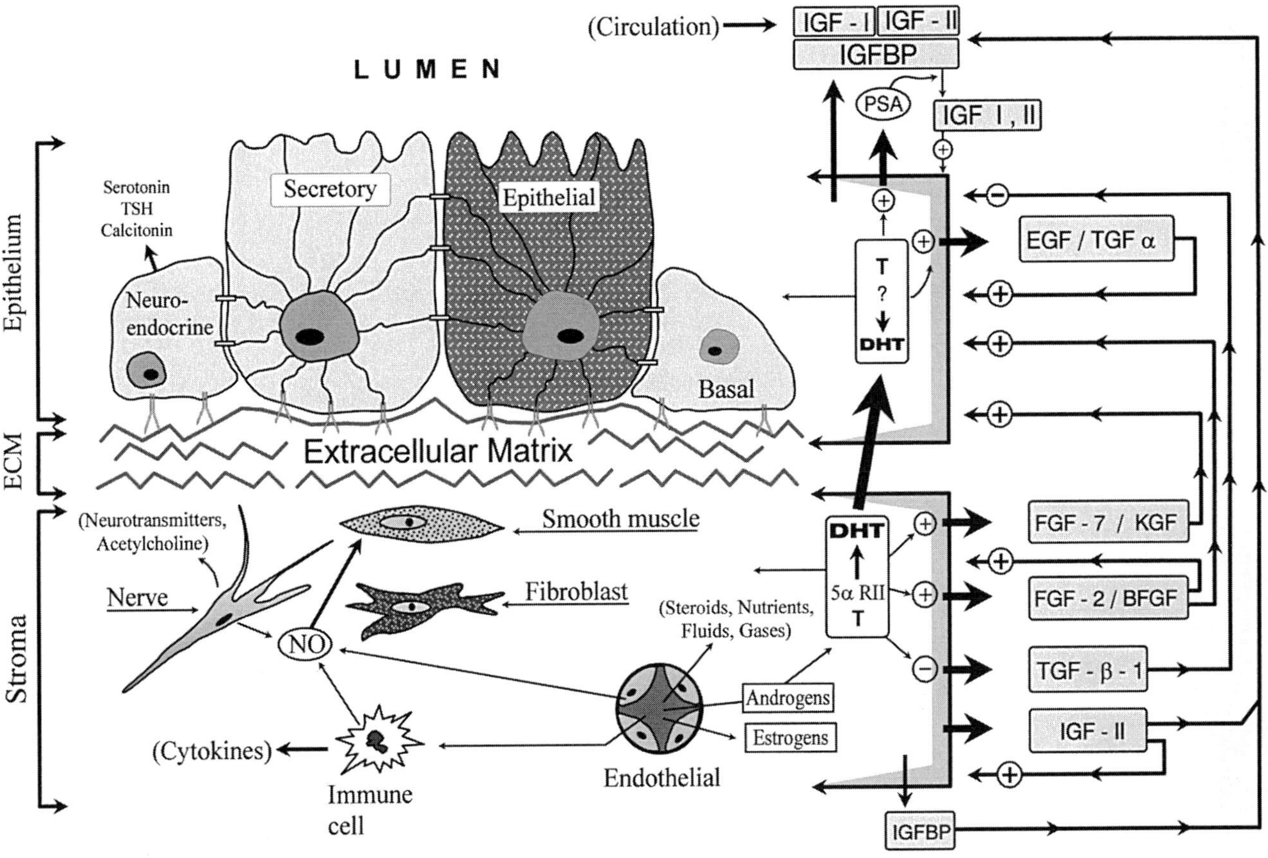

Figure 45–9. A schematic of the types of stromal-epithelial interactions in information transfer and regulation within the prostate. Testosterone and growth factors interact on and between stromal and epithelial cells. The production of growth factors is either stimulated or inhibited by androgens. The growth factors can function on the same cell (autocrine) or on distant cells (paracrine). Nitric oxide (NO) is formed from nerve, endothelial, or macrophages and affects smooth muscle contraction (see text for details of these pathways). Important features of this schematic are (1) three types of prostatic epithelial cells—neuroendocrine, secretory, and basal; (2) five important prostatic stromal cells—smooth muscle, fibroblast, immune cells, endothelial, and nerve; (3) testosterone is converted to DHT by 5-α reductase in the stromal compartment; (4) three sources of NO production in the prostate—nerve, immune cells (macrophages), and endothelial cells; and (5) stromal-epithelial interactions are mediated through various growth factors (see text).

tate growth. Mariotti and Mawhinney (1981) have provided evidence that collagen synthesis and degradation can be important events in accompanying limitations on prostatic growth in animals. At present, it has not been established whether or not collagen has a definite effect on normal prostate growth and function, but several types of collagens are critical components of the extracellular matrix and basement membrane (see Fig. 45–1).

Cell Adhesion Molecules

Cell-to-cell and extracellular matrix interactions are becoming major targets for understanding how the phenotype of a cell is regulated. Transmembrane receptors on the cell surface extend out through the plasma membrane and form a bridge directly connecting the cytoskeleton with proteins and receptors located within the extracellular matrix or on neighboring cells (see Fig. 45–1). The CAMs are divided into four major types: (1) *integrins* that link the cell to the basement membrane and extracellular matrix components through heterodimer interactions; (2) *cadherins* that link the cell to neighboring cells through homotypic polymers; (3) *selectins* that link the cell to carbohydrate moieties primarily on the vascular system; and (4) *immunoglobulin superfamily adhesion molecules*. The most extensively studied of these CAMs in the prostate in order of interest have been E-cadherins that bind prostate epithelial cells to each other, CD-44 that binds cells to the hyaluronic acid ICAM, and CD-71 that binds to transferrin, as well as several of the integrin molecules. These bindings have been surveyed in prostate tumor cell lines in vitro (Rokhlin and Cohen, 1995), but more extensive work needs to be carried out in vivo in the normally developing prostate and in the prostate affected by cancer.

The cadherins are the most important of the cell-to-cell adhesion molecules and are classified into three subtypes that include (1) the E-caderins found in adult epithelial cells (also termed earlier uvomorulin, Cel CAM, 120/80, ARC-1, and L-CAM); (2) N-cadherins found in neural tissues of muscle (also termed A-CAM); and (3) the P-cadherins found primarily in placenta and epithelium (see review by Albelva, 1994). In the prostate cell, for example, E-cadherins extending out of the surface membrane to make contact with the neighboring cell and form a homodimer, and the E-cadherin extending inside the cell by passing through the membrane would form as an organizing center that binds a complex of three cytoplasmic proteins termed catenin-αβ. This complex is localized to the zonula adherins of the cell and participates in junction formation and stabilization of the cytoskeleton. These interlocking matrix systems interact to form a structural network organization that terminates with direct contact with the nuclear matrix that forms tissue specific DNA organization. **The interactions of the tissue matrix regulate many aspects of DNA functions that are involved in growth and differentiation, and the study of this system is at the forefront of molecular cell biology (Getzenberg et al, 1990).**

The CAMs have been implicated as having a major role in tumor progression and metastasis (see review by Albelva, 1994). The repertoire of integrins can vary during the neoplastic process (Van Waes et al, 1995). The αβ4 integrin is expressed at the base of normal epithelial cells in an area that forms the hemidesmosome complex that links it to the basement membrane for its attachment to laminin. αβ4 is absent in LNCaP cells and is down-regulated in PC-3 and DU-145 cells (Rokhlin and Cohen, 1995). Laminin has been proposed to be an important extracellular matrix protein that changes its isoform during the neoplastic transformation, This protein has been studied in prostate carcinoma cell lines (Rabinovitz et al, 1994). In the prostate, there has been differential expression of extracellular matrix molecules in the α6 integrins in normal and neoplastic human prostates. These integrin expressions and patterns could be an important new frontier in cell adhesion and extracellular matrix changes related to cancer (Bonkhoff et al, 1993; Knox et al, 1994). In addition, it has been reported that C-CAM can act as a tumor suppressor in prostate cancer development, and when C-CAM gene is transfected into the PC-3 prostate tumor cell line, it repressed growth (Kleinerman et al, 1995). In addition, P-CAM is lost in prostate cancer and is an excellent basal cell marker in the normal prostate (Jarrard et al 1996).

Most interest in cancer of the prostate has been placed on the study of E-cadherin expression, which has also been shown to suppress tumor cell invasion and metastasis in experimental tumor models and to be reduced in or absent from high-grade prostate cancers (Umbas et al, 1992; Bussemakers et al, 1994). In some cases, the reduction and redistribution of the E-cadherin protein on the periphery of the cell is associated with mutations or deletion of the α-catenin gene in human prostate cancer cells (Morton et al, 1993). It has been reported that E-cadherin expression can be silenced or reduced by DNA hypermethylation of the CpG islands in the promoter region of the E-cadherin gene (Graff et al, 1995; Yoshiura et al, 1995).

In summary, different components of matrix interactions can have either an inhibitory role in negative regulation of normal prostate growth or a positive role in establishing tumor growth. There have been many hypotheses concerning the mechanism of these epithelial-stromal interactions, but they have yet to be fully determined (Muntzing, 1980; Tenniswood, 1986; Getzenberg et al, 1990; Chung et al, 1992; Sikes et al, 1995).

To this point, the discussion, has concerned primarily insoluble elements in inducing stromal-epithelial interactions, but soluble hormones, such as steroids, vitamins, and growth factors, are also important (Sikes et al, 1995). The prostatic stroma cells contain steroid receptors and respond to both androgens and estrogens (see earlier discussion), and the stroma has an androgen-metabolizing ability to form DHT greater than that of the epithelium. Androgens and estrogens can alter the formation of collagen (Coffey and Walsh, 1990) and other extracellular matrix components such as glycosoaminoglycans in the prostate (DeKlerk et al, 1984; DeKlerk and Hunan 1985; Kofoed et al, 1990; Horsfall et al, 1994).

The Role of Vitamin A and D in Normal Prostate Function

We have previously discussed androgens and estrogens stimulating growth, but vitamins such as A and D also affect the prostate because they bind to receptors that are similar to the steroid receptors in protein sequence. They are discussed before introducing the growth factors. Recent considerations of both vitamin A and its retinoid derivatives, as well as vitamin C, vitamin E, and vitamin D, on prostate growth have been reviewed by Kadmon and Thompson (1995).

Vitamin A

It has long been known that vitamin A can protect against the development of prostate cancer in carcinogenic-induced animal models (Lasnitzki, 1955, 1974; Chopra and Wilkof, 1979; Pollard et al, 1991). Vitamin A is a retinol, and the natural and synthetic analogues are called retinoids. There are over six human retinoid receptors (RAR [α, β, γ] and RXR [α, β, γ]), and all six belong to the steroid receptor superfamily. This complex field is exemplified by the fact that the retinoids bind to receptors and can produce a pleotrophic response, including proliferation, differentiation, morphogenesis, programmed cell death, and interactions with extracellular matrix formation and the immune system (Kadmon and Thompson, 1995). Retinoids have the ability to modify growth factor activity, particularly TGF-β, and to induce protein kinase C and other kinase cascades. There is approximately 60 ng/g wet weight of retinoids in the normal prostate, 146 ng/g in BPH, and 75 ng/g in prostatic carcinoma (Kadmon and Thompson, 1995). At present, chemoprevention in prostate cancer trials have used a compound called fenretinide (4-HPR) and 9-*cis*-retinoic acid.

Retinoids can inhibit the growth of both normal and cancerous prostate cells, both in vivo (Pollard et al, 1991) and in vitro (Peehl et al, 1991; Igawa, 1994; Young et al, 1994). It was observed that retinoic acids can antagonize the effects of androgens on LNCaP cells, and this process was modulated by a decrease in the expression of the androgen receptor in a concomitant down-regulation of PSA (Young et al, 1994). In those studies, retinoic acid did not block the binding to the androgen receptor but did affect its expression, and it was postulated that it may also affect other transcription factors (Young et al, 1994). It is of interest that retinoid acid can also affect the expression of other receptors, such as vitamin D3, progesterone, and estrogen receptors. 4HPR also inhibits the growth of PC-3 cells, and it was shown that this factor was the result of a block in the cell cycle transition from G1 to S phase and that this inhibition was associated with the suppression of C-myc gene expression (Igawa et al, 1994). This factor results in suppression of growth without cytotoxicity. 4HPR has been used to effectively treat the Dunning prostatic cancer model (Pienta et al, 1993).

Vitamin D

Vitamin D was originally classified as a vitamin because in the early 1900s, it was determined to be essential for the maintenance of calcium homeostasis and normal skeletal development. On determination of its chemical structure, it was apparent that it was actually not a vitamin but a steroid (see review by Buillon et al, 1995). Indeed, the receptor for vitamin D has been shown to be similar in structure to a steroid receptor and is located on LNCaP cells (Miller et al, 1992). There is conflicting information on the effects 1,25 (OH) vitamin D_3 on prostate cancer cells in culture, with Miller and associates (1992) showing a pronounced mitogenic effect on proliferation, whereas Skowronski and colleagues (1993) have shown that this derivative blocks the proliferation of LNCaP and PC-3 cells. It appears that 1,25 (OH) vitamin D_3 markedly stimulates the levels of insulin growth factor–binding protein 6 in human prostate tumor cells (Drivdahl et al, 1995).

As described earlier in this chapter, although it is evident that the prostate and other sex accessory tissues are clearly hormonally regulated, the role of vitamin D in the normal prostate is only beginning to be elucidated. **Some investigations have revealed that vitamin D is involved in the differentiation of the normal prostate and has a pronounced effect on the organization of the rat prostate with vitamin D receptors in epithelial and stromal cells. Specifically, vitamin D has been found to induce columnar differentiation, resulting in increased secretory capacity in prostate epithelium, and stromal atrophy.** In castrate animals, vitamin D was shown to significantly enhance the growth and differentiation of the prostate, resulting in a prostate that is twice the size of the prostate of an animal that did not receive vitamin D (Getzenberg et al, 1996). Importantly, although changes in the seminal vesicle were noted, they are not of the magnitude of those seen in the prostate. Overall, these studies suggest the importance of vitamin D in prostate growth and differentiation. These findings may further support investigations that demonstrate the importance of vitamin D in the epidemiology of prostate cancer (Schwartz and Hulka, 1990; Hanchette and Schwartz, 1992) where it is reported to be associated with a low incidence of prostate cancer.

Growth Factors and Growth Suppressors

Because the normal adult prostate is not growing rapidly or increasing in size, one would not anticipate an abundance of active growth factors in the normal prostate. However, this is a paradox because many adult tissues that are not rapidly growing still contain very high levels of growth factors that can be demonstrated by extracting the tissues and showing that they contain soluble factors that can stimulate in vitro fibroblast growth (Chung et al, 1992; Sikes et al, 1995). Paradoxically, injecting growth factors intraprostatically can induce some limited growth (Marengo and Chung, 1994).

It has been proposed that many of these prostate growth factors in the normal human prostate may not be active because they are sequestered by binding to components of the extracellular matrix, such as heparin or heparin sulfates that are part of the GAGs. Indeed, it is known that heparin binding to growth factors is one of the most efficient ways to remove and purify many growth factors such as those in the basic FGF family. If the prostate growth factors are sequestered at the extracellular matrix, it is important to know what mechanisms are involved in their binding and in their release. Therefore, simply measuring total growth factor levels in the prostate is, in itself, not sufficient to define their actual biologic activity in the prostate. **In all types of growth, it now appears that there is a balance between factors that activate growth and factors that suppress these growth-promoting factors. These latter inhibitory or braking elements have been termed suppressors. In this regard, the extracellular matrix could be termed a suppressor element in regard to its ability to sequester growth factors.** In addition, extracellular matrix interactions with cells can determine or direct the response of a cell to a mitogen like a growth factor.

In summary, both stromal and epithelial cells themselves can synthesize and respond to growth factors in a reciprocal and interactive manner (see Fig. 45–9); see the reviews by Steiner, 1993 Sikes et al, 1995). Many of these growth factors appear to be under hormonal regulation, particularly in response to androgens, estrogens, and other endocrine factors. Androgens and growth factors can also stimulate the synthesis and degradation of extracellular matrix components that can alter a cell's response to steroids and growth factors. Therefore, the interactions of steroids, growth factors, and the extracellular matrix with the cell is reciprocal and dynamic, and can have either positive or negative effects in regulating cell growth.

Growth Factor Mechanisms

Growth factors are usually large polypeptides that either stimulate or inhibit growth. Regulation of their synthesis, postranslational modification, transport, presentation, and binding to a specific target cell receptor is a multistep process that can vary with each type of growth factor. The cell is signaled to produce synthesis of a growth factor by environmental signals that include cell-to-cell extracellular matrix communications and hormonal levels. The genes for making the growth factors are activated by making messenger RNAs, which can be processed to various forms, which are then translated, usually to an inactive or progrowth factor form. Proteolysis activates the growth factor, which then can either work internally in the cell (intracrine) or be secreted extracellularly to serve as soluble signals either to its own cell in which it was synthesized (autocrine) or to stimulate a nearby cell (paracrine). After being secreted, the growth factor can be sequestered by binding to the extracellular matrix, but on release, the growth factor is capable of binding to specific growth factor receptors that reside on the plasma membrane of the target cell. Once a receptor binds the growth factor, the receptor is activated to become a kinase that enzymatically phosphorylates a protein that initiates a cascade of kinase pathways all the way to the nucleus. The abbreviations of these kinases of different pathways include MEK, JAK, STAT, and ERK. G-proteins (RAS, RHO, RAC) or protein kinase A and C may also be involved. These cell-signaling pathways are complex and involve cross-talk. They all result in sending a signal from the membrane receptor to the nucleus to activate a series of transcription factors that will either activate or silence a group of genes.

Figure 45–9 is an overview of important growth factors in the prostate that may activate (+) or inhibit (−) growth. These growth factors can be stimulated or inhibited in their production by androgens. Testosterone is converted to DHT in the stroma and, by paracrine action, can activate the epithelial cells. This activation often can be secondary through autocrine or paracrine effects such as insulin growth factors (IGF-I, II), which can be bound to plasma-binding proteins that can be regulated in their release by PSA activity. Besides growth factors, nitric oxide and neurogenic factors as well as cytokines can all modulate growth of the prostate (see Fig. 45–9).

HORMONE REVIEW WITH RESPECT TO PROSTATE GROWTH (Table 45–6)

Fibroblast Growth Factor

FGF is a large family of related growth factors (see reviews by Sikes et al, 1995 and Story, 1995). Earlier terms for FGF include prostate growth factor, osteoblastic growth factor, a form of tumor angiogenesis factor, endothelial growth factor, uterine growth factor, seminiferous growth factor, and KGF, just to name a few. Acidic FGF (AFGF) is now termed FGF-1; basic FGF (BFGF) is FGF-2 and keritinocyte FGF (KFGF) is FGF-7. Many believe that androgens induce prostate growth by stimulation of these growth factors to act in either an autocrine or paracrine fashion as shown in Figure 45–9. **FGFs can be isolated from many tissues and derive from cells of embryonic mesoderm or neuroectoderm origin. They can also be found in a wide variety of tumors and are produced by many cells in culture.** In 1979, Jacobs and colleagues identified a prostatic growth factor that they were able to show was a mitogenic factor present in human prostatic extracts (Jacobs et al, 1979; Jacobs and Lawson, 1980; Lawson et al, 1989; Muller et al, 1990; Yan et al, 1993; Culig et al, 1995; Cunha et al, 1995; Story, 1995). All of these earlier growth factors are now categorized as specific members of the FGF family (FGF-1 through FGF-7). FGF-1/AFGF and FGF-7/KFGF may have their greatest roles in the prostate during development and FGF-2/BFGF may have its greatest effect in the adult prostate under androgen stimulation, but these roles have not been fully determined in vivo nor in abnormal growth of the prostate, although there is no doubt that these are powerful factors to be considered.

Epidermal Growth Factor

Sherwood and Lee (1995) have reviewed the importance of EGFs in normal and abnormal growth of the prostate. They compare EGF and TGF-α and conclude the **EGF appears to be the predominant EGF-related growth factor in the normal prostate and in BPH. They believe that these two growth factors are important for maintaining the structural and functional integrity of BPH**. These growth factors are localized to the secretory epithelium, and their secretion is augmented by the presence of androgens. The receptors for EGF (EGFR) are located in the basal neuroendocrine cells and appear to be androgen independent

Table 45–6. PROPERTIES OF GROWTH FACTORS

Type			
Abbreviation	***Name***	**Size**	**Comment**
βFGF	Basic fibroblast growth factor (prostate growth factor, endothelial growth factor, tumor angiogenesis factor, osteoblastic factor)	155 amino acids 17.6 kD	Present in normal prostate. Elevated in BPH. In tissues of mesoderm origin, stromal elements
	Related int-2 oncogene	27 kD	Overexpression produces prostate epithelial hyperplasia but not glandular hyperplasia in transgenic mice
EGF	Epidermal growth factor; urogastrone	67-kD single chain	Controversial in normal human prostate but elevated in cancer. Prevalent in rat v.p.
TGF-α	Transforming growth factor-α; 30% similar to EGF, not related to TGF-β	5.6 kD	Low levels in human prostate, overexpression in transgenic mouse causes epithelial hyperplasia
TGF-β	Transforming growth factor-β; two genes (1 + 2), three combinations, TGF-β-1, TGF-β-2, TGF-β-3	25-kD dimer, disulfide	Inhibitor of epithelial growth; stimulates growth of fibroblast; TGF-β-2 elevated in BPH. Related to MIS and to inhibin and activin
MIS	Müllerian inhibiting substance	140-kD dimer of 2 identical 70-kd units	Causes repression of müllerian ducts
IGF	Insulin-like growth factor I and II somatomedin family	7.5-kD single chain	Related to proinsulin
PDGF	Platelet-derived growth factor	30-kD dimer	Mitogen for connective tissue cells

in the expression of this receptor. The early name of this growth factor was urogastrone, a growth factor that is a cleaved polypeptide of 53 amino acids with three disulfides that was first found in the urine and is now known to be similar to mouse EGF (MW, 16,000). EGF has been reported to be of high concentration (272 ng/ml) in human ejaculate and is produced in the prostate (Gregory et al, 1986).

High levels of FGF (FGF-2/BFGF) are found in all prostates, but EGF level is usually much lower. This has led Storey (1983) to conclude that EGF is not the major growth factor in the human prostate; indeed, messenger RNA for EGF has been difficult to detect in normal or abnormal growth of the human prostate (Mori et al, 1990).

There is still much conflict over the role of EGF in the normal human prostate, but prostate cancer cells in culture (LNCaP) do have significant levels of EGF that are 100 times that of TGF-α when measured intracellularly (Connolly and Rose, 1990). Morris and Dodd (1990) have measured the level of EGF and its receptor EGFR in the human prostate and have shown the highest levels in prostate cancer tissues, thus emphasizing the potential importance of EGF in cancer.

EGFR extends through the plasma membrane. It has a molecular weight of 170,000 and, like basic FGF, the receptor is an enzyme tyrosine kinase (see review by Sherwood and Lee, 1995). The c-erb-B2/neu oncoprotein is a 185-kD transmembrane glycoprotein that is closely related but not identical to EGFR. This protein is located in the cytoplasm and is not amplified in prostate cancer cells as it has been in breast cancer. This oncoprotein receptor has been reviewed in relation to prostate growth by Sikes and associates (1995). The c-erb-B2/neu oncoprotein has been demonstrated to be overexpressed in 11 of 16 human prostate cancer specimens and is transfected in the cells and can cause altered growth (Giri et al, 1993; Kuhn et al, 1993; Zhau et al, 1992). It has been demonstrated that EGFR and the neu oncoprotein may be involved in the progression of human prostate cancers (see the review by Sikes et al, 1995).

Transforming Growth Factor-α

TGF-α is very closely related to EGF (see reviews by Sherwood and Lee, 1995 and Sikes et al, 1995). TGFs were first so named because of their ability to promote cell colony formation in suspension cultures and, therefore, were an initial operational definition, but now the factors are purified. TGF-α is made as a prehormone precursor of 160 amino acids and is then processed by elastase to a smaller 50 amino acid peptide with a molecular weight of 5600. TGF-α is structurally similar to EGF and is believed to bring about most of its effects by interacting with the same EGFr as EGF. Both EGF and TGF-α can serve as transmembrane proteins or be excreted into the extracellular space. Both the free and membrane forms can bind to EGFR. TGF-α has been shown to stimulate the growth of human prostate cancers in culture and may be an autocrine factor in androgen-independent growth (Wilding et al, 1989; Sherwood and Lee, 1995; Sikes et al, 1995).

Transforming Growth Factor-β

TGF-β and its related superfamily in the prostate have been reviewed by Steiner (1995) and Sikes and colleagues (1995). TGF-β, containing 5 isomers, is not related to TGF-α, and the similarity in nomenclature causes some confusion. There are two genes for TGF-β, termed 1 and 2, and they have 70% homology. There are three combinations possible between these two genes when a dimer is formed; thus there is TGF-β1, 2, and 3. Although both TGF-β1 and 2 are expressed in prostate tissue, TGF-β2 has been shown to be significantly increased in expression in BPH as compared with the normal prostate, whereas TGF-β1 was not (Mori et al, 1990). **TGF-β is of paramount interest because it may function as a braking system in negatively regulated normal prostate epithelial cell growth while being a positive factor in stimulating normal stromal cell growth.** These generalizations may be changed in cancers or BPH tissues where the epithelial cells have changed their response to TGF-β, and now instead of inhibiting growth, TGF-β may stimulate growth (Kyprianou and Isaacs, 1988; Steiner and Barrack, 1992; Steiner et al, 1992; Steiner, 1993). In prostate cancer, androgens appear to lose their ability to regulate TGF-β (Steiner et al, 1994).

Other growth factors related to the TGF-β family are MIS activin, inhibin, and bone morphogens. MIS is a 140,00-MW protein that causes regression in the müllerian ducts, and inhibin is a peptide involved in feedback control of follicle-stimulating hormone. Inhibin has been reported to be present in the human prostate and seminal plasma, and is synthesized in the rat ventral prostate under hormonal control (Sheth et al, 1981; Sathe et al, 1986).

Bone Morphogenic Proteins

Prostate cancer cells often metastasize to the bone and produce osteoblastic lesion where new bone elements are laid down. **The growth factors that are capable of inducing bone formation are TGF-β1 and 3, and members of the bone morphogenic protein (BMP) family**. As mentioned earlier, TGF-β1 is overexpressed in prostate cancer cells (see the review by Steiner, 1993), and it is now apparent that normal, BPH, and prostate cancer can also form and secrete bone morphogens (Bentley et al, 1992; Harris et al, 1994; Barnes et al, 1995). These bone morphogens are produced both in human and rat prostate, as well as in the Dunning tumor model. There are several forms of the bone morphogens, and BMP-2, 3, 4 and 6 are the predominant forms identified in prostatic tissue. **The bone morphogens have the ability not only to stimulate the formation of osteoblasts but also are strong growth factors operating in the embryonic period and having the ability to induce LNCaP cells to form a fibroblast-like morphology (Harris et al, 1994). Bone morphogens as well as TGF-β stimulate the proliferation of fibroblasts and inhibit osteoclasts, and through this pathway, they could produce the increased bone formation seen in osteoblastic metastasis.** Bentley and colleagues (1992) suggested that there may be a correlation between the presence of BMP-6 in human prostate cancer and the ability of prostate cells to metastasize to the bone, and Steiner and co-workers (Barnes et al, 1995) showed that BMP-6 messenger RNA and protein expression was higher in prostate cancer compared with adjacent normal prostates and was elevated in higher Gleason grade tissues and that this morphogen was not under androgen control.

Media taken from Dunning rat tumor cell growth has the ability to induce the growth of osteoblasts. Chung and coworkers have studied the ability of human fibroblast, LNCaP, and bone stromal cells to produce factors that induce growth in bone formation both in vitro and in animal models (Chung et al, 1992; Gleave et al, 1992; Thalmann et al, 1994; Wu et al, 1994; Sikes et al, 1995). These investigators have brought attention to the bone-derived growth factor of 70,000 kD as well as ostepontin and a 157,000 protein p-157, which is related to human complement factor H.

Human bone stromal cells also produce hepatocyte growth factor and scatter factor (HGF/SF), which is also a strong mitogen for inducing prostatic epithelial cell growth. In addition, prostatic fibroblasts can produce this growth factor and should serve as a paracrine signal. The HGF/SF receptor is coded by this c-met proto-oncogene, and Pisters and colleagues (1993) has observed the presence of this receptor in basal epithelial layers of normal prostate glands and its absence in luminal cells. HGF was expressed in abundant amounts in prostate cancer cells and in prostate and bone fibroblasts (Pisters et al, 1993; see review Sikes et al, 1995). **In summary, there is a reciprocal stimulation of prostate cells on the growth of the bone.**

Insulin-Like Growth Factors I and II (Somatomedin)

The IGFs involve two protein growth factors (IGF I and IGF II), which are related in sequence to insulin. These growth factors interact with two different types of receptors—type I and type II. In addition, this system is involved in a very complex equilibrium with the ability of the growth factors to interact with six different binding proteins (BP) that are present in both the serum and tissues and are termed IGF-BP. **These IGF-BPs can be altered in expression at various times and in various tissue compartments, as well as the ability of a series of proteases to cleave these binding proteins to release the free form of the IGFs (see review by Peehl et al, 1995). There are many of these proteases, one of the most prominent being PSA, a serine protease.** This attests to the difficulty in analyzing the role of IGFs, binding proteins, and proteases in the regulatory control of both normal and abnormal growth of the prostate. They point out that prostate epithelial cells contain type I IGF receptor and that the prostatic stromal cells synthesize and secrete IGF II. Both the prostate stromal and epithelial cells can secrete a number of the IGF-BPs, with most attention being placed on IGF-BP-III, which is cleaved by PSA. Peehl points out that there are aberrations in the IGF associated with BPH that include an increase in transcription of IGF-II, increased levels of the type I IGF receptor, and an altered pattern of protease expression in the BPH stromal cells. In prostate cancer, IGF-BP-II increases, whereas IGF-BP-III decreases. These complex equilibria and changes in the IGF system with development, growth, and malignant transformation are of potentially great importance because of the strong mitogenic effect of these proteins have on the growth of the prostate (Peehl et al, 1995; Sikes et al, 1995).

Platelet-Derived Growth Factor

Platelet-derived growth factor is expressed in many tissues and is found in the urine, although it is primarily derived from platelets and a modified form is expressed by the c-sis oncogene. Platelet-derived growth factor has a strong mitogenic effect on mesenchymal and connective tissue cells and makes cells competent to respond to other growth factors. It has been shown to be expressed in prostate tumor models and cells in culture (Rijnders et al, 1985; Smith et al, 1995).

The interest in platelet-derived growth factor may have arisen because it is viewed as a mediator of the effects of inflammation on prostate growth, as first proposed by Gleason colleagues (1993). Inflammation is closely associated with BPH (Kohnen et al, 1979). The cause and effect has not been fully determined, but it is intriguing that both activated oxygen and growth factors formed by these types of interactions are associated with inflammation.

Endothelins

There is increased activity in the study of the biologic properties of the peptides called endothelins, of which there are three kinds, endothelin-1, endothelin-2, and endothelin-3. **These peptides have the most potent activity in constricting blood vessels and elevating blood pressure in mammals, and they may have profound effects on the muscular tone of the prostate as well as growth. Human seminal fluid contains the highest concentration of endothelins, where it is about 500 times as high as that present in plasma (Casey et al, 1992; Nelson et al, 1995).** Kobayashi 1994a and colleagues observed that prostate epithelial cells produce endothelin-1 and that the high-affinity endothelin-1 receptors are present in the prostate gland and exceed even the concentration of cholinergic and andronergic binding sites and can function in muscular tone (Langestroer et al, 1993; Kobayashi et al, 1994a, 1994b). Nelson and colleagues (1995) studied the level of endothelin-1 and its relation to prostate cancer and metastasis, as well as its possibility as a serum marker. They reported that immunoreactive endothelin is significantly elevated in men with metastatic prostate cancer and is present in all cell lines of human prostate cancer tested. Nelson also reports that endothelin-1 is a prostate cancer mitogen in vitro and elevates alkaline phosphatase activity in new bone formation. It is apparent that the endothelins and their receptors will become an important new factor in understanding normal and cancerous prostate growth and its effects on bone metastasis and the morbidity of cancer, particularly pain.

Neuroendocrine, Pituitary, Embryonic, and Other Types of Prostate Growth Factors

In addition, there are other identified growth factors that are claimed to originate in the prostate, but as yet, there is no proven growth factor that is unique only to the prostate that could be termed a true prostate-specific factor and that does not exist in any other tissues. It is possible that common growth factors may be altered in processing so as to produce increased specificity for an organ, but this is not established. Earlier, Crabb and co-workers (1986) had reported the complete primary structure of a prostate epithelial growth factor that they have termed prostatropin. Much work will be required to prove that any growth factor is present only in the prostate and to eliminate the possible contamination of other known growth factors. Proteases in the prostate can also clip and modify known growth factors to produce altered forms.

Other potentially important protein growth factors, such as nerve growth factor, bombesin-like growth factors, calcitonin, parathyroid, and thyroid-stimulating hormones are present in the prostate (reviewed by Sikes et al, 1995). Prolactin has been shown to have trophic effects on the increase in DNA synthesis in isolated human BPH tissue (Launoit et al, 1988), and to regulate growth and citrate production. Receptors for many pituitary factors, including prolactin, LHRH, growth hormone, somatostatin, and thyroid-stimulating hormone have been sporadically reported in the prostate, but most of the attention has focused on the prolactin and LHRH receptors (Kadar et al, 1988a, 1988b; Costello and Franklin, 1994). It is still unclear how these endocrine, neuroendocrine, and pituitary factors might act as growth hormones in direct interaction on the prostate cells. Costello and Franklin (1994) reviewed the subject and showed that prolactin function together with DHT as the primary factors in regulating citric acid production by the prostate and that its effects are directed to specific lobes (rat lateral) of the prostate (Grayhack and Lebowitz, 1967).

Grayhack and colleagues have long proposed that there is a second factor released by the testes other than testosterone that may be involved in prostatic growth in both the rat and dog, but this factor has not been isolated and characterized (Dalton et al, 1990).

There is growing interest in how cytokines such as interleukins and tumor necrosis factor may function in the prostate. Particular interest has focused on interleukin-6, which may play a critical role in prostate cancer morbidity such as pain and weight loss (Twillie et al, 1995).

It is important to identify any specific growth factor that mediates the urogenital sinus mesenchyme interactions on prostate epithelial cells. These are termed mesenchymal inductive mediators, and as mentioned previously, they may involve EGF, FGF-7/KGF, and FGF-2/BFGF, as well as TGF-β. Rowley and Tindall (1987) identified such factors from the urogenital sinus and have used differential hybridization to identify early growth response factor-α that functions as a transcription factor and is regulated in a negative manner by androgens but is stimulated by the protein kinase C pathway. They believe that this is a highly conserved factor that may function early in the G1 cell cycle.

THE REGULATION OF PROSTATE GROWTH: BALANCE OF CELL REPLICATION AND CELL DEATH

Throughout life, the prostate responds to endocrine signals as it develops, undergoes a rapid phase of growth at puberty, maintains its size, and then in some cases, develops an abnormal growth with aging that may result in either benign or malignant disease. The kinetics of this process are now being defined in terms of the dynamic interplay of growth-promoting and growth-suppressing factors. The mechanisms of how these factors regulate the cell cycle, DNA synthesis, mitosis, and death have been investigated (see the review of Denmeade et al, 1996). The cell kinetics and dynamics of cell replication and cell death in the human prostate are now being defined in quantitative numbers (Berges et al, 1993). **Resolving the mechanisms that control this normal growth balance is most crucial to understanding the imbalance that occurs in tumor growth.**

DNA Synthesis and Cell Cycle Control

Prostate growth requires cell replication, and cells must first undergo DNA synthesis. This can be determined on human prostatic tissue by the incorporation of precursors into the DNA, such as thymidine (Meyer et al, 1982), iododeoxyuridine (Masters and O'Donoghue, 1983), or 5-bromodeoxyuridine (Nemoto, 1990). Other markers include antibodies against specific nuclear proteins associated with proliferation, such as Ki-67, PCNA, histones, topoisomerase enzymes, or by counting mitotic indices, and all have been used to detect the proliferation of DNA in prostate cells (Berges et al, 1995). These techniques have been very helpful in working out the temporal sequence of events that occur in the growth of the prostate under hormonal stimulation in animal models (Coffey et al, 1968; Sufrin and Coffey, 1973; Lesser and Bruchovsky, 1973; deKlerk et al, 1976; Humphries and Isaacs, 1982; English et al, 1985, 1986, 1987, 1989; Evans and Chandler, 1987). Castration causes a 90% loss in the total number of prostatic epithelial cells and a slower, but less complete, reduction of approximately 40% in the number of stromal cells (deKlerk et al, 1976). In castrated men treated with androgen restoration, there is an initial delay of 1 day before the onset of DNA synthesis, which then reaches a maximum rate at 2 to 3 days and then subsides back to normal levels, even in the continued presence of androgen stimulation (Coffey et al, 1968; Sufrin and Coffey, 1973; deKlerk et al, 1976). It is unknown as to why the rapid synthesis of DNA stops after the gland is restored to its full size. It is believed that a permissive factor involves the number of stem cells and the amount of extracellular matrix and mesenchyme. In development, the growing epithelial cells have the ability to involute into the stroma, folding into three-dimensional tubular glands budding and branching into the final architecture that forms the prostate glandular pattern. **These permissive factors and limitations must include the development of angiogenesis to support the gland and the stromal-epithelial interactions discussed earlier. They are driven overall by available androgens, growth factors and their corresponding receptors, and intracellular signalling events that initiate the replication and death cell cycle regulations and possible regulation of homeotic genes.**

Buttyan and his colleagues (Katz et al, 1989) have studied the sequence of events that occur following testosterone repletion in castrated men that precede the onset of DNA synthesis. They demonstrated that the oncogene c-fos showed the earliest transient rise, increasing threefold within 1 hour, followed by an increase in ras oncogenes with 2 hours, followed by the transient transcription of both myc and myb within 6 to 8 hours. This is typical of many other tissues that are stimulated to grow where similar transient rises in oncogenes precede the onset of DNA synthesis.

Cell Cycle Control

There are many normal expressions of oncogenes during growth and development, and it has been proposed that mutated oncogenes, or aberrant forms, may be at the heart of genetic expression in cancer. Deletion or mutation of genetic material that serves as a negative regulator has been shown to release the brake that holds tissues and growth in check. This type of genetic material has been termed a *suppressor* gene, which means that their absence or blocked function can induce growth. One such suppressor gene implicated in prostatic tissues in culture has been the retinoblastoma gene (Bookstein et al, 1990). The retinoblastoma gene was first discovered in retinoblastoma but is now known to be a general control of the cell cycle of most normal cells and undergoes aberrations in many types of cancer. **When the retinoblastoma gene is hypophosphorylated, it binds to the nuclear matrix and inhibits cell proliferation. When the retinoblastoma protein is phosphorylated, it then releases the brake and allows the cell to move through the rest of the cell cycle. These restriction points in the cell cycle are regulated by a group of gatekeepers that are termed *cyclins*, and are denoted as A, B, C, D or E, according to where they gatekeep throughout the cycle.** There are abnormalities in the regulation of the cyclin expression that occur in many types of human cancers, and they can be autonomously expressed or regulated by growth factors (Chen et al, 1995; see review of Denmeade et al, 1996). When a cell replicates its DNA, it must first stop and assess whether its DNA is damaged. If the DNA is damaged, the cell cycle is blocked at this point because a suppressor factor (p53) is induced that stimulates the cyclin-dependent kinase inhibitors (p16 and p21). These p53-induced cyclin-dependent kinases are inhibitors that arrest cell division. **Thus, a mutation in either p53, p16, or p21 allows the cell cycle to proceed with damaged DNA that can be copied, inducing a tumor cell genetic instability (Koh et al, 1995; Waldman et al, 1995).**

In summary, the decision of a cell to replicate, repair its DNA, differentiate, or senesce and die depends on the regulation of the cell cycle involving activators and suppressors of the cell cycle–dependent kinases and the ability of the cell to repair its DNA and to undergo a successful mitosis. Pathways in the cell cycle and its regulation are altered during aging, senescence, and abnormal growth such as that associated with cancers, and this is a major frontier in understanding sex accessory tissue growth.

Cell Aging, Senescence, and Immortality

Telomeres and telomerase activity are becoming important molecular monitors of both immortality and cancer, and have been studied in human prostate cancers (Sommerfeld et al, 1995, 1996). The Hayflick phenomenon indicates that a cell can undergo a finite number of cell divisions before they senesce and ultimately self-terminate by apoptosis. Cells that do not senesce are termed immortal and can be established as cell lines in culture for very long periods of time. Many of these cells can be passaged in culture for what appears to be an indefinite length of time, but they do not exhibit a malignant phenotype when they are transplanted back in vivo. The cells that are not immortal are limited in their number of doublings, which is approximately 50. These mortal cells shorten their telomeres with each cell cycle until they become unstable (see review of Greider and Blackburn, 1996). Each time a cell cycle occurs, telomeres are shortened because of the end replication problems in the RNA-primed DNA polymerase reaction that causes small telomeric noncoding sequences not to be replicated. These losses continue with each subsequent cell cycle and accumulate. When a critical level of shortening is reached, after approximately 50 to 100 doublings, the cell then becomes unstable and senesces. **Therefore, it has been proposed that telomere length serves as a type of mitotic clock that counts the number of cell cycles. Therefore, as cells replicate, they continue shortening their telomeres until death, unless they find a way to stabilize their telomere lengths and become immortal. This has occurred in immortal cells in culture, where they have short but constant telomere lengths, presumably stabilized due to the induction or activation of the ribonucleoprotein enzyme, termed telomerase, that restores or maintains the length.** Functioning as a reverse transcriptase, telomerase carries its own RNA template for making telomeric DNA. Telomerase carries out direct polymerization for the nucleotides to form new DNA to form the chromosomal end, thus balancing the loss of telomeres that occurs with each cycle. Telomeres are shortened in prostate cancer owing to the extended number of replications, and telomerase is activated; however, this is not the case in BPH (Sommerfeld, et al, 1995, 1996). Recently, Meeker and associates (Sommerfeld et al, 1995, and unpublished information) have observed that telomerase is also a marker of the stem cells in the rat ventral prostate. These telomerase-rich cells are heavily enriched following castration where these stem cells are concentrated. **Thus, germ cells, stem cells, and cancer all have an immortality, as do cells that have been established as cell lines, and in each of these cases, telomerase has been activated to stabilize the shortening of telomeres that occurs with each replication, thus allowing immortality.**

DNA Damage

DNA can be damaged in somatic cells by several pathways. Examples are (1) during the cell cycle by telomere losses, (2) by errors in replication that cannot be repaired by mismatched repair enzymes, (3) by failure of the cell cycle to monitor itself and to inhibit damaged DNA from going through the cycle by aberrations in the suppressor system, (4) by xenophiles and carcinogens in the environment, and (5) by oxidative damage brought about by free radicals such as activated oxygen. Free radicals can be generated in the prostate through oxidative processes, which can result in lipid peroxidation and DNA damage, and through the activity of macrophages and lymphocytes, which can cause spurious damage. **Nitric oxide has become a new and potent free radical–forming agent in the prostate, where Chang and colleagues have shown it to be activated or enriched following castration in the rat lateral prostate and seminal vesicles but not in the ventral prostate or coagulating gland (Chamness et al, 1995). Nitric oxide is formed by the action of nitric oxide synthase (NOS), which can convert arginine to citrulline-forming nitric oxide. NOS can be of neural origin (n-NOS), from endothelial cells (e-NOS) that can affect smooth muscle cells, or induced in macrophages (i-NOS).**

The prostate protects itself against electrophilic attacks from carcinogens by inducing a battery of protective enzymes, of which glutathione *S*-transferases are the most prominent. Nelson and colleagues (1995) have reported that human prostate basal cells contain high levels of glutathione *S*-transferase pi and that in prostate cancer, this activity is uniformly missing in association with cancer lesions removed at the time of radical prostatectomy. Lack of expression of glutathione *S*-transferase pi gene in cancer is likely to be due to methylation of the cytosine residues in the promoter region of the gene. Nelson and colleagues (1994) have drawn attention to the importance of this enzyme in protecting stem cells in the prostate from carcinogenic attack and that these enzymes can be induced by dietary and environmental considerations.

Apoptosis and Cell Death

Apoptosis is a term that is used for a natural programmed type of cell death that is part of the normal process of life and is taken from the Greek word meaning "the falling of leaves from a tree." Apoptosis is a force that keeps cell replication in balance and that maintains the static size of the prostate. It is a dynamic system with marked differences between necrosis and apoptosis, both at the histologic and biochemical levels. The mechanisms of apoptosis, in addition to factors that cause the survival of cells, is one of the most active areas of research in sex accessory tissues. Excellent reviews on prostatic apoptosis and cell death have been made available through the works of Isaacs and colleagues (Isaacs, 1994; Denmeade et al, 1996).

In 1973, Kerr and Searle first drew attention to the fact that histologically, the cells of the prostate appear to undergo apoptosis during castration-induced involution of the rat prostate. This was a follow-up of Kerr's earlier work in 1972 describing apoptosis as a basic biological phenomenon in tissue growth and death (Kerr, et al, 1973). The significance of cell death and apoptosis was reviewed by the works of Stein and Helpap (1981) and Isaacs in 1984, who began to delineate the biochemical pathways and kinetics of prostate cell death (Isaacs, 1984; Kyprianou and Isaacs, 1988, 1989; Isaacs et al, 1992), and by the work of Buttyan and his colleagues (Connor et al, 1988; Buttyan et al, 1988), as well as the work of Tenniswood (Montpetit et al, 1986).

It was long believed that cell death following androgen withdrawal was simply the choking off of an important biologic factor required to maintain the life of the cell. **Now we know that this involution process is an induced and very active biochemical process rather than merely a passive loss of factors**. Lee and associates (1985a) were the first to report that if protein or RNA synthesis is blocked following castration, the rate of prostate gland involution was markedly reduced (Stanisic et al, 1978). Kyprianou and Isaacs (1988) have reported that there is an increase in TGF-β receptors during castration and that this factor may regulate cell death from a growth factor standpoint. Barrack and Berry (1987) have studied DNA synthesis in canine prostates induced to massive growth by the combination of androgens and estrogens, and have shown that there is a decrease in the amount of DNA synthesis per unit amount of DNA required to maintain a large gland when 5α-reduced androgens and estrogens are given simultaneously. This has led them to suggest that estrogens are decreasing the rate of cell death in the prostate in the presence of 5α-reduced androgens and not increasing cell proliferation. What determines the setpoint for determining the level of cells in the prostate and their rates of growth and death is of paramount importance in understanding BPH and prostate cancer. Buttyan and co-workers (1988) have studied the cascade of induction of a series of oncogenes and heat-shock proteins that follows castration and precedes cell loss.

Later, it was reported that a temporal series of proteins that are induced following castration in the prostate and the most actively studied was trpm-2 by the work of Tenniswood and his colleagues (Montpetit et al, 1986). This was followed by the cloning of the gene (Leger et al, 1987, 1988). This trpm-2 protein was dramatically increased 48 hours following castration and was associated with epithelial cell involution of the prostate. The role of trpm-2 is in cell death now appears to be a secondary marker associated with, but not causing, involution. Trpm-2 has been shown to be similar to clusterin, a sulfated glycoprotein-2 normally found in Sertoli cells and present in human seminal plasma, and is suggested to be important in fertility (O'Bryan et al, 1990).

Proteolytic enzymes, such as cathepsin D, are activated during castration-induced involution in the rat prostate (Tanabe et al, 1982; Sensabaugh et al, 1990). Plasminogen activators are also increased following castration (Rennie et al, 1984), and three forms are increased following castration in the prostate epithelial cells (Andreasen et al, 1990).

Several groups have studied the appearance of two-dimensional protein patterns that were altered by castration or androgen treatment (Anderson et al, 1983; Lee et al, 1985b, 1987). The colleagues of Liao (Saltzman et al, 1987) have shown that specific messages and products are required to be synthesized in the prostate during the process of involution. Saltzman has shown that androgen withdrawal causes the production of a 29,000-MW protein and its messenger RNA during the involution of the rat ventral prostate (Saltzman et al, 1987). Chang and associates (1987) have reported that glutathione *S*-transferase is induced following castration; this is an enzyme located at the cell nucleus that appears to be a DNA-binding protein.

For a critical discussion of enzymes and factors that change in prostatic cell death, see the definitive review of Denmeade and co-workers (1996). They reviewed data that indicates that following castration in the rat, the serum testosterone levels fall by 90% within 2 hours and by 98%

within 6 hours. The active DHT decreases 95% in prostate cells by 12 to 24 hours; within 12 hours of castration, the androgen receptor is no longer detected in the nucleus; and by 24 hours, there is very little androgen receptor remaining. Following this dramatic decrease in androgens, there is a much slower involution of the cells that may require the loss of survival factors besides DHT. They suggest that FGF-7 or KGF that is produced in the stromal cells and secondarily stimulates the prostate epithelial cells may be a prime candidate.

It is obvious that the interlocking cell cycles of cell death and cell replication are paramount events in regulating the balance in the prostate. This factor has been reviewed by Denmeade and associates (1996) and Harris and Savil (1995). It is apparent that p53 knockout mice are still capable of undergoing prostate involution following castration, and therefore, p53 is not required for involution but it still may alter the pathway in some noncritical manner. **Most interestingly, cytokines and extracellular matrix can provide exogenous survival signals, and attention is turned to bcl-2, which is a strong survival factor and seems to block cell death. Overexpression of bcl-2 has been proposed to block cell death and increase growth in malignant cells. This process may be involved with a complex pathway involving interaction with c-myc and the binding of bcl-2 to a series of related proteins such as bax to form active or inactive dimers**. Overexpression of bax, which can form heterodimers with bcl-2, can actually promote apoptosis, but this is a complex problem because bcl-2/bax heterodimers favor cell survival and prevent apoptosis, whereas a high level of bax with excess bax homodimers favor cell death. Therefore, the level of expression of bax is critical.

A series of proteases appear to be involved in controlling the onset of cell death, and some of these are in the family of interleukin-1 beta-converting enzyme (ICE), which is a protein of 503 amino acid residues that is very homologous to ICE. This is a cysteine protease related to Ced-3, which is a key factor in cell death in flat worms.

The switching, regulation, and inhibition of apoptosis starting with p53 pathways, survival factors, and the fas pathway are being resolved, and they involve ced-3/ICE–, ced-9/bcl-2– and ced-4–like proteins that have not all been identified. As each of these families is expanded, as bcl-2 now appears to be a family of proteins and ICE is likewise a set of proteins, we must await further resolution before we will be able to fully decipher these complex interactions in detail. **In the meantime, apoptosis is now being used as a quantitative tool in the study of the balance of cell proliferation and cell death in prostate pathology (see the reviews of Gaffney, 1994; Montironi et al, 1994; Wheeler et al, 1994).**

ACKNOWLEDGMENTS

We gratefully acknowledge the expertise of Ruth Middleton in the preparation of the manuscript, and Donald Vindivich for his help in the preparation of the illustrations. We are also grateful for the careful review of this manuscript by the Residents, Fellows, Faculty, and Patrick C. Walsh of the Brady Urological Institute.

REFERENCES

Ablin RJ, Soanes WA, Bronson P, Witebsky E: Precipitating antigens of the normal human prostate. J Reprod Fertil 1970; 22:573–574.

Abrahamsson PA, Wadstrom LB, Alumets J, Falkmer S, Gramelius L: Peptide hormone–serotonin–immunoreactive cells in normal and hyperplastic prostate glands. Pathol Res Pract 1987; 181:675–683.

Abrahamsson PA, Lilja H: Partial characterization of a thyroid-stimulating hormone–like peptide in neuroendocrine cells of the human prostate gland. Prostate 1989; 14:71–81.

Achtstatter TH, Moll R, Moore B, Franke WW: Cytokeratin polypeptide patterns of different epithelial cells from human male urogenital tract. Immunofluorescence and gel electrophoretic studies. J Histochem Cytochem 1985; 33:415–426.

Albelva SM: Role of cell adhesion molecules in tumor progression and metastatic. In Wegner CD, ed: Adhesion Molecules. London, Academic Press, 1994, pp 71–84.

Alexander RB, Greene GL, Barrack ER: Estrogen receptors in the nuclear matrix: Direct demonstration using monoclonal antireceptor antibodies. Endocrinology 1987; 120:1851–1857.

Amelar RD, Hotchkiss RS: The split ejaculate: Its uses in the management of male infertility. Fertil Steril 1965; 16:46–49.

Amelar RD, Dubin L: Semen Analysis. *In* Male Infertility. Philadelphia, W. B. Saunders Company, 1977, pp 105–140.

Amelar RD: Coagulation, liquefaction and viscosity of human semen. J Urol 1962; 87:187–190.

Anderson KM, Liao S: Selective retention of dihydrotestosterone by prostatic nuclei. Nature 1968; 219:277–279.

Anderson DC, Marshall JC, Galuao-Teles A, et al: Gynaecomastia and impotence associated with testosterone binding. Proc Royal Soc Med 1972; 65:787–788.

Anderson KM, Baranowski J, Ekonomous SG, Rubenstein M: A qualitative analysis of acetic proteins associated with regressing, growing or dividing rat ventral prostate cells. Prostate 1983; 4:151–166.

Andreasen PA, Kristensen P, Lund LR, Dano K: Urokinase-type plasminogen activator is increased in the involuting ventral prostate of castrated rats. Endocrinology 1990; 126:2567–2577.

Andrews GS: The histology of the human fetal and prepubertal prostate. J Anat 1951; 85:44–54.

Aragona C, Friesen HG: Specific prolactin binding sites in the prostate and testis of rat. Endocrinology 1975; 97:677–683.

Arcadi JA: Role of ground substance in atrophy of normal and malignant prostatic tissue following estrogen administration in orchiectomy. J Clin Endo Metab 1954; 14:1113–1125.

Armbruster DA: Prostate-specific antigen: Biochemistry, analytical methods, and clinical application. Clin Chem 1993; 39:181–195.

Assimos D, Smith C, Lee C, Grayhack JT: Action of prolactin in regressing prostate: Independent of action mediated by androgen receptors. Prostate 1984; 5:589–595.

Aumuller G: *In* Prostate Gland and Seminal Vesicles, Handbuch der Mikroskopischen Anatomie des Menschen, VII/6. Berlin, Springer-Verlag, 1979.

Aumuller G: Morphology and endocrine aspects of prostatic function. Prostate 1983; 4:195–214.

Aumuller G, Seitz J: Protein secretion and secretory processes in male sex accessory glands. Int Rev Cytol 1990; 121:127–231.

Aumuller G, Seitz J, Lilja H, et al: Species-specificity and organ-specificity of secretory proteins derived from human prostate and seminal vesicle. Prostate 1990; 17:31–40.

Banerjee PP, Banerjee S, Zirkin BR: DNA synthesis occurs throughout the rat ventral prostate during its postnatal development. Biol Reprod 1993a; 48:258–261.

Banerjee S, Banerjee PP, Zirkin BR: Cell proliferation in the dorsal and lateral lobes of the rat prostate during postnatal development. J Androl 1993b; 14:310–318.

Barak M, Calderon I, Abramovici H, et al: The use of a seminal vesicle specific protein (MHS-5 antigen) for diagnosis of agenesis of vas deferens and seminal vesicles in azoospermic men. J Androl 1994; 15:603–607.

Barnes J, Anthony CT, Wall N, Steiner MS: Bone morphogenetic protein-6 expression in normal and malignant prostates. World J Urol 1995; 13:337–343.

Barrack ER: Steroid hormone receptor localization in the nuclear matrix: Interaction with acceptor sites. J Steroid Biochem 1987; 27:115–121.

Barrack ER, Berry JJ: DNA synthesis in the canine prostate: Effects of androgen and estrogen treatment. Prostate 1987; 10:45–56.

decreased endothelin B receptor expression in advanced prostate cancer. Cancer Res 1966; 56:663–668.

Nelson WG, Pienta KJ, Barrack ER, Coffey DS: The role of the nuclear matrix in the organization and function of DNA. Ann Revs Biophys Biophys Chem 1986; 15:457–475.

Nemoto R, Hattori K, Uchida K, et al: S-phase fraction of human prostate adenocarinoma studied with in vivo bromodeoxyuridine labeling. Cancer 1990; 66:509–514.

Neubauer B Bisser T, Jones CD, et al: Antagonism of androgen and estrogen effects in the guinea pig seminal vesicle, epithelium and fibromuscular stroma by keoxifene (LY 156758). Prostate 1989; 15:273–286.

Niemi M, Harkonen M, Larmi TKL: Enzymic histochemistry of human prostate. Arch Pathol 1963; 75:528–537.

O'Bryan MK, Baker HWG, Saunders JR, et al: Human seminal clusterin (SP-40, 40). J Clin Invest 1990; 85:1477–1486.

Oesterling JE: Prostate specific antigen: A critical assessment of the most useful tumor marker for adenocarcinoma of the prostate. J Urol 1991; 145:907–923.

Oesterling JE: PSA leads the way for detecting and following prostate cancer. Contemporary Urol 1993; 5:60–82.

Oesterling JE, Chan DW, Epstein JI, et al: Prostate specific antigen in the preoperative and postoperative evaluation of localized prostatic cancer treated with radical prostatectomy. J Urol 1988; 139:766–772.

Oesterling JE, Epstein JI, Walsh PC: The inability of adrenal androgens to stimulate the adult prostate—an autopsy evaluation of men with hypogonadotropic hypogonadism and panhypopituitarism. J Urol 1986; 136:103–104.

Oesterling JE, Juniewicz PE, Walters JR, et al: Aromatase inhibition in the dog. II. Effects of growth, function and pathology of the prostate. J Urol 1988; 139:832–839.

Olin EH, Fabiana R, Johansson L, Ronquist G: Arachidonic acid 15-lipoxygenase and traces of E protaglands in purified human prostasomes. J Reprod Fertil 1993; 99:195–199.

Oliver JA, Elhilali MM, Belitsky P, MacKinnon KJ: LDH isoenzymes in benign and malignant prostate tissue. The LDH/VI ratio as an index of malignancy. Cancer 1970; 25:863–866.

Pang S, Levine L, Chow D, et al: Dihydrotestosterone and its relationship to testosterone in infancy and childhood. J Clin Endocrinol Metab 1979; 48:821–826.

Parker MG, ed: Nuclear Hormone Receptors: Molecular Mechanisms, Cellular Functions, Clinical Abnormalities. London, Academic Press, 1991.

Partin AW, Oesterling EJ: The clinical usefulness of prostate specific antigen: Update 1994. J Urol 1994; 152:1358–1368.

Peehl DM, Cohen D, Rosenfeld RG: Insulin-growth factor system in the prostate. World J Urol 1995; 13:306–311.

Peehl DM, Wong ST, Stamey TA: Cytostatic effects of serumin on prostate cancer cells cultured from primary tumors. J Urol 1991; 145:624–630.

Phadke AM, Samant NR, Deval SP: Significance of seminal fructose studies in male fertility. Fertil Steril 1973; 24:894–903.

Pienta KJ, Murphy BC, Getzenberg RH, Coffey DS: The tissue matrix and the regulation of gene expression in cancer cell. Adv Mol Cell Biol 1993a; 7:131–156.

Pienta KJ, Nguyen NM, Lehr JE: Treatment of prostatic in the rat with the synthetic retinoid fenretinide. Cancer Res 1993b; 53:224–226.

Pienta KJ, Partin AW, Coffey DS: Cancer as a disease of DNA organization and dynamic cell structure. Cancer Res 1989; 49:2525–2532.

Pisters LL, Troncoso P, Zhau HYE et al: The role of hepatocyte growth factor/scatter factor and its receptor, the c-met protooncogene in human prostatic tumor growth. J Urol 1993; 149:482A.

Pollard M, Luckert PH: Prevention of primary prostate cancer in Lobund-Wistar rats. Cancer Res 1991; 51:3610–3611.

Poulos A, White LG: Phospholipids of human spermatozoa and seminal plasma. J Reprod Fertil 1973; 35:265–272.

Pourian MR, Kvist U, Bjorndahl L, Oliw EH: Rapid and slow hydroxylators of seminal E prostaglandins among men in barren unions. Andrologia 1995; 27:71–79.

Pretlow TG, Nagabhushan M, Sy M, et al: Putative preneoplastic foci in the human prostate. J Cell Biochem 1994; 19(Suppl):224–231.

Price D, Williams-Ashman HG: The accessory reproductive glands of mammals. *In* Young WC, Corner GW, eds: Sex and Internal Secretions. Huntington NY, Robert E. Krieger Publishing Company, 1973, pp 366–448.

Prins GS: Neonatal estrogen exposure induces lobe-specific alterations in adult rat prostate androgen receptor expression. Endocrinology 1992; 130:3703–3714.

Prins GS, Birch L. The developmental pattern of androgen receptor regulation in the rat prostate lobes is altered following neonatal exposure to estrogen. Endocrinology 1995; 136:1303–1314.

Propping D, Tauber PF, Zaneveld LJD, Schumacher GFB: Purification and characterization of two plasminogen activators from human seminal plasma. Fed Proc 1974; 33:289–293.

Purnell DM, Heathfield BM, Trump BF: Immunocytochemical evaluation of human prostatic carcinomas for carcinoembryonic antigen, nonspecific cross-reactivating antigen, beta chronic gonadotropins and prostate-specific antigen. Cancer Res 1984; 44:285–292.

Rabinovitz I, Cress AE, Nagle RB: Biosynthesis and secretion of laminin in S-laminin by human prostate carcinoma cell lines. Prostate 1994; 25:95–107.

Rackley RR, Yang B, Pretlow TG, et al: Differences in the leucine aminopeptidase activity in extracts from human prostatic carcinoma and benign prostatic hyperplasia. Cancer 1991; 68:587–593.

Rajfer J, Coffey DS: Sex steroid imprinting of the immature prostate: Long term effects. Invest Urol 1979a; 16:186–190.

Rajfer J, Coffey DS: Effects of neonatal steroids on male sex tissues. Invest Urol 1979b; 17:3–8.

Randall VA: Role of 5α-reductase in health and disease. Baillieres Clin Endocrinol Metab 1994; 8:405–431.

Reed MJ, Stitch SR: The uptake of testosterone and zinc in vitro by the human benign hypertrophic prostate. J Endocrinol 1973; 58:405–419.

Reese JH, McNeil JE, Redwine EA, et al: Tissue type plasminogen activator as a marker for functional zones, within the human prostate gland. Prostate 1988; 12:47–53.

Reeves DS: Pharmacology of the prostate. *In* Chisolm GD, Williams DI, eds: Scientific Foundations of Urology, 2nd ed. London, Heineman Medical Books, 1982, pp 514–520.

Reigman PHF, Vlietstra RJ, Suurmeijer L, et al: Characterization of the human kallikrein locus. Genomics 1992; 14:6–11.

Rennie PS, Bouffard R, Bruchovsky N, Chang H: Increased activity of plasminogen activators during involution of the rat ventral prostate. Biochem J 1984; 221:171–178.

Rijnders AWM, van der Korput JAGM, van Stenbrugge GJ, et al: Expression of cellular oncogenes in human prostatic carcinoma cell lines. Biochem Biophys Res Commun 1985; 132:548–554.

Rittmaster RS: Finesteride. N Engl J Med 1994; 330:120–125.

Roche PJ, Hoare SA, Parker MG: A consensus DNA-binding site for the androgen receptor. Mol Endocrinol 1992; 2229–2235.

Rohan TE, Howe GR, Burch JE, Jain M: Dietary factors and risk of prostate cancer: A case-control study in Ontario, Canada. Cancer Causes Control 1995; 6:145–154.

Rohr HP, Bartsch G: Human benign prostatic hyperplasia: A stromal disease? Urology 1980; 16:625–633.

Rokhlin OW, Cohen MB: Expression of cellular adhesion molecules on human prostate tumor cell lines. Prostate 1995; 26:205–212.

Romas NA, Kwan DJ: Prostatic acid phosphatase. Urol Clin North Am 1993; 20:581–588.

Romics I, Bach D: Zn, Ca and Na levels in the prostatic secretion of patients with prostatic adenoma. Int Urol Nephrol 1991; 23:45–49.

Rose DP, Connolly JM: Dietary fat, fatty acids and prostate cancer. Lipids 1992; 27:798–803.

Rowley DR, Tindall DJ: Responses of NBT-II bladder carcinoma cells to conditioned medium from normal fetal urogenital sinus. Cancer Res 1987; 47:2955–2960.

Roy AV, Brower ME, Hayden JE: Sodium thymolphthalein monophosphate: A new acid phosphatase substrate with greater specificity for the prostatic enzyme in serum. Clin Chem 1971; 17:1093–1102.

Rui H, Mevag B, Purvis K: Two-dimensional electrophoresis of proteins in various fractions of human split ejaculate. Int J Androl 1984; 7:509–520.

Russell DW, Wilson JD: Steroid 5α-reductase: Two genes/two enzymes. Ann Rev Biochem 1994; 63:25–61.

Saltzman AG, Hiipakka ARA, Chang C, Liao S: Androgen repression of the production of a 29-kilodalton protein and its mRNA in the rat ventral prostate. J Biol Chem 1987; 262:432–5437.

Sansone G, Martino M, Abrescia P: Binding of free and protein-associated zinc to rat spermatozoa. Comp Biochem Physiol (C) 1991; 99:113–117.

Sathe VA, Sheth AR, Sheth NA: Biosynthesis of immunoreactive inhibin-like material (IR-ILM) by rat prostate. Prostate 1986; 8:401–408.

Schoenberg MP, Hakima JM, Wang S, et al: Microsatellite mutation (CAG24›18) in the androgen receptor gene in human prostate cancer. Biochem Biophys Res Commun 1994; 198:74–80.

Schreiter F, Fuchs P, Stockamp K: Estrogenic sensitivity of α-receptors in the urethra musculature. Urol Int 1976; 31:13–19.

Schulze H, Barrack ER: The immunocytochemical localization of estrogen receptors in the normal male and female canine urinary tract and prostate. Endocrinology 1987a; 121:1773–1783.

Schulze H, Barrack ER: The immunocytochemical localization of estrogen receptors in spontaneous and experimentally induced canine prostatic hyperplasia. Prostate 1987b; 11:145–162.

Schwartz GG, Hulka BS: Vitamin D deficiency a risk factor for prostate cancer? Anticancer Res 1990; 10:1307–1322.

Scott WW: The lipids of the prostatic fluid, seminal plasma and enlarged prostate gland of man. J Urol 1945; 53:712–718.

Seamonds B, Yang N, Anderson K, et al: Evaluation of prostate-specific antigen and prostatic acid phosphatase as prostate cancer markers. Urology 1986; 28:472.

Seligman AM, Chauncey HH, Nachlas MM, et al: The colorimetric determination of phosphatases in human serum. J Biol Chem 1951; 190:7–15.

Seligman AM, Sternberger NJ, Paul BD, et al: Design of spindle poisons activated specifically by prostatic acid phosphatase (PAP) and new methods for PAP cytochemistry. Cancer Chemother Rep 1975; 59:233–242.

Sensabaugh JA, Liu X, Patai B, et al: Characterization of castration-induced cell death in the rat prostate by immunohistochemical localization of cathepsin D. Prostate 1990; 16:263–276.

Shellhammer PF, Wright GL Jr: Biomolecular and clinical characteristics of PSA and other candidate prostate tumor markers. Urol Clin North Am 1993; 20:597–606.

Sherwood ER, Lee C: Epidermal growth factor–related peptides in the epidermal growth factor receptor in normal and malignant prostate. World J Urol 1995; 13:290–296.

Sheth AR, Pan SE, Vaze AY, et al: Inhibin in the human prostate. Arch Androl 1981; 6:317–321.

Shimazaki J, Kurihara H, Ito Y, Shida K: Metabolism of testosterone in prostate. Separation of prostatic 17β-ol-dehydrogenase and 5α-reductase. Gunma J Med Sci 1965a; 14:326–333.

Shimazaki J, Kurihara H, Ito Y, Shida K: Testosterone metabolism in prostate. Formation of androstane-17β-ol-3-one and androst-4-ene-3,17α-dione, and inhibitory effect of natural and synthetic estrogens. Gunma J Med Sci 1965b; 14:313–325.

Siiteri PK, MacDonald PC: Role of extraglandular estrogen in human endocrinology. *In* Greep RO, Astwood EB, eds: Handbook of Physiology, Section 7. Endocrinology, Vol II. Baltimore, Williams & Wilkins, 1973, pp 615–629.

Sikes RA, Kao C, Chung LWK: Autocrine and paracrine mediators for prostate growth in cancer progression. *In* McGuire EJ, Bloom D, Catalona WJ, Lipshultz LI, eds. Advances in Urology, Vol 8. St. Louis, Mosby–Yearbook Inc, 1995, pp 21–60.

Silver RI, Wiley EL, Thigpen AE, et al: Cell type specific expression of steroid 5α-reductase II. J Urol 1994a; 152:438–442.

Silver RI, Wiley EL, Davis DL, et al: Expression and regulation of steroid 5α-reductase to prostate disease. J Urol 1994b; 152:433–437.

Sinha AA, Gleason DF, Wilson MJ, et al: Immunohistochemical localization of laminin in basement membranes of normal, hyperplastic and neoplastic human prostate. Prostate 1989; 15:299–313.

Sinowatz F, Gabius HJ, Hellmann KP, et al: Expression of endogenous receptor for neoglycoproteins in Dunning R-3327 rat prostatic carcinoma. Prostate 1990; 16:173–184.

Skowronski RJ, Peehl DM, Feldman D: Vitamin D in prostate cancer: 1,25-hydroxy vitamin D_3 receptor inaction in human prostate cancer cell lines. Endocrinology 1993; 132:1952–1960.

Small EJ, Prins GS: Physiology and endocrinology of the prostate. *In* Vogelzang NJ, Scardino PT, Shipley WU, Coffey DS, eds: Comprehensive Textbook of Genitourinary Oncology. Baltimore, Williams & Wilkins, 1995, pp 600–620.

Smith ER, Hagopian M: Uptake in secretion of carcinogenic chemicals by the dog and rat prostate. *In* Murphy GP, Sandberg AA, Karr JP, eds: The Prostate Cell: Structure and Function, Part B. New York, Alan Liss, 1981, pp 131–163.

Smith RC, Rinker-Schaeffer CW: Understanding molecular biology and carcinogenesis of genitourinary cancers. *In* Vogelzang NJ, Scardino PT, Shipley WU, Coffey DS, eds: Comprehensive Textbook of Genitourinary Oncology Comprehensive Textbook of Genitourinary Oncology. Baltimore, Williams & Wilkins, 1995, pp 68–80.

Smith RG, Syms AJ, Nag A, Lerner S, Norris JS: Mechanisms of the glucocorticoid regulation and growth of the androgen-sensitive prostate-derived R3327 H-G8-A1 tumor cells. J Biol Chem 1985; 260:12454–12463.

Sommerfeld HS, Meeker AK, Piatyszec MA, et al: Telomerase activity: A prevalent marker of malignant human prostate tissue. Cancer Res 1996; 56:218–222.

Sommerfeld HS, Meeker AK, Posadas EM, Coffey DS: Frontiers in prostate cancer. Telomeres and chaos. Cancer 1995; 75:2027–2035.

Stamey TA, Bushby SRM, Bragonje J: The concentration of trimethoprim in prostatic fluid: Nonionic diffusion or active transport? J Infect Dis 1973; 128:686–690.

Stamey TA, Fair WR, Timothy MM, Chung HK: Antibacterial nature of prostatic fluid. Nature 1968; 218:444–447.

Stamey TA, Yang N, Hay AR, et al: Prostate-specific antigen as a serum marker for adenocarcinoma of the prostate. N Engl J Med 1987; 317:909–916.

Stanisic T, Sadlowski R, Lee C, Grayhack JT: Partial inhibition of castration-induced ventral prostate regression with actinomycin D and cyclohexamide. Invest Urol 1978; 16:15–18.

Stauch-Slusher B, Tsai G, Yoo G, Coyle JT: Immunochemical localization of the *N*-acetyl-aspartyl-glutamate (NAAG) hydrolyzing enzyme *N*-acetylated linked dipeptidase (NAALADase). J Comp Neurol 1992; 315:217–229.

Steiner JF: Finasteride: A 5-alpha-reducatse inhibitor. Clin Pharm 1993; 12:15–23.

Steiner MS, Barrack ER: -β, overproduction in prostate cancer: Effects on growth in vivo and in vitro. Mol Endocrinol 1992; 6:15–25.

Steiner MS: Growth factors in urology. A review. Urology 1993; 42:99–110.

Stenman J-H, Leinonen J, Alfthan H, et al: A complex antigen and α1-antichymotrypsin is the major form of prostate-specific antigen in serum of patients with prostate cancer; assay of the complex improves clinical sensitivity for cancer. Cancer Res 1991; 51:222–226.

Stone NN, Fair WR, Fishman J: Estrogen formation in human prostatic tissue from patients with and without benign prostatic hyperplasia. Prostate 1986; 9:311–318.

Storey MT: Regulation of prostate growth by fibroblast growth factors. World J Urol 1995; 13:297–305.

Storey MT, Jacobs SC, Lawson RK: Epidermal growth factor is not the major growth-promoting agent in extracts of prostatic tissues. J Urol 1983; 130:175–179.

Sufrin G, Coffey DS: A new model for studying the effects of drugs on prostatic growth. I. Antiandrogens in DNA synthesis. Invest Urol 1973; 11:45–54.

Sugimura Y, Cunha GR, Donjacour AA, et al: Whole mount autoradiography studies of DNA synthetic activity during postnatal development and androgen-induced regeneration in the mouse prostate. Biol Reprod 1986; 34:985–995.

Suzuki T, Nakajima K, Yamamoto A, Yamanaka H: Metallothionein binding zinc inhibits nuclear chromatin decondensation of human spermatozoa. Andrologia 1995; 27:161–164.

Suzuki T, Suzuki K, Nakajima K, Otaka N, Yamanaka H: Metallothionein in human seminal plasma. Int J Urol 1994; 1:345–348.

Swanson HE, Vanderwer FF, Werff ten Bosch JJ: Sex differences in growth of rats and their modification by a single injection of testosterone propionate shortly after birth. J Endocrinol 1963; 26:197–207.

Syner FN, Moghissi KS, Yanez J: Isolation of a factor from normal human semen that accelerates dissolution of abnormally liquefying semen. Fertil Steril 1975; 26:1064–1069.

Tanabe E, Lee C, Grayhack JT. Activities of cathepsin D in rat prostate during castration-induced involution. J Urol 1982; 127:826–828.

Tauber PF, Zaneveld LJD: Coagulation and liquefaction of human semen. *In* Hafez ESE, Ed: Human Semen and Fertility Regulation in Men. St. Louis, CV Mosby Company, 1976a.

Tauber PF, Zaneveld LJD, Propping D, Schumacher GFB: Components of human split ejaculates. II. Enzymes and proteinase inhibitors. J Reprod Fertil 1976b; 46:165–171.

Tauber PF, Zaneveld LJD, Propping D, Schumacher GFB: Components of human split ejaculate. J Reprod Fertil 1975; 43:249–267.

Tenniswood M: Role of epithelial-stromal interactions in the control of gene expression in the prostate: An hypothesis. Prostate 1986; 9:375–385.

Tenniswood MP, Guenette RS, Lakins J, et al: Active cell death in hormone-dependent tissues. Cancer Metastasis Rev 1992; 11:197–220.

Thalmann GN, Anizinis PE, Chang SM, et al: Androgen independent cancer pogression in bone metastasis in the LNCaP model of human prostate cancer. Cancer Res 1994; 54:2576–2581.

Thompson TC, Chung LWK: Regulation of overgrowth and expression of prostatic binding protein in rat chimeric prostate gland. Endocrinology 1986; 118:2437–2444.

Thompson TC, Zhau H, Chung LWK: Catecholamines are involved in the growth and expansion of prostatic binding protein by the rat ventral prostatic tissue. Prog Clin Biol Res 1987; 239:239–248.

Tilley WD, Marcelli M, McPhaul MJ: Recent studies of the androgen receptor: New insights into old questions. Mol Cell Endocrinol 1990; 68:C7–C10.

Tilley WD, Marcelli M, Wilson JD, McPhaul MJ: Characterization and expression of cDNA in coding the human androgen receptor. Proc Natl Acad Sci USA 1989; 86:327–331.

Tisell LE: Effect of cortisone on the growth of the ventral prostate, the dorsolateral prostate, the coagulating gland and the seminal vesicles in castrated adrenalectomized and in castrated non-adrenalectomized rats. Acta Endocrinol 1970; 64:637–655.

Trachtenberg J, Hicks LL, Walsh PC: Methods for the determination of androgen receptor concentration in human prostatic tissue. Invest Urol 1981; 18:349–354.

Tsai YC, Harrison HH, Lee C, et al: Systematic characterization of human prostatic proteins with 2-dimensional electrophoresis. Clin Chem 1984; 30:2026–2030.

Tullner WW: Hormonal Factors in the Adrenal Dependent Growth of the Rat Ventral Prostate. *In* Vollmer EP, ed: Biology of the Prostate and Related Tissues. National Cancer Institute Monograph 12. Bethesda, Maryland, National Cancer Institute, 1963, p 211.

Tunn S, Senge Th, Schenck B, Neumann F: Biochemical and histological studies on prostates in castrated dogs after treatment with androstanediol, estradiol and cyproterone acetate. Acta Endocrinol 1979; 91:373–384.

Twillie DA, Eisenberg MA, Carducci MA, et al: Interleukin-6: A candidate mediator of human prostate cancer morbidity. Urology 1995; 54:542–546.

Ulvsback M, Lindstrom C, Weiber H, et al: Molecular cloning of a small prostate protein, known as β-microsemenoprotein, PSP 90 or β-inhibin, and demonstration of transcripts in non-genital tissues. Biochem Biophys Res Comm 1989; 164:1310–1315.

Umbas R, Schalken JA, Aalders TW, et al: Expression of the celllular adhesion E-cadherin is reduced or absent in high grade prostate cancer. Cancer Res 1992; 52:5104–5109.

Vafa AZ, Grover PK, Pretlow TG, Resnick ML: Study of activities of arginase, hexosaminidase, and leucine aminopeptidase in prostate fluid. Urology 1993; 42:138–143.

Vane JR, Botting RM: Pharmacodynamic profile of prostacyclin. Am J Cardiol 1995; 75:3a–10a.

Van Waes C, Surh DM, Chen Z, et al: Increase in suprabasillar integrin adhesion molecule expression in human epidermal neoplasm accompanies increased proliferation occurring immortalization and tumor progression. Cancer Res 1995; 55:5434–5444.

Verhoeven G, Swinnen K, Cailleau J, et al: The role of cell-cell interactions in androgen action. J Steroid Biochem Mol Biol 1992; 41:487–494.

Vermeulen A: The physical state of testosterone in plasma. *In* James VHT, Serio M, Maratini L, Eds: The Endocrine Function of the Human Testis, Vol I. New York, Academic Press, 1973, pp 157–170.

Vermeulen A, Verdonck L, Van der Straeten M, Orie N: Capacity of the TeBG in human plasma and influence of specific binding of testosterone on its metabolic clearance rate. J Clin Endocrinol 1969; 29:1470–1480

Vermeulen A: Testicular hormonal secretion and aging in males. *In* Grayhack JT, Wilson JD, Scherbenske MJ, eds: Benign Prostatic Hyperplasia. Proceedings of a workshop sponsored by the Kidney Disease and Urology Program of the NIAMDD, Feb. 20–21, 1975. Washington, DC, U.S. Govt. Printing Office, 1976, pp 77–182.

Vessella RL, Lange PH: Issues in the assessment of PSA immunoassays. Urol Clin N Amer 1993; 20:607–619.

Vignon F, Clavert A, Koll-Back MH, Reville P: On the glandular origin of seminal plasma lipids in man. Andrologia 1992; 24:341–343.

Villoutreix BO, Getzoff ED, Griffin JH: A structural model for the prostate disease marker, human prostate-specific antigen. Protein Science 1994; 3:2033–2044.

Vogelstein B, Pardoll DM, Coffey DS: Supercoiled loops in eukaryotic DNA replication. Cell 1980; 22:79–85.

von Euler US: Zur Kenntnis der pharmakologischen Wirkungen von Natirsekreten und Extrackten mannlicher accessorischer Geschlechtsdrusen. Arch Pathol Pharmakol 1934; 175:78–84.

Waldman T, Kinzler KW, Vogelstein B: P21 is necessary for the p53 mediated g1 arrest in human cancer cells. Cancer Res 1995; 55:5187–5190.

Walensky LD, Coffey DS, Chen T-H, et al: A novel M_r 32,000 nuclear phosphoprotein is selectively expressed in cells competent for self-renewal. Cancer Res 1993; 53:4720–4726.

Walsh PC, Gittes RF: Inhibition of extratesticular stimuli to prostatic growth in the castrate rat by antiandrogens. Endocrinology, 1970; 87:624–627.

Walsh PC, Wilson JD: The induction of prostatic hypertrophy in the dog with androstanediol. J Clin Invest 1976; 57:1093–1097.

Wang MC, Valenzuela LA, Murphy GP, Chu TM: Purification of a human prostate specific antigen. Invest Urol 1979; 17:159–163.

Wang TJ, Hill T, Norton K, et al: Dual monoclonal antibody immunoassay for free PSA. Prostate 1996; 28:10–16.

Watt KWK, Lee PJ, Tinkulu TM, et al: Human prostatic specific antigen: Structural and functional similarities with serum proteases. Proc Natl Acad Sci USA 1986; 83:3166–3170.

Wheeler TM, Rogers E, Aihara M, et al: Apoptotic indexes of biomarker in prostatic interepithelial neoplasia. J Cell Biochem Suppl 1994; 19:202–207.

White IG, Darin-Bennett A, Poulos A: Lipids of Human Semen. *In* Hafez ESE, Ed: Human Semen and Fertility Regulation in Men. St. Louis, CV Mosby Company, 1976, pp 144–152.

White MA: Changes in pH of expressed prostatic secretion during the course of prostatitis. Proc R Soc Med 1975; 68:511–513.

Wilding G, Valvaerius E, Knabbe C, Gelman EP: The role of α in human prostate cancer cell growth. Prostate 1989; 15:1–12.

Williams-Ashman HG: Regulatory features of the seminal vesicle development and function. Curr Top Cell Regul 1983; 22:201–275.

Williams-Ashman HG, Corti A, Sheth AR: Formation and functions of aliphatic polyamines in the prostate gland and its secretions. *In* Goland M, ed: Normal and Abnormal Growth of the Prostate. Springfield, Illinois, Charles C. Thomas Publishers, 1975, pp 222–239.

Williams-Ashman HG, Janne J, Coppoc GC, et al: New aspects of polyamine biosynthesis in eukaryotic organisms. Adv Enzyme Regul 1972; 10:225–245.

Williams-Ashman HG, Pegg AE, Lockwood DH: Mechanisms and regulation of polyamine and putrescine biosynthesis in male genital glands and other tissues of mammals. Adv Enzyme Regul 1969; 7:291–323.

Williams-Ashman HG, Wilson J, Beil R, Lorand L: Transglutaminase reactions associated with the rat semen clotting system. Biochem Biophys Res Commun 1977; 79:1192–1198.

Wilson EM, Colvard DS: Factors that influence interaction of the androgen receptor with nuclei and nuclear matrix. Annals NY Acad Sci 1984; 438:85–99.

Wojno KJ, Epstein JI: The utility of basal cell-specific anti-cytokeratin antibody (34β E12) in the diagnosis of prostate cancer. A review of 228 cases. Am J Surg Pathol 1995; 19:251–160.

Wolff H, Bezold G, Zebhauser M, Meurer M. Impact of clinically silent inflammation on male genital tract organs as reflected by biochemical markers in semen. J Androl 1991a; 12:331–334.

Wolff H, Neubert U, Zebhauser M, et al: *Chlamydia trachomatis* induces an inflammatory response in the male genital tract and is associated with altered semen quality. Fertil Steril 1991b; 55:1017–1019.

Wright GL, Haley C, Beckett ML, Schellhammer PF: Expression of prostate-specific membrane antigen in normal, benign, and malignant prostate tissues. Urol Oncol 1995:1–18–28.

Wu HC, Hsieh JT, Gleave ME et al: Derivation of androgen independent human LCNaP prostate cancer cell sublines: Role of bone stromal cells. Int J Cancer 1994; 57:406–417.

Yacoe ME, Sommer G, Peehl D: In vitro proton spectroscopy of normal and abnormal prostate. Magn Reson Med 1991; 19:429–438.

Yan G, Fukabori Y, Nikolaropoulos S, et al: Heparin-binding keratinocyte growth factor is a candidate stromal to epithelial cell andromedin. Mol Endocrinol 1992; 6:2123–2128.

Yoshiura K, Kanai Y, Ochiai A, et al: Balance of E-cadherin invasion suppressor gene by CpG methylation in human carcinoma. Proc Natl Acad Sci USA 1995; 92:7416–7419.

Young C, Murtha P, Andrews P, et al: Antagonism of androgen action in prostate tumor cells by retinoic acid. Prostate 1994; 25:39–45.

Young CYF, Mertha PE, Andrews PE, et al: Antagonism of androgen action in prostate tumor cells by retinoic acid. Prostate 1994; 25:39–45.

Young HH; Young's Practice of Urology, Vol I. Philadelphia, W. B. Saunders Company, 1926, p 419.

Yu HE, Diamandis E, Sutherland DJA: Immunoreactive prostate-specific antigen levels in female and male breast tumors and its association with steroid hormone receptors and patient age. Clin Biochem 1994a; 27:75–79.

Yu H, Diamandis EP, Levesque MA, et al: Ectopic production of prostate specific antigen by a breast tumor metastatic to the ovary. J Clin Lab Analysis 1994b; 8:251–255.

Yu H, Diamandis EP, Zarghami N, Grass L: Induction of prostate specific

antigen production by steroids and tamoxifen in breast cancer cell lines. Breast Cancer Res Treat 1994c; 32:301–305.
Zaneveld LJD, Chatterton RT: Biochemistry of Mammalian Reproduction. New York, John Wiley & Sons, 1982.
Zaneveld LJD, Tauber PF: Contributions of prostatic fluid components to the ejaculate. *In* The Prostate Cell: Structure and Function, Part A. New York, Alan R Liss, 1981, pp 255–277.
Zhau HYE, Wan DS, Zhou J, et al: Expression of c-erb B-2/neu protooncogene in human prostatic cancer tissue and cell lines. Mol Carcinog 1992; 5:320–327.

46 EPIDEMIOLOGY, ETIOLOGY, PATHOPHYSIOLOGY, AND DIAGNOSIS OF BENIGN PROSTATIC HYPERPLASIA

John D. McConnell, M.D.

Although benign prostatic hyperplasia (BPH) is one of the most common disease processes affecting the aging male, surprisingly little is known about its etiology and pathophysiology. Despite intense research efforts in the last three decades to elucidate the underlying etiology of prostatic growth in older men, cause and effect relationships have not been established. **Previously held notions that the clinical symptoms of BPH (prostatism) are simply due to a mass-related increase in urethral resistance are too simplistic.** It is now clear that **a significant portion of the symptoms are due to obstruction- and age-induced detrusor dysfunction.** Moreover, obstruction may induce a variety of neural alterations in the bladder and prostate that contribute to the symptoms. Undoubtedly, the constellation of cellular pathologies that give rise to the symptoms of BPH are far more complex than we realize. Only by unraveling these complexities, however, will we be able to successfully design alternative strategies to treat and possibly prevent BPH.

EPIDEMIOLOGY

Prevalence and Incidence

No single definition of BPH has gained universal acceptance in clinical or epidemiologic studies. BPH has been variably defined as prostatic enlargement, histologic hyperplasia, lower urinary tract symptoms, diminished uroflow, or urodynamic obstruction, or it has been viewed as and indication for prostatic surgery. Estimates of BPH prevalence depend on the definition of the disease.

Prostate Enlargement and Histologic Hyperplasia

The prostate undergoes significant growth during fetal development, puberty, and in most men, during late middle age. At the end of puberty, the prostate reaches approximately 26 g and is maintained at that weight unless BPH develops (Berry et al, 1984) (Fig. 46–1). At the beginning of the fourth decade, only 8% of men have histopathologic BPH. However, 50% of men aged 51 to 60 and 90% of men over age 80 have histologic evidence of BPH. The age-adjusted histologic incidence of BPH in China is similar (Fang-Liu, 1993). The average weight of the prostate with histologically confirmed BPH at the time of autopsy is 33 ± 16 g (Berry et al, 1984). Logistic growth analysis of BPH lesions removed by enucleation at the Johns Hopkins University Hospital demonstrates that the growth of BPH is most likely initiated before the patient is 30 years of age

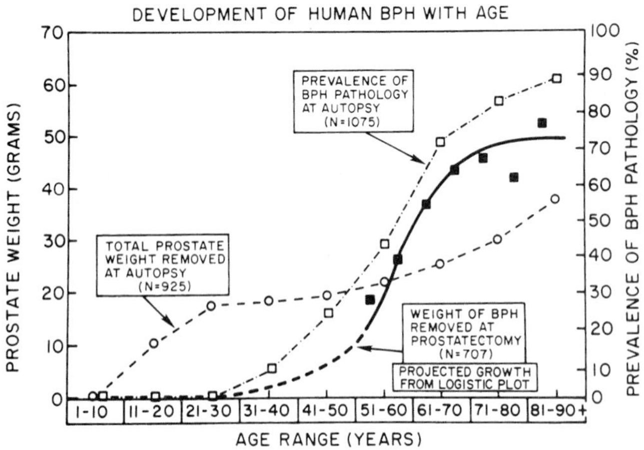

Figure 46–1. Age-related changes in the weight of the prostate removed at autopsy in 925 men, the prevalence of benign prostatic hyperplasia (BPH) pathology at autopsy in 1075 men, and the weight of the adenoma removed at simple perineal prostatectomy in 707 men. The long dashed line indicates the mathematically extrapolated range in this group. (From Berry SJ, Coffey DS, Walsh PC, Ewing LL: J Urol 1984; 132:474.)

(Berry et al, 1984). **In men between 31 and 50 years of age, the estimated doubling time for prostatic weight is 4.5 years, compared with a doubling time of ten years in men between 51 and 70 years of age** and 100 years in patients older than 70 years of age. These data demonstrate that prostatic growth is very slow in elderly men and that symptom progression in this cohort may be due to non-prostatic factors, such as detrusor dysfunction.

A community-based study of BPH in Olmsted County (OC) Minnesota (Girman et al, 1995), using a random sample of white men 40 to 79 years of age with no prior prostate surgery, cancer, or other conditions known to interfere with voiding, demonstrated a median prostate volume (ultrasound estimated) of 26.4 ml, with a 75th percentile of 34.9 ml. The percentage of men with prostatic enlargement of more than 50 ml increased with increasing subject age, regardless of self-reported symptom level. The age-adjusted population-attributable risk for prostatic enlargement (>50 ml) was 15%. Overall, this community-based study demonstrated much smaller increases in prostatic volume from decade to decade than the classic autopsy-based study (Berry et al, 1984). **The average age-related increase in prostatic size in the OC study population was 6 ml per decade.** In a companion study conducted in Shimamaki-mura, Japan, prostate volumes were less than those of the American men in OC, even after adjusting for weight, height, and age (Tsukamoto et al, 1995a).

Symptoms and Uroflow

At age 55, approximately 25% of men note a decrease in the force of their urinary stream (Arrighi et al, 1990). Between 55 and 75 years of age, the probability of this symptom increases linearly to 50% by age 75. In the OC study, the median International Prostate Symptom Score (IPSS) was 6.0 in men 40 to 79 years of age (Girman et al, 1995). **The odds of moderate-to-severe symptoms (IPSS ≥ 8) increased with age from 1.9 for men 50 to 59, to 3.4 (95% CI 1.8–6.1) for men 70 to 79 years old, relative to men 40 to 49 years of age.** Adjusting for age, the odds of moderate-to-severe symptoms were 3.5 times greater for men with prostatic enlargement (>50 ml) than for men with smaller prostates.

The probability of moderate-to-severe symptoms increases with age in Japanese and Scottish men, similar to that seen in men in OC; however, clear population differences have been observed. The probability of moderate symptoms in Japanese men aged 60 to 69 is 45% compared with 37% in the OC population (Tsukamoto, et al 1995b). Age-related increases in symptoms were similar in the Scottish population studied, but the men tended to report a lower degree of bother for a given symptom level than those men studied in OC (Garraway et al, 1991, 1993). **The only nationwide urologic symptom survey conducted, demonstrated that 13% of patients aged 50 to 80 in France have moderate symptoms (IPSS of 18–19) and 1% had severe symptoms (IPSS ≥ 20)** (Sagnier et al, 1995). In all community-based studies reported to date, increases in symptom severity clearly lead to measurable impairment in quality of life.

The age-specific distribution of urinary flow rates in the OC community demonstrated that peak flow rates are age dependent, with median peak flow rates dropping approximately 2 ml/second each decade, from 20.3 ml/second for men aged 40 to 44, to 11.5 ml/second for men 75 to 79 (Fig. 46–2*A*) (Girman et al, 1993). Twenty-four percent of men aged 40 to 44 had peak urinary flow rates less than 15 ml/second, a threshold commonly used to confirm a clinical diagnosis of BPH, compared with 69% of men older than 75 years of age (see Fig. 46–2*B*). Peak flow rates below 10 ml/second were found in 6% of men aged 40 to 44, and 35% of men aged 75 to 79. Voided urine volume decreased significantly with age from a median of 35.5 ml for men aged 40 to 44 to a median volume of 22 ml for men aged 75 to 79, at a decline of approximately 4.3 ml/year.

Correlation Between Prostate Volume, Symptoms, and Peak Urinary Flow Rate

Community-based epidemiologic and clinical studies have demonstrated that the relationship between prostatic size and lower urinary tract symptoms is not linear. Analysis of the baseline data from the OC study demonstrated that age explained only approximately 3% of the variability in symptom scores, whereas prostate volume and peak flow rate explained only an additional 10%. However, the odds of moderate-to-severe symptoms, adjusting for age, were 3.5 times higher for men who had prostate volumes above 50 ml than for those who did not (Girman et al, 1995).

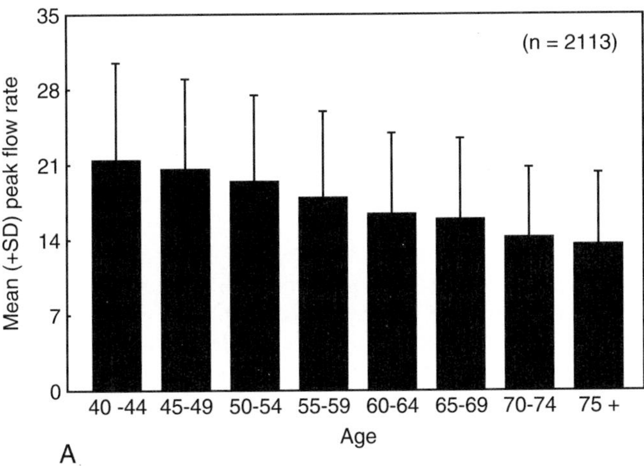

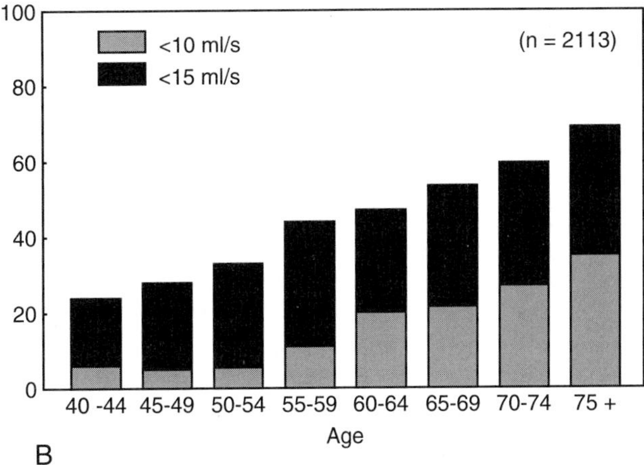

Figure 46–2. Peak urinary flow rate (ml/sec) measured in standing position by Dantec 1000 in private laboratories of randomly selected Olmsted County community men. *A*, mean (plus standard deviation) for each 5-year age category. *B*, Percentage of randomly selected Olmsted County community men with peak flow rates less than 10 ml per second and less than 15 ml per second by 5-year age category. Hatched bars show percentage of men with peak urinary flow rate less than 10 ml per second, and solid bar represents percentage of men with peak urinary flow rate between 10 and 15 ml per second, so that total heights of stacked bars represent percentage with peak urinary flow rate less than 15 ml per second. (From Girman CJ, Panser LA, Chute CG, et al: J Urol 1993; 150:887.)

BPH Prevalence: Case Definition Studies

The diagnosis of BPH is often made by the clinician's combined assessment of prostate size, urinary symptoms, and reduced urinary flow rate. The clinical diagnosis of BPH, made entirely on the basis of a history and physical examination, in the Baltimore Longitudinal Study of Aging parallels the autopsy prevalence of pathologically defined BPH (Guess et al, 1990) (Fig. 46–3). In the Baltimore Longitudinal Study of Aging, 69% of men aged 61 to 70 were given the clinical diagnosis of BPH, whereas the prevalence of pathologic BPH in this decade was estimated to be 70.7%. These results suggest that **the proportion of the male *population* with clinically recognizable prostatism by a given age is about the same as the proportion with pathologic evidence of BPH, despite the poor correlation between symptoms and prostate size or histology in *individual* patients.** A community-based study of men in Central Scotland determined the prevalence of BPH in a population of men aged 40 to 79 based on a clinical definition of BPH that included an enlarged prostate (>20 g) and *either* an elevated symptom score (11 or higher on a scale of 0–48) or a reduced peak urinary flow rate (<15 ml/second) (Garraway et al, 1991). The prevalence of clinically defined BPH ranged from approximately 14% for men in their 40s to 40% for men in their 70s (Table 46–1). Further analysis of this population demonstrated that **51% of men meeting the specified definition of BPH also reported interference with at least one of a number of selected daily activities; about 25% reported interference with daily activities most or all of the time.** Interestingly, only a small minority of the population had sought medical consultation (Guess et al, 1993b). Using a similar definition of *clinical BPH*, the age-adjusted prevalence of the disease may be lower in Japan than in the United States or Scotland (Fig. 46–4) (Barry et al, 1993b). Bosch and associates (1995) found a 19% prevalence of *clinical* BPH (prostate volume > 30 ml and an IPSS > 7) in a community-based study of 502 Dutch men. These authors demonstrated that the observed prevalence of BPH in the population studied could vary

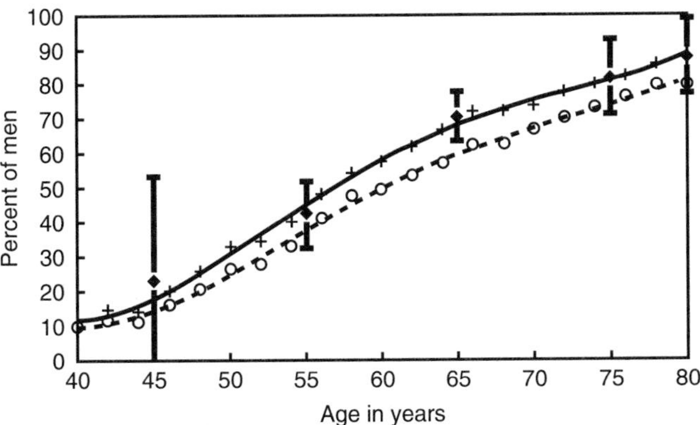

Figure 46–3. Comparison between the age-specific prevalence of prostatism (clinically diagnosed BPH) among men in the BLSA and the age-specific autopsy prevalence (♦) of BPH as published by Berry and associates (1984). Error bars on the autopsy prevalences are ± 1 standard error. The terms cumulative clinical prevalence (+) and point clinical prevalence (0) are defined in the text. (From Guess HA, Arrighi HM, Metter EJ, et al: Prostate 1990; 17:241. Reprinted by permission of John Wiley & Sons, Inc.)

Table 46–1. PREVALENCE OF BPH FOR DIFFERENT AGE GROUPS

Age Group (Years)	No. (BPH/Total)	Prevalence (Per 1000 Men)	95% Confidence Interval (Per 1000 Men)
40–49	38/276	138	97–178
50–59	47/204	237	173–288
60–69	64/149	430	350–509
70–79	28/70	400	285–515

BPH, Benign prostatic hyperplasia.
From Garraway WM, Collins GN, Lee RJ: Lancet 1991; 338:469–471.

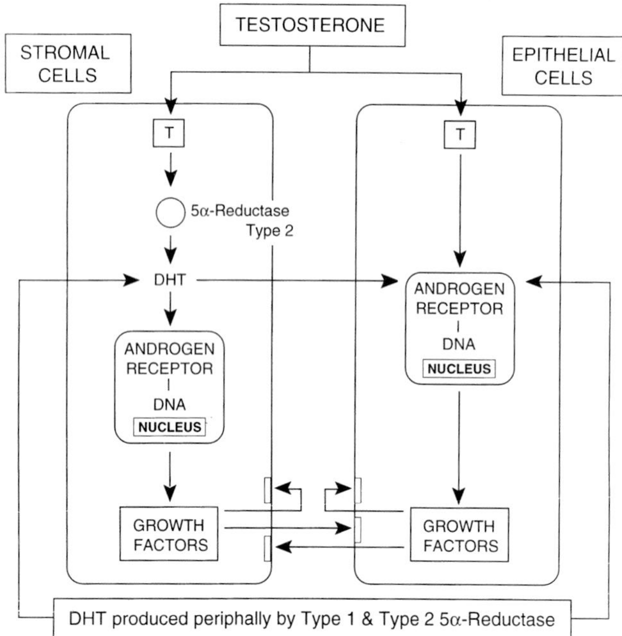

Figure 46–4. Testosterone (T) diffuses into the prostate epithelial and stromal cell. T can interact directly with the androgen (steroid) receptors bound to the promoter region of androgen-regulated genes. In the stromal cell, a majority of T is converted into dihydrotestosterone (DHT), a much more potent androgen, which can act in an autocrine fashion in the stromal cell, or in a paracrine fashion by diffusing into epithelial cells in close proximity. DHT produced peripherally, primarily in the skin and liver, can diffuse into the prostate from the circulation and act in a true endocrine fashion. In some cases, the basal cell in the prostate may serve as a DHT production site, similar to the stromal cell. Autocrine and paracrine growth factors may also be involved in androgen-dependent processes within the prostate.

more than fourfold depending on the clinical definition used. The lowest prevalence rate of 4.3% occurred using a clinical definition of prostate volume greater than 30 ml and an IPSS greater than 7, a peak uroflow less than 10 ml/second, and the presence of a postvoid residual urine volume (PVR) greater than 50 ml.

Etiologic Risk Factors

Age and normal androgen hormone status are the major etiologic risk factors for BPH; the disease is not seen in 20-year-old men or in men castrated before puberty. The autopsy and population-based studies cited earlier demonstrate unequivocal, age-related increases in prostate size and prostatism prevalence. Presumably, prostatic aging is associated with either the acquisition of growth-promoting influences or the loss of growth-inhibiting influences—either of which require a normal androgen milieu.

With the exception of lower prevalence in Japanese men, clear racial differences in the prevalence of BPH histopathology, prostate size, or clinically diagnosed BPH are not apparent (Guess, 1995). The age-specific autopsy prevalence of histologic BPH shows little geographic or racial variation (Isaacs and Coffey, 1989). However, Japanese men have a lower prevalence of prostatic enlargement and lower urinary tract symptoms than men in Minnesota or Scotland (Tsukamoto et al, 1995a). Previously published data suggesting a high prevalence of BPH in Jewish men are likely due to selection bias or differences in health-seeking behavior (Lytton, 1983). Similarly, previous studies suggesting a higher incidence of BPH in black men (Derbes et al, 1937) have been refuted by a well-conducted trial in the Kaiser Permanente System, which showed the age-adjusted relative risk of surgically treated BPH among black men with equal access to care to be identical to that of white men (Sidney et al, 1991a).

Epidemiologic studies have found either no association, a weak inverse association, or a weak biphasic association between smoking and either surgically treated BPH or prostatism. Morrison (1992) concluded that smoking was not causally related to a decreased risk of surgically treated BPH. Seitter and Barrett-Conner (1992) reported no association between smoking and surgically treated BPH in a 12-year follow-up of 929 men. Sidney and colleagues (1991a) found a small but statistically significant negative association between being a current smoker at baseline and the subsequent risk of undergoing surgery for BPH. The authors postulated that this may be due to the hormonal effects of smoking, either on the disease itself, or on the decision to perform surgery for BPH. If a negative effect of smoking on BPH exists, it is unlikely to be due to the hormonal effects of nicotine, which is known to increase serum testosterone (T) levels in humans (Dai et al, 1988) and increase dihydrotestosterone (DHT) in the canine prostate (Meikle et al, 1988). Daniell (1993b) demonstrated that prostatectomy specimens from smokers were smaller than those from nonsmokers. Moreover, the age-adjusted prevalence of smoking was lower among men surgically treated for BPH than among men from a general medical practice. Roberts and colleagues (1994) observed a biphasic association between smoking and prostatism in a community-based study of 2000 men. Moderate smokers were found to have fewer symptoms of prostatism than nonsmokers and men who have never smoked, whereas heavy smokers had symptoms similar to those who had never smoked.

Studies on the relationship between body mass and BPH are conflicting. Obesity may give rise to larger prostate size, but the prevalence of BPH treatment is the same as or lower than in men with normal body mass. The body mass index (kgm^2) was found to be negatively associated with surgically treated BPH in patients followed in a prepaid health plan (Sidney et al, 1991b). In the Veterans Association Normative Aging Study, however, the body mass index was found to be negatively associated with the clinical diagnosis of BPH but not with surgically treated BPH (Glynn et al, 1985). A multivariate analysis of numerous variables demonstrated that the body index effect was independent of age, smoking, and alcohol intake. Although obesity is associated with higher estrogen levels, Daniell (1993a) found that the weight-for-height distribution of men who underwent prostatectomy was similar to that of a control group, despite the fact that the obese men tended to have larger resected weights of tissue. The biologic effect of obesity on the prostate is complex; lower body mass index is associated with higher serum T levels (Eldrup et al, 1987), whereas estrogen levels are higher in obesity.

The majority of autopsy studies examining the relationship between hepatic cirrhosis and BPH have found a somewhat lower autopsy prevalence among men with cirrhosis (Guess, 1995). Most cases of cirrhosis in these studies were induced by alcoholic liver disease, so that the effects of alcoholism cannot be distinguished from the effects of cirrhosis. High alcohol consumption may decrease plasma T levels and increase estrogen levels (Chopra et al, 1973), negatively affecting prostate growth independent of liver disease.

BPH does not appear to be related to vasectomy (Sidney, 1987). Also, vasectomy does not appear to affect prostate size (Jakobsen et al, 1988), and the relative risk of a hospital diagnosis of BPH among men with vasectomy is 0.97 (Guess, 1992).

In summary, epidemiologic studies have failed to reveal clear risk factors, other than aging, that increase the prevalence of BPH. However, the population-based genetic studies, discussed later, demonstrate a positive risk with a family history of the condition.

ETIOLOGY

BPH is only one cause of the lower urinary tract symptoms in aging men commonly referred to as "prostatism." Histopathologically, BPH is characterized by an increased number of epithelial and stromal cells in the periurethral area of the prostate. The observation of new epithelial gland formation—normally seen only in fetal development—gives rise to the concept of "embryonic reawakening" of the stroma cells' inductive potential (Cunha et al, 1983). The precise molecular etiology of this hyperplastic process is uncertain. **The observed increase in cell number may be due to epithelial and stromal proliferation or to impaired programmed cell death, leading to cellular accumulation.** Androgens, estrogens, stromal-epithelial interactions, growth factors, and neurotransmitters may play a role, either singly or in combination, in the etiology of the hyperplastic process.

Hyperplasia

In a given organ, the number of cells, and thus the volume of the organ, depends on the equilibrium between cell proliferation and cell death (Isaacs, 1984). An organ can enlarge not only by an increase in cell proliferation but also by a decrease in cell death. **Although androgens and growth factors stimulate cell proliferation in experimental models, the role of cell proliferation in human BPH must be questioned because there is no clear evidence of an active proliferative process.** Although it is possible that the early phases of BPH are associated with a rapid proliferation of cells, the established disease appears to be maintained in the presence of an equal or reduced rate of cell replication. **Androgens are not only required for normal cell proliferation and differentiation in the prostate but also actively inhibit cell death** (Isaacs, 1987). In the dog, experimental BPH can be produced by androgens combined with estradiol (Walsh and Wilson, 1976; DeKlerk, 1979; Berry et al, 1986a). Despite a significant increase in gland size, there is actually a reduction in the rate of DNA synthesis compared with that of untreated controls (Barrack and Berry, 1987), indicating that androgens and estrogens both inhibit the rate of cell death.

BPH may be viewed as a stem cell disease (Isaacs, 1987). Presumably, dormant stem cells in the normal prostate rarely divide, but when they do, they give rise to a second type of transiently proliferating cell capable of undergoing DNA synthesis and proliferation, thus maintaining the number of cells in the prostate. Once the proliferating cells mature through a process of terminal differentiation, they have a finite life span before undergoing programmed cell death. In this paradigm, **the aging process induces a block in this maturation process so that the progression to terminally differentiated cells is reduced, lowering the overall rate of cell death.** Indirect evidence for this hypothesis comes from the observation that secretion, one parameter of epithelial cell differentiation, decreases with age, suggesting that the number of differentiated cells capable of secretory activity may be decreasing (Isaacs, 1987).

Hormones may exert their influence over the stem cell population not only with advancing age but also during embryonic and neonatal development (Naslund and Coffey, 1986). The size of the prostate may be defined by the absolute number of potential stem cells present in the gland, which, in turn, may be dictated at the time of embryonic development. Studies in animal models have suggested that **early imprinting of prostatic tissue by postnatal androgen surges is critical to subsequent hormonally induced prostatic growth** (Naslund and Coffey, 1986).

The Role of Androgens

Although androgens do not cause BPH, the development of BPH requires the presence of testicular androgens during prostate development, puberty, and aging (McConnell, 1995). Patients castrated before puberty, or who are affected by a variety of genetic diseases that impair androgen action or production, do not develop BPH. It is also known that prostatic levels of DHT, as well as the androgen receptor (AR) remain high with aging, despite the fact that peripheral levels of T are decreasing. Moreover, androgen withdrawal leads to partial involution of established BPH (Peters and Walsh, 1987).

In the brain, skeletal muscle, and seminiferous epithelium, T directly stimulates androgen-dependent processes. **In the prostate, however, the nuclear membrane-bound enzyme steroid 5α-reductase converts the hormone T into DHT, the principal androgen in this tissue** (see Fig. 46–4) (McConnell, 1995). Ninety percent of total prostatic androgen is in the form of DHT, principally derived from testicular androgens. Adrenal androgens may comprise 10% of total prostatic androgen, although the importance of this stored hormone source in the etiology of BPH is negligible. Inside the cell both T and DHT bind to the same high affinity androgen-receptor protein. DHT is a more potent androgen than T owing to its higher affinity for the AR. Moreover, the DHT receptor complex may be more stable than the T receptor complex. The hormone receptor then binds to specific DNA-binding sites in the nucleus, which results in increased transcription of androgen-dependent genes and, ultimately, stimulation of protein symphysis. Conversely, androgen withdrawal from androgen-sensitive tissue results in a decrease in protein symphysis and tissue involution. **Besides inactivation of key androgen-dependent genes (e.g., prostate-specific antigen [PSA]), androgen with-**

drawal leads to the activation of specific genes involved in programmed cell death.

Androgen Receptors

The prostate, unlike other androgen-dependent organs, maintains its ability to respond to androgens throughout life. In the penis, AR expression decreases to negligible rates at the completion of puberty (Roehrborn, 1987; Takane, 1991). Thus, despite high circulating levels of androgen, the adult penis loses its ability for androgen-dependent growth. If the penis maintained high levels of AR throughout life, presumably the organ would grow until the time of death. In contrast, AR levels in the prostate remain high throughout aging (Barrack et al, 1983; Rennie, 1988; Husmann, 1990; Takane, 1991). In fact, there is evidence that suggests that nuclear AR levels may be higher in hyperplastic tissue than in normal controls (Barrack et al, 1983). Age-related increases in estrogen, as well as other factors, may increase AR expression in the aging prostate, leading to further growth (or to a decrease in cell death), despite decreasing levels of androgen in the peripheral circulation and so-called normal levels of DHT in the prostate.

Dihydrotestosterone and Steroid 5α-Reductase

Intraprostatic DHT concentrations are maintained but not elevated in BPH. Initial studies of resected prostatic tissue suggested that prostatic DHT levels were higher in the hyperplastic gland than in normal control tissues. However, the controls used for these early studies were largely accident victims. Ongoing metabolism of DHT after death lowers the level of this androgen in cadaveric tissues. This was clearly shown in a study by Walsh and associates (1983), in which prostatic surgical specimens from men without BPH were used as the control. These investigators demonstrated that DHT levels are the same in hyperplastic glands as in normal glands. However, the aging prostate maintains a high level of DHT, as well as a high level of AR; thus, the mechanism for androgen-dependent cell growth is maintained. There is little question that androgens have at least a permissive role in the development of the disease process.

Two steroid 5α-reductase enzymes have been discovered, each encoded by a separate gene (Russell and Wilson, 1994). Type 1 5α-reductase, the predominant enzyme in extraprostatic tissues, such as skin and liver, is normally expressed in the 5α-reductase deficiency syndrome and is poorly inhibited by finasteride. Type 2 5α-reductase is the predominant, if not sole, prostatic 5α-reductase, although it is also expressed in extraprostatic tissues. Mutations in the type 2 enzyme are responsible for the clinical phenotype observed in the 5α-reductase deficiency syndrome. It is exquisitely sensitive to inhibition by finasteride and epristeride. Clearly, **the type 2 enzyme is critical for the normal development of the prostate and hyperplastic growth later in life.** The role of type 1 5α-reductase in normal and abnormal prostate growth remains to be defined.

Immunohistochemical studies with type 2 5α-reductase–specific antibodies show primarily stromal cell localization of the enzyme (Silver et al, 1994a). Acinar epithelial cells uniformly lack type 2 protein, whereas some basal epithelial cells stain positively. Type 1 5α-reductase protein cannot be detected in BPH or prostate cancer (Silver et al, 1994b), although trace levels of type 1 mRNA have been seen in normal prostates.

These data demonstrate that the **stromal cell plays a central role in androgen-dependent prostatic growth** and suggests a new paracrine model for androgen action in the gland (see Fig. 46–4). In addition, it is likely that **circulating DHT—produced in the skin and liver—may act on prostate cells in a true endocrine fashion.** This factor may have therapeutic implications, given the observation that finasteride and epristeride inhibit only the type 2 enzyme (McConnell et al, 1995).

The Role of Estrogens

Evidence has been found in animal models to suggest that estrogens play a role in the pathogenesis of BPH; the role of estrogens in the development of human BPH, however, is less clear. In the dog, in which estrogens act synergistically with androgens to produce experimental BPH, estrogen appears to be involved in induction of the AR (Moore, 1979). Estrogen may, in fact, sensitize the aging dog prostate to the effects of androgen (Barrack and Berry, 1987). The canine prostate contains an abundance of high-affinity estrogen receptor (Trachtenberg, 1980). In the dog, estrogen treatment stimulates the stroma, causing an increase in the total amount of collagen (Berry and Isaacs, 1984; Berry et al, 1986b).

Serum estrogen levels increase in men with age, absolutely or relative to T levels. There is also suggestive evidence that intraprostatic levels of estrogen are increased in men with BPH. Patients with larger volumes of BPH tend to have higher levels of estradiol in the peripheral circulation (Partin et al, 1991). Although there are relatively low concentrations of classic high-affinity estrogen receptors in human BPH (Ekman et al, 1983), there may be a sufficient amount for biologic activity.

From experimental studies with aromatase inhibitors, it appears that decreases in intraprostatic estrogen in animal models may lead to a reduction in drug-induced stromal hyperplasia (Oesterling et al, 1988). At the present time, however, the role of estrogens in human BPH is not as firmly established as the role of androgens. Species variation and cause-and-effect relationships are problematic.

There are high levels of progesterone receptor in the normal and hyperplastic prostate. However, the role of the progesterone receptor in normal prostatic physiology, as well as in BPH, remains to be defined.

Androgens are clearly not the only important factors for the development of BPH. All mammalian prostates studied have T, DHT, and AR; however, only the dog and humans develop BPH. Interestingly, another glandular organ that remains androgen responsive throughout life, the seminal vesicle, does not develop hyperplasia. Obviously, other mechanisms or cofactors must be present in these two unique species to make them susceptible to the disease. Nonandrogenic substances from the testis, perhaps transmitted through the vas deferens or deferential blood vessels, for example, may play some role (Darras et al, 1992).

Regulation of Programmed Cell Death

Programmed cell death (apoptosis) is a physiologic mechanism crucial to the maintenance of normal glandular hemostasis (Kerr and Searle, 1973). Cellular condensation and fragmentation precede phagocytosis and degradation, during which the apoptotic cell is phagocytosed by neighboring cells and degraded by lysosomal enzymes. Apoptosis occurs without activation of the immune system, but requires both RNA and protein symphysis (Lee, 1981). In the rat prostate, active cell death occurs naturally in the proximal segment of the prostatic ductal system in the presence of normal concentrations of plasma T (Lee et al, 1990). Androgens (presumably T and DHT) appear to suppress programmed cell death elsewhere in the gland. **Following castration, active cell death is increased in the luminal epithelial population as well as in the distal region of each duct.** Tenniswood (1986) has suggested that there is regional control over androgen action and epithelial response, with androgens providing a modulating influence over the local production of growth regulatory factors that varies in different parts of the gland. Members of the transforming growth factor (TGF)-β family are likely candidates for this regulatory step (Martikainen et al, 1990).

In the rat prostate, at least 25 different genes are induced following castration (Montpetit et al, 1986). Normal glandular hemostasis requires a balance between growth inhibitors and mitogens, which respectively restrain or induce cell proliferation but also prevent or modulate cell death. Abnormal hyperplastic growth patterns, such as BPH, might be induced by local growth factor or growth factor receptor abnormalities, leading to increased proliferation or decreased levels of programmed cell death.

Stromal-Epithelial Interaction

There is abundant experimental evidence to demonstrate that **prostatic stromal and epithelial cells maintain a sophisticated paracrine type of communication.** The growth of canine prostate epithelium can be regulated by cellular interaction with the basement membrane and stromal cells. Isaacs (1984), using a marker of canine prostatic epithelial cell function, has demonstrated that epithelial cells grown on plastic quickly lose their ability to secrete this protein. In addition, the cells begin to grow rapidly and change their cytoskeletal staining pattern. In contrast, if the cells are grown on prostatic collagen, they maintain their normal secretory capacity and cytoskeletal staining pattern and do not grow rapidly. This is strong evidence that **one class of stromal cell excretory protein (i.e., extracellular matrix) partially regulates epithelial cell differentiation. Thus, BPH may be due to a defect in a stromal component that normally inhibits cell proliferation, resulting in loss of a normal breaking mechanism for proliferation.** This abnormality could act in a autocrine fashion and lead to proliferation of stromal cells as well.

Further evidence of the importance of stromal-epithelial interactions in the prostate comes from the elegant developmental studies of Cunha, which demonstrate the importance of embryonic prostatic mesenchyme in dictating differentiation of the urogenital sinus epithelium (Cunha et al, 1983). **The process of new gland formation in the hyperplastic prostate suggests a reawakening of embryonic processes in which the underlying prostatic stroma induces epithelial cell development** (Cunha et al, 1983; McNeal, 1990). Many of the prostatic stromal-epithelial interactions observed during normal development and in BPH may be mediated by soluble growth factors or by the extracellular matrix, which itself has growth factor–like properties. This model is even more intriguing, given the cellular localization of 5α-reductase (and thus DHT production) in the prostate stromal cell (Silver et al, 1994b).

As our understanding of stromal-epithelial cell relationships in the prostate increases, it is possible that therapies may be designed to induce regression of established BPH by modulating these autocrine and paracrine mechanisms.

Growth Factors

Growth factors are small peptide molecules that stimulate, or in some cases inhibit, cell division and differentiation processes (Steiner, 1995). Cells that respond to growth factors have on their surface receptors specific for that growth factor, which, in turn, are linked to a variety of transmembrane and intracellular signaling mechanisms. **Interactions between growth factors and steroid hormones may alter the balance of cell proliferation versus cell death to produce BPH** (Fig. 46–5). Story and colleagues (1989) were the first to demonstrate that extracts of BPH stimulate cellular growth. This putative prostatic growth factor was subsequently found on sequence analysis to be basic fibroblastic growth factor (β-FGF). Subsequently, a variety of growth factors have been characterized in normal, hyperplastic, and neoplastic prostatic tissue. In addition to β-FGF, other heparin-binding growth factors (e.g., α-fibroblastic growth factor), TGF-β, and epidermal growth factor (EGF) have been found in normal and BPH tissue. TGF-β is a potent inhibitor of proliferation in normal epithelial cells in a variety of tissues. In models of prostatic cancer, there is evidence to suggest that malignant cells have escaped the growth-inhibitory effect of TGF-β (McKeehan, 1988). Similar mechanisms may be operational in BPH.

There is mounting evidence of an interdependency among growth factors, growth factor receptors, and the steroid hormone milieu of the prostate (Kyprianou and

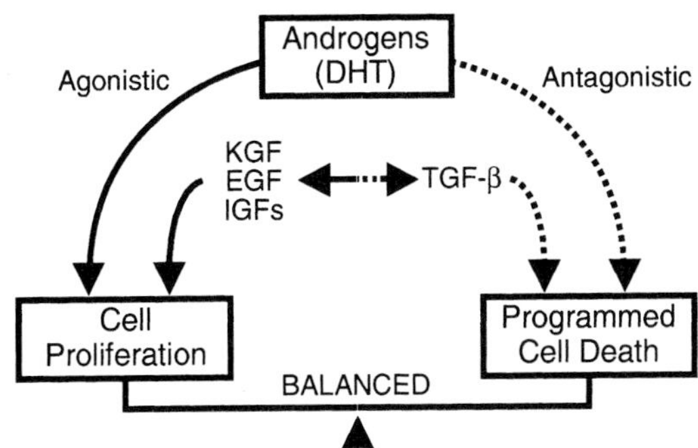

Figure 46–5. Prostate hyperplasia is probably due to an imbalance between cell proliferation and cell death. Androgens play a necessary but probably permissive role. Growth factors are more likely to be sites of primary defects.

Isaacs, 1989; Rennie, 1988). Although data on the absolute level of growth factor and growth factor receptors in hyperplastic as opposed to normal tissue are conflicting, it is likely that growth factors play some role in the pathogenesis of BPH. However, further research is necessary to establish the role of growth factors in a disease process in which cellular proliferation is not obvious.

If cellular proliferation is a component of the BPH process, it appears that growth stimulatory factors such as β-FGF, EGF, keratinocyte growth factor (KGF), and insulin growth factor may play a role, with DHT augmenting or modulating the growth factor effects. In contrast, TGF-β, which is known to inhibit epithelial cell proliferation, may normally exert a restraining influence over epithelial proliferation, which is lost or down-regulated in BPH (Wilding et al, 1989; Sporn and Roberts, 1990, 1991; McKeehan et al, 1984; Roberts et al, 1993). TGF-β1 is a potent mitogen for fibroblasts and other mesenchymal cells, but it is also an important inhibitor of epithelial cell proliferation. TGF-β1 also regulates extracellular matrix synthesis and degradation, and can induce cells to undergo apoptosis. TGF-β also up-regulates the production of basic fibroblast growth factor (bFGF-2), which is known to be an autocrine growth factor for prostate stromal cells (Story et al, 1989, 1993). Thus, up-regulation of TGF-β1 (which is expressed in prostate stromal cells) during BPH favors expansion of the stromal compartment. Interestingly, the observation that TGF-β1 may regulate smooth muscle contractile protein expression suggests that TGF-β isoforms may be physiologic regulators of prostatic smooth muscle function (Orlandi et al, 1994).

KGF, a member of the FGF family (FGF-7), is produced in prostatic stromal cells (Yan et al, 1992). However, cell surface receptors for stromal-derived KGF are expressed exclusively in epithelial cells. As a result, **KGF is the leading candidate for the factor mediating the stromal cell–based hormonal regulation of the prostatic epithelium.** There is direct evidence that KGF plays this role in the androgen-dependent mesenchymal-epithelial interactions involved with development of the seminal vesicle (Alarid et al, 1994). Abnormalities in stromal KGF production or epithelial KGF receptors could promote epithelial cell proliferation.

A unique animal model provides additional evidence that FGF-like factors may be involved in the etiology of BPH. **A transgenic mouse line expressing the int-2 FGF-3 growth factor demonstrates a type of androgen-sensitive epithelial hyperplasia in the male mouse prostate that is histologically similar to human and canine BPH** (Tutrone et al, 1993). Further support for a role of β-FGF in BPH comes from the studies of Begun and co-workers (1995), who demonstrated a two- to threefold elevation of β-FGF in BPH compared with histologically normal glands. To date, this is the only study to demonstrate an alteration in levels of a specific regulatory polypeptide in BPH versus normal tissue.

An additional source of growth factors in human BPH tissue may be the inflammatory cell infiltrates seen in many prostate specimens. Theyer and associates (1992) reported extensive infiltration of human BPH tissues by activated T cells. Peripheral blood- and tumor-infiltrating T-cells are know to express vascular endothelial growth factor, a potent epithelial mitogen (Freeman et al, 1995). T cells are known to produce and secrete a variety of other growth factors, including HB-EGF and β-FGF-2 (Blotnick et al, 1994). Thus, T cells present in the local prostate environment may be capable of secreting potent epithelial and stromal mitogens that promote stromal and glandular hyperplasia.

Genetic and Familial Factors

There is substantial evidence that **BPH has an inheritable genetic component.** Sanda and associates (1994) conducted a retrospective case-control analysis of surgically treated patients with BPH and controls at Johns Hopkins University Hospital. The patients with BPH were men whose resected prostate weights were in the highest quartile (>37 g) and whose age at prostatectomy was in the lowest quartile. **The hazard-function ratio for surgically treated BPH among first-degree male relatives of the patients with BPH as compared with the first-degree male relatives of the controls was 4.2 (95% confidence interval (CI), 1.7–10.2), demonstrating a very strong relationship** (Table 46–2). The results did not appear to be due to differences in health-seeking behavior between the two groups. A segregation analysis showed that the results were most consistent with an **autosomal dominant inheritance pattern.** Using this model, **approximately 50% of men undergoing prostatectomy for BPH at less than 60 years of age could have the inheritable form of disease.** In contrast, only **about 9% of men undergoing prostatectomy for BPH at more than 60 years of age would be predicted to have a familial risk.**

Table 46–2. FAMILY HISTORY OF EARLY ONSET BPH INCREASES RISK OF CLINICALLY SIGNIFICANT BPH

Relatives	Frequency of Clinical BPH (%)*		Odds Ratio (Unadjusted)†	Age-Adjusted Relative Risk of Clinical BPH‡	Significance‡	
	Case Relatives	*Control Relatives*			*Chi-Square*	*P Value*
All first-degree male relatives	28.3	8.6	4.2 (1.7–10.2)	4.4 (1.9–9.9)	13.36	0.0003
Fathers of proband	33.3	13.2	3.3 (1.1–10.2)	3.5 (1.3–9.5)	5.94	0.0148
Brothers of proband	24.2	3.9	8.0 (1.6–40.5)	6.1 (1.3–29.7)	6.85	0.0089

*Percent of informative male relatives with history of prostatectomy (open or transurethral) for BPH (60 case relatives and 105 control relatives).
†Chi-square analysis of proportions; Taylor 95% confidence intervals in parentheses.
‡Cox proportional hazards survival model. Censored outcome—prostatectomy. Time variable—age at death or current age. Values in parentheses indicate 95% confidence intervals.
BPH, Benign prostatic hyperplasia.
From Sanda MG, Beaty TH, Stutzman RE, et al: J Urol 1994; 152:115.

In addition, monozygotic twins demonstrate a higher concordance rate of BPH than do dizygotic twins (Partin et al, 1994).

In a community-based cohort study of more than 2000 men, Roberts and associates (1995) found an elevated risk of moderate-to-severe urologic symptoms in men with a family history of an enlarged prostate and a family history of BPH as compared with those with no history. Recent analysis of the subjects who participated in the U.S. Finasteride Clinical Trial identified 69 men who had three or more family members with BPH, including the proband (Sanda et al, 1994). Regression analysis demonstrated that **familial BPH was characterized by large prostate size, with a mean prostate volume of 82.7 ml in men with hereditary BPH, compared with 55.5 ml in men with sporadic BPH.** Serum androgen levels and the response to 5α-reductase inhibition were similar in patients with familial and sporadic BPH.

These studies clearly demonstrate the presence of a familial form of BPH and suggest the presence of a gene contributing to the pathogenesis of the disease. Preliminary studies demonstrate evidence of DNA mutations (White et al, 1990), DNA hypomethylation (Bedford et al, 1987), and abnormalities of nuclear matrix protein expression (Partin et al, 1993) in human BPH. However, the specific gene or genes involved in familial BPH remain to be elucidated.

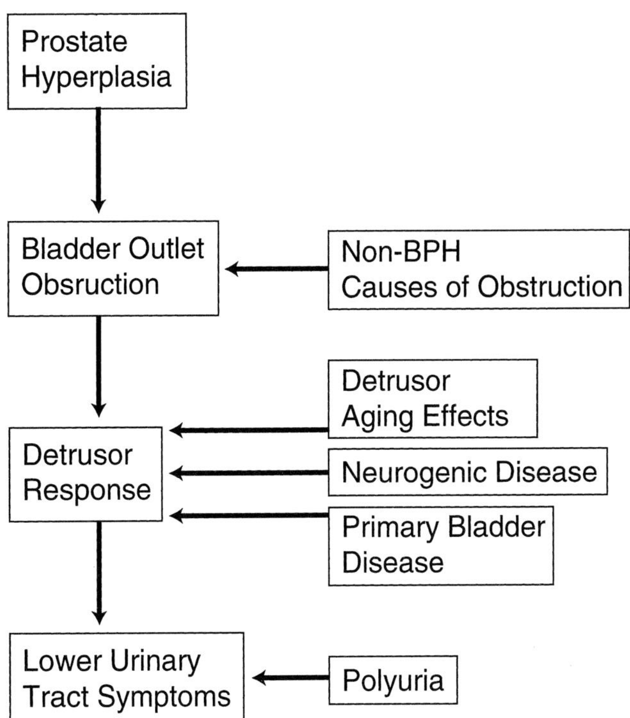

Figure 46–6. The pathophysiology of BPH involves complex interactions between urethral obstruction, detrusor function, and urine production.

Other Factors

Experimental evidence suggests that the testes may produce nonandrogenic substances that may play a role in the pathogenesis of BPH. Rats with intact testes treated with exogenous androgen demonstrate a greater degree of prostatic growth than castrated rats treated with androgen (Dalton et al, 1990; Darras et al, 1992). Similar results have been seen in castrated dogs versus those with testes intact that were treated with exogenous androgen and exogenous T and estradiol combination (Juniewicz et al, 1994). In addition to increases in prostate weight, the incidence of histologic BPH was significantly higher in those dogs with intact testes. To date, a candidate testicular nonandrogenic factor has not been identified. However, Sutkowski and colleagues (1993) have demonstrated that fluid collected from human spermatocele fluid is mitogenic to both human prostatic epithelial and stromal cells in culture.

PATHOPHYSIOLOGY

The pathophysiology of BPH is complex (Fig. 46–6). **Prostatic hyperplasia increases urethral resistance, resulting in compensatory changes in bladder function.** However, the elevated detrusor pressure required to maintain urinary flow in the face of increased outflow resistance occurs at the expense of normal bladder storage function. **Obstruction-induced changes in detrusor function, compounded by age-related changes in both bladder and nervous system function, lead to urinary frequency, urgency, and nocturia, the most bothersome BPH-related complaints.** Thus, an understanding of BPH pathophysiology requires detailed insight into obstruction-induced bladder dysfunction.

Pathology

Anatomic Features

McNeal (1978) demonstrated that **BPH first develops in the periurethral *transition zone* of the prostate.** The transition zone consists of two separate glands immediately external to the preprostatic sphincter. The main ducts of the transition zone arise on the lateral aspects of the urethral wall at the point of urethral angulation near the verumontanum. Proximal to the origin of the transition zone ducts are the glands of the *periurethral zone,* which are confined within the preprostatic sphincter and course parallel to the axis of the urethra. All BPH nodules develop either in the transition zone or in the periurethral region (McNeal, 1978, 1990).

Although early transition zone nodules appear to occur either within or immediately adjacent to the preprostatic sphincter, as the disease progresses and the number of small nodules increase, they can be found in almost any portion of the transition or periurethral zones. However, **the transition zone also enlarges with age, unrelated to the development of nodules** (McNeal, 1990).

One of the unique features of the human prostate is **the presence of the prostatic capsule, which plays an important role in the development of prostatism** (Caine and Schuger, 1987). In the dog, the only other species known to develop naturally occurring BPH, symptoms of prostatism rarely develop because the canine prostate lacks a capsule.

Presumably the capsule transmits the pressure of tissue expansion to the urethra and leads to an increase in urethral resistance. Thus, the clinical symptoms of BPH in humans may be due not only to age-related increases in prostatic size but also to the unique anatomic structure of the human gland. **Clinical evidence of the importance of the capsule can be found in series that clearly document that incision of the prostatic capsule (transurethral incision of the prostate) results in a significant improvement in outflow obstruction, despite the fact that the volume of the prostate remains the same.**

The size of the prostate does not correlate with the degree of obstruction. Thus, other factors such as dynamic urethral resistance, the prostatic capsule, and anatomic pleomorphism are more important in the production of clinical symptoms than the absolute size of the gland. In some cases, predominant growth of periurethral nodules at the bladder neck gives rise to the middle lobe (Fig. 46–7). The middle lobe must be of periurethral origin because there is no transition zone tissue in this area. It is not clear whether middle lobe growth occurs at random in men with BPH or whether there is an underlying genetic susceptibility to this pattern of enlargement.

Histologic Features

BPH is a true **hyperplastic** process. Histologic studies document an increase in the cell number (McNeal, 1990). In addition, thymidine uptake studies in the dog clearly indicate an increase in DNA synthesis (Barrack and Berry, 1987). The term benign prostatic **hypertrophy** is pathologically incorrect.

McNeal's studies (1990) demonstrate that the majority of **early periurethral nodules are purely stromal in character.** These small stromal nodules resemble embryonic mesenchyme with an abundance of pale ground substance and minimal collagen. It is unclear whether these early stromal nodules contain mainly fibroblast-like cells or whether differentiation toward a smooth muscle cell type is occurring. In contrast, **the earliest transition zone nodules represent proliferation of glandular tissue,** which may be associated with an actual reduction in the relative amount of stroma (Fig. 46–8). The minimal stroma seen initially consists primarily of mature smooth muscle, not unlike that of the uninvolved transition zone tissue. These **glandular nodules are apparently derived from newly formed small duct branches** that bud off from existing ducts, leading to a

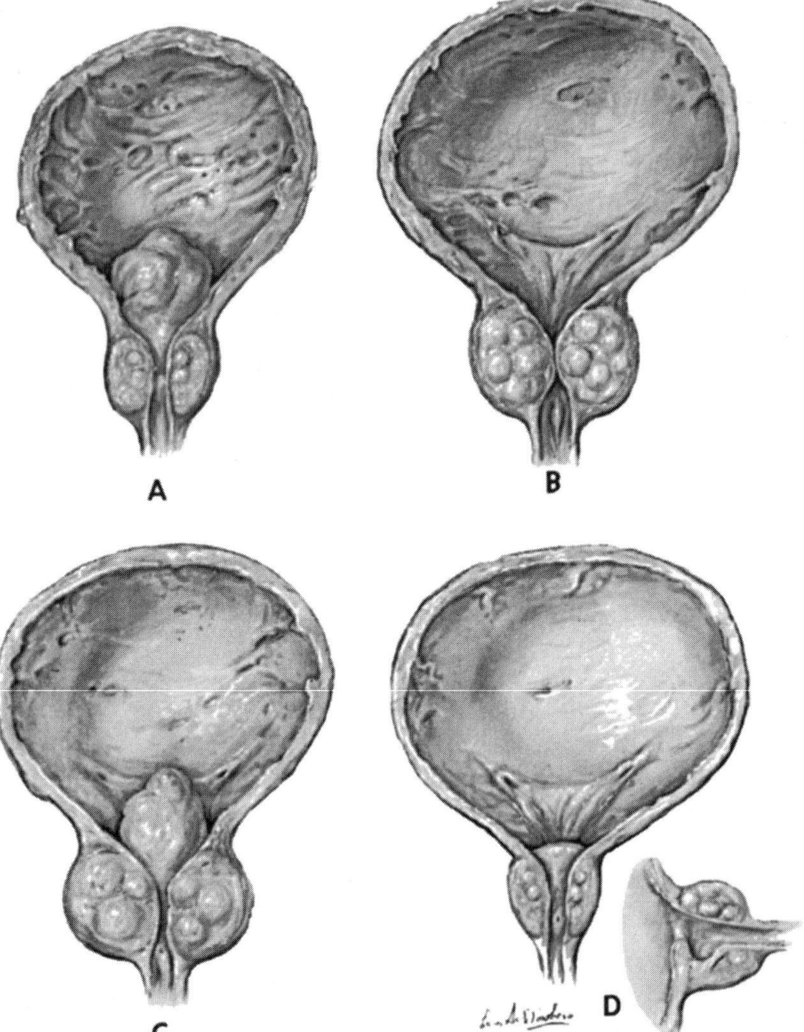

Figure 46–7. Gross appearance of hyperplastic prostatic tissue obstructing the prostatic urethra forming lobes. *A,* Isolated middle lobe enlargement. *B,* Isolated lateral lobe enlargement. *C,* Lateral and middle lobe enlargement. *D,* Posterior commissural hyperplasia (median bar). (After Randall A: A Surgical Pathology of Prostatic Obstruction. Baltimore, Williams & Wilkins, 1931.)

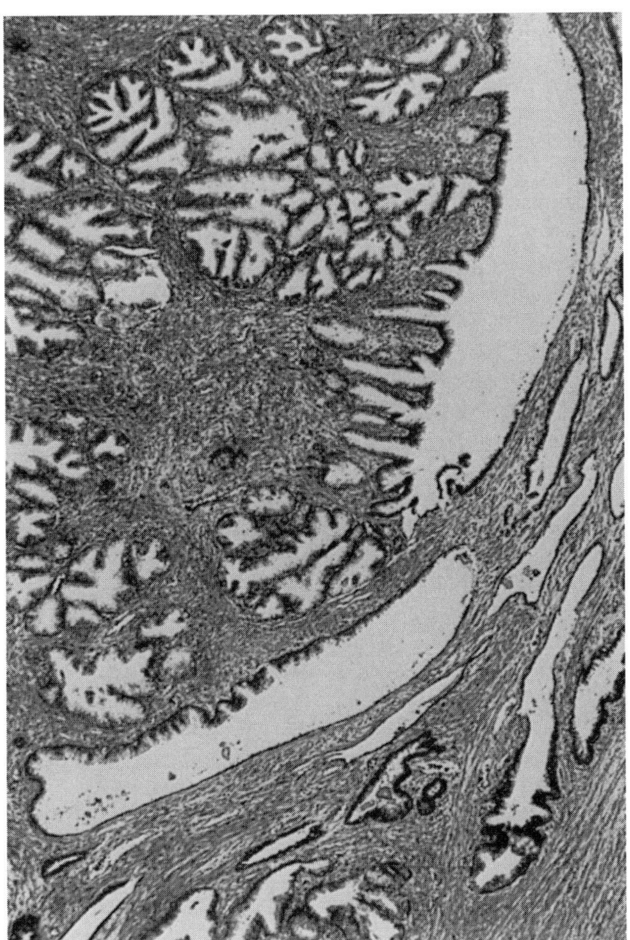

Figure 46–8. Larger glandular nodule *(upper left)* with focus of stromal hyperplasia. Tangent ducts bordering nodule show epithelial hypertrophy and formation of new gland branches, which are seen exclusively on wall of duct that faces nodule, Hematoxylin and eosin; × 70. (From Bostwick DG: Pathology of the Prostate. New York, Churchill Livingstone, 1990.)

totally new ductal system within the nodule. This type of **new gland formation is rare outside** of embryonic development. This proliferative process leads to a tight packing of glands within a given area, as well as an increase in the height of the lining epithelium. There appears to be hypertrophy of individual epithelial cells as well. Again, the observed increase in transition zone volume with age appears to be related not only to an increased number of nodules but to an increase in the overall size of the zone as well.

During the first 20 years of BPH development, the disease may be predominantly characterized by an increased number of nodules, whereas the subsequent growth of each new nodule is generally slow (McNeal, 1990). Then a second phase of evolution occurs where there is a significant increase in large nodules. In the first phase, the glandular nodules tend to be larger than the stromal nodules. In the second phase, when the size of individual nodules is increasing, the size of glandular nodules clearly predominates.

There is significant pleomorphism in stromal-epithelial ratios in resected tissue specimens. Studies from primarily **small resected glands demonstrate a predominance of fibromuscular stroma** (Shapiro et al, 1992b, 1992c) (Fig. 46–9). Larger glands, predominantly those removed by enucleation, demonstrate primarily epithelial nodules (Franks, 1976). However, an increase in stromal-epithelial ratios does not necessarily indicate that this is a stromal disease; stromal proliferation may well be due to epithelial disease.

Importance of Prostatic Smooth Muscle

Regardless of the exact proportion of epithelial to stromal cells in the hyperplastic prostate, there is no question that **prostatic smooth muscle represents a significant volume of the gland** (Shapiro et al, 1992a) (see Fig. 46–8). Although the smooth muscle cells in the prostate have not been extensively characterized, presumably their contractile properties are similar to those seen in other smooth muscle organs. The spatial arrangement of smooth muscle cells in the prostate is not optimal for force generation; however, there is no question that **both passive and active forces in prostatic tissue play a major role in the pathophysiology of BPH** (Shapiro, 1992a). The factors that determine passive tone in the prostate remain to be elucidated. The series elastic elements in the stromal and epithelial cells and (most importantly) the extracellular matrix contribute to passive tissue force—independent of active smooth muscle contraction. However, **stimulation of the adrenergic nervous system clearly results in a dynamic increase in prostatic urethral resistance. Blockade of this stimulation by alpha-receptor blockers clearly diminishes this response.** It is not clear, however, that alpha blockade decreases active tension; certainly, passive tone is not diminished.

Several additional observations on prostatic stromal and smooth muscle cells are important. It is generally assumed that the stromal cells are resistant to the effects of androgen withdrawal. In short-term studies, **androgen ablation appears to affect primarily the epithelial cell population.** In general, however, stromal cells have much slower turnover rates than epithelial cells. If the effect of androgen ablation is primarily to increase cell death rates, a decrease in stromal cell numbers may not be appreciated until a year or more of

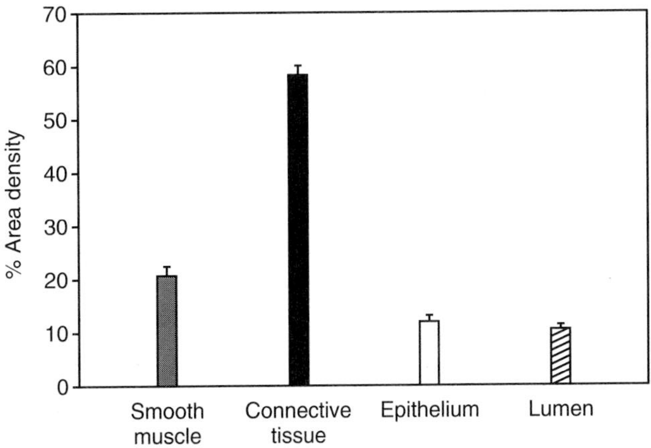

Figure 46–9. Prostate sections obtained from men with symptomatic BPH were analyzed by double immunoenzymatic staining and quantitative image analysis. The percent area density of smooth muscle and connective tissue is significantly greater than glandular epithelium and glandular lumen area density (mean ± SEM). (From Shapiro E, Hartano V, Lepor V: Prostate 1992; 20:259. Copyright 1992, Wiley-Liss Inc. Reprinted by permission of Wiley-Liss, Inc., a division of John Wiley & Sons, Inc.)

therapy. Thus, further study is required to determine whether or not the stromal cell is really resistant to androgen withdrawal. Likewise, it cannot be assumed that hormonal therapy has no effect on the stroma even if stromal cell volumes are not decreased. In a variety of smooth muscle cell systems (e.g., vascular and myometrial), contractile proteins, neuroreceptors, and extracellular matrix proteins are known to be regulated by a variety of hormones and growth factors. Thus, a given therapy may affect stromal cell function without decreasing the absolute number of volume of cells.

Active smooth muscle tone in the human prostate is regulated by the adrenergic nervous system (Schwinn, 1994). Recently, the alpha$_1$-adrenoreceptor nomenclature has been standardized (Hieble et al, 1995) to reconciled differences in nomenclature based on pharmacologic and molecular studies. **Receptor binding studies clearly demonstrate that the alpha$_{1A}$ (previously called alpha$_{1C}$) is the most abundant adrenoreceptor subtype present in the human prostate (Lepor et al, 1993a, 1993b). Moreover, the alpha$_{1A}$-receptor clearly mediates active tension in human prostatic smooth muscle** (Lepor et al, 1993b). Molecular studies demonstrate that the $_{1A}$ mRNA is the most abundant adrenoceptor message in the human prostate (Price et al, 1993). It is still unclear whether or not other factors may regulate smooth muscle contraction. Endothelin and endothelin receptors (Kobayashi et al, 1994a, 1994b) have been reported in human prostate. However, the physiologic role of this potent contractile agent on prostate smooth muscle function remains to be defined.

The role of adrenergic stimulation in the prostate may exceed simple smooth muscle contraction. Adrenergic neurotransmitters are known to regulate expression of contractile protein genes in cardiac myocytes (Kariya et al, 1993) and are known to be involved in the development of cardiac hypertrophy (Matsui et al, 1994). Interestingly, recent evidence suggests that T may regulate the expression of adrenergic receptors, at least in the kidney (Gong et al, 1995). It is possible that adrenergic neurotransmitters may play a role in prostatic smooth muscle cell *regulation* as well as contraction.

The Bladder's Response to Obstruction

Evidence suggests that the bladder's response to obstruction is largely an adaptive one (see Chapter 26). However, it is also clear that many of the clinical symptoms of prostatism are related to obstruction-induced changes in bladder function rather than to outflow obstruction directly. Approximately one third of men continue to have significant voiding dysfunction after surgical relief of obstruction (Abrams et al, 1979). Obstruction-induced changes in the bladder are of two basic types. First, those **changes that lead to *detrusor instability* or decreased *compliance,* which are clinically associated with symptoms of frequency and urgency.** Secondly, those **changes associated with impaired *detrusor contractility,*** which are **associated with further deterioration in the force of the urinary stream, hesitancy, intermittency, increased residual urine,** and (in a minority of cases) detrusor failure. Acute urinary retention should not be viewed as an inevitable result of this process. Many patients presenting with acute urinary retention have more than adequate detrusor function, with evidence of a precipitating event leading to the obstruction.

Much of our knowledge of the detrusor's response to obstruction is based on experimental animal studies. Limited information is available on the natural history of the human bladder's response to obstruction. Gosling and colleagues (1986) has demonstrated that **the major endoscopic detrusor change, trabeculation, is due to an increase in detrusor collagen.** Severe trabeculation is associated with significant residual urine (Barry et al, 1993) (Table 46–3), suggesting incomplete emptying may be due to increased collagen rather than impaired muscle function. Severe trabeculation, however, is seen in fairly advanced disease. In experimental animal models, **the initial response of the detrusor to obstruction is the development of smooth muscle hypertrophy** (Levin et al, 1995). It is likely that this **increase in muscle mass, although an adaptive response to increased intravesical pressure and maintained flow, is associated with significant intracellular and extracellular changes in the smooth muscle cell that lead to detrusor instability.** Obstruction also induces changes in smooth muscle cell contractile protein expression, energy production, and cell-to-cell communication (Levin et al, 1995).

In experimental animal models, unrelieved obstruction is associated with the development of significant increases in detrusor extracellular matrix (collagen) (Levin et al, 1995). This also appears to be the case in the human, although cause-and-effect relationships have not been established (Gosling et al, 1986). In addition to obstruction-induced changes in the smooth muscle cell and extracellular matrix of the bladder, there is increasing evidence that **obstruction may modulate neural-detrusor responses** as well (Steers et al, 1990; Gosling et al, 1986).

Correlations Between Obstruction and Symptoms

As mentioned earlier, population-based studies have **failed to demonstrate any clear relationship between prostatic growth and the development of symptoms. For this reason the term "lower urinary tract symptoms (LUTS)" may be more appropriate than "prostatism."** These observations have been confirmed in prospective clinical trials of patients with BPH. The American Urological Association

Table 46–3. MEAN VALUES OF SEVERAL BPH SEVERITY MEASURES FOR EACH LEVEL OF BLADDER TRABECULATION RECORDED AT CYSTOSCOPY

Degree of Trabeculation (Number of Points)	AUA Score	Flow (ml/second) Peak	Flow (ml/second) Average	Postvoid Residual (ml)	Ultrasound Size (g)
None (11)	17.7	9.4	5.1	111	41.4
Mild (81)	15.8	10.9	5.6	90	44.6
Moderate (88)	17.8	10.0	4.8*	101	56.2*
Severe (15)	15.9	7.5*	3.5*	245*	72.1*

*P < 0.05, using mild trabeculation as the reference category.
AUA, American Urological Association; BPH, benign prostatic hyperplasia.
From Barry MJ, Cockett ATK, Holtgrewe HL, et al: J Urol 1993; 150:351–358.

(AUA) BPH Treatment Outcome Pilot Study demonstrated no significant correlation between the IPSS and prostate size as measured by ultrasound (Table 46–4) (Barry et al, 1993). Prostate size did correlate negatively with peak and average flow rates but not with residual urine.

Numerous studies have shown **minimal to no correlation between the IPSS and the degree of obstruction, as assessed by pressure-flow urodynamic studies.** Yalla and coworkers (1995) demonstrated that the mean IPSS in patients with urodynamically defined obstruction was not statistically different from that in a group with no obstruction. Of the severely symptomatic patients, 22% did not have obstruction. Interestingly, all mildly symptomatic patients had urodynamic evidence of obstruction. No significant correlations were found between the severity of obstruction and the IPSS. In this study, the initial history and physical correctly identified a subgroup of patients who had an 80% probability of physiologic obstruction. Men with significant comorbidities that suggested the probability of alternate diagnoses had obstruction only 58% of the time. Ko and colleagues (1995), in a study of 103 symptomatic men over the age of 22, demonstrated no significant correlation between the IPSS and pressure-flow urodynamic studies with the Schäfer model ($r = 0.025 - 0.137$). The authors concluded that the **IPSS and pressure-flow urodynamic studies measured independent variables, which should not be linked in the evaluation and treatment decision in a patient with prostatism.**

Sophisticated urodynamic measurement of compressive versus constrictive obstruction in men with BPH suggests that prostate volume alone explains only 15% of the variation in urethral resistance (Bosch et al, 1995). The degree of passive and active tone in the periurethral tissue, the configuration of the prostate, and prostatic volume all contribute to urethral resistance. Given this complex relationship, it is not surprising that treatment strategies designed to singly address prostatic size or active smooth muscle contraction have limited efficacy.

Complications of Benign Prostatic Hyperplasia

Little is known about the ultimate complications and morbidity associated with untreated BPH. Internationally, **between 20% and 50% of men undergoing prostate surgery have urinary retention** (McConnell et al, 1994). However, **the likelihood that a patient with a given symptom complex will progress to complete urinary retention** over a given time span is not certain but **is probably in the range of 1% per year.**

Even less is known about the cumulative risk of obstructive uropathy and chronic renal failure among men with BPH. Patients with histologic hyperplasia and urodynamic obstruction but without bothersome symptoms are said to have silent BPH. Although this condition is probably rare, it does occur (McConnell et al, 1994). **It is difficult to identify a clinical indicator that might be useful in predicting which patients will develop serious BPH complications without bothersome symptoms.** Only large-scale screening efforts could identify those few patients with silent prostatism.

A small fraction of patients have urinary tract infections when they are treated for BPH, but it is unknown what risk factors predispose men to this complication. Also unknown is the extent to which a urinary tract infection in men with BPH predisposes them to renal function deterioration.

Bladder decompensation as a result of chronic outlet obstruction may be a long-term complication of untreated BPH in some patients. However, the probability of detrusor muscle decompensation, particularly decompensation not reversible by surgery, in men who are following a strategy of watchful waiting is unknown. Bladder diverticuli may complicate obstruction but are an uncommon cause of additional morbidity.

Bladder stones may occur as a result of bladder outlet obstruction, urinary tract infection, a retained foreign body (such as a fragment of a catheter balloon), and dietary factors. **The prevalence of bladder stones in men who undergo surgery for BPH is approximately 1% to 2%** (McConnell et al, 1994). The incidence of bladder stones over time in men with symptomatic BPH is unknown.

Accurate data on BPH as a primary cause of death are not available for most countries in the world. Mortality ascribed to BPH varies from region to region and from country to country. Ekman (1989) has attempted to use World Health Organization death rates for BPH from 50 countries, presenting the death rates as the number of deaths

Table 46–4. CORRELATION (AND ASSOCIATED P VALUES) BETWEEN MEASURES OF BPH SEVERITY AT BASELINE

	AUA Symptom Score	Global Problem Score	Peak Flow Rate	Postvoid Residual	Prostate Size*	General Health Index	Activity Index	Mental Health Index
AUA symptom score	1.00	—	—	—	—	—	—	—
Global problem score	0.49 (0.0001)	1.00	—	—	—	—	—	—
Peak flow rate	−0.07 (0.27)	0.02 (0.81)	1.00	—	—	—	—	—
Postvoid residual	0.01 (0.84)	−0.09 (0.25)	−0.19 (0.009)	1.00	—	—	—	—
Prostate size*	−0.09 (0.22)	0.03 (0.68)	−0.14 (0.06)	0.7 (0.35)	1.00	—	—	—
General health index	−0.37 (0.0001)	−0.54 (0.0001)	−0.17 (0.02)	0.17 (0.0223)	0.13 (0.076)	1.00		
Activity index	−0.29 (0.0001)	−0.37 (0.0001)	−0.12 (0.10)	0.12 (0.11)	0.13 (0.087)	0.48 (0.001)	1.00	—
Mental health index	−0.29 (0.0001)	−0.48 (0.0001)	−0.11 (0.14)	0.05 (0.47)	0.12 (0.12)	0.66 (0.0001)	0.34 (0.0001)	1.00

*Ultrasound estimate.
AUA, American Urological Association; BPH, benign prostatic hyperplasia.
From Barry MJ, Cockett ATK, Holtgrewe HL, et al: J Urol 1993; 150:351–358.

per 100,000 males aged 45 and older. The reported death rates ranged from 29.7 per 100,000 men over 45 years in East Germany (1984) to 0.5 per 100,000 males older than 45 years in Singapore (1985). The reported rate for the United States is 1.8 per 100,000 (1983). However, lack of uniformity in criteria for attributing deaths to BPH limits the usefulness of these data. **A recent analysis of WHO statistics by Napalkov and associates (1995) clearly demonstrates that the death rate for BPH is significantly lowered by management strategies employed in developed countries.**

Although mortality from BPH is extremely rare in the United States and serious complications are uncommon, the symptoms of prostatism are bothersome to many patients. **If symptoms interrupt normal daytime activities or sleep, create anxiety, or reduce perception of general health, the quality of life can decline significantly. Yet, the degree of bothersomeness may be dramatically different for different patients with the same degree of symptom severity** (Barry et al, 1992a). Because BPH is primarily a quality-of-life disease, and because significant variations do exist in individual patients' perceptions of bothersomeness and treatment risk, **the patient should play a central role in determining the need for treatment.**

DIAGNOSIS

The complex of symptoms commonly referred to as prostatism is not specific for BPH. Aging men with a variety of lower urinary tract pathologies may exhibit similar, if not identical, symptoms. The initial diagnostic challenge in these patients is to establish that the symptoms are due to BPH. This is the primary focus of initial evaluation and diagnostic testing. Fortunately, **nonprostatic causes of symptoms can be excluded in a significant majority of patients on the basis of history, physical examination, and urinalysis.** Additional diagnostic testing is necessary in patients in whom the diagnosis is still unclear after initial evaluation. These tests may also have a modest (but unproven) value in predicting the response to treatment. The following recommendations reflect the consensus opinion for two independent groups who have developed practice guidelines (Cockett et al, 1993; McConnell et al, 1994).

Initial Evaluation

Medical History

A detailed medical history focusing on the urinary tract, previous surgical procedures, general health issues, and fitness for possible surgical procedures must be performed (Cockett et al, 1993; McConnell et al, 1994). Specific areas to discuss when taking the history of a man with BPH symptoms include a history of hematuria, urinary tract infection, diabetes, nervous system disease (e.g., Parkinson's disease or stroke), urethral stricture disease, urinary retention, and aggravation of symptoms by cold or sinus medication. Current prescription and over-the-counter medications should be examined to determine if the patient is taking drugs that impair bladder contractility (anticholinergics) or that increase outflow resistance (alpha sympathomimetics). A history of prior lower urinary tract surgery suggests the possibility of urethral or bladder neck stricture. Use of a voiding diary (recording times and volume) may help identify patients with polyuria or other nonprostatic disorders.

Physical Examination

A digital rectal examination and a focused neurologic examination must be done (Cockett et al, 1993; McConnell et al, 1994). In addition, examination of the external genitalia should be performed to exclude meatal stenosis or a palpable urethral mass. The digital rectal examination and neurologic examination are performed to detect prostate or rectal malignancy, to evaluate anal sphincter tone, and to rule out any neurologic problems that may cause the presenting symptoms. The presence of induration is as important a finding as the presence of a nodule.

Rectal examination establishes the approximate size of the prostate gland. In patients who choose or require invasive therapy such as surgery, estimation of prostate size is important to select the most appropriate technical approach. Digital rectal examination provides a sufficiently accurate measurement in most cases. However, **the size of the prostate should not be considered in deciding whether active treatment is required.** Prostate size does not correlate with symptom severity, degree of urodynamic obstruction, or treatment outcomes (Donkervoort et al, 1975; Bissada et al, 1976; Roehrborn et al, 1986; Simonsen et al, 1987; Meyhoff et al, 1981). If a more precise measurement of prostate size is needed to determine whether to perform open prostatectomy rather than transurethral resection of the prostate (TURP), ultrasound (transabdominal or transrectal) is more accurate than intravenous urography (IVU) or ureterocystoscopy.

Urinalysis

A urinalysis must be done either by using a dipstick test or by examining the spun sediment to rule out urinary tract infection and hematuria, either of which strongly suggest non-BPH pathology as a cause of symptoms (Cockett et al, 1993; McConnell et al, 1994).

There is insufficient evidence that urinalysis is an effective screening procedure for asymptomatic men (Preventative Task Force (US), 1989). Because serious urinary tract disorders are relatively uncommon, the positive predictive value of screening for them is low, and the effectiveness of early detection and intervention is unproved. However, in older men with BPH (who have a higher prevalence of these disorders), the benefits of an innocuous test such as urinalysis clearly outweigh the harm involved. The test permits the selective use of renal imaging and endoscopy for patients with the greatest chance of benefiting from them. More important, urinalysis assists in distinguishing urinary tract infections and bladder cancer from BPH. These conditions may produce urinary tract symptoms (such as frequency and urgency) that mimic BPH.

The positive predictive value of urinalysis for cancer or other urologic diseases is 4% to 26%, depending on the patients screened and the rigor of follow-up studies (Mohr et al, 1986, 1987; Messing et al, 1987). **Urine cytology should be considered in men with severe irritable symp-**

toms, especially if they have a history of smoking. If a dipstick approach is used, a test that includes leukocyte esterase and nitrite tests for the detection of pyuria and bacteriuria should be used.

Serum Creatinine Measurement

Measurement of serum creatinine should be performed in all patients with symptoms of prostatism to exclude renal insufficiency due to the presence of obstructive uropathy (Cockett et al, 1993; McConnell et al, 1994). In a combined analysis of BPH studies, the percentage of patients with renal insufficiency range was 13.6% (range 0.3%–30%) (McConnell et al, 1994). This may be an overestimation, because the reports contain information only on patients eventually receiving treatment. Still, the number of patients with renal insufficiency, in a population of patients seeing a physician for symptomatic prostatism, may be as high as 1 in 10.

It is well established that **BPH patients with renal insufficiency have increased risk for postoperative complications.** The risk is 25% for patients with renal insufficiency, compared with 17% for patients without the condition (Mebust et al, 1989). Moreover, the mortality increases up to sixfold for BPH patients treated surgically if they have renal insufficiency (Holtgrewe and Valk, 1962; Melchior et al, 1974). Of 6102 patients evaluated in 25 studies by IVU before prostate surgery, 7.6% had evidence of hydronephrosis (McConnell et al, 1994). Of these patients, 33.6% had associated renal insufficiency.

Elevated serum creatinine in a patient with BPH is an indication for imaging studies (ultrasound) to evaluate the upper urinary tract. In a retrospective analysis of 345 patients who had undergone prostatectomy, 1.7% (n = 6) had occult and progressive renal damage (Mukamel et al, 1979). These patients had minimal or no urinary symptoms and presumably fit the category of patients with silent prostatism. Measurement of serum creatinine is one modality used to identify such patients. Although renal insufficiency from minimally symptomatic BPH is probably rare, the probability has yet to be defined. Meanwhile, routine creatinine measurement is reasonable.

Serum Prostate-Specific Antigen

Prostate cancer can lead to prostatism by producing urethral obstruction similar to BPH. Moreover, prostate cancer commonly coexists with BPH in the same patient. In most men with a ten year or greater life span, the knowledge of concomitant prostate cancer may well alter management of the BPH component. Conversely, the early detection of small volume prostate cancer in an 80-year-old man is unlikely to be beneficial. **PSA and digital rectal examination increases the detection rate of prostate cancer over digital rectal examination alone** (see Chapter 83). Therefore, measurement of the serum PSA should be performed in patients in whom the identification of cancer would clearly alter BPH management (Cockett et al, 1993; McConnell, 1994). There is significant overlap between the serum PSA values of men with BPH and men with clinically localized prostate cancer. Twenty-eight percent of men with histologically proven BPH have a serum PSA greater than 4.0 ng/ml (McConnell et al, 1994). Serum PSA trends over time (PSA velocity), measurement of free versus complexed PSA, and PSA density (see Chapter 84) may help improve the specificity of PSA in men with BPH.

A special concern relates to men with BPH treated by androgen withdrawal (e.g., with finasteride). Serum PSA is reduced approximately 40% to 50% after 3 to 6 months of treatment. Failure to establish a baseline (pretreatment) PSA level complicates interpretation of future PSA values.

Symptom Assessment

The IPSS, which is identical to the AUA Symptom Index, is recommended as the symptom scoring instrument to be used for the baseline assessment of symptom severity in each patient presenting with prostatism (Cockett et al, 1993; McConnell et al, 1994). When the IPSS system is used, **symptoms can be classified as mild (0 to 7), moderate (8 to 19), or severe (20 to 35).** The symptom score should also be the primary determinant of treatment response or disease progression in the follow-up period. Although other symptom score questionnaires are used, the IPSS is now the standard in the United States and internationally.

The IPSS *cannot* be used to establish the diagnosis of BPH. Men (and women) with a variety of lower urinary tract disorders (e.g., infection, tumor, neurogenic bladder disease) have a high IPSS. However, **the IPSS is the ideal instrument to grade baseline symptom severity, assess the response to therapy, and detect symptom progression in those men managed by watchful waiting.** It should be emphasized that optimal treatment decisions in individual patients also need to take into account how a given level of symptoms affects each patient's quality of life (bothersomeness).

Most patients seeking treatment for BPH do so because of bothersome symptoms that affect the quality of their lives. Tools that quantify those symptoms are important in determining the severity of the disease and documenting the response to therapy, assessing the patient's symptoms, and following them over time to determine the progression of the disease and points of necessary intervention. Such assessment tools also allow comparison of the effectiveness of various interventions. To the patient, of course, relief of symptoms is the single most important outcome—not flowrate, detrusor pressure, or urethral resistance factors.

The IPSS was developed by the Measurement Committee of the AUA (Barry et al, 1992a, 1992b). Each question on the IPSS can yield 0 to 5 points, producing a total symptom score that can range from 0 to 35. This seven-question set is internally consistent (Cronbach's alpha = 0.85) and reliable (test-retest correlation of 0.93). The index correlates strongly with patients' global ratings of their urinary difficulties (r = 0.78) and is sensitive to treatment response.

The AUA score can be divided into mild, moderate, and severe symptom categories (Barry et al, 1992a). Only 1 of 120 men with scores from 0 to 7 was bothered more than a little by his symptoms; these men can be considered the mild symptom group. The majority of the 108 men with symptom scores from 8 to 19 were still bothered not at all or only a little. Only 4 of the 108 men were bothered a lot.

These men can be identified as having moderate symptoms. Most men with scores from 20 to 35 were bothered by their condition some or a lot and can be considered to have severe symptoms.

Clearly, symptom scores alone do not capture the morbidity of a prostate problem as perceived by the individual patient. The impact of symptoms on a patient's lifestyle must be considered as well. **An intervention may make more sense for a moderately symptomatic patient who finds his symptoms very bothersome than for a severely symptomatic patient who finds his symptoms tolerable.** Although the IPSS correlates well with quality-of-life measures (Sagnier et al, 1995), there is still a need for sensitive BPH-specific quality-of-life instruments.

Additional Diagnostic Tests

Additional testing should be considered after the initial evaluation if there is a significant chance the patient's lower urinary tract symptoms may not be due to BPH.

In the Agency for Healthcare Policy and Research's (AHCPR) BPH Guidelines, **patients with a normal initial evaluation and only mild symptomatology on the IPSS (scores of 0 to 7) do not need additional diagnostic evaluation (Fig. 46–10) (McConnell et al, 1994). These patients should be placed in a watchful waiting program and followed. Men who have developed serious complications of BPH should be treated surgically in most cases. Urinary flow rate, PVR, and pressure-flow urodynamic studies are appropriate tests to consider in the evaluation of men with moderate-to-severe symptoms (IPSS symptom score ≥ 8). The value of pressure-flow studies is debated, especially in men who elect watchful waiting or medical therapy as their management option. Ureterocystoscopy should not be performed routinely but is optional during later evaluation if invasive treatment is being strongly considered (McConnell et al, 1994).** In the International Consensus recommendations, urinary flow rate and PVR are recommended tests (Cockett et al, 1993).

It may be appropriate for the physician to offer treatment alternatives to the patient without performing any further diagnostic tests. Especially if the patient chooses watchful waiting or noninvasive therapy, invasive diagnostic tests may not be necessary. Conversely, even if additional diagnostic tests were not performed initially and if the patient elects an invasive treatment option, it may be appropriate for the physician to consider further evaluation.

Diagnostic Tests in Men Who Require BPH Surgery

Both AHCPR and International Consensus Guidelines **recommend surgery if the patient has refractory urinary retention (failing at least one attempt of catheter removal) or any of the following conditions, which are clearly secondary to BPH: recurrent urinary tract infection, recurrent gross hematuria, bladder stones, renal insufficiency, or large bladder diverticula** (see Fig. 46–10) (Cockett et al, 1993; McConnell et al, 1994).

In this situation, the performance of further diagnostic tests is not necessary unless there is reason to suspect that the patient's retention may be due to primary bladder disease. In that case, urodynamic studies (for example, filling cystometry) may be helpful. Pressure-flow urodynamic studies are not possible if the patient cannot urinate. Ureterocystoscopy is appropriate to consider before the operative procedure to help plan the most prudent approach. The presence

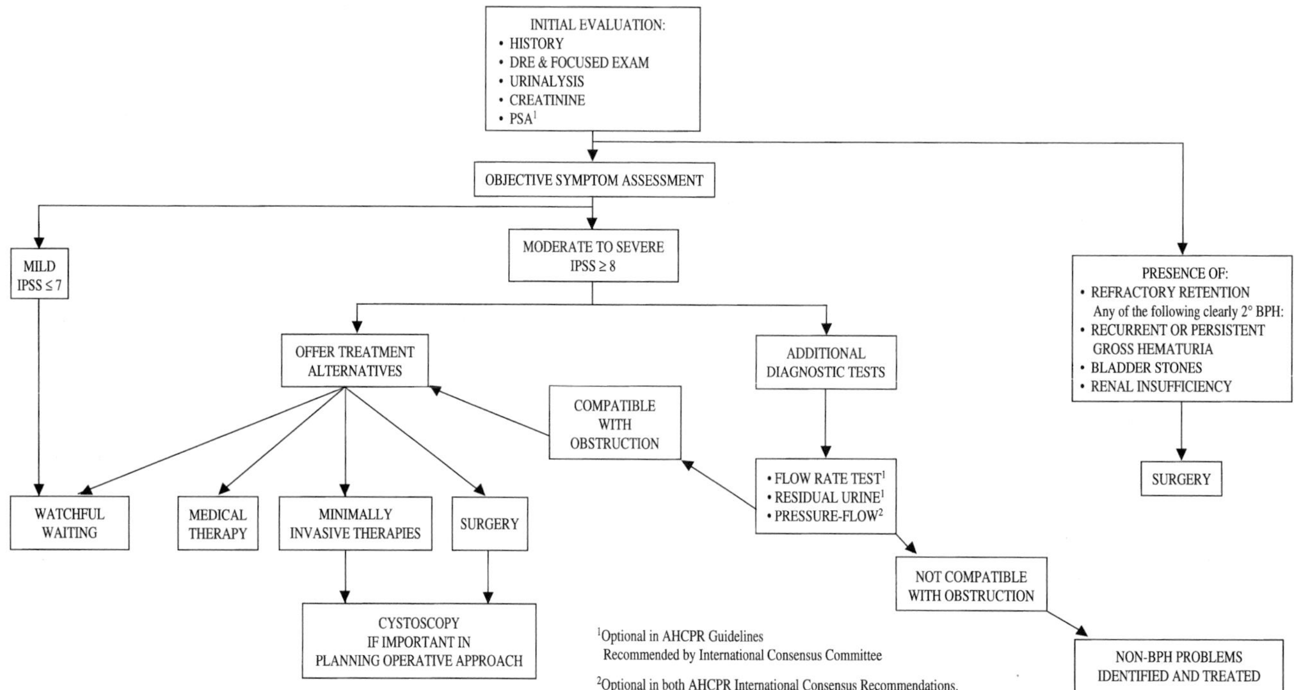

Figure 46–10. Algorithm for the evaluation and treatment of BPH based upon the AHCPR Guidelines (McConnell et al, 1994) and recommendations from the International Consensus meeting (Cockett et al, 1993).

of infection and hematuria in patients should prompt appropriate evaluations for these conditions before treatment of BPH is initiated.

Uroflowmetry

Uroflowmetry is the electronic recording of the urinary flow rate throughout the course of micturition (see Chapters 27 and 31). It is a common, noninvasive urodynamic test used in the diagnostic evaluation of patients presenting with symptoms of bladder outlet obstruction. The results of uroflowmetry are nonspecific for causes of the symptoms. For example, an abnormally low flow rate may be caused by an obstruction (e.g., hyperplastic prostate, urethral stricture, meatal stenosis) or by detrusor hypocontractility. The AHCPR Guideline Panel reached the following conclusions regarding uroflowmetry (McConnell et al, 1994):

- **Flow rate measurements are inaccurate if the voided volume is less than 125 to 150 ml.**
- **Flow rate recording is the single best noninvasive urodynamic test to detect lower urinary tract obstruction. Evidence, however, is insufficient to recommend a given cut-off value to document the appropriateness of therapy.**
- **The peak flow rate (Q_{max}) more specifically identifies patients with BPH than does the average flow rate (Q_{ave}).**
- **Although Q_{max} decreases with advancing age and decreasing voided volume, no age or volume correction is recommended for clinical practice.**
- **Although considerable uncertainty exists, patients with a Q_{max} greater than 15 ml/second appear to have somewhat poorer treatment outcomes after prostatectomy than patients with a Q_{max} of less than 15 ml/second.**
- **A Q_{max} of less than 15 ml/second does not differentiate between obstruction and bladder decompensation.**

Despite its limitations, flow rate recording has demonstrated some sensitivity in diagnosing BPH. Scott and colleagues (1967) and Shoukry and associates (1975) found that Q_{max} correlated better than symptoms with the presence or absence of obstruction as determined by pressure-flow studies. Siroky and colleagues (1979, 1980) concluded that uroflowmetry was able to distinguish physiologically those patients who have obstruction from those who do not. Gleason and co-workers (1982) found that Q_{max} distinguished between normal men and those with BPH, urethral stricture, or prostatitis. However, they also noted that a subgroup of patients with a decompensated detrusor muscle could not be separated from the men with obstruction on the basis of Q_{max} alone. In a similar study, significant differences were noted in both Q_{max} and Q_{ave} between normal volunteers and 16 patients with BPH who were to undergo prostatectomy (Groshar et al, 1991). After prostatectomy, both parameters improved significantly in the 16 patients, and the postoperative values approximated those of the normal population.

Chancellor and colleagues (1991) found that **flow rate recording cannot distinguish between bladder outlet obstruction and impaired detrusor contractility as the cause for a low Q_{max}.** None of eight measured, noninvasive urodynamic parameters was significantly different for 31 patients with outlet obstruction than for 14 patients with impaired detrusor contractility. Abrams and associates (1977, 1979) studied the value of uroflowmetry before prostatectomy. Failure rates for surgery were found to decrease with the addition of flow rate measurement to symptom assessment in preoperative evaluation.

Q_{max} appears to predict surgical outcome in some studies. In one study (Jensen et al, 1984), 53 patients underwent prostatectomy based on clinical indication alone. The study population was divided according to Q_{max} into three groups: Q_{max} less than 10 ml/second, between 10 and 15 ml/second, and greater than 15 ml/second. All three groups experienced improvements in their symptom score after surgery, but **the group with a Q_{max} less than 10 ml/second before treatment had a better overall subjective outcome as assessed by global subjective judgment.**

In a report that included men studied before and 6 months after prostatectomy (Jensen et al, 1988a), patients were divided into three groups: Q_{max} greater than 15 ml/second; Q_{max} between 10 and 15 ml/second; Q_{max} less than 10 ml/second. Subjective evaluation revealed an overall symptomatic improvement rate of 89% after surgery. The difference in success rates for men falling above or below the cut-off value of Q_{max} = 10 ml/second was not significant ($p < 0.2$). When a Q_{max} cut-off of 15 ml/second was used, success rates for men above or below the cut-off value differed significantly.

Unfortunately, not all investigators have used 15 ml/second as the cut-off. McLoughlin and co-workers (1990), using urodynamic testing and a cut-off of 12 ml/second, evaluated 108 men with prostatism before and 1 year after surgery and determined that a Q_{max} less than 12 ml/second as an indicator for obstruction would subject only 3% of patients unnecessarily to TURP. These authors believed that routine pressure-flow studies or cystometrograms were not indicated, but the screening of flow rates, followed by further urodynamic testing in patients with a Q_{max} of greater than 12 ml/second, should be considered.

Very low flow rates do not appear to portend a poor treatment outcome. In one study (Donkervoort et al, 1975) of 84 patients undergoing surgery for symptomatic BPH, patients with a low preoperative Q_{max} (>7 ml/second) improved symptomatically as much as patients with a Q_{max} greater than 7 ml/second.

Neither subjectively assessed symptoms nor quantified symptom score analysis correlate strongly with uroflowmetry measurements; they are independent assessment tools. Patients with a peak flow rate (Q_{max}) greater than 15 ml/second have somewhat poorer outcomes than those with a Q_{max} less than 15 ml/second (although the majority of patients still improve). Other investigators report similar findings for different Q_{max} cut-off values (for example, 12 ml/second). Patients with very bothersome symptoms suggestive of prostatism, but having a Q_{max} greater than 15 ml/second, may benefit from further urodynamic testing (that is, pressure-flow studies) to reduce the number of surgical treatment failures. A Q_{max} less than 15 ml/second does not differentiate between outflow obstruction and detrusor impairment. Apparently, no minimal threshold of Q_{max} reliably diagnoses detrusor failure or predicts a poor surgical outcome. The wide range of Q_{max} cut-offs used by individual health care organizations is not surprising. Every flow rate threshold used can be supported by at least one small study.

Postvoid Residual Urine

Postvoid residual urine is the volume of fluid remaining in the bladder immediately following the completion of micturition. Studies indicate that residual urine normally ranges from 0.09 to 2.24 ml, with the mean being 0.53 ml (Hinman and Cox, 1967). Seventy-eight percent of normal men have residual urine volumes of less than 5 ml, and 100% have volumes of less than 12 ml (Di Mare et al, 1963). The AHCPR BPH Guideline Panel reached the following conclusions regarding PVR (McConnell et al, 1994):

- **Residual urine volume measurement has significant intraindividual variability that limits its clinical usefulness.**
- **Residual urine volume does not correlate well with other signs or symptoms of prostatism.**
- **Large residual urine volumes may predict a slightly higher failure rate with a strategy of watchful waiting. However, the threshold volume defining a poorer outcome is uncertain.**
- **It is uncertain whether residual urine volume predicts the outcome of surgical treatment.**
- **It is uncertain whether residual urine volume indicates impending bladder or renal damage.**
- **Residual urine volume can be measured with sufficient accuracy noninvasively by transabdominal ultrasonography. The measurement variation due to the method used is less than the biologic range of patient PVR variation.**

PVR measurement can be performed by noninvasive (ultrasound) and by invasive (catheterization) methods. The most common method is urethral in-and-out catheterization. Invasive techniques are accurate if performed correctly, but they carry a small risk of discomfort, urethral injury, urinary tract infection, and transient bacteremia (which has not been quantified in the literature). In addition to standard diagnostic ultrasound instruments for abdominal scanning, there is a much smaller, portable, and less expensive device to measure PVR (BladderScan; Bard, Covington, GA). Its reported accuracy is comparable to more expensive ultrasound units and catheterization. With this device, the mean difference between estimated PVR and true PVR (that is, by catheterization) was 6.9 ml in 39 measurements taken in 20 children with neurogenic bladders (Massagli et al, 1990). In 164 measurements in adult patients, the correlation coefficient was $r = 0.79$ (Ireton et al, 1990).

The intraindividual variation in PVR measurement is significant regardless of the techniques used. Although repeated measurements may minimize the error, they are either costly (noninvasive techniques) or uncomfortable (invasive techniques) for the patient. Birch and colleagues (1988) reported that of 30 men with BPH, 66% had wide variations in PVR when three measurements were performed on the same day using five different formulas to calculate the volume. In 34% of patients, there was no difference among the three measurements. In 58%, at least two volumes were significantly different. In 8% of patients, all three were different. In most patients, two measurements were statistically similar, whereas the third one yielded different results. This study proves that the intraindividual variation of the amount of residual urine is greater than the differences between the various formulas used. Bruskewitz and co-workers (1982) found similarly wide variations of the measured amount when they performed repetitive measurements of PVR (repeated 2–5 times) by in-and-out catheterization on 47 men before prostatectomy. They also found no correlation between the amount of residual urine and any ureterocystoscopic or urodynamic findings, symptoms, or the presence or absence of a history of urinary tract infections.

Most clinical studies demonstrate minimal correlation between PVR and baseline measurements of symptoms, flow rate, or urodynamic measures of obstruction (Griffiths and Castro, 1970; Abrams and Griffiths, 1979; Shoukry et al, 1995).

However, Neal and associates (1987) found a significant association in 253 men between PVR, age, below-normal (undefined) Q_{max}, and high urethral resistance. Low voiding pressure, however, did not correlate well with PVR. The authors concluded that outflow obstruction is related to the development of increasing amounts of PVR urine. In the AUA Outcome Study, Barry and colleagues (1993) found a significant correlation between high PVR and low flow rates but no correlation with the IPSS (see Table 46–4).

Traditionally, urologists have assumed that increasing amounts of PVR denote BPH progression and are thus an indication for surgery. This concept underlies the common inclusion of PVR in each individual government's appropriateness criteria. Unfortunately, data are lacking to support the predictive value of PVR. Andersen (1982) studied 104 men with BPH and reported two patterns of BPH progression. The slow course was characterized by the development of high levels of PVR that resulted in decompensation of the detrusor muscle and eventually led to urinary retention. The fast course was associated with uninhibited detrusor contractions (UDCs). The amount of PVR, the presence of UDCs, and symptoms correlated poorly in the study. Nevertheless, Andersen recommended PVR as a safety parameter, when measured longitudinally throughout the clinical course of a patient with prostatism.

Jensen and co-workers (1988d) examined the prognostic value of PVR and 14 other clinical and urodynamic variables in relation to outcome of surgery in 120 men with prostatism. They found that PVR was the second best predictor of outcome after pressure-flow studies. However, the combination of these two predictors did not allow the authors to predict correctly the outcome in any of 14 patients who failed treatment.

Unpublished data from a randomized trial comparing TURP with watchful waiting (Veterans Affairs Cooperative Study Group*), demonstrate that **PVR does not predict the outcome of surgery,** and there appears to be little evidence to support criteria that require a certain amount of PVR before surgery is justified. In this trial, **high PVR did predict a slightly higher failure rate for watchful waiting.** However, the majority of men with large residual urine volume did not require surgery during the three-year duration of the trial.

In summary, **PVR is best viewed as a safety parameter. Men with significant residual urine should be monitored more closely if they elect nonsurgical therapy.** However,

*Bruskewitz, personal communication.

the majority of men with elevated PVRs are apparently not at high risk for complications.

Pressure-Flow Studies

If the initial evaluation, flow rate, and PVR are not sufficiently suggestive of bladder outlet obstruction, further urodynamic assessment by pressure-flow studies should be considered, especially if an invasive treatment is considered (i.e., surgery) or if surgical treatment has failed (Cockett et al, 1993; McConnell et al, 1994). **Pressure-flow studies differentiate between patients with a low Q_{max} secondary to obstruction and those whose low Q_{max} is caused by a decompensated or neurogenic bladder** (see Chapters 27 and 31). Pressure-flow studies may also identify high-pressure obstruction in symptomatic men with normal flow rates. The test-retest reliability of pressure-flow studies appears to be reasonable (Rosier et al, 1995). A new test, micturitional urethral pressure profilometry, correlates well with pressure-flow studies using the Abrams-Griffith or Schäfer nomograms (DuBeau et al, 1995).

Evidence for the usefulness of pressure-flow studies to predict surgical failure is equivocal. Some investigations have reported reduced failure rates, whereas others have reported that pressure-flow studies performed no better than Q_{max} measurements in this regard. Some patients who are excluded from surgery based on the pressure-flow test may still benefit from surgery.

Pressure-flow studies are most useful for distinguishing between urethral obstruction and impaired detrusor contractility. These studies should be performed when the distinction between the two will affect therapeutic decisions. **Patients with a history of neurologic diseases that are known to affect bladder or sphincteric function, as well as patients with normal flow rates (Q_{max} > 15 ml/second) but bothersome symptoms, may also benefit from urodynamic evaluation, especially if surgical therapy is contemplated.**

The value of pressure-flow plots is accepted by many urodynamic experts. Yet, there is little standardization in interpretation of these plots and somewhat arbitrary cut-off values for defining obstruction as opposed to nonobstruction. Investigators have proposed various ways to present the same sets of data and claim superior differentiation between patient groups (Abrams et al, 1979; Jensen et al, 1988b, 1988d; Schäfer et al, 1988, 1989; Spångberg et al, 1991). This variability in data presentation and definition has made it difficult to analyze the evidence that supports the use of pressure-flow studies.

The value of pressure-flow measurement in predicting treatment outcome is uncertain. Bruskewitz and associates (1983) studied prospectively the outcome of patients with urethral resistance either less than or greater than 0.6. The authors concluded that in patients with moderate prostatism, a cut-off value of R = 0.6 does not predict either indirect health outcomes (Q_{max}, detrusor pressure, resistance) or direct health outcomes (symptom score assessment, global subjective symptom assessment) after surgery. In a study by Abrams (1977), **the inclusion of pressure-flow data in the preoperative evaluation and indication for surgery reduced the subjective failure rate to 12% (down from 28%) when patients were certified as candidates for surgery without the urodynamic data.** However, a 28% failure rate is significantly higher than that reported in other TURP series (McConnell, et al, 1994). Jensen and Andersen (1990) recommended invasive urodynamic testing for patients with a Q_{max} greater than 15 ml/second. For the population in their study, this results in an additional 95% of patients excluded from surgery and a decrease in failure rate to 8.3%. The support for this recommendation has to be questioned, however, in light of an earlier study by Jensen and associates (1988d) that found most unsatisfied patients are incorrectly classified preoperatively even with urodynamic testing.

Pressure-flow studies permit more accurate categorization of patients. Abrams and associates (1979) used pressure-flow plots in addition to flow rate measurement. The study found that in about half the cases, the patients with prostatism could be correctly classified as obstructed or nonobstructed by Q_{max} alone but that the addition of the detrusor pressure at Q_{max} allowed correct classification in two thirds of patients. Combining the two parameters into a single urethral resistance factor did not help in the group encompassing two thirds of the patients. The remaining one third of the patients were assessed by pressure-flow plot. In many of these patients, both pressure and Q_{max} were low, indicating a decompensating detrusor muscle as the source for the low Q_{max}.

Schäfer and associates (1988, 1989) used sophisticated, computerized analysis of pressure-flow data to define passive and dynamic urethral resistance measures. They documented that approximately 25% of patients undergoing TURP are not obstructed, based on the investigators' criteria, although these patients may have a low Q_{max}. The improvement rate based on objective measures (Q_{max} and PVR) was 100% in patients categorized as severely obstructed but was lower in the mildly obstructed and nonobstructed patients.

The Schäfer model has been used and expanded by other investigators (Spångberg et al, 1991), but correlation of the objective results with direct health outcomes (symptom improvement) is again lacking. Others have employed computer programs to analyze pressure-flow plots, but they also do not report outcome data (Rollema et al, 1991). These computer-assisted urodynamic assessments need further evaluation before they can be recommended routinely.

Pressure-flow studies provide much more specific insight into detrusor function and the etiology of voiding dysfunction than do flow rate measurements. However, the limited number of outcome-based investigations performed demonstrate a modest additional value of pressure-flow studies over symptom and flow rate evaluation. The benefit of pressure-flow studies is clearest in those patients with significant symptoms who have a Q_{max} greater than 15 ml/second or in whom the initial evaluation suggests bladder dysfunction rather than BPH as the cause of patient symptoms.

Filling Cystometry (Cystometrography)

Filling cystometry adds limited information to the evaluation of most men with prostatism and is not recommended in routine cases (Cockett et al, 1993; McConnell et al, 1994). The test may have value in the evaluation of patients with known or suspected neurologic lesions and prostatism, but pressure-flow studies provide more specific information (Jensen et al, 1988c). In patients with suspected primary bladder or neurologic lesions and who cannot urinate (retention), filling cystometry may be useful.

Filling cystometry, an invasive urodynamic study (see Chapters 27 and 31), provides information on bladder capacity, the presence and threshold of UDCs, and bladder compliance. **UDCs are present in about 60% of men with prostatism and correlate strongly with irritative voiding symptoms** (McConnell et al, 1994). However, UDCs resolve in most patients after surgery. Only about one fourth of patients who have UDCs before treatment retain them afterward. Patients whose symptoms do not improve following surgery are more likely to have persistent UDCs, but preoperative cystometrography does not help identify those patients.

Although filling cystometry may demonstrate a poorly contractile detrusor in men with primary bladder dysfunction, pressure-flow studies provide much more insight into the interaction between bladder contraction and urethral resistance. Filling cystometry may be considered for men in urinary retention who cannot urinate for a pressure-flow study.

Urethrocystoscopy

Urethrocystoscopy is not recommended to determine the need for treatment (Cockett et al, 1993; McConnell et al, 1994). **The test is recommended for men with prostatism who have a history of microscopic or gross hematuria, urethral stricture disease (or risk factors, such as history of urethritis or urethral injury), bladder cancer, or prior lower urinary tract surgery (especially prior TURP). To help the surgeon determine the most appropriate technical approach, urethrocystoscopy may be considered in men with moderate-to-severe symptoms who have chosen (or require) surgical or other invasive therapy.**

Urethrocystoscopy provides visual documentation of the appearance of the prostatic urethra and bladder in men with BPH. Historically, many urologists believed that the visual appearance of the lower urinary tract defines the severity of disease or predicts the outcome of treatment. However, this common urologic procedure has been poorly studied. No data are available on the sensitivity, specificity, or predictive value of the test. Potential benefits of urethrocystoscopy include the ability to demonstrate prostatic enlargement and visual obstruction of the urethra and the bladder neck; identification of specific anatomic abnormalities that alter clinical decision making; identification of bladder stones, trabeculation, cellules, and diverticula; measurement of PVR; and the ruling out of unrelated bladder and urethral pathology. Potential harms include patient discomfort, anesthetic or sedative risk, urinary tract infection, bleeding, and urinary retention. However, the probability of any of these harms occurring is uncertain. Except for discomfort, their occurrence is likely to be infrequent.

The endoscopic appearance of the bladder and prostate is often believed to be helpful in the decision to treat. Although the linkage between the endoscopic appearance of the lower urinary tract and treatment outcome is poorly documented in the literature, available information suggests that the relationship is minimal. **The endoscopic demonstration of obstruction (e.g., so-called kissing lateral lobes) is of no predictive value. Bladder trabeculation may predict a slightly higher failure rate in patients managed by watchful waiting but does not predict the success or failure of surgery.** Urethrocystoscopy may, nevertheless, be useful in determining the technical feasibility of specific invasive therapies. For example, **if urethrocystoscopy reveals a large middle lobe, transurethral incision of the prostate is unlikely to be successful**. The decision to perform an open prostatectomy may be appropriately influenced by the shape of the gland, as well as its size. In all of these cases, however, the patient and his physician have already selected invasive therapy. **Therefore, urethrocystoscopy is performed to select (or rule out) specific techniques, not to determine the need for treatment.**

Imaging of the Urinary Tract

Upper urinary tract imaging is not recommended in the routine evaluation of men with prostatism unless they also have one or more of the following: hematuria, urinary tract infection, renal insufficiency (ultrasound recommended), a history of urolithiasis, or a history of urinary tract surgery (McConnell et al, 1994).

IVU, to image the urinary tract of men with BPH before treatment, was performed by 73.4% of urologists in the United States in the late 1980s (Holtgrewe et al, 1989). The number of urologists using ultrasonography to image the urinary tract is unknown. **IVU is associated with a 0.1% incidence of significant adverse events.** There are no direct adverse events known to be associated with ultrasonography.

Of all renal imaging studies performed in men with BPH, 70% to 75% are entirely normal (McConnell et al, 1994). Only a small fraction of the 25% to 30% of abnormal findings mandate changes in the management of the patient. The incidence of any significant findings is no higher in the urinary tract of men with BPH, compared with age- and sex-matched controls, except for bladder stones, diverticula, and trabeculation indicating the presence of bladder outlet obstruction. Bundrick and Katz (1986) reported a change in management in 2.2% (4 of 180) of patients, based on findings obtained on IVU in a population preselected by excluding men with hematuria, infections, and a history of bladder tumors. Pinck and associates (1980) deferred TURP in favor of a more urgent intervention in 2.5% (14 of 557). These data indicate that a change in management would result in about 10% of the 25% of patients in whom the imaging study is abnormal.

The presence or history of hematuria, renal insufficiency, urinary tract infection, and history of stones or prior urinary tract surgery increases the likelihood that IVU or ultrasonography will demonstrate clinically significant findings (Kreel et al, 1974; Andersen et al, 1977; Wilcox and Mitchell, 1977; Butler et al, 1978; Bauer et al, 1980; Morrison 1980; Christofferson and Moller, 1981; Wasserman et al, 1987; Juul et al, 1989). Donker and Kakiailatu (1978) reported that by screening those men with urinary tract infections, gross hematuria, and renal insufficiency, they would have diagnosed almost all of the abnormal findings in their population of 307 men with BPH. Although there are no conclusive data on the combined incidence of the important clinical predictors listed earlier, approximately one third of all men with BPH have one or another indication for urinary tract imaging.

Assuming that an indication for renal imaging exists, a number of investigators strongly recommend that, instead of IVU, ultrasonography combined with a KUB and a determination of the renal function by measurement of the serum creatinine should be used (Matthews et al, 1982; Lilienfeld et al, 1985; Cascione et al, 1987; Fidas et al, 1987; Hendrikx et al, 1988; Solomon and Van Niekerk, 1988; Stavropoulos et al, 1988).

REFERENCES

Epidemiology

Arrighi HM, Guess HA, Metter EJ, et al: Symptoms and signs of prostatism as risk factors for prostatectomy. Prostate 1990; 16:253.

Barry MJ, Boyle P, Garraway M, et al: Epidemiology and natural history of BPH. *In* Cockett ATK, Aso Y, Chatelain C, et al (eds): Proceedings of the Second International Consultation on Benign Prostatic Hyperplasia (BPH). Channel Islands, Scientific Communications International 1993, p 19.

Berry SJ, Coffey DS, Walsh PC, et al: The development of human benign prostatic hyperplasia with age. J Urol 1984; 132:474.

Bosch JLHR, Kranse R, Van Mastrigt R, et al: Reasons for the weak correlation between prostate volume and urethral resistance parameters in patients with prostatism. J Urol 1995; 153:689–693.

Chopra IJ, Tulchinsky D, Greenway FL: Estrogen-androgen imbalance in hepatic cirrhosis. Ann Intern Med 1973; 79:198.

Dai WS, Gutai JP, Kuller LH, et al: Cigarette smoking and serum sex hormones in men. Am J Epidemiol 1988; 128:796.

Daniell HW: Larger prostatic adenomas in obese men with no associated increase in obstructive uropathy. J Urol 1993a; 149:315.

Daniell HW: More stage A prostatic cancers, less surgery for benign hypertrophy in smokers. J Urol 1993b; 149:68.

Derbes VDP, Leche SM, Hooker CW: Incidence of benign prostate hyperplasia among the whites and negroes in New Orleans. J Urol 1937; 38:383–387.

Eldrup E, Lindholm J, Winkel P: Plasma sex hormones and ischemic heart disease. Clin Biochem 1987; 20:105.

Fang-Liu G: Incidence of benign prostatic hyperplasia and prostate cancer in China. Chinese J Surg 1993; 31:323–326.

Garraway WM, Collins GN, Lee RJ: High prevalence of benign prostatic hypertrophy in the community. Lancet 1991; 338:469–471.

Garraway WM, McKelvie G, Rogers A, et al: Benign prostatic hypertrophy influences on daily living in middle-aged and elderly men. Urology (Italy) 1992; 12:161–164.

Garraway WM, Russell EB, Lee RJ, et al: Impact of previously unrecognized benign prostatic hyperplasia on the daily activities of middle-aged and elderly men. Br J Gen Pract 1993; 43:318.

Girman CJ, Epstein RS, Jacobsen SJ, et al: Natural history of prostatism: Impact of urinary symptoms on quality of life in 2115 randomly selected community men. Urology 1994; 44:825.

Girman CJ, Jacobsen SJ, Guess HA, et al: Natural history of prostatism: Relationship among symptoms, prostate volume and peak urinary flow. J Urol 1995; 153:1510–1515.

Girman CJ, Panser LA, Chute CG, et al: Natural history of prostatism: Urinary flow rates in a population-based study. J Urol 1993; 150:887.

Glynn RJ, Campion EW, Bouchard GR, et al: The development of benign prostatic hyperplasia among volunteers in the Normative Aging Study. Am J Epidemiol 1985; 121:78.

Guess HA: Benign prostatic hyperplasia antecedents and natural history. Epidemiol Rev 1992; 14:131.

Guess HA: Epidemiology and natural history of benign prostatic hyperplasia. Urol Clin North Am 1995; 22:247–261.

Guess HA, Arrighi HM, Metter EJ, et al: The cumulative prevalence of prostatism matches the autopsy prevalence of benign prostatic hyperplasia. Prostate 1990; 17:241.

Guess HA, Chute CG, Garraway WM, et al: Similar level of urologic symptoms have similar impact in Scottish and American men—though Scots report less symptoms. J Urol 1993; 150:1701.

Isaacs JT, Coffey DS: Etiology and disease processes of benign prostatic hyperplasia. Prostate 1989; 2(Suppl 2):33–40.

Jakobsen H, Torp PS, Juul N: Ultrasonic evaluation of age-related human prostatic growth and development of benign prostatic hyperplasia. Scand J Urol Nephrol 1988; 107(Suppl):26.

Lytton B: Interracial incidence of benign prostatic hypertrophy. *In* Hinman F, ed: Benign Prostatic Hypertrophy. New York, Springer-Verlag, 1983, p 22.

Meikle AW, Liu XH, Taylor GN, et al: Nicotine and cotinine effects of 3-alpha hydroxysteroid dehydrogenase in canine prostate. Life Sci 1988; 43:1845.

Morrison AS: Risk Factors for surgery for prostatic hypertrophy. Am J Epidemiol 1992; 135:974.

Roberts RO, Jacobsen SJ, Rhodes T, et al: Cigarette smoking and prostatism: A biphasic association? Urology 1994; 43:797.

Sagnier PP, Macfarlane G, Teillac P, et al: Impact of symptoms of prostatism on bothersomeness and quality of life of men in the French community. J Urol 1995; 153:669.

Seitter WR, Barrett-Connor E: Cigarette smoking, obesity and benign prostatic hypertrophy: A prospective population-based study. Am J Epidemiol 1992; 135:500.

Sidney S: Vasectomy and the risk of prostatic cancer and benign prostatic hypertrophy. J Urol 1987; 138:795.

Sidney S, Quesenberry CP, Sadler MC, et al: Incidence of surgically treated benign prostatic hypertrophy and of prostate cancer among black and white multiphasic examinees in a prepaid health care plan. Am J Epidemiol 1991a; 134:825.

Sidney S, Quesenberry C, Sadler MC, et al: Risk factors for surgically treated benign prostatic hyperplasia in a prepaid health care plan. Urology 1991b; 38(Suppl 1):13.

Tsukamoto T, Kumamoto Y, Masumori N, et al: Japanese men have lower increase in prostate growth and greater decrease in peak urinary flow rate with age than American men. J Urol 1995a; 153:477A.

Tsukamoto T, Kumamoto Y, Masumori N, et al: Prevalence of prostatism in Japanese men in a population-based study with comparison to a similar American study. J Urol 1995b; 154:391–395.

Etiology

Alarid ET, Rubin JS, Young P: Keratinocyte growth factor functions in epithelial induction during seminal vesicle development. Proc Natl Acad Sci USA 1994; 91:1074–1078.

Barrack ER, Berry SJ: DNA synthesis in the canine prostate: Effects of androgen and estrogen treatment. Prostate 1987; 10:45–56.

Barrack ER, Bujnovszky P, Walsh PC: Subcellular distribution of androgen receptors in human normal, benign hyperplastic, and malignant prostatic tissue: Characterization of nuclear salt-resistant receptors. Cancer Res 1983; 43:1107–1116.

Bedford MT, van Helden PD: Hypomethylation of DNA in pathological conditions of the human prostate. Cancer Res 1987; 47:5274.

Begun FP, Story MT, Hopp KA, et al: Regional concentration of basic fibroblast growth factor in normal and benign hyperplastic human prostates. J Urol 1995; 153:839–843.

Berry SJ, Coffey DS, Strandberg JD et al: Effect of age, castration, and testosterone replacement on the development and restoration of canine benign prostatic hyperplasia. Prostate 1986a; 9:295.

Berry SJ, Coffey DS, Ewing LL: Effects of aging on prostate growth in beagles. Am J Physiol 1986b; 250:R1039–R1046.

Berry SJ, Isaacs JT: Prostatic growth and androgen metabolism with aging in the dog versus the rat. Endocrinology 1984; 114:511–516.

Blotnick S, Peoples GE, Freeman MR, et al: T lymphocytes synthesize and export heparin-binding epidermal growth factor–like growth factor and basic fibroblast growth factor, mitogens for vascular cells and fibroblasts: Differential production and release by CD4+ and CD8+ T cells. Proc Natl Acad Sci USA 1994; 91:2890–2894.

Cunha GR, Chung LWK, Shannon JM, et al: Hormone-induced morphogenesis and growth: Role of mesenchymal-epithelial interactions. Recent Prog Horm Res 1983; 39:559.

Dalton DP, Lee C, Huprikar S, et al: Nonadrogenic role of testis in enhancing ventral prostate growth in rats. Prostate 1990; 16:225.

Darras FS, Lee C, Huprikar S, et al: Evidence for a non-androgenic role of testis and epididymis in androgen-supported growth of the rat ventral prostate. J Urol 1992; 148:432.

DeKlerk DP, Coffey DS, Ewing LL, et al: Comparison of spontaneous and experimentally induced canine prostatic hyperplasia. J Clin Invest 1979; 64:842–849.

Ekman P, Barrack ER, Greene GL, et al: Estrogen receptors in human prostate: Evidence for multiple binding sites. J Clin Endocrinol Metab 1983; 57:166–176.

Freeman MR, Schneck FX, Gagnon M, et al: Peripheral blood T lymphocytes and T cells infiltrating human cancers express vascular endothelial growth factor: A potential role for T cells in angiogenesis. Cancer Res 1995; 55:4140–4145.

Husmann DA, Wilson CM, McPhaul MJ, et al: Antipeptide antibodies to two distinct regions of the androgen receptor localize the receptor protein to the nuclei of target cells in the rat and human prostate. Endocrin 1990; 126:2359–2368.

Isaacs JT: Antagonistic effect of androgen on prostatic cell death. Prostate 1984; 5:545.

Juniewicz PE, Berry SJ, Coffey DS, et al: Requirement of testis in establishing sensitivity of canine prostate to develop benign prostatic hyperplasia. J Urol 1994; 152:996.

Kerr JFR, Searle J: Deletion of cells by apoptosis during castration induced involution in the rat prostate. Virchows Arch B Cell Pathol 1973; 13:87–102.

Kyprianou N, Isaacs JT: Expression of transforming growth factor-β in the rat ventral prostate during castration-induced programmed cell death. Mol Endocrinol 1989; 3:1515.

Lee C: Physiology of castration-induced regression in rat prostate. *In* Murphy GP, Sandbreg AA, Karr JP, eds: The Prostatic Cell: Structure and function. New York, Alan R. Liss, Inc., 1981, pp 145–159.

Lee C, Sensibar JA, Dudek SM, et al: Prostatic ductal system in rats: Regional variation in morphological and functional activities. Biol Reprod 1990; 43:1079–1086.

McConnell JD: Prostatic growth: New insights into hormonal regulation. Br J Urol 1995; 76(Suppl 1):5–10.

McKeehan WL, Adams PS, Rosser MP: Direct mitogenic effects of insulin, epidermal growth factor, glucocorticoid, cholera toxin, unknown pituitary factors and possibly prolactin, but not androgen, on normal rat prostate epithelial cells in serum-free, primary cell culture. Cancer Res 1984; 44:1998.

McKeehan WL, Adams PS: Heparin binding growth factor/prostatropin attenuates inhibition of rat prostate tumor epithelial cell growth by transforming growth factor type beta. In Vitro Cell Dev Biol 1988; 24:243.

Martikainen P, Kyprianou N, Isaacs JT: Effect of transforming growth factor-β on proliferation and death of rat prostatic cells. Endocrinology 1990; 127:2963–2968.

Montpetit ML, Lawless KR, Tenniswood M: Androgen repressed messages in the rat ventral prostate. Prostate 1986; 8:25–26.

Moore RJ, Gazak JM, Quebbeman JF, et al: Concentration of dihydrotestosterone and 3α-androstanediol in naturally occurring and androgen induced prostatic hyperplasia in the dog. J Clin Invest 1979; 64:1003.

Naslund JF, Coffey DS: The differential effects of neonatal androgen, estrogen, and progesterone on adult prostate growth. J Urol 1986; 136:1136–1140.

Oesterling JE, Juniewicz PE, Walters JR, et al: Aromatase inhibition in the dog. II. Effect of growth function and pathology of the prostate. J Urol 1988; 139:832–839.

Orlandi A, Rapraz P, Gabbianai G: Proliferative activity and alpha-smooth muscle actin expression in cultured rat aortic smooth muscle cells are differently modulated by transforming growth factor beta-1 and heparin. Exp Cell Res 1994; 214:528–536.

Partin AW, Getzenberg RH, CarMichael MJ, et al: Nuclear matrix protein patterns in human benign prostatic hyperplasia and prostate cancer. Cancer Res 1993; 53:744.

Partin AW, Oesterling JE, Epstein JI, et al: Influence of age and endocrine factors on the volume of benign prostatic hyperplasia. J Urol 1991; 145:405–409.

Partin AW, Page WF, Lee BR, et al: Concordance rates for benign prostatic disease among twins suggest hereditary influence. Urology 1994; 44:646.

Peters CA, Walsh PC: The effect of nafarelin acetate, a luteinizing hormone-releasing hormone agonist, on benign prostatic hyperplasia. N Engl J Med 1987; 317:599–604.

Rennie PS, Bruchovsky N, Goldenberg SL: Relationship of androgen receptors to the growth and regression of the prostate. Am J Clin Oncol 1988; 11(Suppl 2):S13–17.

Roberts RO, Rhodes T, Panser LA, et al: Association between family history of benign prostatic hyperplasia and urinary symptoms: Results of a population-based study. Am J Epidemiol 1995; 142:965–973.

Roberts AB, Sporn MB: Physiological actions and clinical applications of transforming growth factor-beta (TGF-beta). Growth Factors 1993; 8:1–9.

Roehrborn CG, Lange JL, George FW, et al: Changes in amount and intracellular distribution of androgen receptor in human foreskin as a function of age. JCI 1987; 79:44–47.

Russell DW, Wilson JD: Steroid 5α-reductase: Two genes/two enzymes. Annu Rev Biochem 1994; 63:25.

Sanda MG, Beaty IH, Stutzman RE, et al: Genetic susceptibility of benign prostatic hyperplasia. J Urol 1994; 152(1):115–119.

Silver RI, Wiley EL, Thigpen AE, et al: Cell type specific expression of steroid 5α-reductase 2. J Urol 1994a; 152:438–442.

Silver RI, Wiley EL, Davis DL, et al: Expression and regulation of steroid 5α-reductase 2 in prostate disease. J Urol 1994b; 152:433–437.

Sporn MB, Roberts AB: TGF-β: Problems and prospects. Cell Regul 1990; 1:875–882.

Sporn MB, Roberts AB: Interactions of retinoids and transforming growth factor-β in regulation of cell differentiation and proliferation. Mole Endocrinol 1991; 5:3–7.

Steiner MS: Review of peptide growth factors in benign prostatic hyperplasia and urological malignancy. J Urol 1995; 153:1085–1096.

Story MT, Livingston B, Baeten L, et al: Cultured human prostate-derived fibroblasts produce a factor that stimulates their growth with properties indistinguishable from basic fibroblast growth factor. Prostate 1989; 15:355–365.

Story MT, Hopp KA, Meier DA, et al: Influence of transforming growth factor beta 1 and other growth factors on basic fibroblast growth factor level and proliferation of cultured human prostate-derived fibroblasts. Prostate 1993; 22:183–197.

Sutkowski DM, Kasjanski RZ, Sensibar JA, et al: Effect of spermatocele fluid on growth of human prostatic cells in culture. J Androl 1993; 14:233.

Takane KK, Wilson JD, McPhaul MJ: Decreased levels of the androgen receptor in the mature rat phallus are associated with decreased levels of androgen receptor messenger ribonucleic acid. Endocrin 1991; 129(2): 1093–1100.

Tenniswood M: Role of epithelial-stromal interactions in the control of gene expression in the prostate: an hypothesis. Prostate 1986; 9:375–385.

Theyer G, Kramer G, Assman I, et al: Phenogypic characterization of infiltrating leukocytes in benign prostatic hyperplasia. Lab Invest 1992; 66:96–107.

Trachtenberg J, Hicks LL, Walsh PC: Androgen- and estrogen-receptor content in spontaneous and experimentally induced canine prostatic hyperplasia. 1980; 65:1051–1057.

Tutrone RF, Ball RA, Ornitz DM: Benign prostatic hyperplasia in a transgenic mouse: a new hormonally sensitive investigatory model. J Urol 1993; 149:633–639.

Walsh PC, Hutchins GM, Ewing LL: Tissue content of dihydrotestosterone in human prostatic hyperplasia is not supranormal. J Clin Invest 1983; 72:1772–1777.

Walsh PE, Wilson JD: The induction of prostatic hypertrophy in the dog with androstanediol. J Clin Invest 1976; 57:1093–1097.

White JJ, Nuewirth H, Miller CD, Schneider EL: DNA alterations in prostatic adenocarcinoma and benign prostatic hyperplasia: Detection by DNA fingerprint analyses. Mutat Res 1990; 237:37.

Wilding G, Valverius E, Knabbe C, et al: Role of transforming growth factor-α in human prostate cancer cell growth. Prostate 1989; 15:1–12.

Yan G, Fukabori Y, Nikolaropoulost S, et al: Heparin-binding keratinocyte growth factor is a candidate stromal to epithelial cell andromedin. Mol Endocrinol 1992; 6:2123.

Pathophysiology

Abrams PH, Farrar DJ, Turner-Warwick RT, et al: The results of prostatectomy: A symptomatic and urodynamic analysis of 152 patients. J Urol 1979; 121:640–642.

Barrack ER, Berry SJ: DNA synthesis in the canine prostate: Effects of androgen and estrogen treatment. Prostate 1987; 10:45–56.

Barry MJ, Fowler FJ Jr, O'Leary MP, et al and the AUA Measurement Committee: The American Urological Association Symptom Index for benign prostatic hyperplasia. J Urol 1992a; 148:1549–1557.

Barry MJ, Cockett ATK, Holtgrewe HL, et al: Relationship of symptoms of prostatism to commonly used physiological and anatomical measures of the severity of benign prostatic hyperplasia. J Urol 1993; 150:351–358.

Bosch JLHR, Kranse R, Van Mastrigt R, et al: Reasons for the weak correlation between prostate volume and urethral resistance parameters in patients with prostatism. J Urol 1995; 153:689–693.

Caine M, Schuger L: The "capsule" in benign prostatic hypertrophy. U.S.

Department of Health and Human Services, NIH Publication No. 87-2881, 1987, p 221.
Cockett ATK, Khoury S, Aso Y, et al: Proceedings of the 2nd International Consultation on Benign Prostatic Hyperplasia (BPH), Scientific Communication International Ltd., 1993.
Ekman P: BPH epidemiology and risk factors. Prostate 1989; 2(Suppl 2):23–28.
Franks LM: Benign prostatic hypertrophy: Gross and microscopic anatomy. Department of Health Education and Welfare, NIH Publication No. 76-1113-63, 1976.
Gong G, Johnson ML, Pettinger WA: Testosterone regulation of renal α_{2B}-adrenergic receptor mRNA levels. Hypertension 1995; 25:350–355.
Gosling JA, Gilpin SA, Dixon JS, et al: Decrease in the autonomic innervation of human detrusor muscle in outflow obstruction. J Urol 1986; 136:501.
Hieble JP, Bylund DB, Clarke DE, et al: International union of pharmacology x. Recommendation for nomenclature of α_1-adrenoceptors: Consensus update. Pharmacol Rev 1995; 47:267–270.
Kariya KI, Farrance IKG, Simpson PC: Transcriptional enhancer factor-1 in cardiac myocytes interacts with an α_1-adrenergic- and β-protein kinase C-inducible element in the rat β-myosin heavy chain promoter. J Biol Chem 1993; 268:26658–26662.
Ko DSC, Fenster HN, Chambers K, et al: The correlation of multichannel urodynamic pressure-flow studies and American Urological Association Symptom Index in the evaluation of benign prostatic hyperplasia. J Urol 1995; 154:396–398.
Kobayashi S, Tang R, Wang B, et al: Localization of endothelin receptors in the human prostate. J Urol 1994a; 151:763.
Kobayashi S, Tang R, Wang B, et al: The binding and functional properties of endothelin receptor subtypes in the human prostate. Mol Pharmacol 1994b; 45:306.
Lepor H, Tang R, Meretyk S, Shapiro E: Alpha$_1$ adrenoceptor subtypes in the human prostate. J Urol 1993a; 149:640–642.
Lepor H, Tang R, Shapiro E: The alpha-adrenoceptor subtype mediating the tension of human prostatic smooth muscle. Prostate 1993b; 22:301–307.
Levin RM, Monson FC, Haugaard N, et al: Genetic and cellular characteristics of bladder outlet obstruction. Urol Clin North Am 1995; 22:263–283.
Matsui H, Makino N, Yano K, et al: Modulation of adrenergic receptors during regression of cardiac hypertrophy. J Hypertens 1994; 12:1353–1357.
McConnell JD, Barry MJ, Bruskewitz RC, et al: Benign Prostatic Hyperplasia: Diagnosis and Treatment. Clinical Practice Guideline. No. 8, AHCPR Publication No 94-0582. Rockville, MD: Agency for Health Care Policy and Research, Public Health Service, US Department of Health and Human Services, 1994.
McNeal JE: Origin and evolution of benign prostatic enlargement. Invest Urol 1978; 15:340.
McNeal J: Pathology of benign prostatic hyperplasia: Insight into etiology. Urol Clin North Am 1990; 17:477.
Napalkov P, Maisonneuve P, Boyle P: Worldwide patterns of prevalence and mortality from benign prostatic hyperplasia. Urol 1995; 46(3 Suppl A):41–46.
Price DT, Schwinn DA, Lomasney JW, et al: Identification, quantification, and localization of mRNA for three distinct alpha$_1$ adrenergic receptor subtypes in human prostate. J Urol 1993; 150:546–551.
Schäfer W: Principles and clinical application of advanced urodynamic analysis of voiding function. Urol Clin North Am 1990; 17:553.
Schwinn DA: Adrenergic receptors: unique localization in human tissues. Advances in Pharmacology 1994; 31:333–341.
Shapiro E, Hartanto V, Lepor H: Anti-desmin vs anti-actin for quantifying the area density of prostate smooth muscle. Prostate 1992a; 20:259.
Shapiro E, Hartanto V, Lepor H: Quantifying the smooth muscle content of the prostate using double-immuno-enzymatic staining and color assisted image analysis. J Urol 1992b; 147:1167.
Shapiro E, Hartanto V, Lepor H: The response to alpha blockade in benign prostatic hyperplasia is related to the percent area density of prostate smooth muscle. Prostate 1992c; 21:297.
Steers WD, Ciambotti J, Erdman S, et al: Morphological plasticity in efferent pathways to the urinary bladder of the rat following urethral obstruction. J Neurosci 1990; 19:1943.
Yalla SV, Sullivan MP, Lecamwasam HS, et al: Correlation of American Urological Association Symptom Index with obstructive and nonobstructive prostatism. J Urol 1995; 153:674–680.

Diagnosis

Abrams PH: Prostatism and prostatectomy: The value of urine flow rate measurement in the preoperative assessment for operation. J Urol 1977; 117:70–71.
Abrams PH, Farrar DJ, Turner-Warwick RT, et al: The results of prostatectomy: A symptomatic and urodynamic analysis of 152 patients. J Urol 1979; 121:640–642.
Abrams PH, Griffiths DJ: The assessment of prostatic obstruction from urodynamic measurements and from residual urine. Br J Urol 1979; 51:129–134.
Andersen JT, Jacobsen O, Strandgaard L: The diagnostic value of intravenous pyelography in intravesical obstruction in males. Scand J Urol Nephrol 1977; 11:225–230.
Andersen JT: Prostatism III. Detrusor hyperreflexia and residual urine. Clinical and urodynamic aspects and the influence of surgery on the prostate. Scand J Urol Nephrol 1982; 16:25–30.
Barry MJ, Cockett ATK, Holtgrewe HL, et al: Relationship of symptoms of prostatism to commonly used physiological and anatomical measures of the severity of benign prostatic hyperplasia. J Urol 1993; 150:351–358.
Barry MJ, Fowler FJ Jr, O'Leary MP, et al and the AUA Measurement Committee: The American Urological Association Symptom Index for benign prostatic hyperplasia. J Urol 1992a; 148:1549–1557.
Barry MJ, Fowler FJ Jr, O'Leary MP, et al and the AUA Measurement Committee: Correlation of the American Urological Association Symptom Index with self-administered versions of the Madsen-Iverson, Boyarsky and Maine Medical Assessment Program Symptom Indexes. J Urol 1992b; 148:1558–1563.
Bauer DL, Garrison RW, McRoberts JW: The health and cost implications of routine excretory urography before transurethral prostatectomy. J Urol 1980; 123:386–389.
Birch NC, Hurst G, Doyle PT: Serial residual volumes in men with prostatic hypertrophy. Br J Urol 1988; 62:571–575.
Bissada NK, Finkbeiner AE, Redman JF: Accuracy of preoperative estimation of resection weight in transurethral prostatectomy. J Urol 1976; 116:201–202.
Bruskewitz RC, Iversen P, Madsen PO: Value of postvoid residual urine determination in evaluation of prostatism. Urology 1982; 20:602–604.
Bruskewitz RC, Jensen KM-E, Iversen P, Madsen PO: The relevance of minimum urethral resistance in prostatism. J Urol 1983; 129:769–771.
Bundrick TJ, Katz PG: Excretory urography in patients with prostatism. Am J Roentgenol 1986; 147:957–959.
Butler MR, Donnelly B, Komaranchat A: Intravenous urography in evaluation of acute retention. Urology 1978; 12:464–466.
Cascione CJ, Bartone FF, Hussain MB: Transabdominal ultrasound versus excretory urography in preoperative evaluation of patients with prostatism. J Urol 1987; 137:883–885.
Chancellor MB, Blaivas JG, Kaplan SA, Axelrod S: Bladder outlet obstruction versus impaired detrusor contractility: The role of uroflow. J Urol 1991; 145:810–812.
Christofferson I, Moller I: Excretory urography: A superfluous routine examination in patients with prostatic hypertrophy. Eur Urol 1981; 7(2):65–67.
Cockett ATK, Khoury S, Aso Y, et al, eds: Proceedings of the 2nd International Consultation on BPH. Channel Islands, U.K., Scientific Communication International Ltd., 1993.
Di Mare JR, Fish SR, Harper JM, Politano VA: Residual urine in normal male subjects. J Urol 1963; 96:180–181.
Donker PJ, Kakiailatu F: Preoperative evaluation of patients with bladder outlet obstruction with particular regard to excretory urography. J Urol 1978; 120:685–686.
Donkervoort T, Zinner NR, Sterling AM, et al: Megestrol acetate in treatment of benign prostatic hypertrophy. Urology 1975; 6:580–587.
DuBeau CE, Sullivan MP, Cravalho E, et al: Correlation between micturitional urethral pressure profile and pressure-flow criteria in bladder outlet obstruction. J Urol 1995; 154(2 Pt 1):498–503.
Fidas A, Mackinlay JY, Wild SR, Chisholm GD: Ultrasound as an alternative to intravenous urography in prostatism. Clin Radiol 1987; 38:479–482.
Gleason DM, Bottaccini MR, Drach GW, Layton TN: Urinary flow velocity as an index of male voiding function. J Urol 1982; 128:1363–1367.
Griffiths HJL, Castro J: An evaluation of the importance of residual urine. Br J Radiol 1970; 43:409–413.
Groshar D, Embon OM, Koritny ES, et al: Radionuclide assessment of bladder-emptying function in normal male population and in patients before and after prostatectomy. Urology 1991; 37:353–357.
Hendrikx AJM, Doesburg WH, Reintjes AGM, et al: Effectiveness of ultrasound in the preoperative evaluation of patients with prostatism. Prostate 1988; 13:199–208.
Hinman F, Cox CE: Residual urine volume in normal male subjects. J Urol 1967; 97:641–645.

Holtgrewe HL, Mebust WK, Dowd JB, et al: Transurethral prostatectomy: Practice aspects of the dominant operation in American urology. J Urol 1989; 141:248–253.

Holtgrewe HL, Valk WL: Factors influencing the mortality and morbidity of transurethral prostatectomy: A study of 2,015 cases. J Urol 1962; 87:450–459.

Ireton RC, Krieger JN, Cardenas DD, et al: Bladder volume determination using a dedicated, portable ultrasound scanner. J Urol 1990; 143:909–911.

Jensen KM-E, Andersen JT: Urodynamic implications of benign prostatic hyperplasia. Urologe [A] 1990; 29:1–4.

Jensen KM-E, Bruskewitz RC, Iversen P, Madsen PO: Spontaneous uroflowmetry in prostatism. Urology 1984; 24:403–409.

Jensen KM-E, Jørgensen JB, Mogensen P: Urodynamics in prostatism I. Prognostic value of uroflowmetry. Scand J Urol Nephrol 1988a; 22:109–117.

Jensen KM-E, Jørgensen JB, Mogensen P: Urodynamics in prostatism II. Prognostic value of pressure-flow study combined with stop-flow test. Scand J Urol Nephrol Suppl 1988b; 114:72–77.

Jensen KM-E, Jørgensen JB, Mogensen P: Urodynamics in prostatism III. Prognostic value of medium-fill water cystometry. Scand J Urol Nephrol Suppl 1988c; 114:78–83.

Jensen KM-E, Jørgensen JB, Mogensen P: Urodynamics in prostatism IV. Search for prognostic patterns as evaluated by linear discriminant analysis. Scand J Urol Nephrol Suppl 1988d; 114:84–86.

Juul N, Torp-Pedersen S, Nielsen H: Abdominal ultrasound versus intravenous urography in the evaluation of infravesically obstructed males. Scand J Urol Nephrol 1989; 23:89–92.

Kreel L, Elton A, Habershon R, et al: Use of intravenous urography. BMJ 1974; 4:31–33.

Lilienfeld RM, Berman M, Khedkar M, Sporer A: Comparative evaluation of intravenous urogram and ultrasound in prostatism. Urology 1985; 26:310–312.

Massagli TL, Jaffe KM, Cardenas DD: Ultrasound measurement of urine volume of children with neurogenic bladder. Dev Med Child Neurol 1990; 32:314–318.

Matthews PN, Quayle JB, Joseph AEA, et al: The use of ultrasound in the investigation of prostatism. Br J Urol 1982; 54:536–538.

McConnell JD, Barry MJ, Bruskewitz RC, et al: Benign Prostatic Hyperplasia: Diagnosis and Treatment. Clinical Practice Guideline. No. 8, AHCPR Publication No 94-0582. Rockville, MD: Agency for Health Care Policy and Research, Public Health Service, US Department of Health and Human Services, 1994.

McLoughlin J, Gill KP, Abel PD, Williams G: Symptoms versus flow rates versus urodynamics in the selection of patients for prostatectomy. Br J Urol 1990; 66:303–305.

Mebust WK, Holtgrewe HL, Cockett ATK, Peters PC, and Writing Committee: Transurethral prostatectomy: Immediate and postoperative complications. A cooperative study of 13 participating institutions evaluating 3,885 patients. J Urol 1989; 141:243–247.

Melchior J, Valk WL, Foret JD, Mebust WK: Transurethral prostatectomy in the azotemic patient. J Urol 1974; 112:643–646.

Messing EM, Young TB, Hunt VB: The significance of asymptomatic microhematuria in men 50 or more years old: Findings of a home screening study using urinary dipsticks. J Urol 1987; 137:919–922.

Meyhoff HH, Ingemann L, Nordling J, Hald T: Accuracy in preoperative estimation of prostatic size. A comparative evaluation of rectal palpation, intravenous pyelography, urethral closure pressure profile recording and cystourethroscopy. Scand J Urol Nephrol 1981; 15:45–51.

Mohr DN, Offord KP, Owen RA, Melton LJ: Asymptomatic microhematuria and urologic disease. JAMA 1986; 256:224–229.

Mohr DN, Offord KP, Melton LJ: Isolated asymptomatic microhematuria: A cross sectional analysis of test-positive and test-negative patients. J Gen Intern Med 1987; 2:318–324.

Morrison JD: Help or habit? Excretion urography before prostatectomy. Br J Clin Pract 1980; 34:239–241.

Mukamel E, Nissenkorn I, Boner G, Servadio C: Occult progressive renal damage in the elderly male due to benign prostatic hypertrophy. J Am Geriatr Soc 1979;27:403–406.

Napalkov P, Maisonneuve P, Boyle P: Worldwide patterns of prevalence and mortality from benign prostatic hyperplasia. Urology 1995; 46(Suppl 3A):41–46.

Neal DE, Styles RA, Powell PH, Ramsden PD: Relationship between detrusor function and residual urine in men undergoing prostatectomy. Br J Urol 1987; 60:560–566.

Pinck BD, Corrigan MJ, Jasper P: Pre-prostatectomy excretory urography: Does it merit the expense? J Urology 1980; 123:390–391.

Preventive Services Task Force (US): Guide to clinical preventive services: An assessment of the effectiveness of 169 interventions. Baltimore, Williams & Wilkins, 1989, p 419.

Roehrborn CG, Chinn HK, Fulgham PF, et al: The role of transabdominal ultrasound in the preoperative evaluation of patients with benign prostatic hypertrophy. J Urol 1986; 135:1190–1193.

Rollema HJ, van Mastrigt R, Janknegt RA: Urodynamic assessment and quantification of prostatic obstruction before and after transurethral resection of the prostate: Standardization with the aid of the computer program CLIM. Urol Int Suppl 1991; 1:52–54.

Rollema HJ, van Mastrigt R: Objective analysis of prostatism: A clinical application of the computer program CLIM. Neurourol Urodyn 1991; 10:71–76.

Rosier PF, de la Rosette JJ, Koldewijn EL, et al: Variability of pressure-flow analysis parameters in repeated cystometry in patients with benign prostatic hyperplasia. J Urol 1995; 153:1520–1525.

Sagnier PP, MacFarlane G, Teillac P, et al: Impact of symptoms of prostatism on level of bother and quality of life of men in the French community. J Urol 1995; 153(3 Pt 1):669–673.

Schäfer W, Noppeney R, Rhbben H, Lutzeyer W: The value of free flow rate and pressure/flow-studies in the routine investigation of BPH patients. Neurourol Urodyn 1988; 7:219–21.

Schäfer W, Rhbben H, Noppeney R, Deutz F-J: Obstructed and unobstructed prostatic obstruction. A plea for urodynamic objectivation of bladder outflow obstruction in benign prostatic hyperplasia. World J Urol 1989; 6:198–203.

Schäfer W: Principles and clinical application of advanced urodynamic analysis of voiding function. Urol Clin North Am 1990; 17:553.

Scott FB, Cardus D, Quesada EM, Riles T: Uroflowmetry before and after prostatectomy (Pt 2). South Med J 1967; 60:948–952.

Shoukry I, Susset JG, Elhilali MM, Dutartre D: Role of uroflowmetry in the assessment of lower urinary tract obstruction in adult males (Pt 2). Br J Urol 1975; 47:559–566.

Simonsen O, Møller-Madsen B, Dorflinger T, et al: The significance of age on symptoms and urodynamic and cystoscopic findings in benign prostatic hypertrophy. Urol Res 1987; 15:355–358.

Siroky MB, Olsson CA, Krane RJ: The flow rate nomogram II: Clinical correlation. J Urol 1980; 123:208–210.

Siroky MB, Olsson CA, Krane RJ: The flow rate nomogram I: development. J Urol 1979; 122:665–668.

Solomon DJ, Van Niekerk JPDV: Ultrasonography should replace intravenous urography in the pre-operative evaluation of prostatism. S Afr Med J 1988; 74:407–408.

Spångberg A, Teriö H, Ask P, Engberg A: Pressure/flow studies preoperatively and postoperatively in patients with benign prostatic hypertrophy: Estimation of the urethral pressure/flow relation and urethral elasticity. Neurourol Urodyn 1991; 10:139–167.

Stamey TA, Yang N, Hay AR, et al: Prostate-specific antigen as a serum marker for adenocarcinoma of the prostate. N Engl J Med 1987; 317:909.

Stavropoulos N, Christodoulou K, Chamilos E, et al: Evaluation of patients with benign prostatic hypertrophy: IVU versus ultrasound. J R Coll Surg Edinb 1988; 33:140–142.

Wasserman NF, Lapointe S, Eckmann DR, Rosel PR: Assessment of prostatism: Role of intravenous urography. Radiology 1987; 165:831–835.

Wilcox RG, Mitchell JRA: Intravenous urography in the management of acute retention. Lancet 1977; i:1247–1249.

47
NATURAL HISTORY, EVALUATION, AND NONSURGICAL MANAGEMENT OF BENIGN PROSTATIC HYPERPLASIA

Herbert Lepor, M.D.

OVERVIEW

The term benign prostatic hyperplasia (BPH) has very different connotations for the pathologist, radiologist, urodynamicist, practicing urologist, and patient. BPH to the pathologist is a microscopic diagnosis characterized by cellular proliferation of the stromal and epithelial elements of the prostate (Strandberg, 1993). The radiologist makes the diagnosis of BPH in the presence of bladder base elevation on the cystogram phase of the intravenous pyelogram, or an enlarged prostate on diagnostic imaging studies of the male pelvis (Smith and Resnick, 1993). The hallmark of BPH to the urodynamicist is the synchronous observation of elevated voiding pressure and a low urinary flow rate in the absence of other disease processes that cause bladder outlet obstruction (Abrams, 1994). To the practicing urologist, BPH represents a constellation of signs and symptoms that develop in the male population in association with aging and prostatic enlargement presumably due to bladder outlet obstruction (Shapiro and Lepor, 1995). The patient is typically concerned about the impact of BPH on quality of life rather than the presence of cellular proliferation, prostatic enlargement, or elevated voiding pressures. Owing to the diverse connotations of the term BPH, it is necessary to define BPH as microscopic BPH, macroscopic BPH, or clinical BPH. **Microscopic BPH** represents histologic evidence of cellular proliferation of the prostate. **Macroscopic BPH** refers to enlargement of the prostate resulting from microscopic BPH. **Clinical BPH** represents the lower urinary tract symptoms and bladder dysfunction resulting from macroscopic BPH.

Microscopic BPH describes a proliferative process of the stromal and epithelial elements of the prostate (Bartsch et al, 1979). The proliferative process originates in the transition zone and the periurethral glands (McNeal, 1983). Microscopic BPH is rarely identified in males younger than 40 years of age (Berry et al, 1984). The autopsy incidence of BPH is age dependent, the proliferative process being present in approximately 70% and 90% of males in their seventh and ninth decades of life, respectively. The development of microscopic BPH requires aging and testes as the source of androgens (Walsh, 1986). Androgens play a passive role in the proliferative process. The specific biochemical event that initiates and promotes microscopic BPH has yet to be identified and characterized. Growth factors presumably are involved through autocrine and paracrine stromal epithelial interactions (Steiner, 1993). The pathogenesis of BPH is reviewed in Chapter 46.

Macroscopic BPH describes an enlarged prostate. Digital rectal examination provides an estimate of prostate size. The transition zone (inner gland) accounts for the majority of BPH tissue. The transition zone volume can be quantified using transrectal ultrasonography (Lepor et al, 1994) or magnetic resonance imaging (Tempany et al, 1993). There is no consensus regarding the extent of enlargement required to establish the diagnosis of macroscopic BPH. Because prostate size has limited clinical significance, a precise definition of macroscopic BPH is not essential.

The clinical manifestations of BPH include lower urinary tract symptoms, poor bladder emptying, urinary retention, detrusor instability, urinary tract infection, hematuria, and renal insufficiency (Riehmann and Bruskewitz, 1993). Historically, the pathophysiology of clinical BPH was attributed to bladder outlet obstruction secondary to macroscopic enlargement of the prostate gland. This hypothesis has been supported by epidemiologic data suggesting that the prevalence of microscopic BPH, macroscopic BPH, and clinical BPH is age dependent, and therefore these conditions are causally related (Isaacs and Coffey, 1989). This simplistic concept of the pathophysiology of BPH has been challenged by recent reports demonstrating weak or no relationships between prostate size, severity of bladder outlet obstruction, and severity of symptoms (Barry et al, 1993; Bosch et al, 1995; Girman et al, 1995; Yalla et al, 1995).

NATURAL HISTORY

The natural history of a disease process refers to the prognosis of the disease over time (Barry, 1993). The natural history of BPH must be considered when counseling patients about the risks and benefits of treatment versus watchful waiting.

Assessing the Natural History of Benign Prostatic Hyperplasia

There are several caveats relevant to designing and interpreting studies characterizing the natural history of BPH. Ideally, the natural history of BPH should be defined by a large prospective study evaluating subjects at specified follow-up intervals. **Retrospective studies are subject to bias related to patient selection and lack of systematic and meticulous follow-up.** All clinically relevant manifestations of BPH should be ascertained using quantitative outcome measures. **The relevant outcome measures should capture lower urinary tract symptoms, bladder dysfunction (bladder compliance and bladder emptying), bladder outlet obstruction, urinary tract infection, urinary retention, and renal insufficiency.** Defining the natural history of symptoms qualitatively using subjective terms such as slightly improved, or stable or progressive symptoms is of limited clinical utility. The natural history of BPH must be examined over long intervals of time. The natural history analysis should be stratified according to baseline age and disease severity so that prognostic information is applicable to individual patients. Because the severity of lower urinary tract symptoms and bladder outlet obstruction are not necessarily causally related, these features of the disease process should be analyzed independently.

Literature Review of the Natural History of Benign Prostatic Hyperplasia

There exists a paucity of reliable information related to the natural history of BPH. A prospective longitudinal study adequately defining the natural history of BPH has never been reported. The sporadic reports in the literature relevant to the natural history of BPH are reviewed in this section.

Prospective and Retrospective Studies

Clarke (1937) reported the first study of the natural history of BPH. Ninety-three cases of prostatic obstruction uncomplicated by infection or bladder failure were followed over a period of time averaging 4.3 years. **This study demonstrated that the symptoms of BPH are not inevitably progressive and that a significant group of men experience spontaneous resolution of symptoms.**

Craigen and colleagues (1969) reported one of the first

prospective studies on the natural history of BPH. A total of 123 men with lower urinary tract symptoms and no evidence of carcinoma of the prostate or urinary retention were followed for 7 years. **This study demonstrated that only a small percentage (approximately 10%) of men with symptoms (not necessarily BPH) progress to urinary retention and nearly half become totally asymptomatic.** The lack of objective and BPH-related baseline characteristics of the study population precludes generalizing these studies to the natural history of BPH.

Barnes and Marsh (1983) reported a retrospective case review on the natural history of BPH. Of the 208 evaluable patients, 80 (39%) underwent a prostatectomy when followed between 6 months and 13 years (mean follow-up 4.8 years). The indications for prostatectomy in the majority of patients were symptomatic worsening or the lack of spontaneous improvement. **Using prostatectomy as a proxy for disease progression is not appropriate because some patients with stable symptoms underwent prostatectomy.** Of the subjects not undergoing prostatectomy, symptoms were stable or improved in 29% of cases. **This retrospective review provides further evidence that BPH is not necessarily a progressive disease.**

Birkhoff and colleagues (1976) reported a retrospective review of the natural history of BPH in 26 of 156 subjects who initially presented with prostatism between 1951 and 1970. One of the unique features of this study was that a quantitative symptom questionnaire was developed to ascertain symptom progression. Urine flow, postvoid residual volume, renal function, and prostate volume were quantified using uroflowmetry, planimetry of the postvoid film on the intravenous urogram, percent phenolsulfonphthalein excretion, and digital rectal examination, respectively. Although these objective parameters were independently measured, the data were expressed as a composite objective score. The mean symptom score decreased (symptom severity increased) by 2.1 points per year. The mean objective score decreased (disease progression) by 2.4 points per year. **Although there was a general tendency for the group to exhibit slight symptom progression over a 3-year interval, approximately half of the patients were improved or unchanged.**

Ball and co-workers (1981) reviewed the natural history of 107 men with symptoms suggestive of bladder outlet obstruction who, after undergoing routine clinical, radiographic, and urodynamic evaluation, elected not to undergo elective prostatectomy. Fifty-three (50%) of these 107 patients were urodynamically obstructed. These patients were re-evaluated 5 years after the initial examination. Of the 107 patients, 10 (9%) required surgery, 64 (60%) returned for reassessment, and 33 (31%) responded to a postal questionnaire. **Of the 97 patients who did not undergo surgery, symptoms deteriorated in 16, improved in 31, and were unchanged in 50. The group mean peak flow rate (PFR) decreased in the 64 evaluable untreated subjects from 13.1 to 11.9 ml/second.** Despite the mean decrease in PFR, the mean voiding detrusor pressure in 43 evaluable subjects decreased by 4 cm H_2O. **Of these 43 patients, 21 (49%) exhibited a decrease in voiding pressure. These findings suggest that significant and progressive bladder outlet obstruction rarely occurs over 5 years.**

Watanabe (1986) reported a longitudinal study of prostate volume in 4885 Japanese subjects undergoing mass transrectal ultrasonography (TRUS) screening. Only 16 cases were followed with multiple prostate volume measurements over a 7-year interval. The three patients exhibiting significant prostatic growth were all in their sixth decade of life. In a subset of 348 Japanese men undergoing TRUS screening, the mean prostate volume progressively decreased after age 40. These observations are in contrast to the age-dependent prevalence rates of macroscopic BPH reported by Guess and associates (1990) and the autopsy prevalence rates of BPH reported by Berry and colleagues (1984). It is conceivable that this discrepancy between age and prostate volume may reflect racial differences of BPH in whites and Orientals (Lepor et al, in press).

Longitudinal Studies of Aging

Two longitudinal studies of aging have reported age-dependent prevalence rates of BPH. These studies have been extrapolated to provide insights into the natural history of BPH.

The Veterans Administration Normative Aging Study enrolled 2036 healthy male volunteers in a longitudinal study between 1967 and 1970 (Glynn et al, 1985). The clinical diagnosis of BPH was based on the findings of an enlarged or abnormally firm prostate, or a history of symptoms believed not to be related to prostatitis or prostate cancer. The specific criteria for diagnosing BPH were not standardized. The definition of clinical BPH encompassed both symptoms and prostatic enlargement, two unrelated clinical occurrences. **The study does not address the natural history of BPH because only the development and not the progression of the disease was evaluated. The cumulative probabilities that a 40-year-old man would develop clinical BPH or that he would undergo a prostatectomy for BPH by 80 years of age were estimated to be 0.777 and 0.292, respectively.**

The Baltimore Longitudinal Study of Aging represents another large prospective longitudinal study of human aging (Guess et al, 1990). As of December, 1988, 1371 male volunteers were enrolled. Medical examinations performed every 2 years included a digital rectal examination and questions focusing on the presence of urinary symptoms. There were no standardized criteria for assigning the diagnosis of BPH. The age-specific prevalence rates of an enlarged prostate versus both an enlarged prostate and symptoms are compared in Figure 47–1.

Age-Specific Prevalence of Benign Prostatic Hyperplasia: Cross-Sectional Community Studies

Because there exists a paucity of prospective longitudinal BPH natural history studies, the natural history has been inferred from cross-sectional community studies capturing age-specific prevalence rates of prostate enlargement, symptoms, and bladder outlet obstruction. **The Ohmsted County community–based study of urinary symptoms and health status represents the largest and most comprehensive cross-sectional survey of macroscopic and clinical BPH. This study provides reliable age-dependent prevalence rates for symptoms (Chute et al, 1993), prostate size**

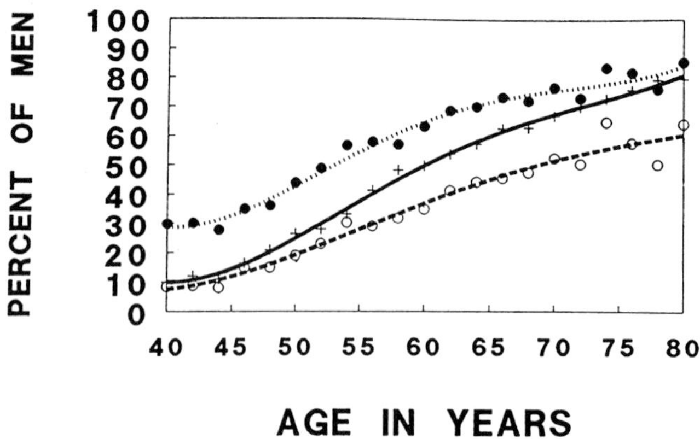

Figure 47–1. Comparison of three different measures of prostatism among men in the Baltimore Longitudinal Study of Aging. The lower line is the percent of men with prostate enlargement on digital rectal examination, the middle line is the percent in whom benign prostatic hyperplasia was diagnosed clinically on the basis of a history and physical examination, and the top line is the percent who had either prostate enlargement, obstructive urologic symptoms, or both. (Reproduced by permission from Guess HA: Prostate 1990; 17:241–246.)

(Oesterling et al, 1993), and PFR (Girman et al, 1993) for white males between the ages of 40 and 79 years of age. The Ohmsted County community–based study demonstrated that the prevalence of lower urinary tract symptoms is age dependent (Chute et al, 1993) (Table 47–1). **The age-dependent prevalence of symptoms has been confirmed in different countries throughout the world, including Scotland (Guess et al, 1993), France (Sagnier et al, 1994), Japan (Tsukamoto et al, 1995), and New Zealand (Nacey et al, 1995)** (see Table 47–1). **Although the prevalence of moderate-to-severe symptoms consistently increases with advancing age,** the age-dependent severity of symptoms varies among different countries. The basis for these differences may be attributed to environmental factors, linguistic differences in the questionnaire, or racial differences in the proliferative disease. Racial differences in the cellular composition of BPH have been reported by Lepor and colleagues (1996).

Community-based studies have also reported the age-dependent prevalence of bladder outlet obstruction using uroflowmetry as a proxy for obstruction (Girman et al, 1993). The mean PFR decreased progressively from 20.3 ml/second in men between the ages of 40 and 44 to 11.5 ml/second in men between the ages of 75 and 79. The percent of men in the Ohmsted County study with PFRs less than 15 ml/second increased from 24% in men aged 40 to 44 years to 69% in men older than 75 years of age (Girman et al, 1993). The age-dependent PFR values observed in Ohmsted County are similar to values previously reported by Garraway and associates (1991).

The age-dependent prevalence of macroscopic BPH has also been inferred from community-based studies. Approximately one quarter of the participants in the Ohmsted County study underwent TRUS. Oesterling and colleagues (1993) reported that the relationship between prostate volume and age was statistically significant ($P < .0001$; $r^2 = .185$). Bosch and associates (1994) reported a weaker correlation ($P < .001$; $r^2 = 0.068$) between prostatic volume and age.

The Ohmsted County and other community-based population studies demonstrate that the percentage of patients exhibiting a threshold American Urological Association (AUA) symptom score greater than 7, PFR less than or equal to 10 ml/second, and prostate volume greater than 50 cm^3 increases in consecutive 10-year age groups, suggesting that bladder outlet obstruction and prostate size are age dependent and causally related. The relationship between two measurable parameters is defined by the square of the correlation coefficient (r^2). The r^2 values of .03 and .07 for the pairwise relationships between age versus prostate volume indicate that age accounts for only 3% to 7% of the variation in prostate volume. Girman and colleagues (1995) did not report the r^2 values for age versus PFR and age versus symptom scores; however, inspection of the scatter plots suggests no clinically significant relationships. Bosch and co-workers (1995) reported that the r^2 values for the International Prostate Symptom Score versus both PFR and age were .008 and .006, respectively. The r^2 values for the pairwise relationships between AUA symptom score versus PFR (0.03), PFR versus prostate size (−.05), and prostate volume versus PFR (−.12) reported by Girman and associates (1995) demonstrate weak and clinically irrelevant relationships between these parameters.

ASSESSING THE EFFECTIVENESS AND SAFETY OF MEDICAL THERAPY FOR BENIGN PROSTATIC HYPERPLASIA

The role of treatment for any disease process depends on the magnitude of the clinical effect and the incidence and severity of treatment-related morbidity. Assessing the effectiveness of medical therapies for BPH requires defining clinically relevant end points, identifying quantitative and reliable clinical outcome measures, eliminating

Table 47–1. PREVALENCE OF MODERATE-TO-SEVERE SYMPTOMS (AUA SYMPTOM SCORE ≥8)

Reference	Number of Subjects	Country	Percent AUA Symptom Score ≥8 According to Age (Years)			
			40–49	*50–59*	*60–69*	*70–79*
Chute et al, 1993	2150	United States	26	33	41	46
Sagnier et al, 1994	2011	France	—	8	14	27
Tsukamoto et al, 1995	289	Japan	41	29	31	56
Nacey et al, 1995	515	New Zealand	13	24	34	33

AUA, American Urological Association.

investigator and patient bias, accounting for the placebo response, and enrolling the proper number of subjects so that only clinically significant changes are statistically significant. Assessing the safety of medical therapies requires a rigorous effort to identify all treatment-related clinical, biochemical, teratogenic, and mutagenic adverse effects related to treatment.

Clinical End Points

The clinically significant consequences of BPH include lower urinary tract symptoms; detrusor dysfunction characterized by detrusor acontractility, detrusor instability, and detrusor fibrosis; incomplete bladder emptying; acute and chronic urinary retention; urinary tract infection; renal insufficiency; and hematuria (Shapiro and Lepor, 1995). **Based on this definition and the presumed pathophysiology of clinical BPH, the clinically relevant end points of therapy have been to decrease bladder outlet obstruction, thereby relieving symptoms, improving bladder emptying, ameliorating detrusor instability, reversing renal insufficiency, and preventing future episodes of urinary tract infection and urinary retention.**

Quantitative Outcome Measures

Symptoms

Symptoms associated with BPH have been termed prostatism (Abrams, 1994b). **Several different quantitative instruments have been developed to determine the severity of BPH symptoms and to assess the symptom response to BPH therapies.** The Boyarsky (1977) and the Madsen-Iverson (1983) Symptom Indices were developed to determine the efficacy of BPH therapies and for selecting candidates for prostatectomy, respectively. Both of these nonvalidated symptom instruments were also widely used to determine the response to BPH medical therapies in the 1980s. **The AUA Symptom Index was developed specifically as an outcome measure in the study of different BPH therapies** (Cockett et al, 1992). **The AUA Symptom Index captures the severity of seven BPH symptoms (Barry et al, 1992a) (see Chapter 4).** The AUA Symptom Index was validated, shown to discriminate between BPH and controls (Barry et al, 1992a), and was highly responsive when used to evaluate patient response to prostatectomy (Barry et al, 1995c). Linear relationships have been observed among the AUA, Madsen-Iversson, and Boyarsky symptom scores, indicating that all three instruments capture the same phenomena (Barry et al, 1992b). In a survey of 500 urologists 1 year after publication of the AUA Symptom Index, 60% were using it to evaluate and follow patients with BPH (Barry and O'Leary, 1995).

An international consultation on BPH recommended adding one BPH-specific quality of life question to the AUA Symptom Index. This modified AUA Symptom Index is termed the International Prostate Symptom Score and is widely used outside the United States in clinical practice and research (Barry and O'Leary, 1995). **Symptom problem and BPH impact indices have been developed and validated. These indices quantify symptom bother and its impact on quality of life (Barry et al, 1995a).**

There is no standardization for reporting changes in symptom scores following treatment. Symptom response has been reported as a percentage of patients achieving a threshold response or as group mean change in a symptom index. Expressing the symptom response as a single threshold response does not discriminate the magnitude of the clinical effect. When the baseline symptom scores are mild or moderate, small and clinically insignificant changes correspond to large percentage changes. When baseline symptom scores are severe, relatively large absolute changes may not be clinically significant. Symptom outcome should be expressed as a percentage of patients achieving threshold responses and group mean changes.

The clinical significance of changes in the AUA Symptom Index have recently been reported by Barry and associates (1995b). One thousand one hundred and sixty-five subjects participating in a randomized double-blind placebo-controlled study of medical therapy completed the AUA Symptom Index at baseline and after 3 months of treatment. The absolute and percent changes in AUA Symptom Index and BPH Impact Index were correlated with five global ratings of symptom improvement (Fig. 47–2). The group mean changes in AUA Symptom Index for subjects rating their improvement as markedly, moderately, or slightly improved, unchanged, or worse were −8.8, −5.1, −3.0, −0.7, and +2.7, respectively. **The relationship between the patients' global ratings of improvement and AUA Symptom Index and BPH Impact Index changes was dependent on the baseline AUA Symptom Index. This important study provides the data required to determine sample sizes and interpret the clinical significance of symptom improvement in BPH clinical trials.**

The developers of the AUA Symptom Index recognized that it was not specific for clinical BPH. Males with chronic prostatitis, urinary tract infection, transitional cell carcinoma, urethral stricture, neurogenic bladder, glucosuria, and congestive heart failure also may have lower urinary tract symptoms. **Lepor and Machi (1993) administered the AUA Symptom Index to a group of men and women between the ages of 50 and 75 years attending a general health fair. The mean AUA Symptom Index and the proportion of subjects with mild, moderate, and severe symptoms were identical in the age-matched male and female groups.** Because the symptoms associated with clinical BPH are not disease or gender specific, it is an oversimplification to assume that lower urinary tract symptoms in aging males with a so-called enlarged prostate and low PFR are due to macroscopic BPH.

Bladder Outlet Obstruction

Experimental animal models of bladder outlet obstruction have demonstrated profound changes in bladder ultrastructure, cellular composition, metabolism, and function (Levin et al, 1995). These experimental observations must be extrapolated cautiously to humans because the response to bladder outlet obstruction depends on the species, as well as the severity and duration of obstruction (Levin et al, 1993). **Animal studies demonstrate that under experimental conditions, bladder outlet obstruction**

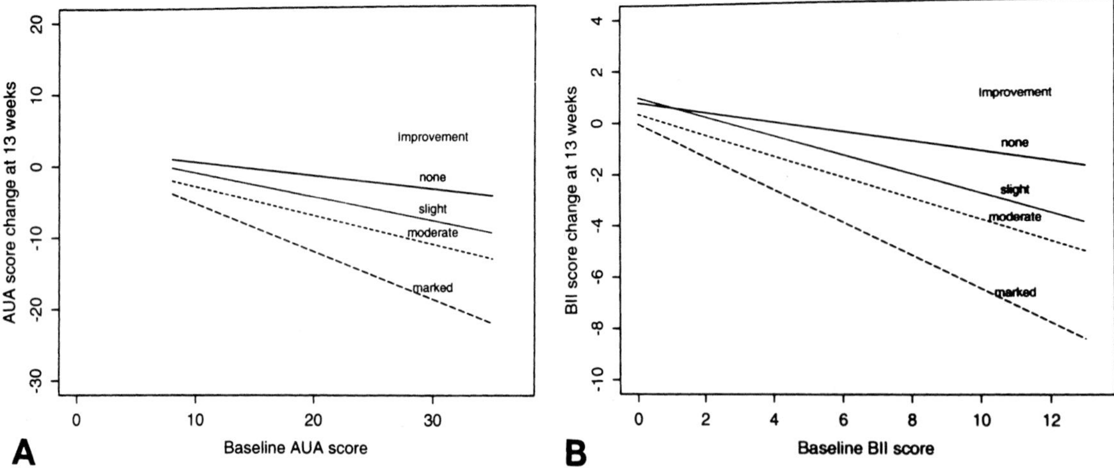

Figure 47–2. Relationship between baseline and absolute change scores for all subjects participating in the Veterans Administration Benign Prostatic Hyperplasia Medical Therapy Study rating global improvement at 13 weeks as none, slight, moderate, or marked. A, AUA Symptom Index, 1120 patients; B, BPH impact index, 1117 patients. (From Barry MJ: J Urol 1995; 154:1770–1774.)

causes alterations likely to adversely affect bladder function. The justification for measuring and treating bladder outlet obstruction in males with BPH is to reverse or prevent these deleterious consequences of bladder outlet obstruction.

There is general agreement among urodynamicists that bladder outlet obstruction is determined most accurately by the synchronous measurement of detrusor pressure and urinary flow (Abrams, 1994a). The sine qua non of bladder outlet obstruction is the simultaneous measurement of elevated voiding pressures and low PFR (Blaivas, 1990). Abrams and Griffiths (1979), Schafer and colleagues (1988), and Rollema (1991) have proposed different methods for analyzing the synchronous pressure flow data.

The primary limitation of urodynamic measurements of bladder outlet obstruction is their lack of clinical relevance. The degree of bladder outlet obstruction is not related to the severity of symptoms. Nitti and colleagues (1994) have shown that patients with BPH classified as obstructed, equivocal, and unobstructed using the Abrams and Griffiths nomogram have the same group mean AUA symptom score. Ko and associates (1995) reported no correlation between AUA symptom scores and the Schafer obstruction scores. There is no evidence that untreated urodynamic obstruction portends clinical progression or detrusor deterioration. Urodynamic testing does not predict symptom improvement following alpha blockage (Witjes et al, 1995), transurethral microwave thermotherapy (Tubaro et al, 1995), or prostatectomy (Jensen et al, 1983).

Because synchronous pressure flow urodynamic measurements do not correlate with severity of bladder dysfunction, severity of symptoms, or response to therapy, it is difficult to justify the routine use of these studies in the evaluation of patients with BPH. Long-term studies are needed to determine whether or not urodynamic measurements predict disease progression. The primary use of urodynamic testing is to discriminate the differential diagnosis of males presenting with multiple etiologies for symptoms.

Uroflowmetry represents a noninvasive and inexpensive measure of bladder outlet obstruction (Siroky, 1990). The lower limit of normal for PFRs ranges between 10 and 15 ml/second (Kaplan and Te, 1995). Ko and colleagues (1995) recently reported no significant correlation between PFR and Schafer nomograms of urethral obstruction or detrusor function. **It is not unusual to find a discrepancy in the diagnosis of bladder outlet obstruction between uroflowmetry and synchronous pressure flow studies** (Gerstenberg et al, 1982). **There are several factors other than bladder outlet obstruction that may result in a low PFR** (Kaplan and Te, 1995). Straining artifacts on machine-read flow rate recordings must be adjusted. Because PFR is dependent on bladder volume (Drach et al, 1979; Siroky et al, 1979), a low PFR may simply result from an inadequate voided value. A reliable uroflow measurement requires a voided volume of approximately 125 ml. A weak detrusor in the absence of bladder outlet obstruction may also be associated with a low PFR. PFRs decrease with advancing age in asymptomatic men (Jorgensen et al, 1986). Despite these limitations, uroflowmetry has become one of the primary outcome measures for clinical investigations of BPH therapies because the test is simple and noninvasive.

The reporting of changes in PFR has not been standardized. At the lower spectrum of PFR, a relatively small absolute change (i.e., 4 to 6 ml/second) corresponds to relatively high-percentage change, whereas at the higher end of PFR, a relatively large absolute change (i.e., 12 to 17 ml/second) corresponds to a relatively modest percent change. The clinical significance of the changes in PFR cannot be defined owing to the lack of correlations with relevant clinical, physiologic, or biochemical outcomes.

Bladder Emptying

Failure to empty the bladder may result from an acontractile bladder or bladder outlet obstruction. The inability to empty the bladder in the aging male patient is often attributed to bladder outlet obstruction secondary to BPH in the absence of primary neurologic diseases, diabetes, or urethral stricture. **Barry and co-workers (1993) reported only a weak correlation between postvoid residual volume and severity of bladder outlet obstruction in males with BPH.** There are no longitudinal studies indicating that postvoid residual volume is age dependent.

The clinical significance of a postvoid residual volume is controversial. Although it appears logical that postvoid residual volume may produce or exacerbate symptoms by decreasing the bladder functional capacity, Barry and associates (1993) reported no correlation between AUA symptom score and postvoid residual volume. It has been suggested that postvoid residual volume may predispose the patient to urinary tract infection and irreversible bladder dysfunction secondary to stasis and overdistention. **There is no data documenting that the incidence of urinary tract infection is related to postvoid residual volume.** Another limitation of postvoid residual volume measurements is variability over short intervals of time (Bruskewitz et al, 1982). It is imperative to measure the postvoid residual volume on several occasions if this parameter will influence treatment decisions.

There is no standardization for reporting changes in postvoid residual volume. Typically, the data are presented as absolute group mean changes. The majority of BPH clinical trials exclude subjects with high baseline postvoid residual volume (> 300 ml) because of the potential risks of randomization to a placebo or ineffective treatment group. **Therefore, the majority of subjects enrolled in clinical trials have clinically insignificant baseline postvoid residual volume. Evaluating the effect of a drug on bladder emptying in men without a significant postvoid residual volume is irrelevant.**

Detrusor Instability

The definition of detrusor instability is the development of a detrusor contraction exceeding 15 cm H_2O at a bladder volume less than 300 ml (Riehmann and Bruskewitz, 1993). Detrusor instability decreases bladder capacity and presumably contributes to irritative symptoms. **Approximately 60% of men who are candidates for transurethral prostatectomy have urodynamic evidence of detrusor instability, which resolves postoperatively in about two thirds of these patients** (Abrams and Griffiths, 1979; Coolsaet and Block, 1986; Cucchi, 1994). The resolution of detrusor instability suggests that bladder outlet obstruction causes detrusor instability. **There is no evidence demonstrating that the severity of bladder outlet obstruction or symptoms is correlated with the presence or absence of detrusor instability (Coolsaet and Block, 1986). In addition, the presence of detrusor instability is unrelated to the subjective outcome following transurethral prostatectomy (Dorflinger et al, 1985).**

The clinical significance of detrusor instability in men with BPH is unresolved. There is no evidence that men with detrusor instability electing watchful waiting are predisposed to experience progression of the disease. The presence of detrusor instability does not reliably predict the response to medical or surgical treatment. **Therefore, assessing detrusor instability has not become a standard outcome measure.**

Urinary Retention

Acute and chronic urinary retention are often attributed to BPH. Episodes of acute retention may be precipitated by sympathomimetic or anticholinergic drugs, or events leading to bladder overdistention. **Acute retention is often considered an absolute indication for intervention. Of 59 Danish patients presenting to an emergency room with acute retention, 73% had recurrent urinary retention within 1 week** (Breum et al, 1982). Taube and Gajraj (1989) reported that 72% of men presenting with acute urinary retention failed a voiding trial. **The natural history of acute urinary retention for those individuals following successful voiding trials is not known.**

The incidence of urinary retention has not been defined in cross-sectional population studies. Because urinary retention is a relatively uncommon event, a study designed to determine whether or not medical therapy prevents urinary retention would require large numbers of patients followed for a long period of time. Another goal of therapy may be to prevent a second episode of urinary retention following a successful voiding trial. In order to test the effectiveness of drug therapy for this indication, subjects successfully completing a voiding trial following an episode of urinary retention would be randomized to active treatment and placebo.

Urinary Tract Infection, Renal Insufficiency, and Hematuria

Unlike other manifestations of BPH, the diagnosis of urinary tract infection, renal insufficiency, and hematuria is not controversial and the requirements for measurement are noninvasive and inexpensive. Because these events are not disease or gender specific, one must be cautious in assuming a causal relationship to BPH. The occurrence of a urinary tract infection in men with a high postvoid residual volume may be due to BPH resulting from urinary stasis. Despite the apparent logic of this assumption, there is no evidence that the occurrence of urinary tract infection in the aging male population is associated with either a postvoid residual volume or bladder outlet obstruction. It is reasonable to assume that renal insufficiency occurs secondary to urinary retention if renal failure is reversed following catheter drainage. Hematuria may be associated with prostatic urethral varicosities.

Because the incidences of urinary tract infection, renal insufficiency, and hematuria are relatively uncommon and are not disease-specific events in the aging male population, it would be extremely difficult to design a prospective study to determine whether any BPH treatment prevents or reverses these events.

Eliminating Bias

Bias may be defined as a systematic error or difference between the true value and that actually attained due to all causes other than sampling ability. The only mechanism that can be used to ensure that the potential bias of the subject and the investigator does not influence the outcome is a double-blind design. Because subjects are typically randomized to receive a drug or its matching placebo, any effect of the investigators' bias would occur equally in the intervention and control groups.

The importance of eliminating bias cannot be overemphasized in BPH clinical trials. Some patients are very enthusiastic about receiving the new treatment. In the absence of a blinded randomization, these patients may be disproportionately directed into the active treatment groups. A subject receiving a known placebo would be reluctant to report any adverse events or clinical response. An investigator may be inclined to censor various outcomes if treatment group assignment is known. Although subjective outcome measures such as symptoms are more likely to be influenced by the placebo response, quantitative outcome measurements such as postvoid residual volume and PFR are also subject to a placebo response.

Sample Size

It is a general misconception that the validity of a clinical trial is directly proportional to the number of subjects enrolled. One of the objectives of a clinical trial is to determine whether or not the difference observed between two different treatment groups is clinically relevant. If the sample size of the clinical trial is properly determined in the early planning phase, a statistically significant outcome represents a clinically significant outcome. Calculation of sample size with provisions for adequate levels of significance and power is an essential part of planning a trial. Enrolling an excessive number of subjects may result in an overpowered study—that is, a small and clinically insignificant difference may be statistically significant. Conversely, enrolling insufficient numbers of subjects may result in an underpowered study—that is, a large and clinically significant difference may not be statistically significant. **The larger the number of subjects enrolled in a study, the smaller is the change that is required to achieve statistical significance.** Therefore, the reader must examine the magnitude of the between group difference and make a judgment about clinical significance.

Adverse Events

In order for a drug to enter into clinical investigation in humans, it must be shown to elicit no significant chemical, behavioral, physiologic, teratogenic, mutagenic, or carcinogenic effects in at least two animal models.

The typical untoward or adverse events captured in a clinical trial include physical findings, laboratory results, and complaints. A comprehensive physical examination and a battery of general laboratory tests are obtained at the beginning of the study to establish a baseline measure and at the completion of the trial to uncover any untoward events. The subjects' complaints are typically recorded at each study visit. The adverse clinical effects may be expected or unexpected.

Complaints may be elicited by means of a checklist or by the subjects' unsolicited recall of an event. **Usually, a greater number of adverse clinical events is recorded with a checklist.** The assessment of adverse events should determine the frequency and severity of the events, and whether or not it was severe enough to terminate a subject's participation in the study.

The majority of clinical trials are powered based on outcome measures and not on adverse events. **There is a tendency for studies to be underpowered as they relate to serious adverse events.**

MEDICAL THERAPY FOR BENIGN PROSTATIC HYPERPLASIA

Medical therapies investigated for BPH include alpha-blockers, androgen suppression, aromatase inhibitors, and plant extracts. Alpha-blockers and androgen suppression are emphasized in this chapter because the safety and efficacy of drugs in these classes have been critically examined. Aromatase inhibitors are briefly reviewed for historic interest. Plant extracts are also reviewed because these agents are widely used in some parts of the world despite the lack of properly designed clinical trials.

The Impact of Medical Therapy

Until recently, prostatectomy was the only widely accepted intervention for BPH. **The enthusiasm for medical therapy has been supported in part by the limitations of prostatectomy that include the morbidity of the surgical procedure, failure to consistently achieve a successful outcome, necessity for retreatment, and the suggestion that prostatectomy increases the risk of delayed life-threatening cardiac events (Lepor, 1993).** Although medical therapies do not achieve the same degree of efficacy as prostatectomy, **the attractive features of medical therapy compared with prostatectomy are that clinically significant outcomes are obtained with fewer, less serious, and reversible side effects** (Lepor, 1993). Because the indication for intervention in the overwhelming majority of patients with BPH is to improve quality of life by relieving symptoms (Mebust et al, 1989), the lower morbidity of medical therapy is of paramount importance in patient-driven treatment decisions.

Medical therapy represents an alternative for individuals who are deemed appropriate candidates for prostatectomy but who lack absolute indications for surgery. Of 1822 patients evaluated for BPH between July 1, 1987 through June 30, 1991 in a single private practice, the percentages of patients undergoing prostatectomy in the first and last years of the 5-year survey were 28% and 8%, respectively (Breslin et al, 1993). **A recent survey of the U.S. Medicare data base revealed that the absolute number of prostatectomies decreased over 30% despite the progressively increasing number of males enrolled in the Medicare program (Holtgrewe, 1995). The decrease in prostatectomy coincides with the acceptance of medical therapy.**

Approximately 30% of white American males older than 50 years of age have moderate to severe symptoms (Chute et al, 1993; Lepor and Machi, 1993). **Based on the demographics of the U.S. population, approximately 8.7 million white men are eligible to discuss BPH treatment options** (Jacobsen et al, 1995). The overwhelming majority of these 9 million men would not elect prostatectomy owing to the risks associated with surgical intervention. **These individuals are potential candidates for medical therapy.**

Selecting Candidates for Medical Therapy

The ideal candidate for medical therapy has symptoms that are bothersome and that impact negatively on quality of life. The finding of a high symptom score alone is not a sufficient indication for medical therapy. The symptoms should be sufficiently bothersome that the patient is willing to make a lifetime commitment to medical therapy, providing the drug is effective and adverse experiences are nonexistent or minimal. Medical therapy should not be offered to individuals presenting with absolute indications for surgical intervention. Individuals presenting with recurrent urinary retention, recurrent urinary tract infections, renal insufficiency, bladder calculi, and recurrent gross hematuria may experience severe and even life-threatening consequences from BPH if they are managed with ineffective or suboptimal therapy. These patients should be offered prostatectomy, the most effective BPH treatment option. It is conceivable that medical therapy, by relieving bladder outlet obstruction, may prevent future episodes of urinary retention and urinary tract infection, and reverse renal insufficiency. Until properly controlled clinical studies unequivocally demonstrate these outcomes, patients presenting with absolute indications for surgery should be discouraged from selecting medical therapy. If informed patients are willing to accept potential risks, medical therapy may be offered with a proviso for careful follow-up and future prostatectomy if medical therapy proves ineffective.

Preventing Benign Prostatic Hyperplasia with Medical Therapy

A potential role of medical therapy is to prevent the development of BPH or its progression. There are numerous factors limiting the enthusiasm for preventing the development of BPH. The clinical manifestations of BPH are rarely life threatening. Effective medical therapy exists, and the natural history is variable and poorly defined. **Because there are no clinical, biochemical, or genetic predictors of disease development or progression, every male is at risk.** Even if the development or progression of BPH was medically preventable, the cost of long-term prophylaxis would likely be prohibitive. **The ability to identify those individuals who are predisposed to develop clinical BPH refractory to medical therapy would provide a rationale for prophylaxis.**

Watchful Waiting

All males with symptomatic BPH do not elect medical or surgical intervention because the symptoms are not bothersome, the complications of treatment are perceived to be greater than the inconvenience due to symptoms, they are reluctant to take a daily pill owing to unrecognized long-term side effects, and the cost of treatment is high. When the patient is reassured that the symptoms are not due to cancer or other serious genitourinary pathology, or that the delay in treatment will not have irreversible consequences, watchful waiting may be the patient-driven treatment of choice. It is unreasonable to discourage an informed patient with severe symptoms and no other consequences of BPH from pursuing watchful waiting despite the safety and effectiveness of medical therapy. Watchful waiting does not imply the total absence of intervention. The severity and distress due to symptoms may be improved through simple measures such as decreasing total fluid intake, especially prior to bedtime; moderating the intake of alcohol- and caffeine-containing products; and following timed voiding schedules.

The impact of watchful waiting was recently examined in a study of 556 subjects with moderate symptoms of BPH randomized to transurethral prostatectomy versus watchful waiting (Wasson et al, 1995). The changes in all outcome measures were significantly greater in the transurethral prostatectomy group. A relevant outcome for patients selecting watchful waiting is disease progression. During 3 years of follow-up, treatment failure was observed in 23 (8.2%) and 47 (17%) subjects randomized to transurethral prostatectomy and watchful waiting, respectively. Treatment failure in the watchful waiting group was due to increasing postvoid residual urine or symptom score in 28 of the 47 cases.

ALPHA-BLOCKADE

Rationale for Alpha-Blockers

The rationale for alpha-blockers in the treatment of BPH is based on the hypothesis that clinical BPH is, in part, due to prostate smooth muscle–mediated bladder outlet obstruction (Caine, 1986). Shapiro and associates (1992) reported that smooth muscle is one of the dominant cellular constituents of BPH, accounting for 40% of the area density of the hyperplastic prostate. Caine and co-workers (1975) reported that the human prostate contracts in the presence of the alpha-adrenergic agonist norepinephrine. Several investigators subsequently demonstrated that **the tension of prostate smooth muscle is mediated by the alpha$_1$-adrenoceptor** (α_1-AR) (Hieble et al, 1985; Lepor et al, 1988; Gup et al, 1989). Lepor and Shapiro (1984) were the first investigators to characterize the α_1-AR in the human prostate. These investigators subsequently reported that **98% of the α_1-AR is localized to the prostate stroma** (Kobayashi et al, 1993). **The most definitive evidence that blockade of prostate α_1-AR relieves bladder outlet obstruction was the observed direct relationship between the area density of prostate smooth muscle and change in the PFR in 26 subjects undergoing prostatic biopsy before initiating terazosin therapy** (Shapiro et al, 1992). Although the prostates of those subjects achieving symptom improvement had a greater group mean area density of smooth muscle compared with nonresponders, a direct relationship between prostate smooth muscle area density and change in symptom scores was not observed. These observations also suggest that nonprostate smooth muscle–mediated α_1-AR events may also be responsible for the effectiveness of alpha-blockade.

Classification of Alpha-Blockers

Alpha-blockers advocated for the treatment of BPH may be classified according to the α_1-AR selectivity and serum elimination half-life (Table 47–2).

Table 47–2. CLASSIFICATION OF ALPHA-BLOCKERS AND RECOMMENDED DOSES

Class of Alpha-Blocker	Dose
Nonselective	
Phenoxybenzamine	10 mg bid
Alpha$_1$	
Prazosin	2 mg bid
Alfuzosin	2.5 mg tid
Indoramin	20 mg bid
Long-Acting Alpha$_1$	
Terazosin	5 or 10 mg qd
Doxazosin	4 or 8 mg qd
Subtype (α_{1a}) Selective	
Tamsulosin	0.4 or 0.8 mg qd

Phenoxybenzamine, a nonselective alpha-blocker, was shown to be highly effective in the management of BPH (Caine et al, 1976; Caine et al, 1978). The disadvantages of phenoxybenzamine were the high incidence and severity of adverse clinical events.

Berthelson and Pettinger (1977) described two subtypes of the α-AR (α_1 and α_2). Prazosin was one of the first α_1-AR antagonists to be investigated for the treatment of BPH (Hedlund et al, 1983). **The efficacy of phenoxybenzamine and prazosin are comparable; however, prazosin is better tolerated, implying that efficacy and toxicity are mediated primarily by the α_1-AR and α_2-AR, respectively** (Lepor, 1989). Prazosin and other alpha$_1$-antagonists, including alfuzosin (Jardin et al, 1991) and indoramin (Ramsay et al, 1985), require at least twice-daily dosing owing to their relatively short serum elimination half-lives.

The next advance in the development of alpha-blockers was the development of drugs with serum elimination half-lives that allowed for once-a-day dosing. Terazosin (Lepor et al, 1992) and doxazosin (Gillenwater et al, 1995) are long-acting alpha-blockers that have been shown to be safe and effective for the treatment of BPH.

Molecular cloning studies have identified three subtypes of the α_1-AR (Lepor, 1996). **Prostate smooth muscle tension is mediated by the α_{1a}-AR** (Forray et al, 1994a). Tamsulosin is an α_1-antagonist investigated for BPH that exhibits some degree of selectivity for the α_{1a}-AR (Foglar et al, 1995). The pharmaceutical industry has developed α_1-antagonists that are 1000-fold selective for the α_{1a}-AR (Forray et al, 1994b). **The impact of these highly selective α_1-AR antagonists will be defined by future clinical trials** (Lepor, 1996).

Interpreting the Literature on Alpha-Blockers

The literature on alpha-blockers has been subjected to meta-analysis (Lepor, 1993a; McConnell et al, 1994; Eri and Tveter, 1995). **These meta-analyses are misleading because all of the alpha-blocker data are combined independent of drug, dose, and study design.**

Study Designs

There are four study designs that have been used to investigate alpha-blockers for BPH: titration to fixed dose, titration to response, randomized dose withdrawal, and titration to maximal dose.

Subjects enrolled in **titration to fixed dose** studies receive one of several predetermined final doses independent of clinical response unless significant adverse effects are encountered. An advantage of this study design is that dose-dependent efficacy and safety of different doses are determined. A disadvantage is the requirement for a large sample size in order to identify statistically significant differences between placebo and all of the treatment groups.

A titration to response design allows the investigators to titrate the dose to a threshold response or maximal dose. An advantage of this design is a smaller sample size because all subjects receiving active treatment are analyzed as a composite group independent of the final dose. A disadvantage of this design is that the maximal therapeutic effect may be underestimated if the titration is not to maximal response. The data are also misleading if it is expressed in terms of group mean changes according to final dose because all nonresponders are titrated to the maximal dose in the absence of toxicity.

A randomized dose withdrawal design begins with an open-label dose titration. All responders are randomized to active drug or placebo. An advantage of this design is the enrichment of responders. A disadvantage is that the results are not generalizable to untreated patients.

A titration to maximal dose design, like titration to response, requires a relatively small sample size because there is only one active treatment group. This study design defines the maximal clinical response achievable in practice, providing that the maximal dose is also the most efficacious tolerable dose.

Comparing Alpha-Blockers

The therapeutic dose range of the different alpha-blockers is highly variable and depends on the potency and pharmacokinetics of the individual drugs. The maximal tolerable and effective doses have not been defined for any alpha-blocker. The relative effectiveness of the different alpha$_1$-blockers can be inferred only by comparing nonconcurrent studies. **Randomized double-blind comparison studies are required to compare different alpha-blockers definitively.**

Alpha$_1$-blockers were initially developed as antihypertensive agents. The literature is inconsistent regarding the effect of alpha$_1$-blockers on blood pressure in BPH subjects. The effect of alpha$_1$-blockers on blood pressure depends on the patient's pretreatment blood pressure. **The effect of alpha$_1$-antagonists on blood pressure is clinically significant only in those subjects who are hypertensive at baseline** (Lepor et al, 1995a; Kirby, 1995). The effects on blood pressure should be reported independently for normotensive and hypertensive subjects.

Review of the Literature

Several reviews have catalogued the extensive clinical experiences with alpha-blockade in BPH (Lepor, 1989;

Lepor, 1993a, 1993b; Lepor, 1995a; Eri and Tveter, 1995; Lepor and Vaughan, 1996). Nonselective and short-acting alpha$_1$-antagonists are used less commonly in clinical practice owing to tolerance and the requirement for multiple daily dosing. Randomized double-blind placebo-controlled studies have reported the safety and efficacy of phenoxybenzamine (Caine et al, 1978; Abrams et al, 1982), prazosin (Hedlund et al, 1983; Martorana et al, 1984; Kirby et al, 1987; LeDuc et al, 1990; Ruutu et al, 1991; Chapple et al, 1992), indoramin (Iacovou and Dunn, 1987; Chow et al, 1990; Scott and Abrams, 1991), and alfuzosin (Ramsay et al, 1985; Carbin et al, 1991; Jardin et al, 1991; Hansen et al, 1994). With the exception of alfuzosin, these studies typically enrolled relatively small numbers of subjects into short-term single-dose studies without quantitative assessment of symptom improvement. **Multicenter randomized double-blind placebo-controlled studies have determined the safety and efficacy of multiple doses of the long-acting alpha$_1$-blockers terazosin and doxazosin and the subtype selective alpha$_{1a}$-antagonist tamsulosin. Subjects enrolled in these studies generally presented with moderate to severe symptoms, postvoid residual volume less than 300 ml, and no absolute indications for surgical intervention.** Representative studies are reviewed to illustrate the safety, efficacy, and most effective use of alpha-blockers in BPH. The reader is referred to the original articles for more comprehensive outcome assessments.

Terazosin

Terazosin is the most extensively investigated alpha$_1$-blocker for BPH. Randomized double-blind placebo-controlled studies demonstrate the efficacy and safety of terazosin for BPH (DiSilverio, 1992; Lepor et al, 1992; Lloyd et al, 1992; Brawer et al, 1993; Roehrborn et al, 1995; Lepor et al, in press) (Table 47–3).

The multicenter, double-blind, parallel-group, randomized placebo-controlled study of once-a-day administration of terazosin to patients with symptomatic BPH reported by Lepor and colleagues (1992) is representative of the expectations of terazosin therapy. Two hundred and eighty-five patients entered the double-blind treatment receiving either placebo or 2, 5, or 10 mg terazosin once daily. **Statistically significant decreases from baseline obstructive, irritative, and total symptom scores were observed for all terazosin treatment groups. The level of improvement in the symptom scores was dose dependent. The 10-mg terazosin treatment group exhibited significantly greater decreases in mean irritative and total symptom scores compared with the placebo group.** The 5- and 10-mg terazosin treatment groups exhibited a significantly greater mean decrease in obstructive scores compared with the placebo group. The percentages of patients experiencing a greater than 30% improvement in the total symptom scores for the placebo and the 2-, 5-, and 10-mg treatment groups were 40%, 51%, 57%, and 69%, respectively (Fig. 47–3). The percentage of patients experiencing greater than 30% improvement in total symptom score in the 10-mg treatment group was significantly greater than that of the placebo group.

A statistically significant improvement from baseline was seen in the peak and mean urinary flow rates for all the treatment groups. The effect of terazosin on PFR was also dose dependent. The 10-mg treatment group exhibited a significantly greater increase from baseline in peak and mean urinary flow rates compared with the placebo group. The percentages of patients experiencing a greater than 30% increase in PFR in the placebo and the 2-, 5-, and 10-mg treatment groups were 26%, 40%, 35%, and 52%, respectively (see Fig. 47–3). A significantly greater proportion of patients in the 10-mg terazosin treatment group exhibited a greater than 30% improvement in PFR compared with the placebo group.

Overall, the adverse events in the four treatment groups were minor and reversible. Although a higher incidence of asthenia, flulike syndrome, and dizziness was observed in the terazosin treatment groups, the differences from placebo were not statistically significant. There was a significantly greater incidence of postural hypotension in the 5-mg terazosin group than in the placebo group. The incidence of syncope for all terazosin-treated patients was less than 0.5%.

Table 47–3. EFFICACY OF TERAZOSIN IN BENIGN PROSTATIC HYPERPLASIA

Reference	Number Enrolled	Randomized Treatment (Months)	Dose (mg)	Group Mean Difference from Placebo	
				PFR (ml/second)	*Symptom Score*
Lepor et al, 1992	285	3	2	+1.1	−1.0
			5	+0.6	−1.3$^{\times}$
			10	+1.9^{+}	−2.3*
DiSilverio, 1992	137	2	2	+1.2	—
			5	+1.5$^{\times}$	—
			10	+1.2	—
Lloyd et al, 1992	132	3	2	−1.2	−2.0
			5	−0.4	−2.1
			10	+0.3	−2.8
Brawer et al, 1993	160	6	Titration to response	+1.4$^{\times}$	−3.5$^{\times}$
Roehrborn et al, 1995	2084	12	Titration to 10	+1.4$^{\times}$	−4.0*
Lepor et al, in press	1229	12	Titration to 10	+1.3*	−3.5*

PFR, Peak flow rate.
$^{\times}P < 0.05$; $^{+}P < 0.01$; $^{*}P < 0.001$.

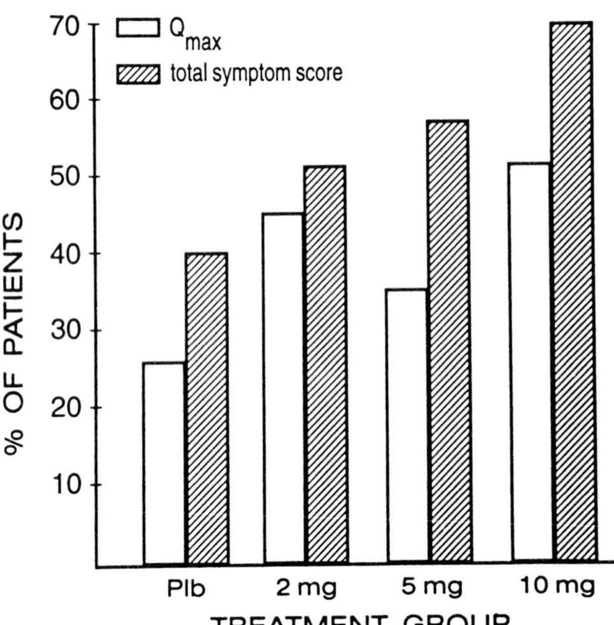

Figure 47–3. Two hundred eighty-five patients were enrolled in a randomized double-blind study comparing placebo and 2 mg, 5 mg, and 10 mg terazosin once daily. Percentages of patients experiencing greater than 30% improvement in total symptom scores and peak urinary flow rates are shown. (From Lepor H: Urology 1993; 42:483–501. Reprinted by permission from Urology.)

The relationships between percentage change in total symptom score and PFR versus baseline age, prostate size, PFR, postvoid residual volume, and total symptom score were examined to identify clinical or urodynamic factors that predicted response to terazosin therapy. **No significant association was observed between treatment effect and any of these baseline factors.**

Lepor (1995a) presented an interim report of 494 patients entered into an open-label extension study demonstrating the durable clinical response of terazosin. Durations of follow-up ranged from 3 to 42 months. The percentages of patients on final terazosin doses of 1, 2, 5, 10, and 20 mg were 7, 12, 26, 34, and 21, respectively. Of the 494 patients, 213 (43.1%) withdrew prematurely: 55 (11%) due to therapeutic failure, 96 (19%) due to adverse events, and 62 (13%) due to administrative reasons.

At all follow-up visits, the group mean PFR was significantly higher than baseline values (Fig. 47–4). At baseline, PFR was 10.0 ml/second. From 3 to 42 months, improvement ranged from 2.3 to 4.0 ml/second. Between 3 and 42 months, at least a 30% improvement in PFR from baseline was observed in 40% to 59% of the patients.

At all follow-up intervals, the group mean Boyarsky symptom scores were significantly lower than at baseline; this was true of the obstructive, irritative, and total score (Fig. 47–5). From 3 months onward, improvement ranged from 4.0 to 5.4 points. Between 3 and 42 months, at least a 30% improvement in total symptom score from baseline was observed in 62.4% to 77.1% of the patients.

Mean changes in blood pressure were analyzed according to whether subjects were normotensive or hypertensive at baseline. In normotensive patients, small, clinically insignificant decreases in blood pressure were noted. Hypertensive patients had larger and clinically significant decreases irrespective of treatment for hypertension. No clinically significant changes in pulse rates were noted. **Terazosin lowered blood pressure primarily in those subjects with hypertension. The ability to treat two common coexisting conditions (BPH and hypertension) is a desirable feature of this drug.**

Doxazosin

Doxazosin is a long-acting alpha$_1$-blocker that has been extensively investigated in subjects with BPH. The half-life of doxazosin is longer than terazosin (22 versus 12 hours). The efficacy, safety, and durability of clinical re-

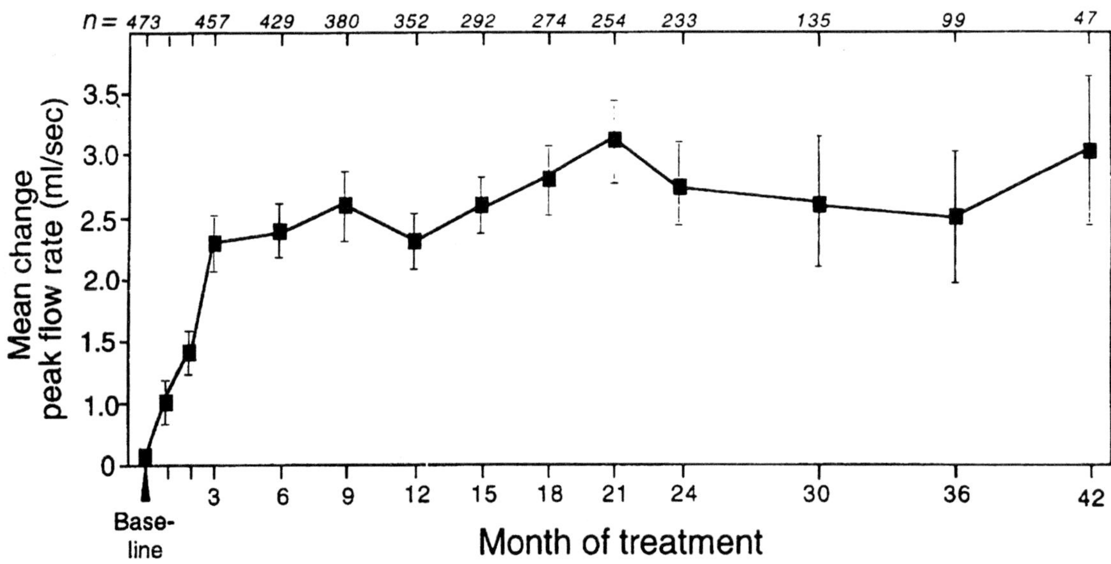

Figure 47–4. Mean change in peak flow rate between baseline and 42 months in terazosin-treated patients. The numbers across the top of the graph indicate the number of patients available at each time interval. All data points were significantly different from baseline at the $P \leq 0.05$ level. (From Lepor H: Urology 1995; 45:406–413. Reprinted with permission from Urology.)

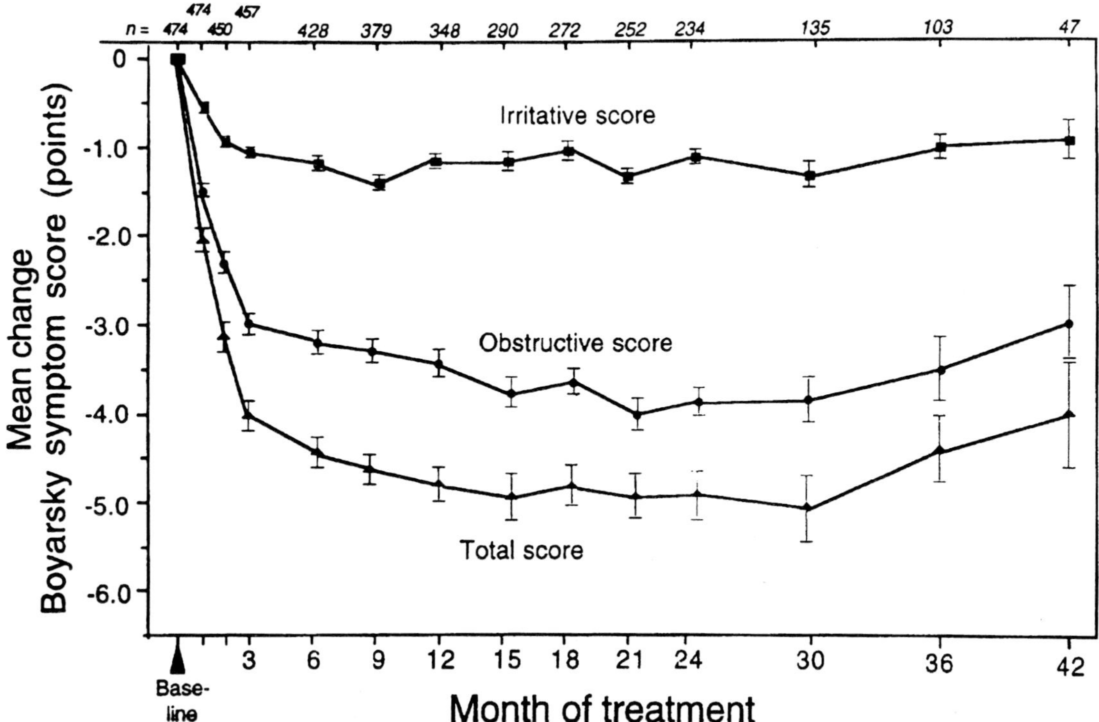

Figure 47–5. Mean change in Boyarsky symptom scores from baseline to 42 months. Baseline scores were 10.5 for total score, 6.2 for obstructive scores, and 4.3 for irritative scores. The numbers across the top of the graph indicate number of patients available at each time interval. All changes were significant at the P ≤ 0.05 level. (From Lepor H: Urology 1995; 45:406–413. Reprinted with permission from Urology.)

sponse of doxazosin have been demonstrated in at least three multicenter randomized double-blind placebo-controlled studies (Chapple et al, 1994; Fawzy et al, 1995; Gillenwater et al, 1995) (Table 47–4) and a long-term open-label extension study (Lepor, 1995b).

Fawzy and associates (1995) reported a 16-week multicenter randomized double-blind placebo-controlled titration to response study in 100 normotensive subjects with BPH. Of the 41 evaluable subjects receiving doxazosin, 88% underwent titration to the maximal dose (8 mg). **The group mean changes in PFR and symptom score were significantly greater in the doxazosin group compared with the placebo group** (see Table 47–4). **The magnitudes of these treatment-related effects are similar to those of terazosin.** The systolic blood pressure changes in normotensive subjects receiving doxazosin are greater than in those receiving terazosin. The treatment-related incidences of dizziness, fatigue, headache, somnolence, hypotension, and nausea were 20%, 8%, 8%, 6%, 8%, and 8%, respectively. The percentages of subjects withdrawing owing to an adverse event were 14% and 2.1% in the doxazosin and placebo groups, respectively. The treatment-related incidence of adverse clinical events in this doxazosin study appears slightly higher than terazosin.

Gillenwater and colleagues (1995) reported a multicenter randomized double-blind placebo-controlled titration to fixed dose study comparing placebo versus 2, 4, 8, and 12 mg of doxazosin in 248 men with mild-to-moderate essential hypertension. The group mean changes in PFR and Boyarsky symptom score are summarized in Table 47–4

Table 47–4. EFFICACY OF DOXAZOSIN IN BENIGN PROSTATIC HYPERPLASIA

Reference	Number Enrolled	Randomized Treatment (Months)	Dose (mg)	Group Mean Difference from Placebo: *PFR (ml/second)*	*Symptom Score*
Chapple et al, 1994	135	3	4	+1.5	NR
Fawzy et al, 1995	100	4	Titration 2–8	+2.2⁺	−3.2*
Gillenwater et al, 1995	248	3.5	2	+1.4	−2.5
			4	+2.2ˣ	−4.7*
			8	+3.2⁺	−3.9*
			12	+3.5⁺	−2.1

NR, Not reported; PFR, peak flow rate.
ˣP < 0.05; ⁺P < 0.01; *P < 0.001.

according to treatment groups. **Because relatively small numbers of subjects were randomized into the individual treatment groups, the failure to demonstrate statistical significance between placebo and some of the active treatment groups reflects the small sample size. The group mean improvement in PFR was dose dependent and statistically significant compared with placebo for all active treatment groups. The group mean improvement in symptom scores compared with placebo was statistically significant for the 4-mg and 8-mg doxazosin groups.** Statistically and clinically significant changes in systolic blood pressure were observed between placebo and the 4-, 8-, and 12-mg doxazosin groups. Lowering of blood pressure was a desirable outcome in these hypertensive patients. The overall treatment-related incidences of dizziness and fatigue were 15% and 10%, respectively. The percentages of subjects withdrawing owing to an adverse event in the doxazosin versus placebo groups were 11.1% and 4.1%, respectively.

Statistically significant changes in symptom scores and PFR relative to baseline have been reported in a long-term open label doxazosin extension study (Lepor, 1995b). The initial improvements in symptom scores and PFR in 450 subjects were maintained for up to 42 months.

A comparison of the nonconcurrent multicenter randomized double-blind placebo-controlled studies of terazosin (see Table 47–3) and doxazosin (see Table 47–4) shows similar efficacy. Although these drugs have not been subjected to a comparative study, it is unlikely that such a trial would demonstrate clinically significant differences.

Tamsulosin

Tamsulosin is the most potent alpha$_1$-antagonist investigated for the management of BPH. One of the unique features of tamsulosin is that it exhibits some degree of specificity for the α_1-AR (Foglar et al, 1995). The efficacy and safety of tamsulosin have been investigated in three multicenter randomized double-blind placebo-controlled studies (Kawabe et al, 1990; Abrams et al, 1995; Lepor, 1995c) (Table 47–5).

Abrams and co-workers (1995) reported a multicenter randomized double-blind placebo-controlled trial in 313 European men with clinical BPH. The patients were randomized in a 2:1 ratio to receive 0.4 mg of tamsulosin or placebo for 9 weeks. The differences in the group mean changes for Boyarsky symptom score and PFR between placebo and 0.4 mg of tamsulosin are shown in Table 47–5. The percentages of subjects exhibiting a 30% improvement in PFR in the placebo and tamsulosin groups were 21% and 30%, respectively. The percentages of subjects exhibiting a 25% reduction in the Boyarsky symptom score in the placebo and tamsulosin groups were 44% and 67%, respectively. The treatment-related incidences of dizziness, abnormal ejaculation, and headache were 3%, 3%, and 2%, respectively. The incidences of postural hypotension, syncope, and tachycardia were 1% in both the placebo and tamsulosin groups. The authors concluded that 0.4 mg of tamsulosin was equally effective and better tolerated than 5 and 10 mg of terazosin and 2 and 4 mg of doxazosin. A comparison of Tables 47–3 to 47–5 shows that 0.4 mg of tamsulosin achieves a therapeutic effect that more closely resembles 2 mg of terazosin and doxazosin. Although the treatment-related incidence of adverse clinical events was exceedingly low in the group treated with 0.4 mg of tamsulosin, these rates are comparable to 2 mg of terazosin (Lepor et al, 1992). Although the absence of a blood pressure–lowering effect of tamsulosin is convincing, the changes in blood pressure were not analyzed according to baseline blood pressure (normotensive versus hypertensive). **The unique features of tamsulosin (efficacy without adverse clinical events, no requirement for dose titration, and no effects on blood pressure) may be attributed to either a relatively low dose and submaximal alpha-blockade achieved by 0.4 mg of tamsulosin or subtype selectivity.**

Lepor and associates (in press) reported a multicenter randomized double-blind placebo-controlled study of 418 American men with clinical BPH randomized to receive placebo, or 0.4 or 0.8 mg of tamsulosin for 1 year. The group mean changes in AUA symptom score and PFR are summarized in Table 47–5. The symptom score and PFR improvements were slightly greater in the 0.8-mg tamsulosin group compared with the 0.4-mg tamsulosin group. **The efficacy of 0.8 mg of tamsulosin appears comparable to 10 mg of terazosin and 8 mg of doxazosin. An interim analysis of this study (Lepor et al, 1995c) reported that the treatment-related incidences of dizziness, headache, and abnormal ejaculation associated with 0.4- and 0.8-mg tamsulosin groups were 4%, 0%, and 6% versus 6%, 0%, and 18%, respectively.** Somnolence was not associated with any tamsulosin dose. The group mean changes in systolic and diastolic blood pressure in the placebo and tamsu-

Table 47–5. EFFICACY OF TAMSULOSIN IN BENIGN PROSTATIC HYPERPLASIA

Reference	Number Enrolled	Randomized Treatment (Months)	Dose (mg)	Group Mean Difference from Placebo: *PFR (ml/second)*	Group Mean Difference from Placebo: *Symptom Score*
Kawabe et al, 1990	270	1	.1	+0.3	NR
			.2	+2.6	NR
			.4	+2.1	NR
Abrams et al, 1995	313	2¼	.4	+1.7ˣ	−1.3⁺
Lepor, in press	418	52	.4	+1.3⁺	−2.9*
			.8	+1.7*	−3.2*

NR = Not reported; PFR, peak flow rate.
ˣ$P < 0.05$; ⁺$P < 0.01$; *$P < 0.001$.

nasteride and placebo were highly statistically significant, this is due, in part, to large sample sizes. Whether these treatment-related benefits are clinically significant or not depends on the expectations of the individual physicians and patients. The long-term safety of finasteride has been demonstrated. The adverse clinical events associated with finasteride are related primarily to sexual function. There is no valid evidence at the present time to support or refute the claim that finasteride alters the natural history of clinical BPH. Finasteride appears to be effective in the management of gross hematuria associated with BPH, especially following prostatectomy.

Antiandrogens have also been investigated for BPH. These studies failed to demonstrate statistically significant treatment-related efficacy. The equivocal efficacy and problematic toxicity of antiandrogens limited the enthusiasm for marketing these drugs for the treatment of BPH.

Table 47–8. COMPARISON OF PLACEBO, FINASTERIDE, TERAZOSIN, AND COMBINATION THERAPY IN BENIGN PROSTATIC HYPERPLASIA

	Placebo	Finasteride	Terazosin	Combination
AUA Symptom Index	−2.6	−3.2	−6.6*	−6.2*
SPI	−1.4	−1.7	-3.9^{+}	-4.2^{+}
BPH II	−0.5	−0.5	-1.2^{+}	-1.7^{+}
Prostate volume (cm^3)	+0.5	6.1*	+0.5	+7.2*
PFR (ml/sec)	+1.4	+1.6	+2.7*	+3.2*

*Difference between final and baseline study visits.

AUA, American Urological Association; BPH II, BPH impact index; PFR, peak flow rate; SPI, symptom problem index.

$^{\times}P < 0.05$; $^{+}P < 0.01$; $^{*}P < 0.001$ (p values relative to placebo).

COMBINATION THERAPY

A review of the existing literature on the medical therapy of BPH suggests that alpha-blockers are more effective than androgen suppression for BPH. Although the adverse clinical events associated with both treatment strategies are relatively uncommon and reversible, the nature of the adverse events associated with alpha-blockers is of greater concern. **The relative safety and efficacy of alpha-blockade and androgen suppression as administered individually or in combination can be determined only from a direct comparative study.** A pilot, nonrandomized study comparing terazosin versus terazosin plus finasteride suggested that some additional benefit may be achieved by adding an antiandrogen to terazosin therapy (Lepor and Machi, 1992).

Veterans Administration Cooperative Study No. 359

A comparison of placebo versus finasteride versus terazosin versus combination (finasteride plus terazosin) therapy has been conducted. **Lepor and co-workers (in press) reported the first multicenter randomized double-blind trial comparing placebo, finasteride, terazosin, and combination therapy (finasteride plus terazosin) in 1229 U.S. veterans with clinical BPH.** All subjects randomized to finasteride received a daily dose of 5 mg. The dose of terazosin was titrated in all patients up to 10 mg, providing that adverse clinical events were not encountered. The dose of terazosin was reduced at the discretion of the investigators to 5 mg when adverse events occurred. **Of the 1229 subjects randomized, 1007 (81.9%) completed the 1-year randomized treatment on assigned study medication.**

The group mean changes between baseline and final study visit for the relevant primary and secondary outcome measures are summarized in Table 47–8. **The mean group differences between finasteride and placebo were not statistically significant for AUA Symptom Index, symptom problem index, BPH impact index, and PFR. The mean group differences between terazosin versus placebo and terazosin versus finasteride for all of the outcome measures other than prostate volume were highly statistically significant in favor of terazosin. The group mean differences between combination therapy and terazosin for all of the outcome measures other than prostate volume were not statistically significant owing to the lack of treatment-related efficacy of finasteride. The Veterans Adminstration study unequivocally demonstrated the superiority of alpha-blockade over androgen suppression for the treatment of clinical BPH over a 1-year interval. Prostate volume decreased approximately 20% in the finasteride and combination groups. The number of subjects withdrawing from the study due to adverse clinical events in the finasteride, terazosin, and combination groups were similar.**

The efficacy of terazosin observed in the Veterans Administration study is in agreement with the literature, whereas the efficacy of finasteride is less than that previously reported. The most likely explanations are differences in the symptom score instrument and baseline prostate volumes in the finasteride studies. The average prostate volume in the Veterans Administration study treatment groups ranged from 36.2 to 38.4 cm^3. These volumes are comparable to the Scandinavian Finasteride Study and clinical investigations of other alpha-blockers, antiandrogens, and minimally invasive therapies. A subset analysis of the Veterans Administration study demonstrated that the group mean changes in AUA symptom scores for placebo and finasteride in men with baseline prostate volumes over 50 cm^3 were −2.0 and −2.9, respectively. The group mean changes in PFR for placebo and finasteride in men with prostate volumes over 50 cm^3 were +0.4 and +2.5 ml/second, respectively. These differences between placebo and finasteride are in agreement with the results of the North American and International Finasteride Trials that enrolled a disproportionate number of men with large prostates. **In the group of men with prostate volumes greater than 50 cm^3, the group mean changes in AUA symptom score and PFR in the terazosin group were –5.8 and 3.9 ml/second, respectively. Terazosin is more effective than finasteride in those subjects with large prostates. The Veterans Administration cooperative medical therapy trial provides compelling evidence supporting the use of selective $alpha_1$-blockers as first-line medical therapy. An algorithm for the medical management of BPH based on**

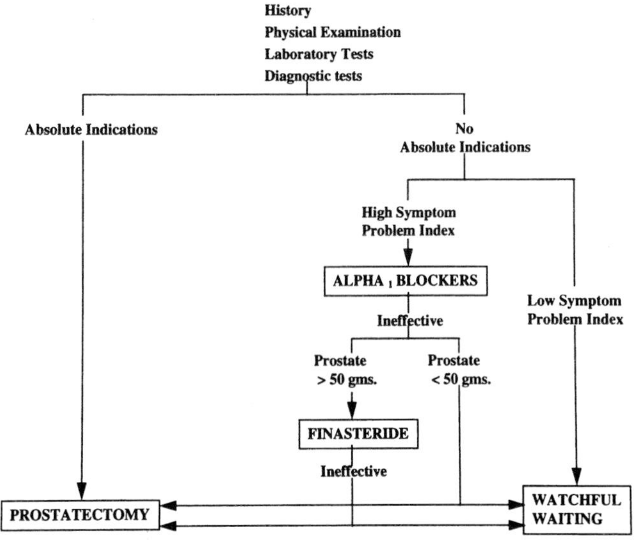

Figure 47–8. Algorithm for medical management of benign prostatic hyperplasia.

the literature and results of the Veterans Administration Medical Therapy Trial is presented in Figure 47–8.

AROMATASE INHIBITORS

Rationale for Aromatase Inhibitors

The rationale for aromatase inhibition is that estrogens may be involved in the pathogenesis of BPH. The estrogenic effect most likely mediates stromal-epithelial interactions that regulate the proliferative activity of the prostate. Several observations support the role of stroma in the development of BPH and the influence of estrogens on prostatic stroma. The inductive potential of prostatic mesenchyme (stroma) is supported by the observation of Cunha and coworkers (1980) in a mouse embryonic animal model. Coffey and Walsh (1990) reported that estrogen treatment of castrated beagles produces a three- to fourfold increase in the total amount of prostatic stroma. Estrogens also greatly enhance the ability of androgens to induce BPH in a canine model (Walsh and Wilson, 1976; DeKlerk et al, 1979). This synergistic effect may be mediated by the ability of estrogens to up-regulate prostatic androgen-receptor content. Stromal hyperplasia can be induced in the prostates of dogs and monkeys treated with aromatizable androgens and prevented by aromatase inhibitors such as atamestane (Habenicht et al, 1987; Habenicht and El Etreby, 1989).

Review of the Literature

Atamestane is a highly selective aromatase inhibitor that lowers both serum and intraprostatic levels of estradiol and estrone (El Etreby et al, 1991). **Gingell and co-workers (1995) reported a multicenter randomized double-blind placebo-controlled study comparing placebo and 400 mg of atamestane in 160 subjects with clinical BPH.** The administration of atamestane resulted in a statistically significant decrease in serum estradiol and estrone levels, and a statistically significant increase in serum testosterone. **No statistically significant group mean differences were observed for changes in Boyarsky symptom score, PFR, or prostate volume between the atamestane and placebo groups.** One of the explanations contributing to the failure of atamestane to achieve clinical efficacy was the increase in testosterone. **The development of atamestane for BPH was suspended because of these negative clinical findings.** The failure to demonstrate that atamestane causes regression of established BPH or clinical improvement does not negate the influence of estrogens in the pathogenesis of BPH.

PHYTOTHERAPY

Phytotherapy refers to the use of plant extracts for medicinal indications. Several plant extracts are widely prescribed throughout the world for the treatment of BPH. Fitzpatrick and Lynch (1995) and Lowe and Ku (in press) have recently reviewed the phytotherapy literature for BPH. The most commonly described plant extracts include the root of *Hypoxis rooperi*, the fruit of *Sabal serulata* (*Serenoa repens*), the bark of *Pygeum africanum*, pollen extract, the seeds of *Cucuibita pepo*, the leaves of the trembling poplar, and the roots of *Echinacea purpurea*. **The mechanisms of action for these phytotherapies are unknown or unproven.** The following modes of action have been suggested: antiandrogenic effect, antiestrogenic effect, decrease in sex hormone–binding globulin, inhibition of growth factors, and interference with metabolism of prostaglandins. **The reported efficacy and safety of these therapies have not been based on multicenter randomized double-blind placebo-controlled studies.**

It is imperative that the safety and efficacy of phytotherapies be investigated using multicenter randomized double-blind placebo-controlled studies. Because the differences between finasteride and placebo for AUA symptom scores and PFR in one large study were not statistically significant (Lepor et al, in press), the efficacy of phytotherapy cannot be established based on showing equivalency to finasteride.

The rationale for phytotherapy in the treatment of BPH is that the placebo effect in some cases is therapeutic and not associated with adverse clinical events. **In an era of medical therapies with proven efficacy and safety, deliberately prescribing a placebo is difficult to justify. It is also unlikely that patients would select phytotherapies if disclosure is made that the mechanism is simply via placebo.**

FUTURE STRATEGIES FOR DRUG DEVELOPMENT FOR BENIGN PROSTATIC HYPERPLASIA

Medical therapies provide relief of symptoms for a significant proportion of men with BPH. The therapeutic response to medical therapy is less than prostatectomy. Therefore, opportunities exist to develop novel strategies that may be more effective than existing therapies. Developing different classes of drugs to relax smooth muscle and targeting nonprostatic factors are potential opportunities.

New Strategies for Altering Dynamic and Static Obstruction

Endothelins are potent vasoconstrictors. Langenstroer and associates (1993) reported that human prostate contains endogenous endothelin and that **endothelin elicits a very potent contraction in the human prostate. The contractile response elicited by endothelin in the human prostate is not abolished by pretreatment with selective alpha$_1$-blockers.** These observations suggest that relaxation of prostatic smooth muscle in BPH may also be achieved by endothelin antagonists. The pharmaceutical industry is actively engaged in efforts to synthesize selective endothelin antagonists. Kobayashi and colleagues (1994) characterized the binding properties of endothelin receptor subtypes in the human prostate. Both ET_A and ET_B receptors are present in the human prostate. The ET_A and ET_B receptors are localized primarily in the stroma and glandular epithelium, respectively. Preliminary studies suggest that both ET_A and ET_B receptors mediate the tension of prostate smooth muscle. **Endothelin antagonists may emerge as another treatment for BPH.**

Nitric oxide is a nonadrenergic noncholinergic mediator of smooth muscle activity. Nitric oxide has been shown to mediate cavernosal smooth muscle activity. **Burnett and colleagues (1995) have reported nitric oxide synthase activity in the prostate using immunohistochemical and biochemical investigations. Takeda et al (1995) have shown that prostate smooth muscle tension is mediated by nitric oxide. These preliminary studies suggest that nitric oxide inhibitors may also play a future role in treating BPH.**

Development of Therapy Directed Toward Unrecognized Factors Resulting in Clinical Benign Prostatic Hyperplasia

It is generally assumed that the clinical manifestations of BPH are the result of bladder outlet obstruction. Therefore, pharmacologic strategies have been directed toward reducing bladder outlet obstruction. **There are several observations that suggest nonprostatic factors may also contribute to clinical BPH.** The severity of clinical prostatism as indicated by symptom scores is poorly correlated with the measure of bladder outlet obstruction. In addition, the changes in symptom scores following therapy for BPH are poorly correlated with changes in PFR and obstruction grade. The discordance between symptom severity and measures of obstruction suggests that nonprostatic factors may be contributing to clinical BPH. **It is the author's belief that several factors such as aging, the hormonal milieu, nonurologic diseases, and prostatic growth affect bladder morphometry, neurologic innervation, bladder outlet obstruction, and renal function, and that these factors collectively contribute to clinical BPH. Our present understanding of the pathophysiology of clinical BPH is rudimentary. Therefore, it is imperative to develop a more comprehensive understanding of the pathophysiology of symptoms. This knowledge will result in more effective use of existing therapies, and will provide the rationale for the next generation of therapeutic modalities.**

REFERENCES

Overview

Abrams P: In support of pressure-flow studies for evaluating men with lower urinary symptoms. Urology 1994; 44:153–155.

Barry MJ, Cockett ATK, Holtgrewe HL, et al: Relationship of symptoms of prostatism to commonly used physiological and anatomical measures of the severity of benign prostatic hyperplasia. J Urol 1993; 150:351–358.

Bartsch G, Muller HR, Oberholzer M, et al: Light microscopic stereological analysis of the normal human prostate and of benign prostatic hyperplasia. J Urol 1979; 122:487–489.

Berry SJ, Coffey DS, Walsh PC, et al: The development of human prostatic hyperplasia with age. J Urol 1984; 132:474–479.

Bosch J, Kranse R, Van Mastrigt R, et al: Reasons for the weak correlation between prostate volume and urethral resistance parameters in patients with prostatism. J Urol 1995; 153:689–693.

Girman CJ, Jacobsen SJ, Guess HA, et al: Natural history of prostatism: Relationship among symptoms, prostate volume and peak urinary flow rate. J Urol 1995; 153:1510–1515.

Isaacs JT, Coffey DS: Etiology and disease process of benign prostatic hyperplasia. Prostate 1989; 2(Suppl):33–50.

Lepor H, Wang B, Shapiro E: Relationship between prostatic epithelial volume and serum prostate-specific antigen levels. Urology 1994; 44:199–205.

McNeal JG: The prostate gland: Morphology and pathobiology. Monogr Urology 1983; 4:3–33.

Riehmann M, Bruskewitz RC: Benign prostatic hyperplasia: Clinical manifestations and indications for intervention. *In* Lepor H, Lawson RK, eds: Prostate Diseases. Philadelphia, W. B. Saunders Company, 1993, pp 108–118.

Shapiro E, Lepor H: Pathophysiology of clinical BPH. Urol Clin North Am 1995; 22:285–290.

Smith ER, Resnick MI: Imaging of the prostate. *In* Lepor H, Lawson RK, eds: Prostate Diseases. Philadelphia, W. B. Saunders Company, 1993, pp 72–86.

Steiner M: The role of peptide growth factors in the prostate. A review. Urology 1993; 42:99–110.

Strandberg JD: Comparative pathology of benign prostatic hyperplasia. *In* Lepor H, Lawson R, eds: Prostate Diseases. Philadelphia, W. B. Saunders Company, 1993, pp 212–225.

Tempany CMC, Partin AW, Zerhouni EA, et al: The influence of finasteride on the volume of peripheral and periurethral zones of the prostate in men with benign prostatic hyperplasia. Prostate 1993; 22:39–42.

Walsh PC: Benign prostatic hyperplasia. *In* Walsh PC, Gittes RF, Perlmutter AD, Stamey TA, eds: Campbell's Urology, 5th ed. Philadelphia, W. B. Saunders Company, 1986, pp 1248–1265.

Yalla SV, Sullivan MP, Lecamwasan HS, et al: Correlation of American Urological Association Symptom Index with obstructive and nonobstructive prostatism. J Urol 1995; 153:674–686.

Natural History

Ball AJ, Feneley RCL, Abrams PH: The natural history of untreated "prostatism." Br J Urol 1981; 53:613–616.

Barnes RW, Marsh C: Progression of obstruction and symptoms. *In* Hinman F, ed: Benign Prostatic Hypertrophy. New York, Springer Verlag, 1983, pp 711–713.

Barry MJ: Epidemiology and natural history of benign prostatic hyperplasia. *In* Lepor H, Lawson RK, eds: Prostate Diseases. Philadelphia, W. B. Saunders Company, 1993, pp 96–107.

Barry MJ, Cockett ATK, Holtgrewe HL, et al: Relationship of symptoms of prostatism to commonly used physiological and anatomical measures of the severity of benign prostatic hyperplasia. J Urol 1993; 150:351–358.

Barry MJ, Fowler FJ, O'Leary MP, et al: The American Urological Association symptom index for benign prostatic hyperplasia. J Urol 1992; 148:1549–1557.

Berry SJ, Coffey DS, Walsh PC, et al: The development of human prostatic hyperplasia with age. J Urol 1984; 132:474–479.

Birkhoff JD, Wiederhorn AR, Hamilton ML, et al: Natural history of benign prostatic hypertrophy and acute urinary retention. Urology 1976; 7:48–52.

Bosch JLHR, Hop WCJ, Niemer AQ, et al: Parameters of prostate volume and shape in a community-based population of men between fifty-five and seventy-four years of age. J Urol 1994; 152:1501–1505.

Bosch J, Kranse R, Van Mastrigt R, et al: Reasons for the weak correlation between prostate volume and urethral resistance parameters in patients with prostatism. J Urol 1995; 153:689–693.

Chute CG, Panser LA, Girman CJ, et al: The prevalence of prostatism: A population-based survey of urinary symptoms. J Urol 1993; 150:85–89.

Clarke R: The prostate and the endocrines: A control series. Br J Urol 1937; 9:254–271.

Craigen AA, Hickling JB, Saunders CRG, et al: Natural history of prostatic obstruction: A prospective survey. J R Coll Gen Pract 1969; 18:226–232.

Garraway WM, Collins GN, Lee RJ: High prevalence of benign prostatic hypertrophy in the community. Lancet 1991; 338:469–471.

Girman CJ, Jacobsen SJ, Guess HA, et al: Natural history of prostatism: Relationship among symptoms, prostate volume and peak urinary flow rate. J Urol 1995; 153:1510–1515.

Girman C, Panser L, Chute C, et al: Natural history of prostatism: Urinary flow rates in a community-based study. J Urol 1993; 150:887–892.

Glynn RJ, Campion EW, Bouchard GR, et al: The development of benign prostatic hyperplasia among volunteers in the Normative Aging Study. Am J Epidemiol 1985; 121:78–90.

Guess HA, Arrighi HM, Metter EJ, et al: The cumulative prevalence of prostatism matches the autopsy prevalence of benign prostatic hyperplasia. Prostate 1990; 17:241–246.

Guess HA, Chute CG, Garraway WM, et al: Similar levels of urological symptoms have similar impact on Scottish and American men although Scots report less symptoms. J Urol 1993; 150:1701–1705.

Isaacs JT, Coffey DS: Etiology and disease process of benign prostatic hyperplasia. Prostate 1989; 2(Suppl):33–50.

Lepor H, Wang B, Shapiro E, et al: Comparison of the cellular composition of BPH in Chinese and American Caucasian males. Urology 1996; 47:38–42.

Nacey JN, Morum P, Delahunt B: Analysis of the prevalence of voiding symptoms in Maori, Pacific Island and Caucasian New Zealand men. Urology 1995; 46:506–511.

Oesterling JE, Jacobsen SJ, Chute CG, et al: Serum prostate-specific antigen in a community-based population of healthy men: Establishment of age-specific reference ranges. JAMA 1993; 270:860–864.

Riehmann M, Bruskewitz RC: Benign prostatic hyperplasia: Clinical manifestations and indications for intervention. *In* Lepor H, Lawson RK, eds: Prostate Diseases. Philadelphia, W. B. Saunders Company, 1993, pp 108–118.

Sagnier PP, Macfarlane G, Richard F, et al: Results of an epidemiological survey employing a modified American Urological Association Index for benign prostatic hyperplasia in France. J Urol 1994; 151:1226–1270.

Tsukamoto T, Kumamoto Y, Masumori N, et al: Prevalence of prostatism in Japanese men in a population-based study with comparison to a similar American study. J Urol 1995; 154:391–395.

Watanabe H. Natural history of benign prostatic hypertrophy. Ultrasound Med Biol 1986; 12:567–571.

Assessing the Effectiveness and Safety of Medical Therapy for Benign Prostatic Hyperplasia

Abrams P: In support of pressure-flow studies for evaluating men with lower urinary symptoms. Urology 1994a; 44:153–155.

Abrams P: New words for old: Lower urinary tract symptoms for "prostatism." BMJ 1994b; 308:929.

Abrams PH: Prostatism and prostatectomy: The value of urine flow rate measurement in the preoperative assessment for operation. J Urol 1977; 117:70.

Abrams PH, Griffiths D: The assessment of prostatic obstruction from urodynamic measurements and from residual urine. Br J Urol 1979; 51:129–134.

Barry MJ, Cockett ATK, Holtgrewe HL, et al: Relationship of symptoms of prostatism to commonly used physiological and anatomical measures of the severity of benign prostatic hyperplasia. J Urol 1993; 150:351–358.

Barry MJ, Fowler FJ, O'Leary MP, et al: The American Urological Association symptom index for benign prostatic hyperplasia. J Urol 1992a; 148:1549–1557.

Barry MJ, Fowler FJ, O'Leary MP, et al: Correlation of the American Urological Association symptom index with self-administered versions of the Madsen-Iversen, Boyarsky, and Maine Medical Assessment Program symptom indexes. J Urol 1992b; 148:1558–1563.

Barry MJ, Fowler FJ, O'Leary MP, et al: Measuring disease-specific health status in men with benign prostatic hyperplasia. Med Care 1995a; 33:AS145–155.

Barry M, Girman C, O'Leary M, et al: Using repeated measures of symptom score, uroflowmetry and prostate specific antigen in the clinical management of prostate disease. J Urol 1995c; 153:99–103.

Barry MJ, O'Leary MP: The development and clinical utility of symptom scores. Urol Clin North Am 1995; 22:229–307.

Barry MJ, Williford WO, Chang Y, et al: Benign prostatic hyperplasia–specific health status measures in clinical research: How much change in the American Urological Association symptom index and the benign prostatic hyperplasia impact index is perceptible to patients? J Urol 1995b; 154:1770–1774.

Blaivas JG: Multichannel urodynamic studies in men with benign prostatic hyperplasia: Indicators and interpretation. Urol Clin North Am 1990; 17:543–544.

Boyarsky S, Jones G, Paulson DF, et al: A new look at bladder neck obstruction by the Food and Drug Administration regulators: Guidelines for investigation of benign prostate hypertrophy. Transactions of the American Academy of Genito-Urinary Surgeons. 1977; 68:29–32.

Breum L, Klarskov P, Munck LK, et al: Significance of acute urinary retention due to infravesical obstruction. Scand J Nephrol 1982; 16:21.

Bruskewitz RC, Iversen P, Madsen PO: Value of post-void residual urine determination in evaluation of prostatism. Urology 1982; 20:602.

Byar DP, Simon RM, Friedewald WT, et al: Randomized clinical trials; perspective on some recent ideas. N Engl J Med 1976; 295:74–80.

Cockett ATK, Barry MJ, Holtgrewe HL, et al: Indications for treatment of benign prostatic hyperplasia. Cancer 1992; 70:280.

Coolsaet BRLA, Block C: Detrusor properties related to prostatism. Neurourol Urodyn 1986; 5:435.

Cucchi A: The development of DI in prostatic obstruction in relation to sequential changes in voiding dynamics. J Urol 1994; 51:1342.

Dorflinger T, Frimodt-Moller PC, Bruskewitz RC, et al: The significance of uninhibited detrusor contractions in prostatism. J Urol 1985; 133:819–821.

Drach GW, Layton TN, Binard WJ: Male peak urinary flow rate: Relationships to volume voided and age. J Urol 1979; 122:210–214.

Gerstenberg TC, Andersen JT, Klarskov AP, et al: High flow infravesical obstruction in men: Symptomatology, urodynamics and the results of surgery. J Urol 1982; 127:943.

Jensen KME, Bruskewitz RC, Iversen P, et al: Predictive value of voiding pressures in benign prostatic hyperplasia. Neurourol Urodyn 1983; 2:117–125.

Jorgensen JB, Jensen KME, Bille-Brahe NE, et al: Uroflowmetry in asymptomatic elderly males. Br J Urol 1986; 58:390–395.

Kaplan SA, Te A: Uroflowmetry and urodynamics. Urol Clin North Am 1995; 22:309–320.

Ko DSC, Fenster HN, Chambers K: The correlation of multichannel urodynamic pressure-flow studies and American Urological Association Symptom Index in the evaluation of benign prostatic hyperplasia. J Urol 1995; 154:396–398.

Lepor H, Machi GM: Comparison of AUA Symptom Index in unselected males and females between 55 and 79 years of age. Urology 1993; 42:36.

Levin RM, Longhurst PA, Monson FC, et al: Experimental studies on bladder outlet obstruction. *In* Lepor H, Lawson RK, eds: Prostate Diseases. Philadelphia, W. B. Saunders Company, 1993, pp 118–130.

Levin RM, Monson FC, Haugaard N, et al: Genetics and cellular characteristics of bladder outlet obstruction. Urol Clin North Am 1995; 22:263–283.

Madsen PO, Iverson P: A point system for selecting operative candidates. *In* Boyarsky S, Hinman F, eds: Benign Prostatic Hypertrophy. New York, Springer Verlag, 1983, pp 763–765.

Nitti V, Kim Y, Combs A: Correlation of the AUA Symptom Index with urodynamics in patients with suspected benign prostatic hyperplasia. Neurourol Urodyn 1994; 13:521–529.

Riehmann M, Bruskewitz RC: Benign prostatic hyperplasia: Clinical manifestations and indications for intervention. *In* Lepor H, Lawson RK, eds: Prostate Diseases. Philadelphia, W. B. Saunders Company, 1993, pp 108–118.

Rollema HJ, Van Mastrigt R: Objective analysis of prostatism: A clinical application of the computer program CLIM. Neurourol Urodyn 1991; 10:71.

Schafer W, Noppeney R, Rubben H, et al: The value of free flow rate and pressure/flow studies in the routine investigation of BPH patients. Neurourol Urodyn 1988; 7:219.

Shapiro E, Lepor H: Pathophysiology of clinical BPH. Urol Clin North Am 1995; 22:285–290.

Shaw LW, Chalmers TC: Ethics in cooperative clinical trials. Ann NY Acad Sci 1970; 169:487–495.
Siroky MB, Olsson CA, Krane RJ: The flow rate nomogram: Development. J Urol 1979; 122:665.
Siroky MB: Interpretation of urinary flow rates. Urol Clin North Am 1990; 17:537.
Taube M, Gajraj H: Trial without catheter following acute retention of urine. Br J Urol 1989; 63:180.
Tubaro A, Carter SS, Rosette J, et al: The prediction of clinical outcome from transurethral microwave thermotherapy by pressure flow analysis: A European multicenter study. J Urol 1995; 153:1526–1530.
Wasson JH, Reda DJ, Bruskewitz RC, et al: A comparison of transurethral surgery with watchful waiting for moderate symptoms of benign prostatic hyperplasia. N Engl J Med 1995; 332:75–79.
Witjes WPJ, de Wildt MJAM, Rosier PFWN, et al: Terazosin treatment in patients with symptomatic benign prostatic hyperplasia. J Urol 1995; 153:273A.

Medical Therapy for Benign Prostatic Hyperplasia

Breslin DS, Muecke EC, Reckler JM, et al: Changing trends in the management of prostate diseases in a single private practice: A 5-year follow up. J Urol 1993; 150:347–350.
Chute CG, Panser LA, Girman CJ, et al: The prevalence of prostatism: A population-based survey of urinary symptoms. J Urol 1993; 150:85–89.
Holtgrewe HL: Economic issues and the management of benign prostatic hyperplasia. Urology 1995; 46(Suppl 3A):23–25.
Jacobsen S, Girman C, Guess H, et al: New diagnostic and treatment guidelines for benign prostatic hyperplasia. Arch Intern Med 1995; 155:477–481.
Lepor H, Machi GM: Comparison of AUA Symptom Index in unselected males and females between 55 and 79 years of age. Urology 1993; 42:36.
Lepor H: Alpha blockade in the therapy of benign prostatic hyperplasia. *In* Lepor H, Lawson RK, eds: Prostate Diseases. Philadelphia, W. B. Saunders Company, 1993, pp 170–181.
Mebust WK, Holtgrewe HL, Cockett ATK, et al: Transurethral prostatectomy: Immediate and postoperative complications. A cooperative study of 13 participating institutions evaluating 3,885 patients. J Urol 1989; 141:243.

Alpha-Blockade

Abrams PH, Shah PJR, Choa RG, et al: Bladder outflow obstruction treated with phenoxybenzamine. Br J Urol 1982; 54:527–530.
Abrams P, Schulman CC, Vaage S, et al: Tamsulosin, a selective alpha$_{1c}$ adrenoceptor antagonist: A randomized, controlled trial in patients with benign prostatic obstruction. Br J Urol 1995; 76:325–336.
Berthelson S, Pettinger WA: A functional basis for the classification of alpha adrenergic receptor. Life Sci 1977; 21:595–600.
Brawer MK, Adams G, Epstein H, et al: Terazosin in the treatment of benign prostatic hyperplasia. Arch Fam Med 1993; 2:929–935.
Caine M: The present role of alpha adrenergic blockers in the treatment of benign prostatic hypertrophy. J Urol 1986; 136:1–6.
Caine M, Perlberg S, Meretyk S: A placebo-controlled double-blind study of the effect of phenoxybenzamine in benign prostatic obstruction. Br J Urol 1978; 50:551–554.
Caine M, Pfau A, Perlberg S: The use of alpha adrenergic blockers in benign prostatic obstruction. Br J Urol 1976; 48:255.
Caine M, Raz S, Zeigler M: Adrenergic and cholinergic receptors in the human prostate, prostatic capsule and bladder neck. Br J Urol 1975; 27:193–202.
Carbin BE, Bauer P, Friskand M, et al: Efficacy of alfuzosine (an alpha-1-adrenoreceptor blocking drug) in benign hyperplasia of the prostate. Scand J Urol Nephrol 1991; 138(Suppl):73–75.
Chapple CR, Stott M, Abrams PH, et al: A 12-week placebo-controlled double-blind study of prazosin in the treatment of prostatic obstruction due to benign prostatic hyperplasia. Br J Urol 1992; 70:285.
Chapple CR, Carter P, Christmas TJ, et al: A three-month double-blind study of doxazosin as treatment for benign prostatic obstruction. Br J Urol 1994; 74:50–56.
Chow W, Hahn D, Sandhu D, et al: Multicentre controlled trial of indoramin in the symptomatic relief of benign prostatic hypertrophy. Br J Urol 1990; 65:36–38.
DiSilverio F: Use of terazosin in the medical treatment of benign prostatic hyperplasia: Experience in Italy. Br J Urol 1992; 70(Suppl):22–26.
Eri LM, Tveter KJ: Alpha blockade in the treatment of symptomatic benign prostatic hyperplasia. J Urol 1995; 154:923–934.
Fawzy A, Braun K, Lewis GP, et al: Doxazosin in the treatment of benign prostatic hyperplasia in normotensive patients: A multicenter study. J Urol 1995; 154:105–109.
Foglar R, Shibata K, Hirasawa A, et al: Use of recombinant alpha$_1$ adrenoceptors to characterize subtype selectivity of drugs for the treatment of prostatic hypertrophy. Eur J Pharmacol 1995; 288:201–207.
Forray C, Bard JA, Wetzel JM, et al: The alpha$_1$ adrenergic receptor that mediates smooth muscle contraction in human prostate has the pharmacologic properties of a cloned human alpha$_{1c}$ subtype. Pharmacology 1994a; 45:703.
Forray C, Chiu G, Wetzel JM, et al: Effects of novel alpha$_{1c}$ adrenergic receptor antagonists on the contraction of human prostate smooth muscle. J Urol 1994b; 151:267A.
Gillenwater JY, Conn RL, Chrysant SG, et al: Doxazosin for the treatment of benign prostatic hyperplasia in patients with mild to moderate essential hypertension: A double-blind, placebo-controlled dose response multicenter study. J Urol 1995; 154:110–115.
Gup DI, Shapiro E, Baumann M, et al: The contractile properties of human prostate adenomas and the development of infravesical obstruction. Prostate 1989; 15:105–114.
Hansen BJ, Nordling J, Mensink HJ, et al: Alfuzosin in the treatment of benign prostatic hyperplasia: Effects on symptom scores, urinary flow rates and residual volume. A multicentre, double-blind, placebo-controlled trial. Scand J Med Nephrol 1994; 157(Suppl):169.
Hedlund H, Andersson KE, Ek A: Effects of prazosin in patients with benign prostatic obstruction. J Urol 1983; 130:275–278.
Hieble JP, Caine M, Zalaznik E: In vitro characterization of the alpha-adrenoceptors in human prostate. Eur J Pharmacol 1985; 107:111–117.
Iacovou JW, Dunn M: Indoramin—an effective new drug in the management of bladder outflow obstruction. Br J Urol 1987; 60:526–528.
Jardin A, Bensadoun H, Delauche-Cavallier MC, et al: Alfuzosin for treatment of benign prostatic hypertrophy. Lancet 1991; 337:1457–1461.
Kawabe K, Ueno A, Takimoto Y, et al: Use of an alpha$_1$ blocker, YM617, in the treatment of benign prostatic hypertrophy. J Urol 1990; 144:908–912.
Kirby RS: Doxazosin in benign prostatic hyperplasia: Effects on blood pressure and urinary flow in normotensive and hypertensive men. Urology 1995; 46:182–186.
Kirby RS, Coppinger SWC, Corcoran MO, et al: Prazosin in the treatment of prostatic obstruction. A placebo-controlled study. Br J Urol 1987; 60:136–142.
Kobayashi S, Tang R, Shapiro E, et al: Characterization of human alpha-1 adrenoceptor binding sites using radioligand receptor binding on slide-mounted tissue sections. J Urol 1993; 150:2002.
LeDuc A, Cariou G, Baron C, et al: A multicenter, double-blind, placebo-controlled trial of the efficacy of prazosin in the treatment of dysuria associated with benign prostatic hypertrophy. Urol Int 1990; 45(Suppl 1):56–62.
Lepor H: Nonoperative management of benign prostatic hyperplasia. J Urol 1989; 141:1283–1289.
Lepor H: Alpha blockade in the therapy of benign prostatic hyperplasia. *In* Lepor H, Lawson RK, eds: Prostate Diseases. Philadelphia, W. B. Saunders Company, 1993a, pp 170–181.
Lepor H: Medical therapy for benign prostatic hyperplasia. Urology 1993b; 42:483–501.
Lepor H: Alpha blockade for the treatment of BPH. Urol Clin North Am 1995a; 22:375–386.
Lepor H: Long-term efficacy and safety of terazosin in patients with benign prostatic hyperplasia. Urology 1995b; 45:406–413.
Lepor H: Prostate selectivity of alpha blockers: From receptor biology to clinical medicine. Eur Urol 1996; 29:12–16.
Lepor H, Auerbach S, Puras-Baez A, et al: A randomized multicenter placebo controlled study of the efficacy and safety of terazosin in the treatment of benign prostatic hyperplasia. J Urol 1992; 148:1467–1474.
Lepor H, Gup DI, Baumann M, et al: Laboratory assessment of terazosin and alpha-1 adrenergic receptor in human benign prostatic hyperplasia. Urology 1988; 32(Suppl 6):21–26.
Lepor H, the Multicenter Study Group: Long-term efficacy and safety of terazosin in patients with benign prostatic hyperplasia. Urology 1995a; 45:406–413.
Lepor H, the Multicenter Study Group: Long-term efficacy and safety of doxazosin for the treatment of benign prostatic hyperplasia. J Urol 1995b; 153:273A.
Lepor H, Shapiro E: Characterization of the alpha-1 adrenergic receptor in human benign prostatic hyperplasia. J Urol 1984; 132:1226–1229.

Lepor H, the Tamsulosin Investigator Group: Clinical evaluation of tamsulosin, a prostate selective alpha$_{1c}$ antagonist. J Urol 1995; 153:274A.

Lepor H, the Tamsulosin Investigator Group: Long-term efficacy of tamsulosin, a prostate selective alpha$_1$ antagonist. J Urol. In press.

Lepor H, Vaughan ED: Medical Management of BPH: Part II. AUA Update Series 1996; 15:26–31.

Lloyd SN, Buckley JF, Chilton CP, et al: Terazosin in the treatment of benign prostatic hyperplasia: A multicentre, placebo-controlled trial. Br J Urol 1992; 70(Suppl 1):17–21.

Martorana G, Giberti C, Damonte P, et al: The effect of prazosin in benign prostatic hypertrophy, a placebo controlled double-blind study. I.R.C.S. Medical Science 1984; 12:11–12.

McConnell JD, Barry MJ, Bruskewitz RC, et al: Benign Prostatic Hyperplasia: Diagnosis and Treatment. Clinical Practice Guideline, No. 8. AHCPR Publication. Rockville, MD, Agency for Health Care Policy and Research Public Health Services, US Department of Health and Human Services, 1994.

Ramsay JWA, Scott GI, Whitfield HN: A double-blind controlled trial of new alpha-1 blocking drug in the treatment of bladder outflow obstruction. Br J Urol 1985; 57:657.

Roehrborn CG, Oesterling JE, Lloyd K, et al: Hytrin community assessment trial: Evaluation of the clinical effectiveness of terazosin vs. placebo in the treatment of patients with symptomatic benign prostatic hyperplasia. J Urol 1995; 153:272A.

Ruutu ML, Hansson E, Juusela HE, et al: Efficacy and side-effects of prazosin as a symptomatic treatment of benign prostatic obstruction. Scand J Urol Nephrol 1991; 25:15–19.

Scott MA, Abrams P: Indoramin in the treatment of prostatic bladder outflow obstruction. Br J Urol 1991; 67:499.

Shapiro E, Hartanto V, Lepor H: Anti-desmin vs. anti-actin for quantifying the area density of prostate smooth muscle. Prostate 1992; 20:259–267.

Androgen Suppression

Andersen JT, Ekman P, Wolf H, et al: Can finasteride reverse the progress of benign prostatic hyperplasia? A two-year placebo controlled study. Urology 1995; 46:631–637.

Berger BM, Naadimuthu A, Boddy A, et al: The effect of zanoterone, a steroidal androgen receptor antagonist, in men with benign prostatic hyperplasia. J Urol 1995; 154:1060–1064.

Bluestein DL, Oesterling JE: Hormonal therapy in the management of benign prostatic hyperplasia. *In* Lepor H, Lawson RK, eds: Prostate Diseases. Philadelphia, W. B. Saunders Company, 1993, pp 182–198.

Cabot AT: The question of castration for enlarged prostate. Ann Surg 1896; 24:265–309.

Caine M, Perlberg S, Gordon R: The treatment of benign prostatic hypertrophy with flutamide (SCH 13521): A placebo-controlled study. J Urol 1975; 114:564–568.

Coffey DS, Walsh PC: Clinical and experimental studies of benign prostatic hyperplasia. Urol Clin North Am 1990; 17:461–475.

Donkervoort T, Zinner NR, Sterling AM, et al: Megestrol acetate in treatment of benign prostatic hyperplasia. Urology 1975; 6:580–587.

Eri LM, Tveter KJ: A prospective placebo-controlled study of the antiandrogen casodex as treatment for patients with benign prostatic hyperplasia. J Urol 1993a; 150:90–94.

Eri LM, Tveter KJ: A prospective placebo-controlled study of the luteinizing hormone–releasing hormone agonist leuprolide as treatment for patients with benign prostatic hyperplasia. J Urol 1993b; 150:359–364.

Finasteride Study Group: Finasteride (MK-906) in the treatment of benign prostatic hyperplasia. Prostate 1993; 22:291–299.

Geller J, Nelson CG, Albert JD, et al: Effect of megestrol acetate on uroflow rates in patients with benign prostatic hypertrophy: Double-blind study. Urology 1979; 14:467–474.

Gormley GJ, Stoner E, Bruskewitz RC, et al: The effect of finasteride in men with benign prostatic hyperplasia. N Engl J Med 1992; 327:1185–1191.

Guess HA, Heyse JF, Gormley GJ: The effect of finasteride on prostate-specific antigens in men with benign prostatic hyperplasia. Prostate 1993; 22:31–37.

Jenkins EP, Andersson S, Imperato-McGinley J, et al: Genetic and pharmacological evidence for more than one human steroid 5 alpha-reductase. J Clin Invest 1992; 89:293.

Juniewicz PE, McCarthy M, Lemp BM, et al: The effect of the steroidal androgen receptor antagonist WIN49596 on the prostate and testes of beagle dogs. Endocrinology 1990; 126:2625.

Keane PF, Timoney AG, Kiely E, et al: Response of the benign hypertrophied prostate to treatment with an LHRH analogue. Br J Urol 1988; 62:163–165.

Lepor H: Medical therapy for benign prostatic hyperplasia. Urology 1993; 42:483–501.

McConnell JD: Hormonal treatment of benign prostatic hyperplasia. Urol Clin North Am 1995; 22:387–400.

McConnell JD: Medical management of benign prostatic hyperplasia with androgen suppression. Prostate 1990; 3(Suppl):49–59.

Meiraz D, Margolin Y, Lev-Ran A, et al: Treatment of benign prostatic hyperplasia w/hydroxyprogesterone-caproate: Placebo-controlled study. Urology 1977; 9:144–148.

Oesterling JH: Benign prostatic hyperplasia. Medical and minimally invasive treatment option. N Engl J Med 1995; 32:99–109.

Ostri P, Swartz P, Myerhoff HH, et al: Antiandrogenic treatment of benign prostatic hyperplasia: A placebo-controlled trial. Urol Res 1989; 17:29–33.

Peters CA, Walsh PC: The effect of nafarelin acetate, a luteinizing-hormone-releasing hormone agonist, on benign prostatic hyperplasia. N Engl J Med 1987; 317:599–604.

Puchner PJ, Miller MI: The effects of finasteride on hematuria associated with benign prostatic hyperplasia: A preliminary report. J Urol 1995; 154:1779–1782.

Schroeder FH, Westerhof M, Bosch RJLH, et al: Benign prostatic hyperplasia treated by castration or the LH-RH analogue buserelin: A report on 6 cases. Eur Urol 1986; 12:318–321.

Scott WW, Wade JC: Medical treatment of benign nodular prostatic hyperplasia with cyproterone acetate. J Urol 1969; 101:81–85.

Shapiro E: Embryologic development of the prostate. Urol Clin North Am 1990; 17:487–493.

Stone NN: Flutamide in treatment of benign prostatic hypertrophy. Urology 1989; 34:64–68.

Stoner E, Members of the Finasteride Study Group: Three-year safety and efficacy data on the use of finasteride in the treatment of benign prostatic hyperplasia. Urology 1994; 43:284–294.

Sufrin G, Coffey DS: A new model for studying the effect of drugs on prostatic growth. I: Antiandrogens and DNA synthesis. Invest Urol 1973; 11:45.

Tammela TLJ, Kontturi MJ: Urodynamic effects of finasteride in the treatment of bladder outlet obstruction due to benign prostatic hyperplasia. J Urol 1993; 149:342–344.

Tammela TLJ, Kontturi MJ: Long-term effects of finasteride on invasive urodynamics and symptoms in the treatment of patients with bladder outflow obstruction due to benign prostatic hyperplasia. J Urol 1995; 154:1466–1469.

Tchetgen M, Oesterling JE: The role of prostate specific antigen in the evaluation of BPH. Urol Clin North Am 1995; 22:333–344.

Thigpen AE, Silver RI, Guileyardo JM, et al: Tissue distribution and ontogeny of steroid 5 alpha-reductase isozyme expression. J Clin Invest 1993; 92:903.

Vaughan ED, Lepor H: Medical management of BPH: Part 1. AUA Update Series 1996; 16:18–24.

Vermeulen A, Giagulli VA, Schepper PD, et al: Hormonal effects of an orally active 4-azasteroid inhibitor or 5 alpha reductase in humans. Prostate 1989; 14:45–53.

Walsh PC, Madden JD, Harrod MJ, et al: Familial incomplete male pseudohermaphroditism, type 2: Decreased dihydrotestosterone formation in pseudovaginal perineoscrotal hypospadias. N Engl J Med 1974; 291:944–949.

White JW: The results of double castration in hypertrophy of the prostate. Ann Surg 1895; 22:1.

Combination Therapy

Lepor H, Machi GM: The combination of terazosin and flutamide for symptomatic BPH. Prostate 1992; 20:89.

Lepor H, Williford WO, Barry M: A randomized placebo controlled trial of terazosin and finasteride monotherapy and terazosin/finasteride combination therapy in men with clinical benign prostatic hyperplasia. N Engl J Med. In press.

Aromatase Inhibitors

Coffey DS, Walsh PC: Clinical and experimental studies of benign prostatic hyperplasia. Urol Clin North Am 1990; 17:461–475.

Cunha GR, Lung B, Reese B: Glandular epithelial induction by embryonic mesenchyme in adult bladder epithelium of BALB/c mice. Invest Urol 1980; 17:302–304.

DeKlerk DP, Coffey DS, Ewing LL, et al: Comparison of spontaneous and experimentally induced canine prostatic hyperplasia. J Clin Invest 1979; 64:842–849.

El Etreby MF, Nishino Y, Habenicht UF, et al: Atamestane, a new aromatase inhibitor for the management of benign prostatic hyperplasia. Journal of Andrology 1991; 12:403–414.

Gingell JC, Knonagel H, Kurth KH, et al: Placebo controlled double-blind study to test the efficacy of the aromatase inhibitor atamestane in patients with benign prostatic hyperplasia not requiring operation. J Urol 1995; 154:399–401.

Habenicht UF, El Etreby MF: Selective inhibition of androstenedione-induced prostate growth in intact beagle dogs by a combined treatment with the antiandrogen cyproterone acetate and the aromatase inhibitor 1-methyl-androsta-1, 4-dien-3, 17-dione (1-methyl-ADD). Prostate 1989; 140:309–322.

Habenicht UF, Schwarz K, Neumann F, El Etreby MF: Induction of estrogen-related hyperplastic changes in the prostate of the cynomolgus monkey *(Macaca fascicularis)* by the androstenedione and its antagonization by the aromatase inhibitor 1-methyl-androsta-1, 4-diene-3, 17-dione. Prostate 1987; 11:313–326.

Walsh PC, Wilson JD: The induction of prostatic hypertrophy in the dog with androstenediol. J Clin Invest 1976; 57:1093–1097.

Phytotherapy

Fitzpatrick JM, Lynch TH: Phytotherapy for urinary tract infection agents in the management of symptomatic benign prostatic hyperplasia. Urol Clin North Am 1995; 22:407–412.

Lowe FC, Ku JC: Phytotherapy for the treatment of BPH: A critical reappraisal. Urology. In press.

Future Strategies for Drug Development in Benign Prostatic Hyperplasia

Burnett AL, McGuire MP, Tillman SL, et al: Characterization and localization of nitric oxide synthase in the human prostate. Urology 1995; 45:435–439.

Kobayashi S, Tang R, Wang B, et al: Localization of endothelin-1 receptors in the human prostate. J Urol 1994; 151:763–766.

Langenstroer P, Tang R, Shapiro E, et al: Endothelin-1 in the human prostate: Tissue levels, source of production, and isometric tension studies. J Urol 1993; 150:495–499.

Takeda M, Tang R, Shapiro E, et al: Effects of nitric oxide on human and canine prostates. Urology 1995; 45:440–446.

An important issue in YAG therapy of BPH is wattage. Wattage settings of between 40 and 70 W resulted in coagulation necrosis, whereas power of more than 70 W produced vaporization of tissue and a significant prostatectomy defect. Other canines treated with 90 W, 95 W, and 100 W power showed similar results without ill effects such as severe bleeding or adjacent organ damage (Kandel and Harrison, 1990). Average treatment time was 45 minutes and reflected a learning curve. No significant bleeding, retention, incontinence, or short-term strictures of the urethra or bladder neck were noted. There was histologic evidence of a healed capsular perforation but no damage to the adjacent rectum or bladder. Vaporization gave an immediate increase in the prostatic urethral lumen, whereas coagulation necrosis did not (Kandel et al, 1992).

Interest in YAG laser treatment of BPH languished for several years but was rekindled by Roth and associates (1990) with the TULIP device, an acronym for transurethral laser-induced prostatectomy.

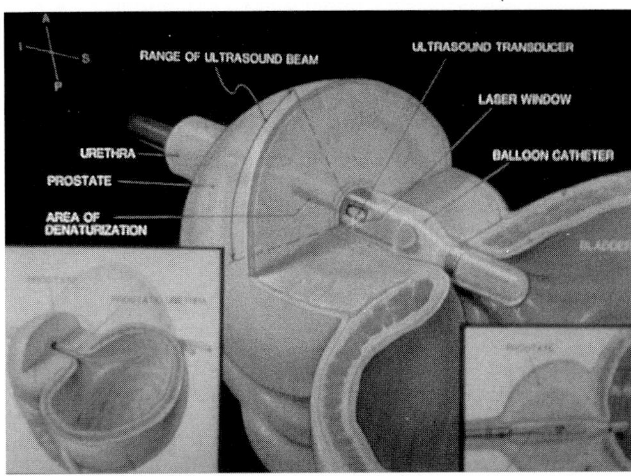

Figure 48–5. TULIP device in place with balloon-inflated, ultrasound scanning of one fourth of the prostate (90° sector), area of denaturization following laser treatment, and position of the laser window in the center of the ultrasound transducer (Courtesy of Intrasonics Corporation, Burlington, MA.)

Side-Firing YAG Lasers Used for Coagulation Necrosis Prostatectomy

The TULIP Device

The TULIP (Intrasonics Corporation, Burlington, MA) system consists of a transurethral probe and an ultrasound imager (Figs. 48–4, 48–5, and 48–6). On its end, a No. 20 Fr metal probe contains a 7.5-MHz imaging ultrasound (US) transducer and a side-firing (90-degree angle) YAG laser window. The ultrasound transducer scans a 90-degree sector of the prostate, and the laser is fired through its window, which is positioned between the two halves of the transducer, while the tissue is imaged in real time. The TULIP probe is enclosed within a sleeve filled with sterile water to provide standoff from tissue and to permit accuracy of US imaging and consistent laser spot size without charring or attenuation. The 36-Fr or 48-Fr balloon is inflated to 2 atm (not enough pressure to dilate the tissue (Roth and Aretz, 1991). The probe is pulled from the bladder neck to the apex under US control, allowing one to measure prostatic tissue depth at various positions in the urethra and to avoid treatment of areas with insufficient depth. The pull rate is approximately 1 mm/second. Almost any standard YAG laser in use in most operating rooms can be adapted for use with the TULIP device. A continuous laser power of up to 60 W is required. Animal study results are shown in Figure 48–7.

Human studies under an FDA protocol were begun at ten academic and private practice centers in 1990. McCullough and associates (1993) reported on the United States National Cooperative Study of 150 TULIP-treated BPH patients. Before therapy the average gland size was 40 g, SS was 19, Qmax was 7 ml/second, and PVR was 117 ml. Six months after therapy the SS had decreased to 6 (68% improvement), Qmax increased to 12 ml/second (78% improvement), and

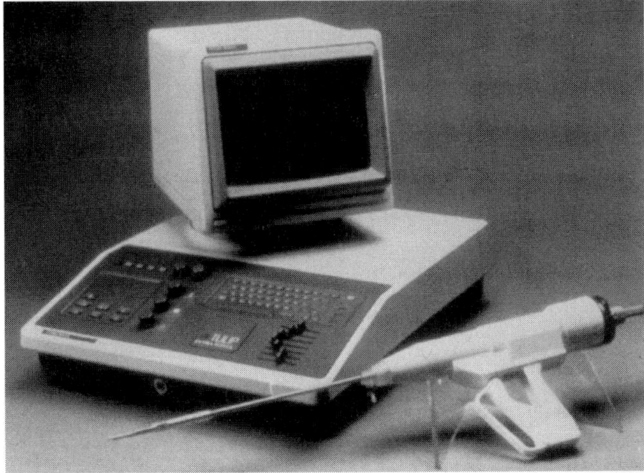

Figure 48–4. TULIP device consisting of probe, keyboard, and ultrasound monitor. (Courtesy of Intrasonics Corporation, Burlington, MA.)

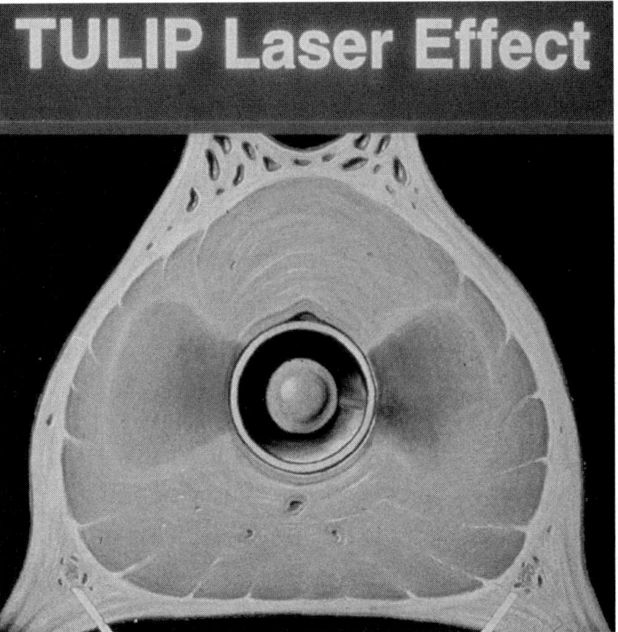

Figure 48–6. TULIP device in place showing laser coagulation in progress. (Courtesy of Intrasonics Corporation, Burlington, MA.)

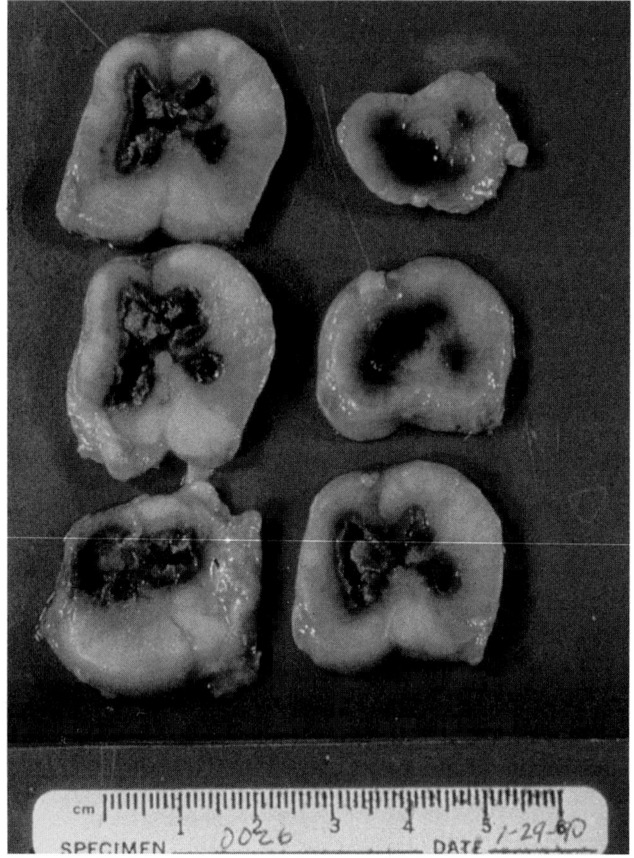

Figure 48–7. Cross sections of benign prostatic hyperplasia (BPH) in canines treated with the TULIP device in four quadrants several weeks after treatment. (From Assimos DG, McCullough DL, Woodruff RD, et al: Canine transurethral laser induced prostatectomy. J Endourol 1991; 5:145–149.)

PVR decreased to 54 ml (53% improvement). Approximately 60 patients were available for 6-month follow-up. The mean hospital stay was 1.2 ± 0.5 days; originally an overnight stay had been mandated in the study. More recently, patients have been treated as outpatients. The actual combined intraoperative ultrasound and laser treatment time averaged 23 ± 13 minutes.

No incontinence or impotence was noted. Three percent of patients experienced retrograde ejaculation, 1% stricture or bladder neck contracture, and approximately 25% urinary tract infection between 1 and 6 months postoperatively. Approximately 4% underwent TURP; no repeat laser treatment was permitted. Patients had to achieve at least a 50% decrease in SS or a score of below 12, and/or at least a 50% improvement in flow rate for treatment to be considered successful. Using these criteria, 81% improved in SS, 56% improved in flow, 49% improved in both, and 87% showed improvement in either.

Subsequent 6-month follow-up data on a larger number of patients were presented at the 1993 AUA meeting by Fuselier and colleagues (1993). In approximately 110 patients, Qmax increased from 7 to 12 ml/second, and SS decreased from 19 to 6. Most investigators place a suprapubic tube or Foley catheter for 1 to 2 weeks postoperatively because the BPH-treated glands swell acutely following laser therapy. In the author's experience, the prostatic lumen continues to

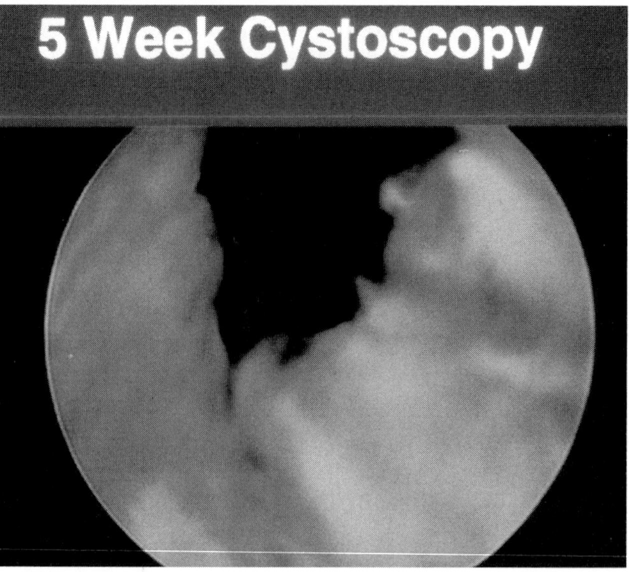

Figure 48–8. Prostatic urethra 5 weeks following TULIP treatment, with coagulated tissue still somewhat edematous. (Courtesy of Intrasonics Corporation, Burlington, MA.)

enlarge for up to 6 months postoperatively and gradually smooths and rounds out (Figs. 48–8 and 48–9). More recently, most operators have begun to make up to eight to ten passes through the prostate and are lasing the bladder neck and middle lobes. The number of joules (watts × seconds) used is increasing.

The TULIP device has been used for BPH treatment in Japan and Europe. Martin and Senge (1993) reported their early experience with 28 TULIP-treated patients in Germany. Preoperatively, SS was 16, and Qmax was 7 ml/second. At 6 months, SS had decreased to 3 and Qmax had increased to 21 ml/second in nine patients. Other recent European

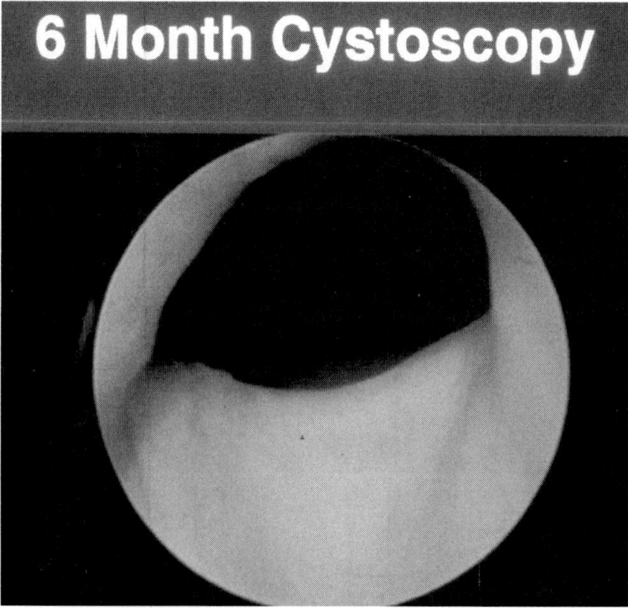

Figure 48–9. Six-month follow-up of the urethra in Figure 48–8 showing smoothed out prostatic urethral lumen. (Courtesy of Intrasonics Corporation, Burlington, MA.)

studies have shown similar efficacy. Schulze and associates (1994) reported a prospective randomized trial of TULIP versus TURP with results favorable to TULIP. Results in a large group of TULIP patients were reported in 1995 (Schulze et al, 1995). Takahashi and co-workers (1994) reported excellent 1-year TULIP results from Japan.

Babayan (1995) recently reported the 2-year follow-up data of the United States National Cooperative Study. The data are reproduced in Table 48–1. The data show that improvements are nearly equivalent to the results obtained by TURP. A second generation TULIP II device has been developed and is being used in Europe and Asia. It is smaller and lighter and uses 360-degree ultrasound imaging. Improved results have been obtained with it (Babayan, 1995).

COMMENTS ON THE TULIP DEVICE. Advocates of the device point out that it is safe and the results are nearly as good as those achieved with TURP and are reproducible; also, the technique can be learned with only a short training period. Most urologists are probably more comfortable using the visually directed lasers.

The TULIP device is not approved for sale in the United States by the FDA but has been approved for marketing by the Ministries of Health and Welfare in France and Japan.

Visual Side-Firing YAG Lasers Resulting in Coagulation Necrosis

Johnson and colleagues (1991) reported on the use of a side-firing YAG laser using a quartz 600-μm fiber with a gold-plated solid metal alloy disk reflector tip designed to reflect the laser beam to a 90-degree angle to the long axis of the fiber. The 7.5-Fr device is inserted in a standard 21-Fr cystoscope through the working channel and is used under direct vision or videocystoscopic control (with proper laser eye precautions). Johnson and colleagues (1991) used 60 W of power and noted that a large prostatectomy defect could be created without significant complications and without capsular perforation. This gold-plated tip device is called the Urolase (Bard Corporation, Covington, GA) (Fig. 48–10).

Costello and associates (1992a) reported on the first Urolase-treated human patients with BPH. Costello and associates (1992b) described their initial experiences in 17 patients, using 60 W of power for 60 seconds at the 6, 3, 9, and 12 o'clock positions. No incontinence, prostatic capsular perforation, or significant adverse events were noted. SS improved more than flow rates. Of the 17 patients, 18% underwent subsequent TURP, and 7 patients were thought to have been left with significant obstructive tissue. Mean Qmax increased from 5 to 9 ml/second (80%), and mean SS dropped from 15 to 4.

Table 48–1. LONG-TERM TULIP THERAPY RESULTS

	Months Post Treatment	Number Patients	Pre-TULIP	Post-TULIP	Percent Change
SS (modified Boyarsky) decrease	3	222	18	8	59
	6	212	19	7	63
	12	188	18	7	62
	24	57	18	6	69
Qmax increase	3	208	7 ml/second	12	66
	6	195	8 ml/second	12	59
	12	171	8 ml/second	12	55
	24	46	7 ml/second	11	68

Modified from Babayan RK: Transurethral ultrasound–guided laser-induced prostatectomy (TULIP): Past, present, and future. J Endourol 1995: 9:141–144.

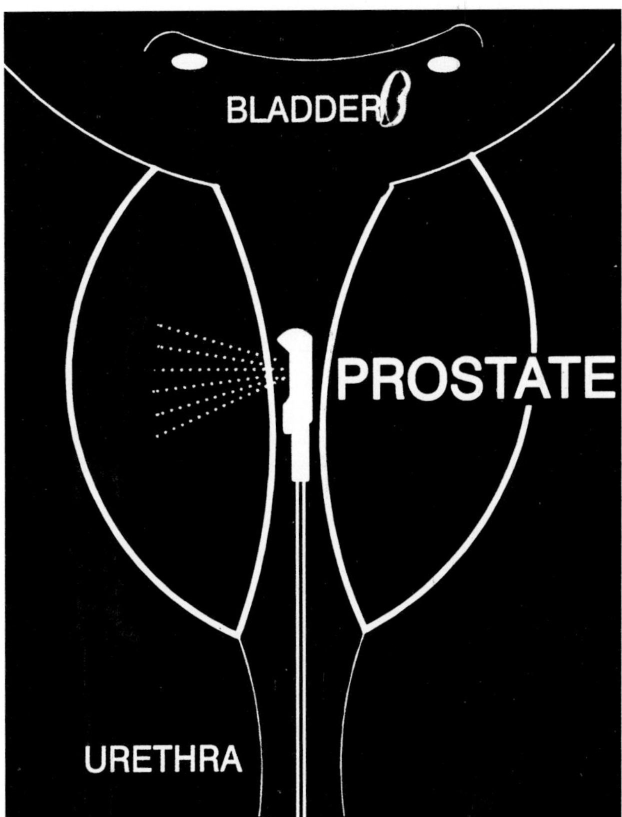

Figure 48–10. Diagram of metal-tipped Urolase fiber with laser energy deflected to 90°. (Courtesy of J. N. Kabalin, M.D., and Bard Company, Covington, GA.)

Kabalin (1993) published an early report on 25 patients with BPH who were entered in a prospective randomized trial of TURP versus Urolase laser prostatectomy. Twelve underwent TURP; they had a mean Qmax of 9 ml/second preoperatively and 23 ml/second at 6 months and an SS (AUA) of 19 preoperatively and 6 postoperatively. Thirteen Urolase-treated patients had a mean Qmax of 9 ml/second at entry into the study and 21 ml/second at 6 months; SS dropped from 21 to 5 at 6 months. The patients were treated at the 3, 6, 9, and 12 o'clock positions with a total mean number of 11,461 joules. PSA levels increased 17-fold from the nadir after TURP and approximately sixfold after laser treatment. In both the Urolase-treated and TURP groups, two patients required postoperative catheters for more than 4 days; in the TURP group there was also one patient with TURP syndrome requiring transfusion and one with extravasation. No patients in either group experienced new-onset erectile dysfunction postoperatively, but 1 of 12 sexually active laser-treated patients had retrograde ejaculation, and nine of ten similar TURP patients had retrograde ejaculation. Two laser-treated patients had residual apical tissue at cystoscopy, and one had residual bladder neck tissue. Kabalin states that each should have had a proximal and distal laser treatment. He believes that the technique can be learned by performing five to ten procedures. Most TULIP operators think that the same is true of the learning curve with that device.

Subsequent laser series have been reported. Cammack and colleagues (1993) described canine experiments with the Urolase. They challenged the standard treatment of 40 to 60 W for 60 seconds at four quadrants, comparing it with their own treatment of 15 W applied for 180 seconds. At the standard high-dose setting, they noted some explosions and fractures in the glands extending to the capsule. In contrast, the low-dose treatments produced equal or better lesion depths (9 to 15 mm) than those obtained with high-dose treatment with no explosions, bleeding, or fractures. Probes were also conserved for longer periods. More recently, in a randomized study in humans, Orihuela and co-workers (1995) compared the two types of treatment just mentioned and found no difference in safety and efficacy.

Dixon and associates (1993) reported a prospective, double-blind, randomized study of Urolase laser prostatectomy (N = 19) versus TURP (N = 23). SS (AUA) decreased from 18 to 10 in the laser-treated group and from 20 to 8 in the TURP group (P = .75, laser versus TURP). Qmax increased from 9 to 12 ml/second in the laser group and from 8 to 17 ml/second in the TURP group (P = .04, laser versus TURP); voided volume in the laser group decreased from 205 to 160 ml after treatment, whereas it increased from 173 to 244 ml in the TURP group (P = .046, laser versus TURP); and PVR declined from 121 to 84 ml in the laser group and from 203 to 80 ml in the TURP group (P = .877, laser versus TURP). These were 3-month follow-up patients.

Winters and colleagues (1993) compared the results of TULIP to those of Urolase in 28 patients treated with each device. Improvement in SS of at least 5 points occurred in about 67% in both groups of patients, and about 14% of patients in each group had postoperative retention. The authors concluded that the treatments were effective and safe.

Costello and Shaffer (1993) reported their Australian experience with 120 patients in a TURP versus Urolase randomized prospective study. They increased the number of joules used from 11,000 in earlier studies to around 21,000 in current studies and shifted away from the 12 and 6 o'clock positions to render more treatments to the lateral lobes and the median lobe. The Qmax of TURP patients increased to 20 ml/second and that of Urolase patients averaged 16 ml/second, whereas SS was reduced to 6 in TURP patients and to 13 in the laser group. The preoperative values of SS and Qmax were not stated. These authors have treated 11 patients receiving warfarin anticoagulation without sequelae. They are comfortable in treating glands of 65 g and less with the Urolase.

Kabalin and colleagues (1993) reported on the national United States cooperative Urolase group. Preliminary data revealed that the SS (AUA) decreased from 21 to 10 (N=48) at 3 months, whereas Qmax increased from 7 to 13 ml/second, and PVR decreased from 156 to 57 ml.

Kabalin (1995a) recently reported a meta-analysis (gleaned from over 20 papers) of YAG laser coagulation prostatectomy with 24-month follow-up. Many of the papers reported on the Urolase device (Bard, Inc., Covington, GA). Two-year mean values were as follows: Qmax increased from 7 ml/second to 19 ml/second, PVR decreased from 197 ml to 97 ml, and (SS) AUA decreased from 22 to 7 (Table 48–2). Kabalin's paper is highly recommended as a resource for reviewing clinical outcomes.

Kabalin (1995b) also reported complications in a large personal series of over 225 patients at Stanford that included urethral stricture in 1% of patients, bladder neck contractures in 4%, and reoperation for residual tissue in 4%. His current treatment schema is depicted in Figures 48–11, 48–12, and 48–13.

Every report seen by this writer on treatment with the Urolase recommends increasing the amount of joules given later in the series from the initial amount (around 11,000 joules). This is also true of the TULIP device. Treatment of the median (middle) lobes had earlier been off limits both to these lasers and to the TULIP device. Now treatment with both devices includes them.

In Kabalin's last 100 patients treated with 40 W for 90 seconds, the mean prostate size was 35 g, the mean energy delivery was 41,000 joules, and the mean operative time was 90 minutes.

COMMENTS ON LASER FIBERS. A number of companies now sell laser fibers. Lack of inclusion of their names and fibers in this article does not imply that they are not equivalent to the ones mentioned. The goal of this article is directed more toward pointing out principles of therapy. The best way to examine these devices is to visit the exhibit areas at urology meetings. There are several variables requiring consideration. The angles of reflection range from 70 to 105 degrees. A variety of tip constructions are available. Fiber sizes range from 400 to 1000 μ. The Lasersonics UltraLine Fiber (Heraeus Lasersonics, Milpitas, CA) (Fig. 48–14) uses an 80-degree quartz fiber without a metal tip. It can be placed directly against tissue (contact) and can vaporize it without damaging the tip, unlike metal tips, which can be fouled and burned up when they come into contact with tissue. Vaporization of a portion of the tissue has a theoretical advantage in that it establishes an immediate partial cavity that has an increased chance of allowing earlier voiding. Then the underlying tissue can be coagulated (Fig. 48–15). The quartz fiber can also be used to incise the bladder neck by direct contact (like a transurethral incision

Table 48–2. COMBINED META ANALYSIS OF COAGULATION LASER PROSTATECTOMY RESULTS

	Months Post Treatment	Number Patients	Pre-Treatment	Post-Treatment	Percent Change
SS (AUA) decrease	0	1559	22	—	—
	3	1050		8	64
	6	1197		8	64
	12	272		7	68
	24	40		7	68
Qmax increase	0	1579	8 ml/	—	—
	3	1050	second	16	100
	6	1176		16	100
	12	273		17	113
	24	40		19	138
PVR decrease	0	1141	197 ml	—	—
	3	857		68	65
	6	786		61	69
	12	267		97	51
	24	40		97	51

Modified from Kabalin JN: ND:YAG laser coagulation prostatectomy for benign prostatic hyperplasia. Part I: Clinical Outcomes. Afri J Urol 1995; 1:112–118.

device is referred to as transurethral microwave thermotherapy (TUMT).

Devonec and co-workers (1993a) reported that the human prostate is more resistant to heat than the canine prostate. Young patients require more heat than the elderly, probably because a better blood supply dissipates heat more readily. Acinar cells are more resistant to heat than smooth muscle. The canine prostate is pear shaped and consists of predominantly glandular tissue, whereas the human prostate is more chestnut shaped, has a better blood supply, and consists of predominantly adenofibromyomatous tissue. Zonal differences are also noted. The anterior portion of the dog prostate is more heat sensitive than the posterior portion. In humans, tissue lateral to the urethra shows the effects of heat more. The transition zone is more heat sensitive than the peripheral zone. These differences seem to be related to different blood supply distributions. In an earlier report, Devonec and associates (1991) described 37 patients whose prostates were heated to 45 to 55°C. Lidocaine local anesthesia was used in a treatment session lasting approximately 1 hour. At a 3-month follow-up, the following results were noted: SS decreased from 12 to 8; Qmax increased from 8 to 11 ml/second, and PVR decreased from 109 to 50 ml. Changes in prostatic volume did not occur. Preoperative PSA values averaged 4.2, but at 1 week those values had increased to 11, lending credence to the concept of damage or necrosis to prostatic tissue secondary to heat. Treated glands revealed preserved urethral tissue 2 to 5 mm thick and coagulation necrosis 5 to 17 mm from the urethral lumen. De la Rosette and associates (1993) reported on 130 patients treated with TUMT. Eleven underwent TURP, three experienced technical failures, and 23 were lost to follow-up. Ninety-three were therefore evaluable as possible successes.

In these patients, mean AUA SS decreased from 17 to 7 at 3, 6, and 12 months. Sixty-three percent of patients had a decrease of 50% or more in SS, and 15% showed no improvement. Average Qmax increased by 1 ml/second, PVR did not change significantly, and prostate volume did not change. PSA values increased to 20 at 1 week and returned to baseline by 3 months, indicating some parenchymal damage. Twenty-six percent of patients experienced urinary retention, which was treated by Foley catheter, usually for a week or less.

Ogden and co-workers (1993) reported a prospective randomized trial of TUMT using a sham control group. Entry criteria included patients with BPH who had two measurements of Qmax of less than 15 ml/second, an SS (Madsen) of more than 8 for 6 months, and a PVR of less than 350 ml. There were 21 patients in the sham control group and 22 treated patients. The TUMT group showed a 70% decrease in Madsen SS (15 to 4), a Qmax increase of 53% (9 to 13 ml/second), and a 92% decrease in PVR (147 to 12 ml). No significant changes in these values were noted in the sham control group. The authors concluded that the improved results in the TUMT group were not due to placebo effect.

Dahlstrand and his group (1993) also reported a randomized study of TUMT (39 patients) versus TURP (44 patients). At 12 months, Qmax increased from 8 to 12 in the TUMT group and from 8 to 18 in the TURP group; Madsen SS decreased from 11 to 3 in the TUMT group and from 13 to 1 in the TURP group. PVR decreased from 105 to 51 ml in the TUMT group and from 116 to 22 ml in the TURP group, and prostate size was unchanged in the TUMT group and decreased 47% in the TURP group. No new impotence was noted in either group, and antegrade ejaculation was preserved in all of the TUMT patients and in 75% of the TURP group. Four TUMT nonresponders underwent subsequent TURP, and three TURP patients underwent subsequent urethrotomy. Bladder capacity increased 10% postoperatively in the TUMT group and 18% in the TURP group. In those patients undergoing urodynamic evaluation, bladder instability was found in 6 of 21 TUMT patients before treatment and in 8 of 21 after, whereas in the TURP group there were 5 of 13 such patients before treatment and 2 after. The TURP group had better results but more major complications.

Dahlstrand and colleagues (1995) reported a 36-month follow-up on the study just mentioned. The previously reported results were durable in both the TURP and TUMT groups. Very little difference in SS and PVR was noted in the two groups. Pressure flow studies have shown a more pronounced decrease in intravesical outflow obstruction after TURP than after TUMT.

Devonec and associates (1993b) reported the results of the Prostasoft I, II, and II-A (ablation) software programs for increasing prostate temperatures. Their results showed that improvement was dose dependent. Thermocoagulation was achieved with temperatures above 45°C and thermoablation with temperatures above 60°C. The Prostasoft I achieved intraprostatic temperatures of between 45 and 50°C. Prostasoft II achieved temperatures of 45 to 60°C, and Prostasoft II-A achieved temperatures of up to 75°C. PSA values increased 277% with the Prostasoft I, 870% with the Prostasoft II, and 1380% with the Prostasoft II-A. At higher temperatures, some analgesia and sedation were required. The urethra was preserved in histologic sections in ten patients given the Prostasoft II protocol. In the Prostasoft II-A ablation group, no tissue was available for histologic analysis, but cavities in the prostate were present in 70% of cases. Presumably the urethra was destroyed in such cases in the treatment area. No damage to the rectum, external sphincter, or ureteral orifices was noted. The authors presume that the mechanism of action of TUMT at the lower power levels is a reduction in urethral resistance and possible alpha-fiber nerve damage.

This author presumes that the Prostasoft II-A protocol results in urethral damage and cavity formation much like the results of laser therapy and, as in laser therapy, requires anesthesia.

Mulvin and his group (1994) reported a study of TUMT versus Foley catheter placement (sham). SS decreased in both groups significantly, as did Qmax and PVR. However, when the treatment group was compared to the sham group, there was no significant difference at 3 months. This study is reminiscent of the study of Lepor and colleagues (1992) of balloon dilation versus catheter placement and makes a strong case for controlled studies of all devices.

Debruyne and co-workers (1993) conducted a study of TUMT therapy versus a sham control group in which they randomized 25 patients to each group. The SS dropped about the same amount at 3 months, and the flow rate increased 4 ml/second in the TUMT group and none in the sham group. By 6 months, the improvement in SS persisted in the treatment group but deteriorated in the sham group.

Table 48–4. U.S. PROSTATRON COOPERATIVE STUDY RESULTS

	Months Post Treatment	Number Patients	Pre-Treatment	Post-Treatment	Percent Change
SS (Madsen)	0	118	14		
decrease	12	118		5	64
Qmax increase	0	104	9 ml/second		
	12	104		11	22
PVR decrease	0	93	127 ml		
	12	93		118	7

Adapted from Blute ML, Tomera KM, Hellerstein DK, et al: Transurethral microwave thermotherapy for management of benign prostatic hyperplasia: Results of the United States Prostatron Cooperative Study. J Urol 1995; 150:1591–1596.

Blute (1994) reported a prospective double-blind study of TUMT versus a sham group performed at the Mayo Clinic. The patients were randomized in a 2:1 ratio of TUMT treatment to sham treatment. PSA levels increased 536% one week after TUMT treatment, but there was no change in the sham group. Although both the TUMT and sham groups showed improvement in SS and Qmax, the results were statistically significant only in the TUMT treated group.

Blute and his group (1995) reported on the United States Cooperative Prostatron trial, Table 48–4. After 1 year, the decrease in SS was 64%, the increase in Qmax was 22%, and the decrease in PVR was 7%. Topical anesthesia was used in 66 patients (56%), IV sedation in 22 (19%), oral sedation in 27 (23%), and combined oral and IV sedation in 3 (3%).

Kirby and colleagues (1993) reported strikingly similar results in 140 men treated in the United Kingdom. SS dropped from 24 to 12 (50%), Qmax increased from 10 to 12 ml/second (20%), and PVR was unchanged.

It should be noted that the United States Prostatron Study uses the lower power software (Prostasoft I). What happens when higher power is used? Perrin and co-workers (1995) reported that when the Prostasoft 2.5 (high-energy) software was compared with the standard Prostocol 2.0, the high-energy group produced a decrease in SS of 62% versus 48% and an increase in Qmax of 71% versus 25%. The urinary retention rate was 78% in the high-energy group versus 23% in the standard group.

Miller and his group (1995) reported on a new device called T3. It is a transurethral thermoablation device with urethral cooling that directs energy preferentially to the lateral and anterior prostate and avoids the rectal area. It produces temperatures of over 70°C in the prostate. Topical and occasionally IV sedation are used. Foley catheters are left in place for 2 to 5 days postoperatively. Three-month data revealed a decrease in SS (AUA) from 20 to 8 (62%), and improvement of more than 50% was noted in 73% of patients. Qmax increased from 9 to 14 (52%), and improvement of more than 50% was noted in 57% of patients.

Comments on Transurethral Thermotherapy

It appears that thermotherapy in the lower temperature range (45° to 50°C) results in a decrease in SS. As the intraprostatic temperatures rise with treatment with higher power devices (e.g., TUMT Prostasoft II-A or Prostocol 2.5 protocols), more tissue is destroyed, cavities are produced, and sedation and analgesia are required. Up to 80% of patients experience urinary retention after thermotherapy at such high power, and results similar to those achieved with laser therapy are noted. Patients with urethral lengths of more than 45 mm and large middle lobes have decreased chances of success with this therapy. The multiple treatments required by the earlier transurethral thermotherapy devices seem to be inefficient with regard to time and are not economically feasible compared with 60- or 90-minute treatments. In the long-term, efficacy and economics will determine which treatment devices will prevail. Whether preservation of the prostatic urethra is a goal worth striving for

Table 48–5. TRANSRECTAL HYPERTHERMIA AND TRANSURETHRAL DEVICES FOR HYPERTHERMIA AND THERMOTHERAPY

Company	Machine	Frequency	Intraprostatic Temperature	Cooling	Prostate Necrosis	No. Sessions
Rectal Probes						
Biodan (Israel)	Prostathermer	915 MHz	42–44°C	Rectal	No	6–10 × 1 hr
Technomatics (Belgium)	Primus	915 MHz	N/A	Rectal	No	6–10 × 1 hr
Bruker	Prosteare	915 MHz	N/A	Rectal	No	N/A
Urethral Probe						
Direx (Israel)	Thermex II	Variable radiofrequency	42–44°C	No	Urethral lesion	1 × 3 hr
	Modified Thermex II	Variable radiofrequency	44–47.9°C	No	Urethral lesion	90 min
BSD	BSD device	915 MHz	42–49°C	No	Urethral lesion	5–10 × 1 hr
EDAP (France)	Prostatron	1296 MHz	45–75°C	Urethral	Urethra preserved at lower temperatures Destroyed with higher temperatures (75°C) Prostate necrosis	60 min

Courtesy of ML Blute, M.D., with modifications by the author.

will also be sorted out with time. **The Prostatron device has been approved by a committee of the FDA**. It is obvious that the use of higher power devices produces cavities similar to those seen after laser therapy. The adage, "more pain, more gain" seems to apply to these higher power regimens. A list of hyperthermia and thermotherapy devices is presented in Table 48–5.

TRANSURETHRAL ELECTROVAPORIZATION OF THE PROSTATE

The VaporTrode (Circon-ACMI Corporation, Stamford, CT) vaporization electrode is an adaptation of an old device, the rollerball electrode, which has been in service in urology for years. The mechanism is described in an article by Kramalowsky and Tucker (1991).

The fundamental electrosurgical energy principle employed is that current density across an electrode is not uniform. The highest current density occurs at the edge of the electrode. The VaporTrode is a grooved rollerball electrode and has eight sites at the edges of the grooves (Fig. 48–21). In the contact area, a thermal reaction raises the temperature of the tissue to more than 100°C, a temperature that vaporizes prostatic tissue. With the *cutting* current turned up to at least 200 W and usually 250 to 280 W, the depth of the vaporization zone is 3 to 4 mm with a zone of coagulation beneath it of 1 to 3 mm. The plain round rollerball electrode is capable of causing vaporization and coagulation depths of only about 50% of the VaporTrode's effects.

The *coagulation* setting can be used with the VaporTrode to coagulate bleeders. The same settings are used that one uses for a routine TURP procedure. The *blend* mode is not used.

Technique

The VaporTrode is used in a routine ACMI resectoscope sheath and resecting mechanism by simply substituting it for the regular loop electrode. Vaporization of the BPH tissue is performed in much the same way as it is in a regular TURP procedure except that the pull speed is one-quarter of the usual TURP cutting pull speed. The tissue is progressively vaporized to a suitable depth using multiple passes (Fig. 48–22). The time required is approximately the same as that needed for a regular TURP.

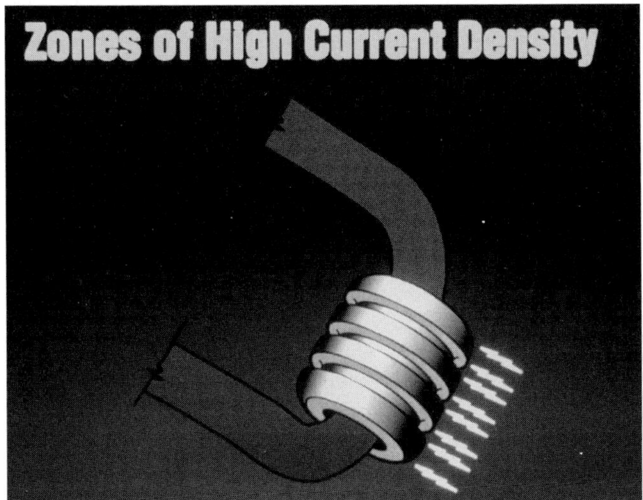

Figure 48–21. VaporTrode tip with eight zones of high current density. (Courtesy of Circon ACMI Corporation, Stamford, CT.)

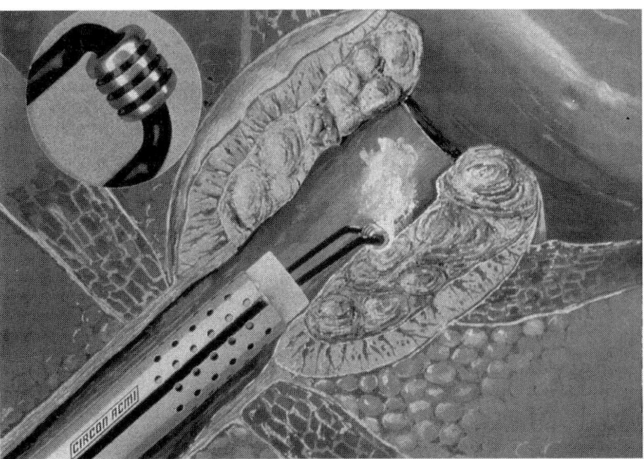

Figure 48–22. VaporTrode vaporizing a 3- to 4-mm zone of BPH. (Courtesy of Circon ACMI Corporation, Stamford, CT.)

A deeper zone of coagulation results in less bleeding and minimal absorption of fluid. Most authors remove the catheter the same day or the next day. Occasionally but infrequently, irrigation is required. The procedure is often performed as an outpatient procedure.

Experimental Data

Perlmutter and his group (1995) studied the effects of TVP on the living canine model. Five male dogs underwent TVP in which a Wolf resectoscope (Wolf Instrument Corporation, Germany was passed through a suprapubic cystostomy in an antegrade fashion. Both silver- and gold-plated Wolf electrosurgical rolling cylinders (similar in appearance to the ACMI VaporTrode device) were used with a Valleylab Force 4B electrosurgical generator (Valleylab, Boulder, CO).

These investigators found that after a single pass of the rolling cylinder coagulation occurred at depths of less than 1.4 mm deep to the vaporization. After multiple passes, the zone was as much as 2.5 mm deep. When temperatures were measured using thermometry probes 5 mm away from the vaporization site, only a 4°C increase was noted. Temperatures were measured in the irrigation fluid as it passed through the prostatic fossa. Within 1 to 2 seconds after electrovaporization, the temperature of the irrigation fluid passing out of the prostate was 5.5°C higher than the temperature of the inflow. No dangerous heat patterns were noted at the capsule or at the level of the rectum or neurovascular bundle. The long-term effects of high amounts of current through these areas is unknown, however.

Clinical Reports

Kaplan and Te (1995) reported preliminary results of TVP in 25 patients with mild to moderate symptoms of prostatism. SS (AUA) decreased from 18 to 4 at 3 months (78%), Qmax increased from 7 to 17 ml/second (143%), and PVR dropped from 58 to 44 ml (24%). The mean operative time was 40 minutes, and there were minimal changes in hematocrit and serum sodium. Three patients had mild hematuria (12%), and one developed a bulbar stricture (4%). The mean interval to catheter removal was 15 hours. There were minimal irritative symptoms, and no one had to be recatheterized.

The authors stressed that the device is cost effective (the only expendable cost is that of the electrode) and that minimal postoperative irritative symptoms occurred. No changes in erections were noted. All patients had retrograde ejaculation. Two patients remained on anticoagulation therapy during this treatment. There were five patients with prostate gland volumes of less than 70 g.

Anesthesia requirements are the same as those for TURP. Stewart and colleagues (1995) reported their initial experience. Qmax increased from 10 to 16 ml/second (60%), and SS (AUA) dropped from 25 to 11 (56%). Estimated blood loss was 135 ml, average hospital stay was 2.6 days, and mean catheter time was 2.0 postoperative days. Fifteen of 25 patients had presented with urinary retention.

Te and his group (1995) reported several additional patients undergoing TVP at Columbia Presbyterian Hospital, Loma Linda, and Boston University. They compared the results of 29 patients who underwent laser vaporization prostatectomy with those of a group undergoing TVP (Fig. 48–23). At 3 months after the procedure, the results were not significantly different statistically in terms of SS (AUA), Qmax, or PVR. However, 20% of the laser group needed recatheterization after the procedure, whereas none of the TVP group needed it. More of the laser group had irritative symptoms (19) than the TVP group (3).

Comments on Transurethral Electrovaporization of the Prostate

This device appears to be a formidable competitor for routine TURP and vaporization laser therapy. Other groups are anecdotally reporting higher rates of irritative symptoms, bleeding, and less effective objective results than are reported here. Longer follow-up time is needed, and many more patients need to be studied in a variety of institutions and the results compared with TURP and laser TURP. The TVP device, which costs about $100 to $200, is less expensive than a laser fiber and uses readily available electrosurgical equipment. It creates an instant lumen, which permits early catheter removal. **Because the device uses a resectoscope and vaporizes only about one third of the depth of a resectoscope loop per pass, up to three times as many passes (causing urethral friction) may be required to obtain the same size cavity as obtained in a routine TURP. This could result in a greater incidence of urethral strictures. This author and some colleagues have noted that in some patients after an initial vaporization cavity has been created, it is difficult to make the cavity any deeper because of the charred tissue. Perhaps new generators will help with this problem. However, this device or a variation of it have the potential to capture a significant part of the TURP market.**

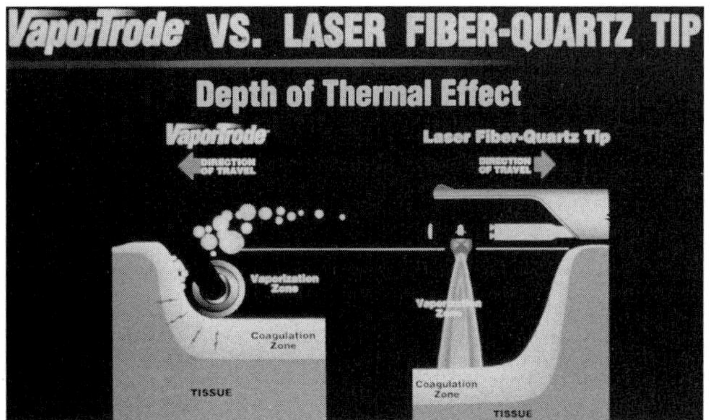

Figure 48–23. VaporTrode depths of vaporization and coagulation versus UltraLine type of laser treatment. (Courtesy of Circon ACMI Corporation, Stamford, CT.)

INTRAURETHRAL STENTS

Urethral stents as a temporary or permanent solution for obstruction are a relatively new treatment modality in urology. In the field of cardiovascular medicine, they have been used to keep open peripheral arteries following dilatation in pioneering work by Dotter (1969), and they have also been used in the coronary as well as the peripheral arteries in the more recent past (Maass et al, 1982; Dotter et al, 1983; Wright et al, 1985). Palmaz and associates (1987) placed stents in renal arteries. Stents have been used to treat iliac artery obstruction (Rousseau et al, 1989), caval obstruction (Furui et al, 1990), bronchial obstruction (Mair et al, 1990), tracheal stenosis (Skapshay et al, 1989), cervical obstruction (Luesley et al, 1990), and lacrimal duct stenosis (Hurwitz, 1989). Spiral stents and polyurethane stents are generally considered temporary stents that should be used for 6 months or less. Mesh stents are considered more permanent.

Spiral Stents

Fabian (1980) introduced the spiral stent to urology. It is a stainless steel wire coil, the body of which is placed in the prostatic urethra with the proximal end, which is tapered, resting in the bladder. The distal end, which is another coil, rests in the bulbar urethra and is connected by a short, straight wire, which extends through the external sphincter, to the coil body. Variable lengths are available from 4.5 to 8.5 cm. Fabricus and colleagues (1983) and Flier and Seppelt (1987) have reported success with the Fabian spiral.

The Fabian spiral is enhanced by plating it with 24K gold. This is called the ProstaKath (Pharma-Plast). The gold plating helps prevent incrustation. The outside diameter is 21 Fr (7 mm). It is inserted using a No. 21 Fr panendoscope with a 30-degree or 0-degree lens with the aid of grasping forceps under direct vision while the patient is under local anesthesia. The length of the spiral is 1 to 1.5 cm longer than the prostatic urethra. It may also be inserted over a catheter guide using ultrasound guidance (Nordling et al, 1989). The stent can be easily removed or repositioned using direct view panendoscopy with the aid of grasping forceps.

The stent does not become epithelialized. It may become dislodged or encrusted and may be associated with infection or intractable frequency, urgency, or incontinence (Harrison and DeSouza, 1990; Nielsen et al, 1989; Nordling et al, 1989).

In the series of Nordling and colleagues (1989), acute or chronic urinary retention (average volume 1000 ml) was relieved successfully in 41 of 45 consecutive patients under local anesthesia with the ProstaKath stent; ultrasound guidance was used in 35 patients (77%) and endoscopic visualization was used in 6 (23%). The authors thought it was a good alternative to an indwelling catheter in patients who were high operative risks.

Thomas and co-workers (1993) also used the ProstaKath stent to treat acute retention; voiding was re-established in 57 of 64 patients. Sixteen patients developed stent-related problems that required further treatment. The authors' results do not support the use of this stent for patients with symptoms of outflow obstruction or chronic retention. Isogawa and Ohmori (1993), however, reported good results in such patients, as did Yasumoto and colleagues (1992). Rodriguez and his group (1991) reported good results in 63% of their cases.

Rosenklide and associates (1991) described some late complications of ProstaKath therapy. The device was inserted in 29 consecutive patients with obstructive BPH. Fifteen patients (52%) showed relief of symptoms. In 14 cases (48%) the spiral was removed. In nine patients, removal was necessary because of urinary retention, and in five, it followed stent dislocation into the bladder. A few stents were severely calcified. These patients had chronic urinary infections that were resistant to antibiotic therapy.

Polyurethane Stents

Nissenkorn (1991) reported on the intraurethral catheter (IUC) indwelling polyurethane stent in a series of patients with BPH who were either at high risk for surgical treatment or refused it. The device is made of Puroflex Urolosoft (Angiomed, Germany) and comes in lengths of 30, 45, and 60 mm. It is a double malecot-like device and measures 16 Fr in diameter; it has a nylon string on the distal end and a flared crown like a trumpet on the bladder end (Fig. 48–24). It is placed under local anesthesia with lidocaine jelly using a No. 22 Fr cystoscope. After placement, the string can be cut. If adjustment or removal is necessary, it can be done with a biopsy forceps. Eighty-five devices were placed in 73 patients, 60 of whom had previous indwelling catheters for a duration of 1 week to 3 years. At 6 months, 63 patients (74%) had successful outcomes. Compared with permanent external catheters, Nissenkorn noted that the patients were much better able to work, ambulate, and have intercourse, and that there was less chance of stricture development. He thought that the most appropriate use for this stent was in patients requiring a temporary Foley catheter for more than a few days.

Sassine and Schulman (1994) described 43 patients treated with the Nissenkorn stent during the last 3 years. The patients were in urinary retention and had a short life expectancy. Approximately 84% (36 of 43 patients) were able to void without incontinence or significant PVR. This stent appears to be a valid alternative to a chronic indwelling catheter.

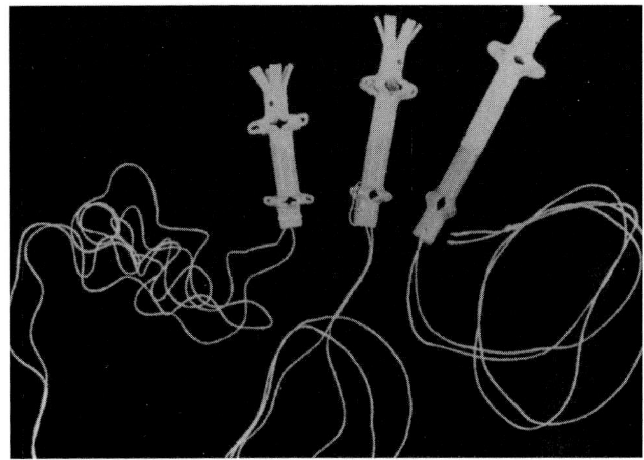

Figure 48–24. Nissenkorn polyurethane stents. (Courtesy of Angiomed, Germany.)

Contraindications to both the spiral stent and the IUC include bladder stones or bladder tumors and recent treatment with extracorporeal shock wave lithotripsy.

Bioresorbable Stents

Kemppainen and his group (1993) described the use of a biodegradable stent made of self-reinforced polylactide (SR-PLLA) in rabbits after urethrotomy. Minimal tissue reaction occurred, and the stents were completely absorbed at 14 months. Petas and his colleagues (1995) reported the use of self-reinforced polyglycolic acid wire mesh to form temporary stents in patients after VLAP. The 8- × 45-mm stent expands 64% in 14 days. Of 30 patients in whom the stent was placed immediately after VLAP, 29 voided by the first or second postoperative day. Four patients went into retention owing to early degradation of the stent or too short a spiral. Stents were seen to be degraded at 4 weeks when viewed cystoscopically. The authors are enthusiastic.

Wire Mesh Stents

There are two wire mesh stents, the Urolume Wallstent (American Medical Systems, Minnetonka, MN) and the Titan Intraprostatic ASI Stent (Boston Scientific, Boston, MA). The Swiss inventor Hans Wallstent invented the Wallstent. This self-expanding stent was developed originally for vascular use by Rousseau and colleagues (1987). Milroy and his group (1988) reported using the device in the human genitourinary tract for treatment of urethral strictures. Sarramon and associates (1989) began using the stent in canine urethras in 1986 and in humans in 1987.

The Urolume Wallstent is a flexible, self-expanding, metal superalloy stent. The ASI stent is made of titanium and must be expanded to its final shape by inflating a balloon inside

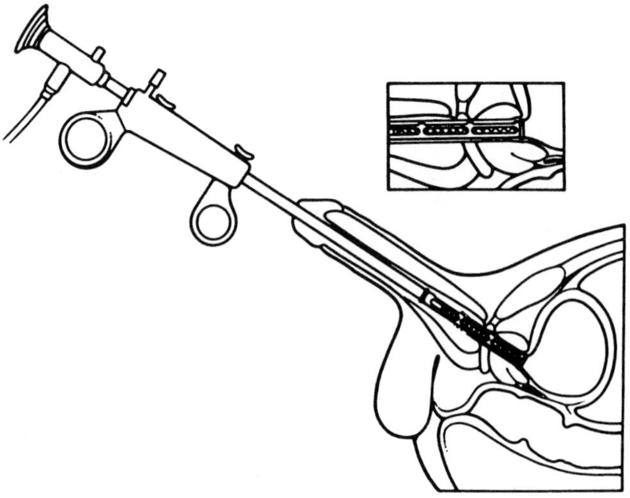

Figure 48–25. Wallstent deployment tool. (Courtesy of American Medical Systems, Minnetonka, MN.)

it after it is seated in place. The balloon is then deflated and removed. The Wallstent is placed in position using a special deployment tool that extrudes the compressed stent into position, and the stent then expands itself.

Urolume Wallstent

This device is made in six lengths of 1.5, 2, 2.5, 3, 3.5, and 4 cm. The deployment tool (No. 21 Fr) (Fig. 48–25) comprises a panendoscope with a 0-degree lens to view the urethra to help place the stent under direct vision (Figs. 48–26 and 48–27) after first measuring the required length with a urethral catheter with 1-cm markings. Local prostatic blocks with lidocaine and IV sedation may be used, or spinal or epidural anesthesia may be used. The stent expands to 42 Fr (14 mm). Generally, no postoperative urethral catheter is required. Radial forces tend to keep the stent in place. After epithelization occurs, cystoscopy can be performed through the stent. The stent can be removed later if necessary by resecting the epithelium with a low-current resectoscope and jarring the stent with grasping forceps. It can then be pulled gently, which lengthens and narrows the lumen, so that it can be extracted through the resectoscope stent (Oesterling, 1991).

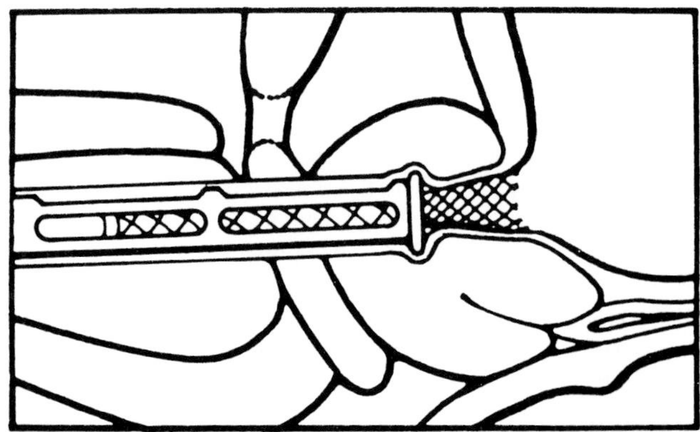

Figure 48–26. Wallstent deployment with stent partially extruding and self-expanding. (Courtesy of American Medical Systems, Minnetonka, MN.)

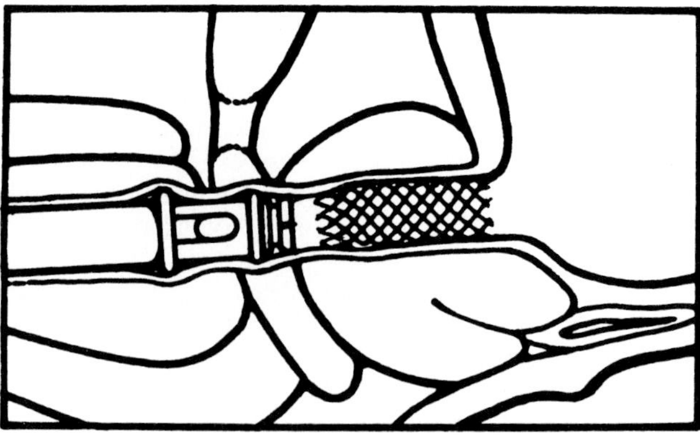

Figure 48–27. Wallstent fully expanded in the prostatic urethra. Tool being withdrawn. (Courtesy of American Medical Systems, Minnetonka, MN.)

Milroy (1991) worked previously with Barrinon in France and found on screening electron microscopy 2 to 12 months later that excellent covering of the stent with epithelium had occurred. Figures 48–28 and 48–29 show the Wallstent in position immediately following placement in the urethra and months later after epithelization. As is true of all stents, the Wallstent was used initially in high-risk patients who were experiencing urinary retention or had severe obstructive symptoms.

Chapple and his associates (1990) used the stent in a group of debilitated patients. The great majority (11 of 12) of the patients were able to urinate in a satisfactory manner. Irritative symptoms, especially urgency, were a transient problem lasting up to 4 to 6 weeks.

McLoughlin and colleagues (1990) used the stent in a similar group of surgically unfit patients, 18 of 19 of whom were in acute urinary retention; the other was in chronic

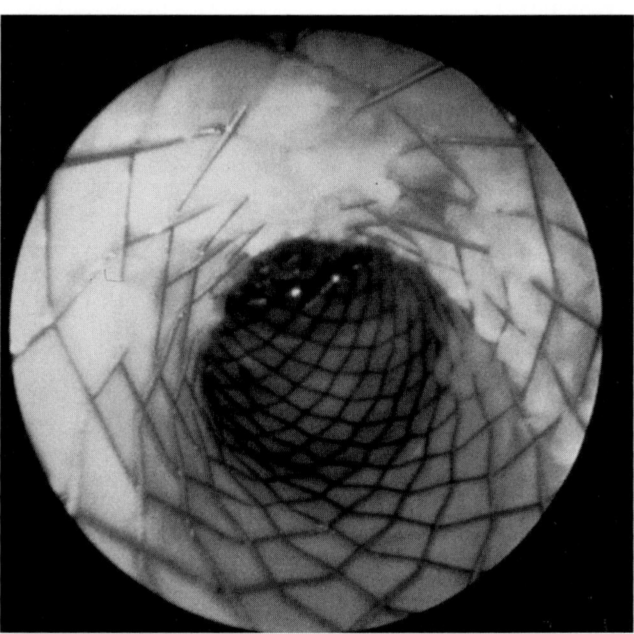

Figure 48–28. Wallstent immediately after placement in the urethra. (Courtesy of American Medical Systems, Minnetonka, MN.)

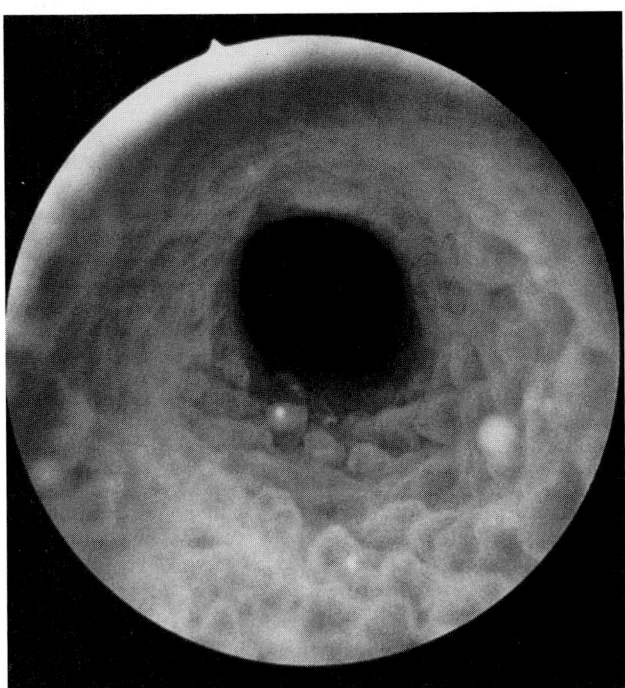

Figure 48–29. Wallstent months after placement, covered with epithelium. (Courtesy of American Medical Systems, Minnetonka, MN.)

retention. Using local anesthesia, all 18 patients with acute urinary retention were able to void immediately after stent deployment.

Oesterling (1991) reported preliminary results in a United States study of 12 patients. After a 3-month follow-up, he reported a 65% decrease in SS, a 99% increase in Qmax, and a decrease of 75% in PVR in a group of patients with obstructive BPH. Eight patients (67%) had irritative voiding symptoms postoperatively.

Milroy (1991) places the stents using transrectal ultrasound guidance or direct endoscopic placement. He favors endoscopic placement. Among 45 patients treated, 42 were fully satisfied and passed urine without difficulty and with reduced PVR. Frequency, urgency, and dysuria during the first 4 to 6 weeks following placement were problems. No erectile dysfunction in these patients was noted, and most of those who were sexually active reported retrograde ejaculation. Five of the 45 stents were removed after deployment.

At the 1993 AUA meeting, Oesterling and Epstein (1993) reported on the North American Urolume Stent Cooperative Study of a group of 95 healthy patients who were candidates for TURP. At 12 months, the SS in these patients had decreased from 15 to 6, Qmax had increased from 9 to 15 ml/second, and PVR had decreased from 129 ml to 24 ml. By 6 months, 55% of the stents had epithelialized.

At the 1995 AUA meeting, Oesterling and his group (Defalco et al, 1995) presented the 3-year results of the North American Urolume Stent Cooperative Study. There were two cohorts. The first was a group of 95 healthy patients, and the second was a group of 31 patients who were in urinary retention. Table 48–6 provides a look at their results.

In a European multicenter study conducted by Milroy and co-workers (1994), similar groups of patients were treated. A nonretention group included 94 patients and the retention group had 46 patients, for a total of 140 men.

Qmax in the nonretention group increased from 9 to 17 ml/second (84%). The mean SS (Madsen) decreased from 16 to 8 (50%). All of the men in acute retention were able to void. Following treatment, their mean Qmax was 14 ml/second, and the mean SS was 3. Stents were removed in 10% of the total group, mainly because of poor placement (80%), and removed because of untoward effects such as irritative symptoms or incrustation.

The Urolume stent continues to be modified, and a third generation stent has now been developed (Bajoria et al, 1995). In their series using the second-generation Urolume, 33% of stents had to be removed, generally because of stent migration or epithelial hyperplasia in the lumen.

Chapple and co-workers (1995) presented a randomized study of the Urolume stent (34 patients) versus TURP (26 patients). A shorter operative time and a shorter hospital stay were required for the Urolume group. SS and Qmax improvements were equivalent. Two stents were removed,

Table 48–6. 36-MONTH FOLLOW-UP NORTH AMERICAN UROLUME STUDY

	Months Post Treatment	Number Patients	Preoperative	Postoperative	Percent Change
Nonretention Cohort					
SS (Madsen) decrease	0	95	14		
	36	95		5	65
Qmax increase	0	95	9 ml/		
	36	95	second	15	67
PVR decrease	0	95	89 ml		
	36	95		54	40
Retention Cohort					
SS (Madsen)	36	31	Retention	5	
Qmax	36	31	Retention	11 ml/second	
PVR	36	31	Retention	46 ml	

13% of all stents were removed.

Modified from Defalco A, Oesterling JE, Epstein H: The North American Experience with the Urolume endourethral prosthesis as a treatment for BPH: Three year results. (Abstract.) J Urol 1995; 153:829.

and there was a slight increase in irritative symptoms in the Urolume group. Only 3-month data were available.

This stent appears to offer an effective means of establishing good flow rates, relieving obstructive symptoms, and decreasing PVR. PSA levels are not altered by the stent (Oesterling, 1995). One can perform cystoscopic maneuvers through it once epithelization has occurred. Removal, when necessary, is not difficult or dangerous. Its long-term effects on the urethra have not been reported; thus, questions such as whether patients will ever need a transurethral resection of overgrown epithelium have not been resolved. Its major drawback appears to be the irritative symptoms precipitated by placement of this foreign body in two thirds of patients during the first 1 to 2 months postoperatively. The stent has been approved by the FDA for use in patients with bulbar urethral strictures but not for those with BPH.

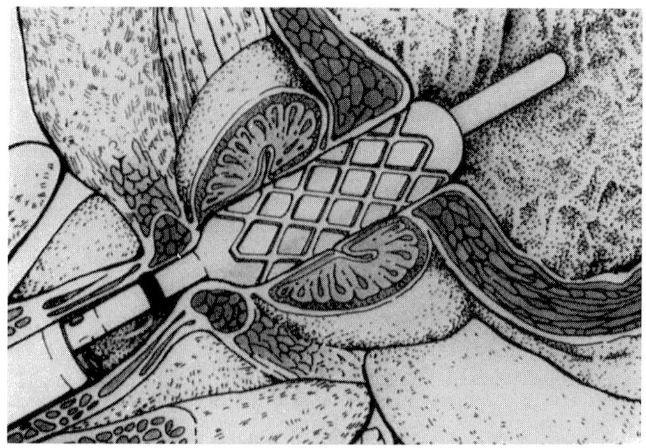

Figure 48–31. ASI Titan stent expanded by high pressure balloon inflation. (Courtesy of Boston Scientific, Boston, MA.)

Intraprostatic Stent—ASI Titan

The Titan stent is made of titanium alloy and has an internal diameter of 33 Fr (11 mm). Various lengths ranging from 1.9 to 5.8 cm are available in 4-mm increments. As mentioned earlier, it is not self-expanding like the Wallstent; thus, it must be expanded by inflating a removable balloon within it.

Its deployment system is also under 0-degree angle cystoscopic guidance under direct vision. Its use requires either IV sedation and local prostatic block or spinal or epidural anesthesia. A noncompliant balloon expands the stent after it is placed in the prostatic urethra (Figs. 48–30, 48–31, 48–32). A removal tool can be used to withdraw displaced stents by pushing the stent into the bladder, grasping the stent with a wire noose, bending and inverting it into a sheath, and pulling it out. No postoperative catheter is required in most patients.

As reported for the Wallstent, early series dealt with high-risk patients from England who were unfit for surgery and were in urinary retention. Kirby and co-workers (1991) reported on 27 men in acute retention. Almost 89% (24 of 27) could void well with a decreased PVR after stent placement. In another series from England, Abrams and colleagues (1991) reported a group of 50 patients in urinary retention. After 1 year the Qmax was 13 ml/second in the 43 patients who were followed. In both of these series, a total of six stents had to be removed; this was accomplished without difficulty. Again, many patients suffered irritative symptoms in the first few weeks after treatment. Parra (1991) reported 14 patients in the United States with obstructive symptoms due to BPH who had a Qmax of around 15 ml/second 6 months after treatment.

Kirby and associates (1992) reported on 30 patients with BPH considered to be unfit for TURP. One year after placement of the stent, 21 men had a mean Qmax of 11 ml/second, and the PVR was 56 ml.

Chiou and colleagues (1993b), reporting on the United States Cooperative Study, described 106 patients, many of whom were high-risk patients in retention. A reduction in SS from 17 to 5 was noted at 6 months, and Qmax increased from 4 to 15. Patients in retention had a Qmax of 14 at 6 months, whereas the PVR of those not in retention decreased from 138 to 66 ml. Thirteen stents were removed. The authors thought that the stent was of considerable use in high-risk patients who have obstruction or are in urinary retention. Miller and colleagues (1993) reported similar results in a larger series of 148 patients from England. Most of these patients were unfit for TURP and in urinary retention. Effective voiding was re-established in 89% of patients. The

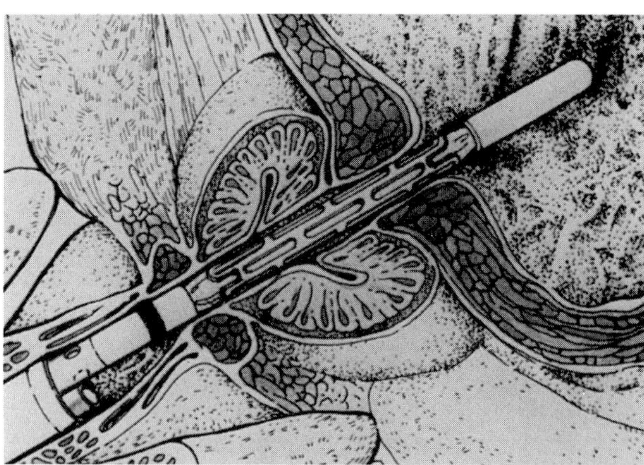

Figure 48–30. ASI Titan stent in place over uninflated expandable balloon. (Courtesy of Boston Scientific, Boston, MA.)

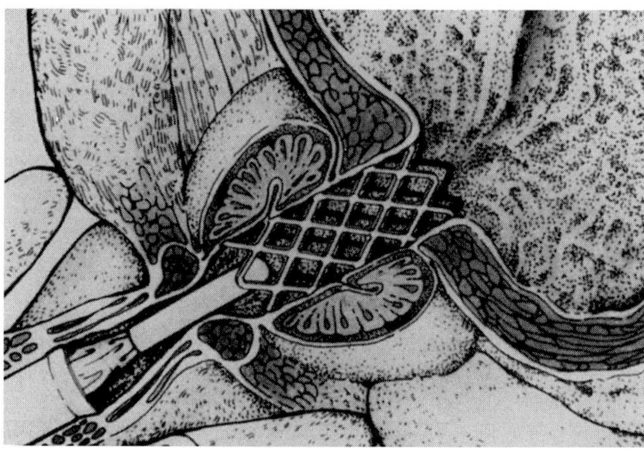

Figure 48–32. ASI Titan stent expanded, and inflation device removed. (Courtesy of Boston Scientific, Boston, MA.)

authors stressed the need to avoid intravesical stent protrusion to prevent incrustation; this is a difficult problem, especially in patients with middle lobe obstruction. They also stressed the judicious use of perioperative antibiotics.

Kaplan and his group (1995) recently reported the long-term results of the North American Trial Stent Study Group. The results are reproduced in Table 48–7. In this study there was a nonretention group and a urinary retention group.

The Titan stent seems to produce results that are slightly inferior to those achieved by the Urolume. Whether one is easier to place or remove is not clear from the literature. This stent has a smaller lumen, with a size of 33 Fr versus 42 Fr for the Urolume. Whether this is important is not known. Obviously, it could be more difficult to perform cystoscopic maneuvers through a No. 33 Fr stent than through a No. 42 Fr, but whether this is a practical problem is also not clear.

Neither the Wallstent nor the Intraprostatic Stent has yet been approved by the FDA for the treatment of BPH.

Thermosensitive Stents

A new stent made of a thermosensitive biocompatible material composed of titanium-nickel (Nitinol, Angiomed, Germany) was reported on by Gottfried and colleagues (1993) at the 1993 AUA meeting. The stent is made of woven material and is placed in the prostatic urethra, where it expands to its ultimate diameter in a few seconds. It is easy to remove atraumatically. Lengths available range from 2 to 8 cm. All 13 patients who had bladder neck obstruction and were in retention were able to void spontaneously after local placement of the stent under endoscopic control. Dysuria was noted for 3 to 5 days. Epithelial overgrowth began at 3 months. The stents were also used in six patients with urethral strictures.

Gottfried and his group (1995b) recently offered further data on this stent. It can be removed atraumatically. It has been used in 54 patients with BPH who were poor operative risks. A group of patients in urinary retention comprised 76% of the series; the nonretention group comprised 24%. After treatment 53 of 54 patients could void. In the nonretention group, Qmax increased from 5 to 16 ml/second, PVR dropped from 194 to 11 ml, and SS (AUA) dropped from 24 to 4 at 6 months.

Comments on All Stents

The ultimate niche that will be achieved by stents in the treatment of BPH is unknown. Certainly, good results have been obtained in several short- and long-term series, especially among patients who are too ill for other procedures such as TURP. Whether stents will be competitive with other minimally invasive treatments for long-term management of the low-risk patients who would normally be candidates for TURP remains to be seen. This writer is a bit concerned about epithelial proliferation within the stent lumen and the rather high rate of stent removal (14% to 33%).

For completeness, it should be emphasized that stents have also been used to treat patients with detrusor sphincter dyssynergia (Oesterling, 1991) instead of sphincterotomy, and patients with Parkinson's disease who exhibited voiding symptoms as a therapeutic trial to see whether they improved (Milroy, 1991).

TRANSURETHRAL NEEDLE ABLATION OF THE PROSTATE

The transurethral needle ablation (TUNA) of the prostate device (VidaMed, Menlo Park, CA) is a vehicle used to place interstitial radiofrequency (RF) needles through the urethra into the lateral prostatic lobes to cause coagulation necrosis (Figs. 48–33 and 48–34). This is accomplished by heating the tissue to around 100°C at RF power of 490 KHz for 4 minutes per lesion. Cavities of 1 cm or greater are created.

Technique

A No. 22 Fr urethral catheter is placed under direct vision in the urethra. Two needles at 60-degree angles to each other

Table 48–7. NORTH AMERICAN TITAN STENT GROUP LONG-TERM RESULTS

	Months Post Treatment	Number Patients	Preoperative	Postoperative	Percent Change
Nonretention Group					
SS (Madsen) decrease	0	85	16		
	24	85		9	44
Qmax increase	0	85	9 ml/second		
	24	85		11 ml/second	22
PVR decrease	0	85	117 ml		
	24	85		74 ml	37
Retention Group					
SS (Madsen)	24	59	Retention	5	
Qmax	24	59	Retention	11 ml/second	
PVR	24	59	Retention	31 ml	

19% of all stents placed were explanted.

Reprinted by permission of the publisher from Kaplan SA, Chiou RK, Morton WJ: Long-term experience utilizing a new balloon expandable prostatic endoprosthesis: The Titan stent. North American Titan Stent Study Group. Urology 1995; 45:224–234. Copyright 1995 by Elsevier Science Inc.

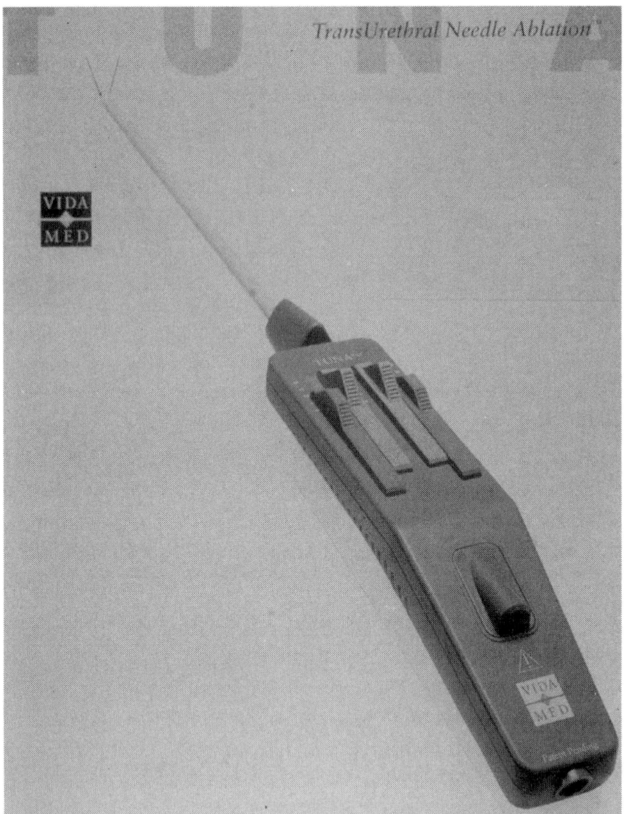

Figure 48–33. TUNA device, through which a panendoscope lens can be placed up through the catheter for placement. (Courtesy of VidaMed Corporation, Menlo Park, CA.)

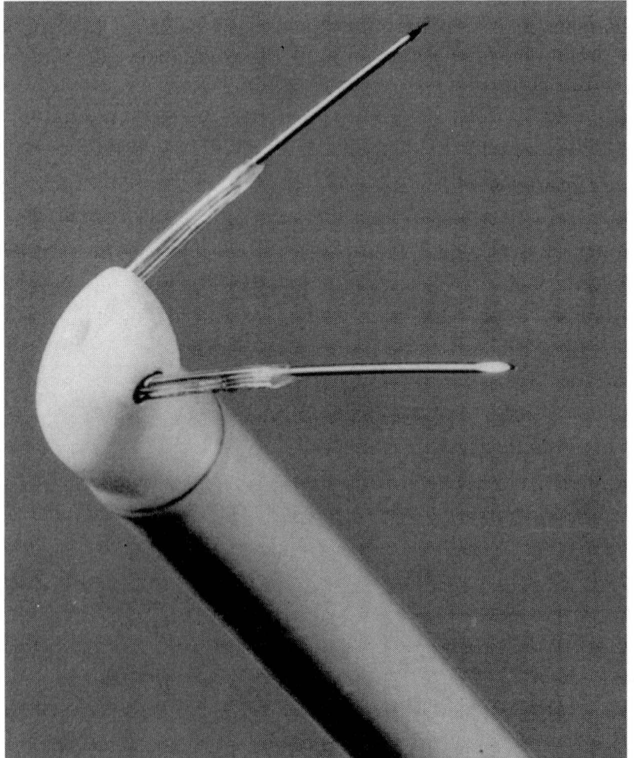

Figure 48–34. TUNA radiofrequency needles deployed with proximal protective sheaths to protect the urethra. (Courtesy of VidaMed Corp., Menlo Park, CA.)

and at a 90-degree angle to the catheter are located at the tip of the catheter and advanced into the prostatic parenchyma by piercing the urethra. Covering shields can be advanced over the proximal needle portion to protect the urethra. Thermosensors at the end of the catheter, on the shields, and in the rectum measure the temperature in the prostate and periprostatic areas. The shaft can be rotated and the prostate can be treated, for example, at the 2, 4, 8, and 10 o'clock positions and moved from the bladder neck toward the verumontanum as the various prostatic zones are treated with the laser. The needles are not seen under direct vision.

Clinical Data

Schulman and Zlotta (1994a) reported treating 80 patients with this technique. Most patients were given urethral gel lidocaine plus IV sedation. The treatments lasted an average of about 30 minutes. Temperatures of proximal lesions (adjacent to the urethra at the shield thermocouple) averaged 45 to 76°C. Urethral and rectal temperatures averaged 41°C. Experiments had previously demonstrated that temperatures were 40°C greater at the tip of the needle than at the shield thermocouple.

Pathologic examination of tissue revealed that coagulation necrosis occurs at the needle tip sites in lesions ranging from 1.2×0.7 cm to 1.7×1 cm.

Results

Although 80 patients were treated, only 14 patients were available for study 3 months after therapy. Mean Qmax increased from 10 to 15 ml/second (50%). Fifty percent of patients achieved at least a 50% improvement. SS decreased from 22 to 7 (68%) at 6 months.

These numbers are small. However, this initial experience was promising. The bladder neck was not treated, and the urethra was spared. Even though intraprostatic temperatures of 100°C are generated, there is little pain, perhaps due to a paucity of sensory endings in the parenchyma and the rapidity of temperature generation to 100°C, according to Schulman's theory.

Goldwasser and colleagues (1993) performed experiments on canines and established that 1-cm cavities could be created in prostate parenchyma using radiofrequency needles without causing damage to the surrounding structures.

Features of Transurethral Needle Ablation of the Prostate

Schulman and Zlotta (1994b) selected the following features of TUNA as advantages compared with TURP and laser TURP: outpatient procedure, local plus IV sedation, short learning curve, size of lesions can be regulated to fit size of prostate, 20% urinary retention rate lasts for only a few days, hematuria and dysuria last only a few days when they occur, no retrograde ejaculation or sexual dysfunction, improvement in Qmax of more than 50% is noted in majority of patients, longer follow-up is required, therapeutic effect occurs gradually over 30 postoperative days, and 20% of patients show no objective response but irritative symptoms are improved. Schulman and Zlotta (1995a) basically covered the same set of patients described in their earlier series (1994a) with a little additional data.

Goldwasser and colleagues (1995) were very positive about the results of therapy. Most of their patients wear a catheter for 1 day and return to work in 2 to 3 days. At 3 months, these authors noted a bladder pressure drop during urination to 55 cm H_2O (from 95 cm H_2O). Qmax increased from 9 to 14 ml/second (56%). SS improved very significantly. However, the median lobe cannot be treated, a definite deficiency in the present writer's opinion. The bladder neck is not treated either, which is also a potential deficiency. Goldwasser and his colleagues stated that the TUNA device is initially very low cost and the only investment of any consequence is in disposables.

Heaton (1995) reported on his preliminary results from Kingston, Ontario. Three (20%) of his 15 patients went into urinary retention and had to be catheterized; two of these problems were caused by clots. Follow-up time was too short to be meaningful (i.e., less than 6 months). Few other problems occurred.

The VidaMed Company (personal communication, 1995) sent this author some literature summarizing their data from a variety of centers around the world. The data is *not* peer reviewed (Table 48–8).

At the 1995 AUA meeting several papers on TUNA were presented. Issa and Kabalin (1995) reported on 12 patients with 3-month data. Their data were comparable to the previous data given by Schulman and Zlotta (1994a, 1994b). Woo and colleagues (1995) reported on 30 patients with only 1-month data. Seven of eight patients not catheterized at the time of the procedure developed urinary retention.

Eardley and associates (1995) reported the early results of a European collaborative trial. Forty-three patients had been entered in this trial. Minimal 3-month data were available and were comparable to Schulman and Zlotta's early data.

Campo and his group (1995) reported the results of 40 patients treated in Italy. Six-month data were available for only a few patients but were in line with others' results. No retrograde ejaculation or erectile dysfunction was noted. SS decreased dramatically from 24 to 5 at 6 months in 15 patients. Qmax increased from 4 to 13 ml/second.

Steele and Sleep (1995) reported on 60 patients treated with TUNA. The mean SS decreased from 20 to 5 at 3 months, and the detrusor muscle pressure at Qmax decreased from 96 cm H_2O to 57 cm H_2O. These results were durable to 6 months.

Schulman and Zlotta (1995b) updated their data on 30 patients to 6 months. Qmax increased from 10 to 15 ml/second (50%), International prostate (IP) (SS) decreased from 21 to 7 (67%). Postoperative urinary retention was noted in 25% of patients. Also, 28 patients who were in retention preoperatively were treated, and 22 (79%) were subsequently able to void.

Table 48–8. TUNA COMBINED STATISTICS

	Months Post Treatment	Number Patients	Pre-operative	Post-operative	Percent Change
IP (SS) decrease	0	254	22		
	3	213		9	59
	6	150		8	64
	12	29		8	64
Qmax increase	0	254	8 ml/second		
	3	219		13	63
	6	136		13	63
	12	35		14	75

Adapted from VidaMed Company, personal communication, 1995.

Comments on Transurethral Needle Ablation of the Prostate

Preliminary data are promising, although very few patients so far have been followed for as long as 12 months. Twenty-five percent of patients develop acute urinary retention. Sexual function is preserved. The median lobes and the bladder neck are not treated. The procedure appears to be safe and is performed under local lidocaine anesthesia and IV sedation. Prospective randomized studies comparing TUNA to laser TUR and TURP as well as to thermotherapy (TUMT) will be of great interest. This writer is concerned about the inability to treat the bladder neck and median lobes because many of the patients he sees in his practice appear to need therapy delivered to those areas.

FINAL COMMENTS

How does one decide which patient is to receive which treatment? To be specific, this author believes that patients who require "minimally invasive" treatment should receive one of the therapies other than balloon dilation or hyperthermia because they are more effective.

Which patients need minimally invasive treatment? Basically, those who have moderate (8 to 18) to severe symptoms (19 to 35) as noted in the AUA SS form. Those who have absolute indications for a TURP or open prostatectomy as described by McConnell and colleagues (1994) in the Agency for Health Care Policy and Research (AHCPR) Guidelines such as refractory retention or any of the following (clearly secondary to BPH)—recurrent urinary tract infection, recurrent or persistent gross hematuria, bladder stones, or renal insufficiency—are generally best treated by a TURP or, if a very large gland is present, an open prostatectomy. For urinary retention alone, stents may be an option in high-risk patients.

Are there special niches for the various treatments? Yes, there are some special niches to which some therapies appear to be better suited. The following list reflects the author's subjective biases but is incomplete:

1. *Thermotherapy (TUMT)—Prostatron:* Patients with less severe symptoms who wish to experience minimal discomfort and treatment bother. Patients suited for the TUNA device might also fall into this niche. Long-term TUNA data are scanty.
2. *Laser therapy:* Patients who are taking anticoagulation therapy and those who do not mind a slower trend of improvement than occurs with a TURP.

3. *SLT laser therapy:* Those with a small prostate gland of 20 to 30 g.

4. *Stents:* Elderly poor-risk patients who have a shortened life-span and are at high risk for anesthesia.

5. Men who wish to preserve antegrade ejaculation can be treated with TUMT, laser, or the TUNA device.

6. Because the TUNA device, the Prostatron, and HIFU generally do not treat the bladder neck or the median lobe very effectively, patients who are deemed candidates for treatment of these areas would be best treated by TVP, laser, or stents.

Other than these niches, patients who in general would be candidates for a routine TURP (i.e., for the usual rather than absolute indications) are also candidates for HIFU, TUMT, laser prostatectomy, TVP, and stents.

The author's observations lead him to believe the following: Urologists feel most comfortable when they can deliver therapy by direct vision. The median or middle lobes should be treated. The author personally prefers a technique that creates an instant channel (more TURP-like) such as that delivered by laser vaporization, VaporTrode, or high-energy TUMT. If one wishes to generate minimal pain during treatment, preservation of the urethra is a goal that can be accomplished by treating with TUMT, the TUNA device, interstitial laser, or even stents. All new treatments should be planned as outpatient-directed therapy.

One cannot be too dogmatic about the indications for these devices because they are constantly changing. Perhaps the best advice is given below:

Be not the first by whom the new are tried
Nor yet the last to lay the old aside.

—Alexander Pope

REFERENCES

Abrams P, Gillatt D, Chadwick D: Intraprostatic stent—experience with the ASI stent to treat bladder outflow obstruction. (Abstract.) J Urol 1991; 145:373.

Aslam M, Lynch MD, O'Donoghue N: Interstitial laser coagulation for the treatment of urinary outflow obstruction. (Abstract.) J Urol 1993; 149:1.

Assimos DG, McCullough DL, Woodruff RD, et al: Canine transurethral laser induced prostatectomy. J Endourol 1991; 5:145–149.

Babayan RK: Transurethral ultrasound-guided laser-induced prostatectomy (TULIP): past, present, and future. J Endourol 1995; 9:141–144.

Baert L, Aneye F, Willemen P, et al: Transurethral microwave hyperthermia for benign prostatic hyperplasia: preliminary clinical and pathological results. J Urol 1990; 144:1383–1387.

Bajoria S, Agarwal SA, White R, et al: Experience with the second generation UroLume prostatic stent. Br J Urol 1995; 75:325–327.

Beisland HO, Sander S: Localized prostate carcinoma treated with TUR and neodymium-YAG laser irradiation. Scand J Urol Nephrol 1991; 138(Suppl) 117–119.

Bihrle R, Foster RS, Sanghvi NT, et al: High intensity focused ultrasound for the treatment of benign prostatic hyperplasia: Early United States clinical experience. J Urol 1994; 151:1571–1575.

Blute ML, Tomera KM, Hellerstein DK, et al: Transurethral microwave thermotherapy: An alternative for the treatment of benign prostatic hypertrophy. One year clinical results of the Prostatron study group. (Abstract.) J Urol 1993; 149:143.

Blute ML, Patterson DE, Segura JW, et al: Transurethral microwave thermotherapy versus sham: A prospective double blind study. (Abstract.) J Urol 1994; 151:752.

Blute ML, Tomera KM, Hellerstein DK, et al: Transurethral microwave thermotherapy for management of benign prostatic hyperplasia: Results of the United States Prostatron Cooperative Study. J Urol 1995; 150:1591–1596.

Burhenne HJ, Chisholm RJ, Quenville NF: Prostatic hyperplasia: Radiological intervention—work in progress. Radiology 1984; 152:655–657.

Bush W: Über die Einflusse welche heftigere Erysipelen zuweilen auf organisierte Neubioldungen haben. Ureh Naturheilke Preues Pjien Westphal 1866; 23:28–30.

Cammack JT, Motamedi M, Torres JH, et al: Endoscopic Neodymium: YAG laser coagulation of the prostate: Comparison of low power versus high power. (Abstract.) J Urol 1993; 149.

Campo B, Muto G, Rigatti P, et al: TUNA: Clinical reliability of a new procedure for prostatic obstruction treatment. J Urol 1995; 153:533A.

Castaneda F, Reddy PK, Wasserman N, et al: Benign prostatic hypertrophy, retrograde transurethral dilation of the prostate urethra in humans. Work in progress. Radiology 1987; 163:645–648.

Cavaliere R, Ciocatto EC, Clovonelle BC, et al: Selective heat sensitivity of cancer cells: Biochemical and clinical studies. Cancer 1969; 20:1351–1381.

Chapple CR, Milroy EJG, Richards D: Permanently implanted urethral stent for prostatic obstruction in the unfit patient: Preliminary report. Br J Urol 1990; 66:58–65.

Chapple CR, Rosario DJ, Wasserfallen M, et al: A randomised study of the Urolume stent vs prostatic surgery. (Abstract.) J Urol 1995; 153:436.

Chiou YK, Chico RK, Lynch B, et al: Randomized comparison of balloon dilation and transurethral incision for symptomatic benign prostatic hyperplasia: Long-term follow-up. (Abstract.) J Urol 1993a; 149:1004.

Chiou RK, Suarez GM, Wadle RW, et al: Use of the "Titan" intraprostatic stent in men with BPH: Preliminary results from the United States National Cooperative Study. (Abstract.) J Urol 1993b; 149:12.

Costa FJ: Lomefloxacin prophylaxis in visual laser ablation of the prostate. Urology 1994; 44:933–936.

Costello AJ, Johnson DE, Bolton DM, et al: YAG laser ablation of the prostate as a treatment for benign prostatic hypertrophy. Lasers Surg Med 1992a; 12:121–124.

Costello AJ, Bowsher WG, Bolton DM: Laser ablation of the prostate in patients with benign prostatic hypertrophy. Br J Urol 1992b; 69:603–608.

Costello A, Shaffer BS: Laser ablation of benign prostatic hypertrophy. Two and a half years' experience with a right angle delivery system. (Abstract.) J Urol 1993; 149:3.

Costello AJ, Bolton DM, Ellis D, et al: Histopathological changes in human prostatic adenoma following neodymium:YAG laser ablation therapy. J Urol 1994; 152:1526–1529.

Cummings JM, Parra RO, Boullier JA: Laser prostatectomy: Initial experience and urodynamic follow-up. Urology 1995; 45:414–420.

Dahlstrand C, Geinsson G, Fall M, et al: Transurethral microwave thermotherapy versus transurethral resection for benign prostatic hyperplasia. Preliminary results of a randomized study. Eur Urol 1993; 23:292–298.

Dahlstrand C, Walden M, Pettersson S: Three-year follow-up of transurethral microwave thermotherapy versus transurethral resection for benign prostatic obstruction. (Abstract.) J Urol 1995; 153:434.

Debruyne FMJ, Bloem FAG, de la Rosette JOMCH, et al: Transurethral thermotherapy (TUMT) in benign prostatic hyperplasia: Placebo versus TUMT. (Abstract.) J Urol 1993; 149:752.

Defalco A, Oesterling JE, Epstein H: The North American experience with the Urolume endourethral prosthesis as a treatment for BPH: Three year results. (Abstract.) J Urol 1995; 153:829.

de la Rosette JJ, Foreling FM, Debruyne FM, et al: Clinical results with microwave thermotherapy of benign prostatic hyperplasia. Eur Urol 1993; 23(Suppl 1):68–71.

de la Rosette JJMCH, Slaa, ET, van Iersel T, et al: Are results of laser treatment irrespective of the type of fiber or technique used? (Abstract.) J Urol 1995; 153:229.

Devonec M, Berger N, Perrin P: Transurethral microwave heating of the prostate—or from hyperthermia to thermotherapy. J Endourol 1991; 5:129–135.

Devonec M, Berger N, Fendler JP: Thermoregulation during transurethral microwave thermotherapy: Experimental and clinical fundamentals. Eur Urol 1993a; 23(Suppl 1):63–67.

Devonec M, Ogden C, Perrin P, et al: Clinical response to transurethral microwave—is thermal dose dependent? Eur Urol 1993b; 23:267–274.

Devonec M, Fendler JP, Nosser M: The clinical response to thermotherapy is dose dependent: From thermocoagulation to thermoablation. (Abstract.) J Urol 1993c; 149:142.

Diesting W: Transurethral dilatation of the prostate: A new method in the treatment of prostatic hypertrophy. Urol Int 1956; 2:158–171.

Dixon C, Machi G, Theune C, et al: A prospective double blind randomized study comparing laser ablation of the prostate and transurethral prostatectomy for the treatment of BPH. (Abstract.) J Urol 1993; 149:6.

Dixon CM, Theune C: Evaluating the cost of lasers for the treatment of benign prostatic hyperplasia. J Endourol 1995; 9:189–193.

Dotter CT: Transluminally placed coilspring endarterial tube grafts: Long-term patency in canine popliteal artery. Invest Radiol 1969; 4:329–332.

Dotter CT, Buschmann RW, McKinney MK, et al: Transluminal expandable nitinol coil stent grafting: Preliminary report. Radiology 1983; 147:259–260.

Dowd J, Smith JJ: Balloon dilatation of the prostate. Urol Clin North Am 1990; 17:671–677.

Dowd J, Smith JJ: Prostatic balloon dilatation in 115 unequivocally obstructed patients. J Endourol 1991; 5:99–104.

Eardley J, Fitzpatrick J, Frick J: TUNA therapy for symptomatic benign prostatic hyperplasia. A collaborative European trial. (Abstract.) J Urol 1995; 153:553.

Fabian KM: Der Intraprostatische "Partielle Katheter" (Urologische Spirale). Urologe [A] 1980; 19:236–238.

Fabricus PG, Matz M, Zepnick N: Endourethral spiral—an alternative to continuous catheterization? Z Arztl Fortbild (Jena) 1983; 77:482–485.

Fabricus PG, Schafer J, Schneller N, et al: Efficacy of transrectal hyperthermia for benign prostatic hyperplasia: A placebo controlled study. (Abstract.) J Urol 1991; 145:363.

Flier G, Seppelt U: Enfaugen mit der urologischen Spirale. Urologe [B] 1987; 27:304–307.

Foster RS, Bihrle R, Sanghvi N, et al: Production of prostatic lesions in canines using transrectally administered high intensity focused ultrasound. Eur Urol 1993a; 23:330–336.

Foster RS, Bihrle R, Sanghvi N, et al: High-energy focused ultrasound in the treatment of prostatic disease. Eur Urol 1993b; 23(Suppl 1):29–33.

Foster RS, Bihrle R, Sanghvi N, et al: High-intensity focused ultrasound for the treatment of benign prostatic hyperplasia. Semin Urol 1994; 12:200–204.

Fournier GR, Jr, Narayan P: Laser effects on prostatic tissue: Review of experimental data. J Endourol 1995; 9:89–92.

Fry FJ: Intense focus ultrasound in medicine. Eur Urol 1993; 23(Suppl 1):2–7.

Fugate D, Sirls LT, Kirkemo A, et al: Detailed cost analysis of high power visual laser assisted prostatectomy vs. transurethral prostatectomy. (Abstract.) J Urol 1995; 153:362.

Furui S, Sawoda S, Irie T, et al: Hepatic IVC obstruction: Treatment of two types with Gianturco expandable metallic stents. Radiology 1990; 176(3):620–621.

Furuya S, Tsukamoto T, Kumamoto Y, et al: Transurethral balloon laser thermotherapy for symptomatic benign prostatic hyperplasia: Preliminary clinical results. J Endourol 1995; 9:145–149.

Fuselier HA, Roth RA, Babayan RK, et al: TULIP—national human cooperative study results. (Abstract.) J Urol 1993; 149:8.

Gelet A, Chapelon JY, Margonari J, et al: High intensity focused ultrasound experimentation on human benign prostatic hypertrophy. Eur Urol 1993; 23:(Suppl 1)44–47.

Gilling PJ, Cass CB, Malcolm AR, et al: Combination holmium and Nd:Yag laser ablation of the prostate: Initial clinical experience. J Endourol 1995; 9:151–153.

Goldenburg SL, Perez-Marrero RA, Lee L: Endoscopic balloon dilation of the prostate: Early experience. J Urol 1990; 144:83–88.

Goldwasser B, Ramon J, Engelberg S, et al: Transurethral needle ablation of the prostate using low level radiofrequency energy: An animal experimental study. Eur Urol 1993; 24:400–405.

Goldwasser B, McConnell JB, Marberger M: BPH: What really works? Symposium. Contemp Urol 1995; April:76–90.

Gomella LG, Lofti MAMR, Rivas DA, et al: Contact laser vaporization techniques for benign prostatic hyperplasia. J Endourol 1995; 9:117–123.

Gottfried HW, Schimers HP, Miller K, et al: New thermosensitive stent for subvesical obstruction. (Abstract.) J Urol 1993; 149:1013.

Gottfried HW, Frohneberg D, de la Rosette JJMCH, et al. Transurethral laser ablation of prostate (TULAP)—experience of a European multicenter study using UltraLine fiber. (Abstract.) J Urol 1995a; 153:230.

Gottfried HW, Schimers HP, Gschwend J, et al: Initial experiences with the thermothermstent in treatment of benign prostatic hyperplasia. Urologe [A] 1995b; 34:110–118.

Harrison NW, DeSouza JV: Prostatic stenting for outflow obstruction. Br J Urol 1990; 65(2):192–196.

Harzman R, Weckesman D: Lokale hyperthermie bei Prostaterkrankungen? Atk Urol 1991; 22:10–14.

Heaton JPW: Radiofrequency thermal ablation of the prostate: The TUNA technique. Techn Urol 1995; 1:3–10.

Hernandez-Granulau J, Eshghi M, Choudhury M, et al: Balloon divulsion of the prostate for treatment of benign prostatic hyperplasia: 18 month follow-up: Is it really worth it? (Abstract.) J Urol 1990; 143:347.

Hurwitz JJ: Teflon tubes for stenting and bypassing the lacrimal drainage pathways. Ophthal Surg 1989; 20:855–859.

Isogawa Y, Ohmori K: Application of urethral stent under metal bougie guidance. Hinyokika Kiyo 1993; 39:231–235.

Issa MM, Kabalin JN: Transurethral needle ablation (TUNA) of the prostate: Report of initial United States clinical trial. (Abstract.) J Urol 1995; 153:535.

Johnson DE, Levinson AK, Greskovich FJ, et al: Transurethral laser prostatectomy using a right angle delivery system. SPIE Proceedings 1991; 1421:36–38.

Kabalin JN: Laser prostatectomy performed with a right angle firing neodymium:YAG laser fiber at 40 watts power setting. J Urol 1993; 150:95–99.

Kabalin JN: Three year experience with neodymium:YAG laser coagulation prostatectomy in 225 patients. (Abstract.) J Urol 1995a; 153:229.

Kabalin JN: ND:YAG laser coagulation prostatectomy for benign prostatic hyperplasia. Part I: Clinical outcomes. Afr J Urol 1995b; 1:112–118.

Kabalin JN: ND:YAG laser coagulation prostatectomy for benign prostatic hyperplasia. Part II. Dosimetry and operative techniques. Afr J Urol 1995c; 1:119–129.

Kabalin JN: Holmium:YAG laser vaporization prostatectomy. (Abstract.) J Urol 1995d; 153:229.

Kabalin JN, Gill HS, Leach GE, et al: Visual laser assisted prostatectomy (VLAP) using urolase right angle fiber. Preliminary reports with 60 watts protocol. (Abstract.) J Urol 1993; 149:4.

Kandel LB, Harrison LH: Commentary: Laser treatment of urethral lesions. *In* Whitehead ED, ed: Current Operative Urology/1990. Philadelphia, J. B. Lippincott, 1990, pp 365–367.

Kandel LB, Harrison LH, McCullough DL, et al: Transurethral laser prostatectomy: Creation of a technique for using the neodymium:yttrium aluminum garnet (YAG) laser in the canine model. (Abstract.) J Urol 1986; 135:110.

Kandel LB, Harrison LH, McCullough DL: Transurethral laser prostatectomy in the canine model. Lasers Surg Med 1992; 12:33–42.

Kaplan SA, Te AE: Transurethral electrovaporization of the prostate: A novel method for treating men with benign prostatic hyperplasia. Urology 1995; 45:566–572.

Kaplan SA, Chiou RK, Morton WJ: Long-term experience utilizing a new balloon expandable prostatic endoprosthesis: The Titan stent. North American Titan Stent Study Group. Urology 1995; 45:224–234.

Kemppainen E, Talja M, Bihhela M, et al: A bioresorbable urethral stent. An experimental study. Urol Res 1993; 21:235–238.

Kingston TE, Nonnenmacher AK, Crowe H, et al: Further evaluation of transurethral laser ablation of the prostate in patients treated with anticoagulant therapy. Aust N Z J Surg 1995; 65:40–43.

Kirby R, Liu S, Eardley I, et al: The use of the ASI titanium stent in the treatment of acute retention due to BPH. (Abstract.) J Urol 1991; 145:389.

Kirby RS, Heard BR, Miller P, et al: Use of the ASI titanium stent in the management of bladder outlet obstruction due to benign prostatic hyperplasia. J Urol 1992; 48:1195–1197.

Kirby RS, Williams G, Witherow R, et al: The Prostatron transurethral microwave device in the treatment of bladder outflow obstruction due to benign prostatic hyperplasia. Br J Urol 1993; 72:190–194.

Klein LA: Two year follow-up of balloon dilatation of the prostate and an algorithm for future patient selection. J Endourol 1991; 2:109–112.

Klein LA, Perez-Marrero R, Bowers GW, et al: Balloon dilatation of the prostate: A multicenter study with one year followup. (Abstract.) J Urol 1989; 141(2):335.

Knapp PM, Newman DM: Transrectal hyperthermia treatments in patients with obstructive benign prostatic hypertrophy (BPH). (Abstract.) J Urol 1991; 145:209.

Koeghane S, Cranston D, Lawrence K, et al: The Oxford laser prostate trial: A prospective randomised controlled trial of contact vaporisation of the prostate versus TURP. (Abstract.) J Urol 1995;153:5;230.

Kramalowsky EV, Tucker RD: The urological application of electrosurgery. J Urol 1991; 146:669–674.

Kurtz SB, Sirls LT, Leach GE: Use of the neodymium:yag laser to control refractory bleeding from the prostate. J Urol 1994; 152:920–921.

Leach GE: Local anesthesia for laser prostatectomy. J Endourol 1995; 5:159–161.

Lepor H, Sypherd IY, Machi G, et al: Randomized double-blind study comparing effectiveness of balloon dilatation of the prostate (BDP) and cystoscopy for the treatment of symptomatic benign prostatic hyperplasia. J Urol 1992; 147:639–644.

Linder A, Braf Z, Lev A, et al: Local hyperthermia of the prostate gland for the treatment of benign prostatic hypertrophy and urinary retention. Br J Urol 1990; 65:201–203.

Lofti MS, Milam D, Albala D: Contact laser vaporization of the prostate and kidney: Applications in minimally invasive therapy including benign prostatic hypertrophy. (Abstract.) J Urol 1993;149:1012.

Luesley DM, Redman CW, Buxton EJ, et al: Prevention of postcone biopsy cervical stenosis using a temporary cervical stent. Br J Obstet Gynaecol 1990; 97:334–337.

Maass D, Kropf L, Ggloff L, et al: Transluminal implantation of intravascular "double helix" spiral prostheses: Technical and biological considerations. Proc Eur Soc Artif Organs 1982; 9:252–257.

Madersbacher S, Kratzik C, Szabo N, et al: Tissue ablation in benign prostatic hyperplasia with high-intensity focused ultrasound. Eur Urol 1993; 23(Suppl 1):39–43.

Madersbacher S, Kratzik C, Susani M, et al: Tissue ablation in benign prostatic hyperplasia with high intensity focused ultrasound. J Urol 1994; 152:1960–1961.

Magin RL, Fridd CW, Bonfiglio TA, et al: Thermal destruction of the canine prostate by high intensity microwaves. J Surg Res 1980; 29:265–275.

Mair EA, Parsons DS, Lally PK, et al: Treatment of severe bronchomalacia with expanding endobronchial stents. Arch Otolaryngol Head Neck Surg 1990; 116(9):1087–1090.

Marberger M: Editorial. Eur Urol 1993; 23(Suppl 1):1.

Martin W, Senge T: TULIP: An alternative to TURP. (Abstract.) J Urol 1993; 149:9.

Matzkin H: Hyperthermia as a treatment modality in benign prostatic hyperplasia. Urology 1994; 43(Suppl):17–20.

McConnell JD, Barry MJ, Bruskewitz RC, et al: Benign prostatic hyperplasia: Diagnosis and treatment. Quick Reference Guide for Clinicians, No. 8. (AHCPR Publication No. 94–0583.) Rockville, MD, Department of Health and Human Services, 1994.

McCullough DL: Editorial comment. J Urol 1990; 144:87–88.

McCullough DL: This month in investigative urology: Transurethral laser treatment of benign prostatic hyperplasia. J Urol 1991; 146:1128–1135.

McCullough DL: Part I. Minimally invasive management of benign prostatic hyperplasia. *In* Walsh PC, Retik AB, Stamey TA, Vaughan ED Jr, eds: Campbell's Urology Update 8. Philadelphia, W. B. Saunders, 1993, pp 1–12.

McCullough DL: Part II. Minimally invasive management of benign prostatic hyperplasia. *In* Walsh PC, Retik AB, Stamey TA, Vaughan ED Jr, eds: Campbell's Urology Update 9. Philadelphia, W. B. Saunders, 1994, pp 1–14.

McCullough DL, Herrera M, Harrison LH, et al: Transurethral balloon dilatation of the prostate (TUBDP)— alternative to transurethral resection of the prostate? (Abstract.) Urology 1989; 141:339.

McCullough DL, Roth RA, Babayan R, et al: Transurethral ultrasound-guided laser-induced prostatectomy: National human cooperative study results. J Urol 1993; 150:1607–1611.

McLoughlin J, Jager R, Abel PD, et al: The use of prostatic stents in patients with urinary retention who are unfit for surgery. Br J Urol 1990; 66:66–70.

Meier AH, Weil EH, van Waalwijk van Doorn ES, et al: Transurethral radiofrequency heating or thermotherapy for benign prostatic hypertrophy: A prospective trial on 65 consecutive cases. Eur Urol 1992; 22:39–43.

Milam DF, Smith JA Jr: Laser prostatectomy devices and their tissue effects. J Endourol 1995; 9:85–88.

Miller PD, Gillatt D, Abrams P: Selection of patients for treatment with ASI prostatic stent. (Abstract.) J Urol 1993; 149:13.

Miller J, Becker HC, Ludwig M: Visual ablation of the prostate (VLAP) in high risk patients—analysis of results and perioperative morbidity. (Abstract.) J Urol 1995a; 153:414.

Miller PD, Parsons K, Ramsey EW: Transurethral microwave thermoablation (TUMT) for benign prostatic hyperplasia using a new device (T3). (Abstract.) J Urol 1995b; 153:532.

Milroy E: Permanent prostate stents. J Endourol 1991; 5(2):75–78.

Milroy EJG, Chapple CR, Cooper JE, et al: A new treatment for urethral strictures. Lancet 1988; 8:1424–1427.

Milroy E, Coulange C, Pansadoro V, et al: The Urolume permanent prostate stent as an alternative to TURP: Long term European results. (Abstract.) J Urol 1994; 151:396.

Moriel EZ, Chertin B, Hadas I: Laser evaporation of the prostate—results and complications in 170 patients. (Abstract.) J Urol 1995; 153:231.

Moseley WG, Goldenburg SL, Marks LS: Balloon dilatation of the prostate: A three year combined center study of 249 patients. (Abstract.) J Urol 1993; 149:1003.

Mulvin D, Creagh T, Kelly D, et al: Transurethral microwave versus transurethral catheter therapy for benign prostatic hyperplasia. Eur Urol 1994; 26:6–9.

Muschter R, Hessel S, Hofstetter A, et al: One year experience in interstitial laser coagulation for benign prostatic hyperplasia. (Abstract.) J Urol 1993; 149:1012.

Muschter R, Hofstetter A, Anson K, et al: Nd:YAG and diode lasers for interstitial laser coagulation of benign prostatic hyperplasia: Experimental and clinical evaluation. (Abstract.) J Urol 1995; 153:229.

Muschter R, Perlmutter AP: The optimization of laser prostatectomy. Part II: Other lasing techniques. Urology 1994; 44:856–861.

Narayan P, Tewari A, Fournier G, et al: Impact of prostate size and techniques of laser prostatectomy (evaporization vs coagulation) on the outcome of therapy for benign prostatic hyperplasia. (Abstract.) J Urol 1995; 153:231.

Nielsen KK, Kroman-Andersen B, Nordling J: Relationship between detrusor pressure and urinary flow rate in males with an intraurethral prostatic spiral. Br J Urol 1989; 3:275–279.

Nissenkorn I: Prostatic stents. J Endourol 1991; 5:79–82.

Nissenkorn I, Rotbard M, Slutzker D, et al: The connection between the length of the heating antenna and volume of the prostate in transurethral thermotherapy for benign prostatic hyperplasia. Eur Urol 1993; 23:307–311.

Nordling J, Holm HH, Karskov P, et al: The intraprostatic spiral: A new device for insertion with the patient under local anesthesia and with ultrasonic guidance with 3 month follow-up. J Urol 1989; 142:756–758.

Oesterling JE: A permanent epithelializing stent for the treatment of benign prostatic hyperplasia. Preliminary results. J Androl 1991; 12:423–428.

Oesterling JE: Benign prostatic hyperplasia: Medical and minimally invasive treatment options. N Engl J Med 1995; 332:99–109.

Oesterling JE, Epstein H: North American Urolume Study Group. (Abstract.) J Urol 1993; 149:10.

Ogden CW, Reddy P, Johnson H, et al: Sham versus transurethral microwave thermotherapy in patients with symptoms of benign prostatic outflow obstruction. Lancet 1993; 341:14–17.

Orihuela E, Cammack T, Motamedi M, et al: Randomized clinical trial comparing low power–slow heating versus high power–rapid heating noncontact neodymium:yttrium-aluminum-garnet laser regimens for the treatment of benign prostatic hyperplasia. Urology 1995; 45:783–789.

Palmaz JD, Kapp DT, Hayoski H, et al: Normal and stenotic renal arteries; experimental balloon-expandable intraluminal stenting. Radiology 1987; 164:705–708.

Parra RO: Titanium urethral stent: An alternative to prostatectomy in the high surgical risk patient. (Abstract.) J Urol 1991; 145:293.

Perlmutter AP, Vaughan ED: Prostatic heat treatments for symptomatic BPH. American Urological Association Update Series, Lesson 36, Vol. 12. Houston, TX, AUA Office of Education, 1993.

Perlmutter AP, Muschter R: The optimization of laser prostatectomy. Part I: Free beam side fire coagulation. Urology 1994; 44:847–855.

Perlmutter AP, Muschter R, Razvi HA: Electrosurgical vaporization of the prostate in the canine model. Urology 1995; 46:518–523.

Perrin P, Devonec M, Houdelette P, et al: Transurethral microwave thermotherapy: Higher energy protocol improves clinical results. (Abstract.) J Urol 1995; 153:434.

Petas A, Talja M, Tammela T, et al: Bioresorbable PGA-urospiral preventing urinary retention in VLAP. (Abstract.) J Urol 1995; 153:534.

Pinto KJ, McCullough DL: Results of side firing yag laser contact (vaporization) and noncontact (coagulation) TURP for BPH—preliminary results of an outpatient procedure. (Abstract.) J Urol 1995; 153:415.

Pow-Sang M, Cowan DF, Orihuela E, et al: Thermocoagulation effect of diode laser radiation in the human prostate: Acute and chronic study. Urology 1995; 45:790–794.

Quinn SF, Dyer R, Smothers R, et al: Balloon dilation of the prostatic urethra. Work in progress. Radiology 1985; 157:57–58.

Reddy PK: Role of balloon dilation in the treatment of benign prostatic hyperplasia. Prostate 1990; (Suppl 3):39–48.

Reddy PK: Balloon dilatation of the prostate: Principles and techniques. J Endourol 1991; 5:93–97.

Reddy PK: Personal communication, 1993.

Reddy PK, Wasserman N, Castaneda F, et al: Balloon dilatation of the prostate for treatment of benign hyperplasia. Urol Clin North Am 1988; 15:529–535.

Richter S, Nissenkom I, Rotbard M, et al: The treatment of benign prostatic hyperplasia causing complete urinary retention through local transurethral hyperthermia. Eur Urol 1992; 22:278–280.

Rodriguez V, Salvador-Bayarri J, Izquierdo de la Torre F: Intraprostatic prostheses. Arch Esp Urol 1991; 44:615–621.

Rosenklide P, Pedersen JF, Meyhoff HH: Late complications of ProstaKath treatment for benign prostatic hypertrophy. Br J Urol 1991; 68:387–389.

Roth RA, Aretz TH: Transurethral ultrasound-guided laser induced prostatectomy (TULIP procedure): A canine prostate feasibility study. J Urol 1991; 146:1128–1135.

Roth RA, Aretz TH, Lage AL: "TULIP": Transurethral laser induced prostatectomy under ultrasound guidance. (Abstract.) J Urol 1990; 143:285.

Rousseau H, Puel J, Joffre F, et al: Self-expanding endovascular prosthesis: An experimental study. Radiology 1987; 164:709–714.

Rousseau H, Joffre F, Rallat C, et al: Iliac artery endoprosthesis: Radiologic and histologic findings after two years. Am J Roentgenol 1989; 153: 1075–1076.

Sadoughi NS: Transurethral ND:YAG laser ablation of the prostate. (Abstract.) J Urol 1993; 149:1009.

Sander S, Beisland HO: Laser in the treatment of localized prostatic cancer. J Urol 1984; 132:280–281.

Sapozink MD, Boyd SD, Astrahan MD, et al: Transurethral hyperthermia for benign prostatic hyperplasia: Preliminary clinical results. J Urol 1990; 143:944–950.

Saranga R, Matzkin H, Braf Z: Local microwave hyperthermia in the treatment of benign prostatic hyperplasia. Br J Urol 1990; 65:349–353.

Sarramon JP, Joffre F, Rischmann P, et al: Wallstent endourethral prosthesis for recurrent urethral strictures. Ann Urol 1989; 23(5):383–387.

Sassine AM, Schulman CC: Intraurethral catheter in high-risk patients with urinary retention: 3 years of experience. Eur Urol 1994; 25:131–134.

Schulman CC, Vanden Bossche M: Hyperthermia and thermotherapy of benign prostatic hyperplasia: A critical review. Eur Urol 1993; 23(Suppl 1)53–59.

Schulman CC, Zlotta AR: Transurethral needle ablation of the prostate (TUNA): Pathological, radiological, and clinical study of a new office procedure for treatment of benign prostatic hyperplasia using low-level radiofrequency energy. Semin Urol 1994a; 12:205–210.

Schulman CC, Zlotta AR: Transurethral needle ablation of the prostate (TUNA): A new anesthesia-free office procedure for treatment of benign prostatic hyperplasia using radiofrequency energy. Urol Int 1994b; 1: 16–17.

Schulman CC, Zlotta AR: Transurethral needle ablation of the prostate for treatment of benign prostatic hyperplasia: Early clinical experience. Urology 1995a; 45:28–33.

Schulman CC, Zlotta AR: Transurethral needle ablation (TUNA) of the prostate: Clinical experience of a new office procedure for treatment of benign prostatic hyperplasia (BPH). (Abstract.) J Urol 1995b; 153:435.

Schulze H, Martin W, Hoch P, et al: TULIP versus TURP—a prospective randomized study. (Abstract.) J Urol 1994; 151:228.

Schulze H, Martin W, Hoch P, et al: Transurethral ultrasound-guided laser-induced prostatectomy: Clinical outcome and data analysis. Urology 1995; 45:241–247.

Servadio C, Leib Z: Hyperthermia in the treatment of prostate cancer. Prostate 1984; 5:205–211.

Servadio C, Leib Z, Lev A: Further observations on the use of local hyperthermia for the treatment of diseases of the prostate in man. Eur Urol 1986; 12:38–40.

Servadio C, Linder A, Lev A, et al: Further observations on the effect of local hyperthermia on benign enlargement of the prostate. World J Urol 1989; 6:204–208.

Servadio C, Braf F, Siegel Y, et al: Local thermotherapy of the benign prostate. A 1-year follow-up. Eur Urol 1990; 18:169–173.

Shanberg AM, Tansey LA, Gaghdassarian R: The use of neodymium YAG laser in prostatectomy. (Abstract.) J Urol 1985; 133:331.

Shumaker BP: Contact laser ablation of the prostate for the treatment of benign prostatic hypertrophy. Semin Urol 1994; 12:170–173.

Shapshay SM, Beamis JF, Dumon JF: Total cervical tracheal stenosis: Treatment by laser, dilation, and stenting. Am J Otol Rhinol Laryngol 1989; 8:890–895.

Sonn DJ, Badlani GH: Contact laser vaporization of the prostate: Sidefire technique. J Endourol 1995; 9:113–116.

Stawarz B, Szmiglielski S, Orgrodnik J, et al: A comparison of transurethral and transrectal microwave hyperthermia in poor risk surgical benign prostatic hypertrophy patients. J Urol 1991; 146:353–357.

Steele GS, Sleep DJ: Transurethral needle ablation of the prostate: Does the pressure flow curve change? (Abstract.) J Urol 1995; 153:435.

Stewart SC, Benjamin D, Weil D, et al: Electro-vaporization of the prostate: A pilot study. (Abstract.) J Urol 1995; 153:437.

Strohmaier WL, Bichler KH, Fluchter SH, et al: Local microwave hyperthermia of benign prostatic hyperplasia. J Urol 1990; 144:913–917.

Susani M, Modersbacher S, Kratzik C, et al: Morphology of tissue destruction by focused ultrasound. Eur Urol 1993; 23(Suppl 1):34–38.

Takahashi S, Homma Y, Minowada S, Aso Y: Transurethral ultrasound-guided laser-induced prostatectomy (TULIP) for benign prostatic hyperplasia: Clinical utility at one-year follow-up and imaging analysis. Urology 1994; 43:802–807.

Te AE, Reis R, Kaplan SA: TVP: A new modification of TURP. Contemp Urol 1995; May:74–83.

Thomas PJ, Britton JP, Harrison NW: The ProstaKath stent: Four years experience. Br J Urol 1993; 71:430–432.

Thomas R: Personal communication, 1993.

Vale JA, Miller PD, Kirby RS: Balloon dilatation of the prostate—should it have a place in the urologist's armamentarium? J R Soc Med 1993; 86:83–86.

Vallencien G, Chartier-Kostler E, Bataille N, et al: Focused extracorporeal pyrotherapy. Eur Urol 1993; 23(Suppl 1):48–52.

van Iersel T, deWildt MJAM, Debruyne FMJ: Are results of laser treatment irrespective of the type of fiber or technique used? (Abstract.) J Urol 1995;153:229.

Van Earps O, Golomb J, Siegel Y, et al: Local hyperthymia in benign prostatic hyperplasia (BPH). (Abstract.) J Urol 1990; 143:902.

Vanden Bossche M, Noel JD, Schulman CC: Transurethral hyperthermia for benign prostatic hypertrophy. World J Urol 1991; 9:2–6.

Vanden Bossche M, Peltier A, Schulman CC: Transurethral radiofrequency heating for BPH at various temperatures with Thermex: Clinical experience. Eur Urol 1993; 23:302–306.

Wasserman NF, Reddy RK, Zhanuy G, et al: Experimental treatment of benign prostatic hyperplasia with transurethral balloon dilation of the prostate: Preliminary study in 73 humans. Radiology 1990; 1:488–494.

Watson G: Comments made at AUA Annual Meeting, San Antonio, Texas, May 15–20, 1993, postgraduate course on BPH, 1993.

Watson G: Heat and the prostate. Eur Urol 1993; 23(Suppl 1):60–62.

Watson GM, Perlmutter AP, Shah TK, et al: Heat treatment for severe, symptomatic prostatic outflow obstruction. World J Urol 1991; 9:7–11.

Weiss JN, Badlani GH, Ravalli JM, et al: Balloon dilatation of the prostate: Urodynamic evaluation. (Abstract.) J Urol 1990; 143:373.

Weiss JN, Badlani GH, Ravalli JM, et al: Urodynamic and symptomatic effects of balloon dilation of the prostate. J Endourol 1991; 5:105–107.

Winters JC, Fuselier HA, Appell RA: ND:YAG prostatectomy—comparison of techniques. (Abstract.) J Urol 1993; 149:7.

Wright KC, Wallace S, Chamsanguej C, et al: Percutaneous endovascular stents: An experimental evaluation. Radiology 1985; 156:69–72.

Yasumoto R, Yoshihara H, Kawashima H: The use of metallic stents in 32 patients with benign prostatic hypertrophy. Preliminary results and 3 months of followup. Nippon Hinyokika Gakkai Zasshi 1992; 83:473–482.

Yerushalmi A, Servadio C, Leib Z, et al: Local hyperthermia for treatment of carcinoma of the prostate: A preliminary report. Prostate 1982; 3:623–630.

Yerushalmi A, Fishelovitz Y, Singer D, et al: Localized deep microwave hyperthermia in the treatment of poor operative risk patients with benign prostatic hyperplasia. J Urol 1985;133:873–876.

Yerushalmi A, Singer D, Katsnelson R, et al: Localized deep microwave hyperthermia in the treatment of BPH: Long term assessment. Br J Urol 1992; 70:178–182.

Zerbib M, Conquy S, Martinacke P, et al: Localized hyperthermia versus sham procedure in obstructive benign hyperplasia of the prostate: A prospective randomized study. J Urol 1992; 147:1048–1052.

49
TRANSURETHRAL SURGERY

Winston K. Mebust, M.D.

TRANSURETHRAL PROSTATECTOMY

History

Transurethral prostatectomy, as we know it today, was developed in the United States in the 1920s and 1930s. Nesbit (1975) pointed out that there were several significant factors important in its development: (1) The invention of the incandescent lamp by Edison in 1879; (2) the cystoscope, developed independently by Nitze and Lieter in 1887; and (3) the development of the fenestrated tube by Hugh Hampton-Young, which allowed the obstructing tissue to be sheared-off blindly. Other important factors were the invention of the vacuum tube in 1908 by deForest that allowed the constant production of high-frequency electrical current that could be used in resecting tissue. In 1926, Bumpus combined the cystoscope and the tubular punch. Also, at that time, Stearns developed the Tungsten loop that could be used for the resection. This was put together by McCarthy in 1932, using a Foroblique lens so that he could resect the tissue under direct vision using a wire loop.

In the 1970s, the development of the fiberoptic lighting system, together with the Hopkins (1976) rod lens wide-angle system, significantly improved visualization for endoscopic surgery. Previously, the optical system was a series of small lenses placed in a rigid tube. In the Hopkins rod lens wide-angle system, the air spaces were replaced by solid glass rods. The spacer tubes were shorter, resulting in minimal obstruction and increased admission of light.

Over the years, transurethral resection of the prostate (TURP), as a treatment modality for obstructing benign prostatic hyperplasia (BPH), gained popularity throughout the world. It is now considered the gold standard for the surgical management of BPH. In the 1986 National Health Survey, 96% of patients had a TURP when they had prostate surgery done for BPH. It was estimated that 350,000 Medicare patients had a TURP that year. However, today there are many medical and surgical alternatives to transurethral prostatectomy, and the number of TURPs has fallen to less than 200,000 per year in the Medicare-age group.

Another factor that may have influenced the incidence of transurethral prostatectomy was the formal development of patient care guidelines for patients with BPH (McConnell et al, 1994). In 1989, the Omnibus Budget Reconciliation Act created the Federal Agency for Health Care Policy and Research (AHCPR). Patient care guidelines were demanded by Congress, and two of the first selected were the diagnosis and management of BPH. **It was the BPH Guideline Panel's recommendation that patients with minimal symptoms should undergo watchful waiting, and that if intervention was to be considered in patients that were more symptomatic, the patient should be informed of the harms and benefits of each therapeutic modality and participate actively in making the decision, not only whether to intervene but which treatment modality would be his choice.** Many patients opted for a less invasive procedure, although less effective than TURP.

Indications for Prostatectomy

In 1968, Lytton and co-workers (1968) estimated that the chance of a 40-year-old man having a prostatectomy in his lifetime was approximately 10%. However, Glynn and colleagues in 1985 raised the estimate to 29%. Arrighi and associates (1991), in reviewing the Baltimore Longitudinal Study on Aging (BLSA), believed that men over age 60 had a 39% chance of requiring surgery in the next 20 years, men 50 to 59 years of age a 24% chance, and men 40 to 49 years of age a 13% chance.

There are very few studies in the natural history of patients who are seen initially because of modest symptoms of prostatism without an absolute indication for intervention (i.e., acute refractory urinary retention, recurrent infections). Ball and co-workers (1981) followed 97 patients for 5 years and found that the patient's symptoms were essentially the same in 52% and worse in only 16.5%. The urodynamic studies revealed little change in that group, and only 1.6% of the patients developed retention. Conversely, Birkhoff and associates (1976) followed 26 patients for 3 years and found a 50% to 70% worsening of the patient's subjective symptoms and 71% deterioration in objective criteria. Further, acute retention was unpredictable.

The most common reasons that intervention is recommended in a patient with symptoms of bladder outlet obstruction and irritability are that the symptoms are moderate to severe, bothersome, and interfere with the patient's quality of life. Mebust and colleagues (1989) noted that 90% of the patients undergoing a TURP had symptoms of prostatism, but 70% had another indication as well (e.g., acute urinary retention occurring in 27%).

In 1989, the American Urological Association (AUA) initiated the Guideline Panel for Diagnosis and Management of Benign Prostatic Hyperplasia. Recognizing the significance of assessing the patient's symptoms, a symptom score was developed by the AUA's Measurement Committee, Winston Mebust, Chairman. Barry (1992) was the senior author of this questionnaire, which came to be known as the "AUA-7 Symptom Index" (Table 49–1). Other scoring systems have been developed such as the Madsen and Iversen (1983), Boyarsky and associates (1977), and the International Continence Society Study on BPH. However, the AUA-7 was validated as to its clarity, test/retest reliability, internal consistency, and criteria validity. The AHCPR took over the AUA BPH Guideline Panel in 1990. The guideline panel subsequently recommended a formal assessment of the patient's symptoms, using any scoring system, but preferring the AUA-7. Patients with mild symptoms (having a score of 0 to 7) were to be assigned to watchful waiting; those with moderate (8 to 19) or severe (20 to 35) symptoms would undergo further testing and/or treatment. **It should be noted that the AUA-7 Symptom Index is not disease specific.** The questionnaire has been given to older women, who obviously do not have a prostate but may have bladder dysfunction, resulting in a significant score on the Symptom Index. The symptom score was considered to be part of the patient's initial evaluation but did not make the diagnosis of BPH.

The AUA-7 Symptom Index was then adopted at the World Health Organization Consultation on BPH in Paris in 1991 (Mebust). In addition to the AUA-7 Symptom Index, one global quality of life question was added—"if you were to spend the rest of your life with your urinary condition, just the way it is now, how would you feel about it?" Responses ranged from "delighted" to "terrible." Therefore, not only should the patient's severity of symptoms be considered in deciding whether intervention is warranted or not but also how much the patient is being bothered by his symptoms and how they affect his overall quality of life. It should be pointed out that patients having symptoms secondary to an obstructing prostate may have a variation in their symptoms over time. Ball and Smith (1982) noted that 31% of the patients they were following had improvement in their symptoms. Recently, there have been efforts to develop a

Table 49–1. AUA-7 SYMPTOM INDEX FOR BENIGN PROSTATIC HYPERPLASIA

	Not at All	Less Than 1 Time in 5	Less Than Half the Time	About Half the Time	More Than Half the Time	Almost Always
1. Over the past month, how often have you had a sensation of not emptying your bladder completely after you finished urinating?	0	1	2	3	4	5
2. Over the past month, how often have you had to urinate again less than two hours after you finished urinating?	0	1	2	3	4	5
3. Over the past month, how often have you found you stopped and started again several times when you urinated?	0	1	2	3	4	5
4. Over the past month, how often have you found it difficult to postpone urination?	0	1	2	3	4	5
5. Over the past month, how often have you had a weak urinary stream?	0	1	2	3	4	5
6. Over the past month, how often have you had to push or strain to begin urination?	0	1	2	3	4	5
7. Over the past month, how many times did you most typically get up to urinate from the time you went to bed at night until the time you got up in the morning?	none	1 time	2 times	3 times	4 times	5 or more times
	AUA Symptom Score = sum of questions A1–A7 = ________					

Modified from McConnell JD, Barry D, Bruskewitz RC, et al: Benign prostatic hyperplasia: Diagnosis and treatment. Clinical practice guideline. Agency for Health Care and Policy Research. Publication No. 94-0582, Feb 1994.

Table 49–2. BENIGN PROSTATIC HYPERPLASIA (BPH) IMPACT INDEX

1. Over the past month, how much physical discomfort did any urinary problems cause you?	none	only a little	some	a lot
2. Over the past month, how much did you worry about your health because of urinary problems?	none	only a little	some	a lot
3. Overall, how bothersome has any trouble with urination been during the past month?	not at all bothersome	bothers me a little	bothers me some	bothers me a lot
4. Over the past month, how much of the time has any urinary problem kept you from doing the kinds of things you would usually do?	none of the time	a little of the time	most of the time	all of the time
		BPH Impact Index = sum of questions B1–B4 = ________		

From Barry MJ, Fowler FJ Jr, O'Leary MP, et al: Measuring disease-specific health status in men with benign prostatic hyperplasia. Medical Care 1995; 33(4) (Suppl):AS145–AS155.

concise questionnaire to evaluate further the degree to which the condition is bothersome or the impact on quality of life of patients with symptoms from BPH (Barry et al, 1995). Such an example is the BPH Impact Index developed by Barry and associates (1995) (Table 49–2).

Although symptoms constitute the primary reason for recommending intervention, in patients with an obstructing prostate, there are some absolute indications. These are acute refractory urinary retention, recurrent infection, recurrent hematuria, and azotemia. A postvoid residual urine has been used by some urologists as an indication, but as pointed out by Bruskewitz and co-workers (1982), there can be extreme variability within a given patient as to the amount of postvoid residual when this factor is assessed repetitively over a period of time. Furthermore, there is no information on the amount of postvoid residual urine that represents the point "that if nothing is done, irreparable damage to the bladder will occur." However, it was believed by the AHCPR BPH Panel (McConnell et al, 1994) that it might be of some use in following patients who are assigned to watchful waiting. In the AHCPR BPH Guideline, the patient's history is taken with focus on the urinary tract. However, many of these patients have other comorbidity problems, and Mebust and colleagues (1989) noted that only 23% did not have a significant medical problem prior to surgery. The most common were pulmonary (14.5%), gastrointestinal (13.2%), myocardial infarction (12.5%), arrhythmia (12.4%), and renal insufficiency (4.5%). Therefore, a general medical evaluation is warranted. A urinalysis is also recommended to be sure that the patient's symptoms are not related to infection. A digital rectal examination should be done, taking into consideration the consistency of the prostate, to help the urologist in determining whether the patient has cancer or not and also for an estimate of size. The size of the prostate might be important in selecting what type of surgical therapy would be warranted (e.g., transurethral incision of the prostate, or in the very large prostate, an open prostatectomy). A serum creatinine is also to be obtained. It was noted by Mebust and colleagues (1989) that patients with a serum creatinine level greater than 1.5% had a 25% incidence of postoperative complications versus 17% in those who had a normal creatinine level.

A number of tests are considered to be optional for the urologist in evaluating the patient with moderate-to-severe symptoms from BPH. Many consider uroflowmetry to be the single best noninvasive urodynamic test to detect lower tract obstruction. However, it should be pointed out that the patient's obstructive symptoms, when evaluated with a formal questionnaire, correlate poorly with uroflowmetry measurements. Further, there is no specific cut-off point at which one can state that the patient is definitely obstructed. **A Qmax less than 15 ml/second does not differentiate between outflow obstruction and detrusor impairment.** Pressure flow studies are recommended as an optional test. This is one of the best ways to evaluate a patient's degree of obstruction and detrusor function, particularly when the diagnosis is unclear. However, it is invasive, is uncomfortable for the patient, requires expensive equipment, and requires considerable experience in performing so that the results are reproducible.

A number of tests are not recommended, such as a filling cystometrogram. Although this test can demonstrate uninhibited bladder contractions, it is invasive and does not give much more information than what can be obtained from the patient's history of bladder irritability symptoms. **Cystoscopy, done routinely in the physician's office as a diagnostic procedure, is not recommended.** The only reason for performing cystoscopy in the urologist's office is if the urologist needs to know the size of the prostate and its configuration in making a recommendation as to the type of therapy that would be useful for this patient (e.g., transurethral incision, if a small prostate or an open prostatectomy, if a very large prostate). If it is critical for the urologist to know the exact size when deciding whether or not the patient should have an open prostatectomy, transrectal ultrasound is more precise than cystoscopy. **Upper tract imaging is also not recommended to be performed routinely.** Rather, it should be reserved for patients with hematuria or renal insufficiency, or for those with a history of urinary infection, urinary tract surgery, or stones.

Anesthesia

Transurethral surgery of the prostate is usually performed under a general or spinal anesthetic. However, Sinha and associates (1986) have reported doing a TURP under local anesthesia. More recently, Birch and colleagues (1991) have recommended performing a TURP under sedation and local anesthesia. However, they pointed out that the gland size should be less than 40 g. Nielsen and associates (1981) noted no difference in blood loss between an epidural or a general anesthetic. McGowan and Smith (1980) evaluated spinal anesthesia versus general anesthesia and found no difference in blood loss, postoperative morbidity, or mortality.

It is the author's feeling that a patient's anesthetic should be tailored to that particular patient. During the procedure, the anesthetist should monitor the patient's tissue oxygen saturation, electrocardiogram, and if warranted, the serum sodium level, in addition to the usual parameters.

Perioperative Antibiotics

Urinary tract infections can be found in 8% to 24% of BPH patients preoperatively. The infection should be treated prior to surgery. The use of prophylactic antibiotics is somewhat controversial. Gibbons and colleagues (1978) found that prophylactic antibiotics did not reduce postoperative infection, but Nielsen and co-workers (1981), Leroy and associates (1992), Viitanen and colleagues (1993), and Prescott and associates (1990) have found them useful. In the AUA Study (Mebust et al, 1989), over 60% of the patients were given prophylactic antibiotics. **It is our recommendation that the patients be given systemic antibiotics prior to the initiation of surgery, and we usually recommend a first-generation cephalosporin.** We then maintain the patient on oral antibiotics for 5 days after catheter removal.

Surgical Technique—General Considerations

Since Creevy and Webb (1947) pointed out the danger of water causing hemolysis, the emphasis has been on using nonhemolytic fluids for irrigation during transurethral prostatectomy. Although water is less expensive, and a TURP can be performed safely using it, probably the majority of urologists today use a nonhemolytic solution. A variety of fluids are available today (e.g., 1.5% glycine, cytol—a combination of sorbitol and mannitol, and mannitol). These are not isotonic fluids but rather nonhemolytic (e.g., 1.5% glycine and have an osmolarity of approximately 200 mOsm/L).

The patient is placed in the lithotomy position with the buttocks just off the end of the table. We prefer Alcock leg holders over knee crutches for leg support. The perineum is not shaved but scrubbed for 5 minutes with a germicidal soap. An O'Connor rectal shield is inserted for manipulation of the gland during surgery.

At the time of surgery, the urethra is calibrated with bougie a boules. The majority of patients calibrate at 28 F or greater, but a significant number are less, as pointed out by Emmett and co-workers (1963). If the distal urethra is inadequate, to accommodate the more commonly selected 28 French resectoscope, a smaller size should be used. For several years, we have successfully used a 24 French resectoscope sheath, even in cases with very large glands. However, if the distal urethra is inadequate, a perineal urethrostomy may be performed by inserting the resectoscope through the more commodious bulbar urethra. The technique of perineal urethrostomy has been described elsewhere (Melchior, 1974). Alternatively, an internal urethrotomy can be performed as advocated by Emmett and colleagues (1963) and Bailey and Shearer (1979). The common area of narrowing is at the postnavicular region, and in this instance, we would perform a dorsal internal urethrotomy using a curved #12 scalpel blade. A generous ventral meatotomy often leads to a splattering or an errant direction of the urinary stream and is to be avoided.

Surgical Technique

Various surgical techniques have been espoused by urologists for removing the prostate adenoma. **However, every surgical technique basically employs the principle that the resection should be performed in a routine step-by-step manner.** The resection technique may vary according to the size or configuration of the prostate but should be based on an orderly plan. All of the techniques use the general principle of resecting ventrally first so that the adenomatous tissue drops down allowing the surgeon to resect from the top downward rather than from the floor upward. However, some surgeons have suggested resecting the floor of the median lobe to improve water flow during the resection.

In our teaching technique, we often resect one lobe of the prostate and the residents resect the other. Today, we use the video camera in almost all transurethral prostatectomies. We find that this helps in teaching residents, but also it reduces the back strain encountered by the surgeon bending over the resectoscope.

Our standard technique was described by Nesbit (1943) over 50 years ago. The Nesbit technique is divided into three stages:

FIRST STAGE. Following the preliminary endoscopy and urethral calibration, the bladder is filled with approximately 150 ml of a nonhemolytic irrigation solution (e.g., 1.5% glycine) (Fig. 49–1*A*). The resection begins at the bladder neck, starting at the 12-o'clock position and carried down to the 9-o'clock position, in a stepwise fashion. The adenoma is resected down to the level where the apparent circular fibers of the bladder neck become visible. Over-resection of the entire neck, or excessive cauterization, may lead to vesical neck contracture. The anterior quadrant, from 12 to 3 o'clock, is now resected. The posterior quadrants are then individually resected, down to the 6-o'clock position. **If, at the completion of the entire resection, the bladder neck appears to be partially obstructing, which is particularly true of glands weighing less than 20 g, we advise incising the bladder neck with a Collings knife at the 6-o'clock position.** This step is recommended by Kulb and associates (1987) to reduce the incidence of postoperative vesical neck contracture.

SECOND STAGE. The adenoma is resected in quadrants (Figs. 49–2*A* to *C*, 49–3*A* to *C*, and 49–4*A* to *C*). The resectoscope is placed in front of the verumontanum. The resection begins at 12 o'clock, so that the lateral lobe tissue falls into the midfossa. The resection is carried down to the prostatic capsule, which is recognized as a rather fibrous structure compared with the granular appearance of the prostatic adenoma. The right lateral lobe and then the left lateral lobe are resected so that the tissue now falls to the floor. With the right lateral lobe on the floor of the prostatic fossa, resection of this fallen lobe is started at the 3-o'clock position approximately. The posterior portion on the floor of the prostatic fossa is resected. Care must be taken not to resect too deeply in the region of the posterior aspect of the vesical neck to prevent undermining of the trigone. The resection is carried

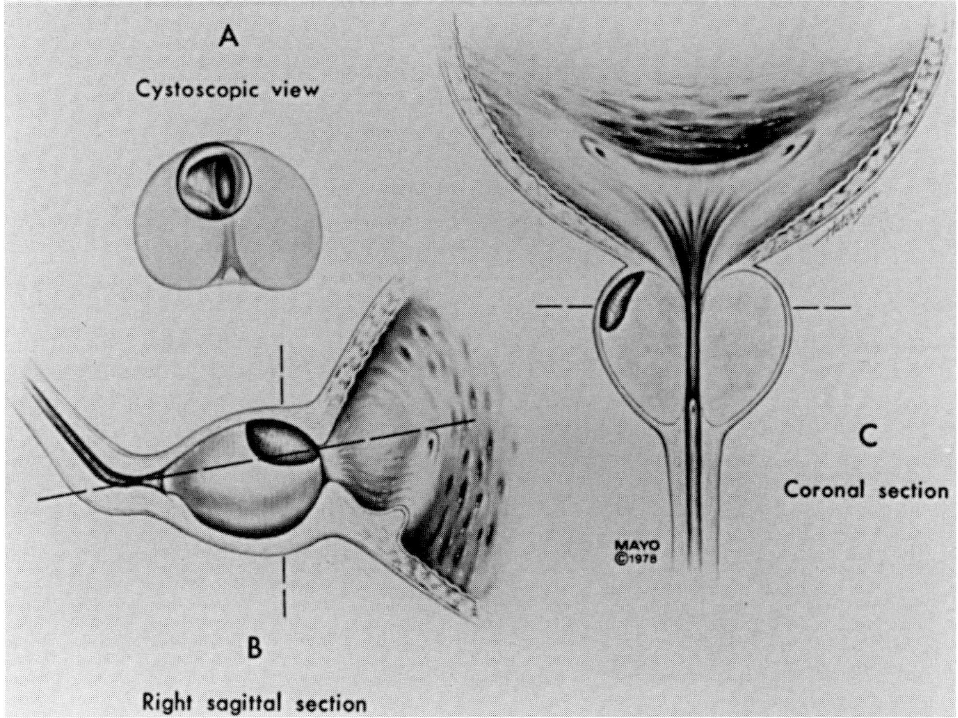

Figure 49–1. First stage of resection of the prostate. The resection is begun at 12 o'clock, and the tissue at the bladder neck and adjacent adenoma is resected in quadrants. (By permission of the Mayo Foundation.)

to the right side of the verumontanum. A similar procedure is started at approximately 9 o'clock. The posterior portion of the lobe is resected to the left side of the verumontanum. The apical portion of the lobe remains. At this stage, therefore, the posterior portions of the lateral lobe, including the floor tissue, have been resected to the verumontanum. As one resects the lower two quadrants in the floor of the prostate, the capsule fibers become less distinct. The resection is performed with an O'Connor rectal shield in place. We employ the Iglesias modification of the Nesbit scope so that one hand is free to palpate the depth of resection as the floor tissue is removed.

THIRD STAGE. The adenoma is removed immediately proximal to the external sphincter mechanism, preserving the verumontanum (Figs. 49–5*A* to *C*, 49–6, and 49–7). The prostatic apex is concave. A sweeping motion is used so that the loop is moved from a lateral-to-medial direction as it approaches the sphincter mechanism. However, Shah and

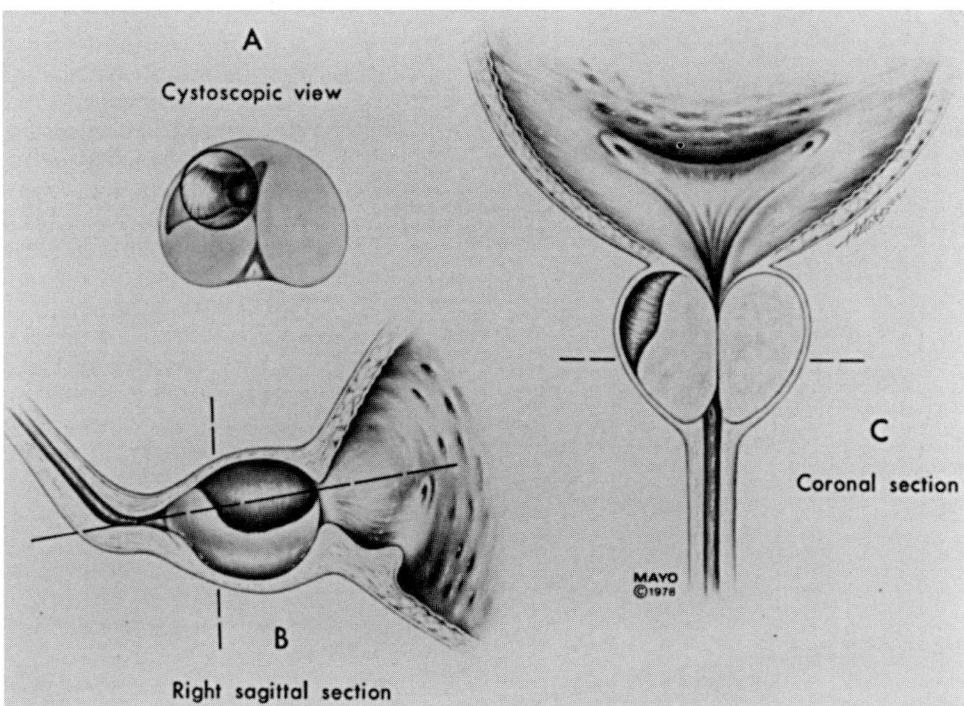

Figure 49–2. The midportion of the gland is resected starting at 12 o'clock, carrying it down to the 9-o'clock position *(A)*. The sagittal and coronal section views are noted *(B* and *C)*. (By permission of the Mayo Foundation.)

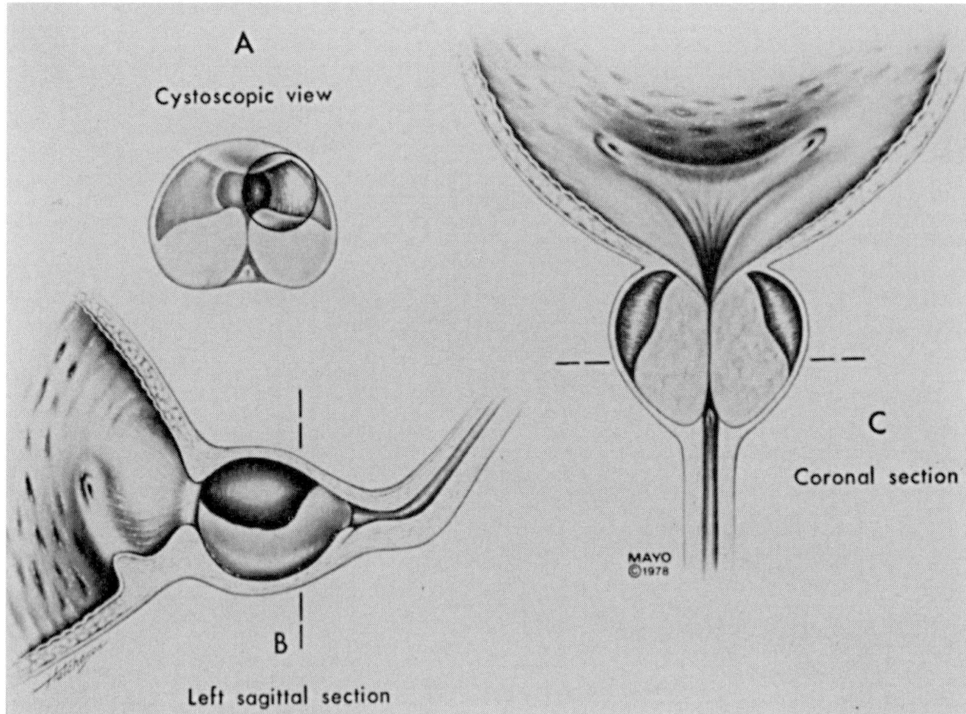

Figure 49–3. The resection is now begun at 12 o'clock, and the left side of the patient's gland in the midfossa is resected down to the 3-o'clock position as noted in *A*. Sagittal and coronal sections are noted *(B* and *C)*. (By permission of the Mayo Foundation.)

co-workers (1979) observed that 10% to 20% of the prostate projects below the verumontanum. Therefore, it may be necessary to leave a small rim of the adenoma to avoid sphincter injury.

Turner-Warwick (1983) has divided the sphincter mechanism into three areas: first, immediately adjacent to the verumontanum; second, from the verumontanum to the capsule; and third, beyond the capsule of the prostate. Injury to the second or third portion of the sphincter mechanism can result in significant urinary incontinence. Therefore, we begin our resection by placing the resectoscope next to the verumontanum. We continue the resection up to the 12-o'clock position, rather than starting at the 12-o'clock position as in the prior two steps.

With the patient in the lithotomy position, the distal portion of the prostate is not always parallel to the surgical table but is tilting slightly toward the cephalad end. The most common area of damage to the external sphincter is at the 12-o'clock position. Thus, care must be taken as one approaches the 12-o'clock position.

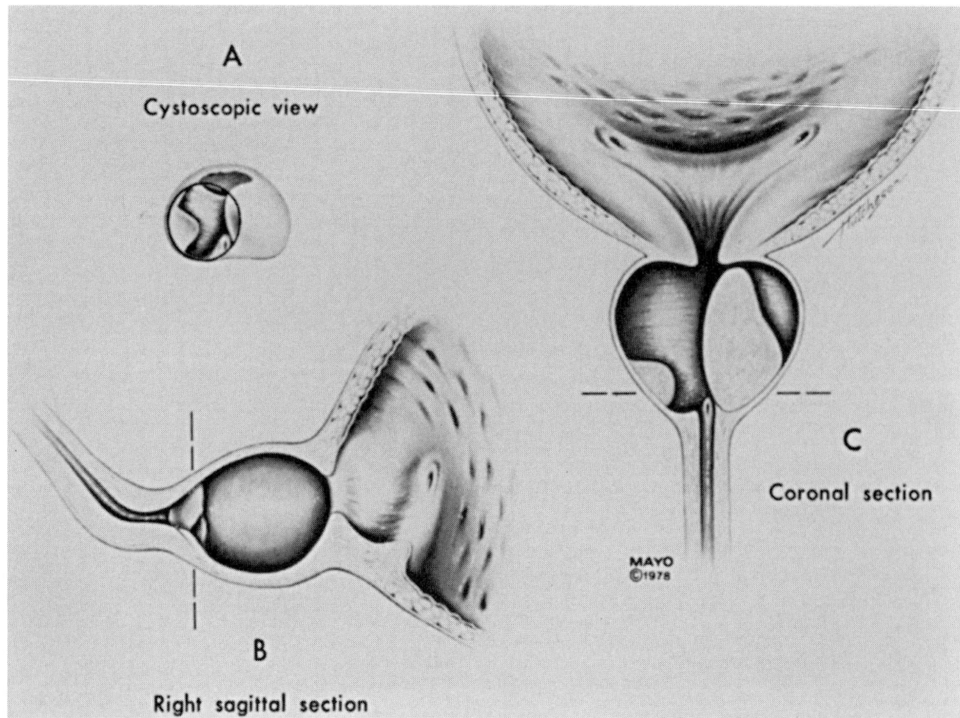

Figure 49–4. The midportion of the gland is resected further from the 9-o'clock to 6-o'clock positions as noted in *A* with sagittal views in *B* and *C*. (By permission of the Mayo Foundation.)

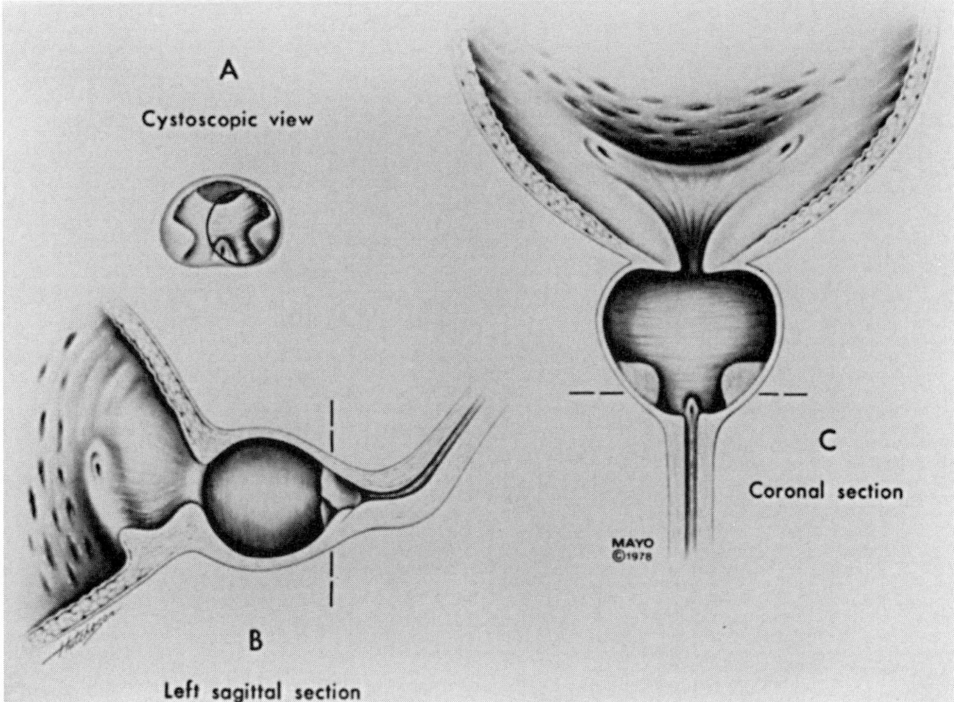

Figure 49–5. The tissue remaining at the apex is now resected. It is begun by initiating the resection next to the verumontanum and carrying it toward the 12-o'clock position. Small amounts of residual tissue at the apex are noted *(A, B,* and *C).* (By permission of the Mayo Foundation.)

When the resection is completed, the surgeon should pull the resectoscope into the urethra, just distal to the verumontanum, and note that there is no falling and obstructing tissue. Some small wings of adenoma may be attached to the sphincter area. These can be judiciously trimmed. Care must be taken not to cut too deeply and thus damage the sphincter mechanism. Occasionally, there is tissue that is nothing more than mucosal tags, which are unimportant. They will slough and will not cause obstruction. When significant tissue drops into the prostatic fossa, with the scope in the distal urethra, it is usually the tissue that remains at the roof of the midfossa area. The surgeon should replace the scope in the midfossa and resect the adenoma down to the fibrous capsule.

Management of Intraoperative Problems

HEMOSTASIS. The amount of intraoperative bleeding depends on the size of the prostate, the length of time

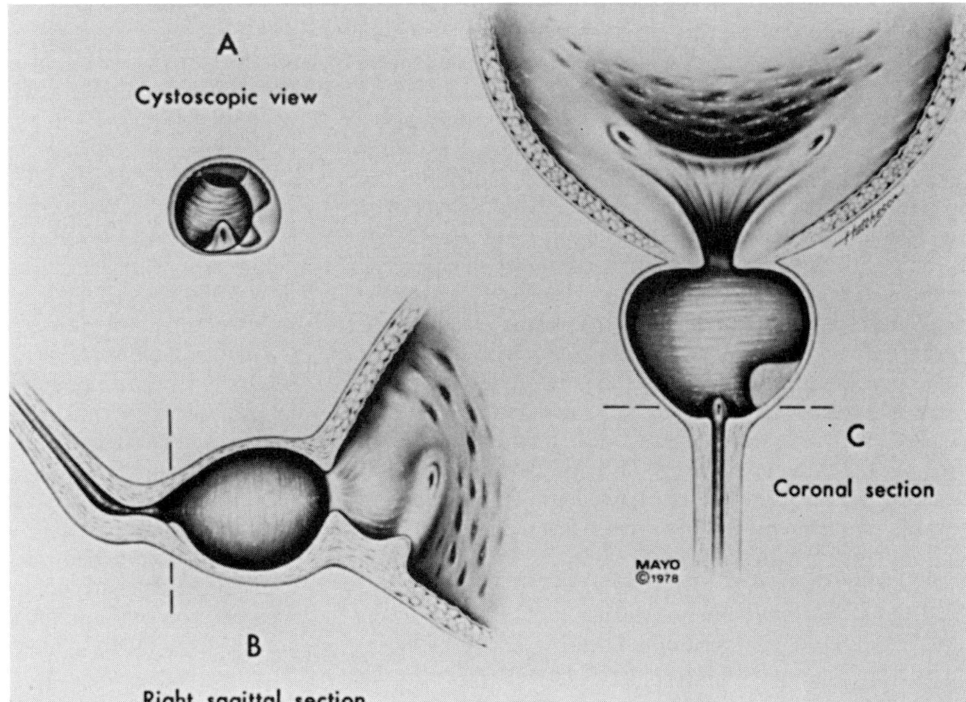

Figure 49–6. Residual tissue is carefully cleared on the patient's right side. (By permission of the Mayo Foundation.)

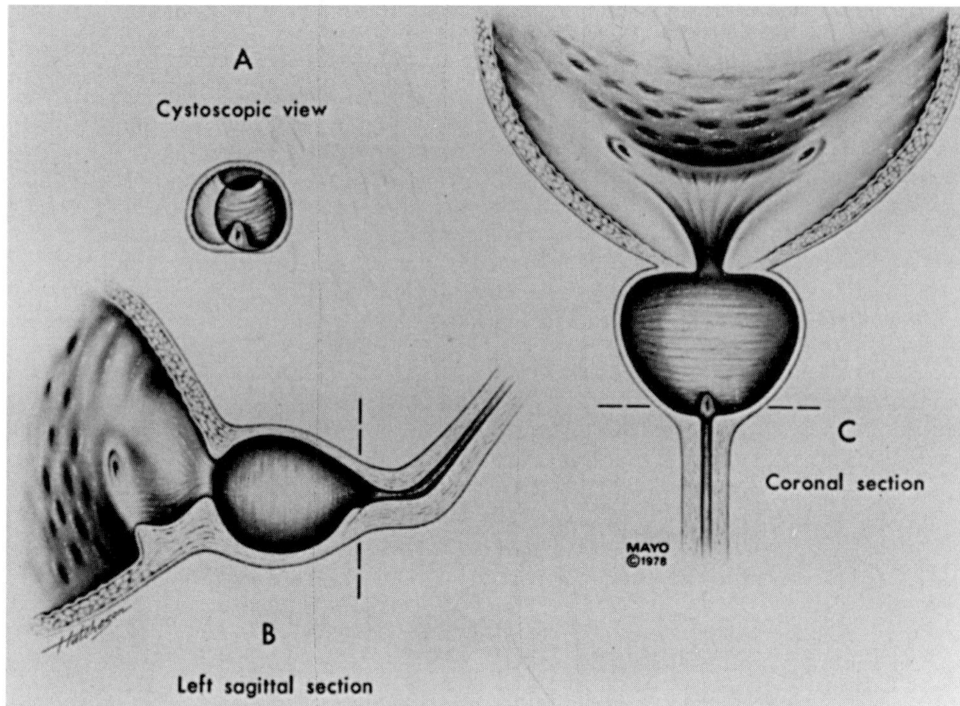

Figure 49–7. The remaining residual tissue is cleared from the patient's left side, leaving an unobstructed view from the verumontanum through the bladder neck into the bladder. (By permission of the Mayo Foundation.)

required to resect the adenoma, and to a degree, the surgeon's skill. Arterial bleeding is controlled by electrocoagulation. This should be done as one completes each stage of the resection, before moving on to the next stage. **After the catheter is inserted, at the end of the surgical procedure, the irrigation fluid should be light pink.** However, if the irrigation fluid has a continued red color, one should suspect arterial bleeding. The surgeon should reinsert the resectoscope and coagulate the arterial bleeding. Venous bleeding is apparent at the end of the procedure, when on irrigating the catheter, the return is initially clear, but then dark blood later oozes from the catheter. **Venous bleeding can be controlled by filling the bladder with 100 ml of irrigating fluid and placing the catheter on traction for 7 minutes at the operating table.** The balloon of the catheter is overinflated to 50 mm of fluid.

Extravasation, or perforation of the prostatic capsule, occurs in about 2% of patients. The symptoms of extravasation are restlessness, nausea, vomiting, and abdominal pain, despite spinal anesthesia. Pain is usually localized to the lower abdomen or back. If extravasation is suspected, the operation should be terminated as rapidly as possible, but hemostasis must be secured. Bleeding must be controlled, even as the extravasation is increased, because simultaneous postoperative management of extravasation and hemorrhage is difficult. Cystography may provide information as to the diagnosis and, to some degree, the extent of the extravasation. **Over 90% of these patients can be managed simply by urethral catheter drainage and cessation of the operative procedure.** If there is extensive extravasation and concern about infecting the perivesical tissue, suprapubic drainage should be instituted.

TRANSURETHRAL RESECTION SYNDROME. In the AUA Cooperative Study (Mebust et al, 1989), transurethral resection (TUR) syndrome occurred in 2% of the patients. The syndrome was characterized by mental confusion, nausea, vomiting, hypertension, bradycardia, and visual disturbance. Usually, the patients do not become symptomatic until the serum sodium concentration reaches 125 mEq. The risk is increased if the gland is larger than 45 g and the resection time is over 90 minutes.

In 1950, several studies were undertaken to determine the amount of fluid absorbed during TURP. Hagstrom (1955) weighed patients preoperatively and postoperatively, and calculated that approximately 20 ml/minute of fluid was absorbed by the patient. However, there was significant patient variation. Oester and Madsen (1969), using a double-isotope technique, demonstrated that the average amount of fluid absorbed by the patient was 1000 cc and that one third of this fluid was absorbed intravenously. Madsen and Naber (1973) demonstrated that pressure in the prostatic fossa and the amount of fluid absorbed was dependent on the height of the fluid by the patient. They noted that when the height of the fluid was changed from 60 to 70 cm, fluid absorption was greater than twofold. They also reported that approximately 300 ml of fluid/minute were needed for a good vision field. This could not be achieved when the fluid level was below 60 cm of water. Harrison and colleagues (1956) believed that the TUR syndrome was related to dilutional hyponatremia. Certainly, the syndrome can be reduced by the administration of 3% saline. However, other factors have been suggested as a possible cause. Glycine is metabolized to glycolic acid and ammonium. Ammonium intoxication has been suggested as a possible cause of the TUR syndrome or direct toxic effect of glycine. **Nevertheless, it is our belief that the TUR syndrome is secondary to dilutional hyponatremia.** This can be corrected by giving the patient 200 ml of 3% saline very slowly over a period of time. Conversely, one can attempt to calculate the amount of water overload by determining the serum sodium preoperatively and postoperatively, knowing the patient's weight, and determining the amount of extracellular fluid. More recently,

Stalberg and co-workers (1992) in patients undergoing a TURP with general anesthesia, the irrigating fluid was tagged with 1% ethanol and the amount of ethanol excreted in the breath measured. This is believed to be a very effective and quick way of determining which patients are becoming overloaded with fluid. In those patients who have a large gland or when the operating time is being prolonged, we will obtain a serum sodium routinely, although the patient is still undergoing surgery. In those patients who demonstrate a drop in serum sodium, we will treat with diuretics (e.g., furosemide [Lasix]). Serum sodium is retained in the postoperative recovery room, and if need be, further diuretics are used.

INTRAOPERATIVE PRIAPISM. During the surgical procedure, a penile erection may occur, which may obviate the surgery, unless a perineal urethrostomy is performed. This usually has been managed by injecting an alpha-adrenergic agent directly into the corpora cavernosa. We would usually dilute the solution of ephedrine or phenylephrine (e.g., 0.3 ml 1% phenylephrine diluted to 3 ml with normal saline for 100 μg/1 ml) (Lee et al, 1995).

Outcomes of Transurethral Prostatectomy

PATIENT SYMPTOMS. In developing the guideline for the diagnosis and management of BPH, the AHCPR panel (McConnell et al, 1994) questioned patients as to what was the most significant factor they considered in deciding on what type of therapy should used in treating their bladder outlet obstruction secondary to BPH. The foremost factor was relief of symptoms.

In reviewing the literature, the AHCPR Guideline Panel used meta-analysis to combine the various clinical studies. They noted that the chance of improvement of patient symptoms following a TURP was 70% to 96% confidence interval (CI), with a mean of 88%. The magnitude or reduction in symptom score was 85%. **This was significantly better than less invasive procedures.**

MORTALITY. Over the past 50 to 60 years, there has been a gradual reduction in the immediate postoperative mortality rate associated with transurethral resection of the prostate. Perrin and colleagues (1976) found a mortality rate of 5%, reported in the 1930s. Holtgrewe and Valk (1962) reported 2.5%; Melchior and associates (1974b), 1.3%; and Mebust and co-workers (1989), 0.2%. This was the mortality rate noted at 30 days. The number of patients in each of these three studies was well over 2000.

Roos and colleagues (1989), using insurance claim data from England, Denmark, and Manitoba, Canada, noted that the death rate at 90 days was significantly higher compared with an open prostatectomy. They noted an early postoperative death rate of 2.9%. This study included almost 40,000 patients. Excluding this study, the mortality rate from other series that were combined using meta-analytic techniques, the probability was 1.18%. However, including the study by Roos and co-workers with other reports, the mean estimate was 1.5% (90% CI—0.5% to 0.3%).

In more recent studies, Ala-Opas and colleagues (1993) found no immediate mortality in a series of over 400 patients undergoing a TURP. Chute and associates (1991), in an epidemiologic study, compared patients who had a TURP with those who did not have a TURP and found that the mortality rate over time was identical. Montorsi and co-workers (1993) compared a group of patients who underwent either TURP or open prostatectomy and found the mortality rate in each group was identical. Concato and colleagues (1992) compared a group of patients retrospectively, undergoing a TURP or prostatectomy, and when correcting for comorbidity, the mortality rate was the same for both groups. However, a chart review had been conducted by Malenka and associates (1990), looking at comorbidity factors in the Canadian population. They could not identify comorbidity factors to account for the apparent difference in mortality rate between TURP and open prostatectomy.

Recently, Fuglsig and co-workers (1994) age-matched a group of patients who had undergone a TURP with those who had not, and the mortality rate for the two groups was identical. The mortality rate could be influenced by many factors, such as the type of hospital where the surgery was performed, the skill of the surgeon, the size of the gland, the operating time, or again, comorbidity factors.

In reviewing the cause of death in the Canadian series, it was secondary to cardiac disease. In the patients who were studied in Denmark, the cause of death was pulmonary complications. **This suggests that the observation by Roos and associates (1989) was truly related to comorbidity being significant in those undergoing TURP as opposed to those who underwent an open prostatectomy.**

The immediate morbidity rate, following a TURP, was reported by Mebust and co-workers (1989) as 18%. This was similar to the rates reported by Holtgrewe and Valk (1962) and Melchior and associates (1974b). Although the incidence was unchanged, in the Mebust report, the incidence of significant complications (e.g., acute pyelonephritis) was not as high as that noted in the previous studies. The most common complications in the immediate postoperative period were failure to void (6.5%), bleeding requiring transfusion (3.9%), and clot retention (3.3%). The AHCPR BPH Guideline Panel (McConnell et al, 1994) found a mean immediate postoperative complication rate of 14.95% with a 90% CI of 5.2% to 30.7%. In recent studies, the immediate postoperative complication rate has been noted by Plentka and associates (1991) (3.1%), Estey and colleagues (1993) (7.8%), and Chute and co-workers (1991) (4.2%). However, these are all retrospective studies.

Wasson and associates (1995) recently reported on a prospective randomized study in which patients were assigned to either watchful waiting or a transurethral resection of the prostate. **Ninety-one percent of the men had no complication during the first 30 days after surgery. Specifically, there was no difference between either group as to the incidence of urinary incontinence or impotence.** The most frequent complications noted were a need for replacement of the urinary catheter (4%), perforation of the prostatic capsule (2%), and hemorrhage requiring transfusion (1%). At the end of 3 years of follow-up, the mortality rate was the same for each group. Twenty-three patients in the treatment group were considered treatment failures, and 47 patients were in the watchful waiting group. The failure rate in the watchful waiting group was 6.1 per 100 person-years of follow-up as compared with 3 per 100 person-years of follow-up in the surgery group (P = .002). The higher rate in the watchful waiting group was largely attributed to a higher incidence of three outcomes: (1) intractable urinary retention (2.9% versus 0.9%); (2) a high volume of residual urine (5% versus 1.1%); (3) a high urinary symptom score (4.3% versus 0.4%). In those undergoing surgery, there was improvement in peak flow rate, reduction in the severity of symptoms, and reduction in the degree to which the symptoms bothered the patient. **The authors noted that the outcomes of surgery were best for the men who were most bothered by urinary symptoms at baseline.** This study refutes the uncontrolled observations in prior retrospective series that transurethral resection frequently leads to incontinence and impotence, and it confirms that the incidence of short-term complications and retreatment after surgery is low.

There are few data on the long-term outcomes of patients undergoing transurethral prostatectomy. In the study conducted by Wasson and colleagues of 280 men undergoing surgery, at 3 years follow-up, nine men had vesical neck contracture requiring endoscopic surgery; nine had a urethral stricture that required dilatation, and eight underwent a second transurethral resection, four because of adenocarcinoma. Bruskewitz and co-workers (1986), in following a series of patients over 3 years, noted that at 1 year, most patients' symptoms improved (84%) and 10% remained approximately the same. At 3 years, 75% had improved and 13% remained the same. The change in symptomatology was the development of urge incontinence occurring in those patients several years after surgery. Only one of the 84 patients required a repeat resection, resulting in an incidence of 2%. However, 10% of the patients developed a vesical neck contracture.

Meyhoff and Nordling (1986) noted that 90% of their patients were considered to have satisfactory results at 5 years after TURP. Flow rates were improved from preoperative values, although there had been a slight decline in flow rates over the 5-year period. They did note an 8% re-resection rate, but all patients were noted to have especially small glands, suggesting that these might have been postoperative vesical neck contractures, as had been noted in the prior studies.

Ala-Opas and associates (1993) found that 92% of the patients were satisfied with the results of their surgery 6.5 years after the procedure had been done. Montorsi and associates (1993), in a group of patients followed for 5 years, found that 95% of the patients were unobstructed and subjectively satisfied as to their urinary status.

OTHER SURGICAL TECHNIQUES FOR TRANSURETHRAL PROSTATECTOMY

CONSTANT FLOW RESECTOSCOPE. In 1975, Iglesias and co-workers introduced the constant flow resectoscope, suggesting that it would allow a continuous resection, clearer vision, and low intraprostatic fossa pressure with decreased fluid absorption (Fig. 49–8). The surgical time should also be decreased. However, Stephenson and colleagues (1980) compared constant flow with the standard interrupted flow and could find no difference in speed of resection, blood loss, or glycine absorption. Similarly, Flechner and Williams (1982) found no difference between the two techniques. Holmquist and colleagues (1979) compared the constant flow rectoscope with constant suprapubic drainage and found constant suprapubic drainage to be superior. However, Gellman (1980) cautioned that it was important to resect the floor tissue first to improve flow characteristics. At this time, the problem seems to be maintaining a constant inflow and outflow, while keeping the pressure low within the prostatic fossa and maintaining good visibility. **Therefore, there does not appear to be a clear-cut advantage to constant flow irrigation, as opposed to the more standard intermittent irrigation, during transurethral prostatectomy.**

TRANSURETHRAL INCISION OF THE PROSTATE. Transurethral incision of the prostate (TUIP) is not a new procedure. Edwards and associates (1985) credit Bottini with describing the technique in 1887, but Hedlund and Ek (1985) credit Guthrie in 1834. However, in 1973, Orandi published the first significant series on TUIP. The procedure seemed to be most useful in those who had a small prostate (which has been called a primary vesical neck contracture, median bar, and sclerosed du Col) and who had obstructive bladder outlet symptoms. Classically, the patient was a younger man, as compared with those undergoing a classic TURP. **The advantage of TUIP was that it was quick, was technically easier, and was associated with less morbidity and a decrease in retrograde ejaculation as compared with TURP.** The incidence of retrograde ejaculation following TURP is anywhere from 50% to 95%; but following a transurethral incision of the bladder neck, it has been reported from 0% to 37%. Turner-Warwick (1979) noted that with one incision, the incidence of retrograde ejaculation was less than 5%; but with two incisions, it was 15%. Hedlund and Ek (1985) reported no difference between one and two incisions.

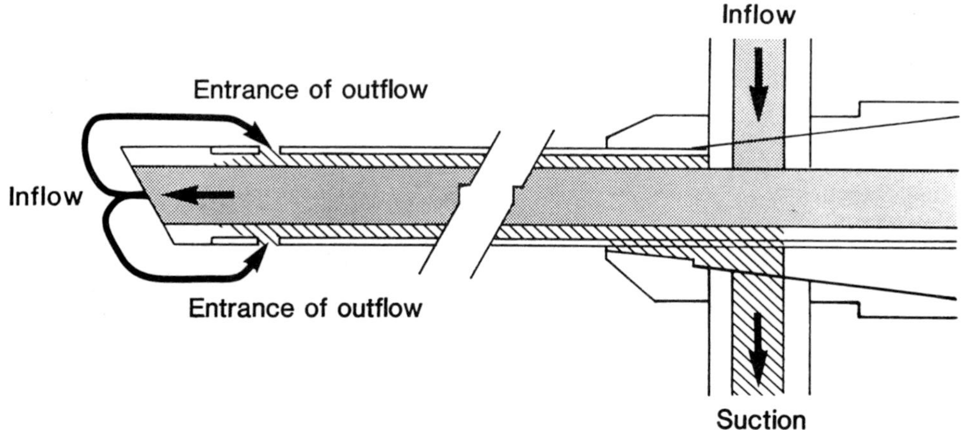

Figure 49–8. Constant flow resectoscope, in which fluid is introduced through the center core and removed through the outer core, using suction.

Few comparative studies have been conducted to determine the differences between TURP and TUIP. Miller and colleagues (1992) reported on 108 patients who underwent a bladder neck incision and compared them with a similar group undergoing TURP. They believed that bladder neck incision was better than TURP in terms of a shorter operative time and shorter duration of catheterization. No other perioperative differences were found. For the 10-year follow-up, there was no difference in the reoperation rates between the two groups. Patient approval was given as 80% initially, and there was some slight drop over the 10-year period of follow-up but no difference between the two groups.

Orandi (1973), in a prospective study over a 2-year period of 132 patients managed with TURP or TUIP, found that the results and complications did favor TUIP but there was no statistical difference. The only apparent difference was the higher incidence of bladder neck contracture after TURP.

Dorflinger and co-workers (1992) randomized 60 patients to either TURP or TUIP. They found that both operations significantly improved symptom scores and maximum flow rates, but the improvement of flow rate was better for the TURP group. Neither operation caused any significant change in sexual activity or erectile potency postoperatively. Retrograde ejaculation was seen in over 50% of the TURP group and in only one patient in the TUIP group. The AHCPR BPH Guideline Panel (McConnell et al, 1994) put these various studies together using meta-analytic techniques, and the results are noted in Table 49–3. There is a slightly better chance of improvement of symptoms and degree of symptom improvement in the TURP group. In the 30- to 90-day mortality rate, the incidence of incontinence and retrograde ejaculation was lower in the TURP group.

The surgical technique is relatively simple. Using a Collings knife, the incision is performed at the 5-o'clock and 7-o'clock position, starting at the ureteral orifice and carrying it to the verumontanum (Fig. 49–9). The incision depth should be to the point where fine filaments of the external capsule are seen. Care must be taken not to cause undue extravasation and not to enter the rectum. With completion of the incisions and with the scope in the more distal urethra, there should be no visual obstruction to the bladder. Additionally, a biopsy of the prostate should be performed to ensure that carcinoma is not overlooked.

TRANSURETHRAL ELECTROVAPORIZATION OF THE PROSTATE. Mebust and co-workers (1972, 1977) used a transurethral probe with direct-vision capabilities to heat and desiccate the prostate. The energy source was the cutting current of the electrosurgical unit. The procedure was chosen for high-risk patients, because it could quickly be performed without blood loss. Sloughing of tissue after the procedure was not a problem, and improved flow rates were obtained. Some patients, however, did experience prolonged pyuria with prostatitis-like symptoms.

This technology has recently undergone re-evaluation by several urologists. Rather than the probe used by Mebust and Damico (1972), a roller ball (Fig. 49–10) is used to vaporize the tissue. The roller ball is put in a resectoscope and using the technique similar to a standard TURP, the ball is rolled over the tissue, resulting in destruction of the

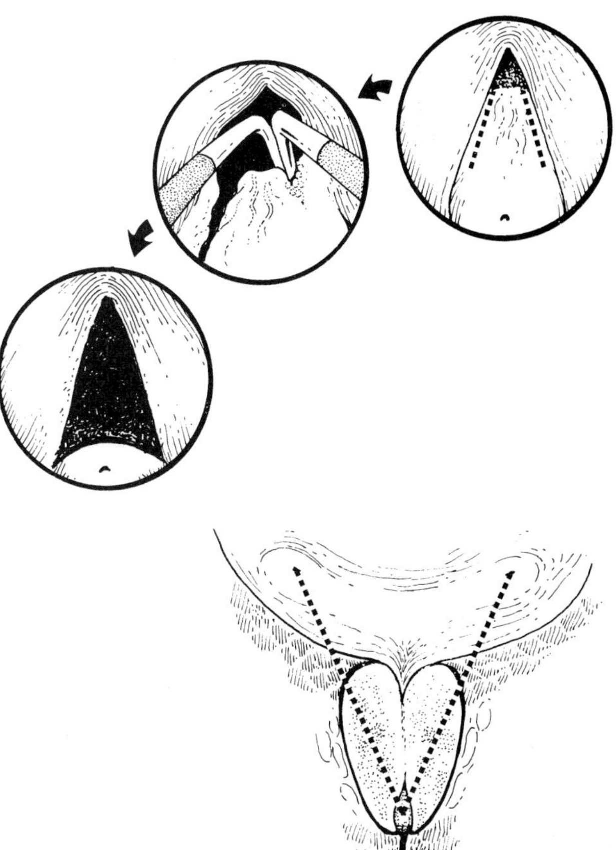

Figure 49–9. Transurethral incision of the prostate. The incision is started at the ureteral orifice and carried through the bladder neck up to the verumontanum. This procedure is done bilaterally. (From Mebust WK: A review of TURP complications and the National Cooperative Study, Lesson 24, Volume VIII, 1989, pp 189–190.)

Table 49–3. TREATMENT OUTCOMES BALANCE SHEET

	TUIP	TURP
Chance of symptom improvement	78–83% (80)	75–96% (88)
Degree of symptom improvement	73%	85%
Morbidity (20% significant)	2.2–33% (14)	5.2–30.7% (16)
Mortality (30–90 days)	0.2–1.5%	0.53–3.31%
Incontinence—total	0.061–1.1%	0.68–1.4%
Operative treatment for surgical complications	1.34–2.65%	0.68–10%
Impotence	3.9–24.5%	3.3–34.8%
Retrograde ejaculation	6–55%	25–99%

TUIP, Transurethral incision of the prostate; TURP, transurethral resection of the prostate.

From Barry MJ, Fowler FJ Jr, O'Leary MP, et al: The American Urological Association's symptom index for benign prostatic hyperplasia. J Urol 1992; 148:1549–1557. Copyright © 1992, Lea & Febiger.

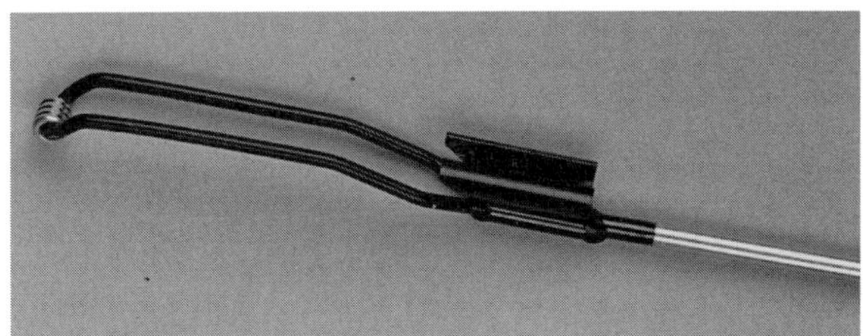

Figure 49–10. ACMI-CIRCON roller ball used to vaporize tissue using the cutting current of the electrosurgical unit with a setting of greater than 200 watts.

obstructing tissue. The preliminary reports seem to be associated with good results. However, this technique will need long-term evaluation to determine if the results are durable and free of complications.

TRANSURETHRAL RESECTION OF BLADDER TUMORS

Bladder cancer is the fourth most prevalent, noncutaneous malignancy in the adult American male. Approximately 52,000 new cases per year will be diagnosed, and there will be approximately 9500 cancer deaths. Of the bladder malignancies, transitional cell carcinoma accounts for 90%, squamous cell carcinoma 5%, and adenocarcinoma approximately 2%; rhabdomyosarcoma was observed in only 1%. Sixty-five percent to 95% of these tumors will present as papillary transitional cell carcinomas. These will be grade I and grade II. In the Melicow (1952) series, 80% were found to be papillary, either with a narrow stalk or a broad base, and 80% on the posterior were lateral walls. These superficial tumors will be confined to the mucosa (Ta) or invading the lamina propria (T1) and are readily managed with transurethral resection.

Surgical Procedures

These superficial tumors are usually managed by transurethral surgery, that is, using a Bugbee electrode, cold-cup biopsy, transurethral resection, or laser fulguration. Transurethral resection is not usually a definitive therapy for transitional cell carcinoma, invasive to the bladder muscle. Barnes and associates (1977) reported a 5-year survival rate for stage B lesions treated by transurethral resection as 31%, but they did not divide them into stages B1 or B2 (T2, T3a lesions). In a series of 46 patients, Jacobsen and co-workers (1987) treated patients with T1 and T2 bladder tumors with radical transurethral resection. During a 6-month period, more than 50% of the tumors recurred, and subsequent progression of the tumors was seen within 24 months in 30% and 50% of the patients with T1 and T2 tumors, respectively.

Conversely, Solsona and co-workers (1992), in a series of 59 patients who were followed for an average of 55 months, found 52.5% had no evidence of recurrence at the average follow-up of 59 months. However, 47.5% had recurrent disease at the average of 51.8 months, ranging from 13 to 106 months. Three of the patients (5%) developed distant metastases at 9, 22, and 30 months. The overall survival at 55.4 months was 83%, with 72.8% of the cases retaining their bladders. However, I should point out that these were a highly select group of patients with muscle-infiltrating bladder cancer managed by a definite transurethral resection of bladder tumor. This is best used in patients with limited life expectancy and small papillary tumors invading the muscle. **The tumor must be completely resected transurethrally, as verified by negative biopsies of tumor depth and periphery. However, it has been our general belief that patients with invasive tumor should be considered for radical cystectomy and some form of urinary diversion.** It may be necessary to do an extensive resection of a sessile, infiltrating tumor to control hematuria, but in general, we usually recommend a transurethral resection as a biopsy procedure, taking multiple and deep bites to confirm the degree of invasion and extent of the tumor.

Preoperative Evaluation

The patient usually presents with hematuria, dysuria, and urinary frequency. Occasionally, a bladder tumor can be an incidental finding, as in a patient undergoing a transurethral resection of an obstructed prostate. Upper tract imaging is usually performed to evaluate the kidneys and ureters, as well as the bladder, as a source of the hematuria. We usually rely on an intravenous pyelogram, but many urologists use a computed tomographic (CT) scan. A CT scan does have the advantage of indicating the size of the bladder tumor and, to a degree, the depth of invasion into the bladder wall.

The definitive diagnosis is made by cystoscopic examination, at which time the urologist should determine the size and position of the lesion, particularly as related to the ureteral orifices and bladder neck, whether the lesion is sessile or papillary, and whether it is multiple or single. Bimanual pelvic examination should be performed (Fig. 49–11). If the mass is palpable but mobile, the carcinoma is usually a more advanced lesion (e.g., T3a lesion); if the mass is immobile, that would suggest a stage T3b lesion. Surgical findings, in addition to the patient's general state of health and history of prior bladder tumors, are then considered to determine the proper surgical procedure.

In patients who are candidates for definitive transurethral resection of the bladder lesion (e.g., superficial papillary lesions), random biopsies should be performed in the bladder as well as in the prostatic fossa. The prostatic fossa biopsy can be performed with a cold-cup biopsy, but more typically, the prostatic urethra will require biopsy by a transurethral resectoscope loop.

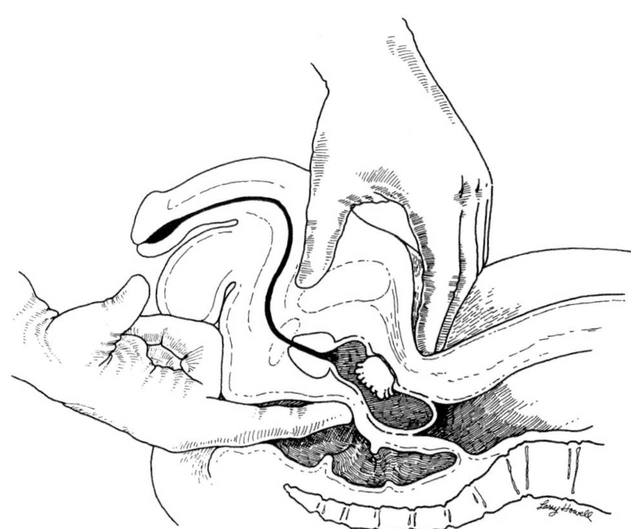

Figure 49–11. Technique of bimanual examination. (From Mebust WK: Transurethral resection of bladder tumors. *In* Crawford DE, Borden TA, eds: Genitourinary Cancer Surgery. Philadelphia, Lea & Febiger, 1982.)

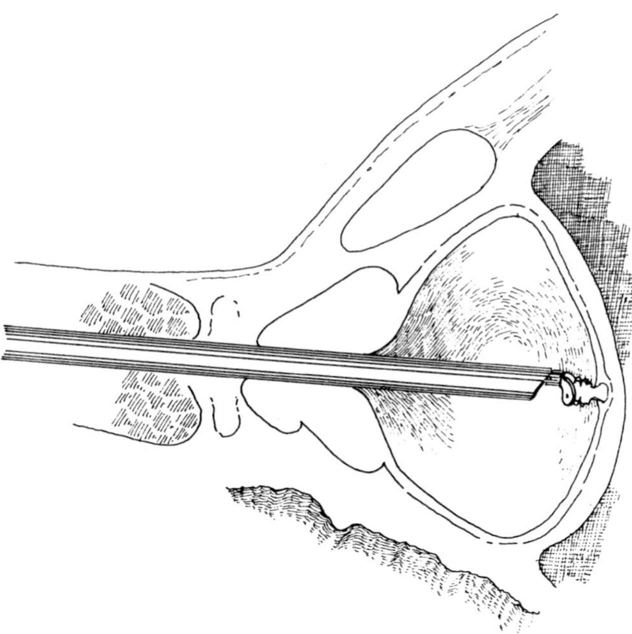

Figure 49–12. Cold-cup biopsy of bladder tumor. (From Mebust WK: Transurethral resection of bladder tumors. *In* Crawford DE, Borden TA, eds: Genitourinary Cancer Surgery. Philadelphia, Lea & Febiger, 1982.)

Surgical Procedures

Water is used as the bladder irrigant during the endoscopic and transurethral surgical procedure because it is cytolytic and theoretically will reduce the incidence of reimplantation of viable tumor cells elsewhere in the bladder. Whether or not antibiotics should be used prophylactically is unclear. Upton and Das (1986), in a small series of patients in a double-blind study, assigned one half to treatment with carbenicillin and the others to treatment with placebo. They found no advantage of preoperative antibiotics. However, Badenoch and colleagues (1990) found that in 18% of men and 75% of women, the tumors were infected with a wide range of bacteria. No correlation was found between tumor infection and histologic grade or stage of the tumor. Infective complications requiring parenteral antibiotics were more frequent in women (25%) but were rarer in men (3%). These authors recommend that women be given prophylactic antibiotics prior to a transurethral resection of their bladder tumor. **It is our general belief that patients undergoing endoscopic surgery should have a prophylactic antibiotic initiated just prior to the procedure, and we usually prefer a first-generation cephalosporin.**

The operation is usually performed with the patient under a spinal or general anesthetic. However, Engberg and associates (1983) reported using local anesthesia. They infiltrate the base of the lesion as well as the urethra. However, they emphasize the need to use a very small cystourethroscope.

At the time of surgery, the surgeon should have available a transurethral resectoscope, a fulgurating (Bugbee) electrode, a cold-cup instrument and a laser. After evaluation of the patient, with the consideration of the diagnostic factors described previously, one of the following surgical procedures may be elected.

COLD-CUP BIOPSY AND FULGURATION. As much as possible of the initial small lesion should be removed with a cold-cup biopsy (Fig. 49–12). The tumor base should be submitted separately so the depth of the invasion can be determined. If necessary, the base can be resected with a resectoscope to help determine the depth of invasion. However, the problem with the resectoscope is the charring effect that occurs with the cautery. **The cold-cup biopsy technique permits the pathologist to examine the specimen that is uncharred by the resectoscope so as to render a better histologic evaluation.** Again, random biopsies are usually performed. A Bugbee electrode or resectoscope may be used to fulgurate the base of the tumor completely. In those patients in whom the histology is known and who are having a recurrence of the tumor 2 to 3 mm in size, the Bugbee electrode can be used as definitive therapy, fulgurating the lesion. The depth of penetration, using the Bugbee electrode, is approximately 2 mm. Conversely, one may wish to use a laser, with which 3 to 4 mm of penetration can be easily obtained. Again, both techniques destroy the lesion, leaving it unavailable for the pathologist to study. The Bugbee electrode and the laser can also be used for those lesions that are between the air bubble and the bladder neck at the 12-o'clock position and are not easily accessible to a resectoscope or a cold-cup biopsy instrument. The Bugbee electrode with the Albarran bridge or the laser with a deflecting unit can be used to destroy these lesions. Not uncommonly, suprapubic pressure is required (Fig. 49–13).

TRANSURETHRAL RESECTION

Papillary Lesions. The majority of papillary transitional cell carcinomas are small (approximately 1 to 3 cm in size) and usually have a low histologic grade. They are usually located on the lateral or posterior wall and are readily amenable to transurethral resection. The lesion is near the bladder neck or ureteral orifice, and the location may complicate the surgical removal. This issue will be discussed later.

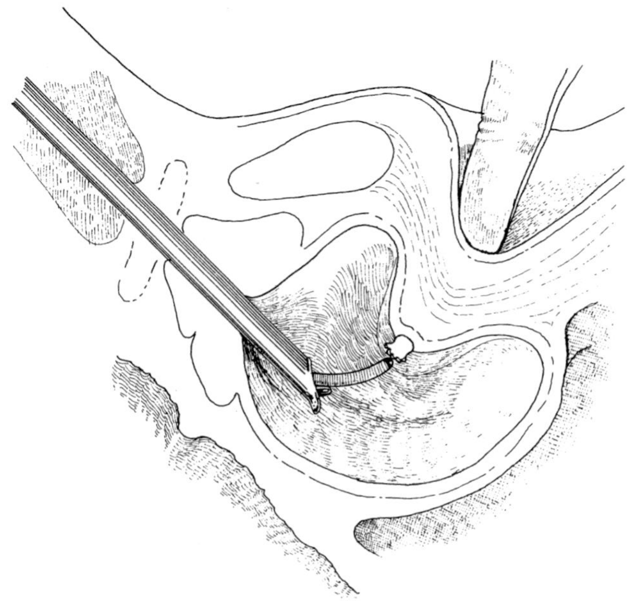

Figure 49–13. Bugbee electrode employed for lesion at 12 o'clock position. (From Mebust WK: Transurethral resection of bladder tumors. *In* Crawford DE, Borden TA, eds: Genitourinary Cancer Surgery. Philadelphia, Lea & Febiger, 1982.)

Resection is usually begun at the anterior portion of the tumor, moving the loop cephalad to caudad, similar to a transurethral resection of benign prostatic hyperplasia (Fig. 49–14). However, a point may be reached where it is more advisable to extend the loop, and with a rocking-type motion, similar to scraping a wall, the loop is brought down and the lesion further removed (Fig. 49–15). **Bleeding vessels should be controlled as the resection proceeds, particularly the larger lesions, so that the surgeon does not become disoriented because of poor visibility caused by the excessive bleeding.** For this reason, the resection is usually begun at the anterior portion of the tumor so that the blood will fall down into the bottom of the bladder and not obscure the surgeon's view. Again, the base should be submitted as a separate entity so the depth of invasion can be determined. If possible, a cold-cup biopsy should be used rather than the resectoscope. However, it may be necessary to also use a resectoscope to be sure the tumor is completely excised. The base of the tumor, and approximately 1 cm around the base of the tumor, should then be carefully fulgurated. When the surgeon is completing the procedure, the resected area should demonstrate clean bladder muscle fibers, rather than a granular appearance of infiltrating tumor.

Multiple Papillary Lesions. Treatment of multiple papillary lesions with transurethral resection depends on their position and size and on the surgeon's skill. In general, we find that it is advisable to remove the smaller lesions initially and to start at the dome of the bladder so that any bleeding goes toward the bladder base and does not obscure the surgeon's vision. The larger lesions are then resected in the manner described earlier.

Sessile Lesions. The finding of a sessile lesion is usually associated with a high-grade infiltrating bladder lesion, as compared with the papillary type. A bimanual pelvic examination is important because if the surgeon feels a mass, this probably indicates a stage T3a lesion or, if the mass is fixed, possibly a stage T3b lesion. For the patient with a sessile lesion, with or without a palpable mass, the surgeon may consider a transurethral resection as a definitive procedure, but not uncommonly, one must consider performing just a biopsy and evaluating the patient for radical cystectomy and diversion.

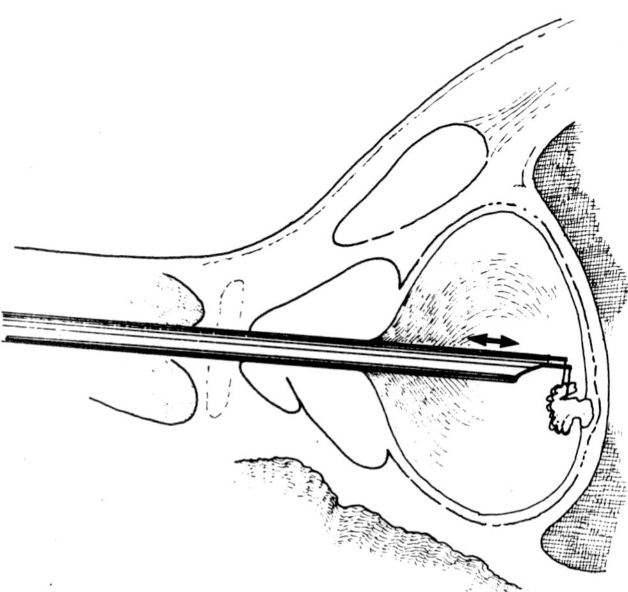

Figure 49–14. Transurethral resection begun at superior portion of the tumor. (From Mebust WK: Transurethral resection of bladder tumors. *In* Crawford DE, Borden TA, eds: Genitourinary Cancer Surgery. Philadelphia, Lea & Febiger, 1982, pp 199–206.)

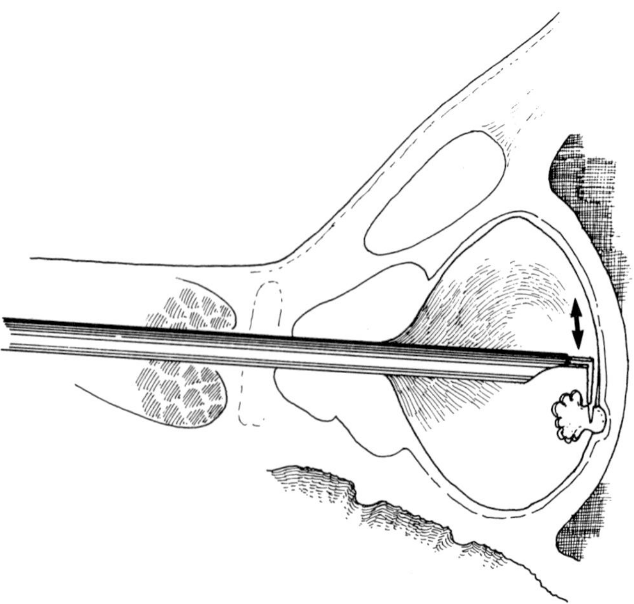

Figure 49–15. Transurethral resection completed with a rocking type of motion. (From Mebust WK: Transurethral resection of bladder tumors. *In* Crawford DE, Borden TA, eds: Genitourinary Cancer Surgery. Philadelphia, Lea & Febiger, 1982, pp 199–206.)

Resections usually begin at the top of the lesion, and the bleeding is controlled as the procedure continues to avoid impairing the surgeon's vision (Fig. 49–16). It may be necessary to remove the bulk of the tumor and then to resect the base and the bladder wall immediately adjacent as separate specimens. If this is to be a definitive procedure, and bladder muscles should appear clean, and in some instances, there may be small areas of perivesical fat observed.

As the surgeon approaches the base of the tumor, the bleeding must be well controlled to allow proper visualization and resection of the base. At this point, all resected tissue must be removed from the bladder with the Ellik evacuator. If the surgeon observes small areas of perivesical fat, the procedure still may be accomplished transurethrally with low-pressure flow of the irrigating fluid. Extravasation may occur but is usually minimal, and if the patient does not have infected urine, bladder drainage with a urethral catheter should be sufficient. However, if there has been significant bleeding and it is obvious that a major perforation has occurred, as indicated by the patient having pain and abdominal rigidity, it may be necessary to insert a perivesical drain, or if by chance it is an intraperitoneal perforation, actual exploration and closure of the defect may be required.

Postoperative Care

At the completion of transurethral resection of the bladder tumor, the bladder irrigation should be crystal clear. All bleeding must be completely controlled. We then

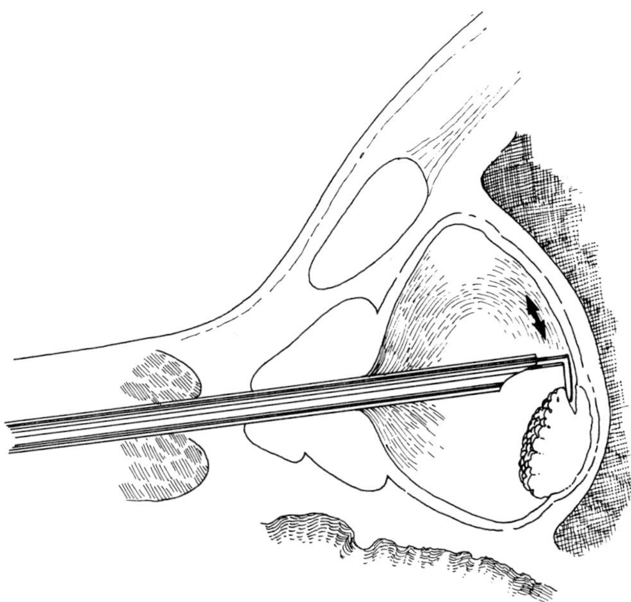

Figure 49–16. Resection of the sessile tumor with the rocking or scraping motion of the resectoscope loop. (From Mebust WK: Transurethral resection of bladder tumors. *In* Crawford DE, Borden TA, eds: Genitourinary Cancer Surgery. Philadelphia, Lea & Febiger, 1982, pp 199–206.)

insert either a two-way catheter for dependent drainage, or more commonly, if we are not concerned about possible extravasation, we use a three-way catheter for irrigation. The catheter is removed when the urine is clear.

Our usual routine in following these patients with superficial carcinoma is to repeat the cystoscopy on a 3- to 4-month basis, which would also include bladder washings for cytology. If the patient remains free of tumor for 1 year, cystoscopic examinations are performed on a 6-month basis for 2 years, and if the results, including cytology, are negative, we examine the patient on a yearly basis. An intravenous pyelogram should be repeated every 2 years to rule out the occurrence of upper tract lesions. Many of the patients who develop recurrences are placed on intravesical chemotherapy, which is dealt with in another section of this text.

Special Surgical Problems

If a neoplasm is found next to the bladder neck in the 12-o'clock position, it can usually be brought into vision by suprapubic pressure. As noted in the prior section, a laser or Bugbee electrode with a deflecting element (i.e., Albarran bridge) can be used to treat these lesions. There is, however, the occasional patient in whose case, because of a tight suspensory ligament of the penis, one cannot get the instrument into proper position. In such cases, we will insert the scope through a perineal urethrostomy.

The bladder tumor may involve a ureteral orifice or overlie the intramural ureter, or both. If this is associated with hydronephrosis, which is noted on upper tract imaging, it usually represents an infiltration into the ureter, as opposed to simply the bulk of the tissue obstructing the ureter. These patients may require a more definitive procedure than a transurethral resection. Whether or not hydronephrosis is present, the tumor should be resected, even if it requires sacrificing the ureteral orifice. Fulguration should be kept to a minimum to prevent stenosis of the orifice.

Rees (1969) noted that 70% of the patients who had the orifice resected developed vesicoureteral reflux. It was his belief that if the urine was sterile, there was no apparent damage to the kidney with the reflux. Recently, De Torres Mateos and colleagues (1987) found that the incidence of reflux, when the orifice was resected, was 77%. However, they noted a statistically significant relationship between the development of upper tract tumors and reflux (20% of the patients with reflux and 0.9% without reflux developed tumors). They recommend a close follow-up of these patients who have reflux with upper tract imaging. **Transurethral removal of lesions that occur on the lateral wall may be hampered by the stimulation of the obturator nerve, resulting in marked adductor spasm of the leg as well as movement of the bladder.** This may result in extravasation of the bladder as the surgeon attempts to remove the lesion. Such patients may be given a general anesthetic, and with a neuromuscular blocking agent (e.g., succinylcholine), the obturator reflex can be prevented. Another solution is to block the nerve with local anesthetic as it exits from the obturator foramen, as described by Augspurger and Donohue (1980). Alternatively, stimulation of the bladder lesion with the coagulation current and then resecting with the neuromuscular junction refractory can permit an unimpaired resection.

Occasionally, patients will present with bladder outlet obstruction symptoms and be scheduled for a standard transurethral resection of his prostate. An unsuspected bladder tumor may be found, and the question is whether one should resect the tumor and prostate at the same time. Vicente and co-workers (1988) found that there was no bladder tumor implantation within the prostatic fossa when a simultaneous resection was performed.

VESICOLITHOLAPAXY AND LITHOTRIPSY

Bladder stones have plagued humanity since the beginning of time. The etiology is probably bladder outlet obstruction, urinary tract infection, and perhaps, diet.

Historically, bladder stones were removed through either a suprapubic incision, "the high operation," or through the perineum, "the low operation." The suprapubic incision was usually associated with a significant mortality because the peritoneum was often violated and the patient developed peritonitis and subsequent death. The "low operation" entailed blindly inserting gorgets into the bladder and blindly extracting the stone. This procedure was also associated with a significant morbidity and mortality. Angeloff (1972), however, reported that the Arabic physicians Albicosis of Cordoba and Avicenna performed blind transurethral stone extractions. However, the first documented blind transurethral lithotripsy was performed by Civiale in 1824.

With the invention of the cystoscope in 1877 by Nitze (Nesbit, 1975), optics were then available for crushing stones under direct vision. The Hendrickson lithotrite (Fig. 49–17) is an example of such an instrument that can mechanically

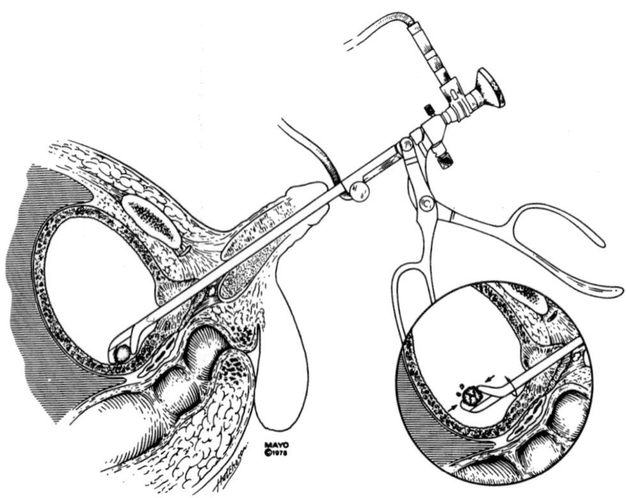

Figure 49–17. Mechanical litholpaxy using the visual Hendrickson lithotrite.

crush a stone under direct vision. **The contraindications to this procedure were patients with small-capacity bladders, multiple stones, large stones (larger than 2 cm) that could not be engaged, and an inadequate urethra.** The procedure was difficult to perform because of the poor water flow through the instrument and subsequent poor visualization within the bladder. The risk of bladder injury was always present. **The technique was to fill the bladder with 150 ml of fluid, grasp the stone, rotate the lithotrite so the stone engaged would be away from the mucosa, and then crush it manually.** This procedure was repeated several times to reduce the stone into small fragments. Fragments were then washed out with an Ellik evacuator. They can also be extracted singly using an alligator-jaw forceps or triradial forceps.

Today, there are four different techniques of endocorporeal lithotripsy. These include the mechanical device (e.g., Lithoclast), the electrohydraulic lithotripsy, ultrasound, and the pulsed-dye laser.

BALLISTIC OR MECHANICAL LITHOTRIPSY. The Lithoclast, developed in Switzerland, is essentially a pneumatic jackhammer. Using compressed air, a probe is mechanically driven into the stone, causing fragmentation. Denstedt and co-workers (1992) reported a series of eight bladder cases in which all the stones were fragmented. The size of the stones averaged 3.8 cm in diameter, and the patients, on average, had three stones in their bladder. Grasso and associates (1994) reported on the Browne Pneumatic Impactor, which also used compressed air to drive a Nitinol wire probe into the stones. This was used with the flexible scope primarily for ureteral calculi. Dretler and Rosen (1993) developed an electromechanical impactor. An electrode was sheathed within the tip of the probe. With discharge of electricity, in a saline-filled compartment, a plasma was developed, resulting in a shock wave, which drove the metal probe into the stones. With the electrode sheathed, there would be little damage to the urothelium. Again, this has been used primarily in ureteral stones.

ELECTROHYDRAULIC LITHOTRIPSY. Bergman and co-workers (1982) and Rouvalis (1970) credit Yutkin for discovering the principle of electrohydraulic lithotripsy (EHL). The URAT 1 was developed by Goligowsky of the Soviet Union in the 1960s. Today, EHL is one of the more commonly used modalities in treating bladder calculi.

Numerous companies manufacture EHL units. The technique involving the EHL is somewhat dependent on the manufacturer's recommendation. The generator usually permits variations in power settings and whether or not the shock impulse is to be single or repetitive. Originally, 1/6-normal saline was recommended as the bladder irrigating fluid, but we have found normal saline is just as useful. The electrode chosen is usually No. 9 Fr, although smaller electrodes are available. The tip of the electrode is placed within 1 to 2 mm of the stone rather than touching the stone. **The tip of the electrode should be at least 1 cm away from the bladder wall to avoid bladder injury and at least 1 cm away from the lens system.** We prefer a short burst of energy to conserve the electrode, and we try to concentrate the shock wave at one location to facilitate breaking the stone. Following breaking the stone, the fragments are removed with the Ellik evacuator. The stones can also be removed manually with grasping forceps through the cystoscope. We recommend that a repeat cystoscopy then be performed in approximately 2 months to be sure that all the stone fragments have been removed.

In a series of 100 patients, Rouvalis (1970) reported that 86% of the patients were older than age 65, 62% had solitary stones and 38% had multiple stones. They reported a 100% success rate with EHL. The composition of the stones was urate, phosphate, or oxalate. The size of stones ranged from 3 to 6 cm in 64% of the cases. Angeloff (1972) reported a success rate of 97%. He believed that the contraindications to EHL were urethral stricture; a large prostate, particularly with a large median lobe; small-capacity bladder; sepsis; and severe renal failure. Bulow and Frohmuller (1981) reported a success rate of 92% and Bergman and co-workers (1982) reported a success rate of 95%.

ULTRASOUND ENDOCORPOREAL LITHOTRIPSY. In 1953, Mulvaney was one of the first specialists to use ultrasound in treating urinary calculi. Using a piezo crystal, electric energy is created into sound waves with 27,000 cycle/minute. Hautmann and colleagues (International Urinary Stone Conference, 1984) reported using ultrasound in 412 patients with bladder stones. Infravesical obstruction occurred in 95.4% of these patients, and the most common was BPH, occurring in 58.9%. The average calculus fragment was 15 g, ranging from 1 to 85 g. Composition of the stones was uric (47.5%), struvite (75%), calcium oxalate (28%), and mixed (17.5%). There were two episodes of perforations in these patients. Today, ultrasound lithotripsy is performed primarily for ureteral calculi.

LASER LITHOTRIPSY. The concept of the use of lasers in stone fragmentation is not particularly new. The first attempt at calculus vaporization using a ruby laser was carried out by Mulvaney and Beck (1968). Initial problems were excessive thermal injury, which limited the clinical applicability of this technique. The next major advancement in technology involved the development of a Q-switched laser. This produced a plasma at the stone surface and not vaporization secondary to thermal action, which had occurred with previous lasers. Another device developed by Watson and associates (1987) was the tunable pulsed-dye laser. **This device also caused fluid vaporization, resulting**

in the formation of a plasma bubble. The mechanical shock wave was then developed. This has been used primarily in ureteral stones. Its principal drawback is the expense of the equipment. Furthermore, there has been difficulty with the pulsed-dye laser in treating pure calcium oxalate monohydrate stones and cystine stones. Its role in treating bladder calculi has not been established.

REFERENCES

Ala-Opas MY, Aitola PT, Metsola TEJ: Evaluation of immediate and late results of transurethral resection of the prostate. Scand J Nephrol 1993; 27:235–239.

Angeloff A: Hydro electrolithotripsy. J Urol 1972; 108:867–871.

Arrighi HM, Metter EJ, Guess HA, et al: Natural history of benign prostatic hyperplasia and risk of prostatectomy. The Baltimore Longitudinal Study of Aging. Urology 1991; 38(1 Suppl):4–8.

Augspurger R, Donohue RE: Prevention of obturator nerve stimulation during transurethral surgery. J Urol 1980; 123:170.

Badenoch DF, Murdoch DA, Tiptaft RC: Microbiological study of bladder tumors, their histology and infective complications. Urology 1990; 35(1):5–8.

Bailey MJ, Shearer RJ: The role of internal urethrotomy in the prevention of urethral stricture following transurethral resection of prostate. Br J Urol 1979; 51:28–31.

Ball AJ, Feneley RCL, Abrams PH: The natural history of untreated prostatism. Br J Urol 1981; 53:613.

Ball AJ, Smith PJB: The long-term effects of prostatectomy: A uroflowmetric analysis. J Urol 1982; 128(3):538–540.

Barnes RW, Dick AL, Hadley HL, Johnson OL: Survival following transurethral resection of bladder carcinoma. Cancer Res 1977; 37:2895.

Barry MJ, Fowler FJ Jr, O'Leary MP, et al: The American Urological Association's symptom index for benign prostatic hyperplasia. J Urol 1992; 148:1549–1557.

Barry MJ, Fowler FJ Jr, O'Leary MP, et al: Measuring disease-specific health status in men with benign prostatic hyperplasia. Medical Care 1995; 33(Suppl):AS145–AS155.

Bergman B, Nygaard E, Osterman G, Tomic R: Vesical calculi: Experience of electrohydraulic lithotripsy with URAT I. Scand J Urol Nephrol 1982; 16:217–220.

Birch BR, Gelister JS, Parker CJ, et al: Transurethral resection of prostate under sedation and local anesthesia (sedoanalgesia). Experience in 100 patients. Urology 1991; 38(2):113–118.

Birkhoff JD, Wiederhorn AR, Hamilton ML, et al: Natural history of benign prostatic hypertrophy and acute urinary retention. Urology 1976; 7:48–52.

Boyarsky S, Jones G, Paulson DF, et al: A new look at bladder neck obstruction by the Food and Drug Administration: Guidelines for investigation of benign prostatic hypertrophy. Trans Am Assoc Genitourin Surg 1977; 68:29–32.

Bruskewitz RC, Iversen P, Madsen PO: Value of post void residual urine determination in evaluation of prostatism. Urology 1982; 20:602.

Bruskewitz RC, Larsen EH, Madsen PO, et al: 3-Year followup of urinary symptoms after transurethral resection of the prostate. J Urol 1986; 136:613–615.

Bulow H, Frohmuller HG: Electrohydraulic lithotripsy with aspiration of the fragments under vision—304 consecutive cases. J Urol 1981; 126:454–456.

Chute CG, Stephenson WP, Guess HA, et al: Benign prostatic hyperplasia: A population-based study. Eur Urol 1991; 20(Suppl 2):11–17.

Concato J, Horwitz RI, Feinstein AR, et al: Problems of co-morbidity in mortality after prostatectomy. JAMA 1992; 267:1077–1086.

Creevy CD, Webb EA: A fatal hemolytic reaction following transurethral resection of the prostate gland: A discussion of its prevention and treatment. Surgery 1947; 21:56–66.

De Torres Mateos JA, Banus Gassoll JM, Palou Redorta J, et al: Vesicorenal reflux and upper urinary tract transitional cell carcinoma after transurethral resection of recurrent superficial bladder carcinoma. J Urol 1987; 138:49–51.

Denstedt JD, Eberwein PM, Singh RR: The Swiss Lithoclast: A new device for intracorporeal lithotripsy. J Urol 1992; 148:1088–1090.

Dorflinger T, Jensen FS, Krarup T, et al: Transurethral prostatectomy compared with incision of the prostate in the treatment of prostatism caused by small benign prostate glands. Scand J Urol Nephrol 1992; 26:333–338.

Dretler SP, Rosen DI: The electromechanical impactor: The results of design modifications. J Urol 1993; 150:1399–1401.

Edwards LE, Bucknall TE, Pittam MR, et al: Transurethral resection of the prostate and bladder neck incision: A review of 700 cases. Br J Urol 1985; 57:168–171.

Emmett JL, Rous SN, Greene LF, et al: Preliminary internal urethrotomy in 1036 cases to prevent urethral stricture following transurethral resection; caliber of normal adult male urethra. J Urol 1963; 89:829.

Engberg A, Spangberg A, Urnes T: Transurethral resection of bladder tumors under local anesthesia. Urology 1983; 22:385–387.

Estey EP, Mador DR, McPhee MS, et al: A review of 1486 transurethral resections of the prostate in a teaching hospital. Can J Surg 1993; 36(1):37–40.

Flechner SM, Williams RD: Continuous flow and conventional resectoscope methods in transurethral prostatectomy: Comparative study. J Urol 1982; 127:257–259.

Fuglsig S, Aagaard J, Jonler M, et al: Survival after transurethral resection of the prostate: A 10-year followup. J Urol 1994; 151:637–639.

Gellman AC: Endoscopic prostatectomy with the continuous flow resection technique. Int Surg 1980; 65; 5:433–436.

Gibbons RP, Stark RA, Correa RJ Jr, et al: The prophylactic use—or misuse—of antibiotics in transurethral prostatectomy. J Urol 1978; 119:381.

Glynn RJ, Campion EW, Bouchard GR, et al: The development of benign prostatic hyperplasia among volunteers in the normative aging study. Am J Epidemiol 1985; 121:78.

Grasso M, Loisides P, Beaghler M, et al: Treatment of urinary calculi in a porcine and canine model using the Browne Pneumatic Impactor. Urology 1994; 44(6):937–941.

Hagstrom RS: Studies on fluid absorption during transurethral prostatic resection. J Urol 1955; 73(5):852–859.

Harrison RH III, Boren JS, Robison JR: Dilutional hyponatremic shock: Another concept of the transurethral prostatic resection reaction. J Urol 1956; 75(1):95–110.

Hedlund H, Ek A: Ejaculation and sexual function after endoscopic bladder neck incision. Br J Urol 1985; 57:164–167.

Holmquist BG, Holm B, Ohlin P: Comparative study of the Iglesias technique and the suprapubic drainage technique for transurethral resection. Br J Urol 1979; 51:378–381.

Holtgrewe HL, Valk WL: Factors influencing the mortality and morbidity of transurethral prostatectomy: A study of 2,015 cases. J Urol 1962; 87:450–459.

Hopkins HH: Optical principles of the endoscope. *In* Berci G, ed: Endoscopy. New York, Appleton-Century-Crofts, 1976, pp 3–26.

Iglesias JJ, Sporer A, Gellman AC, et al: New Iglesias resectoscope with continuous irrigation, simultaneous suction and low intravesical pressure. J Urol 1975; 114:929–933.

International Urinary Stone Conference "2nd 1983—Singapore": Urinary Stone Proceedings of the Second International Urinary Stone Conference, Singapore, 1983. Hautmann R, Terhorst B, Rathert P, et al: Ultrasonic litholapaxy of bladder stones—10 years of experience with more than 400 cases. Melbourne, NY, Churchill Livingstone, 1984, pp 120–124.

Jacobsen F, Lundbeck F, Vaeth M, et al: Transurethral treatment of invasive tumours of the urinary bladder (T_1, T_2): Recurrence and progression. Scand J Urol Nephrol 1987; 104(Suppl):123–125.

Kulb TP, Kamer M, Lingeman JE, et al: Prevention of post-prostatectomy vesical-neck contracture by prophylactic vesical-neck incision. J Urol 1987; 137:230–231.

Lee M, Cannon B, Sharifi R: Chart for preparation of dilutions of α-adrenergic agonists for intracavernous use in treatment of priapism. J Urol 1995; 153:1182–1183.

Leroy A, Humbert G, Fillastre JP, et al: Penetration of lomefloxacin into human prostatic tissue. Am J Med 1992; 92(Suppl 4A):12S–14S.

Lytton B, Emery JM, Harvard BM: The incidence of benign prostatic obstruction. J Urol 1968; 99:639.

Madsen PO, Iversen P: A point system for selecting operative candidates. *In* Hinman F Jr, ed: Benign Prostatic Hypertrophy. New York, Springer-Verlag, 1983, pp 763–765.

Madsen PO, Naber KG: The importance of the pressure in the prostatic fossa and absorption of irrigating fluid during transurethral resection of the prostate. J Urol 1973; 109:446–452.

Malenka DJ, Roos N, Fisher ES, et al: Further study of the increased mortality following transurethral prostatectomy: A chart-based analysis. J Urol 1990; 144:224–227; discussion on page 228.

McConnell JD, Barry MD, Bruskewitz RC, et al: Benign prostatic hyperplasia: Diagnosis and treatment. Clinical practice guideline. Agency for Health Care Policy and Research. Publication No. 94–0582 Feb 1994.

McGowan SW, Smith GFN: Anaesthesia for transurethral prostatectomy: A comparison of spinal intradural analgesia with two methods of general anaesthesia. Anaesthesia 1980; 35:847–853.

Mebust WK, Damico C: Prostatic desiccation: A preliminary report of laboratory and clinical experience. J Urol 1972; 108:601–603.

Mebust WK, Holtgrewe HL, Cockett ATK, Peters PC, and Writing Committee: Transurethral prostatectomy: Immediate and postoperative complications. A cooperative study of thirteen participating institutions evaluating 3,885 patients. J Urol 1989; 141:243–247.

Mebust WK, Roizo R, Schroeder F, et al: Correlations between pathology, clinical symptoms and the course of the disease. The International Consultation on Benign Prostatic Hyperplasia—Proceedings, pp 51–62, 1991, Paris.

Mebust WK, White TG: Immune reactions following desiccation surgery of the canine prostate. Invest Urol 1977; 14:427–430.

Melchior J, Valk WL, Foret JD, et al: Transurethral prostatectomy: Computerized analysis of 2,223 consecutive cases. J Urol 1974a; 112:634–642.

Melchior J, Valk WL, Foret JD, et al: Transurethral resection of the prostate via perineal urethrostomy: Complete analysis of 7 years of experience. J Urol 1974b; 111:640–643.

Melicow MM: Histological study of vesical urothelium interviewing between gross tumors in total cystectomy. J Urol 1952; 68:261.

Meyhoff HH, Nordling J: Long term results of transurethral and transvesical prostatectomy: A randomized study. Scand J Urol Nephrol 1986; 20:27–33.

Miller J, Edyvane KA, Sinclair GR, et al: A comparison of bladder neck incision and transurethral prostatic resection. Aust N Z J Surg 1992; 62:116–122.

Montorsi F, Guazzoni G, Bergamaschi F, et al: Long-term clinical reliability of transurethral and open prostatectomy for benign prostatic obstruction: A term of comparison for nonsurgical procedures. Eur Urol 1993; 23:262–266.

Mulvaney WP: Attempted disintegration of calculi by ultrasonic vibrations. J Urol 1953; 70:704–707.

Mulvaney WP, Beck CW: The laser beam in urology. J Urol 1968; 99:112–115.

Nesbit RM: A history of transurethral prostatectomy. Rev Mex Urol 1975; 35:349–362.

Nesbit RM: Transurethral prostatectomy. Springfield, IL, Charles C Thomas, 1943.

Nielsen OS, Maigaard S, Frimodt-Moller N, et al: Prophylactic antibiotics in transurethral prostatectomy. J Urol 1981; 126:60–62.

1986 National Health Survey. Hyattsville, MD: National Center for Health Statistics 1988;197, Ser 13, No 95.

Oester A, Madsen PO: Determination of absorption of irrigating fluid during transurethral resection of the prostate by means of radioisotopes. J Urol 1969; 102:714–719.

Orandi A: Transurethral incision of the prostate. J Urol 1973; 110:229–231.

Perrin P, Barnes R, Hadley H, et al: Forty years of transurethral prostatic resections. J Urol 1976;116:757–758.

Plentka L, Loghem JV, Hahn E, et al: Comorbidities and perioperative complications among patients with surgically treated benign prostatic hyperplasia. Urology 1991; 38(Suppl 1):43–48.

Prescott S, Hadi MA, Elton RA, et al: Antibiotic compared with antiseptic prophylaxis for prostatic surgery. Br J Urol 1990; 66:509–514.

Rees RM: The effect of transurethral resection of the intravesical ureter during the removal of bladder tumors. Br J Urol 1969; 41:2.

Roos NP, Wennberg JE, Malenka DJ, et al: Mortality and reoperation after open and transurethral resection of the prostate for benign prostatic hyperplasia. Special Article. N Engl J Med 1989; 320(17):1120–1123.

Rouvalis P: Electronic lithotripsy for vesical calculus with "URAT I": An experience of 100 cases and an experimental application of the method to stones in the upper urinary tract. Br J Urol 1970; 42:485–491.

Shah PJR, Abrams PH, Feneley RCL, et al: The influence of prostatic anatomy on the differing results of prostatectomy according to the surgical approach. Br J Urol 1979; 51:549–551.

Sinha B, Haikel G, Lange PH, et al: Transurethral resection of the prostate with local anesthesia in 100 patients. J Urol 1986; 135:719–721.

Solsona E, Iborra I, Ricos JV, et al: Feasibility of transurethral resection for muscle infiltrating carcinoma of the bladder: A prospective study. J Urol 1992; 147:1513–1515.

Stalberg HP, Hahn RG, Jones AW: Ethanol monitoring of transurethral prostatic resection during inhaled anesthesia. Anesth Analg 1992; 75: 983–988.

Stephenson TP, Latto P, Bradley D, et al: Comparison between continuous flow and intermittent flow transurethral resection in 40 patients presenting with acute retention. Br J Urol 1980; 52:523–525.

Turner-Warwick R: The sphincter mechanism: Their relation to prostatic enlargement and its treatment. *In* Hinman F Jr, ed: Benign Prostatic Hypertrophy. New York, Springer-Verlag, 1983, pp 809–828.

Turner-Warwick R: A urodynamic review of bladder outlet obstruction in the male and its clinical implications. Urol Clin North Am 1979; 6:171–192.

Upton JD, Das S: Prophylactic antibiotics in transurethral resection of bladder tumors: Are they necessary? Urology 1986; 27(5):421–423.

Vicente J, Chechile G, Pons R, et al: Tumor recurrence in prostatic urethra following simultaneous resection of bladder tumor and prostate. Eur Urol 1988; 15:40–42.

Viitanen J, Talja M, Jussila M, et al: Transurethral resection of the prostate and related topics. Randomized controlled study of chemoprophylaxis in transurethral prostatectomy. J Urol 1993; 150:1715–1717.

Wasson JH, Reda DJ, Bruskewitz RC, et al: A comparison of transurethral surgery with watchful waiting for moderate symptoms of benign prostatic hyperplasia. N Engl J Med 1995; 332:75–79.

Watson GM, Murray S, Dretler SP, et al: The pulsed dye laser for fragmenting urinary calculi. J Urol 1987; 138:195–198.

50
RETROPUBIC AND SUPRAPUBIC PROSTATECTOMY

Joseph E. Oesterling, M.D.

OVERVIEW

In recent years, a number of new treatment options for benign prostatic hyperplasia have been developed, investigated, and used. These include not only medications, such as terazosin (Hytrin; Lepor et al, 1992), doxazosin (Cardura; Gillenwater et al, 1995), and finasteride (Proscar; Gormley et al, 1992), but also minimally invasive procedures, such as visual laser ablation of the prostate (VLAP; Cocules et al, 1995), electrovaporization of the prostate (EVP; Kaplan and Te, 1995), and transurethral incision of the prostate (TUIP; Kletscher and Oesterling, 1992). Most often, however, these approaches are reserved for men with moderate symptoms and a small to medium-sized prostate gland. Patients with acute urinary retention, persistent or recurrent urinary tract infections, marked hemorrhage from the enlarged prostate, and renal insufficiency as a result of bladder outlet obstruction are indications for prostatectomy, either transurethral resection of the prostate (TURP) or open prostatectomy.

Indications for Open Prostatectomy

Open prostatectomy, whether performed via the retropubic approach or the suprapubic approach, should be considered when the prostate gland is greater than 50 to 75 grams. It is also the procedure of choice for men who have a concomitant bladder condition that requires treatment, such as a symptomatic bladder diverticulum or a large, hard bladder calculus that cannot be managed transurethrally. Consideration should also be given to open prostatectomy when there is a coexisting unilateral or bilateral inguinal hernia. Schlegel and Walsh (1987) have demonstrated that a preperitoneal inguinal herniorrhaphy can be accomplished via the same lower midline incision that is used for the prostatectomy. **Another indication for performing an open prostatectomy rather than TURP is marked ankylosis of the hips that prevents proper placement of the patient in the dorsal lithotomy position.**

When compared with TURP, an open prostatectomy offers the advantages of complete removal of the prostatic adenoma under direct vision and minimal to no risk of the TUR syndrome (dilutional hyponatremia). The disadvantages, as compared with TURP, include the need for a lower midline incision, and as a result, a longer hospitalization and an extended convalescence period. In addition, there may be an increased potential for intraoperative hemorrhage from the prostatic fossa. Thus, an open prostatectomy should be reserved for men fulfilling the inclusion criteria stated earlier. **Contraindications to this operation include a small prostate gland, a previous prostatectomy, previous pelvic surgery preventing access to the prostate gland, and any type of prostate cancer.**

Preoperative Evaluation

In deciding whether or not to perform an open prostatectomy for a man with symptomatic BPH, it is necessary to evaluate the lower urinary tract. Most often, the patient will have already completed the American Urological Association (AUA) symptom questionnaire and had a peak urinary flow rate determination. The postvoid residual urine volume also may have been verified with an abdominal ultrasound. **A cystoscopic examination is not performed routinely in the man with obstructive voiding symptoms (McConnell et al, 1994).** It should only be carried out in men with suspected other conditions, such as a urethral stricture, a bladder calculus, or a bladder diverticulum. It also can be helpful in confirming the presence of a large prostate gland, by assessing the length of the prostatic urethra. For this indication, it is most ideal to perform the cystoscopic examination under anesthesia just prior to surgery, when the pelvic floor musculature is relaxed.

Before either retropubic or suprapubic prostatectomy, prostate cancer must be excluded. **All men should undergo a digital rectal examination and have a serum prostate-specific antigen determination.** If the digital rectal examination detects induration or nodularity, or the serum prostate-specific antigen concentration is elevated, a transrectal ultrasound–guided biopsy of the prostate gland should be performed. A transrectal ultrasound, by itself, is not indicated as a first-line diagnostic test for evaluating the prostate gland to detect early, curable prostate cancer. However, it can be useful in determining prostate size in an effort to substantiate the presence of a large prostate gland.

With regard to evaluating the upper urinary tracts preoperatively, it is only necessary in men with known disease or individuals suspected of having an abnormality, such as hematuria (Oesterling et al, 1993). For individuals who require upper tract evaluation and have normal renal function, a routine intravenous pyelogram with a postvoid drainage film can be obtained. For men with compromised renal function (a creatinine concentration greater than 2.0 mg/dl), renal sonography and/or bilateral retrograde pyelogram is preferred. Computed tomography scan and magnetic resonance imaging scan are not commonly used.

Before performing an open prostatectomy for benign prostatic hyperplasia, the patient should undergo a complete medical evaluation, consisting of a detailed history, a thorough physical examination, and an appropriate laboratory assessment. With most patients being in their late sixties, seventies, and early eighties, the risk for cardiovascular disease, pulmonary conditions, hypertension, diabetes mellitus, malignancies, and coagulopathies is high. Indeed, all major organ systems need close scrutiny; if an abnormality is uncovered, the appropriate subspecialty should be consulted so that recommendations can be instituted in preparation for the procedure. The patient's medications should be reviewed in detail, and careful attention should be given to whether he is taking aspirin; a nonsteroidal anti-inflammatory agent, such as ibuprofen (Motrin); or other agents like warfarin (Coumadin) that can lead to a bleeding diathesis. All such medications must be discontinued before either a retropubic or suprapubic prostatectomy. **Aspirin should be discontinued seven to ten days before surgery, nonsteroidal anti-inflammatory agents two to three days before surgery, and warfarin (Coumadin) three to four days prior to the procedure.** All patients in this age group should have a chest radiograph, an electrocardiogram, routine electrolytes, coagulation studies, and a complete blood count. Knowing the serum creatinine level is especially important for patients in urinary retention. If the value is elevated, surgery should be delayed until the serum creatinine concentration stabilizes. A urinalysis is mandatory, and when there is suspicion of a urinary tract infection, a urine specimen should be sent for culture and sensitivity. If an infection is present, appropriate antimicrobial therapy must be instituted. Usually, a sulfa medication, such as sulfamethoxazole-trimethoprim (Bactrim DS or Septra DS) or a fluoroquinolone (ciprofloxacin, norfloxacin [Noroxin], or floxacin [Floxin]) is highly effective. However, it should be noted that patients who perform clean intermittent catheterization or have an indwelling urethral catheter will have infected urine. For these men, intravenous antibiotic therapy is given perioperatively with the first dose being given before surgery.

Last, the patient must be informed of the benefits and risks associated with open prostatectomy and written informed consent is obtained. Clearly, the benefit to be achieved is improved urination. **Potential risks include urinary incontinence, erectile dysfunction, retrograde ejaculation, urinary tract infection, and the need for a blood transfusion.** Traditionally, 5% to 10% of men undergoing this operation require one or more units of blood. Thus, it may be prudent to have several units of blood available when performing an open prostatectomy. Patients who are concerned about infectious processes associated with blood transfusion can donate several units of their own blood prior to surgery so that it is available at the time of the procedure. **The preferred donation schedule is one unit per week, with the last donation being two weeks prior to surgery.** While donating, the patient should be receiving oral iron supplemental medication (ferrous sulfate or ferrous gluconate). Other potential untoward effects include deep vein thrombosis and pulmonary embolus.

At present, this entire preoperative evaluation is conducted on an outpatient basis before admission.

The Day of Surgery

The patient is kept NPO after midnight and takes a Fleet's enema on rising the morning of surgery. On arrival at the hospital, he reports to the admission's office and, from there, is taken directly to the surgery theater. The type of anesthesia to be used is discussed and finalized with the patient and his family. **Usually, either a long-acting spinal anesthesia or an epidural anesthesia is used.** If either of these two regional anesthesias is medically contraindicated or the patient does not prefer them, general anesthesia with adequate relaxation may be used.

RETROPUBIC PROSTATECTOMY

Retropubic prostatectomy is the enucleation of the hyperplastic prostatic adenoma through a direct incision of the anterior prostatic capsule. This approach to open prostatectomy was made popular by Terrence Millin, who reported the results of the procedure on twenty patients in *Lancet* in 1945. The advantages of this procedure over the suprapubic approach are (1) excellent anatomic exposure of the prostate, (2) direct visualization of the prostatic adenoma during enucleation to ensure complete removal, (3) precise transection of the urethra distally to preserve urinary continence, (4) clear and immediate visualization of the prostatic fossa after enucleation to control all bleeding sites, and (5) minimal to no trauma to the urinary bladder. The disadvantage, as compared with suprapubic prostatectomy, is that direct access to the bladder is not achieved. This may be an important consideration when there is a concomitant bladder diverticulum that requires excision or a large bladder calculus. The suprapubic approach also may be preferred when the obstructive prostatic enlargement primarily involves the median lobe.

Operative Technique

Anesthesia

As indicated earlier, the preferred anesthesia is spinal or epidural. With either approach, the patient can avoid having to wake up from a general anesthesia and being drowsy for several hours or the remainder of the day. Also, it appears that the intraoperative blood loss is less and the frequency of postoperative deep vein thrombosis and pulmonary embolus is reduced with these types of regional anesthesia (Peters and Walsh, 1985). **Usually, general anesthesia is given only when there is a medical contraindication to a regional anesthesia or when the patient simply prefers general anesthesia.**

Proper Positioning of the Patient

The patient is placed on the operating table in the supine position with the umbilicus over the break in the table. If a cystoscopic examination is to be performed, the patient is prepped and draped in the usual manner for a transurethral diagnostic procedure. For convenience and so the patient does not have to be placed in the dorsal lithotomy position, a flexible cystoscopy is preferred. **Following the cystoscopy, the table is hyperextended maximally and placed in twenty degrees of Trendelenburg position.** This maneuver increases the distance between the umbilicus and the pubic symphysis, and gives better exposure to the retropubic space.

Incision and Exposure of the Prostate

After prepping and draping the patient in the usual sterile manner, a No. 22 Fr urethral catheter with a 30-ml balloon is passed into the bladder and connected to a sterile closed-drainage system; 30 ml of water are placed in the balloon. A lower midline incision from the umbilicus to the pubic symphysis is made. It is deepened through the subcutaneous adipose tissue, and the linea alba is incised. **The rectus abdominis muscles are separated in the midline, and the transversalis fascia is incised sharply without entering the peritoneal cavity to expose the space of Retzius.** At the superior aspect of the wound, the posterior rectus abdominis fascia is incised above the semicircular line to the level of the umbilicus. The peritoneum is now mobilized cephalad, starting at the pubic symphysis and sweeping anterolaterally with the two index fingers. The pelvis is inspected for any abnormalities, and the groin areas are examined for indirect and direct inguinal hernias. If such a hernia is identified, it can be repaired using the preperitoneal approach described by Schlegel and Walsh (1987). **As the peritoneum is brought out of the pelvis with blunt dissection, the vas deferens is identified laterally between the bladder and the external iliac vessels. It is dissected free of surrounding tissues and transected between two large hemoclips in order to prevent episodes of epididymitis following the operation.**

A self-retaining Balfour retractor is placed in the incision and opened. A well-padded, malleable blade is connected to the retractor and used to displace the bladder posteriorly and superiorly. Unlike in an anatomic radical retropubic prostatectomy, the balloon of the catheter is not positioned beneath the malleable blade. Instead, it is allowed to rest at the level of the bladder neck and aids in identifying the prostatovesicular junction later in the operation. The anterior surface of the bladder and prostate are exposed. Using DeBakey forceps and Metzenbaum scissors, the preprostatic adipose tissue is gently removed to expose the superficial branch of the dorsal vein complex and the puboprostatic ligaments (Fig. 50–1).

Hemostatic Maneuvers

Prior to proceeding with enucleation of the prostatic adenoma, it is important to achieve complete control of the dorsal vein complex as well as the lateral pedicles at the bladder neck (the main arterial blood supply to the prostate gland). (Walsh and Oesterling, 1990). To accomplish this task, the endopelvic fascia is incised bilaterally and the puboprostatic ligaments are transected bilaterally, just as when performing an anatomic radical retropubic prostatectomy (Reiner and Walsh, 1979). However, in patients with marked prostatic enlargement, this maneuver is usually easier because the enlarged prostate gland protrudes out from beneath the pubic symphysis. With the apex of the prostate released from the inferior surface of the pubic symphysis, the avascular plane between the urethra and the dorsal vein complex can be identified with the right index finger. The urethra, containing the palpable catheter, lies posterior, and the dorsal vein complex is located anteriorly. A right-angle clamp is passed through the avascular plane, and a 0-Vicryl tie is placed around the dorsal vein complex distal to the apex of the prostate (Fig. 50–2). The superficial branch of the dorsal vein at the bladder should be coagulated or ligated.

At this point, attention is focused on securing the lateral pedicles at the prostatovesicular junction. The 30-ml balloon of the catheter is used to identify the junction between the bladder and the prostate. The balloon is then deflated, and a chromic suture on a large CTX needle is used to place a figure-of-eight stitch deep into the prostatovesicular junction at the level where the seminal vesicles approach the prostate gland bilaterally. With this maneuver, the main arterial blood supply to the prostate adenoma is controlled. Having secured the dorsal vein complex earlier, the major sources of hemorrhage for this operation have been eliminated.

Enucleation of the Adenoma

With a sponge stick on the bladder neck to depress the bladder posteriorly, a number 15 blade on a long handle

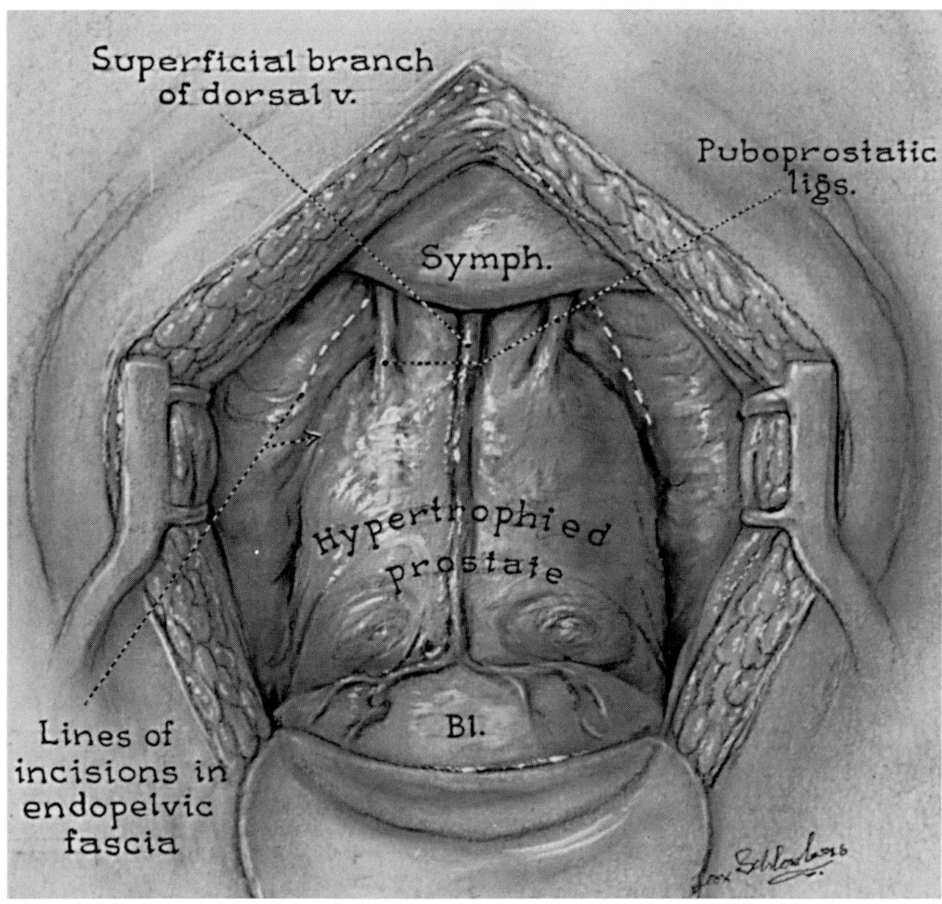

Figure 50–1. Retropubic prostatectomy. The space of Retzius has been opened and the periprostatic adipose tissue has been dissected free from the superficial branch of the dorsal vein complex. The endopelvic fascia is incised bilaterally (dotted lines), and the puboprostatic ligaments are transected bilaterally. (From Walsh PC, Oesterling JE: Improved hemostasis during simple retropubic prostatectomy. J Urol 1990: 143:1203. © By Williams & Wilkins, 1990.)

is used to make a *transverse* capsulotomy in the prostate approximately 1.5 to 2.0 cm distal to the bladder neck (Fig. 50–3). The superficial branch of the dorsal vein complex is transected as the transverse capsulotomy is made. It does not bleed because the dorsal vein complex has already been controlled both proximally and distally. The incision is deepened to the adenoma and extended sufficiently lateral in each direction to allow for complete enucleation. A pair of Metzenbaum scissors is used to dissect the overlying prostatic capsule from the underlying prostatic adenoma. Once a well-defined plane is developed in all directions anteriorly, the right index finger can be inserted between the prostatic adenoma and the capsule to further develop the plane laterally and posteriorly (Fig. 50–4). Next, a pair of Metzenbaum scissors is used to incise the anterior commissure from the bladder neck to the apex, separating the lateral lobes of the prostate anteriorly. The posterior prostatic urethra is exposed, and the right index finger is inserted down to the verumontanum. The mucosa of the urethra overlying the left lateral lobe is divided at the level of the apex without injury to the external urinary sphincter. With the aid of a Babcock clamp, the left lateral lobe is removed safely. This maneuver is then repeated for the right lateral lobe. If a median lobe is present, the overlying mucosa is incised at the level of the bladder neck, and this lobe is removed (Fig. 50–5). In this manner, the entire prostatic adenoma is removed with preservation of a strip of posterior prostatic urethra. **Because the capsulotomy was a transverse rather than longitudinal incision, there is no risk that the incision will inadvertently be extended into the sphincteric mechanism during the enucleation process and cause subsequent urinary incontinence.**

The prostatic fossa is now carefully inspected to ensure that all the adenoma has been removed and that hemostasis is complete. **If hemorrhage is persistent, a chromic suture on a large CTX needle can be used to place a figure-of-eight stitch into the bladder neck at the five- and seven-o'clock positions. When placing these stitches, it is necessary to visualize the ureteral orifices so that they are not incorporated into the stitches.** Indigo carmine dye is readily excreted by the kidneys and can be given intravenously to aid in the visualization of the ureteral orifices if it should be necessary. If the bladder neck has a relatively small opening at the end of the operation, it may be appropriate to perform a wedge resection at the six-o'clock position and advance the bladder mucosa into the prostatic fossa. The maneuver helps prevent the development of a bladder neck contracture.

Closure

After inspecting the bladder and confirming no abnormalities, a No. 24 Fr Malecot suprapubic tube is placed into the dome of the bladder and secured with a 3-0 chromic purse-string stitch. A No. 22 Fr Foley catheter with a 30-ml balloon is inserted through the anterior urethra and prostatic fossa into the bladder. With the suprapubic tube and the urethral catheter in place and hemostasis complete, the pros-

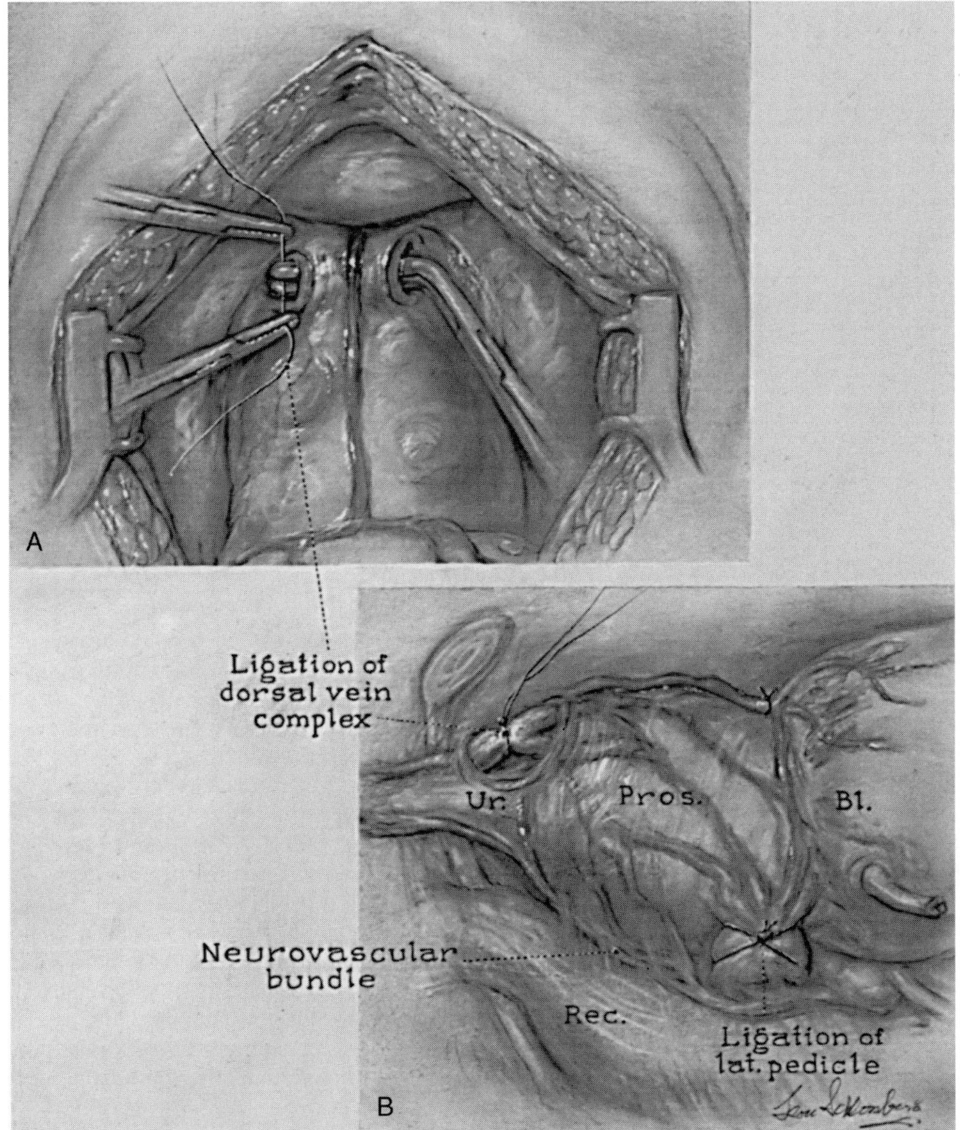

Figure 50–2. Retropubic prostatectomy. *A*, A right-angle clamp is placed through the avascular plane between the urethra posteriorly and the dorsal vein complex anteriorly. A 0-Vicryl tie is grasped and tied around the dorsal vein complex. For this operation, unlike a radical prostatectomy, the dorsal vein complex is not transected. *B*, Using a 2–0 chromic suture on a CTX needle, a figure-of-eight stitch is placed through the prostatovesicular junction just above the level of the seminal vesicles to control the main arterial blood supply to the prostate gland. When placing this stitch, care must be taken to avoid entrapment of the neurovascular bundles located posteriorly and slightly laterally. (From Walsh PC, Oesterling JE: Improved hemostasis during simple retropubic prostatectomy. J Urol 1990: 143:1203. © By Williams & Wilkins, 1990.)

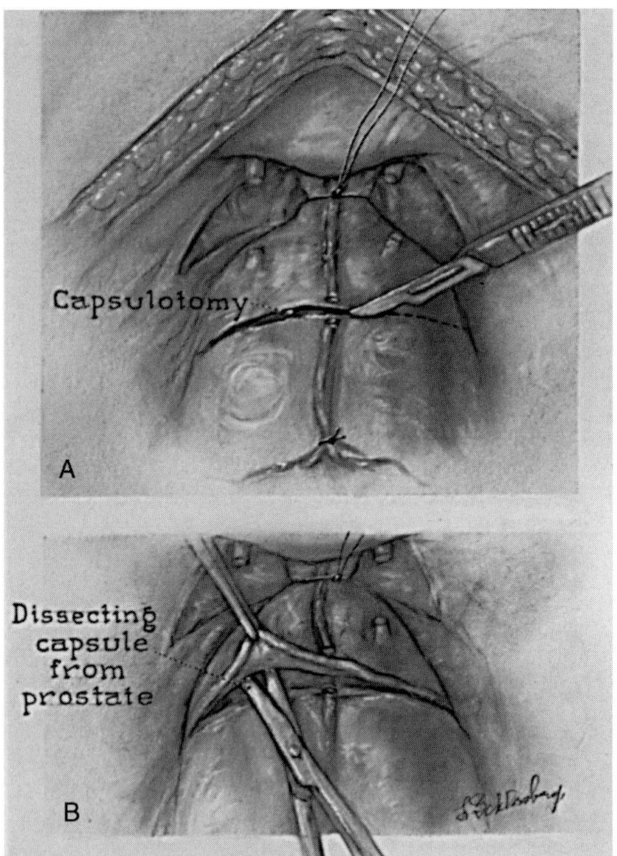

Figure 50–3. Retropubic prostatectomy. *A,* With the superficial branch of the dorsal vein complex secured proximally and distally, a number 15 blade on a long handle is used to make the transverse capsulotomy. *B,* Metzenbaum scissors are used to develop the plane anteriorly between the prostatic adenoma and the prostatic capsule. (From Walsh PC: Retropubic prostatectomy for benign and malignant diseases. In Marshall FF, ed: Operative Urology. Philadelphia, W.B. Saunders Company, 1991, pp 264–289.)

tatic capsule is closed (Fig. 50–6). A 2-0 chromic suture on a 5/8 circle-tapered needle is used to create two running stitches. The two stitches begin laterally and meet in the midline; they are first tied separately and then together to create a watertight closure. Fifty milliliters of water are then placed in the balloon to ensure that the end of the catheter remains in the bladder and does not fall into the prostatic fossa. A small, closed-suction drain is placed via a separate stab incision lateral to the prostate and bladder on each side to prevent hematoma and urinoma formation. The pelvis is irrigated with copious amounts of normal saline solution, and the rectus fascia is reapproximated with a number 2 nylon suture on a TP1 needle in a running fashion. The skin is closed with a running 4-0 Vicryl subcuticular stitch. The suprapubic tube and drains are secured to the abdominal wall, and the urethral catheter is secured to the lower extremity.

Postoperative Considerations

In the recovery room, the output from the pelvic drains, suprapubic tube, and urethral catheter is monitored. In addition, it is routine to verify the hematocrit. **If significant hemorrhage is noted, the urethral catheter should be placed on traction so that the balloon containing 50 ml of water can compress the bladder neck and prostatic fossa.** Constant and reliable traction can be maintained by securing the catheter to an abdominal catheter holder, as described previously by Oesterling (1992; Fig. 50–7). In addition, continuous bladder irrigation should be initiated to prevent clot formation. **For maximal effect, the inflow should be through the urethral catheter and the outflow through the suprapubic tube.** For most patients, these measures are effective and nothing further needs to be instituted. Nevertheless, if excessive bleeding persists after these measures, the urethral catheter can be removed and a cystoscopic inspection of the prostatic fossa and bladder neck can be performed to identify discrete bleeding sites. If marked hemorrhage should continue to persist, the patient should be reexplored. This author has not found measures, such as silver nitrate or alum installations, intravenous ϵ-aminocaproic acid (Amicar), embolization of the hypogastric arteries, or ligation of the hypogastric arteries, to be useful.

On the evening on the day of surgery, the patient is started on a clear liquid diet and asked to perform the dorsiflexion and plantarflexion exercises 100 times per hour while awake and to perform pulmonary exercises. Effective pain management consists of intravenous Ketorolac tromethamine (Toradol), 15 mg intravenous every 6 hours for forty-eight hours, and intravenous morphine sulfate on an as-needed basis via a patient-controlled analgesic pump. However, if significant hematuria is present, Toradol should not be used. **On the first postoperative day, the patient is advanced to a regular diet and asked to ambulate six times per day (two times in the morning, two times in the afternoon, and two times in the evening).** In addition, he continues the dorsiflexion and plantarflexion exercises and appropriate pulmonary exercises. **On the second day after surgery, the pelvic drains are removed if the drainage is less than 75 ml per 24-hour period.** Also, the appropriate discharge instructions are reviewed with the patient at this time in preparation for dismissal on the third day following surgery. The patient goes home with both the urethral catheter and suprapubic tube indwelling.

The urethral catheter is usually removed five days following surgery, and the suprapubic tube is clamped at the same time. If the patient voids well with a minimal postvoid residual urine volume, the suprapubic tube is then removed.

Complications

The overall rate of morbidity and mortality associated with this procedure is extremely low. **Although excessive hemorrhage had been a major concern traditionally, blood loss is now minimal and the need for a blood transfusion is uncommon.** Indeed, controlling the dorsal vein complex distal to the apex of the prostate and ligating the lateral pedicles to the prostate at the prostatovesicular junction markedly reduces venous and arterial bleeding, respectively. Nevertheless, it may still be prudent to have several units of autologous blood available at the time of retropubic prostatectomy. Urinary extravasation also can be of concern in the immediate postoperative period; this most

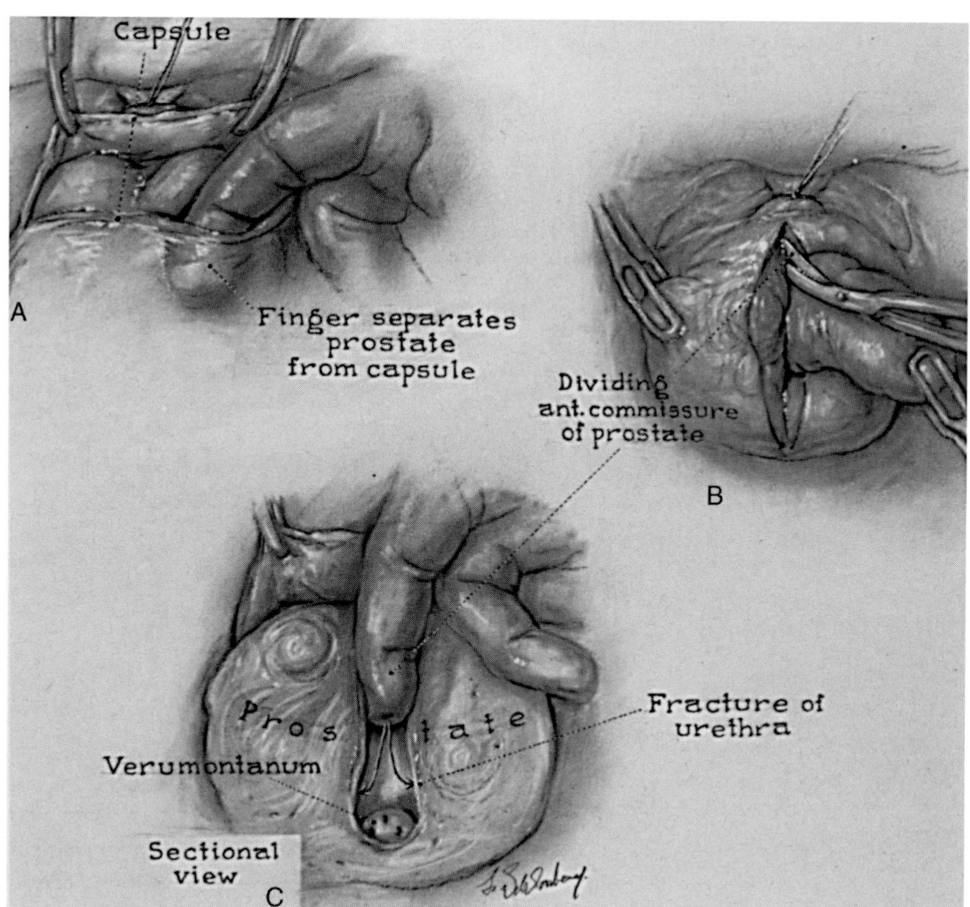

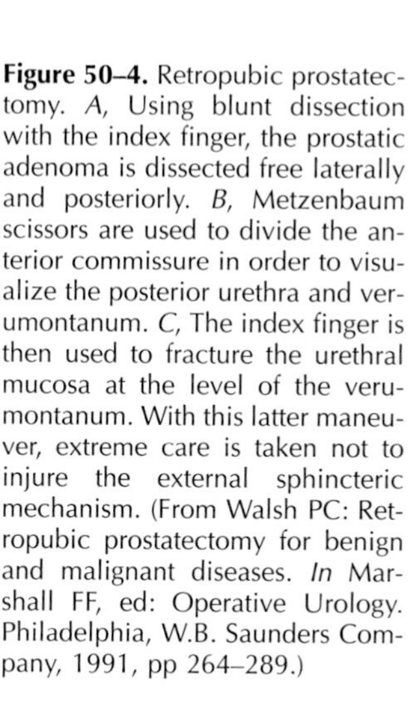
Figure 50–4. Retropubic prostatectomy. *A*, Using blunt dissection with the index finger, the prostatic adenoma is dissected free laterally and posteriorly. *B*, Metzenbaum scissors are used to divide the anterior commissure in order to visualize the posterior urethra and verumontanum. *C*, The index finger is then used to fracture the urethral mucosa at the level of the verumontanum. With this latter maneuver, extreme care is taken not to injure the external sphincteric mechanism. (From Walsh PC: Retropubic prostatectomy for benign and malignant diseases. *In* Marshall FF, ed: Operative Urology. Philadelphia, W.B. Saunders Company, 1991, pp 264–289.)

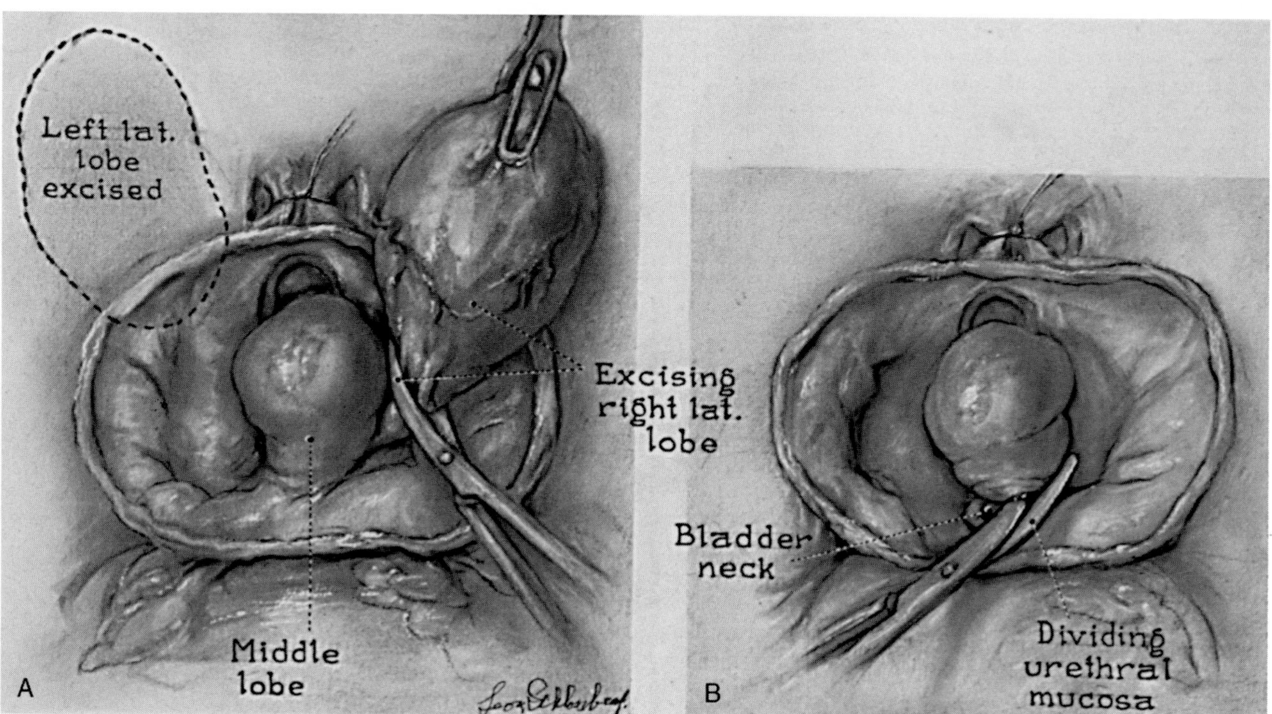

Figure 50–5. Retropubic prostatectomy. *A*, After removal of the left lateral lobe of the prostate, the right lateral lobe is excised with the aid of a tenaculum and Metzenbaum scissors. *B*, Lastly, the median lobe is removed under direct vision. (From Walsh PC: Retropubic prostatectomy for benign and malignant diseases. *In* Marshall FF, ed: Operative Urology. Philadelphia, W.B. Saunders Company, 1991, pp 264–289.)

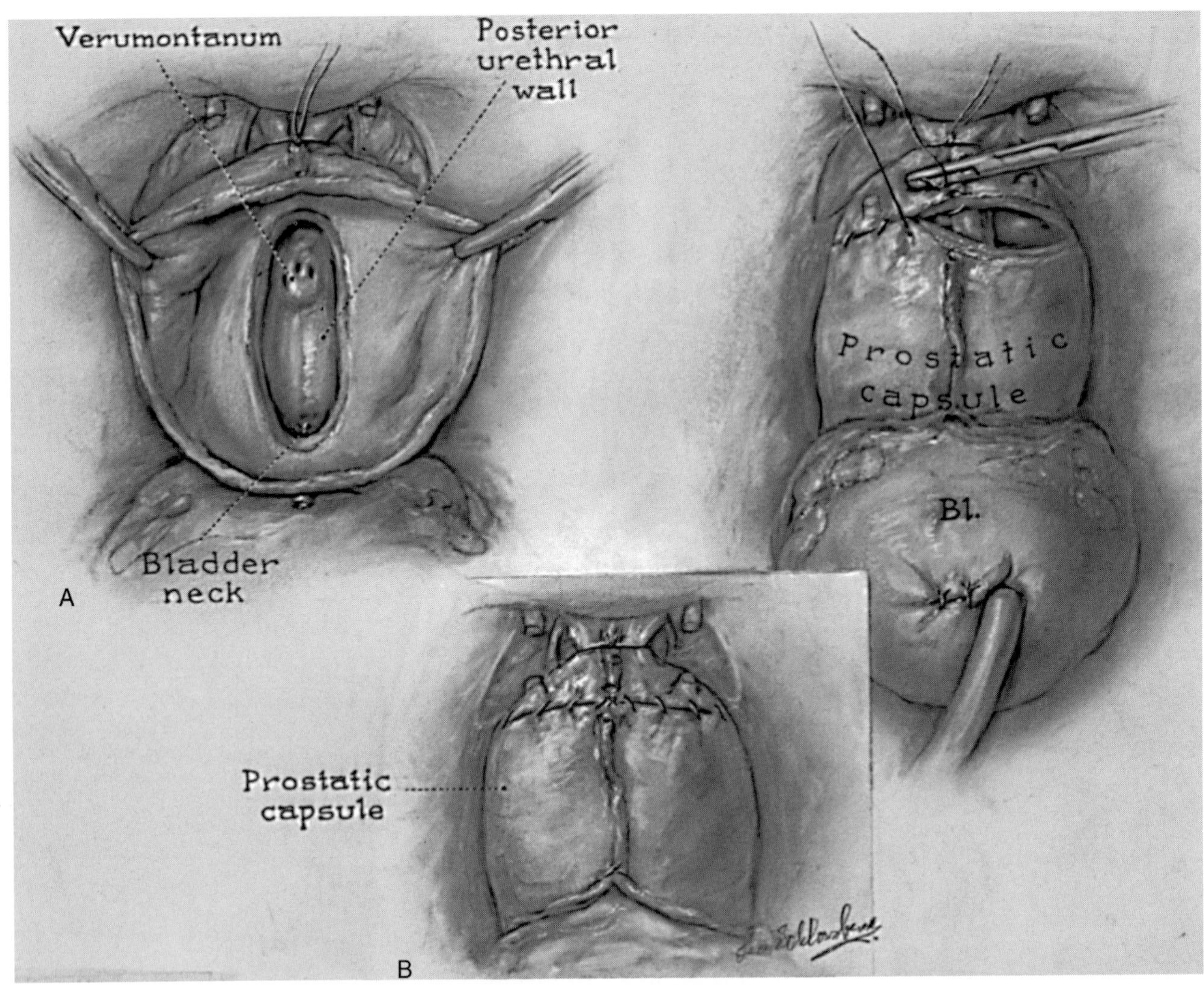

Figure 50–6. Retropubic prostatectomy. *A*, View of the prostatic fossa and posterior urethra after enucleation of all the prostatic adenoma. Note that the verumontanum and a strip of posterior urethra remain intact. *B*, After placement of a urethral catheter and a Malecot suprapubic tube, the transverse capsulotomy is closed with two running, 2-0 chromic stitches. The two stitches are tied first to themselves and then to each other across the midline to create a watertight closure of the prostatic capsule. (From Walsh PC: Retropubic prostatectomy for benign and malignant diseases. *In* Marshall FF, ed: Operative Urology. Philadelphia, W.B. Saunders Company, 1991, pp 264–289. Copyright 1992 by Elsevier Science Inc.)

likely results from an incomplete closure of the prostatic capsulotomy. This untoward effect resolves spontaneously with continued catheter drainage. The drain should be left in place until the capsule seals.

Following a retropubic prostatectomy, urgency and urge incontinence may be present for several weeks to several months, depending on the preoperative bladder status. If the condition is severe, the patient may be given an anticholinergic agent such as oxybutynin (Ditropan). Stress incontinence and total incontinence are rare. With a transverse capsulotomy and precise enucleation of the prostatic adenoma under direct vision, risk of injury to the external sphincter mechanism is minimal. If stress incontinence does result after the procedure, the patient may benefit from transurethral collagen injections for a mild condition or an artificial urinary external sphincter when the situation is more severe.

Late urologic complications also are not common. Acute cystitis rarely occurs as long as the patient voids to completion. Acute epididymitis most often occurs when a bilateral vasectomy is not performed at the time of retropubic prostatectomy. Infected urine can reflux into the ejaculatory ducts, now made more patent by the operation; bacteria traverse the vas deferens to reach the epididymitis. Because of this potential complication, it is advised to perform a bilateral vasectomy at the time of surgery.

Erectile dysfunction occurs in approximately 3% to 5% of patients undergoing an anatomical simple retropubic prostatectomy; it is more common in older men than in younger men. Retrograde ejaculation occurs in approximately 80% to 90% of patients following surgery. The risk of this untoward effect is reduced if the bladder neck is preserved at the time of surgery.

Also, approximately 2% to 3% of patients will develop a bladder neck contracture six to twelve weeks after surgery. This commonly occurs in men who have a relatively small opening at the bladder neck at the end of the operation. As stated earlier, for these men, it may be appropriate to perform a wedge resection at the six o'clock position and advance the bladder mucosa into the prostatic fossa. **However, if a bladder neck contracture does develop, the initial man-**

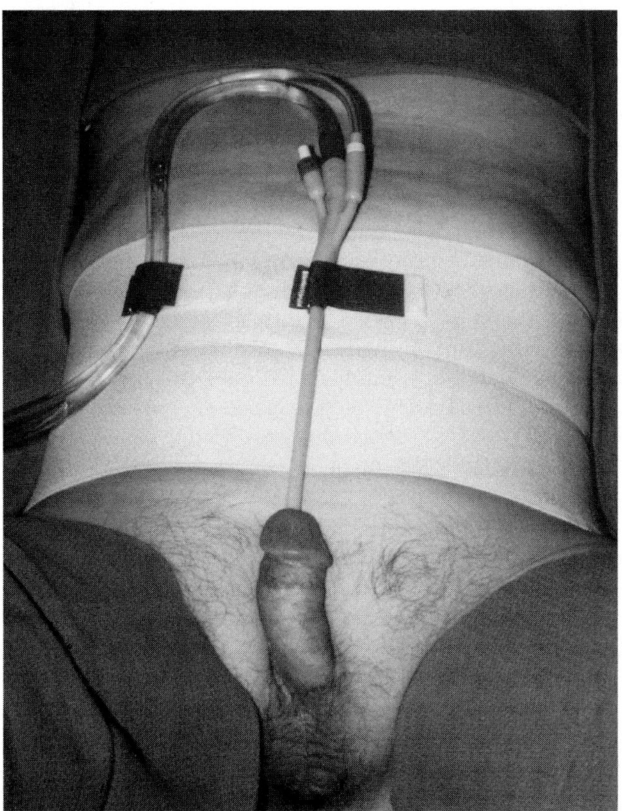

Figure 50–7. Abdominal catheter holder used to provide constant and controlled tension on the urethral catheter. Note that with the use of the Velcro straps, there is no need for adhesive tape, which can be time consuming to place and uncomfortable to the patient. (From Oesterling JE: Abdominal catheter holder to maintain controlled urethral catheter tension post transurethral resection of the prostate. Urology 1992: 40:206, 1992. Copyright 1992 by Elsevier Science Inc.)

agement should be dilatation with urethral sounds or a direct vision incision of the bladder neck, using a Colling's knife to create a No. 22 Fr opening in diameter.

With regard to other nonurologic untoward effects, the most common ones are deep vein thrombosis, pulmonary embolus, myocardial infarction, and a cerebral vascular event. The incidence of any one of these complications is less than 1%, and the overall mortality rate resulting from this operation approaches zero.

SUPRAPUBIC PROSTATECTOMY

Suprapubic prostatectomy is the enucleation of the hyperplastic prostatic adenoma through an extraperitoneal incision of the lower anterior bladder wall. This approach to open prostatectomy was first carried out by Eugene Fuller of New York in 1894; it was later made popular by Peter Freyer of London, England, who described the procedure in *Lancet* in 1900 and then reported results on 1000 patients in 1912. The major advantage of this procedure over the retropubic approach is that it allows for greater visualization of the bladder neck and bladder. As a result, this operation is ideally suited for patients who have (1) a large median lobe protruding into the bladder;(2) a concomitant, symptomatic bladder diverticulum; or (3) a large bladder calculus. It also may be the preferred type of open prostatectomy for very obese men, in whom it is difficult to gain direct access to the prostatic capsule and dorsal vein complex (Culp, 1975). The disadvantage, as compared with the retropubic approach, is that direct visualization of the apical prostatic adenoma is reduced. As a result, the apical enucleation can be less precise, and this factor could affect postoperative urinary continence. Also, not having direct vision of the prostatic fossa after enucleation may make it more cumbersome for achieving complete hemostasis.

Operative Technique

Anesthesia

As for a simple retropubic prostatectomy, the preferred type of anesthesia is spinal or epidural. Only when there is a medical contraindication to regional anesthesia or the patient simply prefers general anesthesia should this type be employed.

Proper Positioning of the Patient

The patient is placed on the operating table in the supine position, with the umbilicus over the break in the table. The table is hyperextended maximally and placed in twenty degrees of Trendelenburg position to increase the distance between the umbilicus and the pubic symphysis, and thereby, facilitate exposure into the pelvis. **After prepping and draping the lower abdomen and external genital area in the usual, sterile manner, a No. 18 Fr catheter is inserted into the bladder and 250 ml of water are instilled. The catheter is removed.**

Incision and Exposure of the Prostate

With the bladder distended, a lower midline incision is made from the umbilicus to the pubic symphysis (Fig. 50–8). It is deepened through the subcutaneous adipose tissue, and the linea alba is incised. The rectus abdominus muscles are separated in the midline, and the transversalis fascia is incised sharply without entering the peritoneal cavity to expose the space of Retzius. At the superior aspect of the wound, the posterior rectus abdominus fascia is incised above the semicircular line to the level of the umbilicus. The peritoneum is then swept cephalad to develop the prevesical space. Also, at this time, the vas deferens on each side is identified laterally between the bladder and the iliac vessels and transected between two large hemoclips.

A self-retaining Balfour retractor is placed in the incision to retract the rectus muscles laterally. The anterior bladder wall is identified, and two 3-0 Vicryl stitches are placed on each side of the midline below the peritoneal reflection. **A small vertical cystotomy is made with a number 15 blade on a long handle. The cystotomy is then extended cephalad and caudally to within 1 cm of the bladder neck (see Fig. 50–8).** After inspecting the bladder, a well-padded, narrow malleable blade is placed in the bladder, connected to the Balfour retractor, and used to retract the bladder cephalad. The bladder neck and prostate gland can now be visualized. A narrow Deaver retractor is now placed over

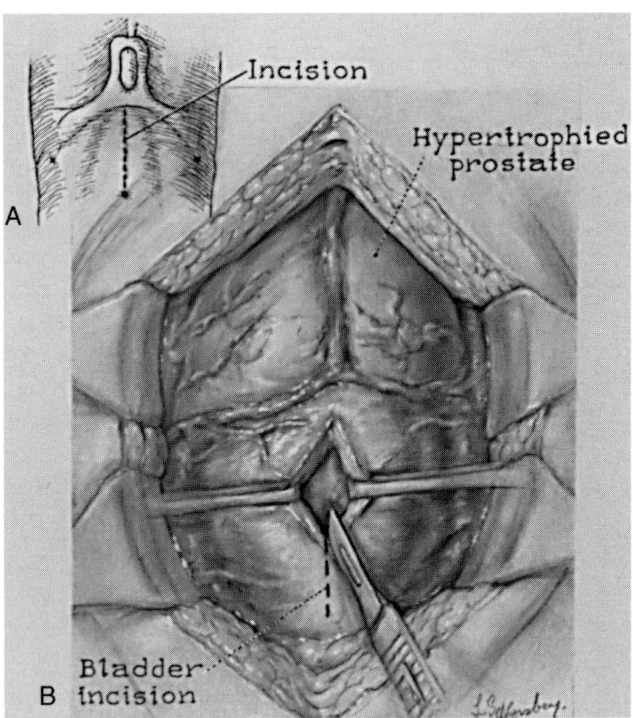

Figure 50–8. Suprapubic prostatectomy. *A*, A lower midline incision is made from the umbilicus to the pubic symphysis. *B*, After developing the prevesical, a small, longitudinal cystotomy is made with a number 15 blade on a long handle. (From Stutzman RE: Suprapubic prostatectomy. *In* Marshall FF, ed: Operative Urology. Philadelphia, W.B. Saunders Company, 1991, pp 259–263.)

the bladder neck and used to further expose this area in the trigone of the urinary bladder.

Enucleation of the Adenoma

A number 15 blade on a long handle is used to create a semicircular incision in the bladder mucosa just distal to the trigone (Fig. 50–9). Care is taken not to violate the trigone or injure the ureteral orifices. Using a pair of Metzenbaum scissors, the plane between the prostatic adenoma and prostatic capsule is developed at the 6-o'clock position (Fig. 50–10). Once a well-established plane is created posteriorly, the prostatic adenoma is dissected circumferentially and inferiorly toward the apex, using blunt dissection (Fig. 50–11). At the apex, the prostatic urethra is transected sharply using a pair of Metzenbaum scissors. With this maneuver, care is taken not to violate the external sphincteric mechanism. At this point, the prostatic adenoma, either as one unit or separate lobes, can be removed from the prostatic fossa.

Hemostatic Maneuvers

On enucleation of the adenoma, the prostatic fossa must be inspected for residual tissue, which can be removed by sharp or blunt dissection. The prostatic fossa also must be examined for discrete bleeding sites, which most often can be controlled with electrocautery. In addition, a hemostatic stitch at the 5- and 7-o'clock positions at the prostatovesicular junction should be placed to ensure control of the main arterial blood supply to the prostate. Using an Allis clamp to grasp the bladder neck and pull it medial, a 0-chromic suture on a large CTX needle is used to place a figure-of-eight stitch on each side at the level of where the seminal vesicles approach the prostate gland (Fig. 50–12). With this maneuver, hemostasis is usually complete. If necessary, indigo carmine dye can be used to aid in identifying the ureteral orifices.

If hemorrhage remains pronounced despite the hemostatic stitches, a number two nylon purse-string suture can be placed around the vesical neck, brought out through the skin, and tied firmly, as described by Malament (1965). With this maneuver, the bladder neck is closed, the prostatic fossa is tamponaded, and the hemorrhage is controlled. It is also possible to placate the prostatic capsule; O'Connor (1982) described using 0-chromic suture on a 5/8 circle needle to place a stitch in the posterior prostatic capsule to prevent further bleeding.

Closure

A No. 22 Fr, urethral catheter with a 30-ml balloon is passed through the urethra into the bladder. In addition, a No. 24 Fr Malecot suprapubic tube is placed into the dome of the bladder and secured with a 3-0 chromic purse-string stitch; it exits the bladder via a separate stab incision (Fig. 50–13). The cystotomy incision is next closed in a single layer, using a 2-0 chromic figure-of-eight stitch. Care is taken to get a small amount of bladder mucosa in the stitch. With this approach, the bladder closure is watertight and

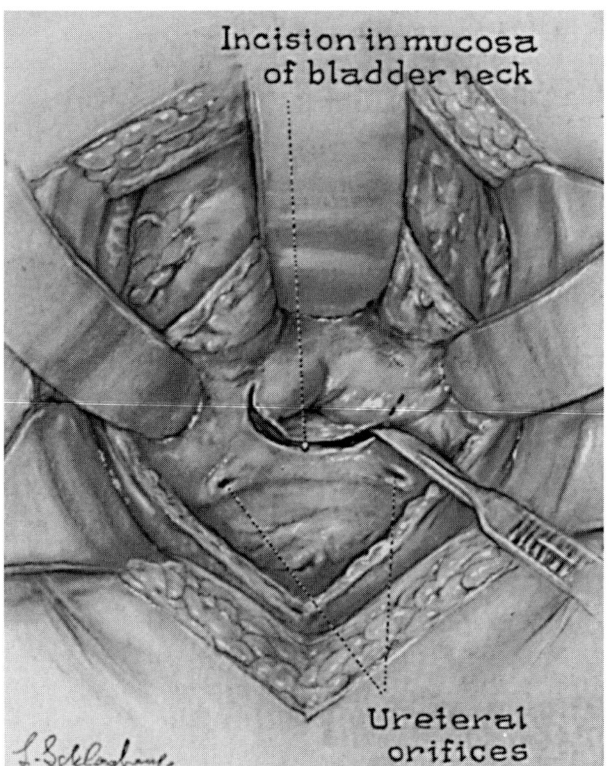

Figure 50–9. Suprapubic prostatectomy. With adequate exposure of the bladder neck, a semicircular incision in the bladder mucosa is made distal to the trigone, using a number 15 blade on a long handle. (From Stutzman RE: Suprapubic prostatectomy. *In* Marshall FF, ed: Operative Urology. Philadelphia, W.B. Saunders Company, 1991, pp 259–263.)

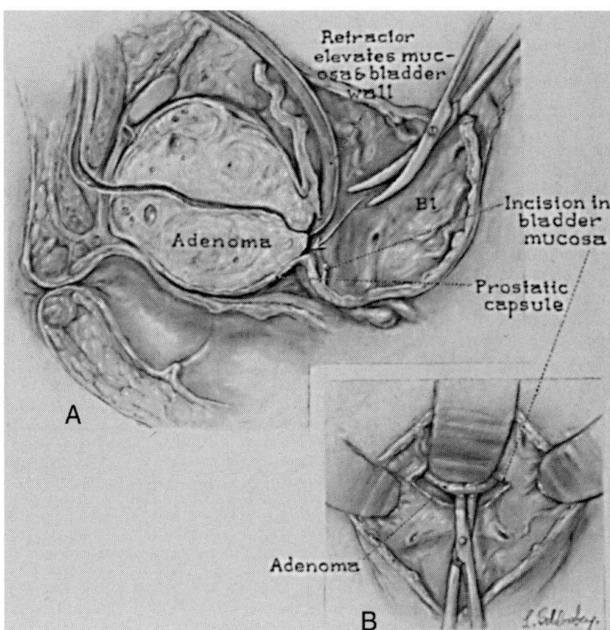

Figure 50–10. Suprapubic prostatectomy. *A,* Starting at the bladder neck posteriorly, Metzenbaum scissors are used to develop the plane between the prostatic adenoma and the prostatic capsule (*lateral view*). *B,* Anterior view of the same maneuver. (From Stutzman RE: Suprapubic prostatectomy. *In* Marshall FF, ed: Operative Urology. Philadelphia, W.B. Saunders Company, 1991, pp 259–263.)

completed in a timely manner. Fifty milliliters of water are placed in the balloon to ensure that the catheter end remains in the bladder and does not fall into the prostatic fossa. The catheter and suprapubic tube are irrigated to confirm a watertight closure and to verify that hemorrhage is minimal. A small, closed-suction drain is placed via a separate stab incision lateral to the bladder on each side. The pelvis is irrigated with copious amounts of normal saline solution, and the rectus fascia is closed with a number 2 nylon suture on a TP1 needle in a running fashion. The skin is closed with a running 4-0 Vicryl subcutaneous stitch. Next, the suprapubic tube and drains are secured to the abdominal wall, and the urethral catheter is anchored to the lower extremity.

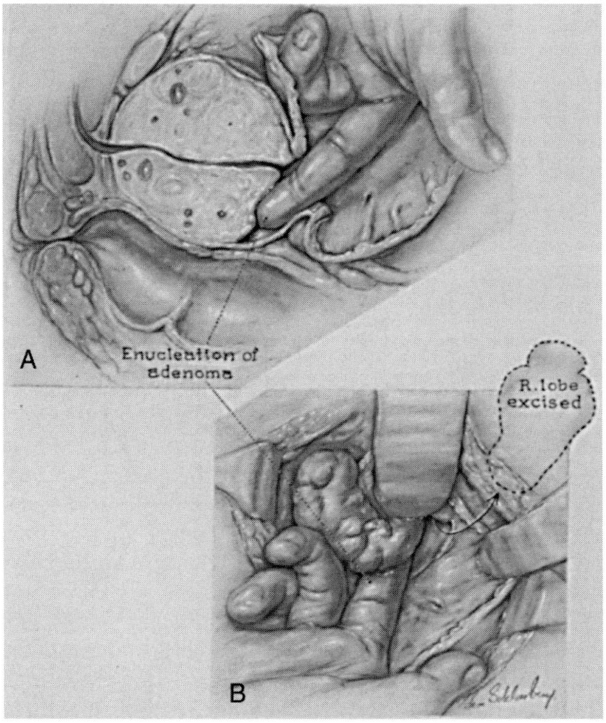

Figure 50–11. Suprapubic prostatectomy. *A,* Using the index finger, the prostatic adenoma is enucleated from the prostatic fossa (*lateral view*). *B,* Anterior view of the same maneuver. With extremely large prostate glands, the left, right, and median lobes should be removed separately. (From Stutzman RE: Suprapubic prostatectomy. *In* Marshall FF, ed: Operative Urology. Philadelphia, W.B. Saunders Company, 1991, pp 259–263.)

Postoperative Considerations

Postoperatively, the care rendered to a patient who has just undergone a suprapubic prostatectomy is similar to that

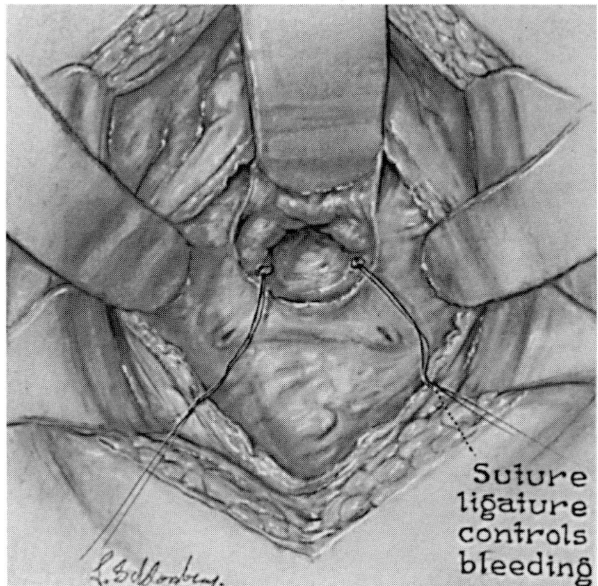

Figure 50–12. Suprapubic prostatectomy. After enucleation of the entire prostatic adenoma, hemostatic stitches consisting of 0-chromic on a CTX needle are placed at the 5-o'clock and 7 o'clock positions at the prostatovesicular junction. (From Stutzman RE: Suprapubic prostatectomy. *In* Marshall FF, ed: Operative Urology. Philadelphia, W.B. Saunders Company, 1991, pp 259–263.)

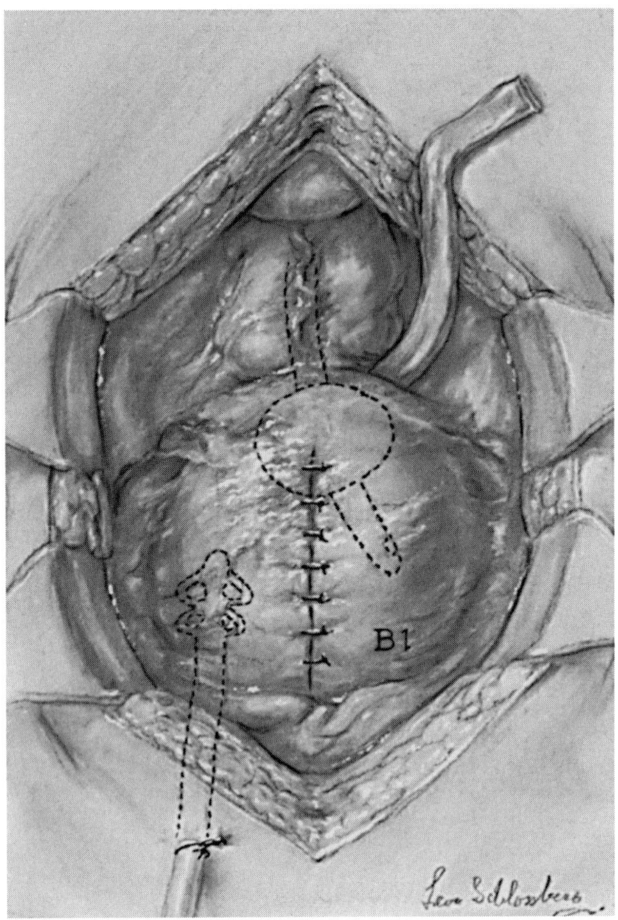

Figure 50–13. Suprapubic prostatectomy. After placing a urethral catheter and a Malecot suprapubic tube, the cystotomy is closed in one layer using 2–0 chromic, figure-of-eight stitches. A closed suction drain is placed on each side of the bladder and exits via separate stab incision. Note that closed drains are now used. (From Stutzman RE: Suprapubic prostatectomy. *In* Marshall FF, ed: Operative Urology. Philadelphia, W.B. Saunders Company, 1991, pp 259–263.)

of a man who is managed with a retropubic prostatectomy. In the recovery room, the output from the pelvic drains, suprapubic tube, and ureteral catheter is monitored; the hematocrit is verified as well. If significant hemorrhage is noted, the urethral catheter should be placed on traction so that the balloon, containing 50 ml of water, can compress the bladder neck and prostatic fossa. Continuous bladder irrigation should be initiated to prevent clot formation. As for a retropubic prostatectomy, if hemorrhage should persist, the urethral catheter can be removed and a cystoscopic examination of the prostatic fossa can be performed; all bleeding sites can be fulgurated.

On the evening of the day of surgery, the patient is started on a clear liquid diet and asked to perform dorsiflexion and plantarflexion exercises one hundred times per hour while awake. Pain management consists of intravenous Toradol, 15 mg every six hours for forty-eight hours, and intravenous morphine sulfate on an as-needed basis via a patient-controlled analgesia pump. However, if significant hematuria is present, Toradol should not be used. **On the first postoperative day, the patient is advanced to a regular diet and allowed to ambulate six times per day (two times in the morning, two times in the afternoon, and two times in the evening).** In addition, he continues the dorsiflexion and plantarflexion exercises and appropriate pulmonary exercises. **On the second day after surgery, the pelvic drains are removed if the drainage is less than 75 ml per 24-hour period.** Also, appropriate discharge instructions are reviewed with the patient at this time in preparation for discharge on the third day following surgery. The patient goes home with both urethral catheter and suprapubic tube indwelling.

The urethral catheter is usually removed five to seven days following surgery, and the suprapubic tube is clamped at the same time. If the patient voids well with minimal postvoid residual urine volume, a cystogram is obtained. If there is no extravasation, the suprapubic tube is removed.

Complications

The complications following a suprapubic prostatectomy are no different than those that can occur after a retropubic prostatectomy. They include excessive hemorrhage and urinary extravasation in the postoperative period and infectious processes, such as cystitis and epididymo-orchitis, on catheter removal. Potential long-term urologic complications include urge or stress urinary incontinence, or both; bladder neck contracture; retrograde ejaculation; and erectile dysfunction. All are very uncommon (2%–3%) except for retrograde ejaculation, which occurs in nearly 100% of the patients. The urge incontinence may be due to bladder instability and usually resolves in four to six weeks; if it persists, oxybutynin (Ditropan) therapy may be initiated. As with any pelvic surgery, there is a risk of deep vein thrombosis and pulmonary embolus. **However, with the use of the sequential pneumatic compression stockings, dorsiflexion and plantarflexion exercises, and early ambulation following surgery, the risk of clot formation approaches zero.**

SUMMARY

Open prostatectomy, whether performed via a retropubic approach or a suprapubic approach, is an excellent treatment option for (1) men with symptomatic benign prostatic hyperplasia due to a markedly enlarged prostate gland; (2) individuals with a concomitant bladder condition, such as a bladder diverticulum or large bladder calculi; and (3) patients who cannot be placed in the dorsal lithotomy position for a transurethral resection of the prostate gland. With improved surgical technique, the procedures are routinely carried out in a precise manner with minimal hemorrhage. **Efficacy, in terms of improvement in symptom score and peak urinary flow rate, is greater than for any other treatment option available for the obstructing prostate gland, including transurethral resection of the prostate (McConnell et al, 1994).** Meanwhile, untoward effects are minimal and the length of hospitalization has been markedly reduced. For most patients, the length of hospital stay is three days or less. Thus, for the properly selected individual, an open prostatectomy is a highly effective operation.

REFERENCES

Cowles RS, Kabalin JN, Childs S, et al: A prospective randomized comparison of transurethral resection to visual laser ablation of the prostate for the treatment of benign prostatic hyperplasia. Urology 1995; 46:155.

Culp DA: Benign prostatic hyperplasia: Early recognition and management. Urol Clin North Am 1975; 2:29.

Freyer PJ: A new method of performing prostatectomy. Lancet 1900; 1:774.

Freyer PJ: One thousand cases of total enucleation of the prostate for radical cure of enlargement of that organ. Br Med J 1912; 2:868.

Fuller E: Six successful and successive cases of prostatectomy. J Cutan Genitourin Dis 1895; 13:229.

Gillenwater, J.Y., Conn, R.L., Chrysant, S.G., et al: Doxazosin for the treatment of benign prostatic hyperplasia in patients with mild to moderate essential hypertension: A double-blind, placebo-controlled, dose-response multicenter study. J Urol 1995; 154:110.

Gormley, G.J., Stoner, E., Bruskewitz, R.C., et al: The effect of finasteride in men with benign prostatic hyperplasia. N Engl J Med 1992; 327:1185.

Kaplan SA, Te AE: Transurethral electrovaporization of the prostate: A novel method for treating men with benign prostatic hyperplasia. Urology 1995; 45:566.

Kletscher BA, Oesterling JE: Transurethral incision of the prostate: a viable alternative to transurethral resection. Semin Urol 1992; 10:265.

Lepor H, Auerbach S, Puras-Baez A, et al: A randomized, placebo-controlled multicenter study of the efficacy and safety of terazosin in the treatment of benign prostatic hyperplasia. J Urol 1992; 148:1467.

Malament M: Maximal hemostasis in suprapubic prostatectomy. Surg Gynecol Obstet 1965; 120:1307.

McConnell JD, Barry MJ, Bruskewitz RC, et al: Benign prostatic hyperplasia: diagnosis and treatment. Quick reference guide for clinicians. No. 8. Rockville, MD: Department of Health and Human Services, 1994 (AHCPR publication number 94-0583.)

Millin R: Retropubic prostatectomy: New extravesical technique: Report on 20 cases. Lancet 1945; ii:693.

O'Connor VJ Jr: An aid for hemostasis in open prostatectomy: Capsular plication. J Urol 1982; 127:448.

Oesterling JE: Abdominal catheter holder to maintain controlled urethral catheter tension post transurethral resection of the prostate. Urology 1992; 40:206.

Oesterling JE, Cooner WH, Jacobsen SJ, et al: The influence of patient age on the serum prostate-specific antigen concentration: An important clinical observation. Urol Clin North Am 1993; 20:687.

Peters C, Walsh PC: Blood transfusion and anesthetic practices in radical retropubic prostatectomy. J Urol 1985; 134:81.

Reiner WG, Walsh PC: An anatomical approach to the surgical management of the dorsal vein and Santorini's plexus during radical retropubic surgery. J Urol 1979; 121:198.

Schlegel PN, Walsh PC: Simultaneous preperitoreal hernia repair during radical pelvic surgery. J Urol 1987; 137:1180.

Walsh PC, Oesterling JE: Improved hemostasis during simple retropubic prostatectomy. J Urol 1990; 143:1203.

IX
PEDIATRIC UROLOGY

51
NORMAL AND ANOMALOUS DEVELOPMENT OF THE URINARY TRACT

Max Maizels, M.D.

This chapter focuses on the embryology of the urinary tract because an understanding of early human development enables the pediatric urologist to become a far better surgeon. This understanding has been hampered because there is little access to personally examine actual embryos. This chapter alleviates this obstacle by showing actual images of human development.

Although many theories of normal or pathologic development have not been tested, they may have become accepted as factual. Although it is plausible that urologic malformations arise from aberrant normal development, this is not necessarily correct (Hamilton and Mossman, 1976a; Currarino and Weisbruch, 1989). For this reason, real data are presented in order to avoid "handing down the tale from one generation to the next without amplification or question" (Aterman, 1990). Furthermore, differences in development among species could lead to incorrect inferences when concepts based on data derived from nonhuman subjects are applied to children. With this in mind, the focus of this chapter remains primarily on human embryology.

In Table 51–1, human development is presented as a time table. For simplicity, the periods of development are presented only by gestational age. When necessary, the gestational age presented herein was derived by interpolation from crown-rump length (Table 51–2; Fitzgerald, 1978).

MORPHOGENESIS OF THE GERM LAYERS

ZYGOTE (CONCEPTION TO FIRST WEEK). Development begins after the sperm fertilizes an ovum. The combined cell, a zygote, begins development by division, cleavage, into about 30 smaller cells, blastomeres. The blastomeres congregate as a hollow sphere, the blastula, which is about the same size as the parent zygote (Fig. 51–1*A*). Darkly colored cells form an inner cell mass, the precursor of the tissues of the embryo.

LAMINAR EMBRYO (SECOND TO THIRD WEEK). The inner cell mass flattens, and the cells separate, or laminate, as two sheets of cells. One sheet, the endoderm, lines the undersurface of the inner cell mass, and the other sheet,

Table 51–1. TIME TABLE OF THE DEVELOPMENT OF THE HUMAN URINARY SYSTEM

Days After Ovulation	Developmental Event
	Period of the Embryo
18	Cloacal membrane at caudal end of primitive streak (Fig. 51–1)
20	Para-axial mesoderm and lateral plate mesoderm (Figs. 51–2 and 51–3); tail end of embryo folds to create cloaca
22	Intermediate mesoderm; pronephric duct present (Fig. 51–4)
24	Nephrotomes of the pronephros disappear Mesonephric ducts and tubules appear (Fig. 51–4)
26	Caudal portions of the wolffian ducts end blindly short of the cloaca
28	Wolffian duct has fused to the cloaca; ureteral buds appear (Figs. 51–5 and 51–6); septation of cloaca begins (Figs. 51–28, 51–30, 51–31)
32	Common excretory ducts dilate and extend into the cloaca (Fig. 51–36); metanephric mesenchyme caps the ureteral buds (Figs. 51–5, 51–6, 51–8, 51–17)
33	Ureteral buds have extended and appear as primitive pelves (Fig. 51–6)
37	Metanephroi are reniform (Fig. 51–7); ureteral bud ampullae divide into cranial and caudal poles (Fig. 51–6); elongate growth of ureter (Fig. 51–21); Chawalla's membrane (Fig. 51–22)
41	Müllerian ducts appear (Figs. 51–50 and 51–55); cloaca partitioning (Fig. 51–28); genital tubercle prominent (Figs. 51–27 and 51–29); lumen of ureter is discrete
44	Urogenital sinus separate from rectum (Fig. 51–28); wolffian ducts and ureters drain separately into the urogenital sinus (Figs. 51–34 to 51–36)
	Indifferent Stage of Embryo Begins
48	First nephrons appear (Fig. 51–8); collecting tubules appear; urogenital membrane ruptures
51	Kidneys in lumbar region (Fig. 51–18); orifices of ureters cranial to those of the wolffian ducts; müllerian ducts descend adjacent to the mesonephric ducts (Figs. 51–34, 51–35, 51–50)
52	Glomeruli appear in the kidney
54	Müllerian ducts are fused behind the urogenital sinus; Müller's tubercle distinct (Fig. 51–34); testis distinguishable
	Period of the Fetus Begins
8 weeks	Primary and secondary urethral grooves (Fig. 51–29*C*)
9 weeks	First likelihood of renal function
	Indifferent Stage of Embryo Ends
10 weeks	Genital ducts of opposite sex degenerate (Fig. 51–54); bladder muscularization
12 weeks	External genitalia become distinctive for sex; male penile urethra forming; feminization of female begins (Fig. 51–49) Urogenital union (Fig. 51–52); apex of bladder separates from allantoic diverticulum; prostate appears (Fig. 51–46); Cowper's glands (Fig. 51–48) and Skene's glands appear
13 weeks	Bladder becomes muscularized
14 weeks	Ureter begins to attain submucosal course in bladder
16 weeks	Mesonephros involuted; glandar urethra forms (Fig. 51–44); sinus vagina (Fig. 51–57)
18 weeks	Ureteropelvic junction apparent (Fig. 51–52)
20–40 weeks	Further growth and development complete the urogenital organs including, among others, testis descent after 26 weeks (Fig. 51–53); differentiation of myometrium (Fig. 51–58)

Table 51–2. CROWN-RUMP LENGTH RELATED TO GESTATIONAL AGE

Age (Weeks)	Length (mm)
4	5
5	8
6	12
8	23
12	56
16	110
20	160
24	200
28	240
32	280
36	310
40	350

After FitzGerald MJT (ed): Abdominal and pelvic organs. *In* Human Embryology. New York, Harper & Row, 1978, p 106.

the ectoderm lines the upper surface. The lamination of the inner cell mass into an endoderm and an ectoderm layer marks the blastoderm. Cleavages of the ectoderm and endoderm enlarge as the amniotic cavity and yolk sac, respectively (Fig. 51–1*B*). During the third week, cells migrating between the ectoderm and endoderm streak the previously smooth surface of the blastoderm (see Fig. 51–1*C* and *D*). These cells accumulate into the mesoderm. At the caudal end of the primitive streak the mesoderm does not separate the endoderm from the ectoderm, and the layers remain apposed in later stages of development as the cloacal membrane (see the section entitled Development of the Cloaca).

SOMITE EMBRYO (THIRD TO SIXTH WEEK). The primordial germ cells are visible in somite embryos (Fig. 51–2).

Thereby, there are three germ layers. During the period of the embryo (to 8 weeks of development), the germ layers form the organs of the body. During the period of the fetus (8 weeks to term), the formed organs mature.

CONCEPTS OF MOLECULAR BIOLOGY

Molecular biologic concepts are overviewed before kidney development is shown (Table 51–3). **Development may be viewed to result from a program of differential gene activation and repression, which modulates cell proliferation and differentiation (Hardman et al, 1994).**

Transcription factors, growth factors, and genes are the molecular controls that underpin kidney development. The strategy of molecular biology research may involve randomly searching cDNA libraries and then conducting in situ hybridization to identify and localize new molecules that may be implicated in development.

Transcription Factors

So-called master genes may encode proteins, which bind DNA and thereby affect DNA transcription. These proteins control differentiation by orchestrating the expression of other genes, which, in turn, encode locally produced growth factors (e.g., insulin-like growth factor [IGF-2]). Oncogenes encode transcription factors, which may be involved in tumorigenesis.

Growth Factors

Growth factors are small proteins, polypeptides, which after release from within cells, may stimulate cell proliferation, inhibition of proliferation, differentiation, and transformation migration. The factors act by binding to specific-cell membrane receptors; the complex may activate a phosphorylation-mediated cascade of intracellular transductional events, which signals the nucleus to synthesize morphogenetic molecules. The factors are likely important in development, because there is an ontogeny during development for the mRNA encoding the factor itself and its receptor; also, perturbing growth factor interactions alter development (Hammerman et al, 1992).

The factors can act as blood-circulating hormones on the cell in which they are synthesized (autocrine), or on nearby (paracrine) or contiguous (juxtacrine) cells.

A synopsis of growth factor families includes the following (Hammerman et al, 1992):

1. IGFs. IGF-proinsulin–like single chain peptide growth factor (IGFs) is present in the blood so it can act as a hormone; it is made in liver. Prenatal renal production of IGF-1 depends on stimulation by growth hormone (GH)–like peptides, whereas postnatal renal production depends on GH itself (GH-IGF-1 axis; Hammerman et al, 1992). IGF-2 is viewed as a fetal growth factor.
2. Epidermal growth factor (EGF) and transforming growth factor (TGF)-αα. EGF/TGF-α peptides act via the same membrane receptor to stimulate tubulogenesis. EGF is known to stimulate proliferation of embryonic lung epithelium. Receptors are found on the end buds of the epithelium comparable to the ureteric bud (Perantoni et al, 1991).
3. TGF-β. This growth factor belongs to a family of dimeric proteins (two disulfide-linked monomers) with five distinct molecular forms (TGF-β1–5). Müllerian inhibiting substance (MIS) is TGF-β5 (Hammerman et al, 1992). The biologic actions are diverse and inhibit or stimulate cell proliferation and migration, differentiation, and extracellular matrix formation. With such extensive activities, the factor is implicated in cell and tissue remodeling characteristic of development.
4. Platelet-derived growth factor. This is a polypeptide dimer. It is a mitogen for connective tissue cells (Hammerman et al, 1992).
5. Fibroblast growth factor (FGF) (acidic and basic). This is grouped within a large family of peptides that binds heparin. FGF may involve vascularization of the nephron.
6. Nerve growth factor (NGF)-β. The NGF-β receptor mRNA, or both, for NGF are identified in kidney, bladder, or during nephron differentiation. Interference with NGF expression inhibits kidney morphogenesis (Hammerman et al, 1992).

Conserved Families of Genes

Genes may show sequences with a specific DNA binding motif (paired box [PAX]) or may be strongly conserved in

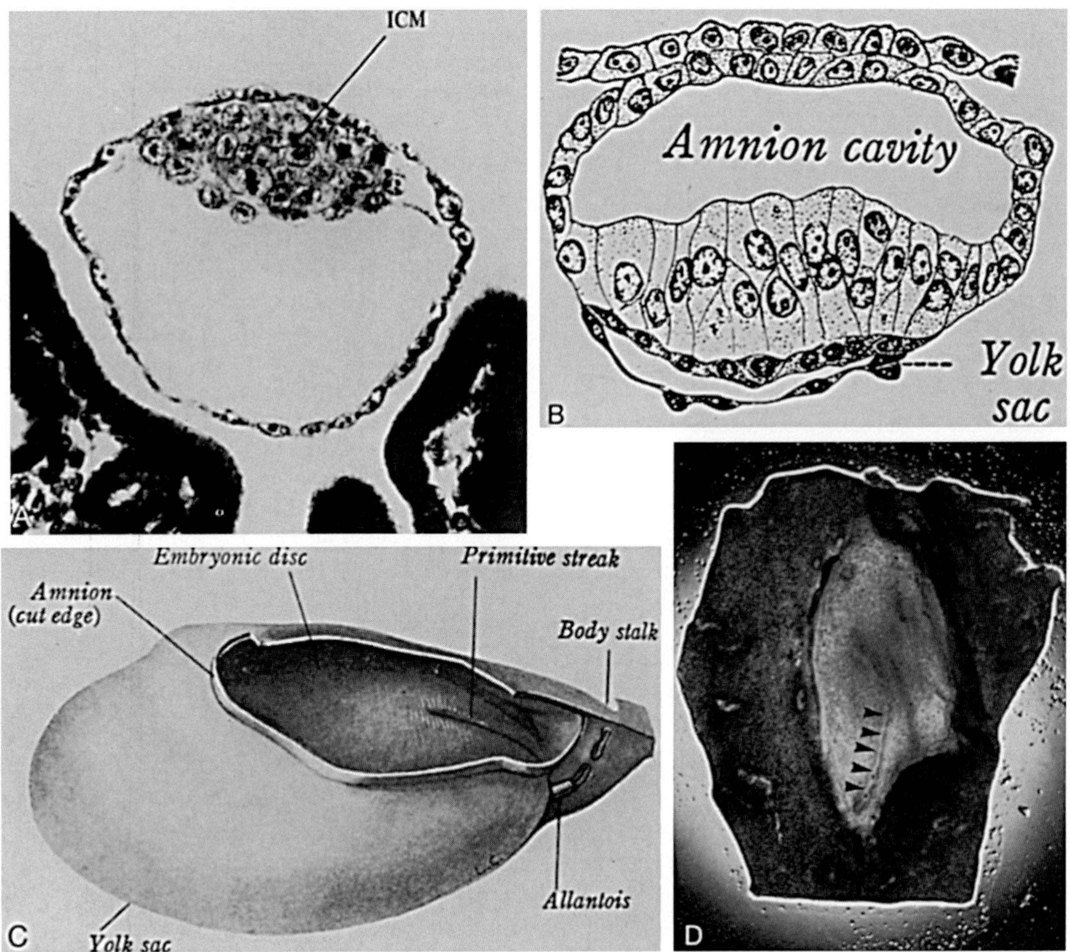

Figure 51–1. Morphogenesis of the germ layers. *A*, Blastocyst consists of cells arranged as a sphere. Some cells aggregate as the inner cell mass (ICM) (blastocyst of bat). (From Austin CR, Short RV: Reproduction in Mammals, Book 2. Embryonic and Fetal Development, 2nd ed. Cambridge, Cambridge University Press, 1973.) *B*, The inner cell mass laminates into endoderm and ectoderm. Clefts above and below the cell layers develop into the amnion cavity and yolk sac, respectively (monkey). (From Arey LB: Developmental Anatomy, Philadelphia, W. B. Saunders Company, 1974.) Cell migration between the endoderm and ectoderm streaks the smooth blastoderm. These migrating cells develop into mesoderm. *C*, Primitive streak of the human. (From Arey LB: Developmental Anatomy. Philadelphia, W. B. Saunders Company, 1974.) *D*, Primitive streak (*arrowheads*) is located in the center of the clear blastoderm (wet mount of the chick embryo viewed by transillumination).

evolution (homeobox [HOX]). The genes encode transcription factors.

Apoptosis

Apoptosis is genetically programmed, active cell death. This is an important mechanism in embryonic morphogenesis, presumably to eliminate unwanted cells (Coles et al, 1993).

Traditionally, cell death is believed to occur by necrosis. Namely, cell injury leads to cell rupture and, thereby, death. The cell contents flood the interstitium and excite an inflammatory response. Apoptosis is another mechanism for cell death; death is programmed to occur as a normal event. In apoptosis, there is transcriptional activation of a calcium-sensitive endonuclease, which degrades DNA. Characteristically, during apoptosis, there is nuclear condensation, shrinkage, and fragmentation; fragmentation of cytoplasm; and cell shrinkage. The cell fragments are rapidly phagocytosed without an accompanying inflammatory response. The absence of an inflammatory response and the rapidity of cell fragment removal have made this process inconspicuous when tissues have been examined by routine histology.

The three suggested varieties of apoptosis could guide urinary tract embryogenesis. The three varieties of apoptosis are (1) phylogenetic apoptosis—cell death associated with vestigial structures (e.g., appendix testis in a male), (2) morphogenetic—cell death associated with sculpting of specific structures (e.g., glans urethra), and (3) histogenic—cell death associated with cell differentiation (e.g., metanephrogenic mesenchyme) (Coles et al, 1993).

OVERVIEW OF THE NORMAL DEVELOPMENT OF THE URINARY SYSTEM

The definitive urinary system results from complex interactions of embryonic mesoderm with itself and with endoderm. This development seems to repeat that of lower vertebrate adults: the pronephros persists in cyclostomes (e.g., lamprey), the mesonephros is the functional kidney of amni-

Table 51–3. SYNOPSIS OF MOLECULAR BIOLOGICAL AGENTS THAT MAY BE INVOLVED IN DEVELOPMENT OF THE URINARY TRACT

Normal Development	Related Maldevelopments
Ureter bud outgrowth	Renal agenesis
Formin	
Ureter bud branching	
Promoted by	
EGF, HGF, TGF-β	
Protein kinase C phosphorylation	
Inhibited by	
NGF receptor and NGF	
Metanephrogenesis	
Promoted by	
EGF, NGF, TGF-α	Polycystic kidney disease
IGF-1 and -2	Abundant in Wilms' tumor (Goodyer et al, 1991)
Transferrin	
Inhibited by	
TGF-β	
Nephron segmentation	
Promoted by	
EGF, TGF-α, IGF-1 and -2	
Inhibited by	
TGF-β	
Vascularization of the nephron	
Heparin-binding growth factors	
FGF-basic (angiogenesis)	
Extracellular matrix proteins	
Collagen I, III	Ratio alters bladder compliance
Fibronectin	Dysplasia
Tenascin	Seaming up urethra
Epithelial basement membrane–specific proteins	
Collagen IV, V	Alport's syndrome
Laminin dysplasia/prevents formation of nephric vesicle	Bud branching (Fouser and Arner, 1993)
Proteoglycans	
Heparin sulfate proteoglycan	
Entactin, cytokeratin	
Fetal uterus	
EGF, FGF, IGF (Glatstein et al, 1994)	
Chromosomal/genic	
Chromosome 11p13	
WT1 gene product targets IGF-2	Wilms' tumor, genitourinary abnormalities, aberrant nephrogenic mesenchyme differentiation (hypoplasia/aplasia/nephroblastomatosis) (Poleev, 1992)
HOX	
Pax	
Renal tubule induction	

EGF, Epidermal growth factor; FGF, fibroblast growth factor; HGF, hepatocyte growth factor; IGF, insulin-like growth factor; TGF, transforming growth factor.

otes (e.g., fish), and the metanephros is the definitive kidney of most birds. These phases are repeated in humans. The first urinary tissue to appear is the pronephros; next, the mesonephros; and finally, the metanephros.

Pronephros

During the fourth week of development, condensed mesoderm adjacent to the midline segments into cubes in tandem, somites (Fig. 51–3). The pronephros appears in the cervical region of the ten-somite embryo between the second and sixth somites (Hamilton and Mossman, 1976a). Cells, presumably derived from the intermediate mesoderm, cluster and then differentiate into pronephric tubules. The tubules do not function. The duct of the pronephric tubules is believed to continue caudally as the mesonephric duct (Fig. 51–4*A*). The pronephros is soon inapparent.

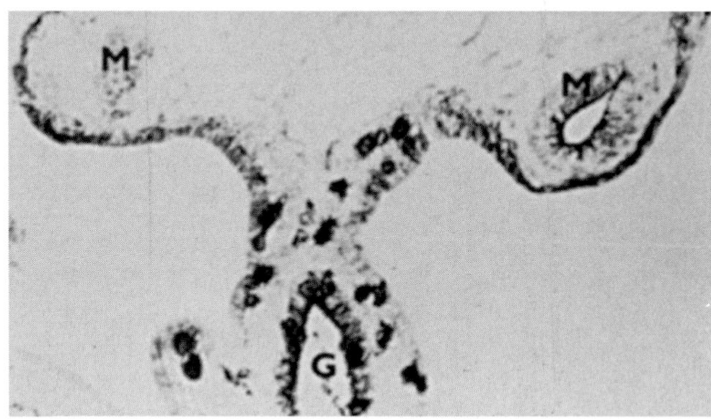

Figure 51–2. Germ cells. Migration of primordial germ cells, which are darkly stained by reaction with alkaline phosphatase, is evident in somite embryos (26 to 44 days). Alkaline phosphatase is lost from the endodermal cells of the allantois and gut but not from the primordial germ cells (28-day-old human embryo). (G, gut; M, mesonephric vesicle; × 37). (From Jirasek JE: Birth Defects 1977; 2:13.)

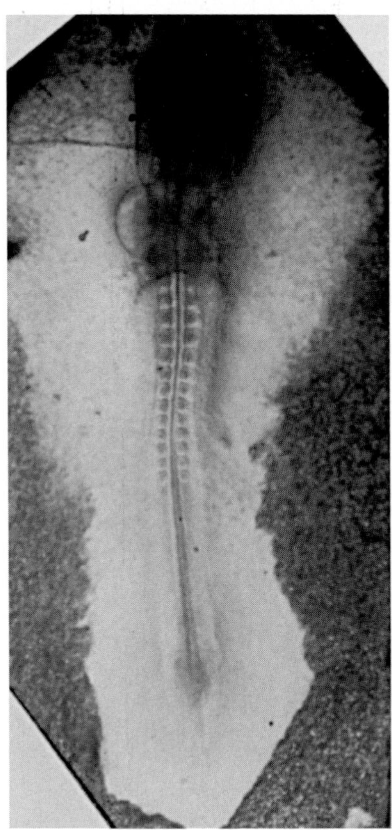

Figure 51–3. Somite stage of development. Mesenchyme condenses as blocklike structures, the somites. A row of somites flanks each side of the midline (wet mount of chick embryo).

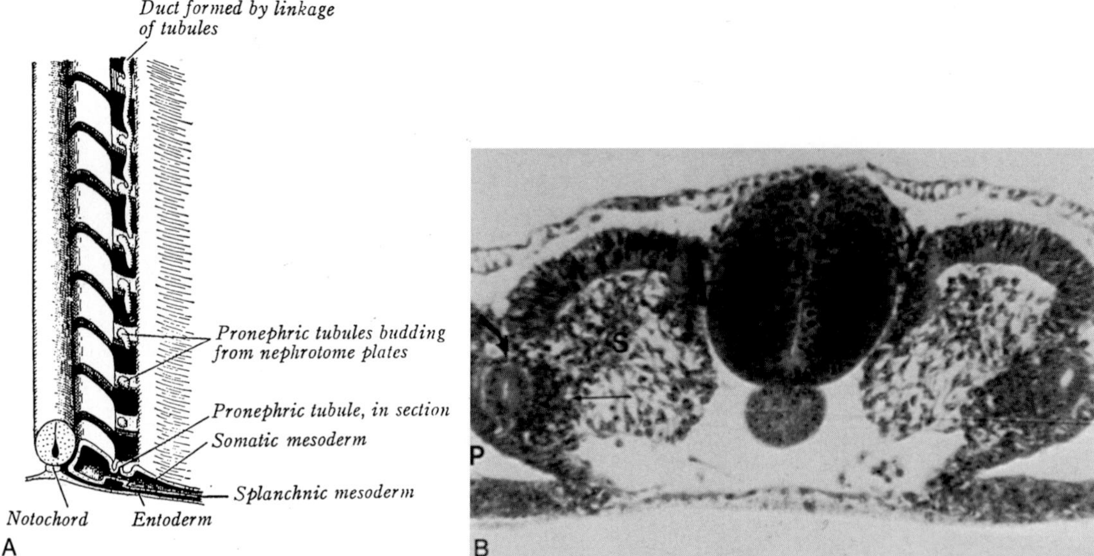

Figure 51–4. Development of the pronephros and mesonephros. *A*, The pronephric duct of lower vertebrates forms by linkage of pronephric tubules. In humans, the pronephric duct probably continues caudally as the mesonephric duct. (From Arey LB: Developmental Anatomy. Philadelphia, W. B. Saunders Company, 1974.) *B*, The mesonephric duct *(curved arrow)* apposes mesoderm *(straight arrow)* intermediate between the somite (S) and the coelom (P). Mesonephric tubules appear after the inductive interaction between the duct and mesoderm (chick embryo). (From Maizels M, Stephens FD: The induction of urologic malformations: Understanding the relationship of renal ectopia and congenital scoliosis. Invest Urol, 1979; 17:209. © The Endocrine Society.)

Mesonephros

The mesonephric (wolffian) duct appears at the level of the cervical somites. By elongate growth of the terminus of the duct, it descends to reach the caudal end of the embryo. The duct descends adjacent to the mesoderm intermediate between the somites and the coelom (primitive peritoneum) (Fig. 51–4*B*). After the duct and mesoderm appose, mesonephric tubules appear. The nephrons of the mesonephros are induced by the advancing ampulla of the mesonephric duct analogous to the induction of nephrons of the kidney during period 3 of ureteric bud development (see the sections entitled Development of the Ureteric Bud and Nephrogenesis). As the mesonephric duct descends, about 40 tubules are induced (Potter, 1972).

By 28 days, the mesonephric duct has contacted the urogenital sinus into which it later drains. By 37 days, the mesonephroi are fully developed; they appear as paired retroperitoneal organs that bulge into the median of the peritoneum (see Figs. 51–5, 51–29, and 51–35). After 10 weeks of development, the caudal mesonephric nephrons degenerate (Felix, 1912a), while the cranial nephrons persist and become incorporated into the genital duct system (see the section entitled Development of the Ducts of the Genitalia).

The human mesonephros is believed to function (Gersh, 1937). Dilatation of the allantois and bulging, followed by rupture of the cloacal membrane, are interpreted to result from hydrostatic pressure generated after secretion of mesonephric urine (Muecke, 1979). Convolution of the tubules and appearance of glomeruli are also evidence of function. Because the mesonephroi of several mammals can excrete marker dyes (e.g., phenol red) (Hamilton and Mossman, 1976a), it is believed the human mesonephros can clear the plasma of unwanted metabolites.

Oyer (1992) has shown mesonephric tissue frequently persists in humans to midgestation. This finding is consistent with anecdotal case reports, which cite embryonic tissue in children. Perhaps such retained rests of embryonic tissue may contribute to extrarenal Wilms' tumor.

It is considered that the mesonephros contributes Sertoli and Leydig cells to the testis or granulosa to the ovary by virtue of anatomic proximity to the gonadal ridge (Oyer, 1992).

Kidney

DEVELOPMENT OF THE URETERIC BUD. After the mesonephric duct drains into the urogenital sinus, the ureteric bud appears. The bud originates as a diverticulum from the posteromedial aspect of the mesonephric duct at the point where the duct bends to enter the cloaca (Fig. 51–6*A*). The most cohesive view of the later development of the ureteric bud derives from microdissections of human embryonic kidneys (Potter, 1972).

There are two patterns of ureteric bud development, which involve either symmetric or asymmetric branching. Branches that are symmetric show similar activities (during period 1, the branchings are symmetric—each branch contributes to form the pelvis and calyces; during periods 1 and 2, the branchings are symmetric—each one induces tubules). Conversely, branches that are asymmetric show different activities (during period 3, the branchings are asymmetric—one branch of the bud induces tubules, the other simply extends toward the cortex). The phrases in italics capsulize development in that period.

PERIOD 1 (5TH TO 14TH WEEK). The initial 4 to 6 *dichotomous branchings* of the ampullae mold the renal pelvis. The metanephrogenic mesenchyme has proliferated

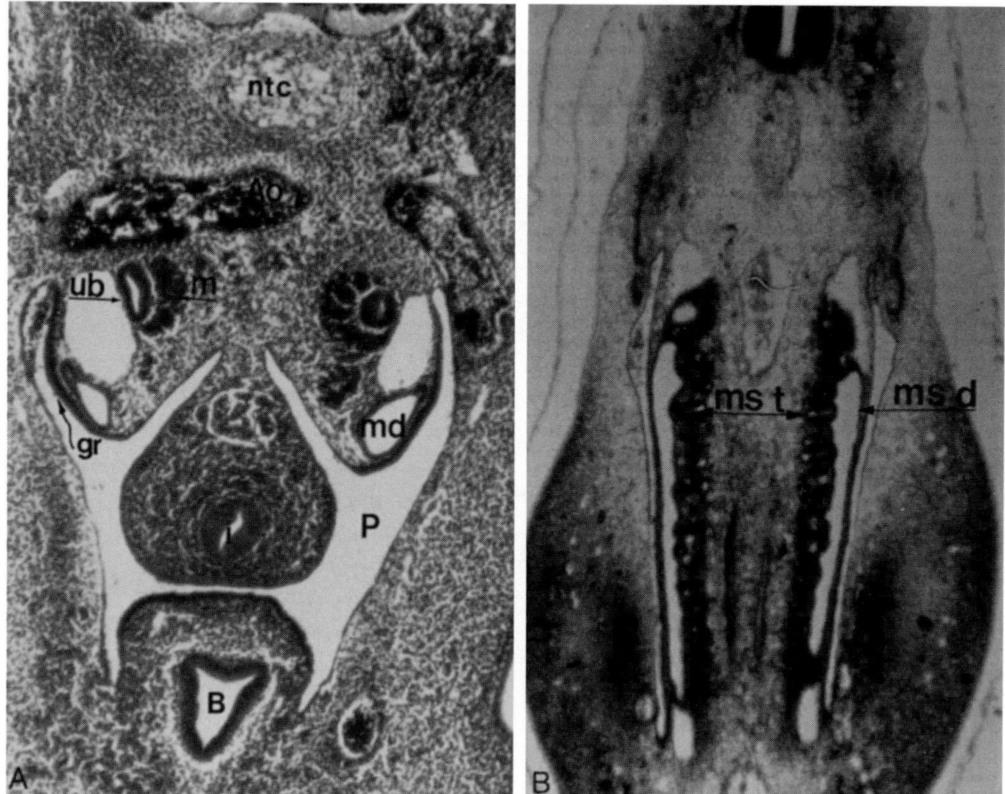

Figure 51–5. Spatial relationship of retroperitoneal and intraperitoneal organs. *A*, Kidney blastema consists of ureteral bud (ub) and its apposed mesenchyme (m). The mesonephric duct (md) is between the renal blastema and gonadal ridge (gr). Note the thickened epithelium. Bladder (B) is an epithelial tube (transverse section of chick embryo) (i, intestine; Ao, aorta; ntc, notochord; P, peritoneum). *B*, Mesonephric tubules (ms t) extend longitudinally along retroperitoneum and drain into mesonephric duct (ms d) (coronal section of chick embryo).

to appose all of the new ampullae of the new ureteric bud branches. The initial branching establishes the inferior and superior poles of the kidney. Branching near the poles of the kidney occurs faster than branching near the midsection. Because of this asynchrony, by 7 weeks, there are about six generations of ampullae at the poles of the kidney and only four generations of ampullae at the midsection of the kidney. The asynchronous branching helps maintain the reniform shape of the kidney (Fig. 51–7) (Hamilton and Mossman, 1976b).

This primitive network of ureteric bud branches dilates and creates the appearance of the pelvis and calyces (Fig. 51–6*B* and *C*). Asymmetric dilatation of the branches may explain the variable appearance of the pelvis and calyces in the newborn.

The subsequent three to five generations of branchings contribute to the calyces. The branchings occur so rapidly that the many branches appear to arise from a common stem. This common stem initially resembles a bulbous chamber (Fig. 51–6*D* and *E*). With later growth, the renal parenchyma projects into this chamber as a conical papilla. This projection converts the bulbous chamber into the cup shape of the definitive calyx (Fig. 51–6*F*). The branchings that occur after 7 weeks are the first to induce nephrons (Fig. 51–8). The bud branching is symmetric. Each branch leads to nephron formation (see the section Nephrogenesis).

The next five to seven generations of branchings of the ampulla of the ureteric bud initiate the collecting ducts. During this interval, branching progresses more slowly. Therefore, as the ampullae extend toward the periphery of the kidney, the collecting ducts laid down close to the calyces are short and wide, whereas the collecting ducts laid down close to the periphery are long and slender.

PERIOD 2 (15TH TO 22ND WEEK). The *ampullae divide infrequently* and a family of nephrons is induced by a single ampulla. Interstitial growth of the collecting ducts causes the ampullae to extend centrifugally toward the surface of the kidney. As each ampulla extends, a family of about four (range of two to eight) nephrons is laid down seriatim as arcades or tiers (Fig. 51–9). The site where the collecting ducts begin centrifugal growth is the corticomedullary junction. The central zone, the medulla, contains the mass of collecting ducts; the peripheral zone, the cortex, contains the nephrons that are attached to collecting ducts. The collecting ducts in the cortex are straight (without branches).

PERIOD 3 (22ND TO 36TH WEEK). As the ampulla grows, it extends further toward the cortex of the kidney. As the ampulla migrates, it *induces about four to six nephrons in series* (see Fig. 51–9). This period of development creates nephrons whose glomeruli lie in the outer half of the cortex. About 75% of the kidney's glomeruli are induced during periods 2 and 3 of development.

PERIOD 4 (32ND TO 36TH WEEK TO ADULTHOOD). The ureteric bud *ampullae cease to induce* new nephrons. The ampullae are inapparent. During this period, the collecting ducts elongate, the proximal tubules convolute, and the loops of Henle penetrate deeper into the medulla. A

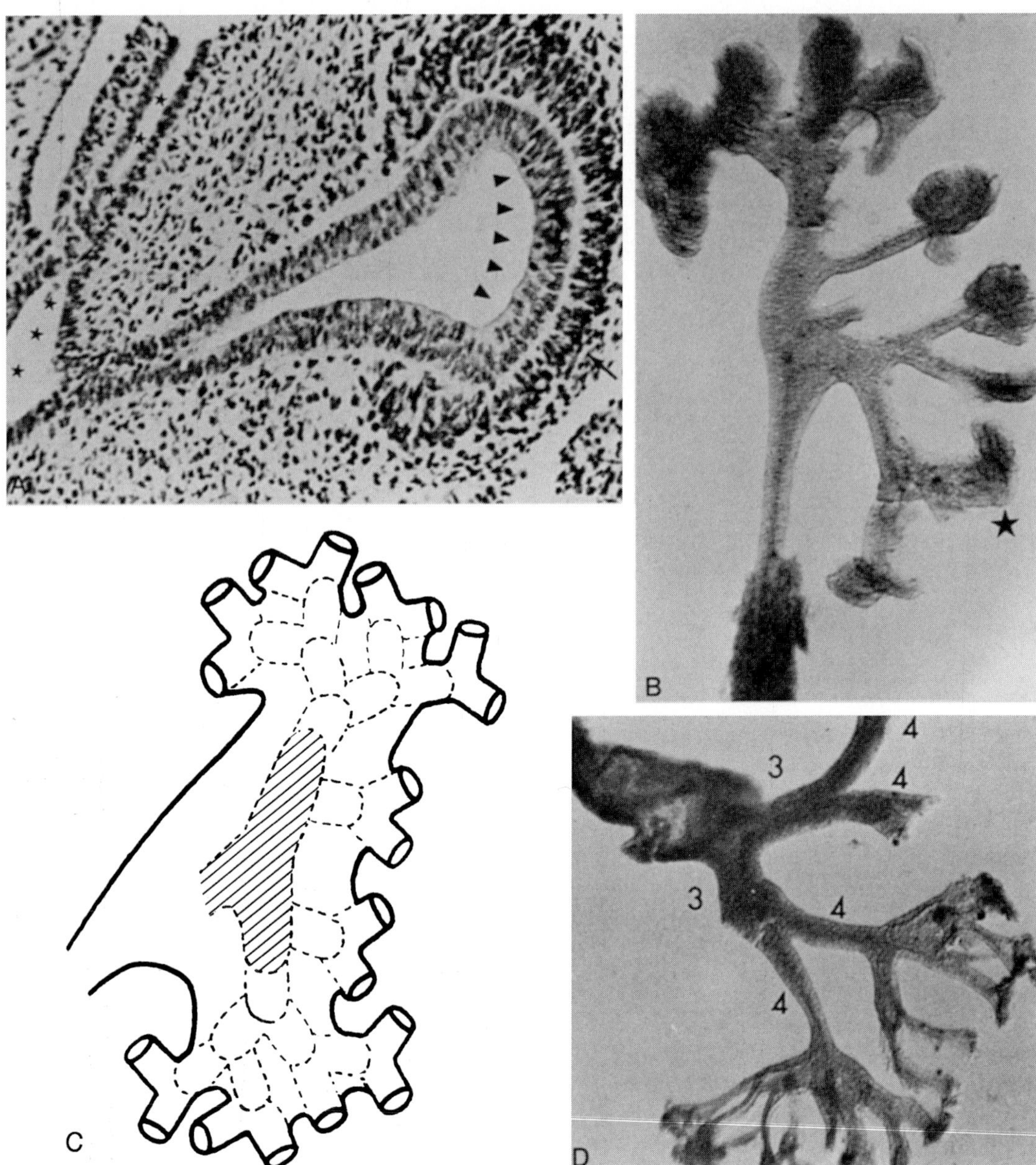

Figure 51–6. Period 1 of the development of the ureteric bud.

A, Ureteric bud *(arrowheads)* arises as a diverticulum from the mesonephric duct *(asterisks).* Metanephric mesenchyme *(black arrow)* surrounds the ampulla of the ureteric bud (28-day-old embryo) (see Fig. 51–4*A*).

B, The ampullae branch dichotomously. The branches then dilate to establish the primitive pelvis and calyces (8-week-old human embryo) *(asterisk,* see *D).*

C, Schematic of *B* to show how dichotomous branchings *(dashed lines)* of the primitive ureteric bud *(hatches)* dilate to create the renal pelvis *(solid outline).*

D, Rapid branchings of the ampullae create a bushlike appearance. The base of the bush becomes a bulbous chamber, a calyx (10-week-old human fetus; numbers refer to generations of ampullary divisions).

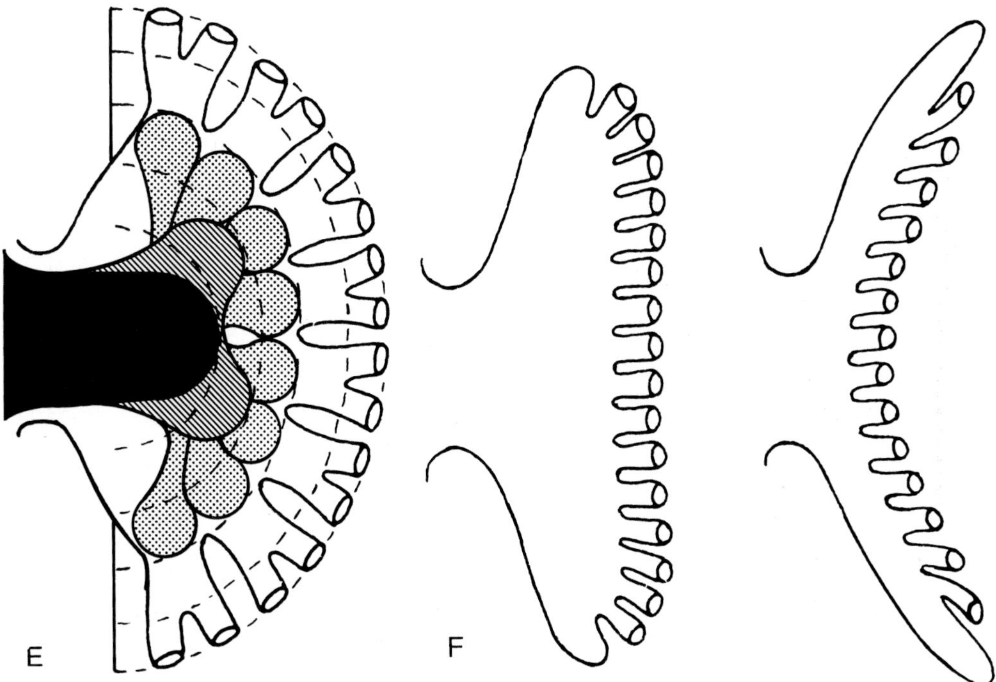

Figure 51–6 *Continued*

E, Schematic of *D* to show development of a calyx. Rapid division of an ampulla *(solid black)* produces multiple short branches of the ureteric bud *(hatches and stippling).* The resultant bulbous chamber is the primitive calyx.

F, Development of a papilla. With secretion of urine and growth of nephrons, the renal tissue flattens the contour of the calyx *(left)* and then intrudes into the lumen of the calyx as the renal papilla *(right).* (From Potter EL: Normal and Abnormal Development of the Kidney. Chicago, Year Book Medical Publishers, 1972.)

typical collecting duct drains about 9 to 11 nephrons. Nephron induction by a branching ureteric bud causes the kidney surface to appear lobular at birth (see Fig. 51–7).

Molecular Biology of Kidney Development

Molecular Biology of Nephric Duct Ascent and Descent

Elongate growth of ducts pervades development of the genitourinary tract with descent of the pronephric, mesonephric, and müllerian ducts toward the cloaca and ascent of the ureter to the lumbar retroperitoneum.

Pronephric duct descent in the axolotl involves elongation by rearrangement of the cells at the tip of the duct. The diameter of the duct tip is narrower than elsewhere, and the cells migrate actively. Poole and Steinberg (1982) concluded that a craniocaudal gradient of adhesion established by the mesoderm guides the migration of the adjacent duct cells. Philopodia mediate the cell contact. The distribution of cell surface alkaline phosphatase activity is consistent with this enzyme being involved in guiding the descent (Zackson and Steinberg, 1988).

Ureteric bud ascent in mammals **initiates topographically near the hind limb bud, so it is considered possible that outgrowth of the limb and ureteric bud may be related phenomena.** This factor may explain why defects of the appendicular skeleton (vertebral defects, imperforate anus, tracheoesophageal fistula, and radial and renal dysplasia [VATER]) are associated with renal anomalies (Van Groesen et al, 1990).

From this perspective, renal agenesis may relate to deficient outgrowth of the ureteric bud (Maas et al, 1992). Mass and colleagues (1992) have pursued heritable renal agenesis in a mouse model (i.e., autosomal recessive renal agenesis and syndactyly and radioulnar fusion), and the condition

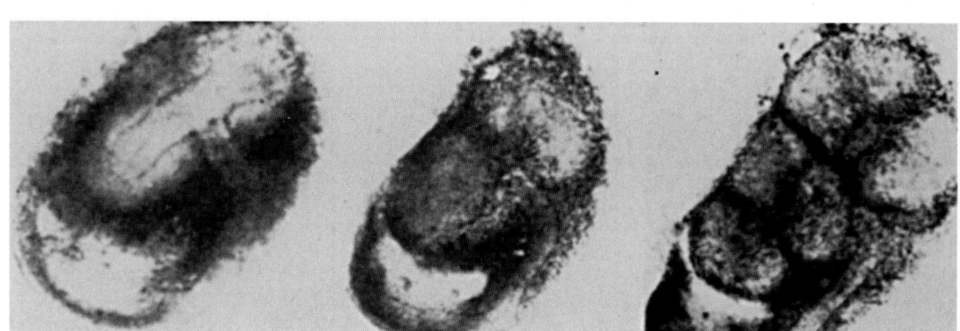

Figure 51–7. Time lapse motion picture prints showing lobular development of mouse kidney in vitro. Branching of the ureteral bud yields lobular renal architecture. (From Saxen L, Toivonen S, Vainio T, Korhonen D: Z Naturforsch 1965; 20b:340.)

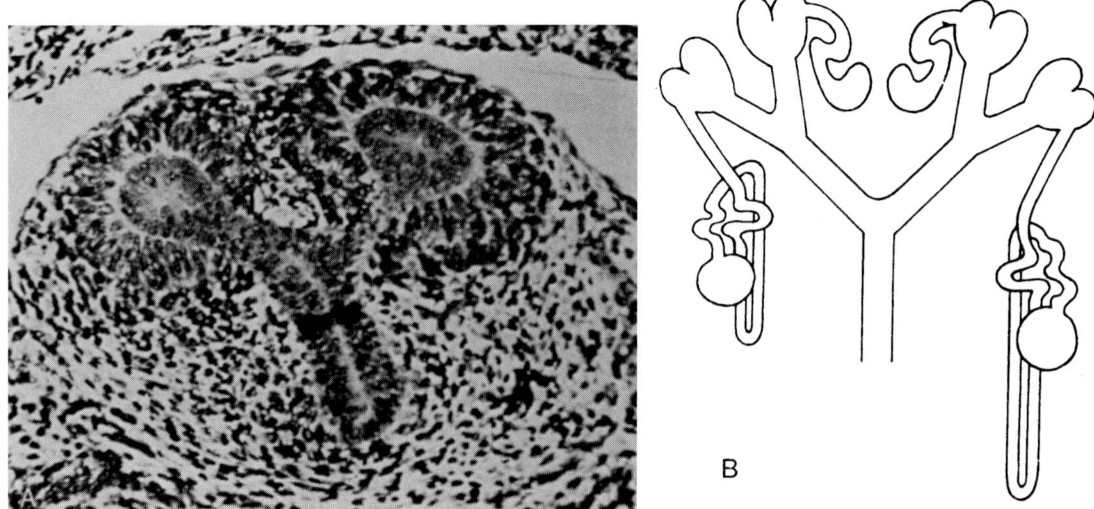

Figure 51–8. Induction of nephrons during period 1 of development of the ureteral bud. *A,* Ampullae branch dichotomously. Each branch remains capped by condensed mesenchyme. *B,* Each branch induces a nephron from its cap of undifferentiated metanephric mesenchyme (schematic). (From Potter EL: Normal and Abnormal Development of the Kidney. Chicago, Year Book Medical Publishers, 1972.)

may involve the gene, formin. The limb deformity likely relates to poor outgrowth of the limb bud ridge. The renal defect result from the same source as the ureteric bud fails to grow out from the wolffian duct and, therefore, does not contact the metanephrogenic mesenchyme (Fig. 51–10). Furthermore, agenesis or hypoplasia results from retarded renal development. Coculture of bud-deficient mesenchymes with potent kidney inducer tissue rescued the induction because the mesenchyme then developed satisfactorily. Molecular responsibility for the failure of induction could not be assigned to either the bud or mesenchyme because gene product transcripts were identified from both components of the blastema. Maas believes that delayed ureteric bud outgrowth desynchronizes the mesonephric duct epithelium interaction with the surrounding mesenchyme. Perhaps close study of the development of the mesonephric duct may provide a more comprehensive explanation of the associated wolffian anomalies seen in cases of renal agenesis in girls (e.g., Mayer-Rokitansky syndrome). Gentamicin reduces the number of glomeruli in vitro, perhaps by interfering with ureteric bud branching (Gilbert et al, 1994).

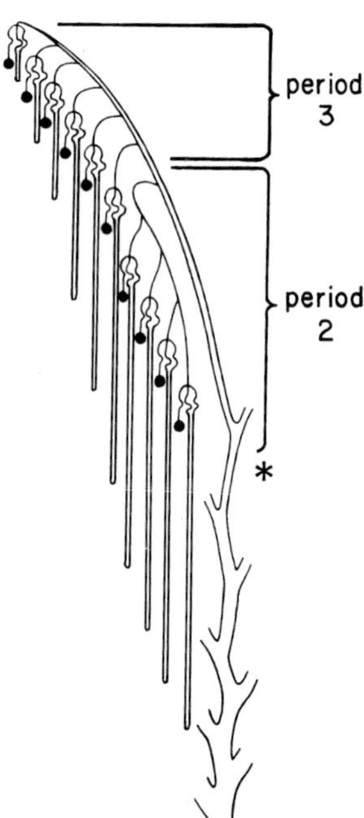

Figure 51–9. Periods 2 and 3 of the development of the ureteric bud. During period 2, as the ampullae migrate toward the cortex, a family of about four nephrons is induced seriatim as "arcades" or tiers by each ampulla. During period 3, a series of about five nephrons are induced, which attach directly to the collecting duct. (*Asterisk* marks site of corticomedullary junction.) (After Potter EL: Normal and Abnormal Development of the Kidney. Chicago, Year Book Medical Publishers, 1972.)

Molecular Biology of Ureteric Bud Branching

The long-held concept that isolated ureteric buds do not grow or branch in vitro has been shaken by Perantoni and colleagues (1991). By culturing ureteric buds bared of their mesenchyme on a surface of gelled type I collagen, the buds branched (Fig. 51–11) (Perantoni et al, 1991). Furthermore, applying leukemia inhibition factor (LIF) blocks nephrogenesis but permits the maintenance of a well-branched and developed duct system (Bard and Woolf, 1992). The mechanisms responsible for ureteric bud branching are speculated by Nigam (1995) to involve positional gradients of growth factors, extracellular matrix, and proteases as the mechanism whereby bud branching is executed. The factors facilitate migratory growth at leading edges of the branch and are inhibitory at branch clefts (Hinchliffe et al, 1992a). The factors are reviewed next (Hardman et al, 1994).

Transcription Factors

Because a branching epithelium is common to many organs (salivary gland, pancreas, lung), it is reasonable to consider that there may be a common branching mechanism. Perhaps, the WT1 gene, which is identified in induced renal

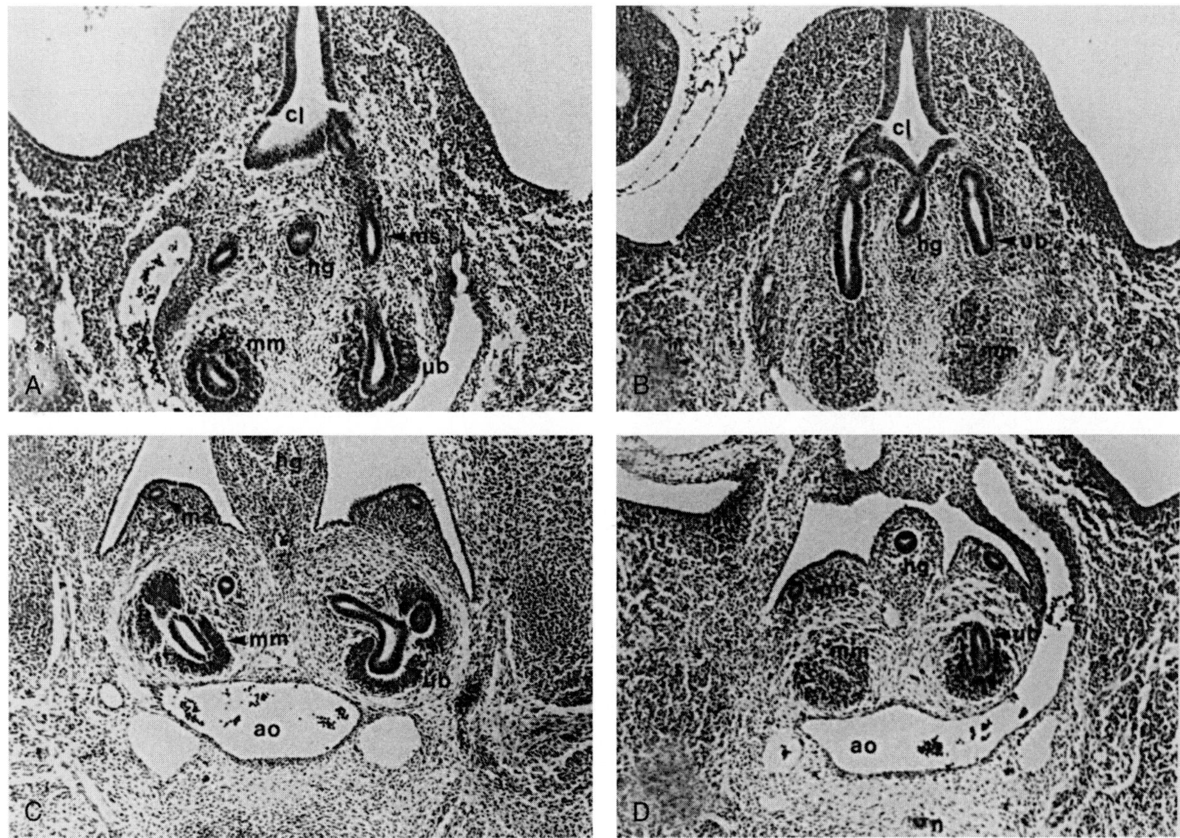

Figure 51–10. Renal agenesis relates to faulty outgrowth of the ureteric bud from the mesonephric. *A*, Normal ureteral bud (ub) contacting metanephrogenic mesenchyme (mm) (hg, hindgut; cl, cloaca). *B*, Renal agenesis is likely in the mutant embryo because the ureteral buds *(arrow)* do not grow out to contact the metanephrogenic mesenchyme (mm) and will likely undergo apoptosis if not induced (*A* and *B*, 12-day mouse embryo). Slightly later in development, the normal embryo shows bilateral well-developed, branched ureteric buds *(C)*, whereas the mutant embryo shows absent or slow bud development despite apposition to the metanephric mesenchyme *(D)* (*C* and *D*, 12.5-day mouse embryo) (ao, aorta). The metanephrogenic mesenchyme is not induced, so renal agenesis develops. (From Maas R, Elfering S, Glaser T, Jepeal L: Deficient outgrowth of the ureteric bud underlies the renal agenesis phenotype in mice manifesting the limb deformit (ld) mutation. Dev Dyn 1994; 199:214–228. Reprinted by permission of John Wiley & Sons, Inc.)

mesenchyme and nephron epithelia, may encode transcription factors, which serve as branching molecules. For example, abolished expression of WT1 in mouse renal mesenchyme is associated with failure of the wolffian duct to branch (Hardman et al, 1994). On the other hand, PAX-2 genes are also expressed within the ureteric bud and its derivatives, but to date there is no evidence that supports their role in branching.

Growth Factors

Growth factors are distributed in mesenchyme of branching organs and are implicated in branching.

EPIDERMAL GROWTH FACTOR. EGF, the adult homologue of the embryonic TGF, caused ureteric bud branching in vitro (Rogers et al, 1993; Hardman et al, 1994). IGF-1 or -2, or NGF added in vitro caused aberrant nephrogenesis with growth failure of both mesenchyme and ureteric bud.

HEPATOCYTE GROWTH FACTOR. The ureteric bud expresses genes that likely encode cell surface receptors, such as for hepatocyte growth factor, the agent involved in organizing the branching of cultured kidney cells. Hepatocyte growth factor enhances renal epithelia proliferation and branching by an unknown mechanism (Hardman et al, 1994). Modulation of protein kinase C phosphorylation influences this process (i.e., inhibition of phosphorylation enhances complexity of branching process, or conversely, activation of phosphorylation inhibits branching) (Santos et al, 1993).

TRANSFORMING GROWTH FACTOR-β. TGF-β can inhibit nephrogenesis and reduce gland growth. TGF-β stains the luminal surface of the ureteric bud. Exogenous TGF-β inhibits bud growth and localizes to branch clefts. In this way, TGF-β may encourage branching by inhibiting epithelial growth locally, at cleft sites (Perantoni et al, 1991). Additionally, because it can inhibit hepatocyte growth factor secretion, perhaps it regulates branching via this interaction (Hardman et al, 1994).

Cell Adhesion and Extracellular Matrix

Perhaps localized deposition of matrix molecules, such as fibronectin, stabilize clefts in the epithelium (Hardman et al, 1994). The activity of growth factors may be modulated by binding to matrix proteoglycans (Hardman et al, 1994). For example, the proteoglycan syndecan binds to FGF and prevents degradation of FGF. As another mechanism, syndecan could co-participate to alter the cytoskeleton and cause

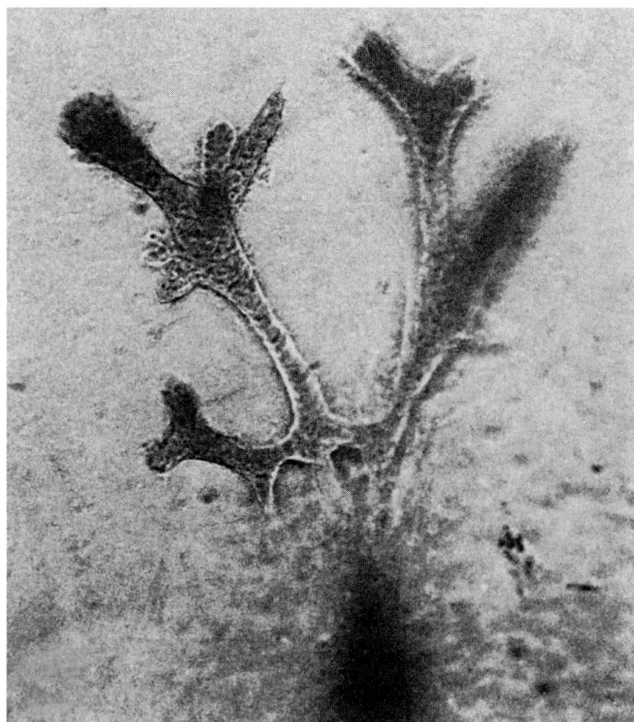

Figure 51–11. Ureteric buds may branch in vitro when grown on a collagen gel support. (Explanted for 4 weeks, × 63). TGF-β may localize to clefts to facilitate branching. (From Perantoni AO, Williams CL, Lewellyn AL: Growth and branching morphogenesis of rat collecting duct anlagen in the absence of metanephrogenic mesenchyme. Differentiation 1991; 48:107–113.)

branching. For example, a purse-string–like contraction of microfilaments at one end of a cell could change the cell shape from a cylinder to a cone and thereby initiate invagination of an epithelium (Hardman et al, 1994). TGF-β may be involved in this process (Hardman et al, 1994).

CLINICAL CORRELATES OF BRANCHING DYSMORPHOGENESIS. Kallmann's syndrome, which involves renal agenesis, shows a mutation of the gene involved with extracellular matrix protein that is homologous with fibronectin, which is called KAL. Because this KAL gene is expressed in the normal fetal kidney, perhaps the lack of renal expression of KAL results in this syndrome.

Theoretically, variations in bud growth, and the timing and location of branching could lead to a spectrum of uropathies of the kidney and ureter (Mellins, 1984), such as a bifid or extrarenal pelvis, the anomalous appearance of the collecting system of a pelvic kidney, or branchings of the ureteric bud that fail to induce nephrons and may coalesce with an adjacent calyx to result in a calyceal diverticulum (Middleton and Pfister, 1974).

Aberrations in branching of the bud during period 1 of development likely engender the anomalous patterns of partial to complete duplication. Septation of the ureteric bud as a bifid, duplex, triplicate, and even partial quadruplication has been reported (Bolkier et al, 1991). Duplication of the vas is viewed to be an extension of the phenomenon (Binderow et al, 1993). Although duplication of the ureter with ectopia may occur in children of either gender, girls may suffer from wetting related to ectopia, whereas boys do not. One case report of a boy who suffered from wetting is an exception to this observation (Ejaz and Malone, 1995).

Apoptosis appears to have a role in the mechanisms of absorption of the common excretory duct into the trigone and the associated migration of the ureter (Gage and Sulik, 1991). Pregnant mice exposed to ethanol during the gestational period that would correspond to late in the fourth week in humans showed fetal hydronephrosis resembling that in infants with fetal alcohol syndrome. Duplication and megaureters also were present.

Molecular Biology of Nephrogenesis

Research has unraveled many of the mechanisms that induce the undifferentiated metanephric mesenchyme of a single phenotype, as viewed by the light microscope, to transform into a specialized epithelium with different phenotypes. Unless otherwise cited, the information presented here largely derives from a review presented by Saxen (1987).

The steps of nephrogenesis are as follows: First, unspecialized mesenchyme is induced and then proliferates. Next, an altered distribution of cytoskeletal and extracellular matrix proteins results in morphogenesis of the tubule. Then, the tubule epithelium segments to acquire different phenotypes, and finally, the nephron becomes vascularized.

Induction of the Nephron

Nephrons are induced by the interaction between an ampulla of the ureteric bud and its adjacent metanephrogenic mesenchyme during period 1 to 3 of ureteric bud branching (see earlier discussion).

Features important to induction are discussed in the following sections.

CLOSE CELL CONTACTS ARE IMPORTANT TO INDUCTION. Grobstein (1956) showed the metanephrogenic blastema will not differentiate into tubules if the metanephrogenic mesenchyme does not closely contact the ureteric bud or another inductor tissue. Cell processes from the ureteric bud will reach out even across the pores of a filter in vitro to the metanephrogenic mesenchyme to initiate induction (Lehtonen et al, 1975). If the tissues are separated to prevent close contact, the ureteric bud does not branch, and the metanephrogenic blastema does not differentiate.

Furthermore, as the basement membrane of the ureteric bud epithelium is discontinuous only where induction occurs, at the tips of the ampullae, close cell contacts with the metanephrogenic mesenchyme are fostered (Saxen et al, 1987). This observation using electron microscopy is supported by the results of immunohistochemical experiments (described in the section entitled Altered Constituents of Cytoskeletal Proteins and Extracellular Matrix Constituents Shift).

Tissues other than the ureteric bud can induce the metanephrogenic blastema to differentiate into tubules (Unsworth and Grobstein, 1970). For example, nervous tissue, especially that of the thoracic spinal cord, can also induce nephrons across a filter (Sariola et al, 1989). The neurons within the tissue are the cells responsible for induction. Nervous tissue treated by immunologic cell lysis to be composed only of glial and undifferentiated cells does not induce tubules, although nervous tissue that contains neurons does induce tubules. This process shows specificity because many other cell types penetrate the filter but do not induce tubules.

NERVE-RELATED ACTIVITIES. Although it is unlikely that neurons themselves are involved in nephrogenesis in vivo, cells expressing neurofilaments are noted around the wolffian duct. Sariola (1988) showed that nerves enter the early developing kidney along the ureter. It has also been demonstrated that antibodies that disturb nerve-mesenchymal binding or antisense oligonucleotides that bind to nerve growth factor receptor mRNA disrupt induction (Bard and Woolf, 1992). Furthermore, cytoskeletal neurofilaments are identified in peritubular stromal cells. They are believed to derive from neural crest rather than mesoderm (Sainio et al, 1994).

APOPTOSIS. Demise of metanephrogenic mesenchyme occurs in the absence of induction by inductor tissue. The inductive process maintains cell integrity and avoids apoptosis of the mesenchyme (Koseki, 1993). Koseki showed that DNA fragmentation was prominent in mesenchymes explanted without inductor. The active fragmentation of the DNA is reduced when apoptosis is inhibited (e.g., by inhibiting protein synthesis or RNA transcription). Also, introduction of inductor tissue to the explant reduced apoptosis. EGF reduced apoptosis but did not lead to differentiation. From these data, induction is believed to involve initial inhibition of apoptosis in the metanephrogenic mesenchyme, which rescues the mesenchyme for differentiation (Koseki et al, 1992; Coles et al, 1993).

PHENOTYPE CONVERSION. Although it is traditionally believed that the metanephrogenic mesenchyme derives from the intermediate mesoderm, startling research by Herzlinger and colleagues (1993) using lineage analysis shows that the ureteric bud epithelium, especially at the tips of the branched bud ampullae, can undergo phenotypic conversion into mesenchyme and contribute to the pool of metanephrogenic mesenchyme. Perhaps, this mechanism is analogous to the phenotypic conversion of the metanephrogenic mesenchyme into tubule epithelium by delamination (see later in text). It is unknown whether or not such conversions occur in vivo (Herzlinger et al, 1993).

PROLIFERATION. Proliferation condenses the induced metanephrogenic mesenchymal cells by two mechanisms. First, persistent direct contact with an inductor tissue (ureteric bud in vivo or spinal cord in vitro) stimulates the metanephrogenic mesenchyme to proliferate. The proliferation is probably mediated by a mitogen, perhaps transferrin. After induction, a burst of DNA synthesis (uptake of radiolabeled thymidine) is observed and cell division follows. Second, after the period of inductive contact, the mesenchymal cells may continue to differentiate without requiring direct contact with an inductor. However, the mesenchyme is now responsive to growth factors within the embryo. The inductive signal appears to spread away from the ureteric bud ampullae via migration of induced metanephrogenic mesenchyme. This would bring the yet uninduced mesenchymal cells that are deep in the renal blastema into contact with the inductor (Saxen, 1987). The number of cells, which have now increased, aggregate, and the renal rudiment grows. Furthermore, the aggregation of cells promotes morphogenesis because there are enough cells to express a new phenotype (i.e., tubular epithelium). Postinductive nephrogenesis may be regulated by mechanisms balanced by local inhibitory and stimulatory growth factors. These may involve local autocrine or paracrine growth factor systems.

CYTOSKELETAL PROTEINS AND EXTRACELLULAR MATRIX CONSTITUENTS SHIFT. It appears that components of extracellular matrix may participate in the initiation of nephron morphogenesis. Using immunohistologic techniques, it was shown that interstitial antigens (see Table 51–3), which are present before induction, are lost during induction (Ekblom et al, 1986). The collagens are lost at the ampullae of the ureteric bud, and fibronectin is lost from the mesenchyme. Fibronectin disappears perhaps because the newly formed cells are unable to elaborate the glycoprotein, or perhaps because proteolytic enzymes in the interstitium degrade it. Because fibronectin has been shown to promote cell mobility, the absence of this product could be responsible for reduced cell mobility, which condenses the mesenchyme. Or it may be that the loss of extracellular matrix permits closer cell apposition and restricts cell mobility, and thereby the cells aggregate. Laminin, which appears intensely after induction, may further encourage aggregation of the cells (Saxen, 1987). The interstitium is now predominated by epithelial-type proteins (see Table 51–3). Perhaps induced metanephrogenic cells synthesize glycoproteins after induction; glycoproteins extruded into the interstitium could then control morphogenesis. The importance of extracellular matrix materials is further strengthened by finding syndecan in the blastema. This is a cell surface proteoglycan, which binds to interstitial proteins (e.g., collagens and fibronectin) and distributes temporally with renal differentiation. Namely, syndecan first appears intensely in the metanephrogenic mesenchyme adjacent to the ureteric bud and precedes the shift in distribution of interstitial glycoprotein described earlier. Syndecan is still present in the differentiating epithelium and is gradually lost as the nephron matures. Syndecan appears to be specific to tubule induction because syndecan is not expressed when metanephrogenic mesenchyme is cultured with tissues that do not show induction (i.e., liver) (Vainio et al, 1989). Mixed species grafting experiments show that syndecan is elaborated by the renal mesenchyme and not from the inductor tissue.

Cell-adhesive molecules (CAMs), such as the neural N-CAM and uvomorulin, may help maintain tubule adhesion. For example, in mouse renal blastema, the metanephrogenic mesenchyme shows N-CAMs before induction. After induction, the N-CAMs are lost and a new CAM, uvomorulin, is expressed. It appears that N-CAMs are important adhesives for predetermined but as yet uninduced nephrogenic mesenchyme. N-CAMs are not expressed as a consequence of induction (Klein et al, 1988).

Just as changes in the distribution of constituents of the extracellular matrix are noted with induction, the distribution of constituents of the cytoskeleton also changes. One such change involves vimentin filaments. These filaments are present in uninduced mesenchyme. Induction of mesenchyme is associated with loss of the filaments. The filaments remain only in undifferentiated mesenchyme between new renal tubules.

MORPHOGENESIS. Inductive interaction in the kidney results in the unique conversion of mesenchyme into an epithelium with a basement membrane. The primitive tubule is the nephric vesicle and emerges from the aggregated metanephrogenic cells. First, a discontinuous basement membrane lines the vesicle. Next, the induced mesenchymal cells condense and the nuclei polarize to a basal position to form an epithelium. It appears that the transition of the mesenchyme to epithelium is also associated with synthesis of large size proteoglycans (Lash et al, 1983). The cells laminate into a comma-shaped, double-layered structure, then swell as a vesicle, and finally connect with the collecting tubule. The tubules then elongate and coil. The two steps of nephrogenesis, change in the extracellular matrix and morphogenesis of tubules, appear metabolically different. For example, inhibitors of DNA, RNA, or protein synthesis impair the morphogenesis of tubules when they are applied to the metanephrogenic blastema during induction but not if they are applied later (Ekblom, 1981).

LINKAGE OF NEPHRON TUBULE TO COLLECTING DUCT. The developing tubule connects with the collecting duct during the S-shaped vesicle stage. Linkage probably relates to local digestion of basement membranes around the duct and confluence of the epithelia (Abrahamson, 1991). In the mouse, genes that express collagen type IV (α 1 and 2) become active during nephrogenesis when this collagen is incorporated into basement membrane formation. The genes become quiescent after nephrogenesis (Sawczuk et al, 1988).

SEGMENTATION. Immunohistochemical studies can identify the glomerulus by podocytes, proximal tubules by the brush border, and the distal tubule by Tamm-Horsfall protein. These studies show that segmentation of the nephron is sequential and proceeds in the following order: glomerulus, proximal, and then distal tubule. The cells that participate in creating the visceral layer of Bowman's capsule flatten and angiogenic cells invade (see the section entitled Vascularization of the Nephron) to create vascular tufts. Potter (1972) counted 822,300 glomeruli in the kidney of a 40-week-old fetus. Glomerular counting of whole fetal kidneys of rats shows that there is an initial phase involving a burst of glomerular differentiation, followed by a second phase of elaboration of tubular development (on basis of tubular length) (Okada and Morikawa, 1988). Glomerular counting in the rabbit also shows a burst of new glomerular development during the early part of gestation (McVary and Maizels, 1989).

Perhaps, abnormal tubular segmentation may account for renal tubular dysgenesis, an autosomal recessive condition characterized by a kidney that contains collecting ducts and glomeruli but not tubules (Swinford et al, 1989).

GLOMERULOGENESIS. Glomerular development may be viewed in two stages—capillary loop stage glomeruli and maturing stage glomeruli.

Capillary Loop Stage Glomeruli. Basement membranes of podocyte and endothelial cells appose, forming a double basement membrane (Fig. 51–12). As the glomerulus matures, podocyte foot processes appear, the endothelium fenestrates, and a single basement membrane emerges. A variety of molecular biologic changes accompany these maturational processes. Glomerular growth is achieved most likely by capillary subdivision, which results in an increased number and length of capillaries (Akoaka et al, 1994).

Splitting and lamination of the normally fused basement membrane is noted in Alport's syndrome, perhaps resulting from an error in collagen type IV synthesis (Bard, 1992).

Maturing Stage Glomeruli. Basement membrane assembly continues and involves mostly the podocytes. Foot process formation is more complex. These activities enhance the surface area for glomerular filtration.

ONTOGENY OF THE RENIN NETWORK. The to-

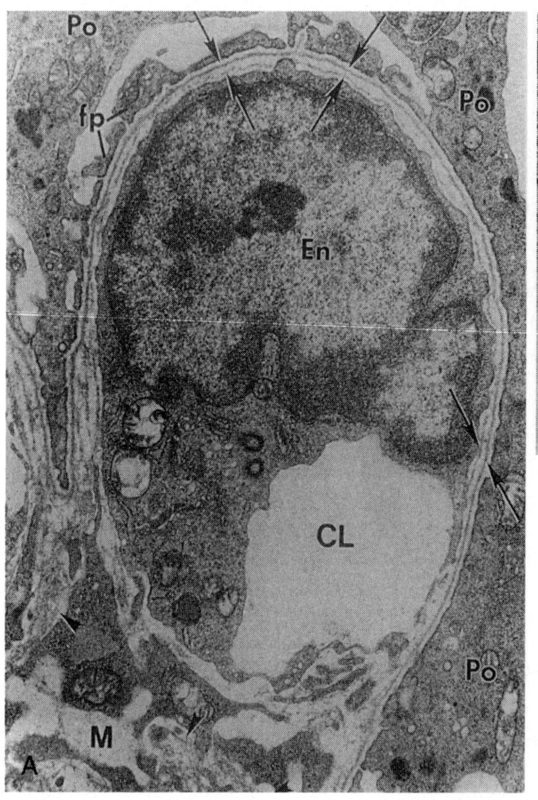

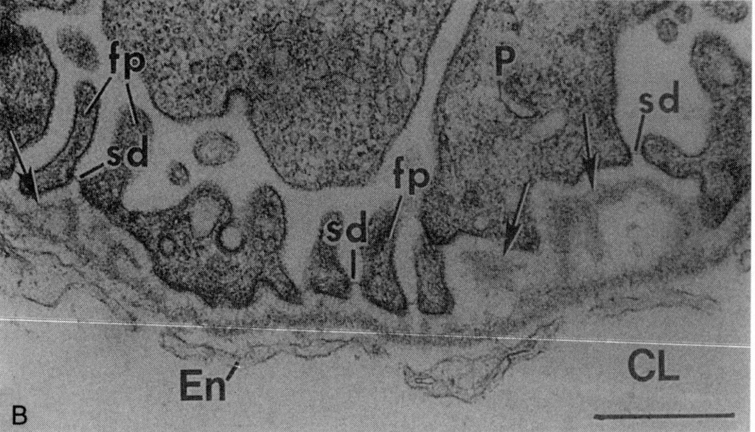

Figure 51–12. Capillary loop (CL) stage glomerulus. *A*, Basement membranes of podocyte and endothelial cells appose forming a double basement membrane. (From Bremer JL: The origin of the renal artery in mammals and its anomalies. Am J Anat 1915; 18:179.) The endothelial cell (En) and podocyte (Po) cell membranes appose (*opposite arrows*) (M, mesangium; fp, foot processus) (Original mag × 19,000; scale bar = 1.5 μm). *B*, Maturing stage glomerulus. Slit diaphragms (sd) expose the endothelium between the podocyte foot processus. The double basement membrane is absent now (newborn rat kidney) (original magnification × 52,000; scale bar = 0.5 μm). (From Abrahamson DR: Glomerulogenesis in the developing kidney. Semin Nephrol 1991; 11:375–389.)

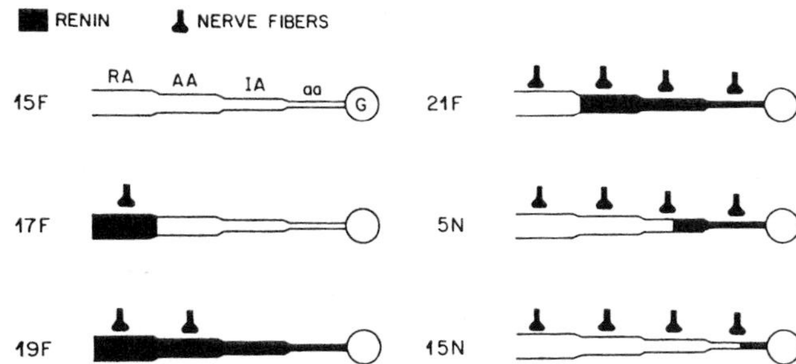

Figure 51–13. Ontogeny in renin and nerve fiber distribution in the developing kidney (RA, renal artery intrarenal branches; AA, arcuate artery; IA, interlobular artery; aa, afferent arteriole; F indicates days of fetal gestation; N indicates days old as a newborn rat). (From Pulilli C, Gomez RA, Tuttle JB, et al: Spatial association of renin-containing cells and nerve fibers in developing rat kidney. Pediatr Nephrol 1991; 5:690–695.)

pography of cells that stain for intracellular renin changes during development. Renin-containing cells (rat stage equivalent to human stage of mid gestation) initially appear within the tunica media of large renal arteries. The topographic pattern moves serially during later stages of development from intrarenal arterial branches, to arcuate arteries, to interlobular arteries, to afferent arterioles of glomeruli in the juxtamedullary region (nerve fiber bundles now are seen surrounding the main renal artery branches) and afferent arterioles of many glomeruli, to later shift to the final distribution within the cells of the juxtaglomerular apparatus (delicate nerve fibers surround the afferent and efferent arterioles, but not renal tubules) (rat stage equivalent to human term) (Fig. 51–13) (Pulilli et al, 1991).

MONITORING GLOMERULOGENESIS. Counting the nonfetal (i.e., not subcapsular) glomeruli along a ray of collecting ducts provides an index of renal development. The count correlates with gestational age to more objectively diagnose hypoplasia or to ascertain somatic growth delay (Fig. 51–14) (Hinchliffe et al, 1992c). For example, asymmetric growth retardation (intrauterine growth retardation) was significantly associated with reduced nephron number at birth (Hinchliffe et al, 1992b). Furthermore, after birth, infants with a history of intrauterine growth retardation who died did not show renal compensation in nephron number or size. Applying this principle of nephron development to cases of vesicoureteral reflux that came to nephrectomy shows that about one half of the patients have less than 25% of normal glomerular counts and are diagnosed as having renal hypoplasia (Hinchliffe et al, 1992a). It is surprising that coexisting obstruction did not correlate with the severity of cortical loss. **Thereby, minimal renal function in cases of vesicoureteral reflux could reflect inherently limited renal function rather than a failure of clinical management.** This represents support for the notion that renal dysgenesis may accompany dysfunction of a ureteric bud that originated from an aberrant site on the wolffian duct (Stephens, 1983).

VASCULARIZATION OF THE NEPHRON. Immune staining for endothelial antigens shows tissue regions adjacent to the metanephric mesenchyme that are avascular and likely are capillary precursors. The spatial relationship between the developing nephrons and the differentiating vasculature is shown (Fig. 51–15) (Kloth et al, 1994). After the nephric vesicle appears, the primitive Bowman's capsule segments from the renal tubule. This begins when mesenchymal cells migrate into the cleft of the vesicle. These cells differentiate into endothelial cells. Primitive capillaries later form and then contain mature erythrocytes (presumably derived from the general circulation). It is speculative but reasonable to consider that growth factors within the basement membrane, such as FGF, stimulate angiogenesis by

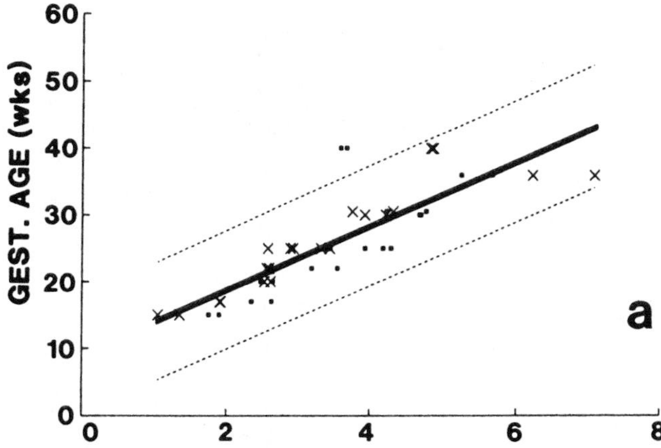

Figure 51–14. Mean medullary ray glomerular count correlated with gestational age. The approximate linear regression equation gestational age = 9 + 5 × (glomerular count) on x axis handily permits diagnosis of appropriate or delayed renal development using histologic material. (Adapted from Hinchliffe SA, Sargent PH, Chan YF, et al: "Medullary ray glomerular counting" as a method of assessment of human nephrogenesis. Pathol Res Pract 1992; 188:775–782.)

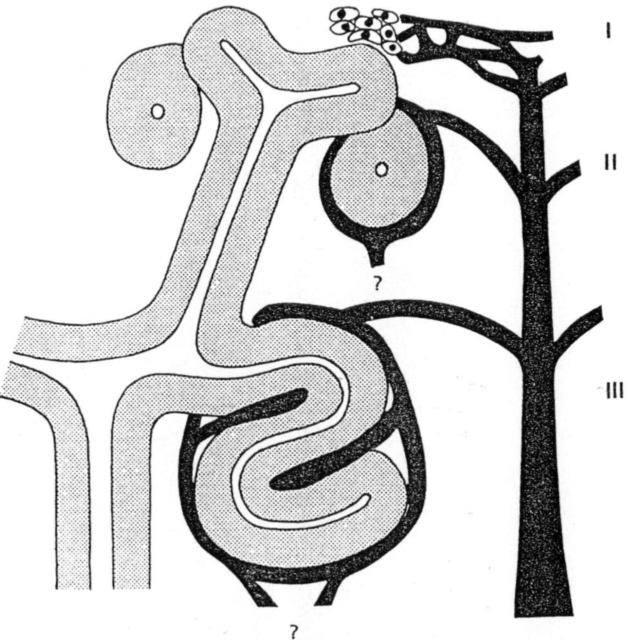

Figure 51–15. Spatial relationship between the developing nephrons and differentiating vasculature is schematized. I, capillary precursors express endothelial antigen adjacent to the ureteral bud ampulla. II, the nephric vesicle is enclosed by vessel-like structures, which stain for epithelial antigen. III, capillary network evident. Venous connections to capillaries are not yet mapped. (From Kloth S, Aigner J, Schmidbauer A, Minuth WW: Interrelationship of renal vascular development and nephrogenesis. Cell Tissue Res 1994; 277:247–257.)

encouraging the migration of precursor endothelial cells into the vascular clefts of the developing glomeruli (Abrahamson, 1991).

It appears that the endothelial cells do not derive from the renal blastema (Abrahamson, 1991). Namely, when mouse metanephric blastema is grafted on the CAM of quail eggs, the glomerular capillaries show the nuclear marker of quail cells while the glomerular podocytes are of mouse origin.

Perhaps the alteration in cellular constituents described earlier promotes vascularization of the nephron. Namely, the degradation of collagen and fibronectin makes split products. These products show angiogenic activity. The nearby mesenchyme may thereby differentiate to vascularize the Bowman's capsule.

Other grafting experiments have shown that the glomerular basement membrane is formed from constituents of both the glomerular epithelium and endothelial cells. The origin of the mesangial cells is unknown. From available immunologic studies, it appears that the mesangial cells, like the glomerular endothelium, do not derive from the renal blastema. Also, explants of murine renal blastema develop Bowman's capsules but do not show capillary endothelium or mesangial cells (Avner et al, 1983).

Other Influences in Nephrogenesis

WT1 GENE. The WT1 gene encodes a transcription factor. This is a large protein with four zinc fingers. It binds DNA sequences that express for molecules likely involved in nephrogenesis. WT1 is noted in uninduced metanephrogenic mesenchyme cells, early nephrons and glomeruli, and Wilms' tumor. From this perspective, WT1 mutations may lead to aberrant induction and perhaps may be involved in cancer. Wilms' tumor originates from metanephrogenic mesenchyme (Hammerman et al, 1992). Chromosome 11p shows deletion of genes. The WT1 transcription product maps to the deletion region. IGF-2 and its mRNA are expressed in high levels in the tumor. Antibody to IGF-1 inhibits growth of the tumor.

HOMEOBOX. Pax 2 is expressed in mesonephros and metanephros. Pax 8 is closely linked to chromosome 2 centromere. Genes controlling these products are likely involved in nephric induction because pax 8 is expressed predominantly in the induced metanephric mesenchyme and pax 2 in the ureter (Fig. 51–16).

TRANSFORMING GROWTH FACTOR-α AND INSULIN-LIKE GROWTH FACTORS 1 AND 2. TGF-α and IGF-1 and IGF-2 are synthesized by the rudimentary kidney and promote tubulogenesis; although TGF-β1 is also produced within the metanephros, it exerts negative control on tubulogenesis, perhaps by localizing to the ampullary tips of the branching ureteric bud. It stimulates formation of extracellular matrix and, thereby, retards induction of new nephrons (Rogers et al, 1993). TGF-α antibodies inhibit nephrogenesis in vitro (Hardman et al, 1994).

HEPATOCYTE GROWTH FACTOR. Hepatocyte growth factor activity may be involved in mesenchyme to epithelial transformation.

TRANSFORMING GROWTH FACTOR-β. TGR-β mouse and rat kidneys cultured with TGF-β show reduced growth differentiation and tubulogenesis.

MORPHOGENESIS OF RENAL DYSPLASIA

Importance of Metanephrogenic Mesenchyme

Metanephrogenic cells are required for normal nephrogenesis, and it appears that the absence of the cells leads to dysplasia (Maizels and Simpson, 1983). Chick renal blastemas that are depleted of condensed metanephrogenic mesenchyme by tissue culture develop further as primitive ducts consistent with those seen in human renal dysplasia (Fig. 51–17).

Sariola (1988) showed that when the mesenchyme does not remain condensed against the ureteric bud, abnormal morphogenesis results. Application of an antibody against the ganglioside G_{D3}, which is on the cell surface of the

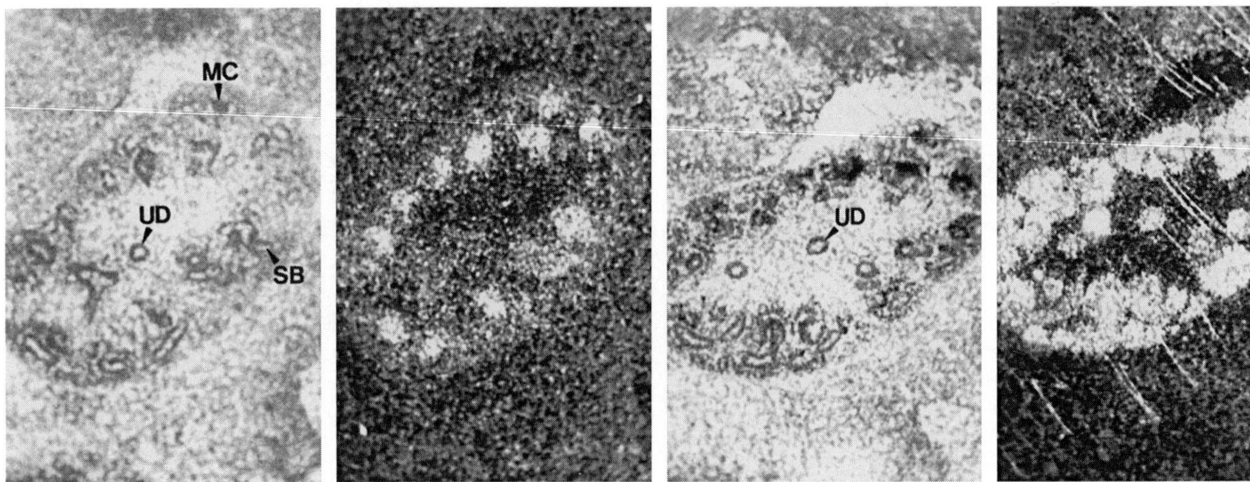

Figure 51–16. Pax 2 and Pax 8 in renal and ureteral development. Pax 8 is expressed in induced metanephrogenic mesenchyme while Pax 2 is also expressed in the ureter (UD). (Mouse 16.5-day post conception embryo, × 100). (From Plachov D, Chowdhury K, Walther C: Pax 8: A murine paired box gene expressed in the developing excretory system and thyroid gland. Development 1990; 110:643–651. Reprinted by permission of the Company of Biologists Ltd.)

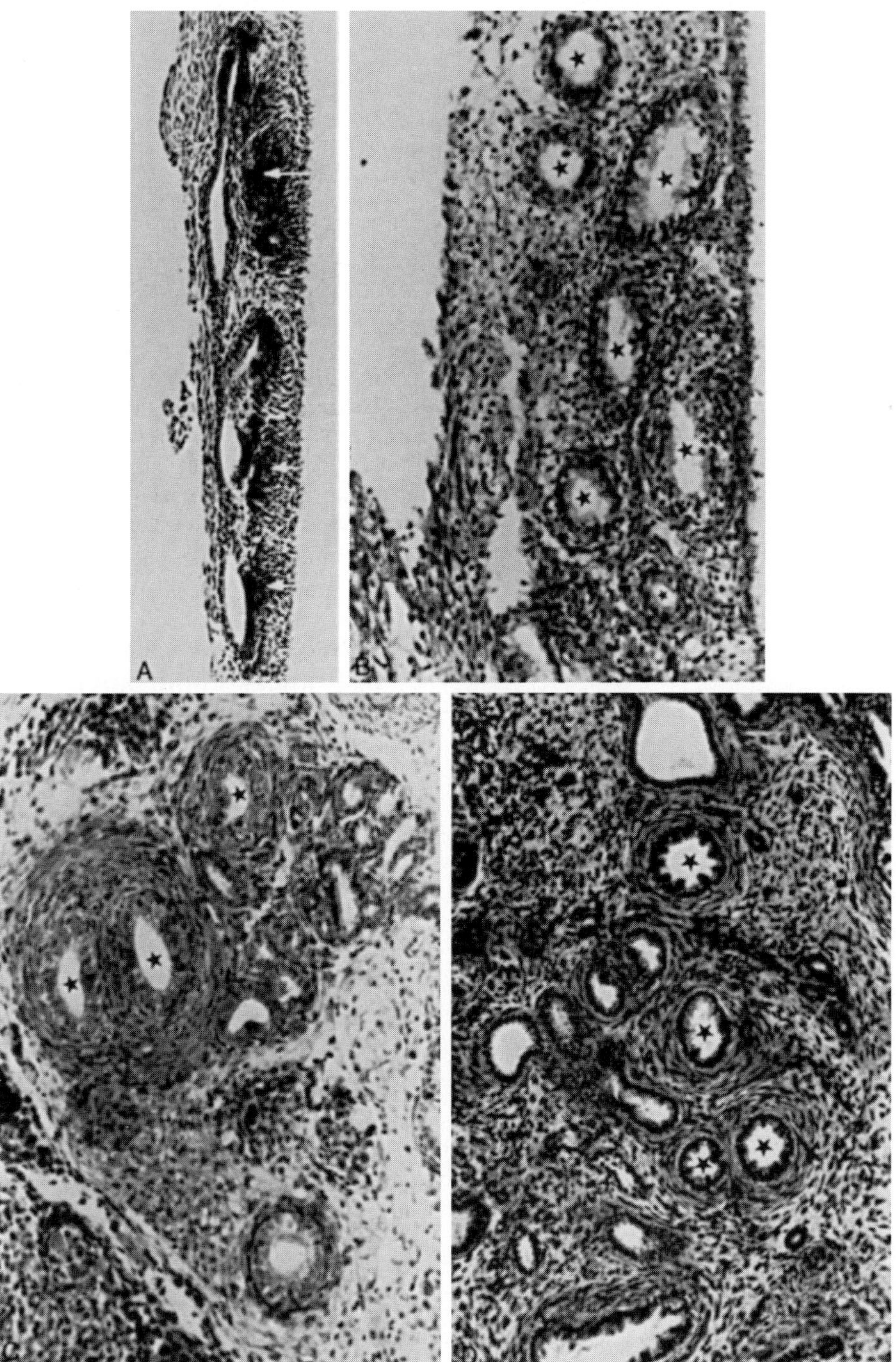

Figure 51–17. Induction of primitive ducts.

A, Longitudinal section of renal blastema microdissected from chick embryo after 8 days of incubation. Visible are segmental branches of the ureteral bud *(short arrows)* and condensed metanephrogenic mesenchyme *(long arrow)*.

B, Renal blastema microdissected from chick embryo and then cultured in vitro. Ureteric bud branches *(asterisks)* are numerous, but the metanephrogenic mesenchyme is no longer condensed or apparent. Renal tubules do not develop in vitro.

C, Renal blastema microdissected from chick embryo; then cultured in vitro to provide branched ureteric buds without condensed metanephrogenic mesenchyme; and, finally, further cultured in ovo, as a graft develops into tissue composed primarily of primitive ducts *(asterisks)*. The ducts are lined with tall epithelium and are surrounded by whorled mesenchymal cells.

D, Nephrectomy specimen in newborn with prune-belly syndrome. Primitive ducts *(asterisks)* typical of renal dysplasia are surrounded by whorled fibromuscular cells and resemble those induced in the chick embryos. (From Maizels M, Simpson SB Jr: Primitive ducts of renal dysplasia induced by culturing ureteral buds denuded of condensed renal mesenchyme. Science 1983; 219:509. Copyright 1983 by the AAAS.)

metanephrogenic mesenchyme, caused both reduced branching of the ureteric bud and tubule epithelium formation during in vitro nephrogenesis of the embryonic kidney. Perhaps, the antibody affected cell-to-cell interactions between the epithelium and mesenchyme.

Renal agenesis in a spontaneous murine mutation may be accounted for by embryos that show absent metanephros or ureteric bud, or both (Mesrobian and Sulik, 1992).

Importance of K^+ in the Extracellular Environment

In vitro differentiation of young renal rudiments (after 7 weeks' gestation) appears to require high local concentrations of potassium (Crocker, 1973). Abnormal ureteric bud branching and nephrogenesis follows in vitro exposure of human renal rudiments to low potassium concentration. There are fewer ureteric bud branches, ampullae, and nephrons. These effects were not seen when older rudiments were cultured. Bud branchings, which contribute to formation of the pelviocalyceal system, were not affected.

Importance of Matrix in the Extracellular Environment

Several experiments show the importance of the matrix. We found it perturbing that the normal shifts in the distribution of major glycoprotein constituents (e.g., fibronectin and laminin) of the interstitium have an impact on later renal development (Spencer and Maizels, 1987). The glutamine analogue DON inhibits synthesis of glycosoaminoglycans and glycoproteins and also inhibits in vitro tubulogenesis in a dose-dependent manner. The effect is specific when DON is applied to the tissues during the induction period. When explants are treated with similar inhibitors and then CAM grafted to observe their further in vivo development, the specimens show primitive ducts (Spencer and Maizels, 1987).

Furthermore, when DON is injected locally into the posterolateral body wall (avoiding the peritoneal cavity) of chick embryos during the induction period of the renal tubules, the kidneys that develop 1 week after injection show halving of the surface area of the tubules compared with controls. Dysplasia did not appear, but the paucity of nephrons resembles hypoplasia (Howe et al, 1989). This view is consistent with the conclusions of Lelongt and associates (1988), who examined the effect of perturbing proteoglycan synthesis in murine renal development. In vitro, the treated kidney showed loose mesenchyme, reduced ureteric bud branching, and fewer nephrons. This resembles the inhibition of antilaminin on murine lung development in vitro: There was less branching of the bronchial tree, the branches were dilated, and there was a dose-dependent slower growth rate than in controls (Schuger et al, 1990).

Lastly, fibroblasts that are altered to express a gene that encodes a glycoprotein secreted by embryonic spinal cord (a known inducer of renal blastema) can induce blastema to make renal tissue, which unaltered fibroblasts cannot (Herzlinger et al, 1994).

Additionally, decreased expression of proteoglycans in extracellular matrix can be induced by addition of mannose to culture medium. The kidney rudiments show dysmorphogenesis, which is seen as disorganization of the ureteric bud branches. The addition of adenosine triphosphate restored the normative appearance. Perhaps, increased endogenous sugars, such as mannose, in vitro, or glucose in vivo in diabetic mothers, alters the extracellular matrix to contribute to a variety of fetal anomalies, including renal agenesis, in diabetics (Liu et al, 1992).

Ekblom and co-workers (1986) concluded that carbohydrates are associated with the actual induction process. Saxen (1987) suggests that the molecules critical to induction (perhaps glycoproteins or carbohydrates, or both) lie at the interphase between the ureteric bud ampulla and metanephrogenic mesenchyme. This may involve growth factors, because in situ hybridization localizes IGF-1 receptor at the tips of the ureteric bud branches. Blocking the receptor reduces in vitro kidney size and disorganizes ureteric bud branching. Because reduced synthesis of extracellular matrix glycoproteins was also noted, perhaps this is the mechanism whereby nephrogenesis is perturbed (Kanwar et al, 1994).

Obstructed Urine Drainage May Not Be of Primary Importance

Clinical observations led to inferences that obstruction of urine drainage may cause renal dysplasia (Bernstein, 1971), but the validity of these inferences has not been well supported by experimental data. Obstruction by suture ligation of the ureter of normal renal blastemas of the chick embryo (Berman and Maizels, 1982) or of mammalian fetuses (Fetterman et al, 1974; Javadpour et al, 1974; Tanagho, 1972) leads to hydronephrosis, not dysplasia. However, abnormal blastemas (e.g., ureteric buds denuded of condensed metanephrogenic mesenchyme) that are obstructed develop dysplasia more often than such abnormal blastemas that develop without ligation of the ureter (Maizels et al, 1983).

The observation made by Gonzalez and co-workers (1990) was unique and showed that complete bladder obstruction applied early in lamb gestation induces bladder dilatation and abdominal wall distention that is comparable to prune-belly syndrome in humans. Furthermore, renal changes consistent with dysplasia were shown.

Clinical Renal Dysplasia

ABNORMAL URETERIC BUD AND METANEPHROGENIC MESENCHYME INTERACTIONS. When the ureters of duplex kidneys drain onto the trigone, their associated renal units are normally formed; on the other hand, when the ureters of duplex kidneys drain outside the trigone (e.g., urethra or bladder diverticulum), the associated renal units are likely to be poorly formed (hypoplasia or dysplasia). Ureters that drain outside the trigone are presumed to have originated from ureteric buds that are defective, perhaps because they were abnormally positioned on the wolffian duct. Malpositioned buds may interact poorly with the metanephrogenic mesenchyme; hypodysplasia may follow (Stephens, 1983). (See also the section entitled Molecular Biology of Nephric Duct Ascent and Descent.)

The notion that obstruction is not required for renal dysplasia to develop is further supported by the observations of Kirillova and colleagues (1982). Microdissection of a human embryo (8 weeks' gestation) showed that the kidney appeared to be a cyst. The ureter was twisted within its mesenchymal coat (see the section entitled Development of the Ureter) but was not obstructed or discontinuous. Histologic sections showed that the cyst was actually the dilated upper ureter, which came to resemble a giant pelvis. Collecting tubules drained into the cyst. Metanephrogenic mesenchyme and tubulogenesis was reduced. This specimen may represent the embryonic progenitor of a unilateral multicystic kidney. It was speculated that an inherently reduced branching of the ureteric bud was responsible. Coalescence of the ureteric bud branches, which were destined to become calyces, led to cyst formation; the paucity of bud ampulla led to only sparse nephrogenesis.

GENETICS. It is likely that genetic problems are interwoven with unilateral and bilateral renal agenesis, especially that associated with müllerian anomalies (as seen in Mayer-Rokitansky syndrome). The gene is single and autosomal dominant with variable expression (Pavanello et al, 1988). Furthermore, almost all females with bilateral renal agenesis associated with Potters syndrome have Mayer-Rokitansky syndrome (Pavanello et al, 1988). The importance of genetic makeup in ureteral abnormalities is emphasized by noting that single ureter vaginal ectopia is likely to be 15 times more common in Japanese than in whites. Furthermore, renal development ectopic ureter is more normal in Japanese than in Caucasians, in whom dysplasia is common (Gotoh, 1983) (see the section entitled Development of the Ducts of the Genitalia, Female).

In summary, it is plausible that dysplasia results from an abnormal interaction between inherently defective metanephrogenic mesenchyme and ureteric bud ampullae. The mesenchyme does not become specialized enough to elaborate tubules and differentiates only into the fibromuscular collar of the primitive duct. Perhaps this mesenchyme may also differentiate heterotopically into cartilage or bone marrow, as is seen clinically and in embryonic renal tissue in amphibians, mice, and birds (Saxen, 1972). The genesis of dysplasia may be accentuated by coexisting renal obstruction (e.g., ureterocele).

Additionally, renal dysplasia could begin with a normal renal blastema that is harmed, perhaps by an adverse environment (e.g., ischemia, toxins). Dysplasia may be induced reliably in the chick model, but there is no model that simulates the multicystic kidney.

Molecular Biology of Renal Compensatory Hypertrophy

TGF-β inhibits the growth of renal tubular cells in vitro. After uninephrectomy, TGF-β is reduced in proximal tubules, perhaps to foster their growth (Kanda et al, 1993). This observation is consistent with the idea that proximal cell hyperplasia is the initial transient response to compensation after uninephrectomy, which is followed by a sustained hypertrophy until the accelerated compensatory growth is complete. Growth hormone stimulates the renal collecting ducts to produce IGF-1, which acts on the proximal tubules and glomeruli to contribute to compensatory renal hypertrophy (Hammerman, 1991). The distal tubular cells show increased TGF-β and may modulate the hyperplasia (Kanda et al, 1993).

ASCENT OF THE KIDNEY

The renal blastema originates at the level of the upper sacral segments in the embryo. The final position of the kidney at the level of the upper lumbar vertebrae in the newborn is attributed to ascent of the renal blastema. **Anatomic studies show that *four mechanisms lead to* normal renal ascent:** (1) caudal growth of the spine, (2) elongate growth of the ureter, (3) molding of the renal parenchyma, and (4) fixation of the kidney to the retroperitoneum, which follows elongate spine growth (Maizels and Stephens, 1979). The kidney also rotates medially on its polar axis, causing the pelvis to face the spine (Fig. 51–18) (Boyden, 1932; Gruenwald, 1941). Additional observations support the findings of these anatomic studies.

Deformed spine growth in the VATER syndrome or induced experimentally is associated with incomplete renal ascent, or ectopia (Brumfield et al, 1991), which is associated with mechanism 4 mentioned earlier. The dependence of renal ascent on elongate growth of the spine may be similar to the passive ascent of the spinal cord. For example, the

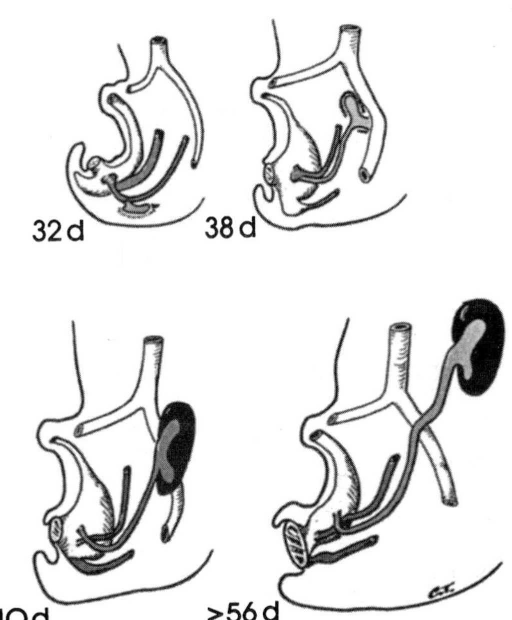

Figure 51–18. Schematic of renal ascent in the human embryo. The ureteric bud has originated from the mesonephric duct and actively elongates to reach the umbilical arteries. By 38 days, the umbilical artery tilts the upper pole of the kidney ventrally. At 40 days, the renal parenchyma elongates, and then by 44 days, the kidney rounds itself to elevate the lower pole of the kidney above the umbilical artery. After 56 days, the kidney fixes to the tissues of the retroperitoneum. Axial growth of the spine elevates the kidney to its final position. (From Maizels M: An Investigation of Urologic Malformations: Experimental Elucidation of Renal Ectopia. Masters' Thesis, Evanston, IL, Northwestern University, 1978.)

Table 51–4. SONOGRAPHIC IDENTIFICATION OF THE FETAL KIDNEY DURING GESTATION

	Sonographic Appearance			
Gestational Age (Weeks)	***Identify (%)***	***Reniform Outline***	***Echogenic Outline***	***Central Complex of Renal Sinus***
<12	10	+	−	−
12–24	80	++	+	+
24–36	100	++	++	++

Ratio of kidney circumference/abnormal circumference is normally constant during pregnancy at 0.27 to 0.3.

From Grannum P, Bracken M, Silverman R, Hobbins JC: Am J Obstet Gynecol, 1980; 136:249.

caudal portion of the spinal cord, called the conus medullaris, ascends from the coccygeal level in the newborn to the lumbar level in the adult because the spine grows faster longitudinally than the spinal cord (Langman, 1969).

Ectopic kidneys located within the bony pelvis are often not reniform. This abnormal shape may reflect the persistence of the normal molding of the renal parenchyma during its failed attempt to hurdle the umbilical artery (mechanism 3) (Friedland and de Vries, 1975).

Congenital crossed renal ectopia, as seen on an intravenous pyelogram, can be distinguished from acquired cross-lateral displacement by imaging the kidneys with a cross-table lateral view on a renogram. The kidney, which becomes displaced across the midline, will be anterior to the great vessels, whereas a kidney that shows congenital crossed ectopia will be aligned with the native kidney posterior to the great vessels (de Jonge et al, 1988).

MORPHOLOGIC DEVELOPMENT OF THE FETAL KIDNEY

As the fetal kidney advances during gestation, it more often resembles its postnatal ultrasound appearance. **This is probably because fat is progressively deposited in the pararenal space and renal sinus (Table 51–4) (Bowie et al, 1983).**

Normative postnatal polar kidney length in children born from 26 weeks' gestation to term was described by de Vries and Levene (1983). The ratio of polar kidney to fetal crown rump length was about 0.78 irrespective of gestational age; the right and left kidneys were of similar length (de Vries and Levene, 1983). The medulla is evident by 27 weeks' gestation (Jeanty et al, 1982).

DEVELOPMENT OF THE GREAT VESSELS AND RENAL VASCULATURE

Three groups of branches of the dorsal aorta appear early in development. They course ventrally (to the intestine), laterally (to the intermediate mesoderm), and dorsolaterally (to the body wall and spine). The lateral branches are well developed only in the areas of the developing mesonephroi. Endothelial branchings continue to originate from the aorta until the aorta has developed a mesodermal coat (tunica media). The branchings create two to three arteries at each segmental level between the mesonephric arteries and the dorsolateral segmental arteries. The arterial branches anastomose as a plexus (Fig. 51–19*A* and *B*). This plexus anastomoses with renal vessels at more cranial segmental levels as the kidneys ascend the retroperitoneum. **Portions of the plexus contribute to the adult pattern of the renal arteries.**

Local mechanical forces may determine which portions of the plexus will involute. For example, in species that have large mesonephroi, the segmental vessels may be pulled ventrally to obliterate the periaortic plexus; in species that have an acute curvature of the caudal trunk, the segmental vessels may be pulled dorsally to obliterate the periaortic plexus. Because human embryos have neither large mesonephroi or an acute curvature of the caudal trunk, the portions of the periaortic plexus that persist may be variable, and thereby, the renal vasculature may also vary (Fig. 51–19*C*) (Bremer, 1915).

Persistence of the embryonic caudal vasculature may tether the rotation of the kidney during lumbar ascent. Nonrotated kidneys with aberrant arterial supply then develop (Nathan and Glezer, 1984).

The development of the renal venous system is undocumented. Sampaio and Aragao (1990) showed that a large vein frequently apposed the anterior and less often the posterior aspect of the ureteropelvic junction (UPJ), an important fact to consider when pyeloplasty is being performed using either open or endoscopic techniques.

Circumcaval ureter results from anomalous development of the inferior vena cava (IVC). The fetal posterior cardinal vein does not regress and becomes a major portion of the infrarenal IVC. Because this segment of the IVC is anterior to the ureter, the ureter is medially displaced. If the medial displacement is below the third lumbar vertebrae, then the ureter becomes kinked and obstructed; if the displacement is higher, kinking may be less prominent and obstruction less likely (Sener, 1993).

FUNCTION OF THE FETAL KIDNEY

The first renal tubules are induced after 7 weeks. Correlations of morphology with renal function of animal embryos have led to projections that the tubules of the human fetus probably function after about 9 weeks of development (Kim et al, 1991). The tubules secrete dyes by 14 weeks (Cameron et al, 1983). Also, by the 14th week of gestation, the loop of Henle is functional and tubular reabsorption occurs (Smith and Robillard, 1989).

In the laboratory, the exteriorized fetus model (Alexander and Nixon, 1961) permits diverse physiologic measurements. The glomerular filtration rate in fetal life is low and likely relates to the kidneys receiving a smaller percent of the cardiac output (3% in utero compared with 17% in newborns), high renal vascular resistance, and low filtration fraction. The rise in glomerular filtration rate during gestation likely relates to the increase in kidney mass rather than to an improved function of the tissues (Smith and Robillard, 1989).

The glomerular filtration rate appears to correlate with gestational age between 27 weeks' gestation to term. The increase in the glomerular filtration rate in the weeks follow-

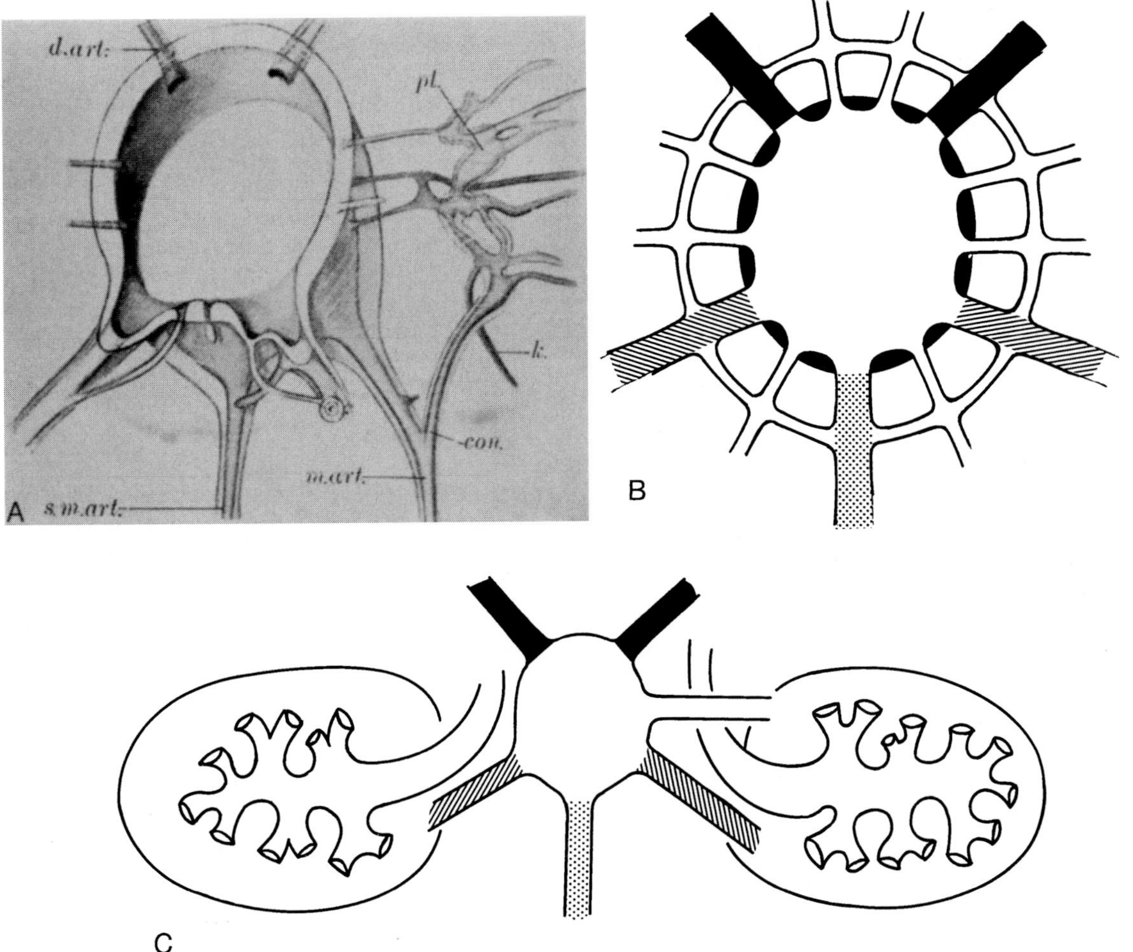

Figure 51–19. Development of renal arteries. *A,* Ventral (s.m. art.); dorsolateral (d. art.); and lateral (m. art.) groups of branches appear at each segmental level of the aorta. A capillary vascular plexus (pl.) exists laterally and supplies the kidney (k). The lateral plexus connects to the mesonephric artery (m. art.) by a thick-walled vessel (con.) and to the aorta by three slender vessels of endothelium only (reconstruction of cat embryo at second lumbar segment). The left side of the drawing is incomplete. (After Bremer JL: Am J Anat 1915; 18:179.) *B,* Schematic of *A. C,* The lateral vascular plexus may be the framework for the variability of the renal arteries. If the plexus involutes, there will be a single renal artery *(left).* If the plexus persists, there may be double or multiple renal arteries *(right).*

ing birth likely relates to the recruitment of superficial cortical nephrons, which thereby increase glomerular perfusion.

The normative pattern of serum creatinine by gestational age at birth is shown in Figure 51–20 (Shimada and Shozou, 1993). Creatinine falls more slowly to the normative value the earlier the gestational age at delivery.

The timing for possible prenatal drainage of urinary obstruction may be evaluated embryologically. Shimada and co-workers (1993) showed that in human fetuses the nephrogenic zone, which should persist normally to term, was absent in cases of severe hydronephrosis by 28 weeks' gestational age; dysplasia was not apparent in specimens around 20 weeks' gestational age. The index of glomerular number (i.e., the radial glomerular count) in cases of severe hydronephrosis was significantly lower than normal at around 30 weeks, whereas it was not different from normal before 20 weeks' gestational age. Because the recoverability of renal development and function in fetal hydronephrosis likely depends on the characteristics of the nephrogenic zone, the authors conclude that prenatal intervention should not be considered until around 20 weeks' gestational age (Atwell et al, 1993; Shimada et al, 1993).

Amniotic fluid volume constituents and volume are believed to mirror kidney function. Although Hippocrates is credited with first suggesting that amniotic fluid derives from fetal urine, other sources are now recognized: during the early weeks of pregnancy by filtration of maternal plasma, by filtration of fetal plasma across the nonkeratinized fetal skin, and during the last trimester from fetal urine (Burghard et al, 1987).

Near term, there is a rise in urea and creatinine concentration and a fall in sodium concentration and osmolality, which are reflective of the increased maturation of fetal renal function. Low molecular weight serum proteins (microglobulins) may be filtered past the immature fetal glomerulus only to be reabsorbed by the proximal renal tubules. When the reabsorptive function of the kidneys increases after the second trimester, the levels of the microglobulins decreases. Should they appear in elevated amounts in the amniotic fluid, this may be viewed as a sign of poor renal function.

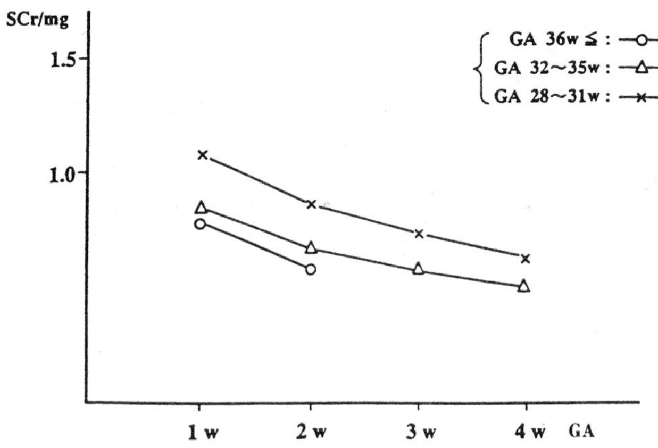

Figure 51–20. Expected postnatal fall in serum creatinine (SCr) by gestational age (GA) at birth. (From Shimada K, Shozou H, Tohda A: Indications for urinary drainage in neonates detected in utero. Nippon Hinyokika Gakkai Zasshi 1993; 84:479–484.)

DEVELOPMENT OF THE URETER

Embryo

After 28 days of development, the ureteric bud appears as an evagination of the mesonephric duct. The primitive ureter ascends the pelvis by a process that involves atresia and recanalization of the lumen (Ruano-Gil et al, 1975; Alcaraz et al, 1991). Between 28 and 35 days of development, the entire length of the ureter is patent. Perhaps, as the cloaca is still imperforate at this stage, mesonephric urine fills the ureter, raises the intraluminal pressure, and maintains this patency. Between 37 and 40 days of development, the lumen of the ureter is not apparent histologically. Perhaps rapid elongate growth of the ureter obliterates the lumen. After this period, the lumen extends cranially and caudally from the midportion of the ureter and soon the entire length of the ureter is apparent again (Fig. 51–21).

These observations may explain why congenital strictures of the ureter are more common at the ureteropelvic junction (UPJ) and ureterovesical junction than elsewhere. Because the ureter lumen at these junctions becomes patent again last, they may be more likely to remain narrow as a stricture. A similar mechanism could account for instances of laryngeal subglottic stenosis (O'Rahilly and Tucker, 1973). As an alternative explanation, cellular debris could obstruct the ureterovesical junction analogous to debris in the cerebral aqueduct causing transient obstruction.

After the common excretory duct is absorbed into the trigone, absorption of the primitive ureter begins. At this period, Alcaraz and associates (1989) identified a ureterovesical membrane between the lumen of the ureter and the chamber of the urogenital sinus (37 days' gestational age). The membrane, probably reflective of Chawalla's membrane, is initially one cell layer thick, then thickens (39 days' gestational age), only to disappear after 39 days' gestational age (Fig. 51–22). **Perhaps, if this membrane persists, it may cause an obstructive uropathy of the lower ureter.**

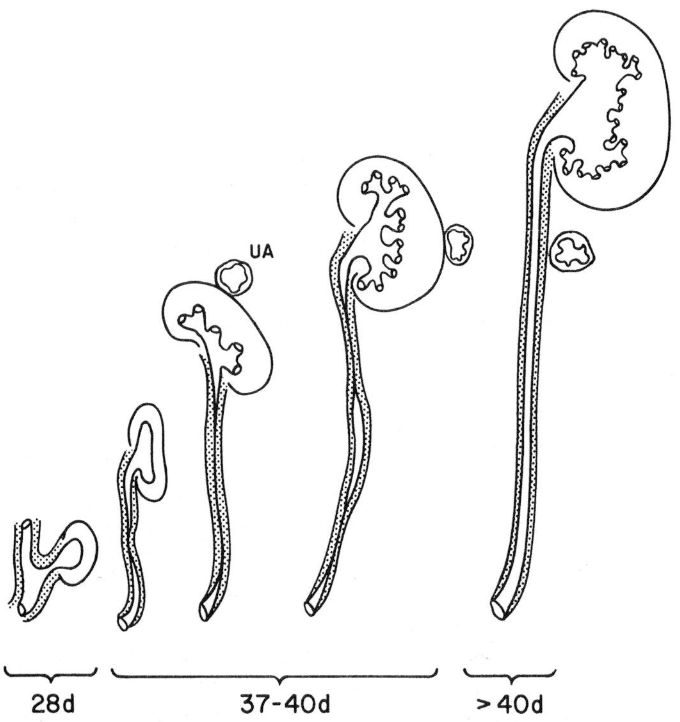

Figure 51–21. Early development of the ureter. At 28 days, the ureteral bud appears from the mesonephric duct. Between 37 and 40 days, the lumen of the ureter is first progressively lost, beginning at its midportion. Then, the lumen of the ureter becomes apparent again, beginning at its midportion. After 40 days, the lumen of the ureter is apparent throughout its length (UA, umbilical artery).

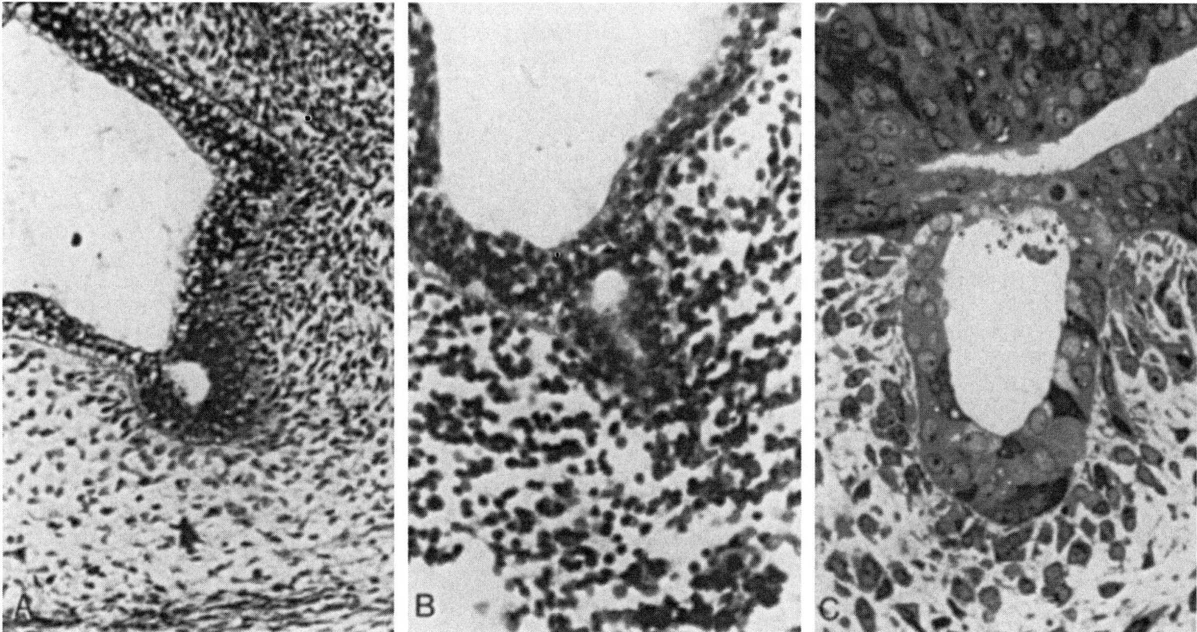

Figure 51–22. Chawalla's membrane in human and rat. The membrane marks the ureterovesical junction in humans (*A*, × 400; *B*, × 640; about 42 days' gestation) and resembles that (*C*) in the rat embryo (× 500; 27 days' gestation). (From Alcaraz A, Vinaixa F, Tejedo-Mateu A, et al: Acta Urol Esp 1989; 13:318.)

Fetus

By 8 weeks of development, the ureter is a patent tube without muscle that has elongated pari passu, with ascent of the kidney in the retroperitoneum. Muscularization of the ureter is described in Table 51–5 (Figs. 51–23 and 51–24). After 10 weeks, the epithelium of the ureter becomes two layered, and by 14 weeks, there is a transitional epithelium. By 18 weeks, the ureter shows intrinsic narrowings at the UPJ, pelvic brim, and ureterovesical junction, and complementary intrinsic dilatations at the spindles of the ureter. It may be that the fetal ureter elongates more than the kidney ascends. The ureter may absorb the excess length by becoming tortuous or folding its wall as pleats, the "fetal folds" of Ostling (1942) (Fig. 51–25).

The first secretion and drainage of renal urine (9 weeks' gestation) precedes muscularization of the upper ureter (12 weeks' gestation) (see Table 51–5) (Matsuno et al, 1984). It may be that urine flow in the ureter mechanically stimulates myogenesis (see the section entitled Development of the Trigone and Bladder).

The distribution of elastica in the human fetal ureter is set after 12 weeks' gestation (Escala et al, 1989). In the adventitia (where the fibers appear first), the elastic fibers are longitudinally oriented; in the muscular layer, the fibers are randomly oriented; and in the submucosa, the fibers radiate from the basement membrane (see Fig. 51–24). During later development, the fibers in each layer increase according to the ratio of 5:1:2, respectively. It is plausible that asynchrony between urine formation and elastic fiber deposition contributes to dilatations of the pelvis and ureter during development.

Cases of UPJ obstruction may show anomalous muscularization as a prominent outer circular and inconspicuous inner longitudinal layer of the ureter (Antonakopoulos, 1985). A sphincteric arrangement of the UPJ muscle in obstruction has also been noted (Antonakopoulos et al, 1985). If this prominent circular disposition of muscle in the fetus does not unravel, UPJ obstruction in the infant may result (Antonakopoulos et al, 1985). In this context, although it is unknown whether or not children with pyloric stenosis exhibit an incidence of urologic anomalies higher than that of the general population (Fernbach and Morello, 1993), cases of pyloric stenosis that also show UPJ obstruction may exhibit a muscular knot at the UPJ, which accounts for the obstruction.

Newborn

The infant grows taller, faster than the ureter elongates. Thereby, the ureter may straighten and unfold its fetal folds (Ostling, 1942). These pleats are not ordinarily obstructive. However, a pleat that intrudes into the lumen of the ureter and becomes fixed by adventitia may obstruct urine drainage as a valve (Fig. 51–26) (Maizels and Stephens, 1980).

DEVELOPMENT OF THE CLOACA

During the period of the laminar embryo, the cloacal membrane is the caudal region of the embryo where ectoderm directly apposes endoderm. Growth of mesenchyme near the cloacal membrane lifts the tail end of the embryo off of the blastoderm. This lifting folds the tail end and creates a chamber, the cloaca, the dilated terminus of the hindgut. The cloaca is lined with endoderm. Further growth of the tail fold flexes the tail end further, and the cloacal membrane comes to be on the ventrum of the embryo. Continued growth of mesenchyme lateral to the cloacal membrane elevates the ectoderm as labioscrotal swellings; continued growth of mesenchyme cranial to the cloacal

Table 51–5. TIME TABLE OF MUSCULAR DEVELOPMENT OF THE HUMAN URINARY TRACT

Gestational Age (Weeks)	Prostate	Urethra	Bladder	Ureter	Pelvis
6	←		No muscle		→
7	← No muscle	→	Muscle in dome and extends caudally	← No muscle	→
		Mesenchyme condenses as rare muscle			
8		U-shaped distribution of muscle	Muscle diffuse in bladder	Ureter drains into the bladder	Dilated chamber
11			←	No muscle	→
		Striated muscle lying outside of and adjacent to smooth muscle cells	Muscle bundles appear	Muscle in upper ureter; superficial ureteral sheath at UVJ	Muscle appears
16	Prostate epithelial buds grow into mesenchyme (Figs. 51–45 and 51–46)	Striated muscle encircles urethra at urogenital diaphragm (muscle is smaller than pelvic floor striated muscle) Enhancement of smooth muscle cell		Upper ureter muscle appears as bundles that have a spiral course	
				Muscle at intramural ureter immature with muscle bundles	
17			Muscle layering is almost complete and advanced beyond that of trigone	Spiral muscle more prominent in ureter (Fig. 51–23). Longitudinal muscle orientation in intravesical ureter and attached to deep periureteral sheath. Waldeyer's sheath separates superficial and deep periurethral sheath.	
21			Bulky middle circular muscle layer	Spiral muscle layer Superficial periureteral sheath at UVJ is well developed	
40	←	Muscularization complete			→
Infants		Muscle fibers show tendency to layer with circular orientation			
Adults		Mesh of fibers oriented as longitudinal, oblique, circular, or radial			
(Antonakopoulos et al, 1985)		Without discrete layers			

Adapted from Matsuno T, Tokunaka S, Koyanagi T: J Urol 1984; 132:148.

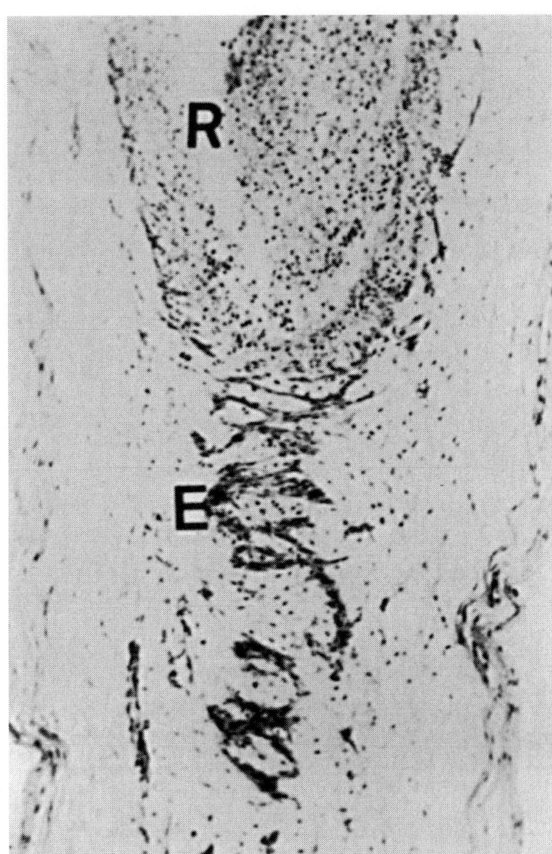

Figure 51–23. Upper ureter of human fetus (17 weeks' gestation). Early muscle bundles (E) course spirally (R, lumen of ureter). (From Matsuno T, Tokunaka S, Koyanagi T: J Urol 1984; 132:148.)

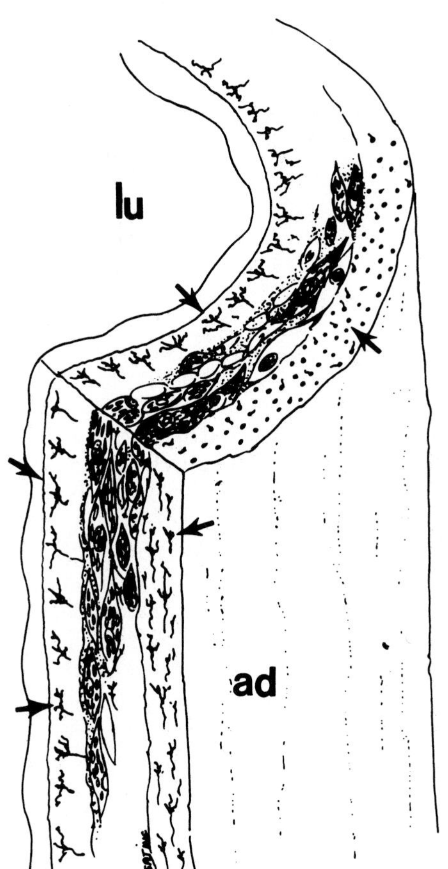

Figure 51–24. Schematic, three-dimensional representation of the elastic fiber orientation of a longitudinal and transverse section of a human fetal ureter (12 weeks' gestation) (lu, ureter lumen; ad, adventitia). (From Escala JM, Keating MA, Boyd G: J Urol 1989; 141:969.)

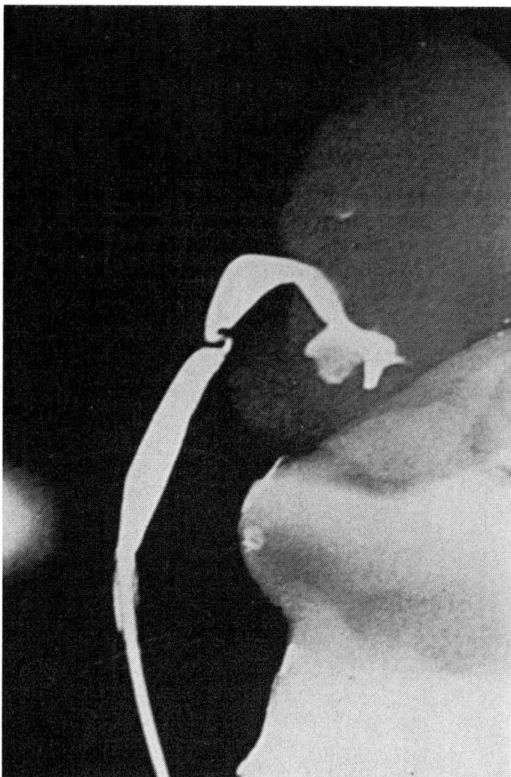

Figure 51–25. Pleats of the ureter. Retrograde pyelogram of a newborn kidney and ureter specimen shows the wall of the ureter folds and pleats of the lumen of the ureter. The pleats probably do not usually obstruct urine drainage.

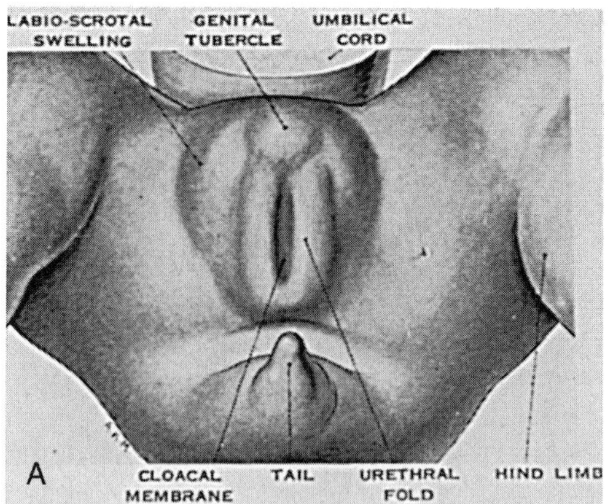

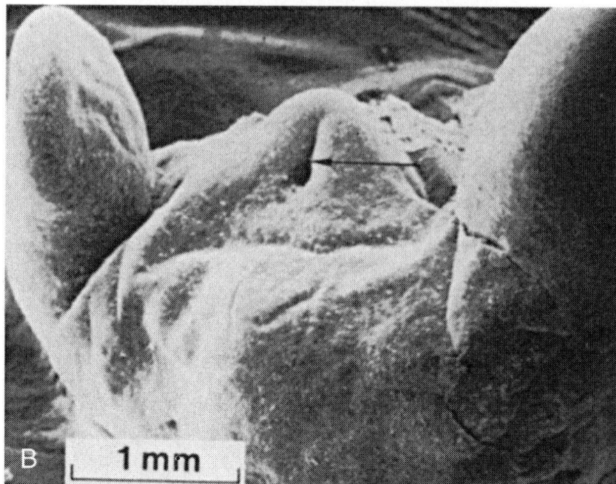

Figure 51–27. *A*, External appearance of the cloaca at about 7 weeks. Growth of the mesenchyme at the caudal end of the embryo lifts the embryo off the blastoderm and creates the tail fold. Further growth and migration of the mesenchyme around the cloacal membrane creates the genital tubercle and the labioscrotal swellings. (From Hamilton WJ, Mossman HW: Human Embryology Prenatal Development of Form and Function. New York, The Macmillan Press Ltd., 1976.) *B*, Scanning electron micrograph of the genital tubercle of the same stage as in *A*. The urethral folds flank the urethral groove *(arrow)*. (See also Fig. 51–29*A* and *C*.) (From Rowsell AR, Morgan BDG: Br J Plast Surg 1987; 40:201.)

membrane elevates the ectoderm as the genital tubercle, the primordium of the phallus (Fig. 51–27). Growth of the mesoderm further cranially makes the infraumbilical body wall prominent.

The classic view holds that **septation of the cloaca** begins at about 28 days of gestation (Stephens, 1983). The urorectal septum, also called Tourneux's fold, extends in the coronal plane toward the cloacal membrane. At the same time, Rathke's plicae appear as two tissue folds from the lateral aspects of the hindgut. These plicae meet each other in the midline, and by 7 weeks' gestation, the cloaca is divided. There is a separate rectum and primitive urogenital sinus (see Figs. 51–28, 51–31, and 51–33*C*). The portion of the primitive urogenital sinus cranial to the mesonephric ducts is the vesicourethral canal, and that caudal to the mesonephric ducts is the urogenital sinus (Fig. 51–29) (Hamilton and Mossman, 1976). Soon, the müllerian ducts poke into the posterior wall of the vesicourethral canal to form Müller's tubercle (see Figs. 51–34 and 51–35). The site that the urorectal septum apposes, the cloacal membrane, marks the perineal body.

A new twist on development of the cloaca was offered by van der Putte (1986). He studied embryos from pigs with hereditary anorectal malformations. Natural markers of the pig cloaca (e.g., specific epithelia identify regions of the

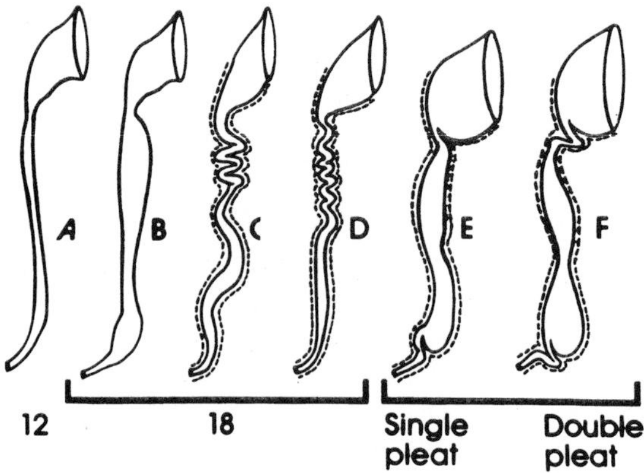

Figure 51–26. Possible embryogenesis of valves of the ureter. *A*, By 12 weeks of gestation, the caliber of the lumen of the ureter is uniform. *B*, At 18 weeks, pelvic and abdominal spindles of the ureter appear. If elongate growth of the ureter occurs faster than that of the trunk, the ureter may become tortuous *(C)* or acquire pleats *(D)*. *E* and *F*, Pleats are normally not obstructive but may persist as valves. (From Maizels M, Stephens FD: Valves of the ureter as a cause of primary obstruction of the ureter: Anatomic, embryologic and clinical aspects. J Urol 1980; 123:742.)

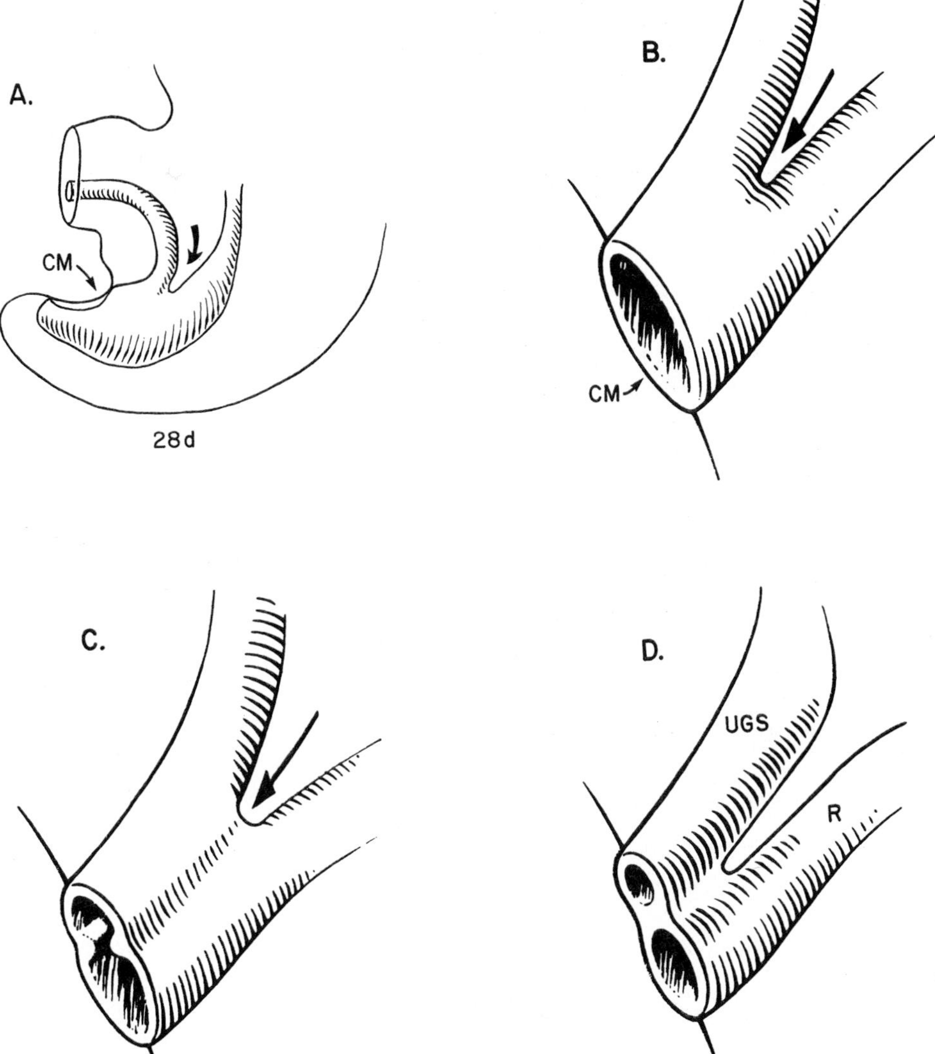

Figure 51–28. Septation of the cloaca. *A,* Lateral view of caudal embryo (CM, cloacal membrane). Septation of the cloaca occurs in a coronal plane as Tourneux's fold *(B)* extends to the cloacal membrane from above, and *(C)* as Rathke's plicae extend toward each other from the sides. *D,* Septation establishes the primitive urogenital sinus (UGS) and rectum (R). (From Stephens FD, Smith ED: Anorectal Malformations in Children. Chicago, Year Book Medical Publishers, 1971.)

cloaca) tracked normal and anomalous development. The septation of the cloaca does not result from fusion of Rathke's and Tourneux's folds, rather there is a shift of the dorsal cloaca toward the cloacal membrane, which carries the urorectal septum caudally (Fig. 51–30). High imperforate anus may relate to excessive mesenchyme in the dorsal part of the cloacal membrane, which prevents rupture of the membrane so there is no anorectal orifice. A rectal fistula is forced to the urinary tract (Figs. 51–31 and 51–32). A similar pushing process is believed to contribute to urethral development in the murine penis (Kluth et al, 1988).

DEVELOPMENT OF THE TRIGONE AND BLADDER

Trigone

After the mesonephric ducts drain into the urogenital sinus, the epithelia of the urogenital sinus (endoderm) and mesonephric duct (mesoderm) are fused. At this time, the ureteric bud evaginates from the mesonephric duct (see the section entitled Development of the Ureter). By 33 days of gestation, the segment of the mesonephric duct beyond the ureteric bud dilates as the common excretory duct, the precursor of the hemitrigone (Alcaraz et al, 1989). The right and left common excretory ducts are absorbed into the urogenital sinus (Hamilton and Mossman, 1976). The mesenchyme of the right and left common excretory ducts is believed to migrate toward the midline because the endodermal mucosa of the bladder does not persist here (Hamilton and Mossman, 1976). The epithelia of both ducts fuse as a triangular area, the primitive trigone. **The terminus of the ureter enters the bladder directly by day 37 (Cutner et al, 1992).** The mesonephric duct orifices grow caudally and flank the paramesonephric ducts at the level of the urogenital sinus. This is the site of the future verumontanum (Figs. 51–33 and 51–34).

The **mechanism of normal absorption of the primitive ureter into the trigone** is inferred from clinical observations of the trigone in duplex kidneys (Fig. 51–35). It is believed that as the common excretory duct is absorbed into the

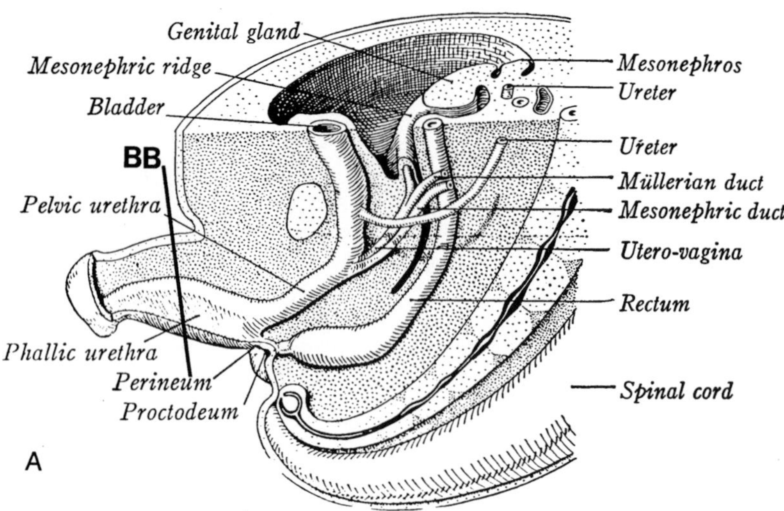

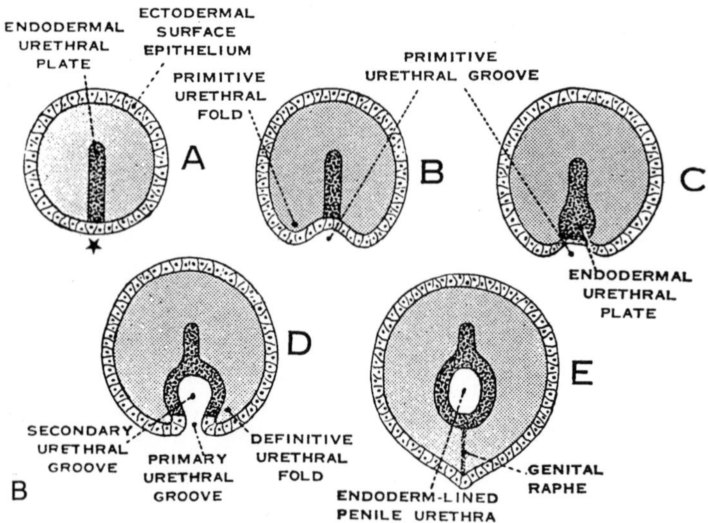

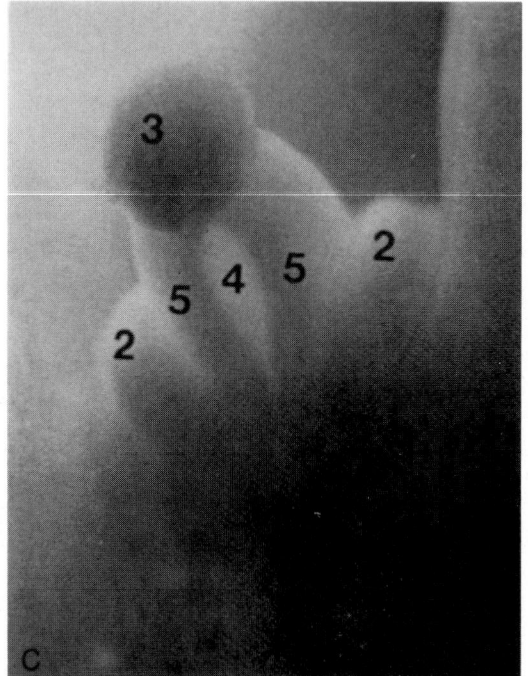

Figure 51–29. Development of the urogenital sinus. *A,* By 9 weeks of development, the urogenital sinus consists of a narrow pelvic part near the bladder and an expanded phallic part near the urogenital membrane (anterior portion of cloacal membrane). (From Arey LB: Developmental Anatomy. Philadelphia, W. B. Saunders Company, 1974.) *B,* Transverse section through phallic part of urogenital sinus (plane BB seen in *A*). The endodermal cells lining the phallic portion of the cloacal membrane (urogenital membrane, *asterisk*) thicken and then degenerate to create the secondary urethral groove. The secondary urethral groove remains as the vestibule in the female and closes as the penile urethra in the male. (From Hamilton WJ, Mossman HW: Human Embryology Prenatal Development of Form and Function. New York, The Macmillan Press Ltd., 1976.) *C,* Transillumination of the phallus of a 9-week-old human fetus viewed from below (2, labioscrotal fold; 3, phallus; 4, urethral groove continuous with urogenital sinus; 5, urethral fold). (From England MA: Color Atlas of Life Before Birth. Chicago, Year Book Medical Publishers, 1983.)

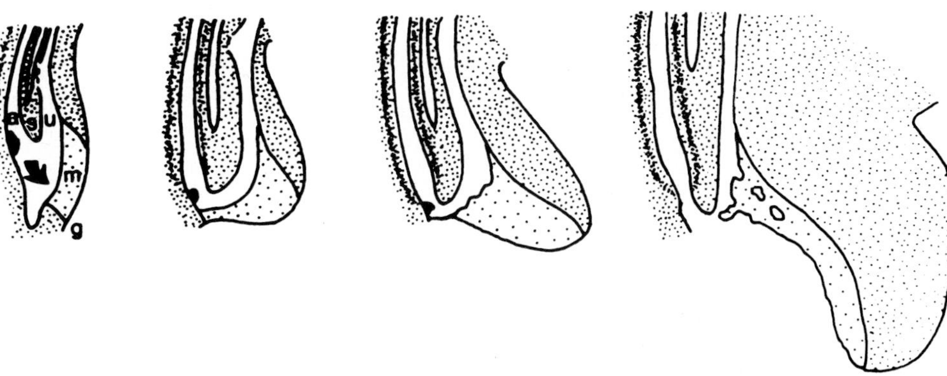

Figure 51–30. Successive stages shown semidiagrammatically in the development of the pig cloaca (11-, 13-, 17-, 25-mm embryos). The epithelial tag (black spot) marks the junction of the gut (g) and dorsal cloacal wall. The tag and dorsal cloaca descend to the cloacal membrane (m), giving the appearance of primary descent of the urorectal septum (s). The membrane (m) ruptures without contacting the septum. (a, anus; u, urethra.) (From van der Putte SCJ: J Pediatr Surg 1986; 21:434.)

urogenital sinus, the orifice of the mesonephric duct moves caudally and the orifice of the ureter moves cranially. Continued growth of the epithelium and mesoderm of the absorbed common excretory ducts separates the ureteral orifices laterally and establishes the framework of the primitive trigone.

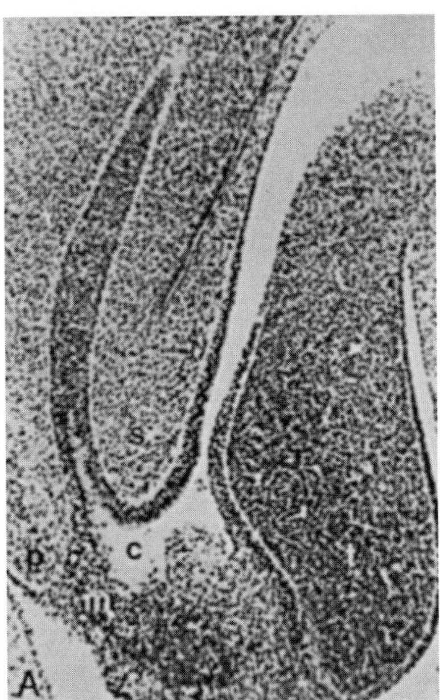

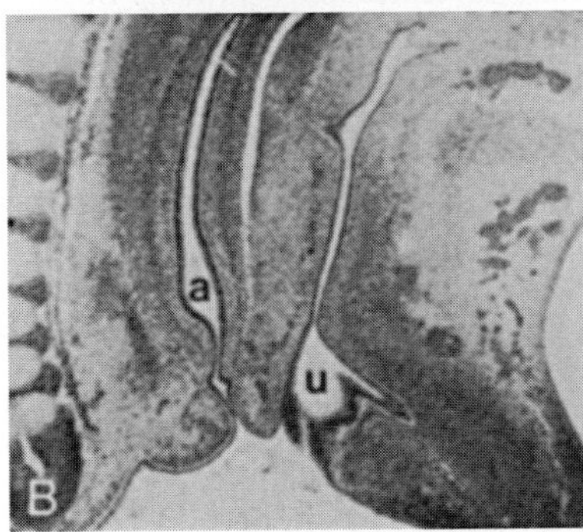

Figure 51–31. Normal development of the human cloaca. *A,* At about 6 weeks of development, the cloaca (c) is bounded by the genital tubercle, urorectal septum (s), postanal swelling (p), and cloacal membrane (midsagittal section, × 120) (cf. 17-mm pig embryo in Fig. 51–30). *B,* At about 7 weeks of development, the cloacal membrane is not evident, and the anorectal (a) and urogenital (u) sinuses show separate openings (midsagittal section, × 30) (cf. 25-mm pig embryo in Fig. 51–30). (From van der Putte SCJ: J Pediatr Surg 1986; 21:434.)

The ureteral orifice, which drains the upper pole of the kidney, rotates posteriorly (clockwise facing the left ureter orifice; counterclockwise facing the right ureter orifice (see Fig. 51–35), so that the orifice lies caudal and medial to the orifice of the lower pole ureter. Weigert and, later, Meyer recognized the regularity of this relationship, which has come to be known as the Weigert-Meyer rule. Similarly, when the orifices of the ureters of duplex kidneys are adjacent to each other on the trigone, they are situated next to each other such that the orifice of the upper pole ureter is medial to the orifice of the lower pole ureter (Stephens, 1982). Because the trigonal musculature does not cross, this is consistent with absorption of the common excretory duct and primitive ureter into the trigone before the trigone muscularizes (Fuss, 1992).

Following this logic, several concepts are plausible. Perhaps the laterally ectopic ureter had originated from a ureteric bud that was abnormally low on the wolffian duct and came to drain further laterally on the trigone than usual. Vesicoureteral reflux would result. Perhaps in caudal ectopy of the ureteral orifice, the ureteric bud had originated abnormally high on the wolffian duct and came to drain on the bladder neck (Mackie and Stephens, 1979) or retained its connection with the wolffian duct (persistent mesonephric duct) (Stephens, 1983).

It is common in instances of clinical vesicoureteral reflux to note that the lateral pillar of the ureteral orifice associated with reflux is not apparent. This observation could reflect a deficiency of Bell's muscle. This muscular deficiency could prevent the ureteral orifice from anchoring to the trigone, so that the orifice could migrate laterally during bladder filling and, thereby, permit vesicoureteral reflux (Fuss, 1992).

Triplicate ureters do not conform regularly to the Weigert-Meyer rule (Stephens, 1983). Inverted Y duplication of the ureter also does not readily conform to these embryologic notions (Ecke and Klatte, 1989).

The separate development of the trigone and bladder accounts for the contiguity of the muscle laminae of the ureter with the trigone and not with the detrusor. This separate development may account for the different pharmacologic responses of the musculature of the bladder neck and trigone from those of the detrusor.

Anomalous differentiation of the common excretory duct may engender an ectopic vas. Namely, the vas issues into the ureter rather than into the verumontanum, so that both the ureter and vas drain into a common duct. Perhaps, this derives from ureteric budding off of the wolffian duct too

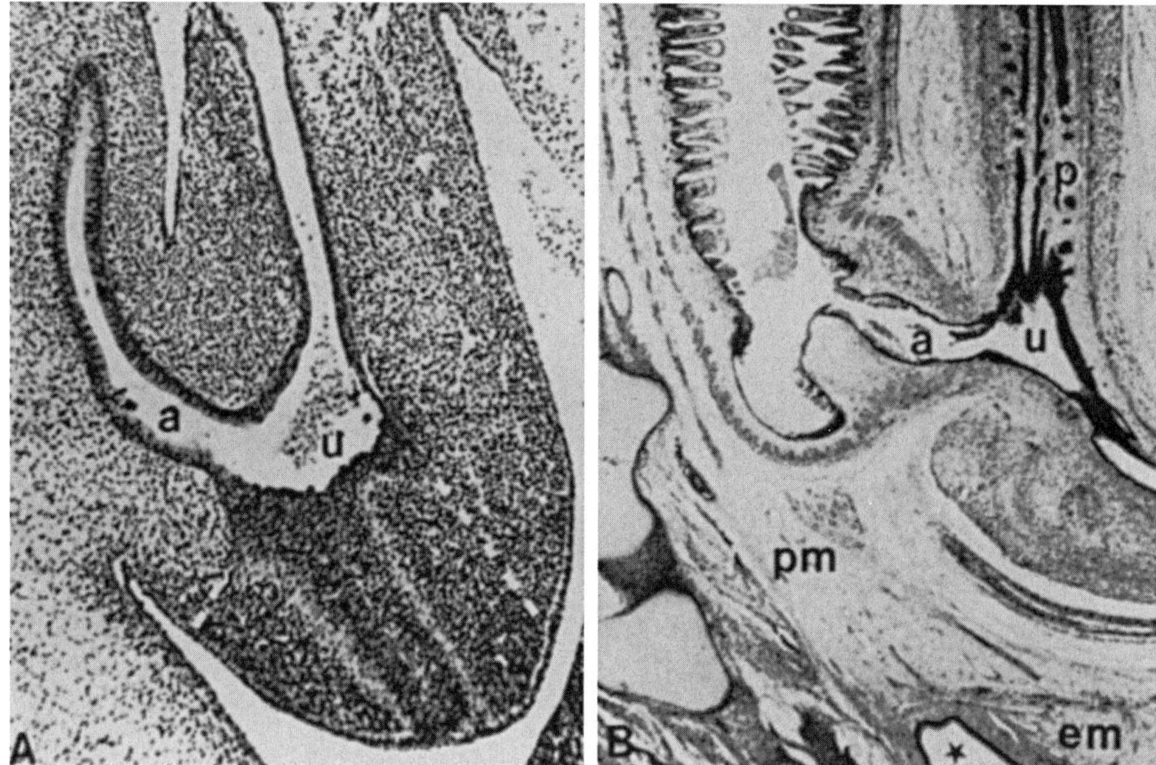

Figure 51–32. Development of high imperforate anus in the pig compared with the human.

A, Anorectal agenesis in a pig (stage is equivalent to before 6 weeks of development in the human) shows persistent communication between the anorectal (a) and urogenital (u) part of the cloaca. Tracking of tissues (see text) leads to the impression that, in this condition, excessive mesenchyme in the dorsal portion of the cloacal membrane may interfere with descent of the dorsal cloaca, and only a single urogenital orifice appears (sagittal section, × 80).

B, Anorectal agenesis in a human at about 19 weeks of development. Anal sinus (a) communicates with urethra (u) distal to the prostate (p). The puborectal (pm) and external sphincter muscles (em) have developed at their normal sites (× 20). (From van der Putte SCJ: J Pediatr Surg 1986; 21:434.)

far cranially, forcing a longer common excretory duct. It follows that if the period of absorption of the common excretory duct into the trigone has elapsed, the duct maybe too long to be entirely absorbed. So this segment remains outside the bladder and still shows its ancestral common drainage between the ureter and vas. This anomaly, albeit rare, should be considered in boys who present with epididymitis or during exploration of a boy's pelvic ureter when the kidney is affected by hydronephrosis. Dissection in this region may sever the vasal connection with the ureter. Although reimplantation of the vas onto the trigone may be considered, fertility is unlikely because the ipsilateral seminal vesicle is routinely absent (Aragona et al, 1992).

The later development of the mesonephric duct as the vas may help explain how an atretic ureter may drain into a seminal vesicle cyst. It is plausible that a ureteric bud failed to separate from the common excretory duct and vas. The ureter might eventually communicate with the ipsilateral

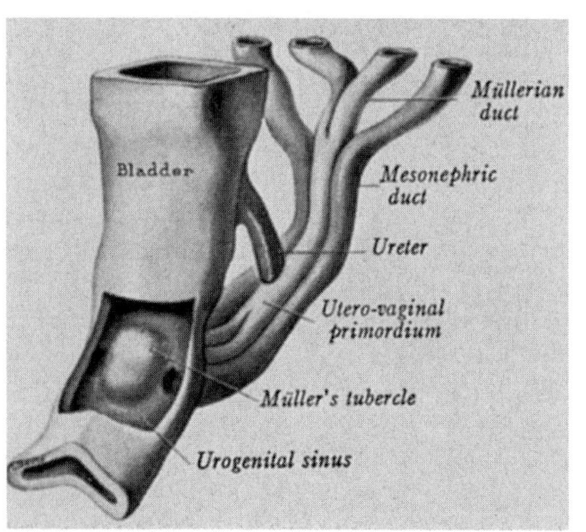

Figure 51–33. Diagrammatic view of the development of the ducts of the genitalia (cf. Fig. 51–25). The paramesonephric ducts descend toward the pelvis medial to the mesonephric ducts. After the mesonephric ducts are absorbed into the trigone, they migrate medially and caudally, flanking the paramesonephric ducts. The termini of these four ducts are at the site of the verumontanum in the male and the cervix in the female (From Arey after Broman. Arey LB: Developmental Anatomy, 7th ed. Philadelphia, W. B. Saunders Company, 1974.)

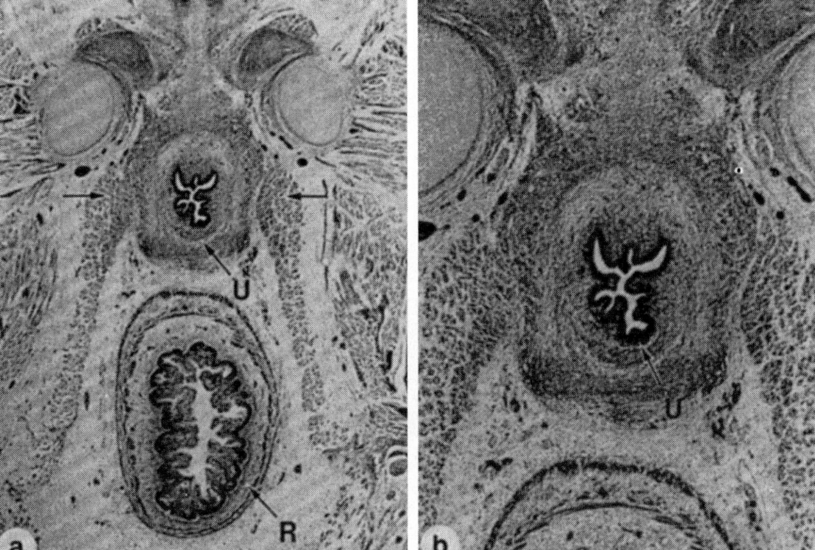

Figure 51–38. Proximity of mesenchyme of urethra and puborectalis makes it plausible that myogenic stem cells migrate through the anlage of cloacal muscle, colonize the urethral wall, and later develop as the striated sphincter. (Ten-week-old human embryo, U, urethra; R, rectum; *arrows*, puborectalis muscle; low-power magnification). (From Bourdelat D, Barbet JP, Butler-Browne GS: Fetal development of the urethral sphincter. Eur J Pediatr Surg 1992; 2:35–38.)

a trough lined by endoderm. The endodermal cells thicken to become the urethral plate. By 8 weeks, the superficial cells of the plate disintegrate. This cell death establishes the superficial, primary, and deep secondary urethral grooves (see Figs. 51–29*B* and *C* and 51–40). The mesenchyme flanking the urethral plate proliferates to form urethral folds. These folds eclipse the urethral groove. The folds do not reach the genital tubercle. From these events, the secondary urethral groove is lined by endoderm and is limited by the secondary urethral fold; the primary urethral groove is lined by ectoderm and is limited by the primary urethral fold.

In normal *male* development, the penis is straight when the phallic urethra is formed. In normal *female* development, the clitoris shows ventral curvature; perhaps, without an underlying urethra, there is no ventral support. In the male, if hypospadias develops, the deficient phallic urethra may permit the ventral curvature to remain as chordee, whereas in the female, if an accessory phallic urethra develops, the ventral curvature may straighten the clitoris and make it prominent (Pietryga and Wozniak, 1992).

Ligaments of the Gonads

At about 8 weeks' gestational age, the inguinal ligament is a thickened placode of the coelom with an underlying condensation of mesenchyme. It is adjacent to but separate from the mesonephros and runs parallel with the paramesonephric duct (Ludwig, 1993) (Fig. 51–41). Shortly after this, the gonadal ligament, another similarly thickened placode, appears at the caudal border of the gonad and is situated between the mesonephric and paramesonephric ducts. The caudal gonadal ligament associates with the genital duct

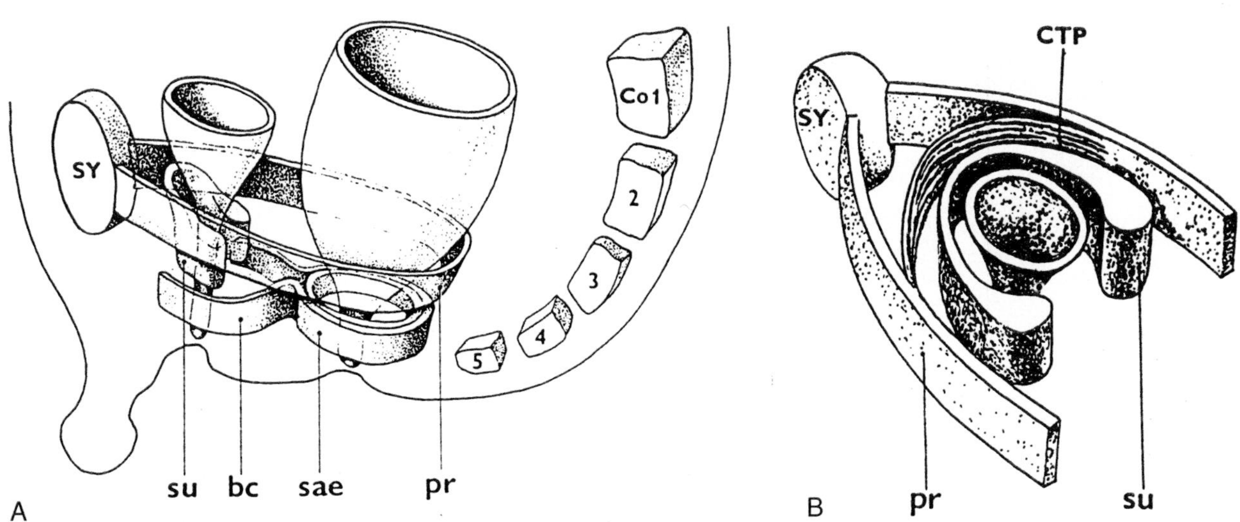

Figure 51–39. *A*, Framework of urethral sphincter at indifferent stage. *B*, A part of the puborectal (pr) muscle fibers originates from the connective tissue plate (CTP) on the ventral aspect of the urethral sphincter (su) at the level of the bladder neck. This arrangement establishes a mechanism whereby the fibers of the puborectalis muscle participate in urinary continence. (bc, bulbocavernosus; sae, sphincter ani externus; sy, symphysis.) (From Tichy M: The morphogenesis of human sphincter urethrae muscle. Anat Embryol 1989; 180:577–582. Copyright © 1989 by Springer-Verlag.)

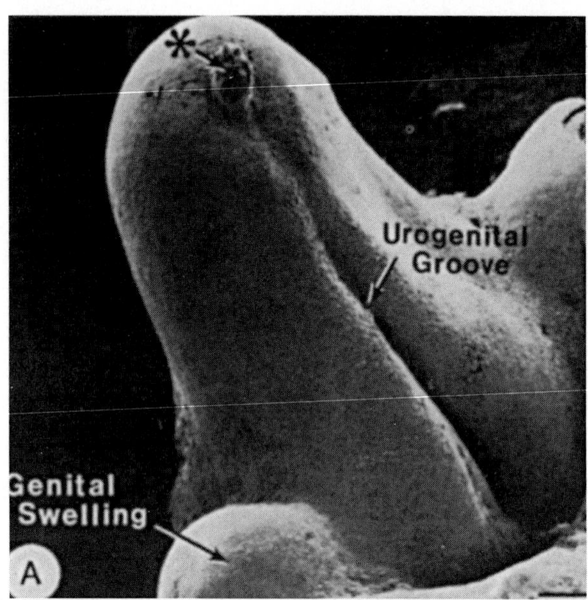

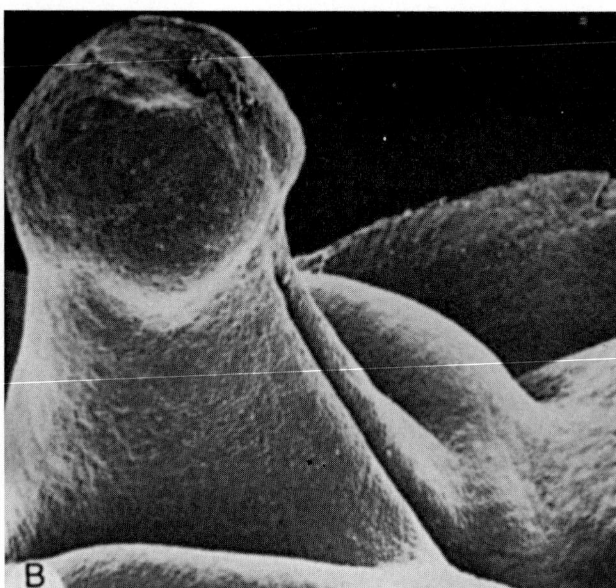

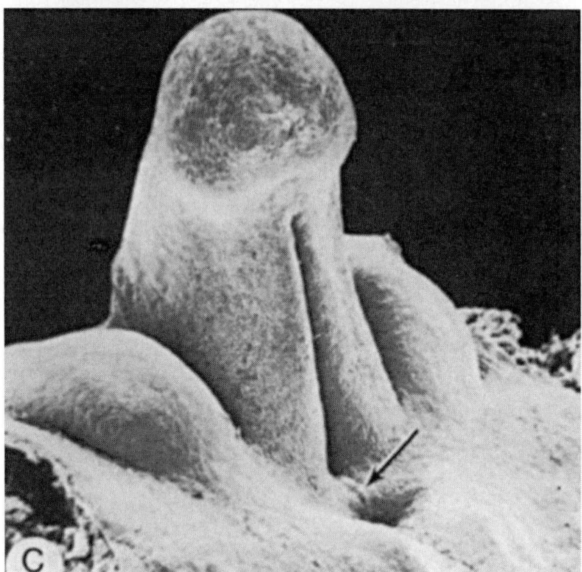

Figure 51–40. Indifferent stage of external genitalia. Ventrum of genital tubercle (8-week-old human embryo) viewed in a scanning electron micrograph. *A*, The urethral groove is between the paired urethral folds. The labioscrotal (genital) swellings are present. An epithelial tag is at the tip of the tubercle *(asterisk)*. *B*, Slightly later, the urethral groove is deeper and the genital swellings more prominent. *C*, Still later, the perineal body *(arrow)* is between the urethral groove and the proctodeal depression (see Fig. 51–29*A*) and *C*). (From Waterman RE: Human embryo and fetus. *In* Hafez ESE, Kenemans P, eds: Atlas of Human Reproduction. Hinghman, MA, Kluwer Boston, Inc., 1982.)

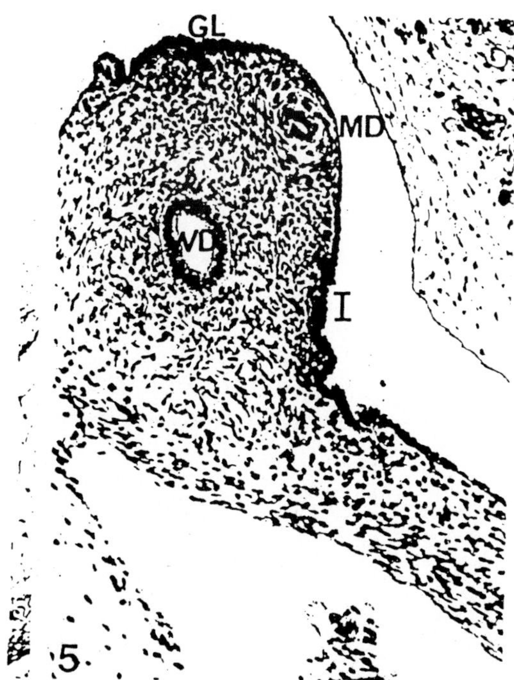

Figure 51–41. Ligaments of the mesonephros and gonad. The inguinal ligament (I) is a placode of coelomic epithelium; the caudal gonadal ligament (GL) is between the wolffian (WD) and müllerian (MD) ducts. (Human male embryo about 11 weeks' gestational age, × 160.) (From Ludwig KS: The development of the caudal ligaments of the mesonephros and of the gonads: A contribution to the development of the human gubernaculum (Hunteri). Anat Embryol 1993; 188:571–577. Copyright © 1993 by Springer-Verlag.)

destined to persist (mesonephric duct in the male and paramesonephric duct in the female).

In female embryos, the site of origin of the caudal gonadal ligament is the boundary between the fallopian tube and the uterus, and develops into the round ligament. Although in male embryos, the caudal gonadal ligament associates closely with the mesonephric duct at the boundary between the epididymal duct and the vas, becoming the gubernaculum (see the section entitled Anatomy of Testis Descent). In this way, the gubernaculum acts primarily on the epididymis. So, with active regression of the gubernaculum, the testis descends via the epididymis as the intermediary.

The anatomic disposition of the gubernaculum at the juncture of the epididymal duct and vas could be the basis for the long-looped vas deferens seen in patients with inguinal or abdominal undescended testis. In such cases, the epididymis remains high but the vas is pulled down through the inguinal canal to the upper scrotum. The anchor point is typically at the juncture of the epididymis and the vas.

Anomalous absorption of the müllerian ducts in the male could lead to cystic anomalies in this region, the formative verumontanum. Such a phenomenon could account in part for müllerian duct cysts and or an enlarged utricle. This anomaly could be the counterpart of retained vaginal cysts in females (Maizels et al, 1983).

Antiandrogen may cause the fetal cranial testis ligament to persist and contribute to undescended testis in the rat.

Just as the persistent cranial end of the mesonephric duct is recognized as the appendix epididymis, embryonal remnants of the mesonephric duct may be identified in an excised hernia sac at infant herniorrhaphy. They may be confused with, but can be differentiated from, the native vas deferens (Popek, 1990).

Thus, the external genitalia at the end of the indifferent stage are characteristic. The genital tubercle is prominent and is flanked laterally by labioscrotal swellings. The ventrum of the tubercle shows the superficial and deep urethral grooves. The paired müllerian ducts have reached the urogenital sinus (Waterman, 1982) and have fused in the midline as the müllerian tubercle. The tubercle protrudes but does not open into the posterior wall of the urogenital sinus. After 10 weeks, the genitalia of the male and female develop differently. Given the high estrogen milieu in pregnancy, absence of estrogen receptors in male fetuses may protect them from estrogen-mediated feminization effects (Jeanty et al, 1982).

The Male Urogenital Sinus

PENIS. By the 10th week, the external genitalia of a boy masculinize. The genital tubercle elongates into a cylindrical phallus. Mesenchyme in the tubercle condenses as the primitive cavernous tissue. At about 12 weeks, an oblique groove appears at the corona of the glans. This groove demarcates the glans from the shaft of the phallus. The organ is now considered to be a penis. A ridge of skin (primitive foreskin) proximal to the groove accentuates the coronal margin. The glans ventrum becomes excavated (analogous to excavation of the endodermal urethral plate) to form the fossa navicularis (Fig. 51–42). The fossa remains filled with desquamated cells. At about 14 weeks' gestation, the penis is bigger; however, the skin on the penile shaft is disproportionately excessive, especially on the dorsum, where it folds on itself "as if it were developing at a much more rapid rate of growth than the differentiating mesoderm into cavernous tissue . . . and appears as if flowing over the dorsum of the glans" (Hunter, 1935).

DEVELOPMENT OF THE SPONGIOSUM. Vasculogenesis is the differentiation of mesenchyme into endothelial precursor, which leads to the morphogenesis of de novo blood vessels (see the section entitled Development of the Great Vessels and Renal Vasculature). This differs from angiogenesis, which is the elaboration of new blood vessels from existing ones, such as mitosis of existing endothelial cells, migration of the endothelial cells to vascular tips, and the sprouting of endothelial buds, as is seen in the vascularization of developing organs (Hara et al, 1994). Angiogenesis is seen postnatally during wound healing or tumorigenesis.

Mesenchymal cells of the phallus appear to accelerate angiogenesis by facilitating cell contacts (Hara et al, 1994). The mesenchymal cells contact neighboring ones or the endothelium of existing capillaries. The mesenchyme organizes into cords, which may connect adjacent capillaries. These cell adherences show immunoreactive fibronectin at the contact areas (Hara et al, 1994).

In hypospadias and especially chordee without hypospadias, a deficiency of corpus spongiosum is evident, perhaps because of failure of this mesenchyme to condense and differentiate into spongy tissue (Altemus and Hutchins, 1991).

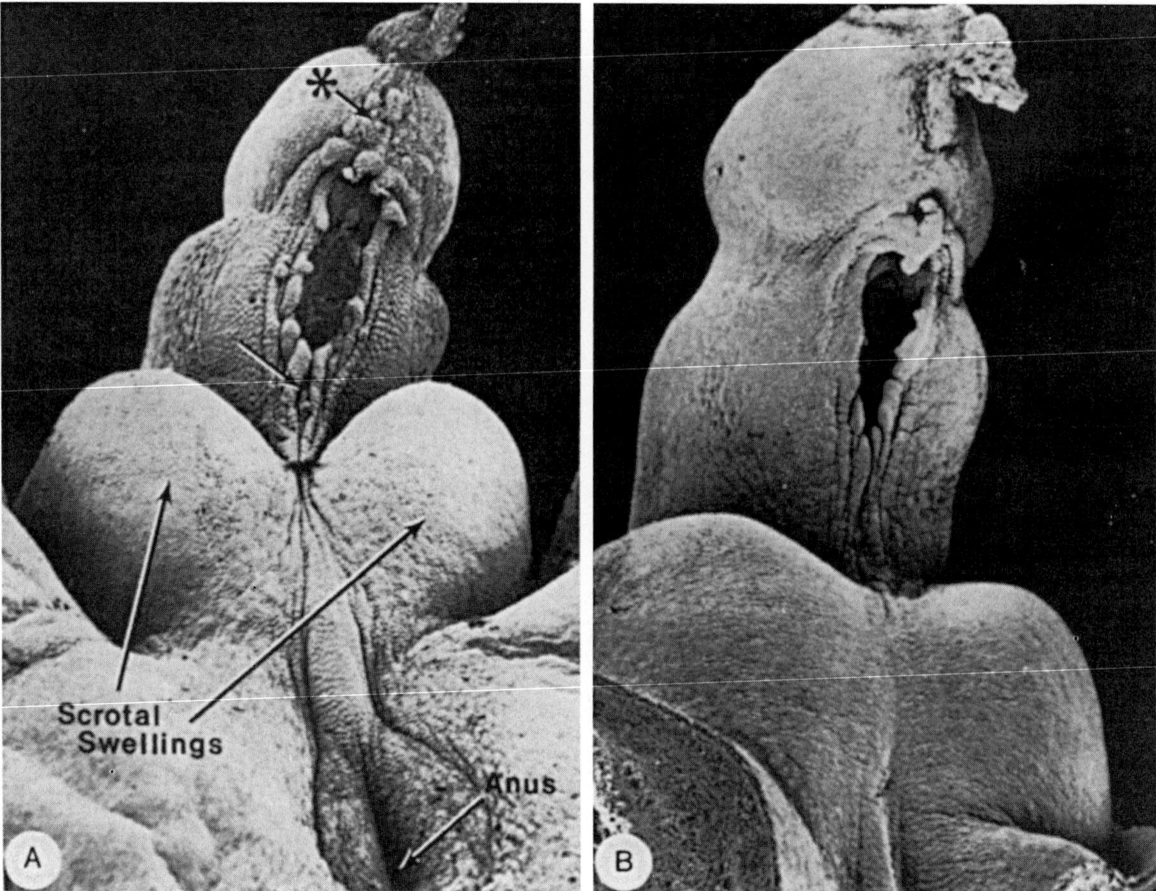

Figure 51–42. Development of the male human genitalia (10 weeks old). Scanning electron micrographs of the ventrum of the genitalia. *A*, The urethral folds are fusing to form the penile urethra. The paired scrotal swellings are converging toward each other. The asterisk marks the urethral plate. The fossa will come to be filled with squames, and the process of fusion of the urethral folds will continue on the glans to complete the glandular urethra during the 4th month. *B*, The urethral folds have fused further to form the penile urethra. The fusion is complete by the end of the 12th week. A sulcus separates the glans from the shaft of the phallus. (From Waterman RE: Human embryo and fetus. *In* Hafez ESE, Kenemans P, eds: Atlas of Human Reproduction. Hinghman, MA, Kluwer Boston, Inc., 1982.)

URETHRA

Penile Urethra. The phallic portion of the urogenital sinus develops into the bulbar and penile urethra. The mesenchyme ventral to the urethral plate epithelium proliferates to fold and approximate the edges of the plate in the midline. The mesenchyme becomes the corpus spongiosum.

The endodermal edges of the secondary urethral groove fuse to tubularize the penile urethra in the 12th week (Fig. 51–43 and see Fig. 51–27*B*). The ectodermal edges of the groove fuse as the median raphe. The penis appears straight (see Fig. 51–43). The scrotal swellings become round, migrate caudally, and fuse to form the scrotum at the base of the penis. By term, the urethra shows an outer circular and an inner longitudinal layer, both of which are contiguous with their respective layers of bladder.

Glanular Urethra. During the 16th week, the glanular urethra appears (Waterman, 1982). Debate regarding the mechanisms involved in formation of the glanular urethra has centered on whether there is ventral fusion of urethral folds or primary excavation of the glans. From a review of the archival histologic material of Hunter (1935) and scanning electron microscopic images of Rowsell and Morgan (Rowsell and Morgan, 1987), it is likely that **both mechanisms are involved.**

The developments of the glans and foreskin likely involve three processes: (1) The fossa navicularis originates from the canalization of a cord of epithelial cells, which had grown in from the tip of the glans (Ruano-Gil et al, 1975). The desquamated cells that cover the glans become a thick layer, and after 20 weeks, the desquamated cells fill the fossa navicularis. (2) The urethral folds (now at the level of the glans corona) extend ventrally to fuse in the midline. This ventral fusion of the folds extends distally to make the floor of the glanular urethra. Ventral fusion of the glanular urethral folds traps the squames, which now appear to plug the glanular urethra. The urethral meatus is now at its definitive glanular position. (3) The foreskin grows ventrally until it completely encircles the glans (Altemus and Hutchins, 1991). The preputial and urethral folds fuse on the ventrum of the glans as the frenulum (Fig. 51–44).

It is plausible that the many anatomic variants of distal shaft hypospadias stem from combinations of anomalous development of these three mechanisms. For example, in patients in whom the glanular urethral folds did not fuse but

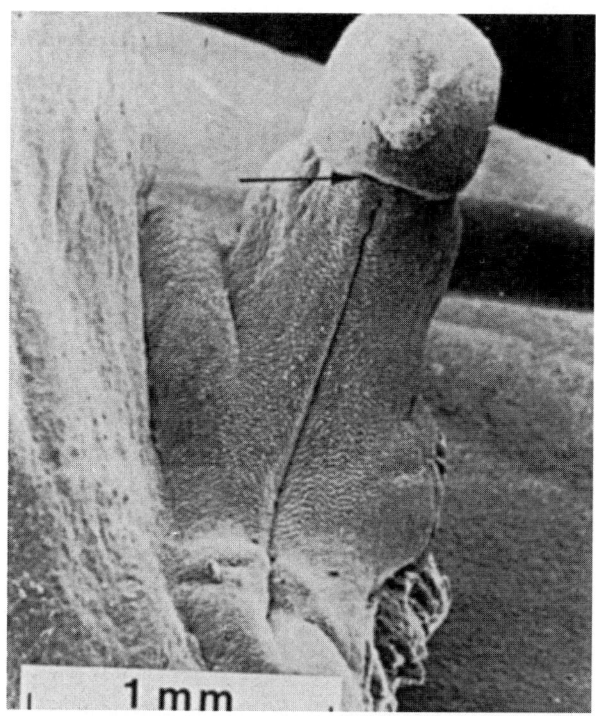

Figure 51–43. Development of male human genitalia (penis) (12 weeks old). The coronal sulcus *(arrow)* separates the glans from the shaft of the penis. The urethral folds have met in the middle on the ventrum of the shaft. An epithelial tag just above the arrow on the glans likely is the site of excavation. (From Rowsell AK, Morgan BDG: Br J Plast Surg 1987; 40:201.)

there was fusion of the preputial folds, the penis would present with hypospadias with a complete foreskin (Hatch et al, 1989). Or, if the glanular urethral folds did not fuse and the glans failed to canalize, the result would be a globular appearance of the glans in some cases of hypospadias.

Failure of fusion of the urethral folds blocks development of the prepuce ventrally, especially the frenulum. These features are typical of hypospadias in boys and of normal development of the clitoral prepuce in girls (Altemus and Hutchins, 1991).

Penile cysts are sometimes referred to as dysembryoplasia involving aberrant fusion of the urethral folds. This is evidenced by noting that segments of epithelium in such a cyst retained below the penile skin demonstrate cytokeratin 13 immunohistochemically (Richard-Lallemand et al, 1994).

However, other rarer anomalies of the urethra do not lend to easy explanation as variants of normal development (Roy-Choudhury and Maji, 1991). Furthermore, the mechanism of urethra formation may vary across species because in the rat, perineal growth appears to push the urethral ostium forward. No urethral folds were noted (Kluth et al, 1988).

Expansion of the epithelial plug in the glans forms the lacuna magna, a site of potential urethral symptoms in boys (Stephens and Fortune, 1993).

Obstruction of the glans due to faulty glans canalization has been noted in fetuses with megalourethra; this could adversely affect the development of the urethra. The condensed mesenchyme destined to form the rigid tunics of the urethra is dispersed, so the urethra yields easily to the obstruction, the lumen dilates, and the wall thins. The mesenchyme, now dispersed, can only make a fibrotic wall rather than healthy spongiosum (Stephens and Fortune, 1993).

Molecular Biology of Seaming the Urethral Lumen. Tenascin, an extracellular matrix glycoprotein that was originally found at the junction between muscle fibers and tendon, is also found in morphogenetically active tissues that are involved with cell adhesion, condensation, and migration (Murakami et al, 1990). Its actions may be mediated via cytoskeletal organization. By immune staining, tenascin was noted in the interstitium of the mesenchyme of the mouse urethral plate during the separation of the urethral plate from the glans. The open, ventral urethra was seamed closed by mesenchyme, which was rich in actin filaments. Tenascin remained in the ventral seam. As tenascin binds to extracellular matrix components, tenascin could mediate cell adhesion to maintain the formation of the newly formed urethra. Also, perhaps, the actin generates mechanical force to participate in formation and closure of the urethral lumen.

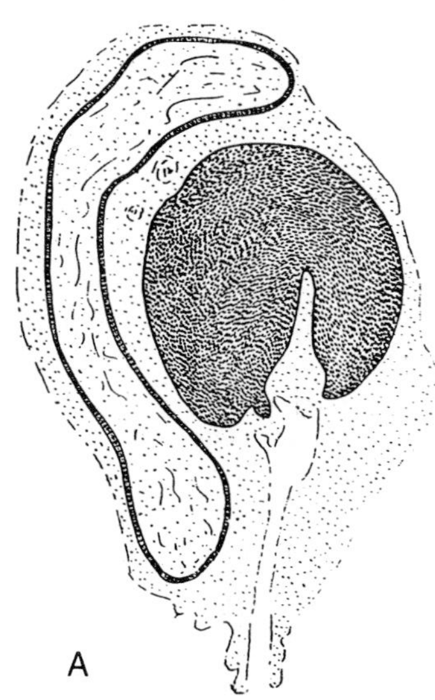

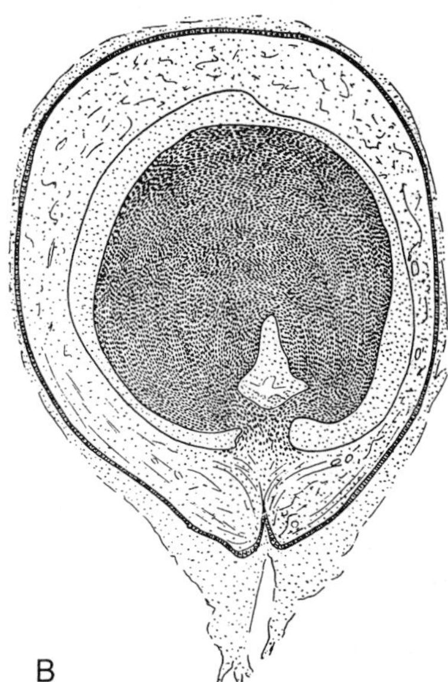

Figure 51–44. Glans penis of the human fetus. *A,* At about 16 weeks' gestation, urethral folds extend ventrally. They will later meet and fuse in the midline. This pattern of fusion traps a plug of squames. *B,* After 20 weeks' gestation, the glandular urethra is complete, and the frenulum marks the site where the preputial and urethral folds fused. (From Hunter RH: J Anat 1935; 70:68.)

PREPUCE. Separation of the prepuce from the glans begins by 6 months of gestation and involves keratinization of the apposed preputial and glanular epithelia (Deibert, 1933). Keratinization begins at opposite sites, the glans corona and distal margin of the prepuce, which extend toward each other. Keratinization leads to pearl formation. The pearl cavitates to create a lumen. When several longitudinally arranged pearls coalesce, the foreskin is separable from the glans. After birth, larger newborns show more preputial glanular separation than smaller ones. Separation should be sufficient by 10 days old to allow mechanical retraction without the likelihood of tearing the epithelia. At surgery for circumcision or hypospadias repair, the degree of pearl formation is variable. When excess preputial skin still remains after circumcision, it may adhere to the underlying glans. Perhaps this occurs in those children in whom pearl formation is deficient and the artificial separation by circumcision was premature. In other children who experience balanitis from infected smegma, perhaps pearl formation is excessive and chemical irritation or bacterial superinfection, or both, follow.

PROSTATE. The pelvic urethra develops into the prostatic and membranous urethra (see Fig. 51–29) (Hamilton et al, 1976b). Prostatic differentiation in the human embryo begins at 8 weeks, with mesenchymal cells under the basal lamina developing into fibroblasts. The testicular Leydig cells are differentiated at this time (Kellokumpu-Lehtinen and Pelliniemi, 1988).

By the tenth week, epithelial outgrowths from the pelvic urethra grow and branch out into the surrounding mesenchyme. By 12 weeks, five groups of tubules have formed the lobes of the prostate (Lowsley, 1912): (1) The middle lobe is made up of about ten branching tubules, which originate on the floor of the urethra between the bladder and the orifices of the ejaculatory ducts. (2) and (3) The lateral lobes originate from about 35 tubules on the lateral walls of the urethra. (4) The posterior lobe originates from the floor of the urethra distal to the ostia of the ejaculatory ducts. The tubules of the posterior lobe grow back behind the lateral lobes from which they are separated by a fibrotic capsule; as the tubules grow out, they push the circular musculature and scatter the fibers. These scattered fibers of circular urethral muscle become the prostate capsule (Wood-Jones, 1901–1902) (Figs. 51–37 and 51–45). The anterior lobe is prominent until 16 weeks of development and then involutes to become insignificant by 22 weeks (Fig. 51–46) (Lowsley, 1912).

Lumens appear in the epithelial buds at the period of maximal testosterone secretion (10 weeks) and contain acid phosphatase. Androgens accelerate the differentiation of a secretory epithelium in vitro after the mesenchyme has begun to differentiate in vivo (Kellokumpu-Lehtinen and Pelliniemi, 1988). The epithelia of the nearby wolffian and müllerian ducts do not appear to contribute to the prostate as the urethra does. All three duct systems (urethra, wolffian, and müllerian) contribute to epithelium of the seminal colliculus. The epithelial cells in the luminal part of the region are columnar, whereas those in the outer part of the prostatic urethra are cuboidal (Kellokumpu-Lehtinen and Pelliniemi, 1988). Through tissue recombinant experiments, Cuhna (1984) showed that depending on the androgen level, mesenchyme but not epithelium of the urogenital sinus induced specific epithelial morphogenesis. During embryonic and neonatal periods, mesenchyme alone exhibits androgen receptor activity. Androgens can accelerate the differentiation of human urethral epithelial cells into secretory prostatic cells in vitro (Kellokumpu-Lehtinen and Pelliniemi, 1988).

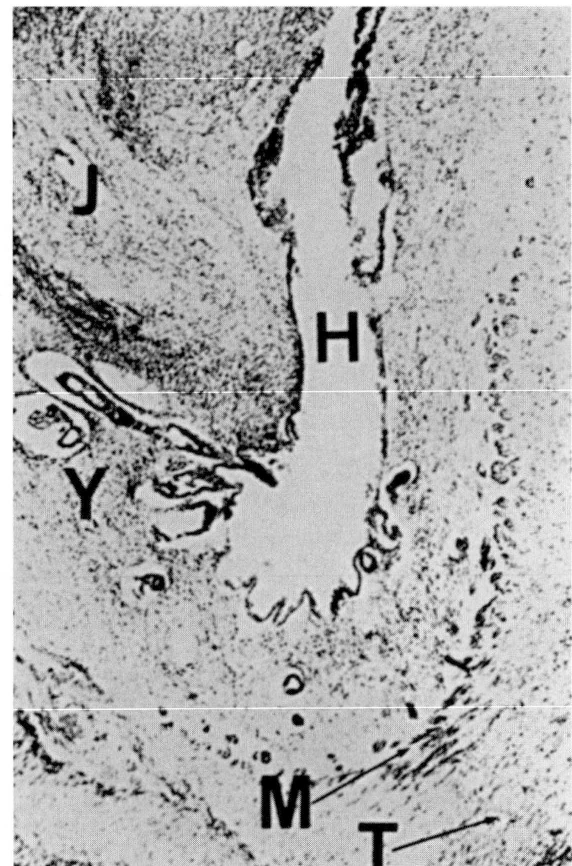

Figure 51–45. Posterior urethra of human fetus at 16 weeks' gestation (sagittal orientation). Prostate buds (Y); striated muscle around the urethra (T), which bounds an inner layer of circular smooth muscle (M); and ejaculatory duct (J) are apparent. (H, lumen of urethra.) (From Matsuno T, Tokunaka S, Koyanagi T: J Urol 1984; 132:148.)

Prostate-specific acid phosphatase, a marker for the development of secondary sexual characteristics, is noted at about 17 weeks' gestational age. Squamous metaplasia, an estrogen-related effect, was also noted in the utricle and large prostatic ducts (Popek et al, 1991).

Postnatal development of the human prostate involves the following factors: (1) In infancy, stratified squamous epithelium initially elicited by maternal estrogens involutes to cuboidal pseudostratified epithelium; (2) in preadolescence (14 years of age), the epithelium is quiescent but acini outgrow in close contact with smooth muscle; and (3) during adolescence, there is maturation involving papillary projections and prostate-specific antigen–positive secretions (Aumuller, 1991).

Prune-belly syndrome may result from deficient mesenchymal and epithelial interactions, perhaps as a primary mesenchymal defect. Pathologic examination of fetal cases show **deficient mesenchyme and ductal development as well as deficient muscle bundle formation of the bladder neck sphincter deficient (mesenchymal maldevelopment).** This condition is distinguished from fetal obstruction by

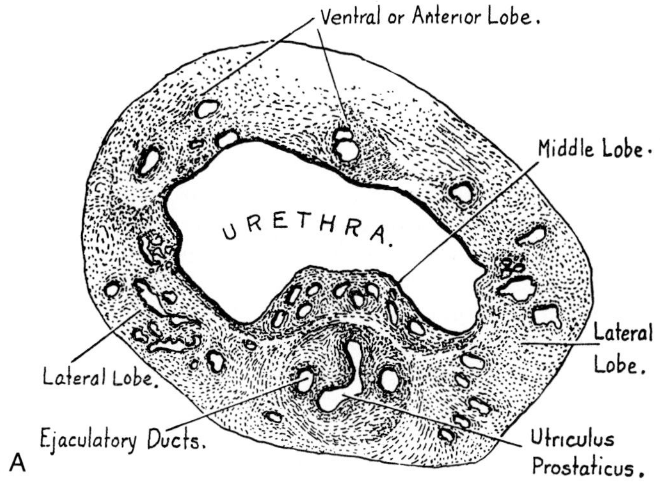

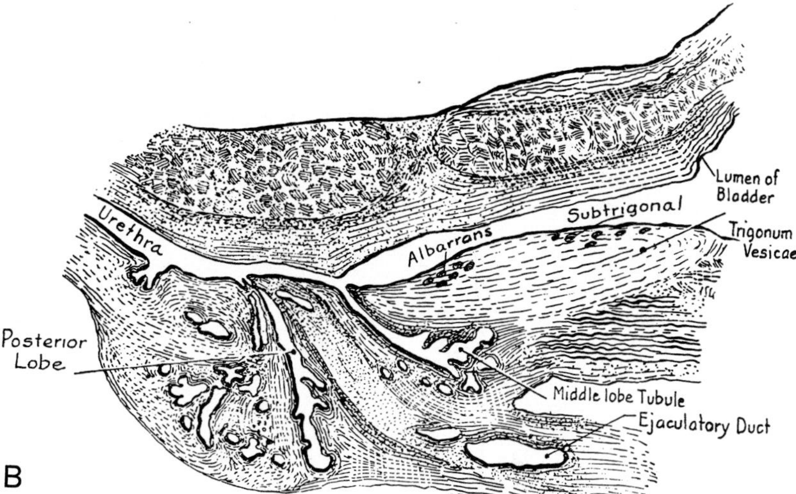

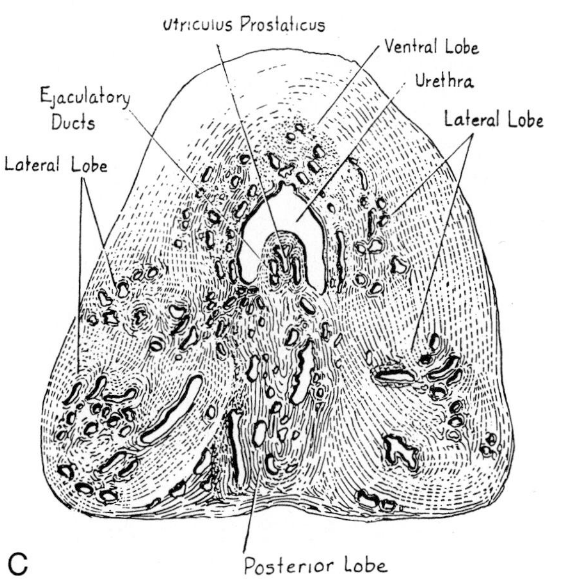

Figure 51–46. Development of the prostate. *A,* At 4 months (transverse section). *B,* At 5 months (longitudinal section). *C,* At 7½ months (transverse section). (From Lowsley OS: Am J Anat 1912; 13:299.)

posterior urethral valves, which show normal, albeit heightened, mesenchymal differentiation in the verumontanum and bladder neck sphincter (Fig. 51–47) (Popek et al, 1991).

Normally, the verumontanum is proximal to the urogenital diaphragm, as a result of the absorption of the fused müllerian ducts into the pelvic urethra. In about 10% of patients with hypospadias, especially severe hypospadias, the verumontanum may be seen by cystoscopy to be at the level of the external sphincter or within the bulbar urethra. This caudal position could result from an abnormal hormonal milieu during development (Ikoma and Shima, 1991).

Molecular Biology of Urogenital Sinus Morphogenesis. The **epithelium of the urogenital sinus and genital tubercle can convert testosterone (produced by the testis) to the more potent androgen dihydrotestosterone (George et al, 1988).** Dihydrotestosterone mediates the differentiation of the derivatives of the urogenital sinus, namely, the prostate (Cunha, 1972; Kellokumpu-Lehtinen and Pelliniemi, 1988), from the pelvic portion of the urogenital sinus, and the external genitalia from the phallic portion of the urogenital sinus (Siiteri and Wilson, 1974). Testosterone mediates the differentiation of the derivatives of the wolffian duct; namely, seminal vesicle, epididymis, and vas deferens (George et al, 1988).

This different responsiveness of target organ to androgen helps explain why in patients in whom the external genitalia cannot convert testosterone to dihydrotestosterone (reductase needed but deficient), they do not masculinize, whereas the internal genitalia in the same patient do masculinize (reductase not needed) (George et al, 1988).

Seminal vesicle induction is an androgen-dependent epithelial-mesenchymal interaction between androgen-receptor–positive mesenchyme and epithelium. In mice, keratinocyte growth factor, a member of FGB, is produced by the mesenchyme and stroma, and likely mediates the androgen-dependent event (Alarid et al, 1994).

COWPER'S GLANDS. Cowper's glands are present by 12 weeks of development. They originate as endodermal buds of the urogenital sinus. The buds penetrate the surrounding compact mesenchyme of the corpus spongiosum. The buds enlarge as racemose glands at the level of the membranous urethra and remain as small glands at the level of the bulbar urethra. After 18 weeks, a glandular epithelium appears (Fig. 51–48).

Cystic anomalies of the gland and duct system engender Cowper's syringocele (Maizels et al, 1983; Brien et al, 1990).

The Female Urogenital Sinus

URETHRA. The pelvic part of the urogenital sinus develops into the lower portion of the definitive urethra and vagina (Hamilton and Mossman, 1976b). Epithelial tubules originate from the primitive urethra after about 11 weeks (Stephens, 1983) to become the paraurethral glands

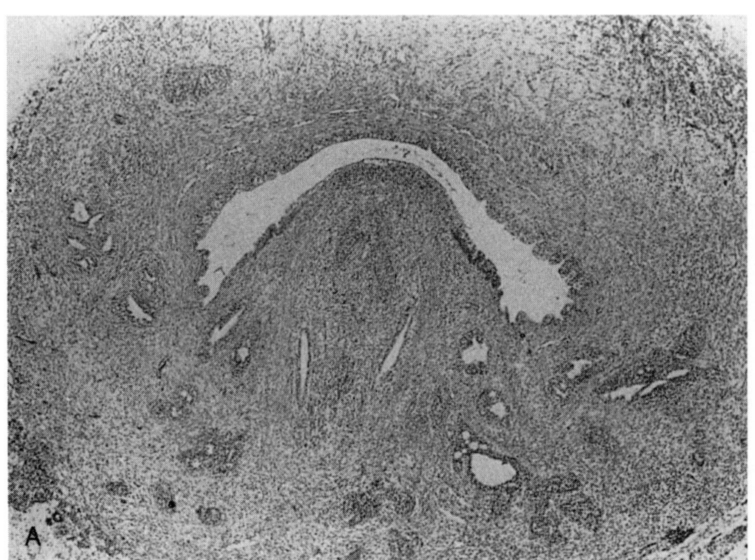

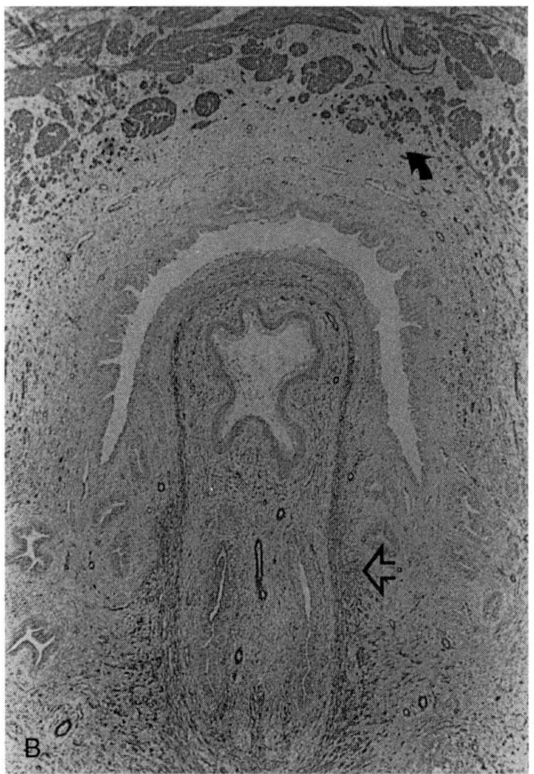

Figure 51–47. Normal human prostate development. *A,* The ejaculatory ducts and solid utricle are visible on the verumontanum (16-week-old fetus, × 10). *B,* By 23 weeks, the utricle is well developed, showing squamous metaplasia, and the ejaculatory ducts issue toward the utricle (× 10). In prune-belly syndrome, deficient mesenchyme makes these structures diminutive. (From Popek EJ, Tyson RW, Miller GJ, Caldwell SA: Prostate development in prune belly syndrome (PBS) and posterior urethral valves (PUV): Etiology of PBS—lower urinary tract obstruction or primary mesenchymal defect? Pediatr Pathol 1991; 11:1–29. Reproduced with permission.)

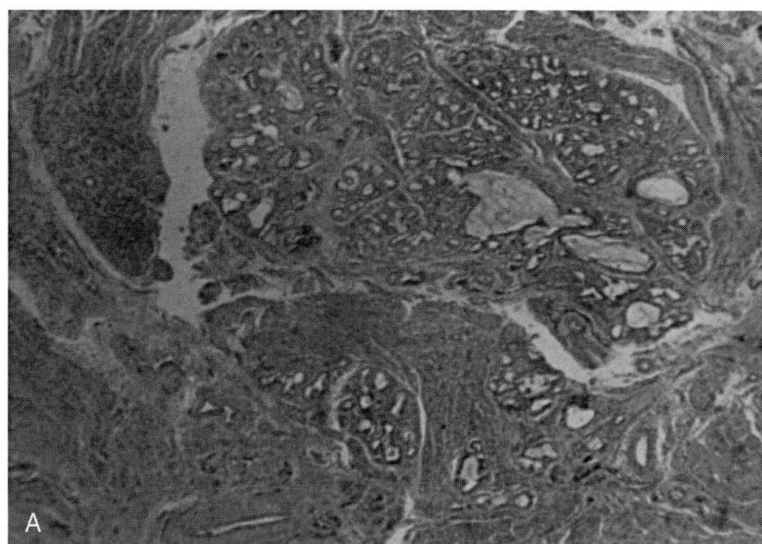

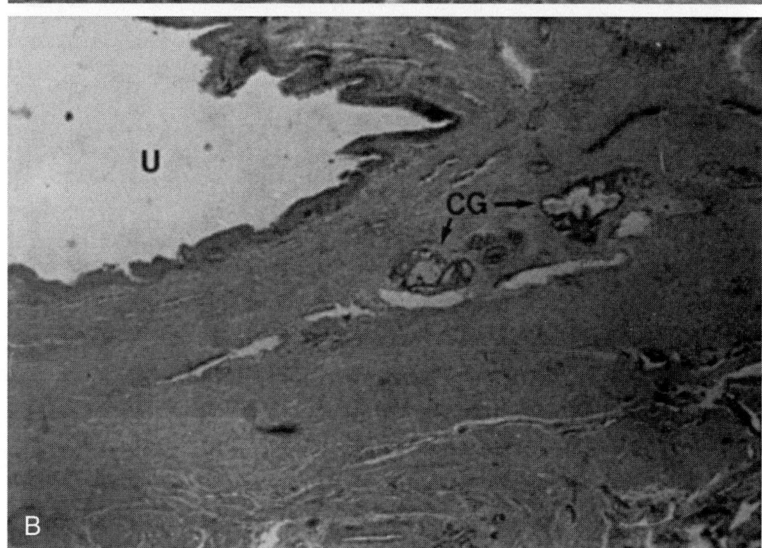

Figure 51–48. Cowper's gland consists of *(A)* glands with racemose drainage at the level of the membranous urethra and *(B)* small glands (CG) near the bulbar urethra (U) (histologic section of stillborn fetus). (Courtesy of FD Stephens.)

of Skene (Hamilton and Mossman, 1976b). These glands are the female homologues of the prostate. Mesenchymal differentiation in the female urethra is less prominent than in the analogous segment in the male (Kellokumpu-Lehtinen and Pelliniemi, 1988).

EXTERNAL GENITALIA. The female embryo at the indifferent phase of genital development begins to feminize the external genitalia in the absence of androgen between 10 and 12 weeks' gestational age (Fig. 51–49). Feminization is mediated by estrogen receptors, which are present only in females. The receptors respond to the high estrogen milieu in pregnancy. Genital swellings grow slowly to cover the superior and lateral aspects of the clitoris (in the male, the swellings grow inferiorly and medially), resulting in a female phenotype. There is a single perineal opening that serves the urethra and vagina. The labia minora are small.

Next, between 20 and 25 weeks' gestational age, fetal ovarian follicular growth starts, likely as a consequence of fetal pituitary FSH, and is associated with the following events. There is rapid ventral outgrowth in the perineum, which brings separate urethral and vaginal openings to the perineum. The labia majora enlarge posteriorly. Then the labia minora grow more than the labia majora, so the labia minora are now prominent and protrude out of the labia majora by 25 weeks' gestational age (as is seen in girls born prematurely). By 26 weeks' gestational age, the labia majora now cover the minora.

The female phenotype is complete by 26 weeks' gestational age. Feminization of genitalia is slower than masculinization, which ends by 14 weeks' gestational age.

HYMEN AND VAGINAL INTROITUS. The embryogenesis of the hymen is important clinically. Examination of newborn girls without major anomalies of the urogenital tract shows that the hymen is uniformly present (Jenny et al, 1987; Mor and Merlob, 1988). This is in contrast to cases with urogenital anomalies (atresia, duplication), in which the hymen is absent.

Variations in the normal skin distribution in the introitus should be kept in mind during examination of girls for sexual abuse. Failure of midline fusion of skin across the posterior fourchette may leave this area covered only by mucosa, which resembles that of the hymen. This mucosa

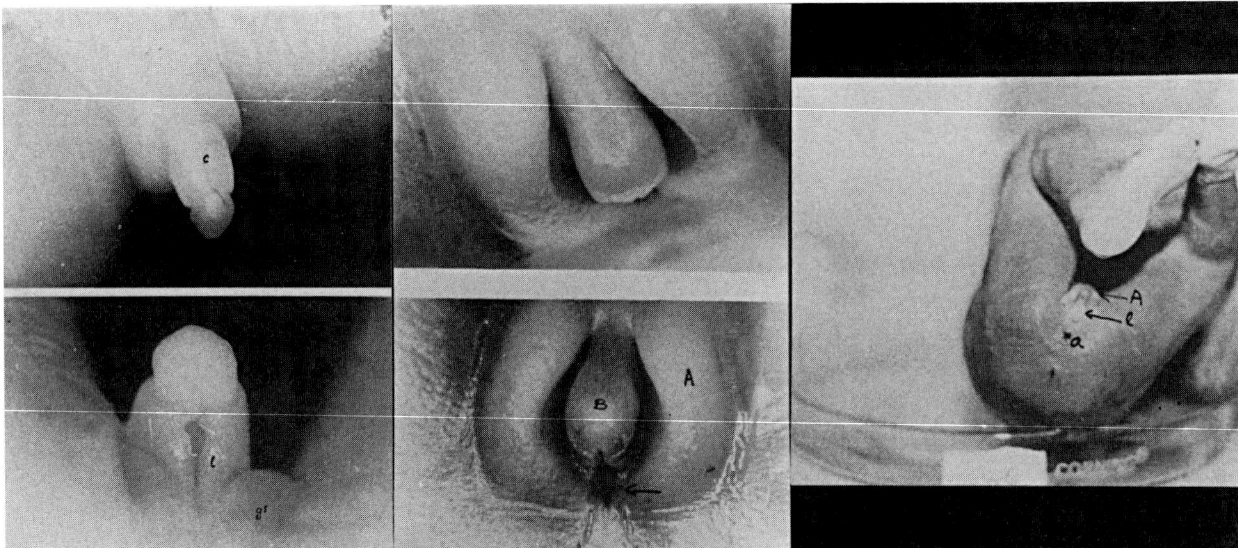

Figure 51–49. Feminization of the external genitalia. *Left panel,* At 12 weeks' gestation, the clitoris (c) is phallus like, the urethral folds (l) are separate up to the base of the clitoris, and the genital swellings (gs) are separate. The urethral folds do not fuse. (From Jirasek JE: Morphogenesis of the genital system in the human. Birth Defects 1977; 15:13.) *Middle panel,* At 22 weeks' gestation, the clitoris (B) is prominent and the genital swellings have migrated up to structure the labia majora (A). *Right panel,* At 26 weeks' gestation, the labia minora (l) protrude out of the labia majora (A) (a, anus.) (In *left* and *middle panels,* top row is dorsal view; bottom row is ventral view.) (From Ammini AC, Pandey J, Vijyaraghavan M, Sabherwal U: Human female phenotypic development: Role of fetal ovaries. J Clin Endocrinol Metab 1994; 79:604–608. © The Endocrine Society.)

extends to the anus. Because the mucosa resembles that of the normal hymen, this appearance of the external genitalia is a congenital anomaly rather than a result of sexual abuse (Adams and Horton, 1989). Estrogen effects may be responsible for edema and hypertrophy of hymenal tissues, which present as hymeneal bands or tags. The bands should involute by a few weeks after birth as the estrogen effects wane (Mor et al, 1983).

VESTIBULE. The phallic portion of the urogenital sinus remains a vestibule because the urethral plate does not extend as far to the genital tubercle as in the male (see Fig. 51–29*A*). The urethra and vagina open into the vestibule (see Fig. 51–49). The labial swellings grow posterior to the vestibule and meet to form the posterior commissure. The swellings also grow lateral to the vestibule to form the labia majora. Urethral folds that flank the urogenital sinus develop into the labia minora (Hamilton and Mossman, 1976b). The phallic part of the urogenital sinus (undersurface of the elongated genital tubercle) contains the urethral grooves, which remain open and thereby contribute to the vaginal vestibule (Bellinger and Duckett, 1982). After the ninth week of development, Bartholin's glands begin as evaginations of the vestibule endoderm and then grow into the labia majora (Stephens, 1983). These glands are the homologues of Cowper's glands in the male. This development is complete by 12 weeks (Waterman, 1982).

Developmental Biology of Masculinized Female Phenotype

Masculinization of female phenotype may occur because genotypic females have androgen receptors. Perhaps, androgen excess could lead to ovarian dysfunction as an additional mechanism behind female pseudohermaphroditism (hypoplastic labia—failure of ovarian function, without clitoromegaly). Masculinization of the female phenotype may include labioscrotal fusion with clitoral hypertrophy (androgen 8–13 weeks' gestational age) or isolated clitoromegaly (androgen after 13 weeks' gestational age) (Ammini et al, 1994). Müllerian inhibiting factor is negligible in the human ovary during gestation (Mor et al, 1983).

A perineal lipoma is commonly noted in an accessory scrotum or, rarely, in an accessory labium majus. The lipoma may have interfered mechanically with normal local morphogenetic migration. These cases do not show associated anomalies. This is distinguished from cases of accessory scrotum and labium without a lipoma, which do show anomalies. Perhaps, such cases without lipoma are more reflective of so-called developmental disorganization of the perineum (Ben-Rafel, 1993; Sule et al, 1994).

Hormonal factors (such as androgen exposure, most commonly from congenital adrenal hyperplasia) may lead the urethral folds to fuse. The union of the folds in utero causes posterior labial fusion in the newborn. It may be that the time period when the folds are exposed to androgen influences the outcome. If the exposure is before 12 to 14 weeks' gestation, posterior fusion and clitoromegaly results. Although exposure after this period results only in clitoromegaly (Klein et al, 1989), a familial form of posterior labial fusion characterized by autosomal dominant inheritance has been described. Knowledge of the embryology helps distinguish posterior labial fusion (a union of the urethral folds in utero) from labial adhesion (an agglutination of the labia minora as a consequence of inflammation). Labial fusion is congenital, does not show a midline raphe, and does not recur after operative correction. Although labial adhesion is rare in the newborn, it shows a midline raphe, which is a result of labial inflammation, and may recur after surgical correction (Klein et al, 1989).

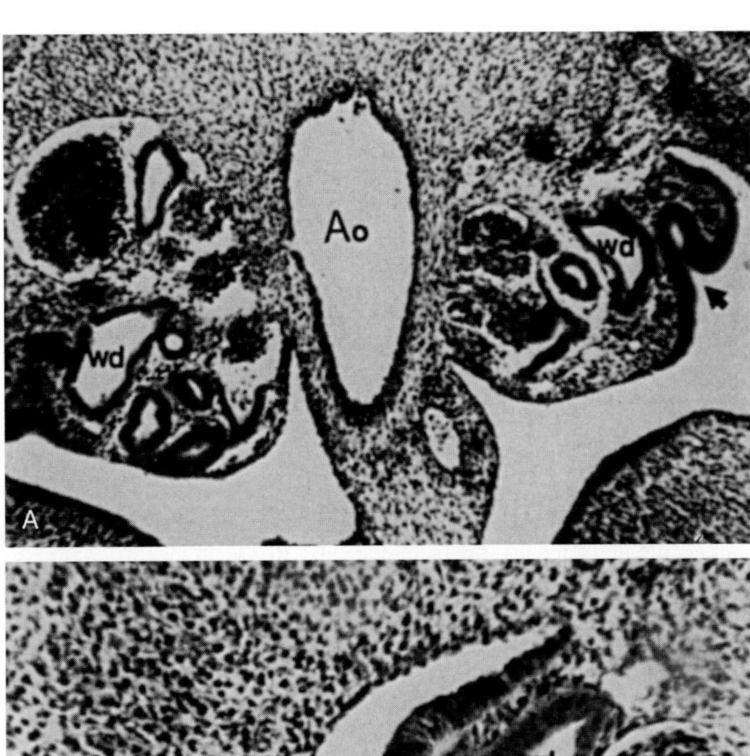

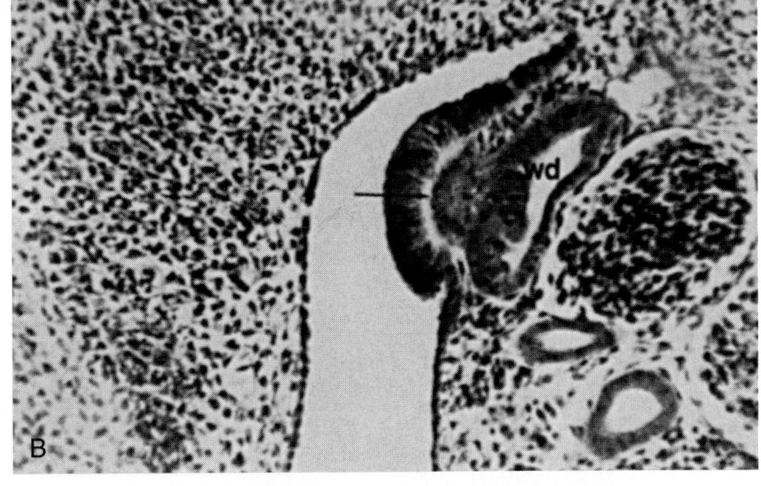

Figure 51–50. Early formation of the müllerian ducts. *A*, The ducts begin as an invagination of the peritoneum *(arrow)* near the developing diaphragm (Ao, aorta). *B*, They descend as a solid core *(arrow)* toward the pelvis alongside the mesonephric duct (wd) (chick embryo). (From Maizels M, Stephens FD: The induction of urologic malformations: Understanding the relationship of renal ectopia and congenital scoliosis. Invest Urol 1979; 17:209.)

Labial fusion has been reported to cause bladder neck obstruction (Wheeler and Burge, 1991).

DEVELOPMENT OF THE DUCTS OF THE GENITALIA

Indifferent Stage

The genital ducts appear during the fifth to sixth weeks. Because genetic males and females appear structurally the same until 10 weeks' gestational age, this period is known as the indifferent stage of sexual development.

The müllerian ducts originate as a funnel-shaped invagination of the coelomic epithelium (peritoneum) near each side of the developing diaphragm (Fig. 51–50). The müllerian duct is also referred to as the paramesonephric duct because it descends to the pelvis lateral and adjacent to the basement membrane of the mesonephric duct (Gruenwald, 1941). The mesonephric and paramesonephric ducts show different ultrastructural characteristics, supporting their different origins (Fig. 51–51) (Lawrence et al, 1992). In the

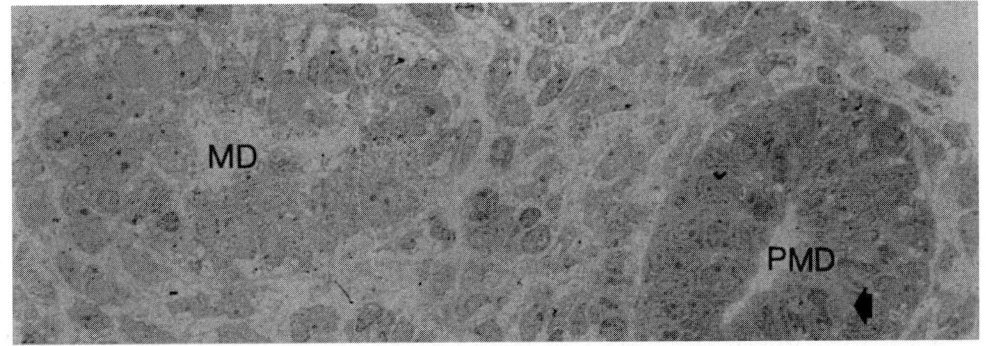

Figure 51–51. The mesonephric duct (MD) appears different from the paramesonephric duct (PMD). This difference supports their different embryologic origins. (Human embryo about 5 weeks' gestational age, × 782.) (From Lawrence WD, Whitaker D, Sugimura H, et al: An ultrastructural study of the developing urogenital tract in early human fetuses. Am J Obstet Gynecol 1992; 167:185–193.)

cranial region, the ducts are separated by mesenchyme; caudally, they are juxtaposed but separate.

The lower segment of the müllerian duct crosses anterior to the mesonephric duct. At about the eighth week of gestation, the medial segments of the müllerian ducts at the level of the bladder fuse to form the uterovaginal primordium (müllerian vagina) (see Figs. 51–34 and 51–35). This primordium (in the female) later merges with an expansion of the urogenital sinus (sinus vagina) to make one contiguous vagina (see the section later that discusses the female) (see Figs. 51–56*A* and 51–57). The uterovaginal primordium protrudes into the dorsal wall of the pelvic portion of the urogenital sinus as Müller's tubercle (see Figs. 51–34 and 51–35). This tubercle lies between and cranial to the mesonephric duct orifices. During the indifferent stage, the mesonephroi begin to degenerate. Between 4 and 8 weeks, the thoracic portions of the mesonephroi degenerate, but newly formed tubules caudally maintain the bulk of the organ in the lumbar region (Felix, 1912d). Of the persisting tubules, the upper 5 to 12 tubules comprise the epigenitalis and a similar number of tubules at the lower portion comprise the paragenitalis. The glomeruli of the epigenitalis degenerate, but their connections to the collecting ducts of the mesonephric duct remain. The ends of the collecting ducts become surrounded by the indifferent gonad. By 8 weeks' gestational age, enzymes necessary for androgen synthesis are present in the human fetal testis. The male gonad differentiates into a testis. The female gonad differentiates into an ovary later, during midgestation (see earlier).

Male

UROGENITAL UNION. After 12 weeks, urogenital union, the fusion of testicular and mesonephric ducts, begins. The rete tubules in the testis connect to the epigenitalis of the mesonephros (Fig. 51–52) (Wood-Jones, 1901–1902). These epigenital ducts now become the efferent ducts (Felix, 1912e, 1912f), and the mesonephric duct becomes the vas deferens. During the fourth month, the efferent ducts adjacent to the testis remain straight, whereas those adjacent to the vas deferens coil. The upper portion of the vas deferens also coils and becomes the epididymis, whereas the lower portion near the müllerian tubercle dilates fourfold to become an ampulla (Felix, 1912g). The lower portion of the vas deferens develops concentric layers of mesenchyme by about 12 weeks, but muscle fibers are not seen until 28 weeks (Felix, 1912g). After 12 weeks, outgrowth of the seminal vesicle bud leads to a septum, which divides the ampulla of the distal portion of the vas deferens into the ejaculatory duct and seminal vesicle (Felix, 1912g).

The remaining mesonephric tubules become vestigial. **Epigenital tubules, which do not participate in urogenital union, remain as the appendix of the epididymis.** The paradidymis comprises the lower group of the lumbar mesonephric tubules (paragenitalis). The paragenitalis degenerates, but tubules between the head of the epididymis and the testis may remain as the organ of Giraldes.

ANATOMY OF TESTIS DESCENT. Heyns (1987) studied **the human anatomy of the gubernaculum and**

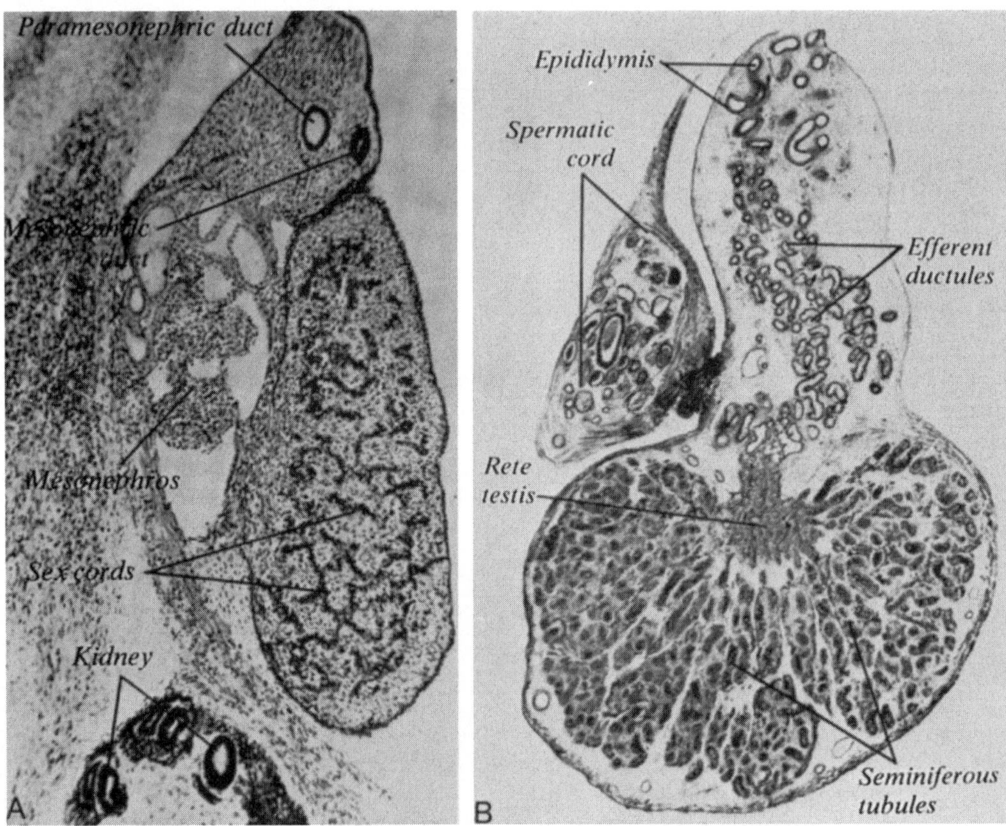

Figure 51–52. Development of the testis and urogenital union. *A*, By 8 weeks, the medullary sex cords have begun to differentiate. The glomeruli of the epigenitalis degenerate, and the collecting tubules will later drain the tubules of the testis. *B*, By 20 weeks, the rete tubules of the testis drain into the coiled efferent ducts. (From FitzGerald MJT: Human Embryology. New York, Harper & Row, 1978.)

testis through dissection of male fetuses. At the stage of the intra-abdominal testis, the epididymis and lower pole of the testis are attached to the gubernaculum (see the discussion of ligaments of the gonads earlier), a cylinder of jelly-like tissue that resembles Wharton's jelly in the umbilical cord. The gubernaculum is covered by peritoneum except posteriorly, where it is adjacent to the mediastinum of the testis (Fig. 51–53). The caudal end of the gubernaculum enters the internal inguinal ring. The inguinal canal is short, with the internal and external rings almost on top of each other. The author has observed the following: (1) Before 23 weeks' gestation, the gubernaculum is above the external ring. (2) The gubernaculum begins to swell, as monitored by wet weight. The swelling peaks at about 28 weeks. (3) The gubernaculum bulges through the external ring. The gubernaculum does not have scrotal extensions (see Fig. 51–53). (4) The testis, epididymis, and gubernaculum move through the inguinal canal as a unit. (5) The gubernaculum becomes smaller and fibrous. By comparison, the wet weight of Wharton's jelly of the umbilicus does not change during this period.

The patent processus advances down by excavating into the gubernaculum. This results in a hollowing out of the gubernaculum and is necessary for testis descent.

Heyns (1987) concludes there are **three anatomic phases of testis descent:** (1) internal descent of the testis toward the internal ring is caused by differential growth of the lumbar vertebral column and pelvis; (2) quick passage of the testis through the inguinal canal is mediated by gubernacular swelling; and (3) descent of the testis from the external ring to the scrotum. The testis descends into the scrotum after 26 weeks' gestation; 60% of males show testis descent by 30 weeks; 93% after 32 weeks (Birnholz, 1983).

MÜLLERIAN DUCTS. The müllerian ducts degenerate after 8 weeks of development when exposed to MIS, which is produced by the Sertoli cells. The degeneration occurs mostly in a craniocaudal direction. In the laboratory, the cranial portion of the duct is more sensitive to the effect of MIS than the caudal portion of the duct (Donahoe et al, 1977), but clinically, regression extends both caudally and cranially (Fig. 51–54). The cranial end of the degenerating müllerian duct may persist as the appendix of the testis (appendix of epididymis) (Fig. 51–55). By 16 weeks, the caudal end of the müllerian duct is degenerated to the level of the ejaculatory ducts (Deibert, 1933). The müllerian vagina does not form, and testosterone inhibits formation of the sinus vagina (Fig. 51–56) (see the section entitled Development of the Ducts of the Genitalia, Female) (Bok and Drews, 1983). At this level, the müllerian ducts are fused as the uterovaginal primordium. This primordium persists as the prostatic utricle (see Fig. 51–46). The utricle becomes large, and a dense layer of stroma surrounds it. The utricle opens into the urogenital sinus in the midline, adjacent to the orifices of the ejaculatory ducts (see Fig. 51–35*b*) (Deibert, 1933). By 22 weeks, the utricle and ejaculatory ducts expand under the floor of the urethra and elevate the wall of the urethra to create the verumontanum (Deibert, 1933). The verumontanum causes the lumen of the prostatic urethra to appear semilunar (see Figs. 51–46*C* and 51–47). Later, the utricle contracts to appear as a small structure on the tip of the verumontanum. By 30 weeks, the seminal vesicles have grown back behind the base of the bladder and the ejaculatory ducts are surrounded by thick musculature.

MOLECULAR BIOLOGY OF MÜLLERIAN DUCT REGRESSION. The mechanisms whereby MIS causes regression of the müllerian ducts are becoming better understood (Josso, 1973; Donahoe et al, 1977). MIS is a polypeptide that is produced by the fetal Sertoli cells. The steroids testosterone, medroxyprogesterone, and progesterone augment the effect of MIS in vitro (Ikawa et al, 1982). This augmentation is believed to be mediated by binding of the steroids to receptors of the mesenchyme that surrounds the müllerian duct. After local absorption of the substance, the mesenchyme may then alter the extracellular matrix by increased hyaluronidase activity or fibronectin lysis. These alterations may facilitate breakdown of the müllerian duct basement membrane (Ikawa et al, 1982; Trelstad et al, 1982). MIS can also act as a hormone (Donahoe et al, 1976). In the rat, only 24 hours of exposure of the müllerian duct to MIS is needed to degenerate the duct (Donahoe, 1977). The gene for MIS is mapped to the short arm of chromosome 19 (Cohen-Haguenaur et al, 1987). In the human testis, MIS is present in high amounts after midgestation, even when müllerian duct regression is complete. Perhaps, other, as yet unrecognized activities for this substance will be found during this period (Voutilainen and Miller, 1987).

The syndrome of hernia uteri inguinale results from a lack of MIS at the end of the indifferent stage of development. The müllerian duct structures (uterus, fallopian tube) persist. This appears in a genotypically and phenotypically normal boy who has cryptorchidism and hernia. Müllerian structures are found inside the hernia sac. The condition is genetically heterologous and may involve an X-linked or an autosomal recessive transmission pattern (Naguib et al, 1989). This syndrome has been described in women who present with an inguinal hernia that contains an ovary, fallopian tube, and unicornuate uterus but is not demonstrated to be related to an aberration of the normal MIS expression (Elliott et al, 1989).

Androgen binding is seen in the developing male rat in the tissue primordia of the glans, corpora, urethral epithelium and its mesenchyme, and prepuce (Murakami, 1987). The female shows much weaker binding in these sites. The fact that the cells that are especially labeled are mesenchymal suggests that as in the prostate, the mesenchymal cells are the targets whereby androgens mediate morphogenesis. Insensitivity to testosterone may explain why in males with the testicular feminization syndrome, in whom there is diminished androgen receptor activity (Cunha, 1972), the distal vagina (sinus vagina formation requires absence of androgen activity) persists, whereas the proximal vagina (müllerian vagina involution is dependent on MIS) does not (Bok and Drews, 1983). Also in this syndrome, the prostate, a derivative of the urogenital sinus (and thereby dependent on androgen), is absent.

Ultrasound examination is accurate in determining the gender of the fetus by visualizing the genitalia (70% of cases at 15 weeks' gestation and 90% of cases after 20 weeks' gestation) (Birnholz, 1983).

Female

UTERUS AND VAGINA. After about 9 weeks' gestation, the septum between the fused müllerian ducts is absent.

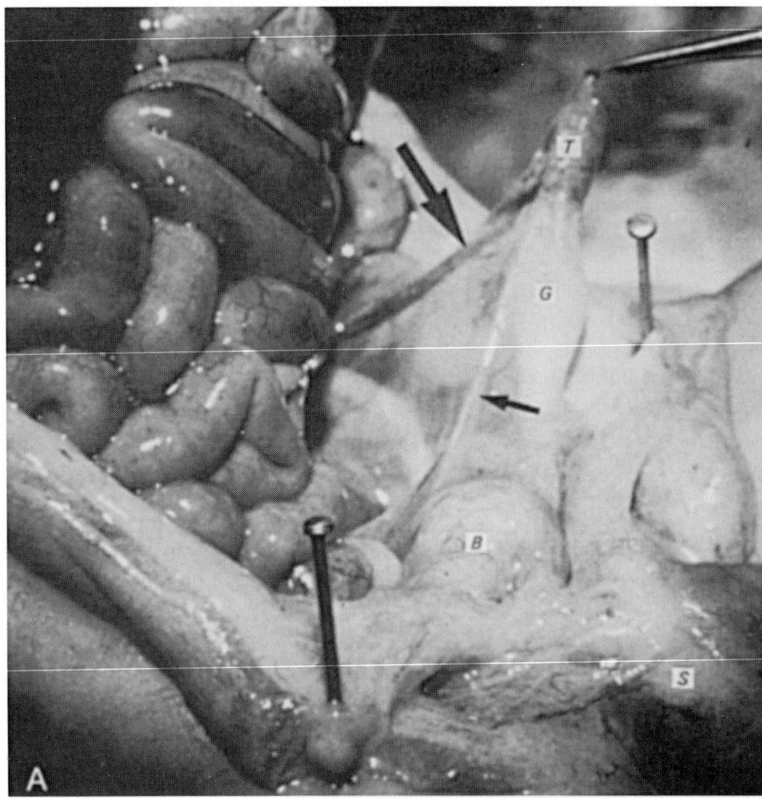

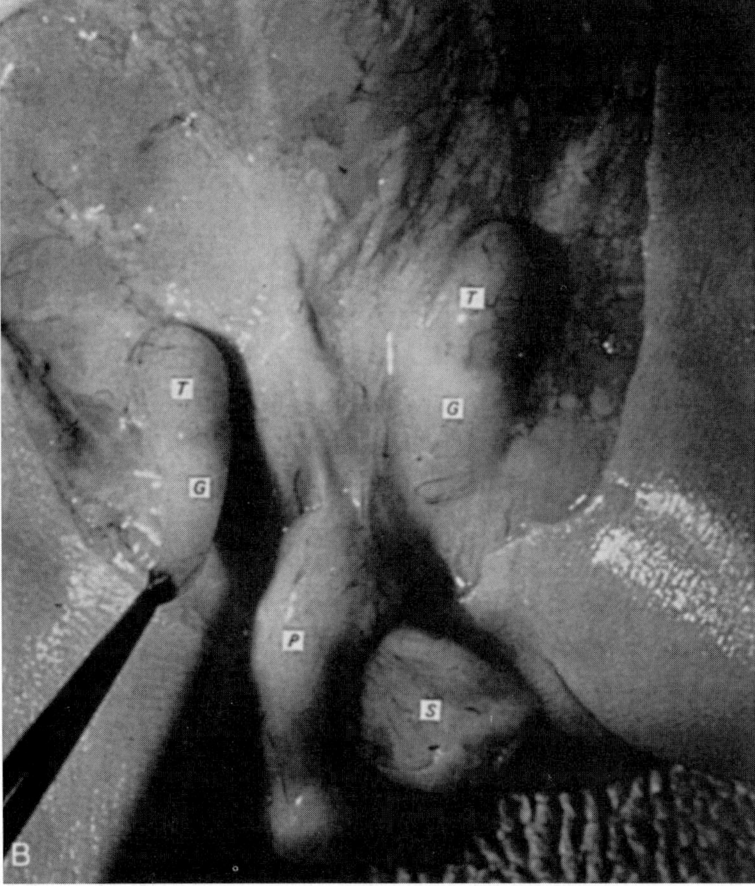

Figure 51–53. Anatomy of testis descent in the human fetus. *A*, At 22 weeks' gestation, testicular vessels *(large arrow)*, vas deferens *(small arrow)*, and gubernaculum (G) are enveloped in a fold of peritoneum (mesorchium). *B*, At 25 weeks' gestation, the skin over the lower anterior abdominal wall and scrotum have been removed. The gubernaculum does not show distal attachments. No extensions to the crural or scrotal area are evident. (T, testis; B, bladder; S, scrotum; P, penis.) (From Heyns CF: J Anat 1987; 153:93.)

Campbell S, Wladimiroff JW, Dewhurst CJ: The antenatal measurement of fetal urine production. J Obstet Gynaecol Br Commonw 1973; 80:680.

Carey MP, Steinberg LH: Vaginal dystocia in a patient with a double uterus and a longitudinal vaginal septum. Aust N Z J Obstet Gynaecol 1989; 29:74.

Chamberlanin PF, Manning FA, Morrison I, Lange IR: Circadian rhythm in bladder volumes in the term human fetus. Obstet Gynecol 1984; 64:657.

Cohen-Haguenaur O, Picard JV, Mattei MG, et al: Mapping of the gene for anti-müllerian hormone to the short arm of human chromosome 19. Cytogenet Cell Genet 1987; 44:2.

Coles HS, Burne JF, Raff MC: Large-scale normal cell death in the developing rat kidney and its reduction by epidermal growth factor. Development 1993; 118(3):777–784.

Coplen DE, Macarak EJ, Levin RM: Developmental changes in normal fetal bovine whole bladder physiology. J Urol 1994; 151:1391–1395.

Crocker JF: Human embryonic kidneys in organ culture: Abnormalities of development induced by decreased potassium. Science 1973; 21:1178.

Cunha GR, Taguchi O, Sugimura Y, et al: Absence of teratogenic effects of progesterone on the developing genital tract of the human female fetus. Hum Pathol 1988; 19:777.

Cunha GR: Androgenic effects upon prostatic epithelium are mediated via trophic influences from stroma. Prog Clin Biol Res 1984; 145:81.

Cunha G: Epithelio-mesenchymal interactions in primordial gland structures which become responsive to androgen stimulation. Anat Rec 1972; 172:179.

Cunha GR, Taguchi O, Sugimura Y, et al: Absence of teratogenic effects of progesterone on the developing genital tract of the human female fetus. Hum Pathol 1988; 19:777.

Cunha GR, Young P, Brody JR: Role of uterine epithelium in the development of myometrial smooth muscle cells. Biol Reprod 1989; 40:861.

Currarino G: Single vaginal ectopic ureter and Gartner's duct cyst with ipsilateral renal hypoplasia and dysplasia (or agenesis). J Urol 1982; 128:988.

Currarino G, Weisbruch GJ: Transverse fusion of the renal pelvis and single ureter. Urol Radiol 1989; 11:88.

Cussenot O, Desgrandchamps F, Teillac P, Lesourd A: Double ureter and congenital diverticulum of the ureter. Surg Radiol Anat 1991; 13:323–326.

Cutner Al, Moscoso G, Cardozo L, et al: Growth of the normal human lower urinary tract from 12 to 21 weeks' gestation. Anat Rec 1992; 234:568–574.

de Jonge MK, Van Nouhys JM, Tjabbes D: How to differentiate between ectopia and displacement in patient with crossed kidney. Urology 1988; 31:450.

de Vries L, Levene MI: Measurement of renal size in preterm and term infants by real-time ultrasound. Arch Dis Child 1983; 58:145.

Deibert GA: The separation of the prepuce in the human penis. Anat Rec 1933; 57:387.

Donahoe PK, Ito Y, Hendren WH III: A graded organ culture assay for detecting of müllerian inhibiting substance. J Surg Res 1977; 23:141.

Donahoe PK, Ito Y, Marfatia S, Hendren WH III: The production of müllerian inhibiting substance by the fetal, neonatal and adult rat. Biol Reprod 1976; 15:329.

Dwoskin JY, Noe HN, Gonzalez ET Jr, et al: Sibling uropathology. Dialogues in Pediatric Urology 1986; 9(6):1–6.

Ecke M, Klatte D: Inverted Y-ureteral duplication with a uterine ectopy as caused of ureteric enuresis. Urol Int 1989; 44:116.

Ejaz T, Malone PS: Male duplex urinary incontinence. J Urol 1995: 153:470–471.

Ekblom P: Determination and differentiation of the nephron. Med Biol 1981; 59:139.

Ekblom P, Vestweber D, Kemler R: Cell-matrix interactions and cell adhesion during development. Annu Rev Cell Biol 1986; 2:27.

Elliott DC, Beam TE, Danapoli TS: Hernia uterus inguinale associated with unicornuate uterus. Arch Surg 1989; 124:872.

Escala JM, Keating MA, Boyd G, et al: Development of elastic fibres in the upper urinary tract. J Urol 1989; 141:969.

Felix W: The Development of the Urinogenital Organs. *In* Keibel F, Mall FP, eds: Manual of Human Embryology, Vol II. Philadelphia, J.B. Lippincott, 1912, a. 866; b. 880; c. 752; d. 815; e. 829; f. 830; g. 938.

Fernbach SK, Morello FP: Renal abnormalities in children with hypertrophic pyloric stenosis—fact or fallacy? Pediatr Radiol 1993: 23:286–288.

Fetterman GH, Ravitch MM, Sherman FF: Cystic changes in fetal kidneys following ureteral ligation. Kidney Int 1974; 5:111.

FitzGerald MJT: Human Embryology. New York, Harper & Row, 1978, p 106.

Fonzo D, Manenti M, Varengo M, et al: Andrological and hormonal findings in subjects with ductus deferens agenesis. Andrologia 1983; 15:614.

Fouser L, Avner ED: Normal and abnormal nephrogenesis. Am J Kid Dis 1993; 21:64–70.

Friedland GW, de Vries P: Renal ectopia and fusion–embryologic basis. Urology 1975; 5:698.

Fritsch H: The connective tissue sheath of uterus and vagina in the human female fetus. Anat Anz 1992; 174:261–266.

Fryns JP, Kleczkowska A, Moerman P, Vandenberghe K: Hereditary hydronephrosis and the short arm of chromosome 6. Hum Genet 1993; 91:514–518.

Fuss FK: Contribution to the trigone musculature in the case of ureteral duplication. J Urol 1992; 147:1363–1364.

Gage JC, Sulik KK: Pathogenesis of ethanol-induced hydronephrosis and hydroureter as demonstrated following in vivo exposure of mouse embryos. Teratology 1991; 44:299–312.

George FW, Peterson KG, Frankel PA, Wilson JD: The androgen receptor in the fetal epididymis is similar to that in the mature rabbit. Proc. Soc, Exp. Biol, Med. 188:500, 1988.

Gersh I: The correlation of structure and function in the developing mesonephros and metanephros. Contrib Embryol 1937; 26:35.

Gilbert T, Gaonach S, Moreau E, Merlet-Benichou C: Defect of nephrogenesis induced by gentamicin in rat metanephric organ culture. Lab Invest 1994; 70:656–666.

Gilsanz V, Cleveland RH: Duplication of the müllerian ducts and genitourinary malformations. Part I: the value of excretory urography. Radiology 1982a; 144:793.

Gilsanz V, Cleveland RH, Reid BS: Duplication of the müllerian ducts and genitourinary malformations. Part II: Analysis of malformations. Radiology 1982b; 144:797.

Glatstein IZ, Choi YM, Osathanondh R, Yeh J: Human fetal uterine cells: Culture, characterization, and analysis of growth factor receptor gene expression. J Clin Endocrinol Metab 1994; 79:126–133.

Glazebrook KN, McGrath FP, Steele BT: Prenatal compensatory renal growth: Documentation with US. Radiology 1993; 189:733–735.

Gonzalez R, Reinberg Y, Burke B, et al: Early bladder outlet obstruction in fetal lambs induces renal dysplasia and the prune-belly syndrome. J Pediatr Surg 1990; 25:342–345.

Goodyer PR, Mulligan L, Goodyer CG: Expression of growth-related genes in human fetal kidney. Am J Kidney Dis 1991; 37:608–610.

Gotoh T, Morita H, Tokunaka S, et al: Single ectopic ureter. J Urol 1983; 129:271.

Grannum P, Bracken M, Silverman R, Hobbins JC: Assessment of fetal kidney size in normal gestation by comparison of ratio of kidney circumference to abdominal circumference. Am J Obstet Gynecol 1980; 136:249.

Greenfield SP, Rutigliano E, Steinhardt G, Elder JS: Genitourinary tract malformations and maternal cocaine abuse. Urology 1991; 37:455–459.

Grobstein C: Trans-filter induction of tubules in mouse metanephrogenic mesenchyme. Exp Cell Res 1956; 10:424.

Gruenwald P: The normal changes in the position of the embryonic kidney. Anat Rec 1943; 85:163.

Gruenwald P: The relation of the growing Mullerian duct to the Wolffian duct and its importance for the genesis of malformations. Anat Rec 1941; 81:1.

Hamilton WJ, Mossman HW: Human Embryology Prenatal Development of Form & Function. New York, The Macmillan Press Ltd, 1976a, p 201.

Hamilton WJ, Mossman HW: The urogenital system. *In* Human Embryology Prenatal Development of Form and Function. New York, The Macmillan Press Ltd, 1976b, pp 377–436.

Hammerman MR: The renal growth hormone/insulin-like growth factor I axis. Am J Kidney Dis 1991; 17;644–646.

Hammerman MR, Rogers SA, Ryan G: Growth factors and metanephrogenesis. Am J Physiol 1992; 262:F523–F532.

Hara K, Doi Y, Nagata N, et al: Role of mesenchymal cells in the neovascularization of the rabbit phallus. Anat Rec 1994: 238:15–22.

Hardman P, Kolatsi M, Winyard PJD, et al: Branching out with the ureteric bud. Exp Nephrol 1994; 2:211–219.

Hatch DA, Maizels M, Zaontz MR, Firlit CF: Hypospadias hidden by a complete prepuce. Surg Gynecol Obstet 1989; 169:233.

Herzlinger D, Abramson R, Cohen D: Phenotypic conversions in renal development. J Cell Sci Suppl 1993: 17:61–64.

Herzlinger D, Qiao J, Cohen D, et al: Induction of kidney epithelial morphogenesis by cells expressing Wnt-1. Dev Biol 1994; 166:815–818.

Heyns CF: The gubernaculum during testicular descent in the human fetus. J Anat 1987; 153:93.

Hinchliffe SA, Chan YF, Jones H, et al: Renal hypoplasia and postnatally acquired cortical loss in children with vesicoureteral reflux. Pediatr Nephrol 1992a; 6(5):439–444.

Hinchliffe SA, Lynch MR, Sargent PH, et al: The effect of intrauterine growth retardation on the development of renal nephrons. Br J Obstet Gynaecol 1992b; 99(4):296–301.

Hinchliffe SA, Sargent PH, Chan YF, et al: "Medullary ray glomerular counting" as a method of assessment of human nephrogenesis. Pathol Res Pract 1992c; 188(6):775–782.

Howe SC, Cromie WJ, Kay NW: Development of an in vitro model for the disruption of extracellular matrix components in the study of congenital renal parenchymal dysmorphism. J Urol 1989; 142:612.

Hulbert WC, Rosenberg HK, Cartwright PC, et al: The predictive value of ultrasonography in evaluation of infants with posterior urethral valves. J Urol 1992; 148(1):122–124.

Hunter RH: Notes on development of prepuce. J Anat 1935; 70:68.

Ikawa H, Hutson JM, Budzik GP, et al: Steroid enhancement of müllerian duct regression. J Pediatr Surg 1982; 17:453.

Ikoma F, Shima H: Caudal migration of the verumontanum. J Pediatr Surg 1991: 26:858–861.

Javadpour N, Graziano AB, Terril R: Experimental induction of patent allantoic duct by intrauterine bladder outlet obstruction. J Surg Res 1974; 17:341.

Jeanty P, Dramaix-Wilmet M, Elkhazen N, et al: Measurements of fetal kidney growth on ultrasound. Radiology 1982; 144:159.

Jenny C, Kuhns MLD, Arakawa F: Hymens in newborn female infants. Pediatrics 1987; 80:399.

Jirasek JE: Morphogenesis of the genital system in the human. Birth Defects 1977; 15(2):13.

Josso N: In vitro synthesis of müllerian inhibiting hormone by seminiferous tubules isolated from the calf fetal testis. Endocrinology 1973; 93:829.

Kanda S, Igawa T, Taide M, et al: Tranforming growth factor-β in rat kidney during compensatory renal growth. Growth Regul 1993; 3:146–150.

Kanwar YS, Liu ZZ, Wada J: Insulin-like growth factor-I receptor in metanephric development. Contrib Nephrol 1994: 107:168–173.

Kellokumpu-Lehtinen P, Pelliniemi LJ: Hormonal regulation of differentiation of human fetal prostate and Leydig cells in utero. Folia Histochem Cytobiol 1988; 26:113.

Kim KM, Kogan BA, Massad CA, Huang, YC: Collagen and elastin in the normal fetal bladder. J Urol 1991; 146:524.

Kirillova IA, Kulazhenko VP, Kulazhenko LG, Novikova IV: Cystic kidney in an 8-week human embryo. Acta Anat 1982; 114:68.

Klein G, Langegger M, Goridis C, Ekblom P: Neural cell adhesion molecules during embryonic induction and development of the kidney. Development 1988; 102:749.

Klein VR, Willman SP, Carr BR: Familial posterior labial fusion. Obstet Gynecol 1989; 73(part 3):500.

Kloth S, Aigner J, Schmidbauer A, Minuth WW: Interrelationship of renal vascular development and nephrogenesis. Cell Tissue Res 1994; 277:247–257.

Kluth D, Lambrecht W, Reich P: Pathogenesis of hypospadias—more questions than answers. J Pediatr Surg 1988; 23(12):1095–1101.

Kogan B, Iwamoto H: Lower urinary tract function in the sheep fetus: Studies of autonomic control and pharmacologic responses of the fetal bladder. J Urol 1989; 141:1019.

Konishi I, Fujii S, Okamura H, Mori T: Development of smooth muscle in the human fetal uterus: an ultrastructural study. J Anat 1984; 139:239.

Koseki C: Cell death programmed in uninduced metanephric mesenchymal cells. Pediatr Nephrol 1993: 7:609–611.

Koseki C, Herzlinger D, Al-Awqati Q: Apoptosis in metanephric development. J Cell Biol 1992; 119:1327–1333.

Langman J: Medical Embryology, 2nd ed. Baltimore, Williams & Wilkins, 1969, p 301.

Lash JW, Saxen L, Ekblom P: Biosynthesis of proteoglycans in organ cultures of developing kidney mesenchyme. Exp Cell Res 1983; 147:85.

Lawrence WD, Whitaker D, Sugimura H, et al: An ultrastructural study of the developing urogenital tract in early human fetuses. Am J Obstet Gynecol 1992; 167:185–193.

Lee JG, Coplen D, Macarak E, et al: Comparative studies on the ontogeny and autonomic responses of the fetal calf bladder at different stages of development: Involvement of nitric oxide on field stimulated relaxation. J Urol 1994: 151:1096–1101.

Lehtonen E, Wartiovaara J, Nordling S, Saxen L: Demonstration of cytoplasmic processes in millipore filters permitting kidney tubule induction. J Embryol Exp Morphol 1975; 33:187.

Lelongt B, Makino H, Dalecki TM, Kanwar YS: Role of proteoglycans in renal development. Dev Biol 1988; 128:256.

Liu ZZ, Carone FA, Dalecki TM, et al: Mannose-induced dysmorphogenesis of metanephric kidney. J Clin Invest 1992; 90:1205–1218.

Liu KW, Fitzgerald RJ: An unusual case of complete urethral duplication in a female child. Aust N Z J Surg 1988; 58:587.

Lowsley OS: The development of the human prostate gland with reference to the development of other structures at the neck of the urinary bladder. Am J Anat 1912; 13:299.

Ludwig KS: The development of the caudal ligaments of the mesonephros and of the gonads: A contribution to the development of the human gubernaculum (Hunteri). Anat Embryol 1993; 188:571–577.

Maas R, Elfering S, Glaser T, Jepeal L: Deficient outgrowth of the ureteric bud underlies the renal agenesis phenotype in mice manifesting the limb deformit (ld) mutation. Dev Dyn 1994; 199;214–228.

Mackie GG, Stephens FD: Duplex kidneys: A correlation of renal dysplasia with position of the ureteral orifice. J Urol 1979; 114:274.

Mackintosh P, Almarhoos G, Heath DA: HLA linkage with familial vesicoureteral reflux and familial pelvi-ureteric junction obstruction. Tissue Antigens 1989; 34:185.

Maizels M, Simpson SB Jr: Primitive ducts of renal dysplasia induced by culturing ureteral buds denuded of condensed renal mesenchyme. Science 1983; 219:509.

Maizels M, Simpson SB Jr, Firlit CF: Simulation of human renal dysplasia in a chick embryo model. Abstract #765. Las Vegas, American Urological Association, Inc., 1983.

Maizels M, Stephens FD: Valves of the ureter as a cause of primary obstruction of the ureter: Anatomic, embryologic and clinical aspects. J Urol 1980; 123:742.

Maizels M, Stephens FD: The induction of urologic malformations: Understanding the relationship of renal ectopia and congenital scoliosis. Invest Urol 1979; 17:209.

Maizels M, Stephens FD, King LR, Firlit CF: Cowper's syringocele—a classification of dilatations of Cowper's gland duct based upon clinical characteristics of 8 boys. J Urol 1983; 129:111.

Markham SM, Waterhouse TB: Structural anomalies of the reproductive tract. (Review.) Curr Opin Obstet Gynecol 1992; 4(6):867–73.

Marra G, Barbieri G, Dell'Agnola CA, et al: Congenital renal damage associated with primary vesicoureteral reflux detected prenatally in male infants. J Pediatr 1994; 124:726–730.

Matsuno T, Tokunaka S, Koyanagi T: Muscualar development in the urinary tract. J Urol 1984; 132:148.

McCandless SE, Uehling D, Friedman AL: Urinary tract malformations in identical twins. J Urol. 1991; 146:145–147

McVary KT, Maizels M: Urinary obstruction reduces glomerulogenesis in the developing kidney: A model in the rabbit. J Urol 1989; 142:646.

Mellins HZ: Cystic dilatations of the upper urinary tract: A radiologist's developmental model. Radiology 1984; 145:291.

Mesrobian HGJ, Sulik KK: Characterization of the upper urinary tract anatomy in the Danforth spontaneous murine mutation. J Urol 1992; 148:752–755.

Middelton AW Jr, Pfister RC: Stone-containing pyelocaliceal diverticulum: Embryogenic, anatomic, radiologic and clinical characteristics. J Urol 1974; 111:2.

Moerman P, Fryns JP, Sastrowijoto SH, et al: Hereditary renal adysplasia: new observations and hypotheses. Pediatr Pathol 1994; 14(3):405–410.

Moore KL: The Developing Human, 2nd ed. Philadelphia, W. B. Saunders Company, 1977.

Moore D, Tudehope D, Lewis B, Masel J: Familial renal abnormalities associated with the oligohydramnios tetrad secondary to renal agenesis and dysgenesis. Aust Paediatr J 1987; 23:137.

Mor N, Merlob P: Congenital absence of the hymen only a rumor? (Letter.) Pediatrics 1988; 82:679.

Mor N, Merlob P, Reisner SH: Tags and bands of the female external genitalia in the newborn infant. Clin Pediatr 1983; 22:122.

Muecke EC: The embryology of the urinary system. *In* Herrison JH, Gittes RF, Perlmutter AD, et al: Campbell's Urology, 4th ed. Philadelphia, W. B. Saunders Company, 1979, p 1286–1307

Murakami R: Autoradiographic studies of the localization of androgen-binding cells in the genital tubercles of fetal rats. J Anat 1987; 151: 209.

Murakami R, Takeda H, Yamaoka I, Sakakura T: Close correlation between the distribution of tenascin and that of actin filaments in the mouse urethral mesenchyme during active morphogenesis. Acta Anat 1990; 138:128–131.

Naguib KK, Teebi AS, Farag TI, et al: Familial uterine hernia syndrome: Report of an Arab family with four affected males. Am J Med Genet 1989; 33:180.

Nathan H, Glezer I: Right and left accessory renal arteries arising from a common trunk associated with unrotated kidneys. J Urol 1984; 132:7.

Newman J, Antonakopoulos GN: The fine structure of the human fetal urinary bladder. Development and maturation: A light, transmission and scanning electron microscopy study. J Anat 1989; 166:135–150.

Nigam SK: Determinants of branching tubulogenesis. Curr Opin Nephrol Hypertens 1995; 4:209–214.

O'Rahilly R, Tucker JA: The early development of the larynx in staged human embryos. Part 1. Embryos of the first five weeks. Ann Otol Rhinol Laryngol 1973; 82(Suppl 7):1–27.

Okada T, Morikawa Y: Histometry of the developing kidney in fetal rats. Nippon Juigaku Zasshi 50:269, 1988.

Okada T, Yamagishi T, Morikawa Y: Morphometry of the kidney in rat pups from uninephrectomized mothers. Anat Rec 1994; 240:120–124.

Ostling K: The genesis of hydronephrosis: Particularly with regard to the changes at the ureteropelvic junction. Acta Chir Scand 1942; 86(Suppl):72.

Oyen R, Gielen J, van Poppel H, Baert L: Seminal vesicle cyst and ipsilateral renal agenesis. Case report. Eur J Radiol 1988; 8:122.

Oyer CE: Juxtagonadal mesonephric glomeruli in fetuses of 11 to 21 weeks of gestation. Pediatr Pathol 1992; 12:683–689.

Pavanello RC, Eigier A, Otto PA: Relationship between Mayer-Rokitansky-Kuster (MRK) anomaly and hereditary renal adysplasia (HRA). Am J Med Genet 1988; 29:845.

Perantoni AO, Williams CL, Lewellyn AL: Growth and branching morphogenesis of rat collecting duct anlagen in the absence of metanephrogenic mesenchyme. Differentiation 1991; 48:107–113.

Pietryga E, Wozniak W: The development of the uterine ligaments in human fetuses. Folia Morphol 1992; 51:181–193.

Pietryga E, Wozniak W: The growth and topography of the human fetal uterus. Folia Morphol 1992; 51:181–193

Plachov D, Chowdhury K, Walther C: Pax8: a murine paired box gene expressed in the developing excretory system and thyroid gland. Development 1990,110:643–651.

Poleev A, Fickenscher H, Mundlos S, et al: PAX8, a human paired box gene: Isolation and expression in developing thyroid, kidney and Wilms' tumors. Development1992; 116(3):611–623.

Poole TJ, Steinberg MS: Evidence of the guidance of pronephric duct migration by a craniocaudally traveling adhesion gradient. Devel Biol 1982; 92:144.

Popek EJ: Embryonal remnants in inguinal hernia sacs. Hum Pathol 1990; 21:339–349.

Popek EJ, Tyson RW, Miller GJ, Caldwell SA: Prostate development in prune belly syndrome (PBS) and posterior urethral valves (PUV): Etiology of PBS–lower urinary tract obstruction or primary mesenchymal defect? Pediatr Pathol 1991; 11(1):1–29.

Potter EL: Normal and Abnormal Development of the Kidney. Chicago, Year Book Medical Publishers, Inc., 1972.

Pulilli C, Gomez RA, Tuttle JB, et al: Spatial association of renin-containing cells and nerve fibers in developing rat kidney. Pediatr Nephrol 1991: 5:690–695.

Rapola J: Kidneys in Meckel's syndrome as a model of abnormal renal differentiation. Int J Dev Biol 1989; 33:177–182.

Richard-Lallemand MA, Choux R, Szekeres G, et al: [Immunohistochemical characterization of a median raphe cyst of the penis.] Ann Pathol 1994; 14(3):174–176.

Rogers SA, Ryan G, Purchio AF, Hammerman MR: Metanephric transforming growth factor β-1 regulates nephrogenesis in vitro. Am Physiol Soc 1993; 264:F996–1002.

Roodhooft AM, Birnholz JC, Holmes LB: Familial nature of congenital absence and severe dysgenesis of both kidneys. N England J Med 1984; 310:1341.

Rowsell AR, Morgan BDG: Hypospadias and the embryogenesis of the penile urethra. Br J Plast Surg 1987; 40:201.

Roy-Choudhury S, Maji BP: Development of the human anterior urethra. J Urol 1991; 146:1085–1093.

Ruano-Gil D, Coca-Payeras A, Tejedo-Mateu A: Obstruction and normal recanalization of the ureter in the human embryo: Its relation to congenital ureteric obstruction. Eur Urol 1975; 1:293.

Sainio K, Nonclercq D, Saarma M, et al: Neuronal characteristics in embryonic renal stroma. Int J Dev Biol 1994; 38:77–84.

Sampaio FJB, Aragao HM: Anatomical relationship between the renal venous arrangement and the kidney collecting system. J Urol 1990; 144:1089–1093.

Santarosa R, Colombel MC, Kaplan S, et al: Hyperplasia and apoptosis. Opposing cellular processes that regulate the response of the rabbit bladder to transient outlet obstructrion. Lab Invest 1994; 70:503–510.

Santava A, Utikalova A, Santavy J: Heredity and origin of duplication of the pelvicalyceal collecting system. Acta Univ Palacki Olomuc Fac Med 1990; 126:209–218.

Santos OF, Moura LA, Rosen EM, Nigam SK: Modulation of HGF-induced tubulogenesis and branching by multiple phosphorylation mechanisms. Dev Biol 1993; 159:535–548.

Sariola H, Aufderheide E, Bernhard H, et al: Antibodies to cell surface ganglioside GD3 perturb inductive epithelial-mesenchymal interactions. Cell 1988; 54:235.

Sariola H, Ekblom P, Henke-Fahle S: Embryonic neurons as in vitro inducers of differentiation of nephrogenic mesenchyme. Dev Biol 1989; 132:271.

Sawczuk IS, Olsson CA, Buttyan R, et al: Gene expression in renal growth and regrowth. J Urol 1988; 140:1145.

Saxen L: Organogenesis of the kidney. *In* Barlow PW, Green PB, Wylie CC, eds: Development & Cell Biology. Mongraph No. 19. Cambridge, Cambridge University press, 1987.

Saxen L, Toivonen S, Vainio T, Korhonen P: Untersuchungen uber die Tubulogenese der Niere. III. Die Analyse der Fruhentwicklung mit der Zeitraffermethode. Z Naturforsch 1965; 20b:340.

Schuger L, O'Shea S, Rheinheimer J, Varani J: Laminin in lung development: Effects of anti-laminin antibody in murine lung morphogenesis. Dev Biol 1990; 137:26.

Sener RN: Nonobstructive right circumcaval ureter associated with double inferior vena cava. Urology 1993; 41:356–360.

Shimada K, Hosokawa S, Tohda A: Histological study of fetal hydronephrosis: Developmental background of prenatal treatment. Nippon Hinyokika Gakkai Zasshi 1993: 84:2097–2102.

Shimada K, Shozou H, Tohda A: Indications for urinary drainage in neonates detected in utero. Nippon Hinyokika Gakkai Zasshi 1993; 84:479–484.

Siiteri PK, Wilson JD: Testosterone formation and metabolism during male sexual differentiation in the human embryo. J Clin Endocrinol Metab 1974; 38:113.

Smith FG, Robillard JE: Pathophysiology of fetal renal disease. Semin Perinatol 1989; 13:305.

Spencer J, Maizels M: Inhibition of protein glycosylation causes renal dysplasia in the chick embryo. J Urol 1987; 138:984.

Stephens FD: Congenital Malformations of the Urinary Tract. New York, Praeger Publishers, 1983.

Stephens FD: Embryopathy of malformations. (Guest Editorial.) J Urol 1982; 127:13.

Stephens FD: Anatomical vagaries of double ureters. Aust N Z J Surg 1958; 28:27.

Stephens FD, Fortune DW: Pathogenesis of megalourethra. J Urol 1993: 149:1512–1516.

Stoll C, Aklembik Y, Roth MP, Dott B, Sauvage P: Risk factors in internal urinary system malformation. Pediatr Nephrol 1990; 4:319–323.

Sule JD, Skoog SJ, Tank ES: Perineal lipoma and the accessory labioscrotal fold: An etiological relationship. J Urol 1994; 151:475–477.

Swinford AE, Bernstein J, Toriello HV: Renal tubular dysgenesis: Delayed onset of oligohydramnios. Am J Med Gent 1989; 32:127.

Tanagho EA: Surgically induced partial ureteral obstruction in the fetal lamb. III. Ureteral obstruction, Invest Urol 1972; 10:35.

Tichy M: The morphogenesis of human sphincter urethrae muscle. Anat Embryol 1989; 180:577–582.

Toaff ME: Origin of the epithelium of atretic hemivaginas. (Letter). Am J Obstet Gynecol 1984; 149:237.

Trelstad RL, Hayashi A, Hayashi K, et al: The epithelial-mesenchymal interface of the male müllerian duct: Basement membrane integrity and ductal regression. Dev Biol 1982; 92:27.

Unsworth B, Grobstein C: Induction of kidney tubules in mouse metanephrogenic mesenchyme by various embryonic mesenchymal tissues. Dev Biol 1970; 21:547.

Vainio S, Lehtonen E, Jalkanen M, et al: Epithelial-mesenchymal interactions regulate the stage-specific expression of a cell surface proteoglycan, syndecan, in the developing kidney. Dev Biol 1989; 134:382.

van der Putte SCJ: Normal and abnormal development of the anorectum. J Pediatr Surg 1986; 21:434.

van Groesen PJ, Beemer FA, van de Kamp JH: Leg duplication and kidney agenesis: Case report and pathogenic considerations. Genet Couns 1990; 1:265–272.

Venyo AKG: Supernumerary fallopian tubes. J Obstet Gynecol 1993; 100:183.

Voutilainen R, Miller WL: Human müllerian inhibitory factor messenger ribonucleic acid is hormonally regulated in the fetal testis and in adult granulosa cells. Mol Endocrinol 1987; 1:604–608.

Waterman RE: Human embryo and fetus. *In* Hafez ESE, Hingham MA, ed: Atlas of Human Reproduction. Hingham, MA, Kluwer Boston, 1982, pp 261–274.

Wheeler RA, Burge DM: Urinary obstruction due to labial fusion. Br J Urol 1991; 67:102

Wladimiroff JW, Campbell S: Fetal urine-production rates in normal and complicated pregnancy. Lancet 1974; i(849):151.

Wlodek ME, Thorburn GD, Hardine R: Bladder contractions and micturition in fetal sheep: Their relation to behavioral states. Am Physiol Soc 1989; 257:r1526–r1532.

Wood-Jones F: The musculature of the bladder and urethra. J Anat Physiol 1901–1902; 36:51.

Zackson SL, Steinberg MS: A molecular marker for cell guidance information in the axolotl embryo. Dev Biol 1988; 127:435.

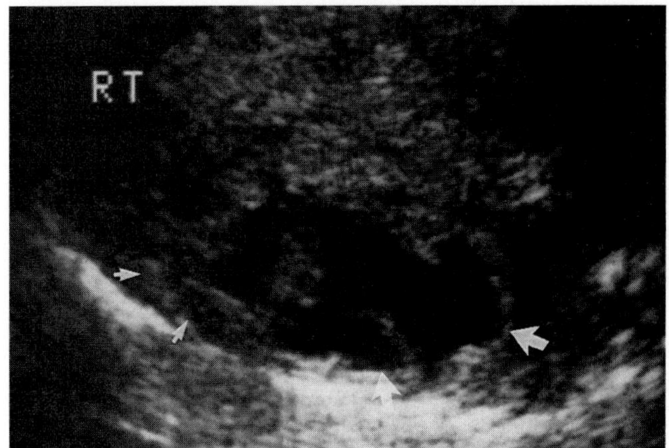

Figure 52–4. Prenatal diagnosis of duplex anomaly. Ultrasound examination at 38 weeks' gestation showing asymmetric hydronephrosis of upper *(large arrows)* and lower *(small arrows)* poles.

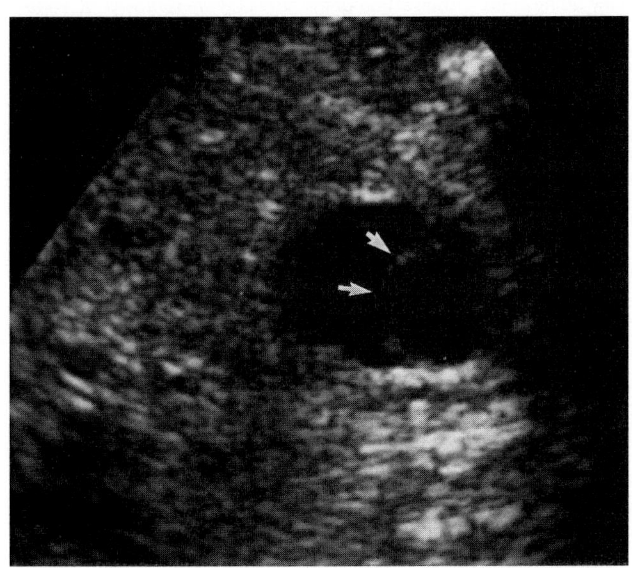

Figure 52–5. Same fetus as above with ureterocele *(arrows)* in bladder.

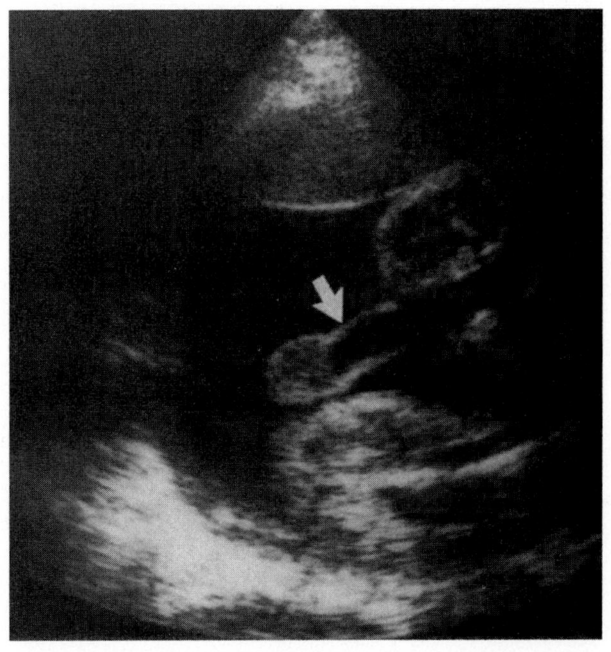

Figure 52–6. Prenatal diagnosis of megalourethra. Ultrasound examination at 33 weeks' gestation showing fluid-filled penile urethra *(arrow)*, normal scrotum, and normal amniotic fluid. The patient had some features of prune-belly syndrome.

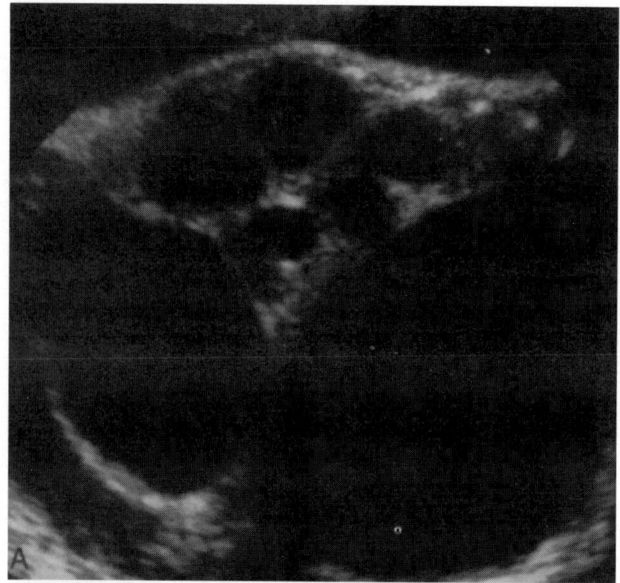

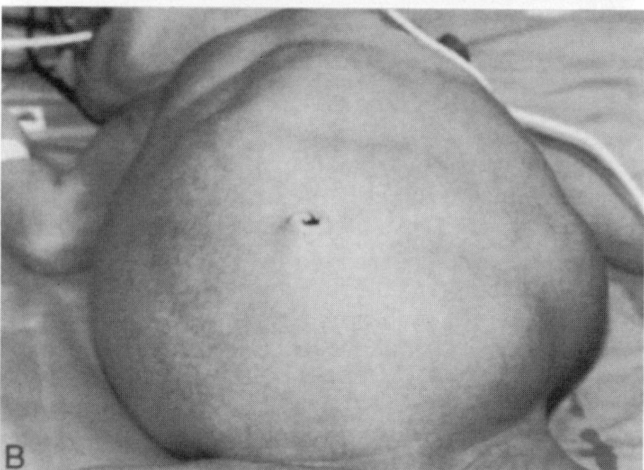

Figure 52–7. Prenatal diagnosis of multicystic dysplastic kidney. *A,* Ultrasound examination at 38 weeks' gestation showing huge multicystic kidney filling entire cross-section of the fetal abdominal cavity. *B,* Picture of neonate with grossly distended abdomen and renal mass visible through the anterior abdominal wall. Infant had moderate respiratory distress from compression of the diaphragm.

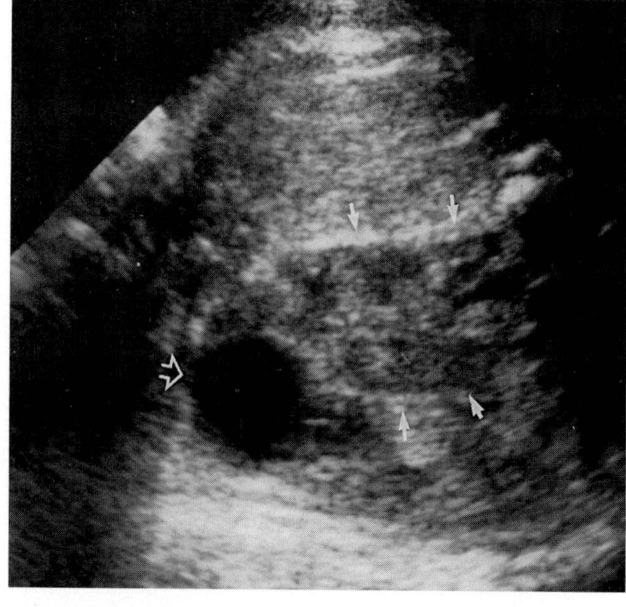

Figure 52–8. Prenatal diagnosis of pelvic kidney. Ultrasound examination at 36 weeks' gestation with kidney *(small arrows)* seen above filled bladder *(open arrow).*

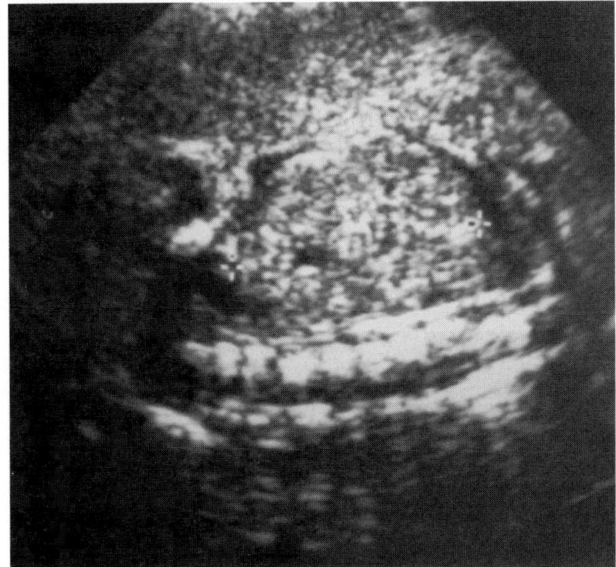

Figure 52–9. Prenatal diagnosis of autosomal recessive polycystic kidney disease. Ultrasound examination at 25 weeks' gestation showing enlarged (37.6 mm) echogenic kidney. Normal kidney length is 30 to 32 mm.

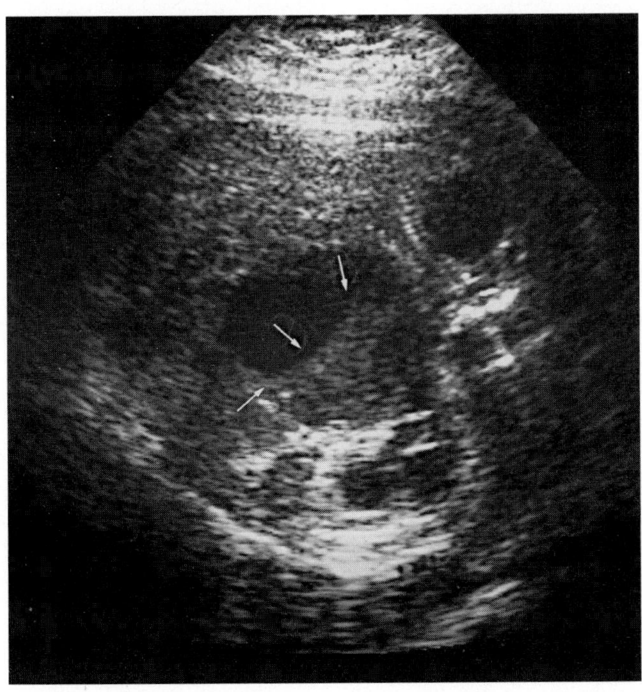

Figure 52–10. Prenatal diagnosis of cloacal anomaly. Ultrasound examination at 34 weeks' gestation showing complex cystic mass in pelvis with fluid-debris line *(arrows)*.

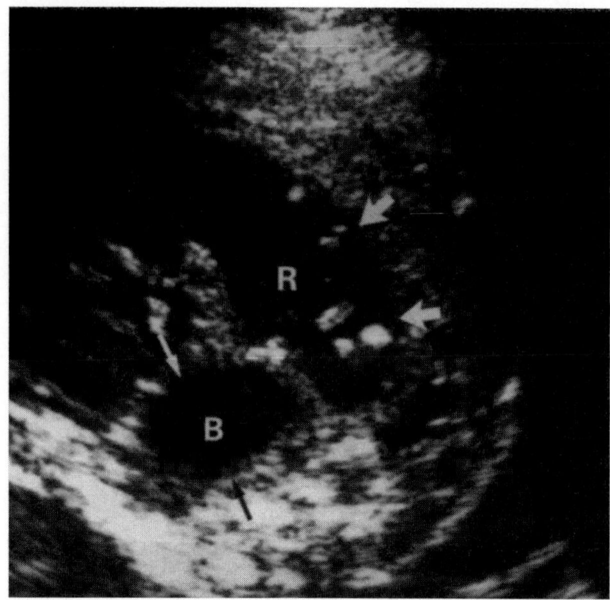

Figure 52–11. Prenatal diagnosis of imperforate anus with rectourinary fistula. Ultrasound examination at 36 weeks' gestation showing dilated rectum (R) *(large arrows)* with intraluminal calcifications posterior to full bladder (B) *(small arrows)*. (From Mandell M, Lillehei CW, Greene M, Benacerraf B: The prenatal diagnosis of imperforate anus: Dilated fetal colon with enterolithiasis. J Pediatr Surg 1992; 27:82–84.

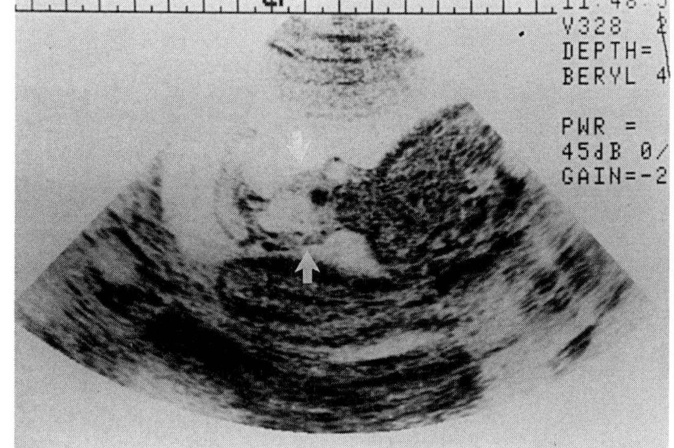

Figure 52–12. Prenatal diagnosis of urachal anomaly. Ultrasound examination at 32 weeks' gestation showing complex urachal cyst *(arrows)*.

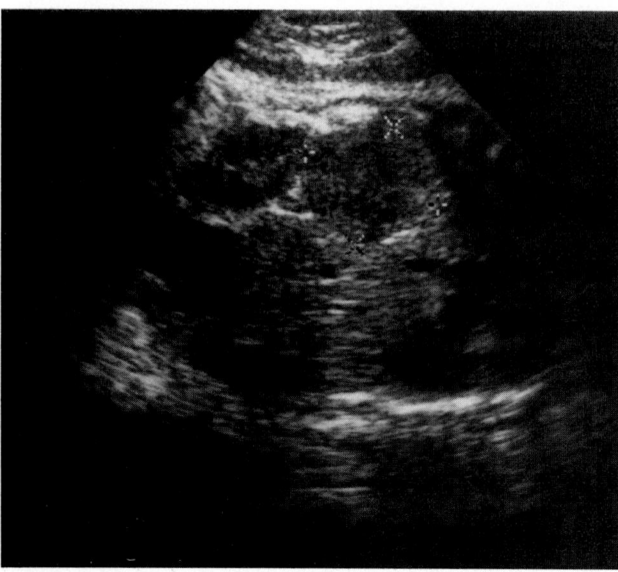

Figure 52–13. Prenatal diagnosis of neuroblastoma. Ultrasound examination at 34 weeks' gestation showing suprarenal solid mass *(calipers)*, which proved to be neuroblastoma.

1995) and mesoblastic nephroma (see Fig. 52–16) (Guillan, 1984) have been diagnosed prenatally.

FETAL INTERVENTION

The management of the fetus, once a fetal genitourinary abnormality is identified, is not standardized and has been controversial over the last decade. **In most cases, this diagnosis leads to additional ultrasound examinations during pregnancy, counseling, and further postnatal evaluation.** As the natural history of the specific defect is elucidated, more information is often available to discuss with the family. A more invasive diagnostic and even therapeutic approach may be indicated, however, if the defect is severe, total renal function is thought to be progressively impaired, oligohydramnios is present, or associated chromosomal and/or multisystem defects are detected.

The number and frequency of repeat gestational ultrasound examinations has changed as more of the in utero history of specific abnormalities is recognized. Obstetric practices also vary, as does the timing of the routine ultrasound examinations. Once a defect is recognized, a specific follow-up recommendation should be considered and communicated to the patient and family. In most cases, if the diagnosis is made in the second trimester, an additional examination is carried out closer to term. The exception to this practice is the finding of fetal bilateral hydroureteronephrosis and an enlarged bladder. We have seen fetuses, between 15 to 20 weeks' gestation, with renal pelvic diameters of less than 1.0 cm, absence of renal cortical cysts, and normal amniotic fluid who have progressed within weeks to severe hydronephrosis, renal hyperechogenicity, and oligohydramnios. In this setting, we therefore recommend a follow-up study within 2 to 4 weeks after the initial findings.

Other, more invasive diagnostic procedures to assess the overall status of the fetus include amniocentesis, PUBS, and chorionic villous sampling. PUBS has become a standard method for rapid fetal sampling as early as 14 to 16 weeks of gestation, whereas chorionic villous sampling has the advantage of allowing chromosomal analysis at 8 to 10 weeks. Newer methods for fetal hematologic analysis may change the relative indications for these procedures in the future (Bianci et al, 1990).

The ability to analyze fetal renal function and predict future renal reserve remains a difficult dilemma. The ultrasound appearance of the fetal renal parenchyma in terms of hyperechogenicity and cysts does provide some indication of abnormal developmental patterns (Mahoney et al, 1984) but does not uniformly predict renal damage (Estroff et al, 1991). **The use of fetal bladder aspiration and observation of refilling and examination of the electrolyte composition and osmolality of the successive fetal urines is the most helpful guide to potential functional reserve** (Crombleholme et al, 1990; Johnson et al, 1994). The use of urinary protein levels, including albumin and β_2-microglobulin, has also shown predictive value of renal function in affected fetuses (Muller et al, 1993; Johnson et al, 1994). Prognostic features for good renal function included a fetal urinary sodium less than 100 mEq/L, chloride less than 90 mEq/L, and an osmolality less than 210 mOsm/L. Diagnostic assessment of fetal renal function based on these published indicators, however is imperfect at best and can be misleading (Wilkins et al, 1987; Elder et al, 1990).

Therapeutic fetal intervention is not new in its concept. Medical treatment of the fetus, via indirect maternal administration, has included thyroid hormone supplementation for hypothyroidism (Weiner et al, 1980), corticosteroid administration for affected females with congenital adrenal hyperplasia to prevent masculinization (Pang et al, 1990) and to improve fetal lung maturity in prematurity (Depp et al, 1980), and treatment for cardiac arrhythmias (Newberger and Keane, 1979). More direct fetal interventional approaches are also not new. Lilley, in 1963, reported the first intrauterine fetal transfusion for severe erythroblastosis. Open hysterotomy was also used for exchange fetal transfusion (Freda and Adamsons, 1964; Acensio et al, 1966) but was discarded as an option over time. The use of ultrasound guidance for direct fetal umbilical vessel cannulation has reduced the risk of this procedure (Seeds and Bowes, 1986). Ultrasound-guided therapeutic aspirations of the fetal chest, abdomen, kidney, and perinephric space have also been reported (Adzick and Harrison, 1994).

Historically, there are some interventions that, although initially promising, have already fallen into disfavor and others that are still in various stages of evaluation. Fetal cephalic shunting for hydrocephalus (Frigoletto et al, 1982) has been of no proven benefit. Open intrauterine surgery, via maternal hysterotomy, has been advocated for congenital diaphragmatic hernia (Harrison et al, 1990), sacral-coccygeal teratomas, and cystic malformations of the lung (Longaker et al, 1991). Despite the remarkable technical advances that these procedures represent, whether they will provide an overall benefit remains to be seen.

The first reported therapeutic fetal intervention for hydronephrosis was performed by specialists from the San Francisco Fetal Treatment Program in the early 1980s. They reported the use of an open hysterotomy for fetal urinary diversion in a 20-week-old fetus. The pregnancy was carried to 35 weeks, but the infant had pulmonary hypoplasia and did not survive (Harrison et al, 1981). They also reported the percutaneous placement of a vesicoamniotic shunt in one of twins at 32 weeks' gestation, who was diagnosed postnatally as having prune-belly syndrome (Golbus et al, 1982). Since that time, many interventions have been performed at various institutions around the world.

Those interventions performed for unilateral hydronephrosis with normal amniotic fluid (Kirkinen et al, 1982; Vintzileos et al, 1983; Newham et al, 1987) have no justification in the absence of maternal indications (Seeds et al, 1984). **The approach to intervention for suspected bladder outlet obstruction has varied in terms of the criteria for selection of candidates for such procedures and the techniques themselves** (Nicolini et al, 1987; Cromblehome et al, 1990). The reviews of an international fetal registry (Manning, 1986; Manning et al, 1990) have shown a decrease in the overall incidence of interventions. Despite the current continued application of these techniques (Johnson et al, 1994), skepticism of the overall results has remained (Colodny, 1987; Elder et al, 1987; Sholder et al, 1988). This is mainly due to the lack of long-term follow-up data, the random selection of patients and criteria for intervention, and the absence of controlled studies.

Despite this lack of consensus on the criteria and indications for fetal intervention for fetal obstructive uropathy, there remain several options to consider. Elective termination of pregnancy is available up to about 23 weeks' gestation. Most major system defects can be noted if the gestational ultrasound examination is performed between 16 to 20 weeks. If severe abnormalities are noted, then this option should be presented, as long it is accessible. As has been previously noted, amniocentesis for karyotyping is critical, given the high incidence of concomitant chromosomal anomalies in this setting.

It has been recognized that **if amniotic fluid is present up to about 27 weeks' gestation, then the profound pulmonary hypoplasia associated with early oligohydramnios is less likely to occur** (Mandell et al, 1992c). In this setting, early delivery after 30 weeks, in the face of severe oligohydramnios, is probably indicated. Exogenous maternal steroid administration (Depp et al, 1980), postnatal synthetic surfactant administration, and intensive respiratory support are critical for improving the perinatal mortality rate in this setting. It is important to state emphatically that early delivery is never indicated in cases of unilateral hydronephrosis or bilateral hydronephrosis without oligohydramnios, unless other obstetric factors would mandate this.

The clinical setting in which fetal intervention involving chronic bladder drainage appears to be most appropriate is the male fetus in the second trimester of gestation (18 to 26 weeks), who presents with several bilateral hydroureteronephrosis, reasonable fetal urinary indicators, and progressive oligohydramnios. **The rationale for fetal urinary drainage is that with severe, early obstruction, both renal and pulmonary development are impaired**. Theoretically, bypassing the obstructed urinary system by shunting urine directly into the amniotic cavity will decompress the kidneys enough to prevent irreversible damage and prevent the development of pulmonary hypoplasia associated with oligohydramnios (Peters et al, 1991a). In terms of the techniques for chronic fetal urinary intervention, both open and closed methods have been described. At this point in time, there

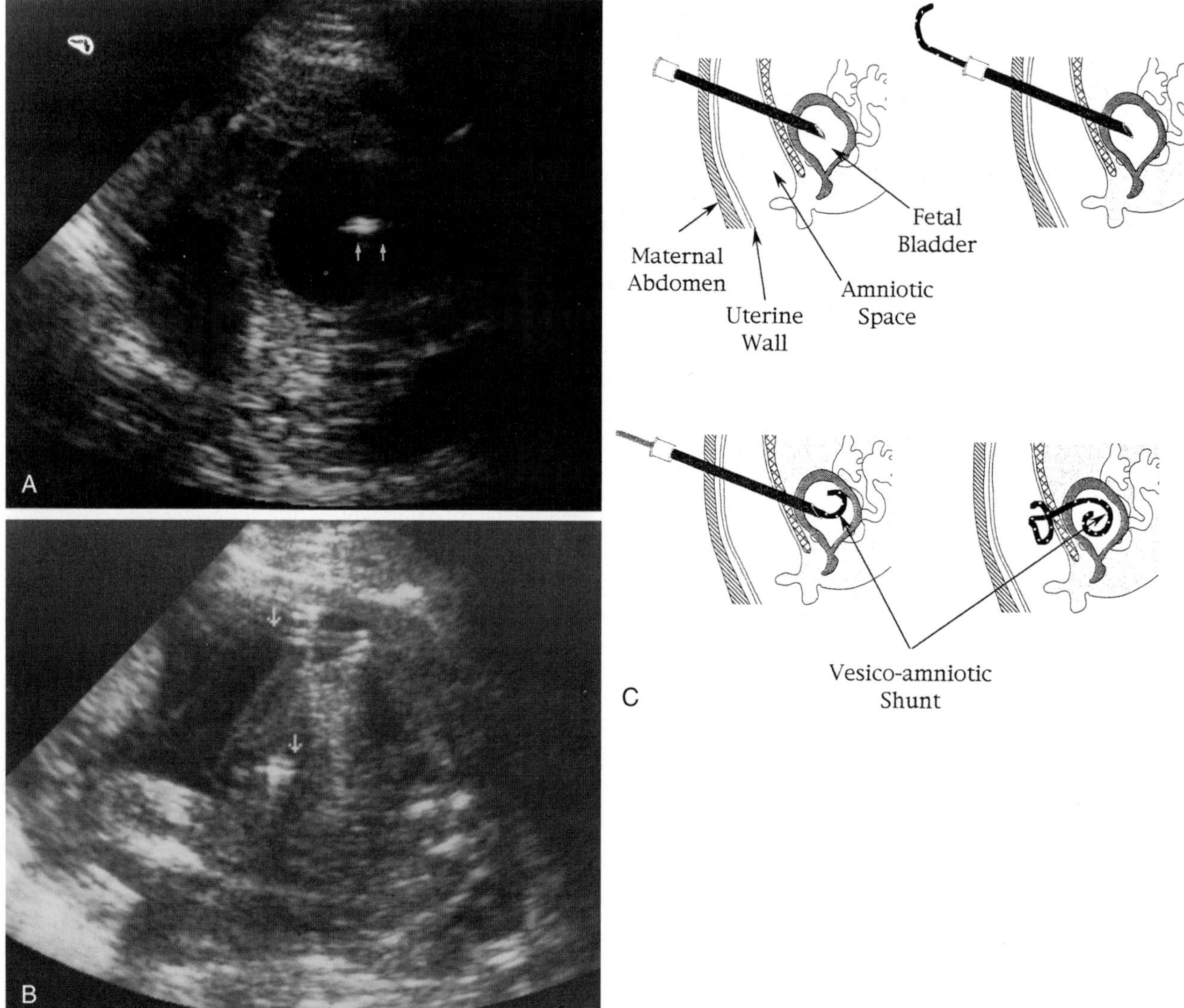

Figure 52–14. Prenatal intervention with vesicoamniotic shunt. *A,* Under ultrasound guidance at 21 weeks' gestation, the trocar *(arrows)* is placed into the fetal bladder percutaneously. *B,* The pigtail shunt is seen in the bladder and on the fetal abdomen. *C,* Schematic diagram of vesicoamniotic shunt being placed in the fetal bladder.

appears to be no advantage to open fetal surgery of the urinary tract despite reports of successful cutaneous ureterostomy and vesicostomy (Longaker et al, 1991).

Percutaneous shunting of the bladder is technically feasible and, in experienced hands, can be performed with relatively low morbidity (Nicolini et al, 1987; Johnson et al, 1994). The use of maternal sedation, local anesthesia, and tocolytic agents is routine, and the fetus can be paralyzed using intramuscular injection of pancuronium (Toma et al, 1990). Under ultrasound guidance, the amniotic space is reconstituted with saline, the fetal bladder is transfixed with a trocar needle, and the vesical amniotic shunt is then placed (Fig. 52–14*A* to *C*). Even if initially technically successful, the shunt often will become obstructed or displaced over time and a second procedure may be necessary. There may also be bowel herniation along the needle tract (see Fig. 52–18) (Robichaux et al, 1991). If amniotic fluid can be reconstituted long enough to allow adequate pulmonary development and postnatal function, then delivery can occur after 32 to 33 weeks.

In addition to these technical considerations, **many questions remain regarding the risks and benefits of fetal urinary intervention for obstructive uropathy** (Sholder et al, 1988; Elder et al, 1987). The risks include misdiagnosis of obstructive uropathy, documented fetal injury, maternal infection, risk to subsequent pregnancies, and inappropriate interventions for non–life-threatening conditions. One of the underpublicized outcomes is the prevention of significant renal impairment in infants who have undergone these procedures in utero. Chronic and late renal insufficiency, and the ultimate need for transplantation should be specifically detailed in the informed-consent procedures.

With the advent of fetal diagnosis and potential therapies, the ethical issues of maternal and fetal rights have been raised (Robertson, 1985). Given the experimental nature of fetal intervention for genitourinary abnormalities, an adversarial relationship between caregivers and family in terms of coercion should never occur. More to the point is the explanation of all the potential risks and benefits, and an honest appraisal of all possible options and outcomes.

POSTNATAL MANAGEMENT

As mentioned in the introduction to this chapter, the major impact of prenatal diagnosis of genitourinary abnormalities has been on the clinical presentation of most patients with congenital uropathies. The majority of infants with obstructive uropathy, including ureteropelvic junction obstruction, obstructive megaureter, ectopic ureterocele and ectopic ureter, as well as increasing numbers of those with vesicoureteral reflux, now present for evaluation and management asymptomatic and in the newborn period (Brown et al, 1987). **This dramatic change in clinical practice has brought about several divergent and sometimes very disparate protocols for diagnostic and therapeutic management.**

Those neonates with prenatal findings of oligohydramnios; cloacal, anorectal or genital malformations; suspected posterior urethral valves; or large abdominal masses are best managed by delivery at or immediate transfer to a tertiary health center and prompt evaluation and treatment. In those male infants with prenatal findings of marked bilateral hydroureteronephrosis and an enlarged bladder or physical findings suggestive of bladder outlet obstruction, an immediate ultrasound examination and voiding cystourethrogram is performed. If posterior urethral valves are confirmed, then a feeding tube is left in place until definitive therapy is instituted. If bilateral reflux or obstructive megaureter is found, then antibiotic prophylaxis is begun.

In the vast majority of cases, however, the neonatal evaluation can be performed safely and electively on an outpatient basis. Our criteria or indications for postnatal evaluation based on prenatal findings is diagrammed in Figure 52–15. It is important to communicate to the primary care physician and the parents that the neonate with prenatally diagnosed hydronephrosis should be discharged home on antibiotic prophylaxis. Our practice is to use amoxicillin, 12 to 15 mg/kg, once a day.

The initial postnatal study is an ultrasound examination, which can be performed in the first several weeks after birth. In most cases, this examination is not performed within the first 1 to 2 days of life, because the rapid changes in renal physiology may underestimate the degree of hydronephrosis (Laing et al, 1984). The examination should consist of longitudinal and transverse images of both kidneys. The examiner should be experienced in neonatal imaging, because prominent hypoechoic renal pyramids can be mistaken for dilated calyces or parenchymal cysts (Haller et al, 1982). A transverse scan of the full bladder is important to obtain in order to visualize dilated ureters posterior to the bladder. This often takes patience and repeat imaging in the neonate. In cases of suspected congenital adrenal hyperplasia, the adrenal glands and the uterus should also be examined.

There has been some controversy over which neonates with a diagnosis of in utero hydronephrosis should undergo voiding cystourethrography. It had been our practice that if the fetal renal pelvic diameter was greater than 8 mm, and caliectasis or ureterectasis was present, then a voiding cystourethrogram (VCUG) was recommended (Steele et al, 1989; Gordon et al, 1990; Mandell et al, 1991). **This study is now performed even if the postnatal ultrasound shows apparent resolution of the fetal hydronephrosis** (Zerin et al, 1993). A more difficult question is whether to perform a

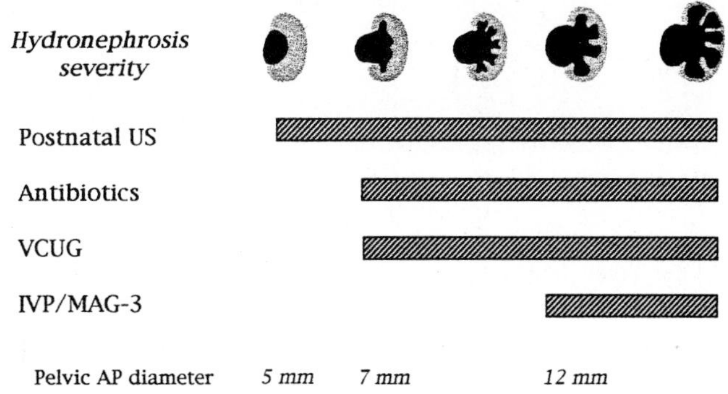

Figure 52–15. Schematic representation of prenatal ultrasound findings as an indication for postnatal evaluation of hydronephrosis.

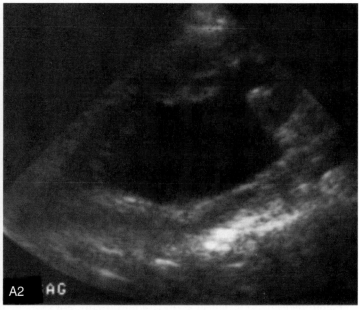

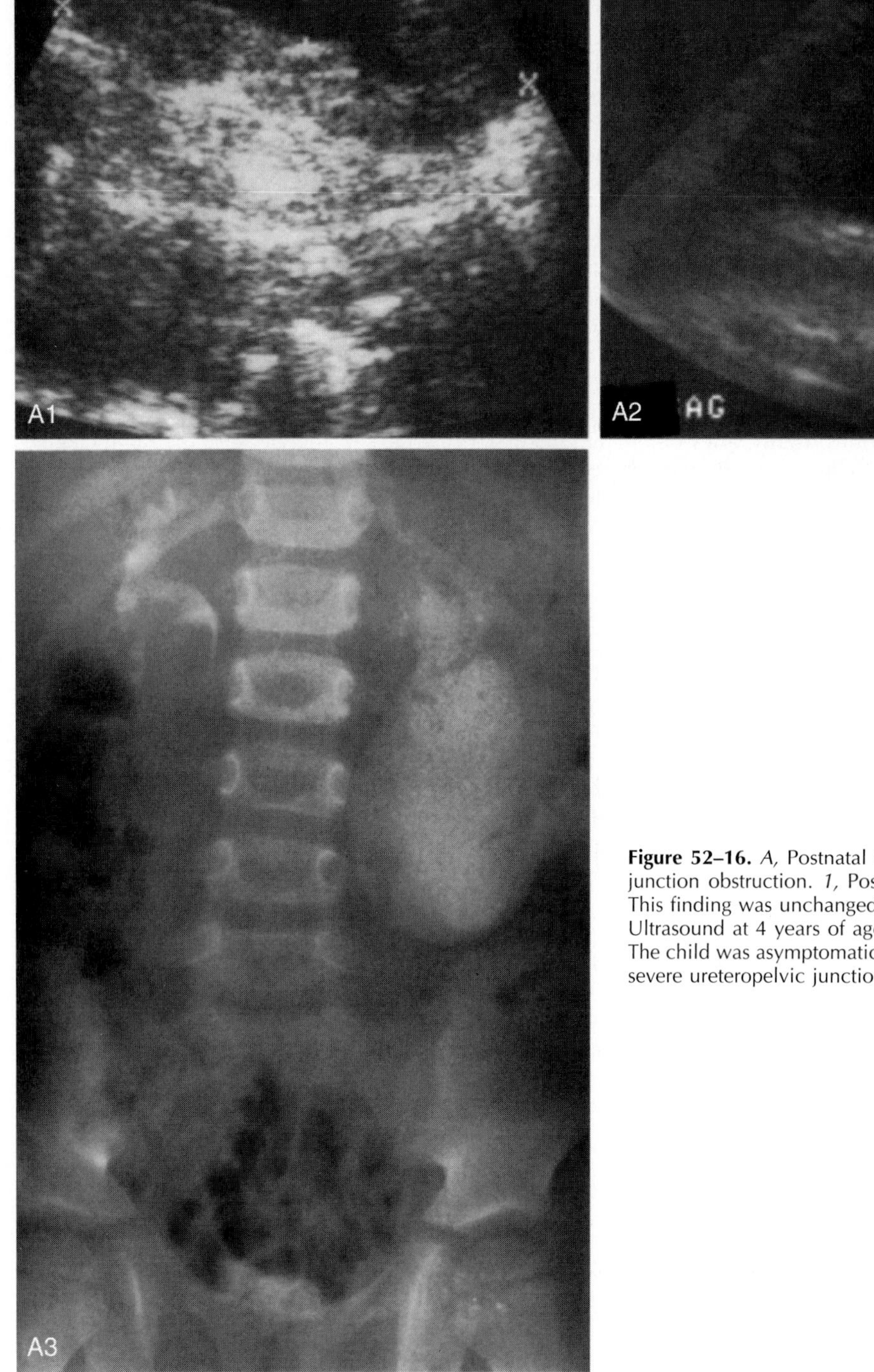

Figure 52–16. *A,* Postnatal follow-up of prenatally diagnosed ureteropelvic junction obstruction. *1,* Postnatal ultrasound showing mild pelvic fullness. This finding was unchanged in degree on subsequent studies for 2 years. *2,* Ultrasound at 4 years of age shows dramatic worsening of hydronephrosis. The child was asymptomatic. *3,* Intravenous urogram at age 4 years showing severe ureteropelvic junction obstruction.

VCUG on all infants with any degree of pelvic dilatation (Marra et al, 1994).

The VCUG should again be performed by a radiologist experienced in dealing with neonates. Oblique views of the ureterovesical junctions and the posterior urethra during voiding are mandatory. If reflux is not seen on the initial filling cycle, then repeat cycles are important if the ureters are very dilated, if voiding is incomplete, or if reflux is strongly suspected (Paltiel et al, 1992). Although a radionuclide examination is used for most follow-up studies, it is our practice to use a standard fluoroscopic technique for the initial examination in both male and female neonates.

If the postnatal ultrasound examination demonstrates significant renal pelvic dilatation (>1.2 cm) and caliec-

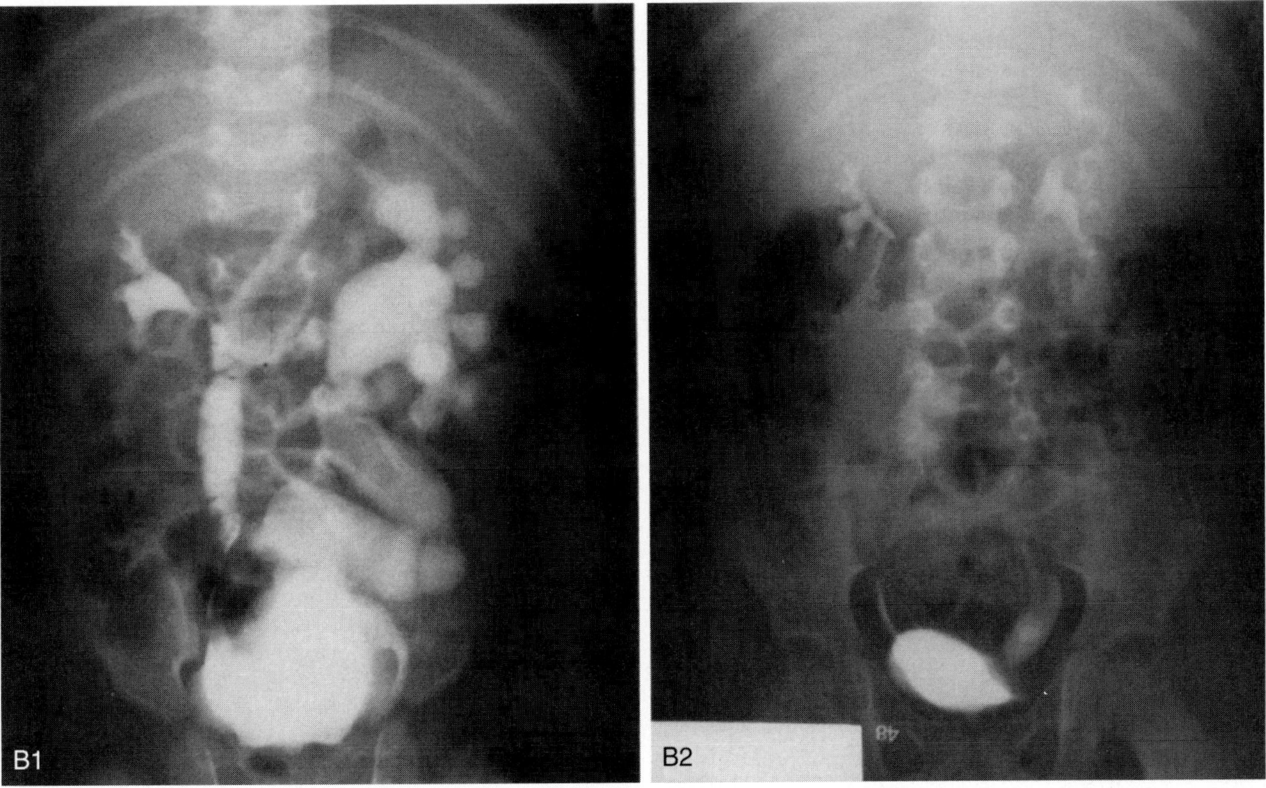

Figure 52–16 *Continued B,* Postnatal follow-up of prenatally diagnosed megaureter. *1,* Initial postnatal intravenous pyelogram showing left hydroureteronephrosis and a tortuous ureter. Renal scan showed no diminution in function. *2,* Follow-up intravenous urogram 20 months later, with no surgery, showing normal upper collecting system with mild distal ureteral dilation.

tasis is noted, a diuretic renal scan is recommended in order to determine the degree of functional obstruction and its effect on the kidneys. There remains a degree of variation in techniques in performing this study, including the age at which the initial and subsequent examinations are performed, the radionuclide agent used, and the exact protocol used during the scan. Owing to the recognized effect of prematurity on the results of renal scans (Koff, 1988), we prefer to perform these studies, in elective situations, in neonates after 1 month of age. Other centers vary in their scheduling of these studies from within the first week to several weeks postnatally (Koff and Campbell, 1992; Maizels et al, 1992). Unfortunately, there is no agreed-on measurement to determine when renal function is too immature to allow an accurate study. If the contralateral normal kidney shows impaired nuclide uptake or excretion, or response to furosemide (Lasix), the scan should be repeated at a later date.

The radionuclide agent used in most of the earlier studies was ^{99m}Tc DTPA (O'Reilly, 1986), but at present, most centers are using ^{99m}Tc MAG-3 (Russell et al, 1988). The radionuclide study should be performed under a protocol, with a bladder catheter, timing of administration, and dose of furosemide standardized (Maizels et al, 1992). Calculated outcomes from designated areas of interest include individual renal differential function (Ransley et al, 1990; Elder and Miraldi, 1988), renal transit time (Whitfield et al, 1978), extraction factor (Heyman and Duckett, 1988), and drainage curves, or t 1/2 (Thrall et al, 1981; O'Reilly, et al, 1979). The halftime, or t 1/2, represents the number of minutes required for half of the radiopharmaceutical to empty after administration of the diuretic. **Despite the standardized formats and graphic presentation of the results, the interpretation and implications of the renal scan remain very subjective**.

Another, more invasive evaluation of the hydrodynamic physiology of the upper urinary tract is the pressure perfusion study of Whitaker (Whitaker, 1979). This study involves antegrade access to the kidney and, in most cases in children, general anesthesia. It has been used as constant volume perfusion and a constant pressure perfusion technique (Woodbury et al, 1989). We now rarely use this technique in the evaluation of neonates and infants.

The therapeutic management strategies of these asymptomatic infants is more diverse at this time than ever. We will not attempt to specifically discuss the treatment protocols for multicystic kidney, ectopic ureterocele and ectopic ureter, vesicoureteral reflux, prune-belly syndrome, anorectal and bladder malformations, or intersex conditions. These conditions are all be carefully outlined in other chapters. It is important to note again, however, the impact of prenatal diagnosis on our clinical practices and plans.

It has been shown that early neonatal correction of obstruction can be performed safely and successfully (Bernstein et al, 1988; Peters et al, 1989). **Whether or not surgical intervention is *necessary* is now the question that is being addressed**. Treatment protocols under evaluation include early surgery for infants who have delayed washout or drainage (t 1/2 $>$ 20 minutes) (King et al, 1984; King and Hatcher, 1991). Others require diminished differential function (<40%) to proceed to surgery, regardless of the t 1/2 (Ransley et al, 1990). Still another approach uses observation only, despite marked reduction in measured glomerular function (Koff and Campbell, 1992). Based on follow-up studies, it appears that indications for operative intervention develop in about 25% or greater of those with moderate reduction in drainage or function followed expectantly (Ransley et al, 1990) (Fig. 52–16*A* and *B*).

Despite the controversies brought about by the prenatal diagnosis of genitourinary abnormalities, the care and well-being of these children has been enhanced by this process. The number of infants with urosepsis has been reduced (Dacher et al, 1992), and the quality of life may be improved. We are continuously evolving in our understanding of these disease processes, and this evolution will certainly benefit our patients.

REFERENCES

Acensio SH, Figueroa-Longo JG, Pelegrina IA: Intrauterine exchange transfusion. Am J Obstet Gynecol 1966; 95:1129.

Adzick NS, Harrison MR: The unborn surgical patient. Curr Probl Surg 1994; 31:1.

Adzick NS, Harrison MR, Glick PL, et al: Experimental pulmonary hypoplasia and oligohydramnios: Relative contributions of lung fluid and fetal breathing movements. J Pediatr Surg 1984; 19:658.

Alcorn D, Adamson TM, Lambert TF, et al: Morphologic effects of chronic tracheal ligation and drainage in the fetal lamb lung. J Anat 1977; 123:649.

Anderson N, Clautice-Engle T, Allan R, et al: Detection of obstructive uropathy in the fetus: Predictive value of sonographic measurements of renal pelvic diameter at various gestational ages. AJR 1995; 164:719.

Aperia A, Broberger O, Thodenius K, et al: Developmental study of the renal response to an oral salt load in preterm infants. Acta Paediatr Scand 1974; 63:517.

Arger BH, Coleman BG, Mintz MC, et al: Routine fetal genitourinary tract screening. Radiology 1985; 156:485.

Arnold AJ, Rickwood AMK: Natural history of pelviureteric obstruction detected by prenatal ultrasonography. Br J Urol 1990; 65:91.

Avni EF, Thoua Y, Lalmand B, et al: Multicystic dysplastic kidney: Natural history from in utero diagnosis and postnatal followup. J Urol 1987; 138:1420.

Barakat AS, Butler MC, Cobb CG, et al: Reliability of ultrasound in the prenatal diagnosis of urinary tract abnormalities. Pediatr Nephrol 1991; 5:12.

Beck AD: The effect of intra-uterine urinary obstruction upon the development of the fetal kidney. J Urol 1971; 105:784.

Benacerraf BR, Saltzman DH, Mandell J: Sonographic diagnosis of abnormal genitalia. J Ultrasound Med 1989; 8:613.

Benacerraf BR, Peters CA, Mandell J: The prenatal evolution of renal cystic dysplasia in the setting of obstructive hydronephrosis and urinoma formation followed sonographically. J Clin Ultrasound 1991a; 19:446.

Benacerraf BR, Peters CA, Mandell J: The prenatal evolution of the nonfunctioning kidney in the setting of obstructive hydronephrosis. J Clin Ultrasound 1991b; 19:446.

Benacerraf BR, Mandell J, Estroff JA, et al: Fetal pyelectasis: A possible association with Down syndrome. Obstet Gynecol 1990; 76:58.

Berhrman RE, Parer JT, deLannoy CW Jr: Placental growth and the formation of amniotic fluid. Nature 1967; 214:678.

Bernstein GT, Mandell J, Lebowitz RL, et al: Ureteropelvic junction obstruction in the neonate. J Urol 1988; 140:1216.

Bianci D, Flint A, Pizzimenti M, et al: Isolation of fetal DNA from nucleated erythrocytes in maternal blood. Proc Natl Acad Sci USA, 87:3279, 1990.

Birnholz JC: Determination of fetal sex. N Engl J Med 1983; 309:942.

Blachar A, Schachter M, Blachar Y, et al: Evaluation of prenatally diagnosed hydronephrosis by morphometric measurements of the kidney. Pediatr Radiol 1994; 24:131.

Bowie JD, Rosenberg ER, Andreotti R, et al: The changing appearance of fetal kidneys during pregnancy. J Ultrasound Med 1983; 2:505.

Broecker BH, Redwine FO, Petres RE: Reversal of acute polyhydramnios after fetal decompression. Urology 1988; 31:60.

Bromley B, Mandell J, Walzer TB, Benacerraf BR: Masculinization of female fetuses with congenital adrenal hyperplasia may already be present at 18 weeks. Am J Obstet Gynecol 1994; 171:264.

Brown T, Mandell J, Lebowitz RL: Neonatal hydronephrosis in the era of sonography. AJR 1987; 148:959.

Carr MC, Benacerraf BR, Mandell J: Prenatal diagnosis of an XY fetus with aphallia and cloacal exstrophy variant. J Ultrasound Med 1994; 13:323.

Carr MC, Benacerraf BR, Estroff JA, Mandell J: Prenatally diagnosed bilateral hyperechoic kidneys with normal amniotic fluid: Postnatal outcomes. J Urol 1995; 153:442.

Ceccherini I, Lituania M, Cordone MS, et al: Autosomal dominant polycystic kidney disease: Prenatal diagnosis by DNA analysis and songraphy at 14 weeks. Prenat Diagn 1989; 9:751.

Cilento BG Jr, Benacerraf BR, Mandell J: Pre and postnatal findings in monochorionic, monoamniotic twins discordant for bilateral renal agenesis/dysgenesis (perinatal lethal renal disease). J Urol 1994a; 151:1034.

Cilento BG Jr, Benacerraf BR, Mandell J: Prenatal diagnosis of cloacal malformation. Urology 1994b; 43:386.

Clemmons JJW: Embryonic renal injury: A possible factor in fetal malnutrition. Pediatr Res 1977; 11:404.

Colodny AH: Antenatal diagnosis and management of urinary abnormalities. Pediatr Clin North Am 1987; 34:365.

Coret A, Morag B, Katz M, et al: The impact of fetal screening on indications for cystourethrography in infants. Pediatr Radiol 1994; 24:516.

Cromblehholme TM, Harrison MR, Golbus MS, et al: Fetal intervention in obstructive uropathy: Prognostic indicators and efficacy of intervention. Am J Obstet Gynecol 1990; 162:1239.

Dacher JN, Mandell J, Lebowitz RL: Urinary tract infection in infants in spite of prenatal diagnosis of hydronephrosis. Pediatr Radiol 1992; 22:401.

Depp R, Boehm JJ, Nosek JA, et al: Antenatal corticosteroids to prevent neonatal respiratory distress syndrome: Risk vs benefit considerations. Am J Obstet Gynecol 1980; 137:338.

Docimo SG, Luetic T, Crone RK, et al: Pulmonary development in the fetal lamb with severe bladder outlet obstruction and oligohydramnios: A morphometric study. J Urol 1989; 142(Part 2):657.

Dungan JS, Fernandez ME, Abbitt PL, et al: Multicystic dysplastic kidney: Natural history of prenatally detected cases. Prenat Diagn 1990; 19:175.

Edelman CM Jr: Maturation of the neonatal kidney. *In* Becker EL, ed: Proceedings of the Third International Congress of Nephrology, Vol 3, 1967 p 1

Elder JS, Miraldi F: Are differential renal functions by renal scan accurate in obstructive uropathy. J Urol 1988; 139:176A.

Elder JS, O'Grady JP, Ashmead G, et al: Evaluation of fetal renal function: unreliability of fetal urinary electrolytes. J Urol 1990; 144:574.

Elder JS, Duckett JW Jr, Synder HM: Intervention for fetal obstructive uropathy, has it been effective? Lancet 1987; 2:1007.

Estroff JA, Mandell J, Benacerraf BR: Increased renal parenchymal echogenicity in the fetus: Importance and clinical outcome. Radiology 1991; 181:135.

Ewigman BG, Crane JP, Frigoletto FD, et al: Effect of prenatal ultrasound screening on prenatal outcome. RADIUS study group. N Engl J Med 1993; 329:874.

Freda VJ, Adamsons K: Exchange tranfusion in utero. Report of a case. Am J Obstet Gynecol 1964; 89:817.

Frigoletto FD, Birnholz JC, Green MF: Antenatal treatment of hydrocephalus by ventricolamniotic shunting. JAMA 1982; 248:2496.

Gardner S, Burton BK, Johnson AM: Maternal serum alpha-fetoprotein screening: A report of the Forsyth County project. Am J Obstet Gynecol 1981; 140:250.

Gearhart JP, Ben-Chaim J, Jeffs RD, Sanders RC: Criteria for the prenatal diagnosis of classic bladder exstrophy. Obstet Gynecol 1995; 85:961.

Glick PL, Harrison MR, Adzick NS, et al: Management of the fetus with congenital hydronephrosis II. Diagnostic assessment and selection for treatment. J Pediatr Surg 1985; 20:376.

Glick PL, Harrison MR, Adzick NS, et al: Correction of congenital hydronephrosis in utero III. Early mid-trimester ureteral obstruction produces renal dysplasia. J Pediatr Surg 1983; 18:681.

Golbus MS, Harrison MR, Filly RA, et al: In utero treatment of urinary tract obstruction. Am. J Obstet Gynecol 1982; 142:383.

Gordon AC, Thomas DF, Arthur RJ, et al: Prenatally diagnosed reflux: A follow-up study. Br J Urol 1990; 65:407.

Grannum P, Bracker M, Silverman R, et al: Assessment of fetal kidney size in normal gestation by comparison of ratio of kidney circumference to abdominal circumference. Am J Obstet Gynecol 1980; 136:249.

Grignon A, Filion R, Filiatrault D: Urinary tract dilatation in utero: Classification and clinical applications. Radiology 1986; 160:645.

Grunewald SM, Crocker EF, Walker AG, Trudinger BJ: Antenatal diagnosis of urinary tract abnormalities: Correlation of ultrasound appearance with postnatal diagnosis. Am J Obstet Gynecol 1984; 148:278.

Guignard JP, Torrado A, DaCunha O, et al: Glomerular filtration rate in the first three weeks of life. J Pediatr 1975; 87:268.

Guillan BB: Prenatal ultrasonic diagnosis of fetal renal tumor. Radiology 1984; 152:69.

Guillan BB, Chang CCN, Yoss BS: Prenatal ultrasonographic diagnosis of fetal adrenal neuroblastoma. J Clin Ultrasound 1986; 14:225.

Gunn TR, Mora JD, Pease P: Antenatal diagnosis of urinary tract abnormalities by ultrasonography after 28 weeks' gestation: Incidence and outcome. Am J Obstet Gynecol, 1995; 172:479.

Haller JO, Berdon WE, Friedman AP: Increased renal cortical echogenicity: A normal finding in neonates and infants. Radiology 1982; 142:173.

Harris RD, Nyberg DA, Mack LA, et al: Anorectal atresia: Prenatal sonographic diagnosis. AJR 1987; 149:395.

Harrison MR, Filly RA, Parer JT, et al: Management of the fetus with a urinary tract malformation. J Am Med Assoc 1981; 246:635.

Harrison MR, Langer JC, Adzick NS, et al: Correction of congenital diaphragmatic hernia in utero: V. Initial clinical experience. J Pediatr Surg 1990; 25:47.

Harrison MR, Ross NA, Noall R, et al: Correction of congenital hydronephrosis in utero I. The model: Fetal urethral obstruction produces hydronephrosis and pulmonary hypoplasia in fetal lambs. J Pediatr Surg 1983; 18:247.

Heyman S, Duckett JW: The extraction factor: An estimate of single kidney function in children during routine radionuclide renography with 99m technetium diethylenetriaminepentaacetic acid. J Urol 1988; 140:789.

Hobbins JC, Romero R, Brannum P, et al: Antenatal diagnosis of renal anomalies with ultrasound I. Obstructive uropath. Am J Obstet Gynecol 1984; 148:868.

Hutton KAR, Thomas DFM, Arthur RJ, et al: Prenatally detected posterior urethral valves: Is gestational age at detection a predictor of outcome? J Urol 1994; 152:698.

Janetschek G, Weitzel D, Stern W: Prenatal diagnosis of neuroblastoma by sonography. Urology 1984; 24:397.

Jeanty P, Dramaiz-Wilnet M, Elkhazen N, et al: Measurement of the fetal kidney growth on ultrasound. Radiology 1982; 144:159.

Johnson MP, Bukowski TP, Reitleman C, et al: In utero surgical treatment of fetal obstructive uropathy: A new comprehensive approach to identify appropriate candidates for vesicoamniotic shunt therapy. Am J Obstet Gynecol 1994; 170:1770.

Keirse MJ, Meerman MB: Antenatal diagnosis of Potter syndrome. Obstet Gynecol 1978; 52 (Suppl): 645.

Kim KM, Kogan BA, Massas CA: Collagen and elastin in the obstructed fetal bladder. J Urol 1991; 146:528.

King LR, Coughlin PWF, Bloch EC, et al: The case for immediate pyeloplasty in the neonate with ureteropelvic junction obstruction. J Urol 1984; 132:303.

King LR, Hatcher PA: Natural history of fetal and neonatal hydronephrosis. Urology 1991; 35:433.

Kirkinen P, Jouppila P, Tounonen S, et al: Repeated transabdominal renocentesis in a case of fetal hydronephrotic kidney. Am J Obstet Gynecol 1982; 142:1049.

Kleiner B, Callen PW, Filly RA: Sonographic analysis of the fetus with ureteropelvic junction obstruction. AJR 148:359, 1987.

Koff SA, McDowell GC, Myard M: Diuretic radionuclide assessment of obstruction in the infant: Guidelines for successful interpretation. J Urol 1988; 140:11657.

Koff SA, Campbell K: Nonoperative management of unilateral neonatal hydronephrosis. J Urol 1992; 148:525.

Laing FC, Burke VD, Wing VW, et al: Postpartum evaluation of fetal hydronephrosis: Optimal timing for followup sonography. Radiology 1984; 152:423.

Lawson TL, Foley WD, Berland LI, Clark KE: Ultrasonic evaluation of fetal kidneys: Analysis of normal size and frequency of visualization as related to stage of pregnancy. Radiology 1981; 138:153.

Lilley AW: Intrauterine tranfusion of fetus in haemolytic disease. BMJ 1963; 2:1107.

Livera LN, Brookfield DS, Eggenton JA, Hawnaur JM: Antenatal ultrasonography to detect fetal renal abnormalities: A prospective screening programme. BMJ 1989; 298:421.

Longaker MT, Golbus MS, Filly RA, et al: Maternal outcome after open fetal surgery: A review of the first 17 human cases. JAMA 1991; 265:737.

Mahony BS, Filly RA, Callen PW, et al: Fetal renal dysplasia: Sonographic evaluation. Radiology 1984; 152:143.

Maizels M, Reisman MF, Flom LS, et al: Grading nephroureteral dilatation detected in the first year of life: Correlation with obstruction. J Urol 1992; 148:609.

Maizels M, Reisman MF, Flom LS, et al: Grading nephroureteral dilatation detected in the first year of life: Correlation with obstruction. J Urol 1992; 148:609.

Mandell J, Blyth B, Peters CA, et al: Structural genitourinary defects detected in utero. Radiology 1991; 178:193.

Mandell J, Bromle B, Peters CA, Benacerraf BR: Prenatal sonographic detection of genital malformations. J Urol 1995; 153:1994.

Mandell J, Lebowitz RL, Peters CA, et al: Prenatal diagnosis of the megacystis-megaureter association. J Urol 1992a; 148:1487.

Mandell J, Lillehei CW, Greene M, et al: The prenatal diagnosis of imperforate anus with rectourinary fistula: Dilated fetal colon with enterolithiasis. J Pediatr Surg 1992b; 27:82.

Mandell J, Paltiel HJ, Peters CA, Benacerraf BR: Prenatal findings associated with a unilateral nonfunctioning or absent kidney. J Urol 1994; 152:176.

Mandell J, Peters CA, Estroff JA, Benacerraf BR: Late onset oligohydramnios associated with genitourinary abnormalities. J Urol 1992c; 148:515.

Mandell J, Peters CA, Estroff JA, et al: Human fetal compensatory renal growth. J Urol 1993; 150:790.

Manning FA: The fetus with obstructive uropathy: The fetal registry. *In* Harrison MR, Golbus MS, Filly RA, eds: The Unborn Patient. Philadelphia, W. B. Saunders Company, 1990, p 394.

Manning FA, Harrison MR, Rodeck C: Catheter shunts for fetal hydronephrosis and hydrocephalus. N Engl J Med 1986; 315:536.

Manning FA, Hill LM, Platt LD: Qualitative amniotic fluid volume determination by ultrasound: Antepartum detection of intrauterine growth retardation. Am J Obstet Gynecol 1981; 139:254.

Marra G, Barbieri G, Moioli C, et al: Mild fetal hydronephrosis indicating vesicoureteral reflux. Arch Dis Child 1994; 70:147.

Marras A, Mereu G, Dessi C, et al: Oligohydramnios and extrarenal abnormalities in Potter syndrome. J Pediatr 1983; 102:597.

McHugo JM, Shafi MI, Rowlands D, et al: Prenatal diagnosis of adult polycystic kidney disease. Br J Radiol 1988; 61:1072.

McVary K, Maizels M: Urinary obstruction reduces glomerulogenesis in the developing kidney: A model in the rabbit. J Urol 1989; 142 (Part 2):646.

Moore ES, deLeon LB, Weiss LS, et al: Compensatory renal hypertrophy in fetal lambs. Pediatr Res 1979; 13:347.

Morse RP, Rawnsley E, Crowe HC, et al: Bilateral renal agenesis in three consecutive siblings. Prenat Diagn 1987; 7:573.

Muller F, Dommergues M, Mandelbrot L, et al: Fetal urinary biochemistry predicts postnatal renal function in children with bilateral obstructive uropathies. Obstet Gynecol 1993; 82:813.

Nakayama DK, Harrison MR, de Lorimier AA: Prognosis of posterior urethral valves presenting at birth. J Pediatr Surg 1986; 21:43.

Newberger JW, Keane JF: Intrauterine supraventricular tachycardia. J Pediatr 1979; 95:780.

Newnham JP, Thomson R, Murphy A, et al: Successful placement of a pyeloamniotic shunt catheter for ureteropelvic junctional obstruction in utero. Med J Aust 1987; 145:540.

Nicolini V, Rodeck C, Fisk N: Shunt treatment for fetal obstructive uropathy. Lancet 1987; 2:1338.

Noe HN, Wyatt RJ, Peeden JN Jr, Rivas MJ: The transmission of vesicoureteral reflux from parent to child. J Urol 1993; 148:1869.

O'Flynn KJ, Gough DCS, Gupta S, et al: Prediction of recovery in antenatally diagnosed hydronephrosis. Br J Urol 1993; 71:478.

O'Reilly PH: Diuresis renography eight years later: Update. J Urol 1986; 136:993.

O'Reilly PH, Lawson RS, Shields RA, et al: Idiopathic hydronephrosis—the diuresis renogram: A new non-invasive method of assessing equivocal pelviureteral junction obstruction. J Urol 1979; 121:153.

Paltiel HJ, Rupich RC, Kiruluta HG: Enhanced detection of vesicoureteral reflux in infants and children using cyclic voiding cystourethrography. Radiology 1992; 184:753.

Pang S, Pollack MS, Marshall RN, Immken L: Prenatal treatment of congenital adrenal hyperplasia due to 21-hydroxylase deficiency. N Engl J Med 1990; 322:111.

Peters CA, Bolkier M, Bauer SB, et al: The urodynamic consequences of posterior urethral valves. J Urol 1990; 144:122.

Peters CA, Carr MC, Lais A, et al: The response of the fetal kidney to obstruction. J Urol 1992a; 148:503.

Peters CA, Docimo SG, Luetic T, et al: Effect of in utero vesicostomy on pulmonary hypoplasia in the fetal lamb with bladder outlet obstruction and oligohydramnios. J Urol 1991a; 146:1178.

Peters CA, Mandell J, Lebowitz RL, et al: Congenital obstructed megaureters in early infancy: Diagnosis and treatment. J Urol 1989; 142:641.

Peters CA, Reid LM, Docimo SG, et al: The role of the kidney in lung growth and maturation in the setting of obstructive uropathy and oligohydramnios. J Urol 1991b; 146:597.

Peters CA, Vasavada S, Dator D, et al: The effect of obstruction on the developing bladder. J Urol 1992b; 148:491.

Petrikovsky BM, Nardi DA, Radis JF, Hoegsberg B: Elevated maternal alpha-feto protein and mild fetal uropathy. Obstet Gynecol 1991; 78:262.

Pocock R, Witcombe J, Andrews H, et al: The outcome of antenatally diagnosed urological abnormalities. Br J Urol 1985; 57:788.

Potter EL: Absence of the ureters and kidneys. Obstet Gynecol 1965; 25:3.

Potter EL: Normal and abnormal development of the kidney. Chicago, Year Book Medical, 1972, p 209.

Queenan JT, Thompson W, Whitfield C, et al: Amniotic fluid volume in normal pregnancy. Am J Obstet Gynecol 1972; 114:34.

Quinlan RW, Cruz AC, Huddleston JF: Sonographic detection of fetal urinary tract anomalies. Obstet Gynecol 1986; 67:558.

Ransley PG, Dhillon HJK, Gordon I, et al: The postnatal management of hydronephrosis diagnosed by prenatal ultrasound. J Urol 1990; 144:584.

Ray D, Berger N, Ensor R: Hydramnios in association with unilateral fetal hydronephrosis. J Clin Ultrasound 1982; 10:82.

Reuss A, Wladimiroff JW, Scholtmeyer RJ, et al: Prenatal evaluation and outcome of fetal obstructive uropathies. Prenat Diagn 1988; 8:93.

Reznik VM, Murphy JL, Mendoza SL, et al: Followup of infants with obstructive uropathy detected in utero and treated surgically postnatally. J Pediatr Surg 1989; 24:1289.

Robertson JA: Legal issues in fetal therapy. Semin Perinatol 1985; 9:136.

Robichaux AG, Mandell J, Greene M, et al: Fetal abdominal wall defect: A new complication of vesicoamniotic shunting. Fetal Diagn Ther 1991; 6:11.

Romero R, Cullen M, Grannum P, et al: Antenatal diagnosis of renal anomalies with ultrasound III: Bilateral renal agenesis. Am J Obstet Gynecol 1985; 151:38.

Roodhooft AM, Birnolz JC, Holmes LD: Familial nature of congenital absence and severe dysgenesis of both kidneys. N Engl J Med 1984; 310:1341.

Rosendahl H: Ultrasound screening for fetal urinary tract malformations. A prospective study in general population. Eur J Obstet Gynecol Reprod Biol 1990; 36:27.

Royer P: The kidney in the newborn. *In* Royer P, Habib R, Mathieu H, et al, eds: Pediatric Nephrology. Philadelphia, W. B. Saunders Company, 1974 p 116.

Rubenstein SC, Benacerraf BR, Retik AB, Mandell J: Fetal suprarenal masses: Sonographic appearance and differential diagnosis. Ultrasound Obstet Gynecol 1995; 5:154.

Rubin MI, Bruck E, Rapoport M: Maturation of renal function in childhood. J Clin Invest 1949; 28:1144.

Rudolph AM, Heyman MA, Teramo KAW, et al: Studies on the circulation of the previable human. Pediatr Res 1971; 5:452.

Russell CD, Thorstad B, Yester MV, et al: Comparison of technetium 99m MAG3 with iodine 131 hippuran by a simultaneous dual channel technique. J Nucl Med 1988; 29:1189.

Sampaio FJB, Aragao AHM: Study of fetal kidney length growth during the second and third trimesters of gestation. Eur Urol 1989; 25:4.

Saunders P, Rhodes P: The origin and circulation of the amniotic fluid. *In* Fairweather DVI, Eskes TKAB, eds: Amniotic Fluid, Research and Clinical Applications. Amsterdam, Excerpta Medica, 1975, p 1018.

Scott J, Renwick M: Antenatal diagnosis of congenital abnormalities in the urinary tract. Br J Urol 1987; 62:295.

Scurry JP, Adamson TM, Cussen LJ: Fetal lung growth in laryngeal atresia and tracheal agenesis. Aust Paediatr 1989; J 25:47.

Seeds JW, Bowes WA: Ultrasound guided fetal intravascular transfusion in severe rhesus immunization. Am J Obstet Gynecol 1986; 154:1195.

Seeds JW, Cefalo RC, Herbert WNP, Bowes WA: Hydramnios and maternal renal failure: Relief with fetal therapy. Obstet Gynecol 1984; 64:265.

Shalev E, Weiner E, Zuckerman H: Prenatal ultrasound diagnosis of intestinal calcifications with imperforate anus. Acta Obstet Gynecol 1983; 65:95.

Sholder AJ, Maizels M, Depp R, et al: Caution in antenatal intervention. J Urol 1988; 139:1026.

Siegel SR, Oh W: Renal function as a marker of human fetal maturation. Acta Paediatr Scand 1976; 65:481.

Skovbo P, Smith-Jensen S: Ultrasound scanning and fetography at polyhydramnios. Acta Obstet Gynecol Scand 1981; 60:51.

Smith FG, Robillard JE: Pathophysiology of fetal renal disease. Semin Perinatol 1989; 13:305.

Steele BT, DeMaria J, Toi A, et al: Neonatal outcome of fetuses with urinary tract abnormalities diagnosed by prenatal ultrasonography. J Can Med Assoc 1987; 137:1171.

Steinhardt GF, Vogler G, Salinas-Madrigal L, et al: Induced renal dysplasia in the young pouch possum. J Pediatr Surg 1988; 23:1127.

Steinhardt GF, Vogler G, Salinas-Madrigal L, et al: Experimental ureteral obstruction in the fetal opossum: Renal functional assessment. J Urol 144 1990; (Part 2):564.

Stephens JD, Sherman S: Determination of fetal sex by ultrasound. N Engl J Med 1983; 309:984.

Thomas DFM, Irving HC, Arthur RJ: Prenatal diagnosis: How useful is it? Br J Urol 1985; 57:784.

Thomas IT, Smith DW: Oligohydramnios, cause of non-renal features of Potter's syndrome, including pulmonary hypoplasia. J Pediatr 1974; 84:811.

Thrall JH, Koff SA, Keyes JW Jr: Diuretic radionuclide renography and scintigraphy in the differential diagnosis of hydronureteronephrosis. Semin Nucl Med 1981; 11:89.

Toma P, Lucigrai C, Dodero P, Lituania M: Prenatal detection of an abdominal mass by MR imaging performed while the fetus is immobilized with pancuronium bromide. AJR 1990; 154:1049.

Townsend RR, Goldstein RB, Filly RA, et al: Sonographic identification of autosomal recessive polycystic kidney disease associated with increased maternal serum/amniotic fluid alpha-fetoprotein. Obstet Gynecol 1988; 72:337.

Vintzileos AM, Nochimson DJ, Walzak MP, et al: Unilateral fetal hydronephrosis: Successful in utero surgical management. Am J Obstet Gynecol 1983; 146:885.

Weiner S, Scharf JL, Bolognese RJ, Librizzi RJ: Antenatal diagnosis and treatment of fetal goiter. J Reprod Med 1980; 24:39.

Whitaker RH: The Whitaker test. Urol Clin North Am 1979; 6:529.

Whitfield HN, Britton KE, Hendry WF, et al: The distinction between obstructive uropathy and nephropathy by radioisotope transit times. J Urol 1978; 50:433.

Wigglesworth JS, Desai R, Guerrini P: Fetal lung hypoplasia: Biochemical and structural variations and their possible significance. Arch Dis Child 1981; 56:606.

Wilkins IA, Chitkara V, Lynch L, et al: The nonpredictive value of fetal urinary electrolytes. Preliminary report of outcomes and correlations with pathologic diagnosis. Am J Obstet Gynecol 1987; 157:694.

Winters WD, Lebowitz RL: Importance of prenatal detection of hydronephrosis of the upper pole. AJR 1990; 155:125.

Woodbury PW, Mitchell ME, Scheidler DM, et al: Constant pressure perfusion: A method to determine obstruction in the upper urinary tract. J Urol 1989; 142:632.

Zedric SA, Duckett JW, Synder HM, et al: Ontogeny of bladder compliance. Neurourol Urodynamics 1990; 9:595.

Zerin JM, Ritchey ML, Chang AC: Incidental vesicoureteral reflux in neonates with antenatally detected hydronephrosis and other renal abnormalities. Radiology 1993; 187:157.

Zerres K, Hansmann M, Mallmann R, Gembruch V: Autosomal recessive polycystic kidney disease: Problems of prenatal diagnosis. Prenat Diag 1988; 8:215.

53
EVALUATION OF THE PEDIATRIC UROLOGIC PATIENT

R. Dixon Walker III, M.D.

One of the strengths of pediatric urology as a subspecialty is that it has a balance between surgical and medical disciplines. The opportunity for diagnosis by history, physical examination, and subsequent radiologic study is still one of the most satisfying in medical practice. An example is the occurrence of observing a schoolgirl who has suffered from incontinence all of her life and is unresponsive to pharmacologic therapy. With a few key questions and a careful examination of the external genitalia, the diagnosis of ectopic ureter is entertained. The diagnosis is then confirmed with a radiologic study and cured by subsequent surgery. Although prenatal ultrasound (US) examination has stolen much of the anticipation of diagnosis from us, much still remains. For the purpose of this chapter, the general approach to diagnosis is divided among problems that present in the neonate, child, and adolescent. There is, of necessity, some overlap with those chapters that deal with more specific problems.

NEONATAL EVALUATION

Consultation with the urologist to the newborn nursery or neonatal intensive care unit requires keen diagnostic skills and cooperation with the pediatrician or neonatalogists so that the best interest of the neonate is determined. **Most often, there is one of three decisions to be made: Is the problem life-threatening or of sufficient magnitude that it requires urgent or emergent evaluation in a tertiary care center? Is the problem one that requires an evaluation that can be performed at the primary or secondary level? Or is the problem one that represents normal or delayed development or an abnormality for which a delay in evaluation and management will be of no consequence?**

After birth, the pediatrician classifies the baby into one of three categories. The normal full-term infant is one with a birth weight of greater than 2500 g and greater than 38 weeks' gestation who is relatively normal on examination. The low-birth-weight infant is one that weighs less than 2500 g and is less than 38 weeks' gestation. The high risk infant is one of exceptionally low birth weight or one that has other abnormalities that place the infant at high risk of mortality (Harper and Yoon, 1987).

A number of levels of concern may be raised by the obstetrician, pediatrician, or nurse. Obstetric problems may include those related to abnormal birth or cesarean section. Breech presentation may be associated with spinal cord injury that results in urinary retention. It may also result in intraperitoneal trauma, including contusion of the kidney manifested by hematuria. Aggressive cesarean section can occasionally result in accidental incision of the abdomen or genitalia.

Calls from the nursery usually center around one of four problems: evaluation of a baby known to have hydronephrosis on prenatal US examination, problems with voiding, abdominal mass, or abnormal genitalia. Although the evaluation and management of each of these problems is covered by other chapters, an overview of evaluation by history and physical examination of problems with voiding, abdominal mass, and abnormalities of the external genitalia are included here. Prenatal hydronephrosis is not covered because the postnatal evaluation predominantly involves radiologic examination.

Many neonates have systemic dysmorphic features, and the urologist may be asked what syndromes are likely to be associated with the genitourinary pathology that is presented. Tables 53–1 and 53–2 list a number of anomalies that might be seen in the newborn or in children. The list is not meant to be exhaustive or complete but rather to introduce the concept of the more common chromosomal, genetic, or nongenetic syndromes. Those who require more detail are directed to the recent reviews by Barakat and colleagues (1986), Walker (1987), and Mininberg (1992).

Genitourinary Examination of the Newborn

The neonate will have already been given a general physical examination by the pediatrician or neonatologist, and the examination by the urologist should focus on the genitouri-

Table 53–1. SYNDROMES ASSOCIATED WITH MULTISYSTEMIC DISEASE

Syndrome	Inheritance	Renal Anomaly	Genital Anomaly	Anomalies in Other Systems
Aarskog-Scott			Shawl scrotum, cryptorchidism	Broad facies, short stature
Beckwith-Wiedemann		Wilms' tumor		Macroglossia, gigantism, hepatoblastoma
Carpenter	AR		Small genitalia	Acrocephaly, polydactyly
Caudal regression		Hydronephrosis, renal agenesis	Vaginal and uterine agenesis	Imperforate anus, LS spine abnormality
Cerebro-oculo-facial	AR	Renal agenesis	Cryptorchidism	Arthrogryposis, microcephaly, cataracts
CHARGE			Small genitalia	Coloboma, heart defects, ear anomalies
Cornelia de Lange			Small genitalia, cryptorchidism	Micromelia, bushy eyebrows
Curran		Renal agenesis		Acral anomalies
Donohue			Enlarged penis or clitoris	Hirsutism, elfin face, thick lips, low-set ears
Drash		Wilms' tumor, glomerulonephritis	Mixed gonadal dysgenesis	
Dubowitz	AR		Hypospadias, cryptorchidism	Eczema, small stature, peculiar facies
Ehlers-Danlos	AR	Hydroureter		Skin hyperextensibility, poor wound healing
Fraser			Hypospadias, cryptorchidism	Cryptophthalmos
G			Hypospadias	Esophageal defect, low-set ears, abnormal facies
Holt-Oram		Renal anomalies		Defects of upper limb
Laurence-Moon-Biedl			Small genitalia	Obesity, retinal pigmentation, polydactyly
Marfan	AD	Renal duplication, hydroureter	Cryptorchidism	Aortic aneurysm, arachnodactyly
Mayer-Rokitansky		Renal agenesis	Duplex uterus, vaginal atresia	
Meckel-Gruber	AR	Renal cysts	Ambiguous genitalia, cryptorchidism	Microcephaly, polydactyly
Menkes		Hydronephrosis, reflux	Cryptorchidism	Kinky hair, CNS abnormality
Ochoa		Neurogenic bladder, hydronephrosis	Cryptorchidism	Aortic aneurysm, arachnodactyly
Opitz	AR		Hypospadias, cryptorchidism	Hypertelorism, mental retardation
Prader-Willi			Cryptorchidism	Hypotonia, obesity, mental retardation
Prune-belly		Hydronephrosis	Cryptorchidism	Hypoplastic abdominal muscle
Roberts	AR	Hydroureter	Hypospadias, large penis, cryptorchidism	Hypomelia, growth retardation
Robinow	AD		Small genitalia, cryptorchidism	Flat face, short forearms
Rubenstein-Taybi	AR		Chordee	Hypoplastic maxilla, broad thumbs and toes
Rudiger	AR	Hydroureter	Small penis	Bicornuate uterus, coarse facies, stub nose
Russell-Silver	AR	Nonspecific renal anomalies	Small penis, hypospadias, cryptorchidism	Short stature, café-au-lait spots, skeletal asymmetry
Seckel	AR		Small genitalia, cryptorchidism	Small head, beak nose
Smith-Lemli-Opitz	AR		Hypospadias, cryptorchidism	Pernicious anemia, mental retardation, syndactyly, microcephaly
VATER		Hydronephrosis, renal dysplasia	Hypospadias	Vertebral anomalies, anal atresia, VSD, TE fistula, radial dysplasia
von Hippel–Lindau		Renal cyst, renal tumor		Pancreatic cyst, cerebral tumor, ichthyosis
Wolfram	AR	Hydroureter		Optic atrophy, deafness, diabetes
Zellwegen	AR	Hydroureter	Hypospadias, cryptorchidism	Hypotonia, hepatomegaly

AD, Autosomal dominant; AR, autosomal recessive; CHARGE, coloboma, heart anomaly, choanal atresia, retardation, and genetic and ear anomalies; CNS, central nervous system; LS, lumbosacral; TE fistula, tracheoesophageal; VATER, vertebral, anal atresia, tracheoesophageal, renal; VSD, ventriculoseptal defect.

Data from Barakat AY, Seikaly MG, Perkaloustian VM: Urogenital abnormalities in genetic disease. J Urol 1986; 136:778–785; Walker RD: Familial and genetic urologic disorders in childhood. AUA Update Series 1987; 6:1–6; Mininberg D: The genetic basis of urologic disease. AUA Update Series 1992; 9:218–223.

Table 53–2. CHROMOSOMAL SYNDROMES ASSOCIATED WITH GENITOURINARY ANOMALIES

Chromosome Number	Clinical Features	Renal Anomalies	Genital Anomalies
4 Autosome Wolf-Hirschhorn syndrome 4-P Trisomy 4-Q	Microcephaly Hemangiomas Hypertelorism Cleft lip/palate Low-set ears	Hydronephrosis	Hypospadias Undescended testicle
8 Autosome Trisomy 8	Large, square head Prominent forehead Widely spaced eyes Slender body and limbs	Hydronephrosis Horseshoe kidney Reflux	Hypospadias Undescended testicle
9 Autosome 9-P Trisomy, 9-P tetrasomy 9-P Monosomy	Small cranium Strabismus Large nose Webbed neck	Renal hypoplasia Pancake kidney	Hypospadias Undescended testicle Infantile male genitalia
10 Autosome 10-Q Syndrome 10-P Syndrome	Microcephaly Oval, flat face Miocropthalmia Short neck	Cystic kidney Hydronephrosis	Undescended testicle Small penis
11 Autosome 11-Q Syndrome	High forehead Flat nose Wide glabella Cleft lip/palate		Micropenis
13 Autosome Patau's syndrome Trisomy 13	Microcephaly Hypertelorism Polydactyly Congenital heart disease	Horseshoe kidney Hydronephrosis Cystic kidney	Undescended testicle
15 Autosome Monosomy 15-Q Prader-Willi syndrome	Obesity Hypotonia Retardation		Hypogonadism Cryptorchidism
18 Autosome Trisomy 18 Edwards' syndrome	Micrognathia Hypertonia Congenital heart disease	Horseshoe kidney Hydronephrosis	Undescended testicle Small penis
20 Autosome 20-P Syndrome	Round face Short nose Dental abnormalities Vertebral abnormalities	Hydronephrosis Polycystic kidney	Hypospadias
21 Autosome Trisomy 21 Down's syndrome	Brachycephalic skull Congenital heart disease Nasal hypoplasia Broad, short hands		Undescended testicle Small penis
22 Autosome Trisomy 22	Microcephaly Preauricular skin tags Low-set ears Beaked nose Cleft palate		Undescended testicle Small penis
Cat's eye syndrome Possibly from both 13 and 22 autosomes	Coloboma Anal atresia Low-set ears Hemivertebrae Congenital heart disease	Renal agenesis Horseshoe kidney Reflux	
Sex chromosome Y Klinefelter's syndrome XXY, XXXY XXXXY	Elongated legs Gynecomastia Eunuchoid body build Sparse body hair		Small penis Small testes
Sex chromosome X Turner's syndrome XO	Short stature Primary amenorrhea Webbed neck Broad chest Coarctation of aorta	Horseshoe kidney	Infantile genitalia

Data from Barakat AY, Seikaly MG, Derkaloustian VM: Urogenital anomalies in genetic diseases. J Urol 1986; 136:778–785; Walker RD: Familial and genetic urologic disorders in childhood. AUA Update Series 1987; 6:1–6; Mininberg D: The genetic basis of urologic disease. AUA Update Series 1992; 9:218–223.

nary system. Inspection of the abdomen usually reveals obvious abnormalities such as prune-belly syndrome or one of the exstrophy complexes. Palpation of the abdomen should primarily note the presence of ascites or intra-abdominal masses. The umbilicus should be examined for drainage that might be consistent with a patent urachus or urachal sinus. The lower spine and buttocks should be inspected for a dimple, sinus, or gluteal atrophy. The external genitalia should be thoroughly examined in both male and female neonates, noting the location of the testicles, the presence of scrotal masses, any abnormalities of the male penis or urethra, and any abnormalities of the labia, urethra, or vagina in the female. The location of the anus, as it relates to any abnormality of the genitalia, should be noted.

Abnormalities of Voiding or Urine Production

Although it is true that some normal infants may not void for 72 hours, this situation is unusual and most infants (93%) normally void within 24 hours (Kramer and Sherry, 1957). If the infant has not voided by 24 hours, this factor should raise a question about underlying abnormalities. Table 53–3 gives the normal volumes expected in a term infant within the first 2 weeks of life (Thomson, 1944). **Oliguria is defined as a urine output of less than 1 ml/kg/hour over an extended time.** Urine output in premature infants may reach levels of 3 to 4 ml/kg/hour. Conditions that may lead to oliguria include congenital nephrotic syndrome, renal vein thrombosis, renal artery thrombosis, renal dysplasia, renal agenesis, obstructive uropathy, prune-belly syndrome, sepsis, autosomal recessive polycystic disease, bilateral multicystic renal disease, and hypovolemia. Many patients with these disorders have associated edema or ascites, particularly males with posterior urethral valves. Laboratory evaluation of these infants should include evaluation for renal failure, acidosis, hyponatremia, and hypokalemia, which can best be initially evaluated with serum creatinine and electrolytes. Electrolyte tables for newborns should be consulted because the serum potassium is often elevated in the first 24 to 48 hours of life and serum creatinine most often reflects the renal function of the mother in the first 24 hours of life. Table 53–4 gives normal levels of fetal electrolytes (Acharya et al, 1965). **It is important to distinguish between prerenal and renal causes of oliguria.**

Table 53–3. URINARY VOLUME IN THE FIRST WEEKS OF LIFE

Day	Volume (ml)	Range
1	20	0–68
2	21	0–82
3	36	0–96
4	65	5–180
5	103	1–217
6	125	42–268
7	147	40–302
10	190	106–320
12	227	207–246

Thomson J: Observations on urine of new-born infants. Arch Dis Child 1944; 19:169–177.

Fractional excretion of sodium (FE Na) that is low for the infant's age may be representative of hypovolemia. Urine should be sent for culture and sensitivity. **From the urologic perspective, an abdominal US examination is essential as the first step in diagnosing a correctable urologic disorder.** Important historical information includes evidence of maternal diabetes, large birth weight, and family history of cystic disease or renal anomaly. Association of the oliguria with hematuria is most suggestive of a vascular abnormality such as renal vein or artery thrombosis.

Notation by the nurse of a distended bladder or poor urinary stream warrants immediate evaluation. Often, the diagnosis is clear, such as in a child with myelodysplasia, in whom urine retention is common after back closure, perhaps due to acute spinal shock (Chiaramonte et al, 1986). A distended bladder may be a sign of a neurogenic bladder without a clear neurologic lesion. **Straining to void in males may be associated with posterior urethral valves and requires evaluation at the first suspicion because of the underlying metabolic abnormalities frequently associated with this condition.** Evaluation of the child with a distended bladder or straining to void includes a thorough neurologic examination by the pediatrician and an US examination and voiding cystourethrogram (VCUG) as an initial radiologic screen of the urinary tract. Drainage from the umbilical area in the newborn may indicate an underlying urachal sinus or patent urachus.

Abdominal Mass

Abdominal masses are now frequently diagnosed on prenatal US examination but are still occasionally discovered on the initial examination by the pediatrician. Most often, the cystic or solid nature of the abdominal mass is best characterized by abdominal US examination.

Examination of the abdomen in patients with a mass remains important. On inspection, one can often note disparity in the symmetry of the abdomen. Palpation of the abdomen may distinguish fluid waves consistent with ascites. Abdominal masses are either cystic or solid. Hydronephrosis frequently does not result in a palpable kidney unless it is large. When it is palpated, the hydronephrotic kidney is smooth and nondescript, whereas the multicystic kidney most often is larger than a comparable hydronephrotic kidney and irregular on palpation. **Masses in the suprapubic area are usually related to the distended bladder and, in males, are suggestive of posterior urethral valves.** Females with lower abdominal masses may have hydrometrocolpos with or without associated hydronephrosis. Solid masses in the neonate are rare, and when they occur in the flank, they are most likely renal hamartoma or neuroblastoma. Solid masses in the pelvis may represent pelvic neuroblastoma or presacral teratoma. **Bilateral flank masses are more often associated with renal insufficiency and can be seen in posterior urethral valves, renal vein thrombosis, or autosomal recessive cystic disease.** When one looks at unexpected renal anomalies diagnosed initially by examination of the neonate, the most common are horseshoe or pelvic kidney, hydronephrosis, and multicystic kidney (Perlman and Williams, 1976).

Table 53–4. SERUM CHEMISTRIES IN TERM INFANTS

Determination	Cord	1–12 Hours	12–24 Hours	24–48 Hours	48–72 Hours
Sodium, mEq/L	147 (126–166)	143 (124–156)	145 (132–159)	148 (134–160)	149 (139–162)
Potassium, mEq/L	7.8 (5.6–12)	6.3 (5.3–7.3)	6.3 (5.3–8.9)	6.0 (5.2–7.3)	5.9 (5.0–7.7)
Chloride, mEq/L	103 (98–110)	100.7 (90–111)	103 (87–114)	102 (92–114)	103 (92–112)

From Acharya PT, Payne WW: Blood chemistry of normal full-term infants in first 48 hours of life. Arch Dis Child 1965; 40:430–435.

Abnormal Genitalia

The range of abnormalities of the external genitalia is discussed in detail in Chapter 69 and is minimally discussed in this chapter. One of the problems often faced is assessing penile size in premature or low-birth-weight neonates. There are several nomograms for measuring newborn penile length. Those by Feldman and Smith (1975) have the advantage of not only setting standards for length but also diameter in premature and full-term infants (Figs. 53–1 and 53–2). **The important determination in a genetic male is whether the phallus is of sufficient length so that the child can be raised as a male. Male infants outside of two standard deviations may be better served with gender reassignment, particularly if the phallus does not respond to androgenic stimulation.** Even if there is a response, there is both clinical and experimental evidence that many of these patients have inadequate penile size as adults. Also, in the male child, the newborn period is an excellent time to examine the testicles because retractile testicles occur less frequently. Caesar and colleagues (1994) have found that some neonates have a cremasteric reflex, but this is still the best time to examine the patient for an undescended testicle. **Undescended testicle is noted in up to 20% of premature males and 3% of full-term males. Of the latter, 1% to 2% of those that are palpable in the groin descend by 3 months of age** (Scorer et al, 1971). Hydrocele is common in newborn males and resolves in most cases by 3 to 6 months of age. Inguinal masses in both males and females may indicate indirect inguinal hernia. **For the female neonate with normal karyotype and a large clitoris or ambiguous genitalia, the most important diagnosis to substantiate is whether the patient has adrenogenital syndrome. Because of the emergent nature of the salt-losing problem associated with this condition, these patients require expeditious evaluation, as outlined in Chapter 70.** Many abnormalities of the genitalia are associated with anomalies in other organ systems, as shown in Tables 53–1 and 53–2.

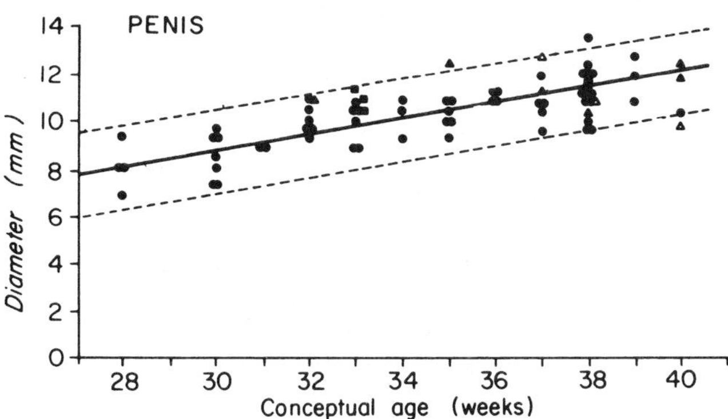

Figure 53–1. Penile diameter in premature and full-term infants. ● Normal premature or full-term infant; ▲ large-for-gestation infant; ■ a twin. (From Feldman KW, Smith DW: Fetal phallic growth and penile standards for newborn male infants. J Pediatr 1975; 86:395–398.)

PRESENTATION OF GENITOURINARY PROBLEMS IN CHILDHOOD

Children are able to present reasonably accurate histories if they are approached with patience and understanding. Parents are also helpful in that they can interpret what their children are saying and can organize their children's complaints. Each family has its own "child language." This language may include childhood neologisms that would not ordinarily be interpretable by the physician. The most common complaints related to the urinary tract that are voiced by the child are either abdominal pain or irritative voiding symptoms. The parents usually provide information on incontinence, fever, hematuria, or abdominal mass. Thus, these presenting symptoms can be roughly placed into four categories: pain, fever, voiding dysfunction, and abdominal mass.

Genitourinary Examination of the Child

The urologic examination of the child should involve having the vital signs taken by the nurse, following which the urologist should perform a thorough examination of the abdomen, back, and buttocks. Physical examination should be performed with the child lying quietly and accompanied by the parent. The child can help by pointing out the area

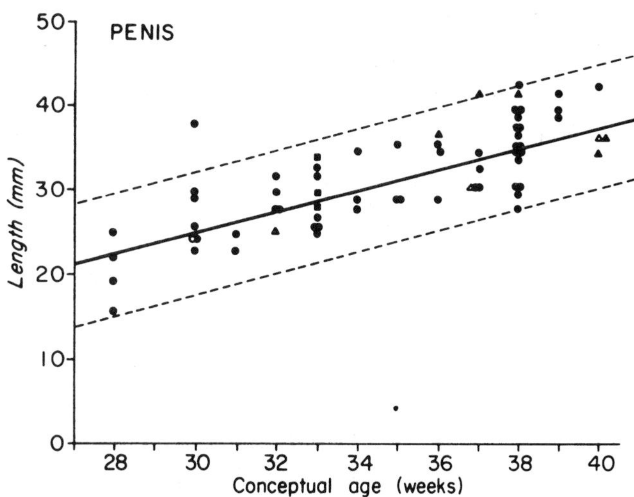

Figure 53–2. Penile length in premature and full-term infants. ● Normal premature or full-term infant; ▲ large-for-gestation infant; ■ a twin. (From Feldman KW, Smith DW: Fetal phallic growth and penile standards for newborn male infants. J Pediatr 1975; 86:395–398.)

of concern. Gentle palpation may elicit tenderness or an abdominal mass. The back and buttocks should be examined for a spinal dimple, sinus, or gluteal atrophy.

The male genitalia should be inspected and palpated. Examination of the genitalia in a female is more delicate, and in most instances, examination by inspection is sufficient. This can be done by having the child placed in a frog-leg position and spreading the labia either by the mother or the child. **Any palpation of the female genitalia should be preceded by a thorough explanation to both parents and child, and gloves should be used.** Most abnormalities of the female genitalia can be noted on inspection. The male genitalia should be inspected and palpated, with notation made of the position of the testicles, evidence of scrotal masses, urethral or penile abnormality, or phimosis.

Pain

In the pediatric urologic literature, pain is most often characterized by its location. From the standpoint of the child and his or her parents, pain is usually abdominal or relates to voiding. Abdominal pain is a common complaint of children and is often nonspecific as to location or degree. Indeed, a great deal of abdominal pain in children does not have a specific etiology and is self-limited. On the other hand, severe abnormalities may be associated with minimal pain. The dilemma for the urologist is to what extent the etiology of the pain should be explored to arrive at an accurate diagnosis. Pain that is severe enough that the child misses school or does not participate in physical activity is significant. Pain associated with systemic symptoms of nausea, anorexia, or fever has a high correlation with underlying disease. Minimal pain, however, may also be associated with severe abnormalities. Thus, all children with abdominal pain need screening to assess the urinary tract. Physical examination may elicit tenderness but is not often helpful in identifying abdominal masses unless the mass is large. **The two principal questions that one must ask in regard to abdominal pain are as follows: Is the pain associated with a congenital or acquired abnormality of the urinary tract? Is the pain associated with urinary tract infection (UTI)?** The best screening test to answer the first question is the abdominal US examination. This test suggests to the urologist whether the patient has an obstructive uropathy, stone, or abdominal mass. **US examination is most insensitive in diagnosing vesicoureteral reflux (VUR), even of high grade.** Urinalysis and urine culture answer the question as to whether there is associated infection or other abnormality in the urine such as microscopic hematuria. Urine can most often be obtained with a midstream clean-catch technique. Catheterization should be reserved for specific indications, such as with a contaminated specimen in a child with suspected pyelonephritis. I prefer to use an unspun specimen for microscopic examination, and notation should be made of bacteria, leukocytes, red blood cells, or casts. All urinalyses with bacteria should be sent for specific culture and sensitivity. Dipstick gives added information about proteinuria and confirms bacteriuria, leukocyturia, and hematuria. The abdominal US examination and urinalysis screen most patients who have underlying abnormalities. **In a review of children whom I have seen with abdominal pain, the only consistent diagnosis that is missed with a normal US examination and urinalysis is VUR.** In most instances, there is a past history of UTI that would have warranted a VCUG that, in turn, would have established the diagnosis. Because of this failure of US examination to diagnose VUR, children with persistent abdominal pain who have no ready explanation for an anomaly in another organ system should have a VCUG to rule out VUR.

Pain with voiding can be categorized by that which is associated with or without UTI. The child may indicate that the pain is associated with irritative voiding symptoms, such as urgency or frequency. The pain may be described as spasmodic or cramping. Urethral dysuria may be associated with initial hematuria or blood spotting found on the child's underwear. Girls may have dysuria because of vaginitis. Physical examination may demonstrate suprapubic or urethral tenderness. In girls, examination may show evidence of vaginitis, labial adhesions, or even sexual abuse. Sexual abuse is of sufficient importance that it will be discussed separately under adolescent problems. Many times, the examination is unrewarding. The two tests that again have the highest yield as a screen are the urinalysis and abdominal US examination. The urine should be examined for evidence of infection or hematuria. Abdominal US examination can diagnose a variety of abnormalities, including bladder stone, foreign body, ureterocele, tumor, or inflammation. VCUG is indicated when urethral pathology is suspected.

Fever

Fever is a common presentation of disease in children. About 1% of children with fever have a UTI (McCarthy, 1988). Fever is a response to a stimulus, usually bacteria or virus, in which pyrogens, released from leukocytes, act through a prostaglandin mediator acting on the thermoregulatory center to increase the temperature from its normal base of 37°C. A high fever may have a role in protecting the body against organisms but also can be deleterious, particularly at high degrees. What constitutes a significant fever is not known, but a temperature greater than 38°C is probably significant. Fever is one of the most important presenting urologic signs because it is so often related to renal pathology. Fever is a sequela of infection. Rarely, there are non-infectious causes of fever, such as necrosis in Wilms' tumor, but these instances are rare. Fever is more commonly related to a complicated rather than an uncomplicated UTI. **A complicated UTI can be defined as one in which, on further diagnostic evaluation, an anomaly is found that places the patient at greater risk of pyelonephritis. In children, most of these anomalies are congenital, and in the series by Smellie and associates (1981), 50% of children with UTI had an underlying abnormality. It is uncommon for children who have a normal urinary tract to have high fever.** The relationship between fever and VUR, the most common congenital abnormality, was evaluated by Woodard and Holden (1976), who found that 90% of children with VUR presented with fever greater than 38.5°C, whereas only 40% of those without VUR had fever of the same magnitude. In a similar study, Levitt and co-workers (1977) found a high incidence of VUR, ureterocele, and obstruction in children with fever. Govan and Palmer (1969) found that 79% of patients with VUR presented with a clinical diagnosis of acute pyelonephritis and fever, whereas 39% of patients without reflux had the same presentation.

Voiding Dysfunction

Children with voiding dysfunction may present with irritative voiding symptoms, obstructive symptoms, incontinence, or hematuria.

Irritative voiding symptoms, such as dysuria, urgency, or frequency, can be multifactorial. Urinalysis and culture rule out UTI, and an US examination of the bladder is appropriate to rule out bladder stone, foreign body, and tumor. These latter causes are not common, and many children with irritative voiding symptoms that are not associated with incontinence have a negative evaluation. **Extraordinary urinary frequency is one of these presentations and has been described by Zoubek and colleagues (1990). These patients are predominately male with a mean age of 5 to 6 years who present with frequency averaging every 30 minutes. After ruling out more serious pathology with urinalysis and US examination, the patients can be treated by reassurance to the parents or with low doses of anticholinergic therapy, although Koff and Byard (1988) did not find this useful. The symptoms are self-limiting, and cystoscopy is contraindicated.** Another group of children who may present with irritative voiding symptoms are girls with vulvovaginitis with or without labial adhesions. Often, the girls are obese, and the vaginitis may be ammoniacal and related to vaginal trapping of urine. Frequently, they may complain of leakage, although they do not have true incontinence. Treatment revolves around allowing for vaginal emptying after voiding, either by having the child face backward on the toilet (which forces the legs apart) or by spreading the legs while facing forward. The ammoniacal dermatitis can be treated with over-the-counter creams used for diaper rash. **Labial adhesions are a common problem. Those that are asymptomatic are self-limited in nature and should be left alone.** Initial treatment of symptomatic patients should be the manual spreading of the labia and application of vitamin A and D ointment by the mother. For adhesions that persist, the use of estrogen creams is helpful, but application should not be continued for more than 2 to 3 weeks. For those who are unresponsive to estrogen cream management and are symptomatic, I recommend lysis of the adhesions under general anesthesia with resection of a thin strip of skin on each side of the labia minora and re-approximation with fine chromic catgut. Postoperatively, the patient is treated daily with antibiotic ointment for 1 week and then vitamin A and D ointment for 1 month. Surgery has been required in less than 5% of patients with labial adhesions but has been successful in resolving the problem in the majority of cases.

Patients who present with obstructive symptoms such as straining to void or retention are likely to have an anatomic reason for their symptoms. Most often obstructive symptoms occur in males, and the diagnosis is established by US examination, VCUG, urodynamic study, and cystoscopy. Diagnoses that should be ruled out include posterior and anterior urethral valves, stricture, urethral sphincter dyssynergia, foreign body or stone, or urethral polyp. Urinary retention is less common in patients with obstruction, and when it does occur, it does so more often with trauma either from stone, foreign body, or in relation to clean intermittent catheterization. **Urinary retention also may be the first presentation for patients with spinal cord tethering or lipoma.** Occasionally, urinary retention may occur in patients who are lazy voiders. Most often these patients are girls who are embarrassed to void at school. Initial therapy is directed at timed voiding, with clean intermittent catheterization (CIC) being used for those who do not respond. Patients with this problem can be returned to normal with retraining.

Incontinence and Hematuria

These two topics are thoroughly covered in Chapters 56, 65, and 66 and are not covered here.

PRESENTATION OF GENITOURINARY PROBLEMS IN ADOLESCENCE

Adolescence is that period of rapid physical, mental, and emotional growth that occurs in the second decade of life. There are many misconceptions by the public regarding adolescence that are important for the physician to resolve in dealing with the patient and his or her parents. Extensive studies have been conducted in normal adolescents, and these studies largely find that tumultuous and disruptive behavior is actually abnormal (Weiner, 1992). For most adolescents, this is a period of adaptation to their parents, friends, the opposite sex, and their surroundings. For the most part, adaptation is achieved by increments rather than through bursts of change. Many of these changes are physical, including the growth spurt as well as sexual maturation. **Some of the emotional changes may be hormonally directed, particularly the more aggressive behavior in males, which appears to be androgen mediated (Susman and Petersen, 1992).** Children with chronic problems who were cared for by their parents now begin facing life with their chronic disease. **The most common chronic condition likely to be seen by the urologists is spina bifida (Blum and Geber, 1992). It is estimated that there are about 11,000 adolescents with spina bifida in the United States.** It is at this age that the patients become concerned about body image, and the desire to become continent leads many of them to request surgery, such as augmentation cystoplasty or undiversion. Patients with spina bifida also become concerned about their sexuality. **Woodhouse (1994) and Bomalski and Teague (1995) have both indicated that satisfactory sexual function can be achieved in a high number of these patients.** End-stage renal failure is also a common chronic disease of adolescence that the urologist may encounter. Patients whose kidneys carried them through childhood may now require transplantation surgery.

Another problem that the urologist may encounter is the mentally impaired child approaching adolescence. These adolescents will require continued self-care and have minimal capacity to be self-sufficient. Diagnoses that may have urologic conditions associated with mental impairment in adolescents include Down's syndrome, Williams' syndrome,

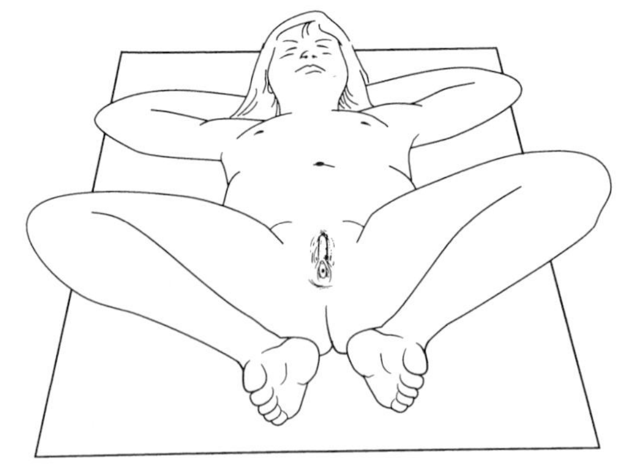

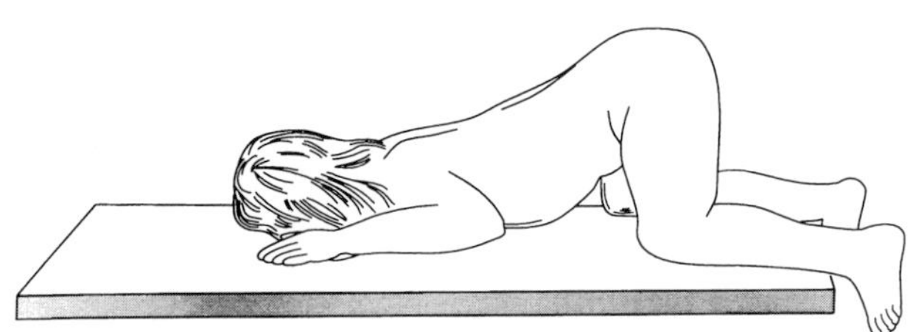

Figure 53–3. Frog-leg position *(top)* and knee-chest position *(bottom).*

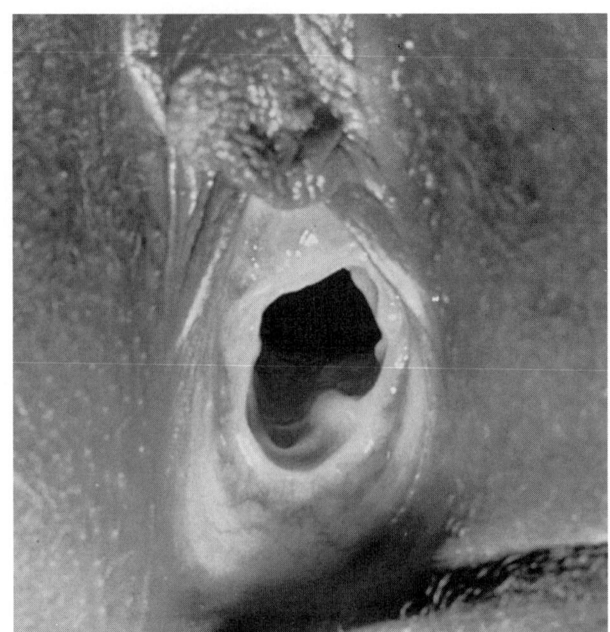

Figure 53–5. Hymen in abused patient showing vaginal dilation.

Prader-Willi syndrome, and some cases of spina bifida and cerebral palsy. The potential for sexual activity in the mentally retarded adolescent needs to be discussed honestly with the parents. **A major problem in this age group is the refractory nature of pharmacologic therapy in the management of incontinence.** An additional problem that the urologist may be asked to face is reconstructive surgery and its role in patient care. Reconstructive surgery that preserves renal function, decreases a risk factor, decreases the number of UTIs, or improves the quality of life for the patient is indicated. Reconstructive surgery that is cosmetic or performed to enhance fertility has to be individualized based on the anticipated goals of the patient.

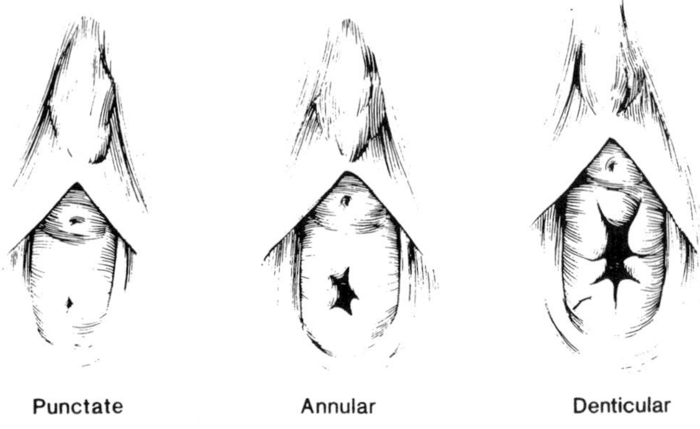

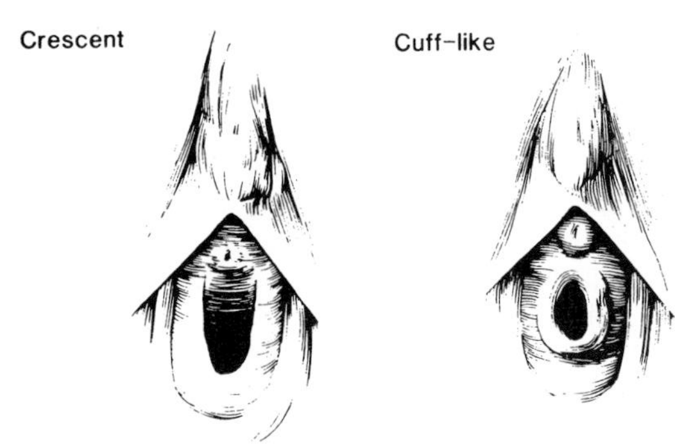

Figure 53–4. Normal hymenal configurations in older children and adolescents. (From Herman-Giddens ME, Frothingham TE: Prepubertal female genitalia: Examination for evidence of sexual abuse. Reproduced by permission of Pediatrics, vol 80, pages 203–208, copyright 1987.)

Another problem that the physician faces in dealing with the adolescent is compliance. In childhood, compliance is dependent on the parent and, despite their diligence, is often poor. In the United States arm of the International Reflux Study, 9% of the patients were lost to follow-up within 5 years (Weiss et al, 1992). Noncompliance often increases in adolescents when the patient begins to take responsibility for taking medication. Methods of assessing noncompliance can be expensive and tedious. **Noncompliance can be in a variety of forms; from failure to take antibacterial therapy, which may affect the patient minimally, to failure to use CIC, which may result in spontaneous perforation and death in a patient with an augmented bladder. Noncompliance in the pediatric urology patient is usually omission of an activity because it interferes with one's time (CIC, timed voiding) or failure to take medication because of side effects that are unacceptable to the patient (such as with steroids for the patient with renal transplant).** Compliance is important, and this factor needs to be established with the patient by making him or her part of the decision-making process and allowing the patient to feel that the system is responsive to his or her needs.

Urologic Aspects of Sexual Abuse

Sexual abuse can occur in any age group, and its inclusion in the adolescent age group is simply because most of the patients present in late childhood or adolescence. **Sexual abuse is defined as any activity with a child for which an individual receives sexual gratification. This may include fondling, exhibitionism, pornography, or intercourse.** United States statutes require physicians to report suspected cases of sexual abuse to appropriate state agencies. **Urologists should suspect sexual abuse in a variety of situations. Four common presentations have been noted: (1) The caretaker may indicate to the physician that there has been sexual abuse. (2) The child may have a complaint directly related to sexual abuse, such as a vaginal discharge or evidence of venereal disease. (3) The child may have a complaint that is not directly related to sexual abuse. Ellsworth and co-workers (1995) have found 18 patients with refractory voiding dysfunction who had evidence of sexual abuse. (4) The child may have no complaints, but evidence of abuse is found on routine examination.** Most often, the urologist is not the most appropriate person to pursue the evaluation of sexual abuse but may need to pursue the presenting complaint. Thus, it is important that the individual be familiar with the normal physical examination of the female genitalia and abnormalities that are consistent with abuse or that are confused with sexual abuse. Examination of the female genitalia is best performed with the patient in the frog-leg position for young children or the knee-chest position for older children (Fig. 53–3). The knee-chest position has the advantage of allowing the hymen to separate with minimal touching. Normal hymenal configurations described by Herman-Giddens and Frothingham are shown in Figure 53–4. **Suspicion of sexual abuse should be considered when the vaginal mucosa is bruised or injected, the vaginal opening is dilated to greater than 3 mm in an infant to a 7-year-old child or 4 mm in a 7- to 13-year-old child, or the hymen is damaged, showing a V notch or cleft** (Fig. 53–5).

Stress Hematuria

Stress hematuria is an infrequent but perplexing problem in the older adolescent or young adult. It is more common in young men but can be seen in either sex. Microscopic

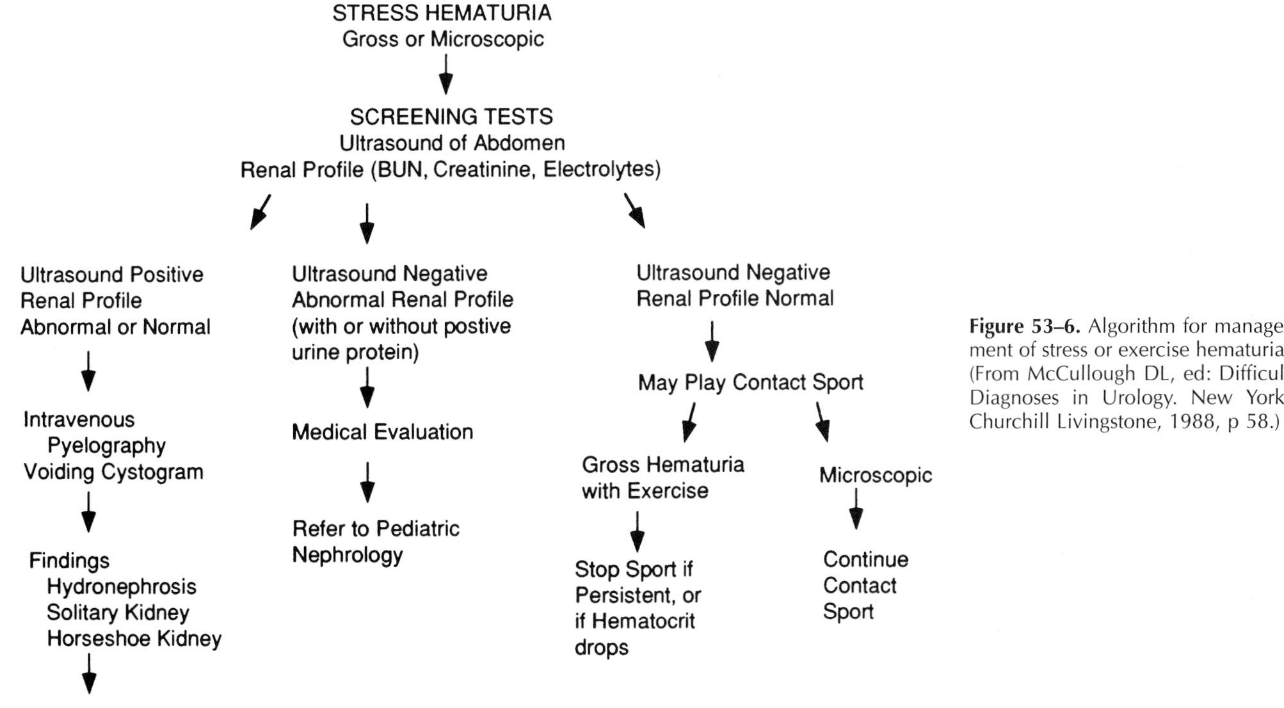

Figure 53–6. Algorithm for management of stress or exercise hematuria. (From McCullough DL, ed: Difficult Diagnoses in Urology. New York, Churchill Livingstone, 1988, p 58.)

Table 53–5. UNSTRETCHED PENIS AND TESTIS SIZE DURING ADOLESCENCE

Age (Years)	Penis Length (cm)	Testis Length (cm)
8–10	4.2 ± 0.8	2.0 ± 0.5
10–12	5.2 ± 1.3	2.7 ± 0.7
12–14	6.2 ± 2.0	3.4 ± 0.8
14–16	8.6 ± 2.4	4.1 ± 1.0

Adapted from Winter JSD, Faiman C: Pituitary-gonadal relations in male children and adolescents. Pediatr Res 1972; 6:126–135.

hematuria is commonly associated with contact sports, particularly hockey and football (Abarbanel et al, 1990). It can be associated with casts and proteinuria and thus resemble a nephritic pattern. Gross hematuria is also common in runners. **In most instances, the student athlete does not have to cease participation in sports.** Figure 53–6 indicates the evaluation of the young person with stress hematuria.

Concerns About Genitalia

In addition to the abnormalities of childhood, such as epispadias or hypospadias, that will persist into adolescence, many boys are concerned about the appearance of their penis. The concealed or buried penis is most often seen in the obese adolescent, and little can be done to improve this situation other that the difficult task of losing weight. Operations for the buried penis that might be performed in early childhood are less successful in this group. Most often, the penis is normal with erection. Boys who are concerned about penile size should be compared with nomograms, such as that shown in Table 53–5, and reassured that it is natural for boys to have a wide range in size.

ACKNOWLEDGMENT

The author wishes to acknowledge the assistance of Dr. Pamela Ellsworth for allowing me to use her material on sexual abuse, and William Tucker for drawing Figure 53–3.

REFERENCES

Neonate

Acharya PT, Payne WW: Blood chemistry of normal full-term infants in first 48 hours of life. Arch Dis Child 1965; 40:430–435.

Barakat AY, Seikaly MG, Der Kaloustian VM: Urogenital abnormalities in genetic disease. J Urol 1986; 136:778–785.

Caesar RE, Kaplan GW: The incidence of the cremasteric reflex in normal boys. J Urol 1994; 152:779–780.

Chiaramonte RM, Horowitz EM, Kaplan GA: Implications of hydronephrosis in newborns with myelodysplasia. J Urol 1986; 136:427–429.

Feldman KW, Smith DW: Fetal phallic growth and penile standards for newborn male infants. J Pediatr 1975; 86:395–398.

Harper RG, Yoon JJ: Transportation of the infant from the delivery room. *In* Harper RG, Yoon JJ, eds: Handbook of Neonatology. Chicago, Year Book Medical Publishers Inc, 1987, pp 40–45.

Kramer I, Sherry SN: The time of passage of the first stool and urine by the premature infant. J Pediatr 1957; 51:373–376.

Mininberg D: The genetic basis of urologic disease. AUA Update Series 1992; 9:218–223.

Perlman M, Williams J: Detection of renal anomalies by abdominal palpation in newborn infants. BMJ 1976; 2:347–349.

Thomson J: Observations on urine of new-born infants. Arch Dis Child 1944; 19:169–177.

Walker, R.D. Familial and genetic urologic disorders in childhood. AUA Update Series 1987; 6:1–6.

Child

Govan DE, Palmer JM: Urinary tract infection in children. The influence of successful anti-reflux operations on morbidity from infection. Pediatrics 1969; 44:677–684.

Koff SA, Byard MA: The daytime urinary frequency syndrome of childhood. J Urol 1988; 140:1280–1281.

Levitt SB, Bekirov HM, Kogan SJ: Proposed selective approach to radiographic evaluation of children with urinary tract infections. *In* Bergsma D, Duckett JW, eds: Urinary System Malformations in Children. New York, Alan R. Liss, Inc., 1977, pp 433–438.

McCarthy PL: Acute infectious illnesses in children. Compr Ther 1988; 14:51–53.

Scorer GC, Farrington GH: Congenital Abnormalities of the Testicle and Epididymis. Butterworth, London, 1971.

Smellie JM, Normand ICD, Katz G: Children with urinary tract infection: A comparison of those with and those without vesicoureteral reflux. Kidney Int 1981; 20:717–722.

Woodard JR, Holden S: The prognostic significance of fever in childhood urinary infections. Clin Pediatr 1976; 15:1051–1054.

Zoubek J, Bloom DA, Sedman AB: Extraordinary urinary frequency. Pediatrics 1990; 85:1112–1114.

Adolescent

Abarbanel J, Benet AE, Lask D, Kimche D: Sports hematuria. J Urol 1990; 143:887–890.

Blum RW, Geber G: Chronically ill youth. *In* McAnarney ER, Kreipe RE, Orr DP, Comerci GD, eds: Textbook of Adolescent Medicine. Philadelphia, W. B. Saunders Company, 1992, pp 222–228.

Bomalski MD, Teagie JL: The long-term impact of urologic management on the quality of life in children with spina bifida. J Urol 1995; 154:778–781.

Ellsworth PI, Mergurian PM, Copenig M: Sexual abuse: Another causative factor in dysfunctional voiding. J Urol 1995; 153:773–776.

Herman-Giddens ME, Frothingham TE: Prepubertal female genitalia: Examination for evidence of sexual abuse. Pediatrics 1987; 80:203–208.

Susman EJ, Petersen AC: Hormones and behavior. *In* McAnarney ER, Kreipe RE, Orr DP, Comerci GD, eds: Textbook of Adolescent Medicine. Philadelphia, W.B. Saunders Company, 1992, pp 125–130.

Weiner IB: Normality during adolescence. *In* McAnarney ER, Kreipe RE, Orr DP, Comerci GD, eds: Textbook of Adolescent Medicine. Philadelphia, W. B. Saunders Company, 1992, pp 86–91.

Weiss R, Duckett J, Spitzer A: Results of a randomized clinical trial of medical versus surgical management of infants and children with Grade III and IV primary vesicoureteral reflux (United States). J Urol 1992; 148:1667–1673.

Winter JSD, Faiman C: Pituitary-gonadal relations in male children and adolescents. Pediatr Res 1972; 6:126–135.

Woodhouse CRJ: The sexual and reproductive consequences of congenital genitourinary anomalies. J Urol 1994; 152:645–651.

54 NEONATAL UROLOGIC EMERGENCIES

David A. Diamond, M.D.
Rafael Gosalbez, M.D.

Neonatal urologic emergencies are those conditions involving the newborn genitourinary system that warrant urgent consultation within the first month of life. During the past decade, this area of urology has changed considerably, owing in large part to three factors. Perhaps the most important has been the advent of prenatal diagnosis, which has enabled us to anticipate urgent problems, such as posterior urethral valves, which can be treated promptly, thereby avoiding the morbidity of delayed diagnosis. A second important factor has been the evolution of neonatal diagnostic imaging, in particular real-time sonography, and nuclear medicine studies. These methods have enabled us, for example, to accurately diagnose the multicystic dysplastic kidney (MCDK) and avoid diagnostic exploration. Third, the ever-increasing capabilities of neonatal intensive care units (NICUs) to sustain premature infants have, as a by-product of their success, produced new types of neonatal urologic emergencies such as neonatal nephrolithiasis.

The purpose of this chapter is to provide the urologist with the fundamental information necessary to provide expert consultation on the major neonatal urologic emergencies.

PRENATAL UROLOGIC ASSESSMENT

Consultation Regarding the Prenatal Diagnosis of Hydronephrosis

A prenatal diagnosis of fetal hydronephrosis is made on one of 500 routine maternal ultrasound examinations (Helin and Persson, 1986; Thomas, 1990). Thus, it is not surprising that this condition has become the most common cause for urologic consultation in the perinatal period.

Ideally, the urologist is consulted soon after the diagnosis of prenatal hydronephrosis is confirmed, thus enabling him or her to counsel the parents as well as the involved physicians. Current diagnostic capabilities allow hydronephrosis to be detected as early as 13 to 14 weeks of gestation (Mahoney et al, 1984). On review of the fetal ultrasound study, certain essential questions should be answered that help determine the emergent nature of the problem at or prior to delivery (Lebowitz and Teele, 1983). It is important to establish the gestational age and sex of the fetus, and the presence of other anomalies. At what gestational age was hydronephrosis diagnosed? Is the hydronephrosis unilateral or bilateral? If it is unilateral, is the other kidney normal? If it is bilateral, are ureters seen? Does the renal parenchyma appear normal or dysplastic with evidence of cortical cysts or increased echogenicity? Does the bladder appear normal, and does it seem to empty? Is a ureterocele present? Perhaps most important, are amniotic fluid levels normal? One series revealing the postnatal findings among 110 neonates with prenatal hydronephrosis is representative of the diagnostic possibilities (Table 54–1).

In two series, postnatal evaluation demonstrated that vesicoureteral reflux occurs in 30% to 40% of patients (Zerin et al, 1993; Marra et al, 1994). Unless one is confronted with the exceedingly rare situation of bilateral hydroureteronephrosis with progressive oligohydramnios, in which case fetal intervention might be contemplated, the urologist is typically uninvolved until the baby is delivered. The majority of cases of hydronephrosis detected prenatally resolve before the end of the pregnancy or within the first year of life (Mandell et al, 1991). Reassuring and advising the parents of the diagnostic possibilities and the orderly sequence of postnatal studies is of great value.

The standard recommendation for a newborn with a diagnosis of prenatal hydronephrosis includes a careful newborn examination and observation of voiding, a postnatal ultrasound after 48 hours of life, and placement of the baby on antibiotic prophylaxis (preferably penicillin G, 20,000 IU/kg or amoxicillin, 10 mg/kg/24 hours) (Laing et al, 1984; Blyth et al, 1993). It is hoped that this approach will minimize the risk of severe urinary tract infection in infancy, which in one study of infants with prenatal hydronephrosis was a minimum of 3% within the first 6 months of life (Daucher et al, 1992). In the setting of unilateral hydronephrosis confirmed postnatally, a voiding cystourethrogram (VCUG) and upper tract imaging study (^{99m}Tc-DTPA or ^{99m}Tc-MAG III renal scan or intravenous pyelogram [IVP]) may be scheduled at 1 month to allow the kidneys to mature (Fig. 54–1). If, however, there is a suggestion of bladder outlet obstruction due to posterior urethral valves, an ectopic ureterocele, or a neuropathic bladder, a VCUG should be performed within the first few days of life. Similarly, a suggestion of high-grade obstruction in a solitary system warrants immediate upper tract imaging.

Rarely does the diagnosis of prenatal hydronephrosis in a newborn represent a true neonatal urologic emergency. However, bladder outlet obstruction with impaired drainage of both upper tracts due to either posterior urethral valves or ureterocele warrants prompt treatment after medical stabilization (Cendron et al, 1994). Similarly, high-grade obstruction of a single system should be treated promptly. One significant concern in the management of these babies is the possibility of pulmonary hypoplasia, secondary to oligohydramnios. Thus, the respiratory status of these babies must be monitored carefully.

Table 54–1. NEONATES WITH PRENATAL HYDRONEPHROSIS STRATIFIED ACCORDING TO DIAGNOSIS BETWEEN 1979 AND 1985

Diagnosis	Percent
Ureteropelvic junction obstruction	48
Distal ureteral obstruction	24
Duplex anomalies with upper pole hydronephrosis	15
Posterior urethral valves	5
Reflux	6
Prune-belly syndrome	1
Miscellaneous	1

After Brown T, Mandell J, Lebowitz R: Neonatal hydronephrosis in the era of sonography. AJR 1987; 148:959–963.

In the rarest of cases, the urologist may be involved in the assessment of the neonate in whom fetal intervention was performed. This procedure should be limited to the few referral centers involved in such work and would typically have entailed placement of a vesicoamniotic shunt (Manning et al, 1986) (Fig. 54–2). On delivery, these newborns must be carefully examined for any complications of shunt placement. Abdominal wall herniation, misplacement of shunts, and shunt migration have all been reported (Crombleholme et al, 1991; Estes and Harrison, 1993). The neonate's pulmonary and renal function should be closely monitored in an NICU setting while undergoing thorough urologic studies.

ANESTHETIC AND PARENTAL BONDING CONSIDERATIONS IN THE NEONATE

In considering neonatal urologic surgery, it is essential to bear in mind that the neonate is not simply a small child. The physiologic and psychologic processes unique to the neonate pose special anesthetic and parental bonding concerns.

Anesthetic Considerations

There is increasing evidence that the physiologic response of neonates to painful stimuli is similar to that of adults (Anand and Hickey, 1987). The sympathetic response to noxious stimulation can have harmful effects on the neonate. Thus, anesthesia is indicated for neonates undergoing surgery unless they are extremely unstable and intolerant of reduced levels of anesthetic agents. In this era of sophisticated neonatal anesthesia support, neonatal urologic surgery may be performed safely, with a 2% risk of major morbidity noted in one series (Parrott and Woodard, 1976).

A major concern in neonatal anesthesia is maintaining adequate oxygenation, which begins with establishing a proper airway. Endotracheal intubation is regarded as virtually mandatory in neonates because of their increased tendency to regurgitation and the possibility of unknown anomalies. Although awake intubation may be used in the unstable neonate, the associated rise in intracranial pressure makes it preferable to anesthetize and paralyze the neonate prior to intubation (Spear, 1992). In the premature infant, a relative deficiency of lung surfactant, known as hyaline membrane disease, results in a form of respiratory distress syndrome. In this syndrome, the instability of smaller airspaces may result in widespread atelectasis, reduction of functional residual capacity, and an impaired ventilation/perfusion ratio. These infants are at increased risk for hypoxemia, hypercapnia, and acidosis. Respiratory support entails constant distending airway pressure or intermittent positive pressure ventilation with positive end-expiratory pressure (Bikhazi and Davis, 1990).

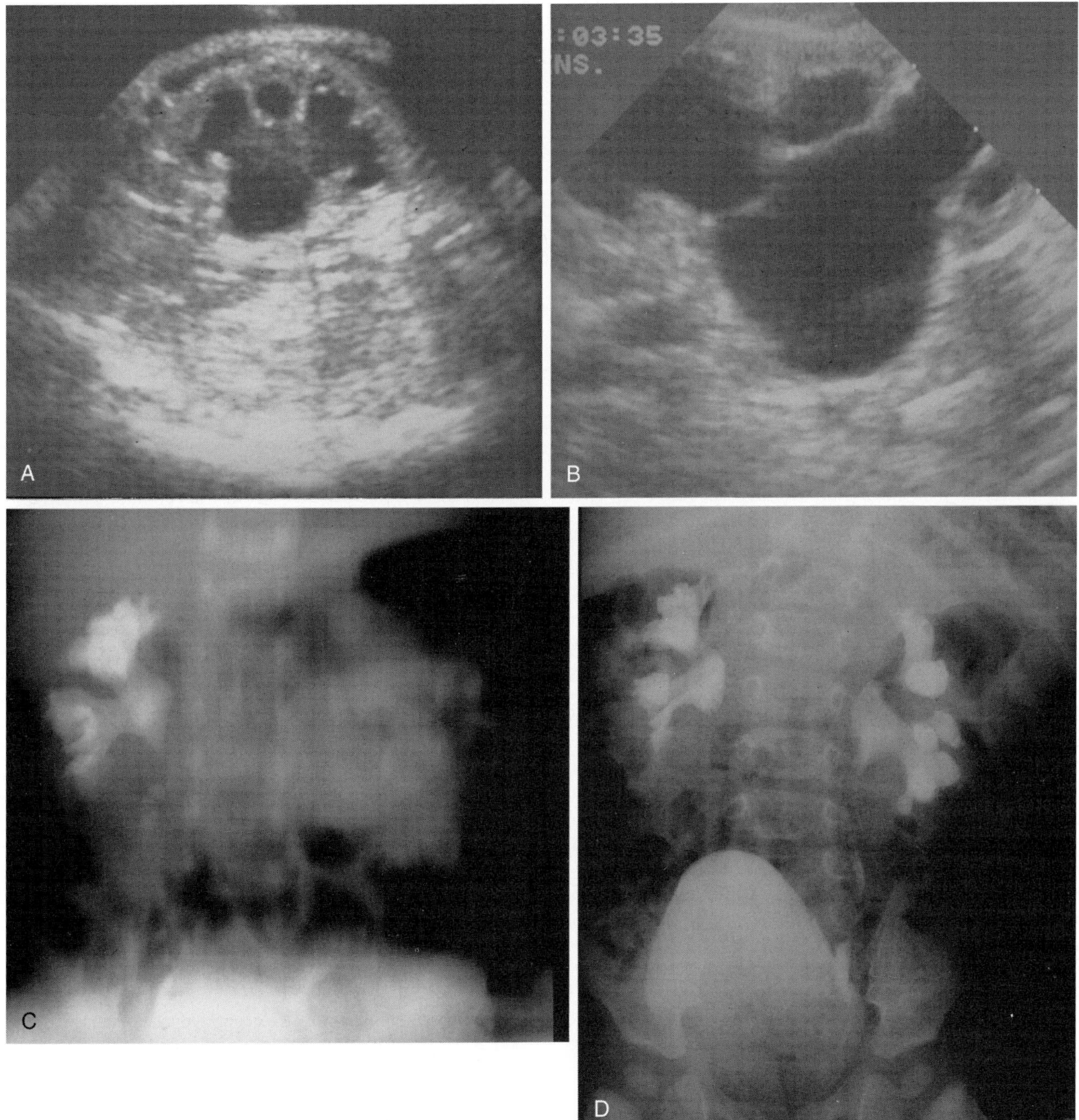

Figure 54–1. *A,* Prenatal ultrasound at 34 weeks demonstrating severe left-sided hydronephrosis. *B,* Newborn ultrasound on day 5 confirming severe left-sided hydronephrosis. *C,* Intravenous pyelogram at 2 weeks demonstrating left ureteropelvic junction obstruction. *D,* Six-month postoperative intravenous pyelogram at age 8 months.

The neonate's oxygen consumption is twice that of the adult, and alveolar oxygen is depleted rapidly owing to the high cardiac output and the neonate's limited pulmonary functional residual capacity. Thus, apnea or airway obstruction may rapidly result in hypoxemia.

Two aspects of the neonate's circulatory status make it particularly susceptible to hypoxemic episodes. The first relates to the syndrome of persistent fetal circulation or persistent pulmonary hypertension of the newborn (PPHN), and the second relates to the oxygen-carrying capacity of the neonatal red blood cell.

PPHN represents a return to a fetal pattern of circulation in the newborn and may result from a variety of causes of severe hypoxemia such as neonatal asphyxia or meconium aspiration (Crone et al, 1991). Because of high pulmonary vascular resistance, there is right to left shunting through the ductus arteriosus or foramen ovale, or both. The mortality rate with persistent fetal circulation is considerable, and only recently has it been successfully managed with cardiorespiratory support from extracorporeal membrane oxygenation (O'Rourke et al, 1989).

Another factor responsible for impaired delivery of oxygen to the tissue in neonates is the admixture of fetal and adult-type hemoglobin (Oski and Delivoria-Padapoulous,

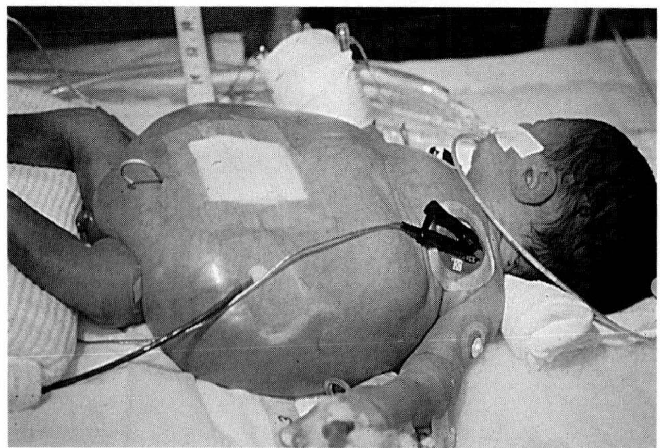

Figure 54–2. Neonate with prune-belly syndrome after fetal intervention with double J vesicoamniotic shunt emanating from the bladder.

1970). At term, fetal hemoglobin (HbF) accounts for 75% to 80% of the total. Fetal hemoglobin has a much lower affinity for the compound 2,3-diphosphoglycerate (DPG), which promotes dissociation of oxygen from hemoglobin, than does adult hemoglobin. Not until 4 to 6 months of age does the child's hemoglobin resemble that of the adult. In addition, DPG levels fall transiently within the first few days of life and begin to rise by the end of the first week. Thus, for the first week of life in particular, the neonate's ability to deliver oxygen to the tissue at a given oxygen tension is compromised.

Cardiac output in the neonate is dependent on blood volume and heart rate. Thus, it is particularly important to hydrate the neonate well preoperatively. Because of the need to minimize dehydration and hypotension, it has been recommended that the last formula be given 6 hours preoperatively, the last breast feeding 4 hours preoperatively, and clear liquids 2 hours prior to surgery (Spear, 1992). A hematocrit and hemoglobin concentration should be obtained, and the infant's electrolyte, glucose, and calcium status should be monitored.

The neonate has a high surface area to body weight ratio and a relatively thin epidermal layer, which allows heat to be lost rapidly to the environment. Thus, hypothermia can develop rapidly, with a resultant increase in metabolic rate and oxygen consumption. In addition, hypothermia results in a leftward shift of the fetal hemoglobin oxygen dissociation curve, impairing the peripheral delivery of oxygen. Cold peripheral vasoconstriction can further impair tissue perfusion. Thus, the importance of transporting the neonate in an incubator, maintaining a warm operating room, using a radiant heater and warm infusates, and wrapping the child appropriately is readily apparent.

Retinopathy of prematurity (ROP), or retrolental fibroplasia, describes the toxic effects of excess oxygen on the developing retinal vessels of premature infants, which in its most severe form may result in blindness. Since the discovery of this relationship in the 1950s, the incidence of ROP declined dramatically before gradually increasing as the capability of salvaging the more vulnerable premature neonate improved. The introduction of accurate transcutaneous oxygen monitoring in the 1980s has been of great value in preventing ROP, such that there are few cases reported in babies greater than 28 weeks of gestation and over 1200 kg. Beyond 44 weeks after conception age, the risk of ROP seems nil (Quinn et al, 1981).

The risk of developing ROP appears multifactorial, and studies have found the use of blood transfusions, duration of Pao_2 of 80 mm Hg or more, and duration of ventilation to be of importance (Merritt et al, 1981). Because ROP has been reported to develop in infants when the only oxygen received was during surgery, it is recommended that intraoperative Pao_2 be maintained at a level no greater than 80 to 90 mm Hg (Betts et al, 1977; American Academy of Pediatrics—American College of Obstetrics and Gynecologists, 1983).

Studies have clearly demonstrated that preterm infants ($<$ 37 weeks' gestational age at birth) are at increased risk for developing postoperative, life-threatening apneic episodes (Steward, 1982; Liu et al, 1983; Welborn et al, 1986). This is believed to be related in part to residual potent inhalational anesthetics, which decrease the ventilatory response to carbon dioxide and may accentuate abnormalities of respiratory control in the preterm neonate. Because apneic episodes may occur up to 12 hours postoperatively in this group of neonates, postoperative observation becomes mandatory. A number of studies have attempted to better define the postconceptual age at which former preterm infants are no longer at risk for postoperative ventilatory dysfunction (Welborn et al, 1990; Kurth and LeBard, 1991). Although the findings of these studies have varied somewhat, it appears clear that former premature infants less than 44 weeks' postconceptual age are at increased risk for developing postoperative ventilatory dysfunction (Malviya et al, 1993). The risk to infants 44 to 60 weeks' postconceptual age remains controversial (Kurth et al, 1987). Thus, one should defer surgery on preterm infants until at least 44 to 46 weeks' postconceptual age, if possible (Welborn, 1990). If not, overnight postoperative apnea monitoring is essential for these patients.

An alternative approach to diminish the risk of postoperative apnea in the former preterm neonate has been the use of spinal and caudal epidural anesthesia (Webster et al, 1991). One study demonstrated spinal anesthesia to be safe and effective for high-risk neonates undergoing outpatient inguinal herniorrhaphy, circumcision, orchidopexy, or cystoscopy without any postoperative apneic episodes (Sartorelli et al, 1992). Although regional anesthesia appears preferable to general anesthesia for the former preterm infant undergoing less than 2 hours of elective, infraumbilical, extraperitoneal surgery, the same guidelines for postoperative apnea monitoring are recommended.

Parental Bonding to the Neonate

Just as the physiology of the neonate is unique, so, too, appears to be the psychologic interaction between child and parent in the neonatal period. A growing body of evidence supports the concept of bonding between parent and neonate, which may begin as early as parental visualization of the fetus on prenatal ultrasound (Fletcher and Evans, 1983; Korsch, 1983). In the neonatal period, the bonding process may be compromised by physical separation of parent and child or by the parental perception of the child as abnormal (Shaheen et al, 1968; Bradbury and Hewison, 1994).

A number of studies have emphasized the importance of allowing children to spend time at home with their parents in order to cement the parental bond (Lampe et al, 1977). Enhanced early exposure of infant to the parent has been associated with a decreased incidence of parenting disorders, including child abuse and neglect (Klaus and Kennell, 1983). A study from the United Kingdom noted that one important risk factor for child abuse was the baby's admission to an NICU (Lynch and Roberts, 1977).

In most major children's centers, the importance of this bonding process is well recognized and rooming in of parents is strongly encouraged. In particular, parental bonding with an ill or premature neonate in an NICU setting is often fostered by a dedicated nursing staff (Haut et al, 1994; Shellabarger and Thompson, 1993). A prospective randomized study comparing a group of babies participating in the rooming in program with a control group found a statistically significant decrease in the number of children in the rooming in program subsequently admitted for parenting inadequacy (O'Connor et al, 1980).

Thus, early discharge of the neonate to home for a period of a few weeks prior to hospitalization is desirable when medically acceptable. If hospitalization is necessary during the neonatal period, the maximization of parental contact with rooming in should be strongly encouraged.

NEONATAL ASSESSMENT AND INITIAL MANAGEMENT OF UROLOGIC EMERGENCIES

Complications of Neonatal Circumcision

The urologist's involvement in neonatal circumcision has traditionally been a limited one, focusing largely on surgical complications, often by inexperienced operators.

The precise incidence of postoperative complications following neonatal circumcision is unknown but appears to be between 0.2% and 2% (Kaplan, 1983; Williams and Kapila, 1993). Although the vast majority of complications are minor, some are devastating. Hemorrhage is the most common complication, occurring in approximately 1% of cases (Warner and Strashin, 1981). It accounted for 53% of complications in one series, and in the majority of cases, it was controlled by conservative measures such as pressure or application of an epinephrine-soaked (aqueous 1:100,000) gauze sponge (Gee and Ansell, 1976). Twenty-five percent of patients with hemorrhage required placement of a hemostatic suture. Hemorrhage is most likely to occur 3 days after birth because of the physiologic depression of plasma levels of vitamin K–dependent clotting factors. These factors return to normal within approximately 1 week, but this depression can be prevented by an injection of vitamin K at birth. Severe hemorrhage has been seen rarely and suggests a bleeding diathesis, such as factor VIII deficiency.

The second most frequent complication of neonatal circumcision is wound infection, although definitions of infection have varied from one series to the next (Wiswell and Geschke, 1989). In general, circumcision wound infections are exceedingly rare, given the rich vascular supply of the penis. If the rare infection is recognized, it should be treated with systemic antibiotics (Uwyyed et al, 1990).

Technical errors in circumcision may result in dehiscence of the repair, denudation of the penile shaft, or injury to the glans. In the event of dehiscence, it is usually practical to allow the defect to heal by secondary intention. Similarly, if a partial denudation of the penile shaft occurs, healing by secondary intention may be appropriate (Sotolongo et al, 1985). If, however, the penile shaft is totally denuded of skin, grafting of the exposed tissue is preferable to avoid undesired scarring and secondary chordee.

Minor injuries to the glans heal well with conservative measures. One must determine that the urethra has not been injured, however. On rare occasions, a glans amputation may result from a blind operative technique and an immediate attempt at reattachment with urethral stenting is warranted. A limited number of case reports describe successful reattachment of the amputated glans with prompt surgical repair (Gluckman et al, 1995).

Urethrocutaneous fistula is a less common complication that may not be recognized in the neonatal period (Lackey, 1968). It is believed to result from crushing of the urethra by the circumcision clamp or entry into the urethra of a hemostatic suture. If the injury is recognized immediately, a primary repair should be performed.

Occasionally, a patient with hypospadias is inadvertently circumcised. The most vulnerable group is those males with the megameatus, intact prepuce variant, in whom the hypospadiac defect is concealed by a circumferential foreskin. If this variant is recognized midway through the procedure, the circumcision should be aborted. One series reported an alarmingly high percentage of hypospadiac males (36%) to have been circumcised (Gee and Ansell, 1976). In two thirds of cases, the hypospadias was unrecognized.

Urinary retention may result from a tight circular bandage and has been associated with reports of circumcision-related urosepsis and acute obstructive uropathy (Berman, 1975; Craig et al, 1994). In this setting, the bandage should be promptly removed and a small feeding tube passed to decompress the bladder.

In addition to urosepsis and meningitis, two devastating complications of circumcision have been reported—necrotizing fasciitis and slough of the entire phallus.

Necrotizing fasciitis has been reported in just a few instances but represents perhaps the most serious complication of an apparently properly performed circumcision (Woodside, 1980). In these cases, aggressive débridement and NICU monitoring have been necessary lifesaving maneuvers.

Sloughing of the penis following circumcision has been infrequently reported. Most commonly, the penile necrosis has resulted from the misuse of electrocautery in association with the Gomco clamp (Azmy et al, 1985; Stefan, 1994). Alternatively, sloughing can occur as a result of injudicious use of epinephrine or prolonged use of a penile tourniquet. In general, these children are best converted to a female phenotype, given the difficulty in creating a functional phallus, although phallic construction has been performed infrequently (Gearhart and Rock, 1989; Gilbert et al, 1993).

Scrotal Mass

The evaluation of the scrotal mass in the neonate entails the same systematic approach that one would employ in an older child; however, the applicable imaging modalities are more limited and the surgical findings are less variable.

One must first distinguish the mass as cystic or solid, which can usually be achieved with transillumination or, if necessary, ultrasound. A cystic scrotal mass invariably represents a hydrocele or, occasionally, an incarcerated hernia, whereas a solid mass represents neonatal testicular torsion until proved otherwise. An incarcerated inguinal hernia warrants prompt surgical correction, not only to preserve bowel integrity but also to avoid ipsilateral cord compression and testicular ischemia.

The differential diagnosis for a solid scrotal mass includes neonatal testicular torsion, scrotal hematoma, testicular tumor, epididymitis, ectopic spleen or adrenal, or torsion of a testicular appendage (Weingarten et al, 1990).

Of all diagnostic possibilities, the most likely is neonatal testicular torsion. Typically the diagnosis is made by the examining pediatrician or nurse within the first 24 to 48 hours in the nursery. The baby is asymptomatic, with scrotal erythema and induration. Because of the small size of the neonate, a technetium testicular scan is rarely helpful. The ultrasound is of limited value as well unless hemorrhagic necrosis is extensive, in which case the diagnosis of a necrotic testis is supported. In one study, the color Doppler ultrasound accurately diagnosed neonatal torsion in nine newborns (Cartwright et al, 1995). However, another preliminary study suggested that testes smaller than 1 cm^3 were particularly difficult to study with Doppler flow (Atkinson et al, 1992). Thus, this diagnostic modality is not yet recommended for definitive assessment of testicular perfusion in the neonate.

The pathogenesis of neonatal testicular torsion remains a mystery. Theories have included difficult labor or breech presentation, high birth weight, and overactive cremasteric reflex (Burge, 1987). In the reported cases, breech presentation has been present infrequently. In one review, the difficulty of labor and birth weight in the population with torsion were found to be no different than those of normals (LaQuaglia et al, 1987). What does seem clear is that neonatal torsion can occur equally commonly on either side and classically entails twisting of the overlying tunica vaginalis in association with the testis and spermatic cord, thus referred to as extravaginal torsion (Fig. 54–3). Extravaginal torsion is a process believed to be unique to the neonatal period in that the testicular tunics become adherent at weeks 4 to 8, preventing their involvement.

Unlike the treatment of testicular torsion in an adolescent, the optimal management of neonatal testicular torsion has remained controversial (Das and Singer, 1990). Perhaps the most important reason is that true salvage of a neonatal testicular torsion is an exceedingly rare event. Another factor is the relatively high anesthetic risk of neonatal surgery, making transfer of the neonate to a tertiary pediatric center desirable (Stone et al, 1995). The third factor is the controversy surrounding the importance of contralateral testicular fixation (Feins, 1983).

In the majority of reports of neonatal testicular torsion, the assessment of the postoperative result is based on physical examination alone. The presence of a normal contralateral testis ensures normal hormonal status, and thus, physiologic evidence of salvage is lacking. In this respect, true salvage has not been convincingly demonstrated.

The importance of contralateral testicular fixation may be best assessed by the study of bilateral neonatal torsion—one of the rarest urologic emergencies of the newborn period. To date, 14 cases have been described, three of which were asynchronous (Gerstmann and Marble, 1980; LaQuaglia et al, 1987; Stone et al, 1995). In no case has testicular salvage been conclusively proved by hormonal studies, but in one case, physical examination at 6 months postoperatively suggested salvage of the asynchronously twisted testis. However, in this case, the torsion was found coincidentally at exploration for a rapidly expanding hydrocele, and thus, its clinical presentation was atypical (Feins, 1983).

Whether or not the contralateral testis is at increased anatomic risk for torsion in the setting of unilateral neonatal torsion is unclear. Nevertheless, the reports of asynchronous neonatal torsion make prompt exploration for the purposes of diagnosis and contralateral fixation (if not salvage) the most prudent approach. In the setting of *bilateral* neonatal torsion, an immediate attempt at detorsion is mandatory and the testes should be left in situ with the hope that some hormonal function will remain.

Epididymitis in the neonate is an exceedingly rare anomaly. However, one report noted that infant males were at relatively high risk for bacteriuria-related epididymitis (Gierup et al, 1975). Of potential importance is the fact that this study from Sweden involved a population of predominantly uncircumcised males. Clinically, epididymitis is indistinguishable from neonatal torsion and exploration is required for diagnosis. The finding of epididymitis, particularly if it is related to urinary infection, warrants a full imaging evaluation with ultrasound and VCUG.

Testicular tumor in the neonate is also a rare anomaly, but its possibility makes an inguinal approach to the clinically indeterminate scrotal mass advisable (Kaplan et al, 1988).

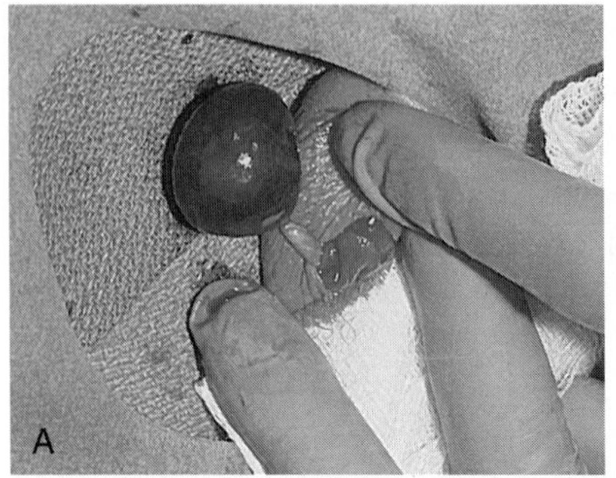

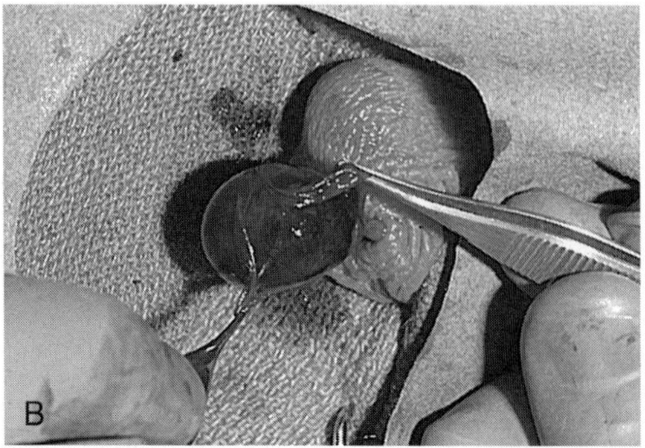

Figure 54–3. *A,* Neonatal testicular torsion involving the tunica vaginalis. *B,* Opening the tunica vaginalis to expose hemorrhagic necrotic contents.

The most recent report of the Prepubertal Testicular Tumor Registry demonstrated gonadal stromal tumors to be the most common neonatal tumor, accounting for 40% of the tumors in this age group (Kay, 1993). These tumors may become clinically apparent as a result of their endocrine manifestations, which in some cases, have entailed ambiguous genitalia (Uehling et al, 1987). Yolk sac tumors composed 30% of neonatal tumors. Follow-up of these patients demonstrated no difference in the disease mortality rate based on age of presentation. Based on the findings of the Prepubertal Testis Tumor Registry study, retroperitoneal lymph node dissection is not routinely recommended for patients with clinical stage I yolk sac tumors but should be reserved for patients with evidence of retroperitoneal disease. Of importance is the knowledge that the tumor marker alphafetoprotein is physiologically elevated at birth, not reaching normal adult levels until 8 months of age. Thus, its use as a clinically significant tumor marker requires age-specific comparison (Masterson et al, 1985). Mature teratoma accounted for 5% of the tumors in the Prepubertal Testis Tumor Registry, and for this tumor, orchiectomy is curative (Giebink and Ruymann, 1974).

Neonatal Abdominal Mass

The diagnosis of an abdominal mass in the newborn has been regarded as a classic neonatal urologic emergency, in that the majority of such masses are genitourinary in origin. Most frequently, such a finding represents a *diagnostic* emergency because the minority of neonatal abdominal masses require immediate surgical intervention.

In evaluating the neonate, the family and maternal history may be of value given the hereditary nature of some lesions (i.e., autosomal recessive polycystic kidney disease) and the diagnostic importance of findings such as oligohydramnios. Prenatal ultrasound studies are of particular value if they are performed to assess the anatomy and development of the mass lesion. Certainly, in the era of prenatal ultrasound, our perspective of the abdominal mass has changed slightly. Some obvious lesions are anticipated, and other more subtle masses may be detectable at delivery, based on prenatal findings.

The physical examination should begin with a general assessment of the neonate to identify findings associated with the mass, such as subcutaneous nodules (neuroblastoma) or dehydration (renal vein thrombosis [RVT]). Palpation of the abdomen is best performed with optimal relaxation of the abdominal wall—ideally with the child asleep—and may be facilitated by flexion of the hips (Perlman and Williams, 1976). During the course of the examination, one should determine the location of the mass; whether it is unilateral or bilateral; and its mobility, size, contour, and consistency. A rectal examination and inspection of the perineum are also important.

Prior to imaging studies, transillumination may be performed in the nursery to distinguish a cystic from a solid lesion (Donn and Faix, 1985). The kidneys are best examined with the infant in the lateral decubitus position and light directed from anterior to posterior. The posterior aspect of the infant is then examined at the costovertebral angle for abnormalities of transillumination.

One should obtain plain films of the abdomen of the neonate in the anteroposterior and lateral projections to demonstrate an intestinal obstruction, soft tissue mass, abnormal calcification, and vertebral anomalies (Hartman and Shochat, 1989).

The ultrasound has supplanted the IVP as the imaging study of choice for the neonatal abdominal mass. It is noninvasive and exceedingly accurate, providing the correct diagnosis in 96% of neonatal abdominal masses in one series (Wilson, 1982). In the event that the neonate cannot be safely transported to the radiology suite, portable state-of-the-art ultrasound equipment may be brought to the nursery.

For the majority of neonates, the combination of physical examination, plain films, and ultrasound provides the diagnosis of the abdominal mass. But in certain settings, additional studies are necessary, including intravenous urography, VCUG, renal scan, computerized tomography, magnetic resonance imaging, and rarely, arteriography (Velchik, 1985; McVicar et al, 1991). The indications for these studies are described in the following discussion.

The differential diagnosis of the neonatal abdominal mass is a broad one, as outlined in Table 54–2. It includes retroperitoneal lesions of the urinary tract and adrenal gland, rarely the pancreas, sacrococcygeal teratoma, and intraperitoneal lesions involving the gastrointestinal tract, liver, and biliary tract and female reproductive tract.

Among all large series of neonatal abdominal masses, certain patterns remain consistent. First, the majority of masses are retroperitoneal (Longino and Martin, 1958; Wedge et al, 1971). Of these masses, the majority of lesions are renal (Melicow and Uson, 1959; Raffensperger and Abousleiman, 1968; Wedge et al, 1971) (Table 54–3).

Renal Masses

Hydronephrosis due to ureteropelvic junction obstruction (UPJ) is the most common cause of the neonatal abdominal mass. Lebowitz noted that UPJ obstruction along with the MCDK accounted for 40% of all neonatal abdominal masses but also found a somewhat higher number of UPJ obstructions than MCDKs presenting as neonatal masses over an equivalent period of time (65 UPJs versus 53 MCDKs) (Lebowitz and Griscom, 1977). The diagnosis of neonatal UPJ obstruction is usually straightforward and ideally can be made on ultrasound examination alone. However, in certain cases, a severe UPJ obstruction must be distinguished from the hydronephrotic variant of MCDK (Sanders and

Table 54–2. CAUSES OF ABDOMINAL MASS IN THE NEWBORN

Cystic	Solid
Hydronephrosis	Neuroblastoma
Multicystic dysplastic kidney	Mesoblastic nephroma
Adrenal hemorrhage	Wilms' tumor
Hydrometrocolpos	Teratoma
Ovarian cyst	Hepatoblastoma
Pancreatic cyst, duplication	Hemangioma (liver)
Choledochal cyst	Hamartoma (liver, pancreas)
Mesenteric/omental cyst	Autosomal recessive polycystic kidney disease
Intestinal duplication	

After Hartman EE, Shochat SJ: Clin Perinatol 1989; 16:123–135.

Table 54–3. DISTRIBUTION OF NEONATAL ABDOMINAL MASSES*

Anatomic System	Percent
Kidney	65
Hydronephrosis (UPJ obstruction, UVJ obstruction, ureterocele)	29
Multicystic kidney	23
Polycystic kidney disease	6
Renal vein thrombosis	2
Solid tumor	5
Ectopy	1
Retroperitoneum	9
Neuroblastoma	6
Teratoma	1
Hemangioma	<1
Abscess	2
Bladder	1
Posterior urethral valves	1
Female genital system	10
Hydrocolpos	6
Ovarian cyst	5
Gastrointestinal	12
Hepatic or biliary	3

UPJ, Ureteropelvic junction; UVJ, Ureterovesical junction.

Data abstracted from Elder JS, Duckett JW Jr: Perinatal urology. *In:* Gillenwater JY, Grayhack JT, Howards SS, Duckett JW Jr, eds: Adult and Pediatric Urology, 2nd ed. St. Louis, Mosby–Yearbook, Inc., 1991, pp 1711–1810.

*Modified from Griscom NT: AJR 1965; 93:447; Raffensperger J, Abousleiman A: Surgery 1968; 63:514; Wedge JJ, Grosfeld JL, Smith JP: J Urol 1971; 106:770; Wilson, DA: Am J Dis Child 1982; 136:147; Emanuel B, White H: Clin Pediatr 1968; 7:529.

Hartman, 1984). A 99m technetium-dimerceptosuccinic acid (Tc-^{99m}DMSA) renal scan should demonstrate some function of the hydronephrotic kidney and usually documents nonfunction of the MCDK (although exceptions have been reported) (Stuck et al, 1982; Carey and Howards, 1988). After making the diagnosis of UPJ obstruction, completion of the urologic work-up should include a VCUG and functional study (IVP or renal scan). The high incidence of bilateral pathology associated with UPJ obstruction appears to have particular relevance to the neonate. In a number of series, UPJ obstructions have been found to occur bilaterally in 20% of neonates, with one series noting a 40% incidence (Williams and Karlaftis, 1966; Uson et al, 1968; Robson et al, 1976; Murphy et al, 1984) (Fig. 54–4). Indeed, Williams found that early evidence of bilaterality was characteristic of infantile UPJ obstruction (Williams and Karlaftis, 1966). Other forms of contralateral pathology that have been well recognized in the setting of UPJ obstruction include MCDK and renal agenesis (Robson et al, 1976).

The pathophysiology of UPJ obstruction was studied by Hanna and colleagues, who demonstrated by electron microscopy that the obstructing segment was histologically abnormal (Hanna et al, 1976). They recognized increased collagen relative to smooth muscle, disorientation of smooth muscle, and increased circular versus longitudinal muscle fibers. This inherently abnormal tissue architecture provides justification for the dismembered approach to surgical repair, when indicated.

Although it seems likely that most UPJ obstructions presenting as an abdominal mass will come to pyeloplasty, the optimal timing of surgical repair remains indeterminate (Bernstein et al, 1988; Sheldon et al, 1992). It is clear that the complication rate of pyeloplasty is highest in the neonatal group—related primarily to delayed anastomotic opening and pyelonephritis (Snyder et al, 1980). Thus, the decision to operate in the neonatal period should be a measured one. In the setting of significant bilateral UPJ obstruction, repair in the neonate should be staged, or if simultaneous bilateral repair is undertaken, nephrostomy drainage should be used.

Multicystic Dysplastic Kidney

The MCDK appears to be the second most common cause of the neonatal abdominal mass. It usually presents as a unilateral lesion, although bilateral MCDKs presenting as bilateral flank masses have been reported (Pathak and Williams, 1964).

The etiology of the MCDK remains somewhat unclear. The primary factor may be abnormal induction of the nephrogenic blastema by the ureteric bud. On the other hand, urinary obstruction early in utero has been demonstrated to result in dysplasia, such that the ureteric atresia classically associated with MCDK may be the predisposing factor (DeKlerk et al, 1977).

The diagnostic evaluation begins with careful palpation—of the sleeping child, if possible. Classically, the MCDK resembles a mobile cluster of grapes in the upper abdomen. An ultrasound examination can confirm this classic configuration (Sanders and Hartman, 1984). The absence

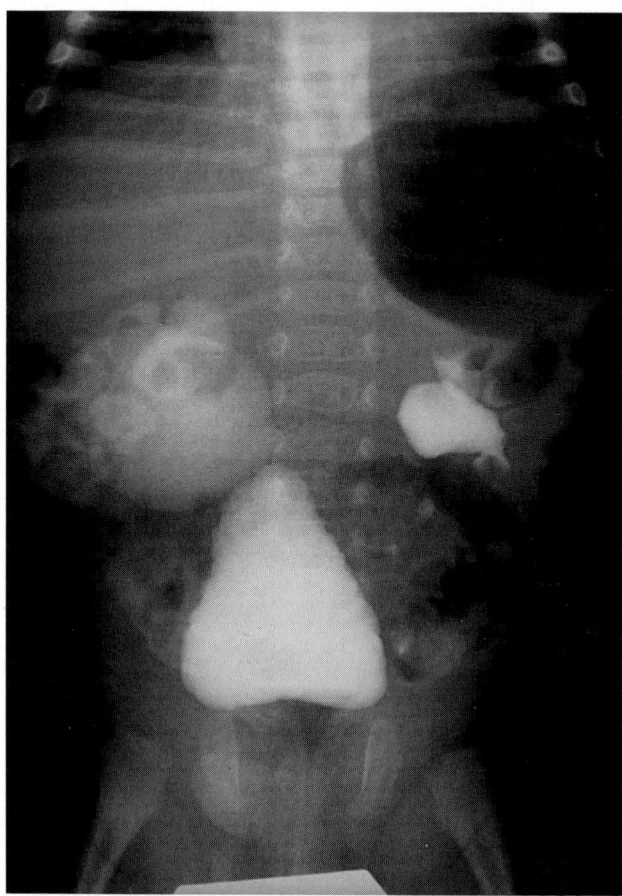

Figure 54–4. Bilateral ureteropelvic junction obstruction presenting as a right abdominal mass. (Reproduced with permission from R. L. Lebowitz.)

of functional parenchyma is confirmed on DMSA renal scan (Velchik,1985) (Fig. 54–5).

Prior to the recent advent of precise ultrasonic imaging and nuclear renal scanning, the diagnosis of MCDK was confirmed at surgery and the kidney removed. In general, the diagnosis can now be made nonoperatively (Gordon et al, 1988). However, occasionally, the distinction between a poorly functioning hydronephrotic kidney and MCDK can be a difficult one. There have been rare reports of scan-documented function in MCDKs; however, nonfunction on DMSA renal scan associated with consistent ultrasonic findings essentially confirms this diagnosis (Stuck et al, 1982) (see Fig. 54–5).

An important aspect of the MCDK is the frequency with which contralateral lesions are found, ranging from 13% to 25% (Pathak and Williams, 1964; DeKlerk et al, 1977). Indeed, the astute observation was made over 30 years ago that the MCDK is harmless but that the danger to the child lies on the other side (Pathak and Williams, 1964). UPJ obstruction is most common, followed by urederovesical junction obstruction and contralateral MCDK. One study demonstrated a considerably higher incidence of contralateral abnormalities if the MCDK was associated with atresia of the lower ureter rather than the upper ureter (DeKlerk et al, 1977). Because of the accuracy in diagnosing the MCDK, surgical removal is no longer mandatory (Gordon et al, 1988). It is advocated by some because of isolated case reports of renal cell carcinoma, Wilms' tumor and an embryonal tumor in an adult, and hypertension (nine cases—only three responding to nephrectomy) (Birken et al, 1985; Dimmick et al, 1989; Susskind et al, 1989). However, the MCDK presenting as a mass may pose other mechanical problems, such as difficulty with feeding, making nephrectomy a more appealing option. The opportunity to follow the MCDK ultrasonographically has supported the notion that over time, the MCDK seems to shrink as cystic fluid is absorbed and, in some cases, to disappear on ultrasound (Avni et al, 1987). Indeed, there is evidence that in some cases, the MCDK may reach its maximum size and begin to involute in utero (Vinocur et al, 1988).

Bilateral Abdominal Mass

Bilateral abdominal masses in the neonate are most commonly due to hydronephrosis (Wedge et al, 1971). Bilateral UPJ obstruction and posterior urethral valves with bilateral hydroureteronephrosis are the most likely entities presenting in this manner. The newborn with prune-belly syndrome presents a special situation in which the deficient abdominal musculature readily allows one to palpate the classically hydronephrotic upper tracts.

Another cause for bilateral abdominal masses in the neonate is autosomal recessive polycystic kidney disease. Often, this diagnosis is suspected on the basis of family history or oligohydramnios and characteristic findings on physical examination including Potter's facies. The ultrasound is diagnostic, demonstrating markedly enlarged and echogenic kidneys and occasionally evidence of hepatic cystic disease.

Solid Neonatal Abdominal Mass

The most common etiology of the solid abdominal mass in the neonate is a neuroblastoma (Hartman and Shochat, 1989). In addition, neuroblastoma is the most common malignancy in the newborn, accounting for half of all neonatal malignant tumors.

On physical examination, neuroblastoma presents as a fixed, irregular mass that often crosses the midline. In patients with the unique stage IV-S disease, abdominal distention secondary to hepatic metastases or subcutaneous nodules may be present (Caty and Shamberger, 1993). Chest and abdominal films may demonstrate paravertebral tumor extension or the punctate calcifications that are typical of neuroblastoma. An ultrasound examination demonstrates a solid, extrarenal mass displacing the kidney laterally and inferiorly. In 75% of cases, urinary vanillylmandelic and homovanillic acid levels are elevated (Schneider et al, 1965).

Of particular importance is the more benign nature of the neuroblastoma in the neonate. The majority of neonates have low-stage or stage IV-S disease, with a 70% overall survival rate (Hartman and Shochat, 1989).

Surgical excision remains the treatment of choice for low-stage and stage IV-S disease, with chemotherapy reserved for stage III and IV neuroblastoma (Weber et al, 1993).

Solid Renal Mass

Congenital mesoblastic nephroma, a benign mesenchymal neoplasm, is the most common intrarenal tumor of the neo-

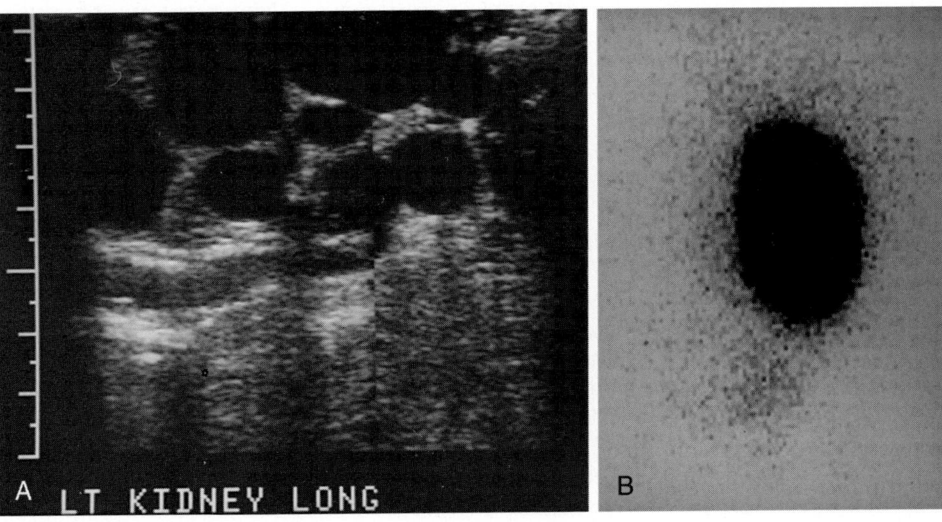

Figure 54–5. *A,* Ultrasound of multicystic dysplastic kidney presenting as abdominal mass. *B,* DMSA renal scan confirming nonfunction. (Reproduced with permission from R. L. Lebowitz.)

nate (Kissane and Dehner, 1992). The National Wilms' Tumor Study noted a 2.8% incidence of mesoblastic nephroma among children with renal tumors and a median age of presentation of 2 months (Howell et al, 1982). A diagnosis may be made on ultrasound, which typically demonstrates a solid intrarenal mass. Atypical forms of mesoblastic nephroma have been described with regard to radiologic features and growth rate of the tumor, but metastasis has not been noted (Zach et al, 1991; Vujanic, 1992) Thus, radical nephrectomy is curative.

A true Wilms' tumor in the neonate is exceedingly rare. Of 3340 patients registered in the National Wilms' Tumor Study from 1969 to 1974, only four cases involved neonates (Hrabovsky et al, 1986). Among these four cases, two appeared to be pure Wilms' tumor, whereas two tumors had elements of both mesoblastic nephroma and Wilms' tumor.

Lower Midline Abdominal Mass

A lower midline abdominal mass in the neonate raises the possibilities of a distended bladder, an ovarian cyst, hydrometrocolpos, and rarely, a sacrococcygeal teratoma. The high likelihood of the distended bladder explaining the mass may be tested with catheterization and attempted drainage. If the distended bladder is ruled out, in the female, hydrometrocolpos is the next most likely explanation.

Hydrometrocolpos is a relatively rare condition that may be suspected on physical examination when a large cystic pelvic mass is found in a female with a hymenal bulge or urogenital sinus (Nguyen et al, 1984).

Two conditions are necessary for hydrometrocolpos to occur. There must be an element of vaginal obstruction as well as abundant secretions from the fetal cervical glands. Vaginal obstruction can result from an imperforate hymen, presenting as an introital bulge. More commonly, it results from a transverse vaginal septum proximal to an atretic vagina associated with persistent urogenital sinus. This condition represents an arrest in embryologic development of the vagina. Fetal cervical secretions result from the high level of circulating maternal estrogens (Diamond, 1988).

In the largest series reported, 65% of patients had a palpable abdominal mass to the umbilicus or xiphoid and 55% presented with acute urinary retention or oliguria (Cook and Marshall, 1964). A cystogram demonstrated the mass to be posterior to the bladder, and rectal examination demonstrated it to be anterior, thus ruling out a sacrococcygeal teratoma or rectal duplication. Over 80% of patients evaluated were found to have hydronephrosis, which was invariably bilateral (Cook and Marshall, 1964). Prior to the advent of abdominal ultrasound, a correct preoperative diagnosis was made in only approximately 50% of cases. Historically, the mortality rate with this lesion exceeded 35% and death was often related to sepsis following laparotomy (Cook and Marshall, 1964).

More recently, the use of ultrasound in association with the cystogram demonstrating anterior compression of the bladder, and a careful perineal examination demonstrating a persistent urogenital sinus, has allowed the accurate preoperative diagnosis of hydrometrocolpos due to a transverse vaginal septum (Hahn-Petersen et al, 1984) (Fig. 54–6). A valuable ultrasound finding appears to be a fluid debris level within the cystic pelvic mass, consistent with mucous secretions (Blask et al, 1991). This affords one the opportunity to drain the hydrometrocolpos through a perineal incision, or percutaneously, thus avoiding the risk of infection associated with laparotomy (Hahn-Petersen et al, 1984).

Neonatal Urinary Ascites

The neonate with ascites is one of the most desperately ill newborns for whom the urologist is consulted. However, neonatal ascites has a variety of etiologies, only some of which are urologic (Griscom et al, 1977). In considering these etiologies, it seems useful to distinguish the child with ascites associated with generalized edema from the child with isolated ascites alone. In the former category, ascites in the neonate is most commonly seen in conjunction with erythroblastosis fetalis. Other etiologies of ascites in conjunction with generalized edema are cardiac disease, such as hypoplastic left-sided heart syndrome, and systemic viral and bacterial infections. In addition, portal hepatic abnormalities may be responsible. Of the causes of isolated neonatal ascites *unassociated* with generalized edema, urinary obstruction and extravasation is the most common etiology (Trulock et al, 1985). Gastrointestinal tract anomalies associated with perforation and peritonitis and chylous ascites are additional causes.

It has long been recognized that bilateral upper tract dilatation was typically associated with urinary ascites. Posterior urethral valves have been responsible for the vast majority of cases, accounting for the 7:1 male-to-female ratio of neonatal urinary ascites (Mann et al, 1974). However, other urologic lesions have been associated with ascites. The majority of these have been lower tract obstructive lesions, including ectopic ureterocele, urethral atresia, and neuropathic bladder (Mann et al, 1974). In addition, a few cases of upper tract obstructive lesions have been associated with neonatal ascites (Wasnick, 1987; Reha and Gibbons, 1989). In most cases related to UPJ obstruction, a solitary functioning kidney has been involved.

Finally, intraperitoneal bladder rupture is a less common but well-recognized cause of neonatal ascites (Redman et al, 1979; Trulock et al, 1985). This entity has been recognized in association with lower tract obstructive lesions and, presumably, the blunt trauma of delivery. Among these reports have been cases of posterior urethral valves and neuropathic bladder due to spina bifida and spinal neuroblastoma. In addition, neonatal blunt rupture of the normal bladder in association with a difficult breech extraction has been reported (Tank et al, 1980). An increasingly recognized entity has been urachal laceration due to attempted umbilical arterial catheterization (Hepworth and Milstein, 1984). This iatrogenic, NICU-related injury has become perhaps the most common cause of neonatal bladder rupture (Diamond and Ford, 1989).

Although the incidence of neonatal urinary ascites is unknown, it would appear to be more common than was previously believed (Garrett and Franken, 1969). For example, in his 1965 review of 104 cases of posterior urethral valves, Williams noted one case of urinary ascites (Williams and Eckstein, 1965). In 1982, Greenfield and associates noted five cases among 59 valve patients presenting over 16 years. Improved NICU care for the sick neonate may account

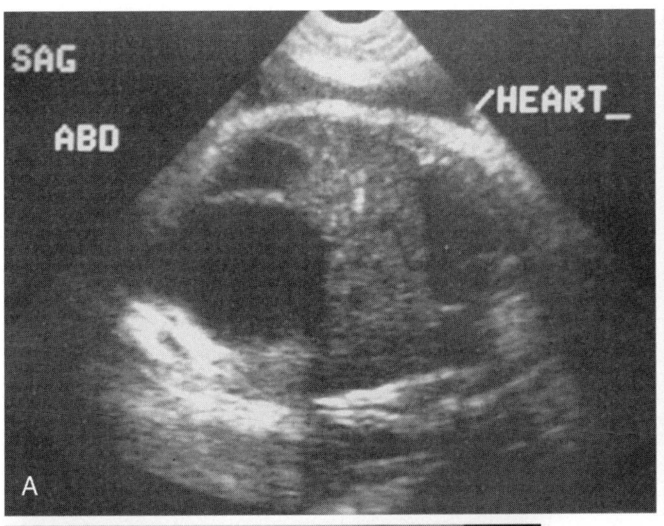

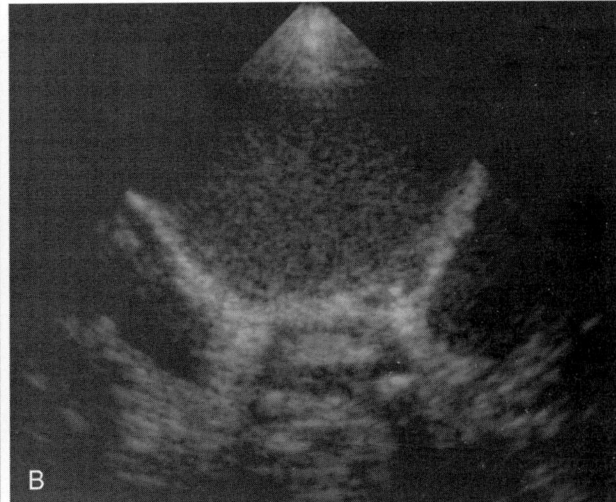

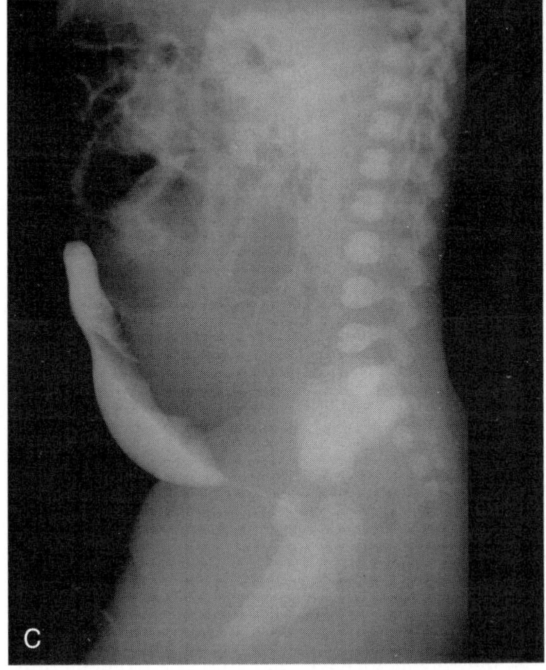

Figure 54–6. Hydrometrocolpos. *A,* Prenatal ultrasound at 38 weeks demonstrating cystic pelvic mass. *B,* Transverse pelvic ultrasound view of cystic mass with characteristic mucoid debris. *C,* Anterior displacement of bladder by distended vagina.

for the increased number of cases. Certainly, the association of neonatal ascites with bladder rupture secondary to the more widespread use of umbilical arterial catheterization is another explanation.

The diagnosis of urinary ascites may be made on the basis of clinical, biochemical, and radiographic evidence (Fig. 54–7). The classic clinical presentation includes progressive abdominal distention with a fluid wave and dullness to percussion over the liver on physical examination. Typically, urine output is disproportionately low relative to fluid intake.

A diagnostic tap of ascites yields straw-colored fluid, which may have an increased blood urea nitrogen (BUN) and creatinine, consistent with urine. However, equilibration of urinary electrolytes with serum through the peritoneal cavity occurs so rapidly that ascitic electrolytes may be nondiagnostic. Serum electrolytes, on the other hand, are consistently diagnostic. Hyponatremia is noted in 70% of cases (Clarke et al, 1993). Serum BUN and creatinine are typically elevated, as is their ratio (BUN/creatinine). In one series, the standard ratio of BUN to creatinine of 10:8 was elevated to greater than 30:1 (Sullivan et al, 1972). The authors attributed this rise to the rapid clearing of urea due to its ability to traverse the peritoneal membrane relative to the larger creatinine molecule. Although other series have consistently demonstrated increased serum BUN and creatinine ratios, not all have achieved the 30:1 ratio noted by Sullivan.

The radiologic evaluation of the child with clinically suspected urinary ascites should confirm the diagnosis and perhaps demonstrate the site of communication between the urinary tract and peritoneum. Evaluation is best begun with an ultrasound and VCUG, which can confirm the presence of obstructive uropathy and occasionally demonstrate urinary extravasation. An IVP or renal scan with DTPA or MAG III may demonstrate the site of upper tract extravasation.

In cases of ascites due to bladder outlet obstruction, distinct radiographic evidence of communication between the upper urinary tract and peritoneum is infrequently noted

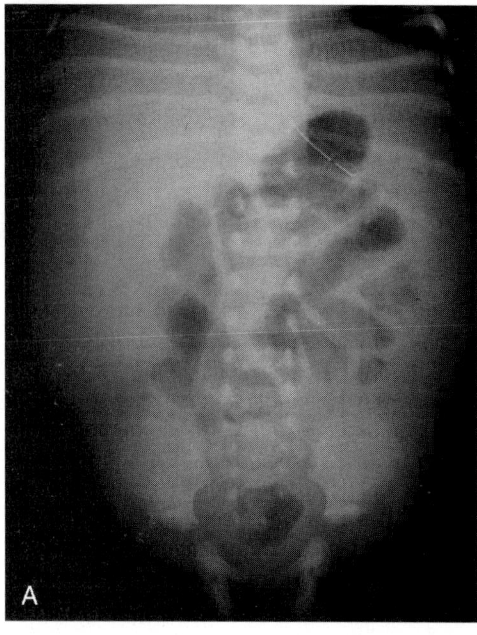

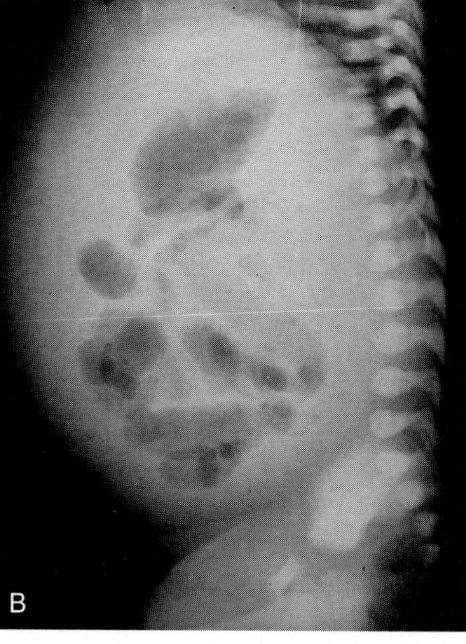

Figure 54–7. *A,* Kidney, ureter, and bladder. *B,* Lateral view of neonate with posterior urethral valves and ascites demonstrating central location of bowel loops and characteristic ground-glass appearance of peritoneum. (Reproduced with permission from A. B. Retik and R. L. Lebowitz.)

(MacPherson et al, 1984). Yet, there is a consensus of opinion that the mechanism responsible for urinary ascites in the setting of obstructive uropathy is forniceal extravasation to the perirenal space and subsequently to the peritoneal cavity. Because urinary ascites is exceedingly rare beyond the neonatal period, the relative thinness of Gerota's fascia in the neonate is believed to be a contributing factor (Adzick et al, 1985).

An important variation of urinary ascites is neonatal urinoma, either alone or associated with ascites secondary to severe obstructive uropathy (Mitchell and Garrett, 1980). Such urinomas typically present as an abdominal mass.

Radiographically, the neonatal urinoma may resemble a duplication anomaly. The subcapsular urinoma typically presents as a C sign by extravasated contrast media, conforming to the contour of the immediately adjacent kidney (MacPherson et al, 1984). A localized perirenal urinoma presents as a rounded, contrast-filled unilocular cystic structure. If the contrast diffuses throughout the perinephric space, to its most dependent locations, then a diffuse perirenal urinoma is diagnosed.

Because these lesions may present as tense masses, the possibility of pulmonary compromise exists (Mitchell and Garrett, 1980). It is recommended that the treatment of urinary ascites be individualized to the pathology and condition of the neonate. For the majority of cases, which are due to bladder outlet obstructive lesions, initial catheter drainage to prevent further accumulation of ascites is adequate management (Krane and Retik, 1974). The ascitic fluid or perirenal collection is absorbed with time. However, if there is respiratory compromise or the suggestion of abscess formation, the urinary collection should be drained directly—often with dramatic improvement in the child's clinical status. If simple catheter drainage is ineffective in improving the child's clinical condition, upper tract decompression by cutaneous ureterostomy or nephrostomy drainage is advised. Direct drainage of the ascites or urinoma may be accomplished at this time.

For *intraperitoneal* bladder rupture, the author's experience with outlet obstructive pathology or lacerations due to umbilical arterial trauma suggests that initial operative management, rather than catheter drainage, is most prudent (Diamond and Ford, 1989).

It has been postulated that urinary ascites represents a so-called protective pop-off mechanism for children with bladder outlet obstructive pathology, allowing for improved overall renal function (Adzick et al, 1985; Rittenberg et al, 1988). Whether there is a differential benefit to the kidney on the side of extravasation is more difficult to determine. Greenfield and co-workers (1982) noted no advantage to the kidney on the side of extravasation, whereas Kay and associates (1980) did note a tissue-sparing effect.

In the setting of neonatal *urinoma,* it is far less clear that such extravasation plays a protective role. In Mitchell's study, kidneys on the side of perirenal extravasation in the face of obstructive uropathy were as likely to have improved function as they were to have impaired function on subsequent studies (Mitchell and Garrett, 1980).

The mortality rates of neonates with urinary ascites have improved remarkably in the past two decades. Scott (1976) noted a 70% mortality rate in 1976, whereas mortality rates in the 1980s dropped to approximately 13% (Kay et al, 1980; Mitchell and Garrett, 1980; Cass et al, 1973; Greenfield et al, 1982). Although a variety of factors are responsible, improved neonatal intensive care is of paramount importance. The most optimistic outcome in this clinical setting argues for aggressive urologic management.

Evaluation of the Newborn with Ambiguous Genitalia

The evaluation and initial management of the newborn with ambiguous genitalia must be regarded as a medical emergency and be handled with great sensitivity toward the family. One's goal should be to make a precise diagnosis of the intersex disorder and to assign a proper sex of rearing. In assessing the newborn with ambiguous genitalia, the family history is often unrevealing, but specific questions may reap large rewards. A history of infant death within the family would suggest the possibility of congenital adrenal hyperplasia (CAH), and infertility, amenorrhea, or hirsutism might also suggest possible familial patterns of intersex states. Certainly, maternal ingestion of progestational or androgenic medication (i.e., danazol) during the pregnancy is of importance. Two delicate areas of relevance are a history of maternal drug abuse during the pregnancy, because cocaine has been associated with genital ambiguity, and finally, consanguinity (Greenfield et al, 1991).

The critical finding on physical examination is that of one or two gonads. This finding rules out female pseudohermaphroditism. Because ovaries do not descend, a distinctly palpable gonad along the pathway of descent is suggestive of a testis. The patient with bilaterally impalpable testes or a unilaterally impalpable testis and hypospadias should be regarded as having an intersex disorder until proved otherwise. In one study, 27% of phenotypic males with cryptorchidism and hypospadias were found to have an intersex disorder (Rajfer and Walsh, 1976).

The examination of the phallus to assess adequacy of size is of paramount importance in considering a male sex of rearing. The average phallic size of the male infant is 3.5 ± 0.4 cm at term; 3.0 ± 0.4 cm at 34 weeks' gestation, and 2.5 ± 0.4 cm at 30 weeks' gestation, measured dorsally from the symphysis pubis to the tip of the stretched glans. In addition, the diameter of the penis in the full-term infant is 1 to 1.5 cm (Feldman and Smith, 1975; Flatau et al, 1975). If an infant's phallic length is less than 2.0 cm, this finding generates concern and may warrant testosterone stimulation (Donahoe et al, 1991).

An additional, important finding on physical examination is that of a uterus, which presents as an anterior midline, cordlike structure on rectal examination. This finding is most readily appreciated within the first few days of life, when the uterus is under the stimulatory effect of placental human chorionic gonadotropin (Donahoe et al, 1991). Further definition of müllerian anatomy can be achieved with ultrasound examination (Horowitz and Glassberg, 1992). The determination of chromosomal sex by means of a karyotype should be performed routinely, although the test requires 48 to 72 hours for preliminary results. Although a buccal smear may provide immediate information regarding chromosomal sex, its inaccuracy limits its usefulness.

Following a history and physical examination, the first evaluation should be biochemical to rule out CAH, in which no gonad is palpable. It is particularly important to diagnose the salt-wasting form, which is the only life-threatening cause of ambiguous genitalia in the newborn period. Thus, one should determine the plasma 17-hydroxyprogesterone level or begin a 24-hour urine collection to measure 17-ketosteroids and pregnanetriol. In the absence of palpable testes, the presence of testicular tissue should be determined by means of a human chorionic gonadotropin stimulation test.

Anatomic definition of the urogenital sinus and ductal structures contributes to the correct diagnosis and is certainly necessary prior to any surgical intervention. The urogenital sinus is imaged by retrograde contrast injection, which also opacifies ductal structures, defines the entry of urethra and vagina into the sinus, and outlines the cervical impression within the vagina. Endoscopy can define these relationships more precisely but is usually not necessary until surgical considerations become imminent. Of particular importance is definition of the relationship between the vaginal opening into the urethra and the external urinary sphincter.

Laparotomy and a longitudinal gonadal biopsy is usually the final clinical step required when a firm diagnosis based on all of the aforementioned data is impossible (Donahoe et al, 1991).

Finally, sophisticated biochemical studies on cultured genital skin fibroblasts may define the precise cellular abnormality responsible for a given intersex disorder, be it an abnormal androgen receptor or an enzyme abnormality. Rarely do they impact on one's initial decision regarding the sex of rearing.

The most common cause of ambiguous genitalia in the newborn period is CAH, secondary to an inborn error of metabolism involving cortisol synthesis. A defect in any one of the five enzymes involved in the cortisol biosynthetic pathway (20,22-desmolase, 3β-hydroxysteroid dehydrogenase, 17α-hydroxylase, 21-hydroxylase, and 11β-hydroxylase) may result in CAH. But the most commonly recognized syndromes result from a deficiency of either terminal enzyme (21-0H, 11β-OH), such that formation of hydrocortisone is impaired, causing a compensatory increase in adrenocorticotrophic hormone secretion. This increase enhances formation of adrenal steroids proximal to the enzymatic defect and results in a secondary increase in the formation of testosterone, the active androgen in CAH (Camacho and Migeon, 1996).

A deficiency in 21-hydroxylase is present in 95% of patients with CAH. The majority of patients with CAH secondary to 21-hydroxylase deficiency exhibit one of the two classic forms of the disease—salt wasting and simple virilization.

In the female with the simple virilizing form of the disorder, female pseudohermaphroditism results. Because the impaired steroidogenesis begins early in life—at the time of formation of the external genitalia (beginning at 10 weeks' gestation)—there is virtually always evidence of some degree of masculinization at birth. This is manifested by enlargement of the clitoris and varying degrees of labial fusion (Fig. 54–8). In addition, the vagina and urethra open into a common urogenital sinus. The enlargement of the clitoris may be so dramatic as to make it appear to be a hypospadiac penis with bilateral cryptorchidism, and cases of complete formation of a masculinized urethra to the tip of an enlarged clitoris have been reported (Diamond, 1995). The severity of the virilization is generally greater in infants who experience salt wasting. The müllerian structures in these patients are typically normal.

In both males and females with the salt-losing variant, symptoms begin within the first few weeks, with failure to regain birth weight, progressive weight loss, and dehydration. Vomiting is prominent and may be so extreme that a mistaken diagnosis of pyloric stenosis may be made.

A deficiency of 11β-hydroxylase accounts for roughly 5% of cases of CAH. Hypertension is a common finding and is believed to be secondary to elevated serum levels of deoxycorticosterone. Virilization occurs in all patients and is as severe as in those with the 21-hydroxylase deficiency.

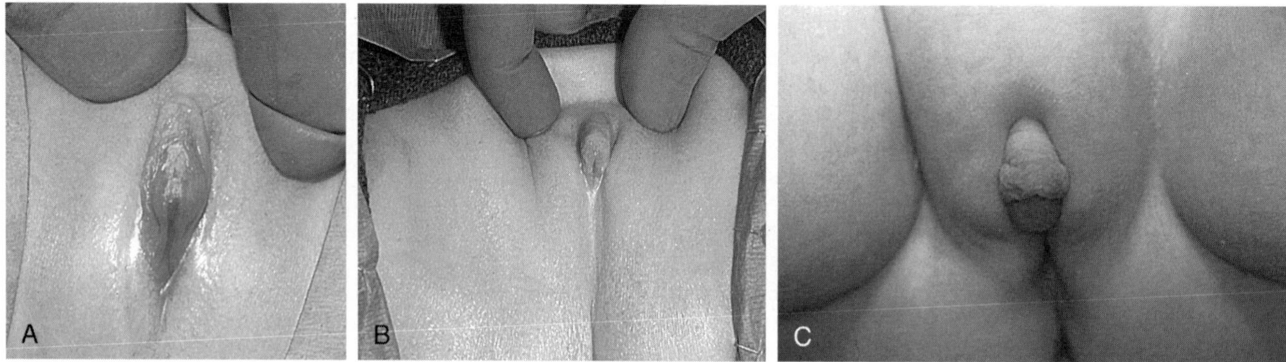

Figure 54–8. *A* to *C*, Congenital adrenal hyperplasia with progressively virilized clitoris and advanced labial scrotal fusion.

Neonatal Intensive Care Unit–Related Complications

Over the past decade, NICUs have provided ever-improving support for the premature and critically ill neonate. This has been a particular advantage for the urologist caring for ill neonates with posterior urethral valves or prune-belly syndrome and for postoperative care of neonates requiring major urologic reconstruction. However, along with the enhanced capabilities of the NICU have come a number of important urologic complications. The three most prominent of these are umbilical arterial catheter–related complications, neonatal nephrolithiasis, and neonatal fungal infection.

Umbilical Arterial Catheter–Related Complications

Catheterization of the umbilical artery is a well-accepted technique for resuscitation and monitoring of the critically ill neonate. With the increasing number of premature infants being admitted to NICUs, umbilical arterial catheterization has been performed with greater frequency. In one series spanning 9 years, 4000 infants treated at one medical center had umbilical arterial catheters (O'Neill et al, 1981). The well-recognized complications of this technique include thrombosis, aortic aneurysm, hemorrhage, necrotizing enterocolitis, infection, hypertension, renal failure, and bladder rupture (Kitterman et al, 1970). Complication rates vary from one series to the next between 1% and 12%, in large part related to the inclusion of autopsy with clinical findings (Kitterman et al, 1970; Marsh et al, 1975; O'Neill et al, 1981). It would appear that clinically apparent complications occur at an approximate rate of 4% (Cochrane et al, 1968).

Thrombosis is the most common complication of umbilical artery catheterization. This becomes relevant to the urologist if the renal arteries become involved selectively or by a larger aortoiliac thrombus. Thrombosis of the renal artery is heralded by hypertension, often severe, and sometimes hematuria and a palpable kidney (Bauer et al, 1975). If there is a strong clinical suspicion, a DTPA flow study can detect major vascular occlusion as well as differential renal perfusion (O'Neill et al, 1981).

In addition to antihypertensive therapy, aggressive surgical management of renal artery thrombosis associated with hypertension is advocated. When the renal process is part of an aortoiliac thrombosis, surgical thrombectomy is indicated (Krueger et al, 1985). If the renal artery is selectively involved, nephrectomy is advocated (Plumer et al, 1975). Often, delay in surgical therapy following a poor response to antihypertensives results in death. In the setting of bilateral renal arterial thrombosis and renal failure, a retroperitoneal approach for thrombectomy has been advocated to afford less complicated subsequent peritoneal dialysis (Lofland et al, 1988).

It is believed that thrombotic complications of the umbilical arterial catheter may be decreased with optimal positioning of the catheter tip, yet the ideal anatomic level of

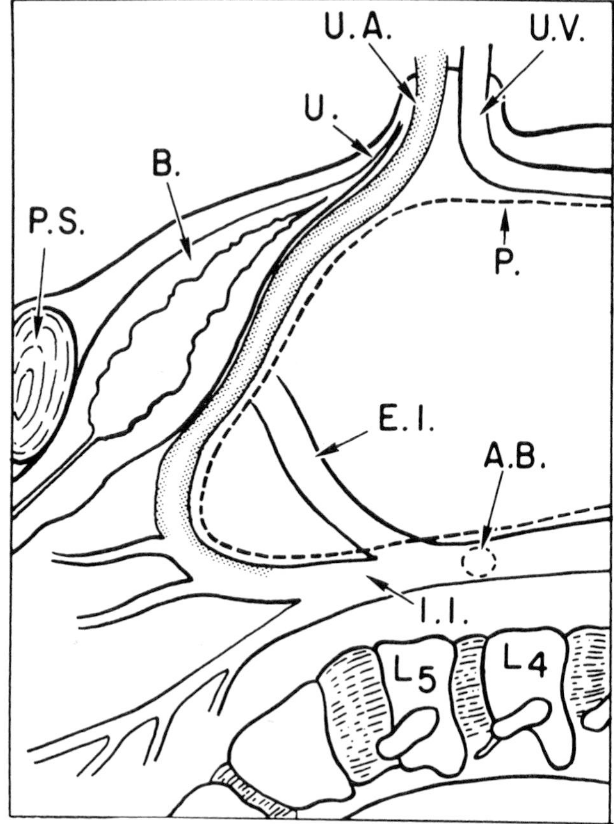

Figure 54–9. Proximity of umbilical artery (UA) and umbilical vein (UV) to urachus (U), bladder (B) and peritoneum (P), pubic symphysis (PS), external iliac artery (EI), aortic bifurcation (AB), and internal iliac artery (II). (Reproduced with permission from Clark JM, Jung AL: Pediatrics 1977; 59:1036–1040.)

the catheter within the aorta remains controversial. Some neonatologists advocate positioning the umbilical arterial catheter above the level of the renal artery, which seems to be associated with fewer overall complications, yet those that do occur involve the visceral vasculature and are more life-threatening (Kitterman et al, 1970). Thus, the majority of vascular surgeons prefer the tip to be positioned in the lower aorta, above the aortic bifurcation, at approximately L-3 (O'Neill et al, 1981).

Rupture of the neonatal bladder due to attempted placement of an umbilical arterial catheter is a more recently recognized complication. It is fairly uncommon, with 11 cases having been described in the literature (Diamond and Ford, 1989). Of these, five cases were associated with an umbilical cutdown and six with an attempt at direct cannulation of the umbilical artery.

The urachus, emanating from the dome of the neonatal bladder, is in close proximity to the umbilical arteries. It is located anteromedial to the arteries and shares with them the umbilical vesical fascia (Clark and Jung, 1977). In addition, the peritoneal reflection on the neonatal bladder dome is adjacent to the urachus (Fig. 54–9). Thus, dissection through the umbilical artery into the urachus can result in a concomitant peritoneal injury, which accounts for the ascites and radiographic finding of intraperitoneal extravasation noted with this lesion (Fig. 54–10). In addition, in the setting of either a cutdown or attempted cannulation, urine is sometimes seen at the umbilicus. Elevated serum BUN and creatinine, due to intraperitoneal urinary extravasation, is the rule (Redman et al, 1979).

Given the rarity of iatrogenic neonatal bladder rupture, its optimal management has not been defined. Among bladder ruptures due to attempted umbilical arterial catheter cannulation, an 18% mortality rate has been noted (Diamond and Ford, 1989). The deaths occurred in two of the three neonates treated nonoperatively. Thus, following a clear diagnosis of this entity with cystographic demonstration of extravasation from the bladder dome, prompt surgical repair is advocated.

Neonatal Nephrolithiasis

Many premature neonates in the NICU receive furosemide for bronchopulmonary dysplasia or congestive heart failure associated with patent ductus arteriosus or other cardiac defects. Over the past 15 years, an increasing number of infants so treated have been noted to develop renal calculi. In one series, ten such cases were noted from approximately 1600 neonatal admissions (Hufnagle et al, 1982). The hypercalciuric effect of furosemide is believed to be responsible for the calcium oxalate and calcium phosphate stones noted in these neonates (Gilsanz et al, 1985).

Renal calcifications are usually bilateral, varying from calcium deposits in the interstitium of renal papilla to staghorn calculi. Ultrasound has demonstrated 2- to 9-mm echogenic foci near the papillary tips in the majority of these infants (Katz et al, 1994). One series noted that calcification appeared after a minimum of 12 days of furosemide at 2 mg/kg/day (Hufnagle et al, 1982). Risk factors for renal calcification in addition to furosemide were an alkaline urine and intermittently decreased urine output (Ezzedeen et al, 1988). Additional risk factors may be low citrate excretion and a decreased glomerular infiltration rate secondary to renal immaturity (Adams and Rowe, 1992).

Metabolic studies of involved neonates on furosemide have consistently demonstrated an elevated urine calcium excretion. In fact, two studies have demonstrated a tenfold increase in urinary calcium excretion after furosemide administration within the first 12 hours of life (Savage et al, 1975; Hufnagle et al, 1982). Contributing to furosemide's sustained diuretic and saluretic effect is its slow elimination, which is dependent on glomerular infiltration rate and tubular secretion, by the immature neonatal kidney (Aranda et al, 1978; Peterson et al, 1980). In addition, the nonrenal mechanisms of furosemide excretion noted in the adult (biliary and intestinal) appear to be inactive in the neonate (Tuck et al, 1983).

The treatment of furosemide-induced neonatal calculi rarely requires surgical intervention. The essential step is to reduce urinary calcium excretion, which can be achieved by withdrawing furosemide and beginning hydrochlorothiazide, which has a hypocalciuric effect (Noe et al, 1984). Effective medical management results in stone dissolution in the vast majority of cases. One group has recommended the prophylactic addition of hydrochlorothiazide to furosemide therapy, which has prevented neonatal calculus formation (Hufnagle et al, 1982).

Genitourinary Candidal Infections in the Neonate

The trend toward aggressive treatment of extremely low-birth-weight babies has led to an increase in the incidence

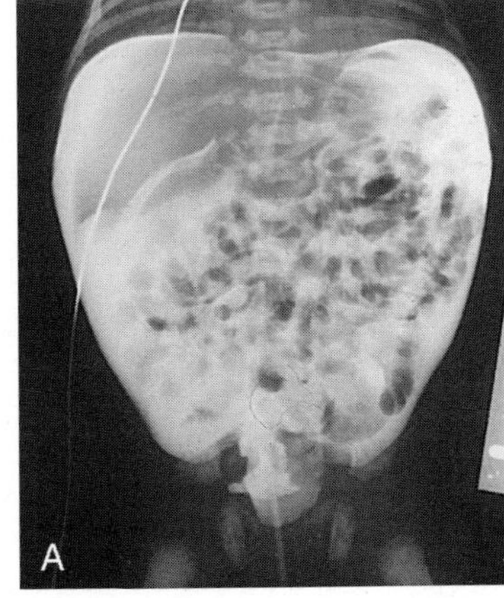

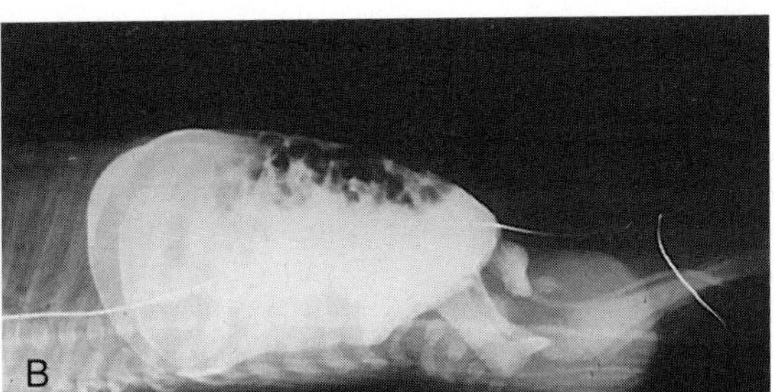

Figure 54–10. Cystographic demonstration of intraperitoneal extravasation following umbilical arterial catheter–related urachal laceration. *A*, Anteroposterior and *B*, cross-table lateral. (Reproduced with permission from Diamond DA, Ford C: J Urol 1989; 142:1543–1544.)

of systemic as well as genitourinary candidiasis in the NICU setting. It is estimated that 10% of neonates less than 1 kg and 4% less than 1.5 kg will have systemic candidiasis (Baley et al, 1981). This is of particular interest to the urologist because the kidney is the target organ most frequently involved (in up to 90%) in *Candida* septicemia (Michigan et al, 1976).

The susceptibility of the kidney to *Candida* seems to be related to a delayed inflammatory response to the fungus relative to other viscera and the ability of the *Candida* to gain access to the protected environment of the renal tubular lumen, in which it proliferates prior to reinvading the renal parenchyma (Pappu et al, 1984).

The neonatal risk factors include extreme immaturity, long-term ventilation, intravascular catheters, repeated courses of antibiotics, and total parenteral nutrition (Smith and Congdon, 1985). However, the diagnosis of candidemia can be a difficult one. Clinically, the suspicion of candidemia should be raised by the picture of bacterial sepsis, with urine or serum cultures positive for *Candida* (Kozinn et al, 1978). Renal candidiasis may be heralded by oliguria or hypertension (Pappu et al, 1984).

The diagnostic criteria for candidemia are indeterminate. Yet the issue is a critical one because of the potential toxicity of antifungal therapy. Some suggest that given *Candida*'s predilection for the urinary tract, a suprapubic aspirate or catheterized specimen of urine growing greater than 10,000 to 15,000 colonies/ml are diagnostic (Kozinn et al, 1978). Others have suggested that the most accurate means of diagnosing candiduria is through two positive cultures of urine sediments separated by 24 hours (Michigan, 1976). All authors seem to agree that a markedly positive urine culture for *Candida* in the setting of an indwelling bladder catheter is nondiagnostic. More recently, the detection of serum *Candida* antigens has been used for early diagnosis. Serum precipitin was reportedly positive in 83% of cases of renal candidiasis, and assays for the *Candida* antigen, mannan, have proved useful for diagnosing and following candiduria and candidemia (Kozinn et al, 1978; Schreiber et al, 1984). The initial management of systemic and urinary candidiasis entails the removal of all predisposing factors, such as intravascular lines, catheters, and broad-spectrum antibiotics. If lines cannot be removed, they should be changed. The mainstay of therapy thereafter entails systemic amphotericin B. The greatest concern with amphotericin B relates to its potential nephrotoxicity (Hermans and Keys, 1983). Thus, many authors suggest the combination of oral 5-fluorocytosine with amphotericin B, which appear to act synergistically (Rabinovich et al, 1974). The recommended duration of treatment varies. Some suggest three negative urine cultures and others the absence of mannan antigen prior to discontinuing therapy (Schreiber et al, 1984; Smith and Congdon, 1985). It is important to remember that the mortality rate of neonates with systemic candidemia is 63%, and thus, this condition must be treated aggressively (Pappu et al, 1984). The greatest challenge to the urologist is the presence of fungal ball formation within the collecting system, resulting in obstruction and often impaired renal function. Ultrasound is particularly useful in the early diagnosis of fungal ball formation. Percutaneous nephrostomy has been used to successfully manage obstructing fungal balls in the neonate (Mazer and Bartone, 1982). This approach avoids a major surgical procedure for the critically ill neonate, and allows the decompression and drainage of the upper tract. It provides one access to fungal material for a firm diagnosis and allows for direct irrigation with amphotericin B of the collecting system (Bartone et al, 1988). In addition, percutaneous guide wire manipulation has been used to disrupt obstructing fungal balls within the collecting system (Bartone et al, 1988). Open pyelotomy and anatrophic nephrolithotomy have been successfully performed in tiny neonates to remove the fungal casts, with placement of formal nephrostomy tubes for subsequent irrigation.

Renal Vein Thrombosis

RVT is the most frequently detected neonatal vascular anomaly. Although its true incidence is unknown, it is found in 1 of 150 to 1 of 250 autopsies.

The pathophysiology of RVT is related to the low arterial and venous pressures in the neonate, resulting in sluggish renal perfusion. Any decrease in the intravascular volume or a hypercoaguable state places the neonate at risk for RVT. Such predisposing clinical situations include dehydration; infection; vascular endothelial damage; a deficiency of antithrombin III, protein C, or protein S; and the presence of anticardiolipin antibodies (Corrigan, 1988; Contractor et al, 1992). The offspring of diabetic mothers are also at increased risk.

Although unilateral RVT rarely progresses to the contralateral side, RVT occurs bilaterally in 20% of patients (Belman et al, 1970). In bilateral cases, the thrombus may be caval in origin, particularly in patients with central venous catheters, or involve both renal veins simultaneously without caval involvement.

Primary RVT occurs suddenly in a previously normal neonate, whereas secondary RVT, which carries a worse prognosis, results from a known cause such as diarrhea with dehydration. In unilateral RVT, the thrombus originates peripherally in the small intrarenal branches of the renal vein (Rosenfield et al, 1980; Gonzalez et al, 1982).

The typical clinical picture is that of a firm, enlarging kidney accompanied by hematuria and proteinuria in an ill neonate. RVT accounts for more than 20% of all cases of neonatal gross hematuria that is due to hemorrhagic renal infarction. Anemia occurs secondary to hemolysis, hematuria, and the trapping of erythrocytes in the thrombus. Thrombocytopenia consistently occurs secondary to trapping of platelets in the thrombotic process. Its absence suggests a late diagnosis and a recovering phase of RVT. Although proteinuria occurs in neonatal RVT, it is not as prominent as in the adult. Azotemia is usually present even in unilateral thrombosis (Belman et al, 1970). Lower extremity edema may be present with inferior vena caval thrombosis.

The diagnosis of RVT cannot be made on clinical grounds alone. Ultrasound has become the standard diagnostic study and demonstrates an enlarged hyperechoic kidney with loss of the corticomedullary junction and sometimes hyperechoic streaks in the interlobular spaces (Lalmand et al, 1990). Direct visualization of the thrombus is diagnostic (Metreweli and Pearson, 1984; Sanders and Jequier, 1989). As the thrombotic process resolves, the kidney decreases in size and becomes more hypoechoic. Prominent collateral circulation and calcifications along the renal vein are late findings (Lund and Seeds, 1993). The vena cava must be carefully imaged and other associated anomalies such as adrenal hemorrhage noted (Veiga et al, 1992; Herman and Siegel, 1993; Orazi et al, 1993; Tran-Minh et al, 1994). Color Doppler imaging has added to the diagnostic capability of ultrasound and is of particular value in following thrombosis during therapy (Stringer et al, 1990; Alexander et al, 1993; Laplante et al, 1993; Fishman and Joseph, 1994). Cavography, although seldom necessary, is diagnostic in virtually all cases and allows for regional delivery of thrombolytic agents.

The treatment of RVT should begin with general supportive measures, including vigorous hydration, electrolyte balance, and broad-spectrum antibiotics. One should treat the underlying cause in secondary cases. Although 90% of patients with unilateral RVT suffer varying degrees of residual renal damage, mortality remains very low (Mocan et al, 1992). Therefore, aggressive anticoagulating or thrombolytic treatment in critically ill neonates that carries a risk for severe hemorrhagic complications is rarely indicated.

Unilateral RVT associated with a caval thrombus and bilateral RVT have more ominous prognoses and frequently lead to chronic renal failure, embolic complications, and death (Duncan et al, 1991). In such cases, treatment with heparin or thrombolytic therapy is indicated. The treatment of choice remains controversial. Heparin has been used extensively in the past for its activity against thrombin formation and platelet aggregation (Gal and Ransom, 1991). In prospective clinical trials, however, heparin has failed to substantially alter the natural history of RVT and complications have been significant (Nuss et al, 1994). The optimum role of heparin in RVT may be as an adjunct to thrombolytic therapy in preventing recurrent thrombosis.

Selective thrombolytic therapy offers the theoretical advantage of minimizing systemic effects while maximizing local fibrinolysis. Treatment should be initiated within 7 days of thrombus formation so that the fibrinolytic pathway can still be activated (Corrigan, 1988). Streptokinase, a nonspecific fibrinolytic protein, was one of the earliest agents used. It has been reported to be effective with reasonable morbidity when delivered locally to neonates and infants. Urokinase is also a nonspecific thrombolytic agent that directly converts plasminogen to plasmin in the circulation and within the thrombus. Regional and systemic urokinase has been used extensively in neonates (Vogelzang et al, 1988; Bromberg and Firlit, 1990; Duncan et al, 1991). Although no prospective studies have been conducted, a retrospective review suggested an improved functional long-term outcome of kidneys treated with urokinase versus those treated with conventional support measures in the neonatal period (Brun et al, 1993). Tissue plasminogen activator is a naturally occurring protein that enhances the binding of plasminogen to fibrin. The activated fibrin-bound plasminogen produces plasmin at the site of the clot, inducing thrombolysis. Because of this selective mechanism, the systemic thrombolytic effects are reduced (Levy et al, 1991). Recombinant tissue plasminogen activator has been used successfully in neonates with RVT (Nowak-Gottl et al, 1992; Dillon et al, 1993). It has also been reported to be successful in cases in which other anticoagulating and thrombolytic therapies had previously failed (Levy et al, 1991). Recombinant tissue plasminogen activator may become the treatment of choice for bilateral RVT and unilateral RVT associated with a vena caval thrombus, and in particular, for those neonates in whom systemic anticoagulation is contraindicated (Nowat-Gottl et al, 1992; Dillon et al, 1993). Surgical thrombectomy no longer has a role in the treatment of RVT.

Even in the most severe cases, aggressive supportive measures, including peritoneal dialysis and thrombolytic therapy, have resulted in excellent survival rates (Pritchard et al, 1985; Bromberg and Firlit, 1990).

Renal Artery Thrombosis

Historically, renal artery thrombosis has been regarded as a rare disorder, most commonly diagnosed in autopsy studies. The most common source of emboli has been the thrombosed ductus arteriosus.

Since the advent of umbilical artery catheterization, the incidence of renal artery thrombosis has increased significantly. In order to maintain patency and decrease the risk of catheter-related thrombosis, intermittent infusion of low-dose heparin or urokinase has become common practice (Bagnall et al, 1989; Ankola and Atakent, 1993; Fletcher et al, 1994).

Because renal artery thrombosis often occurs in conjunction with aortic thrombosis and other severe comorbidities, the clinical presentation is broad. Severe hypertension is common and constitutes a medical emergency. Neonates rapidly develop congestive heart failure, respiratory distress, and central nervous system distress if untreated. Hematuria, azotemia, volume depletion, salt wasting, and proteinuria are commonly present. Signs of lower extremity ischemia may appear with a large aortic thrombus.

The diagnosis is made on clinical grounds and confirmed with real-time and Doppler sonography. Color Doppler sonography may help differentiate between partial and complete vascular occlusion. It is also useful in evaluating the results of anticoagulating or thrombolytic therapy by quantifying the recovery of flow (Colburn et al, 1992; Deeg et al, 1992). Radionucleotide imaging may confirm the diagnosis of renal artery thrombosis and provide a baseline determination of differential renal function. Angiography is the most accurate means of establishing the diagnosis of renal artery thrombosis, but because of its associated risks, angiography is restricted to those cases in which other studies are inconclusive (Colburn et al, 1992).

The treatment of renal artery thrombosis should be individualized. Supportive measures alone or thrombolytic therapy and surgical thrombectomy or revascularization have all been reported with varying degrees of success. Aggressive medical management with antihypertensives, diuretics, and peritoneal dialysis has yielded good results, with recovery of renal function in some cases (Malin et al, 1985). Selective intra-arterial or systemic thrombolysis with streptokinase, urokinase, or recombinant tissue plasminogen activator has been successful as first-line treatment. Surgical thrombectomy is a viable treatment alternative for those neonates with associated aortic thrombosis when thrombolytic therapy is ineffective or contraindicated (Payne et al, 1989; Colburn et al, 1992). Revascularization is an uncommon option in selected cases. Nephrectomy is reserved for those patients with hypertension that is refractory to medical management.

Long-term follow-up of patients with unilateral renal artery thrombosis without azotemia indicates that this is a self-limited process. Hypertension usually resolves, but renal growth may be impaired even when blood flow has been successfully restored (Seibert et al, 1987).

Renal Cortical and Renal Medullary Necrosis

Renal cortical and medullary necrosis results from ischemic injuries to the kidney in the absence of vascular occlusion. Severe perinatal hypoxemia, massive blood loss, septicemia, and hemolytic disease are the main pathophysiologic mechanisms. This disorder is generally fatal, and the diagnosis is rarely made in a live infant. In a recent study, 82 cases of renal cortical and medullary necrosis were found among 1638 infant autopsies (Lerner et al, 1992). The lesion was cortical in 34%, medullary in 28%, and combined in 37%. Forty infants carried the diagnosis of congestive heart failure, and the incidence of prematurity, respiratory distress syndrome, bleeding diathesis, and sepsis was high.

The clinical features include pallor, flaccidity, cyanosis, and oliguria. In the acute stage, thrombocytopenia, anemia, azotemia, and hematuria are common. The diagnosis is established by Doppler ultrasound showing a patent renal artery and vein, and is confirmed by renal biopsy. Unlike adults with cortical necrosis, the juxtamedullary nephrons in infant kidneys are more severely affected than the outer cortical nephrons (Rodriguez-Soriano et al, 1992). This factor may be due to the lower perfusion of the outer renal cortex in infants, which renders it more resistant to ischemia.

Treatment with aggressive supportive measures, including broad-spectrum antibiotics and peritoneal dialysis, has been successful in a small percentage of patients. Among survivors, creatinine clearance is consistently decreased and nephrocalcinosis has been described (Rodriguez-Soriano et al, 1982).

Adrenal Hemorrhage

The large size and vascularity of the neonatal adrenal gland places it at risk for hemorrhagic complications. Adrenal hemorrhage is almost always associated with prolonged labor, perinatal anoxia, bradycardia, sepsis or bleeding disorders, and hypoprothrombinemia. Although 10% of cases are bilateral, the majority of lesions occur on the right side. A likely explanation is that sudden increases in intra-abdominal pressures during prolonged labor or aggressive resuscitative efforts are more readily transmitted from the vena cava to the short right adrenal vein, whereas they are dampened by the longer left adrenal vein. Spontaneous bleeding has been noted prenatally on routine maternal ultrasound during the third trimester (Burbige, 1993). One must maintain a high index of suspicion for a bleeding neuroblastoma.

The clinical features of adrenal hemorrhage include a palpable abdominal mass, jaundice, and anemia. Scrotal hematoma is an unusual clinical presentation (Putnam, 1989; Giacoia and Cravens, 1990) When azotemia and gross hematuria are present, one must suspect a coexistent RVT.

The initial sonographic findings usually demonstrate a sonolucent mass superior to the kidney, sometimes displacing it inferiorly. As the hematoma organizes and is reabsorbed, the sonographic pattern varies and may appear as a complex cystic structure (Cohen et al, 1986). Serial ultrasound examinations show a progressive diminution in size and disappearance of the mass over a period of weeks (Eklof et al, 1986) (Fig. 54–11). On plain x-ray films, peripheral, shell-like calcifications are typical of adrenal hemorrhage, whereas stippled calcifications are suggestive of neuroblastoma. Serial ultrasound examinations and serum and

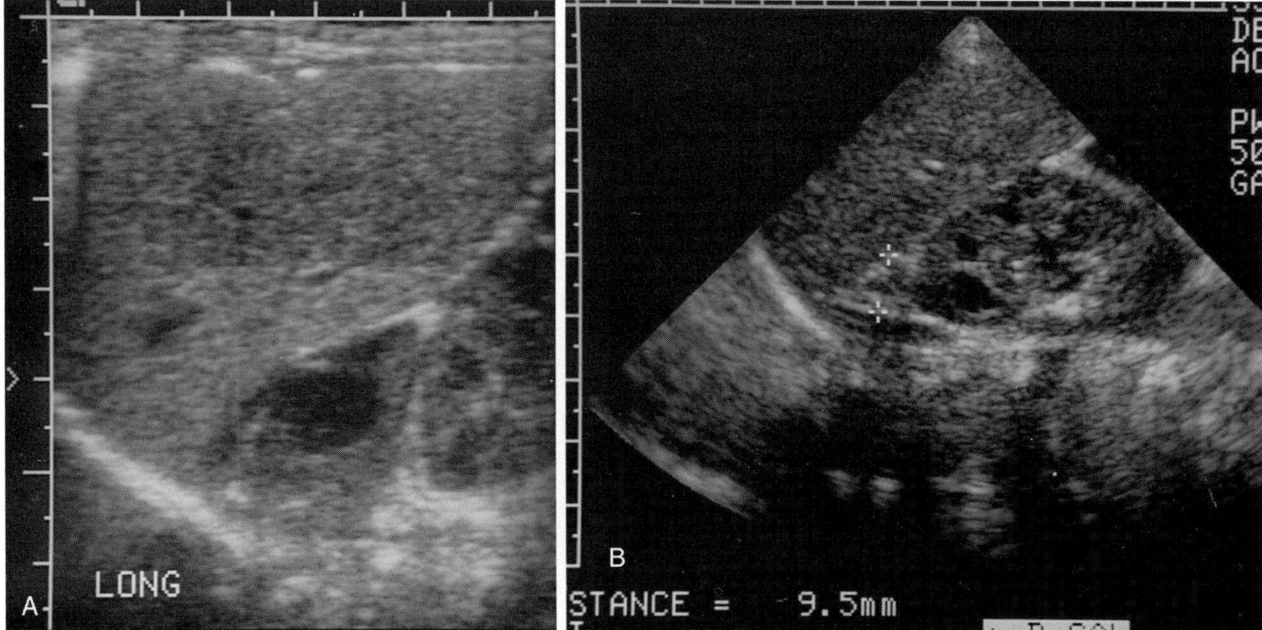

Figure 54–11. *A,* Ultrasound of neonatal adrenal hemorrhage with central sonolucency. *B,* Follow-up study at 2 months demonstrating marked improvement (cursors). (Reproduced with permission from R. L. Lebowitz.)

Weingarten JL, Garofalo FA, Cromie WJ: Bilateral synchronous neonatal torsion of spermatic cord. Urology 1990; 25:135–136.

Neonatal Abdominal Mass

Avni EF, Thoua Y, Lalmand B, et al: Multicystic dysplastic kidney: Natural history from in utero diagnosis and postnatal followup. J Urol 1987; 138:1420–1424.
Bernstein GT, Mandell J, Lebowitz RL, et al: Ureteropelvic junction obstruction. J Urol 1988; 140:1216–1221.
Birkin G, King D, Vane D, Lloyd T: Renal cell carcinoma arising in a multicystic dysplastic kidney. J Pediatr Surg 1985; 20:619–621.
Blask ARN, Sanders RC, Gearhart JP: Obstructed ureterovaginal anomalies: Demonstration with sonography. Radiology 1991; 179:79–83.
Carey PO, Howards SS: Multicystic dysplastic kidneys and diagnostic confusion on renal scan. J Urol 1988; 139:83–84.
Caty MG, Shamberger RC: Abdominal tumors in infancy and childhood. Pediatr Clin North Am 1993; 40:1253–1271.
Cook TT, Marshall VF: Hydrocolpos causing urinary obstruction. J Urol 1964; 92:127–132.
DeKlerk DP, Marshall FF, Jeffs RD: Multicystic dysplastic kidney. J Urol 1977; 118:306–308.
Diamond DA: Hydrometrocolpos. Society for Pediatric Urology Newsletter, March, 1988.
Dimmick JE, Johnson HW, Coleman GU, Carter M: Wilms tumorlet, nodular renal blastema and multicystic renal dysplasia. J Urol 1989; 142:484–485.
Donn SM, Faix RG: Transillumination in neonatal diagnosis. Clin Perinatol 1985; 12:3–20.
Gordon AC, Thomas DFM, Arthur RJ, Irving HC: Multicystic dysplastic kidney: Is nephrectomy still appropriate? J Urol 1988; 140:1231–1234.
Hahn-Petersen J, Kvist N, Neilsen OH: Hydrometrocolpos: Current views on pathogenesis and management. J Urol, 1984; 132:537–540.
Hanna MK, Jeffs RD, Sturgess JM, Barkin M: Ureteral structure and ultrastructure. Part 1. The normal human ureter. J Urol 1976; 116:718–724.
Hanna MK, Jeffs RD, Sturgess JM, Barkin M: Ureteral structure and ultrastructure. Part II. Congenital ureteropelvic junction obstruction and primary obstructive megaureter. J Urol 1976; 116:725–730.
Hartman GE, Shochat SJ: Abdominal mass lesions in the newborn: Diagnosis and treatment. Clin Perinatol 1989; 16:123–135.
Howell CG, Othersen HB, Kiviat NE, et al: Therapy and outcome in 51 children with mesoblastic nephroma: A report of the National Wilms' Tumor Study. J Pediatr Surg 1982; 17:826–830.
Hrabovsky EE, Othersen HB Jr, deLorimier A, et al: Wilms' tumor in the neonate: A report from the National Wilms' Tumor Study. J Pediatr Surg 1986; 21:385–387.
Kissane JM, Dehner LP: Renal tumors and tumor-like lesions in pediatric patients. Pediatr Nephrol 1992; 6:365–382.
Lebowitz RL, Griscom NT: Neonatal hydronephrosis: 146 cases. Radiol Clin North Am 1977; 15:49–59.
Longino LA, Martin LW: Abdominal masses in the newborn infant. Pediatrics 1958; 21:596–604.
McVicar M, Margouleff D, Chandra M: Diagnosis and imaging of the fetal and neonatal abdominal mass: An integrated approach. Adv Pediatr 1991; 38:135–149.
Melicow MM, Uson AC: Palpable abdominal masses in infants and children: A report based on a review of 653 cases. J Urol 1959; 81:705–710.
Murphy JP, Holder TM, Ashcraft KW, et al: Ureteropelvic junction obstruction in the newborn. J Pediatr Surg 1984; 19:642–648.
Nguyen L, Youssef S, Guttman FM, et al: Hydrometrocolpos in neonate due to distal vaginal atresia. J Pediatr Surg 1984; 19:510–514.
Pathak IG, Williams DI: Multicystic and cystic dysplastic kidneys. Br J Urol 1964; 36:318–331.
Perlman M, Williams J: Detection of renal anomalies by abdominal palpation in newborn infants. BMJ 1976; 2:347–349.
Raffensperger J, Abousleiman A: Abdominal masses in children under one year of age. Surgery, 1968; 63:514–521.
Robson WJ, Rudy SM, Johnston JH: Pelviureteric obstruction in infancy. J Pediatr Surg 1976; 11:57–61.
Sanders RC, Hartman DS: The sonographic distinction between neonatal multicystic kidney and hydronephrosis. Radiology 1984; 151:621–625.
Schneider KM, Becker JM, Krasna IH: Neonatal neuroblastoma. Pediatrics 1965; 36:359–366.
Sheldon CA, Duckett JW, Snyder HM III: Evolution in the management of infant pyeloplasty. J Pediatr Surg 1992; 27:501–505.
Snyder HM III, Lebowitz RL, Colodny AH, et al: Ureteropelvic junction obstruction in children. Urol Clin North Am 1980; 7:273–290.
Stuck KJ, Koff SA, Silver TM: Ultrasonic features of multicystic dysplastic kidney: Expanded diagnostic criteria. Radiology 1982; 143:217–221.
Susskind MR, Kim KS, King LR: Hypertension and multicystic kidney. Urology, 1989; 34:362–366.
Uson AC, Cox LA, Lattimer JK: Hydronephrosis in infants and children. JAMA, 1968; 205:71–74.
Velchik MG: Radionuclide imaging of the urinary tract. Urol Clin North Am 1985; 12:603–631.
Vinocur L, Slovis TL, Perlmutter AD, et al: Followup studies of multicystic dysplastic kidneys. Radiology 1988; 167:311–315.
Vujanic GM: Congenital cystic mesoblastic nephroma: A rare cystic renal tumor of childhood. Scand J Urol Nephrol 1992; 26:315–317.
Weber T, Sotelo-Avila C, Gale G: Cystic neuroblastoma in a newborn. J Pediatr Surg 1993; 28:1603–1604.
Wedge JJ, Grosfeld JL, Smith JP: Abdominal masses in the newborn: 63 cases. J Urol 1971; 106:770–775.
Williams DI, Karlaftis CM: Hydronephrosis due to pelvi-ureteric obstruction in the newborn. Br J Urol 1966; 38:138–144.
Wilson DA: Ultrasound screening for abdominal masses in the neonatal period. Am J Dis Child 1982; 136:147–151.
Zach TL, Cifuentes RF, Strom RL: Congenital mesoblastic nephroma, hemorrhagic shock, and disseminated intravascular coagulation in a newborn infant. Am J Perinatol 1991; 8:203–205.

Neonatal Urinary Ascites

Adzick NS, Harrison MR, Flake AW, deLorimier AA: Urinary extravasation in the fetus with obstructive uropathy. J Pediatr Surg 1985; 20:608–615.
Clarke HS Jr, Mills ME, Parres JA, Kropp KA: The hyponatremia of neonatal urinary ascites: Clinical observations, experimental confirmation and proposed mechanism. J Urol 1993; 150:778–781.
Cass A, Khan AU, Smith S, et al: Neonatal perirenal urinary extravasation with posterior urethral valves. J Urol 1973; 18:258.
Diamond DA, Ford C: Neonatal bladder rupture: A complication of umbilical artery catheterization. J Urol 1989; 142:1543–1544.
Garrett RA, Franken EA Jr: Neonatal ascites: Perirenal extravasation with bladder outlet obstruction. J Urol 1969; 102:627–632.
Greenfield SP, Hensle TW, Berdon WE, Geringer AM: Urinary extravasation in the newborn with the posterior urethral valves. J Pediatr Surg 1982; 17:751–756.
Griscom NT, Colodny AH, Rosenberg HK, et al: Diagnostic aspects of neonatal ascites: Report of 27 cases. AJR 1977; 128:961–970.
Hepworth RC, Milstein JM: The transected urachus: An unusual cause of neonatal ascites. Pediatrics 1984; 5:397–400.
Kay R, Brereton RJ, Johnston JH: Urinary ascites in the newborn. Br J Urol 1980; 52:451–454.
Krane RJ, Retik AB: Neonatal perirenal urinary extravasation. J Urol 1974; 111:96–99.
MacPherson RI, Gordon L, Bradford BF: Neonatal urinomas: Imaging considerations. Pediatr. Radiol 1984; 14:396–399.
Mann CM, Leape LL, Holder TM: Neonatal urinary ascites: A report of 2 cases of unusual etiology and a review of the literature. J Urol 1974; 111:124–128.
Mitchell ME, Garrett RA: Perirenal urinary extravasation associated with urethral valves in infants. J Urol 1980; 124:688–691.
Redman JF, Seibert JJ, Arnold W: Urinary ascites in children owing to extravasation of urine from the bladder. J Urol 1979; 122:409–411.
Reha WC, Gibbons MD: Neonatal ascites and ureteral valves. Urology 1989; 33:468–471.
Rittenberg MH, Hulbert WC, Snyder HM III, Duckett JW: Protective factors in posterior urethral valves. J Urol 1988; 140:993–996.
Scott TW: Urinary ascites secondary to posterior urethral valves. J Urol 1976; 116:87–91.
Sullivan MJ, Lackner H, Banowsky LHW: Intraperitoneal extravasation of urine: BUN/serum creatinine disproportion. JAMA 1972; 221:491–492.
Tank ES, Carey TC, Seifert AL: Management of neonatal urinary ascites. Urology 1980; 26:270–273.
Trulock TS, Finnerty DP, Woodard JR: Neonatal bladder rupture: Case report and review of literature. J Urol 1985; 133:271–273.
Wasnick RJ: Neonatal urinary ascites secondary to ureteropelvic junction obstruction. Urology 1987; 30:470–471.

Williams DI, Eckstein HB: Obstructive valves in the posterior urethra. J Urol 1965; 93:236–246.

Evaluation of the Newborn with Ambiguous Genitalia

Camacho AM, Migeon CJ: Testosterone excretion and production rate in adults and in patients with congenital adrenal hyperplasia. J Clin Endocrinol 1996; 26:893–896.

Diamond DA: Intersex disorders *In* Stein BS, Caldamone AA, Smith JA Jr, eds: Clinical Urologic Practice. New York, Norton, 1995, pp 1547–1565.

Donahoe PK, Powell DM, Lee MM: Clinical management of intersex abnormalities. Curr Probl Surg 1991; 28:513–579.

Feldman KW, Smith DW: Fetal phallic growth and penile standards for newborn male infants. J Pediatr 1975; 86:395–398.

Flatau E, Josefsberg Z, Reisner SH, et al: Penile size in the newborn infant. J Pediatr 1975; 87:663–664.

Greenfield SP, Rutigliano E, Steinhardt G, Elder JS: Genitourinary malformations and maternal cocaine abuse. Urology 1991; 37:455–459.

Horowitz M, Glassberg KI: Ambiguous genitalia: Diagnosis, evaluation and treatment. Urol Radiol 1992; 24:306–318.

Rajfer J, Walsh PC: The incidence of intersexuality in patients with hypospadias and cryptorchidism. J Urol 1976; 116:769–770.

Neonatal Intensive Care Unit–Related Complications

Umbilical Arterial Catheter–Related Complications

Bauer SB, Feldman SM, Gellis SS, Retik AB: Neonatal hypertension: A complication of umbilical-artery catheterization. N Engl J Med 1975; 293:1032–1033.

Clark JM, Jung AL: Umbilical artery catheterization by a cutdown procedure. Pediatrics 1977; 59:1036–1040.

Cochrane WD, Davis HT, Smith CA: Advantages and complications of umbilical artery catheterization in the newborn. Pediatrics 1968; 42:769–777.

Diamond DA, Ford C: Neonatal bladder rupture: A complication of umbilical artery catheterization. J Urol 1989; 142:1543–1544.

Kitterman JA, Phibbs RH, Tooley WH: Catheterization of umbilical vessels in newborn infants. Pediatr Clin North Am 1970; 17:895–912.

Krueger TC, Neblett WW, O'Neill JA, et al: Management of aortic thrombosis secondary to umbilical artery catheters in neonates. J Pediatr Surg 1985; 20:328–332.

Lofland GK, Russo P, Sethia B, DeLeval M: Aortic thrombosis in neonates and infants. Ann Surg 1988; 207:743–745.

Marsh JL, King W, Barrett C, Fonkalsrud EW:Serious complications after umbilical artery catheterization for neonatal monitoring. Arch Surg 1975; 110:1203–1208.

O'Neill JA Jr, Neblett WW III, Born ML: Management of major thromboembolic complications of umbilical artery catheters. J Pediatr Surg 1981; 16:972–978.

Plumer LB, Mendoza SA, Kaplan GW: Hypertension in infancy: The case for aggressive management. J Urol 1975; 113:555–557.

Redman JF, Seibert JJ, Arnold W: Urinary ascites in children owing to extravasation of urine from the bladder. J Urol 1979; 122:409–411.

Neonatal Nephrolithiasis

Adams ND, Rowe JC: Nephrocalcinosis. Clin Perinatol 1992; 19:179–195.

Aranda JV, Perez J, Sitar DS, et al: Pharmacokinetic disposition and protein binding of furosemide in newborn infants. J Pediatr 1978; 93:507–511.

Ezzedeen F, Adelman RD, Ahlfors CE: Renal calcification in preterm infants: Pathophysiology and longterm sequelae. J Pediatr 1988; 113:532–539.

Gilsanz V, Fernal W, Reid BS, et al: Nephrolithiasis in premature infants. Radiology 1985; 154:107–110.

Hufnagle KG, Khan SN, Penn D, et al: Renal calcifications: A complication of long term furosemide therapy in preterm infants. Pediatrics, 1982; 70:360–363.

Katz ME, Karlowicz MG, Adelman RD, et al: Nephrocalcinosis in very low birth weight neonates: Sonographic patterns, histologic characteristics and clinical risk factors. J Ultrasound Med 1994; 13:777–782.

Noe HN, Bryant JF, Roy S III, Stapleton SB: Urolithiasis in pre-term neonates associated with furosemide therapy. J Urol 1984; 132:93–94.

Peterson RG, Simmons MA, Rumack BH, et al: Pharmacology of furosemide in the premature newborn infant. J Pediatr 1980; 97:139–143.

Savage ML, Wilkinson AR, Baum JD, Roberton NRC: Furosemide in respiratory distress syndrome. Arch Dis Child 1975; 50:709–713.

Tuck S, Morselli P, Broquaire M, Vert P: Plasma and urinary kinetics of furosemide in newborn infants. J Pediatr 1983; 103:481–485.

Genitourinary Candidal Infections in the Neonate

Baley JE, Annable WL, Kleigman RM: Candida endophthalmitis in the premature infant. J Pediatr 1981; 98:458–461.

Bartone FF, Hurwitz RS, Rojas EL, et al: The role of percutaneous nephrostomy in the management of obstructing candidiasis of the urinary tract in infants. J Urol 1988; 140:338–341.

Hermans PE, Keys TF: Antifungal agents used for deep-seated mycotic infections. Mayo Clinic Proc 1983; 58:223–231.

Kozinn PJ, Taschdjian CL, Goldberg PK, et al: Advances in the diagnosis of renal candidiasis. J Urol 1978; 119:184–187.

Mazer MJ, Bartone FF: Percutaneous antegrade diagnosis and management of candidiasis of the upper urinary tract. Urol Clin North Am 1982; 9:157–164.

Michigan S: Genitourinary fungal infections. J Urol 1976; 116:390–397.

Pappu LD, Purohit DM, Bradford BF, et al: Primary renal candidiasis in two preterm neonates. Am J Dis Child 1984; 138:923–926.

Rabinovich S, Shaw BD, Bryant T, Donta ST: Effects of 5-fluorocytosine and amphotericin B on *Candida albicans* infection in mice. J Infect Dis 1974; 130:28–31.

Schreiber JR, Maynard E, Lew MA: Candida antigen detection in two premature neonates with disseminated candidiasis. Pediatrics 1984; 74:838–841.

Smith H, Congdon P: Neonatal systemic candidiasis. Arch Dis Chil 1985; 60:365–369.

Renal Vein Thrombosis

Alexander AA, Merton DA, Mitchell DG, et al: Rapid diagnosis of neonatal renal vein thrombosis using color doppler imaging. J Clin Ultrasound 1993; 21:468–471.

Bromberg WD, Firlit CR: Fibrinolytic therapy for renal vein thrombosis in the child. J Urol 1990; 143:86–88.

Belman AB, Susmano DF, Burden JJ, et al: Non-operative treatment of unilateral renal vein thrombosis in the newborn. JAMA 1970; 211:1165–1168.

Brun P, Beaufils F, Pillion G et al: Thrombosis of the renal veins. Ann Pediatr 1993; 40:75–80.

Contractor S, Hiatt M, Kosmin M, et al: Neonatal thrombosis with anticardiolipin antibody in baby and mother. Am J Perinatol 1992; 9:409–410.

Corrigan JJ Jr: Neonatal thrombosis and the thrombolytic system: Pathophysiology and therapy. Am J Pediatr Hematol Oncol 1988; 10:83–91.

Dillon PW, Fox PS, Berg CJ, et al: Recombinant tissue plasminogen activator for neonatal and pediatric vascular thrombolytic therapy. J Pediatr Surg 1993; 28:1264–1269.

Duncan BW, Adzick NS, Longaker MT, et al: In utero arterial embolism from renal vein thrombosis with successful postnatal thrombolytic therapy. J Pediatr Surg 1991; 26:741–743,

Duncan RE, Evans AT, Martin LW: Natural history and treatment of renal vein thrombosis in children. J Pediatr Surg 1977; 12:639–645.

Fishman JE, Joseph RC: Renal vein thrombosis in utero: Duplex sonography in diagnosis and follow up. Pediatr Radiol 1994; 24:135–136.

Gal P, Ransom L: Neonatal thrombosis: Treatment with heparin and thrombolytics. DICP 1991; 25:853–856.

Gonzalez R, Schwartz S, Sheldon C, et al: Bilateral renal vein thrombosis in infancy and childhood. Urol Clin North Am 1982; 9:279–283.

Herman TE, Siegel MJ: Special imaging casebook. Denouement and discussion: Neonatal adrenal hemorrhage and renal vein thrombosis. J Perinatol 1993; 8:325–328.

Lalmand B, Avni EF, Nasr A, et al: Perinatal renal vein thrombosis. Sonographic demonstration. J Ultrasound Med 1990; 9:437–442.

Laplante S, Patriquin HB, Robitaille P, et al: Renal vein thrombosis in children: Evidence of early flow recovery with Doppler ultrasound. Pediatr Radiol 1993; 189:37–42.

Levy M, Benson LN, Burrows PE, et al: Tissue plasminogen activator for the treatment of thromboembolism in infants and children. J Pediatr 1991; 118:467–472.

Lund P, Seeds JW: Diagnosis: Renal vein and inferior vena cava thrombosis in a newborn. J Ultrasound Med 1993; 12:248.

Metreweli C, Pearson E: Echographic diagnosis of neonatal renal vein thrombosis. Pediatr Radiol 1984; 14:105–108.

Mocan H, Beattie T, Murphy A: Renal venous thrombosis in infancy: Long term follow up. Pediatr Nephrol 1992; 5:45–49.

Nowak-Gottl U, Schwabe D, Schneider W, et al: Thrombolysis with recombinant tissue-type plasminogen activator in renal venous thrombosis in infancy. Letter to the editor. Lancet 1992; 340:1105.

Nuss R, Hays T, Manco-Johnson M: Efficacy and safety of heparin anticoagulation for neonatal renal vein thrombosis. Am J Pediatr Hematol Oncol 1994; 16:127–131.

Orazi C, Fariello G, Malena S, et al: Renal vein thrombosis and adrenal hemorrhage in the newborn: Ultrasound evaluation of 4 cases. J Clin Ultrasound 1993; 21:163–169.

Pritchard SL, Culham JAG, Rogers PCJ: Low dose fibrinolytic therapy in infants. J Pediatr 1985; 106:594–598.

Rosenfield AT, Zeman RK, Cronan JJ, et al: Ultrasound in experimental and clinical renal vein thrombosis. Radiology 1980; 137:735–741.

Sanders LD, Jequier S: Ultrasound demonstration of prenatal renal vein thrombosis. Pediatr Radiol 1989; 19:133–135.

Stringer DA, Krysil D, Manson C, et al: The value of doppler sonography in the detection of major vessel thrombosis in the neonatal abdomen. Pediatr Radiol 1990; 21:30–33.

Tran-Minh VA, Genin G, Pracros J-P, et al: Coexisting calcified inferior vena cava thrombus and adrenal hemorrhage in the neonate: Report of three cases. Clin Ultrasound 1994; 22:103–108.

Veiga PA, Springate JE, Brody AS, et al: Coexistence of renal vein thrombosis and adrenal hemorrhage in two newborns. Clin Pediatr 1992; 31:174–176.

Vogelzang RL, Moel DI, Cohn RA, et al: Acute renal vein thrombosis: Successful treatment with intraarterial urokinase. Radiology 1988; 169:681–682.

Renal Artery Thrombosis

Ankola PA, Atakent YS: Effect of adding heparin in very low concentration to the infusate to prolong the patency of umbilical artery catheters. Am J Perinatol 1993; 3:229–232.

Bagnall HA, Gomperts E, Atkinson JB: Continuous infusion of low-dose urokinase in the treament of central venous catheter thrombosis in infants and children. Pediatrics 1989; 83:963–966.

Colburn MD, Gelabert HA, Quinones-Baldrich W: Neonatal aortic thrombosis. Surgery 1992; 111:21–28.

Deeg KH, Wolfel D, Rupprecht TH: Diagnosis of neonatal aortic thrombosis by colour coded Doppler sonography. Pediatr Radiol 1992; 22:62–63.

Fletcher MA, Brown DR, Landers S, Seguin J: Umbilical arterial catheter use: Report of an audit conducted by the study group for complications of perinatal care. Am J Perinatol 1994; 2:94–99.

Malin SW, Baumgart S, Rosenberg HK, et al: Non-surgical management of obstructive aortic thrombosis complicated by renovascular hypertension in the neonate. J Pediatr 1985; 106:630–634.

Payne RM, Martin TC, Bower RJ, et al: Management and follow up of arterial thrombosis in the neonatal period. J Pediatr 1989; 114:853–858.

Seibert JJ, Taylor BJ, Williamson SL, et al: Sonographic detection of neonatal artery thrombosis. Clinical correlation. AJR 1987; 148:965–968.

Renal Cortical and Renal Medullary Necrosis

Lerner GR, Kurnetz R, Bernstein J, et al: Renal cortical and renal medullary necrosis in the first three months of life. Pediatr Nephrol 1992; 6:516–518.

Rodriguez-Soriano J, Vallo A, Bilbao F, et al: Different functional characteristics of residual nephrons in infantile versus adult diffuse cortical necrosis. Int J Pediatr Nephrol 1982; 3:71–77.

Adrenal Hemorrhage

Burbige K: Prenatal adrenal hemorrhage confirmed by postnatal surgery. J Urol 1993; 150:1867–1869.

Cohen EK, Daneman A, Stringer DA, et al: Focal adrenal hemorrhage: A new ultrasound appearance. Radiology 1986; 161:631–633.

Eklof O, Mortensson W, Sandstedt B: Suprarenal hematoma versus neuroblastoma complicated by hemorrhage—a diagnostic dilemma in the newborn. Acta Radiol 1986; 27:3–10.

Giacoia GP, Coaveus JD: Neonatal adrenal hemorrhage presenting as scrotal hematoma. J Urol 1990; 143:567–568.

Hosoda Y, Miyano T, Kimura K, et al: Characteristics and management of patients with fetal neuroblastoma. J Pediatr Surg 1992; 27:623–625.

Putnam MH: Neonatal adrenal hemorrhage presenting as a right scrotal mass. (Letter.) JAMA 1989; 261:2958.

Renal Failure in the Neonate

Blowey DL, McFarland K, Alon U, et al: Peritoneal dialysis in the neonatal period: Outcome data. J Perinatol 1993; 8:59–64.

Chevalier RL, Campbell F, Norman A: Prognostic factors in neonatal acute renal failure. Pediatrics 1984; 74:265–272.

El-Dahr SS, Lewy JE: Urinary tract obstruction and infection in the neonate. Clin Perinatol 1992; 19:213–222.

Ellis EN, Arnold WC: Use of urinary indexes in renal failure in the newborn. Am J Dis Child 1982; 136:615–617.

Karlowicz MG, Adelman RD: Acute renal failure in the neonate. Clin Perinatol 1992; 19:139–158.

Kojima T, Kobayashi T, Matsuzaki S, et al: Effects of perinatal asphyxia and myoglobinuria on development of acute, neonatal renal failure. Arch Dis Child 1985; 60:908–912.

Latta K, Krull F, Wilken M, et al: Continous arteriovenous haemofiltration in critically ill children. Pediatr Nephrol 1994; 8:334–337.

Matthews DE, West KW, Rescorla FJ, et al: Peritoneal dialysis in the first 60 days of life. J. Pediatr Surg 1990; 25:110–116.

Merlob P, Litwin A, Lazar L, et al: Neonatal ABO incompatibility complicated by hemoglobinuria and acute renal failure. Clin Pediatr 1990; 29:219–222.

Ronco C, Brendolan A, Bragantini L, et al: Treatment of acute renal failure in newborns by continuous arterio-venous hemofiltration. Kidney Int 1968; 29:908–915.

Rutledge SL, Havens PL, Haymond MW, et al: Neonatal hemodialysis: Effective therapy in the encephalopathy of inborn errors of metabolism. J Pediatr 1990; 116:125–128.

Sadowski RH, Harmon WE, Jabs K: Acute hemodialysis of infants weighing less than five kilograms. Kidney Int 1994; 45:903–906.

Schor N, Ichikawa I, Rennke HG, et al: Pathophysiology of altered glomerular function in aminoglycoside-treated rats. Kidney Int 1981; 19:288–296.

Stapleton FB, Jones DP, Green RS: Acute renal failure in neonates: Incidence, etiology and outcome. Pediatr Nephrol 1987; 1:314–320.

Steele BT, Vigneux A, Blatz S, et al: Acute peritoneal dialysis in infants weighing <1500 gm. J Pediatr 1987; 110:126–129.

Tassilo VL, Salusky JB, Boechart I, et al: Five years' experience with continuous ambulatory or continuous cycling peritoneal dialysis in children. J Pediatr 1987; 111:513–518.

Neonatal Assessment and Initial Management of Major Urologic Conditions

Classic Bladder Exstrophy

Diamond DA, ed: Management of cloacal exstrophy. Dialogues in Pediatric Urology 1990; 13.

Diamond DA, Jeffs RD: Cloacal exstrophy: A 22 year experience. J Urol 1985; 133:779–782.

Gearhart JP, Jeffs RD: Exstrophy of the bladder, epispadias and other bladder anomalies. *In* Walsh PC, Retik AB, Stamey TA, Vaughan ED Jr, eds: Campbell's Urology, 6th ed. Philadelphia, W. B. Saunders Company, 1992, pp 1772–1821.

Howell C, Caldamone AA, Snyder HM III: Optimal management of cloacal exstrophy. J Pediatr Surg 1983; 18:365–369.

Hurwitz RS, Manzoni GAM, Ransley PG, Stephens FD: Cloacal exstrophy: A report of 34 cases. J Urol 1987; 138:1060–1064.

Husmann DA, McLorie GA, Churchill BM: Phallic reconstruction in cloacal exstrophy. J Urol 1989; 142:563–564.

Prune-Belly Syndrome

Adebonojo FO: Dysplasia of the abdominal musculature with multiple congenital anomalies; prune belly or triad syndrome. J Natl Med Assoc 1973; 65:327.

Woodard JR: Prune-belly syndrome *In* Walsh PC, Retik AB, Stamey TA, Vaughan ED Jr, eds: Campbell's Urology, 6th ed. Philadelphia, W. B. Saunders Company, 1992, pp 1851–1871.

Myelomeningocele

Bauer SB: Neurogenic vesical dysfunction in children *In* Walsh PC, Retik AB, Stamey TA, Vaughan ED Jr, eds: Campbell's Urology, 6th ed. Philadelphia, W. B. Saunders Company, 1992, pp 1634–1668.

Cerniglia F: Update: Management of the newborn with myelodysplasia. Dialogues in Pediatric Urology 1994; 17.

Imperforate Anus

Belman AB, King LR: Urinary tract abnormalities associated with imperforate anus. J Urol 1972; 108:823–824.

McLorie GA, Sheldon CA, Fleisher M, Churchill BM: The genitourinary system in patients with imperforate anus. J Pediatr Surg 1987; 22:1100–1104.

Parrott TS, Woodard JR: Importance of cystourethrography in neonates with imperforate anus. Urology 1979; 13:607–609.

55
RENAL FUNCTION IN THE FETUS, NEONATE, AND CHILD

Robert L. Chevalier, M.D.
Stuart S. Howards, M.D.

The development of renal function in the fetus and neonate can be viewed as a continuing evolution of interdependent morphologic and physiologic stages. During gestation, the functional changes are determined by increases in nephron number, growth, and maturation, while homeostasis of the fetus is maintained predominantly by the placenta. At birth, the kidney must suddenly assume this role that was performed by the mother. The kidney's response to this demand is governed to a great extent by its anatomic development (gestational age at delivery), and thus, important functional differences are seen in the premature and full-term neonate.

In this chapter, we review the anatomic and functional aspects of fetal renal development, postnatal functional development, the evaluation of postnatal renal function, and the hormonal control of renal function during development through childhood.

Original studies by Dr. Chevalier were supported by an Established Investigatorship of the American Heart Association and by NIH grants AM25727, HL40209, DK40558, DK44756, DK45179, and HD28810.

ANATOMIC STAGES OF DEVELOPMENT

The major morphogenic stages of the human kidney appear early in development and, except for the last stage, are transitory (Fig. 55–1) (Potter, 1972). **The pronephros appears at 3 weeks, never progresses beyond a rudimentary stage, and involutes by 5 weeks. The mesonephros is seen at 5 weeks of gestation, appears to have transitory function, and degenerates by 11 to 12 weeks. Its major role in renal development is related to the fact that its ductal system gives rise to the ureteric bud.** The ureteric bud is critical for development of the metanephric or definitive kidney. Recent studies have revealed that apoptosis is a primary mechanism responsible for the sequential development of the mammalian kidney. Apoptosis is a physiologic, programmed cell death that normally mediates the deletion of unwanted cells, such as the disappearance of uninduced metanephric mesenchyme (Koseki et al, 1992). **The metanephros begins its inductive phase after 5 weeks of gestation, and in the human, nephrogenesis is completed by**

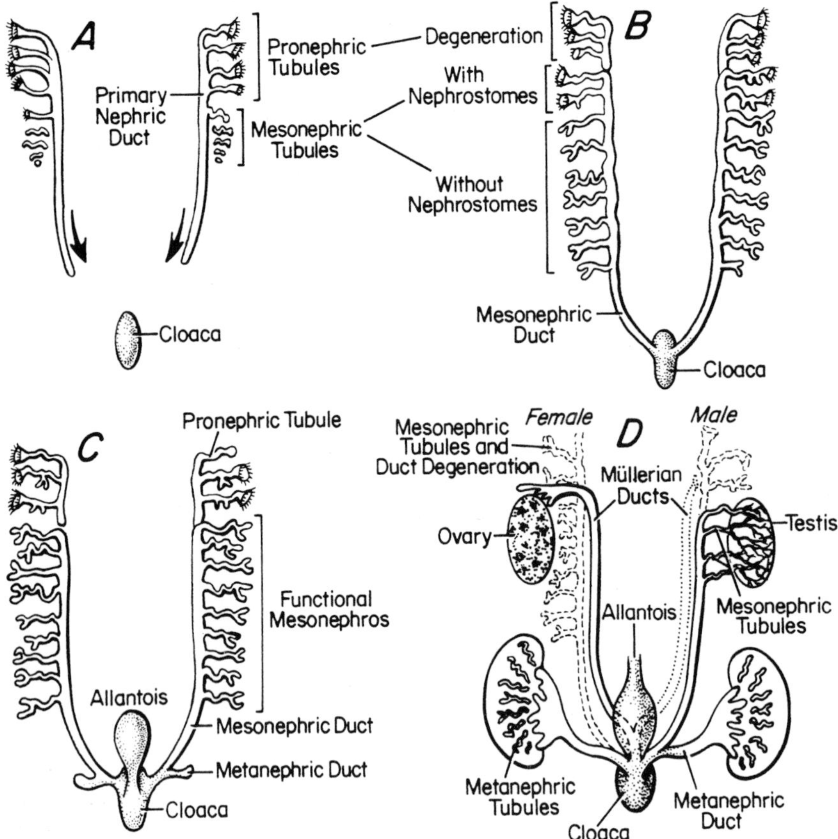

Figure 55–1. Relations of pronephros, mesonephros, and metanephros at various stages of development. To simplify, the tubules have been drawn as if they had been pulled out to the side of the ducts. The first rudimentary pronephros (*A*) is elaborated as a group of tubules emptying on either side into the primary nephric ducts, which extend caudad to discharge ultimately into the cloaca. A little later in development, there arises a second group of tubules more caudal in position than the pronephric tubule. These are mesonephric tubules (A). In their growth, they extend toward the primary nephric ducts and soon open into them (B). The plan, as shown in C, represents approximately the conditions attained by the human embryo toward the end of the fourth week. In D are depicted the conditions after sexual differentiation has taken place: female, left side; male, right side of the diagram. The müllerian ducts (shown in D) arise in human embryos during the eighth week, in close association with the mesonephric ducts. The müllerian ducts are the primordial tubes from which the oviducts, uterus, and vagina of the female are formed. Note that although both mesonephric and müllerian ducts appear in all young embryos, the müllerian ducts become vestigial in the male and the mesonephric ducts become vestigial in the female. (Reprinted with permission from Pattern BM: Human Embryology. New York, McGraw-Hill, 1968, p 450.)

34 to 36 weeks. In the developing metanephric kidney, there is a centrifugal pattern of nephrogenesis and maturation, with the outer cortical nephrons being the last to complete development.

FUNCTIONAL DEVELOPMENT OF THE FETUS

Information regarding the functional development of the metanephric kidney is gained primarily through animal studies. One must be careful in extrapolating such data from species in which there is dissimilarity of structural maturation at comparable gestational ages. **Urine production in the human kidney is known to begin around 10 to 12 weeks.** Salt and water hemostasis, however, is primarily handled by the placenta throughout gestation.

Fetal renal blood flow remains at a relatively low stable rate in utero. The ratio of renal blood flow to cardiac output at 20 weeks is 0.03 compared with the postnatal ratio of 0.2 to 0.3 (Rudolph and Heyman, 1976). This diminished renal blood flow is probably related to several different factors. The number of vascular channels is low early in gestation, and there is increased arteriolar resistance in these channels (Ichikawa et al, 1979; Robillard et al, 1987). Studies in animals have demonstrated a role for renal innervation as well as the renin-angiotensin system (RAS) as chronic modulators of this effect (Robillard et al, 1987). This effect is discussed in greater detail later.

Glomerular filtration rate (GFR) in the fetus is theoretically equal to the single-nephron GFR times the number of functioning glomeruli. This is difficult to determine, however, because **GFR is much higher in juxtamedullary glomeruli compared with subcortical glomeruli (Spitzer and Brandis, 1974).** GFR parallels renal mass and correlates with gestational age because nephrogenesis continues from 10 to 12 weeks of gestation until 34 weeks (Smith and Robillard, 1989).

Fractional excretion of sodium (FE_{Na}) shows a negative correlation with gestational age. **The fetus produces a hypotonic urine with high sodium content and in large volumes.** Potassium excretion increases similarly with gestational age, which may be related to rises in fetal plasma aldosterone concentration. There is a maturational increase in glucose transport of the fetal kidneys. Other tubular functions, such as bicarbonate reabsorption and acid production, are low in the fetus. They are, however, responsive to parathyroid excretion, intravascular volume, and acid infusion, respectively.

EVALUATION OF FETAL RENAL FUNCTION

Human fetal renal blood flow can be measured by color-pulsed Doppler studies, which indicate that blood flow increases from approximately 20 ml/minute at 25 weeks' gestation to more than 60 ml/minute at 40 weeks (Veille et al, 1993). **Hourly human fetal urine production (determined by serial real-time bladder ultrasonography at 2- to 5-minute intervals) increases from 5 ml/hour at 20 weeks'**

gestation to 50 ml/hour at 40 weeks (Rabinowitz et al, 1989). This extraordinary rate of diuresis would extrapolate to approximately 1 L/hour in the adult.

Owing to urinary dilution, human fetal urine sodium is normally below 100 mEq/L, chloride is less than 90 mEq/L, and osmolality is less than 200 mOsm/L (Crombleholme et al, 1990). Although urine values greater than these in fetuses with obstructive nephropathy have been correlated with a poor prognosis, recent reports indicate that sequential fetal urine samples must be obtained, both before and after intrauterine bladder shunting, to improve the predictive value (Evans et al, 1991; Johnson et al, 1994).

More recently, urine total protein less than 20 mg/dl and beta$_2$-microglobulin less than 4 mg/L have been shown to correlate with a favorable prognosis (Johnson et al, 1994). Other indices of tubular function include the measurement of amniotic fluid *N*-acetyl-beta-*D*-glucosaminidase (NAG) (an enzyme present in high concentration in proximal tubular cells) and specific amino acids in fetal urine (Pachi et al, 1993; Eugene et al, 1994). Increased amniotic fluid NAG has been correlated with renal impairment of intrauterine growth retardation (Pachi et al, 1993), and fetal urine valine concentration is increased in fetuses with bilateral renal dysplasia and fetal or neonatal death (Eugene et al, 1994).

POSTNATAL FUNCTIONAL DEVELOPMENT

At birth, several dramatic events occur that alter renal function. The kidney's response to the changing milieu and its success at maintaining homeostasis are heavily influenced by the gestational age at delivery. Intrauterine factors can also significantly affect postnatal renal functional development: Intrauterine growth retardation can permanently reduce the number of functioning nephrons (Merlet-Benichou et al, 1994). This may lead to renal failure presenting at birth (Steele et al, 1988).

In a study of 500 normal neonates, Clark (1977) found that **every infant voided within the first 24 hours of life regardless of gestational age**. After the first 2 days of life, oliguria is generally defined as a urine flow rate less than 1 ml/kg/hour (Anand, 1982). However, infants receiving a restricted solute intake can remain in solute balance with urine flow rates as low as 0.5 ml/kg/hour.

The definition of polyuria is somewhat arbitrary, but any infant or child excreting more than 2000 ml/1.73 m^2 in daily urine output should be evaluated further. It is important to distinguish pollakiuria (urinary frequency) from polyuria in the child, because pollakiuria can be a sign of emotional stress rather than a pathologic process (Asnes and Mones, 1973; Zoubek et al, 1990).

Renal blood flow increases sharply at birth, with a 5- to 18-fold rise noted in different animal studies (Gruskin et al, 1970; Aperia and Herin, 1975). This increase reflects several factors. There is a redistribution of flow from the inner to outer cortex (Aperia et al, 1977) and a drop in renal vascular resistance associated with increased intrarenal prostaglandins (Gruskin et al, 1970).

GFR doubles during the first week in term infants (Guignard et al, 1975). Owing to the dependence of GFR on gestational age, for infants born before 34 weeks, GFR rises slowly. After reaching a postconceptional age of 34 weeks, a rapid rise is then observed. **Factors responsible for this rapid rise include diminished renal vascular resistance (Gruskin et al, 1970) and increasing perfusion pressure, glomerular permeability, and filtration surface (John et al, 1981). In experimental animals, the increase in surface area for filtration accounts for most of the maturational increase in GFR (Spitzer and Brandis, 1974).** Serum creatinine, which reflects maternal levels at birth, also decreases by 50% in the first week of life in term or near-term infants. GFR continues to rise, reaching adult levels by 2 years of age (Rubin et al, 1949). Moreover, in very-low-birth-weight infants, GFR does not catch up to that of age-matched term infants of the same postconceptional age until after 9 months of age (Vanpee et al, 1992).

In the neonate, tubular function changes in association with the rise in GFR. **There remains a blunted response to sodium loading, however, due to a lack of increase in FE$_{Na}$ (Kim and Mandell, 1988).** This problem appears to be related to the high circulating renin, angiotensin, and aldosterone levels and to a diminished renal response to atrial natriuretic peptide (see later). Conversely, **premature infants younger than 35 weeks' gestation who are subjected to sodium deprivation may develop hyponatremia due to tubular immaturity and sodium wasting (Roy et al, 1976; Engelke et al, 1978).** Thus, sodium supplementation is frequently required in premature infants.

In terms of concentrating ability, **the neonate can dilute fairly well (25–35 mOsm/L) but has limited concentrating capacity (600–700 mOsm/L) (Hansen and Smith, 1953).** Concentrating capacity is even more restricted in the premature infant (500 mOsm/L). The factors responsible for this problem include anatomic immaturity of the renal medulla, decreased medullary concentration of sodium chloride and urea, and diminished responsiveness of the collecting ducts to antidiuretic hormone (Stanier, 1972; Schlondorff et al, 1978). By 9 years of age, maximal concentrating ability of very-low-birth-weight infants is not different from that of age-matched term infants (Vanpee et al, 1992).

Acid-base regulation in the neonate is characterized by a reduced threshold for bicarbonate reabsorption (Svenningsen, 1974). Bicarbonate reabsorption is gradually increased with increasing GFR. There is also an inability to respond to an acid load. This improves by 4 to 6 weeks after birth and is accentuated in the premature infant who tends to be slightly acidotic in comparison to the adult.

Glucose transport matures with the rising GFR in the neonate. This is more readily observed in the premature infant because fractional excretion of glucose is higher before 34 weeks of gestation (Arant, 1978).

Calcium and phosphate metabolism also changes shortly after birth. Parathyroid hormone is suppressed at birth, and serum calcium falls. This secondarily causes an increase in parathyroid hormone release. Initially, tubular reabsorption of phosphate is high in the premature infant and remains so until regular feedings commence at term (Arant, 1978).

EVALUATION OF RENAL FUNCTION IN THE INFANT AND CHILD

Glomerular Function

Measurement of GFR in the infant is problematic for a number of reasons. The primary difficulty is obtaining an accurately timed urine collection in the incontinent patient without bladder catheterization. The second is the inherent inaccuracy in measurement of the most readily available index of GFR, plasma creatinine concentration, because precision of the assay in most clinical laboratories is ± 0.3 mg/dl. Thus, calculated GFR in the infant can be overestimated or underestimated by 100% under the best circumstances of sample collections. The third is the rapidly changing GFR with normal growth: GFR factored for adult surface area (1.73 m^2) increases severalfold during the first 2 months of life (Fig. 55–2). Moreover, GFR increases with postconceptional age from 34 to 40 weeks' gestation (Fig. 55–3). Within the first 2 days of life, plasma creatinine concentration reflects maternal levels and may not reflect GFR of the infant. **By 7 days in the term infant, plasma creatinine concentration is normally less than 1 mg/dl, whereas in preterm infants, levels can remain as high as 1.5 mg/dl for the first month of life (Trompeter et al, 1983).** In view of these considerations, it is important to obtain serial values of serum creatinine. A progressive increase in serum creatinine during the neonatal period suggests renal insufficiency regardless of gestational age. Long-term monitoring of GFR in children with urologic abnormalities should account for increasing muscle mass that results in increasing serum creatinine concentration with age. A simple and reliable estimate of creatinine clearance (C_{Cr}) can be derived from the serum creatinine concentration and the patient's height using the empirical formula developed by Schwartz and colleagues (1987):

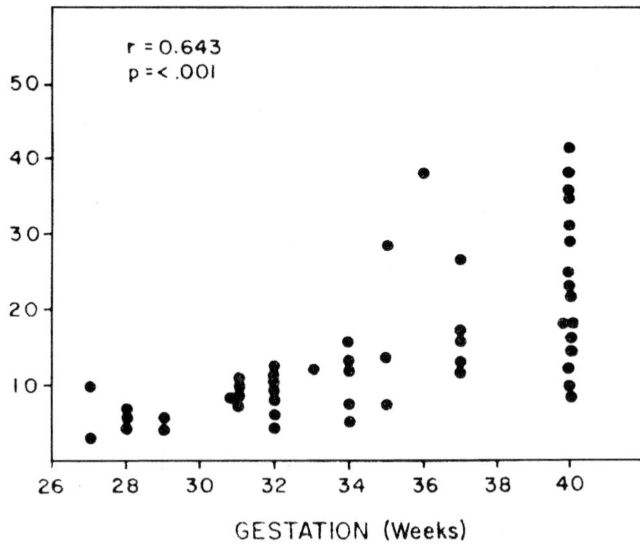

Figure 55–3. Creatinine clearance in relation to gestational age in clinically well infants studied from 24 to 40 hours after birth. (Reproduced from Siegel SR, Oh W: Renal function as a marker of human fetal maturation. Acta Paediatr Scand 1976; 65:481–485.)

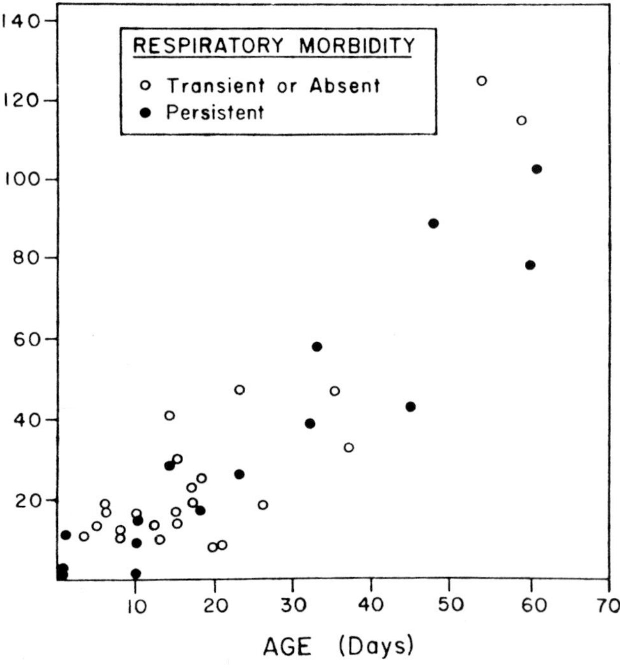

Figure 55–2. Creatinine clearance in relation to postnatal age during the first 60 days of life for preterm infants (birth weight mean = 1380 g, gestational age mean 31 weeks). During the first 10 days of life, creatinine clearance was lower (7.5 ml/min/1.73 m^2) in infants with persistent respiratory morbidity than in those without respiratory dysfunction (14.7 ml/min/1.73 m^2) (P <.05). Beyond the eleventh day, there was no difference between groups. (Reproduced from Ross B, Cowett RM, Oh W: Renal functions of low birth weight infants during the first two months of life. Pediatr Res 1977; 11:1161–1164.)

$$C_{Cr} = k \times L/P_{Cr}$$

where C_{Cr} = creatinine concentration (ml/minute/1.73 m^2), k = a constant (0.33 for preterm, 0.45 for full-term infants, 0.55 for children), and L = body length (cm). **Although C_{Cr} is constant at 80 to 140 ml/minute/1.73 m^2 after 2 years of age, the marked increase during the first 2 years of life should be taken into account when interpreting values for young infants.**

A more accurate determination of GFR can be obtained by creatinine clearance based on a 24-hour urine collection. As with the estimated C_{Cr} described earlier, the value should be corrected for adult surface area by multiplying by 1.73 and dividing by the patient's surface area (SA, derived from a nomogram [Cole, 1984]). Thus,

$$C_{Cr}\ (\text{ml/minute/1.73 m}^2) = \text{"uncorrected"}\ C_{Cr}\ (\text{ml/minute}) \times 1.73/\text{SA}$$

Expression of all pediatric C_{Cr} in this fashion should reduce confusion and ambiguity in comparing the result to expected normal ranges (see Figs. 55–2 and 55–3). It should be emphasized that accuracy of the calculated C_{Cr} depends on adequacy of the timed urine collection.

For more precise measurement of GFR, and to determine the relative contribution of each kidney to total GFR, a radiolabeled tracer that is cleared solely by glomerular filtration can be infused intravenously, and plasma concentration of the isotope can be measured sequentially with concurrent scintigraphy. An agent frequently used for this purpose is 99Tc-diethylenetriaminepentaacetic acid (Tc-DTPA). Although precision of measurement of Tc-DTPA is greater than that of creatinine, and urine collection is not required, adequate venous access and patient cooperation during scintigraphy are necessary. The requirement for patient cooperation may limit the usefulness of the technique in infants and small children. As with C_{Cr}, measurement of GFR by Tc-DTPA clearance should be corrected for adult surface area, as described earlier.

Tubular Function

Sodium Excretion

In the fetus and neonate, external sodium balance is positive as a consequence of sodium accretion necessary for rapid growth. In older infants and children, however, urinary sodium excretion is generally equivalent to sodium intake, as long as the patient is in a steady state. **The 24-hour urine sodium excretion, therefore, reflects the quantity of sodium ingested over the previous day and is normally 1 to 3 mEq/kg/day.** Patients with obligatory renal sodium losses (salt wasting) must increase their sodium intake to compensate for these ongoing losses. A diagnosis of salt-wasting nephropathy must be made while the patient is maintained on a restricted sodium intake (less than 1 mEq/kg/day) for 3 to 5 days. To prevent dangerous volume depletion or hyponatremia, the patient's blood pressure, weight, urine output, and serum sodium concentration should be closely monitored during the study. The 24-hour urine sodium excretion can also be helpful in monitoring compliance of patients on a restricted sodium intake (patients with hypertension, nephrogenic diabetes insipidus, or nephrotic syndrome, for example). The parents of those with sodium excretion greater than 3 mEq/kg/day may be counseled to improve their diets.

Of even greater clinical utility, the fraction of filtered sodium appearing in the urine (FE_{Na}) can be used to isolate the tubular from the glomerular contribution to sodium excretion. This may be used to distinguish prerenal causes of oliguria from renal parenchymal or postrenal etiologies. A timed urine collection is not necessary, because sodium and creatinine concentration can be measured in a random urine sample (U_{Na}, U_{Cr}) and a concurrent plasma sample (P_{Na}, P_{Cr}):

$$FE_{Na} = 100\%(U_{Na} \times P_{Cr})/(P_{Na} \times U_{Cr})$$

In the oliguric neonate (urine flow less than 1 ml/kg/hour), FE_{Na} less than 2.5% suggests a prerenal condition (Mathew et al, 1980), whereas in the older infant or child, a value below 1% is consistent with prerenal oliguria. Similar criteria can be used to differentiate causes of hyponatremia: FE_{Na} is increased in renal sodium wasting, adrenal insufficiency, and the syndrome of inappropriate antidiuretic hormone secretion. In each case, the urine sample must be obtained (by bladder catheterization if necessary) before administration of any drugs affecting urine sodium excretion, such as diuretics.

Urinary Acidification

Although renal insufficiency can interfere with urinary acidification, retention of organic acids due to decreased GFR results in an increase in unmeasured anions. In renal tubular acidosis (RTA), this anion gap is in the normal range (5 to 15 mEq/L) and is defined as

$$\text{Anion gap} = Na^{+}{}_{s} - [Cl^{-}{}_{s} + HCO_3{}^{-}{}_{s}]$$

The diagnosis of RTA should be considered in any infant or child with failure to thrive, because chronic systemic acidosis impairs growth. In addition, RTA can lead to nephrocalcinosis or nephrolithiasis (see later).

A classification of RTA has been developed, based on the nephron segment affected and the transport defect involved. Thus, RTA can result from defective distal tubular acidification (type I), decreased threshold for proximal tubular bicarbonate reabsorption (type II), a combined proximal and distal abnormality (type III), or a distal defect involving impaired potassium secretion (type IV). **During the first 3 weeks of life, the threshold for bicarbonate reabsorption can be as low as 14.5 mEq/L in the normal infant (Brown et al, 1978).** This should not be regarded as RTA, because treatment with alkali has been shown not to alter growth and development (Brown et al, 1978). Congenital hydronephrosis can result in type I or type IV RTA in the infant or child (Hutcheon et al, 1976; Rodriguez-Soriano et al, 1983). **Appropriate evaluation and treatment are important to prevent the sequelae of RTA. These include growth retardation, osteodystrophy, nephrocalcinosis or nephrolithiasis, and polyuria.**

The approach to the infant or child with suspected RTA is shown in Figure 55–4. The presence of metabolic acidosis in the infant can be difficult to ascertain on the basis of

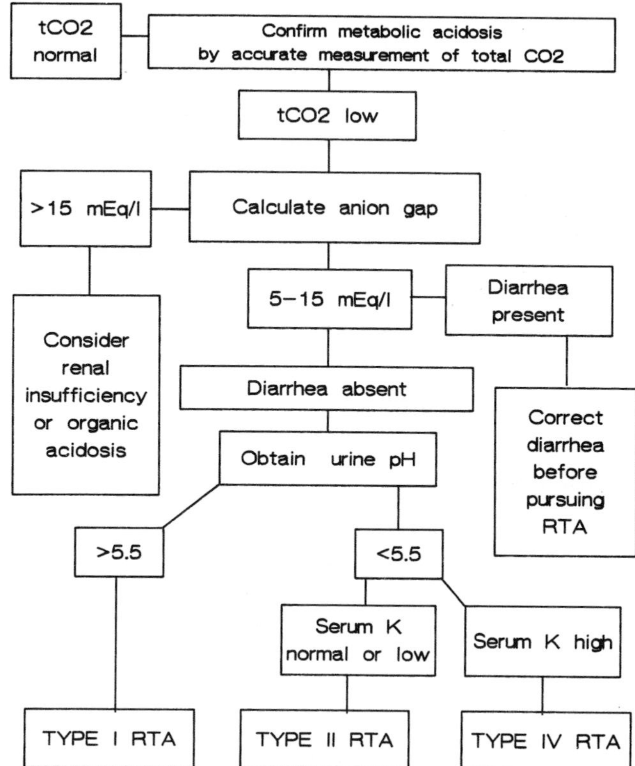

Figure 55–4. Evaluation of suspected renal tubular acidosis in the infant. See text for details.

serum total CO_2, because problems in obtaining the sample (venous access, small sample volume) can result in spuriously low values. Therefore, it is important to obtain the sample from a vein with good blood flow and to transfer it expeditiously to the laboratory in a capped syringe on ice (as with arterial blood for blood gas analysis). Accurate measurement of urine pH is also crucial to making the diagnosis, and a urine sample should be obtained at the time of the blood sample from a freshly voided or bagged specimen. Urine should be withdrawn into a syringe, the air should be expressed, and the sample should be transferred immediately to the laboratory for measurement by pH meter (dipsticks are not sufficiently accurate). **A urine pH below 5.5 in the face of a total CO_2 below normal for the patient's age suggests gastrointestinal bicarbonate loss or a defect in proximal tubular bicarbonate reabsorption with intact distal acidification (type II), while inappropriately high urine pH is consistent with distal or type I RTA. Elevated serum potassium concentration in the face of normal renal function suggests type IV RTA.**

Owing to the difficulty in infants in pursuing bicarbonate infusion to rule out type II, or acid infusion to rule out type I, alternate approaches have been developed to define the type of RTA. The simplest approach is to initiate alkali therapy with sodium bicarbonate or sodium citrate (Shohl's solution or Bictra) at a dose of 3 mEq/kg/day divided in four doses. The aim is to increase serum total CO_2 to the normal range (generally greater than 20 mEq/L) and to raise urine pH above 7.8. Patients with type II RTA or infants with type I may require much greater doses of alkali (10 or more mEq/kg/day) to maintain a normal plasma total CO_2 concentration and to allow a normal growth rate. The fractional excretion of bicarbonate can then be calculated from random paired blood and urine samples as for FE_{Na} (see earlier). In contrast to types I and IV, in which the fractional bicarbonate excretion is less than 15%, the value in type II is greater than 15% owing to the reduced threshold for bicarbonate reabsorption (Chan, 1983). An alternate means to distinguish type II from other forms of RTA is to measure blood and urine P_{CO_2} after correction of acidosis with alkali therapy. In patients with type II RTA, the difference between urine and blood P_{CO_2} is greater than 20 mm Hg, whereas in those with type I, the difference is less than 15 mm Hg (Donckerwolke et al, 1983). A third option used to identify patients with a distal tubular acidification defect (types I or IV) is to calculate the urinary anion gap, as follows:

$$\text{Urinary anion gap (mEq/L)} = Na^+ + K^+ - Cl^-$$

Normal patients and those with intact distal urinary acidification have a negative urinary anion gap, whereas those with types I or IV RTA have a positive gap (Batlle et al, 1988).

Although the above-mentioned studies should permit separation of type II from types I and IV RTA, the latter two forms are usually distinguishable (prior to treatment with alkali) by the presence of hyperkalemia in type IV but not type I RTA. In addition, infusion of furosemide, 1 mg/kg, should result in acidification of urine in patients with type IV RTA but not in those with type I (Stine and Linshaw, 1985).

Although there are a number of causes of RTA in children (Chan, 1983), congenital obstructive nephropathy (Hutcheon et al, 1976; Rodriguez-Soriano et al, 1983) and Fanconi's syndrome should always be considered (see later). Serum electrolytes, calcium, phosphorus, parathyroid hormone, and thyroid function tests should be obtained. A urinalysis should be performed to screen for glucosuria. In addition, the urine amino acid pattern may reveal diffuse aminoaciduria. A 24-hour urine collection should be obtained for calculation of creatinine clearance, protein excretion, calcium excretion, and tubular reabsorption of phosphorus (see later). Sonographic examination of the urinary tract should be performed not only to identify hydronephrosis but also to reveal nephrocalcinosis or nephrolithiasis that can develop in children with type I RTA.

As described earlier, most infants and children with RTA respond well to alkali therapy (sodium bicarbonate or Shohl's solution). Some patients with type IV, however, may have persistent hyperkalemia despite correction of acidosis. This can be managed by administration of chlorothiazide, 10 to 20 mg/kg/day, or polystyrene sodium sulfonate (Kayexalate), 1 g/kg/day. Patients receiving diuretics need to be monitored closely for the development of volume contraction, which can actually reduce potassium excretion. Infants receiving Kayexalate may undergo volume expansion from exchange of sodium for potassium and may develop bowel obstruction from inspissated resin in the intestinal tract. As long as adequate GFR is maintained, most children with RTA due to urologic abnormalities will need treatment to continue indefinitely to ensure normal growth and to prevent complications such as nephrocalcinosis. **The dose of alkali may need to be adjusted every 3 to 6 months in the rapidly growing infant.**

Urinary Concentration

Most disorders of urinary concentration in infants and children are due to renal maldevelopment (renal dysplasia and obstructive nephropathy), interstitial nephritis (pyelonephritis), or renal insufficiency. Additional causes include renal tubular acidosis, sickle cell nephropathy, and medullary cystic disease. These disorders generally result in a mild to moderate impairment in concentration, such that the urine specific gravity is greater than 1.005. Evaluation should include serum electrolytes, blood urea nitrogen (BUN), creatinine, urinalysis and urine culture, renal ultrasonography, and, possibly, voiding cystourethrogram. Infants with diabetes insipidus usually have urine specific gravity consistently less than 1.005.

There is no physiologic definition of polyuria, and screening of urinary concentrating ability may be initiated based on parental concern over excessive voiding frequency. Measurement of urine output and interpretation of thirst in the infant is problematic. For these reasons, the infant with unexplained dehydration or hypernatremia should be screened for a urine-concentrating defect.

A urine specific gravity greater than 1.020 generally rules out a serious abnormality of urinary concentration. In the young infant, overnight fluid restriction can result in dangerous volume depletion and hypernatremia. Such patients should undergo a formal water deprivation test in hospital. This should begin with fluid restriction starting in the morning, with close monitoring of body weight and vital signs until loss of 3% body weight or until the urine osmolality exceeds 600 mOsm in neonates (800 mOsm in older infants or children). If tachycardia or hypotension develop at any time, the test should be terminated.

In patients failing to produce a concentrated urine during water deprivation, fluid should be restricted on a separate day, and desmopressin (DDAVP, 10 μg for infants, or 20 μg for children) is instilled into the nostrils. Urine osmolality should be measured at 2-hour intervals for 4 to 6 hours. Renal response to DDAVP should be considered normal if the urine osmolality exceeds 600 mOsm for neonates or 800 mOsm for older infants and children. Such patients should be evaluated for central diabetes insipidus by a neurologist or endocrinologist.

Calcium Excretion

Urinary calcium excretion in the neonate is most easily assessed by determination of the calcium/creatinine ratio (mg/mg) in a random urine sample. In contrast to the older child, in whom a ratio exceeding 0.2 should be considered abnormal (Moore et al, 1978), the ratio in the infant receiving breast milk can rise to 0.4 in the term infant and to 0.8 in the preterm neonate (Karlen et al, 1985). The most common cause of hypercalciuria in neonates is the administration of calciuric drugs, such as furosemide and glucocorticoids, which are used in the management of bronchopulmonary dysplasia. Such patients may be at risk for the development of nephrocalcinosis or nephrolithiasis (Jacinto et al, 1988). This, in turn, may lead to renal dysfunction later in childhood (Downing et al, 1992). Although it may not be feasible to discontinue glucocorticoids, substitution of chlorothiazide for furosemide may reduce urinary calcium excretion.

Phosphorus, Glucose, and Amino Acid Excretion

Because serum phosphorus concentration is higher in the neonate than in the older infant or child, **any neonate with serum phosphorus level below 4 mg/dl should be evaluated for renal phosphorus wasting.** This evaluation can be accomplished in the neonate by measuring phosphate and creatinine concentration in urine (U_{Cr}, U_{PO4}) and plasma (P_{Cr}, P_{PO4}), and calculating the fractional tubular reabsorption of phosphorus (TRP):

$$\text{TRP} = 100\%[1-(U_{PO4} \times P_{Cr})/(P_{PO4} \times U_{Cr})]$$

After the first week of life in the neonate, the TRP should be greater than 95% in term infants and greater than 75% in preterm infants (Karlen et al, 1985). After the neonatal period, the TRP should be greater than 85%. Values below these ranges suggest a proximal tubular disorder or hyperparathyroidism.

In preterm infants, the threshold for tubular glucose reabsorption is lower than that in the term infant or older child. **The most common cause of glucosuria in hospitalized infants is intravenous infusion of dextrose at rates exceeding the tubular reabsorptive threshold.** Percent glucose reabsorption (μmol/ml) is normally greater than 99% (Rossi et al, 1994).

Similar to glucose handling, the proximal tubule of the neonate is limited in its ability to reabsorb amino acids when compared with the older infant. This results in a generalized aminoaciduria that is normal during the neonatal period. Thus, **in the evaluation of aminoaciduria, it is important to compare results to those of age-matched normal infants (Brodehl, 1978).** Normal values for fractional amino acid reabsorption have been determined for neonates, infants, and children (Rossi et al, 1994).

HORMONAL CONTROL OF RENAL FUNCTION DURING DEVELOPMENT

Renin-Angiotensin System

Fetal and neonatal renal function is significantly modulated by a number of circulating hormones. The best studied is the RAS. Inasmuch as angiotensin II receptors have been identified in the fetal rat by the tenth day of gestation (term equals 21 days) (Jones et al, 1989), and renin appears in the mesonephric and renal arteries by the 15th day (Richoux et al, 1987), a role for the RAS has been postulated in the process of angiogenesis. In the human fetus, renin is present in the transient mesonephros and can be identified as early as the eighth week of gestation in the metanephros (Celio et al, 1985). **By the 19th day of gestation in the rat, renin messenger RNA (demonstrated by in situ hybridization histochemistry) as well as the renin protein (demonstrated by immunocytochemistry) are distributed along arcuate and interlobular arteries (Gomez et al, 1986; Gomez et al, 1989). However, in the early postnatal period, renin becomes localized to the juxtaglomerular apparatus, which persists to adulthood (Gomez et al, 1986). In addition to these developmental changes in distribution of renin, there is an eightfold decrease in the renal renin mRNA content during early development in the rat (Gomez et al, 1988a).** These developmental changes are not irreversible: Inhibition of angiotensin II formation by chronic intake of enalapril in the adult rat causes a redistribution of renin upstream along afferent arterioles and an increase in renal renin mRNA content reminiscent of the fetal pattern (Gomez et al, 1988b; Gomez et al, 1990). In view of these findings, it is possible that as a result of normal maturation, the sensitivity of the renal vasculature to angiotensin II increases, with secondary inhibition of renin gene expression.

Although plasma renin activity (PRA) remains low during fetal life (Pernollet et al, 1979), there is a marked increase in the perinatal period in most mammalian species, including humans (Osborn et al, 1980; Siegel and Fisher, 1980; Wallace et al, 1980; Fiselier et al, 1984). The mechanism underlying this increase in PRA, which is triggered by vaginal delivery (Jelinek et al, 1986), may relate to a rise in prostaglandin synthesis (Joppich and Hauser, 1982) or increased sympathetic nervous activity (Vincent et al, 1980). However, studies in piglets failed to support the belief that increased sympathetic nervous activity is related (Osborn et al, 1980). It is likely that contraction of the extracellular space resulting from physiologic postnatal natriuresis contributes to the perinatal increase in PRA (Aperia et al, 1977).

In addition to developmental changes in renin synthesis, **the adrenal response to angiotensin increases during fetal**

and early postnatal life. In the fetal lamb, furosemide infusion does not increase either PRA or plasma aldosterone concentration (Siegel and Fisher, 1980). In late gestation, however, PRA increases without a mineralocorticoid response, whereas in the neonate, both PRA and aldosterone concentration increase after furosemide infusion (Siegel and Fisher, 1980). Maturation of the mineralocorticoid response can also be demonstrated by angiotensin II infusion, which results in greater plasma aldosterone concentrations in human adults than in fetal sheep (Robillard et al, 1983). The physiologic significance of these events may rest in the response to hemorrhage, which causes a greater increase in PRA, plasma angiotensin II, and aldosterone in late rather than in early gestation in the ovine fetus (Robillard et al, 1982). Because blood pressure is maintained during moderate hemorrhage in late but not in earlier gestation (Robillard et al, 1982), the RAS may play a critical role in modulation of hemodynamics in the perinatal period. **Because of the critical dependence of the fetal and neonatal glomerular capillary pressure on angiotensin-mediated efferent arteriolar tone, fetal or neonatal GFR can fall precipitously following exposure to angiotensin converting enzyme inhibitors (Martin et al, 1992).** Both the potency and duration of action of captopril are significantly greater in the neonate than in older children (O'Dea et al, 1988). Moreover, in response to a reduction in renal mass, the remaining hyperfiltering immature nephrons are even more susceptible to the action of angiotensin converting enzyme inhibitors, which can induce renal failure and further nephron injury.

Atrial Natriuretic Peptide

Atrial natriuretic peptide (ANP) is a newly discovered peptide secreted by cardiac myocytes. It has been shown to possess a number of systemic hemodynamic and renal effects, including an increase in GFR, natriuresis, diuresis, inhibition of renin and aldosterone release, vasorelaxation, and an increase in vascular permeability (Goetz, 1988). Circulating ANP binds to specific receptors coupled to particulate guanylate cyclase, resulting in formation of guanosine 3′,5′-cyclic monophosphate (cyclic GMP), a second messenger responsible for the physiologic effects of ANP (Inagami, 1989). In addition, ANP binds to an even greater number of receptors not coupled to guanylate cyclase. Classified as clearance receptors, these receptors are believed to contribute to the regulation of plasma ANP levels by removal of ANP from the circulation (Inagami, 1989). The precise role of ANP in the regulation of sodium and fluid homeostasis remains unclear at present. However, evidence has accumulated to suggest that ANP plays a role in the physiologic adaptation of the fetus and neonate to its changing environment. ANP is present in the fetal rat heart shortly after completion of organogenesis (Dolan and Dobrozsi, 1987; Toshimori et al, 1987), and ANP mRNA first appears in the ventricles before becoming localized to the atria in the perinatal period (Wei et al, 1987). Compared with the mother, plasma ANP concentration is significantly higher in the fetus (Castro et al, 1988; Yamaji et al, 1988). Because metabolic clearance of ANP by the fetus exceeds that of the adult (Ervin et al, 1988), release of ANP from fetal cardiac myocytes must be far greater than that in adults.

A number of stimuli have been shown to increase fetal plasma ANP levels. Acute volume expansion in the ovine fetus (Ross et al, 1987) and intrauterine blood transfusion in the human fetus (Robillard and Weiner, 1988) raise the plasma ANP concentration. Induction of atrial tachycardia in the fetal lamb results in hydrops and an increase in plasma ANP concentration (Nimrod et al, 1988). Fetal hypoxia has also been shown to result in contraction of circulating volume as well as an increase in ANP levels (Cheung and Brace, 1988). By increasing vascular permeability, ANP may therefore contribute to regulation of blood volume in these pathologic states.

Atrial ANP content decreases in the perinatal period, with a subsequent increase during the first 15 days of postnatal life in the rat (Dolan et al, 1989). This pattern is the opposite of that observed for plasma ANP concentration, which is elevated in the first several days of life, then decreases with maturation (Weil et al, 1986; Kikuchi et al, 1988). It is likely that reduction in atrial ANP during the perinatal period results from increased release into the circulation. In preterm infants, plasma ANP levels are initially even higher than in full-term infants, and the ensuing postnatal decrease in levels is correlated with decreasing atrial size and decreasing body weight (Bierd et al, 1990). Therefore, it is likely that ANP plays a role in physiologic postnatal natriuresis and diuresis. Following the initial postnatal diuresis, however, the neonate enters a state of positive sodium balance necessary for rapid somatic growth.

The renal effects of infused ANP are reduced in the fetus compared with those in the adult (Brace et al, 1989; Hargrave et al, 1989). The natriuretic effect of ANP in the neonate is also reduced (Bräunlich, 1987; Chevalier, 1988), and systemic clearance of ANP is increased compared with that of the adult (Chevalier, 1988). Moreover, compared with the adult, the neonatal renal natriuretic and diuretic response to acute volume expansion is attenuated (Schoeneman, 1980). However, chronic sodium loading of artificially reared preweaned rat pups increases the renal response to acute volume expansion, with an increase in the urinary excretion of cyclic GMP (Muchant et al, 1995). Therefore, it appears that rather than reflecting functional immaturity, the renal response to ANP in the neonate reflects an adaptation to the requirement for sodium conservation during this period.

Vasopressin

Similar to the adult, fetal and newborn sheep have been shown to respond to both osmolar and nonosmolar stimuli for release of arginine vasopressin (AVP) (Leake et al, 1979; Robillard et al, 1979). In spite of the fact that circulating levels of AVP are significantly higher in the fetus than in the adult (Pohjavuori and Fyhrquist, 1980), **the fetal collecting duct appears to be less sensitive to AVP than the adult collecting duct (Robillard and Weitzman, 1980).** This may be due to a reduced density of AVP receptors, which increase during early development (Rajerison et al, 1982). In addition, the tubular effects of vasopressin may be antagonized by increased prostanoid synthesis in early development (Melendez et al, 1990).

In the postnatal period, during which the collecting ducts develop full responsiveness to AVP, excessive or inappropriate AVP secretion due to birth asphyxia, intracerebral hemorrhage, or respiratory distress syndrome can result in severe hyponatremia (Kaplan and Feigin, 1978; Moylan et al, 1978; Stern et al, 1979). Conversely, infants born with nephrogenic diabetes insipidus do not respond to circulating AVP and may develop life-threatening hypernatremia.

Prostaglandins

Maternal serum prostaglandin concentration increases progressively during pregnancy (Reyes and Melendez, 1990). Because prostaglandins cross the placenta, blood levels are also elevated in the fetus and neonate (Reyes and Melendez, 1990). **Maternal administration of nonsteroidal anti-inflammatory drugs (NSAIDs), such as indomethacin, can result in prolonged renal insufficiency and oliguria in the neonate (Buderus et al, 1993; Kaplan et al, 1994).** Prolonged intrauterine exposure to NSAIDs can also impair fetal renal development (Kaplan et al, 1994). Administration of indomethacin to neonates with patent ductus arteriosus also frequently results in decreased GFR and oliguria (Reyes and Melendez, 1990). Caution should be exercised in the administration of NSAIDs to any infant or child with a single functioning kidney or with renal impairment, because such patients are at increased risk for additional nephron injury and deterioration of GFR.

Nitric Oxide

Nitric oxide, a potent endothelium-derived relaxing factor, has multiple effects on renal function, including renal vasodilatation, regulation of tubuloglomerular feedback, and natriuresis (Bachmann and Mundel, 1994). Basal production of nitric oxide in the third-trimester sheep fetus maintains baseline renal blood flow (Bogaert et al, 1993). In the neonatal pig, endogenous nitric oxide synthesis is also responsible for basal vasoconstrictor tone, and this effect is proportionately greater than that in the adult (Solhaug et al, 1993). Renal endothelial nitric oxide production may be increased in early development as a response to increased vasoconstrictor influences described earlier. A counter-regulatory function of renal nitric oxide production has been proposed also following unilateral ureteral obstruction (UUO) in the adult rat, in which endogenous renal nitric oxide activity parallels increased renal vascular resistance (Chevalier et al, 1992).

THE FUNCTIONAL RESPONSE OF THE DEVELOPING KIDNEYS TO MALFORMATION OR INJURY

Reduced Functioning Renal Mass

A reduction in the number of functioning nephrons in early development is most often the result of a congenital malformation or a perinatal vascular accident, such as a renal embolus or renal vein thrombosis. Unilateral ureteral occlusion in the fetal lamb at midtrimester results in a 50% increase in contralateral kidney weight by 1 month (Peters et al, 1993). These findings are corroborated by two prenatal ultrasound studies of human fetuses with unilateral renal agenesis or multicystic kidney. In both reports, the single functioning kidneys were significantly longer than those in the control patients (Glazebrook et al, 1993; Mandell et al, 1993). **Such studies demonstrate unequivocally that compensatory renal growth can begin prenatally.** Because the placenta provides the excretory function for the fetus, an increased excretory burden on the kidney is not required to initiate compensatory growth. Rather, alterations in growth factors or inhibitors presumably modulate the prenatal changes. Perhaps not surprising in view of the rapid growth of the normal kidney in the early postnatal period, **compensatory renal growth in the neonate greatly exceeds that in the adult (Dicker and Shirley, 1973; Shirley, 1976; Hayslett, 1979).** Whereas compensatory increase in renal mass in the adult is largely due to cellular hypertrophy, hyperplasia is also stimulated in the uninephrectomized weanling rat (Karp et al, 1971; Phillips and Leong, 1967). Neonatal glomerular hypertrophy results also from increased glomerular basement membrane surface area and proliferation of mesangial matrix (Olivetti et al, 1980). As in the adult, the majority of the compensatory increase in renal mass in the neonate is due to an increase in tubular volume (Hayslett et al, 1968; Horster et al, 1971).

Previously, compensatory renal growth in the uninephrectomized neonatal rat was thought to involve an increase in nephrogenesis of the remaining kidney (Bonvalet et al, 1972). This was subsequently disproved by careful serial morphologic studies (Kaufman et al, 1975; Larsson et al, 1980). In the guinea pig, approximately 20% of glomeruli are underperfused during the first several weeks of life and cannot be identified by uptake of colloidal carbon (India ink) injected in vivo (Chevalier, 1982a). Following uninephrectomy at birth, however, these glomeruli are recruited within the first 3 weeks of life, resulting in an earlier increase in the number of perfused glomeruli per kidney (Chevalier, 1982a). The prior confusion regarding apparent compensatory nephrogenesis in animals subjected to uninephrectomy during early development is therefore likely due to incorrectly describing newly perfused glomeruli as newly formed glomeruli.

As with the enhanced increase in compensatory renal growth observed in the neonate with reduced renal mass, **the functional adaptation by remaining nephrons is greater in early development than in the adult.** In dogs subjected to 75% renal ablation at birth, GFR increased markedly such that at 6 weeks of age, it was not different from that of sham-operated littermates (Aschinberg et al, 1978). However, dogs undergoing renal ablation at 8 weeks of age had a GFR 6 weeks later that was less than 50% that of sham-operated controls (Aschinberg et al, 1978). Reduced renal mass in the neonatal guinea pig or rat results in acceleration of the normal centrifugal functional nephron maturation, such that the compensatory increase in single nephron GFR is greater in superficial than in deep nephrons (Chevalier, 1982b; Ikoma et al, 1990). These studies indicate that functional as well as morphologic correlates of compensatory renal growth are augmented in early postnatal development.

Sonography permits serial measurement of renal size in the fetus and beyond birth. Such tracking of renal size reflects the function of an abnormal contralateral kidney in infants with two functioning kidneys: An exaggerated rate of increase in renal size is correlated with contralateral renal function contributing less than 15% of total function (O'Sullivan et al, 1992).

Congenital Urinary Tract Obstruction

The response of the developing kidney to ureteral obstruction differs from that of the adult. **Complete UUO during midgestation in the fetal sheep results in dysplastic development of the ipsilateral kidney (Beck, 1971).** When subjected to UUO later in gestation, however, dysplastic changes do not develop (Glick et al, 1983). In the human infant, ureteral atresia in early gestation results in irreversible multicystic dysplasia of the ipsilateral kidney (Griscom et al, 1975). Ureteropelvic junction obstruction presumably develops later in gestation and causes less severe functional renal impairment, which may be minimized by early release of obstruction postnatally (King et al, 1984). These studies illustrate the critical importance of the timing of urinary tract obstruction with respect to renal development and the greater susceptibility to injury of the fetal kidney.

Even in the early postnatal period, the maturing kidney appears to be more susceptible to injury resulting from UUO than the adult kidney. As in uninephrectomy (see earlier), partial UUO in the neonatal guinea pig results in a greater adaptive increase in GFR of the intact opposite kidney than UUO in older animals (Taki et al, 1983). However, despite lower intraureteral hydrostatic pressure in neonatal than adult guinea pigs (Chevalier, 1984), the decrement in GFR due to ipsilateral UUO is more severe in younger than in older animals (Taki et al, 1983), and renal growth of kidneys with partial UUO since birth is arrested by 3 weeks of age (Chevalier et al, 1988). Morphologically, the neonatal guinea pig with ipsilateral partial UUO develops contraction of glomerular volume, glomerular sclerosis, and tubular atrophy (Chevalier et al, 1987). Most importantly, growth arrest cannot be prevented and function is not restored by release of obstruction after 10 days, even though intraureteral pressure is normalized (Chevalier et al, 1988). In contrast, release of obstruction after a similar period in the adult animal does not cause renal atrophy and allows restoration of a normal glomerular perfusion pattern and renal blood flow (Chevalier et al, 1987).

As with UUO in the adult, chronic partial UUO in the neonatal guinea pig results in a marked increase in vascular resistance of the ipsilateral kidney. Whereas normal renal development in the guinea pig is characterized by a progressive increase in renal blood flow and recruitment of perfused glomeruli (Chevalier, 1983; Chevalier, 1982a), these events are prevented by ipsilateral UUO at birth (Chevalier et al, 1987; Chevalier and Gomez, 1989). Normal renal growth and hemodynamic maturation can be restored, however, by removal of the intact opposite kidney at the time of ureteral obstruction (Chevalier and Kaiser, 1984). This factor suggests that growth factors regulated by total functional renal mass can modulate the response of the developing kidney to ipsilateral UUO.

The greater hemodynamic impairment of the neonatal kidney subjected to UUO may relate to the increased renal vascular resistance of the immature kidney and increased activity of the RAS (see earlier). The renin content of the neonatal guinea pig kidney with ipsilateral UUO is increased compared with sham-operated controls, and release of obstruction returns renin content to normal levels (Chevalier and Gomez, 1989). Inhibition of endogenous angiotensin II formation by chronic administration of enalapril to neonatal guinea pigs with UUO restores the normal maturational rise in renal blood flow, the number of perfused glomeruli, and the increase in glomerular volume of the ipsilateral kidney (Chevalier and Peach, 1985; Chevalier et al, 1987). Although administration of enalapril does not restore the renal blood flow of the neonatal guinea pig kidney after release of 5 or 10 days of ipsilateral UUO, enalapril reduces renal vascular resistance of the intact opposite kidney by 40% after release of contralateral UUO (Chevalier and Gomez, 1989). Moreover, the vasoconstrictor response of the intact kidney to exogenous angiotensin II is increased following release of contralateral UUO (Chevalier and Gomez, 1989). These studies indicate a dynamic functional balance between the two kidneys, which appears to be mediated or modulated by the intrarenal RAS.

As discussed earlier, the intrarenal distribution of renin changes dramatically during development. In the fetus and early postnatal period, microvascular renin extends along interlobular and afferent arterioles, becoming localized to the juxtaglomerular region by the 20th postnatal day in the rat (Gomez et al, 1986). **In 4-week-old rats subjected to complete UUO during the first 2 days of life, renal renin content is increased in the obstructed kidney, and immunoreactive renin extends along the afferent arteriole (El-Dahr et al, 1990).** Thus, UUO from birth results in persistence of the fetal or early neonatal pattern even after the time of weaning (21 days). Furthermore, the proportion of juxtaglomerular apparatuses with renin gene expression (identified by in situ hybridization histochemistry) is increased in the obstructed kidney of 4-week-old rats (El-Dahr et al, 1990). In addition to increased renin production and storage, neonatal UUO results in recruitment of renin-secreting cells by the renal cortex (Norwood et al, 1994). Four weeks of UUO in adult rats, however, did not alter the juxtaglomerular localization of renin (El Dahr et al, 1990). These studies indicate that the renal response to UUO is age dependent, with the neonate manifesting a greater activity of the RAS.

Perinatal Ischemia and Hypoxia

Renal dysfunction in the fetus and neonate is often the result of circulatory disturbances in the perinatal period. In response to hemorrhage or hypoxia, renal vascular resistance in the ovine fetus is increased while GFR is maintained, suggesting predominant efferent arteriolar vasoconstriction (Robillard et al, 1981; Gomez et al, 1984). This may be mediated at least in part by angiotensin (Robillard et al, 1982). Catecholamine release may be more important in mediating renal vascular resistance in early fetal life, whereas vasopressin appears to play a greater role in the more mature ovine fetus (Gomez et al, 1984). In the neonatal lamb, hypoxia increases PRA, aldosterone, and vasopressin (Weismann and Clarke, 1981). Although GFR is reduced during hypoxia, the effect does not change during the first month of life (Weismann and Clarke, 1981). The preterm infant, however, may have renal responses to ischemia and hypoxia that are more similar to the fetus than to the neonate.

One of the homeostatic mechanisms for preservation of renal perfusion in the face of hypotension is autoregulation of renal blood flow. Compared with adult rats, **young rats manifest autoregulation of renal blood flow at lower perfusion pressures, commensurate with the lower mean arterial pressure during early development (Chevalier and Kaiser, 1983).** Interestingly, whereas adult rats with prior uninephrectomy maintain autoregulation (albeit at higher levels of renal blood flow), **uninephrectomy at birth impairs autoregulation in young rats (Chevalier and Kaiser, 1983).** These observations raise the possibility that following reduction in functioning renal mass, the neonatal kidney may be at greater risk for renal ischemia in the face of superimposed hypotension. Following temporary complete occlusion of the renal artery, however, the mortality rate has been shown to be greater in adult rats than in young rats (Kunes et al, 1978). Although this study suggests that the neonatal kidney may be more resistant than the adult kidney to certain insults, **perinatal circulatory disorders can result in a variety of persistent glomerular and tubular functional abnormalities (Stark and Geiger, 1990; Dauber et al, 1976).**

Toxic Nephropathy

Neonates are increasingly exposed to a variety of potentially nephrotoxic agents. Fortunately, the developing kidney appears to be more resistant than the adult kidney to a number of toxic agents. Sodium dichromate and uranyl nitrate, both experimental models of toxic acute renal failure, cause less renal injury in young animals than in adult animals (Pelayo et al, 1983; Appenroth and Bräunlich, 1988). More relevant clinically, renal concentrations of aminoglycosides (Marre et al, 1980; Lelievre-Pegorier et al, 1985; Provoost et al, 1985) and cisplatin (Jongejan et al, 1986) are lower in young animals than in adult animals receiving high doses. This may be due to the normally reduced perfusion of superficial cortical nephrons in the developing kidney, such that these nephrons receive a lower dose of toxin. Another possibility is the proportionately greater renal mass compared with body weight in early development. Few studies have addressed the potential long-term impact of toxic renal injury, however. Following uninephrectomy for Wilms' tumor, for example, irradiation and chemotherapy cause greater impairment of compensatory renal growth in young infants than in older infants and children (Mitus et al, 1969; Luttenegger et al, 1975).

Implications of Congenital Renal Disease for Adult Function

Glomerular hyperfiltration and glomerular hypertrophy have been implicated in the progression of most forms of renal insufficiency (Brenner et al, 1982; Fogo and Ichikawa, 1989). **In view of the greater response by remaining nephrons, the neonate with reduced renal mass is theoretically at greater risk than the adult for long-term renal dysfunction.** In this regard, reduced renal mass causes greater proteinuria and glomerular sclerosis in the immature kidney than in the adult kidney (Celsi et al, 1987; Okuda et al, 1987; Ikoma et al, 1990). There is circumstantial evidence that intrauterine growth retardation is also accompanied by a nephron deficit and, in addition to renal insufficiency, may lead to the development of hypertension in adulthood (Brenner and Chertow, 1994). Likewise, congenital unilateral renal agenesis in humans has been associated with focal glomerular sclerosis and progression to renal insufficiency in adulthood (Kiprov et al, 1982; Bhathena et al, 1985; Wikstad et al, 1988). Over 25% of children undergoing unilateral nephrectomy developed renal insufficiency and proteinuria in adulthood (Argueso et al, 1992). The critical question is what is the number of functioning nephrons below which progression is inevitable? In oligomeganephronia, a form of renal hypoplasia in which the number of nephrons is reduced to less than 50%, glomeruli develop marked hypertrophy and sclerosis, leading to renal failure in later childhood (Bhathena et al, 1985; Elema, 1976). These considerations underscore the importance of attempting to maximize functional renal mass in the neonate or infant with renal impairment of any etiology.

REFERENCES

Anatomic Development and Fetal Renal Function

Crombleholme TM, Harrison MR, Golbus MS, et al: Fetal intervention in obstructive uropathy: Prognostic indicators and efficacy of intervention. Am J Obstet Gynecol 1990; 162:1239–1244.

Eugene M, Muller F, Dommergues M, et al: Evaluation of postnatal renal function in fetuses with bilateral obstructive uropathies by proton nuclear magnetic resonance spectroscopy. Am J Obstet Gynecol 1994; 170:595–602.

Evans MI, Sacks AJ, Johnson MP, et al: Sequential invasive assessment of fetal renal function and the intrauterine treatment of fetal obstructive uropathies. Obstet Gynecol 1991; 77:545–550.

Ichikawa I, Maddox DA, Brenner BM; Maturational development of glomerular ultrafiltration in the rat. Am J Physiol 1979; 236:F465–F471.

Johnson MP, Bukowski TP, Reitleman C, et al: In utero surgical treatment of fetal obstructive uropathy: A new comprehensive approach to identify appropriate candidates for vesicoamniotic shunt therapy. Am J Obstet Gynecol 1994; 170:1770–1779.

Koseki C, Herzlinger D, Al-Awqati Q: Apoptosis in metanephric development. J Cell Biol 1992; 119:1327–1333.

Pachi A, Lubrano R, Maggi E, et al: Renal tubular damage in fetuses with intrauterine growth retardation. Fetal Diagn Ther 1993; 8:109–113.

Potter EL: Normal and Abnormal Developmenet of the Kidney. Chicago, Year Book, 1972.

Rabinowitz R, Peters MT, Vyas S, et al: Measurement of fetal urine production in normal pregnancy by real-time ultrasonography. Am J Obstet Gynecol 1989; 161:1264–1266.

Robillard JE, Nakamura KT, Wilkin MK, et al: Ontogeny of renal hemodynamic response to renal nerve stimulation in sheep. Am J Physiol 1987; 252:F605–F612.

Rudolph AM, Heyman M: Circulatory changes during growth in the fetal lamb. Circ Res 1976; 26:289.

Smith FG, Robillard JE: Pathophysiology of fetal renal disease. Semin Perinatol 1989; 13:305.

Spitzer A, Brandis M: Functional and morphologic maturation of the superficial nephrons: Relationship to total kidney function. J Clin Invest 1974; 53:279–287.

Veille JC, Hanson RA, Tatum K, Kelley K: Quantitative assessment of human fetal renal blood flow. Am J Obstet Gynecol 1993; 169:1399–1402.

Postnatal Functional Development

Anand SK: Acute renal failure in the neonate. Pediatr Clin North Am 1982; 29:791–800.

Aperia A, Broberger O, Herin P: Renal hemodynamics in the perinatal period: A study in lambs. Acta Physiol Scand 1977; 99:261.

Aperia A, Herin P: Development of glomerular perfusion rate and nephron filtration rate in rats 17–60 days old. Am J Physiol 1975; 228:1319–1325.

Arant BS Jr: Developmental patterns of renal functional maturation compared in the human neonate. J Pediatr 1978; 92:705–712.

Asnes RS, Mones RL: Pollakiuria. Pediatrics 1973; 52:615–617.

Clark DA: Times of first void and first stool in 500 newborns. Pediatrics 1977; 60:457–459.

Engelke SC, Shah RL, Vasan U, Raye JR: Sodium balance in very low-birth-weight infants. J Pediatr 1978; 93:837–841.

Gruskin AB, Edelmann CM Jr, Yuan S: Maturational changes in renal blood flow in piglets. Pediatr Res 1970; 4:7–13.

Guignard JP, Torrado A, DaCunha O, Gautier E: Glomerular filtration rate in the first three weeks of life. J Pediatr 1975; 87:268.

Hansen JPL, Smith CA: Effects of withholding fluid in the immediate postnatal period. Pediatrics 1953; 12:99.

John E, Goldsmith DI, Spitzer A: Quantitative changes in the canine glomerular vasculature during development: Physiologic implications. Kidney Int 1981; 20:223–239.

Kim MS, Mandell J: Renal function in the fetus and neonate. *In* King LR Jr, ed: Urologic Surgery in Neonates and Young Infants. Philadelphia, W. B. Saunders Company, 1988, pp 41–58

Merlet-Benichou C, Gilbert T, Muffat-Joly M, et al: Intrauterine growth retardation leads to a permanent nephron deficit in the rat. Pediatr Nephrol 1994; 8:175–180.

Roy RN, Chance GW, Radde IC, et al: Late hyponatremia in very low birthweight infants (<1.3 kilograms). Pediatr Res 1976; 10:526–531.

Rubin MI, Bruck E, Rapaport M: Maturation of renal function in childhood: Clearance studies. J Clin Invest 1949; 28:1144.

Schlondorff D, Weber H, Trizna W, Fine LG: Vasopressin responsiveness of renal adenylate cyclase in rewborn rats and rabbits. Am J Physiol 1978; 234:F16–F21.

Spitzer A, Brandis M: Functional and morphologic maturation of the superficial nephrons: Relationship to total kidney function. J Clin Invest 1974; 53:279–287.

Stanier MW: Development of intra-renal solute gradients in foetal and postnatal life. Pfluegers Arch 1972; 336:263.

Steele BT, Paes B, Towell ME, Hunter DJS: Fetal renal failure associated with intrauterine growth retardation. Am J Obstet Gynecol 1988; 159:1200–1202.

Svenningsen NW: Renal acid-base titration studies in infants with and without metabolic acidosis in the postnatal period. Pediatr Res 1974; 8:659.

Vanpee M, Blennow M, Linne T, et al: Renal function in very low birth weight infants: Normal maturity reached during early childhood. J Pediatr 1992; 121(5 PT)1:784–788.

Zoubek J, Bloom DA, Sedman AB: Extraordinary urinary frequency. Pediatrics 1990; 85:1112–1114.

Evaluation of Renal Function in the Infant and Child

Batlle DC, Hizon MH, Cohen E, et al: The use of the urinary anion gap in the diagnosis of hyperchloremic metabolic acidosis. New Engl J Med 1988; 318:594–599.

Brodehl J: Renal hyperaminoaciduria. *In* Edelmann CM Jr, ed: Pediatric Kidney Disease. Boston, Little, Brown, 1978, pp 1047–1079

Brown ER, Stark A, Sosenko I: Bronchopulmonary dysplasia: Possible relationships to pulmonary edema. J Pediatr 1978; 92:982–984.

Chan JCM: Renal tubular acidosis. J Pediatr 1983; 102:327–340.

Cole CH: The Harriet Lane Handbook. Chicago, Year Book, 1984.

Donckerwolke RA, Valk C, van-Wijngaargen-Peterman MJ: The diagnostic value of the urine to blood carbon dioxide tension gradient for the assessment of distal tubular hydrogen secretion in pediatric patients with renal tubular disorders. Clin Nephrol 1983; 19:254–258.

Downing GJ, Egelhoff JC, Daily DK, et al: Kidney function in very low birth weight infants with furosemide-related renal calcifications at ages 1 to 2 years. J Pediatr 1992; 120(4 PT)1:599–604.

Hutcheon RA, Shibuya M, Leumann E, et al: Distal renal tubular acidosis in children with chronic hydronephrosis. J Pediatr 1976; 89:372–376.

Jacinto JS, Modanlou HD, Crade M: Renal calcification incidence in very low birth weight infants. Pediatrics 1988; 81:31–35.

Karlen J, Aperia A, Zetterstrom R: Renal excretion of calcium and phosphate in preterm and term infants. J Pediatr 1985; 106:814–819.

Mathew OP, Jones AS, James E, et al: Neonatal renal failure: Usefulness of diagnostic incices. Pediatrics 1980; 65:57–60.

Moore ES, Coe FL, McMann BJ, Favus MJ: Idiopathic hypercalciuria in children: Prevalence and metabolic characteristics. J Pediatr 1978; 92:906–910.

Rodriguez-Soriano J, Vallo A, Oliveros R: Transient pseudohypoaldosteronism secondary to obstructive uropathy in infancy. J Pediatr 1983; 103:375–380.

Rossi R, Danzebrink S, Linnenburger K, et al: Assessment of tubular reabsorption of sodium, glucose, phosphate and amino acids based on spot urine samples. Acta Paediatr 1994; 83:1282–1286.

Schwartz GJ, Brion LP, Spitzer A: The use of plasma creatinine concentration for estimating glomerular filtration rate in infants, children, and adolescents. Pediatr Clin North Am 1987; 34:571–590.

Stine KC, Linshaw MA: Use of furosemide in the evaluation of renal tubular acidosis. J Pediatr 1985; 107:559–562.

Trompeter RA, Al-Dahhan J, Haycock GB, et al: Normal values for plasma creatinine concentration related to maturity in normal term and preterm infants. Int J Pediatr Nephrol 1983; 4:145–148.

Hormonal Control of Renal Function During Development

Aperia A, Broberger O, Herin P, Zetterstrom R: Sodium excretion in relation to sodium intake and aldosterone excretion in newborn pre-term and full-term infants. Acta Paediatr Scand 1977; 68:813.

Bachmann S, Mundel P: Nitric oxide in the kidney: Synthesis, localization, and function. Am J Kidney Dis 1994; 24:112–129.

Bierd TM, Kattwinkel J, Chevalier RL, et al: The interrelationship of atrial natriuretic peptide, atrial volume, and renal function in premature infants. J Pediatr 1990; 116:753–759.

Bogaert GA, Kogan BA, Mevorach RA: Effects of endothelium-derived nitric oxide on renal hemodynamics and function in the sheep fetus. Pediatr Res 1993; 34:755–761.

Brace RA, Bayer LA, Cheung CY: Fetal cardiovascular, endocrine, and fluid responses to atrial natriuretic factor infusion. Am J Physiol 1989; 257:R580–R587.

Bräunlich H, Solomon S: Renal effects of atrial natriuretic factor in rats of different ages. Physiol Bohemoslov 1987; 36:119–124.

Buderus S, Thomas B, Fahnenstich H, Kowalewski S: Renal failure in two preterm infants: Toxic effect of prenatal maternal indomethacin treatment? Br J Obstet Gynaecol 1993; 100:97–98.

Castro LC, Law RW, Ross MG, et al: Atrial natriuretic peptide in the sheep. J Dev Physiol 1988; 10:235–246.

Celio MR, Groscurth P, Imagami T: Onotogeny of renin immunoreactive cells in the human kidney. Anat Embryol 1985; 173:149–155.

Cheung CY, Brace RA: Fetal hypoxia elevates plasma atrial natriuretic factor concentration. Am J Obstet Gynecol 1988; 159:1263–1268.

Chevalier RL, Gomez RA, Carey RM, et al: Renal effects of atrial natriuretic peptide infusion in young and adult rats. Pediatr Res 1988; 24:333–337.

Chevalier RL, Thornhill BA, Gomez RA: EDRF modulates renal hemodynamics during unilateral ureteral obstruction in the rat. Kidney Int 1992; 42:400–406.

Dolan LM, Young CA, Khoury JC, Dobrozsi DJ. Atrial natriuretic factor during the perinatal period: Equal depletion in both atria. Pediatr Res 1989; 25:339–341.

Dolan LM, Dobrozsi DJ: Atrial natriuretic polypeptide in the fetal rat: Ontogeny and characterization. Pediatr Res 1987; 22:115–117.

Ervin MG, Ross MG, Castro R, et al: Ovine fetal and adult atrial natriuretic factor metabolism. Am J Physiol 1988; 254:R40–R46.

Fiselier T, Monnens L, van Munster P, et al: The renin angiotensin aldosterone system in infancy and childhood in basal conditions and after stimulation. Eur J Pediatr 1984; 143:18–24.

Goetz KL: Physiology and pathophysiology of atrial peptides. Am J Physiol 1988; 254:E1–E15.

Gomez RA, Chevalier RL, Sturgill BC, et al: Maturation of the intrarenal renin distribution in Wistar-Kyoto rats. J Hypertens 1986; 4(Suppl 5):S31–S33.

Gomez RA, Lynch KR, Chevalier RL, et al: Renin and angiotensinogen gene expression in the maturing rat kidney. Am J Physiol 1988a; 254:F582–F587.

Gomez RA, Lynch KR, Chevalier RL, et al: Renin and angiotensinogen gene expression and intrarenal renin distribution during ACE inhibition. Am J Physiol 1988b; 254:F900–F906.

Gomez RA, Lynch KR, Sturgill BC, Elwood JP, Chevalier RL, Carey RM, Peach MJ. Distribution of renin mRNA and its protein in the developing kidney. Am J Physiol 1989; 257:F850–F858.

Gomez RA, Chevalier RL, Everett AD, et al: Recruitment of renin gene–expressing cells in adult rat kidneys. Am J Physiol 1990; 259:F660–F665.

Hargrave BY, Iwamoto HS, Rudolph AM: Renal and cardiovascular effects of atrial natriuretic peptide in fetal sheep. Pediatr Res 1989; 26:1–5.

Inagami T: Atrial natriuretic factor. J Biol Chem 1989; 264:3043–3046.

Jelinek J, Hackenthal R, Hilgenfeldt U, et al: The renin-angiotensin system in the perinatal period in rats. J Devel Physiol 1986; 8:33–41.

Jones C, Millan MA, Naftolin F, Aguilera G: Characterization of angiotensin II receptors in the rat fetus. Peptides 1989; 10:459–463.

Joppich R, Hauser I: Urinary prostacyclin and thromboxane A_2 metabolites in preterm and full-term infants in relation to plasma renin activity and blood pressure. Biol Neonate 1982; 42:179.

Kaplan BS, Restaino I, Raval DS, et al: Renal failure in the neonate associated with in utero exposure to non-steroidal anti-inflammatory agents. Pediatr Nephrol 1994; 8:700–704.

Kaplan SL, Feigin RD: Inappropriate secretion of antidiuretic hormone complicating neonatal hypoxic ischemic encephalopathy. J Pediatr 1978; 92:431–433.

Kikuchi K, Shiomi M, Horie K, et al: Plasma atrial natriuretic polypeptide concentration in healthy children from birth to adolescence. Acta Paediatr Scand 1988; 77:380–384.

Leake RD, Weitzman RE, Weinberg JA, Fisher DA: Control of vasopressin secretion in the newborn lamb. Pediatr Res 1979; 13:257–260.

Martin RA, Jones KL, Mendoza A, et al: Effect of ACE inhibition on the fetal kidney: Decreased renal blood flow. Teratology 1992; 46:317–321.

Melendez E, Reyes JL, Escalante BA, Melendez MA: Development of the receptors to prostaglandin E_2 in the rat kidney and neonatal renal functions. Dev Pharmacol Ther 1990; 14:125–134.

Moylan FMB, Herin JT, Kishnamoorthy K: Inappropriate antidiuretic hormone secretion in premature infants with cerebral injury. Am J Dis Child 1978; 132:399–402.

Muchant DG, Thornhill BA, Belmonte DC, et al: Chronic sodium loading augments the natriuretic response to acute volume expansion in the preweaned rat. Am J Physiol 1995; 269:R15–R22.

Nimrod C, Keane P, Harder J, et al: Atrial natriuretic peptide production in association with nonimmune fetal hydrops. Am J Obstet Gynecol 1988; 159:625–628.

O'Dea RF, Mirkin BL, Alward CT, Sinaiko AR: Treatment of neonatal hypertension with captopril. J Pediatr 1988; 113:403–406.

Osborn JL, Hook JB, Baile MD: Regulation of plasma renin in deleloping piglets. Dev Pharmacol Ther 1980; 1:217–228.

Pernollet MG, Devynck MA, Macdonald GJ, Meyer P: Plasma renin activity and adrenal angiotensin II receptors in fetal newborn, adult, and pregnant rabbits. Biol Neonate 1979; 36:119–127.

Pohjavuori M, Fyhrquist F: Hemodynamic significance of vasopressin in the newborn infant. J Pediatr 1980; 97:462–465.

Rajerison RM, Butten D, Jard S: Ontogenic development of kidney and liver vasopressin receptors. *In* Spitzer A, ed: The Kidney During Development: Morphology and Function. New York, Masson, 1982, pp 249–256

Reyes JL, Melendez E: Effects of eicosanoids on the water and sodium balance of the neonate. Pediatr Nephrol 1990; 4:630–634.

Richoux JP, Amsaguine S, Grignon G, et al: Earliest renin containing cell differentiation during ontogenesis in the rat. Histochemistry 1987; 88:41–46.

Robillard JE, Weitzman RE, Fisher DA, Smith FG Jr: The dynamics of vasopressin release and blood volume regulation during fetal hemorrhage in the lamb fetus. Pediatr Res 1979; 13:606–610.

Robillard JE, Gomez RA, Meernik JG, et al: Role of angiotensin II on the adrenal and vascular responses to hemorrhage during development in the fetal lamb. Circ Res 1982; 50:645–650.

Robillard JE, Weiner C: Atrial natriuretic factor in the human fetus: Effect of volume expansion. J Pediatr 1988; 113:552–556.

Robillard JE, Weismann DN, Gomez RA, et al: Renal and adrenal responses to converting-enzyme inhibition in fetal and newborn life. Am J Physiol 1983; 244:R249–R256.

Robillard JE, Weitzman RE: Developmental aspects of the fetal response to exogenous arginine vasopressin. Am J Physiol 1980; 238:F407–F414.

Ross MG, Ervin MG, Lam RW, et al: Plasma atrial natriuretic peptide response to volume expansion in the ovine fetus. J Pediatr 1987; 157:1292–1297.

Schoeneman MJ, Spitzer, A: The effect of intravascular volume expansion on proximal tubular reabsorption during development. Proc Soc Exp Biol Med 1980; 165:319–322.

Siegel SR, Fisher DA: Ontogeny of the renin-angiotensin-aldosterone system in the fetal and newborn lamb. Pediatr Res 1980; 14:99–102.

Solhaug MJ, Wallace MR, Granger JP: Endothelium-derived nitric oxide modulates renal hemodynamics in the developing piglet. Pediatr Res 1993; 34:750–754.

Stern P, LaRochette FT Jr, Little GA: Role of vasopressin in water imbalance in the sick newborn. Kidney Int 1979; 16:956.

Toshimori H, Toshimori K, Oura C, Matsue H: Immunohistochemical study of atrial natriuretic polypeptides in the embryonic, fetal and neonatal rat heart. Cell Tiss Res 1987; 248:627–633.

Vincent M, Dessary Y, Annat G, et al: Plasma renin activity, aldosterone and dopamine-β-hydroxylase activity as a functon of age in normal children. Pediatr Res 1980; 14:894.

Wallace KB, Hook JB, Bailie MD: Postnatal development of the renin-angiotensin system in rats. Am J Physiol 1980; 238:R432–R437.

Wei Y, Rodi CP, Day ML, et al: Developmental changes in the rat atriopeptin hormonal system. J Clin Invest 1987; 79:1325–1329.

Weil J, Bidlingmaier F, Dohlemann C, et al: Comparision of plasma atrial natriuretic peptide levels in healthy children from birth to adolescence and in children with cardiac diseases. Pediatr Res 1986; 20:1328–1331.

Yamaji T, Hirai N, Ishibashi M, et al: Atrial natriuretic peptide in umbilical cord blood: Evidence for a circulation hormone in human fetus. J Clin Endocrinol Metab 1988; 63:1414–1417.

The Functional Response of the Developing Kidneys to Malformation or Injury

Appenroth D, Bräunlich H: Age dependent differences in sodium dichromate nephrotoxicity in rats. Exp Pathol 1988; 33:179–185.

Argueso LR, Ritchey ML, Boyle ET Jr, et al: Prognosis of children with solitary kidney after unilateral nephrectomy. J Urol 1992; 148(2 Pt 2):747–751.

Aschinberg LC, Koskimies O, Bernstein J, et al: The influence of age on the response to renal parenchymal loss. Yale J Biol Med 1978; 51:341–345.

Beck AD: The effect of intra-uterine urinary obstruction upon the development of the fetal kidney. J Urol 1971; 105:784–789.

Bhathena DB, Julian BA, McMorrow RG, Baehler RW: Focal sclerosis of hypertrophied glomeruli in solitary functioning kidneys of humans. Am J Kidney Dis 1985; 5:226–232.

Bonvalet JP, Champion M, Wanstok F, Berjal G: Compensatory renal hypertrophy in young rats: Increase in the number of nephrons. Kidney Int 1972; 1:391–396.

Brenner BM, Meyer TW, Hostetter TH. Dietary protein intake and the progressive nature of kidney disease: The role of hemodynamically mediated glomerular injury in the pathogenesis of progressive glomerular sclerosis in aging, renal ablation, and intrinsic renal disease. N Engl J Med 1982; 307:652–659.

Brenner BM, Chertow GM: Congenital oligonephropathy and the etiology of adult hypertension and progressive renal injury. Am J Kidney Dis 1994; 23:171–175.

Celsi G, Bohman S-O, Aperia A. Development of focal glomerulosclerosis after unilateral nephrectomy in infant rats. Pediatr Nephrol 1987; 1:290–296.

Chevalier RL: Glomerular number and perfusion during normal and compensatory renal growth in the guinea pig. Pediat Res 1982a; 16:436–440.

Chevalier RL: Functional adaptation to reduced renal mass in early development. Am J Physiol 1982b; 242:F190–F196.

Chevalier RL: Hemodynamic adaptation to reduced renal mass in early postnatal development. Pediatr Res 1983; 17:620–624.

Chevalier RL: Chronic partial ureteral obstruction in the neonatal guinea pig II: Pressure gradients affecting glomerular filtration rate. Pediatr Res 1984; 18:1271–1277.

Chevalier RL, Sturgill BC, Jones CE, Kaiser DL: Morphologic correlates of renal growth arrest in neonatal partial ureteral obstruction. Pediatr Res 1987; 21:338–346.

Chevalier RL, Gomez RA: Response of the renin-angiotensin system to relief of neonatal ureteral obstruction. Am J Physiol 1989; 255:F1070–F1077.

Chevalier RL, Gomez RA, Jones CA: Developmental determinants of recovery after relief of partial ureteral obstruction. Kidney Int 1988; 33:775–781.

Chevalier RL, Kaiser DL: Autoregulation of renal blood flow in the rat: Effects of growth and uninephrectomy. Am J Physiol 1983; 244:F483–F487.

Chevalier RL, Kaiser DL: Chronic partial ureteral obstruction in the neonatal guinea pig I: Influence of uninephrectomy on growth and hemodynamics. Pediatr Res 1984; 18:1266–1271.

Chevalier RL, Peach MJ: Hemodyamic effects of enalapril on neonatal chronic partial ureteral obstruction. Kidney Int 1985; 28:891–898.

Dauber IM, Krauss AN, Symchych PS, Auld PAM: Renal failure following perinatal anoxia. J Pediatr 1976; 88:851–855.

Dicker SE, Shirley DG: Compensatory renal growth after unilateral nephrectomy in the newborn rat. J Physiol 1973; 228:193–202.

El-Dahr S, Gomez RA, Khare G, et al: Expression of renin and its mRNA in the adult rat kidney with chronic ureteral obstruction. Am J Kidney Dis 1990; 15:575–582.

El-Dahr SS, Gomez RA, Gray MS, et al: In situ localization of renin and its mRNA in neonatal ureteral obstruction. Am J Physiol 1990; 258:F854–F862.

Elema JD: Is one kidney sufficient? Kidney Int 1976; 9:308.

Fogo A, Ichikawa I: Evidence for the central role of glomerular growth promoters in the development of sclerosis. Semin Nephrol 1989; 9:329–342.

Glazebrook KN, McGrath FP, Steele BT: Prenatal compensatory renal growth: Documentation with US. Radiology 1993; 189:733–735.

Glick PL, Harrison MR, Noall RA, Villa RL: Correction of congenital hydronephrosis in utero III: Early mid-trimester ureteral obstruction produces renal dysplasia. J Pediatr Surg 1983; 18:681–687.

Gomez RA, Meernik JG, Kuehl WD, Robillard JE: Developmental aspects of the renal response to hemorrhage during fetal life. Pediatr Res 1984; 18:40–46.

Gomez RA, Chevalier RL, Sturgill BC, et al: Maturation of the intrarenal renin distribution in Wistar-Kyoto rats. J Hypertens 1986; 4(Suppl 5):S31–S33.

Griscom NT, Vawter GP, Fellers FX: Pelvoinfundibular atresia: The usual form of multicystic kidney: 44 unilateral and two bilateral cases. Semin Roentgenol 1975; 10:125–131.

Hayslett JP, Kashgarian M, Epstein FH: Functional correlates of compensatory renal hypertrophy. J Clin Invest 1968; 47:774–799.

Hayslett JP: Functional adaptation to reduction in renal mass. Physiol Rev 1979; 59:137–164.

Horster M, Kemler BJ, Valtin H: Intracortical distribution of number and volume of glomeruli during postnatal maturation in the dog. J Clin Invest 1971; 50:796–800.

Ikoma M, Yoshioka T, Ichikawa I, Fogo A: Mechanism of the unique susceptibility of deep cortical glomeruli of maturing kidneys to severe focal glomerular sclerosis. Pediatr Res 1990; 28:270–276.

Jongejan HTM, Provoost AP, Wolff ED, Molenaar JC: Nephrotoxicity of Cis-platin comparing young and adult rats. Pediatr Res 1986; 20:9–14.

Karp R, Brasel JA, Winick M: Compensatory kidney growth after uninephrectomy in adult and infant rats. Am J Dis Child 1971; 121:186–188.

Kaufman JM, Hardy R, Hayslett JP: Age-dependent characteristics of compensatory renal growth. Kidney Int 1975; 8:21–26.

King LR, Coughlin PWF, Bloch EC, et al: The case for immediate pyeloplasty in the neonate with ureteropelvic junction obstruction. J Urol 1984; 132:725–728.

Kiprov DD, Colvin RB, McCluskey RT: Focal and segmental glomerulosclerosis and proteinuria associated with unilateral renal agenesis. Lab Invest 1982; 46:275–281.

Kunes J, Capek K, Stejskal J, Jelinek J. Age-dependent difference of kidney response to temporary ischaemia in the rat. Clin Sci 1978; 55:365–368.

Larsson L, Aperia A, Wilton P: Effect of normal development on compensatory renal growth. Kidney Int 1980; 18:29–35.

Lelievre-Pegorier M, Sakly R, Meulemans A, Merlet-Benichou C: Kinetics of gentamicin in plasma of nonpregnant, pregnant, and fetal guinea pigs and its distribution in fetal tissues. Antimicrob Agents Chemother 1985; 28:565–569.

Luttenegger TJ, Gooding CA, Fickenscher LG: Compensatory renal hypertrophy after treatment for Wilms' tumor. Am J Roentgenol Radium Ther Nucl Med 1975; 125:348–351.

Mandell J, Peters CA, Estroff JA, et al: Human fetal compensatory renal growth. J Urol 1993; 150(2 Pt 2):790–792.

Marre R, Tarara N, Louton T, Sack K: Age-dependent nephrotoxicity and the pharmacokinetics of gentamicin in rats. Eur J Pediatr 1980; 133:25–29.

Mitus A, Tefft M, Fellers FX: Long-term follow-up of renal functions of 108 children who underwent nephrectomy for malignant disease. Pediatrics 1969; 44:912–921.

Norwood VF, Carey RM, Geary KM, et al: Neonatal ureteral obstruction stimulates recruitment of renin-secreting renal cortical cells. Kidney Int 1994; 45:1333–1339.

O'Sullivan DC, Dewan PA, Guiney EJ: Compensatory hypertrophy effectively assesses the degree of impaired renal function in unilateral renal disease. Br J Urol 1992; 69:346–350.

Okuda S, Motomura K, Sanai T, et al: Influence of age on deterioration of the remnant kidney in uninephrectomized rats. Clin Sci 1987; 72:571–576.

Olivetti G, Anversa P, Melissari M, Loud AV: Morphometry of the renal corpuscle during postnatal growth and compensatory hypertrophy. Kidney Int 1980; 17:438–454.

Patten BM: Human Embryology. New York, McGraw-Hill, 1968.

Pelayo JC, Andrews PM, Coffey AK, et al: The influence of age on acute renal toxicity of uranylnitrate in the dog. Pediatr Res 1983; 17:985–992.

Peters CA, Gaertner RC, Carr MC, Mandell J: Fetal compensatory renal growth due to unilateral ureteral obstruction. J Urol 1993; 150(2 Pt 2):597–600.

Phillips TL, Leong GF: Kidney cell proliferation after unilateral nephrectomy as related to age. Cancer Res 1967; 27:286–292.

Provoost AP, Adejuyigbe O, Wolff ED: Nephrotoxicity of aminoglycosides in young and adult rats. Pediatr Res 1985; 19:1191–1196.

Robillard JE, Gomez RA, Meernik JG, et al: Role of angiotensin II on the adrenal and vascular responses to hemorrhage during development in the fetal lambs. Circ Res 1982; 50:645–650.

Robillard JE, Weitzman RE, Burmeister L, Smith FG Jr: Developmental aspects of the renal response to hypoxemia in the lamb fetus. Circ Res 1981; 48:128–138.

Ross B, Cowett RM, Oh W: Renal functions of low birth weight infants during the first two months of life. Pediatr Res 1977; 11:1162–1164.

Shirley DG: Developmental and compensatory renal growth in the guinea pig. Biol Neonate 1976; 30:169–180.

Siegel SR, Oh W: Renal function as a marker of human fetal maturation. Acta Paediatr Scand 1976; 65:481–485.

Stark H, Geiger R: Renal tubular dysfunction following vascular accidents of the kidneys in the newborn period. J Pediatr 1990; 83:933–940.

Taki M, Goldsmith DI, Spitzer A: Impact of age on effects of ureteral obstruction on renal function. Kidney Int 1983; 24:602–609.

Weismann DN, Clarke WR: Postnatal age-related renal responses to hypoxemia in lambs. Circ Res 1981; 49:1332–1338.

Wikstad I, Celsi G, Larsson L, et al: Kidney function in adults born with unilateral renal agenesis or nephrectomized in childhood. Pediatr Nephrol 1988; 2:177–182.

56
RENAL DISEASE IN CHILDHOOD

Shane Roy III, M.D.
H. Norman Noe, M.D.

Disease of the renal parenchyma in a child requires interaction and efficient communication between the pediatric urologist and his nephrologic colleagues. Prompt recognition of such renal disorders can lead to appropriate evaluation and management, which can decrease unnecessary testing and avoid costly or invasive procedures. Close cooperation in this area will lead to the maximum treatment outcome as well as cost-effective management.

Although in many urban areas and medical centers all specialties are represented, many primary care physicians, because of well-established referral patterns, continue to send all children with any form of urinary finding or complaint to the urologist for initial evaluation. Such trust demands skill in the urologist in distinguishing medical renal disease from purely urologic disorders. This requires a thorough knowledge of the signs and symptoms of renal parenchymal diseases and the normal development of renal function during childhood as well as an ability to interpret laboratory data correctly. Thus, in these circumstances, the urologist must not only be concerned with abnormal urologic anatomy but also understand the pathophysiology and potential histopathology pertaining to renal parenchymal disorders.

The purpose of this chapter is to review the renal disorders of childhood from a clinical perspective and to provide guidelines for their evaluation and management. The fundamentals of the history and physical examination as well as basic laboratory studies are discussed, and certain specific renal diseases are defined in relation to children.

HISTORY AND PHYSICAL EXAMINATION

The history often provides enough information to make a presumptive diagnosis or at least to allow a targeted evaluation. The symptoms expressed by the parents or the child may be nonspecific and may include fatigue, malaise, or even abdominal pain and nausea and vomiting. A general sense of ill health may be marked by a history of weight loss or failure to thrive. A prior recent streptococcal illness may be suggestive of glomerulonephritis, or a prior viral illness might precede hematuria with IgA nephropathy. The child may have a concurrent illness that could give rise to a renal parenchymal abnormality, or he or she may be receiving medications that have nephrotoxic effects. **It is especially important to emphasize a family history to uncover diseases that are genetic or familial in nature.**

During the physical examination, certain clues may suggest a renal parenchymal disorder. In many cases, renal disease can be asymptomatic and somewhat insidious, and failure to thrive or small stature may be the only indicator of disease. Height and weight should be determined and, when plotted to allow assessment of any changes in the rate of growth of the child, can be critical. Other findings, such as flank pain, abdominal tenderness, renal enlargement, edema, or the presence of a rash, may be equally nonspecific. In many cases, edema can suggest certain disease processes; for example, dependent edema; labial and scrotal edema, which may be seen more with the nephrotic syndrome;

periorbital edema, which may occur in both the nephrotic syndrome and acute nephritis; and edema of the scalp, forehead, and lower back, which occurs more often in Henoch-Schönlein purpura. The chest should be examined for signs of fluid overload such as rales, pleural effusions, murmurs, or gallops. Funduscopic examination may reveal retinal edema or vascular spasm, particularly in the presence of acute nephritis and hypertension.

An important aspect of the physical examination in children with suspected renal parenchymal disease is the blood pressure. The 1987 report of the Second Task Force on Blood Pressure includes revised blood pressure standards for children grouped by age and sex. Attention to detail must be paid when obtaining the blood pressure in a child. **Cuff size is a major variable, and the appropriate size cuff should be used in all children.** The inflatable bladder within the blood pressure cuff should be long enough to encircle the arm completely, and the cuff should cover three quarters of the upper arm between the elbow and the proximal end of the humerus. The Task Force designation for significant hypertension is a reading above the 95th percentile for age. Elevation of blood pressure above this level has been found to be a major contributor to the progressive nature of certain renal diseases (Still et al, 1967; Mimran, 1988).

LABORATORY DATA

Laboratory evaluation of the patient with suspected renal disease should be based on the differential diagnosis suggested by the history and physical examination as well as the findings on urinalysis. **The main findings that suggest renal parenchymal disease are hematuria and proteinuria.** Additional laboratory studies include the complete blood count (CBC), serum electrolytes, serum creatinine and blood urea nitrogen, C3 and C4 complement, fluorescent antinuclear antibody (FANA), hepatitis B serology, sickle cell prep or hemoglobin electrophoresis (in African-American patients), quantitative urinary protein excretion, and a creatinine clearance measurement. Renal ultrasound with or without Doppler flow study of the renal vessels may also be performed in patients with suspected renal disease. The number of diagnostic studies as well as the rapidity of their performance are determined by the child's symptoms and clinical presentation. In some cases, renal biopsy is indicated depending on the specific disease or the clinical course of the patient.

Urinalysis

The one single laboratory test required for *every* patient in whom a renal parenchymal disorder is suspected is a urinalysis. The urine must be collected carefully by either clean or sterile technique and examined in the fresh state, **preferably by a physician or an experienced technician** to ensure maximum accuracy. The urinalysis includes a gross inspection of the urine, including its volume, concentrated appearance, and color, as well as dipstick and microscopic examination of the urinary sediment. A red or brown hue suggests either fresh or old bleeding associated with nephritis. It must be remembered, however, that the urine may be discolored for a number of reasons other than hematuria.

Dipstick examination of urine can be easily and quickly performed with any of the commercially available reagent strips. These strips are impregnated with individual reagents that give information about urinary constituents such as red blood cells, hemoglobin, protein, nitrites, pH, specific gravity, glucose, bilirubin, ketones, and so on.

Hematuria

Hematuria is the abnormal presence of red blood cells (RBCs) in the urine. It is typically described as either gross or microscopic, the latter being much more common in children. **The presence of blood in any quantity in the urine must always be confirmed by both dipstick reading and microscopic examination.** This is especially important in the evaluation of grossly discolored urine. It should be remembered that many conditions can produce a red urine that may not involve the presence of red blood cells (Table 56–1).

Although microscopic hematuria is more common than gross hematuria in children, it is more arbitrarily defined. Both adults and children normally excrete erythrocytes in their urine, and although the excretion rate in children has not been well established, most practitioners probably agree that rates of up to 50,000 RBC/hour (24-hour collection) are normal (Vehaskari et al, 1979). Because quantitative measurement techniques to determine the excretion rate of RBCs are not practical for office use, the author and his colleagues rely on qualitative measurements using impregnated reagent strips (dipsticks). The dipsticks are very sensitive and can detect as few as 5 to 20 RBCs/ml (50 or more RBCs/ml are required for an abnormal finding) (Norman, 1987).

Dipsticks can actually detect blood in the urine in the physiologic range. Most dipsticks test for hemoglobin on the basis of a pseudoperoxidase reaction in the reagent strip. In addition, some dipsticks test for intact erythrocytes, which are hemolyzed on a specific reagent strip that releases the

Table 56–1. CAUSES OF RED URINE MIMICKING HEMATURIA

- Heme positive (dipstick)
  - Hemoglobinuria
    - Hemolysis
    - Sepsis
    - Dialysis
  - Myoglobinuria
    - Ketoacidosis
    - Myositis
    - Trauma
- Heme negative (dipstick)
  - Drugs
    - Sulfa drugs
    - Nitrofurantoin
    - Salicylates
  - Foods
    - Beets
    - Food coloring
  - Metabolites
    - Homogentisic acid
    - Porphyrin

hemoglobin, which then provides the indicator reaction for blood. Thus, dipsticks are so sensitive that they can detect insignificant amounts of hematuria, necessitating microscopic examination of any urinary sediment in which blood is suspected.

Microscopy of the urinary sediment can be performed using an unspun or centrifuged specimen. The number of intact erythrocytes present per high power field determines the significance of hematuria. Although some disagreement exists about the number of red cells that are significant, most would agree that the presence of more than 5 RBCs per high power field in a spun specimen or 2 RBCs per high power field in an unspun specimen defines significant microscopic hematuria.

The presence of red cell casts on microscopy also strongly suggests glomerular disease in children. These casts are fragile, and low-speed centrifugation or even gravity sedimentation for 30 minutes will enhance the detection rate. Although red cell casts strongly support a diagnosis of glomerular bleeding, they are not always found. **Attention to red cell morphology in patients with suspected renal parenchymal disease has recently been used to enhance the accuracy of diagnosis**.

Red Blood Cell Morphology

Traditionally, localization of the site of hematuria has relied heavily on routine urine microscopy. **The hallmark of glomerular bleeding has been the presence of RBC casts with or without proteinuria**. Unfortunately, many children with glomerular or renal parenchymal disease have neither red cell casts nor proteinuria. Examination of the morphology of the RBCs in the urine has been shown to be very helpful in determining whether these RBCs have a glomerular or nonglomerular origin (Birch and Fairley, 1979; Rizzoni et al, 1983; Crompton et al, 1993; Roth et al, 1991). **Specifically, RBCs that retain their normal biconcave disc shape or are crenated (eumorphic) indicate nonglomerular bleeding, whereas dysmorphic RBCs are most often associated with glomerular bleeding (Fig. 56–1). Dysmorphic cells have distorted irregular outlines as well as variable cell size when examined under high power magnification (Fig. 56–2). Dysmorphic cells have bizarre shapes with irregular outlines, variable size, and cytoplasmic extrusions**. One particular cell type, a doughnut-shaped cell with cytoplasmic extrusions, has been said to be especially associated with glomerular bleeding.

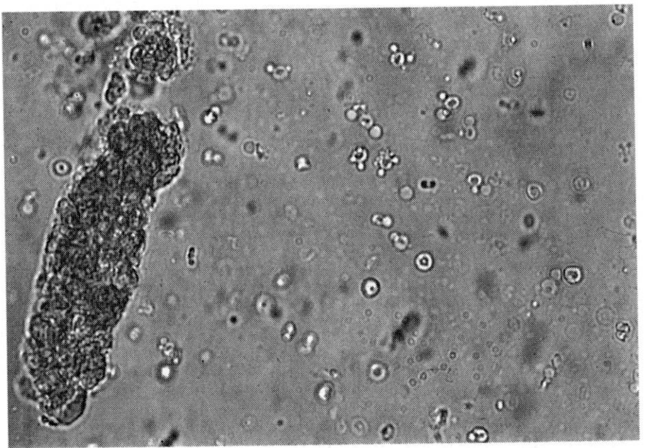

Figure 56–1. Urine from a patient who has poststreptococcal glomerulonephritis demonstrating a red blood cell cast and predominantly dysmorphic red blood cells.

The original reports of urinary red cell morphology relied exclusively on phase-contrast microscopy. Alternatives to this method for determining red cell morphology include Wright's staining of a dry smear of urinary sediment or simple light microscopy performed by an experienced examiner. Although no rigid criteria have been established for correlating RBC dysmorphism with a specific diagnosis, it can be a reliable tool in distinguishing glomerular bleeding. **One study indicated that a rate of 10% dysmorphism was diagnostic of glomerulonephritis and found a diagnostic specificity of 94% and a sensitivity of 92% in such cases (Stapleton et al, 1987)**. Although RBC morphology has proved to be a valuable adjunct to urine microscopy, the presence or absence of dysmorphic cells is not an absolute diagnostic finding. In some conditions the RBC morphology may be inconsistent with the clinical diagnosis. Examples include dysmorphic RBCs seen in nonglomerular disorders such as urinary tract infections, reflux nephropathy, and urolithiasis. However, RBC morphology considered along with other urinary sediment findings (i.e., proteinuria, casts, bacteria, and so on) is frequently all that is needed to localize the bleeding to a glomerular or nonglomerular source. This is especially true in the presence of the appropriate clinical history and physical findings suggestive of renal parenchymal disease. However, if dysmorphic urinary erythrocytes are identified in children with asymptomatic isolated hematuria (without protein or cellular casts), an appropriate evaluation for glomerulonephritis should still be initiated, but, in addition, an examination of the upper urinary tract with renal ultrasound is indicated to exclude urologic causes of hematuria, especially urolithiasis. If, however, all urinary red cells are eumorphic, the initial diagnostic studies should be directed toward discovering a nonglomerular or urologic cause of the hematuria. Such studies involve a urine culture, renal ultrasound, and possibly a voiding cystourethrogram. **If these studies are all normal, particularly in patients with gross eumorphic hematuria, cystoscopy is indicated**.

Proteinuria

Qualitative Detection of Proteinuria

Detection of proteinuria is most commonly made by dipstick (Albustix, Labstix, Multistix). The dye indicator turns a pale to dark green as the urine protein concentration varies from 0 to more than 2000 mg/dl. Only urine with a specific gravity of more than 1.018 should be tested because the dipstick reading for proteinuria is affected by the urine concentration. A strongly alkaline urine can produce a falsely positive dipstick reading for protein.

Quantitative Measurement of Proteinuria

In evaluation of persistent proteinuria or follow-up of parenchymal renal diseases quantitation of urinary protein excretion in a timed urine collection is recommended. Normal urinary protein excretion is less than 4 mg/m^2 per hour, abnormal urinary protein excretion is between 4 and

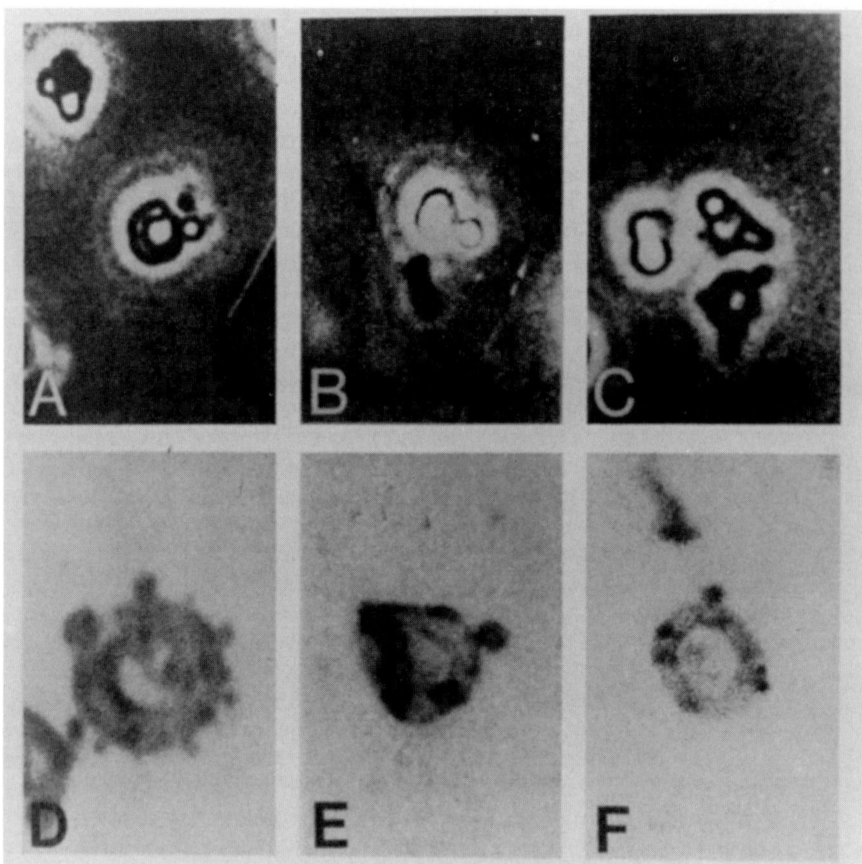

Figure 56–2. Dysmorphic red blood cells viewed by phase microscopy (A, B, and C). Dysmorphic red blood cells (D, E, and F) with Wright's stain.

40 mg/m^2 per hour, and nephrotic range proteinuria is greater than 40 mg/m^2 per hour.

Urinary Protein–Urinary Creatinine Ratio

Measurement of a urinary protein–urinary creatinine (Upr/Ucr) ratio in a random (preferably early morning) urine sample is a reasonably accurate way of assessing and following patients with renal disease. **Upr/Ucr ratios correlate very closely with timed quantitative urinary protein measurements. The normal range for a Upr/Ucr ratio is between 0 and 20 mg protein/mmol creatinine or a ratio of 0 to 0.18 (mg/mg)**. Further estimation of the protein excretion in children with nephrosis also reveals that a Upr/Ucr ratio of less than 0.1 is physiologic, and nephrotic range proteinuria is identified by a Upr/Ucr ratio of greater than 1.0 (mg/mg). When necessary, quantitation of urine protein excretion can be estimated from the linear regression equation: Total protein (g/m^2/day) = 0.63 (Upr/Ucr).

Creatinine Clearance

Clinical estimation of glomerular filtration rate (GFR) is accomplished using a timed urinary creatinine excretion and a plasma creatinine concentration to calculate the creatinine clearance (Ccr). Ccr is less accurate than inulin, ethylenediaminetetra-acetic acid (EDTA), or iothalamate clearances, which require infusion of these markers. GFR corrected for body surface area can also be estimated by the formula

$$GFR = K.HE \div Pcr$$

where K is an empirically derived constant, HE represents body height in centimeters, and Pcr equals plasma creatinine concentration in milligrams per deciliter (Schwartz et al, 1976). K for infants less than 1 year of age is 0.45, for children it is 0.55, for adolescent boys it is 0.7, and for preterm infants it is 0.33. This estimate of Ccr obviates the collection of a timed urine sample with the inherent mistakes associated with its collection.

Urinary Calcium Excretion

Quantitative Urinary Calcium Excretion

The normal value for urinary calcium excretion in 24 hours is less than 4 mg/kg per day in children (Ghazali and Barratt, 1974; Stapleton et al, 1982).

Urinary Calcium–Urinary Creatinine Ratio

Screening for hypercalciuria is performed on a random, preferably fasting, urine sample. **A urinary calcium–urinary creatinine (Uca/Ucr) ratio of less than 0.21 is normal in infants and children (Stapleton et al, 1982)**.

HEMATURIA

Etiology

Gross Hematuria

Among all renal findings, gross hematuria seems to be the most anxiety producing for parents, patients, and physicians. Although hematuria is always alarming, its cause is most often benign, and its course is usually limited. Nonetheless, it is important to ascertain a specific diagnosis in each case to alleviate both family and physician worry that a serious disorder may be overlooked. In the general pediatric population, gross hematuria is uncommon, occurring in approximately 1 of every 1000 visits (Ingelfinger et al, 1977). Among children presenting with acute onset of gross hematuria the causes of such hematuria are most readily detectable. **In Ingelfinger's study (1977), 49% of such patients had either confirmed or suspected urinary tract infections, and only 4% were found to have renal parenchymal disease**. Routine urine cultures are always necessary in any child with hematuria in which white blood cells or bacteria are present on urinalysis. It must be remembered that white blood cells can also suggest inflammation resulting solely from nephritis; if there is a question, a urine culture should always be obtained. A positive culture would most likely occur in a child with a purely urologic or congenital disorder as opposed to a renal parenchymal disease.

Microscopic Hematuria

Microscopic hematuria is more difficult to define and has a prevalence of 1.5% in children and adolescents (Dodge et al, 1976). As mentioned earlier, the presence of hematuria must be confirmed by both dipstick and microscopic examination of the urinary sediment. Microscopic hematuria is defined as the presence in a spun urine specimen of 5 or more RBCs per high power field in two of three urinalyses in an otherwise asymptomatic child. In the symptomatic child in the appropriate clinical situation, however, blood in a single urine sample is sufficient to require an evaluation.

Algorithm for Hematuria Evaluation

There are many causes of hematuria in children. An understanding of the causes allows one to formulate an approach not only to the differential diagnosis of hematuria but also to the most efficient method of evaluation. **Figures 56–3 and 56–4 offer both a differential diagnostic approach to the causes of hematuria in children and a planned evaluation designed to find the source of the hematuria (Fitzwater and Wyatt, 1994). These plans are based on documentation of blood in the urine, urinary RBC morphology, and the presence or absence of proteinuria, all taking into account the history, physical findings, and family history**.

Hematuria with Eumorphic Red Blood Cells

When hematuria with eumorphic RBCs is observed, an investigation for a nonglomerular cause of bleeding is necessary. Causes such as hypercalciuria, nephrolithiasis, nephrocalcinosis, cystitis, trauma, cystic kidney disease, sickle cell disease or trait, tumors, and urinary tract infections must be considered (see Fig. 56–3).

Hypercalciuria; Nephrolithiasis

Hypercalciuria is a common condition and a frequent cause of hematuria in otherwise healthy children. **Hypercalciuria is present in approximately 5% of healthy white children and is the most frequent cause of isolated hematuria in this group. Approximately 30% of children in whom hematuria is isolated (i.e., the urine is noninfected and the hematuria is nonglomerular) are found to be hypercalciuric (Moore, 1981; Stapleton et al, 1984)**. Hypercalciuria may be associated with episodic gross hematuria in the absence of demonstrated renal stones, but there are potential long-term implications for the development of stone disease in a child who has hematuria but has not yet manifested urolithiasis (Roy et al, 1981; Kalia et al, 1981; Noe et al, 1984).

Hypercalciuria may be associated with certain conditions such as immobilization, vitamin D intoxication, and the use of loop diuretics, but in most children it is idiopathic. The mechanism causing the hematuria is unclear but may involve irritation or actual tubular cell injury by calcium-containing crystals. The percentage of children with hypercalciuria who later develop stones is not clear, but it has been shown that two thirds of children with urolithiasis have associated hypercalciuria (Noe et al, 1983).

Urinary findings in the child with hypercalciuria usually are nonspecific with predominantly eumorphic red cells being noted in the urinary sediment. Calcium oxalate crystals may be present, but their presence is inconsistent. Occasionally, dysmorphic cells are seen in the child with established urolithiasis as previously discussed. **Screening for hypercalciuria is performed with a random Uca/Ucr ratio. A ratio of more than 0.21 indicates hypercalciuria in infants and children. Definitive diagnosis of hypercalciuria is established by quantitative measurement of calcium in a 24-hour urine collection. A urinary calcium excretory rate of more than 4 mg/kg per day is abnormal in children (Ghazali and Barratt, 1974; Stapleton et al, 1982).**

Management of hypercalciuria depends on the clinical symptoms. Simple dietary measures include avoidance of dietary excesses of calcium and sodium and increases in fluid intake. Specific therapy with hydrochlorothiazide is reserved for those with clinically significant stone formation. A short course of hydrochlorothiazide often results in the disappearance of microscopic hematuria and can serve as a diagnostic test.

Hematuria with Dysmorphic Red Blood Cells

Postinfectious Glomerulonephritis

Hematuria with symptoms and signs of acute glomerulonephritis including edema, hypertension, oliguria, and

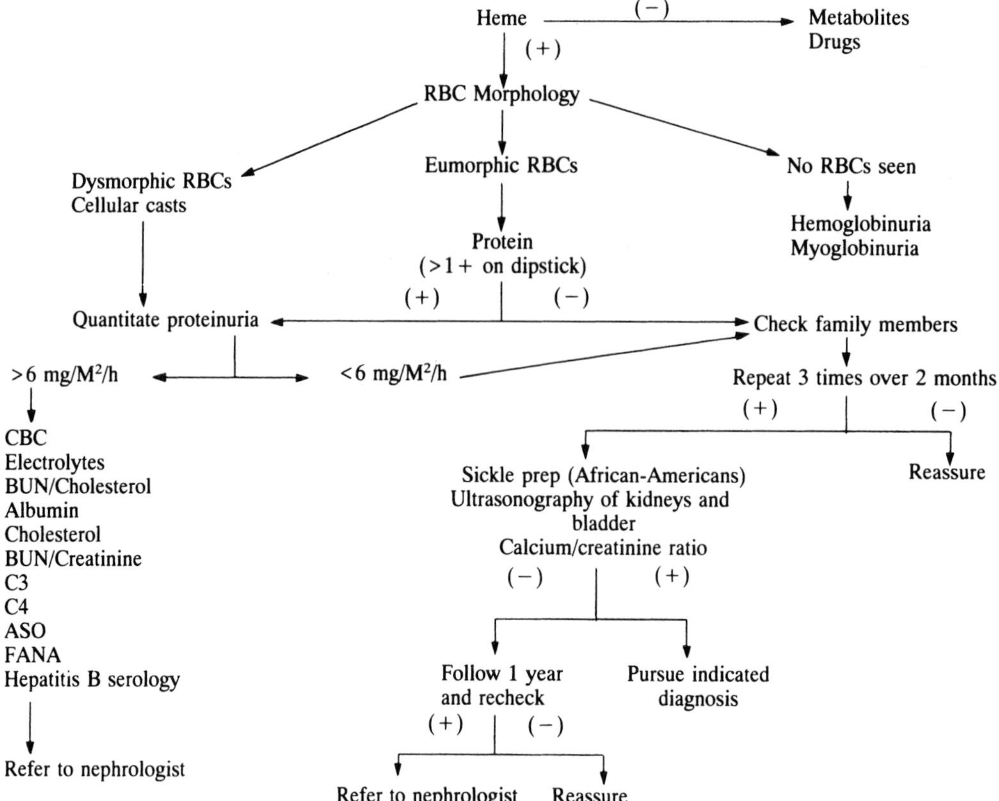

Figure 56–3. Evaluation of hematuria.

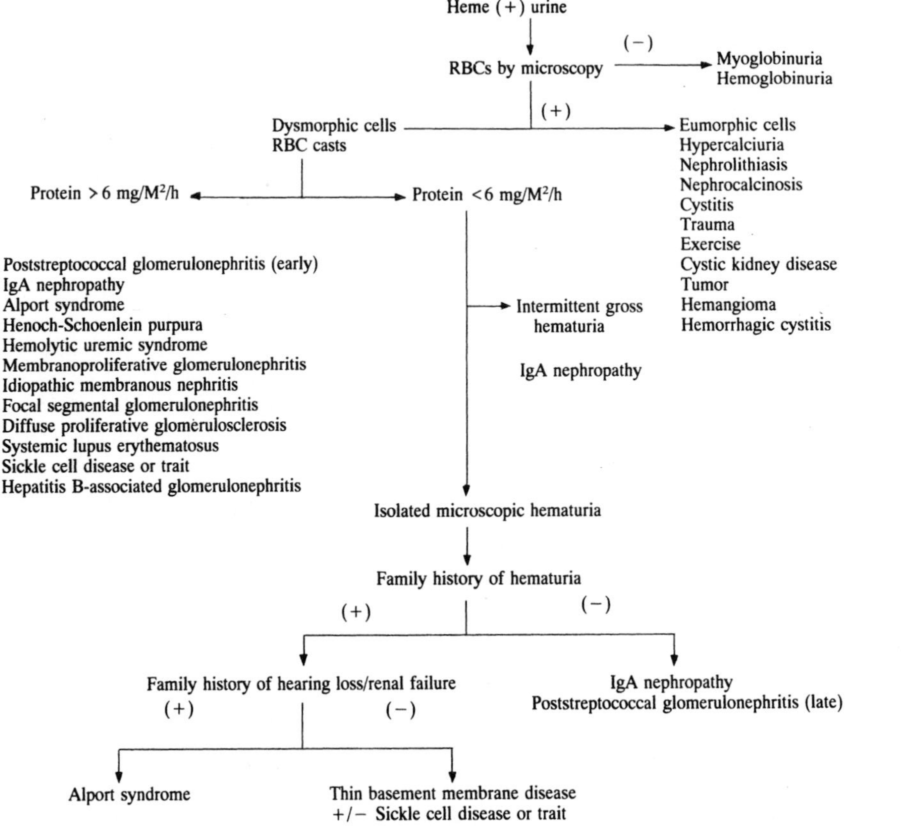

Figure 56–4. Differential diagnosis of hematuria.

the presence of dysmorphic RBCs and RBC casts on urine microscopy requires an investigation to determine the cause. Postinfectious glomerulonephritis, usually following group A beta-hemolytic streptococcal sore throat or pyoderma, is the most common cause of glomerulonephritis in children. A latency period of 7 to 10 days following the occurrence of a group A beta-hemolytic streptococcal sore throat or 21 to 30 days following streptococcal pyoderma occurs prior to the appearance of the common presenting symptoms of edema and brownish cola-colored urine. **A positive antistreptolysin-0 or streptozyme titer and a decreased serum complement (C3) concentration are usually present.** Varying degrees of acute renal insufficiency with oliguria or even anuria requiring intermittent dialysis may be seen. Control of hypertension, management of electrolyte and fluid balance, and treatment of renal functional impairment are necessary during the acute phase of the illness. **Complete recovery of renal function can be expected in more than 90% of cases even in those who have a protracted clinical course requiring peritoneal dialysis or hemodialysis.** Microscopic hematuria and minimal proteinuria may persist for 3 to 6 months. C3 concentrations usually become normal within 2 months of disease onset. **Proteinuria that persists 12 months after disease onset may require a renal biopsy to assess the degree of renal histologic damage.**

IgA Nephropathy

IgA nephropathy is a common cause of glomerulonephritis that is defined immunohistologically by the presence of mesangial deposits of IgA in renal biopsy tissue in the absence of a systemic disease. Patients usually present with recurrent macroscopic hematuria during the course of an upper respiratory infection. IgA nephropathy is most often confused with postinfectious glomerulonephritis. **However, the prodromal period between infection and the appearance of symptoms of nephritis is 7 to 10 days or more in patients with postinfectious glomerulonephritis. Gross hematuria in patients with IgA nephropathy usually appears during an acute infection.** A poor prognosis in patients with IgA nephropathy is indicated by the presence of renal histologic findings of glomerulosclerosis, severe mesangial proliferation, glomerular crescents, and significant interstitial fibrosis associated with renal function impairment, hypertension, male gender, older age at the time of biopsy, and more than 2 g/day of proteinuria (Hogg et al, 1994). **Progressive renal failure may be expected in 30% to 50% of patients after 10 to 20 years of follow-up. No treatment has proved to be of benefit.** Prednisone treatment protocols are currently being evaluated at several centers.

Henoch-Schönlein Purpura

Henoch-Schönlein purpura is a vasculitic syndrome observed primarily in boys between the ages of 2 and 11 years of age. It is manifested by nonthrombocytopenic purpura, colicky abdominal pain, joint pain and swelling, and glomerulonephritis. The diagnosis is confirmed by clinical findings. Renal involvement occurs in 20% to 50% of patients, persistent nephropathy is seen in 1% of all cases, and progression to end-stage renal disease occurs in less than 1%. Children with hematuria alone do not develop chronic renal failure, but 15% of those who have both hematuria and proteinuria may develop renal failure. **In patients who develop nephrotic syndrome with Henoch-Schönlein purpura approximately 50% will develop end-stage renal disease within 10 years. Patients with either a nephritic or nephrotic clinical presentation should be considered for renal biopsy.** No specific treatment is available for Henoch-Schönlein purpura. Steroids can produce favorable results in patients with soft tissue swelling, joint disease, scrotal swelling, and abdominal colic or gastrointestinal hemorrhage. **Neither prednisone nor other immunosuppressants have been proved in a controlled study to benefit patients with Henoch-Schönlein purpura nephritis, but they continue to be used clinically in patients with severe nephritis or nephrotic syndrome.**

Hemolytic-Uremic Syndrome

The hemolytic-uremic syndrome (HUS) is a heterogeneous group of disorders manifested by microangiopathic hemolytic anemia, thrombocytopenia, and acute renal failure. It is the most frequent cause of acute renal failure in children. The vasculopathy involves endothelial damage in small- to medium-sized arteries with fibrin deposition and thrombotic microangiopathy. There are diarrheal and nondiarrheal forms of HUS. The diarrheal form is most common and is associated with cytotoxin-producing organisms such as verotoxin-producing *Escherichia coli* or *Shigella dysenteriae*, which produce Shiga's toxin. Nondiarrheal forms of HUS may be related to infections with *Streptococcus pneumoniae* and many viruses or to autosomal dominant or recessive inheritance, malignancy, renal transplantation, or drugs such as cyclosporine A, oral contraceptives, and chemotherapeutic agents (Kaplan et al, 1990).

Treatment of HUS includes dialysis for renal failure, management of acute renal insufficiency, maintenance of the hemoglobin level at 8 g/dl or higher, and administration of platelet transfusions for symptomatic bleeding. Plasma transfusion for hereditary, prolonged, or recurrent HUS may be considered but should be avoided in patients with pneumococcal-associated HUS (Siegler, 1988). Plasmapheresis, if technically feasible, may be beneficial in patients with recurrent, inherited, or drug-induced HUS.

Prognosis of HUS is poor in patients who have nondiarrheal forms of the disease, are less than a year of age, or have prolonged anuria, severe hypertension, or severe central nervous system disease. Renal transplantation may be necessary following dialysis, but HUS can recur in the transplanted kidney. Recovery of renal function may occur in 65% to 85% of patients with HUS if the hereditary and recurrent forms of HUS are excluded.

Alport's Syndrome

Alport's syndrome consists of hereditary nephritis, high-frequency hearing loss, and ocular abnormalities. Children may present with recurrent or persistent hematuria and proteinuria. **A family history of nerve deafness is usually obtained, and one or more family members may have died from renal failure, undergone dialysis, or re-**

ceived a renal transplant. Gene-mapping studies suggest that clinical subtypes of juvenile-onset end-stage renal disease (ESRD) with deafness, adult-onset ESRD with deafness, and adult-onset ESRD with normal hearing are due to allelic mutations of a single genetic locus on the X chromosome. Also, there is strong evidence that a genetic defect in type IV collagen is responsible for the glomerular basement membrane defects found in renal biopsy tissue from these patients (Kashtan et al, 1990). **The nephritis is progressive in nature, especially in males, and leads to renal failure in the second to third decade of life.**

Systemic Lupus Erythematosus

Systemic lupus erythematosus (SLE) is a multisystem autoimmune disease characterized by widespread inflammation that most often affects females in the second or third decades of life. SLE affects Orientals, African-Americans, Hispanics, and whites in decreasing order of prevalence. **The classic disease onset is marked by fever, rash, arthritis, varying degrees of renal involvement, and decreased C3 and C4 complement. Renal involvement is a major cause of morbidity and mortality. Eighty percent of pediatric patients with SLE are female, and the peak age of onset is 12 years. From 60% to 80% of children have renal involvement at the time of diagnosis, and renal involvement occurs in most of the rest within 2 years**.

The histologic forms of SLE nephropathy are mesangial lupus nephritis (or minimal glomerular involvement), membranous lupus nephropathy, focal glomerulonephritis (FGN), and diffuse proliferative glomerulonephritis (DPGN), which is the most severe form. **Hematuria and proteinuria are almost always observed at diagnosis in children with DPGN (88%), and at least half have massive proteinuria leading to the nephrotic syndrome**. Renal insufficiency is most often seen in patients with DPGN. Membranous nephropathy is usually associated with the nephrotic syndrome, and 50% of patients have microscopic hematuria. Children with FGN have hematuria and mild proteinuria.

SLE may be treated with prednisone, azathioprine, chlorambucil, or cyclophosphamide. Patients with DPGN are treated with an initial course of methylprednisolone followed by high doses of prednisone. Patients with changes in renal function, urinary protein excretion, C3 and C4, and anti-DNA antibody concentration receive follow-up care. If clinical or laboratory improvement after several weeks of treatment fails to occur, or if unacceptable steroid side effects appear, intravenous cyclophosphamide therapy can be considered. **Recent studies in both adults and children demonstrate gratifying improvement in renal function following low-dose oral prednisone, seven monthly doses of intravenous cyclophosphamide, and additional intravenous cyclophosphamide every 3 months for 18 to 24 months**. Longer follow-up observations of patients receiving treatment with this latter protocol are ongoing.

Crescentic Glomerulonephritis

Crescentic glomerulonephritis may be associated with most forms of primary glomerulonephritis or with systemic diseases such as SLE, Henoch-Schönlein purpura, and systemic vasculitis. Patients with a rapidly progressive clinical course usually have large epithelial crescents in more than 50% of their glomeruli on renal biopsy. Children with poststreptococcal crescentic glomerulonephritis usually recover after only symptomatic therapy. **However, children with systemic vasculitis have a worse prognosis, which may be favorably influenced by treatment with plasmapheresis, corticosteroids, or alkylating agents**.

Anti-neutrophil cytoplasmic autoantibodies (ANCA) are found in the circulation of patients with necrotizing systemic vasculitis (polyarteritis nodosa and Wegner's granulomatous) and idiopathic pauci-immune glomerulonephritis. Few if any immune deposits are observed by immunofluorescence microscopy in these patients.

The presence of anti-glomerular basement membrane (GBM) antibodies in patients with lung hemorrhage (Goodpasture's syndrome) and without lung hemorrhage (anti-GBM disease) aid in diagnosing anti-GBM-mediated glomerulonephritis. Anti-DNA autoantibodies, anti-streptococcal antibodies, and serum cryoglobulins differentiate lupus glomerulonephritis, poststreptococcal glomerulonephritis, and cryoglobulinemic glomerulonephritis, respectively, as forms of immune complex glomerulonephritis.

Sickle Cell Nephropathy

Specific renal functional abnormalities such as increased total renal blood flow, decreased flow in the vasa recta, decreased maximum urine osmolality in response to water deprivation, abnormal lowering of urine pH in response to acid loading, and increased tubular secretion of uric acid occur in patients with sickle cell disease. **The features of the clinical entity referred to as sickle cell nephropathy include hematuria, papillary necrosis, glomerulopathy, nephrogenic diabetes insipidus, incomplete renal tubular acidosis, hyperuricemia, and asymptomatic bacteriuria.**

Hematuria is a common renal abnormality in patients with sickle cell anemia. Heterozygotes are affected more frequently than homozygotes probably because there are many more heterozygotes in the population. **Males are affected more often, and the hematuria most frequently arises from the left kidney. Bed rest and hydration should be tried first as treatment. If hematuria is prolonged for 1 to 2 weeks or if transfusion is necessary, alkalinization, aminocaproic acid, or intravenous diuresis should be tried.**

Patients with sickle cell disease may develop the nephrotic syndrome, which can progress to renal failure. Glomerular pathology includes reduplication of the basement membrane with mild mesangial proliferation, focal glomerulosclerosis, or immune complex glomerulonephritis. The authors (Roy et al, 1976) and others have reported acute poststreptococcal glomerulonephritis in several patients with sickle cell disease.

Thin Glomerular Basement Membrane Disease

Recurrent or permanent microhematuria may occur in a familial form. This finding has also been referred to as benign recurrent hematuria or benign familial hematuria to differentiate it from Alport's syndrome, which has a much worse prognosis. In some children benign familial hematuria is accompanied by thin glomerular basement membranes and lamina densa (1233 ± 51 Å and 682 ± 31 Å, respectively, as opposed to the normal dimensions of 1863 ± 31 Å and 1402 ± 40 Å). In one study of 43 patients with isolated microhematuria and abnormal findings on renal biopsy, the only abnormality in 17 patients was thin glomerular capillary basement membranes (Trachtman et al, 1984). The presence of microhematuria in other family members who do not have a history of renal disease or neurosensory deafness or did not die from renal disease is usual, but urinalyses must be performed on these family members. RBC casts are common, but proteinuria is usually absent or minimal.

The results of one well-designed and performed study (Trachtman et al, 1984) in children suggest that a renal biopsy is necessary in children with microhematuria only if there is a positive family history of hematuria in a first-degree relative or if the child has had at least one episode of gross hematuria. In this study, the findings in nearly 75% of renal biopsy specimens were abnormal, and IgA nephropathy and Alport's syndrome were present in 60% of cases. The renal biopsy in a child with isolated microscopic hematuria nearly always shows a normal morphology or nonspecific alterations of unknown clinical relevance.

PROTEINURIA

Isolated Proteinuria

Transient Proteinuria

Proteinuria on a routine screening urinalysis is not uncommon in the pediatric population. It may be related to a febrile illness, exercise, congestive heart failure, seizures, or exposure to cold. **In a study of 8954 schoolchildren between the ages of 8 and 15 years, proteinuria was present in one of four urine specimens in 10.7% of the children and in at least two of four specimens in 2.5% (Vehaskari et al, 1982).** Proteinuria may indicate a completely benign condition or may be the first clue to a significant renal parenchymal disease such as the nephrotic syndrome or glomerulonephritis. Proteinuria is initially detected most often by a semiquantitative dipstick analysis or by the turbidimetric sulfosalicylic acid method. **In an otherwise asymptomatic child, the test for proteinuria should be repeated two or more times. If only the first urine sample is positive for protein, routine medical care is recommended, and the proteinuria is considered isolated or transient.**

Orthostatic Proteinuria

If two or more urine samples are positive for protein, testing to demonstrate orthostatic proteinuria is recommended. The child should void at bedtime and discard the sample. A urine sample is then obtained before the patient arises in the morning or after as little ambulation as possible. A second sample is collected later in the day and labeled specimen number 2. The specific gravity of the first urine sample should be 1.018 or greater. If specimen 1 is free of protein and specimen 2 is positive for protein, the orthostatic test is positive. This test should be repeated to confirm the presence of orthostatic proteinuria. If both samples of urine contain protein, a systematic evaluation for other causes of proteinuria is necessary.

Persistent Asymptomatic Proteinuria

Persistent proteinuria exists when at least 80% of urine specimens contain excessive amounts of protein. The first step in evaluating a child with persistent proteinuria is to quantitate the urinary protein excretion by means of a timed urine sample (12- or 24-hour collection) or with a random Upr/Ucr ratio. Urinary protein excretion of more than 4 mg/m^2 per hour is abnormal, and a level above 40 mg/m^2 per hour is in the nephrotic range. A Upr/Ucr ratio (mg/mg) of above 0.18 is abnormal, and above 2.0 it is in the nephrotic range. Further quantitation of proteinuria using linear regression analysis may be obtained from the equation, Total protein (g/m^2/day) = 0.63 (Upr/Ucr).

In patients with a confirmatory test for orthostatic proteinuria and more than 1.0 g/day of urinary protein excretion and in those with a nonconfirmatory test for orthostatic proteinuria the following studies should be performed: serum electrolytes, BUN, serum creatinine, serum albumin, serum complement (C3), urine culture, and renal ultrasound. A renal biopsy may also be considered depending on the results of this evaluation.

Studies in children with persistent asymptomatic proteinuria have reported either a good prognosis, minimal histologic changes on renal biopsy, or significant renal histologic changes associated with the possibility of progressive renal failure. Among 53 children who underwent renal biopsy because of persistent asymptomatic proteinuria, significant glomerular abnormalities were observed in 47% (Yoshikawa et al, 1991). Focal segmental glomerulosclerosis (FSGS) in 15 patients, with chronic renal failure in 7 of these 15 patients, was observed. A worse prognosis in children with FSGS plus the nephrotic syndrome than in those with FSGS and persistent asymptomatic proteinuria has been reported (Roy and Stapleton, 1987). However, patients in this latter category occasionally progress to chronic renal failure during follow-up. Effective treatment in many patients with persistent asymptomatic proteinuria may not be possible. It is reasonable to recommend a renal biopsy when excessive asymptomatic proteinuria has persisted for more than 6 to 12 months. This will allow a more accurate prognosis to be made in anticipation of potential specific treatment in the future.

Proteinuria with Glomerular Diseases

Nephrotic Syndrome

The nephrotic syndrome in children is defined as the presence of edema, hypoalbuminemia (<2.5 g/dl), hypercholesterolemia, and urinary protein excretion of greater than 40 mg/m^2 per hour. Other laboratory abnormalities such as hyponatremia, hypocalcemia (low albumin-bound calcium with normal ionized calcium concentration), and coagulation abnormalities are commonly present. Recognized histologic forms of childhood nephrotic syndrome are minimal change disease (MCNS), FSGS, membranoproliferative glomerulonephritis (MPGN), mesangial-proliferative glomerulonephritis (MESP-GN) and membranous glomerulonephritis (MEMB-GN) (Kelsch and Sedman, 1993).

Minimal Change Nephrotic Syndrome

Children with the nephrotic syndrome present with edema or with proteinuria discovered during a routine office visit. MCNS accounts for 60% to 90% of children with the nephrotic syndrome. Evaluation of these patients should include measurements of serum electrolytes, BUN, creatinine, C3 and C4 complement, streptozyme titer, antinuclear antibody titer, and hepatitis B antibiody titer. Children with MCNS almost always have a normal C3. **A renal biopsy is necessary in children with the nephrotic syndrome who are less than 1 year or over 10 years of age, children with a low C3 level or a positive anti-nuclear antibody test, and those in whom the disease has a major "nephritic" component.** Recommended treatment is daily prednisone (60 mg/m^2 per day) for 4 to 6 weeks followed by a dose of 40 mg/m^2 on alternate days for 4 to 6 weeks and tapering doses for 4 weeks thereafter (Brodehl, 1991). **Approximately 93% of children with MCNS respond to prednisone, 71% have a subsequent relapse, and 44% have multiple relapses. Steroid-resistant patients should have a renal biopsy, and patients with multiple relapses may require a biopsy prior to a course of either cyclophosphamide or chlorambucil.**

Focal Segmental Glomerulosclerosis

Children with the nephrotic syndrome who fail to respond to a 2-month course of prednisone require a renal biopsy. **Many of these nephrotic children are found to have FSGS, especially those who are over 8 to 10 years of age.** FSGS discovered on renal biopsy generally carries a poor prognosis and may progress to renal failure. Up to 30% of patients with FSGS who receive a renal transplant may develop a recurrence of FSGS in the renal transplant.

Membranoproliferative Glomerulonephritis

MPGN is diagnosed most often during the initial evaluation of patients with nephrotic syndrome because 70% to 80% have a low C3 concentration and are candidates for renal biopsy. They tend to have a nephritic clinical picture rather than the typical nephrotic syndrome at initial presentation. Approximately half of these patients will progress to end-stage renal disease after 10 years of follow-up. Prednisone (40 mg/m^2 on alternate days) is usually recommended for children with MPGN and is continued for years.

Membranous Nephropathy

Idiopathic membranous nephropathy is rarely seen in children. The secondary form of MEMB-GN may be seen in patients with lupus erythematosus, hepatitis B infection, or gold therapy for severe rheumatoid arthritis; on rare occasions it appears de novo in renal transplant patients. As many as half the children with primary membranous nephropathy sustain a spontaneous remission. A course of prednisone is indicated for patients with membranous nephropathy and clinically overt nephrotic syndrome or renal insufficiency.

Membranous nephropathy in North American children secondary to hepatitis B surface antigenemia is not common. In one report (Southwest Pediatric Nephrology Study Group, 1985) 7 of 11 children were male and black, and the mean age of 5.3 years was somewhat less than that of children with idiopathic membranous nephropathy. Eight of ten patients had elevated aspartate aminotransferase levels, all 11 children at some stage of their illness had low serum C3 concentrations, and 10 of 11 had the nephrotic syndrome.

Mesangial Proliferative Glomerulonephritis

Mesangial proliferative glomerulonephritis has an unpredictable clinical course. Some patients may respond to prednisone in a manner similar to those with MCNS, whereas others fail to respond to steroids or alkylating agents and progress to renal insufficiency. Some patients undergo a remission of the nephrotic syndrome without any treatment.

Congenital Nephrotic Syndrome

If the nephrotic syndrome is diagnosed in a child less than 1 year of age, a renal biopsy is indicated. If edema and proteinuria are noted in the first 3 months of life, the congenital nephrotic syndrome (CNS) should be suspected. Cytomegalic inclusion disease and syphilis must be excluded. CNS does not respond to steroids and must be managed conservatively. Long-term management may include daily intravenous albumin infusions, bilateral nephrectomy, dialysis, and early renal transplantation. These children are prone to pneumococcal sepsis, peritonitis, clotting abnormalities, and malnutrition. On rare occasions a spontaneous remission of CNS occurs, so aggressive therapy such as bilateral nephrectomy, dialysis, and transplantation should be delayed until a serious life-threatening complication of CNS occurs.

Proteinuria with Tubulointerstitial Diseases

Reflux Nephropathy

Proteinuria in the presence of a history of a past urinary tract infection or unexplained febrile illness treated with antibiotics should alert the physician to the fact that reflux nephropathy may exist. These children are usually hypertensive. Renal ultrasound may not demonstrate cortical scarring, and therefore a dimercaptosuccinic acid (DMSA) scan should be obtained. Especially in older children, vesicoureteral reflux may have resolved by the time renal scarring is demonstrated.

Acute Tubulointerstitial Nephritis

ATIN is characterized by diffuse or focal inflammation and edema of the renal interstitium with secondary involvement of the tubules and minimal or no glomerular changes. **Clinically, patients may have mild to severe renal failure, normal or decreased urinary output, mild hematuria, decreased urinary concentration, proteinuria, pyuria, white blood cell casts, and, in up to 86% of patients with drug-induced ATIN, eosinophiluria as documented by Hassel's stain. Eosinophiluria is evident in less than 5% of patients with nonsteroidal anti-inflammatory drug (NSAID)–induced ATIN.**

Immune-Mediated Acute Tubulointerstitial Nephritis

The major clinical manifestations of immune-mediated ATIN are those of tubular dysfunction and include proteinuria with glomerular dysfunction, proximal renal tubular acidosis or Fanconi's syndrome with proximal tubular dysfunction, distal renal tubular acidosis, hyperkalemia or sodium wasting with distal tubular dysfunction, and decreased concentrating capacity with medullary and papillary dysfunction. A histologic form of ATIN showing linear immunofluorescence of the tubular basement membrane with IgG and complement is known as anti-tubular basement membrane disease. Sarcoidosis, Sjögren's syndrome, and tubulointerstitial nephritis–uveitis syndrome are other examples of immune-mediated ATIN. **When findings are inconclusive for prerenal azotemia, the clinical picture is not characteristic of ATIN, and obstructive nephropathy has been excluded, a renal biopsy may be required for diagnosis.**

Drug-Related Acute Tubulointerstitial Nephritis

Systemic manifestations of an allergic process such as rash, fever, and eosinophilia may accompany ATIN in patients with drug-induced ATIN. The drugs most commonly associated with ATIN are antibiotics (methicillin, penicillin, ampicillin, cephalosporins, sulfonamides, rifampin), nonsteroidal anti-inflammatory drugs (fenoprofen, naproxen, ibuprofen), and diuretics.

Infection-Related Acute Tubulointerstitial Nephritis

Streptococcal diseases, diphtheria, toxoplasmosis, brucellosis, syphilis, rickettsia, Epstein-Barr virus infections, and other conditions have also been implicated in the etiology of ATIN. Resolution of ATIN often occurs with removal of the inciting factors such as drugs or with treatment of the causative infections. **In biopsy-proven ATIN in which renal failure has persisted for more than 1 week after removal of the inciting factors or when no inciting factors can be found, a short course of high-dose prednisone therapy is recommended (Neilson, 1989).** If the biopsy already shows significant interstitial scarring, less chance of benefit from steroid therapy can be expected. Lack of response to steroids after 3 to 4 weeks is an indication to discontinue therapy. Cyclophosphamide is very effective in animal models of ATIN. **In patients who fail to respond to steroids and have minimal or no fibrosis on biopsy, cyclophosphamide is suggested for 3 to 4 months if the GFR improves.**

RENAL TUBULAR DISORDERS

Nephrogenic Diabetes Insipidus

The inability of a male child to form concentrated urine after receiving the antidiuretic hormone arginine vasopressin suggests a diagnosis of X-linked nephrogenic diabetes insipidus (NDI). In neonates the symptoms of NDI are seen in the first weeks of life and include polyuria, polydipsia, irritability, poor feeding, poor weight gain, fever, and dehydration. Later in childhood obstipation, nocturia, enuresis, poor growth, and mental retardation are seen. Long-standing polyuria may lead to the development of megaureter and hydronephrosis, which can mimic lower urinary tract obstruction. Plasma vasopressin levels are usually normal or slightly elevated in affected children.

Secondary forms of NDI must be excluded such as drug-induced disease (lithium and tetracyclines), analgesic nephropathy, sickle cell disease, hypokalemia, hypercalcemia, obstructive uropathy, renal dysplasia, chronic pyelonephritis, amyloidosis, sarcoidosis, and chronic uremic nephropathy.

A combination of hydrochlorothiazide and amiloride will decrease urine volume, increase urine osmolality, and conserve potassium in patients with NDI. The efficiency of this therapy in patients with NDI is attributed to reduction of the extracellular sodium concentration with enhancement of sodium reabsorption.

Miscellaneous Tubular Disorders

Cystinosis

Low serum bicarbonate, potassium, and phosphate concentrations associated with glucosuria, aminoaciduria, hyperchloremic metabolic acidosis, and rickets characterize the proximal tubulopathy known as Fanconi's syndrome. In the past the most common cause of Fanconi's syndrome in children was infantile nephropathic cystinosis. These children have blond hair, photophobia, depigmentation of the retina, short stature, rickets, and renal insufficiency by 10 years of age. This syndrome is caused by an abnormal efflux of cystine out of the lysosome of most cells of the body. In addition to bicarbonate, phosphate, and vitamin D (calcitriol) supplementation, cysteamine, a cystine-depleting agent, may slow the eventual progression to renal failure.

Ifosfamide Toxicity

Acquired forms of Fanconi's syndrome may occur following exposure to heavy metals (lead, cadmium, mercury), antibiotics (gentamicin, outdated tetracycline, cephalosporin), ifosfamide, and during the final stages of the nephrotic syndrome secondary to FSGS. Ifosfamide has been used with increasing frequency in the treatment of solid tumors, especially Wilms tumor, in children. One report (Burk et al, 1990) describes five children with Wilms tumor who developed Fanconi's syndrome after a total ifosfamide dose of 70 to 108 g/m^2. In addition to the tubulopathy a marked decline in glomerular filtration was observed in these patients. **Appropriate monitoring of these patients before**

each course of ifosfamide and close attention to the total drug dose given during treatment are recommended.

Renal Glucosuria

Renal glucosuria is defined by the presence of glucosuria when the plasma glucose concentration is less than 120 mg/dl. The loss of a glucose transport system is the cause of the glucosuria. The glucose threshold is significantly reduced. Glucosuria is usually found unexpectedly by a glucose-specific dipstick urine test. Because isolated glucosuria is frequently familial, siblings and parents should also be tested with a glucose-specific urinary test. Glucosuria may also be caused by an overflow mechanism secondary to hyperglycemia that occurs in patients with diabetes mellitus receiving intravenous dextrose solutions, epinephrine injections, and glucocorticoid administration. **Treatment is not indicated for isolated glucosuria.**

Bartter's Syndrome

A tubular syndrome caused by reduced sodium chloride reabsorption in the thick ascending limb of Henle's loop is known as Bartter's syndrome. **Signs and symptoms associated with the syndrome are usually the consequence of hypokalemia. Patients initially present with weakness, fatigue, neuromuscular irritability, muscle cramps, polyuria, polydipsia, and failure to thrive in infancy.** Moderate to severe hypokalemia and metabolic alkalosis establish the diagnosis. Elevated plasma renin activity, elevated plasma aldosterone levels, and normal blood pressure are also noted. Inability to concentrate urine is another feature caused by the severe hypokalemia. Bartter's syndrome must be distinguished from surreptitious vomiting and diuretic use or abuse. Therapy consists of potassium chloride replacement in conjunction with either spironolactone or amiloride.

REFERENCES

History and Physical Examination

Mimran A: Renal function in hypertension. Am J Med 1988; 84(Suppl 1B):69–75.

Still JL, Cottom D: Severe hypertension in childhood. Arch Dis Child 1967; 42:34–39.

Laboratory Data

Birch DF, Fairley KF: Hematuria: Glomerular or nonglomerular? Lancet 1979; 2:845–846.

Crompton CH, Ward PB, Hewitt IK: The use of urinary red cell morphology to determine the source of hematuria in children. Clin Nephrol 1993; 39:44–49.

Ghazali S, Barratt TM: Urinary excretion of calcium and magnesium in children. Arch Dis Child 1974; 49:97–101.

Norman ME: An office approach to hematuria and proteinuria. Pediatr Clin North Am 1987; 34:545–560.

Rizzoni G, Braggion F, Zacchelo G: Evaluation of glomerular and nonglomerular hematuria by phase-contrast microscopy. J Pediatr 1983; 103:370–374.

Roth S, Renner E, Rathert P: Microscopic hematuria: Advances in identification of glomerular dysmorphic erythrocytes. J Urol 1991; 146:680–684.

Schwartz GJ, Haycock G, Edelmann CM Jr, Spitzer A: A simple estimate of glomerular filtration rate in children derived from body length and plasma creatinine. Pediatrics 1976; 58:258–263.

Stapleton FB: Morphology of urinary red blood cells: A simple guide to localizing the site of hematuria. Pediatr Clin North Am 1987; 34:561–569.

Stapleton FB, Noe HN, Jerkins GR, Roy S III: Urinary excretion of calcium following an oral calcium loading test in healthy children. Pediatrics 1982; 69:594–597.

Vehaskari VM, Rapola J, Koskimies O, et al: Microscopic hematuria in school children: Epidemiology and clinicopathologic evaluation. J Pediatr 1979; 95:676–684.

Hematuria

Dodge WF, West EF, Smith EH, Bunce H: Proteinuria and hematuria in school children: Epidemiology and early natural history. J Pediatr 1976; 88:327–347.

Fitzwater DS, Wyatt RJ: Hematuria. Pediatr Rev 1994; 15:102–109.

Ghazali S, Barratt TM: Urinary excretion of calcium and magnesium in children. Arch Dis Child 1974; 49:97-101.

Hogg RJ, Silva FG, Wyatt RJ, et al: Prognostic indicators in children with IgA nephropathy—Report of the Southwest Pediatric Nephrology Study Group. Pediatr Nephrol 1994; 8:15–20.

Ingelfinger JR, Davis AE, Grupe WE: Frequency and etiology of gross hematuria in a general pediatric setting. Pediatrics 1977; 59:557–561.

Kalia A, Travis LB, Brouhard BH: The association of idiopathic hypercalciuria and asymptomatic gross hematuria in children. J Pediatr 1981; 99:716–719.

Kaplan BS, Cleary TG, Obrig TG: Recent advances in understanding the pathogenesis of the hemolytic uremic syndromes. Pediatr Nephrol 1990; 4:276–283.

Kashtan CE, Kleppel MM, Butkowski RJ, et al: Alport syndrome, basement membranes and collagen. Pediatr Nephrol 1990; 4:523–532.

Moore ES: Hypercalciuria in children. Contrib Nephrol 1981; 27:20–32.

Noe HN, Stapleton FB, Jerkins GR, Roy S III: Clinical experience with pediatric urolithiasis. J Urol 1983; 129:1166–1168.

Noe HN, Stapleton FB, Roy S III: Potential surgical implications of unexplained hematuria in children. J Urol 1984; 132:737–738.

Roy S III, Murphy WM, Pitcock JA, Rimer RL: Sickle-cell disease and poststreptococcal acute glomerulonephritis. Am J Clin Pathol 1976; 66:986–990.

Roy S III, Stapleton FB, Noe HN, Jerkins GR: Hematuria preceding renal calculus formation in children with hypercalciuria. J Pediatr 1981; 99:712–715.

Siegler RL: Management of hemolytic uremic syndrome. J Pediatr 1988; 112:1014–1020.

Stapleton FB, Noe HN, Jerkins GR, Roy S III: Urinary excretion of calcium following an oral calciium loading test in healthy children. Pediatrics 1982; 69:594-597.

Stapleton FB, Roy S III, Noe HN, Jerkins GR: Hypercalciuria in children with hematuria. N Engl J Med 1984; 310:1345–1348.

Trachtman H, Weiss RA, Bennett B, Greifer I: Isolated hematuria in children: Indications for a renal biopsy. Kidney Int 1984; 25:94–99.

Proteinuria

Brodehl J: Conventional therapy for idiopathic nephrotic syndrome in children. Clin Nephrol 1991; 35:S8–15.

Kelsch R, Sedman AB: Nephrotic syndrome. Pediatr Rev 1993; 14:30–38.

Neilson EG: Pathogenesis and therapy of interstitial nephritis. Kidney Int 1989; 35:1257–1270.

Roy S III, Stapleton FB: Focal segmental glomerulosclerosis in children: Comparison of nonedematous and edematous patients. Pediatr Nephrol 1987; 1:281–285.

Southwest Pediatric Nephrology Study Group: Hepatitis B surface antigenemia in North American children with membranous glomerulonephropathy. J Pediatr 1985; 106:571–578.

Vehaskari VM, Rapola J: Isolated proteinuria: Analysis of a school-age population. J Pediatr 1982; 101:661–668.

Yoskikawa N, Kitagawa K, Ohta K, et al: Asymptomatic constant isolated proteinuria in children. J Pediatr 1991; 119:375–379.

Renal Tubular Disorders

Burk CD, Restaino I, Kaplan BS, Meadows AT: Ifosfamide-induced renal tubular dysfunction and rickets in children with Wilms tumor. J Pediatr 1990; 117:331–335.

57 URINARY TRACT INFECTIONS IN INFANTS AND CHILDREN

Linda M. Dairiki Shortliffe, M.D.

OVERVIEW

During the last decade new imaging techniques and biologic probes have given further insight into the pathogenesis and natural history of urinary tract infections (UTIs) in children. In infants, UTIs are a common cause of fever and are probably the most common cause of renal parenchymal loss. For this reason, the goal of managing UTIs in children is based on identifying and modifying, if possible, factors that may increase risk of renal parenchymal and functional loss from the time of the index infection into the future. This chapter focuses on host and bacterial mechanisms by which bacteria gain access to the bladder and kidney, examines the short- and long-term complications of renal infection, and discusses means of preventing renal damage.

Incidence and Epidemiology of Pediatric Urinary Tract Infections

More boys than girls get UTIs during the first year of life (Asscher et al, 1973; Winberg et al, 1974), and during that period, uncircumcised boys have as high as ten times the risk of circumcised boys of having a UTI (Rushton and Majd, 1992a; Wiswell and Hachey, 1993). About 2.7% of boys and 0.7% of girls have bacteriuria by 1 year of age (Wettergren et al, 1980). This incidence decreases below 1% in school-age boys (ranging between 0.03%–1.2% during the school years) but rises to 1% to 3% in school-age girls (Asscher, 1975; Savage, 1975; Bailey, 1979).

Classification of Urinary Infections

UTIs have been classified in many ways: complicated versus uncomplicated, upper versus lower tract, persistent infections versus reinfections, and symptomatic versus asymptomatic. For practical purposes, **pediatric UTIs may be categorized into four types** (Stamey, 1975)**: (1) first infections, (2) unresolved bacteriuria arising during therapy, (3) bacterial persistence at an anatomic site, and (4) reinfections.** In infants and children, the first occurrence of a UTI should be considered complicated because of the management and treatment implications surrounding these infections.

UTIs may be unresolved because of inadequate therapy related to bacterial resistance to the selected therapeutic agent, inadequate antimicrobial urinary concentration due to poor renal concentration or gastrointestinal malabsorption, or an infection involving multiple organisms. Unresolved infections can usually be treated successfully once proper culture and antimicrobial sensitivity patterns are obtained.

In infants and children, sources of urinary tract bacterial persistence are usually found early because radiologic evaluation should be performed early. The discovery of urinary tract sources of bacterial persistence that are surgically correctable are obviously important (Table 57–1). Most UTIs are, however, reinfections with the same or a different organism.

Infections that are asymptomatic or "covert," as designated by Savage (Savage, 1975), and found only on screening urinary culture when a child is being examined for reasons unrelated to urinary infection can still be classified within these four types.

Table 57–1. SURGICALLY CORRECTABLE CAUSES OF BACTERIAL PERSISTENCE IN CHILDREN

Infection stones
Infected nonfunctioning or poorly functioning kidneys or renal segments
Infected ureteral stumps following nephrectomy
Vesicointestinal or urethrorectal fistula
Vesicovaginal fistula
Infected necrotic papillae in papillary necrosis
Unilateral medullary sponge kidney
Infected urachal cyst
Infected urethral diverticulum or periurethral gland

BACTERIA

The most common bacteria infecting the urinary tract are the gram-negative Enterobacteriaceae, usually *Escherichia coli* (Kunin et al, 1964; Bergström, 1972; Winberg et al, 1974). Specific cell wall O-antigens that can be identified by serotyping have shown that specific *E. coli* serotypes (e.g., 01, 02, 04, 06, 07, and 075) are associated with pediatric UTIs (Kunin et al, 1964; Winberg et al, 1974).

Another bacterial trait that may increase its virulence for the urinary tract is surface structures called pili or fimbriae. The bacterial fimbriae mediate bacterial adherence to uroepithelial cells and red blood cell agglutination, both of which can be used to characterize virulence. Red blood cell agglutinating characteristics of the *E. coli*, called hemagglutination, can be blocked by different sugars (Duguid et al, 1978; Svanborg Edén and Hanson, 1978). Using this characteristic, Källenius and associates discovered that pyelonephritogenic *E. coli* cause mannose-resistant hemagglutination (MRHA) of human red blood cells (Källenius et al, 1981). Characterization of this reaction showed that the terminal glycolipid of the human red cell P blood-group antigen is a receptor that binds P fimbriae on these *E. coli*. Therefore, **two important markers for *E. coli* virulence are MRHA characteristics and P blood group–specific adhesins (P fimbriae or P pili)** (Källenius et al, 1981; Väisänen et al, 1981).

The importance of these two virulence markers has been supported by research examining their association with clinically diagnosed pyelonephritis and cystitis. In one study, most *E. coli* strains causing pediatric clinical pyelonephritis had both MRHA and P fimbriae (MRHA 91% [29 of 32], P fimbriae 81%) (Väisänen et al, 1981), and P fimbriae were absent on less virulent strains. Similarly, Kallenius and associates found P fimbriae on 94% (33 of 35) of *E. coli* causing acute pyelonephritis, 19% (5 of 26) of *E. coli* causing acute cystitis, 14% (5 of 36) of *E. coli* causing asymptomatic bacteriuria, and 7% (6 of 82) of *E. coli* from the feces of healthy children (Källenius et al, 1981).

More recently, when pyelonephritis and cystitis have been more clearly defined by findings of renal inflammation (observed on DMSA renal scan), the distinctions differentiating between upper and lower tract bacteria are less clear. It may be that P-fimbriated *E. coli* are more likely to cause fever than non–P-fimbriated *E. coli,* whether or not the kidney is involved (Majd et al, 1991; Jantausch et al, 1992). This characteristic of P-fimbriation is supported by the finding that urinary interleukin-6 response is higher in children infected with P-fimbriated *E. coli* than in those infected by other organisms (Benson et al, 1994). It has been suggested, moreover, that UTIs caused by P-fimbriated strains may need longer antimicrobial courses than those caused by other strains (Tambic et al, 1992). Other less well-characterized virulence factors may involve the hydrophobic properties of *E. coli* and the iron-binding capability of the bacteria associated with aerobactin production (Jacobson et al, 1988, 1989b).

NATURAL HISTORY OF URINARY TRACT INFECTIONS IN CHILDREN

The natural history of the pediatric UTI is unpredictable and incompletely understood. Although a child's risk factors and the bacterial virulence may partially predict the course of a UTI, these factors alone have not been useful in predicting which individuals will develop pyelonephritis, renal scarring, or parenchymal and functional loss from a single or recurrent urinary infection. About 3% of girls and 1% of boys develop a prepubertal UTI (Winberg et al, 1974), and of these children, 17% or more develop infection-related renal scarring. Of those with scarring, 10% to 20% become hypertensive, and a rare child develops progressive renal dysfunction culminating in end-stage renal disease (Fig. 57–1).

Although it has been recognized that the pathogenesis of UTIs in adults and children differs, UTIs in children have often been studied without regard for age and other pediatric specific factors. For this reason, the course of a pediatric UTI has remained confusing. Research has shown, however, that host factors such as genetics, native immunity, sex, circumcision status, diet, gut, and periurethral colonization alter the course of UTIs in children.

Symptoms

UTI is a common cause of pediatric bacterial infection (Crain and Gershel, 1990; Bonadio et al, 1993; Hoberman et al, 1993). Fever accounts for about 20% of pediatric office visits (Eggli and Tulchinsky, 1993), and **UTI causes about 4.1% to 7.5% of these febrile episodes. In children under age 2, symptoms of UTI are vague and generalized**—fever, irritability, poor feeding, vomiting, diarrhea, and ill appearance (Ginsburg and McCracken, 1982) (Table 57–2). Specifically in febrile infants from birth to 8 to 10 weeks, neither clinical symptoms nor laboratory tests can be used to predict a presumptive UTI nor eliminate likelihood of a UTI even if other sites of infection are suggested clinically (Crain and Gershel, 1990). **Febrile infants who are not suspected of having a urinary source of infection are as likely to have a urinary source as those who are suspected of having a urinary source** (5.1% versus 5.9%), and 3.5% of infants with another possible source, such as otitis media, also have a UTI (Hoberman et al, 1993).

Table 57–2. SYMPTOMS OF 100 INFANTS WITH ACUTE URINARY TRACT INFECTIONS

Symptom	Percent
Fever	67
≥38°C	100°C
≥39°C	57
Irritable	55
Poor feeding	38
Vomiting	36
Diarrhea	31
Abdominal distention	8
Jaundice	7

Modified from Ginsburg CM, McCracken GHJ: Urinary tract infections in young infants. Pediatrics, 1982;69(4):409–412. Reproduced by permission of PEDIATRICS, vol 69, Pages 409–412. Copyright 1982.

The older, toilet-trained, talking child may indicate symptoms, such as dysuria, suprapubic pain, voiding dysfunction, or incontinence, that better localize the problem to the urinary tract, but many of these children still do not describe urinary tract symptoms. In children without localizing signs or with symptoms only vaguely referable to the urinary tract, suspicion must be high to avoiding missing the diagnosis.

Cystitis and Pyelonephritis

The progression from cystitis to pyelonephritis and the relationship between these entities is difficult to determine

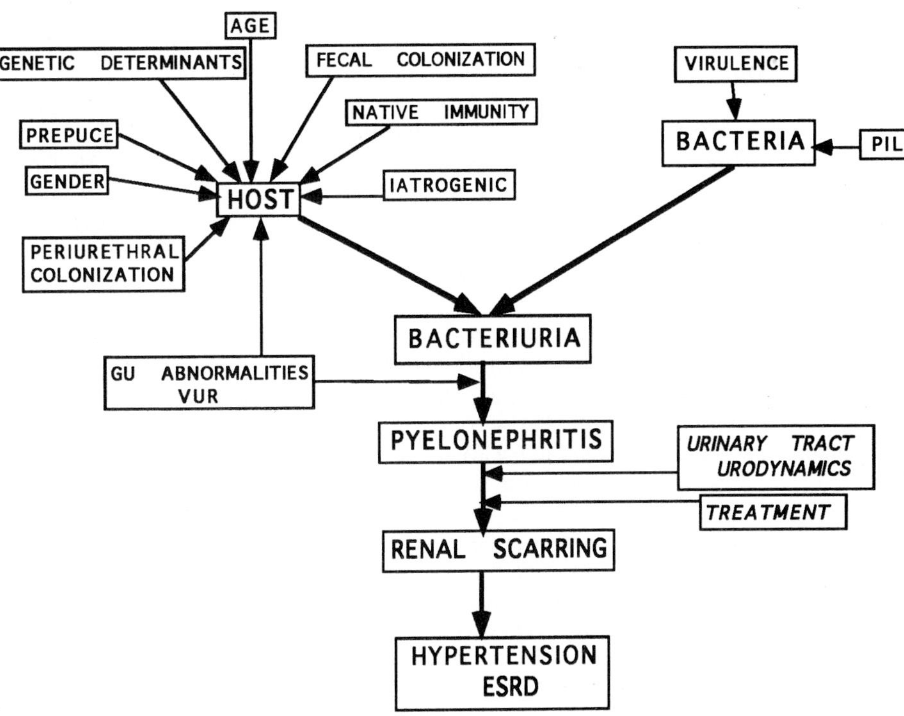

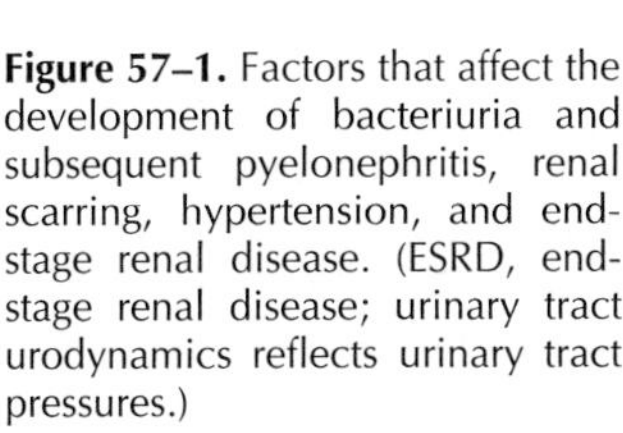

Figure 57–1. Factors that affect the development of bacteriuria and subsequent pyelonephritis, renal scarring, hypertension, and end-stage renal disease. (ESRD, end-stage renal disease; urinary tract urodynamics reflects urinary tract pressures.)

because simple techniques with which to localize the level and extent of urinary tract bacteria are lacking. Although **ureteral catheterization has been the gold standard for localizing upper and lower tract bacteriuria,** this method requires invasive cystoscopy and is an impractical way of following the course of infection (Stamey, 1980). It cannot, moreover, reveal the extent of renal inflammation. The Fairley bladder washout localization technique requires urethral catheterization during acute infection and washing the bladder with sterile water to determine whether the source of bacteria is from the bladder or is supravesical. This technique also cannot be performed or repeated easily during the course of a UTI. **In localization studies using the Fairley or ureteral catheterization technique, however, clinical symptoms correlate poorly with location of bacteria.** In one such study, fewer than half the patients (the majority children) with fever and flank pain had upper tract bacteria (34 of 73), whereas almost 20% (83 of 473) who were asymptomatic had upper tract bacteria (Busch and Huland, 1984).

The discoveries that early renal cortical lesions from pyelonephritis can be detected by technetium 99m dimercaptosuccinic acid (DMSA) nuclear scan and that these lesions correlate with histopathologic areas of acute renal inflammation in animals models have advanced knowledge of the natural history of urinary tract bacteriuria (Parkhouse et al, 1989; Wikstad et al, 1990; Zafaranloo et al, 1990; Giblin et al, 1993). When DMSA lesions are used as the standard for diagnosing acute pyelonephritis, about 50% to 86% of children (about 60% of kidneys) with febrile UTIs and other clinical signs have pyelonephritis (Verber and Meller, 1989; Rushton and Majd, 1992b; Benador et al, 1994; Jakobsson et al, 1994). About half (40%–75%) of these lesions persist on DMSA scans performed 2 months to 2 years later (Rushton and Majd, 1992b; Benador et al, 1994). This factor suggests that as many as 40% to 50% of young children who have febrile UTIs suffer renal scarring.

Renal Scarring

Previously, the coarse renal scarring detected radiologically by calyceal deformity and renal parenchymal thinning over localized or multiple calyces has been called reflux nephropathy. Now that it is clear that such scarring is as likely to occur with or without reflux, this kind of scarring would probably be better termed pyelonephritogenic scarring.

Using older imaging techniques before DMSA, about 17% of school children with screening bacteriuria (bacteriuria found on cultures performed for screening rather than for symptoms) have renal scarring (Asscher et al, 1973; Newcastle Asymptomatic Bacteriuria Research Group, 1975; Savage, 1975). This correlates with Winberg's observation that 4.5% of children had radiologic renal scars after their first symptomatic UTI and 17% had scars after the second symptomatic UTI (Winberg et al, 1974). Although the percentage of scars in these studies may underestimate scarring because current studies using DMSA scintigraphy suggest that the incidence of scarring after symptomatic UTI could be almost twice this rate, these data emphasize that children with both covert and symptomatic UTIs risk significant renal scarring. Although, by definition, the natural history and pathogenesis of scarring in covert or asymptomatic bacteriuria cannot be known, these scars may actually reflect injury from previous undiagnosed bacteriuric episodes and the child's predisposition for recurrent infections.

In most children with UTI in whom renal scars are found, the scars are found on the first set of imaging studies and remain unchanged irrespective of the child's future clinical course (Verber and Meller, 1989). It has been hypothesized that the young kidney is more prone to damage, and as such, the initial UTI in the neonate or young child younger than 4 or 5 years old causes whatever renal damage will occur, and this initial response determines the kidney's future course. This theory is supported by the higher prevalence of early cortical DMSA defects observed in children younger than age 2 years who have UTIs than in those who are older (Ditchfield et al, 1994b).

Although older children may have less risk of scarring from infection than those younger than 5 years, vulnerability for scarring persists until puberty (10–15 years old) at least (Smellie et al, 1985; Shimada et al, 1989). Recent studies using DMSA-detected renal scarring suggest that new or progressive renal scarring may be more common than was previously thought and that up to 7.3% of children with recurrent or persistent bacteriuria and reflux may scar (Shimada et al, 1989; Verber and Meller, 1989; Jakobsson et al, 1994), and almost all young children with recurrent pyelonephritis may suffer renal scarring (Jakobsson et al, 1994). Earlier studies have also linked new or progressive renal scarring to uncontrolled recurrent UTIs and vesicoureteral reflux (Filly et al, 1974; Smellie et al, 1985). Filly and associates found that in girls younger than age 10 who had recurrent UTIs and vesicoureteral reflux, renal scars progressed and developed clubbing or scarring in an area that was previously normal or developed a focal parenchymal decrease of at least 3 mm between examinations in 43% (17 of 40) of kidneys, and two of 16 normal kidneys developed new scars (Filly et al, 1974). Some of the scars took up to 2 years from the episode of pyelonephritis to evolve maximally.

Conversely, radiologic evaluation of girls with nonobstructive reflux grades of 2 to 4 out of 5 without recurrent infections has shown no renal damage for up to 10 years (Holland et al, 1990). This supports earlier animal and clinical data that given normal urinary tract urodynamics, vesicoureteral reflux alone does not cause renal damage or impaired renal growth (Ransley and Risdon, 1978; Smellie et al, 1981; Ransley et al, 1984). **If no infections occur, no association between the severity of vesicoureteral reflux and impaired renal growth has been demonstrated in an otherwise normal urinary tract** (Smellie et al, 1981). Moreover, adults who have acute nonobstructive pyelonephritis and normal urinary tracts rarely develop focal renal cortical scarring, and papillary or calyceal distortion or generalized renal shrinkage rarely occurs (Davidson and Talner, 1978).

Associated Urinary Tract Abnormalities

From previous epidemiologic data, 5% to 10% of children with UTIs have obstructive urinary tract lesions

and an additional 21% to 57% have vesicoureteral reflux (Kunin et al, 1964; Abbott, 1972; Asscher et al, 1973; Winberg et al, 1974; Newcastle Asymptomatic Bacteriuria Research Group, 1975). When only children with pyelonephritis diagnosed by DMSA are examined, 25% to 83% may have vesicoureteral reflux, with many studies showing reflux absent in over half the children with pyelonephritis (Tappin et al, 1989; Jakobsson et al, 1992; Rushton and Majd, 1992b; Ditchfield et al, 1994a).

Children with febrile UTIs and reflux have a high incidence of acute DMSA defects. Which of these acute defects results in scar is still debatable, but the risk of scarring increases with grade of reflux (Jakobsson et al, 1992). Older investigations have documented scars in 5% to 20% of kidneys with grade 1 reflux and in 50% or more of kidneys with grade 5 reflux (Govan et al, 1975; Ozen and Whitaker, 1987; Skoog et al, 1987). Conversely, when renal scarring is used as the index and children with renal scarring are examined, about 60% have vesicoureteral reflux (Asscher et al, 1973; Newcastle Asymptomatic Bacteriuria Research Group, 1975; Savage, 1975). In at least 25% of children, the urinary tract is normal other than the presence of scarring (Ditchfield et al, 1994b). **These data confirm that vesicoureteral reflux is only one factor involved in the ascent of bacteria into the kidney and the subsequent risk of renal scarring. There is no documented association between vesicoureteral reflux and risk of bacteriuria.**

Recurrent Urinary Tract Infections

Recurrent UTIs are common, and the natural history has been well documented by Winberg and colleagues (1974). In boys who become infected before they are 1 year old, 18% develop a recurrent infection, but recurrences developing more than a year after the initial infection are rare. In contrast, if the initial infection occurs in an older boy, 32% will become reinfected. About 26% of girls who have an initial neonatal infection develop a recurrence, and similar to infant boys, recurrences after a year from the neonatal infection are rare. Girls who have their first infection after the neonatal period have a 40% recurrence rate, with the majority of recurrences occurring within the first 3 months and two thirds occurring within the first year. Although the risk of recurrent infection in these girls drops with each infection-free subsequent year, 8% had their first recurrence over 4 years after their original infection, so the risk never totally disappeared. For a girl who has had UTIs, Winberg found **the risk of another UTI occurring within a year of the last UTI is proportional to the number of previous infections** (i.e., the more infections a girl has, the more likely she is to get another). His data show that the risk of getting another UTI within a year of the previous one is greater than 25% with one previous UTI, greater than 50% with two previous UTIs, and almost 75% after three previous UTIs (Winberg et al, 1974). **This recurrence rate did not change, whether the initial infection was symptomatic or asymptomatic, or pyelonephritis or cystitis; in fact, about a third of the recurrences were asymptomatic.**

The low recurrence of UTI in neonates and young boys and high recurrence rates for older girls and boys support the importance of variable host risk factors. First, neonates may be affected by hematogenous infection and age-related factors, such as the immature immune system or unstable gut flora. Second, when a UTI occurs after the immune system attains maturity and fecal flora is stable, the child may have other biologic factors that influence the risk for UTI.

Covert or Asymptomatic Urinary Tract Infection

When patients with covert or asymptomatic infections are diagnosed on screening urinary cultures, they often have symptoms related to the lower urinary tract when they are carefully interviewed. They may have nocturnal or diurnal enuresis, or both, squatting, and urgency, and at least 20% have a history of previous UTI (Kunin et al, 1962; Savage et al, 1975). These symptoms were not the reason they had the urinalysis or culture, however. About 50% of these children have normal urinary tracts, as defined by intravenous urography (IVU) and voiding cystourethrogram (VCUG) (Kunin et al, 1962; Savage et al, 1975). Although a majority of infants who have covert bacteriuria may clear their bacteriuria without treatment (Jodal, 1987), other investigators have found that only about 30% of school-age girls clear their infections spontaneously without treatment (Verrier-Jones et al, 1975; Lindberg et al, 1978). **Whether they are treated when diagnosed or not, the majority of these girls have or will develop persistent infections or reinfections** (Savage, 1975; Verrier-Jones et al, 1975; Jodal, 1987).

Voiding Dysfunction and Constipation

Symptoms of nocturnal and diurnal incontinence are common in children with recurrent UTIs. Epidemiologic studies have shown that nocturnal enuresis alone is unassociated with UTIs, but diurnal enuresis or a combination of diurnal and nocturnal enuresis is associated with pediatric UTIs, even when the enuretic episodes are as infrequent as once a week (Hansson, 1992). Interestingly, this study also revealed that 7-year-old girls who were 3 years or older when they had their first UTI were more likely to have symptoms associated with voiding dysfunction than those who had UTIs when they were younger than 3 years (Hansson, 1992). Furthermore, when followed prospectively, almost 20% of children who experienced a recurrent UTI developed new diurnal enuresis with the onset of the recurrent UTI, and this persisted as long as 12 months later, even though the urine remained clear (Sørensen et al, 1988).

Urodynamic testing in neurologically normal children with recurrent urinary infections and incontinence has shown abnormal cystometry and voiding patterns (Kass et al, 1979; Koff et al, 1979; Bauer et al, 1980; Koff, 1982; Kondo et al, 1983; Qvist et al, 1986; Hansson, 1992; Passerini-Glazel et al, 1992; vanGool et al, 1992a). In 35 such children, Bauer and associates (1980) found that 12 (34%) had normal filling cystometry, nine (26%) had large hypotonic bladders, nine (26%) had small capacity hypertonic bladders with increased intravesical filling pressure and sustained uncontrolled detrusor contraction at a low volume, and five (14%) had hyperreflexic bladders showing uninhibited detrusor contractions during filling. Voiding dysfunction has also been described with staccato (interrupted) urinary flows during voiding, showing increased pelvic floor activity during voiding with resulting incomplete bladder emptying (Bauer et al, 1980; Hansson, 1992; Kjølseth et al, 1993; Passerini-Glazel et al, 1992; vanGool et al, 1992a).

In addition to bladder filling and voiding dysfunction, **many of these children have bowel dysfunction with constipation** (O'Regan et al, 1985). When 47 girls with normal urinary tracts but recurrent UTIs (with or without incontinence) and cystometry-proven bladder instability were studied by digital rectal examination and rectal manometry, all had signs of functional constipation. Importantly, these findings were present even when constipation or encopresis was specifically denied.

Although these findings do not establish causality between UTIs and voiding dysfunction, it can be seen that UTIs may initiate symptoms of bladder dysfunction with variable persistence. In some situations, treatment of constipation or voiding abnormalities, or both, has resulted in decreased frequency of urinary infections (Kass et al, 1979; Koff et al, 1979; Bauer et al, 1980; Koff, 1982; O'Regan et al, 1985; vanGool et al, 1992a, 1992b; Kjølseth et al, 1993). This suggests that bacteriuria provokes abnormal detrusor activity.

PATHOGENESIS OF BACTERIURIA AND RENAL SCARRING

Although acute renal infection has been caused by hematogenous dissemination in animals and may occur in infants or under special circumstances, it is generally accepted that the vast majority of human UTIs are caused by periurethral bacteria ascending into the urinary tract (Kaijser and Larsson, 1982). The bacteria then infects the bladder, ureter, renal pelvis, and kidney. Although research has emphasized the importance of pyelonephritis because of its potential to cause renal damage, **bacterial infection of the collecting system also causes bladder and ureteral inflammation and changes that alter urinary tract urodynamics** (Hinman, 1971; Boyarsky and Labay, 1972). Although the mechanism of ureteral dilation observed during acute infection is unclear, animal studies show that UTIs can cause abnormally elevated renal pelvic pressures, especially if vesicoureteral reflux is absent (Issa and Shortliffe, 1992) This supports the clinical observation that infection with certain so-called pyelonephritogenic *E. coli* may cause the temporary ureteral dilation seen in children with acute pyelonephritis and otherwise normal upper collecting systems (Mårild et al, 1989a).

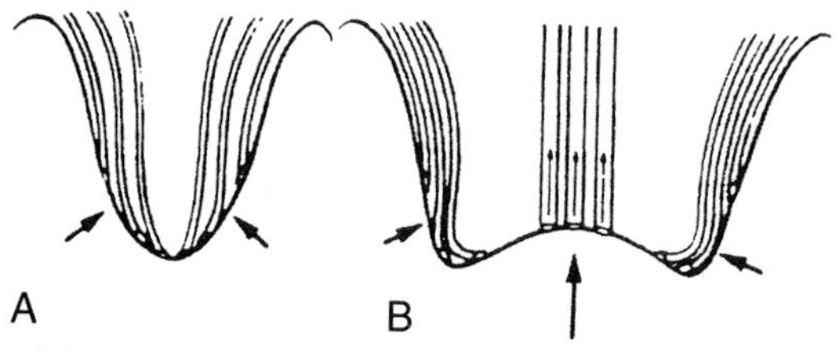

Figure 57–2. Papillary anatomy. *A,* A schematic drawing of a simple convex papilla that does not normally allow intrarenal reflux. *B,* A concave papilla that allows intrarenal reflux. (From Ransley, PG: Intrarenal reflux: anatomical, dynamic, and radiological studies. Part 1. Urol Res 1977; 5:61.)

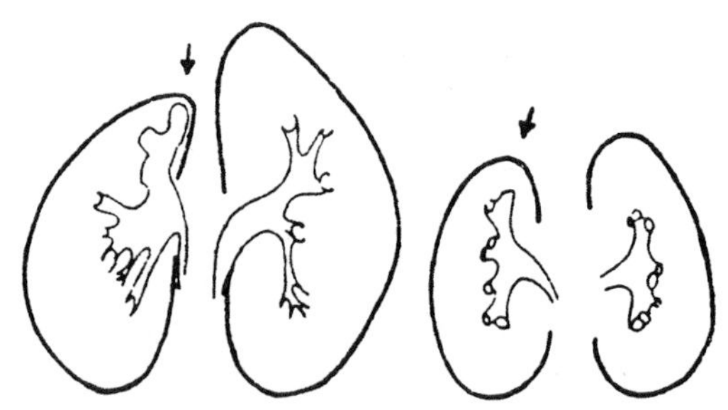

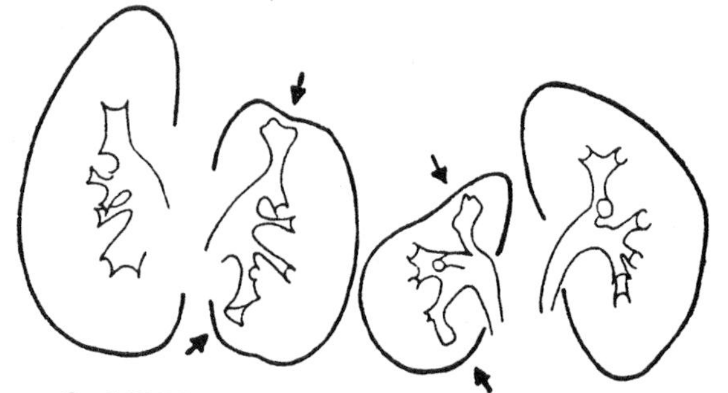

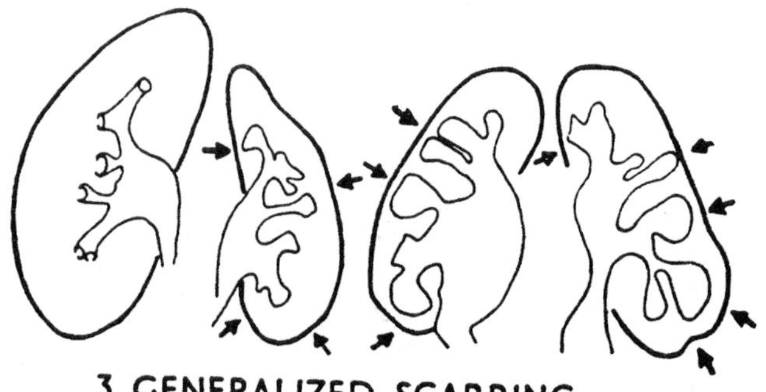

Figure 57–3. The common areas of renal scarring as characterized by parenchymal thinning over a deformed calyx as examined from intravenous pyelograms. The extent of scarring may be related to single polar scars; multiple areas of upper, lower, and medial scars; or generalized scarring as depicted. (Reproduced by permission from Hodson CJ: Natural history of chronic pyelonephritic scarring. BMJ 1965; 2: 191–194.)

The reason why children's kidneys scar and adults' kidneys rarely do is not known. Renal scarring appears to be affected by at least four factors: intrarenal reflux, urinary tract pressure, host immunity, age, and treatment. In 1974, Rolleston and associates found that areas of renal scarring were associated with foci of intrarenal reflux (pyelotubular backflow) observed on voiding cystourethrography in children younger than age 4 years who had vesicoureteral reflux (Hodson, 1965; Rolleston et al, 1974). Calyces allowing reflux contained papillae fused with adjacent papillae that caused the papillary ducts to open at right angles rather than at oblique angles more resistant to reflux (Ransley and Risdon, 1974) (Fig. 57–2). These compound papillae were found most commonly at the renal poles, the areas in which clinical renal scarring is most commonly observed clinically (Hannerz et al, 1987). The common patterns of scarring are shown in Figure 57–3.

otitis media in children (Duncan et al, 1993) or infants with cleft palate (Paradise et al, 1994).

As expected, children with specific immune deficiency syndromes have altered immunity and often have increased risk of bacteriuria and progression of infection. About 20% of children infected with the human immunodeficiency virus get bacterial UTIs with both common and opportunistic organisms (Grattan-Smith et al, 1992).

Fecal Colonization

Human fecal flora depends on the surrounding microbial ecology, native immunity, and microbe-altering drugs and foods. The importance of abnormal fecal colonization in neonates is emphasized by studies showing that fecal colonization with specific pyelonephritogenic bacteria may occur in a neonatal nursery or hospital, with subsequent bacteriuria or pyelonephritis occurring several months later (Tullus, 1986).

The development of multiply antibiotic–resistant organisms in the gut through the use of antibiotic agents is well recognized. **Because the fecal flora is commonly responsible for perineal and periurethral colonization, the importance of responsible antibiotic use cannot be overestimated.** In one study, antibiotic treatment of schoolgirls with phenoxymethylpenicillin for intercurrent infections, usually otitis media, caused recolonization and bacteriuria with strains more likely to be symptomatic (Hansson et al, 1989b).

Genitourinary Anatomic Abnormalities

Historically, UTIs have been a marker for genitourinary tract anatomic abnormalities in children. **Specific genitourinary abnormalities, especially nonfunctioning segments, may serve as a nidus of bacterial infection and cause bacterial persistence because of the difficulty in achieving urinary antimicrobial concentrations adequate to treat UTIs in a poorly concentrating renal segment** (see Table 57–1). Similarly, conditions of genitourinary partial obstruction or renal functional impairment may create increased risk of renal damage because of poor or inadequate treatment. Although the particularly severe sequela of chronic UTI and inflammation, xanthogranulomatous pyelonephritis, is usually rare in children, it may occur in young children with obstruction and UTI, especially in those associated with genitourinary abnormalities and renal nonfunction (Stamey et al, 1977; Zafaranloo et al, 1990; Cousins et al, 1994; Hammadeh et al, 1994).

Several special conditions that may alter a child's risk for UTI are discussed.

Vesicoureteral Reflux

Vesicoureteral reflux is discussed fully in Chapter 61. It is common in children with UTIs, but no correlation between reflux and susceptibility to UTIs has been found (Winberg et al, 1974). Epidemiologic surveys have shown that 21% to 57% of children who have had bacteriuria are subsequently found to have vesicoureteral reflux (Kunin et al, 1964; Abbott, 1972; Asscher et al, 1973; Newcastle Asymptomatic Bacteriuria Research Group, 1975). Reflux may resolve spontaneously (Bellinger and Duckett, 1984; Skoog et al, 1987). In one study, when UTIs were prevented, 87% of grade 1 reflux, 63% of grade 2, 53% of grade 3, and 33% of grade 4 resolved over about 3 years (Bellinger and Duckett, 1984). In groups in which it resolves, the rate of spontaneous resolution is about 30% to 35% each year (Skoog et al, 1987).

Peripubertal Girls with Persistent Vesicoureteral Reflux

The question whether girls approaching puberty who have persistent vesicoureteral reflux have a risk for increased renal damage is problematic. If primary vesicoureteral reflux persists as a girl approaches puberty, it becomes statistically less likely each year to resolve spontaneously. For this reason, some have recommended that girls approaching puberty undergo surgical correction of reflux to avoid the risks of pyelonephritis during future pregnancies. Whether these girls are actually at increased risk of morbidity and should undergo routine correction of reflux is unclear.

Although the prevalence of bacteriuria in pregnant women is the same as that in nonpregnant women (Shortliffe, 1991), **the likelihood that the bacteriuria may progress to pyelonephritis is greatly increased.** Thirteen and a half to sixty-five percent of pregnant women who are bacteriuric on a screening urinary culture develop pyelonephritis during pregnancy if they are left untreated (Sweet, 1977), whereas uncomplicated cystitis in a nonpregnant woman rarely progresses to pyelonephritis. The reason for this increased risk of pyelonephritis may be related to the hydronephrosis of pregnancy that occurs from hormonal and mechanical changes. Increased compliance of the bladder and collecting system, bladder enlargement, and an enlarging uterus may cause some anatomic displacement of the bladder and ureters (Hsia and Shortliffe, 1995).

Although little data are available about vesicoureteral reflux during pregnancy, there are no data to suggest that pregnancy causes vesicoureteral reflux. In one series in which 321 women had a single-film VCUG during the third trimester of pregnancy or immediately postpartum, only nine (2.8%) had vesicoureteral reflux (Heidrick et al, 1967). Although 6.2% (20 of 321) of these women had asymptomatic bacteriuria, only one of these 20 women had vesicoureteral reflux. Therefore, **few of the pregnant women with bacteriuria who developed pyelonephritis had reflux.**

On the other hand, of the nine women who had reflux, three had experienced pyelonephritis during a pregnancy. In another series, 21 of 100 pregnant women (27 refluxing renal units in 21 patients) with asymptomatic bacteriuria were found to have vesicoureteral reflux postpartum, mostly low grade (67% into the ureter only), and 17% of these women also had renal scarring (Williams et al, 1968). Although some have inferred that this scarring was caused by the bacteriuria during pregnancy, this percentage is similar to that found for the percentage of children with screening bacteriuria who have renal scarring (Asscher et al, 1973; Newcastle Asymptomatic Bacteriuria Research Group, 1975; Savage, 1975). Because these women were not evaluated radiologically before their pregnancy, it is unknown when they developed the scars, and it is most likely that they were present since childhood. These data suggest that postpubertal females who have vesicoureteral reflux and a predisposition for frequent UTIs will continue to have this predisposition for infections into adulthood and during pregnancy.

Although the use of ureteral reimplantation to prevent vesicoureteral reflux may decrease the likelihood of ascending pyelonephritis under normal circumstances, under the physiologic changes that occur during pregnancy, the nonrefluxing orifice may not offer the expected protection from pyelonephritis should bacteriuria occur. Unless the postsurgical nonrefluxing ureteral orifice is less likely to allow pyelonephritis during pregnancy than the normal nonrefluxing ureteral orifice, which seems unlikely, correction of the reflux would not protect a woman from pyelonephritis. Therefore, both the persistent reflux and the girl's predisposition for bacteriuria should be assessed before surgical correction of reflux is considered. **If vesicoureteral reflux is surgically corrected, moreover, these girls should not be assured that pyelonephritis during pregnancy is impossible**, because most episodes of pyelonephritis occurring during pregnancy occur in nonrefluxing kidneys. Their urine should still be screened for bacteriuria during pregnancy.

Finally, **before a woman with known pyelonephritogenic nephropathy and possible renal insufficiency is counseled about pregnancy, her renal function should be evaluated carefully.** Although data on the outcome of pregnancies with varying degrees of renal insufficiency is limited, a normal pregnancy is rare if the preconception serum creatinine exceeds 3 mg/dl (about 30 ml/minute clearance) (Davison and Lindheimer, 1978). Other data documenting increased pregnancy complications of prematurity, hypertension, and worsening renal insufficiency have caused some to recommend that conception is ill advised in women with less than 50% of normal renal function (serum creatinine greater than 1.7 mg/dl or less than about 50 ml/min clearance) (Bear, 1976).

Neurogenic Bladder

Children who have neurogenic bladders with abnormally elevated bladder pressures have a risk for increased renal damage from UTIs from the elevated urinary tract pressures and the increased instrumentation commonly required for neurogenic bladders. A neurogenic bladder with chronically or intermittently elevated bladder pressures may cause secondary vesicoureteral reflux from decompensation of the ureterovesical junction resulting from the elevated pressure (Hutch, 1952). If this does not occur, the elevated bladder pressures associated with a neurogenic bladder may also cause effective ureterovesical obstruction. This obstruction increases the risk of renal damage associated with UTIs. As discussed earlier in this chapter, intermittent elevations in bladder pressure associated with physiologic bladder dynamics in the immature bladder may exacerbate vesicoureteral reflux and the risks associated with it.

Children with neurogenic bladder may be more likely to face the risk of the effects of bacteria and possible renal damage because of their lack of ability to spontaneously clear the urinary tract of bacteria. Clean intermittent catheterization programs are useful for emptying the neurogenic bladder, but these catheterization procedures introduce bacteria. Although conclusions from previous studies involving clean intermittent catheterization in children are limited because they focused on both sexes, wide age ranges, different forms of neurogenic bladder, short follow-up time, different prophylactic antimicrobial status, and differing definitions of bacteriuria, they all agree that bacteriuria and even pyuria occurs in most children and in 40% to 80% of the urinary specimens sampled (Taylor et al, 1985; de la Hunt et al, 1989; Joseph et al, 1989; Johnson et al, 1994; Schlager et al, 1995). Few of these children have fever or symptoms, however (Geraniotis et al, 1988; Joseph et al, 1989; Schlager et al, 1995). One study with more than 5 years of follow-up study noted several episodes of urinary calculi and epididymitis (de la Hunt et al, 1989), so the long-term natural history of children on clean intermittent catheterization programs must be studied more extensively.

Although prophylactic antibiotics may decrease bacteriuria associated with catheterization in the short term (Johnson et al, 1994), the actual benefit of such antibiotic use is unproved.

Iatrogenic Factors

Although there are no reliable data regarding risk of catheter-induced infections in children, in adult women, the incidence of catheter-induced UTI ranges from 1% to 20%, depending on the circumstances of catheterization (Stamey, 1980). It has been documented that nosocomial UTIs frequently complicate hospitalization in children, especially when urethral catheterization has taken place (Dele Davies et al, 1992; Lohr et al, 1994). This may be a reason why antimicrobial prophylaxis should be given when urethral manipulation occurs. Children who get hospital-acquired UTIs, who have urinary tract abnormalities, who have recently undergone instrumentation, or who have had recent antimicrobial treatment are more likely to have infections caused by unusual and more antibiotic-resistant organisms (Ashkenazi et al, 1991).

In school-age boys, urethral self-manipulation with water injection or self-instrumentation has been reported to cause UTIs (Labbé, 1990). About 25% of children who are victims of sexual abuse may complain of dysuria and urinary frequency, but these children rarely have UTIs (Klevan and DeJong, 1990).

DIAGNOSIS OF URINARY TRACT INFECTION

Clinical Symptoms

Rapid diagnosis of UTIs so that early diagnosis can be made and rapid antimicrobial treatment can be initiated is the key to preventing renal damage. As discussed earlier in this chapter, symptoms of UTI in infants may be vague and nonlocalizing, made manifest only by signs of generalized illness—fever, irritability, poor feeding, vomiting, and diarrhea. In seriously ill infants and young children, one must suspect UTI and obtain a urinary specimen even if signs may point elsewhere. Older children may describe symptoms, such as dysuria, suprapubic pain, intermittent voiding dysfunction, and incontinence, that can be localized to the urinary tract.

Physical Examination

There are no signs specific for UTI in the infant. If there is a gross genitourinary anatomic abnormality, a renal mass may be palpable, as found in children with xanthogranulomatous pyelonephritis or infected severe hydronephrosis. Palpation in the suprapubic and flank areas may cause pain in the older child, but generalized abdominal or upper quadrant pain may also be present. Perineal examination rarely shows an ectopic ureteral opening, ureterocele, or urethral discharge in girls. In boys, testicular examination may reveal epididymitis.

Diagnostic Tests

Urinary Specimen

Good urinary specimens with which to make the diagnosis of UTI may be difficult to obtain in children, and the reliability of the diagnosis is related to the quality of the specimen. Routinely, there are four ways that urinary specimens are obtained in children. They are listed in order of least to most reliable for UTI diagnosis (Hardy et al, 1976): (1) plastic bag attached to the perineum—a bagged specimen, (2) midstream void, (3) catheterized aspirate, or (4) suprapubic bladder aspirate. Even after extensive skin cleansing, a plastic bag specimen usually reflects the perineal and rectal flora and often leads to indeterminate results. Although a midstream-voided specimen in a circumcised boy, older girl, or older uncircumcised boy who can retract his foreskin may reliably reflect bacteriuria, such specimens obtained in young girls and uncircumcised boys usually reflect periurethral and preputial organisms and cells. A catheterized specimen is reliable if the first portion of urine that may contain urethral organisms is discarded and the specimen is taken from later flow through the catheter; however, this method has the disadvantages of being traumatic and may introduce urethral organisms into a sterile bladder (Dele Davies et al, 1992; Lohr et al, 1994).

The most reliable urinary specimen for culture is obtained by suprapubic bladder aspiration. This specimen can be obtained safely in children and even premature infants with a full bladder by cleansing the skin and percutaneously introducing a 21- or 22-gauge needle 1 to 2 cm above the pubic symphysis until urine is obtained by aspirating the fluid into a sterile syringe (Barkemeyer, 1994). Because urine does not cross the urethra, urethral or periurethral organisms are absent; skin contamination should be nil. Organisms present in a suprapubic aspirate are pathognomonic of bacteriuria. The main drawback of suprapubic aspiration is that needle aspiration may be distasteful or inconvenient, or both, to the older child, parent, or physician, and these considerations may be important (Kramer et al, 1994a).

Generally, if a UTI is suspected in a child who is not yet toilet-trained, only a catheterized or needle-aspirated specimen is acceptable for diagnosis because bagged urinary specimens have an unacceptably high false-positive rate. Under special collection circumstances, when the perineum is cleaned well and the bag removed and processed promptly after voiding, a bagged specimen or even a diaper specimen showing no bacterial growth may be useful in eliminating bacteriuria as a possibility (Ahmad et al, 1991). Plastic bag specimens are unreliable and unacceptable for diagnosis of UTI in high-risk populations and infants younger than 2 months old (Crain and Gershel, 1990).

Urinalysis

The gold standard for the diagnosis of UTI is quantitative urinary culture. Although this standard appears clear, the specimen quality and test and culture interpretations leading to UTI diagnosis are unclear and have been debated. Because it may take 24 hours or more before bacterial colony-forming units (cfu) may grow and the culture is complete, indirect urinary tests that may be performed with routine urinalysis to detect the presence of bacteria or by-products have been sought for more rapid diagnosis. Four determinations from the urinalysis have been advocated as useful for supporting a diagnosis of UTI: (1) microscopic urinary examination for white blood cells—pyuria, (2) microscopic urinary examination for bacteria, (3) urinary leukocyte esterase, and (4) urinary nitrite.

Although there are many confounding factors, generally the microscopic identification of bacteria in the urine is more sensitive and specific for diagnosing UTI than for the identification of pyuria (Hallender et al, 1986; Lohr, 1991). Identification of bacteria under high dry magnification (450–570 magnification) usually represents about 30,000 bacteria/ml.

Urinary leukocyte esterase detects urinary esterases produced by the breakdown of white cells in the urine, and so it is dependent on the presence of white blood cells, which may or may not be present with the infection. The test may be less reliable in infants (Hoberman et al, 1994). Dietary nitrates that are reduced to nitrite by many gram-negative urinary bacteria may be measured by the **urinary nitrite test**. Serious drawbacks of this test are that bacterial reduction to nitrate may take several hours, so this test is most useful only on first morning-voided specimens, and most gram-positive bacteria do not produce this reduction. Although both tests may be performed by dipstick in the urine, the tests are more unreliable when the bacterial count is below 100,000 cfu/ml.

Although there is no test or combination of urinary tests that meets the gold standard of culture, combinations of these tests may help predict patients in whom culture will be positive. In febrile children younger than 2 years of age, Hoberman and associates found that catheter-obtained specimens had a positive predictive value for UTI diagnosis of 88.3% if microscopic examination showed bacteria and $\geq$10 white blood cells/mm^3 but emphasized that UTI in these children is best defined by a urinary leukocyte count of $\geq$10/mm^3 and $\geq$50,000 cfu/ml on culture (Hoberman et al, 1994). Interestingly, in febrile children 3 to 24 months old, a risk-benefit analysis, based on the current literature with the goal of preventing the majority of cases of end-stage renal disease and hypertension, concludes that both urinalysis and culture are needed to optimize prevention (Kramer et al, 1994b). In the general child population, others have shown that when urinary specimens are properly collected and promptly processed, the combination of positive leukocyte esterase and nitrite testing, and microscopic confirmation of bacteria has 100% sensitivity for detection of UTI. Also, when leukocyte esterase and nitrite tests are negative, the negative predictive value approaches 100% (Wiggelinkhuizen et al, 1988; Lohr et al, 1993). The arguments for and against relying on urinalysis characteristics for the presumptive diagnosis of a UTI are well summarized by Lohr (1991).

The finding of urinary sediment red and white blood cell casts are even less reliable.

Urinary Culture

What constitutes a significant UTI is unclear. It is controversial whether colonization of the urinary tract occurs (benign bacteriuria) or whether colonization represents specimen contamination or infection. As has already been discussed, **the technique by which the urinary specimen is collected is related to its reliability for UTI diagnosis** (Table 57–4) (Hellerstein, 1982). Although ≥100,000 cfu/ml of voided urine is the traditional definition for a clinically significant UTI (Kass and Finland, 1956), other studies have shown that ≤10,000 or fewer organisms on a voided specimen may indicate a significant UTI (Stamm et al, 1982; Bollgren et al, 1984). In febrile children younger than 2 years of age, Hoberman and associates showed that ≥50,000 cfu/ml in catheterized specimens constitutes a significant UTI (Hoberman et al, 1994). It should be noted, however, that in most of these studies, only 0.001 ml of urine was cultured, so that the minimal limit of detection was ≥1000 cfu. Cultured colony forming units per milliliter may be low because of hydrational dilution, frequent voiding preventing bacterial multiplication in the bladder, and bacterial growth characteristics.

Table 57–4. CULTURE CRITERIA FOR UTI DIAGNOSIS*

Method of Collection	Colony Count (Pure Culture)	Probability of Infection (%)
Suprapubic aspiration	Gram-negative bacilli: any number Gram-positive cocci: > than a few thousand	>99
Catheterization	$>10^5$	95
	10^4–10^5	Infection likely
	10^3–10^4	Suspicious; repeat
	$<10^3$	Infection unlikely
Clean-voided (male)	$>10^4$	Infection likely
Clean-voided (female)	3 specimens: $>10^5$	95
	2 specimens: $>10^5$	90
	1 specimen: $>10^5$	80
	5×10^4–10^5	Suspicious; repeat
	1–5 × 10^4	Symptomatic; suspicious; repeat
	1–5 × 10^4	Asymptomatic; infection unlikely
	$<10^4$	Infection unlikely

*Compiled from the data of many investigators including: Aronson AS, Gustafoson B, Svenningsen NW: Acta Paediatr Scand 62:396, 1973. Boshell BR, Sanford JP: Ann Intern Med 48:1040, 1958. Kass EH: Trans Assoc Am Physicians 69:56, 1956. Kass EH: Arch Intern Med 100:709, 1957. Pryles CV, Steg NL: Pediatrics 23:441, 1959. Pryles CV, Atkin MD, Morse TS, et al: Pediatrics 24:983, 1959. Pryles CV, Luders D, Alkan MK: Pediatrics 27:17, 1961. Stamey TA: Urinary Tract Infections. Baltimore, The Williams & Wilkins Co, 1972, pp. 1–29.

From Hellerstein S: Recurrent urinary tract infections in children. Pediatr Infect Dis 1982; 1(4):271–281. Copyright © 1982, Williams & Wilkins.

Tests Indicating Renal Involvement

Complete blood counts (Kramer et al, 1993), erythrocyte sedimentation rates, C-reactive protein, urinary concentrating ability (Åbyholm and Monn, 1979), urinary tubular enzymes (Johnson et al, 1990; Tomlinson et al, 1994), antibody-coated bacteria, urinary antibodies, and interleukin-6 (Benson et al, 1994) have been examined as possible simple and noninvasive markers of renal infection (Buyan et al, 1993), but none has proved reliable enough to differentiate upper and lower tract infections or severity of infection to become widely available. These tests have been performed primarily on experimental bases.

MANAGEMENT OF PEDIATRIC URINARY TRACT INFECTIONS

The therapeutic strategy in managing pediatric UTIs is, first, to minimize renal damage during the acutely diagnosed UTI and, second, to minimize risk of future renal damage from subsequent infections. Rapid recognition of a UTI and rapid, appropriate antimicrobial treatment are the keys to preventing renal damage. As discussed earlier, clinical and experimental data show that early antimicrobial treatment appears to be the most effective means of preventing renal scarring and subsequent complications.

Treatment of Acute Urinary Tract Infections

Treatment depends on the child's age and the severity of the illness. The child younger than 2 to 3 months of age with a presumptive UTI, who looks severely systemically ill or has a fever, or flank or abdominal pain, and is unable to take fluids, and the immune-compromised child should be treated with parenteral broad-spectrum antimicrobial agents (e.g., aminoglycoside and ampicillin or a third-generation cephalosporin, or aminoglycoside and cephalosporin [see Table 57–5]) and considered for hospitalization or outpatient parenteral or oral treatment, depending on the child's clinical status.

In appropriate infants and young children with presumptive UTI who are taking fluids, have cooperative and reliable parents, and with whom daily contact is possible, some of the newer third-generation cephalosporins, such as ceftriaxone, allow once-daily outpatient parenteral therapy (Gordon, 1991; Baskin et al, 1992). Most of these third-generation cephalosporins have a broad spectrum, treat even Enterobacter species and *Pseudomonas aeruginosa*, and conveniently

Table 57–5. PARENTERAL ANTIMICROBIAL DRUGS USEFUL FOR TREATING PEDIATRIC URINARY TRACT INFECTIONS

Aminoglycosides	***Cephalosporins***
Gentamicin*	Cefazolin
Tobramycin*	Cefotaxime
Penicillins	Ceftriaxone
Ampicillin	Ceftazidime
Ticarcillin	

*Indicates dosage change required for azotemia

require only once- or twice-daily dosing, but enterococcus is still resistant to most cephalosporins. Because the antimicrobial spectrum varies slightly for each of these drugs, the environment and local ecology may determine drug selection.

Generally, parenteral treatment is continued for 2 to 4 days until the fever is gone and bacterial sensitivities are available to allow treatment with a drug with a narrower spectrum and the child is clinically improved (afebrile with sterile urine and able to take fluids). The child may then be switched to an appropriate oral antimicrobial agent that attains adequate serum levels. Although the duration of treatment is debatable, in most studies involving treatment of febrile UTIs in young children, the total duration of therapy has extended from 7 to 14 days.

Less ill older infants and young children who have presumptive UTIs and are capable of taking fluids and oral medications may be treated with an antimicrobial agent that has a broad spectrum for genitourinary pathogens (Table 57–6). Although the newer oral cephalosporins eliminate most gram-positive and gram-negative organisms and most often can be given only once or twice a day, many enterococcus, *Pseudomonas,* and *Enterobacter* species may be resistant to them (Fennell et al, 1980; Ginsburg et al, 1982; Dagan et al, 1992; Stutman, 1993). In adults, the newer quinolones are useful because of their broader antimicrobial spectrum and special activity against *P. aeruginosa*, but in children, use of this drug is limited because some studies have shown quinolone-induced cartilage toxicity in young animals. With careful monitoring, limited quinolone use has shown no cartilage-related toxicities, and an abnormal urinary tract with upper UTI with *P. aeruginosa* may be a potential indication for use of the drug (Schaad, 1991). On the other hand, nitrofurantoin attains high urinary concentrations and low serum concentrations and, consequently, may be a poor choice to treat a severe systemic and renal infection but ideal for treating a bladder UTI. When culture and sensitivity information are available, the antimicrobial agent should be re-evaluated and changed, if necessary, with treatment continuing for 7 to 14 days.

Table 57–6. ORAL ANTIMICROBIAL DRUGS USEFUL IN TREATING PEDIATRIC URINARY TRACT INFECTIONS

Penicillins	***Cephalosporins***
Ampicillin	Cephalexin
Amoxacillin	Cefaclor
Augmentin (amoxacillin/clavulanate)	Cefixime
	Cefadroxil
	Cefpodixime
Sulfonamides	Cefprozil
Sulfisoxazole	Loracarbef
Trimethoprim-sulfamethoxazole	***Other***
	Nitrofurantoin
	Nalidixic acid

*Indicates dose adjustment required with azotemia

In school-age children who do not appear systemically ill and have a clinically uncomplicated bladder infection, **many oral broad-spectrum antimicrobial agents that are well tolerated will cure the "uncomplicated" UTI in a course of 3 to 5 days and there are no advantages to continuing therapy for a longer period of time** (Lohr et al, 1981; Copenhagen Study Group of Urinary Tract Infections in Children, 1991; Jójárt, 1991; Gaudreault et al, 1992). In some of these children, single-dose treatment, particularly with intramuscular aminoglycoside, may be curative and cause less fecal antimicrobial resistance (Grimwood, 1988; Khan, 1994), but in unselected children, single doses may not be as effective as 3 to 5 days of treatment (Madrigal et al, 1988; Khan, 1994).

After this immediate treatment, the child should receive daily administration of a prophylactic antimicrobial agent until full radiologic evaluation of the urinary tract may be conveniently performed in the next few days to weeks.

Prophylactic Antimicrobial Agents

Urinary prophylactic antimicrobial agents are effective in varying degrees in preventing bacteriuria under certain circumstances. In children, these agents are most commonly used to prevent UTI in the situations listed in Table 57–7.

Although a number of agents may be used for treatment of a UTI, fewer agents have been studied for low-dose prophylaxis in children. **The ideal prophylactic agent should have low serum levels, have high urinary levels, have minimal effect on the normal fecal flora, be well tolerated, and be inexpensive. The potency of these antimicrobial agents is based on the general susceptibility of most fecal Enterobacteriaceae to these agents at urinary levels.** Because these agents are generally concentrated in the urine, the urinary drug levels should be much higher than the drug levels found simultaneously in the serum, gut, or tissue, and if the levels are sufficiently low, antimicrobial resistance patterns in the gut should not develop. This characteristic of the prophylactic antimicrobial agents is most likely dose related, so that inappropriately high dosing for prophylaxis is less effective rather than more effective be-

Table 57–7. REASONS FOR URINARY TRACT PROPHYLAXIS

Vesicoureteral reflux
Unstable urinary tract abnormality (e.g., partial urinary tract obstruction)
Normal urinary tract but frequent reinfections
Awaiting radiologic evaluation after urinary tract infection
Urethral instrumentation
Clean intermittent catheterization
Immunosuppressed or immunocompromised
Infants with first UTI before 8–12 weeks

cause bacterial resistance will develop (Martinez et al, 1985). The parent who doubles or triples the dose of prophylactic antimicrobial agent each time their child develops the slightest symptom or cold may be destroying the prophylactic value of the agent. In addition, general patient compliance with prophylaxis may be difficult (Smyth and Judd, 1993).

Because urinary prophylaxis is usually initiated following treatment of an infection for which long-term (10 days), high-dose treatment was given, the fecal flora may already be resistant to the drug being administered and many of the prophylactic agents. The child who is very susceptible to urinary infections may then become reinfected with a type of bacteria resistant to the prophylactic agent before the gut is repopulated with more normal flora. This accounts for frustrating breakthrough infections that occur soon after the child is placed on prophylactic antimicrobial agents or after treatment of other frequent infections, such as otitis media. The period of greatest risk of recurrent infection is usually the first few weeks after any full-dose treatment. For this reason, the antimicrobial agent being administered should not necessarily be the prophylactic agent.

In children with normal urinary function, useful agents for urinary prophylaxis that have been studied are nitrofurantoin, cephalexin, and trimethoprim-sulfamethoxazole (Brendstrup et al, 1990). Amoxacillin, sulfisoxazole, and trimethoprim alone may also be useful urinary tract prophylactic antimicrobial agents, but they have not been as well studied in children. In the continent child, urinary tract prophylactic antimicrobial drugs should be given once nightly, when they will be excreted into the urine and remain there overnight (Table 57–8).

Nitrofurantoin

Nitrofurantoin is an effective urinary prophylactic agent because its serum levels are low, its urinary levels are high, and it produces minimal effect on the fecal flora (Winberg et al, 1973). Its effectiveness is based on urinary excretion of the antimicrobial once a day, and it has been found to be effective in girls at doses of 1.2 to 2.4 mg/kg each evening (Lohr et al, 1977; Holmberg et al, 1980). When renal function is reduced to less than half normal, the efficacy of nitrofurantoin may be reduced.

The majority of nitrofurantoin drug reactions occur in adults, and it has caused acute allergic pneumonitis, neuropathy, and liver damage (Holmberg et al, 1980). Long-term treatment has been associated with rare cases of pulmonary fibrosis. It should not be used in children with glucose-6-phosphate dehydrogenase deficiency because it is an oxidizing agent and can cause hemolysis. About 10% of blacks in the United States, Sardinians, non-Ashkenazi Jews, Greeks, Eti-Turks, and Thais may have a glucose-6-phosphate deficiency, and in these people, regeneration of glutathione, which is partially responsible for maintaining red blood cell integrity, is impaired by the enzyme deficiency. When nitrofurantoin is given, it oxidizes the hemoglobin to methemoglobin, which is degraded (Thompson, 1969).

Table 57–8. ORAL ANTIMICROBIAL AGENTS USEFUL FOR PEDIATRIC URINARY TRACT PROPHYLAXIS

Drug	Daily Dosage	Age Limitations
Useful and Tested		
Nitrofurantoin	1–2 mg/kg/day	>1 month
Trimethoprim-sulfamethoxazole	(trimethoprim) 2–3 mg/kg/day	>2 months
Cephalexin	2–5 mg/kg/day	
Possibly Useful		
Amoxacillin	5 mg/kg/day	>2 months
Sulfisoxazole	25–50 mg/kg/day	>2 months ?
Trimethoprim	2 mg/kg/day	

? Indicates little data

Cephalexin

Cephalexin has been studied in adults as a prophylactic agent (Martinez et al, 1985). Although resistance by fecal Enterobacteriaceae has developed in many patients taking full-dose cephalexin (500 mg qid), patients taking low doses (one quarter to one eighth of the adult daily dose, 250 to 125 mg/day) do not appear to develop resistance. Cephalexin at one quarter or less of the treatment dose per weight may then be a useful pediatric prophylactic agent.

Trimethoprim-Sulfamethoxazole

Trimethoprim-sulfamethoxazole has been a successful combination drug in the treatment of UTIs, and it has been useful for prophylaxis at a dose of approximately 2 mg/kg of trimethoprim (Grüneberg et al, 1976; Stamey et al, 1977). **Trimethoprim has an unusual characteristic in that it diffuses into the vaginal fluid and, therefore, decreases vaginal bacterial colonization in women also** (Stamey and Condy, 1975). Because the trimethoprim-sulfamethoxazole contains a sulfonamide, it probably should not be used for the first few months of life, because sulfonamides may compete for bilirubin-binding sites on albumin and cause neonatal hyperbilirubinemia and kernicterus.

Trimethoprim

Although most of the studies have been conducted in adult women, trimethoprim (dose approximately 2 mg/kg once nightly) has been found to be as effective as trimethoprim-sulfamethoxazole and nitrofurantoin in preventing recurrent UTIs (Stamm et al, 1980).

Nalidixic Acid

Nalidixic acid had been used to treat children before the advent of more powerful quinolones; however, testing of the newer quinolones (e.g., norfloxacin, cinoxacin) have shown that these drugs may be contraindicated in prepubertal children because they have caused cartilage erosion in weight-bearing joints and arthropathy in immature animals. In limited groups of children treated with quinolones, no such effects have been noted (Schaad, 1991).

Radiologic Evaluation

Imaging studies are basic to urinary tract evaluation for infection. The goal of management in UTIs is to minimize renal damage from the acute infection and the future risk of renal damage. With the multiple imaging modalities available, however, the most efficient and rational order and selection of studies must be made with this goal in mind. **Radiologic imaging can be used to (1) evaluate and localize the acute urinary infection, (2) detect renal damage from the acute infection, (3) identify genitourinary anatomy that increases risk of future renal damage from infection, and (4) evaluate changes in the urinary tract over time. Deciding which studies are necessary in a child with a presumptive or diagnosed UTI depends on whether or not potential radiologic findings would change the child's clinical management** (Fig. 57–4).

Early Imaging

Early urinary tract imaging is important in a seriously ill or febrile child in whom the site of infection is unclear, or who has unusual circumstances. Circumstances such as newly diagnosed azotemia; a poor response to appropriate antimicrobial drugs after 3 to 4 days of administration; an unusual infecting organism (tuberculosis or urea-splitting organism such as *Proteus*); known partial obstruction, such as a ureterocele; ureteropelvic junction obstruction; megaureters; nonfunctioning or poorly functioning renal units; or a history of diabetes, calculi, papillary necrosis, or a neuropathic bladder may warrant early urinary tract imaging.

If treatment depends on localizing the infection to the kidney, an early imaging study should be performed. This is particularly important in the severely ill hospitalized child who improves on initial parenteral treatment but for whom urinary cultures are inadequate or indeterminate for bacterial infection. An acute DMSA scan may show whether acute renal inflammation is present and whether treatment is justified or not. If, on the other hand, UTI appears highly likely and antimicrobial treatment will be started regardless of radiologic findings, early DMSA scintigraphy is probably unnecessary.

Definition of Renal Morphology and Identification of Urinary Tract Abnormalities

Because UTIs in infants and young children may serve as a marker for anatomic abnormalities, after the initial UTI has been adequately treated, the child should be maintained on antimicrobial prophylaxis and radiologic studies should be performed to delineate the urinary tract. Although there is controversy whether studies should be performed after the first or recurrent episode, if obstructive lesions are found in 5% to 10% of children and reflux occurs in 21% to 57% (Kunin et al, 1964; Abbott, 1972; Asscher et al, 1973; Newcastle Asymptomatic Bacteriuria Research Group, 1975), **early detection of these abnormalities merits full radiologic urinary tract evaluation after the first infection in young children. This evaluation usually consists of some form of renal and upper collecting system examination and a VCUG.**

As was emphasized previously, the child's kidney is prone to renal scarring, and evaluation of the renal morphology and documentation of any anomalies or scarring may be important to the child's management. Early studies of the kidney, however, may cause overestimation of renal size resulting from initial edema or lack of appreciation of renal scarring, because mature renal scars may take up to 2 years to be shown by certain imaging techniques (Filly et al, 1974; Troell et al, 1984; Gordon, 1986; Conway, 1988; Johansson et al, 1988b). As a result, later studies may show smaller or scarred kidneys that may be misinterpreted and cause inappropriate changes in patient management.

Obviously, obstruction and other anatomic abnormalities demonstrated by radiologic evaluation may require other

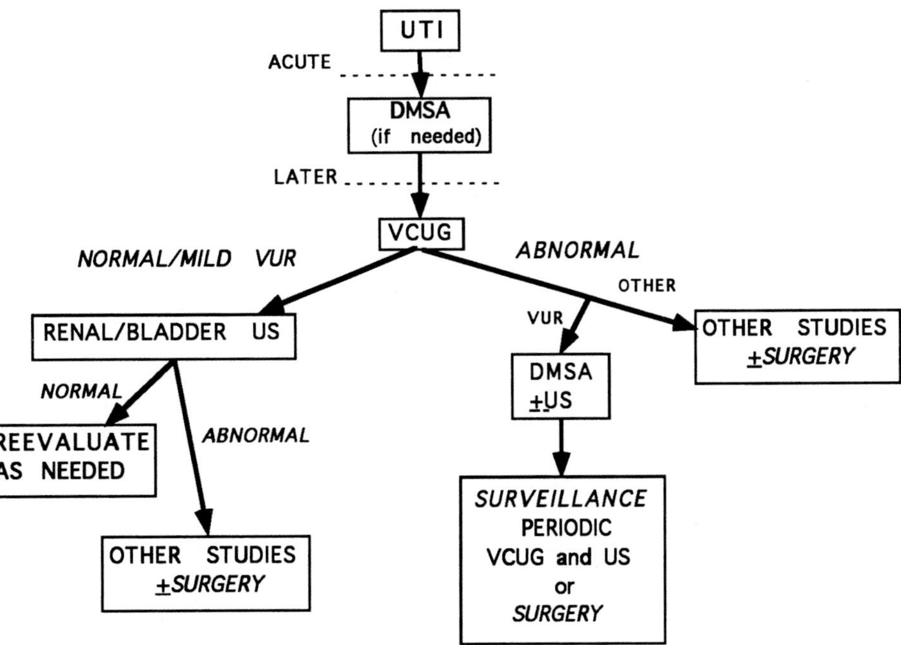

Figure 57–4. Flow diagram of possible imaging studies used to evaluate infants and children with urinary tract infections.

forms of evaluation specific to their diagnosis before definitive management is instituted. These situations must be evaluated and treated individually.

Follow-Up Evaluation

When a child who has a UTI has no abnormality found after urinary tract radiologic evaluation, no further studies are prescribed. If the collecting systems were normal but one or both kidneys showed massive generalized or focal edema with areas of possible hypoperfusion during the acute infection, a subsequent study should be performed to examine the kidney for signs of renal scarring or shrinkage. In this way, children who need to be re-examined for later renal dysfunction may be identified.

If a child has recurrent symptomatic pyelonephritis and no reflux was found on previous fluoroscopic VCUG, a nuclear VCUG may be more sensitive and may reveal the reflux, although it may be less likely to define it (Kogan et al, 1986; Macpherson and Gordon, 1986).

Imaging Techniques in Pediatric Urinary Tract Infections

Imaging techniques that are useful for evaluating children with UTIs are discussed in this section. The radiologic follow-up of children diagnosed to have vesicoureteral reflux is discussed in Chapter 61.

Voiding Cystourethrography

The VCUG is the most important examination in assessing vesicoureteral reflux in children and, as such, is important for assessing UTIs. The VCUG may be performed either with fluoroscopy and iodinated contrast or with nuclear imaging agents (usually technetium 99m pertechnetate) using similar techniques (e.g., direct radionuclide cystography), but these studies give different information. The traditional fluoroscopic VCUG may show urethral and bladder abnormalities and vesicourethral reflux. The radionuclide VCUG may be more sensitive for reflux detection but offers poorer spatial resolution so that urethral lesions, degree of reflux, and details of the collecting system may not be realized. In both fluoroscopic and radionuclide VCUGs, detection of vesicoureteral reflux depends on the child voiding and the technical performance of the study (Fairley and Roysmith, 1977; Lebowitz, 1986; Macpherson and Gordon, 1986).

The main advantage of radionuclide VCUG has been the lower radiation exposure of 1 to 5 mrad (ovarian dose) compared with 27 to 1000 mrad (previously reported ovarian exposure depending on equipment) (Cleveland et al, 1992; Lebowitz, 1992). With modern imaging technology and a tailored examination, however, the fluoroscopic VCUG has been performed with 1.7 to 5.2 mrad (Kleinman et al, 1994), and this imaging study, if available, may offer advantages of greater anatomic resolution over the radionuclide VCUG. In general, the radionuclide VCUG may be most useful for vesicoureteral reflux screening, for evaluating the UTI in older children who have lower risk of reflux, and for periodic reflux re-evaluation (Lebowitz, 1992). The radionuclide VCUG should not be used to evaluate infections in infants or young boys in whom the risk of genitourinary abnormality is high and urethral visualization important, nor in any child in whom imaging resolution of the lower urinary tract is important.

Indirect radionuclide VCUG is performed as part of a renal imaging study. The radionuclide is injected intravenously, and the study is performed when the kidneys and upper collecting systems are cleared of the radiopharmaceutical agent and bladder is filled maximally with it. The child is then asked to void. Although this method avoids catheterization, compared with the direct radionuclide VCUG, there is increased radiation exposure and decreased resolution because of body radionuclide background. Because it detects only about 60% of the reflux compared with the direct VCUG, there are few reasons to perform this test (Eggli and Tulchinsky, 1993).

The VCUG may be performed as soon as the urine is sterile. Studies have shown UTIs do not cause reflux, and even if reflux were associated with inflammation, this would be important to know and could alter management (Lebowitz, 1986). **Whether the VCUG is performed during treatment, immediately after, or a few weeks afterward is not important as long as the child has normal renal function, responds rapidly to antimicrobial treatment, is voiding normally (without urinary frequency), and is maintained on prophylactic antimicrobial treatment to keep urine sterile in the interval between the herald infection and the radiologic evaluation.**

If the VCUG is performed as the initial radiologic study, subsequent imaging may be planned depending on the VCUG results (Hellström et al, 1989). If the VCUG is normal or shows a ureterocele or vesicoureteral reflux, an ultrasound examination of the kidney and bladder usually demonstrates other urinary tract structural abnormalities or anomalies, such as dysplasia or obstruction, if they exist. In general, renal and bladder ultrasound detect children who may need urgent urologic surgery (Alon et al, 1986; Honkinen et al, 1986; Lindsell and Moncrieff, 1986; Macpherson and Gordon, 1986; Alon et al, 1989). If, however, vesicoureteral reflux appears to be the primary diagnosis, DMSA scintigraphy may be the most useful study with which to detect renal scars.

Renal and Bladder Ultrasonography

Routine renal ultrasonography is not as sensitive as DMSA in detecting the subtle changes associated with acute UTI (Verboven et al, 1990; Björgvinsson et al, 1991; Eggli and Tulchinsky, 1993; MacKenzie et al, 1994; Mucci and Maguire, 1994). Ultrasonography may show enlarged swollen kidneys, focal enlargement from edema and inflammation (focal pyelonephritis or lobar nephronia), and ureteral widening (Silver et al, 1976; Alon et al, 1986; Honkinen et al, 1986; Lindsell and Moncrieff, 1986; Macpherson and Gordon, 1986; Hellström et al, 1987; Conway, 1988; Johansson et al, 1988a, 1988b; Alon et al, 1989), but even color Doppler sonography has poor sensitivity for detecting the small areas of inflammation and resulting hypoperfusion that are seen on DMSA (Eggli and Eggli, 1992). Renal and bladder sonography, however, is more likely to detect perinephric fluid collections or anatomic abnormalities, especially those involving urinary tract dilation, than either DMSA or IVU (MacKenzie et al, 1994). Pediatric renal and bladder ultrasonography may be, however, more dependent on the skill and experience of the ultrasonographer with children than is DMSA scintigraphy (Patel et al, 1993).

Nuclear Renography

The fact that nuclear scintigraphy can accurately detect areas of acute renal inflammation and chronic scarring has changed the imaging of pediatric UTIs over the past 5 years. Because about 60% of injected DMSA is bound to the proximal renal tubular cells and excreted only slowly in the urine, it is a good cortical imaging agent (Jakobsson et al, 1992). Because technetium 99m glucoheptonate, on the other hand, is partially concentrated and excreted and is partially bound to the renal tubule, some visualization of the collecting system and cortical definition is observed. DMSA imaging is the commonly used agent when cortical definition alone is needed (Björgvinsson et al, 1991; Eggli and Tulchinsky, 1993).

In acute pyelonephritis, nuclear scintigraphy usually shows either uptake defects or renal swelling. The uptake defects may appear as wedge-shaped polar or lateral renal defects or as scattered uptake defects within the kidney (Wallin and Bajc, 1993). Later, after the acute episode has resolved, the scans show (1) a normal pattern, (2) generally diminished uptake and small kidney volume, (3) diminished uptake in the medial kidney, or (4) polar defects with diminished uptake in the renal poles (Wallin and Bajc, 1994). **DMSA is clearly more sensitive than renal sonography or even IVU in detecting renal scarring.** Because recurrent pyelonephritis appears to occur in the same areas, however, it may be difficult to differentiate new and old or progressive renal scarring unless serial studies have been performed (Björgvinsson et al, 1991; Rushton and Majd, 1992b).

Newer radionuclide technology using pinhole images and high-resolution computed tomography (single photon emission computed tomography) may give greater renal anatomic detail, resolution, and scar detection, but the complete impact of these additions on routine studies is still being examined (Eggli and Tulchinsky, 1993).

In children in whom severe renal scarring has occurred and the glomerular filtration rate (GFR) may need to be estimated, the radionuclide renogram has been found to give an accurate estimate of GFR even in young children (Gates, 1982; Shore et al, 1984; Rehling et al, 1989).

Intravenous Urography

Although the traditional means of evaluating the upper urinary tract and documenting renal scarring was IVU with renal tomography (see Fig. 57–3), in most situations DMSA scintigraphy has replaced the role of IVU. DMSA scintigraphy is more sensitive for detecting renal scars but shows less resolution in defining the scars. An IVU still defines collecting system abnormalities in more detail than either DMSA or ultrasonography. It is probably most useful in defining the collecting system in patients with confusing situations or in whom calyceal detail may be important.

Computed Tomography and Magnetic Resonance Imaging

No studies have directly compared the sensitivity and specificity of DMSA and computed tomography or magnetic resonance imaging in detecting renal lesions in acute or chronic pyelonephritis. For routine evaluation of UTI, neither modality is practical, but in children with complicated infections, either computed tomography or magnetic resonance imaging may be useful in defining renal abnormalities and the extent of disease when other modalities do not and is probably as sensitive as DMSA scintigraphy in detecting renal scars (June et al, 1985; Montgomery et al, 1987).

TREATMENT OF COVERT OR ASYMPTOMATIC BACTERIURIA

Treatment of covert bacteriuria is controversial because of its usually benign prognosis and intermittent lower tract symptoms. As has been discussed, covert bacteriuria is rarely totally asymptomatic. Although the UTI may not be the reason the covert infection was discovered, the associated symptoms such as incontinence elicited later may be troublesome enough to warrant treatment. Treatment of the infection alone, however, may not obviate symptoms of voiding dysfunction. Controlled studies involving older children with treated and untreated covert bacteriuria show that treatment makes little difference in the rate of future reinfections; over half of patients will have recurrent infections regardless of whether they are treated or not, and the risk of any renal damage in these older children is very low (Savage, 1975; Verrier-Jones et al, 1975; Lindberg et al, 1978; Jodal, 1987).

There is evidence that *E. coli* causing covert bacteriuria may belong to strains of *E. coli* that show self-agglutination, loss of surface antigens, and less overall pathogenicity (Lindberg et al, 1975; Hansson et al, 1989b). Some studies have suggested that urinary tract colonization with a strain of *E. coli* causing asymptomatic bacteriuria may prevent colonization with an *E. coli* causing symptoms, and that treatment may actually lead to later acute symptomatic pyelonephritis (Hansson et al, 1989a, 1989b). For this reason, **in difficult cases of recurrent asymptomatic infection, follow-up without further antimicrobial treatment might be considered.**

TREATMENT OF RECURRENT URINARY TRACT INFECTIONS

Because host uroepithelial characteristics are probably independent of gross urinary tract abnormalities or reflux, recurrent UTIs occur regardless of whether or not the urinary tract is normal. Children with urinary tract anatomic abnormalities or vesicoureteral reflux may be treated with prophylactic antimicrobial agents in an attempt to minimize the risk of infections (see Chapter 61). Unfortunately, there are no routinely available tests that can be used to predict which patients have a biologic predisposition for UTIs. Routine bacterial biotyping and sensitivity data obtained from culture, moreover, do not necessarily provide data relating to bacterial virulence. For this reason, management of the possibility of recurrences in these patients depends on the child's age and the severity of the symptoms. In the majority of children with normal urinary tracts who have mainly bladder irritative symptoms associated with their UTIs (the so-called uncomplicated infections), there is evidence that 3 days of an appropriate antimicrobial agent to which the organism is sensitive (Lohr et al, 1981; Madrigal et al, 1988; Copenhagen Study Group of Urinary Tract Infections in Children, 1991; Jójárt, 1991) or even a single dose of a parenteral antimicrobial agent (e.g., aminoglycoside) are effective treatments (Principi et al, 1977; Vigano et al, 1985; Grimwood, 1988). Longer antimicrobial courses of 10 to 14 days have not been proved to be more effective in these cases and may cause an increased number of side effects and antimicrobial resistance in the fecal bacteria (Hansson et al, 1989b; Copenhagen Study Group of Urinary Tract Infections in Children, 1991).

If the child gets frequent recurrent infections (e.g., two or more over a 6-month period), urinary prophylactic antimicrobial treatment over a limited period may be worthwhile, because the child has then established herself or himself as having a biologic predisposition for infections. Antimicrobial agents taken at a prophylactic dosage usually successfully decrease the rate of infections during the period of prophylaxis. When the antimicrobial agent is stopped, however, the child may extend into a period of remission from infection but often eventually returns to an increased basic susceptibility for urinary infections (Winberg et al, 1974; Kraft and Stamey, 1977).

MANAGEMENT OF URINARY INCONTINENCE ASSOCIATED WITH URINARY TRACT INFECTIONS

When symptoms of voiding dysfunction accompany recurrent UTIs, it is probably worth observing the child while he or she is receiving prophylactic antimicrobial agents to observe any change in the voiding pattern while the urine is sterile. If symptoms of incontinence persist, the addition of an anticholinergic agent, such as oxybutynin, and bladder rehabilitation, including timed voidings and biofeedback techniques, may be helpful in relieving incontinence and decreasing the frequency of UTIs (Kass et al, 1979; Koff et al, 1979; Qvist et al, 1986; Passerini-Glazel et al, 1992; vanGool et al, 1992b; Kjølseth et al, 1993). In addition, **if constipation is found or even suspected, there may be an improvement in voiding patterns if this problem is treated** (O'Regan et al, 1985). With the acute onset of bowel and bladder dysfunction in a child, the possibility of a tethered cord or other neurologic abnormalities must be eliminated.

OTHER GENITOURINARY TRACT INFECTIONS

Acute Hemorrhagic Cystitis

Acute hemorrhagic cystitis accompanied by frequency, urgency, and dysuria in children has been associated with UTIs caused by adenovirus 11 (Numazaki et al, 1968; Mufson et al, 1973; Numazaki et al, 1973) and occasionally *E. coli* (Loghman-Adham et al, 1988–1989). **Adenovirus is the most common cause of viral acute hemorrhagic cystitis in children.** In a series of 69 infants and children with acute hemorrhagic cystitis, adenovirus 11 was recovered from the urine in 10 (14.5%), adenovirus 21 from the urine of 2 (2.9%), and *E. coli* from 12 (17.4%), but the remainder (over 60%) had no infectious agents isolated from the urine (Mufson et al, 1973).

Polyomaviruses have caused both hemorrhagic and nonhemorrhagic cystitis in children. In addition, **BK, a DNA virus of the polyomavirus genus, has been found in the urine of bone marrow transplantation patients and other immunosuppressed patients having late-onset hemorrhagic cystitis** (1–5 months after transplantation) causing both symptomatic (hematuria and dysuria) and asymptomatic infections (Apperley et al, 1987).

Because viral cultures are rarely performed, children with symptoms of acute hemorrhagic cystitis most often have no growth on routine urinary culture. Although no antimicrobial treatment is indicated with viral cystitis, radiologic evaluation should still be performed to eliminate other causes for hematuria as well.

Epididymitis, Epididymo-orchitis, and Orchitis

Epididymitis is an important clinical syndrome because of its differential diagnosis and management. Although in some earlier series prepubertal epididymitis was diagnosed rarely (Anderson and Giacomantonio, 1985), **more recent series using newer imaging modalities have diagnosed epididymitis almost as frequently as acute testicular torsion.** Epididymitis is often difficult to distinguish from other pediatric acute scrotal processes, especially acute testicular torsion, and occurs almost as frequently (15%–45%) (Caldamone et al, 1984; Knight and Vassy, 1984; Mendel et al, 1985; Yazbeck and Patriquin, 1994). Although the differential diagnosis and evaluation of the acute scrotum is discussed in Chapter 72 (Congenital Anomalies of the Testis), the etiology and evaluation of epididymitis is related to UTI in many of these cases.

Although there is some overlap, pediatric epididymitis occurs in somewhat of a bimodal age distribution. It occurs in very young boys and again in greater numbers after puberty (Gierup et al, 1975; Knight and Vassy, 1984; Anderson and Giacomantonio, 1985; Likitnukul et al, 1987; Siegel et al, 1987; Melekos et al, 1988). This is a useful distinction clinically because the etiologies and management differ.

Symptoms and Signs

The symptoms and signs of acute epididymitis cannot be differentiated from those of any acute scrotal condition. Characteristics that may be useful for comparison with acute torsion of the testes are a history of more gradual onset, dysuria, urethral discharge, as well as a history of urethral manipulation, recent urinary tract surgery (hypospadias, ureteral reimplantation), catheterization, neurogenic bladder, imperforate anus, or known lower tract genitourinary anatomic abnormalities (ureteral or vasal ectopia, bladder exstrophy) (Mandell et al, 1981; Knight and Vassy, 1984; Umeyama et al, 1985; Siegel et al, 1987; de la Hunt et al, 1989; Stein et al, 1994).

When it is examined, the scrotum in usually inflamed and swollen; there may be localized epididymal pain; 18% to 33% of boys have fever (Doolittle et al, 1966; Gierup et al, 1975; Knight and Vassy, 1984; Anderson and Giacomantonio, 1985; Siegel et al, 1987), 24% to 73% have pyuria (Doolittle et al, 1966; Knight and Vassy, 1984; Anderson and Giacomantonio, 1985; Siegel et al, 1987), and 17% to 73% have peripheral leukocytosis (Doolittle et al, 1966; Gierup et al, 1975; Gislason et al, 1980; Knight and Vassy, 1984; Anderson and Giacomantonio, 1985; Siegel et al, 1987). Although these symptoms are more likely to be associated with epididymitis than acute testicular torsion, none of these symptoms are diagnostic. Pyuria and bacteriuria are rarely found in torsion, however (Doolittle et al, 1966; Gierup et al, 1975; Knight and Vassy, 1984; Anderson and Giacomantonio, 1985; Siegel et al, 1987).

As discussed in Chapter 72, color flow Doppler ultrasound of the scrotum and radionuclide scans of the testes have been helpful in confirming or following epididymitis (Mendel et al, 1985; Mueller et al, 1988; McAlistar and Sisler, 1990; Atkinson et al, 1992; Yazbeck and Patriquin, 1994). Ultrasonography may show an enlarged epididymis of mixed echogenicity surrounded by reactive fluid. Color flow Doppler sonography usually shows increased testicular flow except when there is such extensive swelling that ischemia may occur. Similarly, nuclear scintigraphy usually shows increased perfusion and increased radiotracer deposition in the affected side of the scrotum. Although nuclear scintigraphy may be somewhat more sensitive in detecting flow, especially in prepubertal boys (Atkinson et al, 1992), sonography has better anatomic resolution and may also indicate epididymal or testicular abscesses (McAlistar and Sisler, 1990).

Pathogenesis

In young boys and infants, epididymitis is more likely to be related to genitourinary abnormalities (abnormal connections) or systemic hematogenous dissemination than in older boys (Williams et al, 1979). Urethral and urinary cultures from the prepubertal male are likely to show either nothing or gram-negative organisms and thus be referred to as nonspecific epididymitis, whereas in postpubertal sexually active boys, the cause may involve sexually transmitted organisms (e.g., *Neisseria gonorrhoeae* or *Chlamydia trachomatis*). Similar to the pathogenesis of renal abscess, data support two means of bacterial access to the epididymitis and testes: hematogenous dissemination and urinary tract–related infection. In young boys and infants, hematogenous pathogenesis is supported by reports in which *Haemophilis influenzae* type b has been cultured from epididymal abscesses concurrent with other sites of infection, such as the ear, while the urinalysis remains normal (Weber, 1985; Greenfield, 1986; Lin et al, 1988). Because organisms such as *H. influenzae* may require special culture techniques that are not ordinarily used for urinary cultures, this may also account for the 40% to 84% of cultures from boys diagnosed to have epididymitis without an identifiable organism (Knight and Vassy, 1984; Cabral et al, 1985; Likitnukul et al, 1987). The fact that ascending UTI or bacteria may cause epididymitis and epididymo-orchitis is supported by the observation that the boys who have pyuria and bacteriuria are more likely to have a urinary tract abnormality and appear at a younger age (Siegel et al, 1987).

Management

Epididymitis should be treated according to the likelihood of the causative organism. Specifically, in the young child who has pyuria and possible bacterial epididymitis, initial broad-spectrum antimicrobial coverage similar to that used to treat a UTI in an ill child should be used. Once the culture results and antimicrobial sensitivities are available, the most specific and most cost-effective agent with few side effects that achieves good tissue and urinary levels should be selected. **During or after treatment of the acute urinary and epididymal infections, radiologic evaluation of the urinary tract should be performed, as with any UTI.** Two studies report a high likelihood of genitourinary anatomic abnormalities, in particular abnormal connections between the urinary tract and bowel or genital duct system, when a child has bacterial epididymitis and a UTI (Siegel et al, 1987; Anderson et al, 1989). In both studies, boys with negative urinary cultures had normal urinary tracts. Whether or not all boys with epididymitis, including those with negative urethral and urinary cultures, need a full radiologic evaluation of the urinary tract is unclear from current data. It does appear prudent, however, to perform a VCUG and renal and bladder ultrasound study on prepubertal boys with documented urinary infections and perhaps those in whom epididymal abscesses are found, although these abscesses may be related to hematogenous spread.

Epididymitis Associated with Unusual Organisms

Whenever scrotal masses are considered, tuberculous epididymitis must also be considered as the most common form of urogenital tuberculosis (Cabral et al, 1985). Whereas this form of epididymitis is more likely to be confused with a malignancy rather than a cause of an acute scrotal mass because it usually involves painless swelling, this can be an important cause of epididymitis when dealing with patients from areas in which tuberculosis may be endemic. Although there is evidence for both local urinary spread and hematogenous spread of tuberculosis to the epididymis, in the reported pediatric cases of tuberculous epididymitis, there were usually other signs of hematogenous involvement and the urine may or may not be positive for the organism (Cabral et al, 1985).

RENAL FUNCTION AND ESTIMATION OF GLOMERULAR FILTRATION RATE

Plasma creatinine cannot give the same estimation of renal function in a child that it can in an adult because the plasma creatinine changes with age and size (Donckerwolcke et al, 1970; Schwartz et al, 1976a, 1976b). GFR, on the other hand, when corrected for body surface area, does not change appreciably after age 2 years (Counahan et al, 1976). For this reason, several estimates of GFR from plasma creatinine and body height have been developed for use in following serial renal function in children and in calculating drug doses of nephrotoxic agents (Counahan et al, 1976; Schwartz et al, 1976a; Morris et al, 1982). A formula for estimating GFR in children is GFR (ml/minute/1173 sq m^2) = 0.55 × body length (cm)/plasma creatinine (mg/dl) (Schwartz et al, 1976a). This formula has compared favorably with inulin and creatinine clearances performed simultaneously. Normal values for plasma creatinine and urea for children of various ages are presented in Tables 57–9 and 57–10.

CONSIDERATIONS IN TREATING CHILDREN WITH BACTERIURIA AND RENAL SCARRING

Rational treatment of infants and children with UTIs is based on an understanding of bacterial and host risk factors. After a child with bacteriuria and renal scarring has been identified, management consists of minimizing renal damage from the infection and assessing potential risk factors for preventing further renal infection–related damage.

When a renal scar has been identified, the child and parents need to be educated about the future possibilities of hypertension, proteinuria, and progressive nephropathy. In moderate to severe renal scarring with renal insufficiency, early nephrologic consultation for evaluation and surveillance for hypertension, proteinuria, acid-base balance, and dietary counseling of low protein may improve or stabilize renal function and improve body growth. In addition, the young woman with renal insufficiency from pyelonephritogenic nephropathy and recurrent UTIs may desire pregnancy counseling.

Although familial screening for vesicoureteral reflux may not be routine at all institutions, families in whom a member has vesicoureteral reflux or renal scarring must be made aware of the familial risk of vesicoureteral reflux and UTIs and the need for early diagnosis, treatment, and evaluation of UTIs in other family members.

Table 57–9. DISTRIBUTION OF PLASMA CREATININE CONCENTRATIONS FOR BOYS AND GIRLS BY AGE

Age (years)	Females			Males			P
	n	$\bar{x}$	*s*	*n*	$\bar{x}$	*s*	
1	8	0.35	0.05	9	0.41	0.10	<.2
2	13	0.45	0.07	18	0.43	0.12	<.7
3	24	0.42	0.08	30	0.46	0.11	<.1
4	28	0.47	0.12	49	0.45	0.11	<.5
5	44	0.46	0.11	50	0.50	0.11	<.1
6	44	0.48	0.11	62	0.52	0.12	<.1
7	50	0.53	0.12	59	0.54	0.14	<.9
8	61	0.53	0.11	60	0.57	0.16	<.1
9	61	0.55	0.11	52	0.59	0.16	<.1
10	46	0.55	0.13	58	0.61	0.22	<.1
11	57	0.60	0.13	56	0.62	0.14	<.5
12	54	0.59	0.13	67	0.65	0.16	<.1
13	41	0.62	0.14	53	0.68	0.21	<.2
14	30	0.65	0.13	44	0.72	0.24	<.2
15	22	0.67	0.22	40	0.76	0.22	<.2
16	16	0.65	0.15	24	0.74	0.23	<.2
17	12	0.70	0.20	22	0.80	0.18	<.2
18–20	15	0.72	0.19	19	0.91	0.17	<.005

n, sample number; $\bar{x}$, mean plasma creatinine concentration (mg/dl); s, standard deviation; P, significance of difference between male and female means.

From Schwartz GJ, Haycock MB, Spitzer A: Plasma creatinine and urea concentration in children: Normal values for age and sex. J. Pediatr, 1976; 88:828–830.

Table 57–10. DISTRIBUTION OF PLASMA UREA CONCENTRATIONS FOR BOYS AND GIRLS BY AGE

Age (years)	Females			Males			P
	n	$\bar{x}$	*s*	*n*	$\bar{x}$	*s*	
1	8	4.91	1.23	9	4.82	1.71	<.9
2	13	6.23	2.47	18	4.93	2.12	<.2
3	24	5.08	1.29	30	5.07	1.58	<.9
4	28	4.57	2.02	49	4.78	1.40	<.6
5	44	4.68	1.36	50	5.52	1.74	<.02
6	44	4.81	1.63	62	5.23	1.56	<.2
7	50	4.67	1.39	59	5.44	1.74	<.02
8	61	5.02	1.61	60	4.84	1.69	<.6
9	61	5.16	1.85	52	5.60	2.68	<.4
10	46	4.67	1.82	58	5.55	3.00	<.1
11	57	4.51	1.62	56	5.04	1.73	<.1
12	54	4.23	1.18	67	5.18	1.46	<.001
13	41	4.82	1.71	53	5.24	1.65	<.3
14	30	5.38	2.18	44	5.11	1.90	<.7
15	22	4.87	2.11	40	5.35	1.62	<.4
16	16	4.77	1.59	24	5.18	1.48	<.5
17	12	4.56	1.64	12	5.67	1.59	<.1
18–20	15	5.41	1.46	19	5.48	1.26	<.9

n, sample number; $\bar{x}$, mean plasma urea concentration (mM/l); s, standard deviation; P, significance of difference between male and female means.

From Schwartz GJ, Haycock MB, Spitzer A: Plasma creatinine and urea concentration in children: Normal values for age and sex. J Pediatr 1976; 88:828–830.

REFERENCES

Abbott GD: Neonatal bacteriuria: A prospective study in 1460 infants. BMJ 1972; 1:267.

Åbyholm G, Monn E: Intranasal DDAVP-Test in the study of renal concentrating capacity in children with recurrent urinary tract infections. Eur J Pediatr 1979; 130:149–154.

Ahmad T, Vickers D, Campbell S, et al: Urine collection from disposable nappies. Lancet 1991; 338:674–676.

Alon U, Berant M, Pery M: Intravenous pyelography in children with urinary tract infection and vesicoureteral reflux. Pediatrics 1989; 83(3):332–336.

Alon U, Pery M, Davidai G, Berant M: Ultrasonography in the radiologic evaluation of children with urinary tract infection. Pediatrics 1986; 78(1):58–64.

Anderson P, Giacomantonio J: The acutely painful scrotum in children: Review of 113 consecutive cases. Can Med Assoc J 1985; 132:1153–1155.

Anderson P, Giacomantonio J, Schwarz R: Acute scrotal pain in children: Prospective study of diagnosis and management. Can J Surg 1989; 32(3):29–32.

Andriole VT: The role of Tamm-Horsfall protein in the pathogenesis of reflux nephropathy and chronic pyelonephritis. Yale J Biol Med 1985; 58:91–100.

Apperley J, Rice S, Bishop J, et al: Late-onset hemorrhagic cystitis associated with urinary excretion of polyomaviruses after bone marrow transplantation. Transplantation 1987; 43:108–112.

Ashkenazi S, Even-Tov S, Samra Z, Dinari G: Uropathogens of various childhood populations and their antibiotic susceptibility. Pediatr Infect Dis J 1991; 10:742–746.

Tambic T, Oberiter V, Delmis J, Tambic A: Diagnostic value of a p-fimbriation test in determining duration of therapy in children with urinary tract infections. Clin Ther 1992; 14(5):667–671.

Tappin D, Murphy A, Mocan H, et al: A prospective study of children with first acute symptomatic *E. coli* urinary tract infection. Early 99m-technetium dimercaptosuccinic acid scan appearances. Acta Paediatr Scand 1989; 78:923–929.

Taylor C, Hunt G, Matthews I: Bacterial study of clean intermittent catheterisation in children. Br J Urol 1985; 58:64–69.

Thompson RB: A Short Textbook of Haematology. Philadelphia, J. B. Lippincott Company, 1969.

Tomlinson P, Smellie J, Prescod N, et al: Differential excretion of urinary proteins in children with vesicoureteric reflux and reflux nephropathy. Pediatr Nephrol 1994; 8:21–25.

Torres VE, Velosa JA, Holley KE, et al: The progression of vesicoureteral reflux nephropathy. Ann Intern Med 1980; 92:776–784.

Troell S, Berg U, Johansson B, Wikstad I: Ultrasonographic renal parenchymal volume related to kidney function and renal parenchymal area in children with recurrent urinary tract infections and asymptomatic bacteriuria. Acta Radiol [Diagn] (Stockh) 1984; 25(5):411–416.

Tulassy T, Miltényi M, Dobos M: Alterations of urinary carbon dioxide tension, electrolyte handling and low molecular weight protein excretion in acute pyelonephritis. Acta Scand 1986; 75:415–419.

Tullus K: Fecal colonization with p-fimbriated *Escherichia coli* in newborn children and relation to development of extraintestinal *E. coli* infections. Acta Paediatr Scand 1986; 334(Suppl):1–35.

Umeyama T, Kawamura T, Hasegawa A, Ogawa O: Ectopic ureter presenting with epididymitis in childhood: Report of 5 cases. J Urol 1985; 134:131–133.

Väisänen V, Elo J, Tallgren LG, et al: Mannose-resistant haemagglutination and P antigen recognition are characteristic of *Escherichia coli* causing primary pyelonephritis. Lancet 1981; 2:1366–1369.

vanGool, JD, Vijverberg MAW, deJong TPVM: Functional daytime incontinence: Clinical and urodynamic assessment. Scand J Urol Nephrol 1992a; 141(Suppl):58–69.

vanGool JD, Vijverberg MAW, Messer AP, et al: Functional daytime incontinence: Non-pharmacological treatment. Scand J Urol Nephrol 1992b; 141(Suppl):93–103.

Verber I, Meller S: Serial 99mTc dimercaptosuccinic acid (DMSA) scans after urinary infections presenting before the age of 5 years. Arch Dis Child 1989; 64:1533–1537.

Verboven M, Ingels M, Delree M, Piepsz A: 99mTc-DMSA scintigraphy in acute urinary tract infection in children. Radiatr Radiol 1990; 20:540–542.

Verrier-Jones ER, Meller ST, McLachlan MSF, et al: Treatment of bacteriuria in schoolgirls. Kidney Int 1975; 4(Suppl):S85–S89.

Vigano A, Dalla-Villa A, Bianchi C, et al: Single-dose netilmicin therapy of complicated and uncomplicated lower urinary tract infections in children. Acta Paediatr Scand 1985; 74:584–588.

Walker RD: Renal functional changes associated with vesicoureteal reflux. Urol Clin North Am 1990; 17(2):307–316.

Wallace DMA, Rothwell DL, Williams DI: The long-term follow-up of surgically treated vesicoureteric reflux. Br J Urol 1978; 50:479–484.

Wallin L, Bajc M: Typical technetium dimercaptosuccinic acid distribution patterns in acute pyelonephritis. Acta Paediatr 1993; 82:1061–1065.

Wallin L, Bajc M: The significance of vesicoureteric reflux on kidney development assessed by dimercaptosuccinate renal scintigraphy. Br J Urol 1994; 73:607–611.

Weber T: *Hemophilus influenzae* epidodymo-orchitis. J Urol 1985; 133:487.

Wettergren B, Fasth A, Jacobsson B, et al: UTI during the first year of life in a Göteborg area 1977–79. Pediatr Res 1980; 14:981.

Wiggelinkhuizen J, Maytham D, Hanslo D: Dipstick screening for urinary tract infection. S Afr Med J 1988; 74:224–228.

Wikstad I, Hannerz L, Karlsson A, et al: 99m Tc DMSA renal cortical scintigraphy in the diagnosis of acute pyelonephritis in rats. Pediatr Nephrol 1990; 4:331–334.

Williams C, Litvak A, McRoberts J: Epididymitis in infancy. J Urol 1979; 121:125–126.

Williams GL, Davies DKL, Evans KT, Williams JE: Vesicoureteric reflux in patients with bacteriuria in pregnancy. Lancet 1968; 2:1202–1205.

Winberg J, Anderson HJ, Bergström T, et al: Epidemiology of symptomatic urinary tract infection in childhood. Acta Paediatr Scand 1974; S252: 1–20.

Winberg J, Bergström T, Lidin-Janson G, Lincoln K: Treatment trials in urinary tract infection (UTI) with special reference to the effect of antimicrobials on the fecal and periurethral flora. Clin Nephrol 1973; 1:142.

Winberg J, Bollgren I, Gothefors L, et al: The prepuce: A mistake of nature? Lancet 1989; 1:598–599.

Wiswell T, Hachey W: Urinary tract infections and the uncircumcised state: An update. Clin Pediatr 1993; 32(3):130–134.

Wiswell TE, Enzenauer RW, Holton ME, et al: Declining frequency of circumcision: Implications for changes in the absolute incidence and male to female sex ratio of urinary tract infections in early infancy. Pediatrics 1987; 79(3):338–342.

Wiswell TE, Miller GM, Gelston HM, et al: Effect of circumcision status on periurethral bacterial flora during the first year of life. J Pediatr 1988; 113(3):442–446.

Wiswell TE, Roscelli JD: Corroborative evidence for the decreased incidence of urinary tract infections in circumcised male infants. Pediatrics 1986; 78(1):96–99.

Yazbeck S, Patriquin H: Accuracy of Doppler sonography in the evaluation of acute conditions of the scrotum in children. J Pediatr Surg 1994; 29(9):1270–1272.

Yoder MC, Polin RA: Immunotherapy of neonatal septicemia. Pediatr Clin North Am 1986; 33:481–501.

Zafaranloo S, Gerard P, Bryk D: Xanthogranulomatous pyelonephritis in children: Analysis by diagnostic modalities. Urol Radiol 1990; 12:18–21.

58 ANOMALIES OF THE KIDNEY AND URETEROPELVIC JUNCTION

Stuart B. Bauer, M.D.

Congenital anomalies of the upper urinary tract comprise a diversity of abnormalities, ranging from complete absence to aberrant location, orientation, and shape of the kidney as well as aberrations of the collecting system and blood supply. This wide range of anomalies results from a multiplicity of factors that interact to influence renal development in a sequential and orderly manner. Abnormal maturation or inappropriate timing of these processes at critical points in development can produce any number of deviations in the development of the kidney and ureter.

The embryology of the urinary tract is described in Chapter 51. The reader is encouraged to review this material in order to appreciate the complexity of renal and ureteral development and the factors involved in the formation of an abnormality.

The classification of renal and ureteral anomalies used in this chapter is based on kidney structure rather than function. The chapter is divided into two sections, comprising anomalies of the kidney and the ureteropelvic junction. Anomalies of the kidney may be classified as follows:

I. Anomalies of number
    A. Agenesis
        1. Bilateral agenesis
        2. Unilateral agenesis
    B. Supernumerary kidney
II. Anomalies of volume and structure
    A. Hypoplasia
    B. Multicystic kidney
    C. Polycystic kidney
        1. Infantile
        2. Adult
    D. Other cystic disease
    E. Medullary sponge kidney
    F. Medullary cystic disease
III. Anomalies of ascent
    A. Simple renal ectopia
    B. Cephalad renal ectopia
    C. Thoracic kidney
IV. Anomalies of form and fusion
    A. Crossed ectopia with and without fusion
        1. Unilateral fused kidney (inferior ectopia)
        2. Sigmoid or S-shaped kidney
        3. Lump kidney
        4. L-shaped kidney
        5. Disc kidney
        6. Superior ectopic (unilateral fused) kidney
    B. Horseshoe kidney
V. Anomalies of rotation
    A. Incomplete
    B. Excessive
    C. Reverse
VI. Anomalies of renal vasculature
    A. Aberrant, accessory, or multiple vessels
    B. Renal artery aneurysms
    C. Renal arteriovenous fistula

ANOMALIES OF THE KIDNEY

Anomalies of Number

Agenesis

Bilateral Agenesis

Of all the anomalies of the upper urinary tract, bilateral renal agenesis (BRA) has the most profound effect on the individual. Fortunately, it occurs infrequently when compared with other renal abnormalities. Although BRA was first recognized in 1671 by Wolfstrigel, it was not until Potter's eloquent and extensive description of the constellation of associated defects that the full extent of the syndrome could be appreciated and easily recognized (Potter, 1946a, 1946b, 1952). Subsequently, many investigators have attempted to understand all the facets of this syndrome and to explain them by employing one unifying etiology (Fitch and Lachance, 1972). But there is no unanimity regarding this topic, and controversy still exists concerning the exact mechanism of formation.

INCIDENCE. The anomaly is quite rare, with only slightly more than 500 cases cited in the literature. Potter (1965) estimated that BRA occurs once in 4800 births, but in British Columbia the incidence is 1 in 10,000 births (Wilson and Baird, 1985). Davidson and Ross (1954) noted a 0.28% incidence in autopsies of infants and children, whereas Stroup and colleagues (1990) detected an incidence of 3.5 per 100,000 in the Center for Disease Control and Prevention (CDC) Birth Defects Monitoring Program. As with most anomalies, there is a significant male predominance (nearly 75%). Neither maternal age nor a specific complication of pregnancy nor any maternal disease appears to influence its development (Davidson and Ross, 1954). The anomaly has been reported in two infants of an insulin-dependent diabetic mother (Novak and Robinson, 1994), in several sets of siblings (Rizza and Downing, 1971; Dicker et al, 1984), and even in monozygotic twins (Thomas and Smith, 1974; Cilento et al, 1994). Interestingly, in three pairs of monozygotic twins, one sibling was anephric whereas the other had normal kidneys (Kohler, 1972; Mauer et al, 1974; Cilento et al, 1994). It has been suggested that an autosomal recessive inheritance pattern exists (Dicker et al, 1984). There is a genetic predisposition to this syndrome with a high level of penetrance because when siblings and parents of an index child with BRA were screened, 4.5% had unilateral renal agenesis (Roodhooft et al, 1984), and 3.5% had BRA (McPherson et al, 1987). This figure is 1000 times higher than what has been reported in the general population (Stroup et al, 1990). Some investigators have suggested that this anomaly may be an autosomal dominant trait with variable penetrance (Kovacs et al, 1991; Murugasu et al, 1991; Moerman et al, 1994).

EMBRYOLOGY. Complete differentiation of the metanephric blastema into the adult renal parenchyma requires the presence and orderly branching of a ureteral bud. This occurs normally between the fifth and seventh weeks of gestation after the ureteral bud arises from the mesonephric or wolffian duct. It is theorized that induction of ureteral branching into major and minor calyces depends on the presence of a normal metanephric blastema (Davidson and Ross, 1954). The absence of a nephrogenic ridge on the dorsolateral aspect of the coelomic cavity or the failure of a ureteral bud to develop from the wolffian duct leads to agenesis of the kidney. The absence of both kidneys, therefore, requires a common factor causing renal or ureteral maldevelopment on both sides of the midline.

It is impossible to say which of these two factors is most important. Certainly no kidney can form in the absence of a metanephric blastema, but the presence of a ureteral bud and orderly branching are also necessary for the renal anlage to attain its ultimate morphology. In an extensive autopsy analysis, Ashley and Mostofi (1960) found many clues to the multifactorial nature of this developmental process and shed some light on the causes of BRA. Most anephric children in their series had at least a blind-ending ureteral bud of varying length. Thus, the embryologic insult in some cases was thought to affect the ureteral bud just as or shortly after it arose from the mesonephric duct. Even with complete ureteral atresia, structures of wolffian duct origin (vas deferens, seminal vesicle, and epididymis) were usually present and normally formed, suggesting that the injury occurred at about the time the ureteral bud formed (the fifth or sixth week of gestation). With complete absence of the ureter, a rudimentary kidney was discovered in only a few instances, supporting the concept of the interdependency of the two processes. Conversely, in some instances the ureter was normal in appearance up to the level of the ureteropelvic junction, where it ended abruptly. In those cases, no recognizable renal parenchyma could be identified. In a small number of autopsies the gonads were absent as well, indicating an abnormality or insult that took place prior to the fifth week and involved the entire urogenital ridge (Carpentier and Potter, 1959). Although the nephric and genital portions of the urogenital ridge are closely aligned on the dorsal aspect of the coelomic cavity, an extensive lesion affecting the entire area is necessary to produce both conditions in the developing fetus. Therefore, absence of one or both kidneys may result from one of several causes.

DESCRIPTION. The kidneys are completely absent on gross inspection of the entire retroperitoneum. Occasionally, there might be a small mass of poorly organized mesenchymal tissue containing primitive glomerular elements. Tiny vascular branches from the aorta penetrate this structure, but no identifiable major renal artery is present (Ashley and Mostofi, 1960) (Fig. 58–1).

In addition to the absence of functioning kidneys, each ureter may be wholly or partially absent. Complete ureteral atresia is observed in slightly more than 50% of affected individuals (Ashley and Mostofi, 1960). The trigone, if de-

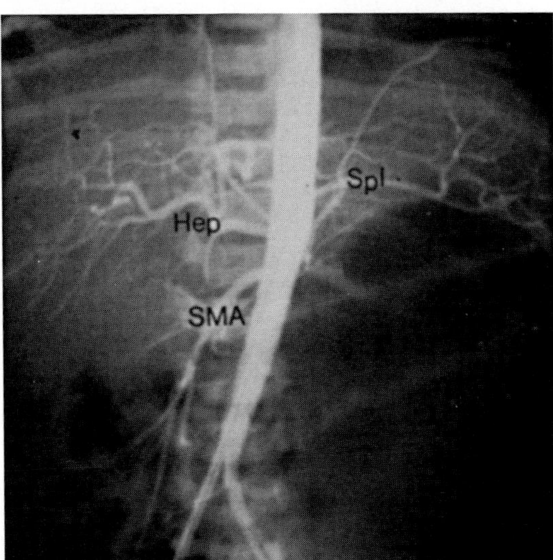

Figure 58–1. Aortogram via an umbilical artery catheter in a newborn with Potter's facies outlines major branches of the aorta but fails to demonstrate either renal artery or kidney.

veloped, is poorly formed owing to failure of the mesonephric duct structures to be incorporated into the base of the bladder. The bladder, when present (in about 50% of cases), is usually hypoplastic owing to the lack of stimulation by fetal urine production. Alternatively, it has been postulated that ureteral bud and wolffian duct structures migrating into the ventral cloacal region are needed to initiate bladder development; their absence and not the *lack* of urine is the cause of arrested development (Levin, 1952; Katz and Chatten, 1974).

ASSOCIATED ANOMALIES. Other findings associated with BRA have been extensively described by Potter (1946) following an exhaustive investigation of these unfortunate individuals. The infants have low birth weights, ranging from 1000 to 2500 g. At birth, oligohydramnios (absent or minimal amniotic fluid) is present. In addition, the characteristic facial appearance and deformity of the extremities set these children apart from normal newborns. The infants generally look prematurely senile and have "a prominent fold of skin that begins over each eye, swings down in a semi-circle over the inner canthus and extends onto the cheek" (Potter, 1946a and b). It is Potter's contention that this facial feature is a sine qua non of nonfunctioning renal parenchyma. He even suggests that its absence confirms the presence of kidneys (Fig. 58–2*A*). In addition to this finding, the nose is blunted, and a prominent depression between the lower lip and chin is evident. The ears appear to be somewhat low set and drawn forward, and are often pressed against the side of the head, making the lobes seem unusually broad and exceedingly large (Fig. 58–2*B*). The ear canals are not dislocated, but the appearance of the ear lobes gives the impression that the ears are displaced downward. The legs are often bowed and clubbed, with excessive flexion at the hip and knee joints. Occasionally, the lower extremities are completely fused as well (sirenomelia) (Bain et al, 1960).

The skin can be excessively dry and appears too loose for the body. This may be secondary to severe dehydration or loss of subcutaneous fat. The hands are relatively large and clawlike.

It is thought that these characteristic facial abnormalities and limb features are caused by the effects of oligohydramnios rather than by multiple organ system defects (Fitch and Lachance, 1972; Thomas and Smith, 1974). Compression of the fetus against the internal uterine walls without any cushioning effect from amniotic fluid could explain all the findings of this syndrome. Urine from the developing kidney is the major source of amniotic fluid, accounting for greater than 90% of its volume by the third trimester (Thomas and Smith, 1974), but the skin, gastrointestinal tract, and central nervous system also contribute small amounts, particularly before urine production begins at 14 weeks. Thus, the absence of kidneys severely reduces the amount of amniotic fluid produced during the latter stages of pregnancy.

Pulmonary hypoplasia and a bell-shaped chest are com-

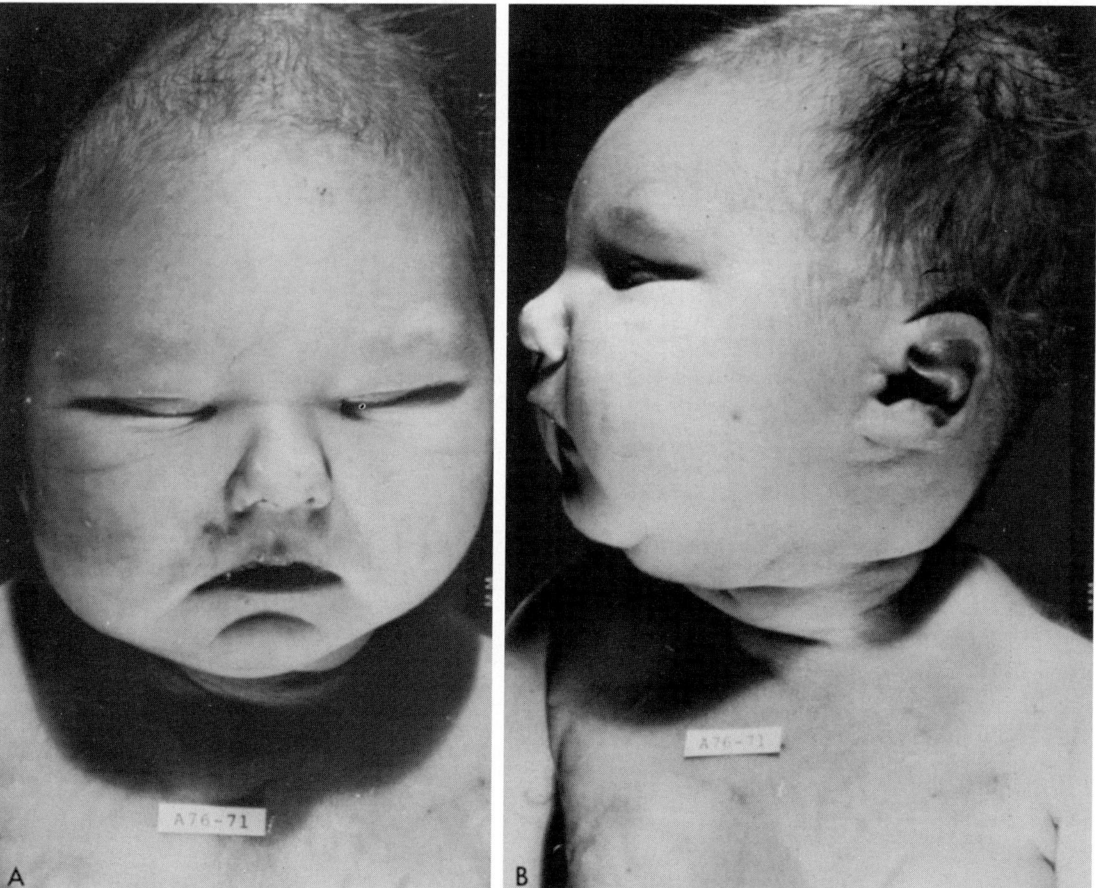

Figure 58–2. An anephric child who lived 2 days has typical Potter's facial appearance. *A*, Note the prominent fold and skin crease beneath each eye, blunted nose, and depression between lower lip and chin. *B*, The ears give an impression of being low-set because lobes are broad and drawn forward, but actually the ear canals are located normally.

mon associated conditions. Originally, these findings were thought to be secondary to uterine wall compression of the thoracic cage as a result of the oligohydramniotic state (Bain and Scott, 1960). Subsequently, it was believed that the amniotic fluid itself was responsible for pulmonary development (Fitch and Lachance, 1972). However, this theory was discounted when it was discovered that there is a significant reduction in the number of airways generated as well as a decrease in acini formation (Hislop et al, 1979). Pulmonary airway divisioning occurs between the 12th and 16th weeks of gestation (Reid, 1977). A reduction in the number of divisions implies interference with this process before the 16th week of gestation. The contribution from the kidneys to the amniotic fluid volume before this time is small, if any. Therefore, the oligohydramnios seen in cases of BRA is a later finding in pregnancy, occurring long after the structural groundwork of the lung has been laid out. Hislop and associates (1979) suggested that the anephric fetus fails to produce proline, which is needed for collagen formation in the bronchiolar tree. The kidney is the primary source of proline (Clemmons, 1977). Thus, pulmonary hypoplasia may result from an absence of renal parenchyma and not from diminished amniotic fluid. This hypothesis is supported by the finding of normal lungs in two babies with prolonged leakage of amniotic fluid beginning at a time when one would have expected pulmonary hypoplasia if the amniotic fluid alone were responsible for the defect (Perlman et al, 1976; Cilento et al, 1994).

In the male, penile development is usually normal, but a few cases of penile agenesis have occurred (O'Connor et al, 1993). Hypospadias is rare, but its occurrence is not related to the presence or absence of testes. In 43% of cases, however, the testes are undescended (Carpentier and Potter, 1959). These authors did not find any infants without testes, but Ashley and Mostofi (1960) noted testicular agenesis in 10%. The vas deferens is normal in most cases. The presence of vasa implies that whatever caused the renal agenesis influenced the ureteral bud only after it formed or that the insult affected only the nephrogenic ridge.

Although this syndrome occurs uncommonly in females, they have a relatively high incidence of genitourinary anomalies when it does affect them (Carpentier and Potter, 1959). The ovaries are frequently hypoplastic or absent. The uterus is usually either rudimentary or bicornuate; occasionally, it is absent entirely, as in sirenomelia. Finally, the vagina is either a short blind pouch or completely absent.

The adrenal glands are rarely malpositioned or absent (Davidson and Ross, 1954), but they can appear flattened or "lying down" on ultrasonography (Hoffman et al, 1992). Anomalies of other organ systems are not unusual. The legs are frequently abnormal, with clubbed or even fused feet producing sirenomelia. A lumbar meningocele with or without the Arnold-Chiari malformation is not infrequently observed (Davidson and Ross, 1954; Ashley and Mostofi, 1960). Other malformations include abnormalities of the cardiovascular and gastrointestinal systems, which are present in up to 50% of infants.

DIAGNOSIS. The characteristic Potter facies and the presence of oligohydramnios are pathognomonic and should alert one to this severe urinary malformation. Amnion nodosum—small white keratinized nodules found on the surface of the amniotic sac—may also suggest this anomaly (Bain et al, 1960; Thompson, 1960). Ninety percent of newborns void during the first day of life (Sherry and Kramer, 1955; Clark, 1977). Failure to urinate in the first 24 hours is not uncommon and should not arouse one's suspicion. Anuria after the first 24 hours without distention of the bladder should suggest renal agenesis (Williams, 1974). However, most infants with renal agenesis who are born alive suffer from severe respiratory distress within the first 24 hours of life. When this becomes the focus of attention, the anuria may go unnoticed, and the renal anomaly is thought of only secondarily.

When the association is made, excretory urography may be attempted but is generally fruitless. Renal ultrasonography is probably the easiest way to identify the kidneys and bladder in order to confirm the presence or absence of urine within these structures. A clue to absent kidneys is the presence of flattened adrenal glands in their normal location (Hoffman et al, 1992). If abdominal ultrasonography is inconclusive, a renal scan can be performed. The absence of uptake of the radionuclide in the renal fossa above background activity will confirm the diagnosis of BRA. Umbilical artery catheterization and aortography can be undertaken if other modalities are unavailable or are not diagnostic. They will define the absence of renal arteries and kidneys.

As the use of maternal ultrasonic screening becomes more pervasive, these unfortunate babies are being diagnosed in the second and third trimesters when severe oligohydramnios is noted and no kidney tissue can be detected. Termination of the pregnancy has been considered when the clinician is certain of the diagnosis (Rayburn and Laferla, 1986).

PROGNOSIS. Nearly 40% of affected infants are stillborn. Most of the children born alive do not survive beyond the first 24 to 48 hours because of respiratory distress associated with pulmonary hypoplasia. Those infants who do not succumb at this time generally remain alive for variable periods depending on the rate at which renal failure develops. The longest surviving child lived 39 days (Davidson and Ross, 1954).

Unilateral Agenesis

Fortunately, complete absence of one kidney occurs more commonly than does BRA. In general, there are no telltale signs (as with BRA) that suggest an absent kidney (Campbell, 1928). The diagnosis is usually not suspected and remains undetected unless careful examination of the external and internal genitalia uncovers an abnormality that is associated with renal agenesis or an imaging study performed for other reasons reveals only one kidney. Prenatal ultrasonography improves the detection rate of this condition and reveals that some cases are due to involution of a multicystic or dysplastic kidney before birth (Mesrobian et al, 1993; Hitchcock and Burge, 1994).

INCIDENCE. The clinically silent nature of this anomaly precludes a completely accurate account of its incidence. Most autopsy series, however, suggest that unilateral renal agenesis (URA) occurs once in 1100 births (Doroshow and Abeshouse, 1961). In a survey of excretory urograms performed at the Mayo Clinic, the clinical incidence approached 1 in 1500 (Longo and Thompson, 1952), but Wilson and Baird (1993) noted a 1 in 5000 occurrence in British Columbia. Recently, ultrasonic screening of 280,000 school children in Taipei revealed an incidence of unilateral agenesis of 1 in 1200 (Shieh et al, 1990). With the increased use of prenatal ultrasonic screening, the incidence of unilateral renal agenesis may be found to be actually higher than previously reported.

The higher incidence of bilateral renal agenesis noted in males is not nearly as striking in the unilateral condition, but males still predominate in a ratio of 1.8:1 (Doroshow and Abeshouse, 1961). This is not surprising considering the timing of embryologic events. Wolffian duct differentiation occurs earlier in the male than does müllerian duct development in the female, taking place closer to the time of ureteral bud formation. Thus, it is postulated that the ureteral bud is influenced more by abnormalities of the wolffian duct than by those of the müllerian duct.

Absence of one kidney occurs somewhat more frequently on the left side. A familial tendency has been noted (Arfeen et al, 1993; Selig et al, 1993) and has been reported in siblings within a single family and even monozygotic twins (Kohn and Borns, 1973; Uchida et al, 1990). In a study of several families, McPherson and colleagues (1987) noted a familial pattern of inheritance and concluded that an autosomal dominant transmission with a 50% to 90% penetrance existed in this study group. This inheritance pattern has been confirmed by others who evaluated families with more than one affected individual (Biedel et al, 1984; Roodhooft et al, 1984; Battin et al, 1993).

EMBRYOLOGY. The embryologic basis for URA does not differ significantly from that described for the bilateral type. The fault lies most probably with the ureteral bud. Complete absence of a bud or aborted ureteral development prevents maturation of the metanephric blastema into adult kidney tissue.

It is unlikely that the metanephros is responsible because the ipsilateral gonad (derived from adjacent mesenchymal tissue) is rarely absent, malpositioned, or nonfunctioning (Ashley and Mostofi, 1960). The high incidence of absent or malformed proximal mesonephric duct structures in the male and müllerian duct structures in the female strengthens the argument that the embryologic insult affects the ureteral bud primarily early in its development and even influences its precursor, the mesonephric duct. The abnormality most likely occurs no later than the fourth or fifth week of gestation, when the ureteral bud forms and the mesonephric or wolffian duct in the male begins to develop into the seminal vesicle, prostate, and vas deferens. The müllerian duct in the female at this time starts its medial migration, crossing over the degenerating wolffian duct (sixth week) on its way to differentiating into the fallopian tube, uterine horn and body, and proximal vagina (Woolf and Allen, 1953; Yoder and Pfister, 1976).

Magee and colleagues (1979) proposed an embryologic classification based on the timing of the faulty differentiation (Fig. 58–3). If the insult occurs before the fourth week (type I), nondifferentiation of the nephrogenic ridge with retardation of the mesonephric and müllerian components results, leading to complete unilateral agenesis of genitourinary structures. The individual has a solitary kidney and a unicornuate uterus. In type II anomalies, the defect occurs early in the fourth week of gestation, affecting both the mesonephric and ureteral buds. The maldeveloped mesonephric duct prevents cross-over of the müllerian duct and subsequent fusion. As a consequence, a didelphic uterus with obstruction of the ipsilateral horn and the vagina is produced. If the insult occurs after the fourth week (type III), the mesonephric and müllerian ducts develop normally; only the ureteral bud and metanephric blastema are affected. Normal genital architecture is present despite the absence of one kidney.

With the discovery on prenatal screening that multicystic and dysgenetic kidneys can involute completely before birth, the cause of every case of URA cannot be attributed to one of the mechanisms cited earlier. In fact, the presence of the splenic flexure of the bowel in its normal location and not in the left renal fossa suggests that a dysplastic or multicystic kidney may have started to form in the proper location but involuted before delivery.

ASSOCIATED ANOMALIES. The ipsilateral ureter is completely absent in slightly more than half the patients (Fortune, 1927; Collins, 1932; Ashley and Mostofi, 1960). Many of the remaining individuals have only a partially developed ureter. In no instance is the ureter totally normal. Partial ureteral development is associated with either complete luminal atresia or patency of a variable degree. A hemitrigone (in association with complete ureteral agenesis) or an asymmetric trigone (in the presence of a partially developed ureter) is recognizable at cystoscopy. Segmental ureteral atresia on one side has been associated with contralateral ureteral or renal ectopia (Limkakeng and Retik, 1972). Except for ectopia or malrotation, anomalies of the contralateral kidney are very infrequently encountered (Longo and Thompson, 1952). Contralateral reflux into the collecting system has been found in 30% of those tested (Atiyeh et al, 1993).

Ipsilateral adrenal agenesis is rarely encountered with unilateral agenesis and is noted in less than 10% of autopsy reports (Fortune, 1927; Collins, 1932; Ashley and Mostofi, 1960) and in 17% of affected individuals evaluated by computed tomography (Kenney et al, 1985). This is not surprising in view of the different embryologic derivations of the adrenal cortex and medulla, which arise separately from the metanephros.

Genital anomalies, on the other hand, are much more frequently observed. Despite the predominance of males with URA, a greater number of reproductive organ abnormalities seem to occur more regularly in females, amounting to at least 25% to 50% of cases compared with 10% to 15% in males. Although a genital anomaly is easier to detect in the female, which may account for the difference in incidence between the two sexes, a more plausible explanation may be related to the difference in timing and interaction of the male and female genital ducts with the developing mesonephric duct and ureteral bud. The incidence of genital organ malformations in both sexes varies from 20% to 40% (Smith and Orkin, 1945; Doroshow and Abeshouse, 1961; Thompson and Lynn, 1966).

Regardless of the sex, both the ipsilaterally and contralaterally positioned testes or ovaries are usually normal. But structures derived from the müllerian or wolffian duct are most often anomalous. In the male, the testes and globus major, which contains the efferent ductules and arises from mesonephric tubules, are invariably present; all structures proximal to that point that develop from the mesonephric duct (the globus minor, vas deferens, seminal vesicle, am-

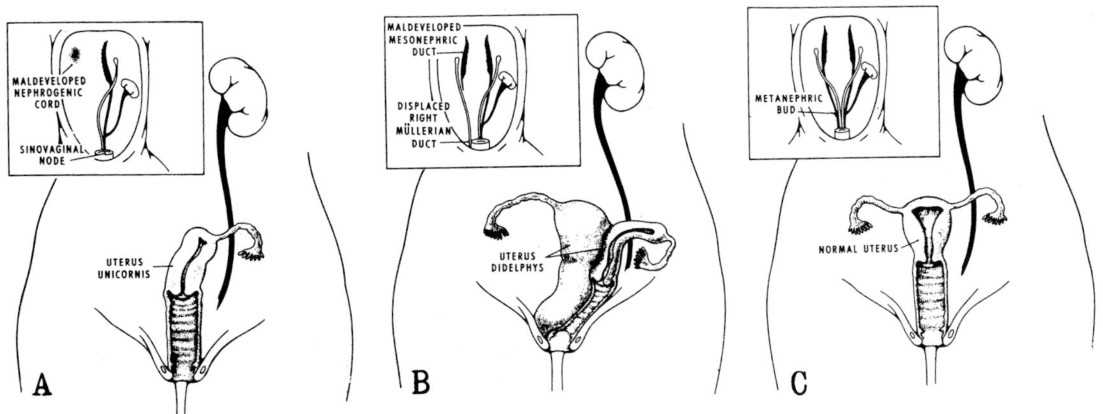

Figure 58–3. A proposed categorization of genital and renal anomalies in females. (From Magee MC, Lucey DT, Fried FA: J Urol 1979;121:265.)

pulla, and ejaculatory duct) are frequently absent, with an incidence approaching 50% (Radasch, 1908; Collins, 1932; Charny and Gillenwater, 1965; Ochsner et al, 1972). In a recent survey and review of the literature (Donohue and Fauver, 1989) of adult males with absence of the vas deferens, 79% were found to have an absent kidney on the ipsilateral side; left-sided lesions predominated in a ratio of 3.5:1. Occasionally, the mesonephric duct structures may be rudimentary or ectopic rather than absent (Holt and Peterson, 1974). Seminal vesicle cysts are but one example of this (Furtado, 1973; Beeby, 1974); six cases were noted among 119 boys (5%) found to have URA during ultrasonic screening of school children (Shieh et al, 1990). Rarely has ipsilateral cryptorchidism been noted.

In the female, a variety of anomalies may result from incomplete or altered müllerian duct development caused by mesonephric duct maldevelopment. Approximately one third of women with renal agenesis have an abnormality of the internal genitalia (Thompson and Lynn, 1966). Conversely, 43% of women with genital anomalies have URA (Semmens, 1962). Most common of these anomalies is a true unicornuate uterus with complete absence of the ipsilateral horn and fallopian tube or a bicornuate uterus with rudimentary development of the horn on the affected side. The fimbriated end of the fallopian tube, however, is usually fully formed and corresponds in its development to the globus major in the male (Shumacker, 1938).

Partial or complete midline fusion of the müllerian ducts may result in a double (didelphic) or septate uterus with either a single or a duplicated cervix (Radasch, 1908; Fortune, 1927). Complete duplication or separation of the vagina, proximal vaginal atresia associated with a small introital dimple, and even complete absence of the vagina have been reported (Woolf and Allen, 1953; D'Alberton et al, 1981). Obstruction of one side of a duplicated system is not uncommon, and unilateral hematocolpos or hydrocolpos associated with a pelvic mass or pain, or both, has been described in pubertal girls (Weiss and Dykhuizen, 1967; Vinstein and Franken, 1972; Gilliland and Dick, 1976; Wiersma et al, 1976; Yoder and Pfister, 1976) (Fig. 58–4). In rare instances, this anomalous condition has been mistaken for a large or infected Gartner's duct cyst. Sometimes a true Gartner's duct cyst is found in prepubertal girls in association with an ectopic ureter that is blind-ending at its proximal end or one that is connected to a rudimentary kidney (Currarino, 1982). Six percent of girls with URA had a Gartner's duct cyst on mass screening of school children (Shieh et al, 1990).

Radiologic investigation of the upper urinary tract in individuals with anomalies of the internal genitalia often leads to discovery of an absent kidney on the affected side (Bryan et al, 1949; Phelan et al, 1953). In fact, because URA is so frequently associated with anomalies of the internal female genitalia, the clinician should evaluate the entire genitourinary system in any girl with one or more of the above mentioned abnormalities.

In addition, anomalies of other organ systems are found

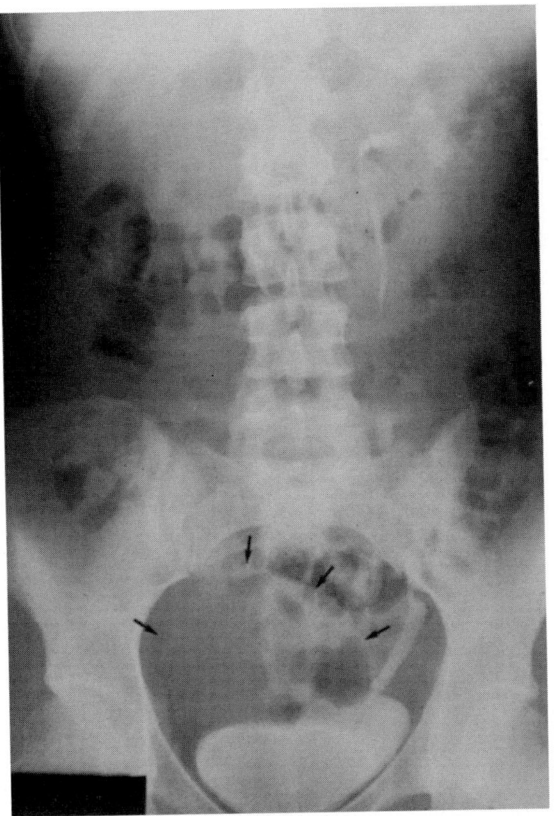

Figure 58–4. A 16-year-old girl with a solitary left kidney had abdominal pain and a pelvic mass that proved to be an obstructed duplicate vagina with hematocolpos.

frequently in affected individuals. The more common sites involve the cardiovascular (30%), gastrointestinal (25%), and musculoskeletal (14%) systems (Emanuel et al, 1974) (Fig. 58–5). They include septal and valvular cardiac defects; imperforate anus and anal or esophageal strictures or atresia; and vertebral or phalangeal abnormalities (Jancu et al, 1976). Several syndromes are associated with URA—Turner's syndrome, Poland's syndrome (Mace et al, 1972), DiGeorge's anomaly when associated with insulin-dependent diabetes mellitus in the mother (Wilson et al, 1993; Novak and Robinson, 1994), and dysmorphogenesis (Say and Gerald, 1968). Thirty percent of children with the VATER syndrome (V, vertebral; A, imperforate anus; TE, tracheoesophageal atresia; R, renal) have renal agenesis (Barry and Auldist, 1974). Thus, a comprehensive review of all organ systems should be undertaken when more than one anomaly is discovered or when specific complexes of anomalies associated with renal agenesis are present. In a small number of children the constellation of defects is incompatible with life, and gestational or neonatal death ensues.

DIAGNOSIS. In general, there are no specific symptoms heralding an absent kidney. Most reports are composed of surveys from autopsy series. The contralateral kidney does not appear to be more prone to disease because it is solitary, unless the absent kidney is really secondary to a multicystic dysplastic organ that was unrecognized at birth, in which case there may be mild ureteropelvic junction obstruction in the remaining functioning kidney. One report evaluating the late effects of URA on the solitary kidney revealed proteinuria in 20%, hypertension in 47%, and diminished renal function in 13% of middle-aged patients (Argueso et al, 1992).

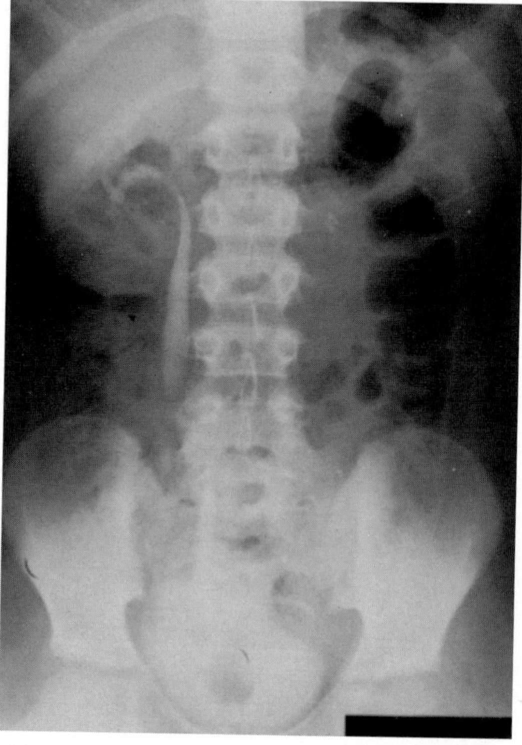

Figure 58–5. A 4-year-old girl had an excretory urogram because of imperforate anus and duplicate vagina. Note absence of left kidney and medial placement of the splenic flexure. At cystoscopy, a hemitrigone was noted.

The diagnosis, however, should be suspected during a physical examination when the vas deferens or body and tail of the epididymis are missing or when an absent, septate, or hypoplastic vagina is associated with a unicornuate or bicornuate uterus (Bryan et al, 1949). Radiologically, an absent left kidney can be surmised when a plain film of the abdomen demonstrates the gas pattern of the splenic flexure of the colon in a medial position because the colon now occupies the area normally reserved for the left kidney (Mascatello and Lebowitz, 1976) (see Fig. 58–5). When this characteristic gas pattern is present, it is a very reliable sign. A similar finding showing the hepatic flexure positioned in the right renal fossa suggests congenital absence of the right kidney (Curtis et al, 1977). A diagnosis of agenesis usually can be confirmed by renal ultrasonography or excretory urography, which reveals an absent kidney or nephrogram (respectively) on that side and compensatory hypertrophy of the contralateral kidney (Hynes and Watkin, 1970; Cope and Trickey, 1982). However, a multicystic kidney can easily be mistaken for true agenesis in an older individual because the cysts involute as the fluid is absorbed during the first several months of life. The colonic gas pattern will not occupy a position closer to the midline if a multicystic kidney was present during gestation, so this provides an excellent clue to the diagnosis when no kidney can be detected by ultrasonography later in life. Prenatal and perinatal ultrasonography reveals a characteristic appearance of the adrenal gland—flattened or lying down—when the kidney has never formed, alerting the clinician to URA (Hoffman et al, 1992).

Failure of one kidney to "light up" during the total body image phase of a radionuclide technetium scan is compatible with the diagnosis of an absent kidney but may not be infallible. Radionuclide imaging of the kidney using an isotope that traces renal blood flow clearly differentiates URA from other conditions in which renal function may be severely impaired, as in cases of severe obstruction or high-grade reflux. Isotope scanning and ultrasonography have largely replaced arteriography in defining agenesis. Fluoroscopic monitoring of the renal fossa at the end of cardiac catheterization or renal ultrasonography at the end of echocardiography has demonstrated an absent kidney on occasion.

Cystoscopy, if performed, usually reveals an asymmetric trigone or hemitrigone, suggesting either partial or complete ureteral atresia and renal agenesis. Cystoscopy has been relegated to a minor diagnostic role since the development of other, more sophisticated and noninvasive radiographic studies (Kroovand, 1985).

PROGNOSIS. There is no clear-cut evidence that patients with a solitary kidney have an increased susceptibility to other diseases. Most reviews dealing with this subject were conducted in the preantibiotic era, and they report a high incidence of "pyelitis," nephrolithiases and ureterolithiasis, tuberculosis, and glomerulonephritis. The increased ability to prevent infection and its sequelae has reduced the incidence of morbidity and mortality among patients with a solitary kidney. In Ashley and Mostofi's series (1960), only 15% of patients died as a result of renal disease, which in almost every case would have been bilateral had two kidneys been present initially. Renal trauma resulted in death in 5%;

some patients in this group might have lived had there been two kidneys (because the source of the autopsy material included many military personnel, the potential risk of injury was accentuated, however). In other words, URA with an otherwise normal contralateral kidney is not incompatible with normal longevity and does not predispose the remaining contralateral kidney to greater than normal risk (Gutierrez, 1933; Dees, 1960). One should be prudent, however, in advising individuals to participate in contact sports or strenuous physical exertion.

Rugui and co-workers (1986) found an increased occurrence of hypertension, hyperuricemia, and decreased renal function but no proteinuria in a small group of patients with congenital absence of one kidney. Only one patient had a renal biopsy, and this showed focal glomerulosclerosis similar to that found in the remaining kidney in patients with the hyperfiltration syndrome noted after unilateral nephrectomy. Thus, they concluded that URA may carry the same potential risk factor. Focal glomerulosclerosis has been confirmed in six other individuals with URA (Nomura and Osawa, 1990). Argueso and associates (1992) assessed 157 middle-aged patients with congenital URA and noted hypertension and proteinuria in 47% and 19%, respectively, but mild renal insufficiency in only 13%. Despite this, survival was not impaired in this group of people.

Supernumerary Kidney

Parenchymal development is controlled in part by an as yet unidentified substance that acts to limit the amount of functioning renal tissue. It is, therefore, interesting to find that nature has created, albeit rarely, a condition in which the individual has three separate kidneys and an excessive amount of functioning renal parenchyma. In such instances, the two main kidneys are usually normal and equal in size, whereas the third is small. The supernumerary kidney is truly an accessory organ with its own collecting system, blood supply, and distinct encapsulated parenchymal mass. It may be either totally separate from the normal kidney on the same side or connected to it by loose areolar tissue (Geisinger, 1937). The ipsilateral ureters may be bifid or completely duplicated. The condition is not analogous to a single kidney with ureteral duplication in which each collecting system drains portions of one parenchymatous mass surrounded by a single capsule.

INCIDENCE. The true incidence of this anomaly cannot be calculated because of its very infrequent occurrence. Approximately 80 cases have been reported since it was first described in 1656; it represents a very rare anomaly of the urinary system (Sasidharan et al, 1976; McPherson, 1987). It affects males and females equally but has a higher predilection for the left side (N'Guessan and Stephens, 1983). Campbell (1970) recorded one case involving bilateral supernumerary kidneys, an anomaly that has even been observed in other animal species (i.e., cow and pig).

EMBRYOLOGY. The sequence of interdependent events involved in ureteral bud formation and metanephric blastema development, which is required for the maturation of the normal kidney, probably also allows for the occurrence of a supernumerary kidney. It is postulated that a deviation involving both of these processes must take place to create the anomaly. A second ureteral outpouching off the wolffian duct or a branching from the initial ureteral bud appears to be a necessary first step. Next, the nephrogenic anlage may divide into two metanephric tails, which separate entirely when induced to differentiate by the separate or bifid ureteral buds (N'Guessan and Stephens, 1983). The twin metanephroi develop only when the bifid or separate ureteral buds enter them. N'Guessan and Stephens do not accept that this condition is the result of widely divergent bifid or separate ureteral buds. Geisinger (1937) proposed that the separate kidneys may be caused either by fragmentation of a single metanephros or by linear infarction producing separate viable fragments that develop only when a second ureteral bud is present.

DESCRIPTION. The supernumerary kidney is a distinct parenchymatous mass that may be either completely separate or only loosely attached to the major kidney on the ipsilateral side. In general, it is located somewhat caudad to the dominant kidney, which is in its correct position in the renal fossa. Occasionally, the supernumerary kidney lies either posterior or craniad to the main kidney, or it may even be a midline structure anterior to the great vessels and loosely attached to each of the other two kidneys (Fig. 58–6).

The supernumerary kidney is reniform in shape but is generally smaller than the main ipsilateral organ. In about one third of cases, the kidney or its collecting system is abnormal. In almost half the reported cases the collecting system is severely dilated with thinned parenchyma, indicating an obstructed ureter.

The ureteral inter-relationships on the side of the supernumerary kidney are variable (Kretschmer, 1929). Convergence of the ipsilateral ureters distally to form a common stem and a single ureteral orifice occurs in 50% of cases (Exley and Hotchkiss, 1944; N'Guessan and Stephens, 1983). Two completely independent ureters, each with its own entrance into the bladder, are seen in the other 50% of cases. The Weigert-Meyer principle, however, usually is obeyed, but in 10% of cases the caudal kidney has a ureter that does not follow the rule and enters the trigone below the ipsilateral

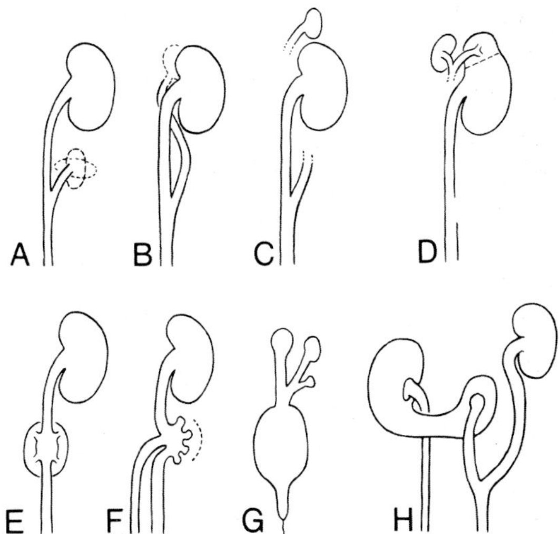

Figure 58–6. Various patterns of urinary drainage when ureters form a common stem. All kidney positions are relative only and are depicted on the left side for ease of interpretation. Dashed lines indicate that detail was not defined. (From N'Guessan G, Stephens FD: J Urol 1983;130:649.)

ureter (Tada et al, 1981) (Fig. 58–7). Rarely, the supernumerary kidney has a completely ectopic ureteral opening into the vagina or introitus (Rubin, 1948; Carlson, 1950). Individual case reports have described calyceal communications between the supernumerary and dominant kidney or fusion of the dominant kidney's ureter with the pelvis of the supernumerary kidney (Kretschmer, 1929) to create a single distal ureter, which then enters the bladder (see Fig. 58–6). The vascular supply to the supernumerary kidney is, as one might expect, very anomalous, and depends on its position in relation to the major ipsilateral kidney. Although some investigators believe that the blood supply to the individual parenchymal masses should also be separate to consider this a true supernumerary kidney (Kaneoya et al, 1989), this view is not held universally.

ASSOCIATED ANOMALIES. Usually, the ipsilateral and contralateral kidneys are normal. Except for an occasional ectopic orifice from the ureter draining the supernumerary kidney, no genitourinary abnormalities are present in any consistent pattern. Few of the case reports describe anomalies of other organ systems.

SYMPTOMS. Although this anomaly is obviously present at birth, it is rarely discovered in childhood. It may not produce symptoms until early adulthood, if at all. The average age at diagnosis in all reported cases was 36 years. Pain, fever, hypertension, and a palpable abdominal mass are the usual presenting complaints. Urinary infection or obstruction, or both, are the major conditions that lead to an evaluation. Ureteral ectopia from the supernumerary kidney may produce urinary incontinence, but this is extremely rare owing to the hypoplastic nature of the involved renal element (Shan, 1942; Hoffman and McMillan, 1948).

A palpable abdominal mass secondary to development of carcinoma in the supernumerary kidney has been noted in two patients. In 25% of all reported cases, however, the supernumerary kidney remains completely asymptomatic and is discovered only at autopsy (Carlson, 1950).

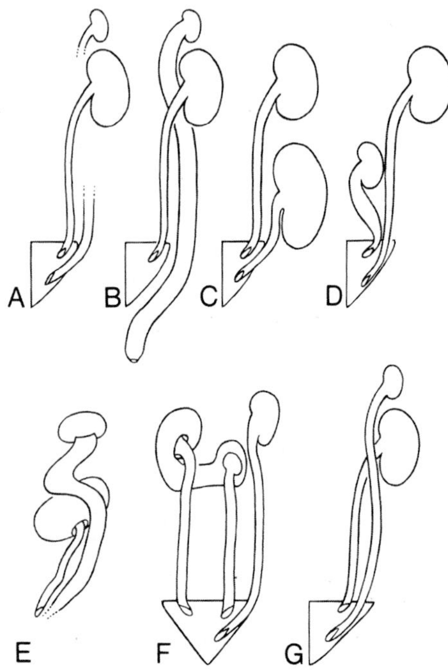

Figure 58–7. Various patterns of urinary drainage of supernumerary and ipsilateral kidneys when ureters are completely separated. All kidney positions are relative only and are depicted on the left side for ease of interpretation. Dashed lines indicate that detail was not defined. (From N'Guessan G, Stephens FD: J Urol 1983;130:649.)

DIAGNOSIS. When the supernumerary kidney is normal and asymptomatic, it is usually diagnosed when excretory urography or abdominal ultrasonography is performed for other reasons. The kidney may be inferior and distant enough from the ipsilateral kidney so that it does not disturb the latter's architecture (Conrad and Loes, 1987). If it is in close proximity, its mere presence may displace the major kidney or its ureter very slightly.

When the supernumerary organ is hydronephrotic, it may distort the architecture of the normal ipsilateral kidney and ureter, a condition that is detectable by ultrasonography. If the collecting system is bifid, the dominant kidney on that side is usually involved in the same disease process. When the ureters are separate, the ipsilateral kidney may show the effects of an abnormal supernumerary kidney. Voiding cystourethrography, ultrasonography, computed tomography with contrast, and even retrograde pyelography may be needed to help delineate the pathologic process. Radionuclide imaging provides information about relative function in the supernumerary and normal kidneys (Conrad and Loes, 1987). Cystoscopy reveals one or two ureteral orifices on the ipsilateral side, depending on whether or not the ureters are completely duplicated and, if so, to what extent ureteral ectopia exists in or outside the bladder. Occasionally, a supernumerary kidney may not be accurately diagnosed until the time of surgery or autopsy.

Anomalies of Volume and Structure

These anomalies, as outlined at the beginning of this chapter, are discussed in Chapter 51.

Anomalies of Ascent

Simple Renal Ectopia

When the mature kidney fails to reach its normal location in the renal fossa, the condition is known as renal ectopia. The term is derived from the Greek "ek" (out) and "topos" (place), meaning literally out of place. Renal ectopia is to be differentiated from renal ptosis, in which the kidney initially is located in its proper place (and has normal vascularity) but moves downward in relation to body position. The ectopic kidney, on the other hand, has never resided in the appropriate location.

An ectopic kidney can be found in one of the following positions: pelvic, iliac, abdominal, thoracic, and contralateral or crossed. Only the ipsilateral retroperitoneal location of the ectopic kidney is discussed here. Thoracic kidney and crossed renal ectopia (with and without fusion) will be dealt with subsequently.

INCIDENCE. Renal ectopia has been known to exist since it was described by sixteenth century anatomists, but it did not achieve clinical interest until the mid nineteenth century. In recent times, with greater emphasis on diagnostic acumen and uroradiologic visualization including prenatal imaging, this condition has been noted with increasing frequency.

The actual incidence among autopsy series varies from 1 in 500 (Campbell, 1930) to 1 in 1200 (Stevens, 1937; Thompson and Pace, 1937; Anson and Riba, 1939; Bell, 1946), but the average occurrence is about 1 in 900 (Abeshouse and Bhisitkul, 1959). With increasing clinical detection, the incidence among hospitalized patients has approached the autopsy rate (Abeshouse and Bhisitkul, 1959). Autopsy studies reveal no significant difference in incidence between the sexes. Clinically, renal ectopia is more readily recognized in females because they undergo uroradiologic evaluation more frequently than males owing to their higher rate of urinary infection and/or associated genital anomalies (Thompson and Pace, 1937).

The left side is favored slightly over the right. Pelvic ectopia has been estimated to occur once in 2100 to once in 3000 autopsies (Stevens, 1937). A solitary ectopic kidney occurs in 1 in 22,000 autopsies (Stevens, 1937; Hawes, 1950; Delson, 1975). At last count in 1973, 165 cases of a solitary pelvic kidney have been recorded (Downs et al, 1973). Bilateral ectopic kidneys have been observed even more rarely and constitute only 10% of all patients with renal ectopia (Malek et al, 1971).

EMBRYOLOGY. The ureteral bud first arises from the wolffian duct at the end of the fourth week of gestation. It then grows craniad toward the urogenital ridge and acquires a cap of metanephric blastema by the end of the fifth week. At this point, the nephrogenic tissue is opposite the upper sacral somites.

As elongation and straightening of the caudal end of the embryo commence, the developing reniform mass either migrates on its own, is forcibly extruded from the true pelvis, or appears to move as the tail uncurls and differential growth between the body and tail of the embryo occurs. Whatever the mechanism or driving force for renal ascent, it is during this migration that the upper ureteral bud matures into a normal collecting system and medial rotation of the renal pelvis takes place. This process of migration and rotation is completed by the end of the eighth week of gestation. Factors that may prevent the orderly movement of the kidney include the following: ureteral bud maldevelopment (Campbell, 1930); defective metanephric tissue that by itself fails to induce ascent (Ward et al, 1965); genetic abnormalities; and maternal illnesses or teratogenic causes because genital anomalies are common (Malek et al, 1971). A vascular barrier that prevents upward migration secondary to persistence of the fetal blood supply has also been postulated (Baggenstoss, 1951), but the existence of an "early" renal blood supply does not prevent the affected kidney's movement to its ultimate position. More probably, it is the end result, not the cause, of renal ectopia.

DESCRIPTION. The classification of ectopia is based on the position of the kidney within the retroperitoneum: the *pelvic* kidney is opposite the sacrum and below the aortic bifurcation; the *lumbar* kidney rests near the sacral promontary in the iliac fossa and anterior to the iliac vessels; and the *abdominal* kidney is so named when it is above the iliac crest and adjacent to the second lumbar vertebra (Fig. 58–8). No single location is most likely for the ectopic kidney (Dretler et al, 1971).

The ectopic kidney is generally smaller than normal and may not conform to the usual reniform shape owing to the presence of fetal lobulations. The axis of the kidney is slightly medial or vertical, but it may be tilted as much as 90 degrees laterally so that it lies in a true horizontal plane. The renal pelvis is usually anterior (instead of medial) to the parenchyma because the kidney has rotated incompletely. As a result, 56% of ectopic kidneys have a hydronephrotic collecting system. Half of these are due to obstruction at either the ureteropelvic (70%) or ureterovesical (30%) junction, 25% are due to reflux grade 3 or greater, and 25% are secondary to malrotation alone (Gleason et al, 1994).

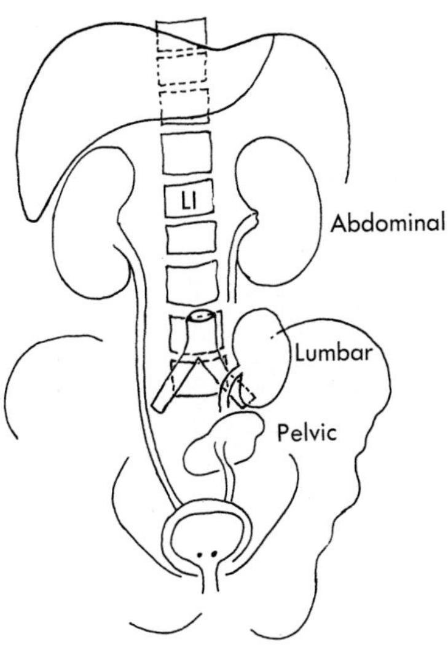

Figure 58–8. Incomplete ascent of kidney: The kidney may halt at any level of the ascent from the pelvis. (From Gray SW, Skandalakis JE: Embryology for Surgeons. Philadelphia, W. B. Saunders Company, 1972.)

The length of the ureter usually conforms to the position of the kidney, but occasionally it may be slightly tortuous. It is rarely redundant, unlike a ptotic kidney, in which the ureter has achieved its full length before the kidney drops (Fig. 58–9). The ureter usually enters the bladder on the ipsilateral side with its orifice situated normally. Therefore, cystoscopy will not distinguish renal ectopia from a normal kidney. The arterial and venous network is predictable only by the fact that it is anomalous; its vascular pattern is dependent on the ultimate resting place of the kidney (Anson and Riba, 1939). There may be one or two main renal arteries arising from the distal aorta or the aortic bifurcation, with one or more aberrant arteries coming off the common or external iliac or even the inferior mesenteric artery. The kidney may be supplied entirely by multiple anomalous branches, none of which arises from the aorta. In no instance does the main renal artery arise from the level of the aorta that would be the proper origin for a normally positioned kidney.

ASSOCIATED ANOMALIES. Although the contralateral kidney is usually normal, it is associated with a number of congenital defects. Malek and colleagues (1971) and Thompson and Pace (1937) found the incidence of contralateral agenesis to be rather high, suggesting that a teratogenic factor affecting both ureteral buds and metanephric blastemas may be responsible for the two anomalies. Bilateral ectopia is seen in a very small number of patients (Fig. 58–10). Hydronephrosis secondary to obstruction or reflux may be seen in as many as 25% of nonectopic contralateral kidneys (Gleason et al, 1994).

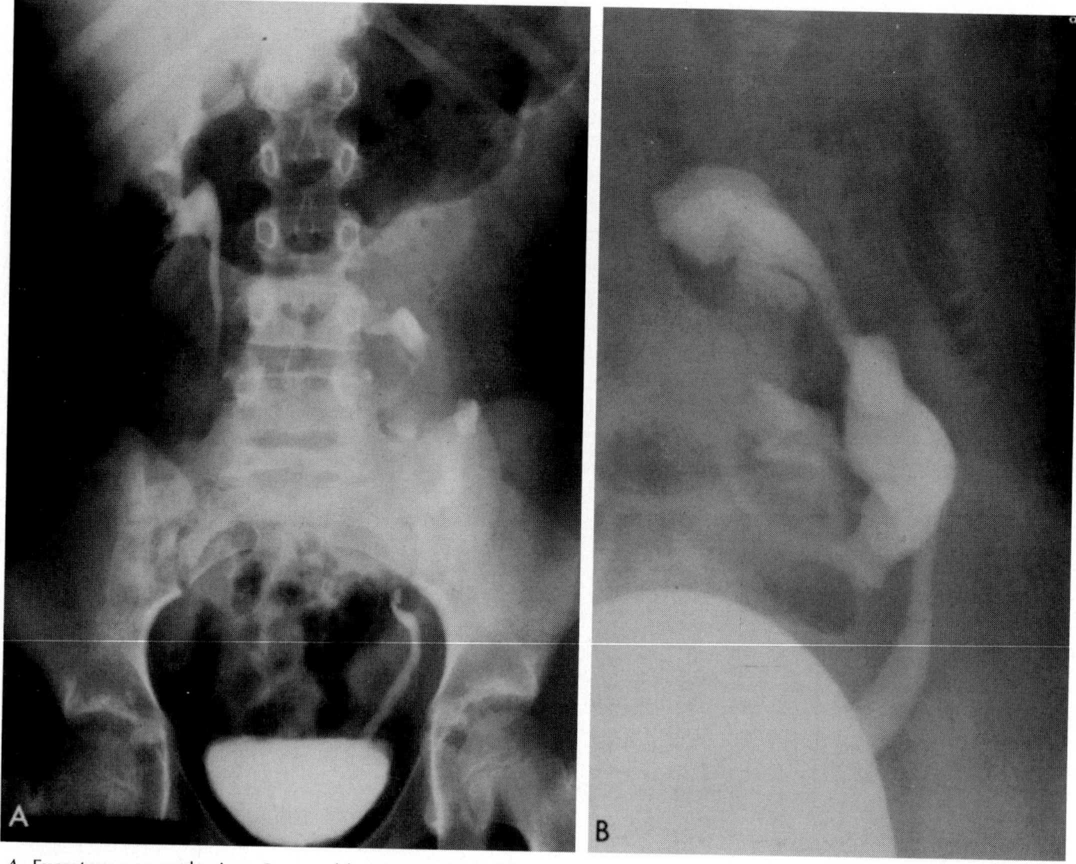

Figure 58–9. *A*, Excretory urography in a 9-year-old girl investigated for recurrent urinary tract infection shows a left lumbar kidney. *B*, Voiding cystourethrography demonstrates reflux to the ectopic kidney. At cystoscopy, the ureteral orifice was located at the bladder neck.

The most striking feature is the association of genital anomalies with ectopia. The incidence varies from 15% (Thompson and Pace, 1937) to 45% (Downs et al, 1973), depending on how carefully the patient is evaluated. Twenty to sixty-six percent of females have one or more of the following abnormalities of the reproductive organs: bicornuate or unicornuate uterus with atresia of one horn (McCrea, 1942); rudimentary or absent uterus and proximal and/or distal vagina (Tabisky and Bhisitkul, 1965; D'Alberton et al, 1981); and duplication of the vagina. In males, 10% to 20% have a recognizable associated genital defect; undescended testes, duplication of the urethra, and hypospadias are the most common problems (Thompson and Pace, 1937).

Rarely, the adrenal gland is absent or abnormally positioned. Twenty-one percent of patients have anomalies of other organ systems (Downs et al, 1973); most of these involve the skeletal or cardiac system.

DIAGNOSIS. With the increasing use of radiography, ultrasonography, and radionuclide scanning to visualize the urinary tract, the incidence of fortuitous discovery of an

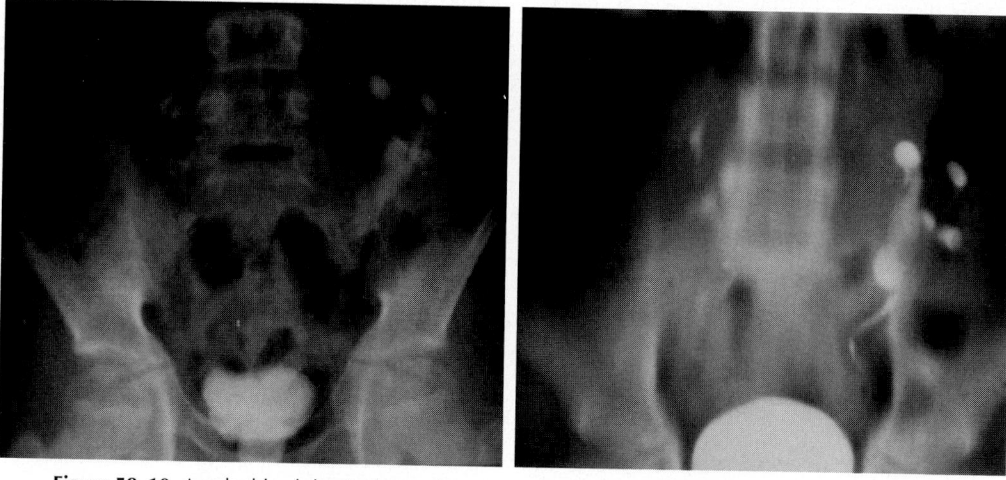

Figure 58–10. A palpable abdominal mass in an 8-year-old girl proved to be bilateral pelvic kidneys.

asymptomatic ectopic kidney is also increasing. The steady rise in reported cases in recent years attests to this fact.

Most ectopic kidneys are clinically asymptomatic. A vague abdominal complaint of frank ureteral colic secondary to an obstructing stone is still the most frequent symptom leading to discovery of the misplaced kidney. The abnormal position of the kidney results in a pattern of direct and referred pain that is atypical for colic and may be misdiagnosed as acute appendicitis or as pelvic organ inflammatory disease in the female. It is rare to find symptoms of compression from organs adjacent to the ectopic kidney. Renal ectopia may also present initially with urinary infection or a palpable abdominal mass. A rare case of ureteral ectopia associated with an ectopic kidney and causing urinary incontinence has been reported (Borer et al, 1993). The difficulty in diagnosing this condition was related to the poor function of the ectopic kidney. DMSA scintigraphy or computed tomography with contrast will delineate these unusual cases (Chang et al, 1992).

Malposition of the colon (as discussed in the earlier section on renal agenesis) may be a clue to the ectopic position of a lumbar or pelvic kidney. The diagnosis is easily made when excretory urography or renal ultrasound fails to reveal a kidney in its proper location. The fact that many of these kidneys overlie the bony pelvis, obscuring the collecting system, can lead to a misdiagnosis with failure to recognize the true position of the kidney.

Nephrotomography during an excretory urogram (if the diagnosis is suspected early enough), ultrasonography, radionuclide scanning, or retrograde pyelography usually satisfies the diagnostician. Cystoscopy alone is rarely useful because the trigone and ureteral orifices are invariably normal unless the ureteral orifice is also ectopic—a rare event. Arteriography may be helpful in delineating the renal vascular supply in anticipation of surgery on the ectopic kidney. This is especially important in cases of solitary ectopia.

PROGNOSIS. The ectopic kidney is no more susceptible to disease than the normally positioned kidney except for the development of hydronephrosis or urinary calculus formation (Gleason et al, 1994). This is due in part to the anteriorly placed pelvis and malrotation of the kidney, which may lead to impaired drainage of urine from a high insertion of the ureter to pelvis or an anomalous vasculature that partially blocks one of the major calyces or the upper ureter. In addition, there may be an increased risk of injury from blunt abdominal trauma because the low-lying kidney is not protected by the rib cage.

Renovascular hypertension secondary to an anomalous blood supply has been reported, but a higher than normal incidence is yet to be proved. Anderson and Harrison (1965), in a review of pregnant women with renal ectopia, could find no increased occurrence of difficult deliveries or maternal or fetal complications related to the ectopic kidney (Anderson and Harrison, 1965; Delson, 1975). Dystocia from a pelvic kidney is a very rare finding, but when it does occur, early recognition is mandatory, and cesarean section is indicated. Although two cases of cancer in an ectopic kidney have been reported, there does not appear to be an increased risk for malignant transformation. No deaths have been directly attributable to the ectopic kidney, but in at least five instances a solitary ectopic kidney has been mistakenly removed, with disastrous results, because the kidney was thought to represent a pelvic malignancy (Downs et al, 1973); this should not happen today with the multiplicity of imaging techniques available for accurate diagnosis of the condition.

Cephalad Renal Ectopia

The mature kidney may be positioned more craniad than normal in patients who have had a history of omphalocele (Pinckney et al, 1978). When the liver herniates into the omphalocele sac with the intestines, the kidneys continue to ascend until they are stopped by the diaphragm. In all reported cases, both kidneys were affected and lay immediately beneath the diaphragm at the level of the tenth thoracic vertebra (Fig. 58–11). The ureters are excessively long but otherwise normal. An angiogram in these patients demonstrates that the origin of the renal artery is more cephalad than normal, but no other abnormality of the vascular network is present. Patients with this anomaly usually have no symptoms referable to the malposition, and urinary drainage is not impaired.

Thoracic Kidney

A very rare form of renal ectopia exists when the kidney is positioned considerably higher than normal. Intrathoracic ectopia denotes either a partial or complete protrusion of the kidney above the level of the diaphragm into the posterior

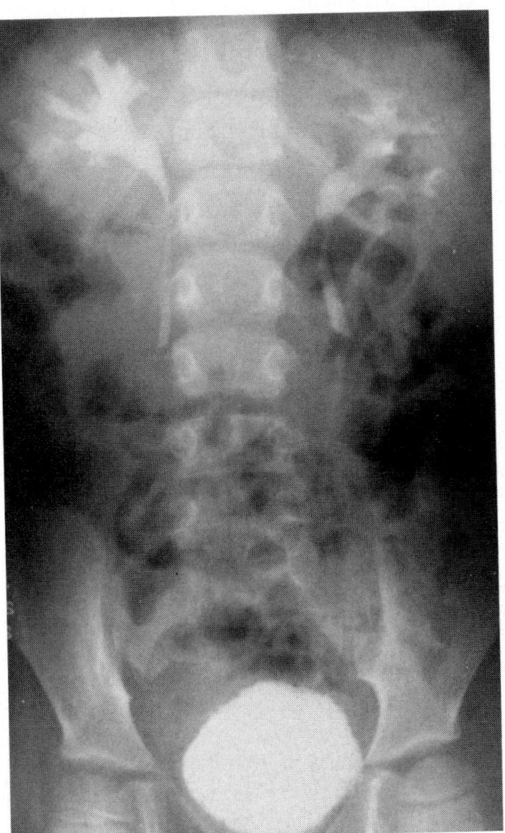

Figure 58–11. This 6-year-old boy had an omphalocele at birth. At the time, the liver was noted to be in the sac. An excretory urogram following a urinary tract infection revealed the kidneys located more cephalad than usual and opposite T10.

mediastinum. Less than 5% of all patients with renal ectopia have an intrathoracic kidney (Campbell, 1930). This condition must be differentiated from a congenital or traumatic diaphragmatic hernia, in which other abdominal organs as well as the kidney have advanced into the chest cavity.

INCIDENCE. Prior to 1940, all reports of this condition were noted as part of autopsy series (DeCastro and Shumacher, 1969). Since 1940, however, at least 140 patients have been reported in the literature (Donat and Donat, 1988); four of these reports have involved bilateral kidneys (Berlin et al, 1957; Hertz and Shahin, 1969; Lundius, 1975; N'Guessan and Stephens, 1984; Liddell et al, 1989). There appears to be a slight left-sided predominance of 1.5:1, and the sex ratio favors males 2:1 (Lozano and Rodriguez, 1975). This entity has been discovered in all age groups, from a neonate (Shapira et al, 1965) to a 75-year-old man evaluated for prostatic hypertrophy (Burke et al, 1967).

EMBRYOLOGY. The kidney reaches its adult location by the end of the eighth week of gestation. At this time, the diaphragmatic leaflets are formed as the pleuroperitoneal membrane separates the pleural from the peritoneal cavity. Mesenchymal tissues associated with this membrane eventually form the muscular component of the diaphragm. It is uncertain whether the delayed closure of the diaphragmatic anlage allows protracted renal ascent above the level of the future diaphragm or whether the kidney overshoots its usual position because of accelerated ascent prior to normal diaphragmatic closure (Spillane and Prather, 1952; Burke et al, 1967; N'Guessan and Stephens, 1984). Recently, delayed involution of mesonephric tissue has been proposed as a causative factor (Angulo et al, 1992) because intrathoracic kidneys occur in only 0.25% of patients with a diaphragmatic hernia (Donat and Donat, 1988). Renal angiography has demonstrated either a normal take-off site (Lundius, 1975) or a more cranial origin (Franciskovic and Martincic, 1959) from the aorta for the renal artery supplying the thoracic kidney.

DESCRIPTION. The kidney is situated in the posterior mediastinum and generally has completed the normal rotation process (Fig. 58–12). The renal contour and collecting system are normal. The kidney usually lies in the posterolateral aspect of the diaphragm in the foramen of Bochdalek. The diaphragm at this point thins out, and a flimsy membrane surrounds the protruding portion of the kidney. Thus, the kidney is not within the pleural space, and there is no pneumothorax (N'Guessan and Stephens, 1984). The lower lobe of the adjacent lung may be hypoplastic secondary to compression by the kidney mass. The renal vasculature and the ureter enter and exit from the pleural cavity through the foramen of Bochdalek.

ASSOCIATED ANOMALIES. The ureter is elongated to accommodate the excessive distance to the bladder, but it never enters ectopically into the bladder or other pelvic sites. The adrenal gland has been mentioned in only two reports; in one it accompanied the kidney into the chest (Barloon and Goodwin, 1957), and in the other it did not (Paul et al, 1960). However, N'Guessan and Stephens (1984) analyzed ten cases and found that the adrenal gland was below the kidney in its normal location in the majority of patients. In unilateral cases, the contralateral kidney was usually normal. No consistent anomalies have been described in other organ systems; however, one child did have trisomy 18 (Shapira et al, 1965), another patient had multiple pulmonary and cardiac anomalies in addition to the thoracic kidney (Fusonie and Molnar, 1966), and a third had vertebral anomalies and supernumerary ribs (Angulo et al, 1992).

SYMPTOMS. The vast majority of individuals remain asymptomatic. Pulmonary symptoms are exceedingly rare, and urinary symptoms are even more infrequent. Most cases are discovered through routine chest radiographs or at the time of thoracotomy for a suspected mediastinal tumor (De-Noronha et al, 1974).

DIAGNOSIS. The diagnosis is most commonly made following a routine chest x-ray study in which the affected hemidiaphragm is elevated slightly. A smooth rounded mass extending into the chest is seen near the midline on an anteroposterior film and along the posterior aspect of the diaphragmatic leaflet on a lateral view. Excretory urography or renal scintigraphy (Williams et al, 1983) usually suffices to clarify the diagnosis. In some instances, retrograde pyelography may be needed. Rarely, when arteriography has been employed to delineate a cardiac or pulmonary anomaly, it has revealed a thoracic kidney at the same time (Fusonie and Molnar, 1966).

PROGNOSIS. Neither autopsy series nor clinical reports suggest that a thoracic kidney can cause serious urinary or pulmonary complications. Because the majority of these patients are discovered fortuitously and have no specific symptoms referable to the misplaced kidney, no treatment is necessary once the diagnosis has been confirmed.

Anomalies of Form and Fusion

Crossed Ectopia With and Without Fusion

When a kidney is located on the side opposite that from which its ureter inserts into the bladder, the condition is known as crossed ectopia. Ninety percent of crossed ectopic kidneys are fused to their ipsilateral mate. Except for the horseshoe anomaly, they account for the majority of fusion defects. The various renal fusion anomalies associated with ectopia are discussed in this section, whereas horseshoe kidney, the most common form of renal fusion, is presented separately.

Fusion anomalies of the kidney were first logically categorized by Wilmer (1938), but McDonald and McClellan (1957) refined and expanded this classification to include crossed ectopia with fusion, crossed ectopia without fusion, solitary crossed ectopia, and bilaterally crossed ectopia (Fig. 58–13). The fusion anomalies have been designated as (1) unilateral fused kidney with inferior ectopia, (2) sigmoid or S-shaped, (3) lump or cake, (4) L-shaped or tandem, (5) disc, shield, or doughnut, and (6) unilateral fused kidneys with superior ectopia (Fig. 58–14). Although this classification has little clinical significance, it does impose some order on understanding the embryology of renal ascent and rotation.

INCIDENCE. The first reported case of crossed ectopia was described by Pamarolus in 1654. Abeshouse and Bhisitkul conducted the last significant review of the subject in 1959 and collected exactly 500 cases of crossed ectopia with and without fusion. Subsequently, numerous case reports have been published.

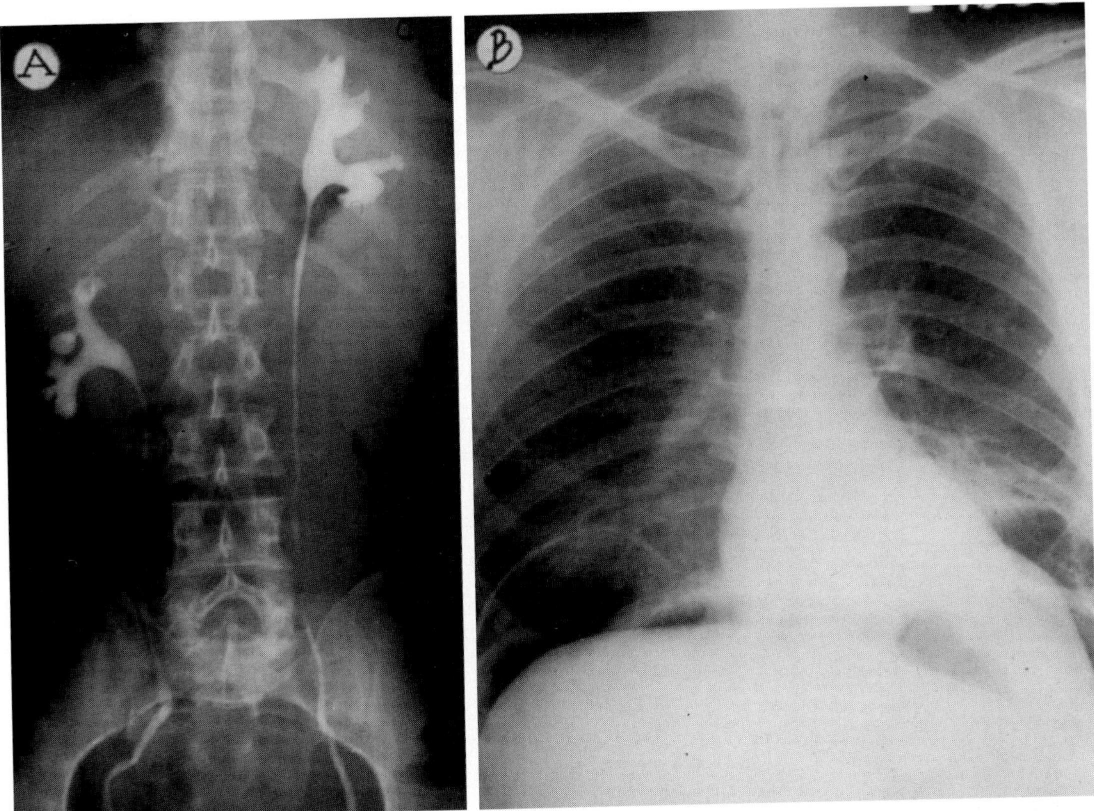

Figure 58–12. Radiograph of a thoracic kidney. The left kidney lies above the diaphragm. *A*, Diagnostic urogram. *B*, Diagnostic pneumoperitoneum. (From Hill JE, Bunts RC: J Urol 1960;84:460.)

Sixty-two patients with crossed ectopia without fusion have been reported (Diaz, 1953; Winram and Ward-McQuaid, 1959), representing approximately 10% of all crossed ectopic kidneys (Lee, 1949). The anomaly occurs more commonly in males in a ratio of 2:1, and left-to-right ectopia is seen three times more often than the right-to-left type (Lee, 1949).

Solitary crossed ectopia has been reported in 34 patients (Miles et al, 1985; Gu and Alton, 1991). Males predominate by a ratio of 2:1. Generally, solitary crossed ectopia involves migration of the left kidney to the right side with absence of the right kidney; this type predominates by a ratio of almost 2:1 over the right-to-left type (Kakei et al, 1976). In most cases, the kidney fails to ascend and rotate completely. Bilateral crossed renal ectopia has been described in five patients (McDonald and McClellan, 1957; Abeshouse and Bhisitkul, 1959) and is considered the rarest form.

Abeshouse and Bhisitkul (1959) compiled 443 reports of crossed ectopia with fusion and estimated its occurrence at 1 in 1000. This figure varies with the type of fusion anomaly; the unilaterally fused kidney with inferior ectopia is the most common variety, whereas fusion with superior ectopia is the least common. The autopsy incidence has been calculated at 1 in 2000 (Baggenstoss, 1951). Crossed ectopia with fusion

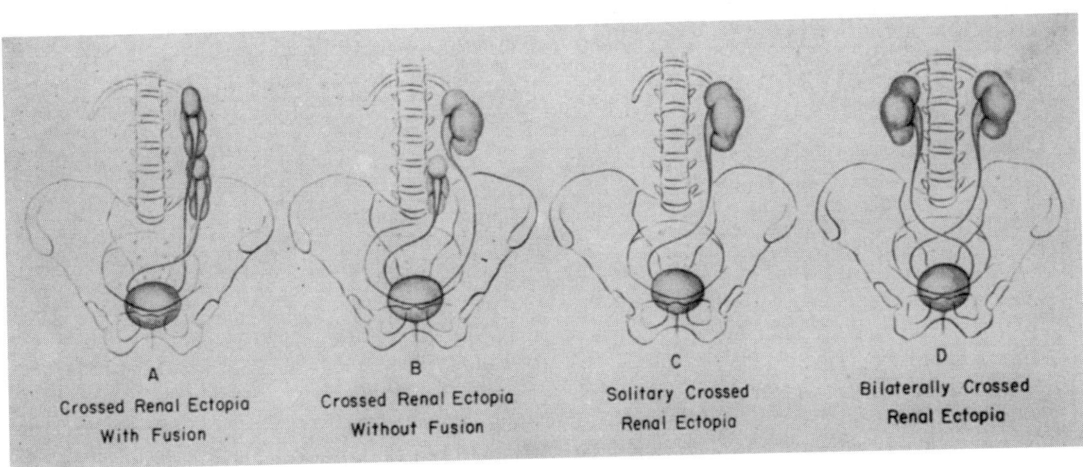

Figure 58–13. Four types of crossed renal ectopia.

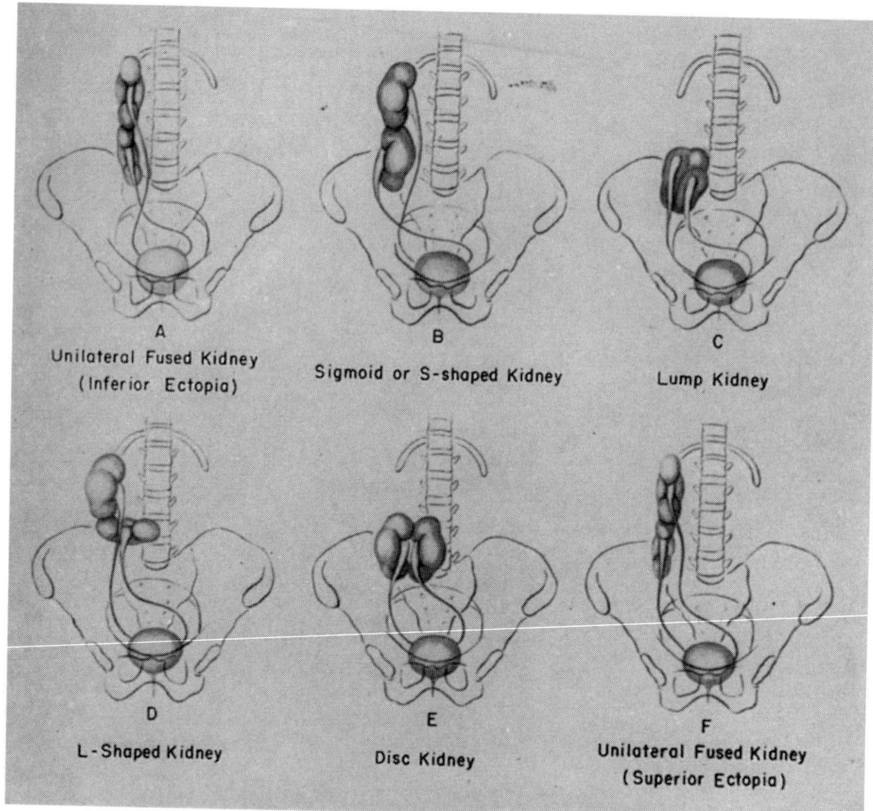

Figure 58–14. Six forms of crossed renal ectopia with fusion.

has been discovered in newborns (Bauer, 1977) and also in a 70-year-old man undergoing urologic evaluation for benign prostatic hypertrophy. There is a slight male predominance (3:2), and a left-to-right cross-over occurs somewhat more frequently than its counterpart.

EMBRYOLOGY. The ureteral bud enters the metanephric blastema, while the latter is situated adjacent to the anlage of the lumbosacral spine. During the next 4 weeks the developing kidney comes to lie at the level of L1–L3 vertebrae. Because the factor or factors responsible for the change in kidney position during gestation are still undetermined, the reasons for crossed ectopia are similarly uncertain. Wilmer in 1938 suggested that cross-over occurs as a result of pressure from abnormally placed umbilical arteries that prevent cephalad migration of the renal unit, which then follows the path of least resistance to the opposite side.

Potter (1952) and Alexander and associates (1950) theorized that crossed ectopia is strictly a ureteral phenomenon, with the developing ureteral bud wandering to the opposite side and inducing differentiation of the contralateral nephrogenic anlage. Ashley and Mostofi (1960) deduced that strong but undetermined forces are responsible for renal ascent and that these forces attract one or both kidneys to their final place on the opposite side of the midline.

Cook and Stephens (1977) postulated that cross-over is the result of malalignment and abnormal rotation of the caudal end of the developing fetus, with the distal curled end of the vertebral column being displaced to one side or the other. This results either in malpositioning of the cloaca and wolffian duct structures, which lie to one side of the vertebral column, allowing one ureter to cross the midline and enter the opposite nephrogenic blastema, or in transplantation of the kidney and ureter to the opposite side of the midline during "normal" renal ascent (Hertz et al, 1977; Maizels and Stephens, 1979).

Kelalis and colleagues (1973) implicated teratogenic factors because they noted an increased incidence of associated genitourinary and other organ system anomalies. Finally, genetic influences may play a role because similar anomalies have occurred within a single family (Greenberg and Nelsen, 1971; Hildreth and Cass, 1978).

Fusion of the metanephric masses may occur when the renal anlage is still in the true pelvis prior to or at the start of cephalad migration, or it may occur during the latter stages of ascent. The extent of fusion is determined by the proximity of the developing renal anlage to one another. Following fusion, advancement of the kidneys toward their normal location is impeded by midline retroperitoneal structures—the aortic bifurcation, the inferior mesenteric artery, and the base of the small bowel mesentery (Joly, 1940).

DESCRIPTION. Fusion of a crossed ectopic kidney is related to the time at which it comes in contact with its mate. The crossed kidney usually lies caudad to its normal counterpart on that side. It is likely that migration of each kidney begins simultaneously, but ascent of the ectopic renal unit probably lags behind because of cross-over time. Thus, it is the superior pole of the ectopic kidney that generally joins with the inferior aspect of the normal kidney. Ascent continues until either the uncrossed kidney reaches its normal location or one of the retroperitoneal structures prevents further migration of the fused mass. The final shape of the fused kidneys depends on the time and extent of fusion and the degree of renal rotation that has occurred. No further rotation is likely once the two kidneys have joined (Fig.

58–15). Therefore, the position of each renal pelvis may provide a clue to the chronology of the congenital defect. An anteriorly placed pelvis suggests early fusion, whereas a medially positioned renal pelvis indicates that fusion probably occurred after rotation was completed.

Ninety percent of crossed ectopic kidneys are fused with their mates. When they are not fused, the uncrossed kidney generally resides in its normal dorsolumbar location and is oriented properly, whereas the ectopic kidney is inferior and lies in either a diagonal or horizontal position with an anteriorly placed renal pelvis. The two kidneys are usually separated by a variable but definite distance, and each is surrounded by its own capsule of Gerota's fascia. In every case of crossed ectopia without fusion, the ureter from the normal kidney enters the bladder on the same side, while that of the ectopic kidney crosses the midline at the pelvic brim and enters the bladder on the contralateral side.

In cases of solitary crossed ectopia, the kidney is usually located somewhat lower than normal but in the opposite renal fossa at the level of L1–L3 and is oriented anteriorly, having rotated incompletely on its vertical axis (Alexander et al, 1950; Purpon, 1963; Gu and Alton, 1991). When the kidney remains in the pelvis or ascends only to the lower lumbar region, it may assume a horizontal lie with an anteriorly placed pelvis because it has failed to rotate fully (Tabrisky and Bhisitkul, 1965). Here, too, the ureter crosses the midline above the S2 vertebra and enters the bladder on the opposite side (Gu and Alton, 1991). The contralateral ureter, if present, is often rudimentary (Caine, 1956). The patient with bilateral crossed ectopia may have perfectly normal-appearing kidneys and renal pelves; however, the ureters cross the midline at the level of the lower lumbar vertebrae (Abeshouse and Bhisitkul, 1959).

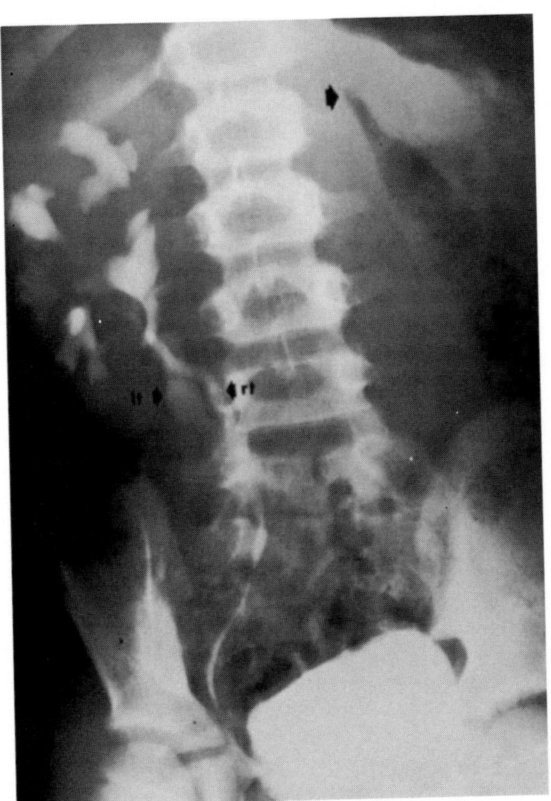

Figure 58–15. An 8-year-old boy with a left-to-right crossed, fused ectopia, in which the two kidneys lie abreast of one another. Splenic flexure lies in empty right renal fossa.

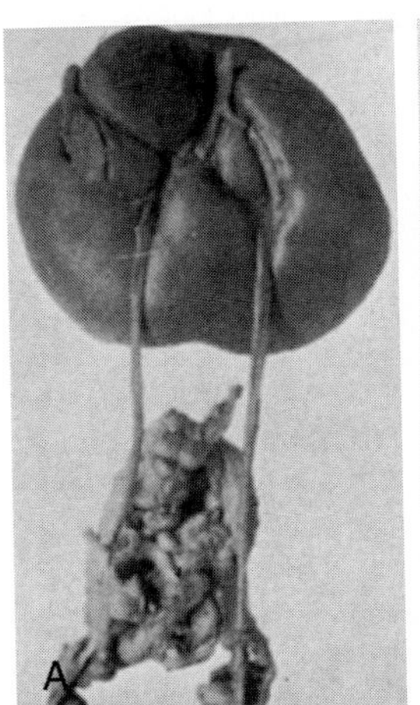

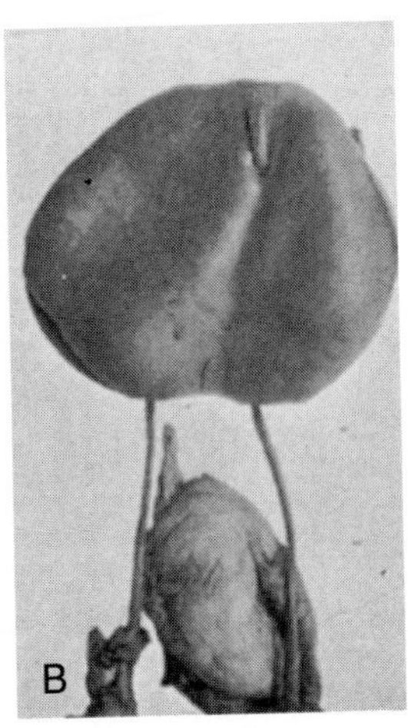

Figure 58–16. *A*, Lump kidney showing the unusual anatomy, with the anterior blood supply coming from above and the ureters leaving from below. *B*, Posterior view of *A*, with the blood supply entering from above and a deep grooving of the parenchyma indicating where the kidney pressed against the spine. (Courtesy of Dr. H. S. Altman.)

Inferior Ectopic Kidney. Two thirds of all unilaterally fused kidneys involve inferior ectopia. The upper pole of the crossed kidney is attached to the inferior aspect of the normally positioned mate. Both renal pelves are anterior; thus, fusion probably occurs relatively early.

Sigmoid or S-Shaped Kidney. The sigmoid or S-shaped kidney is the second most common anomaly of fusion. The crossed kidney is again inferior, and the two kidneys are fused at their adjacent poles. Fusion of the two kidneys occurs relatively late, after complete rotation on the vertical axis has taken place. Thus, each renal pelvis is oriented correctly and faces in opposite directions from one another. The lower convex border of one kidney is directly opposite the outer border of its counterpart, and there is an S-shaped appearance to the entire renal outline. The ureter from the normal kidney crosses downward anterior to the outer border of the inferior kidney, and the ectopic kidney's ureter crosses the midline before entering the bladder.

Lump Kidney. The lump or cake kidney is a relatively rare form of fusion (Fig. 58–16). Extensive joining has taken place over a wide margin of maturing renal anlage. The total kidney mass is irregular and lobulated. Generally, ascent progresses only as far as the sacral promontory, but in many instances the kidney remains within the true pelvis. Both renal pelves are anterior and drain separates areas of parenchyma. The ureters do not cross.

L-Shaped Kidney. The L-shaped or tandem kidney occurs when the crossed kidney assumes a transverse position at the time of its attachment to the inferior pole of the normal kidney (Fig. 58–17). The crossed kidney lies in the midline or in the contralateral paramedian space anterior to the L4 vertebra. Rotation about the long axis of the kidney may produce either an inverted or a reversed pelvic position. The ureter from each kidney enters the bladder on its respective side.

Disc Kidney. Disc, shield, doughnut, or pancake kidneys, as labeled by various authors, are kidneys that have joined

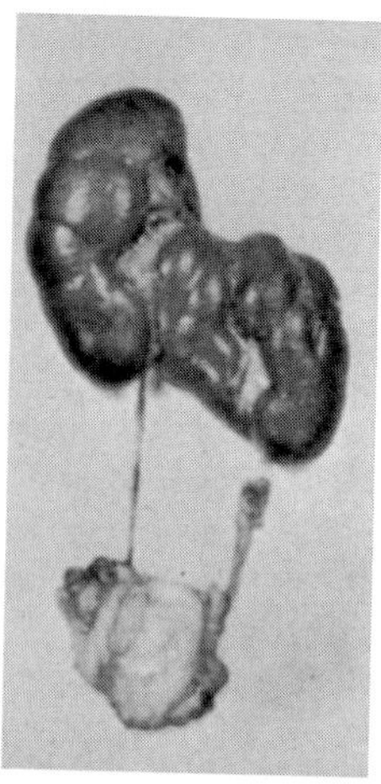

Figure 58–17. Renal fusion. L-shaped kidney in a 1-year-old child in whom a considerable portion of the left renal segment lies across the lower lumbar spine. On each side, the pelvic outlet faces anteriorly. (From Campbell MF: *In* Campbell MF, Harrison JH, eds: Urology, Vol. 2, 3rd ed. Philadelphia, W. B. Saunders Company, 1970.)

at the medial borders of each pole to produce a doughnut or ring-shaped mass; when there is more extensive fusion along the entire medial aspect of each kidney, a disc or shield shape is created. The lateral aspect of each kidney retains its normal contour. Thus, this type of fusion differs from the lump or cake kidney in that the reniform shape is better preserved owing to a somewhat less extensive degree of fusion. The pelves are anteriorly placed, and the ureters remain uncrossed. Each collecting system drains its respective half of the kidney and does not communicate with the opposite side (Fig. 58–18).

Superior Ectopic Kidney. The least common variety of renal fusion is the crossed ectopic kidney that lies superior to the normal kidney. The lower pole of the crossed kidney is fused to the upper pole of the normal kidney. Each renal unit retains its fetal orientation with both pelves lying anteriorly, suggesting that fusion occurred very early.

Regardless of the type of fusion encountered, the vascular supply to each kidney is variable and unpredictable. The crossed ectopic kidney is supplied by one or more branches from the aorta or common iliac artery (Rubinstein et al, 1976). The normal kidney frequently has an anomalous blood supply, with multiple renal arteries originating from various levels along the aorta. In one rare instance, Rubinstein discovered that one renal artery had crossed the midline to supply the tandem ectopic kidney. The solitary crossed ectopic kidney generally receives its blood supply from the side of the aorta or iliac artery on which it is positioned (Tanenbaum et al, 1970).

ASSOCIATED ANOMALIES. In all fusion anomalies the ureter from each kidney is usually not ectopic. Except for solitary crossed ectopia, in which there may be a hemitrigone or a poorly developed trigone with the rudimentary or absent ureter on the side of the ectopic kidney, most patients with crossed ectopia have a normal trigone with no indication that an anomaly of the upper urinary tract is present (Magri, 1961; Tanenbaum et al, 1970; Yates-Bell and Packham, 1972). An ectopic ureteral orifice from the crossed renal unit has been observed in about 3% of cases (Abeshouse and Bhisitkul, 1959; Magri, 1961; Hendren et al, 1976). Occasionally, the ureter from the uncrossed renal segment of a fusion anomaly may have an ectopic orifice (Hendren et al, 1976). In one instance, Malek and Utz (1970) discovered an ectopic ureterocele associated with the uncrossed kidney. Vesicoureteral reflux into the collecting system of the ectopic kidney has been noted frequently (Kelalis et al, 1973). Currarino and Weisbruch (1989) collected 10 cases of midline renal fusion in which a single ureter divided into two pelves that stretched across the midline, each draining one half of the total parenchymatous mass. In 4 of the 10 cases a second ureter was present that drained a separate duplex system on either the right or left side. Most of the affected individuals had an imperforate anus and abnormal vertebrae, or both.

Most orthotopic units are normal. If an abnormality exists, it usually involves the ectopic kidney and consists of cystic dysplasia, ureteropelvic junction obstruction (29%), reflux (15%), or carcinoma (Abeshouse and Bhisitkul, 1959; Gerber et al, 1980; Caldamone and Rabinowitz, 1981; Macksood and James, 1983; Nussbaum et al, 1987; Gleason et al, 1994).

The highest incidence of associated anomalies occurs in children with solitary renal ectopia; these anomalies involve both the skeletal system and the genital organs (Miles et al, 1985; Gleason et al, 1994). The anomalies seem to be related more to renal agenesis than to the ectopic anomaly per se. Fifty percent of patients with solitary crossed renal ectopia have a skeletal anomaly, and 40% have a genital abnormality (Gu and Alton, 1991). The most common is either cryptorchidism or absence of the vas deferens in the male, or

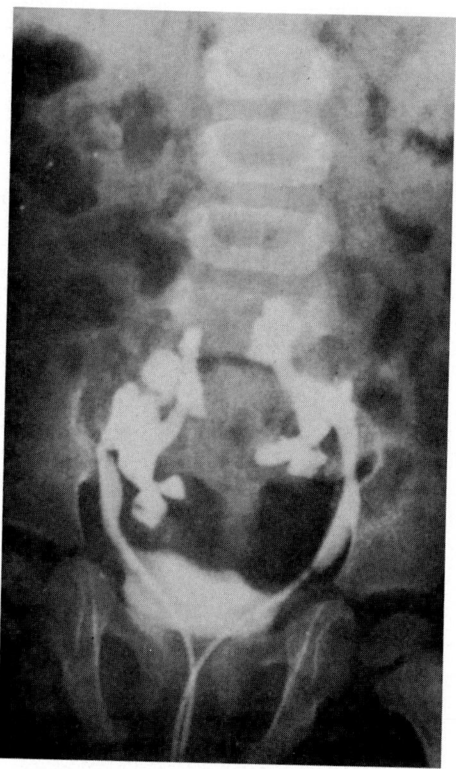

Figure 58–18. Pelvic fused kidney in a 2-year-old girl examined because of the low abdominal mass thought to be an ovarian cyst. (From Campbell MF: *In* Campbell MF, Harrison JH, eds: Urology, Vol. 2, 3rd ed. Philadelphia, W. B. Saunders Company, 1970.)

vaginal atresia or a unilateral uterine abnormality in the female (Yates-Bell and Packham, 1972; Kakei et al, 1976). Imperforate anus has also been observed in 20% of patients with solitary crossed ectopia.

In general, the occurrence of an associated anomaly in patients with crossed renal ectopia, excluding solitary crossed ectopia, is low; the most frequent entities are imperforate anus (4%), orthopedic anomalies (4%), skeletal abnormalities, and septal cardiovascular defects.

SYMPTOMS. Most individuals with crossed renal ectopia have no symptoms. The defects are often discovered incidentally at autopsy, during routine perinatal ultrasound screening, or following bone scanning. If manifestations do occur, signs and symptoms usually develop in the third or fourth decades of life and include vague lower abdominal pain, pyuria, hematuria, and urinary tract infection (Gleason et al, 1994). Hydronephrosis and renal calculi have been discovered in conjunction with some of these symptoms. It is believed that the abnormal kidney position and the anomalous blood supply may impede drainage from the collecting system, creating a predisposition to urinary tract infection and calculus formation.

In one third of the patients, an asymptomatic abdominal mass may be the presenting sign (Abeshouse and Bhisitkul, 1959; Nussbaum et al, 1987). In a few individuals, hypertension has led to the discovery of an ectopic fusion anomaly (Abeshouse and Bhisitkul, 1959), and in one case this was attributable to a vascular lesion in one of the anomalous vessels (Mininberg et al, 1971).

DIAGNOSIS. In the past, the usual method of detection was excretory urography, but ultrasonography and radionuclide scanning (for unrelated reasons) have uncovered more asymptomatic cases recently. Nephrotomography can be used when necessary to define the renal outlines further (Dretler et al, 1971). Cystoscopy and retrograde pyelography are useful in mapping out the collecting system and pattern of drainage. Renal angiography may be required prior to extensive surgery on the ectopic or normal kidney to delineate the anomalous blood supply to the kidneys.

PROGNOSIS. Most individuals with crossed renal ectopia have a normal longevity and prognosis. However, some patients with a potentially obstructive collecting system are at risk for developing urinary tract infection, a renal calculus, or both (Kron and Meranze, 1949). Boatman and colleagues (1972) noted that one third of their symptomatic patients required a pyelolithotomy for an obstructing stone. Stubbs and Resnick (1977) reported a struvite staghorn calculus in a patient with crossed renal ectopia. Urinary infection in association with either vesicoureteral reflux or hydronephrosis has been implicated in the formation of these calculi.

Horseshoe Kidney

The horseshoe kidney is probably the most common of all renal fusion anomalies. It should not be confused with asymmetric or off-center fused kidneys, which may give the impression of being horseshoe-shaped. The anomaly consists of two distinct renal masses lying vertically on either side of the midline and connected at their respective lower poles by a parenchymatous or fibrous isthmus that crosses the midplane of the body. It was first recognized during an autopsy by DeCarpi in 1521, but Botallo in 1564 presented the first extensive description and illustration of a horseshoe kidney (Benjamin and Schullian, 1950). In 1820, Morgagni described the first diseased horseshoe kidney, and since then more has been written about this condition than about any other renal anomaly. Almost every renal disease has been described in the horseshoe kidney.

INCIDENCE. Horseshoe kidney occurs in 0.25% of the population, or about 1 in 400 (Dees, 1941; Nation, 1945; Bell, 1946; Glenn, 1959; Campbell, 1970). As in other fusion anomalies, it is found more commonly in males by a 2:1 margin. The abnormality has been discovered clinically in all age groups ranging from prenatal life to 80 years, but in autopsy series it is more prevalent in children (Segura et al, 1972). This early age prevalence is related to the high incidence of multiple congenital anomalies associated with the horseshoe kidney, some of which are incompatible with long-term survival.

Horseshoe kidneys have been reported in identical twins (Bridge, 1960) and among several siblings within the same family (David, 1974). From the rarity of these reports and the relative frequency of the anomaly, it is doubtful that these observations represent a particular genetic predisposition, but they might be the result of genetic expression with a low degree of penetrance (Leiter, 1972).

EMBRYOLOGY. The abnormality originates between the fourth and sixth weeks of gestation, after the ureteral bud has entered the renal blastema. In view of the ultimate spatial configuration of the horseshoe kidney, the entrance of the ureteral bud must take place prior to rotation and considerably before renal ascent ensues. Boyden (1931) described a 6-week-old embryo with a horseshoe kidney, the youngest fetus ever discovered with this anomaly. He postulated that at the 14-mm stage (4½ weeks), the developing metanephric masses lie close to one another; any disturbance in this relationship may result in joining at their inferior poles. A slight alteration in the position of the umbilical or common iliac artery could change the orientation of the migrating kidneys, thus leading to contact and fusion (Fig. 58–19). It has been postulated that an abnormality in the formation of the tail of the embryo or another pelvic organ could account for the fusion process (Cook and Stephens, 1977). Recently, Domenech-Mateu and Gonzales-Compta (1988), after studying a 16-mm human embryo, suggested that posterior nephrogenic cells may migrate abnormally to form an isthmus or connection between the two developing kidneys to create the horseshoe shape.

Whatever the actual mechanism responsible for horseshoe kidney formation, the joining occurs before the kidneys have rotated on their long axis. In its mature form, the pelves and ureters of the horseshoe kidney are usually anteriorly placed, crossing ventrally to the isthmus (Fig. 58–20). Very rarely, the pelves are anteromedial, suggesting that fusion occurred somewhat later after some rotation had already taken place. In addition, migration is usually incomplete, and the kidneys lie lower in the abdomen than normal. It is presumed that the inferior mesenteric artery prevents full ascent by obstructing the movement of the isthmus.

DESCRIPTION. There are several variations in the basic shape of the horseshoe kidney. In 95% of patients, the kidneys join at the lower pole; in a small number, however, an isthmus connects both upper poles instead (Love and Wasserman, 1975).

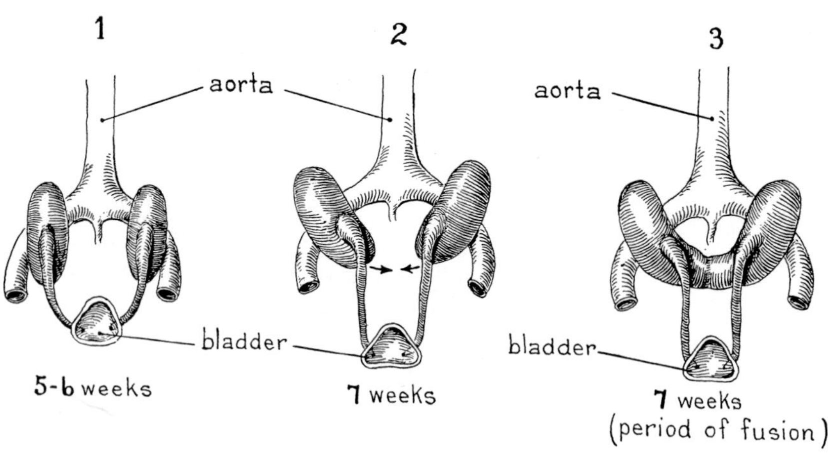

Figure 58–19. Embryogenesis of horseshoe kidney. The lower poles of the two kidneys touch and fuse as they cross the iliac arteries. Ascent is stopped when the fused kidneys reach the junction of the aorta and interior mesenteric artery. (From Benjamin JA, Schullian DM: J Hist Med Allied Sci 1950;5:315, after Gutierrez, 1931.)

Generally, the isthmus is bulky and consists of parenchymatous tissue with its own blood supply (Glenn, 1959; Love and Wasserman, 1975). Occasionally, it is just a flimsy midline structure composed of fibrous tissue that tends to draw the renal masses close together. It is located adjacent to the L3 or L4 vertebra just below the origin of the inferior mesenteric artery from the aorta. As a result, the paired kidneys tend to be somewhat lower than normal in the retroperitoneum. In some instances, the anomalous kidneys are very low, anterior to the sacral promontory or even in the true pelvis behind the bladder (Campbell, 1970). In general, the isthmus lies anterior to the aorta and vena cava, but it is not unusual for it to pass between the inferior vena cava and the aorta or even behind both great vessels (Jarmin, 1938; Meek and Wadsworth, 1940; Dajani, 1966).

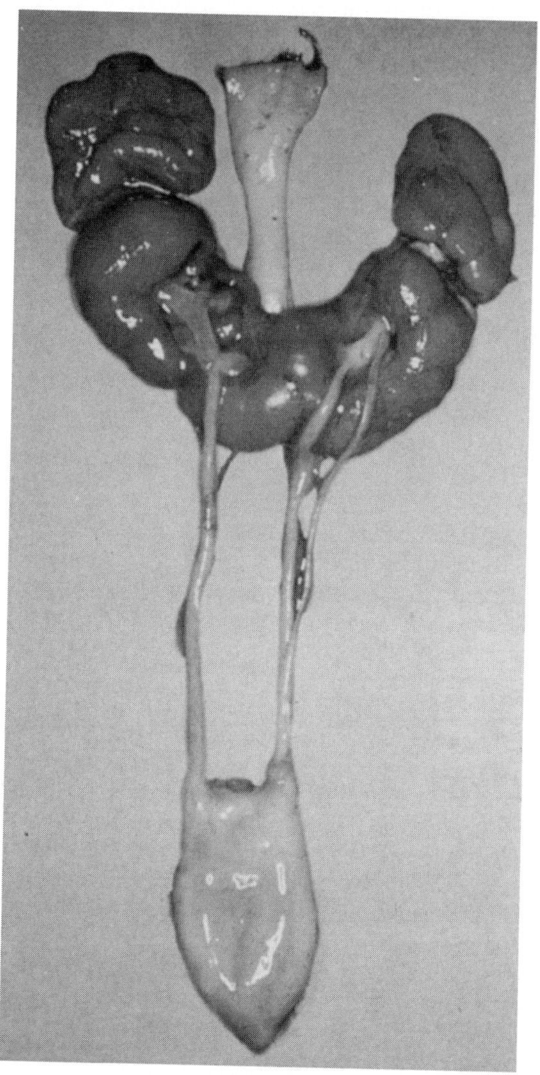

Figure 58–20. Specimen of a horseshoe kidney in a neonate who had multiple anomalies, including congenital heart disease. Note the thick parenchymatous isthmus.

The calyces, normal in number, are atypical in orientation. Because the kidney fails to rotate, the calyces point posteriorly, and the axis of each pelvis remains in the vertical or obliquely lateral plane (on a line drawn from the lower to the upper poles). The lowermost calyces extend caudally or even medially to drain the isthmus and may overlie the vertebral column.

The ureter may insert high on the renal pelvis and lie laterally, probably as the result of incomplete renal rotation. It courses downward and has a characteristic bend as it crosses over and anterior to the isthmus, a deviation that is proportionate to the thickness of the midline structure. Despite upper ureteral angulation, the lower ureter usually enters the bladder normally and rarely is ectopic.

The blood supply to the horseshoe kidney can be variable (Fig. 58–21). In 30% of cases, it consists of one renal artery to each kidney (Glenn, 1959), but it may be atypical with duplicate or even triplicate renal arteries supplying one or both kidneys. The blood supply to the isthmus and lower poles is also very variable. The isthmus and adjacent parenchymal masses may receive a branch from each main renal artery, or they may have their own arterial supply from the aorta originating either above or below the level of the isthmus. Not infrequently, this area may be supplied by branches from the inferior mesenteric, common or external iliac, or sacral arteries (Boatman et al, 1971; Kolln et al, 1972). Three cases of retrocaval ureter and isthmus have been reported (Eidelman et al, 1978; Hefferman et al, 1978).

ASSOCIATED ANOMALIES. The horseshoe kidney, even though it produces no symptoms, is frequently found in association with other congenital anomalies. Boatman and associates (1972) discovered that nearly one third of the 96 patients they studied had at least one other abnormality. Many newborns and young infants with multiple congenital

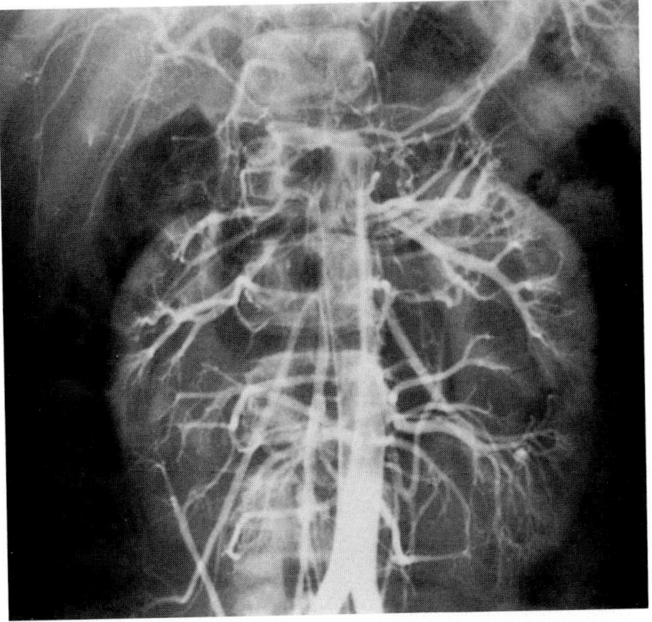

Figure 58–21. Arteriogram in a patient with a horseshoe kidney showing multiplicity of arteries supplying kidney arising from aorta and common iliac arteries. (From Kelalis PP: *In* Kelalis PP, King LR, eds: Clinical Pediatric Urology. Philadelphia, W. B. Saunders Company, 1976.)

anomalies have a horseshoe kidney. Judging from autopsy reports, the incidence of other anomalies is certainly greater in patients who die at birth or in early infancy than in those who reach adulthood (Zondek and Zondek, 1964). This implies that horseshoe kidney may occur more often in patients with another serious congenital anomaly. The organ systems most commonly involved include the skeletal, cardiovascular (primarily ventriculoseptal defects [Voisin et al, 1988]), and central nervous systems. Horseshoe kidney is found in 3% of children with neural tube defects (Whitaker and Hunt, 1987). Anorectal malformations are frequently encountered in these patients. Horseshoe kidney may also be seen in 20% of patients with trisomy 18 and in as many as 60% of females with Turner's syndrome (Smith, 1970; Lippe et al, 1988).

Boatman and his colleagues (1972) also discovered an increased occurrence of other genitourinary anomalies in patients with a horseshoe kidney. Hypospadias and undescended testes each occurred in 4% of males, and bicornuate uterus or septate vagina (or both) were noted in 7% of the females.

Duplication of the ureter occurs in 10% of patients (Zondek and Zondek, 1964; Boatman et al, 1972); in some cases, this has been associated with an ectopic ureterocele. Vesicoureteral reflux has been noted in more than half the patients (Segura et al, 1972; Pitts and Muecke, 1975). Cystic disease, including multicystic dysplasia in half of the upper pole of one side (Novak et al., 1977; Boullier et al, 1992) and adult polycystic kidney disease, has been reported in patients with horseshoe kidneys (Gutierrez, 1934; Campbell, 1970; Pitts and Muecke, 1975; Correa and Paton, 1976).

SYMPTOMS. Nearly one third of all patients with a horseshoe kidney remain asymptomatic (Glenn, 1959; Kolln et al, 1972). In most instances, this anomaly is an incidental finding at autopsy (Pitts and Muecke, 1975). When symptoms are present, however, they are related to hydronephrosis, infection, or calculus formation. The most common symptom that reflects these conditions is vague abdominal pain that may radiate to the lower lumbar region. Gastrointestinal complaints may be present as well. The so-called Rovsing's sign—abdominal pain, nausea, and vomiting on hyperextension of the spine—has been observed infrequently. Signs and symptoms of urinary tract infection occur in 30% of patients, and calculi have been noted in 20% to 80% (Glenn, 1959; Kolln et al, 1972; Pitts and Muecke, 1975; Evans and Resnick, 1981; Sharma and Bapna, 1986). Five to 10% of horseshoe kidneys are detected following palpation of an abdominal mass (Glenn, 1959; Kolln et al, 1972). Recently, horseshoe kidneys have been detected following angiography for evaluation of an abdominal aortic aneurysm (Huber et al, 1990; deBrito et al, 1991).

Ureteropelvic junction obstruction causing significant hydronephrosis occurs in as many as one third of individuals (Whitehouse, 1975; Das and Amar, 1984). The high insertion of the ureter into the renal pelvis, its abnormal course anterior to the isthmus, and the anomalous blood supply to the kidney may individually or collectively contribute to this obstruction.

DIAGNOSIS. Except for the possibility of a palpable midline abdominal mass (Grandone et al, 1985), the horseshoe kidney does not by itself produce symptoms. The clinical features from a diseased kidney, however, are often vague and nonspecific. The anomalies, therefore, may not be suspected until a renal ultrasonogram or an excretory urogram is obtained. Prenatal ultrasonography can now detect horseshoe kidneys before birth (Van Every, 1992; Sherer and Woods, 1992). The classic radiologic features are then easily recognized, and a diagnosis is readily made (Fig. 58–22). Findings that suggest a horseshoe kidney singly or collectively include the following: kidneys that are somewhat low lying and close to the vertebral column; a vertical or outward axis, so that a line drawn through the midplane of each kidney bisects the midline inferiorly; a continuation of the outer border of the lower pole of each kidney toward and across the midline; the characteristic orientation of the collecting system, which is directly posterior to each renal pelvis, with the lowermost calyx pointing caudally or even medially; and the high insertion of the ureter into the pelvis

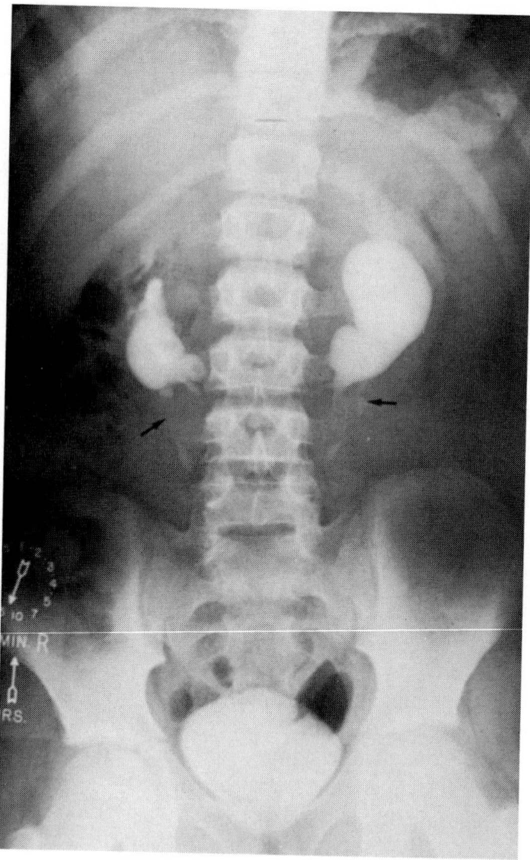

Figure 58–22. Excretory urogram in an 11-year-old boy evaluated for nocturnal incontinence reveals a horseshoe kidney. Note vertical renal axis and medial orientation of the collecting system. The ureters (*arrows*) are laterally displaced and bow over the isthmus.

and the anteriorly displaced upper ureter that appears to drape over a midline mass. However, obstruction due to either a calculus or a ureteropelvic junction stricture may obscure the radiologic picture (Love and Wasserman, 1975; Christoffersen and Iversen, 1976). Other studies, such as retrograde pyelography or computed tomography, may be necessary to confirm the diagnosis.

PROGNOSIS. Although Smith and Orkin (1945) believed that horseshoe kidneys are almost always associated with disease, subsequent investigators have not found this to be so. Glenn (1959) followed patients with horseshoe kidneys for an average of 10 years after discovery and found that nearly 60% remained symptom free. Only 13% had persistent urinary infection or pain, and 17% developed recurrent calculi. Operations to remove these stones or relieve obstruction were necessary in only 25%. In his series, no patients benefited from division of the isthmus for relief of pain; this idea has now been largely repudiated (Glenn, 1959; Pitts and Muecke, 1975).

Many patients with a horseshoe kidney have other congenital anomalies, some of which are incompatible with life beyond the neonatal period or early infancy. Excluding that group, survival is not reduced merely by the presence of this anomaly. Often, a horseshoe kidney is found incidentally, and it is rarely a cause of mortality (Dajani, 1966; Boatman et al, 1972).

Many disease processes have been associated with a horseshoe kidney, but this only reflects the relative frequency of the congenital defect. One hundred and fourteen cases of renal carcinoma within a horseshoe kidney have been reported (Buntley, 1976; Hohenfellner et al, 1992); more than half of these cancers were hypernephromas. However, renal pelvic tumors and Wilms' tumor each account for 25% of the total. Overall, 13 of 2961 Wilms' tumors in the National Wilms' Tumor study occurred in horseshoe kidneys, mostly on the left side, rarely in the isthmus, and practically all with favorable histologic findings. This incidence of Wilms' tumor in horseshoe kidneys is more than twice that expected in the general population (Mesrobian et al, 1985). Except for renal pelvic tumors, a surprisingly high number of these cancers appear to have arisen in the isthmus (Blackard and Mellinger, 1968). For this reason, it has been suggested that teratogenic factors are responsible for abnormal migration of nephrogenic cells that form an isthmus, leading to the horseshoe shape and the increased potential of carcinoma development in this portion of the kidney (Domenech-Mateu and Gonzales-Compta, 1988; Hohenfellner et al, 1992).

It has been suggested that the increased occurrence of chronic infection, obstruction, and stone formation may be instrumental in producing the higher than expected incidence of renal pelvic tumors in this group (Shoup et al, 1962; Castor and Green, 1975). Wilms' tumor, which is also commonly seen, frequently originates in the isthmus as well (Beck and Hlivko, 1960), often creating a very bizarre radiologic picture (Walker, 1977). The incidence of tumors in horseshoe kidneys seems to be increasing compared with the occurrence of tumors in the general population (Dische and Johnston, 1979). Survival from these tumors is related to the pathology and stage of the tumor at diagnosis and not to the renal anomaly (Murphy and Zincke, 1982).

Because it is located above the pelvic inlet, a horseshoe kidney should not adversely affect pregnancy or delivery (Bell, 1946). Glomerulocystic disease has been reported in children younger than 1 year of age but does not appear to be related specifically to the horseshoe anomaly (Craver et al, 1993). The development of renal failure associated with adult polycystic kidney disease is no greater in the presence of a horseshoe kidney (Correa and Paton, 1976). Finally, the last Transplantation Registry report failed to reveal any patient with a horseshoe kidney receiving a renal transplant (Advisory Committee to the Human Transplant Registry, 1975). Since then, however, several individuals have been successfully transplanted (Garg, 1990).

Anomalies of Rotation

The adult kidney, as it assumes its final position in the renal fossa, orients itself so that the calyces point laterally and the pelvis faces medially. When this alignment is not exact, the condition is known as malrotation. Most often, this inappropriate orientation is found in conjunction with another renal anomaly, such as ectopia with or without fusion or horseshoe kidney. This discussion centers on malrotation as an isolated renal entity. It must be differentiated from other conditions that mimic it as the result of extraneous forces such as an abnormal retroperitoneal mass.

INCIDENCE. The true incidence of this developmental anomaly cannot be accurately calculated because minor de-

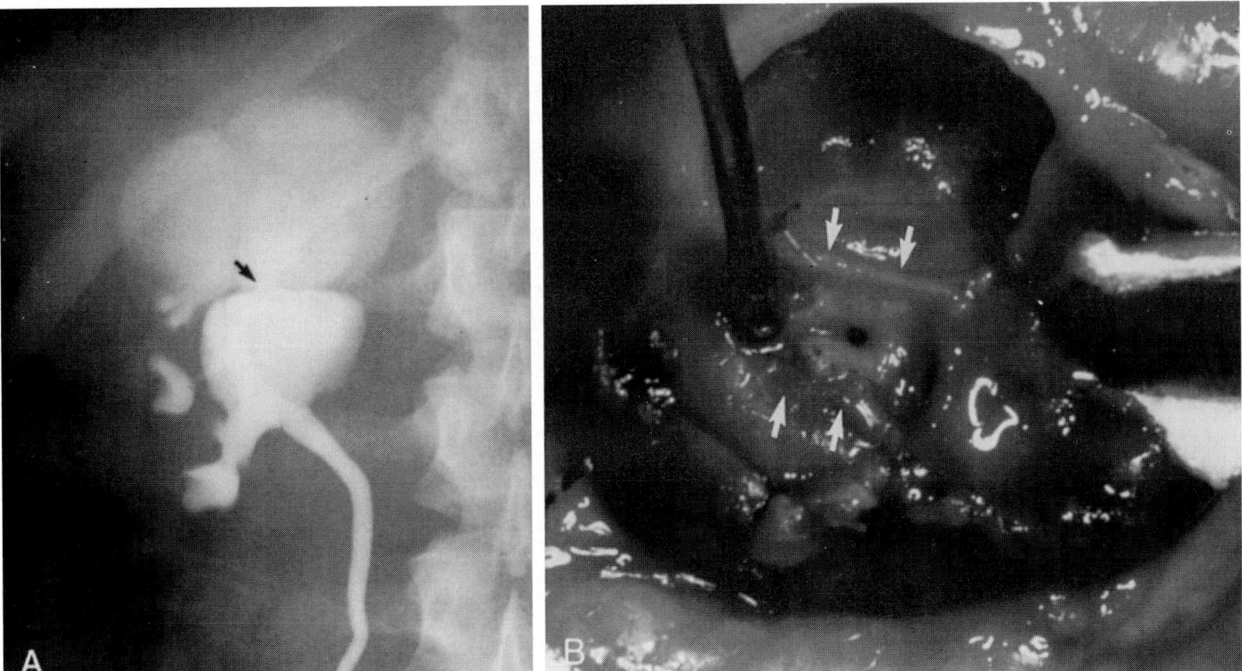

Figure 58–27. *A,* A 14-year-old girl with right flank pain underwent an excretory urogram, and this retrograde pyelogram revealed dilated upper calyces and a narrow upper infundibulum (*arrow*). *B,* At surgery, the infundibular channel was found sandwiched between two segmental arteries (*arrows*).

ered a rare occurrence until selective renal angiography came into vogue. Since then, the overall incidence has been calculated to be between 0.1% and 0.3%. Abeshouse (1951), in a comprehensive review, classified renal artery aneurysms as follows: saccular, fusiform, dissecting, and arteriovenous. The saccular aneurysm, a localized outpouching that communicates with the arterial lumen by a narrow or wide opening, is the most common type, accounting for 93% of all aneurysms (McKeil et al, 1966; Stanley et al, 1975; Hageman et al, 1978; Zinman and Libertino, 1982). When the aneurysm is located at the bifurcation of the main renal artery and its anterior and posterior divisions or at one of the more distal branchings, it is considered congenital in origin and is called the fusiform type (Poutasse, 1957). The presence of similar aneurysms at branching points in the vasculature of other organ systems attests to this possible origin (Lorentz et al, 1984). Acquired aneurysms may be located anywhere and result from inflammatory, traumatic, or degenerative factors. A localized defect in the internal elastic tissue and the media allows the vessel to dilate at that point. It is a true aneurysm because its walls are composed of most of the layers that comprise the normal artery (Poutasse, 1957). The outpouchings may vary in size from 1 to 2 cm up to 10 cm (Gerritano, 1957), but 90% are less than 2 cm in diameter.

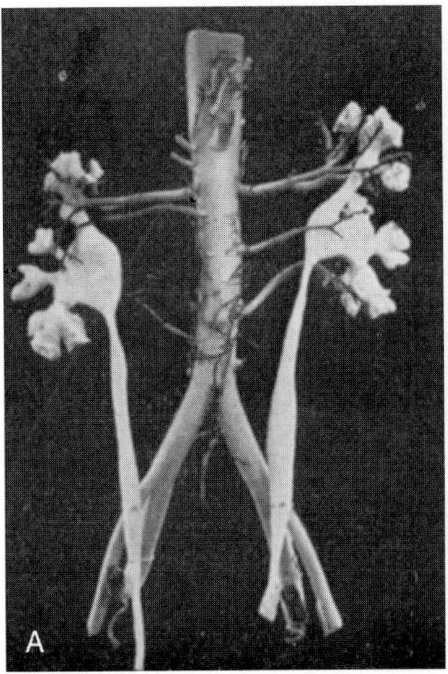

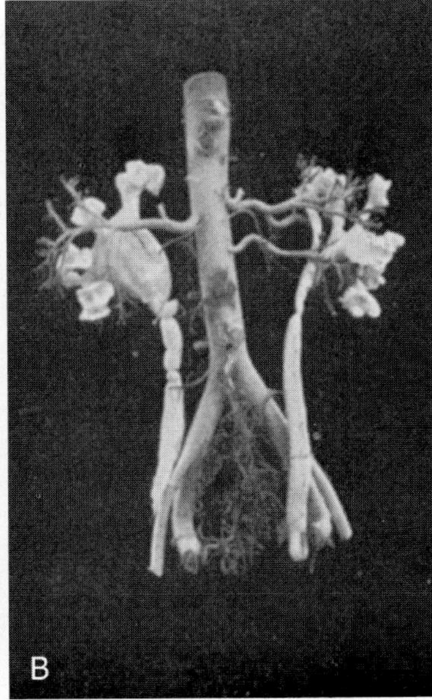

Figure 58–28. Accessory renal vessels demonstrated by celluloid corrosion preparation.

A, In a full-term fetus. The renal pelves and ureters are shown in relationship to the main arterial distribution. On each side there are two accessory renal vessels above and one below, the lower one on the left being in proximity to the ureterovesical junction.

B, In an 8-month-old fetus, the kidney on the right had one renal artery but the organ on the left had an accessory branch to the lower renal pole. Yet, the location of the lower accessory vessel on the left does not suggest that it might cause ureteral obstruction. On the right, there are early hydronephrosis, secondary kinking, and narrowing at the ureterovesical junction. (Courtesy of Dr. Duncan Morison.)

Most renal artery aneurysms are silent, especially those in children (48%) (Sarker et al, 1991). Some produce symptoms at a later age in relation to their size because they have a tendency to enlarge with time. Pain (15%), hematuria, microscopic and macroscopic (30%), and hypertension (55%) secondary to compression of adjacent parenchyma or to altered blood flow within the vascular tree can occur (Glass and Uson, 1967; Bulbul and Farrow, 1992). The hypertension is renin mediated, secondary to relative parenchymal ischemia (Lorentz et al, 1984).

The diagnosis may be suspected when a pulsatile mass is palpated in the region of the renal hilum or when a bruit is heard on abdominal auscultation. A wreathlike calcification in the area of the renal artery or its branches (30%) is indicative (Silvis et al, 1956), but this finding is often missed on a plain abdominal radiograph (Bulbul and Farrow, 1992). Excretory urography may be suggestive of a vascular lesion in 60% of cases, but selective renal angiography (Cerny et al, 1968), digital subtraction angiography or, more recently, color Doppler ultrasonography (Bunchman et al, 1991; Okamato et al, 1992) or magnetic resonance angiography (Takebayashi et al, 1994) is needed to confirm the diagnosis.

Many asymptomatic renal artery aneurysms come to light following the discovery and work-up of hypertension. Fifty percent are diagnosed when a renal arteriogram is performed for other reasons (Zinman and Libertino, 1982). Generally, excision is recommended if (1) the hypertension cannot be easily controlled; (2) incomplete ringlike calcification is present; (3) the aneurysm is larger than 2.5 cm (Poutasse, 1975); (4) the patient is female and is likely to become pregnant because rupture during pregnancy is a strong possibility (Cohen and Shamash, 1987); (5) the aneurysm increases in size on serial angiograms; or (6) an arteriovenous fistula is present. The likelihood of spontaneous rupture (in about 10% of cases) with its dire consequences dictates attentive treatment in the foregoing situations.

Renal Arteriovenous Fistula

Although rare, renal arteriovenous fistulas have been discovered with increasing frequency since they were first described by Varela in 1928. Two types exist, congenital and acquired (Maldonado et al, 1964); acquired fistulas (secondary to trauma, inflammation, renal surgery, or postpercutaneous needle biopsy) accounts for the recent increased incidence. Only the congenital variant is discussed here.

Less than 25% of all renal arteriovenous fistulas are of the congenital type. They are easily identifiable by their cirsoid configuration and multiple communications between the main or segmental renal arteries and venous channels (Crummy et al, 1965; Cho and Stanley, 1978). Although they are considered congenital (because similar arteriovenous malformations can be found elsewhere in the body), they rarely present clinically before the third or fourth decade. Females are affected three times as often as males, and the right kidney is involved slightly more often than the left (Cho and Stanley, 1978). The lesion is generally located in the upper pole (45% of cases), but not infrequently it may be found in the midportion (30%) or lower pole (25%) of the kidney (Yazaki et al, 1976). A total of 91 cases had been reported (Takaha et al, 1980) at the time of the last review.

The exact cause remains an enigma, but the condition is thought to be either present at birth or the result of a congenital aneurysm that erodes into an adjacent vein and slowly enlarges (Thomason et al, 1972). The pathophysiology involved in the shunting of blood, which bypasses the renal parenchyma and rapidly joins the venous circulation and returns to the heart, results in a varied clinical picture. The myriad symptoms are based on the size of the arteriovenous malformation and the length of time it has existed (Messing et al, 1976).

The hemodynamic derangement often produces a loud bruit (in 75% of cases). Diminished perfusion of renal parenchyma distal to the fistulous site leads to relative ischemia and renin-mediated hypertension (40% to 50%) (McAlhany et al, 1971). The increased venous return and high cardiac output with concomitant diminution in peripheral resistance may result in left ventricular hypertrophy and eventually in high-output cardiac failure (50%) (Maldonado et al, 1964). In addition, the arteriovenous fistula usually is located close to the collecting system. As a result, macroscopic and microscopic hematuria may occur in more than 75% of affected individuals (Messing et al, 1976; Cho and Stanley, 1978). Although flank or abdominal pain may be present, a mass is rarely felt (10%).

Excretory urography may reveal diminished or absent function in either one segment or the entire portion of the involved kidney (DeSai and DeSautels, 1973), an irregular filling defect in the renal pelvis or calyces (secondary to either clot or encroachment by the fistula), and calyceal distortion or obstruction distal to the site of the lesion (Gunterberg, 1968). Despite these specific radiographic features, an abnormality may be noted in only 50% of excretory urograms. Doppler ultrasound is a more accurate and noninvasive test, but selective renal arteriography or digital subtraction angiography is the most definitive method for diagnosing the lesion. A cirsoid appearance with multiple small tortuous channels, prompt venous filling, and an enlarged renal and possibly gonadal vein are pathognomonic for a renal arteriovenous fistula (DeSai and DeSautels, 1973).

The symptomatic nature of this lesion, which causes progressive alterations in the cardiovascular system, often dictates surgical intervention. The congenital variant rarely behaves like its acquired counterpart, which may disappear spontaneously after several months. Nephrectomy, partial nephrectomy, vascular ligation (Boijsen and Kohler, 1962), selective embolization (Bookstein and Goldstein, 1973), and balloon catheter occlusion (Bentson and Crandall, 1972) have been employed to obliterate the fistula.

Calyx and Infundibulum

Calyceal Diverticulum

A calyceal diverticulum is a cystic cavity lined by transitional epithelium, encased within the renal substance, and situated peripheral to a minor calyx, to which it is connected by a narrow channel. This abnormality, first described by Rayer in 1841, may be multiple, with the upper calyx being most frequently affected.

An incidence of 4.5 per 1000 excretory urograms has been reported (Timmons et al, 1975). A similar incidence has been noted in both children and adults, with no predilection for either side or sex. Most diverticula occur adjacent to an upper or occasionally a lower pole calyx and have been labeled type I. Type II diverticula are larger and communicate with the renal pelvis directly. They tend to be more symptomatic than type I lesions (Wulfsohn, 1980).

Congenital and acquired factors have been suggested to explain the formation of calyceal diverticula. The similarity in incidence in children and adults is consistent with an embryologic etiology (Abeshouse, 1950; Mathieson, 1953; Devine et al, 1969; Middleton and Pfister, 1974). At the 5-mm stage of the embryo, some of the ureteral branches of the third and fourth generation, which ordinarily degenerate, may persist as isolated branches, resulting in the formation of a calyceal diverticulum (Lister and Singh, 1973).

A localized cortical abscess draining into a calyx has also been postulated as an etiologic factor. Other proposed causes include obstruction secondary to stone formation or infection within a calyx, progressive fibrosis of an infundibular stenosis, renal injury, achalasia, and spasm or dysfunction of one of the supposed sphincters surrounding a minor calyx. Small diverticula are usually asymptomatic and are found incidentally at excretory urography or renal ultrasonography. Over time, these diverticula tend to become progressively distended with trapped urine (Schneck et al, 1994). Infection, milk of calcium (crystallization of calcium salts without actual stone formation) (Patriquin et al, 1985), and true stone formation are complications of stasis or obstruction that can produce symptoms (Lister and Singh, 1973; Siegel and McAlister, 1979). Hematuria, pain, and urinary infection may be seen in the presence of stones. In the Mayo Clinic series (Timmons et al, 1975), 39% of patients with calyceal diverticula had calculi. One child in our series developed an abscess in her infected diverticulum that required percutaneous drainage (Ellis et al, 1990; Schneck et al, 1994).

The diagnosis is made by excretory urography; delayed films are helpful in demonstrating pooling of contrast material in the diverticulum. Retrograde pyelography (Fig. 58–29) and, more recently, computed tomography with contrast and magnetic resonance imaging are sometimes useful in making the diagnosis and defining the precise anatomy. Ultrasonography shows a fluid-filled area more centrally located near the collecting system than a simple renal cyst. When the diverticulum is filled with microcalculi, ultrasound characteristically demonstrates a layering effect within the diverticulum with clear fluid above and echo-dense debris without shadowing below (Patriquin et al, 1985). In fact, ultrasonography may offer a more definitive diagnosis because it is easier to image the milk of calcium within the diverticulum as the patient changes position. Milk of calcium appears as a crescent-shaped density on excretory urography that changes as the patient assumes different positions. Reflux may be found in as many as two thirds of the children, which may explain why some present with urinary infection (Amar, 1975).

In general, patients who are asymptomatic do not require treatment. Persistent pain, resistant urinary infections, hematuria, and milk of calcium or true calculus formation are indications for surgery (Siegel and McAlister, 1979); if feasible, partial nephrectomy is the treatment of choice.

Hydrocalycosis

Hydrocalycosis is a very rare cystic dilatation of a major calyx with a demonstrable connection to the renal pelvis; it is lined by transitional epithelium. It may be caused by a congenital or acquired intrinsic obstruction such as a parapelvic cyst (Fig. 58–30).

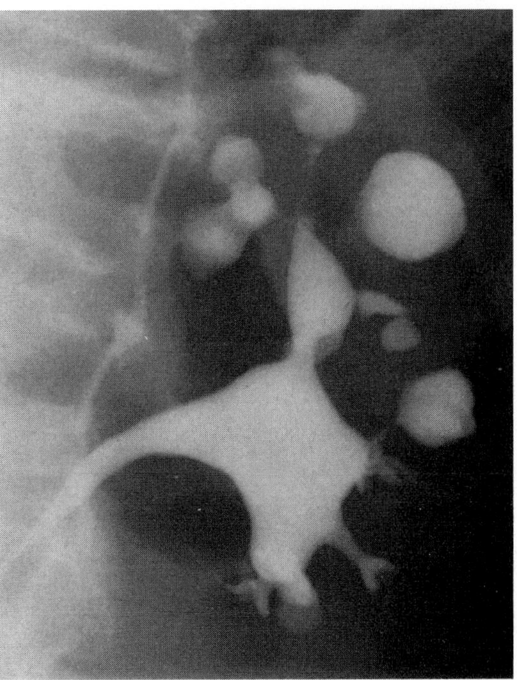

Figure 58–29. A 13-year-old girl with hematuria had a retrograde pyelogram demonstrating multiple calyceal diverticula.

Dilatation of the upper calyx due to obstruction of the upper infundibulum by vessels or stenosis has been described (see Fig. 58–27) (Fraley, 1966; Johnston and Sandomirsky, 1972). Cicatrization of an infundibulum may result from infection or trauma. Conversely, hydrocalycosis has been reported to occur with no obvious cause (Williams and Mininberg, 1968). It has been postulated (Moore, 1950; Williams and Mininberg, 1968) that achalasia of a ring of muscle at the entrance of the infundibulum into the renal pelvis causes a functional obstruction.

Mild upper calyceal dilatation due to partial infundibular obstruction is relatively common but usually asymptomatic. The most frequent presenting symptom is upper abdominal or flank pain. On occasion, a mass may be palpated. Stasis can lead to hematuria or urinary infection, or both.

Hydrocalycosis must be differentiated from multiple dilated calyces secondary to ureteral obstruction, calyceal clubbing as a result of recurrent pyelonephritis or medullary necrosis, renal tuberculosis, a large calyceal diverticulum, and megacalycosis. These entities can be differentiated using a combination of excretory urography, findings at surgery, histopathology of removed tissue, and bacteriology.

Hydrocalycosis due to vascular obstruction is usually treated by dismembered infundibulopyelostomy, thus changing the relationship of the infundibulum to the vessel. When the cystic dilatation is due to an intrinsic stenosis of the infundibulum, an intubated infundibulotomy or partial nephrectomy may be performed. Percutaneous treatment of these narrowed areas has also been successful and is probably the approach of choice today (Lang, 1991). Although clinical improvement is apparent in most instances, the radiologic appearance often is not altered significantly.

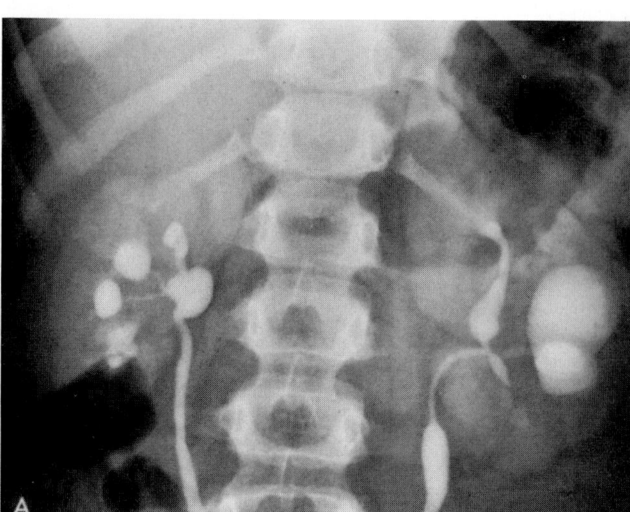

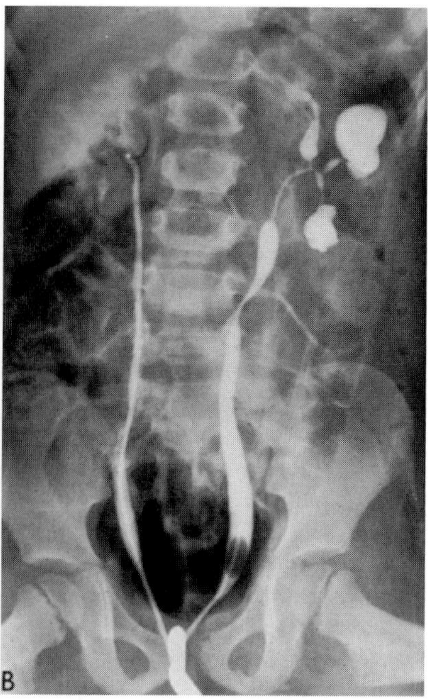

Figure 58–30. Hydrocalycosis of infundibulopelvic stenosis in a 3-year-old boy with bilaterally ectopic ureteral orifices (at the vesical neck) and other congenital anomalies, who presented with urinary infection. Reflux was not demonstrable, and the patient has remained uninfected on suppressive treatment. There has been no urographic change for 5 years. *A*, Long-term excretory urogram. Right infundibular and left infundibulopelvic stenosis. *B*, Retrograde ureteropyelogram (bilateral). Mildly dilated left ureter. Note diffuse tubular backflow on right. (From Malek RS: *In* Kelalis PP, King LR, eds: Clinical Pediatric Urology. Philadelphia, W. B. Saunders Company, 1976.)

Megacalycosis

Megacalycosis is best defined as nonobstructive enlargement of calyces due to malformation of the renal papillae (Fig. 58–31). It was first described by Puigvert in 1963. The calyces are generally dilated and malformed and may be increased in number. The renal pelvis is not dilated nor is its wall thickened, and the ureteropelvic junction is normally funneled with no evidence of obstruction. The cortical tissue around the abnormal calyx is normal in thickness and shows no signs of scarring or chronic inflammation. The medulla, however, is underdeveloped and assumes a falciform crescent appearance instead of its normal pyramidal shape. The collecting tubules are not dilated but are definitely shorter than normal, and they are oriented transversely rather than vertically from the corticomedullary junction (Puigvert, 1963). A mild disorder of maximum concentrating ability has been reported (Gittes and Talner, 1972), but acid excretion is normal after an acid load (Vela Navarrete and Garcia Robledo, 1983). Other functions of the kidney—glomerular filtration, renal plasma flow, and isotope uptake—are not altered either (Gittes, 1984).

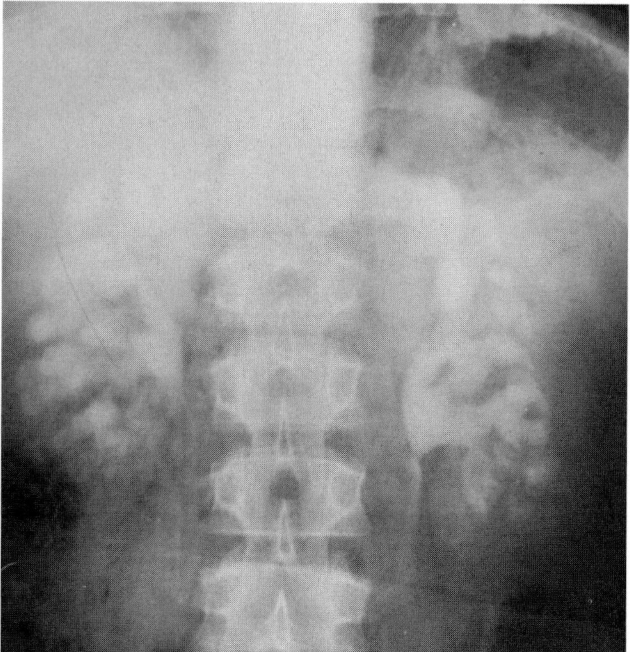

Figure 58–31. Bilateral megacalyces discovered in an 11-year-old boy with abdominal pain and hematuria. He had no history of urinary infection, and voiding cystography did not demonstrate vesicoureteral reflux.

Megacalycosis is most likely to be congenital. It occurs predominantly in males in a ratio of 6:1 and has been found only in whites. Bilateral disease has been seen almost exclusively in males, whereas segmental unilateral involvement occurs only in females. This suggests an X-linked partially recessive gene with reduced penetrance in females (Gittes, 1984). There has been one report of two affected brothers, but the entity is not thought to be familial (Briner and Thiel, 1988).

It has been theorized by Puigvert (1964) and endorsed by Johnston and Sandomirsky (1972) that megacalycosis results from a transient delay in the recanalization of the upper ureter after the branches of the ureteral bud hook up with the metanephric blastema. This produces a short-lived episode of obstruction when the embryonic glomeruli start producing urine. The fetal calyces may dilate and then retain their obstructed appearance despite the lack of evidence of obstruction in postnatal life (Gittes and Talner, 1972). The increased number of calyces frequently seen in this condition may be an aborted response by the branching ureteral bud to the obstruction.

Primary hypoplasia of juxtamedullary glomeruli has been suggested as a cause by Galian and associates (1970), which explains nicely the reason for the lack of concentrating ability; this theory, however, has not been corroborated by others.

The abnormality is noticed in children, usually when x-ray studies are performed following a urinary tract infection or as part of an evaluation when other congenital anomalies are present. Adults frequently present with hematuria secondary to renal calculi, which leads to excretory urographic investigation.

The calyces are dilated and usually increased in number, but the infundibuli and pelvis may not be enlarged. Although the ureteropelvic junction does not appear to be obstructed, there may be segmental dilatation of the distal third of the ureter (Kozakewich and Lebowitz, 1974). Megacalycosis associated with an ipsilateral segmental megaureter has been described in 12 children (Mandell et al, 1987). It occurred mostly in males and was predominantly left sided. A ureter of normal caliber was interposed between the two entities (Fig. 58–32). Not infrequently, this anatomic picture has been mistaken for congenital ureteropelvic or ureterovesical junction obstruction, and surgery has been performed to correct the suspected defect. Postoperatively, the calyceal pattern remains unchanged.

Diuretic renography reveals a normal pattern of uptake and washout of the isotope, and the Whitaker test fails to generate high pressures in the collecting system. Thus, an obstructive picture cannot be proved. Long-term follow-up of patients with this anomaly does not reveal any progression of the anatomic derangement or functional impairment of the kidney (Gittes, 1984).

Unipapillary Kidney

The unipapillary kidney is an exceptionally rare anomaly in humans. Only six cases have been reported (Neal and Murphy, 1960; Sakatoku and Kitayama, 1964; Harrison et al, 1976; Morimoto et al, 1979; Toppercer, 1980). This anomaly is present not uncommonly in monkeys, rabbits, dogs, marsupials, insectivores, and monotremes. The cause is thought to be a failure of progressive branching after the first three to five generations (which create the pelvis) of the ureteral bud (Potter, cited by Harrison et al, 1976). The solitary calyx drains a ridgelike papilla. Nephrons attach to fewer collecting tubules, which then drain directly into the pelvis.

The kidney is smaller than normal but usually is in its correct location. The arterial tree, although sparse, has a normal configuration. The opposite kidney is frequently absent. Genital anomalies are often present. The condition is frequently asymptomatic and is discovered fortuitously in most instances.

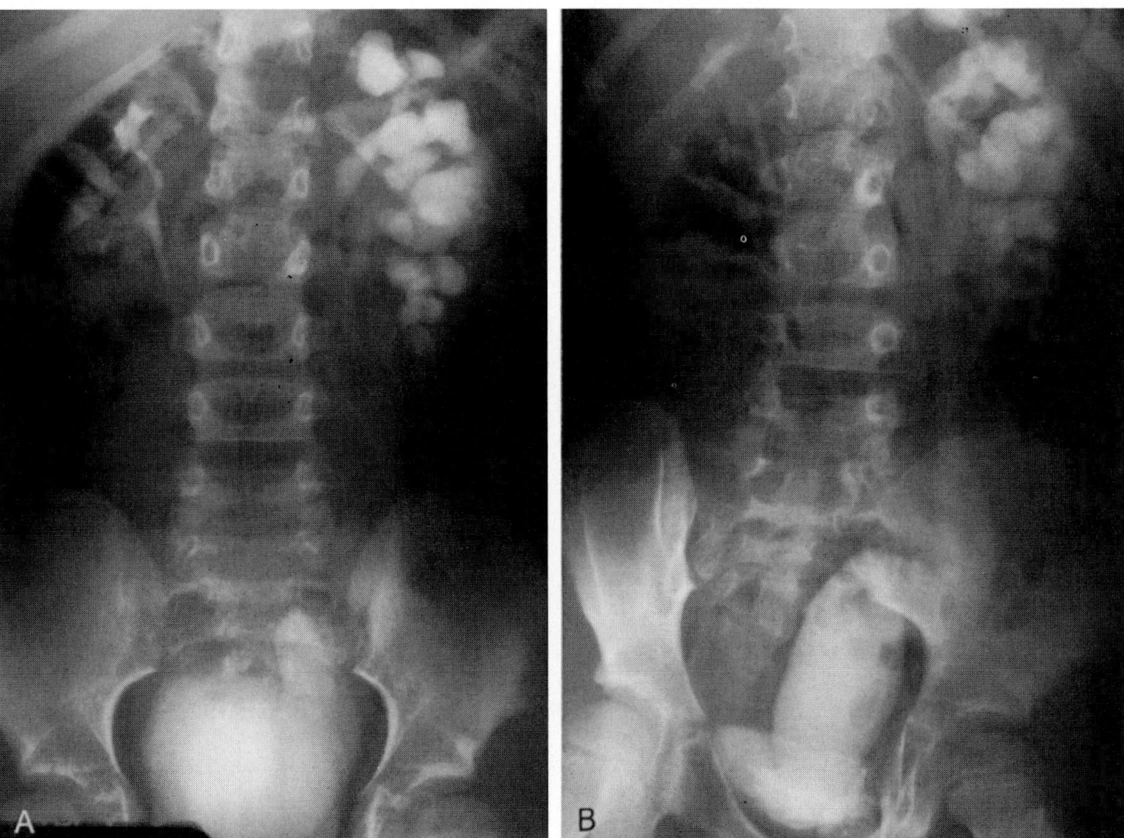

Figure 58–32. An 8-year-old boy with urinary infection was found to have left-sided megacalycosis and a distal megaureter (*A* and *B*). Note the normal caliber upper ureter. A voiding cystogram revealed no reflux, and a diuretic renogram did not demonstrate any obstruction.

Extrarenal Calyces

Extrarenal calyces is an uncommon congenital anomaly in which the major calyces as well as the renal pelvis are outside the parenchyma of the kidney (Fig. 58–33). This entity was originally reviewed by Eisendrath in 1925 and then more extensively by Malament and co-workers in 1961. The kidney is usually discoid, with the pelvis and the major and minor calyces located outside the renal parenchyma. The renal vessels have an anomalous distribution into the kidney, usually at the circumferential edge of the flat widened hilum. Malament and co-workers considered this condition the result of an abnormal nephrogenic anlage or a too early and rapidly developing ureteral bud.

Extrarenal calyces usually do not produce symptoms, although failure of normal drainage may lead to stasis, infection, and calculi. Sometimes, the calyces are blunted, mimicking the radiographic changes usually seen with pyelonephritis or obstruction. This condition should be distinguished from these entities. Surgery is reserved for cases in which infection or obstruction is demonstrated.

Anomalous Calyx (Pseudotumor of the Kidney)

A number of normal variants of the pyelocalyceal system in the kidney have been described. One such entity presents as a localized mass, usually situated between the infundibula of the upper and middle calyceal groups, and is called a hypertrophied column of Bertin (Fig. 58–34). The column may be sufficiently large to compress and deform the adjacent pelvis and calyces, suggesting a mass on excretory urography; this is the so-called pseudotumor. The individual calyces, however, are normally shaped and developed.

It is important to differentiate this calyceal anomaly from true disease of the calyx and from a parenchymal tumor. A renal scan shows normal uptake of the radioisotope in this area (Parker et al, 1976), and renal ultrasound shows a normal echogenic pattern of parenchyma in the area in question.

Infundibulopelvic Dysgenesis

Infundibulopelvic stenosis most likely forms a link between cystic dysplasia of the kidney and the grossly hydronephrotic organ (Kelalis and Malek, 1981; Uhlenhuth et al, 1990). This condition includes a variety of roentgenographically dysmorphic kidneys with varying degrees of infundibular or infundibulopelvic stenosis that may be associated with renal dysplasia (Fig. 58–35). Although not called as such, the first case involving the entire pelvis and all the infundibula of both kidneys was reported by Boyce and Whitehurst in 1976. Rayer had described a focal form of the disease in 1841, and several reports noting narrowing of one or two infundibula appeared between 1949 and 1976 (Uhlenhuth et al, 1990). These reports tried to link the focal form to cystic dysplasia secondary to obstruction, in which multicystic kidney disease is the severest form in the spectrum. Uhlenhuth and colleagues (1990) believe that this phenomenon is the result of extensive dysgenesis of the pyelocalyceal system, although renal function is preserved.

Infundibulopelvic stenosis is usually bilateral and is commonly associated with vesicoureteral reflux, suggesting an abnormality of the entire ureteral bud (Kelalis and Malek, 1981). It usually presents with urinary infection, hypertension, or flank pain. Sometimes, an asymptomatic child with multiple anomalies is evaluated and found to have this condition. Despite extensive dysmorphic features, kidney function is either normal or is only slightly affected when these patients are first diagnosed (Kelalis and Malek, 1981). Long-term follow-up, however, reveals that progressive renal deterioration is common, leading to severe renal insufficiency or end-stage renal disease, especially in all patients with bilateral involvement (Husmann et al, 1994). Biopsies in patients with renal failure demonstrate lesions consistent with hyperfiltration injury. Progressive hydronephrosis is not thought to be responsible for the deterioration in renal function based on histologic assessment of renal tissue adjacent to the dilated calyces. Therefore, infundibulotomy is not recommended unless there is a specific need (e.g., caliceal stones) (Husmann et al, 1994).

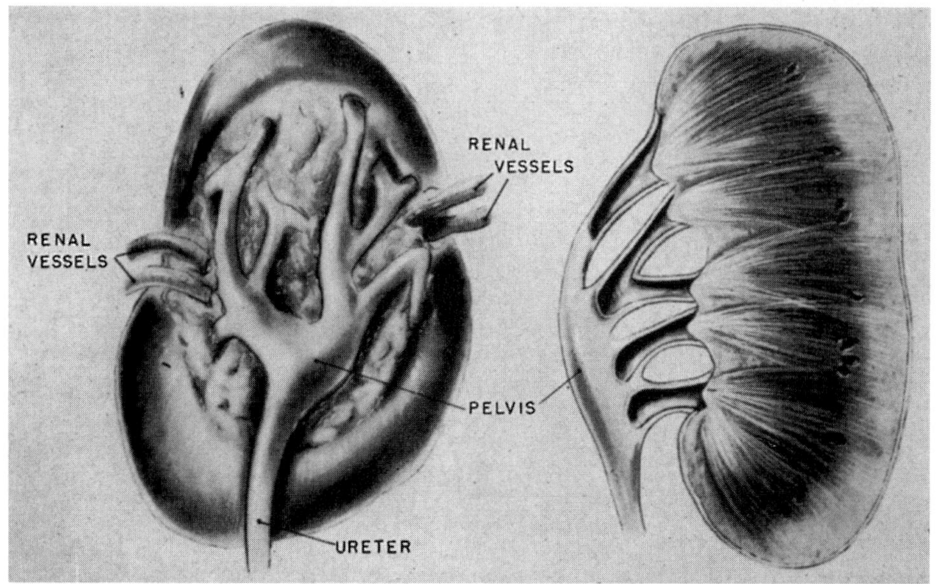

Figure 58–33. Extrarenal calyces. These represent delayed rather than insufficient ureteral growth. (From Malament M, Schwartz B, Nagamatsu GR: Am J Roentgenol 1961;86:823.)

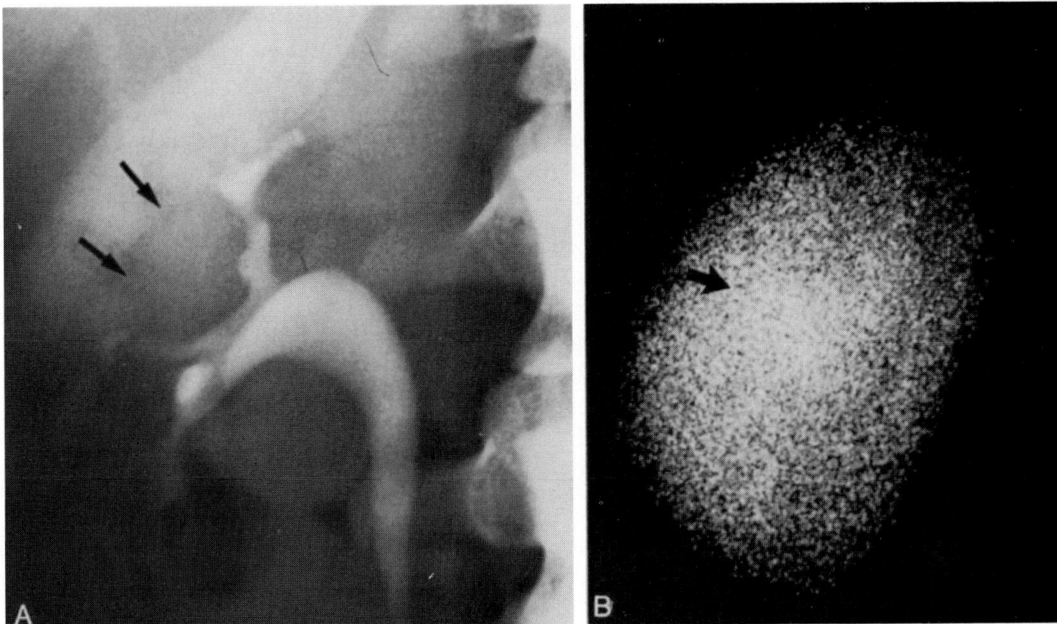

Figure 58–34. *A,* This child has a mass effect with splaying of the middle calyces. *B,* A renal scan demonstrates normal uptake in the area (*arrow*), suggesting the pseudotumor is really a hypertrophied column of Bertin.

Pelvis

Extrarenal Pelvis

An extrarenal pelvis is of clinical importance only when drainage is impaired. This anomaly is sometimes associated with a variety of kidney abnormalities, including malposition and malrotation, that predispose to urinary stasis, infection, and calculus disease.

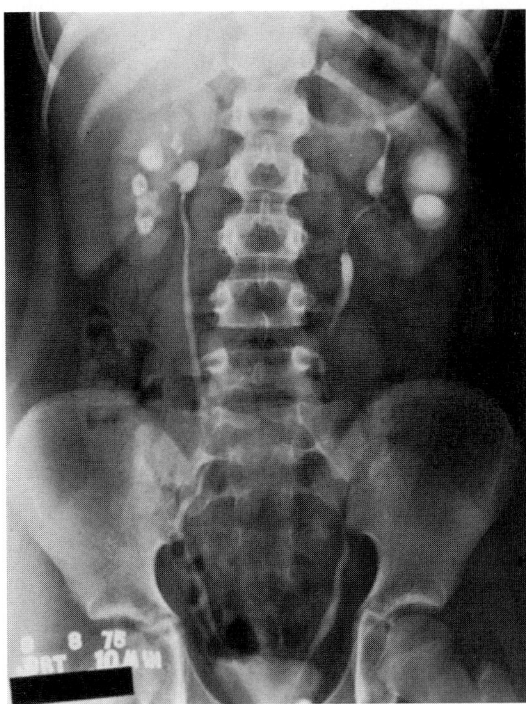

Figure 58–35. Excretory urogram in an 18-year-old male with one urinary tract infection shows severe stenosis of the infundibula and left ureteropelvic junction and a milder form of infundibulopelvic dysgenesis in the right kidney. Vesicoureteral reflux was absent on voiding cystourethrography. (Courtesy of Dr. Panos Kelalis.)

Bifid Pelvis

Approximately 10% of normal renal pelves are bifid, the pelvis dividing first at or just within its entrance to the kidney to form two major calyces. Bifid pelvis should be considered a variant of normal. No increased incidence of disease has been reported in patients with this entity. When further division of the renal pelvis occurs, triplication of the pelvis may result, but this is extremely rare.

ANOMALIES OF THE URETEROPELVIC JUNCTION

Anomalies of the ureteropelvic junction may be classified as follows:

I. Ureteropelvic junction obstruction
   - A. Intrinsic
   - B. Extrinsic
   - C. Secondary

Ureteropelvic Junction Obstruction

Hydronephrosis due to congenital ureteropelvic junction obstruction is one of the more common anomalies seen in childhood. It is defined as an impediment to urinary flow from the renal pelvis into the ureter. Inefficient drainage of urine at this point leads to progressive dilation of the collecting system and a further dimunition in the efficiency of pelvic emptying (Whitaker, 1975; Koff et al, 1986; Koff, 1990). Initially, the muscle of the renal pelvis hypertrophies, and glomerular filtration diminishes to accommodate the obstructive process. Eventually, when the limit of kidney compromise is reached, the structure of the renal parenchyma changes, and impairment of function ensues.

Only primary congenital ureteropelvic junction obstruction is considered in this chapter. Other conditions that delay proximal urinary drainage and secondarily affect the ureteropelvic junction are discussed elsewhere in the text.

INCIDENCE. Ureteropelvic junction obstruction is seen in all pediatric age groups. At one point, about 25% of cases were discovered within the first year of life (Fig. 58–36) (Williams and Kenawi, 1976), but today, with the widespread use of prenatal ultrasonographic imaging of fetuses, nearly all cases are discovered and diagnosed in the perinatal period (Brown et al, 1987). In fact, ureteropelvic junction obstruction is *the* most common cause of dilatation of the collecting system in the fetal kidney, accounting for 80% of all dilations of the collecting system and far exceeding the incidence of multicystic dysplastic kidneys (Colodny et al, 1980; Brown et al, 1987). Relatively few cases are noted after puberty and into adulthood; of those that are, the cause is usually an aberrant vessel to the lower pole parenchyma crossing over the ureteropelvic junction area (Lowe and Marshall, 1984). The obstruction occurs more commonly in males (Williams and Karlaftis, 1966; Kelalis et al, 1971; Johnston et al, 1977), especially in the newborn period, when the ratio exceeds 2:1 (Robson et al, 1976; Williams and Kenawi, 1976; Johnston et al, 1977). Left-sided lesions predominate, and in the neonate more than two thirds occur on this side. Bilateral ureteropelvic junction obstruction is present in 10% to 40% of cases (Fig. 58–37) (Nixon, 1953; Uson et al, 1968; Robson et al, 1976; Williams and Kenawi, 1976; Johnston et al, 1977; Lebowitz and Griscom, 1977); bilaterality is more commonly found in the newborn or infant less than 6 months of age (Perlmutter et al, 1980; Snyder et al, 1980). Unilateral and bilateral ureteropelvic junction obstruction affecting members of more than one generation has been reported in several families (Cohen et al, 1978). A dominant autosomal pattern of inheritance with variable penetrance has been suggested but not proved.

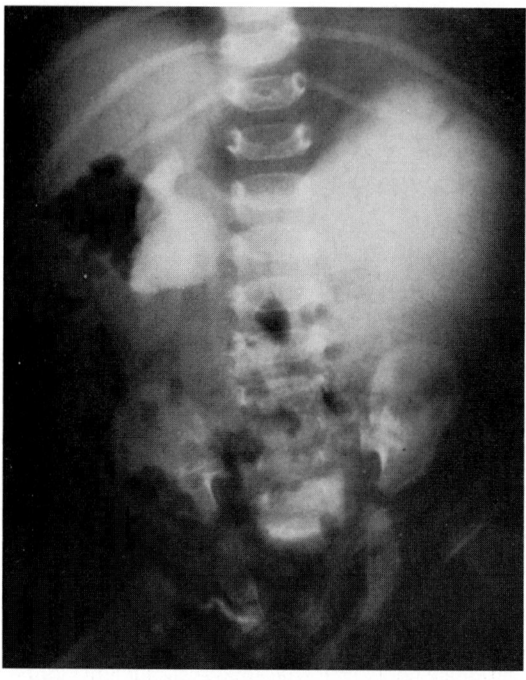

Figure 58–36. Palpation of a smooth, soft abdominal mass that transilluminated in a 3-year-old boy led to this excretory urogram, which at 6 hours reveals a ureteropelvic junction obstruction with severe hydronephrosis. An intrinsic narrowing at the ureteropelvic junction was found at surgery.

ETIOLOGY. The exact cause of ureteropelvic junction obstruction remains an enigma despite investigations along embryologic (Osathanondh and Potter, 1963; Allen, 1973; Ruano-Gil et al, 1975), anatomic (Nixon, 1953; Johnston, 1969), functional (Whitaker, 1975), and histologic (Murnaghan, 1958; Notley, 1968; Hanna et al, 1976) lines. Hydronephrosis is most often due to a narrowing at the ureteropelvic junction (Allen, 1973; Lebowitz and Griscom, 1977). A localized area of developmental arrest, produced by fetal vessels compressing the ureter, has been suggested by Allen (1973) and Osathanondh and Potter (1963). Ruano-Gil and colleagues (1975) showed that the embryonic ureter goes through a solid phase with subsequent recanalization. Failure of complete canalization of the upper end of the ureter may be the cause of ureteropelvic junction obstruction.

Intrinsic. An intrinsic lesion within the ureteropelvic wall may sometimes be the cause of obstruction even in the absence of a gross anatomic cause. Murnaghan (1958) demonstrated an interruption in the development of the circular musculature of the ureteropelvic junction. Whitaker (1975) incorporated these findings and theorized that the renal pelvis cannot effectively create a bolus of fluid at its junction with the ureter when it is not funnel shaped. During an episode of diuresis, the pelvis distends more and loses its already poorly funneled appearance, so that emptying is further impeded (Whitaker, 1975). Notley (1968) and Hanna and associates (1976) learned from electron microscopic studies of the ureteropelvic junction that although the muscle cell orientation is normal, there is an excessive amount of collagen fibers and ground substance between and around the muscle cells. As a result, muscle fibers are widely separated, and their points of connection, or nexuses, are attenuated. Many cells are actually atrophic. These findings are thought to be responsible for a functional discontinuity of the ureteropelvic muscular contractions that result in inefficient emptying and apparent ureteropelvic junction obstruction. Recently, Starr and associates (1992) noted a significant increase in the lamina muscularis and in the number of inner longitudinal muscle bundles of the ureteropelvic junction complexes of obstructed kidneys in infants less than 1 year old (compared with age-matched normals), thus suggesting a dramatic response by the muscle layers to obstruction. Koff and colleagues (1986) showed in experimentally induced obstructions in dogs that resistance to flow is fixed and pressure dependent when an intrinsic obstruction exists, whereas in cases of extrinsic obstruction the exit flow is not related linearly to the intrapelvic pressure. In fact, with increasing pressure during a period of diuresis the exit flow may plateau or even diminish, accentuating the obstruction even more (Koff, 1990).

Less common causes of intrinsic ureteropelvic junction obstruction include valvular mucosal folds (Maizels and Stephens, 1980), persistent fetal convolutions (Leiter, 1979), and upper ureteral polyps (Colgan et al, 1973; Gup, 1975;

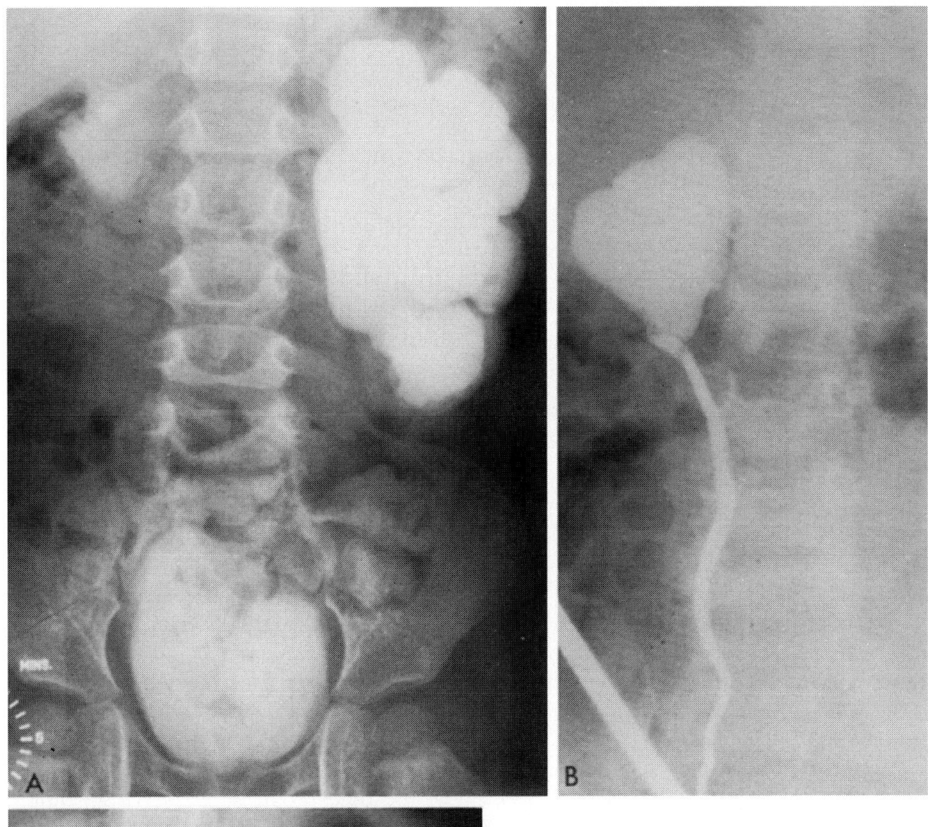

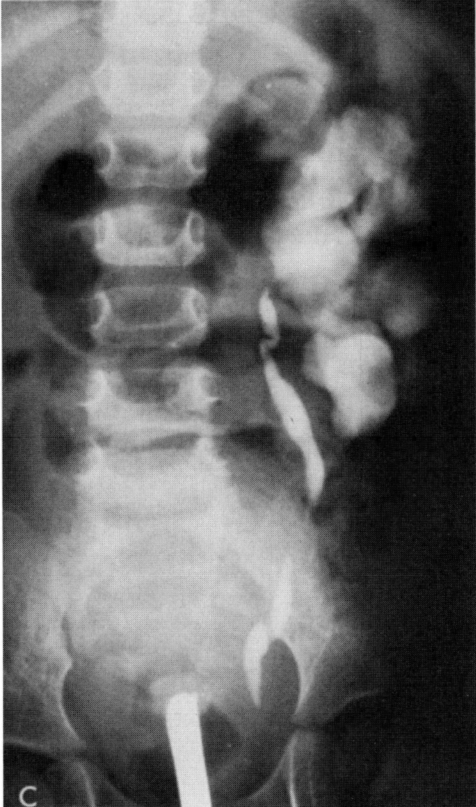

Figure 58–37. *A,* An excretory urogram in a 2-year-old girl with recurrent urinary tract infection demonstrates bilateral ureteropelvic junction obstruction. *B* and *C,* Bilateral retrograde pyelograms confirm the diagnosis.

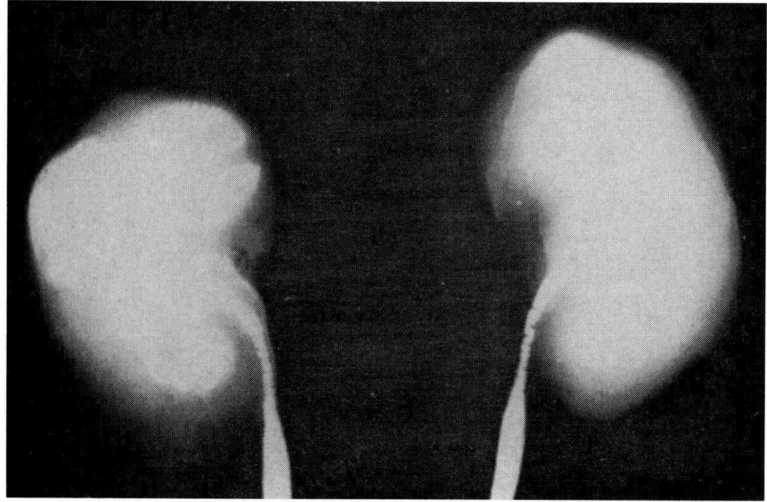

Figure 58–38. Congenital mucosal folds are outlined on a retrograde injection of this specimen taken from an 8-month-old gestational age stillborn fetus. The convolutions do not distend during the injection.

Williams and Kenawi, 1976; Williams et al, 1980; Thorup et al, 1981).

Congenital folds are a variant of ureteral valves and are a common finding in the upper ureter of fetuses after the fourth month of development, a finding that may persist until the newborn period (Fig. 58–38). They are mucosal infoldings with an axial offshoot of adventitia that does not flatten out when the ureter is distended or stretched (Fig. 58–39). The exterior surface of the ureter has a smooth appearance owing to adventitial bridges (Johnston, 1969). The epithelial folds are secondary to differing growth rates of the ureter and the body of the child, with excessive ureteral length occurring early in gestation. This provides a "length reserve" for the ureter, which traverses a shorter distance in the newborn than in the adult (Östling, 1942). Others have thought that congenital folds may represent a phenomenon similar to the persistence of Chwalla's membrane in the lower ureter, which may produce a ureteral valve subsequently (Mering et al, 1972). Östling thought that folds were a precursor of actual ureteropelvic junction obstruction because they are frequently discovered in babies who have a contralateral ureteropelvic obstruction. Ordinarily, folds are not obstructive and disappear with the person's linear growth (Leiter, 1979). They are rarely seen in the older child or adult. Exaggerated or persistent fetal folds containing muscle or high insertion of a valvular leaflet at the ureteropelvic junction, however, may indeed become obstructive (Maizels and Stephens, 1980). This type of obstruction sometimes can be relieved by dissecting the folds and eliminating the kinking (Johnston, 1969), but more com-

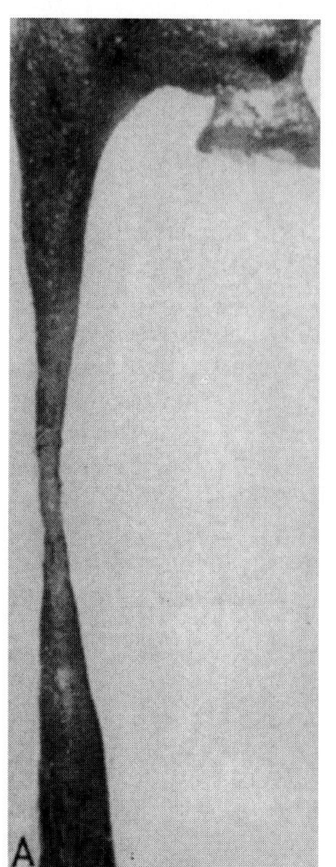

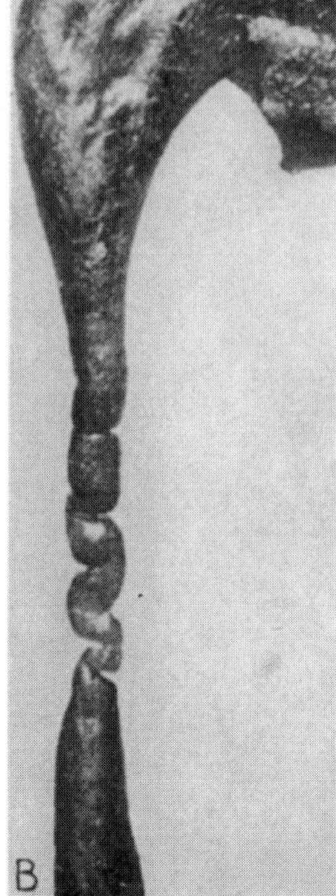

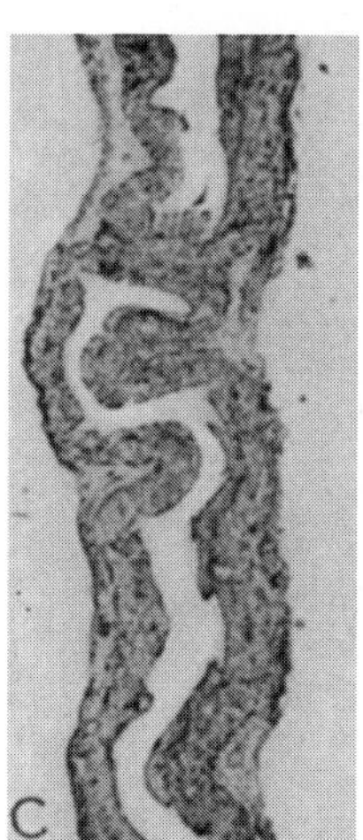

Figure 58–39. Embryologic considerations in the genesis of ureteral folds, kinks, and strictures.

A, Cast of the ureter and the renal pelvis in a newborn. There is physiologic narrowing of the upper ureter below, which is the normal main spindle of the ureter. No ureteral folds are present.

B, Cast of the ureter and the renal pelvis in the newborn. The ureteral folds proceed alternatively from the opposite sides.

C, Ureteral kinks that appear as muscular folds with axial offshoots of the loose adventitia. (Courtesy of Dr. Karl Östling.) (From Campbell MF: *In* Campbell MF, Harrison JH, eds: Urology, Vol. 2, 3rd ed. Philadelphia, W. B. Saunders Company, 1970.)

Maizels, 1992). These people may have a normal excretory urogram when they are asymptomatic, but an obstructed picture results during an episode of pain (Malek, 1983) (Fig. 58–48). To help define these less clear cut conditions, a fluoroscopic pressure-flow study can be performed by injecting contrast medium through a percutaneously placed nephrostomy tube and recording intrapelvic pressures during the constant infusion (Whitaker, 1973; Krueger et al, 1980). Alternatively, a furosemide-induced diuresis during an excretory urogram or renal scan (Koff, 1982) can be done to determine the efficiency of pelvic emptying (Segura et al, 1974). The diuresis created during the test may also produce flank pain if the patient has a history of it (Nesbit, 1956). The intermittent nature of the signs and symptoms in these patients is usually associated with a vessel crossing the ureteropelvic junction, which causes the obstruction.

It is imperative to obtain a voiding cystourethrogram in every patient with ureteropelvic junction obstruction to rule out the possibility of obstruction secondary to vesicoureteral reflux (Whitaker, 1976; Lebowitz and Blickman, 1983).

PROGNOSIS. As more kidneys with ureteropelvic junction obstruction are detected in the perinatal period, a debate has raged regarding the timing of surgical correction. Early in the 1980s prenatal decompression was thought to be mandatory if salvageable renal function was the goal (Manning, 1987). This proved to be unnecessarily aggressive treatment, and now it is universally accepted that prenatal intervention is warranted only in cases of bilateral progressive obstruction associated with increasing oligohydramnios. Even in these cases, this treatment is controversial because it has not been proved that renal function and, secondarily, pulmonary function is retained (Mandell et al, 1990).

Several investigators have shown that early but not immediate postnatal intervention is safe, reliable, and effective in allowing the affected kidney to regain a considerable portion of its potentially recoverable renal function (Perlmutter et al, 1980; Roth and Gonzales, 1983; King et al, 1984; Tapia and Gonzalez, 1995). This is especially true for children younger than 1 year old in whom renal function was reduced to less than 45% in the obstructed kidney preoperatively (Tapia and Gonzalez, 1995). These investigators also showed that somatic growth was affected as well, with 72% of children younger than 1 year being below the 50th percentile in height preoperatively, but only 40% were below that percentile postoperatively.

On the other hand, Ransley (1990), Cartwright and colleagues (1992), and MacNeily and associates (1993) showed that little deterioration in renal function occurred in children with moderate obstruction who were followed nonoperatively for 5 to 7 years. One third of these children underwent pyeloplasty at a later age because of the secondary effects of obstruction (i.e., calculus disease, pain, and urinary infection). Even newborns with moderately severe degrees of obstruction with normal (Koff and Campbell, 1992) or diminished (Koff and Campbell, 1994) function do not seem to lose more function when followed nonoperatively. But these findings are not universally accepted because Homsy and colleagues (1990) noted a 20% decrease in drainage when babies with obstructed kidneys by diuretic renography criteria (T 1/2 washout of more than 20 minutes and residual isotope in the pelvis of more than 25% at 30 minutes) were followed nonoperatively (Fig. 58–49). Thus, controversy exists between those who favor careful observation (Duckett, 1993) and those who favor early corrective surgery (Woodard, 1993). This dilemma may not be resolved until a prospective randomized trial of surgery versus observation is undertaken in affected babies (Allen, 1992).

When the diagnosis is not made until later in childhood or early adulthood, severe chronic obstruction may lead to progressive loss of renal function. With severe stasis and recurrent infections, stone formation sometimes occurs. Renin-mediated hypertension secondary to obstruction may also develop. Repair of the obstruction is warranted to mitigate against the long-term sequalae of this condition.

Even in older individuals most obstructed kidneys can be salvaged by pyeloplasty. A quantitative renal scan using technetium-99-labeled DMSA that determines individual renal function is sometimes helpful in deciding whether to perform a nephrectomy or pyeloplasty, especially when the excretory urogram reveals a kidney with poor concentrating ability and nonvisualization on delayed postinjection films. Most affected kidneys that provide at least one third of

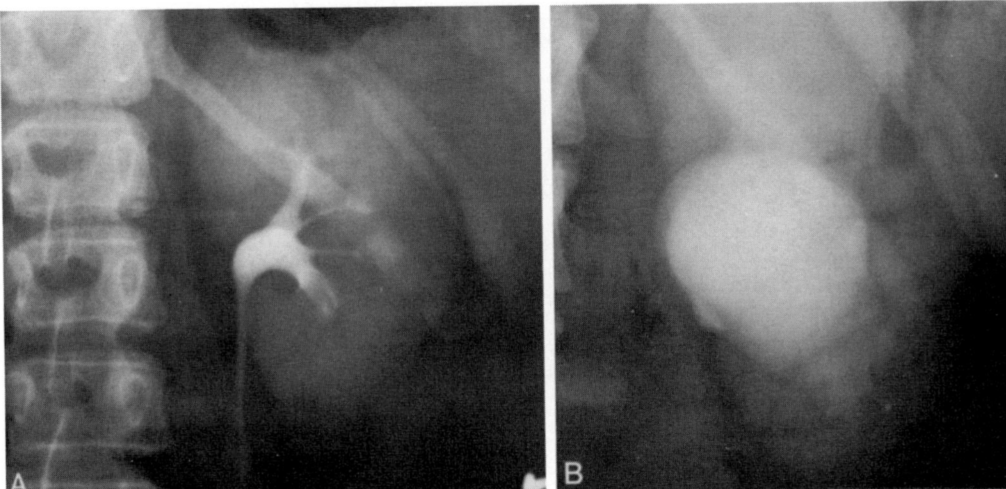

Figure 58–48. *A* and *B*, A 16-year-old boy with intermittent flank pain has a normal collecting system when asymptomatic but severe obstruction when symptomatic.

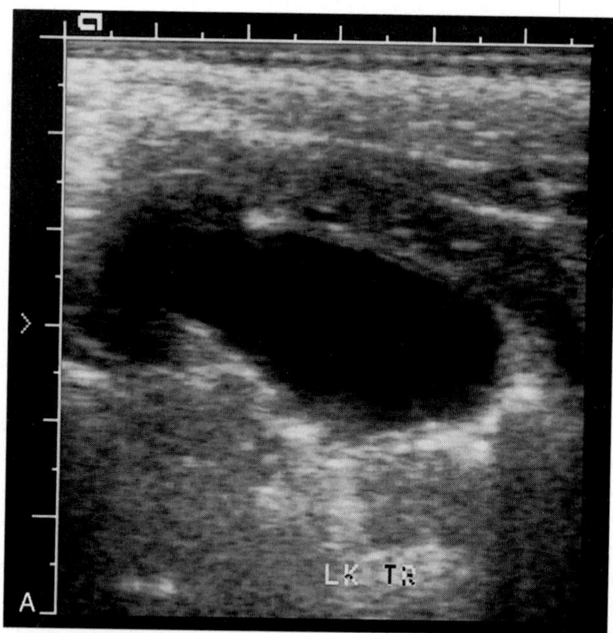

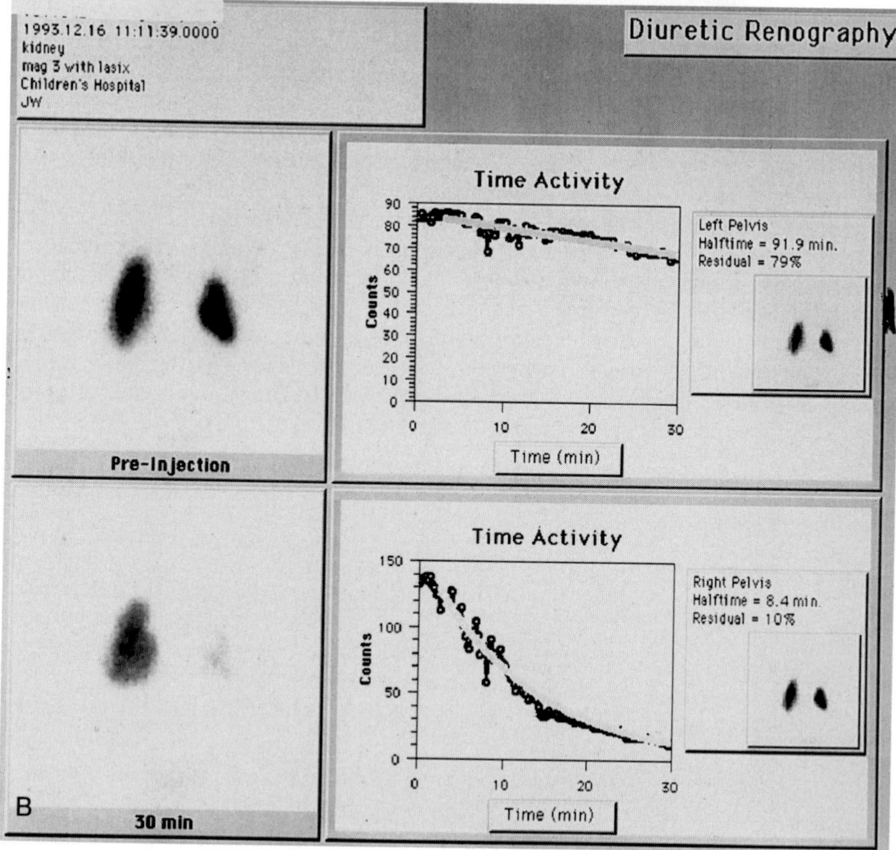

Figure 58–49. *A,* Postnatal renal ultrasound in a newborn girl with prenatally detected hydronephrosis reveals a markedly enlarged left renal pelvis, dilated calyces, and thinned parenchyma.

B, An MAG-3 Lasix renogram demonstrated prolonged washout of radionuclide of the left kidney (as compared with the right kidney) with a calculated T 1/2 time greater than 20 minutes and a residual amount of radioactivity after 30 minutes of more than 50% of the excreted dose.

overall renal function can be saved. Even poorly functioning kidneys (between 10% and 25% function) show some improvement after surgery (Parker et al, 1981; Belis et al, 1982). Only rarely do such kidneys have less than 10% of overall renal function at presentation, and these should probably be removed. The techniques of surgical correction are discussed elsewhere in the text.

REFERENCES

Anomalies of Number

Bilateral Agenesis

Ashley DJB, Mostofi FK: Renal agenesis and dysgenesis. J Urol 1960;83:211.

Bain AD, Scott JS: Renal agenesis and severe urinary tract dysplasia: A review of 50 cases, with particular reference to associated anomalies. Br Med J 1960;1:841.

Bain AD, Beath MM, Flint WF: Sirenomelia and monomelia with renal agenesis in amnion nodosum. Arch Dis Child 1960;35:250.

Carpentier PJ, Potter EL: Nuclear sex and genital malformation in 48 cases of renal agenesis with special reference to nonspecific female pseudohermaphroditism. Am J Obstet Gynecol 1959;78:235.

Cilento BG Jr, Benacerraf BR, Mandell J: Prenatal and postnatal findings in monochorionic, monoamniotic twins discordant for bilateral renal agenesis-dysgenesis (perinatal lethal renal disease). J Urol 1994; 151:1034–1035.

Clark DA: Times of first void and first stool in 500 newborns. Pediatrics 1977;60:457.

Clemmons JJW: Embryonic renal injury: a possible factor in fetal malnutrition. Pediatr Res 1977;11:404.

Davidson WM, Ross GIM: Bilateral absence of the kidneys and related congenital anomalies. J Pathol Bacteriol 1954;68:459.

Dicker D, Samuel N, Feldberg D, Goldman JA: The antenatal diagnosis of Potter syndrome—a lethal and not so rare malformation. Eur J Obstet Gynecol Reprod Biol 1984;18:17.

Fitch N, Lachance RC: The pathogenesis of Potter's syndrome of renal agenesis. Can Med Assoc J 1972;107:653.

Hislop A, Hey EJ, Reid L: The lungs in congenital bilateral renal agenesis and dysplasia. Arch Dis Child 1979;54:32.

Hoffman CK, Filly RA, Allen PW: The "lying down" adrenal sign: A sonographic indicator of renal agenesis or ectopia in fetuses and neonates. J Ultrasound Med 1992;11:533.

Katz SH, Chatten J: The urethra in bilateral renal agenesis. Arch Pathol 1974;97:269.

Kohler HG: An unusual case of sirenomelia. Teratology 1972;6:659.

Kovacs T, Csecsei K, Toth L, Papp Z: Familial occurrence of bilateral renal agenesis. Acta Paediatr Hung 1991;31:13.

Levin H: Bilateral renal agenesis. J Urol 1952;67:86.

Mauer SM, Dobrin RS, Vernier RL: Unilateral and bilateral renal agenesis in monoamniotic twins. J Pediatr 1974;84:236.

McPherson E, Carey J, Kramer A, et al: Dominantly inherited renal adysplasia. Am J Med Genet 1987;26:863.

Moerman P, Fryns JP, Sastrowijoto SH, et al: Hereditary renal adysplasia: New observations and hypotheses. Pediatr Pathol 1994;14:405.

Murugasu B, Cole BR, Hawkins EP, et al: Familial renal dysplasia. Am J Kidney Dis 1991;18:490.

Novak RW, Robinson HB: Coincident DiGeorge anomaly and renal agenesis and its relation to maternal diabetes. Am J Med Genet 1994;50:311.

O'Connor TA, LaCour ML, Friedlander ER, Thomas R: Penile agenesis associated with urethral and bilateral renal agenesis. Urology 1993; 41:564.

Perlman M, Williams J, Hirsh M: Neonatal pulmonary hypoplasia after prolonged leakage of amniotic fluid. Arch Dis Child 1976;51:349.

Potter EL: Bilateral renal agenesis. J Pediatr 1946a;29:68.

Potter EL: Facial characteristics in infants with bilateral renal agenesis. Am J Obstet Gynecol 1946b;51:885.

Potter EL: Pathology of the Fetus and the Newborn. Chicago, Year Book Medical Publishers, 1952.

Potter EL: Bilateral absence of ureters and kidneys. A report of 50 cases. Obstet Gynecol 1965;25:3.

Rayburn WF, Laferla JJ: Mid-gestational abortion for medical or genetic indications. Clin Obstet Gynecol 1986;13:71.

Reid L: The lung: its growth and remodeling in health and disease. Am J Roentgenol 1977;129:777.

Rizza JM, Downing SE: Bilateral renal agenesis in two female siblings. Am J Dis Child 1971;121:60.

Roodhooft AM, Birnholz JC, Holmes LD: Familial nature of congenital absence and severe dysgenesis of both kidneys. N Engl J Med 1984;310:1341.

Selby GW, Parmelee AH Jr: Bilateral renal agenesis and oligohydramnios. J Pediatr 1976;48:70.

Sherry SN, Kramer I: The time of passage of first stool and first urine by the newborn infant. J Pediatr 1955;46:158.

Sirtori M, Ghidini A, Romero R, Hobbins JC: Prenatal diagnosis of sirenomelia. J Ultrasound Med 1989;8:83.

Stroup NE, Edmonds L, O'Brien TR: Renal agenesis and dysgenesis: Are they increasing? Teratology 1990;42:383–395.

Thomas IT, Smith DW: Oligohydramnios, cause of the nonrenal features of Potter's syndrome, including pulmonary hypoplasia. J Pediatr 1974; 84:811.

Thompson VM: Amnion nodosum. J Obstet Gynaecol Br Commonw 1960;67:611.

Williams DI: Personal communication, 1974.

Wilson RD, Baird PA: Renal agenesis in British Columbia. Am J Med Genet 1985;21:153.

Wolf EL, Berdon WE, Baker DH, et al: Diagnosis of oligohydramnios-related pulmonary hypoplasia (Potter syndrome): Value of portable voiding cystourethrography in newborns with respiratory distress. Radiology 1977;125:769.

Unilateral Agenesis

Anders JM: Congenital single kidney with report of a case. The practical significance of the condition with statistics. Am J Med Sci 1910;139:313.

Anderson EE, Harrison JH: Surgical importance of the solitary kidney. N Engl J Med 1965;273:683.

Arfeen S, Rosborough D, Luger M, Nolph KD: Familial renal agenesis and focal and segmental glomerulosclerosis. Am J Kidney Dis 1993;21:663.

Argueso LR, Ritchey ML, Boyle ET Jr, et al: Prognosis of patients with unilateral renal agenesis. Pediatr Nephrol 1992;6:412.

Ashley DJB, Mostofi FK: Renal agenesis and dysgenesis. J Urol 1960;83:211.

Atiyeh B, Husmann D, Baum M: Contralateral renal anomalies in patients with renal agenesis and noncystic renal dysplasia. Pediatrics 1993;91:812.

Barry JE, Auldist AW: The VATER Association. Am J Dis Child 1974;128:769.

Battin J, Lacombe D, Leng JJ: Familial occurrence of hereditary renal adysplasia with müllerian anomalies. Clin Genet 1993;43:23.

Beeby DI: Seminal vesicle cysts associated with ipsilateral renal agenesis: Case report and review of literature. J Urol 1974;112:120.

Biedel CW, Pagon RA, Zapata JO: Müllerian anomalies and renal agenesis: Autosomal dominant urogenital adysplasia. J Pediatr 1984;104:861.

Bryan AL, Nigro JA, Counseller VS: One hundred cases of congenital absence of the vagina. Surg Gynecol Obstet 1949;88:79.

Campbell MF: Congenital absence of one kidney: Unilateral renal agenesis. Ann Surg 1928;88:1039.

Charny CW, Gillenwater JY: Congenital absence of the vas deferens. J Urol 1965;93:399.

Collins DC: Congenital unilateral renal agenesis. Ann Surg 1932;95:715.

Cope JR, Trickey SE: Congenital absence of the kidney: problems in diagnosis and management. J Urol 1982;127:10.

Currarino G: Single vaginal ectopic ureter and Gartner's duct cyst with ipsilateral renal hypoplasia and dysplasia (or agenesis). J Urol 1982; 128:988.

Curtis JA, Sadhu V, Steiner RM: Malposition of the colon in right renal agenesis, ectopia and anterior nephrectomy. Am J Roentgenol 1977; 129:845.

D'Alberton A, Reshini E, Ferrari N, Candiani P: Prevalence of urinary tract abnormalities in a large series of patients with uterovaginal atresia. J Urol 1981;126:623.

Dees JE: Prognosis of the solitary kidney. J Urol 1960;83:550.

Donohue RE, Fauver HE: Unilateral absence of the vas deferens. JAMA 1989;261:1180.

Doroshow LW, Abeshouse BS: Congenital unilateral solitary kidney: Report of 37 cases and a review of the literature. Urol Surv 1961;11:219.

Emanuel B, Nachman RP, Aronson N, Weiss H: Congenital solitary kidney: A review of 74 cases. Am J Dis Child 1974;127:17.
Fortune CH: The pathological and clinical significance of congenital one-sided kidney defect with the presentation of three new cases of agenesis and one of aplasia. Ann Intern Med 1927;1:377.
Furtado AJL: The three cases of cystic seminal vesicle associated with unilateral renal agenesis. Br J Urol 1973;45:536.
Gilliland B, Dick F: Uterus didelphys associated with unilateral imperforate vagina. Obstet Gynecol 1976;48(Suppl 1):5s.
Gutierrez R: Surgical aspects of renal agenesis: With special reference to hypoplastic kidney, renal aplasia and congenital absence of one kidney. Arch Surg 1933;27:686.
Hitchcock R, Burge DM: Renal agenesis: An acquired condition. J Pediatr Surg 1994;29:454.
Hoffman CK, Filly RA, Callen PW: The "lying down" adrenal sign: A sonographic indicator of renal agenesis or ectopia in fetuses and neonates. J Ultrasound Med 1992;11:533.
Holt SA, Peterson NE: Ectopia of seminal vesicle: Associated with agenesis of ipsilateral kidney. Urology 1974;4:322.
Hynes DM, Watkin EM: Renal agenesis—roentgenologic problem. Am J Roentgenol 1970;110:772.
Jancu J, Zuckerman H, Sudarsky M: Unilateral renal agenesis associated with multiple abnormalities. South Med J 1976;69:94.
Kenny PJ, Robbins GL, Ellis DA, Spert BA: Adrenal glands in patients with congenital renal anomalies: Computed tomography appearance. Radiology 1985;155:181.
Kohn G, Borns PF: The association of bilateral and unilateral renal aplasia in the same family. J Pediatr 1973;83:95.
Kroovand RL: Cystoscopy. *In* Kelalis PP, King LR, Belman AB, eds: Clinical Pediatric Urology. Philadelphia, W. B. Saunders, 1985.
Limkakeng AD, Retik AB: Unilateral renal agenesis with hypoplastic ureter: Observations on the contralateral urinary tract and report of four cases. J Urol 1972;108:149.
Longo VJ, Thompson GJ: Congenital solitary kidney. J Urol 1952;68:63.
Mace JW, Kaplan JM, Schanberger JE, Gotlin RW: Poland's syndrome: Report of seven cases and review of the literature. Clin Pediatr 1972;11:98.
Magee MC, Lucey DT, Fried FA: A new embryologic classification for uro-gynecologic malformations: The syndromes of mesonephric duct induced müllerian deformities. J Urol 1979;121:265.
Mascatello V, Lebowitz RL: Malposition of the colon in left renal agenesis and ectopia. Radiology 1976;120:371.
McPherson E, Carey J, Kramer A, et al: Dominantly inherited renal adysplasia. Am J Med Genet 1987;26:863.
Mesrobian HG, Rushton HG, Bulas D: Unilateral renal agenesis may result from in utero regression of multicystic renal dysplasia. J Urol 1993;150:793.
Nomura S, Osawa G: Focal glomerular sclerotic lesions in a patient with urinary oligomeganephronia and agenesis of the contralateral kidney: A case report. Clin Nephrol 1990;33:7.
Novak RW, Robinson HB: Coincident DiGeorge anomaly and renal agenesis and its relation to maternal diabetes. Am J Med Genet 1994;50:311.
Ochsner MG, Brannan W, Goodier EH: Absent vas deferens associated with renal agenesis. JAMA 1972;222:1055.
Phelan JT, Counseller VS, Greene LF: Deformities of the urinary tract with congenital absence of the vagina. Surg Gynecol Obstet 1953;97:1.
Radasch HE: Congenital unilateral absence of the urogenital system and its relation to the development of the Wolffian and Muellerian ducts. Am J Med Sci 1908;136:111.
Roodhooft AM, Birnholz JC, Holmes LD: Familial nature of congenital absence and severe dysgenesis of both kidneys. N Engl J Med 1984;310:1341.
Rugui C, Oldrizzi L, Lupo A, et al: Clinical features of patients with solitary kidneys. Nephron 1986;43:10.
Say B, Gerald PS: A new polydactyly/imperforate-anus/vertebral anomalies syndrome? Lancet 1968;1:688.
Selig AM, Benacerraf B, Greene MF, et al: Renal dysplasia, megalocystis and sirenomelia in four siblings. Teratology 1993;47:65.
Semmens JP: Congenital anomalies of the female genital tract: functional classification based on review of 56 personal cases and 500 reported cases. Obstet Gynecol 1962;19:328.
Shieh CP, Hung CS, Wei CF, Lin CY: Cystic dilatations within the pelvis in patients with ipsilateral renal agenesis or dysplasia. J Urol 1990;144:324.
Shumacker HB: Congenital anomalies of the genitalia associated with unilateral renal agenesis. Arch Surg 1938;37:586.
Smith EC, Orkin LA: A clinical and statistical study of 471 congenital anomalies of the kidney and ureter. J Urol 1945;53:11.
Thompson DP, Lynn HB: Genital anomalies associated with solitary kidney. Mayo Clin Proc 1966;41:538.
Uchida S, Akiba T, Sasaki S, et al: Unilateral renal agenesis associated with various metabolic disorders in three siblings. Nephron 1990;54:86.
Vinstein AL, Franken EA Jr: Unilateral hematocolpos associated with agenesis of the kidney. Radiology 1972;102:625.
Weiss JM, Dykhuizen RF: An anomalous vaginal insertion into the bladder: A case report. J Urol 1967;98:60.
Whitaker RH, Hunt GM: Incidence and distribution of renal anomalies in patients with neural tube defects. Eur Urol 1987;13:322.
Wiersma AF, Peterson LF, Justema EJ: Uterine anomalies associated with unilateral renal agenesis. Obstet Gynecol 1976;47:654.
Wilson RD, Baird PA: Renal agenesis in British Columbia. Am J Med Genet 1993;21:153.
Wilson TA, Blethen SL, Vallone A, et al: DiGeorge anomaly with renal agenesis in infants of mothers with diabetes. Am J Med Genet 1993;47:1078.
Woolf RB, Allen WM: Concomitant malformations: The frequent simultaneous occurrence of congenital malformations of the reproductive and urinary tracts. Obstet Gynecol 1953;2:236.
Yoder IC, Pfister RC: Unilateral hematocolpos and ipsilateral renal agenesis: Report of two cases and review of the literature. Am J Roentgenol 1976;127:303.

Supernumerary Kidney

Campbell MF: Anomalies of the kidney. *In* Campbell MF, Harrison JH, eds: Urology, Vol. 2, 3rd ed. Philadelphia, W. B. Saunders, 1970, p 1422.
Carlson HE: Supernumerary kidney: A summary of fifty-one reported cases. J Urol 1950;64:221.
Conrad GR, Loes DJ: Ectopic supernumerary kidney. Functional assessment using radionuclide imaging. Clin Nucl Med 1987;12:253.
Exley M, Hotchkiss WS: Supernumerary kidney with clear cell carcinoma. J Urol 1944;51:569.
Geisinger JF: Supernumerary kidney. J Urol 1937;38:331.
Hoffman RL, McMillan TE: Discussion. Trans South Central Sec, American Urology Assoc 1948;82.
Kaneoya F, Botoh B, Yokokawa M: Unusual duplication of renal collecting system mimicking supernumerary kidney. Nippon Hinyokika Bakkai Zasshi 1989;80:270.
Kretschmer HL: Supernumerary kidney. Report of a case with review of the literature. Surg Gynecol Obstet 1929;49:818.
McPherson RI: Supernumerary kidney: Typical and atypical features. Can Assoc Radiol J 1987;38:116.
N'Guessan G, Stephens FD: Supernumerary kidney. J Urol 1983;130:649.
Rubin JS: Supernumerary kidney with aberrant ureter terminating externally. J Urol 1948;61:405.
Sasidharan K, Babu AS, Rao MM, Bhat HS: Free supernumerary kidney. Br J Urol 1976;48:388.
Shan JH: Supernumerary kidney with vaginal ureteral orifice. J Urol 1942;47:344.
Tada Y, Kokado Y, Hashinaka Y, et al: Free supernumerary kidney: a case report and review. J Urol 1981;126:231.

Anomalies of Ascent

Simple Renal Ectopia

Abeshouse BS, Bhisitkul I: Crossed renal ectopia with and without fusion. Urol Int 1959;9:63.
Anderson EE, Harrison JH: Surgical importance of the solitary kidney. N Engl J Med 1965;273:683.
Anderson GW, Rice GG, Harris BA Jr: Pregnancy and labor complicated by pelvic ectopic kidney. J Urol 1951;65:760.
Anderson GW, Rice GG, Harris BA Jr: Pregnancy and labor complicated by pelvic ectopic kidney anomalies. A review of the literature. Obstet Gynecol Surv 1949;4:737.
Anson BJ, Riba LW: The anatomical and surgical features of ectopic kidney. Surg Gynecol Obstet 1939;68:37.
Baggenstoss AH: Congenital anomalies of the kidney. Med Clin North Am 1951;35:987.
Bell ET: Renal Diseases. Philadelphia, Lea & Febiger, 1946.
Borer JG, Corgan FJ, Krantz R, et al: Unilateral single vaginal ectopic

ureter with ipsilateral hypoplastic pelvic kidney and bicornuate uterus. J Urol 1993;149:1124.
Campbell MF: Renal ectopy. J Urol 1930;24:187.
Chang TD, Carr MC, Bauer SB: Occult manifestations of extravesical ectopic ureters causing incontinence. Presented at the Annual Meeting of the New England Section of the American Urological Association, Toronto, Canada, September 15, 1992. (Abstract No. P30.)
D'Alberton A, Reschini E, Ferrari N, Candiani P: Prevalence of urinary tract abnormalities in a large series of patients with uterovaginal atresia. J Urol 1981;126:623.
Delson B: Ectopic kidney in obstetrics and gynecology. NY State J Med 1975;75:2522.
Downs RA, Lane JW, Burns E: Solitary pelvic kidney: Its clinical implications. Urology 1973;1:51.
Dretler SP, Olsson CA, Pfister RC: The anatomic, radiologic and clinical characteristics of the pelvic kidney, an analysis of 86 cases. J Urol 1971;105:623.
Fowler HA: Bilateral renal ectopia. A report of four additional cases. J Urol 1941;45:795.
Gleason PE, Kelalis PP, Husmann DA, Kramer SA: Hydronephrosis in renal ectopia: Incidence, etiology and significance. J Urol 1994;151:1660.
Hawes CJ: Congenital unilateral ectopic kidney: A report of two cases. J Urol 1950;64:453.
Malek RS, Kelalis PP, Burke EC: Ectopic kidney in children and frequency of association of other malformations. Mayo Clin Proc 1971;46:461.
McCrea LE: Congenital solitary pelvic kidney. J Urol 1942;48:58.
Stevens AR: Pelvic single kidneys. J Urol 1937;37:610.
Tabisky J, Bhisitkul I: Solitary crossed ectopic kidney with vaginal aplasia: A case report. J Urol 1965;94:33.
Thompson GJ, Pace JM: Ectopic kidney: A review of 97 cases. Surg Gynecol Obstet 1937;64:935.
Ward JN, Nathanson B, Draper JW: The pelvic kidney. J Urol 1965;94:36.

Cephalad Renal Ectopia

Pinckney LE, Moskowitz PS, Lebowitz RL, Fritzsche P: Renal malposition associated with omphalocele. Radiology 1978;129:677.

Thoracic Kidney

Ang AH, Chan WF: Ectopic thoracic kidney. J Urol 1972;108:211.
Angulo JC, Lopez JI, Vilanova JR, Flores N: Intrathoracic kidney and vertebral fusion: A model of combined misdevelopment. J Urol 1992;147:1351.
Barloon JW, Goodwin WEJ: Thoracic kidney: Case reports. J Urol 1957;78:356.
Berlin HS, Stein J, Poppel MH: Congenital superior ectopia of the kidney. Am J Roentgenol 1957;78:508.
Burke EC, Wenzl JE, Utz DC: The intrathoracic kidney. Report of a case. Am J Dis Child 1967;113:487.
Campbell MF: Renal ectopy. J Urol 1930;24:187.
DeCastro FJ, Shumacher H: Asymptomatic thoracic kidney. Clin Pediatr 1969;8:279.
DeNoronha LL, Costa MFE, Godinho MTM: Ectopic thoracic kidney. Am Rev Respir Dis 1974;109:678.
Donat SM, Donat PE: Intrathoracic kidney: A case report with a review of the world's literature. J Urol 1988;140:131.
Franciskovic V, Martincic N: Intrathoracic kidney. Br J Urol 1959;31:156.
Fusonie D, Molnar W: Anomalous pulmonary venous return, pulmonary sequestration, bronchial atresia, aplastic right upper lobe, pericardial defect and intrathoracic kidney. An unusual complex of congenital anomalies in one patient. Am J Roentgenol 1966;97:350.
Gray SW, Skandalakis JE: The diaphragm. *In* Embryology for Surgeons. Philadelphia, W. B. Saunders, 1972, pp 359–366.
Hertz M, Shahin N: Ectopic thoracic kidney. Isr J Med Sci 1969;5:98.
Hill JE, Bunts RC: Thoracic kidney: Case reports. J Urol 1960;84:460.
Liddell RM, Rosenbaum DM, Blumhagen JD: Delayed radiologic appearance of bilateral thoracic ectopic kidneys. Am J Roentgenol 1989; 152:120.
Lozano RH, Rodriguez C: Intrathoracic ectopic kidney: Report of a case. J Urol 1975;114:601.
Lundius B: Intrathoracic kidney. Am J Roentgenol 1975;125:678.
N'Guessan G, Stephens FD: Congenital superior ectopic (thoracic) kidney. Urology 1984;24:219.
Paul ATS, Uragoda CG, Jayewardene FLW: Thoracic kidney with report of a case. Br J Surg 1960;47:395.
Robbins JJ, Lich R, Jr: Thoracic kidney. J Urol 1954;72:133.
Shapira E, Fishel E, Levin S: Intrathoracic kidney in a premature infant. Arch Dis Child 1965;40:86.
Spillane RJ, Prather GC: Right diaphragmatic eventration with renal displacement. Case report. J Urol 1952;68:804.
Williams AG, Christie JH, Mettler SA: Intrathoracic kidney on radionuclide renography. Clin Nucl Med 1983;8:408.

Anomalies of Form and Fusion

Crossed Renal Ectopia With and Without Fusion

Abeshouse BS: Crossed ectopia with fusion: Review of literature and a report of four cases. Am J Surg 1947;73:658.
Abeshouse BS, Bhisitkul I: Crossed renal ectopia with and without fusion. Urol Int 1959;9:63.
Alexander JC, King KB, Fromm CS: Congenital solitary kidney with crossed ureter. J Urol 1950;64:230.
Ashley DJB, Mostofi FK: Renal agenesis and dysgenesis. J Urol 1960; 83:211.
Baggenstoss AH: Congenital anomalies of the kidney. Med Clin North Am 1951;35:987.
Bauer SB: Personal communication, 1977.
Bissada NK, Fried FA, Redman JF: Crossed-fused renal ectopia with a solitary ureter. J Urol 1975;114:304.
Boatman DL, Culp DA Jr, Culp DA, Flocks RH: Crossed renal ectopia. J Urol 1972;108:30.
Caine M: Crossed renal ectopia without fusion. Br J Urol 1956;28:257.
Caldamone AA, Rabinowitz R: Crossed fused renal ectopia, orthotopic multicystic dysplasia and vaginal agenesis. J Urol 1981;126:105.
Campbell MF: Renal ectopy. J Urol 1930;24:187.
Cass AS, Vitko RJ: Unusual variety of crossed renal ectopy with only one ureter. J Urol 1972;107:1056.
Cook WA, Stephens FD: Fused kidneys: Morphologic study and theory of embryogenesis. *In* Bergsma D, Duckett JW, eds: Urinary System Malformations in Children. New York, Allen R. Liss, 1977.
Currarino G, Weisbruch GJ: Transverse fusion of the renal pelves and single ureter. Urol Radiol 1989;11:88.
Diaz G: Renal ectopy: Report of a case with crossed ectopy without fusion, with fixation of kidney in normal position by the extraperitoneal route. J Int Coll Surg 1953;19:158.
Dretler SP, Olsson CA, Pfister RC: The anatomic, radiologic and clinical characteristics of the pelvic kidney: An analysis of eighty-six cases. J Urol 1971;105:623.
Gerber WL, Culp DA, Brown RC, et al: Renal mass in crossed-fused ectopia. J Urol 1980;123:239.
Gleason PE, Kelalis PP, Husmann DA, Kramer SA: Hydronephrosis in renal ectopia: Incidence, etiology and significance. J Urol 1994;151:1660.
Glenn JF: Fused pelvic kidney. J Urol 1958;80:7.
Greenberg LW, Nelsen CE: Crossed fused ectopia of the kidneys in twins. Am J Dis Child 1971;122:175.
Gu L, Alton DJ: Crossed solitary renal ectopia. Urology 1991;38:556.
Hendren WH, Donahoe PK, Pfister RC: Crossed renal ectopia in children. Urology 1976;7:135.
Hertz M, Rabenstein ZJ, Shalrin N, Melzer M: Crossed renal ectopia: clinical and radiologic findings in 22 cases. Clin Radiol 1977;28:339.
Hildreth TA, Cass AS: Cross renal ectopia with familial occurrence. Urology 1978;12:59.
Joly JS: Fusion of the kidneys. Proc R Soc Med 1940;33:697.
Kakei H, Kondo A, Ogisu BI, Mitsuya H: Crossed ectopia of solitary kidney: A report of two cases and a review of the literature. Urol Int 1976;31:40.
Kelalis PP, Malek RS, Segura JW: Observations on renal ectopia and fusion in children. J Urol 1973;110:588.
Kretschmer HL: Unilateral fused kidney. Surg Gynecol Obstet 1925;40:360.
Kron SD, Meranze DR: Completely fused pelvic kidney. J Urol 1949; 62:278.
Lee HP: Crossed unfused renal ectopia with tumor. J Urol 1949;61:333.
Looney WW, Dodd DL: An ectopic (pelvic) completely fused (cake) kidney associated with various anomalies of the abdominal viscera. Ann Surg 1956;84:522.
Macksood MJ, James RE Jr: Giant hydronephrosis in ectopic kidney in a child. Urology 1983;22:532.
Magri J: Solitary crossed ectopic kidney. Br J Urol 1961;33:152.
Maizels M, Stephens FD: Renal ectopia and congenital scoliosis. Invest Urol 1979;17:209.

Malek RS, Utz DC: Crossed, fused, renal ectopia with an ectopic ureterocele. J Urol 1970;104:665.
McDonald JH, McClellan DS: Crossed renal ectopia. Am J Surg 1957;93:995.
Miles BJ, Moon MR, Bellville WD, Keesling VJ: Solitary crossed renal ectopia. J Urol 1985;133:1022.
Mininberg DT, Roze S, Yoon HJ, Pearl M: Hypertension associated with crossed renal ectopia in an infant. Pediatrics 1971;48:454.
Nussbaum AR, Hartman DS, Whitley N, et al: Multicystic dysplasia and crossed renal ectopia. Am J Roentgenol 1987;149:407.
Pathak IC: Crossed renal ectopia without fusion associated with giant hydronephrosis. J Urol 1965;94:323.
Potter EL: Pathology of the Fetus and the Newborn. Chicago, Year Book Medical Publishers, 1952.
Purpon I: Crossed renal ectopy with solitary kidney: A review of the literature. J Urol 1963;90:13.
Rubinstein ZJ, Hertz M, Shahin N, Deutsch V: Crossed renal ectopia: Angiographic findings in six cases. Am J Roentgenol 1976;126:1035.
Shah MH: Solitary crossed renal ectopia. Br J Urol 1975;47:512.
Srivastava RN, Singh M, Ghai OP, Sethi U: Complete renal fusion ("cake"/ "lump" kidney). Br J Urol 1971;43:391.
Stubbs AJ, Resnick MI: Struvite staghorn calculi in crossed renal ectopia. J Urol 1977;118:369.
Tabrisky J, Bhisitkul I: Solitary crossed ectopic kidney with vaginal aplasia: A case report. J Urol 1965;94:33.
Tanenbaum B, Silverman N, Weinberg SR: Solitary crossed renal ectopia. Arch Surg 1970;101:616.
Thompson GJ, Allen RB: Unilateral fused kidney. Surg Clin North Am 1934;14:729.
Wilmer HA: Unilateral fused kidney: A report of five cases and a review of the literature. J Urol 1938;40:551.
Winram RG, Ward-McQuaid JN: Crossed renal ectopia without fusion. Can Med Assoc J 1959;81:481.
Yates-Bell AJ, Packham DA: Giant hydronephrosis in a solitary crossed ectopic kidney. Br J Surg 1972;59:104.

Horseshoe Kidney

Advisory Committee to the Renal Transplant Registry: The twelfth report of Human Renal Transplant Registry. JAMA 1975;233:787.
Beck WC, Hlivko AE: Wilms' tumor in the isthmus of a horseshoe kidney. Arch Surg 1960;81:803.
Bell R: Horseshoe kidney in pregnancy. J Urol 1946;56:159.
Benjamin JA, Schullian DM: Observation on fused kidneys with horseshoe configuration: The contribution of Leonardo Botallo (1564). J Hist Med Allied Sci 1950;5:315.
Blackard CE, Mellinger GT: Cancer in a horseshoe kidney. Arch Surg 1968;97:616.
Boatman DL, Cornell SH, Kolln CP: The arterial supply of horseshoe kidney. Am J Roentgenol 1971;113:447.
Boatman DL, Kolln CP, Flocks RH: Congenital anomalies associated with horseshoe kidney. J Urol 1972;107:205.
Boullier J, Chehval MJ, Purcell MH: Removal of a multicystic half of a horseshoe kidney: Significance of pre-operative evaluation in identifying abnormal surgical anatomy. J Pediatr Surg 1992;27:1244.
Boyden EA: Description of a horseshoe kidney associated with left inferior vena cava and disc-shaped suprarenal glands, together with a note on the occurrence of horseshoe kidneys in human embryos. Anat Rec 1931; 51:187.
Bridge RAC: Horseshoe kidneys in identical twins. Br J Urol 1960;32:32.
Buntley D: Malignancy associated with horseshoe kidney. Urology 1976;8:146.
Campbell MF: Anomalies of the kidney. *In* Campbell MF, Harrison JH, eds: Urology, Vol. 2, 3rd ed. Philadelphia, W. B. Saunders, 1970, pp 1447–1452.
Castor JE, Green NA: Complications of horseshoe kidney. Urology 1975;6:344.
Christoffersen J, Iversen HG: Partial hydronephrosis in a patient with horseshoe kidney and bilateral duplication of the pelvis and ureter. Scand J Urol Nephrol 1976;10:91.
Cook WA, Stephens FD: Fused kidneys: Morphologic study and theory of embryogenesis. *In* Bergsma D, Duckett JW, eds: Urinary Systems Malformations in Children. New York, Allen R. Liss, 1977.
Correa RJ Jr, Paton RR: Polycystic horseshoe kidney. J Urol 1976;116:802.
Craver RD, Ortenberg J, Baliga R: Glomerulocystic disease: Unilateral involvement of a horseshoe kidney in trisomy 18. Pediatr Nephrol 1993;7:375.
Dajani AM: Horseshoe kidney: A review of twenty-nine cases. Br J Urol 1966;38:388.
Das S, Amar AD: Ureteropelvic junction obstruction with associated renal anomalies. J Urol 1984;131:872.
David RS: Horseshoe kidney: A report of one family. Br Med J 1974;4:571.
deBrito CJ, Silva LA, Fonseca Filho VL, Fernandes DC: Abdominal aortic aneurysm in association with horseshoe kidney. Int Angiol 1991;10:122.
Dees J: Clinical importance of congenital anomalies of upper urinary tract. J Urol 1941;46:659.
Dische MR, Johnston R: Teratoma in horseshoe kidneys. Urology 1979;13:435.
Domenech-Mateu JM, Gonzales-Compta X: Horseshoe kidney: A new theory on its embryogenesis based on the study of a 16-mm human embryo. Anat Rec 1988;222:408.
Eidelman A, Yuval E, Simon D, Sibi Y: Retrocaval ureter. Eur Urol 1978;4:279.
Evans WP, Resnick MI: Horseshoe kidney and urolithiasis. J Urol 1981;125:620.
Garg RK: Personal communication, 1990.
Glenn JF: Analysis of 51 patients with horseshoe kidney. N Engl J Med 1959;261:684.
Grandone CH, Haller JO, Berdon WE, Friedman AP: Asymmetric horseshoe kidney in the infant: Value of renal nuclear scanning. Radiology 1985;154:366.
Gutierrez R: The Clinical Management of Horseshoe Kidney: A Study of Horseshoe Kidney Disease, Its Etiology, Pathology, Symptomatology, Diagnosis and Treatment. New York, Paul B. Hoeber, 1934.
Hefferman JC, Lightwood RG, Snell ME: Horseshoe kidney with retrocaval ureter: Second reported case. J Urol 1978;120:358.
Hohenfellner M, Schultz-Lampel D, Lampel A, et al: Tumor in the horseshoe kidney: Clinical implications and review of embryogenesis. J Urol 1992;147:1098.
Huber D, Griffin A, Niesche J, et al: Aortic aneurysm in the presence of a horseshoe kidney. Aust NZ J Surg 1990;60:963.
Jarmin WD: Surgery of the horseshoe kidney with a postaortic isthmus: Report of two cases of horseshoe kidney. J Urol 1938;40:1.
Kolln CP, Boatman DL, Schmidt JD, Flocks RH: Horseshoe kidney: A review of 105 patients. J Urol 1972;107:203.
Leiter E: Horseshoe kidney: Discordance in monozygotic twins. J Urol 1972;108:683.
Lippe B, Geffner ME, Dietrich RB, et al: Renal malformations in patients with Turner syndrome: Imaging in 141 patients. Pediatrics 1988;82:852.
Love L, Wasserman D: Massive unilateral nonfunctioning hydronephrosis in horseshoe kidney. Clin Radiol 1975;26:409.
Meek JR, Wadsworth GH: A case of horseshoe kidney lying between the great vessels. J Urol 1940;43:448.
Mesrobian H-GJ, Kelalis PP, Hrabovsky E, et al: Wilms' tumor in horseshoe kidneys: A report from the National Wilms' Tumor Study. J Urol 1985;133:1002.
Murphy DM, Zincke H: Transitional cell carcinoma in the horseshoe kidney: Report of 3 cases and review of the literature. Br J Urol 1982;54:484.
Nation EF: Horseshoe kidney, a study of thirty-two autopsy and nine surgical cases. J Urol 1945;53:762.
Novak ME, Baum NH, Gonzales ET: Horseshoe kidney with multicystic dysplasia associated ureterocele. Urology 1977;10:456.
Pitts WR, Muecke EC: Horseshoe kidneys: A 40 year experience. J Urol 1975;113:743.
Roy JB, Stevens RK: Polycystic horseshoe kidney. Urology 1975;6:222.
Segura JW, Kelalis PP, Burke EG: Horseshoe kidney in children. J Urol 1972;108:333.
Sharma SK, Bapna BC: Surgery of the horseshoe kidney—an experience of 24 patients. Aust NZ J Surg 1986;56:175.
Sherer DM, Woods JR Jr: Antenatal diagnosis of horseshoe kidney. J Ultrasound Med 1992;11:274.
Shoup GD, Pollack HM, Dou JH: Adenocarcinoma occurring in a horseshoe kidney. Arch Surg 1962;84:413.
Silagy JM: The horseshoe kidney and its disease. J Mt Sinai Hosp 1952;18:297.
Smith DW: Recognizable patterns of human malformation; genetic embryologic and clinical aspects. Major Problems in Clinical Pediatrics. 7. Philadelphia, W. B. Saunders, 1970, p 50.
Smith EC, Orkin LA: A clinical and statistical study of 471 congenital anomalies of the kidney and ureter. J Urol 1945;53:11.

Van Every MJ: In utero detection of horseshoe kidney with unilateral multicystic dysplasia. Urology 1992;40:435.
Voisin M, Djernit A, Morin D, et al: Cardiopathies congenitales et malformations urinaires. Arch Mal Coeur 1988;81:703.
Walker D: Personal communication, 1977.
Whitaker RH, Hunt GM: Incidence and distribution of renal anomalies in patients with neural tube defects. Eur Urol 1987;13:322.
Whitehouse GH: Some urographic aspects of the horseshoe kidney anomaly—a review of 59 cases. Clin Radiol 1975;26:107.
Zondek LH, Zondek T: Horseshoe kidney in associated congenital malformations. Urol Int 1964;18:347.

Anomalies of Rotation

Campbell MF: Anomalies of the kidney. *In* Campbell MF, ed: Urology, Vol. 2, 2nd ed. Philadelphia, W. B. Saunders, 1963, p 1589.
Felix W: The development of the urogenital organs. *In* Keibel F, Mall FP, eds: Manual of Human Embryology, Vol. 2. Philadelphia, J. B. Lippincott, 1912, p 752.
Gray SW, Skandalakis JE: The kidney and ureter. *In* Embryology for Surgeons. Philadelphia, W. B. Saunders, 1972, p 480.
Mackie GG, Awang H, Stephens FD: The ureteric orifice: The embryologic key to radiologic status of duplex kidneys. J Pediatr Surg 1975;10:473.
Smith EC, Orkin LA: A clinical and statistical study of 471 congenital anomalies of the kidney and ureter. J Urol 1945;53:11.
Weyrauch HM Jr: Anomalies of renal rotation. Surg Gynecol Obstet 1939;69:183.

Anomalies of Renal Vasculature

Aberrant, Accessory, or Multiple Vessels

Anson BJ, Daseler EH: Common variations in renal anatomy, affecting the blood supply, form and topography. Surg Gynecol Obstet 1961;112:439.
Anson BJ, Kurth LE: Common variations in the renal blood supply. Surg Gynecol Obstet 1955;100:157.
Fraley EE: Dismembered infundibulopyelostomy: Improved technique for correcting vascular obstruction of the superior infundibulum. J Urol 1969;101:144.
Fraley EE: Vascular obstruction of superior infundibulum causing nephralgia. A new syndrome. N Engl J Med 1966;275:1403.
Geyer JR, Poutasse EF: Incidence of multiple renal arteries on aortography. JAMA 1962;182:118.
Graves FT: The aberrant renal artery. J Anat 1956;90:553.
Graves FT: The anatomy of the intrarenal arteries and its application to segmental resection of the kidney. Br J Surg 1954;42:132.
Gray SW, Skandalakis JE: Anomalies of the kidney and ureter. *In* Embryology for Surgeons. Philadelphia, W. B. Saunders, 1972, p 485.
Guggemos E: A rare case of an arterial connection between the left and right kidneys. Ann Surg 1962;156:940.
Merklin RJ, Michele NA: The variant renal and suprarenal blood supply with data on the inferior phrenic, ureteral and gonadal arteries. A statistical analysis based on 185 dissections and review of the literature. J Int Coll Surg 1958;29:41.
Nathan J: Observation on aberrant renal arteries curving around and compressing the renal vein: Possible relationship to orthostatic proteinuria and to orthostatic hypertension. Circulation 1958;18:1131.
Pick JW, Anson BJ: The renal vascular pedicle. J Urol 1940;44:411.
Sampaio FJB, Aragao AHM: Anatomical relationship between the intrarenal arteries and the kidney collecting system. J Urol 1990;143:679.
Sampaio FJB, Aragao AHM: Anatomical relationship between the renal venous arrangement and the kidney collecting system. J Urol 1990a; 144:1089.
Takebayashi S, Ohno T, Tanaka K, et al: MR angiography of renal vascular malformations. J Comp Assist Tomog 1994;18:596.
White RR, Wyatt GM: Surgical importance of aberrant renal vessels in infants and children. Am J Surg 1942;58:48.

Renal Artery Aneurysms

Abeshouse BS: Renal aneurysm: Report of two cases and review of the literature. Urol Cutan Rev 1951;55:451.
Bulbul MA, Farrow GA: Renal artery aneurysms. Urology 1992;40:124.
Bunchman TE, Walker HS, Joyce PF, et al: Sonographic evaluation of renal artery aneurysm in childhood. Pediatr Radiol 1991;21:312.
Cerny JC, Chang CY, Fry WJ: Renal artery aneurysms. Arch Surg 1968;96:653.
Cohen JR, Shamash FS: Ruptured renal artery aneurysms during pregnancy. J Vasc Surg 1987;6:51.
Gerritano AP: Aneurysm of the renal artery. Am J Surg 1957;94:638.
Glass PM, Uson AC: Aneurysms of the renal artery: A study of 20 cases. J Urol 1967;98:285.
Hageman JH, Smith RF, Szilagyi DE, Elliot JP: Aneurysms of the renal artery: Problems of prognosis and surgical management. Surgery 1978; 84:563.
Lorentz WB Jr, Browning MC, D'Souza VJ, et al: Intrarenal aneurysm of the renal artery in children. Am J Dis Child 1984;138:751.
McKeil CF Jr, Graf EC, Callahan DH: Renal artery aneurysms: A report of 16 cases. J Urol 1966;96:593.
Poutasse EF: Renal artery aneurysm: Report of 12 cases, two treated by excision of the renal aneurysm and repair of renal artery. J Urol 1957;77:697.
Poutasse EF: Renal artery aneurysms. J Urol 1975;113:443.
Rhodes JF, Johnson G Jr: Renal artery aneurysm. J Urol 1971;105:155.
Sarker R, Coran AG, Cilley RE, et al: Arterial aneurysms in children: Clinicopathologic classification. J Vasc Surg 1991;13:47.
Silvis RS, Hughes WF, Holmes FH: Aneurysm of the renal artery. Am J Surg 1956;91:339.
Stanley JC, Rhodes EL, Gewertz GL, et al: Renal artery aneurysms: significance of macroaneurysms exclusive of dissections and fibrodysplastic mural dilations. Arch Surg 1975;110:1327.
Zinman L, Libertino JA: Uncommon disorders of the renal circulation: renal artery aneurysm. *In* Breslin DJ, Swinton NW, Libertino JA, Zinman L, eds: Renovascular Hypertension. Baltimore, Williams & Wilkins, 1982, pp 110–114.

Renal Arteriovenous Fistula

Bentson JR, Crandall PH: Use of the Fogarty catheter in arteriovenous malformations of the spinal cord. Radiology 1972;105:65.
Boijsen E, Kohler R: Renal arteriovenous fistulae. Acta Radiol 1962;57:433.
Bookstein JJ, Goldstein HM: Successful management of post biopsy arteriovenous fistula with selective arterial embolization. Radiology 1973; 109:535.
Cho KJ, Stanley JC: Non-neoplastic congenital and acquired renal arteriovenous malformations and fistula. Radiology 1978;129:333.
Crummy AB Jr, Atkinson RJ, Caruthers SB: Congenital renal arteriovenous fistulas. J Urol 1965;93:24.
DeSai SG, DeSautels RE: Congenital arteriovenous malformation of the kidney. J Urol 1973;110:17.
Gunterberg B: Renal arteriovenous malformation. Acta Radiol 1968;7:425.
Maldonado JE, Sheps SG, Bernatz PE, et al: Renal arteriovenous fistula. Am J Med 1964;37:499.
McAlhany JC Jr, Black HC, Hanback LD Jr, Yarbrough DR III: Renal arteriovenous fistulas as a cause of hypertension. Am J Surg 1971; 122:117.
Messing E, Kessler R, Kavaney PB: Renal arteriovenous fistula. Urology 1976;8:101.
Takaha M, Matsumoto A, Ochi K, et al: Intrarenal arteriovenous malformation. J Urol 1980;124:315.
Thomason WB, Gross M, Radwin HM, et al: Intrarenal arteriovenous fistulas. J Urol 1972;108:526.
Yazaki T, Tomita M, Akimoto M, et al: Congenital renal arteriovenous fistula: Case report, review of Japanese literature and description of nonradical treatment. J Urol 1976;116:415.

Calyx and Infundibulum

Abeshouse BS: Serous cysts of the kidney and their differentiation from other cystic diseases of the kidney. Urol Cutan Rev 1950;54:582.
Amar A: The clinical significance of renal caliceal diverticulum in children: Relation to vesicoureteral reflux. J Urol 1975;113:255.
Briner V, Thiel G: Hereditares Poland syndrom mit megacalicose der rechten niere. Schweitzerische Med Wochenschr 1988;118:898.
Boyce WH, Whitehurst AW: Hypoplasia of the major renal conduits. J Urol 1976;116:352.
Dacie JE: The "central lucency" sign of low bar dysmorphism (pseudotumour of the kidney). Br J Radiol 1976;49:39.
Devine CJ Jr, Guzman JA, Devine PC, Poutasse EF: Calyceal diverticulum. J Urol 1969;101:8.

Eisendrath DN: Report of case of hydronephrosis in kidney with extrarenal calyces. J Urol 1925;13:51.
Ellis JH, Patterson SK, Sonda LP, et al: Stones and infection in renal caliceal diverticula: Treatment with percutaneous procedures. Am J Roentgenol 1990;156:995.
Fraley EE: Vascular obstruction of superior infundibulum causing nephralgia—new syndrome. N Engl J Med 1966;275:1403.
Galian P, Forest M, Aboulker P: La megacaliose. Nouv Presse Med 1970;78:1663.
Gittes RF: Congenital magacalices. Monogr Urol 1984;5:(1):1.
Gittes RF, Talner LB: Congenital megacalyces vs. obstructive hydronephrosis. J Urol 1972;108:833.
Harrison RB, Wood JL, Gillenwater JY: A solitary calyx in a human kidney. Radiology 1976;121:310.
Husmann DA, Kramer SA, Malek RS, Allen TD: Infundibulopelvic stenosis: A long-term follow-up. J Urol 1994;152:837.
Johnston JH, Sandomirsky SK: Intrarenal vascular obstruction of the superior infundibulum in children. J Pediatr Surg 1972;7:318.
Kelalis PP, Malek RS: Infundibulopelvic stenosis. J Urol 1981;125:568.
Kleeman FJ: Unilateral megacalicosis. J Urol 1973;110:387.
Kozakewich HPW, Lebowitz RL: Congenital megacalices. Pediatr Radiol 1974;2:251.
Lang EK: Percutaneous infundibuloplasty: Management of calyceal diverticula and infundibular stenosis. Radiology 1991;181:871.
Lister J, Singh H: Pelvicalyceal cysts in children. J Pediatr Surg 1973;8:901.
Malament M, Schwartz B, Nagamatsu GR: Extrarenal calyces: Their relationship to renal disease. Am J Roentgenol 1961;86:823.
Mandell GA, Snyder HM 3rd, Haymen SK, et al: Association of congenital megacalycosis and ipsilateral segmental megaureter. Pediatr Radiol 1987;17:28.
Mathieson AJM: Calyceal diverticulum: A case with a discussion and a review of the condition. Br J Urol 1953;25:147.
Middleton AW Jr, Pfister RC: Stone-containing pyelocaliceal diverticulum: Embryogenic, anatomic, radiologic and clinical characteristics. J Urol 1974;111:1.
Moore T: Hydrocalycosis. Br J Urol 1950;22:304.
Morimoto S, Sangen H, Takamatsu M, et al: Solitary calix in siblings. J Urol 1979;122:690.
Neal A, Murphy L: Unipapillary kidney: An unusual developmental abnormality of the kidney. J Coll Radiol Aust 1960;4:81.
Parker JA, Lebowitz R, Mascatello V, Treves S: Magnification renal scintigraphy in differential diagnosis of septa of Bertin. Pediatr Radiol 1976;4:157.
Patriquin H, Lafortune M, Filiatrault D: Urinary milk of calcium in children and adults: Use of gravity-dependent sonography. Am J Roentgenol 1985;144:407.
Puigvert A: Megacaliosis: Diagnostico diferencial con la hidrocaliectasia. Med Clin 1963;41:294.
Puigvert A: Megacalicose—Diagnostic differential avec l'hydrocaliectasia. Helv Chir Acta 1964;31:414.
Rao DVN, Sharma SK, Rao NS, Bapna BC: Extrarenal calyces with complications: A case report. Aust NZ J Surg 1972;42:178.
Sakatoku J, Kitayama T: Solitary unipapillary kidney: Presentation of a case. Acta Urol Jpn 1964;10:349.
Schneck FX, Bauer SB, Peters CA, Kavoussi LR: Natural history and management of calyceal diverticula in children. Presented at the annual meeting of the American Urological Association, San Francisco, May 15, 1994. Abstract No. 185.
Siegel MJ, McAlister WH: Calyceal diverticula in children: Unusual features and complications. Radiology 1979;131:79.
Timmons JW Jr, Malek RS, Hattery RR, DeWeerd J: Caliceal diverticulum. J Urol 1975;114:6.
Toppercer A: Unipapillary human kidney associated with urinary and genital abnormalities. Urology 1980;16:194.
Uhlenhuth E, Amin M, Harty JI, Howerton LW: Infundibular dysgenesis: A spectrum of obstructive renal disease. Urology 1990;35:334.
Vela Navarrete R, Garcia Robledo J: Polycystic disease of the renal sinus: Structural characteristics. J Urol 1983;129:700.
Webb JAW, Fry IK, Charlton CAC: An anomalous calyx in the mid-kidney: An anatomical variant. Br J Radiol 1975;48:674.
Williams DI, Mininberg DT: Hydrocalycosis: Report of three cases in children. Br J Urol 1968;40:541.
Wulfsohn M: Pyelocaliceal diverticula. J Urol 1980;123:1.

Anomalies of the Ureteropelvic Junction

Allen TD: Congenital ureteral stricture. J Urol 1970;104:196.
Allen TD: Congenital ureteral strictures. *In* Lutzeyer W, Melchior H, eds: Urodynamic. Upper and Lower Urinary Tract. Berlin, Springer-Verlag, 1973, pp 137–147.
Allen TD: The swing of the pendulum. J Urol 1992;148:534.
Amar AD: Congenital hydronephrosis of lower segment in duplex kidney. Urology 1976;7:480.
Belis JA, Belis TE, Lai JCW, et al: Radionuclide determination of individual kidney function in the treatment of chronic renal obstruction. J Urol 1982;127:898.
Belman AB, Kropp KF, Simon NM: Renal pressor hypertension secondary to unilateral hydronephrosis. N Engl J Med 1968;278:1133.
Bernstein GT, Mandell J, Lebowitz RL, et al: Ureteropelvic junction obstruction in the neonate. J Urol 1988;140:1216.
Brown T, Mandell J, Lebowitz RL: Neonatal hydronephrosis in the era of ultrasonography. AJR 1987;148:959.
Carr MC, Peters CA, Retik AB, Mandell J: Urinary levels of the renal tubular enzyme N-acetyl-beta-D-glucosaminidase in the unilateral obstructive uropathy. J Urol 1994;151:442.
Cartwright PC, Duckett JW, Keating MA, et al: Managing apparent ureteropelvic junction obstruction in the newborn. J Urol 1992;148:1224.
Cohen B, Goldman SM, Kopilnick M, et al: Ureteropelvic junction obstruction: its occurrence in 3 members of a single family. J Urol 1978;120:361.
Colgan JR III, Skaist L, Morrow JW: Benign ureteral tumors in childhood: A case report and a plea for conservative management. J Urol 1973; 109:308.
Colodny AH, Retik AB, Bauer SB: Antenatal diagnosis of fetal urologic abnormalities by intrauterine ultrasonography; therapeutic implications. Presented at Annual Meeting of the American Urological Association, San Francisco, May 18, 1980.
Conway JJ, Maizels M: The "well tempered" diuretic renogram: A standard method to examine the asymptomatic neonate with hydronephrosis or hydroureteronephrosis. J Nucl Med 1992;33:2041.
Dejter SR Jr, Eggli DF, Gibbons MD: Delayed management of neonatal hydronephrosis. J Urol 1988;140:1305.
Dowling KJ, Harmon EP, Ortenberg J, et al: Ureteropelvic junction obstruction: The effect of pyeloplasty on renal function. J Urol 1988;140:1227.
Duckett JW: When to operate on neonatal hydronephrosis. Urology 1993;42:617.
Ericsson NO, Rudhe U, Livaditis A: Hydronephrosis associated with aberrant renal vessels in infants and children. Surgery 1961;50:687.
Foote JW, Blennerhassett JB, Wiglesworth FW, MacKinnon KJ: Observations on the ureteropelvic junction. J Urol 1970;104:252.
Fourcroy JL, Blei CL, Glassman LM, White R: Prenatal diagnosis by ultrasonography of genitourinary abnormalities. Urology 1983;22:223.
Fung LCT, Steckler RE, Khoury AE, et al: Intrarenal resistive index correlates with renal pelvis pressure. J Urol 1994;152:607.
Grignon A, Filiatrault D, Homsy Y, et al: Ureteropelvic junction stenosis: Antenatal ultrasonographic diagnosis, postnatal investigation and follow-up. Radiology 1986;160:649.
Grossman IC, Cromie WJ, Wein AJ, Duckett JW: Renal hypertension secondary to ureteropelvic junction obstruction. Urology 1981;17:69.
Gup A: Benign mesodermal polyp in childhood. J Urol 1975;114:610.
Hanna MK, Jeffs RD, Sturgess JM, Barkin M: Ureteral structure and ultrastructure. Part II. Congenital ureteropelvic junction obstruction and primary obstructive megaureter. J Urol 1976;116:725.
Homsy YL, Saad S, Laberge I, et al: Transitional hydronephrosis in the newborn and infant. J Urol 1990;144:579.
Hutch JA, Hinman F Jr, Miller ER: Reflux as a cause of hydronephrosis and chronic pyelonephritis. J Urol 1962;88:169.
Johnston JH: The pathogenesis of hydronephrosis in children. Br J Urol 1969;41:724.
Johnston JH, Evans JP, Glassberg KI, Shapiro SR: Pelvic hydronephrosis in children: A review of 219 personal cases. J Urol 1977;117:97.
Joseph DB, Bauer SB, Colodny AH, et al: Lower pole ureteropelvic junction obstruction and incomplete duplication. J Urol 1989;141:896.
Juskiewenski S, Moscovici J, Bouissou F, et al: Le syndrome de la junction pyelo-ureterale chez l'enfant. A propos de 178 observations. J d'Urologie 1983;89:173.
Kass EJ, Majd M, Belman AB: Comparison of the diuretic renogram and pressure profusion study in children. J Urol 1985;134:92.
Kass EJ, Fink-Bennett D: Radioisotopic evaluation of the dilated urinary tract. Urol Clin North Am 1990;17:273.
Kelalis PP, Culp OS, Stickler GB, Burke EC: Ureteropelvic obstruction in children: Experiences with 109 cases. J Urol 1971;106:418.
King LR, Coughlin PWF, Bloch EC, et al: The case for immediate pyeloplasty in the neonate with ureteropelvic junction obstruction. J Urol 1984;132:725.

Koff SA: Ureteropelvic junction obstruction: role of newer diagnostic methods. J Urol 1982;127:898.
Koff SA: Pathophysiology of ureteropelvic junction obstructions. Urol Clin North Am 1990;17:263.
Koff SA, Campbell KD: Non-operative management of unilateral neonatal hydronephrosis. J Urol 1992;148:525.
Koff SA, Campbell KD: The non-operative management of unilateral neonatal hydronephrosis: Natural history of poorly functioning kidneys. J Urol 1994;152:593.
Koff SA, Hayden LJ, Cirulli C: Pathophysiology of ureteropelvic junction obstruction: Experimental and clinical observations. J Urol 1986;136:336.
Krueger RP, Ash JM, Silver MM, et al: Primary hydronephrosis: Assessment of diuretic renography, pelvis perfusion pressure, operative findings and renal and ureteral histology. Urol Clin North Am 1980;7:231.
Lebowitz RL, Blickman JG: The coexistence of uretero-pelvic junction obstruction and reflux. Am J Roentgenol 1983;140:231.
Lebowitz RI, Griscom NT: Neonatal hydronephrosis: 146 cases. Radiol Clin North Am 1977;15:49.
Leiter E: Persistent fetal ureter. J Urol 1979;122:251.
Lowe FC, Marshall SF: Ureteropelvic junction obstruction in adults. Urology 1984;23:331.
MacNeily AE, Maizels M, Kaplan WE, et al: Does early pyeloplasty really avert loss of renal function? A retrospective review. J Urol 1993;150:769.
Maizels M, Stephens FD: Valves of the ureter as a cause of primary obstruction of the ureter: Anatomic, embryologic and clinical aspects. J Urol 1980;123:742.
Malek RS: Intermittent hydronephrosis. The occult ureteropelvic junction obstruction. J Urol 1983;130:863.
Mandell J, Peters CA, Retik AB: Current concepts in the perinatal diagnosis and management of hydronephrosis. Urol Clin North Am 1990;17:247.
Manning FA: Fetal surgery for obstructive uropathy: Rational considerations. Am J Kidney Dis 1987;10:259.
Mering JH, Steel JR, Gittes RF: Congenital ureteral valves. J Urol 1972;107:737.
Munoz AI, Pascual y Baralt JF, Melendez MT: Arterial hypertension in infants with hydronephrosis. Am J Dis Child 1977;131:38.
Murnaghan GF: The dynamics of the renal pelvis and ureter with reference to congenital hydronephrosis. Br J Urol 1958;30:321.
Nesbit RM: Diagnosis of intermittent hydronephrosis: Importance of pyelography during episodes of pain. J Urol 1956;75:767.
Nixon HH: Hydronephrosis in children: A clinical study of seventy-eight cases with special reference to the role of aberrant renal vessels and the results of conservative operations. Br J Surg 1953;40:601.
Notley RG: Electron microscopy of the upper ureter and the pelviureteric junction. Br J Urol 1968;40:37.
O'Reilly PH, Lawson RS, Shields RA, Testa HJ: Idiopathic hydronephrosis—the diuresis renogram: a new noninvasive method of assessing equivocal pelvioureteral junction obstruction. J Urol 1979; 121:153.
Osathanondh V, Potter EL: Development of the kidney as shown by microdissection. Arch Pathol 1963;76:271.
Östling K: The genesis of hydronephrosis. Acta Chir Scand 1942; 86:Suppl. 72.
Palmer JM, Lindfors KK, Ordorica RC, Marber DM: Diuretic Doppler sonography in postnatal hydronephrosis. J Urol 1991;146:605.
Parker RM, Rudd TG, Wonderly RK, Ansell JS: Ureteropelvic junction obstruction in infants and children: functional evaluation of the obstructed kidney preoperatively and postoperatively. J Urol 1981;126:509.
Perlmutter AD, Kroovand RL, Lai YW: Management of ureteropelvic obstruction in the first year of life. J Urol 1980;123:535.
Platt JF, Rubin JM, Ellis JH: Distinction between obstructive and nonobstructive pyelocaliectasis with duplex Doppler sonography. Am J Roentgenol 1989;153:997.
Ransley PA, Dhillon HK, Gordon I, et al: The postnatal management of hydronephrosis diagnosed by prenatal ultrasound. J Urol 1990;144:584.
Robson WJ, Rudy SM, Johnston JH: Pelviureteric obstruction in infancy. J Pediatr Surg 1976;11:57.
Roth DR, Gonzales EJ Jr: Management of ureteropelvic junction obstruction in infants. J Urol 1983;129:108.
Ruano-Gil D, Coca-Payeras A, Tejedo-Maten A: Obstruction and normal re-canalization of the ureter in the human embryo: its relation to congenital ureteric obstruction. Eur Urol 1975;1:287.
Segura JW, Hattery RR, Hartman GW: Fluoroscopic evaluation of intermittent ureteropelvic junction obstruction after furosemide stimulation. J Urol 1974;112:449.
Shopfner CE: Ureteropelvic junction obstruction. Am J Roentgenol 1966;98:148.
Snyder HM III, Lebowitz RL, Colodny AH, et al: Ureteropelvic junction obstruction in children. Urol Clin North Am 1980;7:273.
Squitieri AP, Ceccarelli FE, Wurster JC: Hypertension with elevated renal vein renins secondary to ureteropelvic junction obstruction. J Urol 1974;111:284.
Starr NT, Maizels M, Chou P, et al: Microanatomy of and morphometry of the hydronephrotic "obstructed" renal pelvis in asymptomatic infants. J Urol 1992;148:519.
Stephens FD: Ureterovascular hydronephrosis and the "aberrant" renal vessels. J Urol 1982;128:984.
Tapia J, Gonzalez R: Pyeloplasty improves renal function and somatic growth in children with ureteropelvic junction obstruction. J Urol 1995;154:218.
Thorup J, Pederson PV, Clausen N: Benign ureteral polyps as a cause of hydronephrosis in a child. J Urol 1981;126:796.
Uehling DT, Gilbert E, Chesney R: Urologic implications of the VATER association. J Urol 1983;129:352.
Ulmsten U, Diehl J: Investigation of ureteric function with simultaneous intraureteric pressure recordings and ureteropyelography. Radiology 1975;117:283.
Uson AC, Cox LA, Lattimer JK: Hydronephrosis in infants and children. I. Some clinical and pathological aspects. JAMA 1968;205:323.
Whitaker RH: Methods of assessing obstruction in dilated ureters. Br J Urol 1973;45:15.
Whitaker RH: Some observations and theories on the wide ureter and hydronephrosis. Br J Urol 1975;47:377.
Whitaker RH: Reflux induced pelviureteric obstruction. Br J Urol 1976; 48:555.
Williams DI, Karlaftis CM: Hydronephrosis due to pelviureteric obstruction in the newborn. Br J Urol 1966;38:138.
Williams DI, Kenawi MM: The prognosis of pelviureteric obstruction in childhood: A review of 190 cases. Eur Urol 1976;2:57.
Williams PR, Fegetter J, Miller RA, Wickham JEA: The diagnosis and management of benign fibrous ureteric polyps. Br J Urol 1980;52:253.
Woodard JR: Hydronephrosis in the neonate. Urology 1993;42:620.

59

RENAL DYSPLASIA AND CYSTIC DISEASE OF THE KIDNEY

Kenneth I. Glassberg, M.D.

Renal dysgenesis is maldevelopment of the kidney that affects its size, shape, or structure. **Dysgenesis is of three principal types: dysplastic, hypoplastic, and cystic.** Imprecise language use has confused discussions of these disorders; to avoid perpetuating this confusion, the author begins by outlining the terminology adopted in 1987 by the Section on Urology of the American Academy of Pediatrics, which provided precise definitions of dysgenesis, dysplasia, hypoplasia, hypodysplasia, aplasia, and agenesis (Table 59–1), which are discussed in this chapter. Note particularly that whereas dysplasia is always accompanied by hypoplasia, the converse is not true; hypoplasia may occur in isolation. When both conditions are present, the term hypodysplasia is preferred (Schwarz et al, 1981a). The author updates the 1987 American Academy of Pediatrics classification of cystic diseases of the kidney and includes the most recent genetic findings.

Table 59–1. CLASSIFICATION OF HYPOPLASIA AND HYPODYSPLASIA

Hypoplasia
True ("oligonephronia")
With normal ureteral orifice
With abnormal ureteral orifice
Oligomeganephronia
Segmental (Ask-Upmark kidney)
Hypodysplasia
With normal ureteral orifice
With obstruction
Without obstruction
With abnormal ureteral orifice
Lateral ectopia
Medial or caudal ectopia with ureterocele
With urethral obstruction
Prune-belly syndrome

RENAL AGENESIS

Renal agenesis refers to absent kidney development and can occur secondary to a wolffian duct, ureteral bud, or metanephric blastema defect. Bilateral agenesis occurs in 1 in 4000 births and has a male predominance (Potter, 1965). Because the placenta filters the fetus's blood, it is not the lack of kidney tissue that causes early death but rather the lack of urine production and oligohydramnios. Affected babies are born with immature lungs and pneumothorax, Potter's facies (hypertelorism, prominent inner canthal folds, and recessive chin), and orthopedic defects secondary to intrauterine compression. The actual incidence of agenesis cannot be determined by imaging studies because aplastic kidneys can be misinterpreted as agenesis because they lack function and are too small to be visualized on any study. Most cases of bilateral agenesis are sporadic, and many are associated with other congenital anomalies including urogenital sinus defects.

Unilateral agenesis is more common, with an incidence of 1 in 450 to 1000 births (Kass and Bloom, 1992). Because it may be secondary to a wolffian duct abnormality and the wolffian duct lies adjacent to the müllerian duct, renal agenesis may be associated with malformation of the ipsilateral uterine horn or fallopian tube or absence of the ipsilateral ovary in the female, or with absence of the ipsilateral testicle, vas deferens, or seminiferous tubules in the male. **The pseudonym Mayer-Rokitansky-Küster-Hauser syndrome refers to a group of associated findings that include unilateral renal agenesis or renal ectopia, ipsilateral müllerian defects, and vaginal agenesis.**

On rare occasions when either unilateral or bilateral agenesis is associated with a group of other renal abnormalities within a family, the term familial renal adysplasia is used.

DYSPLASIA

A dysplastic kidney contains focal, diffuse, or segmentally arranged primitive structures, specifically primitive ducts, as a result of abnormal metanephric differentiation. **"Dysplasia" is, therefore, a histologic diagnosis.** The condition may affect all or only part of the kidney, and in a duplex system one segment may be normal and the other dysplastic. The kidney may be of normal size or small and may be grossly normal or deformed. **Cysts of various sizes may or may not be present. When they are present, the condition is called cystic dysplasia. When the entire kidney is dysplastic with a preponderance of cysts, that kidney is referred to as a multicystic dysplastic kidney.** This condition is discussed in a subsequent section of this chapter. **Aplastic dysplasia** is represented by a nubbin of nonfunctioning tissue, not necessarily of reniform shape, that meets the histologic criteria for dysplasia. In utero and postnatal follow-up by ultrasound has shown that some multicystic kidneys shrink with time into such nubbins. **Some instances of aplasia may thus represent the involuted stage of a multicystic kidney.**

Dysplasia may be associated with an absent renal pelvis or ureter; with atresia, stenosis, or tortuosity of the ureter; or with a normal, atretic, or absent ureterovesical junction. The appearance of a grossly abnormal collecting system with or without ureteral anomalies on intravenous urography is sometimes described as renal dysplasia, but such features may occur in the absence of dysplasia. Williams (1974) has suggested that the term renal dysmorphism rather than renal dysplasia be applied to abnormalities noted radiographically or grossly without histologic proof of primitive structures.

Etiology

The origin of renal dysplasia is unclear. Normal renal development is initiated by penetration of metanephric blastema by a ureteric bud at the proper time and place. **According to the Mackie and Stephens (1975) "bud" theory, abnormal ureteric budding can lead not only to an ectopic orifice but also to inappropriate penetration of the blastema, causing renal dysplasia.** These investigators provided supportive evidence from studies of duplex systems, which showed a high correlation between the degree of lateral ectopia of the lower pole orifice and the extent of dysplasia of the lower pole segment.

Once renal function begins, obstruction can distort development secondary to the physical and chemical effects of poor drainage. It was long assumed that obstruction is a significant factor in dysplasia (Beck, 1971; Bernstein, 1971). Certainly, some evidence exists for the role of obstruction. For example, when both kidneys drain poorly, as in patients with posterior urethral valves, both kidneys may be dysplastic, whereas only the ipsilateral kidney is affected in cases of unilateral obstruction. Also in favor of a role for obstruction is the dysplasia observed in the upper pole of duplex systems when there is an associated obstructed ectopic ureter or ureterocele. The ipsilateral lower pole in such cases is not dysplastic, but the upper pole orifice is ectopic.

According to Mackie and Stephens (1975), an ectopic orifice is a sign of abnormal ureteric budding and metanephric development (i.e., dysplasia). However, some of these findings could also be explained as an embryologic abnormality that causes both obstruction and dysplasia. Moreover, one form of widespread dysplasia, namely, the type associated with multicystic disease, usually develops before urine formation. Potter suggested in 1972 that a teratogenic force acts at various sites to produce the combination of ureteral atresia and multicystic renal disease.

Growing awareness of the importance of the interactions between epithelial cells and mesenchyme in the control of normal development and growth has shed light on the origin of renal dysgenesis. In the chick embryo, simple ureteral ligation alone does not induce renal dysplasia (Berman and Maizel, 1982), whereas reduction of the condensed metanephrogenic mesenchyme is likely to lead to dysplasia (Maizel and Simpson, 1983). Moreover, ligation of the ureter seems to facilitate the dysplastic development of blastemas already deficient in mesenchyme (Maizel and Simpson, 1986). Spencer and Maizel (1987) found that inhibition of the glycosylation of extracellular matrix, which alters the interaction of epithelial and mesenchymal cells, can lead to dysplasia in the absence of obstruction.

The question of the etiology of dysplasia has assumed more than theoretical importance since the advent of fetal surgery. If obstruction is an epiphenomenon of dysplasia rather than its cause, then operations on a fetus to relieve obstruction are unlikely to be of value in preventing severe renal dysplasia or aplasia.

Histology

The histologic definition of renal dysplasia has evolved since the seminal work by Ericsson and Ivemark (1958a, 1958b), who sought to identify the structures that could arise only from embryonic maldevelopment, not from secondary events. They concluded that primitive ducts and cartilage were such unique features. Although the first part of their definition is still accepted, the second part is not. Ericsson and Ivemark (1958b), like some other investigators (Biglar and Killingsworth, 1949; Bernstein, 1971); considered all renal cartilage to be representative of aberrant development of the metanephric blastema and thus dysplastic. However, foci of hyaline cartilage have been found in normal kidneys (Potter, 1972) and in otherwise normal kidneys suffering

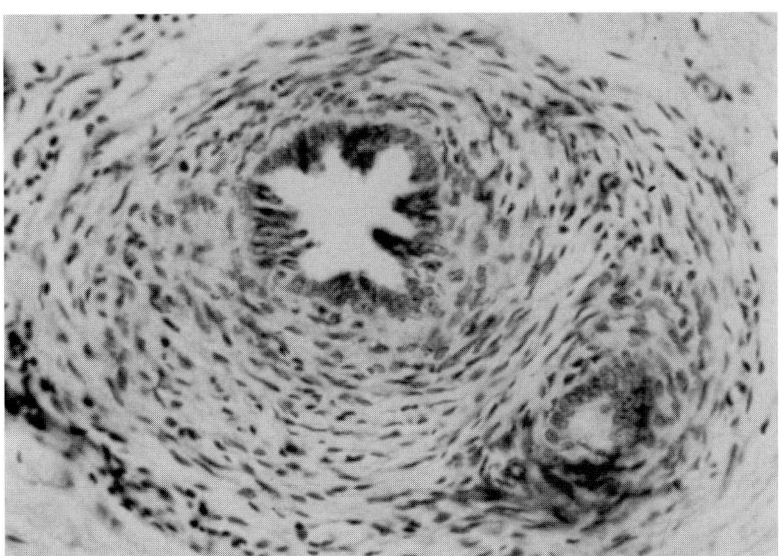

Figure 59–1. Primitive duct lined with columnar epithelial cells. Note concentric arrangement of spindle mesenchymal cells around the duct. Special staining is required to demonstrate smooth muscle cells. (Courtesy of C. K. Chen, M.D.)

from chronic inflammation (Taxy and Filmer, 1975). The present definition, therefore, does not specify nests of metaplastic cartilage as an absolute criterion for dysplasia.

Primitive ducts, which are lined by cuboidal or tall columnar epithelium (often ciliated) and surrounded by concentric rings of connective tissue containing collagen and a few smooth muscle cells but no elastin, are undeniable evidence of dysplasia (Fig. 59–1) (Ericsson and Ivemark, 1958b; Bernstein, 1971). The ducts are of various sizes and can be found in many sites, principally in the medulla and sometimes in the medullary rays. As a rule, the more severely deformed the kidney, the more extensive the primitive ducts (Ericsson, 1974), and in less severe cases, only the peripelvic area may be affected. These structures resemble the aberrant ductules of the fallopian tube and may be remnants of the mesonephric duct (Eisendrath, 1935; Ericsson, 1954).

Several other histologic findings may (but need not) accompany the primitive ducts. Primitive ductules, which are smaller than the primitive ducts, are surrounded by connective tissue devoid of smooth muscle cells. Primitive tubules and glomeruli may be seen also; these resemble structures seen in human kidneys that are regenerating after neonatal renal necrosis (Bernstein and Meyer, 1961), in scars from renal biopsies (Bernstein, 1971), and in animal kidneys after trauma (Bernstein, 1966). Cysts and loose, disorganized mesenchyme and fibrous tissue are other possible features.

Familial Adysplasia

Renal agenesis, renal dysplasia, multicystic dysplasia, and renal aplasia usually appear as isolated sporadic occurrences. On rare occasions, this group of anomalies may appear in many family members but heterogeneously. In other words, one family member may have renal agenesis while another has renal dysplasia, and still another has a multicystic dysplastic or aplastic kidney. When all or part of this group of anomalies is seen in one family, an encompassing term for these four entities is used: familial renal adysplasia.

When the disorder is familial it usually is transmitted as an autosomal dominant disease (Buchta et al, 1973; McPherson et al, 1987). The fact that all of the entities of renal adysplasia can appear in one family suggests that one primary defect leads to this spectrum of anomalies. That primary defect may be either a ureteric bud abnormality or a defect of the metanephric blastema. Curry and associates (1984) make a case for investigating by ultrasound family members and subsequent pregnancies when there is a history of bilateral renal adysplasia and Potter's syndrome. Bernstein (1991) goes further and suggests giving parents an option for investigative studies of family members when a child with even one adysplastic kidney is identified. Incidentally, noncystic dysplastic kidneys not associated with reflux are associated with a 14% incidence of vesicoureteral reflux into the contralateral ureter (Atiyeh et al, 1993).

HYPOPLASIA AND HYPODYSPLASIA

Hypoplasia and hypodysplasia have been subclassified as shown in Table 59–1. The subdivision according to the nature of the ureteral orifice acknowledges the bud theory but is not necessarily intended to be an endorsement of this theory. Hypodysplastic kidneys most often occur in conjunction with ectopic ureteral orifices, with the extent of dysplasia correlating with the degree of ectopia (Schwarz et al, 1981a, 1981b, 1981c). However, hypodysplastic kidneys are seen in a few patients with normal ureteral orifices. In such cases, obstruction may or may not be present.

Renal Hypoplasia

To avoid perpetuating the confusion that has attended the use of the term hypoplasia, the author restricts its use to **small kidneys that have less than the normal number of calyces and nephrons but are not dysplasic or embryonic.** The truly hypoplastic kidney may have a normal nephron density despite its small size.

Hypoplasia is not a specific condition; rather, it is a group of pathologic conditions with the same feature—an abnormally small kidney. It should be distinguished from renal aplasia, in which the kidney is rudimentary and the ureter atretic, and from renal agenesis, in which the kidney does not develop at all.

Hypoplasia may be bilateral or unilateral. In unilateral cases, the other kidney usually shows greater compensatory growth than is characteristic in patients with renal atrophy as a result of acquired disease. Hypoplasia can be associated with reflux, and the term reflux nephropathy is now applied to all types of abnormality associated with reflux. Segmental "hypoplasia" (Ask-Upmark kidney) probably is a type of reflux nephropathy.

Because of the similarity of the word oligonephronia (literally translated as a decreased number of nephrons) to oligomeganephronia, which is a specific clinical entity (see following discussion), the former term should not be used.

True Hypoplasia

True hypoplasia is a congenital condition with no apparent familial tendency or gender predilection. The incidence is unknown because many investigators fail to distinguish among the various causes of a small kidney. In a series of 2153 consecutive autopsies, Rubenstein and co-workers (1961) found a 2.5% incidence of true hypoplasia.

Clinical Features

Clinical manifestations of true renal hypoplasia may be severe or absent. In patients with bilateral true hypoplasia or unilateral true hypoplasia with contralateral aplasia or agenesis, renal insufficiency, dehydration, or failure to thrive may be present. Often, these patients are premature infants who have developmental abnormalities of other organs, particularly the central nervous system. Respiratory problems are a common cause of death in these infants. At the other extreme, in patients with unilateral hypoplasia and contralateral hypertrophy, the diagnosis usually is made incidentally during an evaluation for some other urinary problem or for hypertension.

The urine is of low specific gravity when the condition is bilateral.

Histopathology

For the diagnosis of hypoplasia to be made, the renal parenchyma must be normal and without dysplasia, although Bernstein (1968) has described tubular degeneration, focal cortical scarring, and healed focal necrosis. The characteristic feature is the size of the kidney.

Evaluation

Ultrasound may be useful in demonstrating the presence and site of these kidneys, although it does not reveal the type of hypoplasia (Goldberg et al, 1975). Intravenous urography shows nonappearance or a small shadow; retrograde pyelography reveals a normal-caliber ureter and a reduced number of calyces. Reports by Porstman (1970) and Templeton and Thompson (1968) indicate the finding of a uniformly narrow renal artery on arteriography, in contrast to the tapered vessel seen in acquired atrophy, such as that secondary to pyelonephritis.

Differential diagnosis must take into account solid dysplasia (Potter's type IIB), segmental hypoplasia (Ask-Upmark kidney), oligomeganephronia, and acquired disease (chronic atrophic pyelonephritis, renal ischemia, and glomerulonephritis). Renal biopsy is the only way of proving the diagnosis.

Oligomeganephronia

The combination of a marked reduction in the number of nephrons and hypertrophy of each nephron was described in 1962 by Habib and colleagues and Royer and colleagues and termed oligomeganephronia. It is usually a bilateral condition, although a few instances of unilateral oligomeganephronia associated with contralateral renal agenesis have been reported (Griffel et al, 1972; Lam et al, 1982; Forster and Hawkins, 1994).

There are probably two types of oligomeganephronia: one that appears in association with variable malformation defects and the other a solitary sporadic entity that comprises the majority of cases. Among the multiple defects that have been reported with oligomeganephronia are ocular, auditory, and skeletal anomalies (e.g., lobster-claw deformity of the hands and feet) as well as mental retardation. Park and Chi (1993) reported on two such patients. They found that both patients had a 4p deletion-type chromosomal anomaly and suggested that perhaps many other cases with multiple malformations associated with oligomeganephronia may actually be part of a similar 4p deletion-type syndrome.

Clinical Features

Oligomeganephronia is a congenital but nonfamilial disorder that affects boys more often than girls (3:1). It frequently is associated with low birth weight (<2500 g). The condition usually is discovered soon after the child's birth or, if not, then usually by age 2 years. Infants most frequently are brought to medical attention because of vomiting, dehydration, intense thirst, and polyuria. The creatinine clearance is abnormal (10 to 50 ml/minute per 1.73^2), and the maximum specific gravity of the urine is 1.007 to 1.012. Moderate proteinuria may be present, but this is more likely to be a later finding.

Renal function remains below normal although stable for many years, but polydipsia and polyuria can worsen, and growth is severely retarded in many cases. As the patient enters his or her teens, the creatinine clearance begins to drop rapidly. Marked proteinuria (2 g/24 hours) is common, and the characteristic metabolic features of renal failure—disturbed acid-base balance and abnormal calcium and phosphorus metabolism—are seen. The blood pressure usually is normal. At this point, hemodialysis is required to maintain the patient's life.

Histopathology

The kidneys are smaller than normal (average weight at autopsy is 20 to 25 g) and are not always the same size. Van Acker and colleagues (1971) suggested that because of the reduced number of nephrons, those that exist increase in size to compensate for the deficiency in number. The kidneys are pale and firm with a granular cortical surface and no clear distinction between the cortex and the medulla. The number of renal segments is reduced, generally to five or six, although unirenicular and birenicular kidneys have been described (Bernstein, 1968). The renal artery is small.

The particular histologic features of a case depend on the duration of the disease. In patients 2 to 3 years of age, the characteristic findings are a reduced number of nephrons, enormously enlarged glomeruli (sevenfold to tenfold the normal volume), juxtaglomerular bodies, and proximal tubules elongated to four times their normal length, often with multiple diverticuli (Fig. 59–2). In older children, interstitial fibrosis and atrophy become more prominent, and the glomeruli become increasingly hyalinized until they are destroyed. The end-stage kidney closely resembles that observed in glomerulonephritis except for persisting enlargement of the glomeruli. Dysplasia is not seen.

Evaluation

The kidneys may concentrate contrast medium adequately for an intravenous urogram, producing a picture of small kidneys, usually with normally formed calyces, although Morita and associates (1973) have described a case with dysmorphic calyces. The small kidneys also can be identified by sonography (Scheinman and Abelson, 1970).

Oligomeganephronia may resemble juvenile nephronophthisis–medullary cystic disease complex in its clinical features, but the latter condition generally appears later in life, and defects of tubular function precede glomerular insufficiency (Herdman et al, 1967). Moreover, juvenile nephronophthisis–medullary cystic disease is familial; other cases are found in the relatives of 50% to 80% of affected persons (Habib, 1974). The kidneys in juvenile nephronophthisis are small but not as small as those seen in oligomeganephronia.

Simple bilateral renal hypoplasia may be confused with oligomeganephronia (Carter and Lirenman, 1970). Segmental hypoplasia (Ask-Upmark kidney) is nearly always accompanied by severe hypertension, which is not seen in oligomeganephronia.

Treatment

High fluid intake and correction of salt loss and acidosis are the initial steps. Daily dietary protein should be limited to 1.5 g/kg during the stable phase (Royer et al, 1962). Frank renal failure is managed by dialysis and transplantation. The allograft may come from a living related donor because the disease is not familial.

Ask-Upmark Kidney (Segmental "Hypoplasia")

In 1929, Ask-Upmark described distinctive small kidneys in eight patients, seven of whom had malignant hypertension. Six of these patients were adolescents.

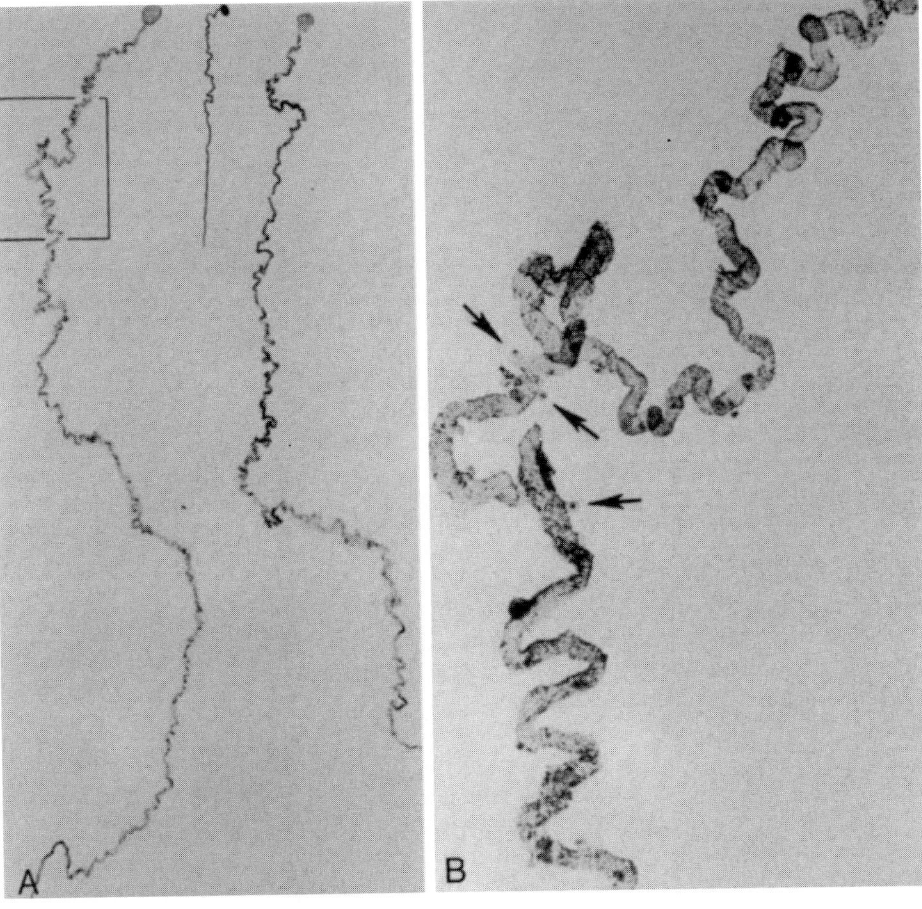

Figure 59–2. *A,* Mosaic photograph of two typical proximal tubules dissected from the kidney of a patient with oligomeganephronia. The silhouette in the top center is a diagrammatic representation to scale of an average proximal tubule from a kidney of an age-matched control.

B, Enlargement of the inset in *A,* showing the diverticula along the course of the nephron. (From Fetterman GH, Habib R: Congenital bilateral oligonephronic renal hypoplasia with hypertrophy of nephrons [oligomeganephronic]. Am J Clin Pathol 1969; 52:199–207. Reproduced with permission of the American Society of Clinical Pathologists.)

ETIOLOGY

Although the Ask-Upmark kidney was originally thought to be a developmental lesion because of the youth of the first patients, findings suggest otherwise. The presence of fibrotic glomeruli and chronic inflammatory cells, as described by Habib and associates (1965) and by Rauber and Langlet (1976), led both Johnston and Mix (1976) and Shindo and co-workers (1983) to suggest that the Ask-Upmark kidney is the result of reflux and ascending pyelonephritis. This hypothesis is supported by the data of Arant and co-workers (1979), who found that 16 of 17 affected patients had vesicoureteral reflux and that signs of reflux had been present in more than 50% of the previously described cases in which appropriate studies had been done.

Chronic pyelonephritis secondary to reflux may be the cause even if no inflammatory cell infiltrates are found. For example, Heptinstall (1979) showed that such cells may disappear from the tissues with time. Hodson (1981) demonstrated in pigs that acute lesions of pyelonephritis may be followed by a histologic picture similar to that of Ask-Upmark kidney, in which glomeruli, collecting ducts, and inflammatory cells have disappeared. Hodson was able to produce histologically similar lesions with sterile high-pressure reflux. The presence of glomerular traces in periodic acid-Schiff (PAS)–stained sections of Ask-Upmark kidneys in areas grossly without glomeruli is further evidence of an acquired rather than a developmental lesion.

Despite these data, the etiology of Ask-Upmark kidney is not yet clear. Some of these kidneys do contain dysplastic elements, indicating a developmental contribution (Bernstein, 1975).

CLINICAL FEATURES

Most patients are 10 years or older at diagnosis, although the lesion has been reported in a premature infant (Valderrama and Berkman, 1979) and in a 13-month-old infant (Mozziconacci et al, 1968). Girls are twice as likely as boys to be affected (Royer et al, 1971; Arant et al, 1979).

Severe hypertension is a prominent symptom. Headache is common, either alone or together with hypertensive encephalopathy (Rosenfeld et al, 1973). Retinopathy is discovered in half the patients (Royer et al, 1971).

Proteinuria and some degree of renal insufficiency may be present if the disease is bilateral. Approximately half of the patients in the series described by Royer and associates (1971) had these signs at diagnosis.

HISTOPATHOLOGY

The Ask-Upmark kidney is smaller than normal—12 to 35 g (Royer et al, 1971). **Its distinctive feature is one or more deep grooves on the lateral convexity, underneath which the parenchyma consists of tubules resembling those in the thyroid gland.** Usually, the hypoplastic segments are easily distinguished from adjacent areas. The medulla consists of a thin band, and remnants of the corticomedullary junction and arcuate arteries are seen. Arteriosclerosis is common, and juxtaglomerular hyperplasia may be seen (Bernstein, 1968; Meares and Gross, 1972; Kaufman and Fay, 1974; Arant et al, 1979).

TREATMENT

In patients with unilateral disease, partial or total nephrectomy may control the hypertension (Royer et al, 1971; Meares and Gross, 1972). Failure of this measure suggests an unrecognized scar or generalized arteriosclerosis in the remaining kidney (Arant et al, 1979). Bilateral disease with renal insufficiency usually is managed medically, although dialysis and transplantation may be needed. Correction of reflux may prevent further renal damage but probably will have no effect on the hypertension.

Renal Hypodysplasia

Hypodysplasia may be associated with a normal or abnormal ureteral orifice, ureterocele, urethral obstruction, and prune-belly syndrome.

Hypodysplasia with Normal Ureteral Orifice

WITH OBSTRUCTION

Primary obstructive megaureter and ureteropelvic junction obstruction usually are associated with small but normal-appearing and normally situated ureteral orifices. Generally, this kidney has suffered diffuse damage because of hydronephrosis, although in a few cases, small areas or even the entire kidney is hypodysplastic or shows multicystic dysplasia (Fig. 59–3).

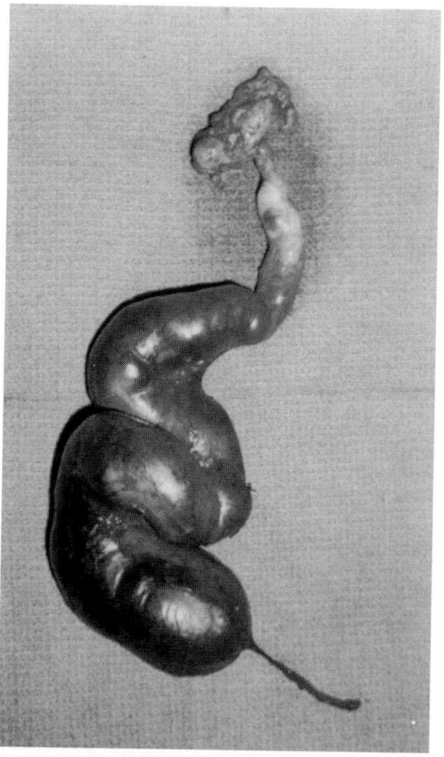

Figure 59–3. Small hypodysplastic kidney found in association with a severely obstructed primary megaureter. (From Glassberg KI, Filmer RB: Renal dysplasia, renal hypoplasia and cystic disease of the kidney. *In* Kelalis P, King LR, Belman AB, eds: Clinical Pediatric Urology. Philadelphia, W. B. Saunders Company, 1985, pp 922–971.)

Clinical Features

Neonates present mostly on the basis of renomegaly. When the disease is severe, stillbirth or significant respiratory distress can occur. For example, of the first 29 reported cases in newborns, seven were stillborn infants, four of whom died of dystocia (McClean et al, 1964; Mehrizi et al, 1964; Blyth and Ockenden, 1971; Kaye and Lewy, 1974; Bengtsson et al, 1975; Ross and Trovers, 1975; Stickler and Kelales, 1975; Stillaert et al, 1975; Fellows et al, 1976; Ritter and Siaforikas, 1976; Begleiter et al, 1977; Kaplan et al, 1977; Loh et al, 1977; Euderink and Hogewind, 1978; Wolf et al, 1978; Shokeir, 1978; Fryns and van den Berghe, 1979; Proesmans et al, 1982). Of the 20 patients who survived the neonatal period, 13 died within 9 months, eight of renal failure, usually in association with hypertension. Nevertheless, five of the seven patients who were alive at the time they were reported, at the ages of 3 months to 9 years, had good renal function.

In children who present after 1 year of age, the principal signs and symptoms are related to hypertension and enlarged and impaired kidneys (e.g., proteinuria, hematuria). Now that the families of DPK patients are being screened by sonography, large numbers of asymptomatic children with renal cysts are being identified before full-blown disease develops.

Typically, symptoms or signs first occur between the ages of 30 and 50 years (Glassberg et al, 1981). These include microscopic and gross hematuria, flank pain, gastrointestinal symptoms (perhaps secondary to renomegaly or associated colonic diverticula), and renal colic secondary either to clots or stone and hypertension. Microscopic or gross hematuria is seen in 50% of patients, and in 19% to 35% of patients it may be the presenting symptom (Multinovic, 1984; Delaney et al, 1985; Zeier et al, 1988; Gabow et al, 1992). In Gabow and associates' series (1992), 42% of patients had at least one episode of gross hematuria, the age at the first episode being 30 years ± 1 year. Only in 10% of patients did the first episode occur before the age of 16 years. In general, they found that increased episodes of gross hematuria were associated with higher serum creatinine levels. Because these patients with DPK have increased renal mass, erythropoietin levels are increased, making anemia unusual even when end-stage renal disease is present (Gabow, 1993).

As blood pressure screening has become more widespread, hypertension more than hematuria has become the principal form of presentation. For example, in a series from Heidelberg, Germany (Zeier et al, 1988), as many as 81% of patients with DPK presented with hypertension. Among the Heidelberg patients with a normal serum creatinine concentration, 30% were found to be hypertensive. Antihypertensive medication instituted early resulted in fewer complications, particularly with regard to the incidence of cerebral hemorrhage. Other series suggest that the incidence of hypertension is about 60% prior to the onset of renal failure (Nash, 1977; Gabow et al, 1984; Valvo et al, 1985; Gabow et al, 1990). The hypertension seems to be renin mediated and secondary to stretching of the intrarenal vessels around cysts, causing distal ischemia (Gabow, 1993).

As noted earlier, the polycystic condition in DPK is not confined to the kidneys. **Hepatic cysts, usually identified incidentally by sonography, help in making the diagnosis of DPK. These cysts are more likely to be found in adults than in children. Such cysts were found by CT scanning in almost 60% of one series of adults (mean age 49)** (Thomsen and Thaysen, 1988). Hepatic cysts often grow, but they seldom produce any clinically important effects. New ones may appear as the patient grows older (Thomsen and Thaysen, 1988). In rare instances, enlargement of hepatic cysts leads to portal hypertension and bleeding esophageal varices (Campbell et al, 1958). When secondary portal hypertension appears, differentiating DPK from RPK can be difficult. In RPK portal hypertension is seen much more frequently and is always secondary to congenital hepatic fibrosis. However, congenital hepatic fibrosis, on very rare occasions, may accompany DPK as well (Cobben et al, 1990). When congenital hepatic fibrosis accompanies DPK, the clinical course is quite variable just as it is in RPK. In three DPK families in which at least one family member had congenital hepatic fibrosis, the genetic defect was localized to PKD1 on the 16th chromosome, clearly supporting a diagnosis of DPK rather than RPK (Cobben et al, 1990). In these three families, congenital hepatic fibrosis was not transmitted vertically with DPK but instead was found only in siblings.

Approximately 10% to 40% of patients have berry aneurysms, and approximately 9% of these patients die because of subarachnoid hemorrhages (Hartnett and Bennett, 1976; Grantham, 1979; Wakabayashi et al, 1983; Sedmon and Gabow, 1984; Ryu, 1990). Now with magnetic resonance imaging (MRI), even small berry aneurysms can be detected. Using MRI, Huston and associates (1993) found that families with a previous history of intracranial aneurysms had a higher incidence of berry aneurysms compared with families without a positive history. In their series 6 of 27 patients (27%) with a family history and 3 of 56 patients (5%) without a family history were found to have aneurysms. The problem is what to do with these aneurysms when they are diagnosed because they average only 6.1 mm in size. Although small aneurysms (i.e., less than 1 cm) have a lower risk of rupture, patients with small aneurysms have a greater risk of rupture when there is a positive family history of ruptured intracranial aneurysms or the presence of DPK (Huston et al, 1993).

However, not all intracranial hemorrhages in patients with DPK are subarachnoid bleeding secondary to berry aneurysms; in some patients, hemorrhage follows the rupture of intracerebral arteries, which is the usual type of intracranial hemorrhage seen in patients with hypertension who do not have DPK. For example, in Ryu's series (1990), a cerebral artery rupture accounted for the hemorrhage in eight patients and a ruptured berry aneurysm in only three. In 10 of these 11 patients, hypertension was present, and funduscopy suggested previous hypertension in the remaining one. Now, with earlier detection and treatment of hypertension, one can expect fewer deaths from intracranial hemorrhage.

Intracerebral bleeding has been reported in at least one child with DPK. This child also had hypertrophic pyloric stenosis (Proesmans et al, 1982), a condition that has been reported in association with DPK in a set of identical twins and their father (Loh et al, 1977). Hypertrophic pyloric stenosis also has accompanied RPK (Gaisford and Bloor, 1968; Lieberman et al, 1971; McGonigle et al, 1981). Other

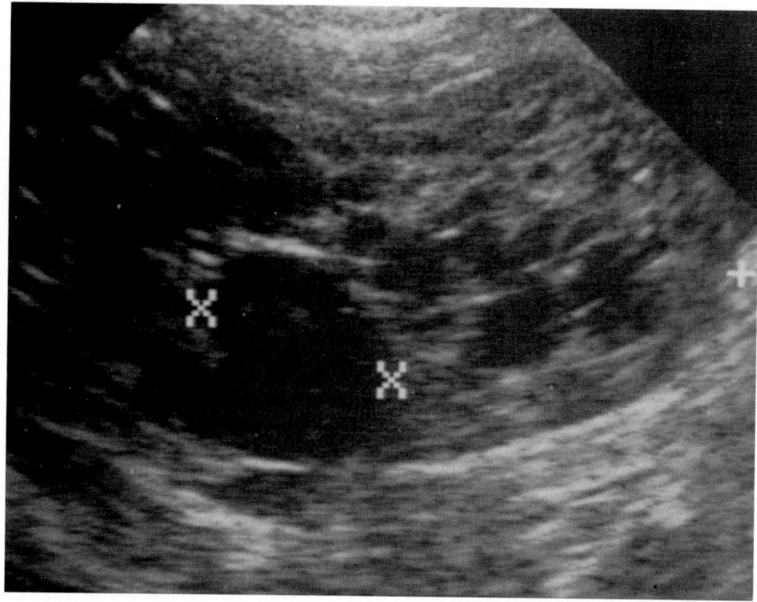

Figure 59–8. Asymmetric presentation of autosomal dominant polycystic kidney disease in a 9-year-old boy with hematuria. Sonogram demonstrates right kidney with multiple cysts. No cysts were identified in left kidney. Subsequently, the diagnosis was made in the patient's brother and mother. Cysts can be expected to develop in the right kidney with time.

abnormalities associated with DPK are mitral valve prolapse and colonic diverticulosis (Scheff et al, 1980); Hossack et al, 1986; Kupin et al, 1987. Patients who have diverticulosis are more likely to have hepatic cysts and symptomatic berry aneurysms (Kupin et al, 1987).

When DPK presents clinically, it usually is found with bilateral cysts. However, the disease can present asymmetrically, with cysts on only one side at first or with a unilateral renal mass (Fig. 59–8).

A variant form of DPK probably exists in which the renal cysts are located primarily in Bowman's space. The cytogenetic study of Reeders and associates (1985) provided evidence that such a condition is a form of DPK. They found that a fetus with cystic disease predominantly of the glomeruli had the same genetic linkages on chromosome 16 as did its DPK-affected mother. Bernstein and Landing (1989) suggest that glomerulocystic kidneys in members of families with DPK are variants; the glomerular cysts may be an early stage of DPK gene expression (Fig. 59–9). One caution: this condition should not be referred to as "glomerulocystic kidney disease" to avoid confusing it with sporadic glumerulocystic kidney disease, a condition that seems to be histologically identical to DPK in infants except for the absence of affected family members (Bernstein, 1993) and other disorders associated with glomerular cysts, which are discussed later in this chapter.

HISTOPATHOLOGY

The renal cysts range from a few millimeters to a few centimeters in diameter and appear diffusely throughout the cortex and medulla with communications at various points along the nephron (Kissane, 1974). Frequently, the epithelial lining resembles the segment of the nephron from which the

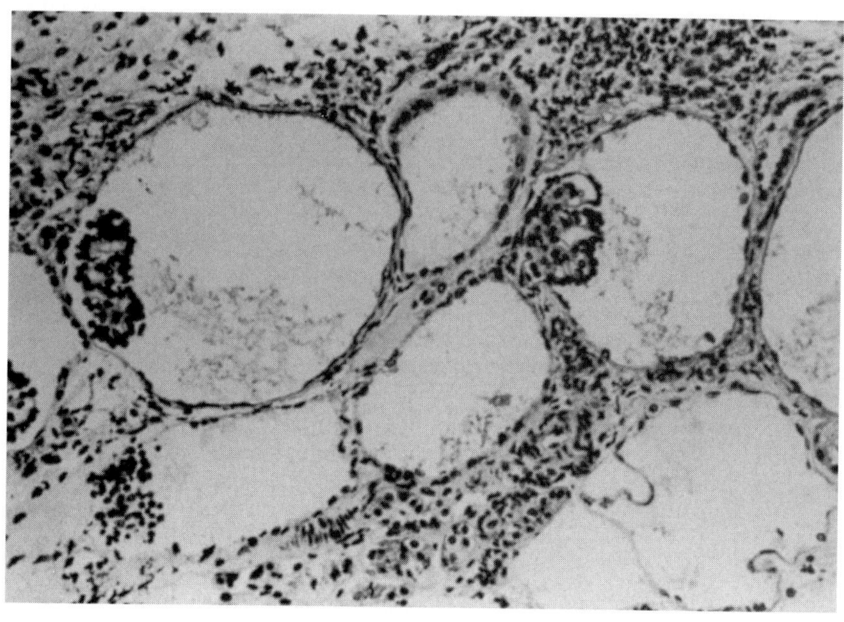

Figure 59–9. Glomerular cysts with a pattern compatible with that of autosomal dominant polycystic kidney disease in early childhood (× 190). (From Bernstein J, Gardner KD: Cystic disease and dysplasia of the kidneys. *In* Murphy WM, ed: Urological Pathology. Philadelphia, W. B. Saunders Company, 1989, pp 483–524.)

cyst is derived (Kaplan and Miller, unpublished data), and it often is active in secretion and reabsorption (Gardner, 1988).

Epithelial hyperplasia or even adenoma formation in the cyst wall is common, and the basement membrane of the wall is thickened. Arteriosclerosis is present in more than 70% of patients with preterminal or terminal renal failure, and interstitial fibrosis, with or without infiltrates, is common (Zeier et al, 1988). This fibrosis may be secondary to infection or to an inflammatory reaction set off by spontaneously rupturing cysts.

Gregoire and co-workers (1987) found a 91% incidence of hyperplastic polyps in kidneys removed from DPK patients either at autopsy or prior to transplantation. Some of the autopsies were performed on patients with normal renal function, yet polyps were still found. However, there was a greater predominance of polyps in patients with renal failure and in those on dialysis. Because hyperplastic epithelium is seen in both chronic renal failure and DPK, a uremic toxin not removed by dialysis may be involved.

Association with Renal Cell Carcinoma

The incidence of renal adenomas is almost as high in DPK as in end-stage renal disease associated with acquired renal cystic disease (i.e., one in four to five patients). However, **whereas end-stage renal disease is associated with an increased incidence of renal cell carcinoma, especially when associated with acquired renal cystic disease (three to six times the incidence seen in the general population), the incidence of renal cell carcinoma in patients with DPK is no higher than that in the general population.** That the incidence of renal cell carcinoma is not increased in DPK is also surprising in view of the frequent finding of epithelial hyperplasia. For example, two other conditions, tuberous sclerosis and von Hippel-Lindau disease, are associated with epithelial hyperplasia (and adenomas as well) and have an increased incidence of renal cell carcinoma (tuberous sclerosis, 2% and von Hippel-Lindau, 35–38%). Although it is recognized that there is no increased incidence of renal cell carcinoma in DPK patients, it is hard to account for certain findings considered typical of a predisposition to renal cell carcinoma that are seen more frequently in DPK patients than in the general population. For example, renal cell carcinoma in DPK is more often concurrently bilateral (12% versus 1% to 5% in the general population), multicentric (28% versus 6%), and sarcomatoid in type (33% versus 1% to 5%) (Keith et al, 1994).

Three factors may have contributed to the impression of a higher incidence of renal cell carcinoma in DPK. First, the chance association of these two rather common lesions is expected to be frequent. Second, some cases of simultaneous DPK and renal cell carcinoma probably in fact represent cancers in patients with von Hippel-Lindau disease or tuberous sclerosis. Third, the epithelial hyperplasia of DPK, which is a precancerous lesion in other conditions, may have been considered precancerous in DPK as well, although available data do not at present justify this view (Jacobs et al, 1979; Zeier et al, 1988).

Evaluation

To make the diagnosis, it is important to have a history of the patient's family spanning at least three generations. Questions should be asked about renal disease, hypertension, and strokes. Abdominal sonography may reveal renal cysts as well as cysts in other organs. When there is no family history to support a diagnosis of DPK, a presumptive diagnosis can be made if bilateral renal cysts are present and two or more of the following are present as well: bilateral renal enlargement, three or more hepatic cysts, cerebral artery aneurysm, and a solitary cyst of the arachnoid, pineal gland, pancreas, or spleen (Grantham, 1993).

When DPK is manifested in utero or in infancy, 50% of affected kidneys are large with identifiable macrocysts (Pretorius et al, 1987). However, the kidneys may appear identical to those seen in RPK, having no apparent macrocysts and showing only enlargement and homogeneous hyperechoic features. In such situations, one must look for a parent with DPK to confirm the diagnosis.

On intravenous urography, the calyces may be stretched by cysts. However, the picture may simulate that of RPK, with medullary streaking of contrast medium. In adults, intravenous urography usually reveals bilateral renal enlargement, calyceal distortion, and a bubble or Swiss cheese appearance in the nephrogram phase. A CT scan may be helpful in some cases and often is superior to sonography for detecting cysts in organs other than the kidney (Fig. 59–10).

According to Gabow and associates (1989b), patients with DPK have a reduced maximum urine osmolality (680 ± 14 mOsm) after overnight water deprivation and administration of vasopressin, a finding that may be helpful in identifying other family members with the disease. However, within the next few years cytogenetic screening should be readily available to identify the gene defects on chromosomes 4 and 16.

Examination of Family Members and Genetic Counseling

Because DPK is an autosomal dominant condition, 50% of the children of affected adults will be affected. Therefore, when the disease is diagnosed, the patient's children should be examined by ultrasound. Before 1970, diagnosis of DPK before age 25 was rare. With ultrasound, the possibility of making the diagnosis in affected individuals before this age is at least 85% (Table 59–7). When genetic studies are used, the diagnostic accuracy approaches 100%.

Gabow and co-workers (1989a) identified DPK in 16 of 59 children under the age of 12, and the disease was suspected in another ten. Bear and colleagues (1984), who studied 61 children sonographically, found DPK in only 2 of 18 children younger than age 10 but in 14 of 43 children between 10 and 19 years of age. Similarly, Sahney and associates (1983) found the disease in only one of five children younger than age 15 but in 16 of 19 children aged 16 to 25 years. This last figure points out the fact that the 50% incidence of affected offspring is an average, not a guarantee.

Bear and co-workers (1984) calculated that the chance that an asymptomatic relative between the ages of 10 and 19 years has DPK is 28% if an ultrasound scan is negative and that, in a similar individual aged 20 to 29 years, the risk is 14%. Other investigators have found rates of 32% to 50% in siblings and children younger than age 20 (Walker et al,

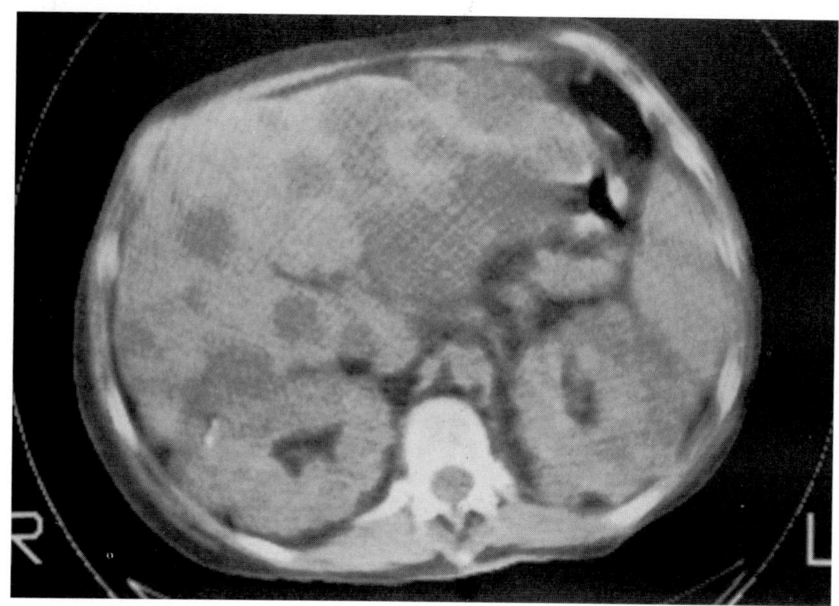

Figure 59–10. CT Scan of an adult male patient with autosomal dominant polycystic kidney disease. Bilateral renal cysts are seen in enlarged kidneys with calcification. Large asymptomatic cysts are seen throughout the liver as well.

1984; Sedman et al, 1987; Taitz et al, 1987). When patients with a known PKD1 defect were selected for renal sonographic screening, 40 of 48 individuals (83%) were found to have cysts prior to age 30 years and all (i.e., individuals) had them after age 30 (Parfrey et al, 1992).

At present, family members of an individual with DPK cannot obtain insurance before the age of 25 years because of the possibility of the disease (Dalgaard and Norby, 1989). Between the ages of 25 and 35, insurance is available but at higher rates, and after the age of 35, insurance can be obtained at normal rates if a sonogram has been negative. Now, with definitive cytogenetic diagnosis available, it may be time for insurance companies to revise their criteria of insurability.

Treatment and Prognosis

Men tend to have more renal involvement than women, manifesting with hypertension and renal insufficiency earlier than women (Grantham, 1993). However, women seem to have more severe cystic involvement of the liver, which causes pain and requires treatment more often than that in men (Grantham, 1993).

Table 59–7. INCIDENCE OF RENAL CYSTS IN SIBLINGS AND OFFSPRING OF PATIENTS WITH DPK*

Reference	Age at Study (Years)	No. with Cysts/ No. Studied (%)
Bear et al	<10	2/18 (11)
Gabow et al	<12	26/59 (40)
Taitz et al	<14	10/22 (45)
Sahney et al	<15	1/5 (20)
Walker et al	5–17	11/22 (50)
Bear et al	10–19	14/43 (34)
Sedman et al	<19	49/154 (32)
Bear et al	20–29	26/62 (42)
Sahney et al	<26	17/24 (70)

*DPK, autosomal dominant polycystic kidney disease.

More than 60% of patients with DPK who do not yet have renal impairment have hypertension (Gabow et al, 1984), which can worsen renal function, cause cardiac disease, and predispose the patient to intracranial hemorrhage. The complications of DPK, thus, can be reduced significantly by controlling the blood pressure.

The rate of renal deterioration seems to correlate with the rate of cyst growth, supposedly because the enlarging cysts cause pressure atrophy. However, histologic studies by Zeier and co-workers (1988) revealed no evidence of pressure atrophy, nor did these investigators find evidence of glomerular hyperperfusion, which had been thought to damage the remaining glomeruli after some had been destroyed.

Fifty to seventy percent of patients with DPK at some time have loin or back pain (Grantham, 1992). The pain can be colicky, acute, or chronic. Colicky pain is secondary to the passage of either stones or clots. Acute pain may be secondary to infection or hemorrhage into a cyst or to subcapsular bleeding. Chronic loin pain requiring narcotics is probably related to distention of cysts and the renal capsule. Rovsing in 1911 described an operation that involved unroofing the cysts to relieve the pain. The procedure fell into some dispute because of reports that renal function could deteriorate following such a procedure. More recent reports, however, are repopularizing the procedure. Ye and associates (1986) reported that the incidence of relief of pain following Rovsing's operation was 90.6% after 6 months and 77.1% after 5 years, whereas Elzinga and associates (1992) found that 80% of patients were pain free at 1 year and 62% at 2 years. Of significance was the finding that renal function did not deteriorate following the procedure in either series; in fact, in the former study there was a significant improvement in renal function in some patients. When pain does return following an unroofing procedure, it often is less severe than it was preoperatively and requires narcotics infrequently (Elzinga et al, 1992). Percutaneous cyst aspiration with or without instillation of a sclerosing agent such as alcohol (Bennett et al, 1987; Everson et al, 1990) or even laparoscopic unroofing (Elzinga et al, 1993) also can play a therapeutic role. However, aspiration alone is more likely to be associated with reaccumulation of cyst fluid.

Upper tract urinary infections are common in patients with DPK, especially women. Schwab and co-workers (1987) divided these cases into parenchymal and cyst infections. In their series, **87% of cyst infections and 91% of parenchymal infections occurred in women.** When a gram-negative enteric organism was the cause, 100% of the infections were seen in women. Presumably, in women the infection is an ascending one. Schwab and co-workers (1987) found that parenchymal infections responded better than cyst infections to treatment, even when the organism causing the cyst infection was proved to be sensitive to the antibiotic used. In their experience, **the only dependable antibiotics were those that were lipid soluble, namely, trimethoprim-sulfamethoxazole and chloramphenicol. Chloramphenicol produced better results. The fluoroquinolones, which are also lipid soluble, are proving useful (Bennett et al, 1990). If a patient with suspected pyelonephritis does not respond to an antibiotic and if the antibiotic used is not lipid soluble, one must consider whether the infection may be present in a noncommunicating cyst** (Gabow, 1993).

Symptomatic children generally are in the terminal stages of the disease, but their survival may be extended by supportive care for complications. As in affected adults, dialysis and transplantation may be appropriate. In the past, allografts from siblings were ruled out because of the frequency of DPK in such donors. However, now that siblings can be screened, this ban may no longer be appropriate.

Presymptomatic patients with DPK should be monitored with blood pressure measurements and tests of renal function. The advantages of such monitoring include the ability to prevent or control infection and hypertension, to identify potential kidney donors from among the family, to offer advice on marriage and childbearing, and to provide prenatal diagnosis. The question of abortion of an affected fetus is an issue that the parents and the physician must consider in view of the improved prognosis for such patients.

In earlier reports of DPK, the prognosis was quite poor, the mean life expectancy ranging from 4 to 13 years after clinical presentation. Life expectancy was even shorter if the disease became apparent after the age of 50 years (Braasch and Schacht, 1933; Roll and Odell, 1949; Dalgaard, 1957). Death usually was attributable to uremia, heart failure, or cerebral hemorrhage (Dalgaard, 1957).

Churchill and associates (1984) calculated that patients with sonographically identifiable DPK have a 2% chance of developing end-stage renal failure by age 40, a 23% chance by age 50, and a 48% chance by age 73. Because of our greater ability to deal with problems such as urinary infection, calculi, hypertension, and renal failure, the outlook for patients with DPK appears to be improving dramatically.

Juvenile Nephronophthisis–Medullary Cystic Disease Complex

Juvenile nephronophthisis was first described by Fanconi and colleagues in 1951. Medullary cystic disease was first reported by Smith and Graham in 1945. Although the two conditions are similar anatomically and clinically, they have a different mode of transmission and a different clinical onset.

Although juvenile nephronophthisis is the more common condition and is responsible for approximately 10% to 20% of cases of renal failure occurring in children (Cantani et al, 1986), this relatively high incidence does not appear to correlate with the low incidence (1 in 50,000 births) reported by Lirenman and associates (1974). A frequency of less than 1 in 100,000 has been reported for medullary cystic disease by Reeders (1990). Both conditions have been known by other names, such as uremic medullary cystic disease, salt-losing enteropathy, and uremic sponge kidney.

Although either condition can occur sporadically, juvenile nephronophthisis usually is inherited as an autosomal recessive trait and becomes manifest between the ages of 6 and 20 years, whereas medullary cystic disease usually is inherited in autosomal dominant fashion and presents after the third decade. The recessive transmission of juvenile nephronophthisis is supported by the frequency of consanguineous marriages among the parents of affected children (Bernstein and Gardner, 1979b; Cantani et al, 1986). Antignac and associates (1993) demonstrated by linkage analysis and Hildebrandt and associates (1993) confirmed that the gene defect for juvenile nephronophthisis is located on chromosome 2.

Clinical Features

Juvenile nephronophthisis and medullary cystic disease both cause polydipsia and polyuria in more than 80% of cases but not to the extent observed in patients with diabetes insipidus (Gardner, 1984a; Cantani et al, 1986). The polyuria is attributable to a severe renal tubular defect associated with an inability to conserve sodium. The polyuria is resistant to vasopressin, and a large dietary salt intake frequently is necessary. Proteinuria and hematuria usually are absent. In children, growth gradually slows, and malaise and pallor may appear in advanced disease. These latter findings are secondary to anemia, which may be attributable to a deficiency of erythropoietin production by the failing kidneys (Gruskin, 1977). Renal failure generally ensues 5 to 10 years after initial presentation (Cantani et al, 1986).

Juvenile nephronophthisis often is associated with disorders of the retina (particularly retinitis pigmentosa), skeletal abnormalities, hepatic fibrosis, and Bardet-Biedl syndrome—a combination of obesity, mental retardation, polydactyly, retinitis pigmentosa, and hypogenitalism. Sixteen percent of patients with juvenile nephronophthisis have associated retinitis pigmentosa (Hildebrandt et al, 1993). When the two entities coexist, the condition is referred to as renal-retinal or Senior-Løken syndrome. However, if one member in a family with juvenile nephronophthisis has retinal disease, that does not mean that others in the family with nephronophthisis necessarily also have retinal disease. Alstrom's syndrome, a nephropathy accompanied by blindness, obesity, diabetes mellitus, and nerve deafness, may be a form of juvenile nephronophthisis (Bernstein, 1976).

Extrarenal abnormalities classically have been associated only with juvenile nephronophthisis. However, Green and co-workers (1990) described two sisters who presented with medullary cystic disease when they were in their mid-30s. Both had a history of congenital spastic quadriparesis.

HISTOPATHOLOGY

Early in the disease course, the kidneys may be of normal size (Cantani et al., 1986). In clinically manifest cases, the kidneys nearly always demonstrate interstitial nephritis, with round-cell infiltrates and tubular dilatation with atrophy. The corticomedullary junction is poorly defined. Atrophy begins in the cortex, but later the entire organ becomes very small and has a granular surface.

Cysts are present in the kidneys of many patients, particularly those with medullary cystic disease (incidence: 85% versus 40% in patients with juvenile nephronophthisis) (Mongeau and Worthen, 1967). These cysts, which range in diameter from 1 mm to 1 cm, usually appear at the corticomedullary junction and, less often, in the medulla, generally within the distal convolutions and the collecting ducts (Fig. 59–11) (Cantani et al, 1986). Biopsies do not always reveal cysts, however, both because affected areas may be missed and because cysts tend to appear only with renal failure in the recessive disease. In the dominant disorder, medullary cysts are sometimes seen prior to the development of renal failure (Lirenman et al, 1974; Stelle et al, 1980; Garel et al, 1984; Cantani et al, 1986; Kleinknecht and Habib, 1992). Similar findings of tubulointerstitial nephritis with medullary cysts have been reported in Bardet-Biedl syndrome (or Laurence-Moon-Bardet-Biedl syndrome)—namely, obesity, mental retardation, hypogenitalism, polydactyly, and retinitis pigmentosa—as well as in Jeune's syndrome.

Some have suggested that the primary defect in juvenile nephronophthisis and medullary cystic disease is a defect of the tubular basement membrane. On histopathology, alternating areas of thickening and thinning of the tubular basement membrane are seen (Cohen and Hoyer, 1986). However, this finding is seen more consistently in juvenile nephronophthisis than in medullary cystic disease (Kleinknecht and Habib, 1992) (Table 59–8). Cohen and Hoyer (1986) reported no abnormalities in the glomerular capillaries or Bowman's capsule and theorized that the interstitial damage was secondary to leakage of Tamm-Horsfall protein through the thin areas of the basement membrane. Kelly and Neilson (1990) were impressed by the number of inflammatory cells seen in the interstitium with medullary cystic disease. Particularly in the early stages, a heavy infiltrate of mononuclear cells is seen. The role of these cells is not clear. Do they represent a response to tubular leakage, antigen, or tissue damage, or do they play a primary role in the development of the cysts? Renal failure may be associated with a large mononuclear cell infiltrate and little evidence of cysts (Bernstein and Gardner, 1983; Neilson et al, 1985).

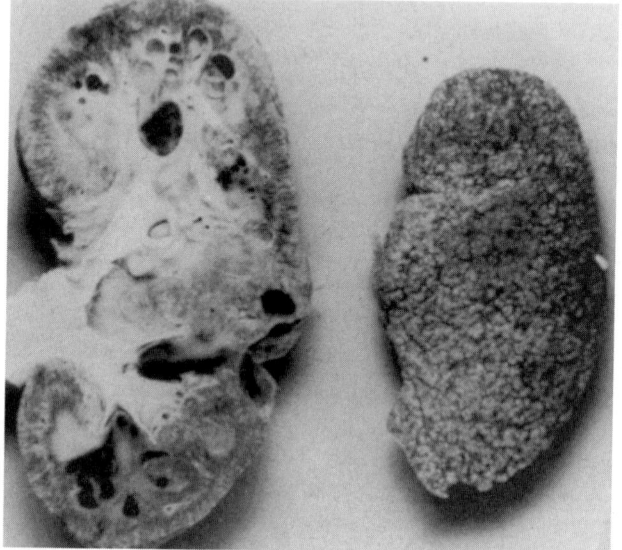

Figure 59–11. The gross appearance of the sectioned and subcapsular surface of a kidney from a patient with medullary cystic disease. Note that the cysts are concentrated at the corticomedullary junction, not at the papillae as in medullary sponge kidney. (From Kissane JM: Pathology of Infancy and Childhood, 2nd ed. St. Louis, C. V. Mosby Company, 1975.)

Table 59–8. MEDULLARY CYSTIC DISEASE–JUVENILE NEPHRONOPHTHISIS COMPLEX*

	Juvenile Nephronophthisis	Medullary Cystic Disease
Inheritance	Autosomal recessive (chromosome 2)	Autosomal dominant (chromosome ?)
Incidence	1:50,000	1:100,000
End-stage renal disease	By age 13 years	20–40 years
Medullary cysts	Develop after renal failure	May develop before onset of renal failure
Tubular basement	Thickened	May not be thickened
Symptoms	Polyuria, polydipsia, anemia, growth retardation (usually after age 2)	Polyuria, polydipsia, anemia; may have hematuria and proteinuria (symptoms usually appear after patient is fully grown)

*Both have tubulointestinal nephritis and small kidneys with granular surface; medullary cysts are not essential for diagnosis and are not present in all cases.

In some patients with juvenile nephronophthisis, especially those with hepatic disease, glomerular cysts have been detected. These lesions are rarely seen in other forms of nephronophthisis (Bernstein and Landing, 1989). Therefore, if glomerular cysts are discovered in a renal biopsy from a patient with juvenile nephronophthisis, hepatic biopsy is advisable. Hepatic biopsy is particularly important if renal transplantation is being considered because hepatic fibrosis may lead to portal hypertension (Bernstein and Landing, 1989).

EVALUATION

In the early stages of the disease, intravenous urography may show a normal or slightly shrunken kidney (Habib, 1974; Chamberlin et al, 1977). Homogeneous streaking of the medulla may be found, presumably secondary to retention of contrast medium within dilated tubules, or ring-shaped densities at the bases of papillae, again perhaps representing contrast-filled tubules (Olsen et al, 1988). In

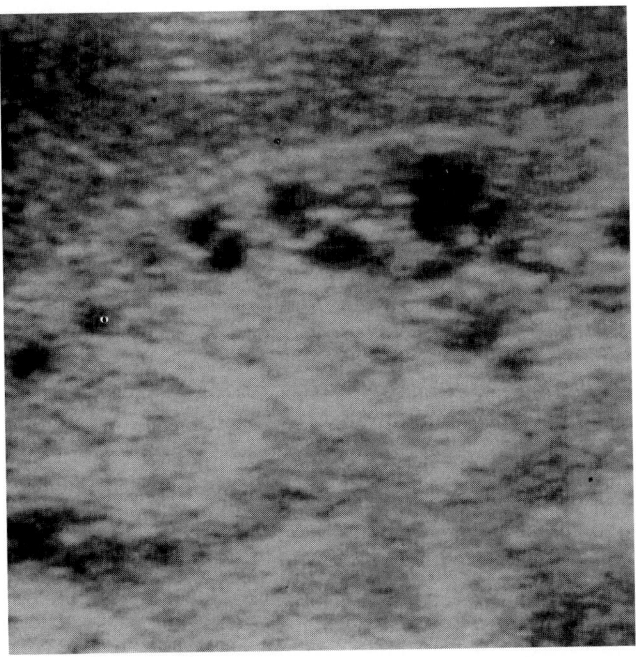

Figure 59–12. Renal sonogram of right kidney in a patient with medullary cystic disease. Note small to medium-size cysts located predominantly at outer edge of medulla and a few well within the medulla. The hyperechogenicity is secondary to the tubulointerstitial fibrosis. (From Resnick JS, Hartman DS: Medullary cystic disease. *In* Pollack HM, ed: Clinical Urography. Philadelphia, W. B. Saunders Company, 1990, pp 1178–1184.)

the late stages of the disease, intravenous urography is of little value. Calcifications are not seen.

Sonography may show smaller than normal kidneys in juvenile nephronophthisis. Cysts may be seen on imaging studies if they are large enough (Rosenfeld et al, 1977), but early in the disease cysts are rarely visible. For example, Garel and associates (1984) demonstrated medullary cysts in 17 of 19 patients with end-stage disease but not in twins who had only mild uremia. The parenchyma may appear hyperechogenic secondary to tubulointerstitial fibrosis (Resnick and Hartman, 1990) (Fig. 59–12).

McGregor and Bailey (1989) described the CT appearance of juvenile nephronophthisis in a 19-year-old patient. In this case, cysts approximately 0.5 cm in diameter were apparent throughout the medulla, although no cysts were visible by sonography. These investigators recommended CT rather than sonography for investigating relatives of known cases. Even though the cysts may be prominent and may help in diagnosis, renal failure probably results, not from the cysts, but from the tubulointerstitial changes.

Treatment

Sodium replacement is indicated early in the course of the disease. Later, dialysis and transplantation will have to be considered. Allografts apparently are not susceptible to the same process that destroyed the native kidney because there is no evidence of serum antibodies to the basement membrane or other renal structural proteins (Cantani et al, 1986; Cohen and Hoyer, 1986).

Congenital Nephrosis

Congenital nephrosis is predominantly of two types. The more common is referred to as the Finnish type (CNF) and has, as the name suggests, been reported principally in Finland, where the incidence is 1 in 8200 (Norio, 1966; Lanning et al, 1989). The other type, described by Habib and Bois in 1973, is referred to as diffuse mesangial sclerosis (DMS). The CNF type is recessive (Norio, 1966), whereas only 10 of the 30 reported cases of DMS were familial (Habib et al, 1989). Both conditions are associated with dilatation of the proximal convoluted tubules. The term "microcystic disease," is now rarely used.

Clinical Features

CNF usually is discovered because of an enormously enlarged and edematous placenta, which accounts for more than 25% of the birth weight (Norio and Rapola, 1989). In DMS, the placenta usually is not enlarged.

In infants with CNF, proteinuria is present in the first urinalysis. Edema usually develops within the first few days and always develops by the age of 3 months. Essentially, these infants starve because of their severe loss of protein in the urine; without treatment, they probably would die of sepsis before renal failure kills them. Without dialysis, half the patients die by the age of 6 months, and the rest die before their fourth birthday (Huttunen, 1976).

In DMS, the onset of symptoms is variable, and the diagnosis is usually made by the age of 1 year. All children have terminal renal failure by the age of 3 years.

Habib and colleagues (1985) have demonstrated that the nephropathy of Drash syndrome (nephrotic syndrome and Wilms' tumor with or without male pseudohermaphroditism) is, in fact, DMS. Of the 35 cases of DMS diagnosed by Habib and co-workers (1989), 13 were associated with Drash syndrome.

Histopathology

CNF and DMS are both characterized by normal-sized kidneys, initially with pronounced proximal tubular dilatation. DMS is distinctive in that the glomeruli have an accumulation of PAS-positive and silver phosphate-staining mesangial fibrils. With advanced disease, the glomerular tufts sclerose and contract (Norio and Rapola, 1989; Habib et al, 1989). Diffuse hypertrophy of the podocytes is also found.

CNF is characterized by a proliferation of the glomerular mesangial cells. In both DMS and CNF, as in all types of nephrosis, there is fusion of the glomerular podocytes. Interstitial fibrosis is present in both conditions but is more pronounced in DMS (Norio and Rapola, 1989).

Evaluation

The diagnosis of CNF can be made at about 6 weeks of gestation because of the greatly elevated levels of amniotic alpha-fetoprotein (AFP) secondary to fetal proteinuria. The use of AFP to diagnose DMS in utero has not been demonstrated.

In the later stages of disease postnatally, ultrasonography reveals enlarged kidneys with cortices that are more echogenic than those of the liver or spleen. The pyramids are small and hazy, and the corticomedullary junction is indistinct or absent. In one study, the kidneys continued to enlarge, and the corticomedullary junction became more effaced as the disease become worse (Lanning et al, 1989).

TREATMENT

After the kidneys have failed, transplantation is curative. Neither type of disease responds to steroids.

Familial Hypoplastic Glomerulocystic Kidney Disease (Cortical Microcystic Disease)

In 1982, Rizzoni and co-workers described two families in which a mother and two daughters were affected by what these investigators called hypoplastic glomerulocystic disease. Melnick and associates (1984) described the same condition under the name cortical microcystic disease, and Kaplan and colleagues (1989a) reported it in a mother and son. This condition is autosomal dominant.

The diagnosis of familial hypoplastic glomerulocystic disease requires four features. First, stable or progressive chronic renal failure must be present. Second, the kidneys must be small or of normal size with irregular calyceal outlines and abnormal papillae. Third, the condition must by present in two generations of a family. Last, histologic evidence of glomerular cysts must be found. These cysts are thin-walled and tend to be subcapsular. Tubular atrophy with some normal glomeruli and tubules in the deeper cortex is also observed. Marked prognathism is present in some patients (Kaplan et al, 1989a; Rizzoni et al, 1982).

Multiple Malformation Syndromes Including Renal Cysts

Renal cysts are a feature of several syndromes characterized by multiple malformations (Table 59–9). Tuberous sclerosis and von Hippel-Lindau disease are autosomal dominant disorders and are the ones most likely to be encountered by urologists. Meckel's syndrome, Jeune's asphyxiating thoracic dystrophy, and Zellweger's cerebrohepatorenal syndrome are some of the more common autosomal recessive syndromes. Many of these conditions involve glomerular cysts, and some have cystic dysplasia as a feature. The most frequently encountered syndromes are listed in Table 59–9.

TUBEROUS SCLEROSIS

Bourneville described tuberous sclerosis in 1880. Since then, the disorder has been reported in between 1 in 9000 and 1 in 170,000 infants (Kuntz, 1988).

Classically, tuberous sclerosis is described as part of a triad of epilepsy (80% of cases), mental retardation (60% of cases), and adenoma sebaceum (75% of cases) (Lagos and Gomez, 1967; Pampigliana and Moynahan, 1976). The lesions of adenoma sebaceum are flesh-colored papules of angiofibroma and are especially prevalent in the malar area. An earlier skin lesion that is a white papule in the shape of an "ash leaf" is sometimes identified (Shepherd et al, 1991). An examination of the skin with ultraviolet light may reveal cutaneous lesions earlier and should be part of a diagnostic evaluation.

The hallmark lesion of the central nervous system is a superficial cortical hamartoma of the cerebrum, which sometimes looks like hardened gyri, creating the appearance of a tuber (root). Hamartomas often affect other organs as well, especially the kidneys and eyes. Periventricular subependymal nodules also occur frequently.

The kidneys of these patients may be free of lesions (Stillwell et al, 1987) or may display cysts, angiomyolipomas, or both (Fig. 59–13).

CYTOGENETICS

Although it is transmitted as an autosomal dominant trait in 15% to 25% of cases, in the remainder, tuberous sclerosis occurs either sporadically or as an example of the genetic condition with variable or incomplete penetrance.

Two genes, one on chromosome 9 (TSC1) and one on

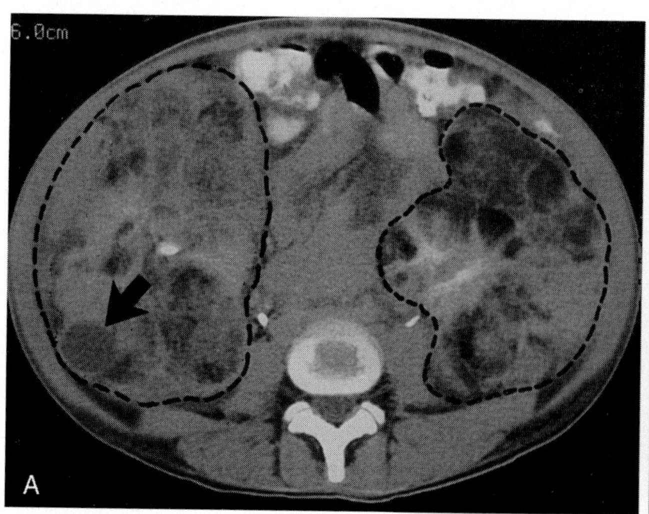

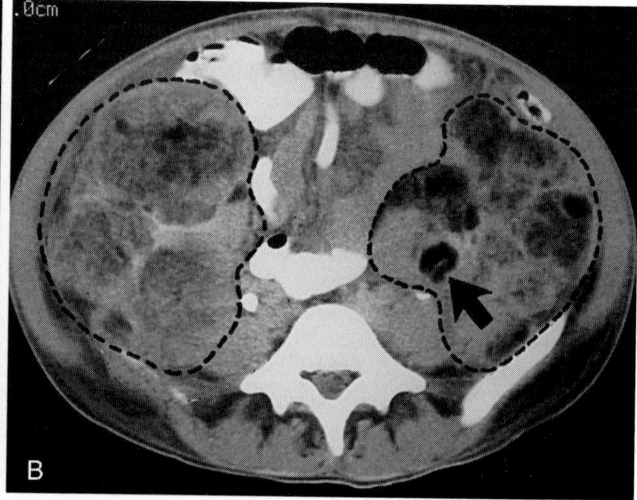

Figure 59–13. A 24-year-old woman known to have tuberous sclerosis since early childhood. Enhanced CT scan demonstrates bilateral renomegaly with multiple renal cysts and angiomyolipomas. *A,* Arrow points to a cyst with a CT value of +10 HU. *B,* Arrow points to an angiomyolipoma with a negative CT value (−50 HU) secondary to its high fat content.

Table 59–9. MULTIPLE MALFORMATION SYNDROMES ASSOCIATED WITH RENAL CYSTS*

	Features	Cyst Characteristics	Other Renal Lesions	Renal Sequelae
Mendelian (single gene) disorders				
Autosomal dominant				
Tuberous sclerosis	Adenoma sebaceum, elipepsy, mental retardation, cranial calcifications	Variable size; eosinophilic hyperplastic lining†	Angiomyolipomas (more common than cysts), renal cell carcinoma (2% incidence)	Occasionally masses compress or obstruct kidney, leading to renal failure
von Hippel-Lindau disease	Cerebellar hemangioblastomas, retinal angiomatosis, pheochromocytoma, cysts of pancreas and epididymis	Variable size; hyperplastic lining	Renal cell carcinoma (35%–38% incidence)	Rarely, masses compress or obstruct kidney, leading to renal failure
Autosomal recessive				
Meckel's syndrome	Microcephaly, polydactyly, posterior encephalocele	Large with fibromuscular collars that probably arise from collecting ducts	Dysplasia, hypoplasia	Possible renal failure
Jeune's asphyxiating thoracic dystrophy	Small chest, respiratory failure	From subcapsular cortical microcysts to dysplasia with cystic component; generalized dilatation of various segments of nephron (similar to DPK‡)	Dysplasia	Possible renal failure or chronic nephritis
Zellweger's cerebrohepatorenal syndrome	Hypotonia, high forehead, hepatomegaly	From glomerular microcysts to 1-cm cortical cysts	—	Rarely, mild azotemia; usually no manifestations
Ivemark's syndrome (renal-hepatic-pancreatic dysplasia)	Biliary dysgenesis, dilated intrahepatic ducts, pancreatic dysplasia	Diffuse, microscopic to large	Dysplasia	Possible renal failure
X-linked dominant disorders				
Orofaciodigital syndrome I	Hypertrophic lingular and buccal frenula; cleft lip, palate, and tongue; hypoplasia of alinasal cartilage, brachydactyly, syndactyly, alopecia	Develop with age	—	Hypertension, renal failure
Chromosomal disorders				
Trisomy 13 (Patau's syndrome)	Any cystic changes usually are not clinically significant. Findings are variable, but cysts generally are microscopic (dysplastic cysts, subcortical cysts, glomerular cysts).			
Trisomy 18 (Edwards' syndrome)				
Trisomy 21 (Down's syndrome)				

*Adapted from Glassberg KI: Cystic disease of the kidney. Probl Urol 1988; 2:157, and Glassberg KI: Renal cystic diseases. Curr Probl Urol 1991; 1:137.
†May resemble DPK in imaging studies.
‡DPK = autosomal dominant polycystic kidney disease.

chromosome 16 (TSC2), have been identified as being responsible for the autosomal dominant transmission of tuberous sclerosis (Kandt et al, 1992; Brook-Carter et al, 1994). However, in a review of ten previously reported cases (in addition to one new case in whom severe bilateral cystic disease was diagnosed by the age of 4 months), in six of the infants there was no family history of tuberous sclerosis, in three no family history was available, and in only one was the disease found to be familial (Campos et al, 1993). In another study (Brook-Carter et al, 1994), in six patients with tuberous sclerosis and a known history of diffuse bilateral cystic disease in early infancy, all six were found to have deletions not only at the TSC2 gene site on chromosome 16 but also in the adjacent PKD1 gene, the gene responsible for autosomal dominant polycystic kidney disease. In all six patients, signs of tuberous sclerosis were not present in the parents or other family members, suggesting that in these six patients, the disease probably represents a new mutation. It is interesting that of the 11 cases reviewed by Campos and colleagues (1993) and of the six studied by Brook-Carter and associates (1994) with diffuse bilateral cystic disease in early infancy, the disease was identified as familial in only one child (Fig. 59–14).

HISTOPATHOLOGY

The renal cysts are of a unique histologic type in that they have a lining of hypertrophic, hyperplastic eosinophilic cells (Bernstein and Meyer, 1967; Stapleton et al, 1980). These cells have large, hyperchromatic nuclei, and mitoses are seen occasionally. The cells often aggregate into masses or tumorlets (Bernstein et al, 1986; Bernstein and Gardner, 1989). Later in the disease, the cyst walls may atrophy into a thickened, unidentifiable lining (Mitnick et al, 1983). In a

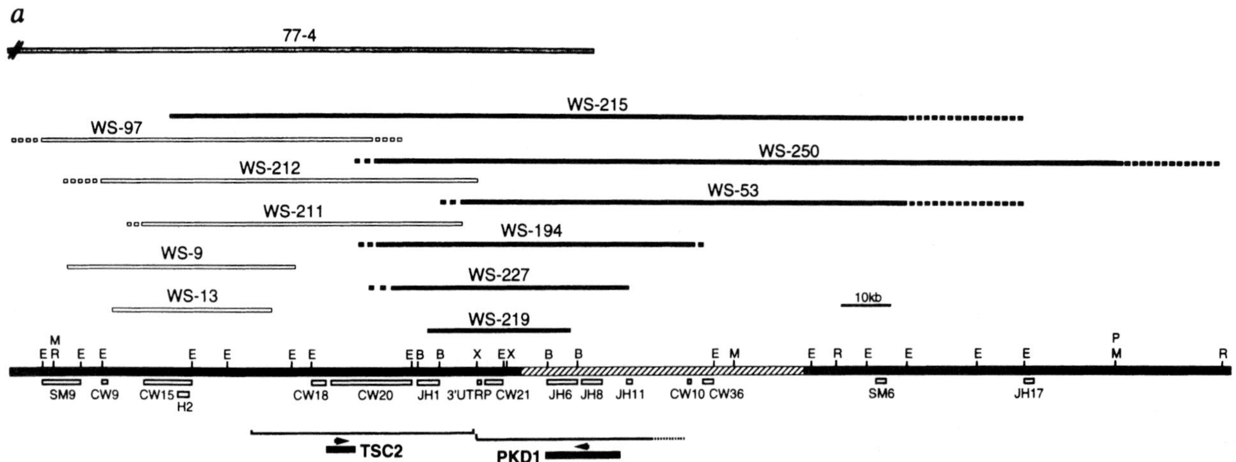

Figure 59–14. A map of a segment of chromosome 16 that includes one of the genes associated with tuberous sclerosis (TSC 2) and one associated with autosomal dominant polycystic kidney disease (PKD1). The positions of DNA probes *(open boxes)* and the TSC2 and PKD 1 genes *(solid boxes)* are illustrated below the chromosomal segment map. Above the segment map, the open boxes represent deletions in patients who have tuberous sclerosis without evidence of perinatal polycystic kidneys. The six closed boxes represent deletions in patients with tuberous sclerosis who have evidence of perinatal polycystic kidneys but not autosomal dominant polycystic kidney disease. Because the parents or other family members of all six patients do not have signs of tuberous sclerosis, the condition might represent a new mutation. The gray bar represents patient 77-4, who has both tuberous sclerosis and autosomal dominant polycystic kidney disease. (From Brook-Carter PA, Peral B, Ward CJ, et al: Deletion of the TSC 2 and PKD 1 gene associated with severe infantile polycystic kidney disease—a contiguous gene syndrome. Nature Genet 1994; 8:328.)

few patients, predominantly glomerular cells have been seen (Bernstein and Gardner, 1989). The cystic disease can lead to renal failure with or without the presence of angiomyolipomas. The probable mechanism is compression of the parenchyma by the expanding cysts. Hypertension may also be present.

Angiomyolipomas occur in 40% to 80% of patients (Chonko et al, 1974; Gomez, 1979). They are rarely identified before the age of 6 years but are common after age 10 (Bernstein et al, 1986). By themselves, these lesions probably do not cause renal failure (Okada et al, 1982; Bernstein et al, 1986). Also, belying their aggressive histologic appearance, which is characterized by pleomorphism and mitoses, no evidence of metastases has been presented.

EVALUATION

Sometimes both renal cysts and angiomyolipomas can be identified by sonography in tuberous sclerosis, the former lesions being sonolucent and the latter having a fluffy, white appearance. When renal cysts are present without angiomyolipomas, the sonographic appearance of the kidneys in tuberous sclerosis is very similar to that in DPK. Therefore, it is not that unusual for a patient in whom cysts typical of DPK are identified to be diagnosed as such only to develop the stigmata of tuberous sclerosis a few years later. To help make the diagnosis, abdominal CT scans can be useful in demonstrating angiomyolipomas that may be present in the kidney or other organs, findings that are compatible with tuberous sclerosis, as well as in revealing cysts in other organs, findings that are compatible with DPK. Magnetic resonance imaging (MRI) or CT of the head may demonstrate the classic cranial calcifications associated with tubers or gliosis (Okada et al, 1982). Ultraviolet light examination of the skin may reveal cutaneous lesions before they become manifest grossly and should be part of the differential diagnosis.

CLINICAL FEATURES AND PROGNOSIS

Renal cysts develop in approximately 20% of patients and frequently are identified first in childhood. However, they lead to serious renal compromise in less than 5% of patients (Stillwell et al, 1987; Bernstein, 1993). The cysts probably originate from nephrons lined with hyperplastic cells that may be present even at birth (Bernstein, 1993).

Because more patients with tuberous sclerosis now survive their central nervous system lesions than in the past, the urologist is more likely to be called on for management of the renal problems (Stillwell et al, 1987). In a recent report, Shepherd and associates (1991) found that renal disease was the leading cause of death (11 of 40 deaths). Of 355 patients they followed at the Mayo Clinic, 49 have died, 9 from nontuberous sclerosis–related disease, 10 from brain tumors, 4 from lymphangiomatosis of the lung, 13 from causes secondary to status epilepticus or bronchiopneunomia, and 11 from renal disease. Of these 11 patients, 2 died from metastatic renal cell carcinoma, 2 from massive hemorrhage associated with renal angiomyolipomas, and 6 from renal failure secondary to the cysts, angiomyolipomas, or both.

ASSOCIATION WITH RENAL CELL CARCINOMA

The numerous reports of renal cell carcinoma in patients with tuberous sclerosis make it clear that this association is more than coincidental and may be as frequent as 2% (Bernstein et al, 1986; Bernstein, 1993). **However, the incidence of renal cell carcinoma is considerably less than that seen in other conditions involving hyperplastic epithelial cells, specifically von Hippel-Lindau disease and acquired renal cystic disease of chronic renal failure, but more frequent than that seen in another condition with hyperplastic cells, autosomal dominant polycystic kidney disease, which may not even have an increased incidence.**

These cancers appear in patients younger than would be expected (7 to 39 years) and may be single or multiple and unilateral or bilateral (Bernstein and Gardner, 1989). **The karyotype of the cells near the tumor is similar to that of the tumor itself, and it is reasonable to suspect**

that the lining of the cysts evolves into the cancer (Ibrahim et al, 1989).

Von Hippel-Lindau Disease

Von Hippel-Lindau disease is an autosomal dominant condition manifested by cerebellar hemangioblastomas, retinal angiomas, cysts of the pancreas, kidney, and epididymis, pheochromocytoma, and renal cell carcinoma.

CYTOGENETICS

The gene associated with the transmission of von Hippel-Lindau disease is located on chromosome 3 (Latif et al, 1993). **The penetrance probably is 100%** (Jennings and Gaines, 1988), **and therefore, the condition can be expected to appear in 50% of the offspring or siblings of affected persons.**

Until cytogenetic evaluation is readily available for members of the patient's family, the genetic nature of the condition mandates careful screening and follow-up of family members. Ophthalmoscopic examination for retinal angiomas is useful, and an abdominal CT scan should be obtained when the patient is between the ages of 18 and 20 years. If no disease is found, re-evaluation is recommended at 4-year intervals (Levine et al, 1990). If cysts or small indeterminate lesions are identified, CT examination should be repeated every 2 years, perhaps with narrow-screen collimation (Levine et al, 1990). The goal is to identify the disease early so that malignancies can be identified before they metastasize.

HISTOPATHOLOGY

When present, renal cysts and tumors often are multiple and bilateral. The cysts usually simulate simple benign cysts, with flattened epithelium that some investigators consider precancerous. When Poston and associates (1995) studied cysts that were surgically removed along with specimens of renal cell carcinoma, they found that cysts larger than 2 cm were more likely to have components of renal cell carcinoma than smaller cysts. Frank cancer usually appears between the ages of 20 and 50 years (Jennings and Gaines, 1988). Loughlin and Gittes (1986) found that the hyperplastic lining cells frequently resembled the clear-cell type of renal cell carcinoma, the most common type in these patients. Ibrahim and co-workers (1989) studied the cysts adjacent to carcinomas and found, much as in tuberous sclerosis, that the karyotype resembled that of the tumors. This similarity is evidence that the hyperplastic cells of the cyst lining are precursors of the carcinomas.

Solomon and Schwartz (1988) believe that a spectrum of pathology is found within the kidneys of patients with von Hippel-Lindau disease. At one extreme is a simple cyst with a single layer of bland epithelium. The next step is a typical proliferative cyst with layers of epithelial cells: in the ensuing step, there are complex neoplastic projections into the cyst lumen. If one agrees with the arbitrary distinction between adenoma and carcinoma on the basis of size, the next stage would be adenoma. Finally, there is the full-blown renal cell carcinoma. In some cases, one might stretch the spectrum two steps further: sclerosing renal cell carcinoma with residual foci of malignant epithelium, and completely hyalinized fibrotic nodules lacking epithelial foci. The latter condition may represent the end point of evolution of the renal cell carcinoma. All of these stages may be found within a single kidney (Solomon and Schwartz, 1988).

EVALUATION

Sonography is useful in diagnosing the typical benign cystic features of von Hippel-Lindau disease: absence of internal echoes, well-defined margins, and acoustic enhancement. On CT scans, sharp, thin walls are seen around homogeneous contents without enhancement after contrast injection. Because multiple lesions (cysts, tumors, or both) are often present, CT frequently is more useful than sonography. CT often is useful in examining the adrenal glands for pheochromocytomas.

When the lesions are small, it is impossible to distinguish tumors from cysts. In such cases, patients should have regular CT scans using narrow-screen collimation (Levine et al, 1982). With larger lesions, and whenever renal cell carcinoma is suspected, renal angiography with magnification or subtraction is advisable (Kadir et al, 1981; Loughlin and Gittes, 1986). This type of study helps to reveal any additional tumors and indicates the appropriateness of conservative surgery (Kadir et al, 1981; Loughlin and Gittes, 1986). Intra-arterial administration of epinephrine is sometimes helpful because it causes vasoconstriction of the normal vessels but has no effect on tumor neovascularity.

CLINICAL FEATURES: ASSOCIATION WITH RENAL CELL CARCINOMA

Renal cysts are the most common malformation and are seen in 76% of patients (Levine et al, 1982). **Renal cell carcinoma occurs in 35% to 38% of affected individuals** (Fill et al, 1979; Levine et al, 1982). **The renal cysts as well as the tumors usually are asymptomatic, although large tumors may cause pain or a mass.** Hematuria may follow rupture of the tumor into the pelvicalyceal system.

Pheochromocytoma occurs in 10% to 17% of individuals and appears to be confined to specific families (Horton et al, 1976; Levine et al, 1982). Patients may present with seizures or dizziness secondary to hemangioblastomas of the central nervous system. Cerebellar hemangioblastomas usually become symptomatic between 15 and 40 years of age (Jennings and Gaines, 1988). Some patients suffer blurred vision secondary to the retinal angiomas.

Because of the high incidence of renal cell carcinoma in patients with von Hippel-Lindau disease, the urologist's primary role is careful surveillance so that small tumors can be identified and treated before they metastasize. Annual or perhaps biannual CT examinations are advised.

TREATMENT

Frydenberg and associates (1995) recommend conservative surgery—that is, excision or partial nephrectomy—for small low-grade tumors but more aggressive surgery for the tumors that are larger than 5 cm. The outlook is poorer with bilateral tumors. Low-grade bilateral tumors can be treated cautiously like unilateral tumors with close monitoring. Patients with bilateral high-grade tumors are probably served best with bilateral nephrectomy (Frydenberg et al, 1993). The most important need in improving survival is careful surveillance to identify tumors early and even more careful surveillance following surgery because of the multicentric characteristics of the tumor.

Classically, the survival rate after nephrectomy has been only 50%. However, in the closely monitored series of seven patients treated by Loughlin and Gittes (1986), six patients were followed for 4 months to 8 years, and only one death from metastatic disease was reported.

Nongenetic Cystic Disease

Multicystic Kidney (Multicystic Dysplasia)

Historically, the terms multicystic and polycystic were used interchangeably in discussing the kidney. However, in 1955, Spence stressed that these terms designated completely different entities. He included them separately in his classification, and subsequent investigators have done likewise.

The multicystic kidney represents a severe form of dysplasia that is sometimes described as multicystic dysplasia. The kidney does not have a reniform configuration, and no calyceal drainage system is present. Typically, the kidney appears to be a "bunch of grapes," with little stroma between the cysts (Fig. 59–15*A*). Renal size is highly variable, from slightly less than normal to enormous, filling most of the abdomen. When the cysts are small, even microscopic, and stroma predominates, the condition is referred to as solid cystic dysplasia (Fig. 59–15*B*). And when an identifiable renal pelvis is associated with what appears to be a multicystic dysplastic kidney, the condition is referred to as the hydronephrotic form of multicystic kidney (Fig. 59–15*C*) (Felson and Cussen, 1975).

ETIOLOGY

In the view of Felson and Cussen (1975), the multicystic kidney is an extreme form of hydronephrosis secondary to the atresia of the ureter or renal pelvis, which is a frequent concomitant condition. The fact that the left kidney is the one more often affected supports this view because this is the kidney more often associated with primary obstructive megaureter (Glassberg, 1977) and ureteropelvic junction obstruction (Johnston et al, 1977). In testing this hypothesis,

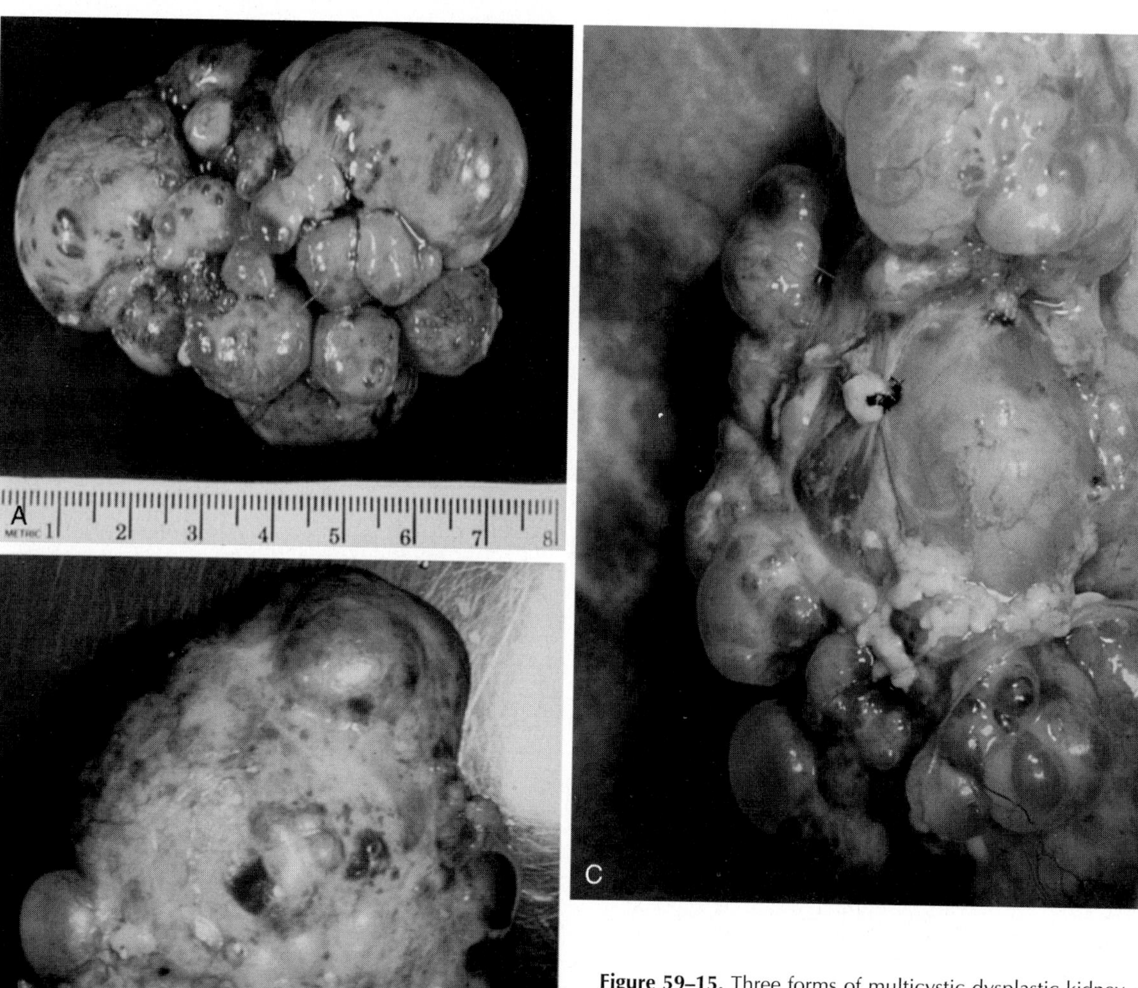

Figure 59–15. Three forms of multicystic dysplastic kidney. *A,* A *typical multicystic kidney* having the appearance of a bunch of cysts. The kidney was composed almost entirely of cysts with very little stroma; *B,* nonfunctioning *solid cystic dysplastic kidney,* which differs from classic multicystic kidney in having smaller and fewer cysts and being composed predominantly of stroma; and *C, hydronephrotic form of multicystic kidney,* which has a medial pelvis that typically is larger than any of the cysts in its associated kidney.

several investigators have attempted to establish an animal model by ligating the ureter at various points in gestation (Beck, 1971; Tanagho, 1972; Fetterman et al, 1974). This approach is not effective in mid or late gestation; early ligation of the fetal lamb ureter produces renal dysplasia but not multicystic dysplasia (Beck, 1971). However, Berman and Maizel (1982) were unable to obtain similar results in the chick. Similarly, other investigators have been able to induce dysplasia, but no one as yet has been able to induce a multicystic dysplastic kidney.

Other theories have been offered by Hildebrandt (1894) and by Osathanondh and Potter (1964). Hildebrandt (1894) suggested that failure of the union between the ureteric bud and the metanephric blastema leads to cystic dilatation in the latter; this hypothesis, like the obstructive view, is supported by the high incidence of concomitant ureteral atresia. Osathanondh and Potter (1964) postulated that Potter type IIA kidneys, the type with large cysts, result from an ampullary abnormality in which the ampullae stop dividing early and therefore produce fewer generations of tubules. In this view, the last generation of tubules produced is cystic and does not induce metanephric differentiation, and the occasional normal or nearly normal nephron is the result of a rare normal ampulla and collecting tubules.

Clinical Features

Multicystic dysplasia is the most common type of renal cystic disease, and one of the most common causes of an abdominal mass, in infants (Longino and Martin, 1958; Melicow and Uson, 1959; Griscom et al, 1975). Widespread prenatal ultrasound evaluation has greatly increased the frequency with which the condition is identified. Although the pathogenetic process leading to a multicystic kidney probably is operative by the eighth week in utero, the mean age at the time of antenatal diagnosis is about 28 weeks, with a range of 21 to 35 weeks (Avni et al, 1987). The reason is not apparent. In less severely affected patients, the condition may be an incidental finding during evaluation of an adult for abdominal pain, hematuria, hypertension, or an unrelated condition. At any age, the condition is more likely to be found on the left (Friedman and Abeshouse, 1957; Fine and Burns, 1959; Porkkulainen et al, 1959; Pathak and Williams, 1964; Griscom et al, 1975) and is slightly more common in males.

The contralateral system frequently is abnormal as well. For example, contralateral ureteropelvic junction obstruction is found in 3% to 12% of infants with multicystic kidney, and contralateral vesicoureteral reflux is seen even more often, being identified in 18% to 43% of infants (Heikkinen et al, 1980; Atiyeh et al, 1992; Flack and Bellinger, 1993; Wacksman and Phipps, 1993; Al-Khaldi et al, 1994). **The high incidence of reflux makes voiding cystourethrography advisable in the evaluation of these children, especially because the reflux affects the only functioning kidney.**

When a diagnosis of multicystic kidney is made in utero by ultrasound, the disease is found to be bilateral in 19% to 34% of cases (Kleiner et al, 1986; Khaldi et al, 1994). Those with bilateral disease often have other severe deformities or polysystemic malformation syndromes (Khaldi et al, 1994). In bilateral cases, the newborn has the classic abnormal facies and oligohydramnios characteristic of Potter's syndrome. The bilateral condition is incompatible with survival, although one infant reportedly survived for 69 days (Kishikawa et al, 1981). Another association, between multicystic kidney and contralateral renal agenesis, likewise is incompatible with life. The association of any of the following entities—renal agenesis, renal dysplasia, multicystic dysplastic kidney, and renal aplasia—within one family has been referred to as familial renal adysplasia (see earlier discussion).

Involution sometimes occurs in the multicystic kidney, either antenatally or postnatally (Hashimoto et al, 1986; Avni et al, 1987). **This involution may be so severe that the affected kidney disappears from subsequent sonograms. In such cases, the kidney may be only a "nubbin," and the condition is referred to as "renal aplasia" or "aplastic dysplasia"** (Bernstein and Gardner, 1989; Glassberg and Filmer, 1992). **Previously, aplastic kidneys, which often are associated with atretic ureters, were thought to be a separate entity. Now, with the experience of following multicystic kidneys sonographically, it is apparent that most aplastic kidneys represent involuted multicystic organs.**

In a few cases, multicystic dysplasia involves a horseshoe kidney (Greene et al, 1971; Walker et al, 1978; Borer et al, 1995) or one pole of a duplex kidney.

Histopathology

Multicystic kidneys with large cysts tend to be large with little stroma, whereas those with small cysts generally are smaller and more solid. The blood supply likewise is variable, ranging from a pedicle with small vessels to no pedicle at all (Parkkulainen et al, 1959). Usually, the ureter is partly or totally atretic, and the renal pelvis may be absent. Griscom and associates (1975) referred to the form without a renal pelvis as pyeloinfundibular atresia and reported finding no evidence of communication between the cysts. However, others have shown distribution of contrast medium among the cysts by means of connecting tubules (Saxton et al, 1981). We have found these tubules by probing gross specimens and by injecting contrast medium into one of the cysts and visualizing the connections between the cysts radiographically (Fig. 59–16). Felson and Cussen (1975) referred to the variety with a renal pelvis as the **"hydronephrotic type"** and demonstrated connections between the cysts and the renal pelvis.

Microscopically, the cysts are lined by low cuboidal epithelium. They are separated by thin septa of fibrous tissue and primitive dysplastic elements, especially primitive ducts. Frequently, immature glomeruli are present, and on occasion, a few mature glomeruli are seen.

Evaluation

Renal masses in infants most often represent either multicystic kidney disease or hydronephrosis, and it is important to distinguish the two, especially if the surgeon wishes to remove a nonfunctioning hydronephrotic kidney or repair a ureteropelvic junction obstruction while leaving a multicystic organ in situ. In newborns, ultrasonography generally is the first study performed. In a few cases, it is

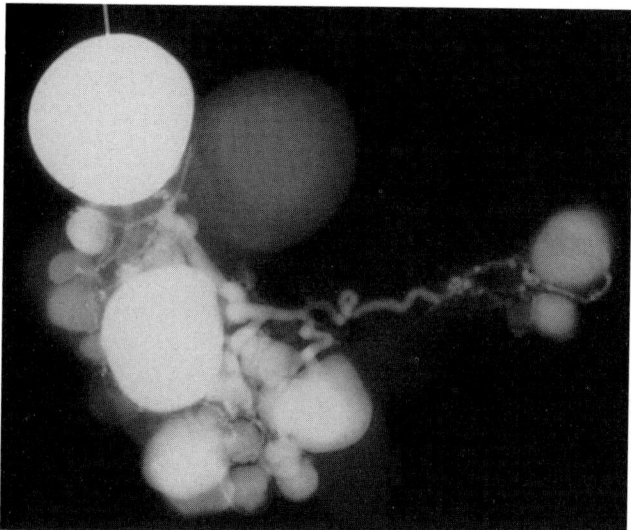

Figure 59–16. Contrast study of a multicystic kidney representing one component of a horseshoe kidney removed at surgery. Contrast injected into one cyst demonstrates communication between the cysts by tubular structures. (From Borer JG, Glassberg KI, Kassner G, et al: Unilateral multicystic dysplasia in one component of a horseshoe kidney: Case report and review of the literature. J Urol 1994; 152:1568, 1994.)

difficult to distinguish multicystic kidney disease from severe hydronephrosis (Gates, 1980; Hadlock et al, 1981). **In general, however, the multicystic kidney has a haphazard distribution of cysts of various sizes without a larger central or medial cyst. In comparison, in ureteropelvic junction obstruction, the cysts or calyces are organized around the periphery of the kidney, and connections usually can be demonstrated between the peripheral cysts and a central or medial cyst representing the renal pelvis (Fig. 59–17). When there is an identifiable renal sinus, the diagnosis is more likely to be hydronephrosis than multicystic kidney.**

A particular diagnostic problem arises in the unusual hydronephrotic form of multicystic kidney disease. Among 14 patients with multicystic kidneys, Felson and Cussen (1975) retrospectively identified 4 who, on intravenous urography, were found to have the calyceal crescents typical of severe hydronephrosis. This feature is thought to represent contrast medium in tubules compressed and displaced by dilated calyces (Dunbar and Nogrady, 1970). All four of these kidneys had small amounts of parenchyma and glomeruli, but no correlation could be made between the parenchymal tissue and the appearance of crescents. In all four kidneys, communications between the cysts were found, and communications with the renal pelvis were found in the three kidneys in which this structure was present.

In these difficult cases, radioisotope studies may be helpful. Hydronephrotic kidneys generally show some function on a dimercaptosuccinic acid (DMSA) scan, whereas renal concentration is seldom seen in multicystic kidneys. Angiography reveals an absent or small renal artery in the multicystic kidney, but this study is rarely indicated. Cystoscopy may reveal a hemitrigone and absent ureteral orifice on the affected side; however, more often, an orifice is present, but retrograde urography demonstrates ureteral atresia. Again, this study is seldom performed.

In a few cases, diagnostic studies are not performed until the patient is older. In these instances, the plain abdominal film often reveals renal calcifications. These deposits usually appear as annular or arcuate shadows (Felson and Cussen, 1975).

As discussed earlier, voiding cystourethrography is indicated in the work-up because of the high incidence of reflux into the single functioning kidney.

Treatment and Prognosis

It has often been stated that the multicystic kidney can be ignored unless its bulk is inconvenient (Pathak and Williams, 1964; Griscom et al, 1975), and that attention should be directed instead to identifying any abnormalities of the contralateral urinary tract. Certainly, the need in the past to explore some multicystic kidneys to rule out malignancy, such as cystic Wilms' tumor and congenital mesoblastic nephroma, has largely been erased by new diagnostic tools. Kidneys that do contain malignancies are likely to be explored because of the retention of some function as seen by excretory urography or nuclear medicine studies (Walker et al, 1984); therefore, routine exploration solely to rule out malignancy is inappropriate.

A nonfunctioning hydronephrotic kidney could be mistaken for a multicystic kidney, although complete nonfunction on a nuclear medicine study is unusual in kidneys affected by ureteropelvic junction obstruction. Even if the correct diagnosis is missed in such a case, however, it is unlikely to have significant consequences because a totally nonfunctioning hydronephrotic kidney is rarely salvageable and probably will cause no problems other than a predisposition to infection or hyperkalemia.

Of greater concern is the potential for malignant degeneration in a multicystic kidney. In only one report has the diagnosis of multicystic kidney been made prior to the diagnosis of an associated cancer (Oddoni et al, 1994). Eight other patients have been described who developed cancer in previously "unrecognized" multicystic dysplastic kidneys. Wilms' tumor was diagnosed in three of these nine patients: in one patient at age 10 months (Raffensberger and Abouselman, 1968), in the patient just mentioned with the previously diagnosed multicystic kidney at 18 months (Oddoni et al, 1994), and in a third child at age 4 years (Hartman et al, 1986). An embryonal cell tumor of the kidney was reported in a fourth patient (Gutter and Hermanck, 1957). In the remaining four, renal cell carcinoma was reported in patients aged 15 to 68 years (Barrett and Wineland, 1980; Burgler and Hauri, 1983; Birken et al, 1985; Shirai et al, 1986; Rackley et al, 1994).

However, it is not clear how many of these nine patients truly had a multicystic kidney. For example, the entity in the case reported by Rackley and associates (1994), entitled "Renal Cell Carcinoma in a Regressed Multicystic Dysplastic Kidney," may not have been such. There is every reason to believe that the kidney that developed an adenocarcinoma in this report was a dysplastic one, not a "typical" multicystic dysplastic one. This patient was reported to have an ipsilateral ureterocele as well. Ureteroceles may be associated with dysplastic kidneys, and some may even have small cysts, but none in this author's experience have been associated with a "typical" multicystic kidney. In some of

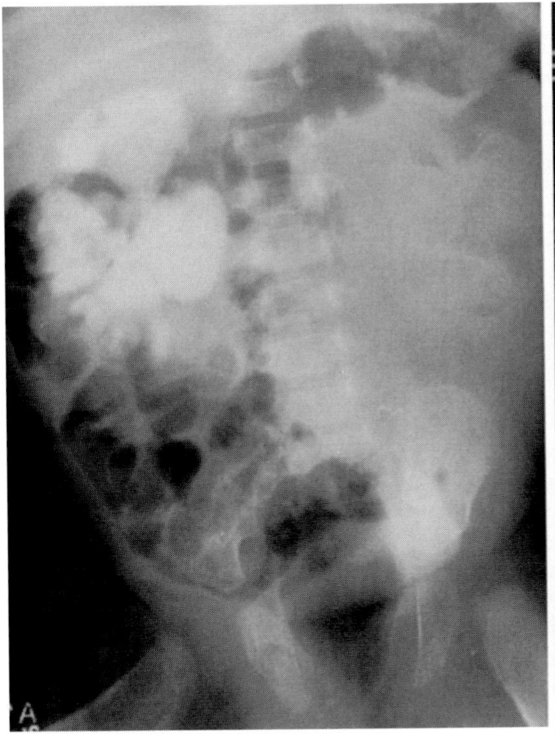

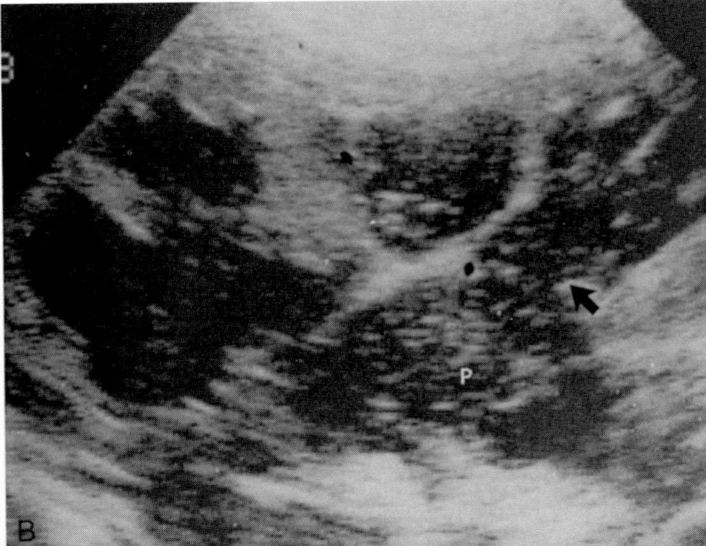

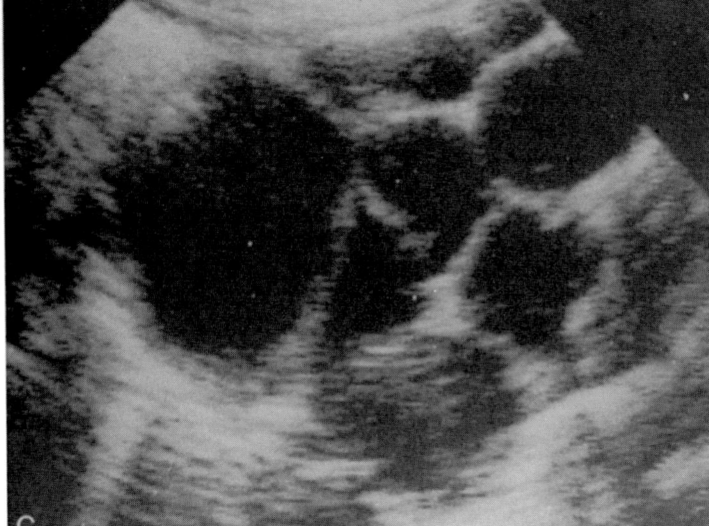

Figure 59–17. Female neonate with fetal alcohol syndrome.

A, Intravenous urogram reveals a right ureteropelvic junction obstruction and nonfunctioning left kidney.

B, Sonogram of right kidney demonstrates regular arrangement of peripheral calyces with infundibular connections *(arrow)* to a medial pelvis (P). Echogenic areas represent pelvicalyceal *Candida.*

C, In comparison, note the left contralateral multicystic kidney with large cysts arranged in a haphazard manner without any evidence of connections to or the presence of a large central or medial cyst. (Gross specimen appears in Figure 59–15*A.*)

the other cases the illustrations do not seem to represent typical multicystic kidneys. Nevertheless, in a few of the reports, the ipsilateral ureter was either atretic or absent, suggesting that these were indeed examples of multicystic dysplasia.

Two reports in the literature might be interpreted as reinforcing the arguments in favor of prophylactic surgical removal. Dimmick and co-workers (1989) and Noe and co-workers (1989) described a total of 120 patients, of whom five had nephrogenic rests of nodular renal blastema. In addition, one of the patients in the series of Dimmick and co-workers (1989) had Wilms' tumorlets in the hilar region. Although these findings suggest a hazard in leaving a multicystic kidney in situ, one must realize that it is unusual for nodular renal blastema or even Wilms' tumorlets to develop into frank Wilms' tumor. For example, nodular renal blastema has been reported in approximately 0.25% to 0.5% of normal kidneys (Bennington and Beckwith, 1975; Bove and McAdams, 1976; Beckwith, 1986) yet the incidence of Wilms' tumor in the general population is much lower. Thus, although nodular renal blastema and Wilms' tumorlets may be part of a nephroblastomatosis–Wilms' tumor spectrum, the majority of these lesions involute in time without ever becoming malignant.

Trying to predict what percentage of multicystic kidneys will develop Wilms' tumors, Noe and associates (1989) used Beckwith's estimated 1% incidence of Wilms' tumor development in nodular renal blastema. They then calculated, using a 5% incidence of nodular renal blastema in multicystic kidneys, that one would have to perform 2000 nephrectomies for multicystic kidney disease to prevent one Wilms' tumor. Accordingly, one must weigh the risk of surgery against that of Wilms' tumor. If one elects to monitor without surgery, the cost-benefit ratio or even the effectiveness of long-term follow-up must be considered. Because nodular renal blastema occurs most often in the hilum (Dimmick et al, 1989), and because most kidneys that shrink lose only cyst fluid, leaving the dysplastic tissue, follow-up by sonography is unlikely to be helpful (Colodny, 1989).

In an effort to determine whether there is a relationship between multicystic dysplasia and neoplasia, Jung and co-workers (1990) performed flow cytometric analyses on specimens from 30 patients. No evidence of tetraploidy or aneuploidy, as would be expected in a preneoplastic condition,

Table 59–10. NATIONAL MULTICYSTIC KIDNEY REGISTRY—SONOGRAPHIC FOLLOW-UP

Follow-up (Year)	No. of Children	Not Identifiable	Smaller	Larger	Unchanged
<1/2	191	13 (7%)	110 (58%)	18 (9%)	50 (26%)
1/2–1	145	15 (10%)	66 (45%)	5 (3%)	59 (41%)
1–3	334	45 (13%)	147 (44%)	14 (4%)	128 (38%)
3–5	97	22 (23%)	24 (26%)	7 (7%)	44 (46%)
>5	63	16 (25%)	23 (37%)	1 (2%)	23 (37%)

With permission, J. Wacksman, M.D., Chairperson, National Multicystic Kidney Registry, April, 1995.

was found. This report is comforting to the surgeon who does not routinely remove multicystic kidneys. Still, one must be aware that some malignant cells retain a diploid karyotype.

Another management question in multicystic kidney disease is the frequency of hypertension. Gordon and associates (1988) reviewed this topic in a thoughtful article. They noted that since 1966, only nine well-documented cases of hypertension in association with multicystic kidneys in situ have been published. In three of these cases, the hypertension resolved after nephrectomy (Burgler and Hauri, 1983; Chen et al, 1985; Javadpour et al, 1970). However, in a series of 20 patients older than 11 years who had multicystic kidney disease, two had hypertension, and in neither of these patients was the blood pressure controlled by nephrectomy (Ambrose, 1976). Other reports suggest that the incidence of hypertension may be greater than that actually reported in the literature (Emmert and King, 1994; Hannah, 1995).

A large number of patients have now been followed for more than 5 years by the National Multicystic Kidney Registry (Table 59–10) (Wacksman, 1995). When the status of neonatal multicystic kidneys is followed over a period of time, the vast majority either become smaller or stay the same size, and only a very small percentage become larger. If the kidney becomes larger, depending on the surgeon's inclinations, consideration can be given to removal. When the kidney stays the same size, it actually becomes smaller in proportion to the size of the child as he or she gets older. Most kidneys that become smaller do so during the first year of follow-up, and an increasing number of those that become smaller disappear from view with time on ultrasound examination. None of the multicystic kidneys in the Registry has developed a tumor during follow-up. However, one must realize that a number of kidneys were removed at the time of entering the study by the decision of the individual surgeon, and a smaller number have been removed later on because of increasing size during follow-up. As a result, it cannot be determined whether the kidneys that were selected for nephrectomy had a greater potential for malignancy or hypertension. Hypertension has developed in only five of the patients in the Registry, and from the data it is not clear in how many of the five the hypertension was thought to be secondary to the multicystic kidney. Occasional urinary tract infections have been seen, but it is not clear whether the multicystic kidney had anything to do with the infections either, particularly because many of these patients also have contralateral reflux.

Questions still must be answered. Does the disappearance of a multicystic kidney on imaging studies mean that there is no longer a potential risk? For example, when these kidneys disappear from view, it means only the fluid within the cysts has disappeared; the cells still remain. How is it necessary to follow those patients who are not operated on, because many inevitably will be lost to follow-up? From Ambrose's experience (1976) it appears that flank pain as an adult is the chief risk of a multicystic kidney that is left in situ, and in such cases the pain usually responds to nephrectomy.

In summary, the available literature offers no proof that the incidence of either tumor or hypertension is higher in individuals with retained multicystic kidneys than in individuals with normal kidneys.

Benign Multilocular Cyst (Cystic Nephroma)

A multilocular cystic lesion in a child's kidney may be a benign multilocular cyst, a multilocular cyst with partially differentiated Wilms' tumor, a multilocular cyst with nodules of Wilms' tumor, or a cystic Wilms' tumor (Fig. 59–18). These four lesions form a spectrum, with the benign multilocular cyst at one extreme and the cystic Wilms' tumor at the other. In adults, there are fewer clinical cases supporting the existence of an entity lying between a benign multilocular cyst and a cystic adenocarcinoma or some other cystic renal tumor.

A multilocular cyst is not a renal segment affected by multicystic kidney disease; these conditions differ clinically, histologically, and radiographically. However, controversy continues about whether the multilocular cyst is a segmental

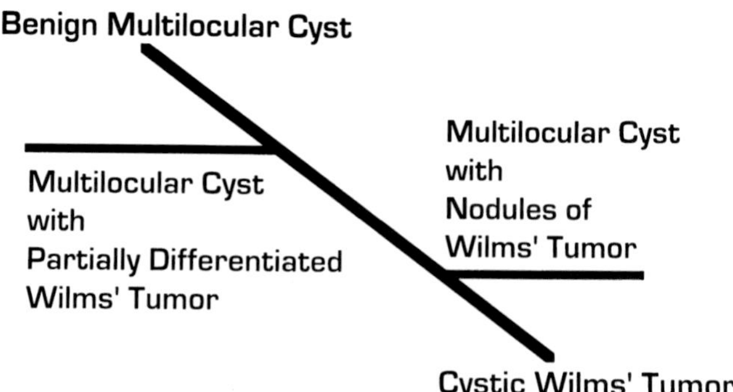

Figure 59–18. The spectrum of multilocular cystic lesions in children ranges from the classic benign multilocular cyst to cystic Wilms' tumor. The specific diagnosis of any of these individual entities cannot be made by imaging studies, but only by histopathologic evaluation. The multilocular cyst with partially differentiated Wilms' tumor differs from a benign multilocular cyst principally by the histologic finding of blastemal cells in the septa.

form of renal dysplasia (Powell et al, 1951; Osathanondh and Potter, 1964; Johnson et al, 1973), a hamartomatous malformation (Arey, 1959), or a neoplastic disease (Boggs and Kimmelsteil, 1956; Christ, 1968; Fowler, 1971; Gallo and Penchansky, 1977). The confusion arises in part from the variability of the histologic picture; the appearance of the primitive stroma, the maturity of tubular and even on occasion muscle elements, and the degree of epithelial atypia differ not only from patient to patient but also within the same lesion.

Past use of many nonspecific terms, such as lymphangioma, partial or focal polycystic kidney, multicystic kidney, and cystic adenoma, makes it difficult to identify relevant published cases for review (Aterman et al, 1973). Edmunds used the term cystic adenoma in 1892 in what was probably the first published description of this lesion. The author favors the term benign multilocular cyst because the descriptor benign separates this lesion from other multilocular cystic lesions, and the term multilocular cyst clearly describes the gross appearance of the lesion. Joshi and Beckwith (1989) prefer the term cystic nephroma because this term implies a benign but neoplastic lesion.

Clinical Features

The great majority of patients present before the age of 2 years or after 40 years. **The patient is more likely to be male if younger than 2 years and female if older than 2 years.** When Castillo and associates (1991) reviewed the literature up until 1990, they found 187 cases of benign multilocular cysts. Sixty-seven percent of children 24 months of age or younger were male, but of patients over 24 months old, 75% were female.

The signs and symptoms differ according to the age at presentation. In children, an asymptomatic flank mass is the most common finding, whereas most adults present with either a flank mass, abdominal pain, or hematuria. The bleeding is secondary to herniation of the cyst through the transitional epithelium into the renal pelvis (Uson and Melicow, 1963; Aterman et al, 1973; Madewell et al, 1983).

Seven cases of bilateral benign multilocular cysts of the kidney have been described (Castillo et al, 1991), in one of which the lesion recurred after excision (Geller et al, 1979). Also, at least two instances are known in which multilocular cysts arose in kidneys known to have been normal previously (Uson and Melicow, 1963; Chatten and Bishop, 1977). Such cases support a neoplastic theory of the origin of this lesion.

Histopathology

These lesions are bulky and are circumscribed by a thick capsule. Normal renal parenchyma adjacent to the lesion frequently is compressed by it. The lesion may extend beyond the renal capsule into the perinephric space or renal pelvis. The loculi, which range in diameter from a few millimeters to centimeters in diameter, do not intercommunicate. They contain clear straw-colored or yellow fluid and are lined by cuboidal or low columnar epithelial cells. In some cases, eosinophilic cuboidal cells project into the cyst lumen, creating a hobnail appearance (Madewell et al, 1983). The definition of multilocular cystic kidney given by Powell and co-workers (1951) and Boggs and Kimmelsteil (1956) requires a normal epithelial lining for the diagnosis. Joshi and Beckwith (1989) also define the septa of a benign multilocular cyst as being composed of fibrous tissue in which well-differentiated tubules may be present but poorly differentiated tissues and blastemal cells are not present.

When Castillo and associates (1991) reviewed the literature on multilocular cysts they included lesions that had interlocular septa containing tissue of two different types: (1) fibrous tissue only or (2) embryonic-type tissue. Adults in general had only the first type, whereas children, principally those under the age of 3 years, had either type. Joshi and Beckwith (1989) refer to the embryonic type as an immature form and prefer the term cystic partially differentiated nephroblastoma (Joshi, 1980) because histologically this form is different from the first group, which they believe is the typical benign multilocular cyst. To make the diagnosis of a cystic partially differentiated nephroblastoma, blastemal cells must be present. Often varying amounts of poorly differentiated tissues such as tubules, glomeruli, mesenchyme, skeletal muscle, and, rarely, cartilage are admixed with the blastemal cells (Joshi and Beckwith, 1989). Supportive evidence that the second variety should not be called a benign multilocular cyst lies in the histories of Joshi and Beckwith's (1989) 18 patients with cystic partially differentiated nephroblastoma; one patient had a contralateral anaplastic Wilms' tumor, and another had two local recurrences following nephrectomy.

As noted earlier, authorities consider benign multilocular cysts to be at one end of a spectrum. Within that spectrum lies cystic partially differentiated nephroblastoma (Fig. 59–19). The author prefers the term multilocular cyst with partially differentiated Wilms' tumor to cystic partially differentiated nephroblastoma because two of the other entities within the spectrum are described with the term Wilms' tumor. For example, when nodules of Wilms' tumor are present, Joshi (1980) designates the lesion as multilocular cyst with nodules of Wilms' tumor. The term cystic Wilms' tumor is reserved for the rare cases of tumor in which cysts are lined by epithelial cells. This entity should not be confused with Wilms' tumors that have sonolucent or radiolucent cyst-like spaces attributable to tumor necrosis.

Although in children there may be a continuum from benign multilocular cyst to cystic Wilms' tumor, and although all of these lesions may be derived from similar cells or tissues, no evidence suggests that one entity transforms into another. Interestingly, none of the genetically determined conditions associated with Wilms' tumor (e.g., hemihypertrophy, aniridia) has accompanied a multilocular cyst (Banner et al, 1981).

In adults there are only rare cases to support such a continuum. For example, if an adult is identified with a multilocular cystic lesion, it almost always is either a benign multilocular cyst, a cystic adenocarcinoma, a cystic oncocytoma, or some other type of cystic tumor. However, rare cases of multilocular cyst with evidence of adenocarcinoma within them have been reported. Taxy and Marshall (1984) reported on three patients with unusual multilocular cysts. In two patients the loculi were lined by cells with clear cytoplasm suggestive of malignancy or at least atypical hyperplasia, and in the third case papillary proliferations and

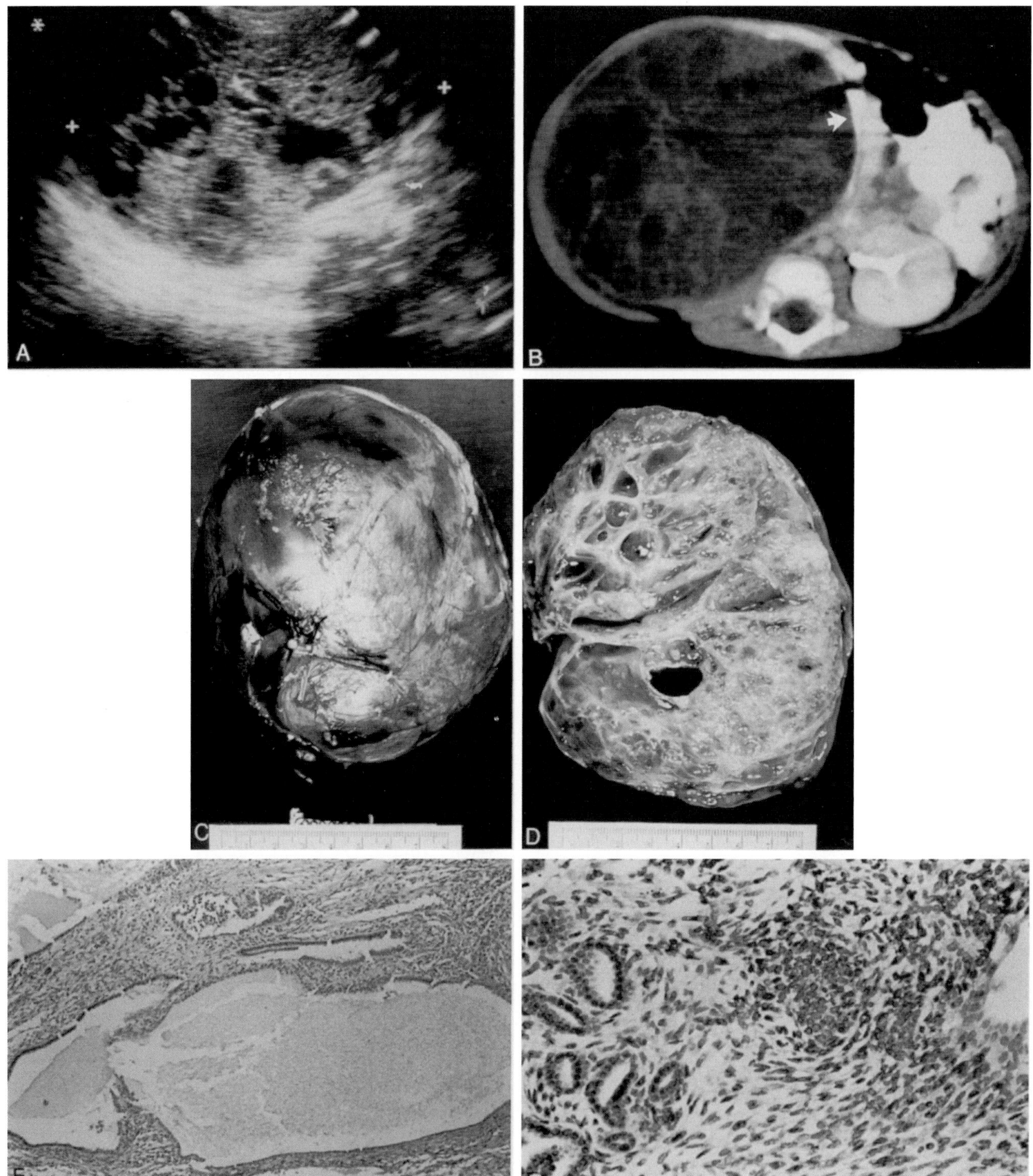

Figure 59–19. A 4-year-old girl with a right-sided abdominal mass.

A, Renal sonogram with multiple cysts throughout the left kidney.

B, On contrast-enhanced CT scan, a large, smoothly outlined left renal mass is seen with fine septa throughout the mass. Residual preserved parenchyma and pelvicalyceal system are compressed medially and pushed to the contralateral side *(arrow).*

C, Uncut gross specimen reveals a smooth-walled, encapsulated renal mass.

D, Cross section of mass reveals multiple noncommunicating loculations.

E, On histology, a hypocellular cystic area is seen with monotonous stroma (× 100).

F, Between loculi, nests of blastematous cells are visualized along with tubular elements *(left),* making the diagnosis of multilocular cyst with partially differentiated Wilms' tumor (× 200). (Courtesy of C. K. Chen, M.D.)

septal invasion by clear cells were interpreted as adenocarcinoma.

EVALUATION

A number of tests may be useful including the following: intravenous urography, sonography, CT, MRI, cyst puncture with aspiration and double-contrast cystography, and arteriography. Ultrasound and CT can distinguish multicystic kidney and multilocular cyst, but neither study is sufficiently reliable to distinguish multilocular cyst, multilocular cyst with foci of Wilms' tumor or adenocarcinoma, mesoblastic nephroma, cystic Wilms' tumor, and clear-cell sarcoma. Typically, the septa are highly echogenic with sonolucent loculi, although if there is debris in a loculus, it may appear more solid. On CT, the septa are less dense than normal parenchyma; when myxomatous material is present, the density is equal to that of solid structures (Wood et al, 1982). Calcification is rarely visible in such lesions in children (Madewell et al, 1983).

In the few cases in which angiography was performed, vascular, hypovascular, and hypervascular patterns were seen (Davides, 1976; Madewell et al, 1983; De Wall et al, 1986). A tumor blush and neovascularity that sometimes was extensive were apparent in some cases (Madewell et al, 1983).

Clear to yellow fluid is recovered by cyst puncture. Contrast will opacify only those loculi through which the needle has passed, because the loculi do not communicate (Madewell et al, 1983).

TREATMENT

Two questions must be answered in selecting the treatment for a multilocular cystic kidney: (1) Is the contralateral urinary tract normal? and (2) Is the abnormal kidney involved with Wilms' tumor? At least four of the cystic tumors in the National Wilms' Tumor Study (NWTS) metastasized (Beckwith and Palmer, 1978); thus, these lesions clearly have malignant potential, although they appear to be less aggressive than classic Wilms' tumor.

The treatment for a multilocular cyst in most children is nephrectomy. If pathologic review shows cystic Wilms' tumor, further treatment should be given according to the NWTS recommendations for the appropriate stage of disease. However, if the focus of tumor does not exceed 2 cm, nephrectomy alone may be sufficient. If enucleation or partial nephrectomy is chosen, recurrence is possible. However, with more Wilms' tumors being treated by local excision, the case for enucleation or partial nephrectomy combined with close follow-up by sonography and CT is stronger, even if malignancy is found within the lesion. In comparison, if a clear-cell sarcoma is found after enucleation, the remaining ipsilateral renal tissue should be removed because of the aggressiveness of this cancer. The recurrence of a multilocular cyst not containing malignancy probably reflects inadequate excision of the initial lesion.

In adults, more often larger amounts of renal tissue are apparently preserved, making partial nephrectomy more feasible. In a report by Castillo and associates (1991), 24 of 29 patients underwent renal-sparing surgery, including 2 who were children.

Simple Cysts

A simple cyst is a discrete finding that may occur well within a kidney or on its surface. It is usually oval to round in shape, has a smooth outline bordered by a single layer of flattened cuboidal epithelium, and is filled with transudate-like clear or straw-colored fluid. It is not connected to any part of the nephron, although it may originate initially from a portion of the nephron. Simple cysts may be singular or multiple, unilateral or bilateral.

Simple cysts may present anytime from soon after birth to old age. Between birth and 18 years of age the incidence of simple renal cysts is fairly stable, ranging from 0.1% to 0.45% with an average incidence of 0.22% (McHugh et al, 1991). However, in adults the frequency rises with age. Using CT, Loucks and McLachlan (1981) demonstrated a 20% incidence of cysts by age 40 years and approximately a 33% incidence of cysts after age 60. On autopsy, Kissane and Smith (1975) identified a 50% incidence of simple renal cysts after age 50. Most reports show no gender predilection; however, in at least two studies, men were affected more frequently than women (Bearth and Steg, 1977; Tada et al, 1983).

CLINICAL FEATURES

In both children and adults, cysts rarely call attention to themselves. Instead, they are discovered incidentally on sonography, CT, or urography performed for a urinary tract or other pelvic or abdominal problem. However, cysts can produce an abdominal mass or pain, hematuria secondary to rupture into the pyelocalyceal system, and hypertension secondary to segmental ischemia (Rockson et al, 1974; Lüscher et al, 1986; Papanicolaou et al, 1986). Cysts can cause calyceal or renal pelvic obstruction as well (Wahlqvist and Grumstedt, 1966; Evans and Coughlin, 1970; Hinman, 1978; Barloon and Vince, 1987). They may or may not increase in size with time. Of 23 cysts in 22 children who underwent sonographic follow-up for up to 5 years, McHugh and associates (1991) found that 17 cysts (74%) remained unchanged in size.

Over an 18-year period, Papanicolaou and co-workers (1986) treated 25 patients who had suffered spontaneous or traumatic rupture of a known cyst, a large number of cases considering the rarity of cyst rupture. Most of these ruptures (21) were spontaneous; three followed blunt trauma, and one was iatrogenic. The cyst ruptured into a calyx in 12 patients. In one patient, the rupture was into the renal pelvis, through the parenchyma but not the capsule. In another, the cyst ruptured through the parenchyma and capsule. In five patients, the rupture was both calyceal and perinephric, and in the remaining four patients, the site of rupture could not be determined. In 21 patients, hematuria was present, and in 17 patients, flank pain was present. The diagnosis was made by high-dose drip infusion nephrotomography in 22 patients, by CT in two, and by retrograde pyelography in one. In 11 patients, the cyst communication closed spontaneously, and in eight, the cyst cavity was obliterated on follow-up studies. Two patients had persistent calyceal communication with 2 months or less of follow-up.

Cysts can rupture into the pelvicalyceal system, maintain a communication, and become a pseudocalyceal diverticlum. The reverse is also possible; closure of the communication of a diverticulum can create a simple cyst (Mosli et al, 1986; Papanicolaou et al, 1986). These two sequences of events can be distinguished only by histologic examination. Theoretically, diverticula should have linings of transitional epithelium, whereas simple cysts should be lined by a single layer of flattened or cuboidal epithelium.

Hypertension caused by cysts has been confirmed in several reports. For example, in two children with simple cysts and hypertension, the blood pressure normalized after surgical decompression of the cysts (Babka et al, 1974; Hoard and O'Brien, 1976). Also, Lüscher and co-workers (1986) identified 22 published cases of renal cysts and hypertension. Surgical removal or aspiration of the cyst was therapeutic in ten patients and yielded improvement in two others with a mean follow-up of 1 year. Ten of the 15 patients who were studied by renal vein renin assays had elevated activity, suggesting local tissue or arterial compression by the cyst. This hypothesis is easily believable if one realizes that a simple cyst can have a pressure as high as 57 cm H_2O and that the lesions in this series of cases generally were large, most exceeding 6 cm in diameter and containing several hundred milliliters of fluid (Amis et al, 1982; Lüscher et al, 1986).

Histopathology

Simple cysts vary considerably in size, ranging from less than 1 cm to greater than 10 cm. The majority are less than 2 cm in diameter, however (Tada et al, 1983). The wall is fibrous and of varying thickness and has no renal elements. The cyst lining is a single layer of flattened or cuboidal epithelium.

Because cysts are increasingly common with age, they have been considered an acquired lesion. Bearth and Steg (1977) found greater ectasia and cystic dilatation of the distal tubules and collecting ducts in patients over the age of 60 years and considered these changes to be precursors of macroscopic cysts.

Evaluation

One can safely make the diagnosis of a classic benign simple cyst by sonography when the following criteria are met: (1) absence of internal echoes; (2) sharply defined, thin, distinct wall with a smooth and distinct margin; (3) good transmission of sound waves through the cyst with consequent acoustic enhancement behind the cyst; and (4) spherical or slightly ovoid shape (Goldman and Hartman, 1990). If all of these criteria are satisfied, the chances of malignancy being present are negligible (Fig. 59–20) (Lingard and Lawson, 1979; Livingston et al, 1981).

When some of these criteria are not met—for example, when there are septations, irregular margins, calcifications, or suspect areas—further evaluation by CT or perhaps needle aspiration or MRI is indicated (Bosniak, 1986). A cluster of cysts is another indication for further study because they may be hiding a small carcinoma. CT is better than sonography in defining such a camouflaged lesion (Bosniak, 1986). Peripelvic cysts often require CT confirmation because they frequently are interspersed between structures of the collecting system and hilum, which can create artificial echoes (Bosniak, 1986).

The CT criteria for a simple cyst are similar to those used in sonography: (1) sharp, thin, distinct, smooth walls and margins; (2) spherical or ovoid shape; and (3) homogeneous content. The density ranges from −10 to +20 Hounsfield units (HU), similar to the density of water, and no enhancement should occur after the intravenous injection of contrast medium. Bosniak (1986) states that he has not seen a tumor with a density of less than 20 HU on a contrast-enhanced scan, but a truly benign cyst can have fluid with a density of greater than 20 HU. In these cases, intravenous contrast injection is particularly helpful.

When the cyst fluid is hyperdense (i.e., between 20 and 90 HU), it still is likely to be a simple cyst if no enhancement occurs when intravenous contrast agent is injected and if the other criteria of CT and sonography are met. Hyper-

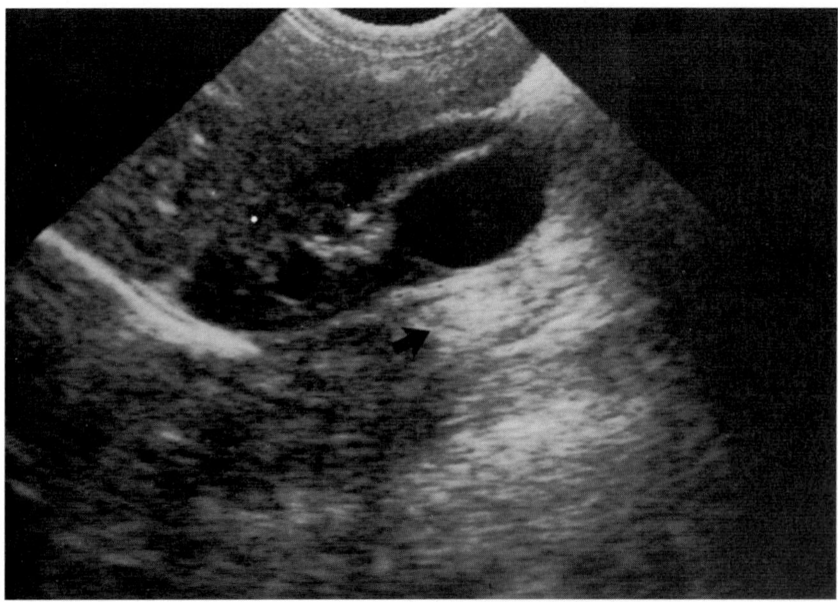

Figure 59–20. Two renal cysts in an 8-year-old boy. Note evidence of enhancement of sound wave transmission through the larger oval cyst by the hyperechogenicity (whiteness) of the image behind the cyst. Family history or even sonographic evaluation of family should be considered to rule out autosomal dominant polycystic kidney disease, especially when more than one cyst is present. In children, it is not unusual for autosomal dominant polycystic kidney disease to first present with one or two cysts.

for some unrelated problem, such as a renal mass, benign prostatic hyperplasia, or hypertension. Rarely is such hypertension attributable to the medullary sponge kidney unless there is pyelonephritis.

Another possible sign is the formation of urinary stones. Yendt (1990) found the incidence of medullary sponge kidney in patients who formed stones before age 20 to be twice as high as that in all other age groups combined. The incidence of medullary sponge kidney in stone-formers differs widely in the reported series, ranging from 2.6% to 21%. The incidence appears to be higher in female than in male stone-formers (Palubinskas, 1961; Lavan et al, 1971; Parks et al, 1982; Sage et al, 1982; Wikstrom et al, 1983; Vagelli et al, 1988; Yendt, 1990). Urinary tract infections likewise seem to be more common in female patients (Parks et al, 1982).

One third to one half of the patients with medullary sponge kidney have hypercalcemia (Ekstrom et al, 1959; Harrison and Rose, 1979; Parks et al, 1982; Yendt, 1990). The etiology does not appear to be the same in all cases. Maschio and co-workers (1982) found a renal calcium leak in eight patients and increased calcium absorption in two. Yendt (1990) found elevated parathyroid hormone levels in 2 of 11 patients with medullary sponge kidney.

In the absence of infections, the stones passed by patients with medullary sponge kidney are composed of calcium oxalate either alone or in combination with calcium phosphate.

Although medullary sponge kidney is not considered a genetic disease, there are a small number of isolated reports of autosomal dominant and autosomal recessive inheritance. In addition, medullary sponge kidney has been reported in association with rare congenital anomalies such as hemihypertrophy, Beckwith-Wiedemann syndrome, (macroglossia, omphalocele, and gigantism), Ehler-Danlos syndrome, anodontia, and Caroli's disease. Beetz and associates (1991) reported on a case of bilateral medullary sponge kidney in 14-year-old girl with Beckwith-Wiedemann syndrome, hemihypertrophy, and Wilms' tumor. Twenty other cases have been reported with congenital hemihypertrophy and fewer with Beckwith-Wiedemann syndrome (Gardner, 1992).

Histopathology

The principal finding is dilated intrapapillary collecting ducts and small medullary cysts, which range in diameter from 1 to 8 mm and give the cross-sectioned kidney the appearance of a sponge. The cysts are lined by collecting duct epithelium (Bernstein, 1990) and usually communicate with the collecting tubules. The cysts and the dilated collecting ducts may have concretions adherent to their walls. Ekstrom and co-workers (1959) found these concretions to be composed of pure apatite (calcium phosphate) in seven of ten patients and of apatite and calcium oxalate in the remaining three. The cysts contain a yellow-brown fluid and desquamated cells or calcified material.

Diagnosis

In general, intravenous urography is more sensitive than CT in detecting mild cases of medullary sponge kidney. In 75% of patients, the disease is bilateral (Kuiper, 1976), but, in some, only one pyramid may be affected. **The urographic features of the disorder are as follows: (1) enlarged kidneys, sometimes with calcification, particularly in the papillae; (2) elongated papillary tubules or cavities that fill with contrast medium; and (3) papillary contrast blush and persistent medullary opacification** (Gedroyc and Saxton, 1988). In some cases, the papillae resemble bunches of grapes or bouquets of flowers, whereas in others, discrete linear stripes appear that can be counted readily.

On occasion, the intravenous urogram of an older child or young adult with one of the milder forms of RPK mimics the appearance of medullary sponge kidney (Yendt, 1990). In these instances, one should evaluate the liver before making a diagnosis.

When nephrocalcinosis is found, one must rule out other hypercalciuric states, such as hyperparathyroidism, sarcoidosis, vitamin D intoxication, multiple myeloma, tuberculosis, and milk alkali syndrome. In these conditions, the calcium deposits are in collecting ducts of normal caliber, whereas in medullary sponge kidney, the calcifications occur in dilated ducts (Levine and Grantham, 1990).

Given that the cysts are small, sonography is not expected to be helpful. However, because children have less renal sinus fat and overlying muscle than adults, sonographic resolution is better, and hyperechoic papillae are seen on occasion (Patriquin and O'Regan, 1985). The hyperechogenicity is secondary to the multiple interfaces created by the dilated ducts and small cysts and to any intraductal calcification.

Gedroyc and Saxton (1988) described two groups of patients in whom additional renal anomalies were detected by ultrasound examination. One group had multiple cortical cysts; the other group had cavities deep in the medulla, which often communicated with the calyces.

Although, at present, urography generally is more sensitive in detecting medullary sponge kidney than CT, newer scanners can identify the tubular ectasia using bone-detail algorithms and window settings (Boag and Nolan, 1988). Thus, CT may be advantageous when bowel gas obscures the kidneys on urography or when renal function is poor.

Treatment and Prognosis

It is the complications of medullary sponge kidney that require management: calculus formation and infection. As noted earlier in this section, many of these patients have hypercalciuria. Thiazides are effective for lowering hypercalciuria and limiting stone formation. If thiazides cannot be used, inorganic phosphates may be appropriate. For those patients with renal lithiasis, thiazides should be administered even if hypercalciuria is not present (Yendt, 1990). Yendt (1990) reports that these drugs prevent calcium stones and arrest the growth of stones already present. If thiazides are ineffective or not tolerated, inorganic phosphates should be tried (Yendt, 1990). However, the latter should not be used in patients with urinary tract infections caused by urease-producing organisms because of the risk of struvite stones (Yendt, 1990).

Because infections are not unusual, especially if stones are present, cultures should be obtained frequently in patients with medullary sponge kidney, and long-term prophylaxis should be considered in some cases. Infections by coagulase-positive staphylococci are common in patients with stones and should be treated even when the colony count in the cultures is less than 100,000/ml (Yendt, 1990).

Stones can now be removed by extracorporeal lithotripsy and percutaneous nephrolithotomy. Therefore, open surgery is rarely necessary.

Kuiper (1976b) estimated that 10% of symptomatic patients with medullary sponge kidney have a poor long-term prognosis because of nephrolithiasis, septicemia, and renal failure. However, this figure is probably lower now because of the more effective treatment available for hypercalciuria and renal lithiasis and because of the better antibiotics available and the selective use of prophylaxis.

Sporadic Glomerulocystic Kidney Disease

Glomerulocystic disease is a specific entity, but the term has often been applied as a catchall to include all conditions in which there are glomerular cysts. The term glomerulocystic means that cysts of the glomeruli or Bowman's space are present diffusely and bilaterally. However, cysts of the glomeruli are present in many forms of renal cystic disease, and they may or may not be the predominant pathology. Thus, the presence of glomerular cysts does not prove that the patient has glomerulocystic disease.

Table 59–11 shows the Bernstein and Landing classification of conditions with glomerular cysts as modified by Glassberg and Filmer (1992) to make it compatible with the AAP classification. The diagnosis of sporadic glomerulocystic disease should be made only when the disorder conforms to the 1941 definition of Roos and the 1976 definition of Taxy and Filmer. That is, glomerulocystic disease is a noninheritable condition producing bilaterally enlarged kidneys containing small cysts, predominantly of Bowman's space. Characteristically, no other family members are affected, and no associated anomalies are present, although in the case described by Taxy and Filmer (1976), subcapsular hepatic cysts were present. Sporadic glomerulocystic disease clearly is different from familial hypoplastic glomerulocystic disease. It is not an inherited disorder, and the kidneys are larger.

The patients evaluated by Bernstein and Landing (1989) after referral and those they found described in the literature differ in age of presentation, clinical course, and renal morphology. These investigators suggest that, in some of the published cases, features of other syndromes were overlooked or family members were inadequately screened for DPK. They have recommended the use of the term sporadic glomerulocystic disease to show that the condition is not genetic.

Bernstein (1993) believes that sporadic glomerulocystic kidney disease in young infants is indistinguishable from DPK when the latter is seen in infants and glomerular cysts are a major histologic finding. The only difference clinically or histologically between the two is that no family history can be identified in the sporadic entity. Bernstein goes as far as to question whether sporadic glomerulocystic kidney disease represents a new mutation of classic DPK rather than a different disease. He concludes that the question is currently unanswerable.

Table 59–11. CONDITIONS ASSOCIATED WITH GLOMERULAR CYSTS

Sporadic glomerulocystic kidney disease
Familial hypoplastic glomerulocystic disease
Autosomal dominant polycystic disease
Juvenile nephronophthisis in association with hepatic fibrosis
Multiple malformation syndromes
- Zellweger's syndrome
- Trisomy 13
- Meckel's syndrome
- Short-rib polydactyly (Majewski type)
- Tuberous sclerosis
- Orofaciodigital syndrome type I
- Brachymesomelia renal syndrome
- Renal-hepatic-pancreatic dysplasia

Acquired Renal Cystic Disease

In 1977, Dunhill and co-workers described acquired renal cystic disease (ARCD) in patients in renal failure. **At first, ARCD was thought to be confined to patients receiving hemodialysis. However, it shortly became apparent that the disorder is almost as common in patients receiving peritoneal dialysis** (Thompson et al, 1986) **and that it may develop in patients with chronic renal failure who are being managed medically without any type of dialysis** (Fisher and Horvath, 1972; Ishikawa et al, 1980; Kutcher et al, 1983; Miller et al, 1989). **Thus, ARCD appears to be a feature of end-stage kidneys rather than a response to dialysis.** Ishikawa (1985) has suggested that the term uremic acquired cystic disease be applied to this entity (Fig. 59–25).

The incidence of ARCD differs among institutions, perhaps as a result of population differences or diagnostic criteria. For example, Feiner and co-workers (1981) require that at least 40% of the kidney be affected by cysts, whereas Basile and co-workers (1988) require only 20% involvement. Judging the extent of involvement is likewise subjective. Some reports include patients with only one cyst, whereas Thompson and co-workers (1986) grade ARCD according to the number of cysts involved, from grade 1 (less than 5 cysts bilaterally) to grade 4 (greater than 14 cysts bilaterally).

The significance of ARCD lies in two areas: (1) the symptoms it may produce (pain and hematuria), and (2) the high incidence of benign and malignant renal tumors that accompany the condition. The incidence of renal tumors warrants special consideration.

INCIDENCE: ASSOCIATION WITH RENAL CELL CARCINOMA

In 1984, Gardner identified 160 patients with ARCD among 430 patients receiving long-term hemodialysis, an incidence of 34% (Gardner, 1984b). This incidence represents an overall figure because the incidence of ARCD rises with time on dialysis and perhaps also with the duration of chronic renal failure and the age of the patient. For example, Ishikawa and co-workers (1980) found ARCD in 44% of patients who had been receiving hemodialysis for less than 3 years but in 79% of those who had been receiving hemodialysis for a longer time. In a later study, the same group found a higher incidence of ARCD with age, particularly in men (Ishikawa et al, 1985). They suggested that a sex-

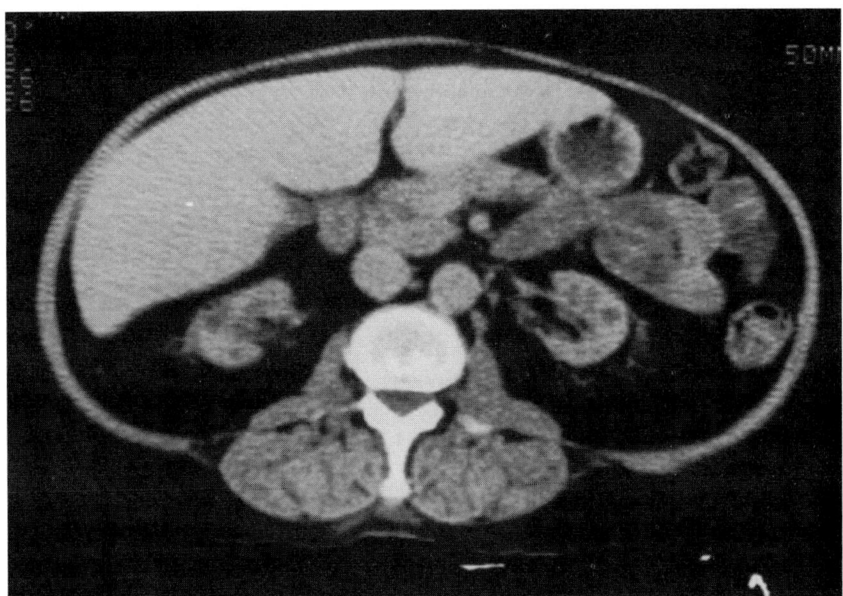

Figure 59–25. Small kidneys with multiple small cysts in a hemodialysis patient with acquired renal cystic disease.

related endogenous growth factor combined with a uremic metabolite was important. Hughson and co-workers (1986) found a 2.9:1 male-to-female ratio for ARCD, which is striking when one considers that the number of male patients undergoing dialysis only slightly exceeds the number of female patients.

ARCD can occur in children as well. Of 22 children with end-stage renal disease on dialysis for a period of 7 to 49 months, Hakim and associates (1994) found multiple cysts in three children and a single cyst in another two. Because simple cysts in children are rare, the two with a single cyst probably represent ARCD, as do the other three, making a 23% incidence of ARCD in this group of children with end-stage renal disease.

The incidence of ARCD appears to be higher in patients with end-stage kidneys secondary to nephrosclerosis than in those in whom renal failure was the result of diabetes (Fallon and Williams, 1989; Miller et al, 1989). However, the lower incidence of ARCD in diabetic patients may well be a result of their shorter survival time on dialysis (Fallon and Williams, 1989).

Renal neoplasms, principally adenomas, occur in 10% of patients receiving chronic hemodialysis, and when ARCD is present, the incidence of neoplasms is even higher, ranging from 20% to 25% (Gardner and Evan, 1984). When renal cell carcinoma is associated with ARCD, it frequently occurs at an earlier age than in the general population, often in the third or fourth decade. In these cases, the cysts are pronounced. When renal cell carcinoma appears after the age of 60 years in an ARCD patient, there usually are fewer cysts (Hughson et al, 1986).

In Japan, the incidence of renal cell carcinoma among dialysis patients is several to 20 times higher than it is in the general population (Odaka, 1988; Ishikawa, 1993), **whereas in the United States it is three to six times higher based on an annual incidence of 8 per 100,000 among the general population in the United States** (Resseguie et al, 1978; Levine et al, 1991). **In Michigan there is a fivefold increase of renal cell carcinoma in dialysis patients, correlating well with the overall U.S. statistic** (Port et al, 1989). **Perhaps the difference in incidence of renal cell carcinoma in Japan and the United States is due to the stronger push in Japan toward routine screening of the kidneys by CT after 3 years of dialysis. According to Levine and associates (1991), CT screening at approximately $600 per study would amount to a cost of $36 million a year, making the cost of such mass screening almost prohibitive.**

Renal cell carcinoma occurring in end-stage renal disease (ESRD) is different biologically in a number of ways from classic renal cell carcinoma: (1) the age of occurrence averages 5 years younger in patients with ESRD; (2) the male-to-female ratio is significantly greater in ESRD patients with renal cell carcinoma compared to that in the general population with renal cell carcinoma (7:1 for ESRD vs. 2:1 for the general population); and (3) the incidence of renal cell carcinoma in ESRD is three to six times that of the general population and may be as high as ten times the incidence in blacks (Matson and Cohen, 1990; Cohen, 1993). These differences probably reflect the high incidence of epithelial hyperplasia, renal cysts, and adenomas seen in patients with ESRD.

Etiology

As noted earlier, the initial view that ARCD is a consequence of hemodialysis per se has been shown to be incorrect. However, if uremic toxins are the principal risk factor, why are there different incidences of ARCD at various institutions? It is possible that different durations of predialysis medical therapy or different dialysis regimens are important, but no data have been collected on this point.

A number of findings suggest a role for toxins. First, the cysts, adenomas, and carcinomas usually are multiple and bilateral, as are the carcinomas induced experimentally in rats by toxins. Second, there is a decline in the incidence of renal cell carcinoma and a regression of the cysts after successful transplantation (Ishikawa et al, 1983), suggesting that some cystogenic or carcinogenic toxin of uremia is being eliminated by the allograft. Third, if transplantation fails and dialysis is resumed, the cysts return.

Clinical Features

The most common presentation of ARCD is loin pain, hematuria, or both. Bleeding, whether into the kidney or into the retroperitoneum, may be secondary to renal cysts or to renal cell carcinoma. Feiner and co-workers (1981) suggested that cystic bleeding is secondary to rupture of unsupported sclerotic vessels in the wall. If the cyst communicates with the nephron, hematuria may result. In some patients, bleeding follows heparinization during dialysis. Also, in some cases, the serum hemoglobin concentration is elevated secondary to increased renal production of erythropoietin (Shalhoub et al, 1982; Ratcliffe et al, 1983; Mickisch et al, 1984).

Histopathology

The cysts develop predominantly in the cortex, although the medulla may be affected, and generally they are bilateral (Fig. 59–26). They average 0.5 to 1.0 cm in diameter, but some have been reported to reach 5.0 cm (Miller et al, 1989). The cysts are filled with clear, straw-colored or hemorrhagic fluid and often contain calcium oxalate crystals (Miller et al, 1989). Some resemble simple retention cysts, with a flat epithelial lining.

The nuclei of the epithelial cells in these cases are round and regular, without prominent nucleoli (Hughson et al, 1980). However, some cysts (atypical or hyperplastic) are lined by epithelial cells with larger, irregular nuclei that contain prominent nucleoli and may show mitotic activity. This hyperplastic lining is thought by some workers to be a precursor of renal tumors. Moreover, some hyperplastic cysts have papillary projections, and to some observers, the distinction between cyst and neoplasm becomes blurred when papillary hyperplasia predominates.

Feiner and co-workers (1981) found that the cysts begin as dilatations or outpouchings of the nephrons. One theory suggests that calcium oxalate crystals precipitate along the nephron lining, disrupting it and causing outpouchings that dilate as they become obstructed by further crystallization (Rushton et al, 1981; Hughson et al, 1986). That oxalate crystals may be a factor in cyst formation is conceivable because crystals have been implicated in the development of cysts in rats given ethylene glycol (Rushton et al, 1981).

The renal adenomas usually are multiple and often are bilateral. Miller and colleagues (1989) performed autopsies on 155 patients with end-stage renal disease and found 25 to have small renal cortical nodules (adenomas). These nodules were multiple, and all were smaller than 2.5 cm in diameter. They usually arose from the walls of the atypical (hyperplastic) cysts.

The cells were either oriented into papillary projections or arranged as solid nodules with tubule formation. The cells were smaller than those found in renal cell carcinoma, with cytoplasm that was either granular and eosinophilic (oncocytes) or pale staining. The nuclei typically appeared small, rounded, and uniform with insignificant nucleoli. Anaplasia and mitosis were absent. In three of these cases, lesions of 3.0 to 3.5 cm were found, all of which were renal cell carcinoma. The cells in these lesions were usually of the clear cell type, with wrinkled nuclei and prominent nucleoli. They were arranged in solid or tubular patterns.

Differentiating these renal tumors into adenomas and carcinomas is arbitrary at times. In Bell's classic 1935 article, renal tumors larger than 3 cm in diameter were considered carcinomas, whereas the smaller ones were considered adenomas. However, even in Bell's work, tumors as small as 1 cm were associated with metastases in a few cases. Also, although the majority of renal cell carcinomas in patients with ARCD are larger than 2.0 to 3.0 cm, some have measured only 1.0 to 1.5 cm (Feiner et al, 1981; Chung-Park et al, 1983; Hughson et al, 1986). The smallest renal cell carcinoma associated with known metastases was 1.2 cm in diameter (Ishikawa, 1988a, 1988b). In sum, most renal nodules that are smaller than 1 cm in diameter are adenomas, and most that are more than 3 cm in diameter are carcinomas. Tumors between 1 and 3 cm in diameter must be considered a gray zone.

It is not clear whether renal adenomas undergo malignant transformation. The large incidence of renal adenomas in the general population and the even larger incidence in uremic patients, combined with the low incidence of renal cell

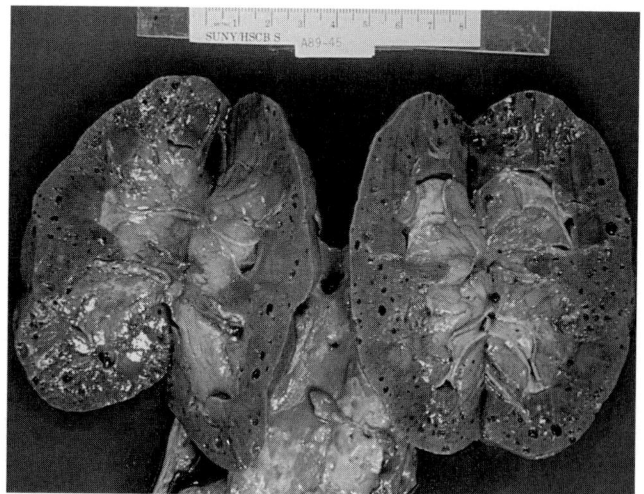

Figure 59–26. Kidneys on autopsy from a 55-year-old man who was on chronic hemodialysis demonstrating acquired renal cystic disease with numerous small, diffuse renal cysts.

PARAPELVIC AND RENAL SINUS CYSTS

Definitions

A number of terms have been used for cysts adjacent to the renal pelvis or within the hilum: peripelvic cysts, parapelvic cysts, renal sinus cysts, parapelvic lymphatic cysts, hilus cysts, cysts of the renal hilum, and peripelvic lymphangiectasis. Some peripelvic cysts are, in fact, simple cysts that arise from the renal parenchyma but happen to abut the renal pelvis, with or without obstruction. Clearly, these are not cysts of the renal sinus. The terms peripelvic and parapelvic generally describe cysts around the renal pelvis or renal sinus. Cysts derived from the renal sinus have no parenchymal etiology.

To avoid confusion, the terms peripelvic and parapelvic should be used only to describe location. The author prefers to use these terms only as adjectives to describe simple parenchymal cysts adjacent to the renal pelvis or hilum, i.e., a peripelvic simple parenchymal cyst (Fig. 59–32). The term renal sinus cyst should be reserved for all other cysts in the hilum, i.e., those that are not derived from the renal parenchyma but rather from the other structures of the sinus, such as arteries, lymphatics, and fat.

Renal Sinus Cysts

The predominant type of renal sinus cyst appears to be one derived from the lymphatics. Most often, these cysts are multiple, and often they are bilateral. The majority appear after the fifth decade, and they may be associated with inflammation, obstruction, or a calculus (Jordan, 1962; Kutcher et al, 1982).

One etiologic theory suggests that lymphatic cysts are secondary to obstruction. Kutcher and associates (1982) note that lymphatic cysts or ectasia also are found in other abdominal organs; these investigators refer to the condition in the renal sinus as peripelvic multicystic lymphangiectasia. In their patient, the cysts were lined by endothelial cells, and the fluid contained lymphocytes. The intrarenal lymphatics also were dilated, with focal cyst formation. These cysts can cause obstruction or even extravasation of contrast medium during urography (Kutcher et al, 1982).

A condition previously described in the Spanish literature (Paramo and Segura, 1972; Vela-Navarrete et al, 1974; Paramo, 1975), but only recently described in the English literature has been called polycystic disease of the renal sinus (Vela-Navarrete and Robledo, 1983)—a problematic term because of the possible confusion with polycystic disease of the kidney. **Vela-Navarrete and Robledo (1983) described 32 patients with this condition, some in multiple generations of a family** (Vela-Navarrete, personal communication, 1990). This entity sounds very much like the case reported by Kutcher and colleagues (1982) and is similar to others reported in association with renal calculi.

Vela-Navarrete and Robledo (1983) found nephrotomography and CT particularly useful in defining the lesions. Sonography was less helpful, perhaps because of the limitations of the equipment then available. On nephrotomography, radiolucencies are identifiable in the renal sinus, along with

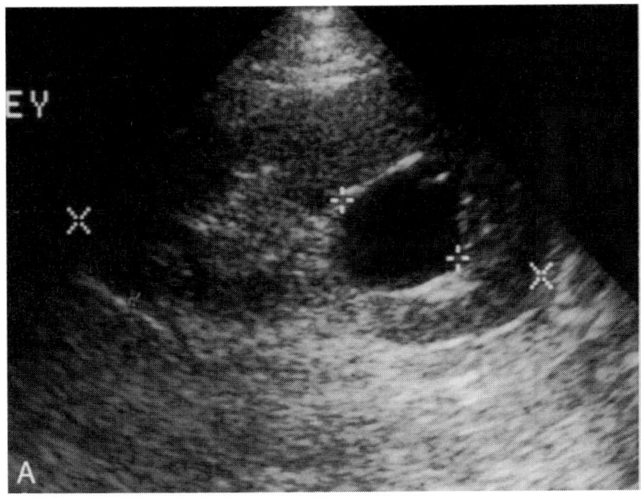

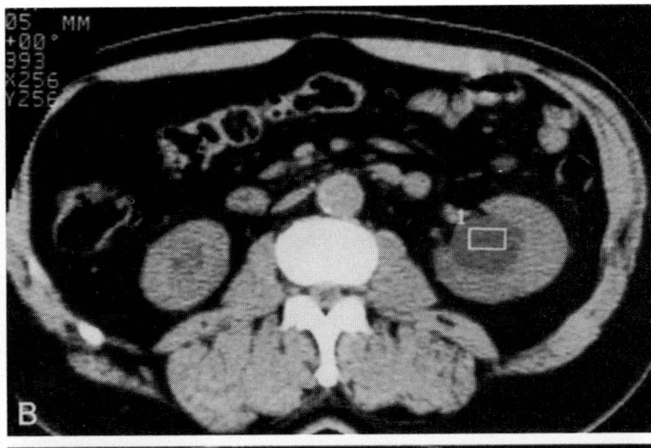

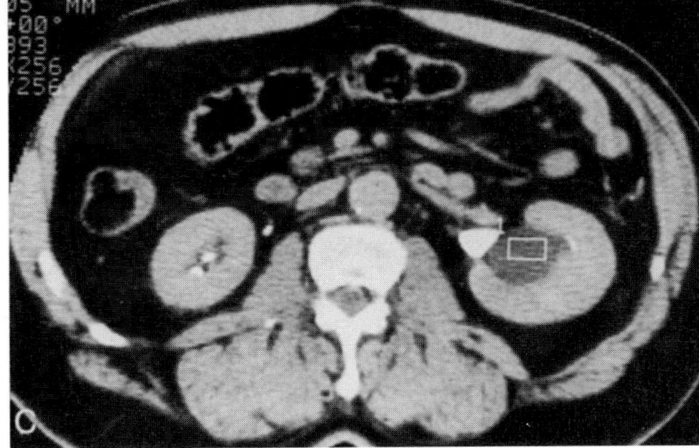

Figure 59–32. Simple cyst with peripelvic location. *A,* Renal sonogram reveals a centrally located left renal cyst. *B,* On precontrast CT scan, the cyst measures 3 HU. *C,* After contrast, the cyst is calibrated to 2 HU. Note how the cyst is situated between a calyx and the renal pelvis. This is a simple parenchymal cyst in a peripelvic location and should not be confused with a renal sinus cyst.

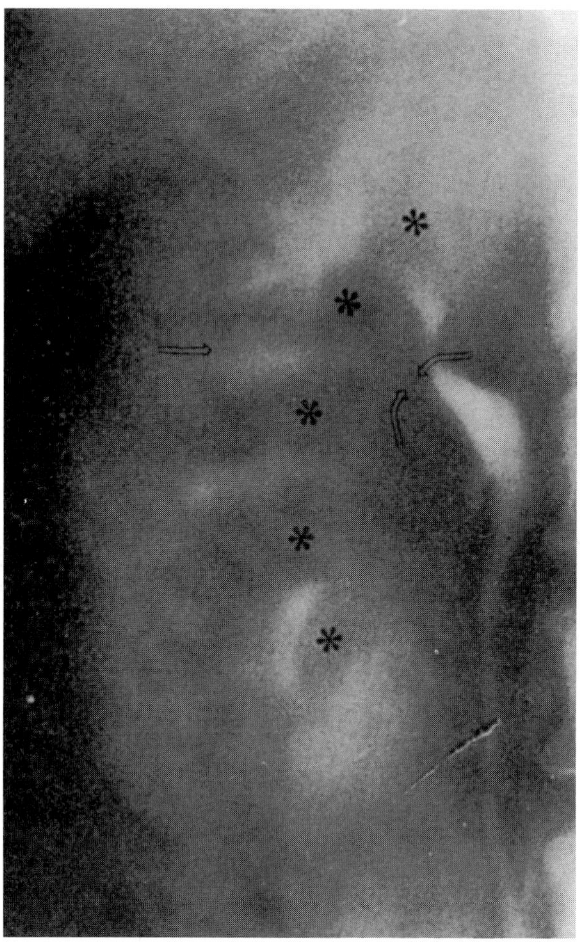

Figure 59–33. "Polycystic disease of the renal sinus" simulating renal pelvic lipomatosis. Nephrotomography demonstrating multiple renal lucencies in the renal sinus *(asterisks)* with medial displacement of the renal pelvis and elongation and stretching of infundibuli *(arrows)*. (From Vela-Navarrete R, Robledo AG: Polycystic disease of the renal sinus: Structural characteristics. J Urol 1983; 129:700.)

stretching of the infundibula. Thus, the appearance is similar to that of renal sinus lipomatosis, leading Vela-Navarrete and Robledo (1983) to suggest that many cases of lipomatosis would be identified as polycystic disease of the renal sinus if CT were used (Fig. 59–33). On CT, the cysts can be seen within the renal sinus as they displace the calyces peripherally (Fig. 59–34). The columns of Bertin may appear attenuated. In the Spanish series, 9 of the 32 patients had small renal calculi visible on plain film.

In five patients in the Spanish series, the lesions were explored. Multiple cysts were found, ranging in size from 2 to 4 cm in diameter and intertwined with stretched infundibula. The fluid was clear, with a plasma-like chemical composition. Histologically, the cyst walls were suggestive of a lymphatic vessel.

This entity has a benign natural history except for the small calculi. These concretions may be secondary to stasis.

Serous cysts have also been reported in the renal sinus. Barrie (1953) suggested that these lesions are secondary to fatty tissue wasting in the renal sinus. Because the space left by the atrophied fat cannot collapse, it fills with transudate. However, no recent reports of serous cysts have been published, and this author suspects that earlier cases were, in fact, lymphatic cysts.

Androulakakis and co-workers (1980) reported eight patients with parapelvic cysts, which they described as extraparenchymal. However, it is not clear how the cysts were identified as such. All lesions were said to be single cysts, but the description suggests that multiple cysts were present in some cases.

From a review of the literature, including CT findings in current cases, it appears that most multiple cystic structures in the area of the renal sinus will turn out to be lymphatic cysts, whereas most singular cysts will be found to be derived from the renal parenchyma. Continued study of cases by CT should clarify the nature of parapelvic and renal sinus cysts.

CONCLUSION

Bilateral renal cystic disease creates a dilemma in diagnosis at any age. The differential diagnosis includes RPK, DPK, tuberous sclerosis, von Hippel-Lindau disease, bilateral simple cysts, and acquired renal cystic disease (Table 59–12). **The cysts in RPK may present at any time**

Table 59–12. DIFFERENTIAL DIAGNOSIS: BILATERAL RENOMEGALY AND RENAL CYSTS

Autosomal recessive polycystic kidney disease
Autosomal dominant polycystic kidney disease
Tuberous sclerosis
von Hippel-Lindau disease
Bilateral simple cysts
Acquired renal cystic disease

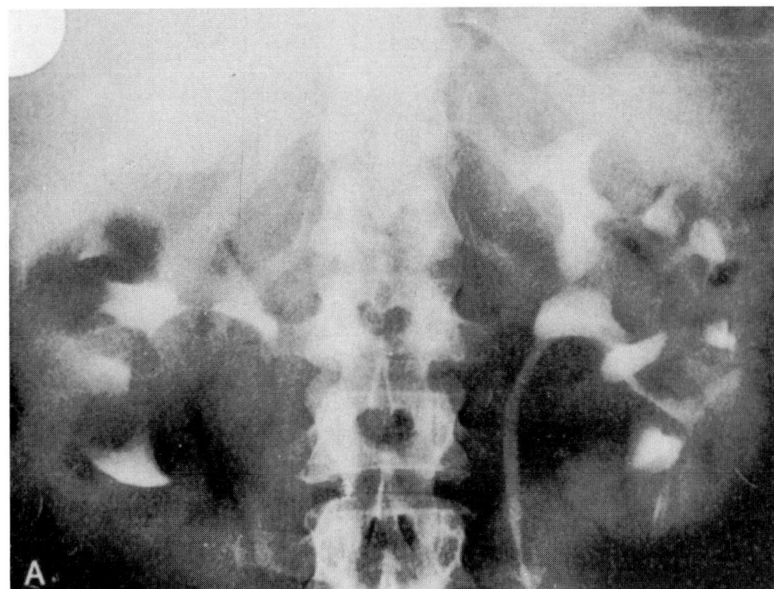

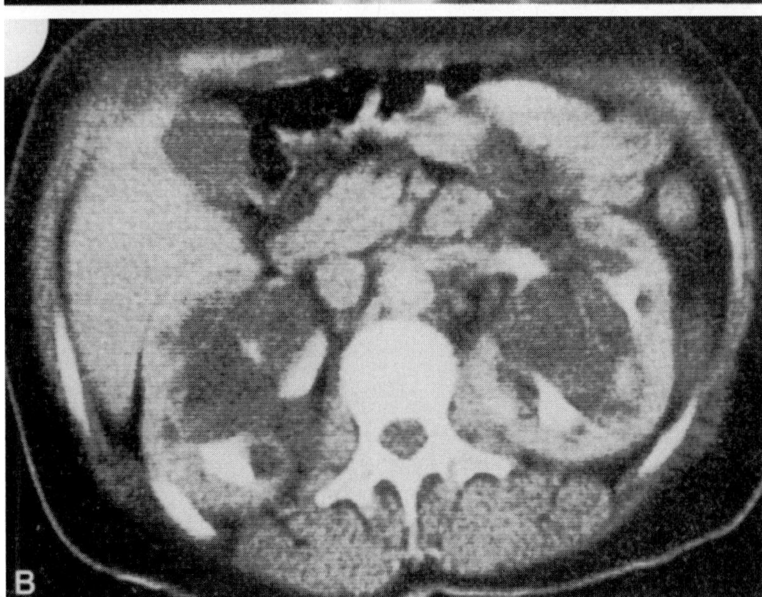

Figure 59–34. "Polycystic disease of the renal sinus," a form of renal sinus cysts. *A,* Intravenous urogram with enlargement of both kidneys, stretching of infundibuli, and trumpet-shaped calyces. *B,* CT scan in midportion of kidneys demonstrates multiple sinus cysts with peripheral displacement of renal pelvis and calyces. (From Vela-Navarrete R, Robledo AG: Polycystic disease of the renal sinus: Structural characteristics. J Urol 1983; 129:700.)

from in utero to the age of 20 years, in DPK from in utero to autopsy, in tuberous sclerosis from in utero to anytime in life but usually before the age of 30, and in von Hippel-Lindau disease infrequently in the first few years of life but almost always by the age of 30; bilateral simple cysts may present at any age but particularly after age 35, and acquired renal cystic disease may become evident after end-stage kidney disease develops.

ACKNOWLEDGMENTS

The author wishes to thank his secretary, Cloyette Harris, for her help in the preparation of this chapter.

REFERENCES

Al-Khaldi N, Watson AR, Zuccollo J, et al: Outcome of antenatally detected cystic dysplastic kidney disease. Arch Dis Child 1994;70:520.

Ambrose SS: Unilateral multicystic renal disease in adults. Birth Defects 1976;13:349.

Amesur NR, Roy HG: Para-pelvic cyst of the kidney. Indian J Surg 1963;25:45.

Amis ES, Jr, Cronan JJ, Yoder IC, et al: Renal cysts: Curios and caveats. Urol Radiol 1982;4:199.

Anderson JC: Hydronephrosis. Springfield, IL, Charles C Thomas, 1963.

Androulakakis PA, Kirayiannis B, Deliveliotis A: The parapelvic renal cyst: A report of 8 cases with particular emphasis on diagnosis and management. Br J Urol 1980;52:342.

Antignac C, Arduy CH, Beckman JS, et al: A gene for familial juvenile nephronophthisis (recessive medullary cystic disease) maps to chromosome 2p. Nature Genet 1993;3:342.

Arant BS, Sotero-Avila C, Bernstein J: Segmental hypoplasia of the kidney (Ask-Upmark). J Pediatr 1979;95:931.

Arey JB: Cystic lesions of the kidney in infants and children. J Pediatr 1959;54:429.

Ask-Upmark E: Über juvenile maligne Nephrosklerose und thr Verhaltnis zu Störungen in der Nierenentwicklung. Acta Pathol Microbiol Scand 1929;6:383.

Aterman K, Boustani P, Gillis DA: Solitary multilocular cysts of the kidney. J Pediatr Surg 1973;8:505.

Atiyeh B, Husmann D, Baum M: Contralateral renal abnormalities in multicystic-dysplastic kidney disease. J Pediatr 1992;121:65.

Atiyeh B, Husmann D, Baum M: Contralateral renal abnormalities in patients with renal agenesis and noncystic renal dysplasia. Pediatrics 1993;9:812.

Avner ED, Ellis D, Jaffe R, et al: Neonatal radiocontrast nephropathy simulating infantile polycystic kidney disease. Pediatrics 1982;100:85.

Avner ED, Sweeney WE, Jr, Ellis D: In vitro modulation of tubular cyst regression in murine polycystic kidney disease. Kidney Int 1989; 36:960.

Avni E, Thova Y, Lalmand B, et al: Multicystic dysplastic kidney: Natural history from in utero diagnosis and postnatal followup. J Urol 1987;138:1420.

Babcock DS: Medical diseases of the urinary tract and adrenal gland. *In* Haller JO, Shkolnik A, eds: Ultrasound in Pediatrics. New York, Churchill Livingstone, 1981, p 113.

Babka JC, Cohen MS, Sode J: Solitary intrarenal cyst causing hypertension. N Engl J Med 1974;291:343.

Banner MP, Pollack HM, Chatten J, et al: Multilocular renal cysts: Radiological-pathologic correlation. AJR 1981;136:239.

Barloon JT, Vince SW: Caliceal obstruction owing to a large parapelvic cyst: Excretory urography, ultrasound and computerized tomography findings. J Urol 1987;137:270.

Barrett DM, Wineland RE: Renal cell carcinoma in multicystic dysplastic kidney. Urology 1980;15:152.

Barrie JH: Paracalyceal cysts of the renal sinus. Am J Pathol 1953; 29:985.

Bartholomew TH, Solvis TL, Kroovand RL, et al: The sonographic evaluation and management of simple renal cysts in children. J Urol 1980;123:732.

Bear JC, McManamon P, Morgan J, et al: Age at clinical onset and at ultrasonographic detection of adult polycystic disease. Am J Med Genet 1984;18:45.

Bear JC, Parfrey PS, Morgan JM, et al: Autosomal dominant polycystic kidney disease: New information for genetic counselling. Am J Med Genet 1992;43:548.

Bearth K, Steg A: On the pathogenesis of simple cysts in the adult: A microdissection study. Urol Res 1977;5:103.

Beck AD: The effect of intra-uterine urinary obstruction upon the development of the fetal kidney. J Urol 1971;105:784.

Beckwith JB: Wilms tumor and other renal tumors in childhood: An update. J Urol 1986;136:320.

Beckwith JB, Kiviat NB: Multilocular renal cysts and cystic renal tumors [editorial]. AJR 1981;136:435.

Beckwith JB, Palmer NF: Histopathology and prognosis of Wilms' tumor: Results from First National Wilms' Tumor Study. Cancer 1978; 41:1937.

Beetz R, Schofer O, Riedmiller H, et al: Medullary sponge kidneys and unilateral Wilms' tumour in a child with Beckwith-Wiedemann syndrome. Eur J Pediatr 1991;150:489.

Begleiter ML, Smith TH, Harris DJ: Ultrasound for genetic counselling in polycystic kidney disease. Lancet 1977;2:1073.

Beitzke H: Über Zysten in Nierenmark. Charite-Ann, 1908;32:285.

Bell ET: Cystic disease of the kidneys. Am J Pathol 1935;11:373.

Beneventi FA: Hydrocalyx: Its relief by retrograde dilatation. Am J Surg 1943;61:244.

Bengtsson U, Hedman L, Svalander C: Adult type of polycystic kidney disease in a newborn child. Acta Med Scand 1975;197:447.

Bennett WM, Elzinga LW, Barry JM: Management of cystic kidney disease. *In* Gardner KD, Jr, Bernstein J, eds: The Cystic Kidney. Boston, Kluwer Academic, 1990, pp 247–275.

Bennett WM, Elzinga L, Golper TA, et al: Reduction of cyst volume for symptomatic management of autosomal dominant polycystic kidney disease. J Urol, 1987;137:620.

Bennington JL, Beckwith JB: Tumors of the kidney, renal pelvis and ureter. *In* Atlas of Tumor Pathology, Series 2, Fascicle 12. Washington, DC, Armed Forces Institute of Pathology, 1975, p 33.

Berdon WE, Schwartz RH, Becker J, et al: Tamm-Horsfall proteinuria. Radiology 1969;92:714.

Berman DJ, Maizel M: Role of urinary obstruction in the genesis of renal dysplasia: A model in the chick embryo. J Urol 1982;128:1091.

Bernstein J: Experimental study of renal parenchymal maldevelopment (renal dysplasia). Presented at the 3rd International Congress of Nephrology. Washington, DC, September, 1966.

Bernstein J: Developmental abnormalities of the renal parenchyma: Renal hypoplasia and dysplasia. Pathol Annu 1968;3:213.

Bernstein J: The morphogenesis of renal parenchymal maldevelopment (renal dysplasia). Pediatr Clin North Am 1971;18:395.

Bernstein J: The classification of renal cysts. Nephron 1973;11:91.

Bernstein J: Developmental abnormalities of the renal parenchyma–renal hypoplasia and dysplasia. *In* Sommers SC, ed: Kidney Pathology Decennial 1966–1975. New York, Appleton-Century-Crofts, 1975, pp 11–17, 36–37.

Bernstein J. A classification of renal cysts. *In* Gardner KD, Jr, ed: Cystic Disease of the Kidney. New York, John Wiley & Sons, 1976, p 7.

Bernstein J: The multicystic kidney and hereditary renal adysplasia. Am J Kidney Dis 1991;18:495.

Bernstein J: Glomerolocystic kidney disease nosological considerations. Pediatr Nephrol 1993;7:464.

Bernstein J, Gardner KD, Jr: Cystic disease of the kidney and renal dysplasia. *In* Harrison JH, Gittes RF, Perlmutter AD, et al, eds: Campbell's Urology, 4th ed: Philadelphia, W.B. Saunders, 1979a, p 1399.

Bernstein J, Gardner KD, Jr: Familial juvenile nephronophthisis: Medullary cystic disease. *In* Edelman CM, Jr, ed: Pediatric Kidney Disease. Boston, Little, Brown, 1979b, p 580.

Bernstein J, Gardner KD: Hereditary tubulointerstitial nephropathies. *In* Cotran R, Brenner B, Stein J, eds: Tubulointerstitial Nephropathies. New York, Churchill Livingstone, 1983, pp 335–357.

Bernstein J, Gardner KD, Jr: Cystic disease of the kidney and renal dysplasia. *In* Walsh PC, Gittes RF, Perlmutter AD, et al, eds: Campbell's Urology, 5th ed: Philadelphia, W.B. Saunders, 1986, p 1760.

Bernstein J, Gardner KD: Cystic disease and dysplasia of the kidneys. *In* Murphy WM, ed: Urological Pathology. Philadelphia, W.B. Saunders, 1989, p 483.

Bernstein J, Landing BH: Glomerulocystic kidney disease. Prog Clin Biol Res 1989;305:27.

Bernstein J, Meyer R: Congenital abnormalities of the urinary system: II. Renal cortical and medullary necrosis. J Pediatr 1961;59:657.

Bernstein J, Meyer R: Parenchymal maldevelopment of the kidney. *In* Kelley VC, ed: Brenneman-Kelley, Practice of Pediatrics, Vol. 3. New York, Harper & Row, 1967, pp 1–30.

Bernstein J, Robbins TO, Kissane JM: The renal lesion of tuberous sclerosis. Semin Diagn Pathol 1986;3:97.

Bernstein J, Slovis TL: Polycystic diseases of the kidney. *In* Edelman CM, ed: Pediatric Kidney Disease, 2nd ed: Boston, Little Brown, 1992, pp 1139–1153.

Biglar JA, Killingsworth WP: Cartilage in the kidney. Arch Pathol 1949;47:487.

Birken G, King D, Vane D, et al: Renal cell carcinoma arising in a multicystic dysplastic kidney. J Pediatr Surg 1985;20:619.

Blyth H, Ockenden BG: Polycystic disease of kidneys and liver presenting in childhood. J Med Genet 1971;8:257.

Boag GS, Nolan R: CT visualization of medullary sponge kidney. Urol Radiol 1988;9:220.

Boggs LK, Kimmelsteil P: Benign multilocular cystic nephroma: Report of two cases of so-called multilocular cyst of the kidney. J Urol 1956;76:530.

Bonal J, Caralps A, Lauzurica R, et al: Cyst infection in acquired renal cystic disease. Br Med J 1987;295:25.

Bosniak MA: The current radiological approach to renal cysts. Radiology 1986;158:1.

Bosniak MA: The small (≤3.0 cm) renal parenchymal tumor: Detection, diagnosis and controversies. Radiology 1991;179:307.

Bosniak MA: Commentary. Difficulties in classifying cystic lesions of the kidney. Urol Radiol 1991a;13:91.

Bourneville DM: Sclérose tubereuse des circonvolutions cérébrales idote et épilepsie hémiplegique. Arch Neurol (Paris) 1880;1:81.

Bove KE, McAdams AJ: The nephroblastomatosis complex and its relationship to Wilms' tumor: A clinicopathologic treatise. Perspect Pediatr Pathol 1976;3:185.

Braasch WF, Schacht FW: Pathological and clinical data concerning polycystic kidney. Surg Gynecol Obstet 1933;57:467.

Bree BL, Raiss GJ, Schwab RE: The sonographically ambiguous renal mass: Can surgery be avoided? Radiology 1984;153(Suppl.):212.

Bretan PN, Busch MP, Hricak H, et al: Chronic renal failure: A significant risk factor in the development of acquired renal cysts and renal cell carcinoma. Cancer 1986;57:1871.

Breuning MH, Reeder ST, Brunner H, et al: Improved early diagnoses of adult polycystic kidney disease with flanking DNA markers. Lancet 1987;2:1359.

Brooke-Carter PT, Peral B, Ward CJ, et al: Deletion of the TSC2 and PKD1 genes associated with severe infantile polycystic kidney disease—a contiguous gene syndrome. Nature Genet 1994;8:328.
Bucciarelli E, Sidoni A, Alberti PF, et al: Congenital nephrotic syndrome of the Finnish type. Nephron 1989;53:177.
Buchta RM, Viseskul C, Gilbert EF, et al: Familial bilateral renal agenesis and hereditary renal adysplasia. Z Kinderheilkd 1973;115:111.
Burgler W, Hauri D: Vitale Komplikationen bei multizystischer Nierende Generation (multizystischer Dysplasie). Urol Int 1983;38:251.
Cacchi R, Ricci V: Sur une rare maladie kystique multiple des pyramides rénales le "rein en éponge." J Urol Nephrol (Paris) 1949;55:497.
Campbell GS, Bick HD, Paulsen EP: Bleeding esophageal varices with polycystic liver: Report of three cases. N Engl J Med 1958;259:904.
Campos A, Figueroa ET, Gunaselcaran S, et al: Early presentation of tuberous sclerosis as bilateral renal cysts. J Urol 1993;149:1077.
Cantani A, Bamonte G, Ceccoli D, et al: Familial nephronophthisis: A review and differential diagnosis. Clin Pediatr 1986;25:90.
Carone FA, Maiko H, Kanwar YS: Basement membrane antigens in renal polycystic disease. Am J Pathol 1988;130:466.
Carone FA, Rowland RG, Perlman SG, et al: The pathogenesis of drug-induced renal cystic disease. Kidney Int 1974;5:411.
Carter JE, Lirenman DS: Bilateral renal hypoplasia with oligomeganephronia: Oligomeganephronic renal hypoplasia. Am J Dis Child 1970;120:537.
Castillo O, Boyle ET, Kramer SA: Multilocular cysts of the kidney: A study of 29 patients and review of the literature. Urology 1991; 37:156.
Chamberlin BC, Hagge WW, Stickler GB: Juvenile nephronophthisis and medullary cystic disease. Mayo Clin Proc 1977;52:485.
Chatten J, Bishop HC: Bilateral multilocular cysts of the kidney. J Pediatr Surg 1977;12:749.
Chen YH, Stapleton FB, Roy S, et al: Neonatal hypertension from a unilateral multicystic dysplastic kidney. J Urol 1985;133:664.
Cho C, Friedland GW, Swenson RS: Acquired renal cystic disease and renal neoplasms in hemodialysis patients. Urol Radiol 1984;6:153.
Chonko AM, Weiss JM, Stein JH, et al: Renal involvement in tuberous sclerosis. Am J Med 1974;56:124.
Christ ML: Polycystic nephroblastoma. J Urol 1968;98:570.
Chung-Park M, Ricanati E, Lankerani M, et al: Acquired renal cysts and multiple renal cell and urothelial tumors. Am J Clin Pathol 1983; 141:238.
Churchill DN, Bear JC, Morgan J, et al: Prognosis of adult onset polycystic kidney disease re-evaluated. Kidney Int, 1984;26:190.
Cobben JM, Breuning MH, Schoots C, et al: Congenital hepatic fibrosis in autosomal-dominant polycystic kidney disease. Kidney Int 1990;38:880.
Cohen AH, Hoyer JR: Nephronophthisis: A primary tubular basement membrane defect. Lab Invest 1986;55:564.
Cohen EP: Epidemiology of acquired cystic kidney disease. *In* Gabow PA, Grantham JJ, eds: Proceedings of the Fifth International Workshop on Polycystic Kidney Disease. Kansas City, Missouri, The PKR Foundation, 1993, pp 81–84.
Cole BR, Conley SB, Stapleton FB: Polycystic kidney disease in the first year of life. J Pediatr 1987;111:693.
Colodny AH: Comments in discussion. J Urol 1989;142:489.
Crocker JF, Brown DM, Vernier RL: Developmental defects of the kidney: A review of renal development and experimental studies of maldevelopment. Pediatr Clin North Am 1971;18:355.
Curry CJR, Jensen K, Holland J, et al: The Potter sequence: A clinical analysis of 80 cases. Am J Med Genet 1984;19:679.
Cussen LJ: Cystic kidneys in children with congenital urethral obstruction. J Urol 1971;106:939.
Dalgaard OZ: Bilateral polycystic disease of the kidneys: A follow-up of two hundred eighty-four patients and their families. Acta Med Scand [Supp] 1957;38:1.
Dalgaard OZ, Norby S: Autosomal dominant polycystic kidney disease in the 1980's. Clin Genet 1989;36:320.
Dalton D, Neiman H, Grayhack JJ: The natural history of simple renal cysts: A preliminary study. J Urol 1986;135:905.
Daniel WW, Jr, Hartman GW, Witten DM, et al: Calcified renal masses: A review of 10 years' experience at the Mayo Clinic. Radiology 1972; 103:503.
Darmady EM, Offer J, Woodhouse MA: Toxic metabolic defect in polycystic disease of kidney. Lancet 1970;1:547.
Darmis F, Nahum H, Mosse A, et al: Fibrose hépatique congénitale à progression clinique renal. Presse Med 1970;78:885.
Dauost MC, Bichet DG, Somlo S: A French-Canadian family with autosomal dominant polycystic kidney disease (ADPKD) unlinked to ADPKD1 or ADPKD2. J Am Soc Nephrol 1993;4:262.
Davides KC: Multilocular kidney disease. J Urol 1976;116:246.
Delaney VB, Adler S, Bruns FJ, et al: Autosomal dominant polycystic kidney disease: Presentation, complications and progression. Am J Kidney Dis 1985;5:104.
Delano BG, Lazar IL, Friedman EA: Hypertension: Late consequences of kidney donation [Abstract]. Kidney Int 1983;23:168.
DeWall JG, Schroder FH, Scholmeijer RJ: Diagnostic work up and treatment of multilocular cystic kidney: Difficulties in differential diagnosis. Urology 1986;28:73.
Dimmick J, Johnson HW, Coleman GU, et al: Wilms tumorlet, nodular renal blastema and multicystic renal dysplasia. J Urol 1989;142:484.
Dunbar JS, Nogrady MG: The calyceal crescent: A roentgenographic sign of obstructive hydronephrosis. Am J Roentgenol 1970;110:520.
Duncan PA, Sagel I, Farnsworth PB: Medullary sponge kidney and partial Beckwith-Wiedemann syndrome. NY State J Med 1979;79:1222.
Dunhill MS, Milard PR, Oliver DO: Acquired cystic disease of the kidneys: A hazard of long-term intermittent maintenance hemodialysis. J Clin Pathol 1977;30:368.
Edmunds W: Cystic adenoma of kidney. Trans Pathol Soc Lond 1892; 43:89.
Eisendrath DN: Clinical importance of congenital renal hypoplasia. J Urol 1935;33:331.
Ekstrom T, Engfeldt B, Langergren C, et al: Medullary Sponge Kidney. Stockholm, Almquist and Wiksells, 1959.
Elfenbein JB, Baluarte HJ, Gruskin AB: Renal hypoplasia with oligomeganephronia. Arch Pathol 1974;97:143.
Elzinga LW, Barry JM, Torres VT, et al: Cyst decompress surgery for autosomal dominant polycystic kidney disease. J Am Soc Nephrol 1992;2:1219.
Emmert GK, Jr, King LR: The risk of hypertension is underestimated in the multicystic dysplastic kidney: A personal perspective. Urology 1994;44:404.
Emmett JL, Witten DM: Clinical Urography: An Atlas and Textbook of Roentgenologic Diagnosis, 3rd ed, vol. 2. Philadelphia, W.B. Saunders, 1971, p 1013.
Ericsson NO: Ectopic ureterocele in infants and children: Clinical study. Acta Chir Scand [Suppl] 1954;97:1.
Ericsson NO: Renal dysplasia. *In* Johnston JH, Goodwin WE, eds: Reviews in Paediatric Urology. Amsterdam, Excerpta Medica, 1974, p 25.
Ericsson NO, Ivemark BI: Renal dysplasia and pyelonephritis in infants and children I. Arch Pathol 1958a;66:255.
Ericsson NO, Ivemark BI: Renal dysplasia and pyelonephritis in infants and children: II. Primitive ductules and abnormal glomeruli. Arch Pathol 1958b;66:264.
Eshghi M, Tuong W, Fernandez R, et al: Percutaneous (endo) infundibulotomy. J Endourol 1987;1:107.
Euderink F, Hogewind BL: Renal cysts in premature children: Occurrence in a family with polycystic kidney disease. Arch Pathol Lab Med 1978;102:592.
European Dialysis and Transplant Association: Report. Proc Eur Dial Transplant Assoc 1978;15:36.
European Polycystic Disease Consortium: The polycystic kidney disease 1 gene encodes a 14kb transcipt and lies within a duplicated region of chromosome 16. Cell 1994;77:881.
Evans AT, Coughlin JP: Urinary obstruction due to renal cysts. J Urol 1970;103:277.
Everson GT, Emmett M, Brown WR, et al: Functional similarities of hepatic cysts and biliary epithelium: Studies of fluid constituents and in vivo secretion in response to secretin. Hepatology 1990;11:557.
Fallon B, Williams RD: Renal cancer associated with acquired cystic disease of the kidney and chronic renal failure. Semin Urol 1989;7:228.
Fanconi G, Hanhart E, Ailbertini A, et al: Die familiäre juvenile Nephronophthise (die idiopathische parenchymatose Schrumptniere). Helv Paediatr Acta 1951;6:1.
Fayemi AD, Ali M: Acquired renal cysts and tumor superimposed on chronic primary diseases: An autopsy study of 24 patients. Pathol Res Pract 1980;68:73.
Feiner HD, Katz LA, Gallo GR: Acquired renal cystic disease of kidney in chronic hemodialysis patients. Urology 1981;17:260.
Fellows RA, Leonidas JC, Beatty EC, Jr: Radiologic features of "adult type" polycystic kidney disease in the neonate. Pediatr Radiol 1976;4:87.

Felson B, Cussen LJ: The hydronephrotic type of congenital multicystic disease of the kidney. Semin Roentgenol 1975;10:113.

Fetterman GH, Ravitch MM, Sherman FE: Cystic changes in fetal kidneys following ureteral ligation: Studies of microdissection. Kidney Int 1974;5:111.

Fill WL, Lamiel JM, Polk NO: The radiographic manifestations of von Hippel-Lindau disease. Radiology 1979;133:289.

Filmer RB, Carone FA, Rowland RG, et al: Adrenal corticosteroid-induced renal cystic disease in the newborn hamster. Am J Pathol 1973;72:461.

Fine MG, Burns E: Unilateral multicystic kidney: Report of six cases and discussion of the literature. J Urol 1959;81:42.

Fisher ER, Horvath B: Comparative ultrasound study of so-called renal adenoma and carcinoma. J Urol 1972;108:382.

Flack CE, Bellinger MF: The multicystic dysplastic kidney and contralateral reflex: Protection of the solitary kidney. J Urol 1993;150:1873.

Forster SV, Hawkins EP: Deficient metanephric blastema—A cause of oligomeganephronia. Pediatr Pathol 1994;14:935.

Fowler M: Differentiated nephroblastoma: Solid, cystic or mixed. J Pathol 1971;105:215.

Friedland GW, deVries PA, Nino-Murcin M, et al: Congenital anomalies of the papillae, calyces, renal pelvis, ureter and ureteral orifice. *In* Pollack HM, ed: Clinical Urography. Philadelphia, W.B. Saunders, 1990, p 653.

Friedman H, Abeshouse BS: Congenital unilateral multicystic kidney: A review of the literature and a report of three cases. Sinai Hosp J (Baltimore) 1957;6:51.

Frydenberg M, Malek R, Zincke H: Conservative renal surgery for renal cell carcinoma in von Hippel-Lindau disease. J Urol 1993;149:461.

Fryns JP, van den Berghe H: "Adult" form of polycystic kidney disease in neonates. Clin Genet 1979;15:205.

Gabow PA: Autosomal dominant polycystic kidney disease. N Engl J Med 1993;329:332.

Gabow PA, Chapman AB, Johnson AM, et al: Renal structure and hypertension in autosomal dominant polycystic kidney disease. Kidney Int 1990;38:1177.

Gabow PA, Duley I, Johnson AM: Clinical profiles of gross hematuria in autosomal polycystic kidney disease. Am J Kidney Dis 1992;20:140.

Gabow PA, Grantham JJ, Bennett WN, et al: Gene testing in autosomal dominant polycystic kidney disease: Results of National Kidney Foundation Workshop. Am J Kidney Dis 1989a;13:85.

Gabow PA, Ikle W, Holmes JH: Polycystic kidney disease: Prospective analysis of non-azotemic patients and family members. Ann Intern Med 1984;101:238.

Gabow PA, Kaehny WD, Johnson AM, et al: The clinical utility of renal concentrating capacity in polycystic kidney disease. Kidney Int 1989b;35:675.

Gabow PA, Schrier RW: Pathophysiology of adult polycystic kidney disease. Adv Nephrol 1989;18:19.

Gaisford W, Bloor K: Congenital polycystic disease of kidney and liver: Portal hypertension, portacaval anastomosis. Proc R Soc Med 1968;61:304.

Gallo GE, Penchansky L: Cystic nephroma. Cancer 1977;39:1322.

Gardner KD, Jr: Composition of fluid in twelve cysts of a polycystic kidney. N Engl J Med 1969;281:985.

Gardner KD, Jr: Juvenile nephronophthisis and renal medullary cystic disease. *In* Gardner KD, Jr, ed: Cystic Disease of the Kidney. New York, John Wiley & Sons, 1976, pp 173–185.

Gardner KD, Jr: Juvenile nephronophthisis–renal medullary cystic disease. Dialogues Pediatr Urol 1984a;7(5):3.

Gardner KD, Jr: Acquired renal cystic disease and renal adenocarcinoma in patients on long-term hemodialysis. N Engl J Med 1984b;310:390.

Gardner KD, Jr: Pathogenesis of human cystic renal disease. Annu Rev Med 1988;39:185.

Gardner KD, Jr: Medullary sponge kidney. *In* Edelman CM, ed: Pediatric Kidney Disease. Boston, Little, Brown, 1992, pp 1641–1646.

Gardner KD, Evan AP: Cystic kidneys: An enigma evolves. Am J Kidney Dis 1984;3:403.

Garel LA, Habib R, Pariente D, et al: Juvenile nephronophthisis: Sonographic appearance in children with severe uremia. Radiology 1984; 151:93.

Gates GF: Ultrasonography of the urinary tract in children. Urol Clin North Am 1980;7:215.

Gedroyc WMW, Saxton HM: More medullary sponge variants. Clin Radiol 1988;39:423.

Gehrig JJ, Gottheiner TI, Swenson RS: Acquired cystic disease of the end-stage kidney. Am J Med 1985;79:609.

Geller RA, Pataki KI, Finegold RA: Bilateral multilocular renal cysts with recurrence. J Urol 1979;121:808.

Glassberg KI: The dilated ureter: Classification and approach. Urology 1977;9:1.

Glassberg KI: Cystic disease of the kidney. Probl Urol 1988;2:157.

Glassberg KI, Filmer RB: Renal dysplasia, renal hypoplasia and cystic disease of the kidney. *In* Kelalis PP, King LR, Belman AB, eds: Clinical Pediatric Urology, 3rd ed: Philadelphia, W.B. Saunders, 1992.

Glassberg KI, Hackett RE, Waterhouse K: Congenital anomalies of the kidney, ureter and bladder. *In* Kendall AR, Karafin L, eds: Harry S. Goldsmith's Practice of Surgery: Urology. Hagerstown, Harper & Row, 1981, p 1.

Glassberg KI, Stephens FD, Lebowitz RL, et al: Renal dysgenesis and cystic disease of the kidney: A report of the Committee on Terminology, Nomenclature and Classification, Section on Urology, American Academy of Pediatrics. J Urol 1987;138:1085.

Goldberg BB, Kotler MM, Ziskin MC, et al: Diagnostic Uses of Ultrasound. New York, Grune & Stratton, 1975.

Goldman SM, Hartman DS: The simple renal cysts. *In* Pollack HM, ed: Clinical Urography. Philadelphia, W.B. Saunders, 1990, p 1603.

Gomez MR: Tuberous Sclerosis. New York, Raven Press, 1979.

Gordon AC, Thomas DFM, Arthur RJ, et al: Multicystic dysplastic kidney: Is nephrectomy still appropriate? J Urol 1988;140:1231.

Gordon RL, Pollack HM, Popky GL, et al: Simple serous cysts of the kidney in children. Radiology 1979;131:357.

Grantham JJ: Polycystic renal disease. *In* Early LE, Gottschalk CW, eds: Strauss and Welt's Disease of the Kidney, 3rd ed: Boston, Little, Brown, 1979, p 1123.

Grantham JJ: Polycystic kidney disease: A predominance of giant nephrons. Am J Physiol 1983;244:F3.

Grantham JJ: Renal pain in polycystic kidney disease: When the hurt won't stop. J Am Soc Nephrol 1992a;2:1161.

Grantham JJ: Polycystic kidney disease: Hereditary and acquired. Adv Intern Med 1993;38:409.

Grantham JJ, Dunoso VS, Evan AP, et al: Viscoelastic properties of tubule basement membranes in experimental renal cystic diseases. Kidney Int 1987;32:187.

Grantham JJ, Geiser JL, Evan AP: Cyst formation and growth in autosomal dominant polycystic kidney disease. Kidney Int 1987;31:1145.

Grantham JJ, Geiser JL, Evan AP: Cyst formation and growth in dominant polycystic kidney disease. Am J Kidney Dis 1991;17:634.

Grantham JJ, Uchic M, Cragoe EJ, Jr, et al: Chemical modification of cell proliferation and fluid secretion in renal cysts. Kidney Int 1989; 35:1379.

Green A, Kinirons M, O'Meara Y, et al: Familial adult medullary cystic disease with spastic quadriparesis: A new disease association. Clin Nephrol 1990;33:231.

Greene LF, Feinzaig W, Dahlin DC: Multicystic dysplasia of the kidney: With special reference to the contralateral kidney. J Urol 1971;105:482.

Griffel B, Pewzner S, Berandt M: Unilateral "oligomeganephronia" with agenesis of the contralateral kidney, studied by microdissection. Virchows Arch [A] 1972;357:179.

Griscom NT, Vawter FG, Fellers FX: Pelvoinfundibular atresia: The usual form of multicystic kidney; 44 unilateral and two bilateral cases. Semin Roentgenol 1975;10:125.

Gross M, Breach PD: The simultaneous occurrence of renal carcinoma and cyst: Problems in management. South Med J 1971;64:1059.

Gruskin AB: Pediatric nephrology for the urologist. *In* Kendall AR, Karafin L, eds: Harry S. Goldsmith's Practice of Surgery: Urology. Hagerstown, Harper & Row, 1977, p 1.

Guay-Woodford LM, Muecher G, Hopkins SD, et al: The severe perinatal form of autosomal recessive polycystic kidney disease maps to chromosome 6p21.1-p12: Implications for genetic counseling. Am J Hum Genet 1995;56:110.

Gutter W, Hermanek P: Maligner Tumor der Nierengegend unter dem Bilde der Knolleniere (nierenblastem Zysten). Urol Int 1957;4:164.

Habib R: Renal dysplasia, hypoplasia and cysts. *In* Strauss J, ed: Pediatric Nephrology: Current Concepts in Diagnosis and Management. New York, Intercontinental Medical Book Corp, 1974, p 209.

Habib R, Bois E: Heterogeneite des syndromes nephrotiques a debut precoce de nourisson (syndrome nephrotique "infantile"): Etude anatomoclinique et genetique de 37 observations. Helv Paediatr Acta 1973;28:91.

Habib R, Courtecuisse V, Ehrensperger J, et al: Hypoplasie segmentaire du rein avec hypertension arterielle chez l'enfant. Ann Pediatr (Paris) 1965;12:262.

Habib R, Courtecuisse V, Mathieu H, et al: Un type anatomo clinique particular, d'insuffisance renale chronique de l'enfant: l'Hypoplasie oligonephronique congenitale bilaterale. J Urol Nephrol (Paris) 1962; 68:139.

Habib R, Gubler M, Niavdet P, Gagnadoux M: Congenital/infantile nephrotic syndrome with diffuse mesangial sclerosis: Relationships with Drash syndrome. *In* Bartsocas CS, ed: Genetics of Kidney Disorders: Progress in Clinical and Biological Research, Vol. 305. New York, Alan R. Liss, 1989, p 193.

Habib R, Loirat C, Gubler MD, et al: The nephropathy associated with male pseudohermaphroditism and Wilson's tumor (Drash syndrome): A distinctive glanular lesion—report of 10 cases. Clin Nephrol 1985;24:269.

Hadlock FP, Deter RL, Carpenter P, et al: Sonography of fetal urinary tract abnormalities. AJR 1981;137:261.

Hakim LS, Adler H, Glassberg KI: Acquired renal cystic disease (ARCD) in the pediatric patient. J Urol 1994;151:330A.

Hamberger J, Richet G, Crosnier J, et al: Nephrology. Philadelphia, W.B. Saunders, 1968, p 1087.

Hanna MK: The multicystic dysplastic kidney (letter to the editor). Urology 1995;45:171.

Harrison AR, Rose GA: Medullary sponge kidney. Urol Res 1979;7:197.

Hartman DS: Cysts and cystic neoplasms. Urol Radiol 1990;12:7.

Hartman GE, Smolik LM, Shochat SJ: The dilemma of the multicystic dysplastic kidney. Am J Dis Child 1986;140:925.

Hartman DS, Weatherby E, III, Laskin WB, et al: Cystic renal cell carcinoma: CT findings simulating a benign hyperdense cyst. AJR 1992; 159:1235.

Hartnett M, Bennett W: External manifestations of cystic renal disease. *In* Gardner KD, Jr, ed: Cystic Disease of the Kidney. New York, John Wiley & Sons, 1976, pp 201–219.

Hashimoto B, Filly R, Cullen P: Multicystic dysplastic kidney in utero: Changing appearance on US. Radiology 1986;159:107.

Heikkinen ES, Herva R, Lanning P: Multicystic kidney: A clinical and histologic study of 13 patients. Ann Chir Gynaecol 1980;69:15.

Henneberry MO, Stephens FD: Renal hypoplasia and dysplasia in infants with posterior urethral valves. J Urol 1980;123:912.

Heptinstall RH: Discussion. *In* Hodson J, Kincaid-Smith P, eds: Reflux Nephropathy. New York, Masson, 1979, p 253.

Herdman RC, Good RA, Vernier RL: Medullary cystic disease in two siblings. Am J Med 1967;43:335.

Hildebrandt F, Singh-Sawhney I, Schnieders B, et al: Mapping of a gene for familial juvenile nephronophthisis: Refining the map and defining flanking markers on chromosome 2. Am J Hum Genet 1993;53:1256.

Hildebrandt O: Weiterer Beitrag zur patologischen Anatomie der Nierengeschwulste. Arch Klin Chir 1894;48:343.

Hinman JAF: Obstructive renal cysts. J Urol 1978;119:681.

Hoard TD, O'Brien DP, III: Simple renal cyst and high renin hypertension cured by cyst decompression. J Urol 1976;115:326.

Hodson CR: Reflux nephropathy: A personal historical review. AJR 1981;137:451.

Holmberg G, Hietala S: Treatment of simple renal cysts by percutaneous puncture and instillation of bismuth-phosphate. Scand J Urol Nephrol 1989;23:207.

Horton WA, Wong V, Eldridge R: Von Hippel-Lindau disease: Clinical and pathological manifestations in nine families with 50 affected members. Arch Intern Med 1976;136:769.

Hossack KF, Leddy CL, Schrier RW, et al: Incidence of cardiac abnormalities associated with autosomal dominant polycystic kidney disease (ADPKD) [Abstract]. Am Soc Nephrol 1986;19:46A.

Hubner W, Pfaf R, Porpaczy P, et al: Renal cysts: Percutaneous resection with standard urologic instruments. J Endourol 1990;4:61.

Hughson MD, Buckwald D, Fox M: Renal neoplasia and acquired cystic kidney disease in patients receiving long term dialysis. Arch Pathol Lab Med 1986;110:592.

Hughson MD, Henniger GR, McManus JF: Atypical cysts, acquired renal cystic disease, and renal cell tumors in end stage dialysis kidneys. Lab Invest 1980;42:475.

Hulbert JC, Hunter D: Percutaneous techniques for intrarenal marsupialization of difficult symptomatic renal cysts. Presented at the 85th Annual Meeting of the American Urological Association. New Orleans, May, 1990.

Hulbert JC, et al: Percutaneous techniques for the management of caliceal diverticula containing calculi. J Urol 1986;135:225.

Huseman R, Grudy A, Welling D, et al: Macropuncture study of polycystic disease in adult human kidneys. Kidney Int 1980;18:375.

Huston J, Torres VE, Wiebers DO: Value of magnetic resonance angiography for detection of intracranial aneurysms in autosomal dominant polycystic kidney disease. J Am Soc Nephrol 1993;3:1871.

Huttunen JR: Congenital nephrotic syndrome of Finnish type: Study of 75 patients. Arch Dis Child 1976;51:344.

Ibrahim RE, Weinberg DS, Weidner N: Atypical cysts and carcinomas of the kidneys in the phacomatoses: A quantitative DNA study using static and flow cytometry. Cancer 1989;63:148.

Ishikawa I: Uremic acquired cystic disease. Urology 1985;26:101.

Ishikawa I: Development of adenocarcinoma and acquired cystic disease of the kidney in hemodialysis patients. *In* Miller RW, et al, eds: Unusual Occurrences as Clues to Cancer Etiology. Tokyo, Japan Scientific Society Press, 1988a, p 77.

Ishikawa I: Adenocarcinoma of the kidney in chronic hemodialysis patients. Int J Artif Organs 1988b;11:61.

Ishikawa I: Letter to the editor. J Urol 1993;149:1146.

Ishikawa I, Onouchi Z, Saito Y, et al: Sex differences in acquired cystic disease of the kidney on long term dialysis. Nephron 1985;39:336.

Ishikawa I, Saito Y, Onouchi Z, et al: Development of acquired cystic disease and adenocarcinoma of the kidney in glomerulonephrotic chronic hemodialysis patients. Clin Nephrol 1980;14:1.

Ishikawa I, Snikura N, Shinoda A: Cystic transformation in native kidneys in renal allograft recipients with long-standing good function. Am J Nephrol 1991;11:217.

Ishikawa I, Yuri T, Kitada H, et al: Regression of acquired cystic disease of the kidney after successful renal transplantation. Am J Nephrol 1983;3:310.

Ivemark BI, Oldefelt P, Zetterstrom B: Familial dysplasia of kidneys, liver and pancreas: A probably genetically determined syndrome. Acta Paediatr 1959;48:1.

Jackman RJ, Stevens JM: Benign hemorrhagic renal cyst: Nephrotomography, renal arteriography and cyst puncture. Radiology 1974;110:7.

Jacobs C, Reach I, Degoulet P: Cancer in patients on hemodialysis. N Engl J Med 1979;300:1279.

Javadpour N, Chelouhy E, Moncada L, et al: Hypertension in a child caused by a multicystic kidney. J Urol 1970;104:918.

Jennings CM, Gaines PA: The abdominal manifestations of von Hippel-Lindau disease and a radiological screening protocol for an affected family. Clin Radiol 1988;39:363.

Johnson DE, Ayala AG, Medellin H, et al: Multilocular renal cystic disease in children. J Urol 1973;109:101.

Johnston JH: The pathogenesis of hydronephrosis in children. Br J Urol 1969;41:724.

Johnston JH, Evans JP, Glassberg KI, et al: Pelvic hydronephrosis in children: A review of 219 personal cases. J Urol 1977;117:97.

Johnston JH, Mix LW: The Ask-Upmark kidney: A form of ascending pyelonephritis? Br J Urol 1976;48:393.

Jordan WP, Jr: Peripelvic cysts of the kidney. J Urol 1962;87:97.

Joshi VV: Cystic partially differentiated nephroblastoma: An entity in the spectrum of infantile renal neoplasia. Perspect Pediatr Pathol 1980;5:217.

Joshi VV, Beckwith JB: Multilocular cyst of the kidney (cystic nephroma) and cystic partially differentiated nephroblastoma. Cancer 1989;64:466.

Jung WH, Peters CA, Mandell JA, et al: Flow cytometric evaluation of multicystic dysplastic kidneys. J Urol 1990;144:413.

Kääriäinen H: Polycystic kidney disease in children: A genetic and epidemiological study of 82 Finnish patients. J Med Genet 1987;24:474.

Kadir S, Kerr WS, Athanasoulis CA: The role of arteriography in the management of renal cell carcinoma associated with von Hippel-Lindau disease. J Urol 1981;126:316.

Kandt RS, Haines JL, Smith M, et al: Linkage of an important gene locus for tuberous sclerosis to a chromosome 16 member for polycystic kidney disease. Nature Genet 1992;2:37.

Kangarloo H, Fine RN: Ultrasonography of cystic renal dysplasia. Int J Pediatr Nephrol 1973;4:205.

Kaplan BS, Gordon I, Pincott J, et al: Familial hypoplastic glomerulocystic kidney disease: A definite entity with dominant inheritance. Am J Med Genet 1989a;34:569.

Kaplan BS, Kaplan P, de Chadarevian JP, et al: Variable expression of autosomal recessive polycystic kidney disease and congenital hepatic fibrosis within a family. Am J Med Genet 1988;29:639.

Kaplan BS, Kaplan P, Rosenberg HK, et al: Polycystic kidney disease in childhood. J Pediatr 1989b;115:867.

Kaplan BS, Rabin I, Nogrady MG, et al: Autosomal dominant polycystic renal disease in children. J Pediatr 1977;90:782.

Kass EJ, Bloom D: Anomalies of the urinary tract. *In* Edelman CM, ed: Pediatric Kidney Disease. Boston, Little, Brown, 1992, pp 2023–2035.

Kaufman J, Fay R: Renal hypertension in childhood. *In* Johnston JH, Goodwin WE, eds: Reviews in Pediatric Urology. Amsterdam, Excerpta Medica, 1974, p 201.

Kaye C, Lewy P: Congenital appearance of adult type (autosomal dominant) polycystic kidney disease. J Pediatr 1974;85:807.

Kelly CJ, Neilson EG: The interstitium of the cystic kidney. *In* Gardner KD, Jr, Bernstein J, eds: The Cystic Kidney. The Netherlands, Kluwer Academic Publishers, 1990, pp 43–53.

Kerr DNS, Warrick CK, Hart-Mercer J: A lesion resembling medullary sponge kidney in patients with congenital hepatic fibrosis. Clin Radiol 1962;13:85.

Khoury Z, Brezis M, Mogle P: Familial medullary sponge kidney in association with congenital absence of teeth (anodontia). Nephron 1988;48:231.

Kishikawa T, Toda T, Ito H, et al: Bilateral congenital multicystic dysplasia of the kidney. Jpn J Surg 1981;11:198.

Kissane JM: Congenital malformations. *In* Heptinstall RH, ed: Pathology of the Kidney, 2nd ed: Boston, Little, Brown, 1974, p 69.

Kissane JM, Smith MG: Pathology of Infancy and Childhood, 2nd ed: St. Louis, C.V. Mosby, 1975, p 587.

Kleiner B, Filly R, Mack L, et al: Multicystic dysplastic kidney: Observations of contralateral disease in the fetal population. Radiology 1986;161:27.

Kleinknecht C, Habib R: Nephronophthisis. *In* Cameron S, Davison AM, Grünfeld JP, et al, eds: Oxford Textbook of Clinical Nephrology. New York, Oxford University Press, 1992, pp 2188–2197.

Kossow AS, Meek JM: Unilateral polycystic kidney disease. J Urol 1982;127:297.

Kuiper JJ: Medullary sponge kidney. Perspect Nephrol Hypertens 1976a; 4:151.

Kuiper JJ: Medullary sponge kidney. *In* Gardner KD, ed: Cystic Diseases of the Kidney. New York, John Wiley & Sons, 1976b, p 151.

Kuntz M: Population studies. *In* Gomez MR, ed: Tuberous Sclerosis, 2nd ed. New York, Raven Press, 1988, p 214.

Kupin W, Norris C, Levin NW, et al: Incidence of diverticular disease in patients with polycystic kidney disease (PCKD). Presented at the 10th International Congress of Nephrology. London, July, 1987.

Kutcher R, Amodio JR, Rosenblatt R: Uremic renal cystic disease: Value of sonographic screening. Radiology 1983;147:833.

Kutcher R, Manadevia P, Nussbaum MK, et al: Renal peripelvic multicystic lymphangiectasia. Urology 1982;30:177.

Lagos JC, Gomez MR: Tuberous sclerosis: Reappraisal of a clinical entity. Mayo Clin Proc 1967;42:26.

Lam M, Halverstadt D, Altshuler G, et al: Congenital oligomeganephronia in a solitary kidney: Report of a case. Am J Kidney Dis 1982;1:300.

Lanning P, Uhari M, Kouvalainan K, et al: Ultrasonic features of the congenital nephrotic syndrome of the Finnish type. Acta Paediatr Scand 1989;78:717.

Latif F, Tory K, Gnarra J, et al: Identification of the von Hippel-Lindau disease tumor suppressor gene. Science 1993;260:317.

Laucks SP, Jr, McLachlan MSF: Aging and simple renal cysts of the kidney. Br J Radiol 1981;54:12.

Lavan JN, Neale FC, Posen S: Urinary calculi: Clinical, biochemical and radiological studies in 619 patients. Med J Aust 1971;2:1049.

Lee JKT, McLennan BL, Kissane JM: Unilateral polycystic kidney disease. AJR 1978;130:1165.

Lenarduzzi G: Repert pielografico poco commune (dilatazione delle vie urinarie intrarenali). Radiol Med 1939;26:346.

Levine E, Collins DL, Horton WA, et al: CT screening of the abdomen in von Hippel-Lindau disease. AJR 1982;139:505.

Levine LA, Gburek BM: Acquired cystic disease and renal adenocarcinoma following renal transplantation. J Urol 1994;151:129.

Levine E, Grantham JJ: Radiology of cystic kidneys. *In* Gardner KD, Jr, Bernstein J, eds: The Cystic Kidney. The Netherlands, Kluwer Academic Publishers, 1990, p 171.

Levine E, Grantham JJ, Slusher SL, et al: CT of acquired cystic disease and renal tumors in long-term dialysis patients. AJR 1984;142:125.

Levine E, Hartmann DS, Smirnidtopoulos JG: Renal cystic disease associated with renal neoplasms. *In* Pollack HM, ed: Clinical Urography. Philadelphia, W. B. Saunders, 1990, pp 1126–1150.

Levine E, Huntrakoon M: Unilateral renal cystic disease. J Comput Assist Tomogr 1989;13:273.

Levine E, Slusher SL, Grantham JJ, et al: Natural history of acquired renal cystic disease in dialysis patients: A prospective longitudinal CT study. AJR 1991;156:501.

Levine E, Weigel JW, Collins DL: Diagnosis and management of asymptomatic renal cell carcinoma in von Hippel-Lindau syndrome. Urology 1983;21:146.

Lieberman E, Salinas-Madrigal L, Gwinn JL, et al: Infantile polycystic disease of the kidneys and liver: Clinical, pathological and radiological correlations and comparison with congenital hepatic fibrosis. Medicine 1971;50:277.

Lingard DA, Lawson TI: Accuracy of ultrasound in predicting the nature of renal masses. J Urol 1979;122:724.

Lirenman DS, Lowry RB, Chase WH: Familial juvenile nephronophthisis: Experience with eleven cases. Birth Defects 1974;10:32.

Livingston WD, Collins TL, Novick DE: Incidental renal masses. Urology 1981;17:257.

Loh JP, Haller JO, Kassner EG, et al: Dominantly inherited polycystic kidneys in infants: Association with hypertrophic pyloric stenosis. Pediatr Radiol 1977;6:27.

Longino LA, Martin LW: Abdominal masses in the newborn infant. Pediatrics 1958;21:596.

Loughlin KR, Gittes RF: Urological management of patients with von Hippel-Lindau disease. J Urol 1986;136:789.

Lundin PM, Olow I: Polycystic kidneys in newborns, infants and children: A clinical and pathological study. Acta Paediatr Scand 1961;50:185.

Lüscher TF, Wanner C, Siegenthaler W, et al: Simple renal cyst and hypertension: Cause or coincidence? Clin Nephrol 1986;26:91.

MacDougall ML, Welling LW, Wiegmann TB: Renal adenocarcinoma and acquired cystic disease in chronic hemodialysis patients. Am J Kidney Dis 1987;9:166.

Mackie GG, Stephens FD: Duplex kidneys: A correlation of renal dysplasia with position of the ureteral orifice. J Urol 1975;114:274.

Madewell JE, Goldman SM, Davis CJ, Jr: Multilocular cystic nephroma: A radiographic pathologic correlation of 58 patients. Radiology 1983; 146:309.

Mahony BS, Filly RA, Callen PW, et al: Fetal renal dysplasia: Sonographic evaluation. Radiology 1984;152:143.

Maizel M, Simpson SB, Jr: Primitive ducts in renal dysplasia induced by culturing ureteral buds denuded of condensed renal mesenchyme. Science 1983;209:509.

Maizel M, Simpson SB, Jr: Ligating the embryonic ureter facilitates the induction of renal dysplasia. Dev Biol, Part B 1986;445.

Marotti M, Hricak H, Fritzche P, et al: Complex and simple cysts: Comparative evaluation with MR imaging. Radiology 1987;162:679.

Maschio G, Tessitore N, D'Angelo A: Medullary sponge kidney and hyperparathyroidism: A puzzling association. Am J Nephrol 1982;2:77.

Matson MA, Cohan EP: Acquired kidney cystic disease: Occurrence, prevalence, and renal cancers. Medicine 1990;69:217.

McClean RH, Goldstein G, Conrad FU, et al: Myocardial infarctions and endocardial fibro-elastosis in children with polycystic kidneys. Bull Johns Hopkins Hosp 1964;115:92.

McClennan BL, Stanley RJ, Melson GL, et al: CT of the renal cyst: Is a cyst puncture necessary? AJR 1979;133:671.

McGonigle RJS, Mowat AP, Benwick M, et al: Congenital hepatic fibrosis and polycystic kidney disease: Role of portacaval shunting and transplantation in three patients. Q J Med 1981;50:269.

McGregor AI, Bailey R: Nephronophthisis-cystic medulla complex: Diagnosis by computerized tomography. Nephron 1989;53:70.

McPherson E, Carey J, Kramer A, et al: Dominantly inherited renal adysplasia. Am J Med Genet 1987;26:863.

McHugh K, Stringer DA, Hebert D, et al: Simple renal cysts in children: Diagnosis and follow-up with US. Radiology 1991;178:383.

Meares EM, Jr, Gross DM: Hypertension owing to unilateral renal hypoplasia. J Urol 1972;108:197.

Mebrizi A, Rosenstein BJ, Pusch A, et al: Myocardial and endocardial fibro-elastosis in children with polycystic kidneys. Bull. Johns Hopkins Hosp. 1964;115:92.

Melicow MM, Uson AC: Palpable abdominal masses in infants and children: A report based on a review of 653 cases. J Urol 1959;81:705.

Melnick SC, Brewer DB, Oldham JS: Cortical microcystic disease of the kidney with dominant inheritance: A previously undescribed syndrome. J Clin Pathol 1984;37:494.

Mery J, Simon P, Horuttle T, et al: A propos de deux observations de maladie polycystique rénale de l'adulte associée au syndrome oral-facial-digital. J Urol (Paris) 1978;84:892.

Meyer WM, Jonas D: Endoscopic percutaneous resection of renal cysts. Presented at the 8th World Congress on Endourology and ESWL. Washington, DC, August-September, 1990.

Mickisch O, Bommer J, Blackman J, et al: Multicystic transformation of kidneys in chronic renal failure. Nephron 1984;38:93.

Miller LR, Soffer O, Nasser VH, et al: Acquired renal cystic disease in end stage renal disease: An autopsy study of 155 cases. Am J Nephrol 1989;9:322.

Mitnick JS, Bosniak MA, Hilton S: Cystic renal disease in tuberous sclerosis. Radiology 1983;147:85.

Mongeau JG, Worthen HG: Nephronophthisis and medullary cystic disease. Am J Med 1967;43:345.

Morgan C, Jr, Rader D: Laparoscopic unroofing of a renal cyst. J Urol 1992;148:1835.

Morita T, Wenzl J, McCoy J, et al: Bilateral renal hypoplasia with oligomeganephronia: Quantitative and electron microscopic study. Am J Clin Pathol 1973;59:104.

Mosli H, MacDonald P, Schillinger J: Caliceal diverticulum developing into simple renal cyst. J Urol 1986;136:658.

Mozziconacci P, Attal C, Boisse J, et al: Hypoplasie segmentaire du rein avec hypertension artéielle. Ann Pediatr 1968;15:337.

Muther RS, Bennett WM: Cyst fluid antibiotic concentration in polycystic kidney disease: Differences between proximal and distal cysts. Kidney Int. 1981;20:519.

Mutinovic J, Fialkow PJ, Agoda LY, et al: Autosomal dominant polycystic kidney disease: Symptoms and clinical findings. Am J Med 1984;53:511.

Myall GF: The incidence of medullary sponge kidney. Clin Radiol 1970;21:171.

Nash DA Jr: Hypertension in polycystic kidney disease without renal failure. Arch Intern Med 1977;137:1571.

Neilson EG, McCafferty E, Mann R, et al: Murine interstitial nephritis III. J Immunol 1985;134:2375.

Neumann HPH, Zerres K, Fischer CL, et al: Late manifestations of autosomal-recessive polycystic kidney disease in two sisters. Am J Nephrol 1988;8:194.

Nicholas JL: An unusual complication of calyceal diverticulum. Br J Urol 1975;47:370.

Noe HN, Marshall JH, Edwards OP: Nodular renal blastema in the multicystic kidney. J Urol 1989;127:486.

Noe HN, Raghavaiah NV: Excision of pyelocalyceal diverticulum under renal hypothermia. J Urol 1982;127:294.

Norio R: Heredity in the congenital nephrotic syndrome: A genetic study of 57 Finnish families with a review of reported cases. Ann Paediatr (Finn.) 1966;12(Suppl. 27):1.

Norio R, Rapola J: Congenital and infantile nephrotic syndromes. *In* Bartsocas CS, ed: Genetics of Kidney Disorders: Progress in Clinical and Biological Research, Vol. 305. New York, Alan R. Liss, 1989, pp 179–192.

Odaka M: Present status of chronic hemodialysis therapy in Japan. Jap Soc Dial Ther 1978;1.

Oddone M, Marino C, Sergi C, et al: Wilms' tumor arising in a multicystic kidney. Pediatric Radiol 1994;24:236.

Okada RD, Platt MA, Fleischman J: Chronic renal failure in patients with tuberous sclerosis: Association with renal cysts. Nephron 1982;30:85.

Olsen A, Hansen Hojhus J, Steffensen G: Renal medullary cystic disease. Acta Radiol 1988;29 (Fasc 5):527.

Osathanondh V, Potter EL: Pathogenesis of polycystic kidneys: Historical survey. Arch Pathol 1964;77:459.

Ostling K: The genes of hydronephrosis. Acta Chir Scand [Suppl] 1942;72.

Palubinskas AJ: Medullary sponge kidney. Radiology 1961;76:911.

Pampigliana G, Moynahan EJ: The tuberous sclerosis syndrome: Clinical and EEG studies in 100 children. J Neurol Neurosurg Psychiatry 1976; 39:666.

Papanicolaou N, Pfister RC, Yoder IC: Spontaneous and traumatic rupture of renal cysts: Diagnosis and outcome. Radiology 1986;160:99.

Paramo PG: Patologia qúistica renal. Acta Assoc Esp Urol 1975;7:1.

Paramo PG, Segura A: Hilioquisosis renal. Rev Clin Esp 1972;126:387.

Parfrey SP, Bear JC, Morgan J, et al: The diagnosis and prognosis of autosomal dominant polycystic kidney disease. N Engl J Med 1990; 323:1085.

Park SH, Chi JGP: Oligomeganephronia associated with 4p deletion type chromosomal anomaly. Pediatr Pathol 1993;13:731.

Parkkulainen KV, Hjeldt L, Sirola K: Congenital multicystic dysplasia of kidney: Report of nineteen cases with discussion on the etiology, nomenclature and classification of cystic dysplasia of the kidney. Acta Chir Scand [Suppl] 1959;244:5.

Parks JH, Coe FL, Strauss AL: Calcium nephrolithiasis and medullary sponge kidney in women. N Engl J Med 1982;306:1088.

Pathak IG, Williams DI: Multicystic and cystic dysplastic kidneys. Br J Urol 1964;36:318.

Patriquin HB, O'Regan S: Medullary sponge kidney in childhood. AJR 1985;145:315.

Penn I: Tumor incidence in renal allograft recipients. Transplant Proc 1979;11:1047.

Perey DYE, Herdman RC, Good RA: Polycystic renal disease: A new experimental model. Science 1967;158:494.

Peters DJM, Spruit L, Saris JJ, et al: Chromosome 4 localization of a second gene for autosomal dominant polycystic kidney disease. Nature Genet 1993;5:359.

Pieke SA, Kimberling WJ, Kenyon KG, et al: Genetic heterogenicity of polycystic kidney disease: An estimate of the proportion of families unlinked to chromosome 16. Am J Hum Genet 1989;45:458.

Plas EG, Hübner WA: Percutaneous resection of renal cysts: A long-term follow-up. J Urol 1993;149:703.

Pollack HM, Banner MP, Arger PH, et al: Comparison of computed tomography and ultrasound in the diagnosis of renal masses. *In* Rosenfeld AT, ed: Genitourinary Ultrasonography. New York, Churchill Livingstone, 1979, p 25.

Porstman W: Renal angiography in children. Prog Pediatr Radiol 1970;3:51.

Port FK, Ragheb NE, Schwartz SH, et al: Neoplasms in dialysis patients: A population-based study. Am J Kidney Dis 1989;14:199.

Poston DO, Jaffes GS, Lubensky IA, et al: Characterization of the renal pathology of a familial form of renal cell carcinoma associated with von Hippel Lindau's disease. J Urol 1993;153:22.

Potter EL: Bilateral absence of ureters and kidneys: A report of 50 cases. Obstet Gynecol 1965;25:3.

Potter EL: Normal and Abnormal Development of the Kidney. Chicago, Year Book Medical Publishers, 1972.

Powell T, Schackman R, Johnson HD: Multilocular cysts of the kidney. Br J Urol 1951;23:142.

Pretorius DH, Lee ME, Manco-Johnson ML, et al: Diagnosis of autosomal dominant polycystic kidney disease in utero and in the young infant. J Ultrasound Med 1987;6:249.

Proesmans W, Van Damme B, Basaer P, et al: Autosomal dominant polycystic kidney disease in the neonatal period: Association with a cerebral arteriovenous malformation. Pediatrics 1982;70:971.

Raboy A, Hakim LS, Ferzli G, et al: Extraperitoneal endoscopic surgery for benign renal cysts. *In* Das S, Crawford EW, eds: Urologic Laparoscopy. Philadelphia, W.B. Saunders, 1994, pp 145–149.

Rackley RR, Angermeier KW, Levin H, et al: Renal cell carcinoma arising in a regressed multicystic dysplastic kidney. J Urol 1994;152:1543.

Raffensberger J, Abouselman A: Abdominal masses in children under one year of age. Surgery 1968;63:514.

Rall JE, Odell HM: Congenital polycystic disease of the kidney: Review of the literature and the data on 207 cases. Am J Med Sci 1949;298, 394.

Ratcliffe PJ, Dunhill MS, Oliver DO: Clinical importance of acquired cystic disease of the kidneys in patients undergoing dialysis. Br Med J 1983;287:1855.

Rauber G, Langlet ML: Hypoplasies segmentaires du rein: Distinction de deux formes histologiques. Nouv Presse Med 1976;5:1759.

Ravden MI, Zuckerman HL, Kay CJ, et al: Evaluation of solitary simple renal cysts in children. J Urol 1980;124:904.

Reeders ST: The genetics of renal cystic disease. *In* Gardner KD, Jr, Bernstein J, eds: The Cystic Kidney. The Netherlands, Kluwer Academic Publishers, 1990, pp 117–146.

Reeders ST, Breuning MH, Comey G, et al: Two genetic markers closely linked to adult polycystic kidney disease on chromosome 16, Br Med J 1986a;292:851.

Reeders ST, Bruening MH, Davies KE, et al: A highly polymorphic DNA marker linked to adult polycystic kidney disease on chromosome 16. Nature 1985;317:542.

Reeders ST, Keeres K, Gal A, et al: Prenatal diagnosis of autosomal dominant polycystic kidney disease with a DNA probe. Lancet 1986b;2:6.

Resnick JS, Brown DM, Vernier RL, Jr: Normal development and experimental models of cystic renal disease. *In* Gardner KD, Jr, ed: Cystic Diseases of the Kidney. New York, John Wiley & Sons, 1976, p 221.

Resnick JS, Hartman DS: Medullary cystic disease of the kidney. *In* Pollack HM, ed: Clinical Urography. Philadelphia, W. B. Saunders, 1990, pp 1178–1184.

Ressequire LJ, Nobrega FT, Farrow GM, et al: Epidemiology of renal and ureteral cancer in Rochester, Minnesota 1950–1978, with special reference to clinical and pathologic features. Mayo Clin Proc 1978;53:503.

Richter S, Karbel G, Bechar L, et al: Should a benign renal cyst be treated? Br J Urol 1983;55:457.

Ritter R, Siafarikas K: Hemihypertrophy in a boy with renal polycystic disease: Varied patterns of presentation of renal polycystic disease in his family. Pediatr Radiol 1976;5:98.

Rizzoni G, Loirat C, Levy M, et al: Familial hypoplastic glomerulocystic kidneys: A new entity? Clin Nephrol 1982;18:263.

Rockson SG, Stone RA, Gunnels JC, Jr: Solitary renal cyst with segmental ischemia and hypertension. J Urol 1974;112:550.

Roos A: Polycystic kidney: Report of a case. Am J Dis Child 1941;61:116.

Rosenfeld AT, Siegel NJ, Kappleman MB: Grey scale ultrasonography in medullary cystic disease of the kidney and congenital hepatic fibrosis with tubular ectasia: New observations. AJR 1977;129:297.

Rosenfeld JB, Cohen L, Garty I, et al: Unilateral renal hypoplasia with hypertension (Ask-Upmark kidney). Br Med J 1973;2:217.

Ross DG, Travers H: Infantile presentation of adult-type polycystic kidney disease in a large kindred. J Pediatr 1975;87:760.

Royer P, Habib R, Broyer M, et al: Segmental hypoplasia of the kidney in children. Adv Nephrol 1971;1:145.

Royer P, Habib R, Mathieu H, et al: L'Hypoplasie renale bilaterale congenitale avec reduction du nombre et hypertrophie des nephrons chez l'enfant. Ann Pediatr (Paris) 1962;38:133.

Rubenstein M, Meyer R, Bernstein J: Congenital abnormalities of the urinary system: I. A postmortem survey of developmental anomalies and acquired congenital lesions in a children's hospital. J Pediatr 1961;58:356.

Rushton GH, Spector M, Rogers AL, et al: Developmental aspects of calcium oxalate tubular deposits and calculi induced in rat kidneys. Invest Urol 1981;19:52.

Ryynanen M, Dolata MM, Lampainen E, et al: Localization of mutation producing autosomal dominant polycystic kidney disease without renal failure. J Med Genet 1987;24:462.

Ryu S: Intracranial hemorrhage in patients with polycystic kidney disease. Stroke 1990;21:291.

Sage MR, Lawson AD, Marshall VR, et al: Medullary sponge kidney and urolithiasis. Clin Radiol 1982;33:435.

Sahney S, Sandler MA, Weiss L, et al: Adult polycystic disease: Presymptomatic diagnosis for genetic counseling. Clin Nephrol 1983;20:89.

Sanders RC: Renal cystic disease. *In* Resnick MI, Sanders RC, eds: Ultrasound in Urology. Baltimore, Williams & Wilkins, 1979, p 97.

Scheff RT, Zuckerman G, Harter H, et al: Diverticular disease in patients with chronic renal failure due to polycystic kidney disease. Ann Intern Med 1980;92:202.

Scheinman JI, Abelson HT: Bilateral renal hypoplasia with oligonephronia. J Pediatr 1970;76:369.

Schwab SJ, Bander SJ, Klahr S: Renal infection in autosomal dominant polycystic kidney disease. Am J Med 1987;82:714.

Schwarz RD, Stephens FD, Cussen LJ: The pathogenesis of renal hypodysplasia: I. Quantification of hypoplasia and dysplasia. Invest Urol 1981a;10:94.

Schwarz RD, Stephens FD, Cussen LJ: The pathogenesis of renal hypodysplasia: II. The significance of lateral and medial ectopy of the ureteric orifice. Invest Urol 1981b;19:97.

Schwarz RD, Stephens FD, Cussen LJ: The pathogenesis of renal hypodysplasia: III. Complete and incomplete urinary obstruction. Invest Urol 1981c;19:101.

Sedman A, Bell P, Manco-Johnson M, et al: Autosomal dominant polycystic kidney disease in childhood: A longitudinal study. Kidney Int 1987; 31:1000.

Sedman A, Gabow PA: Autosomal dominant polycystic kidney disease. Dialogues Pediatr Urol 1984;7:4.

Segal AJ, Spitzer RM: Pseudo thick-walled renal cyst by CT. AJR 1979;132:827.

Shalhoub RJ, Rajan U, Kim VV, et al: Erythrocytosis in patients on long-term hemodialysis. Ann Intern Med 1982;97:686.

Shindo S, Bernstein J, Arant BS, Jr: Evolution of renal segmental atrophy (Ask-Upmark kidney) in children with vesico-ureteral reflux: Radiographic and morphologic studies. J Pediatr 1983;102:847.

Shirai M, Kitagawa T, Nakata H, et al: Renal cell carcinoma originating from dysplastic kidney. Acta Pathol Jpn 1986;36:1263.

Shokeir MHK: Expression of "adult" polycystic renal disease in the fetus and newborn. Clin Genet 1978;14:61.

Siegel MJ, McAlister WH: Simple renal cysts in children. J Urol 1980;123:75.

Smith CH, Graham JB: Congenital medullary cysts of the kidneys with severe refractory anemia. Am J Dis Child 1945;69:369.

Solomon D, Schwartz A: Renal pathology in von Hippel-Lindau disease. Hum Pathol 1988;19:1072.

Sommer JT, Stephens FD: Morphogenesis of nephropathy with partial ureteral obstruction and vesicoureteral reflux. J Urol 1981;125:67.

Spence HM: Congenital unilateral multicystic kidney: An entity to be distinguished from polycystic kidney disease and other cystic disorders. J Urol 1955;74:893.

Spence HM, Singleton R: Cysts and cystic disorders of the kidney: Types, diagnosis, treatment. Urol Surv 1972;22:131.

Spencer JR, Maizel M: Inhibition of protein glycosylation causes renal dysplasia in the chick embryo. J Urol 1987;138:94.

Squiers EC, Morden RS, Bernstein J: Renal multicystic dysplasia: An occasional manifestation of the hereditary renal adysplasia syndrome. Am J Med Genet [Suppl] 1987;3:279.

Stapleton FB, Hilton S, Wilcox J, et al: Transient nephromegaly simulating infantile polycystic disease of the kidneys. Pediatrics 1981;67:554.

Stapleton FB, Johnson D, Kaplan GW, et al: The cystic renal lesion in tuberous sclerosis. J Pediatr 1980;97:574.

Starer F: Partial hydronephrosis due to pressure from normal renal arteries. Br Med J 1968;1:98.

Steele BT, Lirenman DS, Beattie CW: Nephronophthisis. Am J Med 1980;68:531.

Stephens FD: Congenital Malformations of the Urinary Tract. New York, Praeger Publishers, 1983.

Stephens FD, Cussen LG: Renal dysgenesis: A "urologic" classification. *In* Stephens FD, ed: Congenital Malformations of the Urinary Tract. New York, Praeger Publishing, 1983, pp 463–475.

Stickler GB, Kelalis PP: Polycystic kidney disease: A recognition of the "adult" form (autosomal dominant) in infancy. Mayo Clin Proc 1975;50:547.

Stillaert J, Baert A, Van Damme B, et al: A propos du rein polykystique. *In* Kuss R, Legrain M, eds: Seminaries d'Uronephrologie in Pitiere-Salpetriere, 1975. Paris, Masson et Cie, 1975, p 159.

Stillwell TJ, Gomez MR, Kelalis PP: Renal lesions in tuberous sclerosis. J Urol 1987;138:477.

Tada S, Yamagishi J, Kobayashi H, et al: The incidence of simple renal cyst by computed tomography. Clin Radiol 1983;150:207.

Taitz LS, Brown CB, Blank CE, et al: Screening for polycystic kidney disease: Importance of clinical presentation in the newborn. Arch Dis Child 1987;62:45.

Tanagho EA: Surgically induced partial urinary obstruction in the fetal lamb: III. Ureteral obstruction. Invest Urol 1972;10:35.

Taxy JB, Filmer RB: Metaplastic cartilage in nondysplastic kidneys. Arch Pathol 1975;99:101.

Taxy JB, Filmer RB: Glomerulo-cystic kidney. Arch Pathol Lab Med 1976;100:186.

Templeton AW, Thompson IM: Aortographic differentiation of congenital and acquired small kidneys. Arch Surg 1968;97:114.

Thompson BJ, Jenkins DAS, Allan PL, et al: Acquired cystic disease of the kidney: An indication for transplantation? Br Med J 1986;293:209.

Thomsen HS, Thaysen JH: Frequency of hepatic cysts in adult polycystic kidney disease. Acta Med Scand 1988;224:381.

Timmons JW, Jr, Malek RS, Hattery RR, et al: Calyceal diverticulum. J Urol 1975;114:6.

Uson AC, Melicow MM: Multilocular cysts of the kidney with intrapelvic herniation of a "daughter" cyst: Report of 4 cases. J Urol 1963;89:341.

Vagelli G, Ferraris V, Calbrese G, et al: Medullary sponge kidney and calcium nephrolithiasis [Abstract]. Urol Res 1988;16:201.

Valderrama E, Berkman JI: The Ask-Upmark kidney in a premature infant. Clin Nephrol 1979;11:313.

Van Acker KJ, Vincke H, Quatacker J, et al: Congenital oligonephronic renal hypoplasia with hypertrophy of nephrons (oligonephronia). Arch Dis Child 1971;46:321.

Vela-Navarrete R, Garcia de la Péna E, Alverez Villalobos C, et al: Quistes nonefrogénicos del seno renal: Expreividad radiográphica y consideraciones diagnóticas. Rev Clin Esp 1974;132:29.

Vela-Navarrete R, Robledo AG: Polycystic disease of the renal sinus: Structural characteristics. J Urol 1983;129:700.

Wahlqvist L, Grumstedt B: Therapeutic effect of percutaneous puncture of simple renal cyst: Follow-up investigation of 50 patients. Acta Chir Scand 1966;132:340.

Wakabayashi T, Fujita S, Onbora Y, et al: Polycystic kidney disease and intracranial aneurysms: Early angiographic diagnosis and early operation for the unruptured aneurysm. J Neurosurg 1983;58:488.

Walker FC, Loney LC, Rout ER, et al: Diagnostic evaluation of adult polycystic disease in childhood. AJR 1984;142:1273.

Walker RD, Fennell R, Garin E, et al: Spectrum of multicystic renal dysplasia: Diagnosis and management. Urology 1978;11:433.

Weinreb JC, Arger PH, Coleman BG, et al: Cystic renal mass evaluation: Real-time versus static imaging. J Clin Ultrasound 1986;14:29.

Westberg G, Zachrisson L: Proceedings of the Swedish Society of Medical Radiology 1975;4.

Wikstrom B, Backman U, Danielson BG: Ambulatory diagnostic evaluation of 38 recurrent renal stone formers: A proposal for clinical classification and investigation. Klin Wochenschr 1983;61:85.

Williams DI: Urology in Childhood. New York, Springer-Verlag, 1974, p 79.

Williams G, Blandy JP, Tressider GC: Communicating cysts and diverticula of the renal pelvis. Br J Urol 1969;41:163.

Wolf B, Rosenfield AT, Taylor KJW, et al: Presymptomatic diagnosis of adult onset polycystic kidney disease by ultrasonography. Clin Genet 1978;14:1.

Wood BP, Muurahainen N, Anderson VM, et al: Multicystic nephroblastoma: Ultrasound diagnosis (with a pathologic-anatomic commentary). Pediatr Radiol 1982;12:43.

Yendt ER: Medullary sponge kidney. *In* Gardner KD, Jr, Bernstein J, eds: The Cystic Kidney. The Netherlands, Kluwer Academic Publishers, 1990, p 379.

Zeier M, Geberth S, Ritz E, et al: Adult dominant polycystic kidney disease: Clinical problems. Nephron 1988;49:177.

Zerres K, Hansmann M, Mallman R, et al: Autosomal recessive polycystic kidney disease: Problems of prenatal diagnosis. Prenat Diagn 1988;8:215.

60
ANOMALIES OF THE URETER

Richard N. Schlussel, M.D.
Alan B. Retik, M.D.

TERMINOLOGY

Ureteral anomalies are some of the most significant anomalies in all of pediatric urology because they directly affect overall renal function. These congenital problems may present acutely or insidiously. Similarly, if they are incorrectly treated, the adverse outcome may not be appreciated for years. Appropriate management is predicated on knowledge of the relevant embryology, anatomy, and physiology, as well as all the variants thereof. Finally, the urologist entrusted with the care of these children must be familiar with the many reconstructive techniques available so that an optimal outcome can be achieved.

The study of ureteral anomalies has yielded a rich array of terms and descriptions. Many of these terms and categories have been put forth by some of the founders of pediatric urology. Because all of medicine is predicated on effective communication, we summarize classifications used in the past, define current common usages, and propose a standard rational nomenclature that, it is hoped, will allow for accurate communication.

Because ureteral anomalies are at times associated with duplications of the kidney, it is prudent to review renal terminology. A duplex kidney is one that has two separate pelvicalyceal systems. A duplex kidney has an upper pole and a lower pole. These ureters may join at any point. If they join at the level of the ureteropelvic junction, the configuration is termed a bifid system. If the ureters join more distally but are still proximal to the bladder level, the configuration is termed bifid ureters (Fig. 60–1*A*). Double ureters are ureters that drain their respective poles and empty separately into the genitourinary tract. This represents a complete duplication (Fig. 60–1*B*). A ureter that drains the upper or lower pole should be referred to as the upper pole ureter or the lower pole ureter, respectively.

Ectopia is derived from the Greek ex (out) and topos (place); therefore, any ureter whose orifice terminates anywhere other than the normal trigonal position is considered ectopic. Lateral ectopia implies an orifice more cranial and lateral than normal. Caudal ectopia implies that the orifice is more medial and distal than the normal position. Such an orifice may theoretically be found between the normal orifice position and the bladder neck. However, in general practice, an ectopic ureter is meant to imply a ureter whose orifice terminates even more caudally, such as in the urethra or outside of the urinary tract.

Ericsson characterized ureteroceles as either simple or ectopic. A simple ureterocele was defined as one that lies completely within the bladder, whereas those that extended to the bladder neck or distally to the urethra were considered to be ectopic (Ericsson, 1954). Stephens (1958, 1964, 1971,

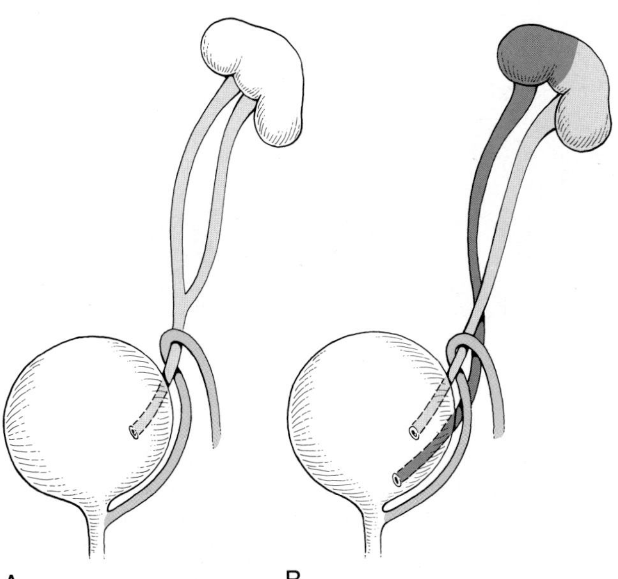

Figure 60–1. *A,* A bifid ureter is depicted as the upper pole and lower pole ureters join proximal to the bladder. *B,* Double ureters are seen as the upper pole ureter and lower pole ureter empty separately into the bladder.

1983) described ureteroceles as either stenotic, sphincteric, or sphincterostenotic, or as a cecoureterocele. A stenotic ureterocele is one whose narrowed or pinpoint opening is found inside the bladder (Fig. 60–2). If a ureterocele had an orifice distal to the bladder neck, it was termed sphincteric (Fig. 60–3). If a ureterocele had an orifice that was both stenotic and distal to the bladder neck, it was considered a sphincterostenotic ureterocele (Fig. 60–4*A*). A cecoureterocele has an intravesical orifice and a submucosal extension that dips into the urethra. This type of ureterocele can distend with urine and obstruct the urethra (Fig. 60–4*B*).

Several terms for ureteroceles in common usage are confusing. They are listed not to encourage their use but to clarify their intended meaning. A simple ureterocele is frequently used to mean a single-system ureterocele. The adult ureterocele has the same implication. An orthotopic ureterocele is a term used for a ureterocele contained within the bladder. Often, the phrase ectopic ureterocele is used to explain a ureterocele associated with a duplicated system.

Obviously, these terms are not completely clear because they are nondescriptive and sometimes inaccurate. In an effort to eliminate this ambiguity and confusion, the Committee on Terminology, Nomenclature and Classification of the Section of Urology of the American Academy of Pediatrics proposed standardized terms that are both descriptive and accurate (Glassberg et al, 1984). According to this classification, a ureterocele is intravesical if the ureterocele is contained in the bladder in its entirety, and it is ectopic if any portion of the ureterocele extends to the bladder neck or the urethra (Fig. 60–5). Ureteroceles are classified further according to the number of systems (single or duplex) and the type of orifice involved (e.g., stenotic, sphincteric, or sphincterostenotic, or as a cecoureterocele). Therefore, by way of example, the ureterocele seen in Figure 60–6 would be categorized as an intravesical ureterocele of a left single system with a stenotic orifice, and the ureterocele shown in Figure 60–4*A* would be categorized as an ectopic ureterocele of a duplicated left system. Such classifications lead to little doubt, and their use should be encouraged.

EMBRYOLOGY

An understanding of normal renal development is critical to an appreciation of how ureteral anomalies evolve and if they are clinically significant. At 4 weeks' gestation, an outpouching arises from the distal mesonephric duct. This outpouching is the ureteric bud, and it interacts with a mass of mesenchyme that is the metanephric blastema. This interaction results in the ureteric bud's branching and developing into the calyces, renal pelvis, and ureter. The meta-

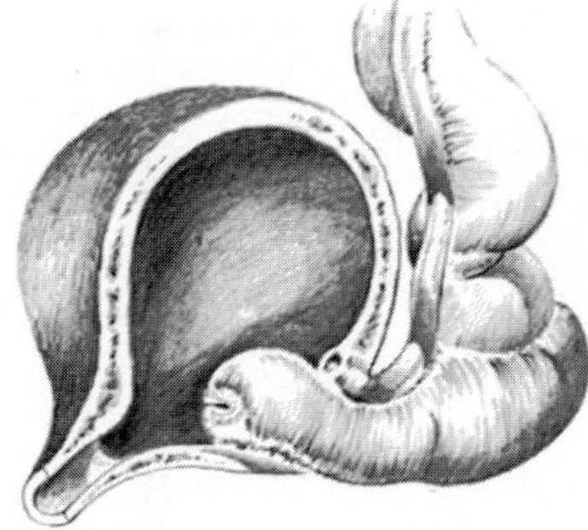

Figure 60–2. Stenotic ectopic ureteroceles—orifice may be located at the tip or at the superior or inferior surface of the ureterocele.

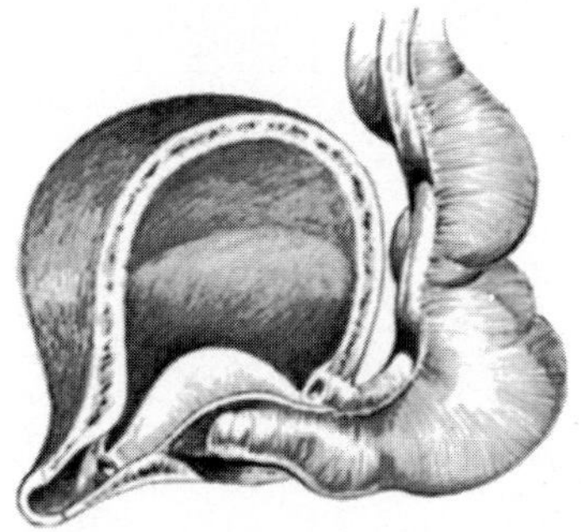

Figure 60–3. Sphincteric ectopic ureteroceles.

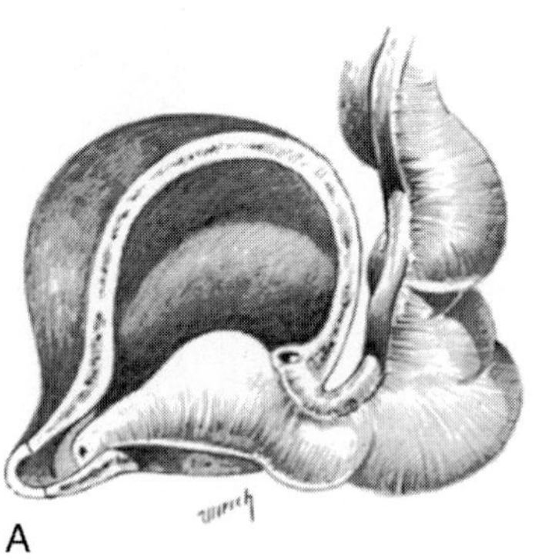

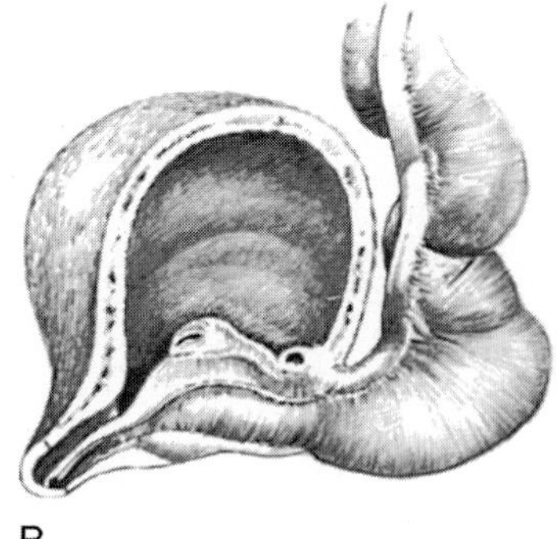

Figure 60–4. *A,* Sphincterostenotic ectopic ureterocele. *B,* Cecoureterocele—lumen extends distal to the orifice as a long tongue beneath the ureteral submucosa. The orifice communicates with the lumen of the bladder and is large and incompetent.

nephric blastema is induced to form all elements of the nephron, including the collecting duct, distal convoluted tube, loop of Henle, proximal convoluted tubule, and glomerulus. The segment of mesonephric duct distal to the ureteric bud is the common excretory duct (Fig. 60–7). This duct eventually is absorbed into the developing bladder and becomes part of the trigone. The point of origin of the ureteric bud is the ureteral orifice. When the common excretory duct is absorbed into the bladder, the ureteral orifice begins to migrate in the bladder in a cranial and lateral direction (Langman, 1975; Moore, 1977) (Fig. 60–8).

If the ureteric bud arose off the mesonephric duct more distally than normally, the ureteral orifice would enter the bladder earlier than usual and hence have a greater period for cranial and lateral migration (Mackie and Stephens, 1975b; Tanagho, 1976; Schwartz et al, 1981). This would result in lateral ectopia. If the ureteric bud arose more proximally on the mesonephric duct than normally, the result would be a ureteral orifice that would have less time in the bladder to undergo its normal migration and hence would result in a ureteral orifice more medial and caudal than is usual (Fig. 60–9). An even further proximal ureteric bud position on the mesonephric duct may result in the ureteral orifice's remaining on the mesonephric duct, with the end result being that the orifice would terminate outside the bladder altogether. In the male, the embryologic equivalents of the mesonephric duct are the epididymis, vas deferens, seminal vesicles, and prostate. In the female, the mesonephric duct proximal to the ureteric bud becomes the epoöphoron, oophoron, and Gartner's duct. An ectopic ureter draining into any of these female structures can rupture into the adjoining fallopian tube, uterus, upper vagina, or vestibule.

The interaction of the ureteric bud with the metanephric blastema is critical to the correct ontogeny of the ureter and collecting system and the future kidney. Examination of the developing kidney reveals close cell-to-cell interactions between the ureteric bud and the metanephric blastema (Saxen, 1987). Experimental models have shown that if these interactions are altered or disrupted, they will result in failure of the blastema to differentiate into normal nephrons (Grobstein, 1956; Kirrilova et al, 1982; Sariola et al, 1988).

In clinical practice, it appears that renal units drained by ureters that terminate in positions other than the trigone do, in fact, have problems with proper development. Recalling the embryology of the trigone and ureteral orifice, it is likely that an abnormal ureteral orifice position reflects an abnormal point of origin of the ureteric bud from the mesonephric duct. This ureteric bud would then be poorly positioned for the necessary interactions with the metanephric blastema. Therefore, these clinical and experimental observa-

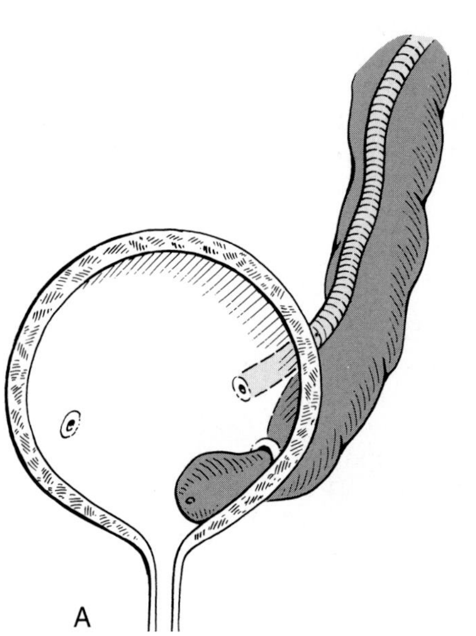

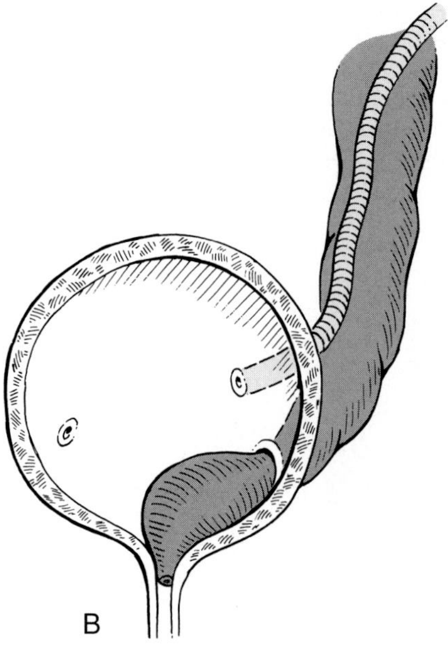

Figure 60–5. *A,* An intravesical ureterocele located entirely within the bladder. *B,* The distal portion of an ectopic ureterocele extends outside the bladder and into the urethra.

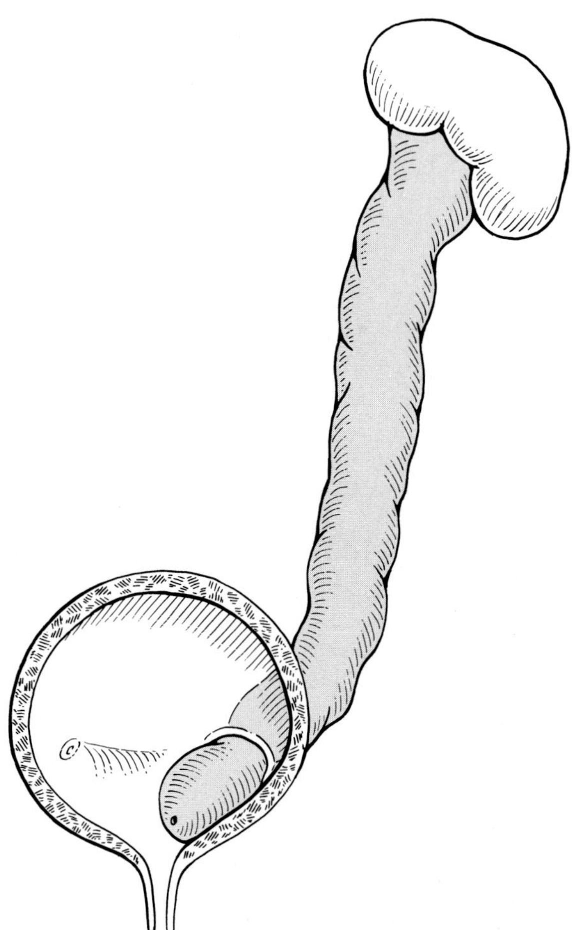

Figure 60–6. A single-system intravesical ureterocele.

tions combine to support the commonly held notion that dysplasia is the product of inadequate ureteric bud-to-blastema interaction (Mackie and Stephens, 1975b).

Following its emergence from the mesonephric duct, the ureteric bud can become a split or bifid structure. The splitting creates two separate collecting systems that join in an eventual common ureter (Fig. 60–10). As mentioned previously, this anatomic arrangement is termed a duplex kidney with a bifid ureter. The ureter distal to the bifurcation has arisen from a normal position on the mesonephric duct, and hence, its single ureteral orifice is in the normal trigonal location.

If two separate ureteric buds originate from the mesonephric duct, two complete and separate interactions will develop between the ureter and the metanephric blastema. The result is two separate renal units and collecting systems, ureters, and ureteral orifices. Using our prior terminology, this complete duplication is synonymous with the duplex systems drained by double ureters (Fig. 60–11). The final position of the ureteral orifices has important clinical implications. Both Weigert (1877) and Meyer (1946) noted that there is a constant trigonal relationship between the upper and lower pole orifices. When performing a cystoscopic examination, it is important to remember this counterintuitive concept, that is, the so-called lower or distally placed orifice is in fact the orifice of the upper pole and the so-called higher or

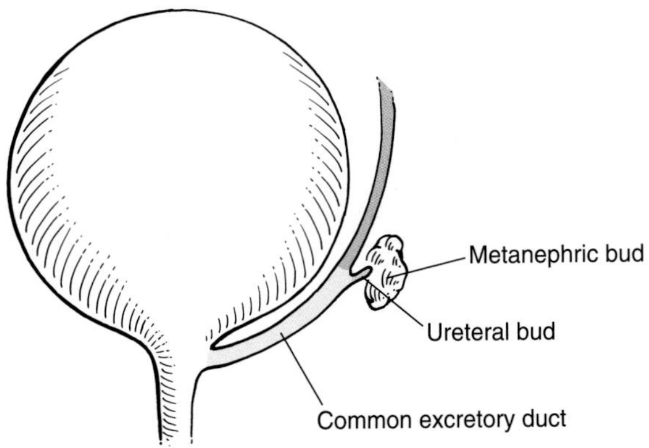

Figure 60–7. The structures of the urinary tract originate from the primitive metanephric blastema and the ureteral bud, which arises from the mesonephric duct. The common excretory duct is the portion of the mesonephric duct distal to the ureteral bud.

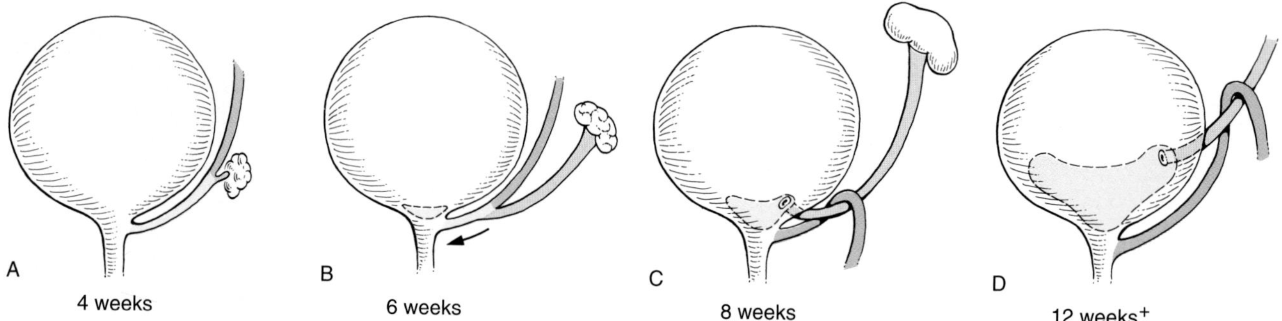

Figure 60–8. The ureteral bud further develops into the ureter and induces the metanephric blastema to differentiate and become the kidney. The common excretory duct is progressively absorbed into the bladder and becomes the trigone. The mesonephric duct will become the vas deferens in the male.

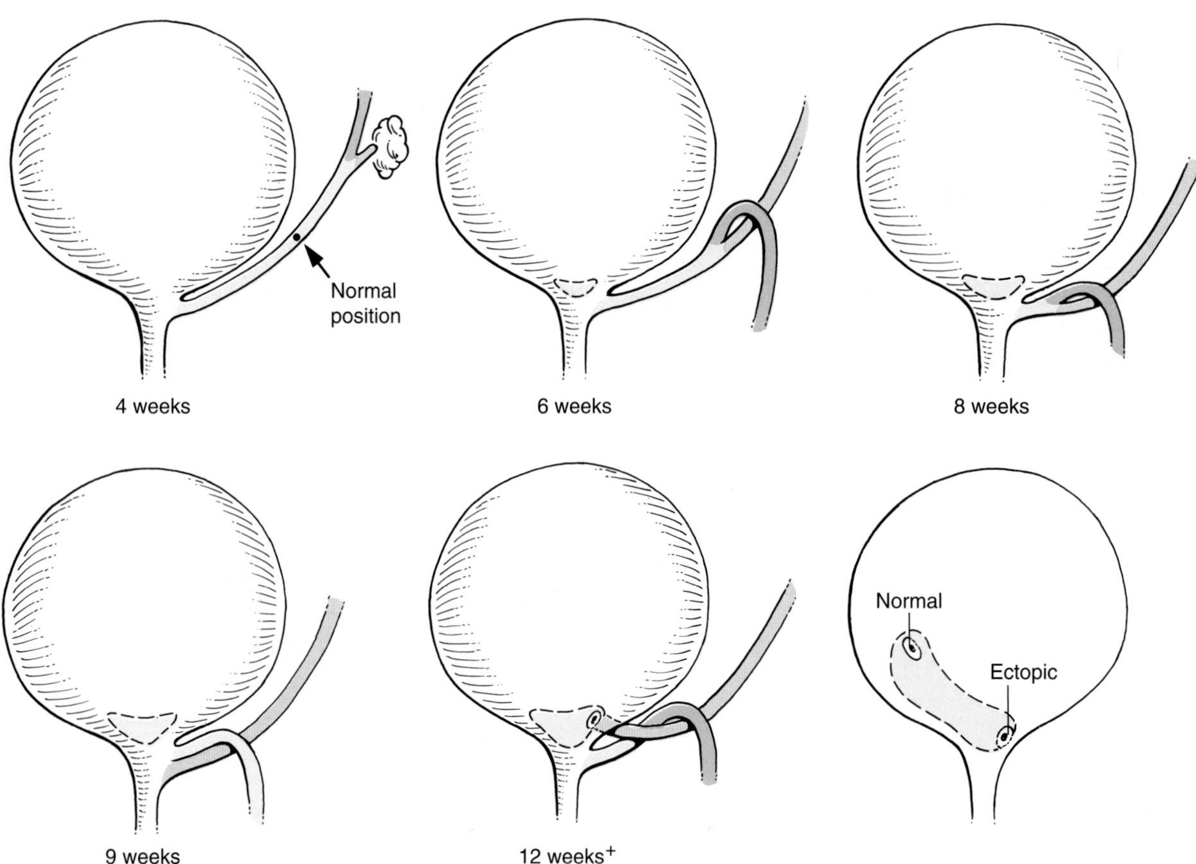

Figure 60–9. Caudal ectopia occurs because of a high origination of the ureteral bud. The ureteral orifice will have less time to be absorbed into the bladder and will have a caudal, medial trigone location or be extravesically located along the path of the mesonephric duct remnants.

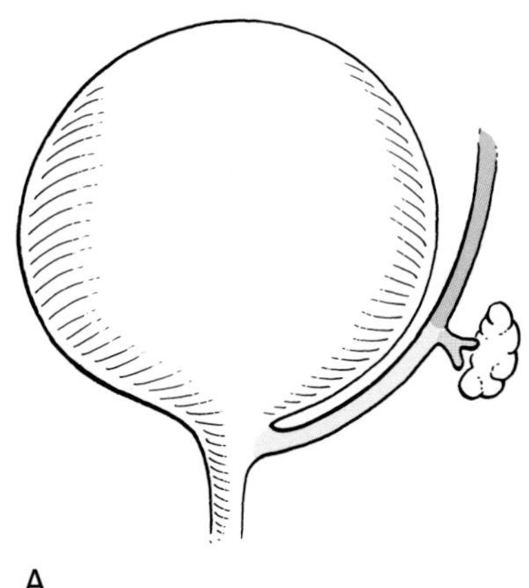

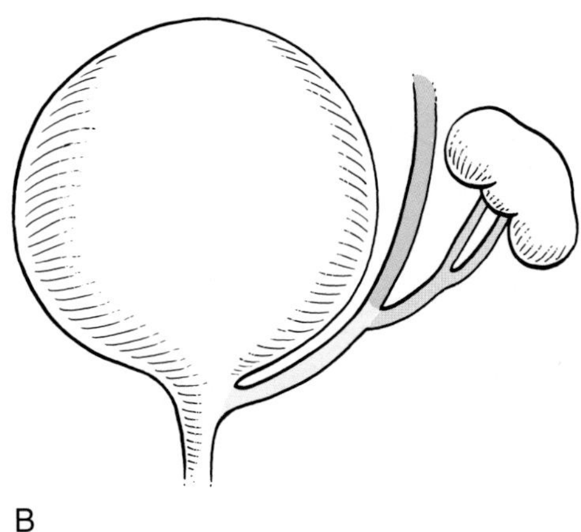

Figure 60–10. Ureteral bud (gray) branching after it arises from the mesonephric duct (red) will create a bifid ureter.

cranial orifice is the lower pole orifice. The lower pole orifice is more cranial and lateral to the caudad medial upper pole orifice. To achieve these positions, the two ureters and orifices rotate 180 degrees clockwise on their longitudinal axes (Fig. 60–12). The Weigert-Meyer rule of complete duplicated systems yields a fairly constant anatomy that is important for radiologic, cystoscopic, and reconstructive considerations.

One could consider any and all congenital anomalies of the ureter to fall into one of the categories in which we have organized this chapter: anomalies of termination, anomalies of structure, anomalies of number, and anomalies of position.

ANOMALIES OF TERMINATION

Lateral Ectopia

Primary reflux is defined as reflux that occurs in the absence of predisposing associated conditions, such as myelomeningocele, detrusor-sphincter-dyssynergia, posterior urethral valves, or ureteroceles. This reflux is due in large part to the abnormal development noted previously that results in lateral ectopia (Cussen, 1979).

The laterally placed ureteral orifice is a result of the ureteric bud's originating from a more caudal point on the mesonephric duct than is usual. As the portion of the mesonephric duct that is distal to the ureteric bud (the common excretory duct) begins to be absorbed into the bladder, it brings the ureteric bud with it. The ureteral orifice begins its cranial and lateral migration on entering the bladder. If the orifice has a prolonged period to undergo such migration (such as when the ureteric bud originates closer to the bladder), the orifice will ultimately reside more cranially and laterally than is normal. Eventually, we find a ureter whose submucosal course is short and nearly perpendicular to the bladder wall as opposed to the normally long and oblique submucosal course (Ambrose and Nicolson, 1962; Stephens and Lenaghan, 1962). A decreased, shorter submucosal course prevents the normal operation of the so-called flap-valve mechanism, and vesicoureteral reflux ensues (Fig. 60–13). The degree of reflux correlates with the degree of laterality and inversely with the length of the submucosal ureter.

Another factor in primary reflux is the frequently found abnormality of a poorly developed trigone. As previously stated, in primary reflux, the ureteric bud arises from the mesonephric duct more caudally than normally, resulting in a short common excretory duct. Because the common excretory duct was shortened, its mesenchymal contribution to the muscular development of the trigone is decreased. Thus the trigone is not only large but also poorly muscularized. Because there has been less time for the common mesenchyme to accumulate around the developing ureteric bud, the intramural ureter will also be deficient in musculature. The normal arrangement has been compared to a hammer

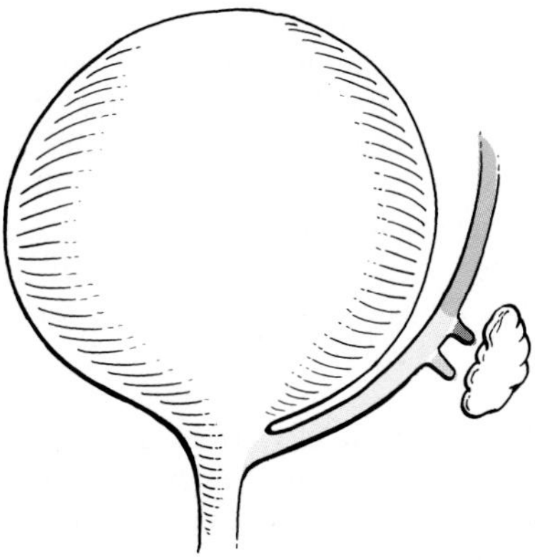

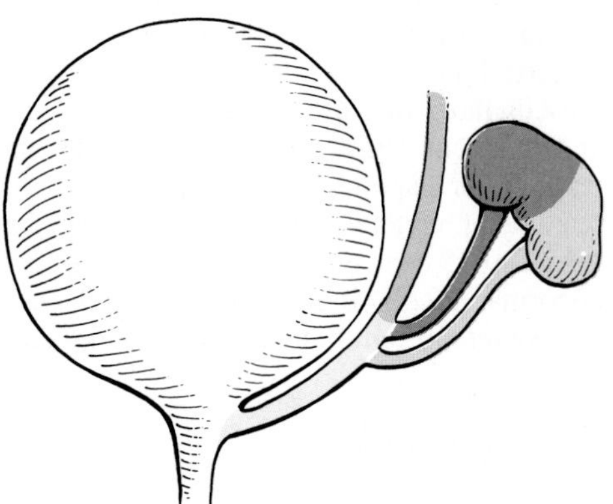

Figure 60–11. Two separate ureteral buds coming off the mesonephric duct will develop into an upper pole and its ureter (black) and a lower pole and its ureter (gray), each having distinct ureteral orifices in the bladder.

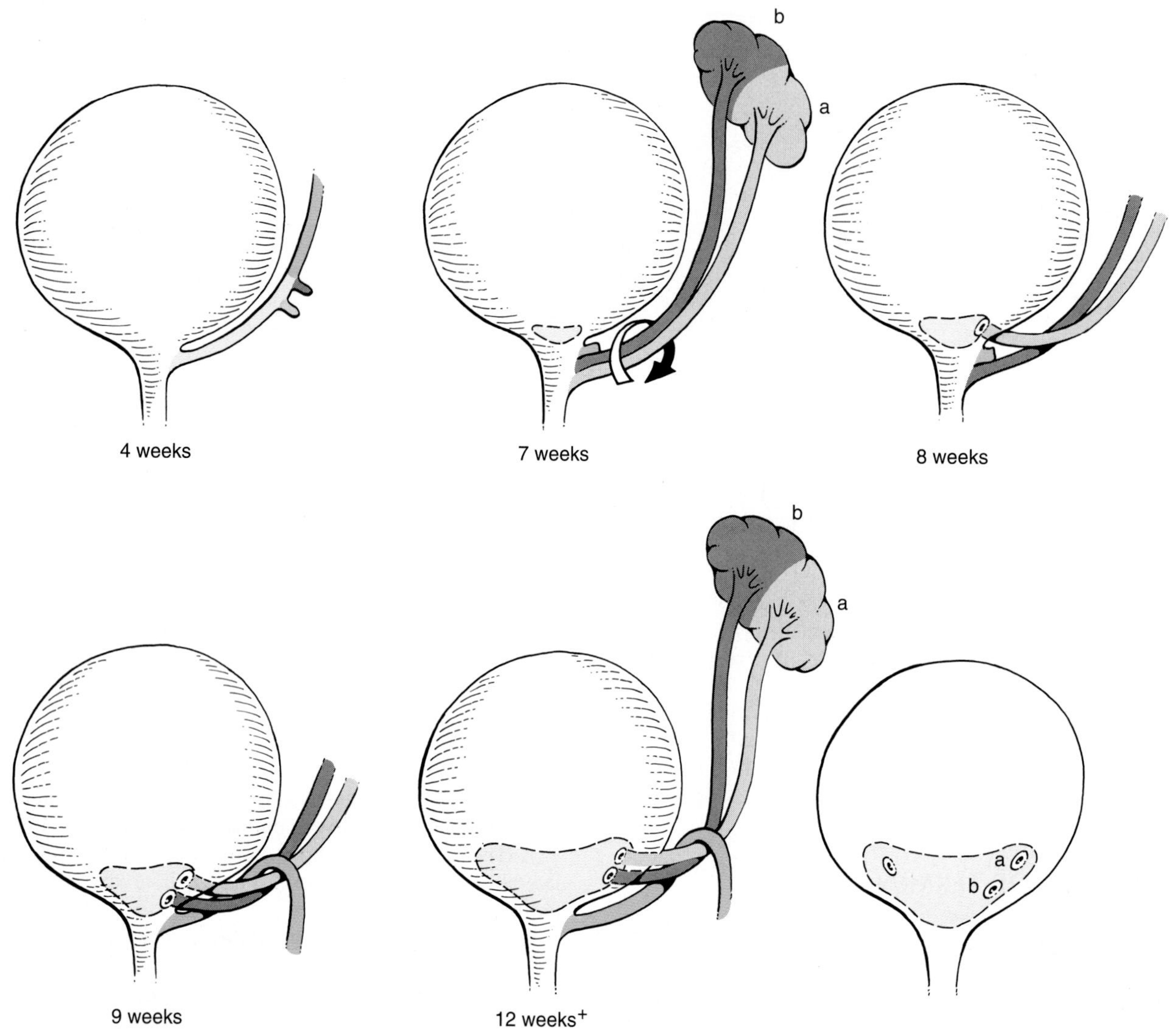

Figure 60–12. The Weigert-Meyer rule is depicted, with the upper pole ureter (black) and the lower pole ureter (gray) rotating on their long axes to yield an upper pole orifice (b) that is medial and caudal to the lower pole orifice (a).

and anvil, with the intravesical urine being the hammer compressing the ureter against the bladder wall musculature, which is the anvil. This altered development also affects the flap valve mechanism by denying the ureter sufficient muscular backing against which it can be compressed.

In addition, because there has been less time for the common mesenchyme to accumulate around the developing ureteric bud, the intramural ureter will also be deficient in musculature. Because of the altered trigonal development and the poor attachments of the ureter, the orifice can be patulous or gaping. It is owing to the combined effects of the lateral ureteral orifice position, the ureter's shortened submucosal course, the poorly developed trigone, and the abnormal morphology of the ureteral orifice that primary vesicoureteral reflux develops (Tanagho et al, 1965).

Ectopic Ureters

As mentioned previously, in the strictest sense, a ureter whose orifice is laterally and cranially located in the bladder could be considered ectopic. However, the term ectopic ureter has universally been used to describe a ureter that terminates at the bladder neck or distally into one of the aforementioned mesonephric duct structures. We employ this general terminology in the following discussion.

The true incidence of an ectopic ureter is uncertain, because many cause no symptoms. Campbell (1970) noted ten examples in 19,046 autopsies in children (one in 1900) but thought that some had been overlooked. Of all ectopic orifices, 80% are associated with a duplicated collecting system. In females, more than 80% are duplicated, whereas in males, the majority of ectopic ureters drain single systems (Schulman, 1976; Ahmed and Barker, 1992). This is particularly true when ectopic ureteroceles are excluded from consideration.

Ectopic ureters appear more commonly in females—clinically, from 2 to 12 times more frequently—with the lesser frequency probably reflecting the incidence more accurately (Eisendrath, 1938; Mills, 1939; Burford et al, 1949; Lowsley and Kerwin, 1956). Ellerker (1958) noted 366 females and 128 males in his review of 494 ectopic ureters,

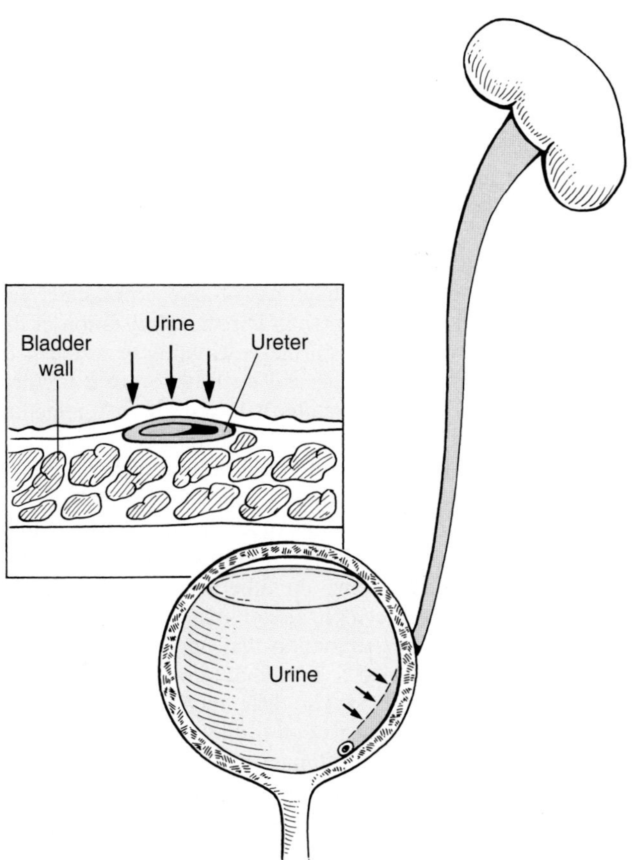

Figure 60–13. Bladder dynamics schematically depict the urine compressing the ureter between the bladder mucosa and the bladder wall muscle, which creates the flap-valve mechanism that prevents reflux.

including autopsies, for a female-to-male ratio of 2.9:1. Between 7.5% and 17% of ectopic ureters appear bilaterally (Eisendrath, 1938; Ellerker, 1958; Ahmed and Barker, 1992). A small percentage involve a solitary kidney. With unilateral ectopic ureter, a contralateral ureteral duplication is not uncommon. Various other abnormalities, including imperforate anus and tracheoesophageal fistula, may be found in association with the ectopic ureter (Ahmed and Barker, 1992).

The distribution of ectopic ureters is itemized by location in Table 60–1. In the male, the posterior urethra is the most common site of the termination of the ectopic ureter. Drainage into the genital tract involves the seminal vesicle three times more often than the ejaculatory duct and vas deferens combined (Riba et al, 1946; Ellerker, 1958; Lucius, 1963; Sullivan et al, 1978; Squadrito et al, 1987). In the female, the urethra and vestibule are the most common sites. The age at diagnosis ranges widely, with many examples not detected during life (Ellerker, 1958).

The earlier reports failed to provide adequate descriptions of the upper tracts, but later reports emphasize that the more remote the ureteral opening, the greater the degree of renal maldevelopment (Schulman, 1976). With duplicated systems, this means hypoplasia or dysplasia of the upper pole segment. In ten cases of ectopic ureter that drained a single system and opened into the male seminal tracts, the kidney was not visualized radiographically in all (Rognon et al, 1973). Of 16 single renal ducts drained by an ectopic ureter, renal dysplasia was present in seven (Prewitt and Lebowitz, 1976). The anomalous single kidney may be ectopic as well. The ectopic ureter itself is also abnormal, usually to a greater degree in the single system than in the duplicated system. Usually, the ureter is variably dilated and drainage is impaired (Williams and Royle, 1969). Muscle cells may show severe alterations on ultrastructure studies. Whether these changes are developmental or acquired is not yet known (Hanna et al, 1977).

Clinical presentation of an ectopic ureter usually differs in males and females. This reflects the differing termination of the ectopic ureters in the two genders. Recalling the embryology of ureteral ectopia, when the ureteric bud arises more proximally on the mesonephric duct than it normally should, the ureteral orifice will remain on the mesonephric duct caudally and will not be absorbed in the bladder. In the female, these parts of the mesonephric duct will become the epoöphoron, oophoron, and Gartner's duct. If an ectopic ureter drains into any of these respective female structures, they can rupture or be incorporated into any of the nearby müllerian duct structures, such as the vagina, uterus, cervix, or fallopian tubes (Fig. 60–14). Therefore, in the female, an ectopic ureteral orifice may be within (e.g., the bladder neck or proximal urethra) or outside the realm of the urinary sphincter, making ectopic ureters one of the more important causes of urinary incontinence in girls (Freedman and Rickwood, 1994). Continuous incontinence in a girl with an otherwise normal voiding pattern after toilet training is the classic symptom of an ectopic ureteral orifice.

On occasion, incontinence becomes apparent at a later age and may be confused with stress incontinence, incontinence associated with neurogenic bladder dysfunction, or psychogenic incontinence. A persistent vaginal discharge from an ectopic orifice located in the vagina is another clinical sign (Acien et al, 1990; See and Mayo, 1991; Gharagozloo and Lebowitz, 1995). Most ectopic ureters are associated with acute or recurrent urinary tract infection. A patient may also present with failure to thrive and chronic infection. Ectopic ureters draining into the proximal urethra often experience reflux, and urge incontinence is common. An ectopic ureter may be severely obstructed, causing massive hydronephrosis and hydroureter, and it may present as an abdominal mass (Uson et al, 1972) or be detected on prenatal ultrasonographic evaluation.

Table 60–1. LOCATION OF 494 ECTOPIC URETERS (INCLUDING AUTOPSIES)

	Number	Percent
128 Males		
Posterior urethra	60	47
Prostatic utricle	13	10
Seminal vesicle	42	33
Ejaculatory duct	7	5
Vas deferens	6	5
366 Females		
Urethra	129	35
Vestibule	124	34
Vagina	90	25
Cervix or uterus	18	5
Gartner's duct	3	<1
Urethral diverticulum	2	<1

From Ellerker AG: Br J Surg 1958; 45:344.

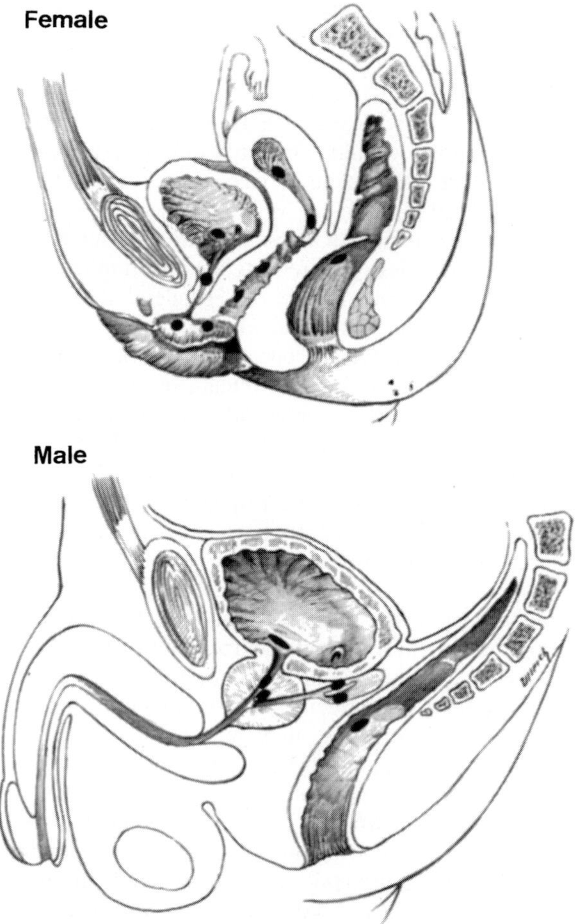

Figure 60–14. Sites of ectopic ureteral orifices in girls and boys.

In males, the mesonephric duct structures eventually form the epididymis, vas deferens, and seminal vesicles. Therefore, an ectopic ureter in the male can drain into the bladder neck, prostatic urethra, or the aforementioned wolffian duct structures (see Fig. 60–14). All of these locations are proximal to the external sphincter. Hence, males with ectopic ureters do not suffer from urinary incontinence as females do.

Because their ectopic ureters drain most commonly into the prostatic urethra and bladder neck, males most often present with urinary tract infection. They may also experience urgency and frequency. In some instances, the ureter ends in the wolffian duct remnants (seminal vesicles, vas deferens, or epididymis), predisposing the individual to epididymitis (Williams and Sago, 1983; Umeyama et al, 1985). Therefore, prepubertal males with epididymitis should prompt the physician to consider the presence of an ectopic ureter. In males, the symptoms may not be as obvious as incontinence in females; males may complain of constipation, pelvic pain, and discomfort during ejaculation, and they may even be infertile (Squadrito et al, 1987). A stone may form in the ectopic ureter. It is most important to remember that boys will be continent because the ectopic ureter always drains proximal to the external sphincter. Urgency and frequency in males, due to the ectopic ureter's draining into the prostatic fossa, should not be mistaken for incontinence.

Diagnosis

Prenatal sonographic diagnosis of ectopic ureters has become common. The condition is identifiable by virtue of the hydronephrosis produced by the obstruction. If this is isolated to the upper pole of a duplex system and the bladder is normal, the diagnosis is relatively straightforward. In other situations, prenatal findings serve to initiate a postnatal evaluation, which will specifically identify the condition.

In a girl, sometimes the diagnosis of an ectopic ureter can be made by physical examination. Direct visualization of the vulva may reveal continuous urinary dribbling or wetness. In the absence of neurogenic vesical dysfunction or a urethral sphincter defect, an ectopic ureter is likely. Often, a punctum or orifice is apparent in the urethrovaginal septum (Fig. 60–15). Perineal and genital skin maceration may reflect the irritating effect of urine continually bathing this area.

The ultrasonographic findings of an ectopic ureter include the dilated pelvis and collecting system of the upper pole and a dilated ureter behind an otherwise normal bladder (Fig. 60–16). A large ectopic ureter may press against the bladder and create an indentation that appears much like a ureterocele and is termed a pseudoureterocele (Diard et al, 1987; Sumfest et al, 1995). The difference is that an ectopic ureter is clearly extravesical with a thick septum of bladder muscle between the ureteral lumen and bladder lumen. This finding is in contrast to a ureterocele, in which the septum is thin and delicate and the ureteral lumen is partially intravesical. Sumfest and associates (1995) noted that their patients had ectopic ureteral drainage into mesonephric duct cysts; these mesonephric duct cysts can rupture into the vagina or bladder. The renal parenchyma associated with a

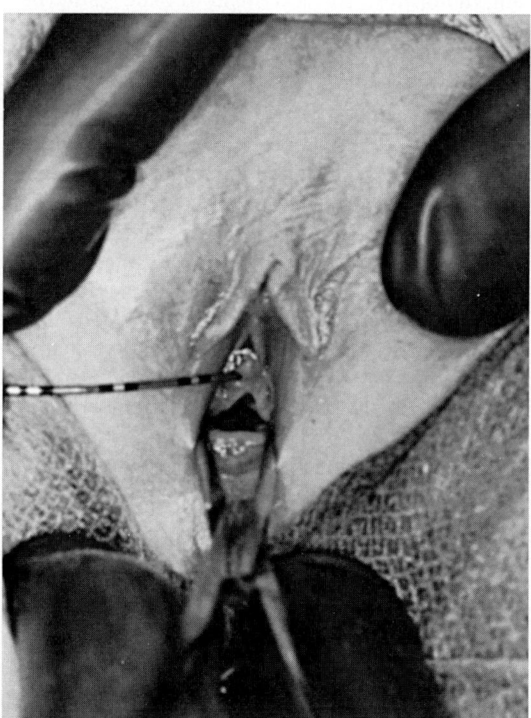

Figure 60–15. Photograph at the time of cystoscopy of an ectopic ureteral orifice in the urethrovaginal septum. A ureteral catheter is in the orifice.

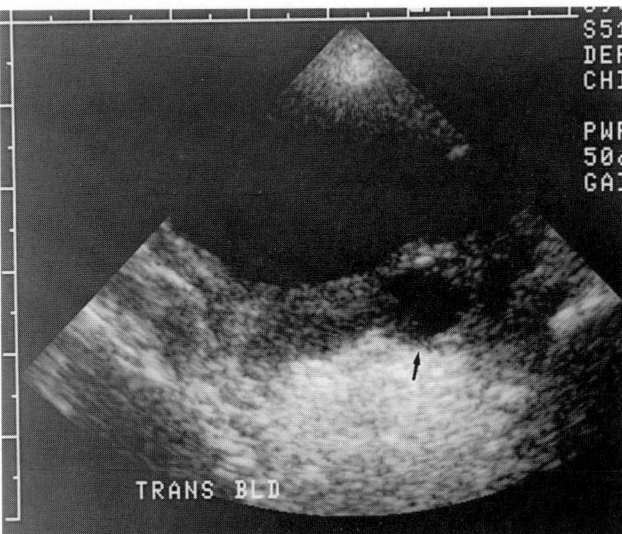

Figure 60–16. Distal ureteral dilatation is seen sonographically as a round hypoechoic area behind the bladder *(arrow)*.

ectopic ureter is often thinner than that of a normally draining lower pole (Nussbaum et al, 1986).

In most instances, the diagnosis of an ectopic ureter is confirmed by excretory urography (Figs. 60–17 and 60–18). The usual radiographic feature is a nonvisualizing or poorly visualizing upper pole of a duplex system that may be massively hydronephrotic. The upper pole displaces the lower pole downward and outward, the so-called drooping lilly appearance. When the upper pole does not excrete contrast and make the duplicated system readily apparent, there are several other clues to suggest that a duplicated system is present. First, the calyces of a lower pole are fewer in number than in the normal kidney. Second, the axis of the lowest to uppermost calyx does not point toward the midline. Third, the uppermost calyx of the lower pole unit is usually farther from the upper pole border than is the lowest calyx from the corresponding lower pole limit. In addition, the lower pole pelvis and the upper portion of its ureter may be farther from the spine than on the contralateral side, and the lower pole ureter may also be scalloped and tortuous secondary to its wrapping around a markedly dilated upper pole ureter (similar to the findings of upper pole hydroureteronephrosis seen in the child with a ureterocele in Figure 60–31). When an ectopic ureter drains a nonvisualizing, diminutive, dysplastic renal unit, these typical radiologic features may not be demonstrated. Care must be taken to identify exactly which kidney is responsible for the ectopic ureter and the incontinence because there often are bilateral duplicated systems. Failure to do so may result in removing the wrong upper pole and the patient's experiencing the same symptoms postoperatively! Particular attention should be paid to the contralateral kidney on excretory urography to avoid missing bilateral ureteral ectopia. This is reported to occur in 5% to 15% of cases (Malek et al, 1972; Mandell et al, 1981) but was noted in 25% of cases in one series (Campbell, 1951).

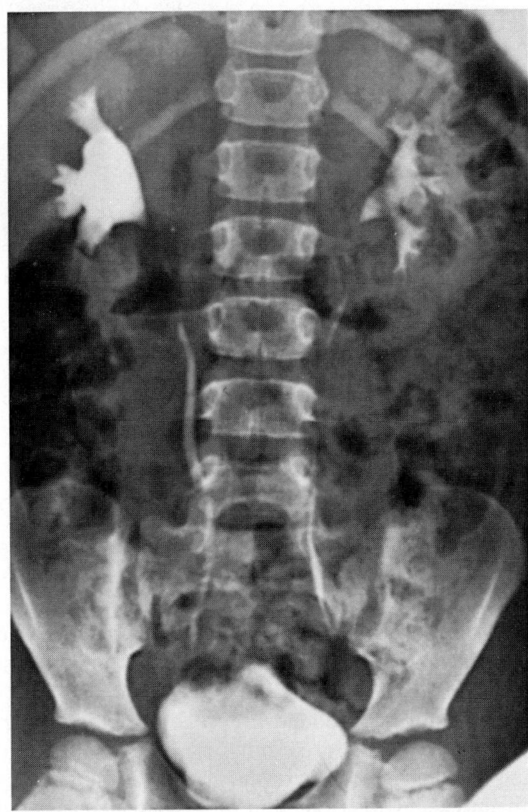

Figure 60–17. Excretory urogram in a 5-year-old girl with urinary incontinence shows a nonvisualizing upper pole on the right side displacing the lower pole downward and outward. Also, note that the right renal pelvis and upper ureter are farther from the spine than on the left.

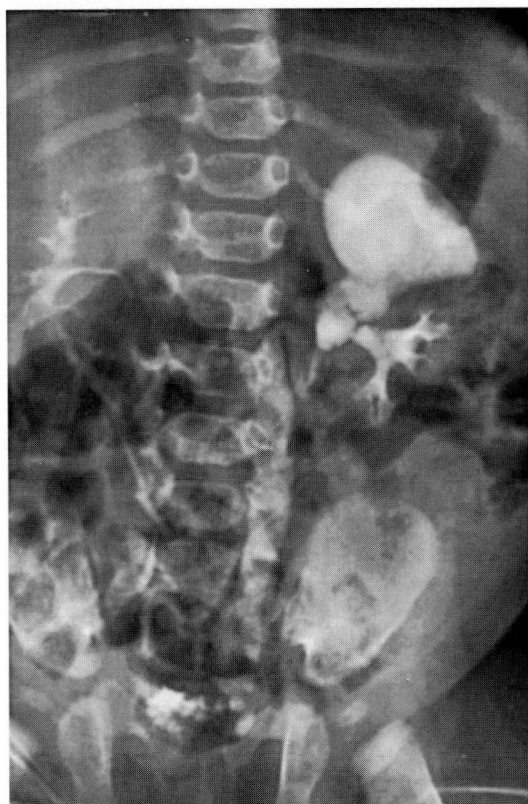

Figure 60–18. Excretory urogram in a 4-month-old girl with a urinary tract infection reveals a left renal duplication with hydronephrosis and hydroureter of the upper pole system.

The functional status of the upper pole renal segment of duplex systems may be evident on excretory urography, but more precise assessment may become important if upper pole salvage is considered. Isotopic renal scanning using ^{99m}technetium-dimercaptosuccinic acid (^{99m}Tc-DMSA) has proved to be the most adequate, although differentiating between the function of the upper and lower poles may be difficult.

Voiding cystourethrography demonstrates reflux into the lower pole ureter in at least half of the cases. More importantly, reflux into the ectopic ureter may be demonstrated at different phases of voiding, providing evidence of the location of the orifice (Fig. 60–19). If the reflux into the ectopic ureter is seen before voiding, the orifice is proximal to the bladder neck; reflux only with voiding suggests an orifice in the urethra. The last finding may be evident only with several cycles of voiding monitored fluoroscopically (Wyly and Lebowitz, 1984). Sphincteric orifices may not produce reflux at all.

Occasionally, the renal parenchyma is difficult to locate and may be identified only by alternate imaging studies (Giles et al, 1982; Gharagozloo and Lebowitz, 1995). In such cases in which an ectopic ureter is strongly suspected because of incontinence yet no definite evidence of the upper pole renal segment is found (Simms and Higgins, 1975), computed tomography or magnetic resonance imaging has demonstrated the small, poorly functioning upper pole segment (Braverman and Lebowitz, 1991) (Fig. 60–20).

Ectopic ureteral orifices may be identified at the time of cystourethroscopy and vaginoscopy. Careful inspection of the vestibule, urethra, and vagina sometimes reveals the ectopic orifice. Often, the orifice is difficult to identify amidst the various mucosal folds of these structures. The authors have not found the intravenous injection of indigo carmine to be particularly helpful because of the delayed function of the segment drained by the ectopic ureter. It has been suggested that two oral doses of phenazopyridine (Pyridium) given the night before and the morning of cystoscopy improve visualization of the ectopic ureter (Weiss et al, 1984). Filling the bladder with a dye solution, such as methylene blue or indigo carmine, is sometimes helpful in detecting the elusive ectopic orifice. If a clear fluid continues to drain into the vulva, one can be certain that an ectopic orifice is present. Deep flank palpation at the time of the examination may result in expression of urine and thereby reveal the orifice location.

Sometimes, the diagnosis must be made by exclusion, that

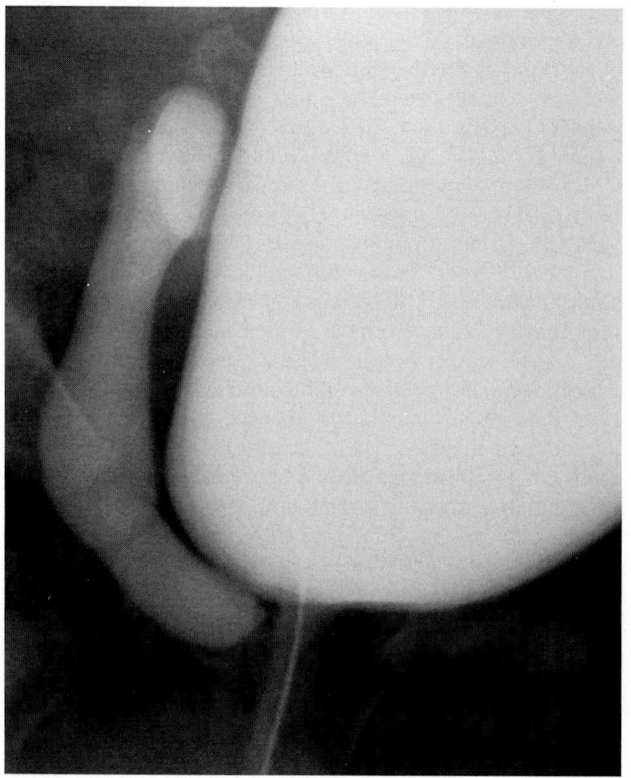

Figure 60–19. A cystogram demonstrates reflux into an ectopic ureter that enters the urethra immediately distal to the bladder neck.

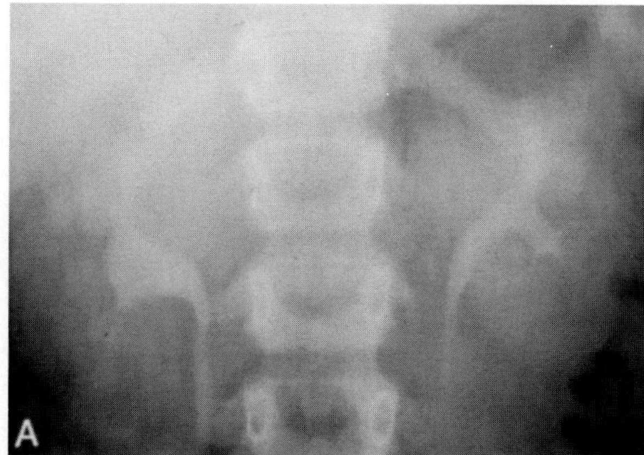

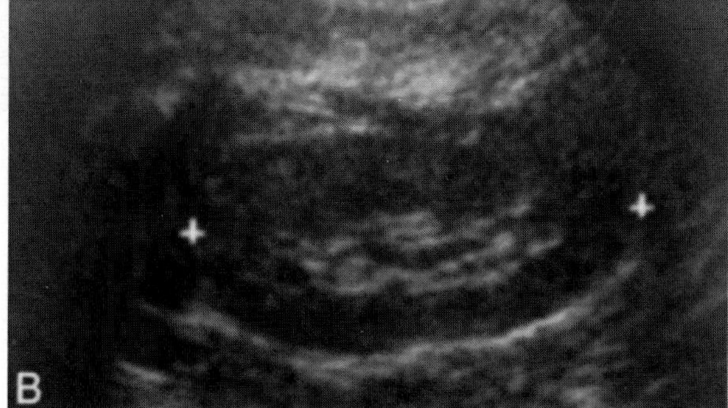

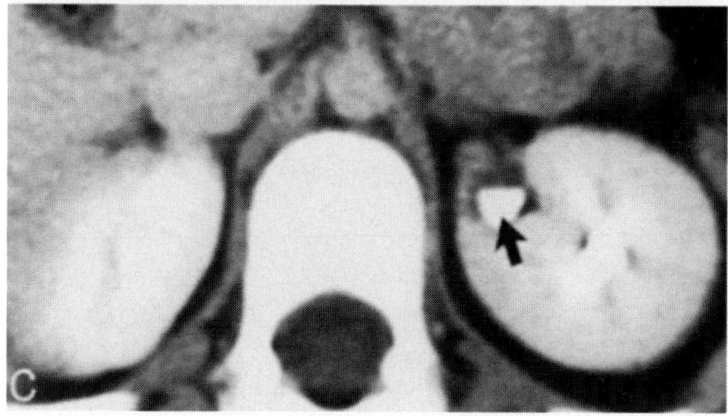

Figure 60–20. *A,* Excretory urogram in 10-year-old girl with constant wetting. No definite evidence for an upper pole segment is present. *B,* Left renal ultrasound in the same patient, also without a clear indication of the presence of an upper pole segment. *C,* Contrast-enhanced computed tomography image in this girl specifically demonstrating the small upper pole segment *(arrow)* associated with the ectopic ureter. Upper pole nephrectomy cured the wetting.

Leadbetter (Leadbetter, 1985), Kropp (Kropp and Angwafo, 1986), or Salle (Rink et al, 1994) procedures. It is often helpful to employ vesicourethral suspension at the same time. Increased exposure using symphyseal splitting has been helpful during these reconstructions (Peters and Hendren, 1989). The success rate is higher in boys than in girls. Bladder capacity often increases in the child who gains satisfactory control. Enterocystoplasty to increase bladder capacity may be necessary in selected cases.

ANOMALIES OF STRUCTURE

Megaureters

By its broadest definition, a megaureter is a large ureter. It is due to obstruction, reflux, or a combination of the two (Pfister et al, 1971; Retik et al, 1978). Each of these states may have several primary or secondary causes (Table 60–2). The term megaureter is sometimes used to exclusively describe a dilated ureter secondary to a ureterovesical junction obstruction. We believe that the classification based on etiology is more descriptive and less likely to lead to misunderstanding.

The primarily obstructed megaureter may be due to an intrinsic stenosis or narrowing of the distalmost portion of the ureter. However, more commonly, it is due to an aperistaltic segment that results in a functional obstruction (Sripathi et al, 1991). This statement is consistent with the operative findings of normal calibration of these ureteral orifices. Primary obstructed megaureter occurs three and a half to five times more often in males. It is two to three times more common on the left side and is bilateral in 15% to 25% of patients. In a few cases, there is contralateral agenesis or dysplasia (Johnston, 1967; Williams and Hulme-Moir, 1970; Pfister et al, 1971). Megaureter may coexist with ureteropelvic junction obstruction (Waltzer, 1983; McGrath et al, 1987; Peters et al, 1989). Familial megaureter has been described in a mother and her adult daughter but is exceedingly rare (Tatu and Brennan, 1981).

Pathology

A number of histologic findings in the undilated segment and the adjacent portion of the dilated ureter have been described by different investigators. Some specimens appear normal by light microscopy, whereas in others, the musculature of the proximal end of the undilated segment may be disorganized, abnormal, or absent. An excessive amount of circular fibers has been described (Murnaghan, 1957; Tanagho et al, 1970). The ureteral musculature is normally organized in a feltlike network of opposing helixes except for the mainly longitudinal pattern of the intramural segment. In some megaureters, the undilated distal segment has an excessively tight helix, which results in a predominantly circular orientation (McLaughlin et al, 1973; Hanna et al, 1976).

The most distal portion has a marked fusiform or bulbous dilation, which abruptly changes into a short, undilated ureteral segment, 0.5 to 4 cm in length, which enters the bladder (Williams and Hulme-Moir, 1970; Pfister et al, 1971). In many cases, the area of abrupt transition between the dilated and normal-sized ureter shows faulty muscular development, with a segment partially or completely deficient in muscle. The muscle that is found is maloriented. An excessive amount of collagen tends to occur within the undilated segment of ureter and in its adventitia as well (Gregoir and Debled, 1969; MacKinnon et al, 1970).

Table 60–2. A PROPOSED CLASSIFICATION

Megaureter (Wide) Examples

Reflux megaureter		Obstructed megaureter		Nonreflux-nonobstructed megaureter	
Primary	Secondary	Primary	Secondary	Primary	Secondary
E X A M P L E S					
Primary reflux megaureter †Prune-belly	Urethral obstruction Neuropathic bladder	Intrinsic obstruction: -stenosis -adynamic segment	Urethral obstruction Neuropathic bladder Extrinsic obstruction: -retroperitoneal tumor	‡Nonreflux-nonobstructed megaureter	Polyuria Infection Remaining wide after relief of distal obstruction

†Some conditions (e.g., prune-belly, ureteroceles, ectopic ureters) may appear under several other columns.
‡As proved not to be obstructed.
Note: An occasional megaureter may show reflux and apparent obstruction.
Adapted from Report of Working Party to Establish an International Nomenclature for the Large Ureter. *In* Bergsma D, Duckett JW Jr, eds: Urinary System Malformations in Children. Birth Defects: Original Article Series, Vol 13, No 5. New York, Alan R. Liss, 1977.

Regardless of whether or not light microscopic studies show obvious pathology, ultrastructural studies have consistently revealed an increase in collagen between the muscle bundles of the obstructing segment and between the individual muscle cells (Notley, 1972; Hanna et al, 1976). The adjacent muscle cells in the most distal portion of the dilated segment are abnormal as well (Hanna et al, 1976). Hanna and associates (1976) noted a progressive improvement in muscle cell morphology extending more proximally up the dilated portion of the megaureter; muscular hypertrophy and hyperplasia are marked (Cussen, 1971). In the absence of an anatomic stenosis, obstruction may be due to failure of peristaltic transmission through the distal ureteral segment. Although various workers have blamed this on a preponderance of circular fibers, increased collagen, or focal muscle absence, the common mechanism appears to be attenuation or frank disruption of muscular continuity, either grossly or at the cellular level; this separates nexuses and thus prevents spread of the action potential (Hanna et al, 1976). Lee and colleagues (1992) performed quantitative histologic analysis of dilated ureters. They found that although the tissue collagen–to–smooth muscle ratio in primary obstructed ureters is higher than in controls, this difference is not statistically significant. Primary refluxing megaureters had a tissue collagen–to–smooth muscle ratio that was significantly higher than in controls.

Hofmann and colleagues (1986) reported increased acetylcholinesterase activity in the juxtavesical segment of obstructed megaureters adjacent to the narrow segment. Hertle and Nawrath (1985) observed an altered (tonic) response to norepinephrine in isolated strips of obstructed megaureter as opposed to increased phasic activity of normal ureters. They ascribed this response to an increased fraction of intracellularly stored calcium in megaureters.

Tokunaka and Koyanagi, with various other associates, have published a series of articles involving light and electron microscopic studies in nonrefluxing megaureter, further defining the pathogenesis of the condition (Tokunaka et al, 1980, 1981, 1982, 1984; Tokunaka and Koyanagi, 1982). They identified two groups of nonrefluxing megaureters: a larger group (group 1), with relatively normal histopathology of the dilated segment and abnormalities limited to the intravesical segment, and a smaller group (group 2), with abnormalities involving the dilated portion of the ureter. In group 1, the abnormal findings of the intravesical ureter included deranged muscle bundle orientation and increased connective tissue. A generously developed bulky periureteral sheath appeared to contribute to obstruction, especially with bladder filling. The kidneys of these megaureters were normal or showed hydronephrosis without dysmorphism. In group 2, the length of the distal narrowed segment was variable, in some cases extending extravesically. Histology was normal. The dilated portion of the ureter, in contrast, was abnormal with a marked reduction of muscle cells, which were small and widely separated in a collagen matrix. Muscle bundles were absent, nexuses were attenuated, and no thick myofilaments were present. Extending ultrastructural observations to a variety of congenital disorders, this group reported muscle dysplasia in the dilated portion of the ureter in different kinds of megaureters: eight of 34 nonrefluxing megaureters, one of 22 refluxing megaureters, and four of 23 single-system and four of nine duplex ectopic ureters. Extensive dysplasia of the entire ureter was associated with severe renal dysplasia or hypoplasia. For single and duplex ureteroceles, in all but one case, muscle dysplasia was limited to the ureterocele dome (present in 17 of 19 cases) and spared the involved ureter.

In the megaureter secondarily obstructed from posterior urethral valves, muscular hypertrophy and hyperplasia tend to be more marked than in intrinsic obstruction. In either case, hypertrophy and hyperplasia are a response to an increased workload and appear in utero.

The favorable results often achieved with corrective surgery of obstructed megaureter in infancy (Peters et al, 1989) may be related to the greater number of mesenchymal cells still present at that age that can continue to differentiate into muscle postoperatively. Chronic or recurrent infection may damage the muscle cells of the megaureter, altering the expected histologic findings and interfering with muscle cell function (Hanna et al, 1977). Keating and colleagues (1989) suggested that many of the prenatally detected primary obstructed megaureters are not actually obstructed and will improve with observation. Longer follow-up and improvements in the ability to diagnose neonatal obstruction are necessary to enhance our understanding of this issue.

Ureteroceles

Few entities in pediatric urology present the clinical challenge of ureteroceles. Ureteroceles have varied effects in regard to obstruction, reflux, continence, and renal function; hence, each ureterocele must be managed on an individual basis and not by a simple algorithm. It is imperative for the treating physician to be acquainted with the multiple presentations, radiologic appearances, and treatment options of ureteroceles, as well as the complications to avoid. Such knowledge yields the best possible clinical results.

Embryology

A ureterocele is a cystic dilatation of the terminal ureter. How this develops has been the subject of several discussions. At 37 days' gestation, Chwalle's membrane, a two-layered cell structure, transiently divides the early ureteric bud from the urogenital sinus (Chwalle, 1927). The stenotic orifice commonly seen in the ureterocele has led several researchers to postulate that this dilatation results from incomplete dissolution of Chwalle's membrane. Others have theorized that the affected intravesical ureter suffers from abnormal muscular development. Without the appropriate muscular backing, the distal ureter assumes a balloon morphology (Tokunaka et al, 1981). A third theory implicates a developmental stimulus responsible for bladder expansion acting simultaneously on the intravesical ureter (Stephens, 1971). Incontrovertible evidence does not exist to uphold any of these theories, which, in fact, have very little effect on clinical practice.

Diagnosis

As with ectopic ureters, ureteroceles are increasingly diagnosed by prenatal ultrasound. The prenatal ultrasound is capable of demonstrating both the hydronephrosis and the intravesical cystic dilatation. If they are diagnosed prenatally, the physician is alerted to perform a more comprehensive postnatal evaluation and to administer prophylactic antibiotics at birth.

Ureteroceles have a particular predilection for race and gender (Brock and Kaplan, 1978; Mandell et al, 1980; Cobb et al, 1982; Caldamone and Duckett, 1984; Scherz et al, 1989; Monfort et al, 1992; Rickwood et al, 1992). They occur most frequently in females (4:1 ratio) and almost exclusively in Caucasians. Approximately 10% are bilateral. Eighty percent of all ureteroceles arise from the upper poles of duplicated systems. Single-system ureteroceles are sometimes called simple ureteroceles and are usually found in adults. These single-system ureteroceles are less prone to the severe obstruction and dysplasia associated with duplicated systems.

However, many ureteroceles are still diagnosed clinically. The most common presentation is that of an infant who has a urinary tract infection or urosepsis (Gonzales, 1992; Monfort et al, 1992; Retik and Peters, 1992; Coplen and Duckett, 1995). We have seen patients whose ultrasound and intraoperative findings revealed frank pus in the obstructed upper pole collecting system. For this reason, all children with a ureterocele (or less specifically, any significant hydronephrosis) should be given prophylactic antibiotics. Stasis of urine in this obstructed system can lead not only to infection but also to calculus formation (Thornbury et al, 1977; Rodriguez, 1984; Moskovitz et al, 1987). Some children may present with a palpable mass in their abdomen, which is a hydronephrotic kidney. The ureterocele, if ectopic, can prolapse out of the urethra and present as a vaginal mass (Fig. 60–26).

If the ureterocele is large enough, it can obstruct the bladder neck or even the contralateral ureteral orifice and result in hydronephrosis of that collecting system. Ectopic ureteroceles can cause incontinence by hindering the normal sphincteric function at or distal to the bladder neck. Infrequently, a child with a ureterocele can present with hematuria. Ureteroceles may have an insidious clinical course and

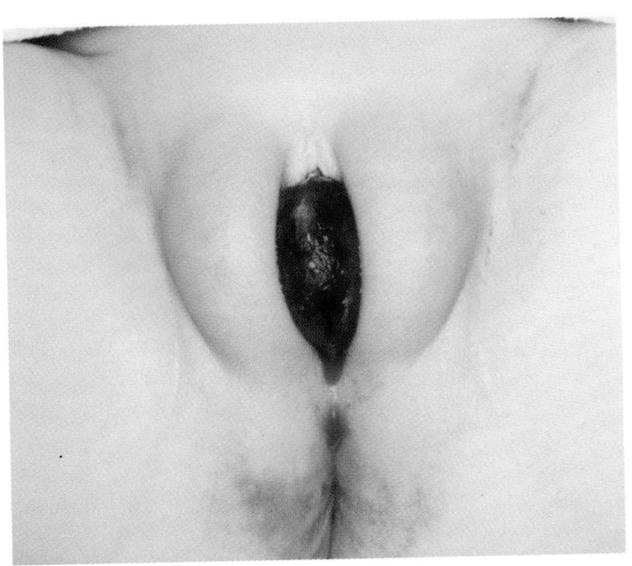

Figure 60–26. A prolapsed ureterocele presented as an interlabial mass in a 3-week-old female.

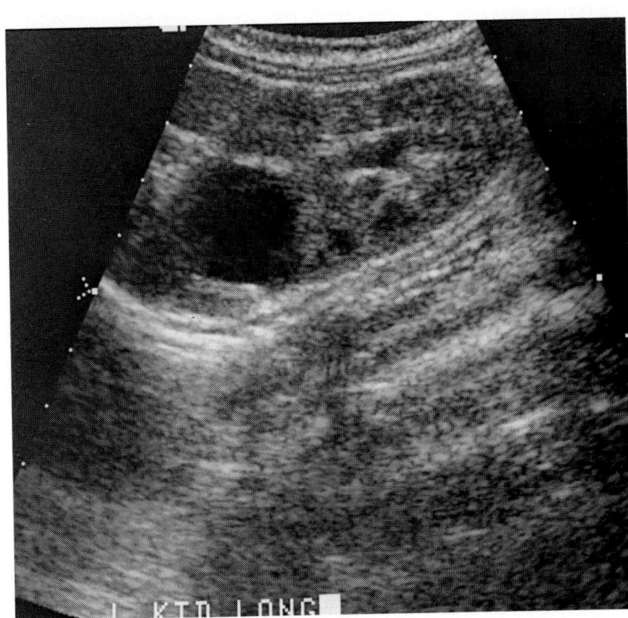

Figure 60–27. Sonographic appearance of upper pole hydronephrosis due to a ureterocele.

result in no specific urologic symptoms but manifest themselves only as a failure to thrive, or as abdominal or pelvic pain. Usually, lengthy evaluation of other organ systems ensues before the problem is correctly localized to the urinary tract.

Imaging studies now available afford us a great deal of insight into the effects of the ureterocele on normal anatomy and physiology. The first study obtained in these evaluations is usually an ultrasound scan (Geringer et al, 1983b; Cremin, 1986; Teele and Share, 1991). Most commonly, the ureterocele is associated with a duplicated collecting system. Sonographically, one can see two separate renal pelves surrounded by their echogenic hila. This duplex kidney is larger than a kidney associated with a single collecting system. A dilated ureter emanates from a hydronephrotic upper pole (Fig. 60–27). This finding should signal the examiner to image the bladder to determine whether or not a ureterocele is present. If the lower pole is associated with reflux, or if the ureterocele has caused delayed emptying from the ipsilateral lower pole, this lower pole may likewise be hydronephrotic. Similarly, the ureterocele may impinge on the contralateral ureteral orifice or obstruct the bladder neck and cause hydronephrosis in the opposite kidney. The upper pole parenchyma drained by the ureterocele will exhibit varying degrees of thickness and echogenicity. Increased echogenicity correlates with dysplastic changes. The bladder frequently displays a thin-walled cyst that is the ureterocele (Fig. 60–28).

However, there are several pitfalls in ultrasound diagnosis. If the bladder is overdistended, the ureterocele may be effaced and go unnoticed. At times, the bladder may be empty, in which case it is difficult to discriminate between the wall of the ureterocele and the wall of the bladder. In such instances, the empty bladder with a ureterocele may be interpreted as simply a partially filled bladder. The dilated ureter should be seen posterior to the bladder. On occasion, a large ureterocele is associated with a diminutive ureter and collecting system. The corresponding upper pole paren-

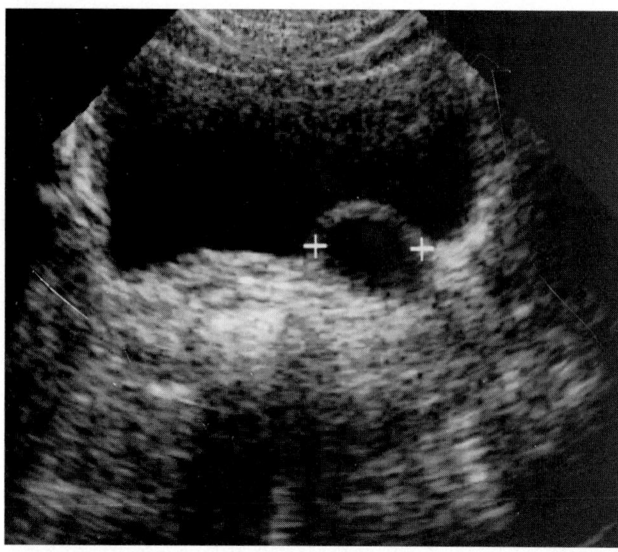

Figure 60–28. An intravesical ureterocele in a 2-month-old female is outlined by the two crosshatches on an ultrasound image.

chyma can be so small as to be nonvisualized. The diagnosis of ureterocele may be overlooked because the duplicated collecting system cannot be identified. This entity has been termed both the nonobstructive ectopic ureterocele (Bauer and Retik, 1978) and ureterocele disproportion (Share and Lebowitz, 1989) (Fig. 60–29).

On occasion, the dilated ureter of an ectopic ureter may be seen immediately posterior to the bladder and impinge on the bladder wall and appear as if the dilated ureter is intravesical. This may give the false impression of a ureterocele, the pseudoureterocele referred to previously (Diard et al, 1987; Sumfest et al, 1995). The difference between the two entities is that a ureterocele is separated from the bladder space by its thin wall, whereas the ectopic ureter has the thicker bladder wall separating it from the intravesical space. A mesonephric duct cyst that communicates with an ectopic ureter can open into the bladder and mimic a ureterocele on radiographic studies (Sumfest et al, 1995).

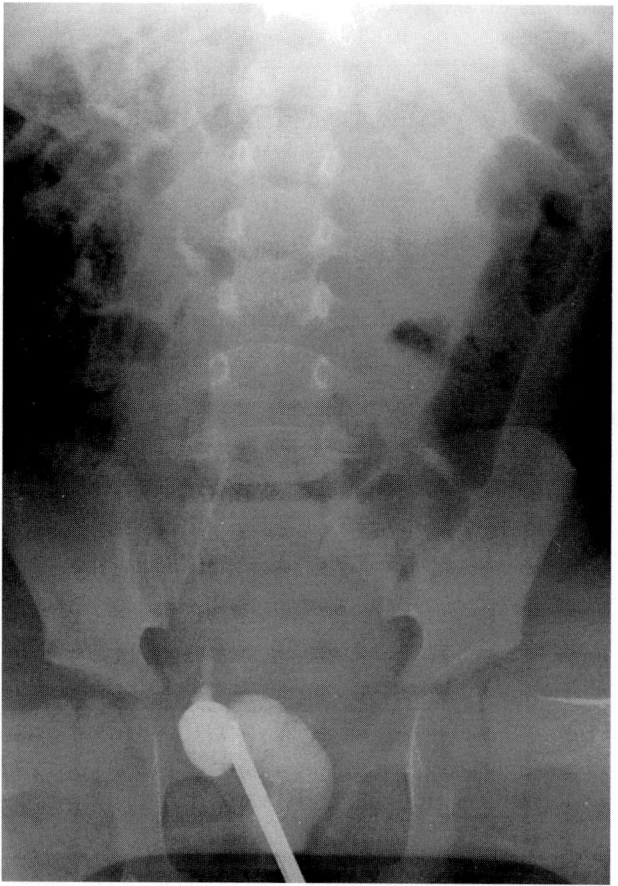

Figure 60–29. Ureterocele disproportion demonstrated via retrograde pyelography. Note the disparity between the large ureterocele and the thin ureter and nondilated collecting system.

Intravenous pyelography is a valuable imaging study in the evaluation of a ureterocele. There are several hallmarks of a urogram in a patient with a ureterocele (Geringer et al, 1983a; Muller et al, 1988), and these findings are similar to those mentioned in the discussion on ectopic ureters. In the great majority of cases, the upper pole functions poorly and excretes contrast in a delayed fashion or not at all. This upper pole is deviated laterally from the spine because of its hydronephrosis. This same upper pole hydronephrosis is responsible for pushing the lower pole laterally and inferiorly (Fig. 60–30). Because only the lower pole calyces are seen, the number of calyces is less than the complement of a normal kidney.

Whereas the upper pole ureter is infrequently seen on the intravenous pyelogram because of the lack of contrast excretion, its presence may be inferred from its effect on the lower pole ureter. The lower pole ureter can be seen as laterally deviated, taking a serpiginous course, and notched. These characteristics all result from its association with the dilated, tortuous upper pole ureter (Fig. 60–31). As mentioned earlier in the section on ultrasonography, hydronephrosis may be seen in the contralateral kidney as a result of obstruction by the ureterocele.

Voiding cystourethrography can demonstrate the size and location of the ureterocele as well as the presence or absence of vesicoureteral reflux. Assessing the severity of such reflux is critical to future management. Reflux into the ipsilateral lower pole is commonly seen (Feldman and Lome, 1981; Caldamone and Duckett, 1984) (Fig. 60–32). Sen and associates (1992) reported reflux in 80 of 148 (54%) ipsilateral lower pole ureters. Rickwood and co-workers (1992) noted that 15 of 23 patients (65%) had ipsilateral lower pole reflux.

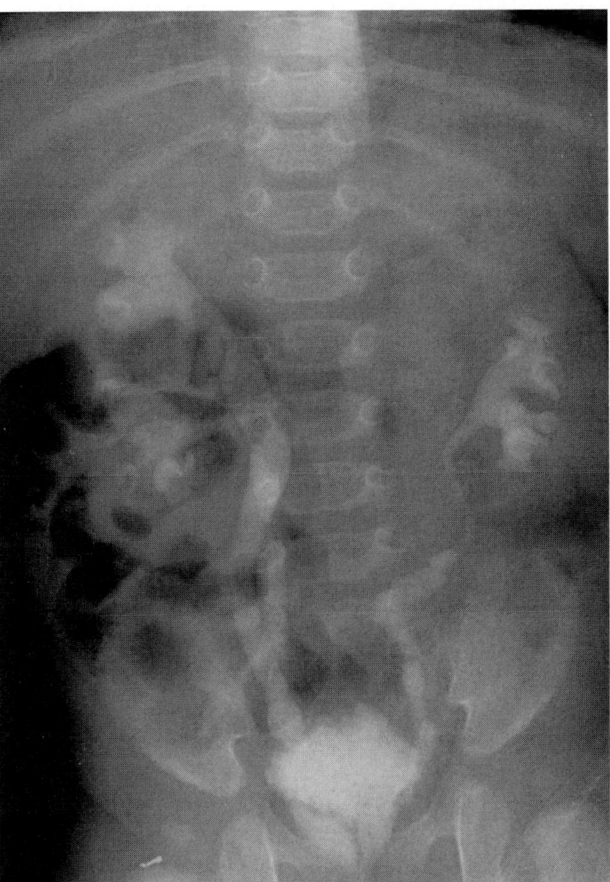

Figure 60–31. An intravenous pyelogram reveals the effects of left upper pole hydronephrosis due to its obstructing ureterocele. The left upper pole is not visualized, the left lower pole ureter takes a serpiginous course around the dilated upper pole ureter, and there is contralateral hydronephrosis owing to the ureterocele obstructing the bladder neck.

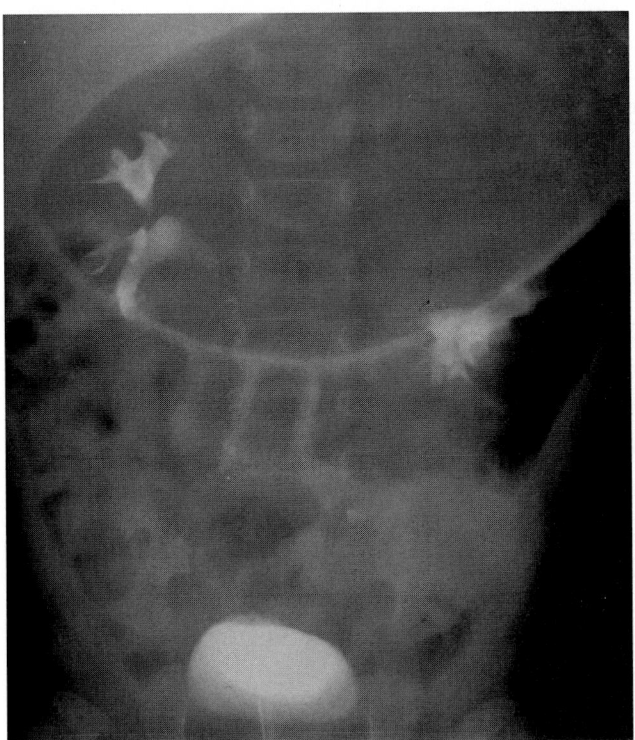

Figure 60–30. Left upper pole hydronephrosis causes lower pole displacement inferiorly and laterally, which is referred to as the drooping lily sign.

Forty percent of patients with ureteroceles in Monfort's series had reflux (Monfort et al, 1992). Reflux may also be seen in the contralateral system if the ureterocele is large enough to distort the trigone and the opposite ureteral submucosal tunnel. In Sen's series, 35 of 127 patients (28%) had reflux in the contralateral unit. Reflux into the ureter of the ureterocele may be present but is uncommon.

Images should be obtained from early in the filling phase because some ureteroceles may efface later in filling and may not be seen. The ureterocele may evert into the ureter and appear to be a diverticulum (Fig. 60–33). When it is performed diligently, cystography demonstrates the ureterocele in the bladder. It appears as a smooth, broad-based filling defect, located near the trigone. It is frequently eccentrically located, and the superior portion of the ureterocele may be angled to one side, thereby giving a clue as to which side the ureterocele is associated with (Fig. 60–34). However, on cystogram the ureterocele is often centrally placed, and it may not be helpful in this regard. In such instances, cystoscopy may shed light on the issue. If the cystoscopic findings are inconclusive, the answer can be obtained by injecting contrast into the ureterocele; this method should define the side from which the ureterocele emanated (Fig. 60–35). Injection of contrast into the uretero-

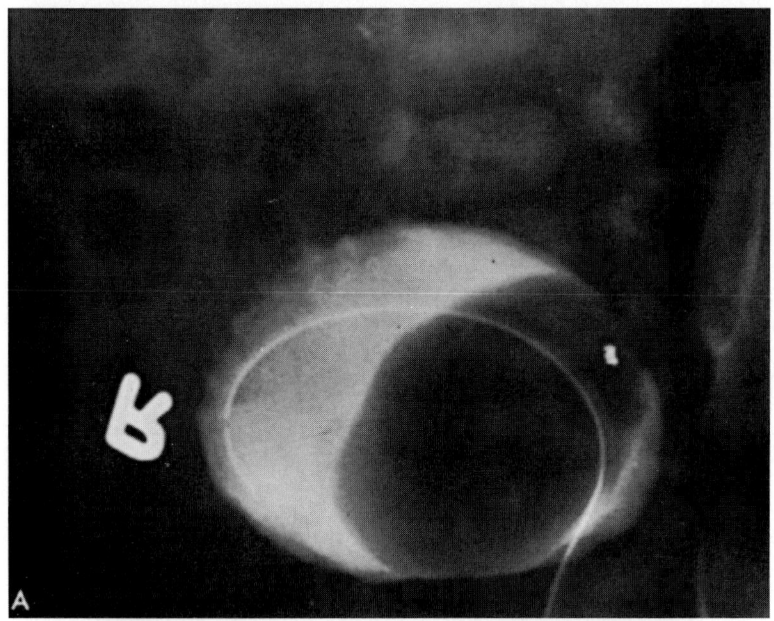

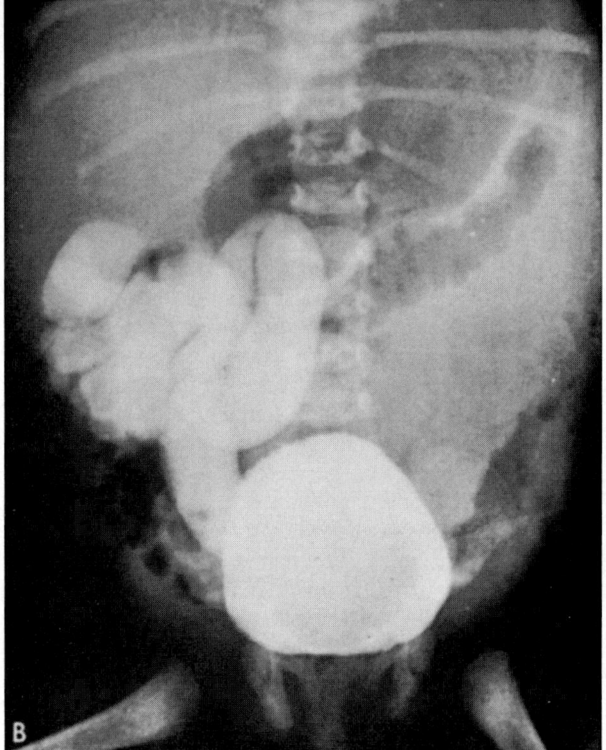

Figure 60–32. *A,* Cystogram outlines a *left* ureterocele. *B,* Postvoiding film shows reflux to the *right* lower pole. This girl had *bilateral* ureteroceles, with the right one being a small subtrigonal one that was not demonstrated on the cystogram.

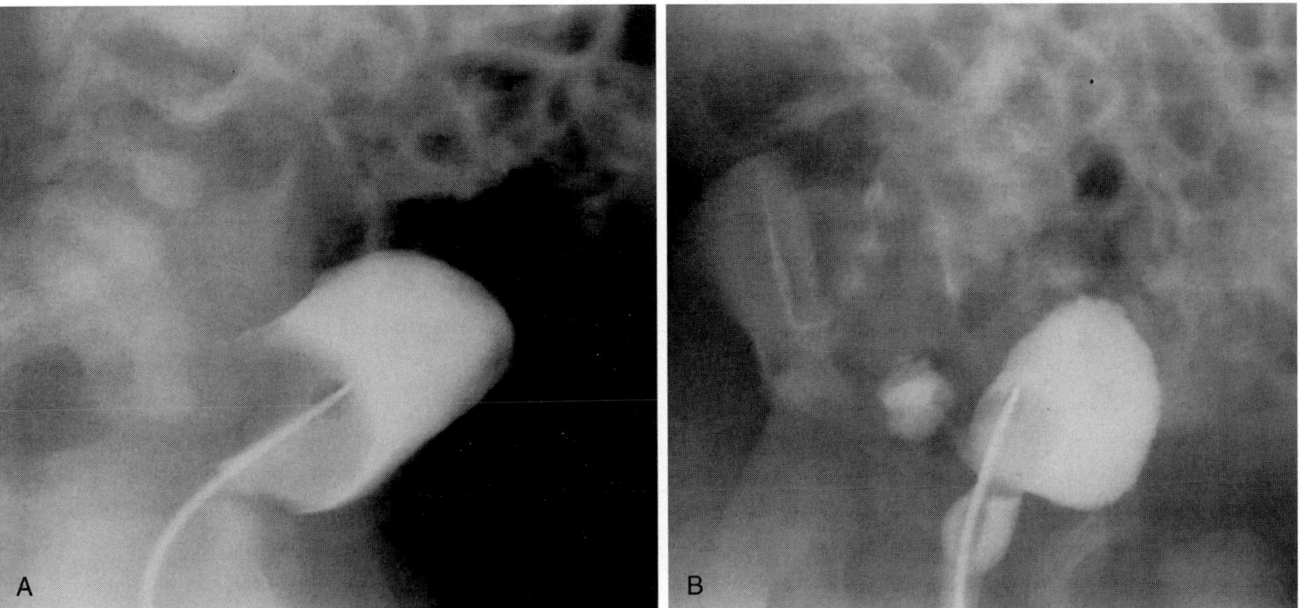

Figure 60–33. A ureterocele seen on a cystogram during early filling *(A)* may be mistaken during late filling for a diverticulum as the ureterocele everts into its own ureter *(B).*

cele can verify the diagnosis of ureterocele disproportion when the upper tract findings are difficult to interpret. Such information is obviously necessary in planning the surgical approach.

Nuclear scans with agents such as DMSA and DTPA can give valuable estimates of upper pole contribution to overall renal function as well as degrees of obstruction (Arap et al, 1984). It is important to trace the regions of interest correctly and consistently in order to obtain accurate information. This information is often helpful in determining whether the upper pole moiety is worth saving.

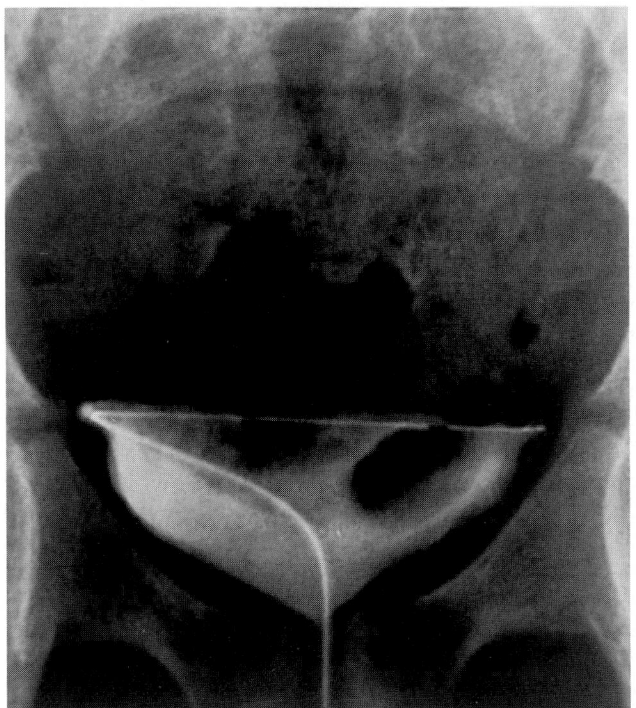

Figure 60–34. A smooth lateral filling defect is the classic appearance of a ureterocele on a cystogram.

Treatment

It should once again be stressed that before any surgical intervention, the surgeon must obtain as much information as possible regarding the patient's altered anatomy and physiology. Only then can a rational treatment plan be devised.

Ureteroceles have a broad spectrum of presentation, anatomy, and pathophysiology; thus, each child must be treated individually. No single method of surgical repair suffices for all cases. The goals of therapy should be clearly defined and factored into the clinical decisions. These goals are preservation of renal function; elimination of infection, obstruction, and reflux; and maintenance of urinary continence. Minimizing surgical morbidity is a goal that must be included in this consideration. The management of a ureterocele associated with an upper pole of a duplicated system has generated much debate. Although the goals of treatment as stated earlier could certainly generate a consensus, the means to achieving those goals have not necessarily been agreed on.

A primary concern is the preservation of renal parenchyma if at all possible. This goal is achieved by correcting obstruction and preventing reflux with its risks of renal parenchymal damage from infection. At times, it is necessary to balance one against the other, because relieving the obstruction of a ureterocele may induce reflux in either or both poles of the involved duplication. In other instances, the same action may cause existing lower pole reflux to resolve. Several means of achieving these goals of therapy are available. Because there are a sizable number of permutations where one considers all the possible combinations and degrees of ipsilateral and contralateral reflux, ipsilateral and contralateral obstruction, varying degrees of salvageable function, infection, and age, one can easily see why most people

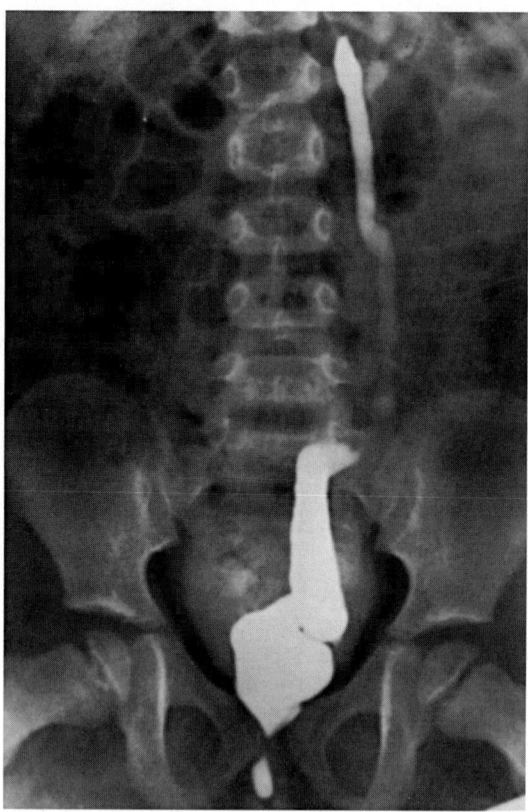

Figure 60–35. Endoscopic injection of a ureterocele outlines the upper pole and the distal extent of the ureterocele.

believe that when dealing with ureteroceles each case must be managed on an individual basis.

In most instances, the upper pole contributes little, if at all, to overall renal function. The aim therefore is to deal with this offending unit in a manner that is geared not only toward alleviating obstruction and its potential for recurrent infection but also toward the cessation of reflux that is present in about half of the cases.

There are two general schools of thought in this regard. One group of surgeons advocates the so-called upper tract approach; this approach consists of upper pole nephrectomy and partial ureterectomy, or less commonly, when significant upper pole function is present, a ureteropyelostomy (Mandell et al, 1980; Cendron et al, 1981; Feldman and Lome, 1981; Caldamone et al, 1984; Reitelman and Perlmutter, 1990). With either of these procedures, the ureterocele should decompress, and with return of the trigone to a more normal configuration, resolution of the ipsilateral lower pole reflux may occur. The advantages of this approach are avoidance of the morbidity of a second surgical procedure and, it is hoped, elimination of a potentially difficult bladder neck and urethral dissection. If a second procedure is eventually required, it can be performed in an older child on an elective basis (King et al, 1983). Mandell and associates (1980) treated 18 patients in this manner. In 14 of these patients, a one-stage procedure was planned; only 3 patients (21%) required reoperation (the indications being persistent lower pole reflux, reflux into the ureteral stump, and failure of ureterocele decompression). They are proponents of the upper pole approach because it meets the goals of a low reoperative rate and resolution of the problems described earlier. They do state, however, that if a patient has high-grade reflux into the ipsilateral lower pole ureter, a combination of upper pole nephroureterectomy, ureterocele excision, and lower pole ureteral reimplantation may be necessary. This combined approach would be recommended because these severe degrees of reflux are less likely to disappear spontaneously and would likely require a second procedure.

Another scenario that should prompt consideration for a single-stage repair at the kidney and bladder level is the case of lower pole reflux associated with a large everting ureterocele and a poorly functioning upper pole. This, too, will unlikely result in reflux resolution because the muscular backing necessary for ureteral compression is usually lacking in everting ureteroceles.

Caldamone and associates (1984) had a similar rate for secondary procedures using the upper tract approach. Of 36 patients managed in this way (including four patients who underwent ureteropyelostomy), only seven (19%) needed secondary procedures, four had bladder outlet obstruction, and three had persistent reflux associated with poor renal growth, renal scarring, or recurrent urinary tract infections. Interestingly, ten of their patients had delayed reflux, that is, reflux that appeared after an upper tract procedure in a patient with no preoperative reflux. Only three of these ten patients had spontaneous resolution of the reflux. These authors concluded that most patients can be managed with an upper urinary tract approach alone.

Likewise, Perlmutter and associates (Kroovand and Perlmutter, 1979; Reitelman and Perlmutter, 1990) direct their attention to removal of the upper pole of the kidney. They combine this procedure with a total ureterectomy to the level of the bladder to prevent possible problems from a retained stump (e.g., a pyoureter or a diverticulum). When the upper pole merits salvage, they perform either an ipsilateral ureteropyelostomy or a distal ureteroureterostomy. In most instances, there is a reasonable chance for resolution of the reflux after decompression of the ureterocele.

One of the more extensive experiences in the literature is that of Scherz and colleagues (1989). They reported their clinical observations in 60 patients with ectopic ureteroceles (defined as either a ureterocele associated with an upper pole of a duplicated system or a ureterocele in an ectopic position). They also compared the need for further surgery in patients treated with the upper urinary tract approach alone versus those who had a combined upper and lower urinary tract approach. The combined approach uses two incisions to achieve upper pole heminephrectomy, partial ureterectomy, and intravesical excision and marsupialization of the ureterocele, along with correction of reflux when present. Of 19 evaluable patients who had the upper urinary tract approach alone, nine (47%) required reoperation for recurrent reflux or infection. In contrast, of 28 patients who were treated with the combined approach, only four (14%) required reoperation, all for reflux. These authors believe that marsupialization is less likely to cause sphincter damage than enucleation. They also emphasize the need for passing a large catheter antegrade through the bladder neck to ascertain that all mucosal lips that might act as obstructing valves have been removed. They believe that the combined approach is a superior one because of its lower reoperative rate. With the exception of the acutely ill child with urosepsis, Hendren and Mitchell (1979) are also advocates of a complete repair, namely, upper pole nephrectomy, ureterocele excision, and ureteral reimplantation.

Gotoh and colleagues (1988) have reported on using the presence or absence of radiographic eversion of the ureterocele, the separation between the upper and lower orifices, and the upper pole function to determine the means of correction. In cases with eversion and separation of the orifices, upper pole function was always absent. When the orifices were adjacent, function was absent in one third of cases. Upper pole nephrectomy was performed with an extravesical resection of the ureterocele and repair of the bladder wall, without lower pole reimplantation.

The reports of Decter and associates (1989) and Gonzales (1992) reiterate the need to consider each case individually. Essentially, they proceed with an upper tract approach in infants who have low-grade or no reflux in the ipsilateral lower pole. In those infants who will likely need a secondary procedure (such as those with high-grade reflux or a prolapsed ureterocele), or in septic patients not responding to antibiotic therapy, they advocate initial decompression of the ureterocele via endoscopic incision.

Our intravesical approach to the ureterocele begins with a transverse incision of the ureterocele between two stay sutures (Fig. 60–36). Proximally, a plane is obtained between the ureterocele wall and the wall of the bladder. The ureterocele is dissected off the bladder to the point where it joins the lower pole ureter. Then the ureters are dissected as a unit, the upper pole ureter is tapered as needed, and both ureters are reimplanted submucosally. Amar (1978) advocates submucosal saline injection to facilitate creation of the submucosal tunnel. The distal portion of the ureterocele is dissected in the same plane to the level of the bladder neck, where it is resected. The detrusor muscle is plicated if it is attenuated and it appears that it may offer insufficient backing. Bladder mucosal flaps are raised to cover the area of the removed ureterocele.

Once again, several technical points regarding ureterocele excision and common sheath reimplantation deserve mention. Separation of the duplicated ureters during intravesical dissection should be discouraged because it can lead to sacrifice of the common blood supply running longitudinally between the two ureters. Plication of the detrusor muscle underlying the ureterocele may be necessary to shore up any areas of muscle deficiency. Further, the distal portion of the ureterocele may extend below the bladder neck. Extreme care must be taken in this part of the dissection to avoid injury to the sphincter mechanisms.

A commonly held belief is that an upper pole drained by a ureterocele is compromised by atrophy and dysplasia to such an extent that it rarely has any significant function. However, with the increased use of prenatal sonography, more ureteroceles are coming to clinical attention at an earlier stage and potentially at a time when upper pole function can be salvaged (Monfort et al, 1992). Treatment options to effect salvage are either upper pole to lower pole ureteropyelostomy or ureteroureterostomy, ureterocele excision with common sheath reimplantation, or transurethral incision of the ureterocele.

Upper pole biopsy at the time of renal exploration may aid in assessing whether the tissue is dysplastic or viable (Coplen and Duckett, 1995). Prior to that procedure, radiographic imaging can provide information regarding the presence of function. An intravenous pyelogram that demonstrates an upper pole that excretes contrast either parri passu with the lower pole or even in only a slightly delayed fashion is suggestive of parenchyma with recoverability. Similarly, a nuclear medicine renal scan with an agent such as DMSA, which binds to the functional nephron tubules, can demonstrate an upper pole that may have salvageable renal parenchyma despite obstruction. The goal in these cases is to create effective drainage of the upper pole collecting system.

One option used to achieve this goal is the upper urinary tract anastomotic techniques of ureteroureterostomy or ureteropyelostomy. This results in the upper pole system's draining into the lower pole system. Such high anastomoses are preferable to a distal ureteroureterostomy because the latter is prone to the travel of urine boluses down one ureter and then at the ureteral-ureteral junction retrograde up the other ureter. This phenomenon is sometimes referred to as the yo-yo effect. It can detrimentally affect urinary drainage and lead to stasis, infection, and ureteral dilatation.

When performing the upper tract anastomoses, dissection should be limited to an absolute minimum, especially medially, in order to prevent disruption of either ureter's blood supply. The upper pole ureter may be considerably larger than the lower pole ureter. A generous longitudinal ureterotomy made in the lower pole ureter is performed to overcome such disproportion, and the anastomosis is performed in an end-to-side fashion. The distal portion of the upper pole ureter should be aspirated with a fine feeding tube to decompress the ureterocele. The distal upper pole ureter is resected as far inferiorly as possible, with care taken to stay directly on this ureter's wall and avoid the vasculature of the adjacent lower pole ureter. If the ureterocele does not reflux, the resection is taken as distally as the wound allows and the remnant lower portion of ureter may be left open.

Ureterocele excision and common sheath reimplantation also achieves the goal of upper tract drainage. The technical aspects of this approach have been described earlier. The disadvantage of this approach compared with the flank upper pole to lower pole anastomoses just described is that the bladder approach has the added morbidity of hematuria, bladder spasm, and several days of bladder drainage with a catheter. In addition, the dissection of the ureterocele bed may be a more involved one and has the potential problems of bladder neck injury.

Descriptions of ureterocele incisions date back to Zielinski's technique of a low transverse incision (Zielinski, 1962) and a longitudinal ureterocele incision proposed by Hutch and Chisholm (1966). These so-called meatotomies were performed via open surgery.

Recently, there has been an increased interest in the endoscopic treatment of ureteroceles (Cobb et al, 1982; Monfort et al, 1992; Blythe et al, 1993; Coplen and Duckett, 1995). Although this modality has been satisfactory in achieving decompression (Wines and O'Flynn, 1972; Tank, 1986), transurethral resection of the ureterocele often led to massive reflux of the involved system. As a result, this procedure fell out of favor, except in cases of sepsis when urgent relief of obstruction was needed. However, improvements in equipment and refinements in technique have led to a re-evaluation of the role of ureterocele incision. Blythe and co-authors (1993) describe their technique of using a No. 3 Fr Bugbee

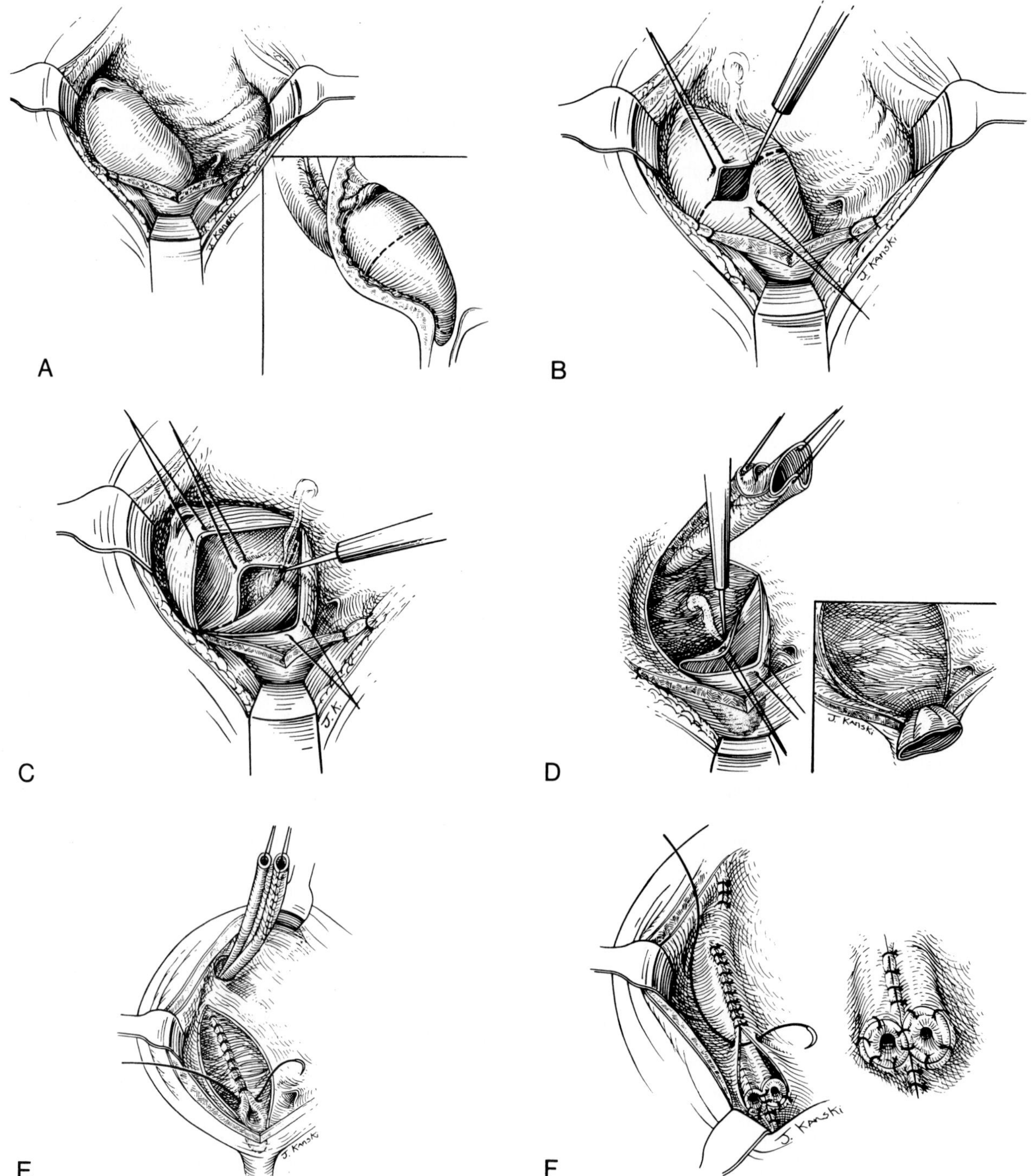

Figure 60–36. Technique for excision of ectopic ureterocele and common sheath reimplantation of upper and lower pole ureters.

A, Appearance of right-sided ureterocele with open bladder, viewed from below. Note proximity of the contralateral ureteral orifice. *Inset,* Cutaway side view demonstrating the close association of the two polar ureters with a common vascular supply. The dotted line indicates the planned initial incision of the ureterocele.

B, After stay sutures are placed, the ureterocele is incised with electrocautery in a transverse direction, exposing the inner cavity of the ureterocele.

C, The posterior mucosal wall of the ureterocele is incised transversely, revealing the often thinned posterior muscular wall of the bladder. This incision will then be continued around the bladder mucosal edge of the ureterocele, including the orifice of the lower pole ureter. Stay sutures are important to provide adequate exposure.

D, The upper and lower pole ureters have been mobilized and are retracted into the bladder. The distal aspect of the ureterocele is being mobilized in a similar fashion. The bladder mucosal surface will also be incised around the edge of the ureterocele to permit complete removal of the ureterocele. *Inset,* The fully mobilized distal ureterocele is retracted caudally, revealing its narrowing attachment at the bladder neck.

E, The dilated upper pole ureter associated with the ureterocele has been tapered and remains in continuity with the lower pole ureter. Both have been brought into the bladder through a newly formed muscular hiatus to provide adequate tunnel length for the ureteral reimplantation. The thinned-out posterior bladder wall has been repaired with multiple interrupted sutures to provide adequate muscular backing for the ureters. The bladder mucosa surrounding the ureterocele defect has been mobilized to permit covering of the ureters.

F, Left, The ureters have been reimplanted into the new ureteral tunnel, have been sutured distally after spatulation, and are being covered with bladder mucosa. The lower pole orifice is medial. *Right,* Final appearance of the ureteral orifices following completion of the reimplantation.

electrode to puncture the ureterocele near its base and proximal to the bladder neck. The new opening should have an intravesical position while the bladder is empty to avoid obstruction by the bladder neck. By using such a technique, obstruction is relieved while the roof of the ureterocele should collapse onto the floor of the bladder and act as a flap valve mechanism to prevent reflux. Using this technique, 73% of their patients needed no further procedures. However, when analyzing their data further, they concluded that intravesical ureteroceles fared better than ectopic ureteroceles with regard to decompression (93% versus 75%), preservation of upper pole function (96% versus 47%), newly created reflux (18% versus 47%), and need for secondary procedures (7% versus 50%). Based on these findings, they recommend ureterocele incision in all neonates as well as in older children with either an intravesical ureterocele, a ureterocele associated with a functioning upper pole, or a single-system ureterocele.

The authors have endoscopically incised ureteroceles in selected cases with similar success. In this series, ureterocele incision resulted in partial or complete decompression of all ureteroceles. More importantly, the radiographic appearance of the upper tract improved in 20 of 22 cases. Five of 12 children who had reflux into the ipsilateral lower pole had their reflux resolve following ureterocele incision, and three others had their reflux decrease in grade. Transurethral incision of the ureterocele resulted in reflux into the ureterocele ureter in 44% of the cases; this induced reflux was equivalent for ectopic and intravesical ureteroceles as well as single and duplicated systems. One third of the patients underwent a second operative procedure, primarily for reflux. One could argue that this minimally invasive outpatient procedure is of benefit to the remainder of the patients who require no further surgery.

We have made several observations based on our experience with transurethral incisions of ureteroceles. When performing routine cystoscopy in a female, it is acceptable to blindly pass the cystoscope sheath and obturator into the bladder via the urethra. However, blind passage of a cystoscope in a child with a ureterocele may result in a tearing of the ureterocele. Therefore, we pass the cystoscope under direct vision. In addition, we try to instill a minimum of irrigation so as not to collapse the ureterocele. The entire bladder is inspected to ascertain the position of the ipsilateral lower pole ureteral orifice and the contralateral ureteral orifice.

Our preferred method of incising the ureterocele is similar to the one described by Rich and colleagues (1990), that is, a transverse incision through the full thickness of the ureterocele wall using the cutting current. Making the incision as distally on the ureterocele and as close to the bladder floor as possible lessens the chance of postoperative reflux into the ureterocele. One can either use a Bugbee electrode or the metal stylet of a ureteral catheter, which is extended just beyond the catheter. We favor the latter instrument because it has a finer tip and allows for more precision. We also prefer to perform the incision under video projection because this magnification enhances accuracy.

In institutions where subureteric Teflon injections are an accepted means of treating reflux, an entirely endoscopic approach has been tried whereby the ureterocele is incised with electrocautery; if reflux occurs in the upper pole or persists in the lower pole, it is managed with Teflon injections (Diamond and Boston, 1987; Yachia, 1993).

Single-System Ureteroceles

Although the single-system ureterocele usually presents in adults, it is sometimes seen in children. The ureterocele in these cases is almost always intravesical and occupies the proper trigonal position. Although most simple ureteroceles have obstructing pinpoint orifices, unobstructed ureteroceles do exist. The degree of obstruction is probably not significant in most adult cases and likewise tends to be less severe than the obstruction seen in duplicated systems in children (Sen et al, 1992).

The ureterocele may vary in size from a tiny cystic dilatation of the submucosal ureter to that of a large balloon that fills the bladder. Histologically, the wall of the ureterocele contains varying degrees of attenuated smooth muscle bundles and fibrous tissue. The ureterocele is covered by vesical mucosa and lined with ureteral mucosa.

Most children with simple ureteroceles present with symptoms of urinary tract infection. Prenatal ultrasonography has detected other asymptomatic cases. Stasis and infection predispose the patient to stone formation in the ureterocele and upper urinary tract. Rarely, large simple ureteroceles prolapse through the bladder neck, causing urinary obstruction.

Excretory urography often demonstrates the characteristic cobra-head (or spring-onion) deformity—an area of increased density similar to the head of a cobra with a halo or less dense shadow around it (Fig. 60–37). The halo represents a filling defect, which is the ureterocele wall, and the oval density is contrast excreted into the ureterocele from the functioning kidney. Larger ureteroceles often fail to fill early with contrast material, resulting in a sizable filling defect in the bladder. These findings are associated with varying degrees of hydronephrosis and hydroureter. The upper urinary tract changes associated with a simple ureterocele are usually not as severe as those associated with an ectopic ureterocele. At cystoscopy, the ureterocele usually expands rhythmically with each peristaltic wave that fills it and then shrinks as a thin jet of urine drains, usually continuously, through the small orifice.

Single-system ureteroceles more readily lend themselves to transvesical excision and reimplantation, with any muscular defect corrected as necessary. These ureteroceles are also more amenable to endoscopic incision (Rich et al, 1990) and are less likely to exhibit postoperative reflux in the incised ureterocele.

Prolapsing Ureteroceles

A ureterocele that extends through the bladder neck and the urethra, and presents as a vaginal mass in girls is termed a prolapsing ureterocele (Orr and Glanton, 1953). This mass can be distinguished from other interlabial masses (such as rhabdomyosarcoma, urethral prolapse, hydrometrocolpos, and periurethral cysts) by virtue of its appearance and location (Witherington and Smith, 1979; Nussbaum and Lebowitz, 1983). The prolapsed ureterocele has a smooth round wall in comparison to the grapelike cluster that typifies rhabdomyosarcoma (see Fig. 60–26). The ureterocele occa-

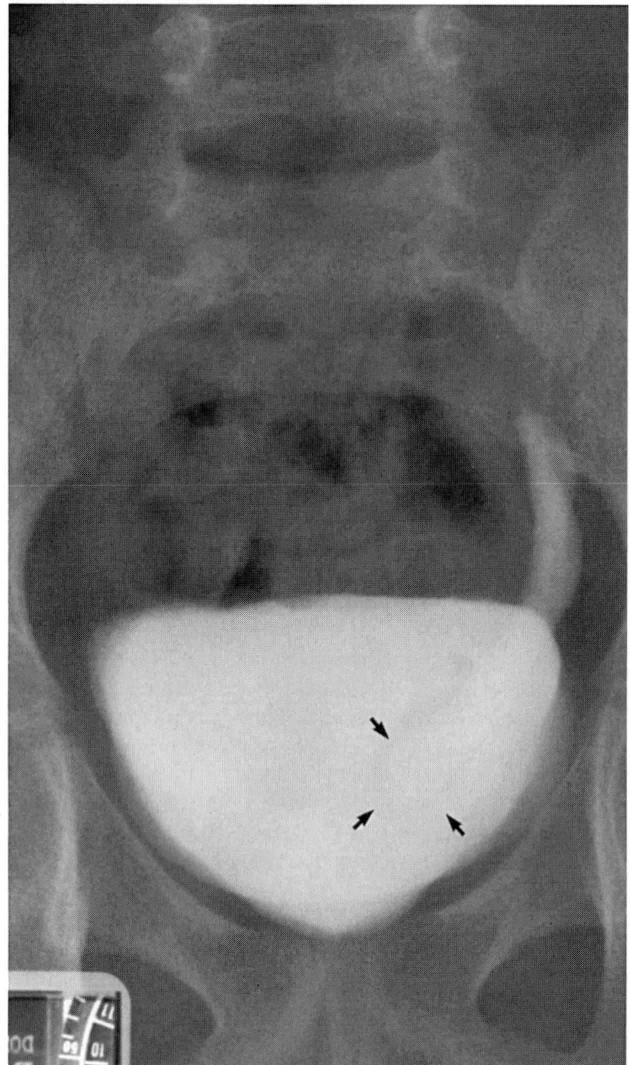

Figure 60–37. Contrast in the ureterocele from a functioning renal unit looks like a cobra head on intravenous pyelogram due to the filling defect of the ureterocele wall.

sionally has a tense, congested, and even necrotic appearance. The color may vary from pink to bright red to the necrotic shades of blue, purple, or brown. The ureterocele usually slides down the posterior wall of the urethra, and hence, the urethra can be demonstrated anterior to the mass and can be catheterized. The vagina (and the corresponding masses that emanate from it such as hydrometrocolpos) is posterior to the ureterocele.

The prolapse can be intermittent and may cause vesical obstruction and, therefore, bilateral renal obstruction. Alternatively, the children may be able to void around the ureterocele. In the former scenario, the patient may have varying degrees of hydronephrosis and azotemia, and may be septic.

The short-term goal is to decompress the ureterocele. The prolapsing ureterocele may be manually reduced back into the bladder; however, even if this is successful, the prolapse is likely to recur. Upper pole nephrectomy (as previously described) combined with aspiration of the ureterocele from above is usually effective in achieving decompression. However, this decompression may not occur rapidly enough in the acutely ill child. In an effort to decompress the ureterocele rapidly, one can make a transverse incision in the ureterocele at the level of the vagina. Because the wall of the ureterocele may be thick, the incision should be appropriately deep. This maneuver is not uniformly successful because the bladder neck in its resting state is closed and this may keep the intravesical ureterocele, which is proximal to the point of incision and proximal to the bladder neck, distended.

Therefore, if incision at the level of the vagina is not effective, endoscopic incision of the ureterocele in its intravesical portion may be necessary. If all of the abovementioned measures fail and the child remains in extremis, open surgical unroofing or marsupialization of the ureterocele is indicated. Common sheath ureteral reimplantation to correct the ensuing reflux can be carried out on an elective basis when the child is older.

Ureteral Stenosis and Stricture

Congenital anatomic narrowing or narrowing of the ureteral lumen as detected by calibration is referred to as congenital ureteral stenosis and congenital ureteral stricture, but developmentally, the term stricture should refer only to obstructions involving a histologic lesion in the ureter. Cussen (1971), in his series of 147 ureteral lesions, noted 81 (55%) with ureteral stenosis. His histologic studies of the stenotic zone revealed normal transitional epithelium, a diminished population of otherwise normal-appearing smooth muscle cells, and no increase in fibrous tissue in the wall of the stenotic zone. Ultrastructural studies were not conducted.

The cause of congenital ureteral stenosis is not certain, but ultrastructural studies such as those of Notley (1972) and Hanna and associates (1976, 1977) may provide the answer. Developmentally, simple narrowing probably results from a disturbance in embryogenesis around the 11th to 12th weeks, with disturbed development of the mesenchyme contributing to the ureteral musculature (Allen, 1977). A spectrum of histologic abnormalities, with or without demonstrable anatomic narrowing, may occur at the zone of obstruction (Hanna et al, 1976). The reader is referred to the previous discussion of megaureter for a description of the reported ultrastructural abnormalities. Three areas of the ureter are particularly liable to ureteral stenosis. They are, in order of decreasing frequency, the distal ureter just above the extravesical junction, the ureteropelvic junction, and rarely, the midureter at the pelvic brim (Allen, 1970; Campbell, 1970). More than one area of segmental stenosis may be present in the same ureter with a widened length of ureter between the segments, suggesting a developmental defect that affects the entire ureteric bud.

The clinical manifestations and treatment of ureteral stenosis and stricture involving the ureteropelvic junction are included in the section on ureteropelvic junction obstruction.

Ureteral Valves

Ureteral valves are uncommon causes of ureteral obstruction consisting of transverse folds of redundant mucosa that contain smooth muscle (Wall and Wachter, 1952). These

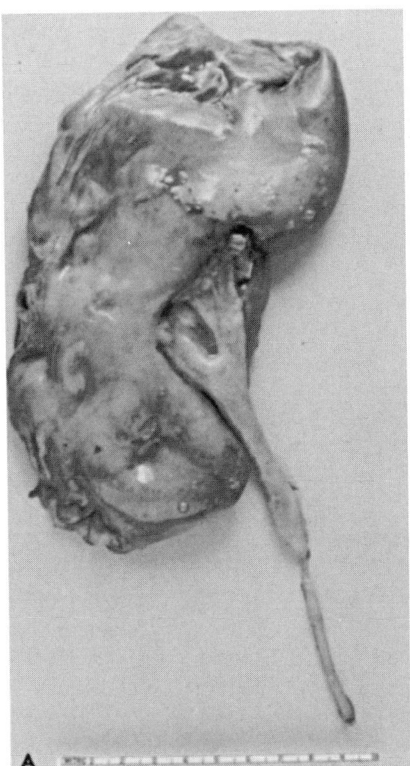

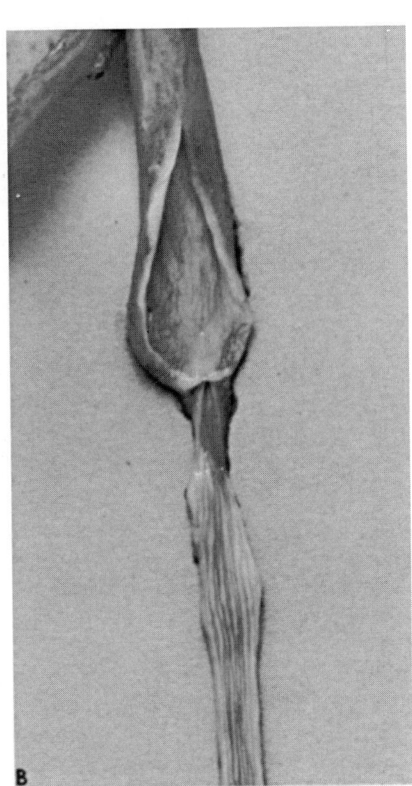

Figure 60–38. Congenital ureteral valve. *A,* Extended view. *B,* Long section showing greatly dilated ureter above the valve and normal size below. (From Simon HB, et al: J Urol 1955; 74:336.)

are single annular or diaphragmatic lesions with a pinpoint opening (Figs. 60–38 and 60–39). The ureter is dilated above the obstruction and normal below it. As determined in a review of 40 congenital ureteral valves, the valves are distributed throughout the length of the ureter, although least commonly in the middle third or the pelviureteral junction (Dajani et al, 1982). Presenting symptoms include flank pain, urinary tract infection, incontinence, hypertension, and hematuria. The valves appear to occur equally in boys and girls, and equally on the right and left sides (Sant et al, 1985).

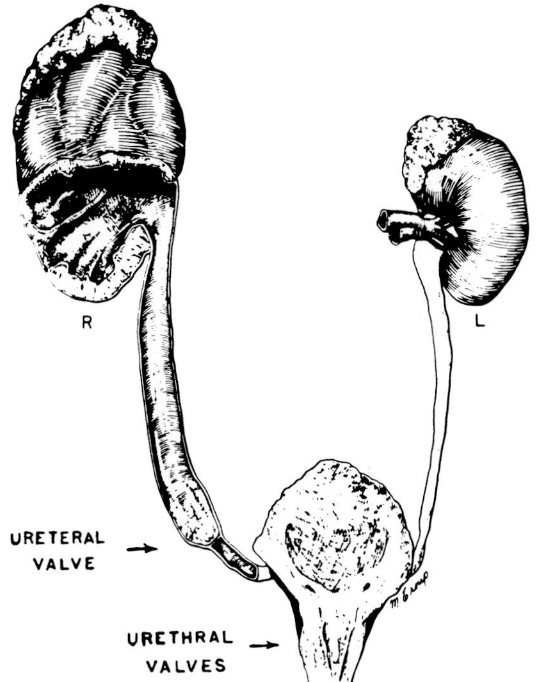

Figure 60–39. Complete diaphragm obstructing the right ureter, with hydroureter and hydronephrosis above. (From Roberts RR: J Urol 1956; 76:62.)

Transverse, nonobstructing mucosal folds are present in 5% of ureters in newborns and gradually disappear with growth (Wall and Wachter, 1952). They may be one of the normal findings described by Ostling (1942) and Kirks and associates (1978). Cussen (1971, 1977) has identified what he termed ureteral valves in 46 of 328 abnormal ureters from infants and children at surgery or at autopsy. Unlike the diaphragmatic valves described previously, these are cusps demonstrated by perfusing the upper ureter with fixative, dilating the lumen, flattening the mucosa, and accentuating the valves. In a patient with valvular obstruction, Cussen noted that the long axis of the distal ureter was eccentric relative to the long axis of the dilated proximal segment, with the fold being an eccentric cusp (Fig. 60–40). He also noted that these flaps could be found in the presence of a normal or stenotic distal ureter. In Cussen's series of 328 intrinsic ureteral lesions, he reported 24 primary valves with no distal obstruction, that is, the ureteral valves were considered the cause of obstruction. A total of 19 valves were reported to be in association with a more distal obstruction; these valves were thought to be either primary or secondary.

Others have observed ureteral obstructions from eccentric cusps, believed to be distinct from secondary folds and kinks associated with ureteral dilation and elongation (Maizels and Stephens, 1980; Gosalbez et al, 1983). The cusp need not contain smooth muscle (Gosalbez et al, 1983; Reinberg et al, 1987). However, Williams (1977) believed that eccentric

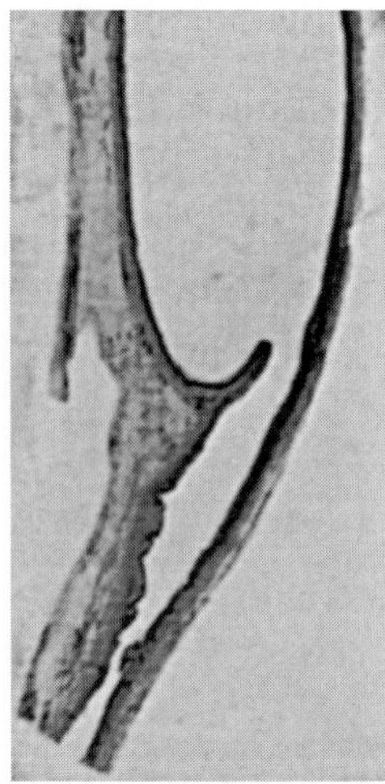

Figure 60–40. A 12-year-old girl with obstructing distal congenital ureteral valve in an ectopic, duplicated ureter. (Courtesy of Dr. Laurence R. Wharton.)

obstructing valves may be more infrequent than Cussen reported. Many of the apparent valves may be artifacts of distention because the dilated ureter at its junction with the undilated segment assumes a kinked and eccentric position resulting from elongation and pull of the surrounding adventitia.

In summary, diaphragmatic annular valves are a rare, although definite, form of ureteral obstruction. Eccentric, cusplike flaps or folds can be obstructing but can also be secondary to the elongation and tortuosity that occurs with ureteral distention at the site of an underlying anatomic or functional obstruction. It has been postulated that several of these anomalies may appear transiently in utero and may be responsible for the milder forms of hydronephrosis that are found postnatally to be nonobstructive. If the lesion is in fact obstructive, an intravenous pyelogram and a retrograde pyelogram should be obtained because these studies deliver the most complete anatomic information about the ureter. Resection of this obstructing lesion with primary reanastomosis is then curative. The involved kidney may be devoid of significant function and require nephrectomy (Sant, 1985).

Spiral Twists and Folds of the Ureter

Campbell (1970) observed this anomaly only twice in 12,080 autopsies in children (Fig. 60–41). He ascribed it to failure of the ureter to rotate with the kidney. This explanation may be simplistic, because the illustration shows more than one twist. Obstruction and hydronephrosis may result from spiral twists. The condition may arise from one of a number of possible persistent manifestations of normal fetal upper ureteral development, as described by Ostling (1942) (Figs. 60–41 and 60–42). These manifestations include ureteral mucosal redundancy, and apparent folds and convolutions that may have a spiral appearance. Radiographic evidence of such findings is often present in the excretory urograms of otherwise normal newborns. However, most of these folds gradually disappear with normal growth of the infant. Occasionally, ureteral convolutions that are enclosed by investing fascia persist as a form of ureteropelvic obstruction (Gross, 1953).

Persistent fetal folds are described in a previous paragraph. An isolated single fold or kink demonstrated radiographically with an otherwise normal upper urinary tract

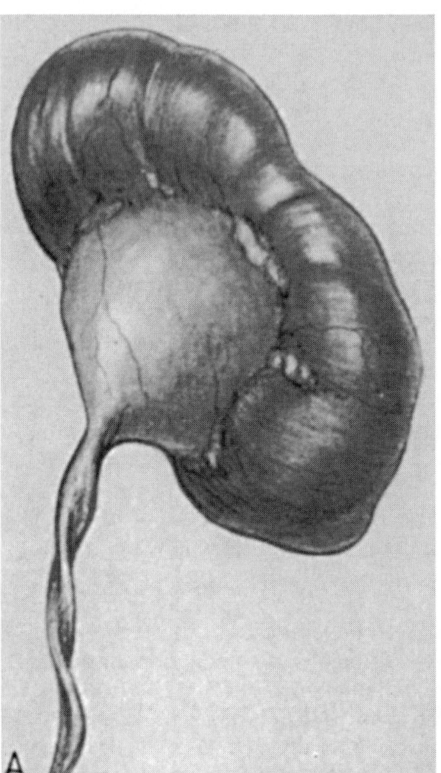

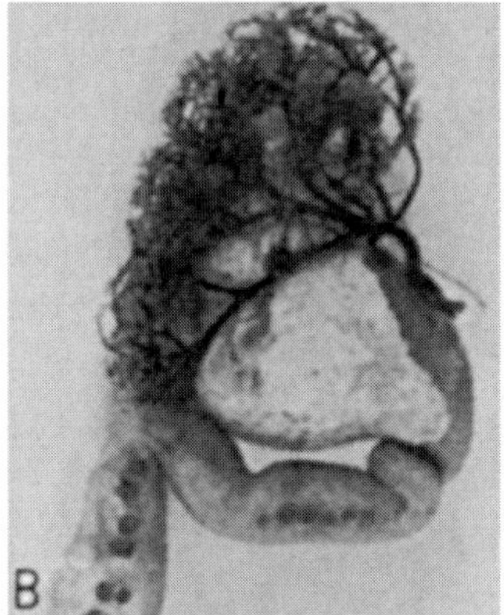

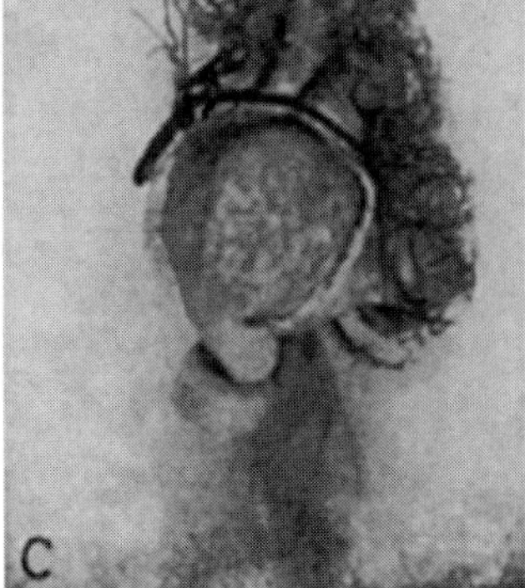

Figure 60–41. Torsion (spiral twists) of the ureter. *A*, Observed in an infant at autopsy. There is secondary hydronephrosis. *B* and *C*, Corrosion specimens from late fetal life. *B*, Anterior view. *C*, Lateral view from pelvic aspect. (Courtesy of Dr. Karl Östling.)

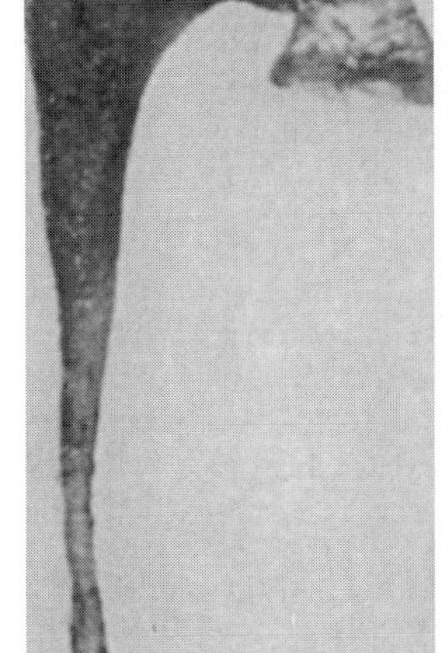

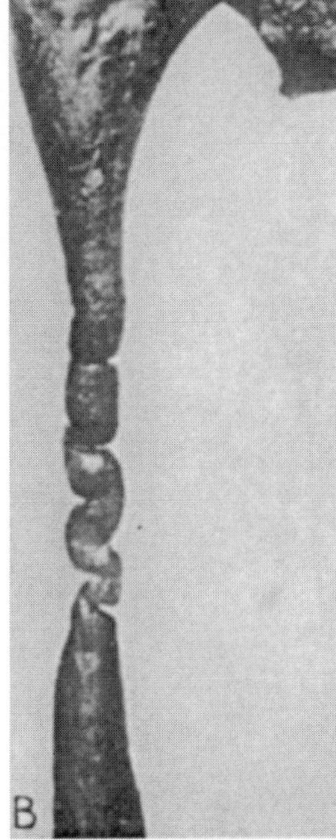

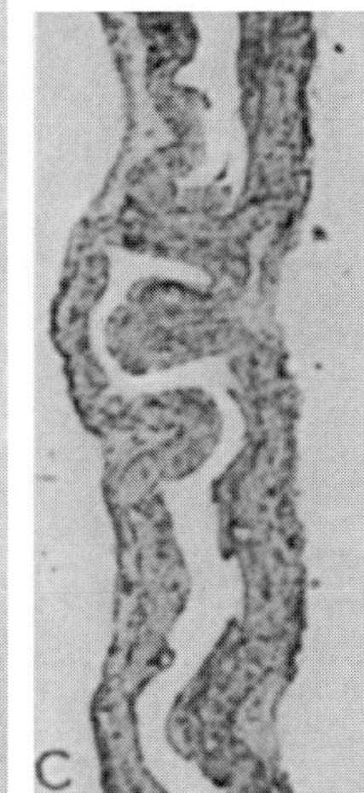

Figure 60–42. Embryologic considerations in the genesis of ureteral fold, kinks, and strictures.

A, Cast of the ureter and the renal pelvis in a newborn. There is physiologic narrowing of the upper ureter, below which is the normal main spindle of the ureter. No ureteral folds are present.

B, Cast of the ureter and the renal pelvis in the newborn. The ureteral folds proceed alternately from the opposite sides.

C, Ureteral kinks that appear as muscular folds with xial offshoots of the loose adventitia. (Courtesy of Dr. Karl Östling.) (From Campbell MF: *In* Campbell MF, Harrison JH, eds: Urology, Vol 2, 3rd ed. Philadelphia, W. B. Saunders Company, 1970.)

may be acquired, nonobstructing, and reversible, and represents acute or intermittent elongation of the ureter with distal obstruction or reflux. Campbell (1970) believed that isolated primary obstructing congenital kinks could occur as an uncommon disorder, but the example he presented did not demonstrate convincing obstruction. Nevertheless, this sort of deformity is often one manifestation of ureteropelvic junction obstruction in association with ensheathment by dense fibrous bands (Gross, 1953).

Ureteral Diverticula

Diverticula of the ureter have been classified by Gray and Skandalakis (1972) into three categories: (1) abortive ureteral duplications (blind-ending bifid ureters) (see Blind-Ending Duplication of the Ureter), (2) true congenital diverticula containing all tissue layers of the normal ureter, and (3) acquired diverticula representing mucosal herniations. Congenital diverticula are very uncommon and have been reported as arising from the distal ureter above the ureterovesical junction, midureter, and ureteropelvic junction (Culp, 1947; McGraw and Culp, 1952). These diverticula can become very large, and secondary hydronephrosis can ensue. The patient may present with abdominal pain or renal colic and a palpable cystic mass. McGraw and Culp's patient, a 64-year-old woman, had a cystic lesion at surgery, extending from under the right costal margin to the pelvic brim.

A typical diverticulum in a 20-year-old man is shown in Figure 60–43. Even small diverticula may be symptomatic. Sharma and co-workers (1981) reported on two patients—a man with repeated infections and a girl with intermittent colic. Fluoroscopy in the second patient demonstrated stasis and peristaltic dysfunction with back and forth ureter to diverticulum reflux. She was cured by diverticulectomy.

As discussed in the section on blind-ending duplications, congenital diverticula below the level of the ureteropelvic junction arise from premature cleavage of the ureteric bud with abortive development of the accessory limb. Those from the ureteropelvic junction region arise from primitive calyceal formation that similarly failed to encounter metanephric tissue (Gray and Skandalakis, 1972).

Single acquired diverticula may be associated with strictures or calculi and may follow trauma (Culp, 1947). Multiple diverticula that are small in size (under 5 mm) have been ascribed to the effect of chronic infection (Holly and Sumcad, 1957; Rank et al, 1960). However, Norman and Dubowy (1966) reported two cases of multiple diverticula that were demonstrable by retrograde ureteropyelography. Such lesions, demonstrable only by supraphysiologic pressures, may be congenital variants with weaknesses of the ureteral wall rather than acquired conditions (Hansen and Frost, 1978). However, the published reports do not contain histologic observations to support either hypothesis. Large diverticula can generally be removed without sacrificing the kidney.

Congenital High Insertion of the Ureter

This rare malformation may drain an otherwise normal and unobstructed kidney (Fig. 60–44). Most high insertions, however, are encountered with ureteropelvic junction obstruction, as is discussed elsewhere in this text.

ANOMALIES OF NUMBER

The reported incidence of ureteral duplication varies widely among different series, depending in part on whether

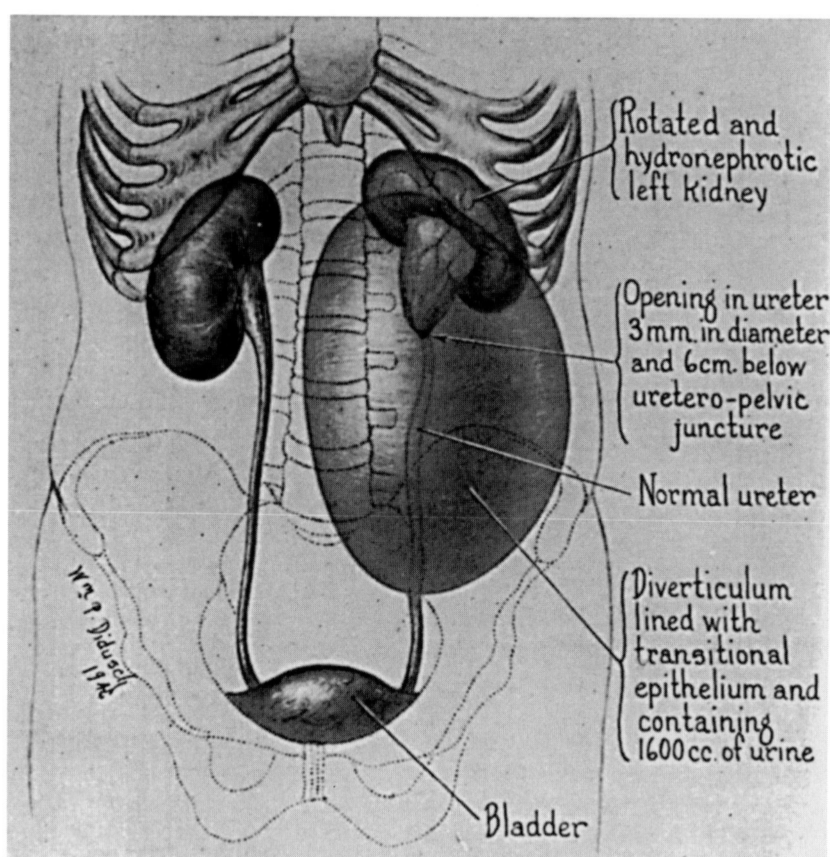

Figure 60–43. Congenital diverticulum of left ureter containing 1600 ml of urine. The kidney was hydronephrotic. (From Culp OS: J Urol 1947; 58:309.)

the survey was based on autopsy or clinical data and on the composition of patient material, and on whether or not bifid pelves were separately recorded (Fig. 60–45). Because it is generally recognized that clinical series usually contain a disproportionate number of duplication anomalies, unselected autopsy data are more accurate in predicting the true incidence. At least two large autopsy series have provided data not too dissimilar regarding partial and complete ureteral duplication (Nation, 1944; Campbell, 1970) (Table 60–3). Nation (1944) reviewed 230 cases of duplication; 121 of these were clinical. He identified 109 cases in approximately 16,000 autopsies, an incidence of one in 147, or 0.68%. Campbell's personal series of 51,880 autopsies in adults, infants, and children included 342 ureteral duplications, an incidence of one in 152, or 0.66%, but only 61 of the 19,046 children had this abnormality, one in 312, or 0.32%. Because

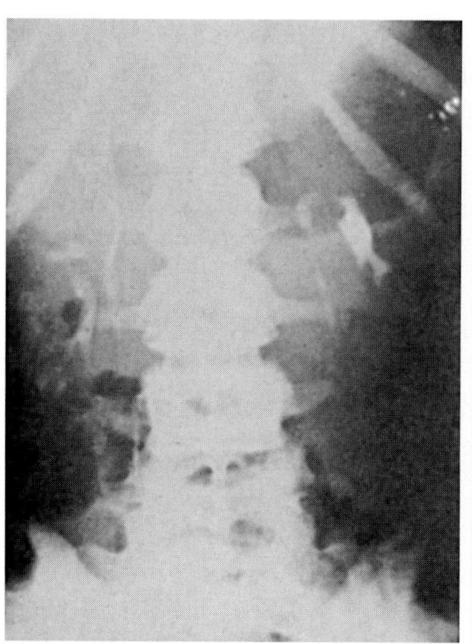

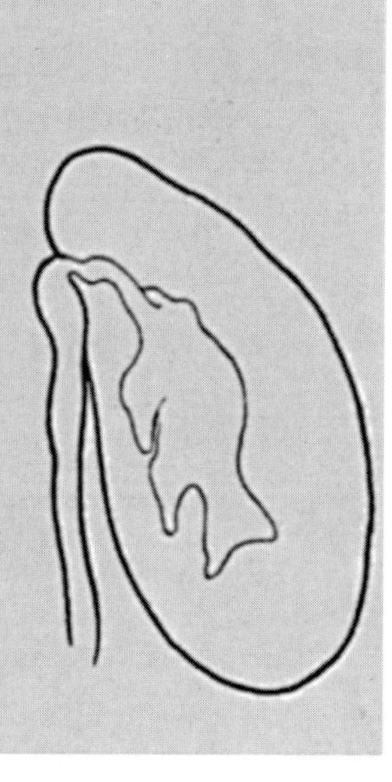

Figure 60–44. A 4-year-old girl with high ureteropelvic insertion and no obstruction.

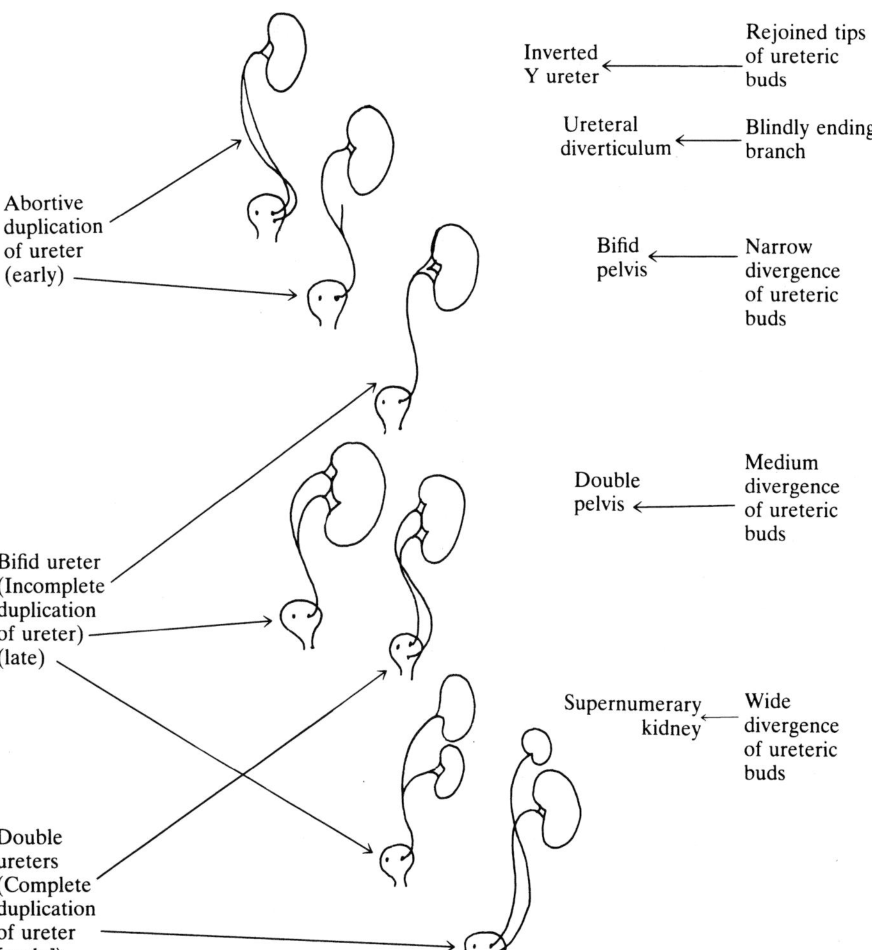

Figure 60–45. Gradations in ureteral and kidney duplications. (From Gray SW, Skandalakis JE, eds: Embryology for Surgeons. Philadelphia, W. B. Saunders Company, 1972.)

the anomaly should be found with equal frequency in unselected autopsies on adults or children, Campbell concluded that some of the duplications in children had been overlooked. Combining Nation's autopsy series and Campbell's adult series, the projected incidence of duplication is one in 125, or 0.8%.

Despite a wealth of information about sex differences in the incidence of duplication in clinical series (the anomaly is identified in women at least two times more frequently than in men), there are no reliable data on sex differences in unselected series. Campbell's autopsy data do not document such a difference. Of Nation's 109 autopsy cases, 56 were female and 53 male. However, only 40% of the 16,000 autopsies were performed in women. Calculating a correction for this difference, one could project a female-to-male ratio of 1.6:1, or 62%. These statistics, however, may not be reliable in view of the small number of cases recorded.

However, clinical and autopsy data are in substantial agreement about other aspects of duplication (see Table 60–3). Unilateral duplication occurs about six times more often than bilateral duplication, with the right and left sides being involved about equally. Excluding bifid pelvis, there does not appear to be a difference in the literature in the incidence of bifid ureter versus double ureters. A small percentage of individuals with bilateral duplications have a mixed condition, such as bifid ureter on one side and double ureters on the other.

Genetics

Evidence exists that duplication may be genetically determined by an autosomal dominant trait with incomplete penetrance (Cohen and Berant, 1976). In parents and siblings of probands with duplication, the incidence of duplication increases from the predicted one in 125 to one in eight (Whitaker and Danks, 1966) or one in nine (Atwell et al, 1974). Two reports of geographic foci suggest that environmental factors can also play a role (Philips et al, 1987; Barnes and McGeorge, 1989).

Position of Orifices

In double ureters, the two orifices are characteristically inverted in relation to the collecting systems they drain. The orifice to the lower pole ureter occupies the more cranial and lateral position, and that of the upper pole ureter has a caudal and medial position (see Fig. 60–12). As mentioned previously, this relationship is so consistent that it has been termed the Weigert-Meyer law, which is based on the original description of Weigert (1877) as modified by Meyer (1946). When the two orifices are not immediately adjacent, the orifice from the upper pole can be found anywhere along a predictable pathway, which Stephens (1958, 1963) has called the ectopic pathway (see Fig. 60–46).

Table 60–3. URETERAL DUPLICATION: CLINICAL, RADIOGRAPHIC, AND AUTOPSY STUDIES

Author, Year	Data Base		No. Duplications	Female	Male	Unilateral	Bilateral	Complete	Partial	Unilateral Complete/Partial	Bilateral Complete/Partial	Bilateral Mixed
Archangelskj, 1926		R	619			502 (80%)	117 (20%)					
	110	A	3 (2.7%)									
Colosimo, 1938	1500	X	50 (3.3%)	(68%)								
Nation, 1944	16000	A	109 (0.68%)	* (63%)	*							
		C	121	88 (73%)	33							
			230 total			177 (77%)	53 (23%)	102 (44%)	118 (51%)	78 (44%)/99 (56%)	35 (45%)/19 (36%)	10 (4.3%)
Nordmark, 1948	4744	X	138 (2.8%)			119 (86%)	19 (14%)	70 (51%)	65 (47%)	59/60	11/5	3 (2.1%)
Payne, 1959		C	141	87 (62%)	54	120 (85%)	21 (15%)	45	78 + 18 bifid pelvis			
	5000	X	83									
Johnston, 1961		C	73									
		A	9									
			82 total	57 (70%)	25			63 (77%)	19 (33%)			
Kaplan and Elkin, 1968	(Partial dupls. only)	X	51	33 (65%)	18	43 (84%)	8 (16%)					
Campbell, 1970	51880	A	342 (0.65%)			293 (85%)	53 (15%)	101 (30%)			4	"one in five cases"
	(19046 child)		61 (0.32%)									
	(32834 adult)		281 (0.85%)									
Timothy et al, 1971		C	46	39 (85%)	7			24 (52%)	16 (35%)	13/15	11/1	6 (13%)
Privett et al, 1976	5196 (1716 child) (3480 adult) (2896 male) (2300 female)	X	91 (1.8%)	63 (66%)	32	79 (85%)	16 (15%)	33 (29%) (but 21 not known)	57 (52%)			

A = Autopsy.
C = Clinical.
R = Review.
X = X-ray.
* = See text.

Rare exceptions to the Weigert-Meyer law have been observed, in which the upper pole orifice is cranial, although it is still medial to the orthotopic orifice. Stephens (1958) collected four examples from the literature and added seven more. Stephens studied the positional relationship between the lower portions of the ureters and noted that it, too, varies according to the terminal position of the upper pole orifice. With the rare cranially placed upper pole orifice, the ureter lies anterior to the lower pole ureter, with the ureters being uncrossed. With a medial orifice, the upper pole ureter lies medially, and with a caudally placed orifice, it spirals in an anterior-to-medial direction around the lower pole ureter as it descends, terminating posterior to the lower pole orifice. Ahmed and Pope (1986) documented a case of uncrossed complete ureteral duplication and reflux into the upper pole, which fits this pattern.

An embryonic hypothesis to explain the exception to the Weigert-Meyer law was proposed by Stephens (1958) and is based on the premise that an upper pole orifice located craniomedially arises from a junctional ureteric bud—one that bifurcated immediately—rather than from a second bud. The embryology is diagrammed in Figure 60–46.

Associated Findings

The distribution of the renal mass drained by each ureter in duplication varies somewhat. On average, about one third of the renal parenchyma is served by the upper collecting system. In a detailed radiographic review, Privett and associates (1976) reported a number of observations about duplication. The mean total number of calyces for single-system kidneys was 9.4, and for duplex units it was 11.3, with a mean of 3.7 calyces in the upper collecting system and 7.6 in the lower collecting system. These investigators also observed that 97% of the single-system kidneys in their series were radiographically normal, whereas 29% of the duplex units had scarring or dilatation, or both. Reflux also was more common in the duplex units in patients who had voiding cystograms. Two of 17 nonduplex units generated reflux (12%) compared with 13 of 31 duplex units (42%).

Hydronephrosis of the lower pole segment is not infrequent and is generally associated with severe reflux into that unit. However, primary ureteropelvic junction obstruction can involve the lower pelvis (Dahl, 1975; Christofferson and Iversen, 1976; Privett et al, 1976).

Other anomalies are encountered with increased frequency. In Nation's (1944) series, 27 (12%) had other urinary tract anomalies, with just over half of these being on the same side. The anomalies included renal hypoplasia and aplasia (today these conditions would probably be termed dysplasia) and various ureteral anomalies, among them ectopic insertion of the upper pole ureter in four cases (3% of the complete duplications). Coexisting urologic anomalies were encountered in 29 of Campbell's (1970) series of 342 duplications. Nonurologic anomalies were found in 63 cases. These were not recorded in detail, but most of the urologic anomalies were, as in Nation's series, a variety of ipsilateral renal and ureteral lesions; 22 were anomalies of the contralateral kidney. The nonurologic lesions mainly involved the gastrointestinal tract plus a few cardiopulmonary lesions. Both of these series, however, were autopsy series. Rarely,

URETER DUPLICATION

normal development

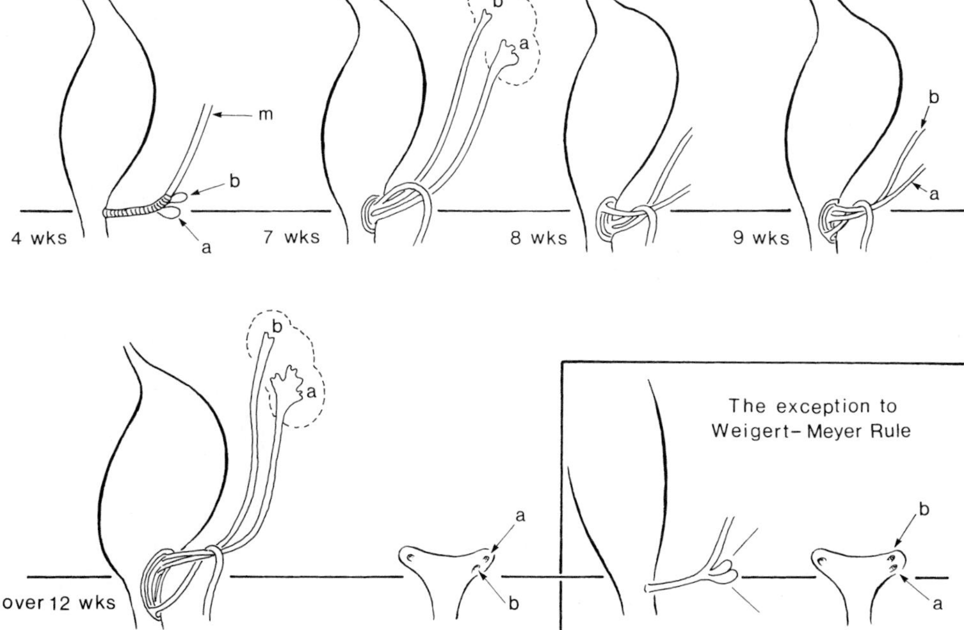

Figure 60–46. Simplified diagram of the changing position of the ureters and mesonephric duct in the development of complete duplication. a, lower pole ureter; b, upper pole ureter; m, mesonephric duct. (Redrawn from Tanagho EA: Urology 1976; 7:451.)

the pelvicalyceal systems communicate, presumably from later fusion of the ureteric buds during pelvicalyceal expansion (Braasch, 1912; Beer and Mencher, 1938).

The increased incidence of duplications in investigations of childhood urinary infections is well established. Campbell (1970) reported a personal series of 1102 children with pyuria, 307 of whom proved to have ureteropelvic anomalies. Of these, 82 (27%) were duplications, or 7.5% of the total group. Kretschmer (1937) reviewed 101 cases of hydronephrosis in infancy and childhood, and noted 24 nonureteral anomalies, over half of which were duplications.

Based on three cases of duplication with some form of ureteral ectopy, coexistent renal dysplasia, and nodular renal blastema, Cromie and colleagues (1980) raised the possibility that this pattern of findings might be more than a coincidental association, accounting for an increased risk of neoplasm (Pendergrass, 1976). This concept deserves further investigation.

Bifid ureter is often clinically unimportant, but stasis and pyelonephritis do occur. When the Y junction is extravesical, free to-and-fro peristalsis of urine from one collecting system to the other may appear, with preferential retrograde waves passing into slightly dilated limbs instead of down the common stem. This results in stasis that is more marked when the Y junction is more distal, when the bifid limbs are wide, or when the Y junction is large. Increased urinary reprocessing from vesicoureteral reflux may enhance this phenomenon, and loin pain can result. About one quarter of the patients studied with nuclear renography by O'Reilly and co-workers (1984) had significant urodynamic abnormalities. Treatment by ureteroneocystostomy is effective when the junction is sufficiently close to the vesical wall that resection of the common sheath or common stem permits placement of both orifices within the bladder. Reimplantation of the common stem may be effective when vesicoureteral reflux is severe and the Y junction is higher up. In the absence of reflux, ureteropyelostomy or pyelopyelostomy with resection of one ureteral limb, preferably the upper limb, down to the Y junction is effective in eliminating regurgitation of urine (Lenaghan, 1962; Kaplan and Elkin, 1968).

Blind-Ending Duplication of the Ureter

Rarely, a ureteral duplication does not drain a renal segment; hence, the term blind-ending. Less than 70 of these anomalies have been reported, although they occur considerably less infrequently than the published data indicate. Most blind-ending ureteral duplications involve one limb of a bifid system; even more unusual is one involving complete duplication (Szokoly et al, 1974; Jablonski et al, 1978). Although the Y junction in the bifid type may be at any level, most are found in the midureter or distal ureter. Blind-ending segments are diagnosed three times more frequently in women than in men and twice as often on the right side (Schultze, 1967; Albers et al, 1971). The condition has been reported in twins (Bergman et al, 1977) and in sisters (Aragona et al, 1987). Many of these blind segments cause no problems. Symptomatic patients most often complain of vague abdominal or chronic flank pain, sometimes complicated by infection or calculi, or both (Marshall and McLoughlin, 1978). The majority of cases are not diagnosed until the third or fourth decade of life.

Because the blind segment does not always fill on excretory urography, retrograde pyelography may be required for diagnosis (Fig. 60–47). At times, however, urinary stasis from disordered peristalsis (ureteroureteral reflux) may be demonstrated (Lenaghan, 1962), with secondary dilatation of the branch. This may be the cause of the pain (van Helsdingen, 1975). Because the lesion is more common in women and on the right side, the propensity for dilation of the right urinary tract with pregnancy might explain the relatively late onset of symptoms.

Embryology

The embryogenesis of blind-ending ureteral duplication is similar to that for duplications in general. It is postulated

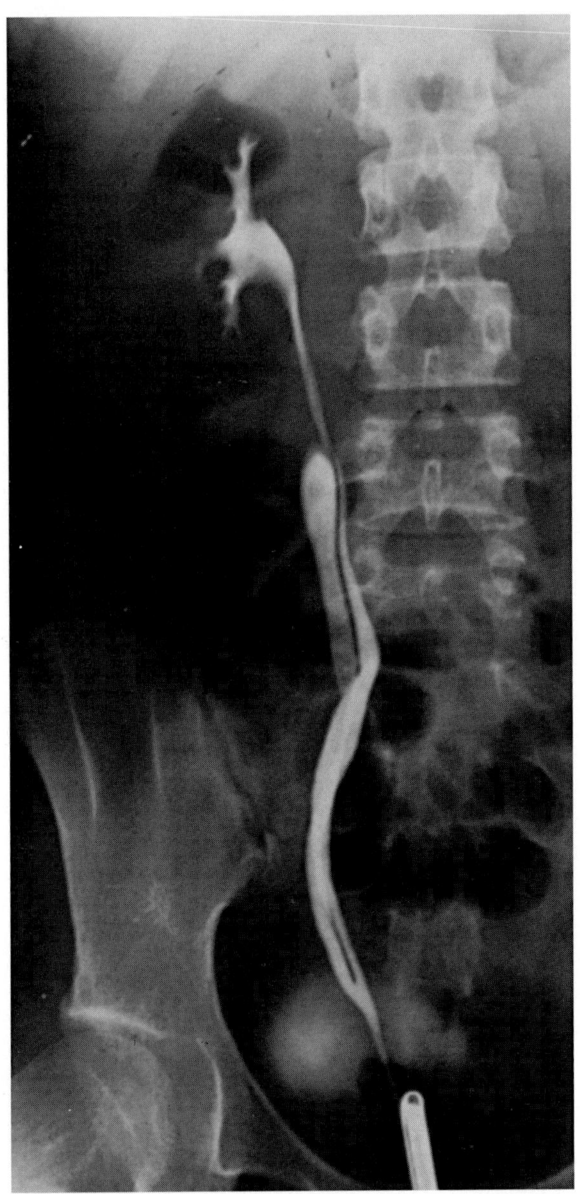

Figure 60–47. Retrograde pyelogram. Blind-ending duplication in an 18-year-old girl noted in evaluation of transitory hematuria. Only the distal portion of this blind-ending duplication has been visualized on intravenous pyelogram.

ation is borne out by similar studies of children with infections and with asymptomatic bacteriuria (Smellie et al, 1975; Walker et al, 1977). An explanation for this finding is based on the spontaneous resolution of reflux that occurs in many children with interval growth of the bladder and elongation of ureteral tunnel length (see later in this chapter).

RACE. It should be noted that the majority of studies on reflux come from North America, Northern Europe, and Scandinavia. **White girls are ten times more likely to have reflux than their black American counterparts** (Askari and Belman, 1982), and black girls are less likely to have reflux when evaluated for urinary infection. However, once reflux is discovered, its grade and chances of spontaneous resolution are similar in both races (Skoog and Belman, 1991). Others have suggested an increased risk in fair-skinned children with blue eyes and blond hair (Manley, 1981) or red-haired children alone (Urrutia and Lebowitz, 1983). The prevalence of reflux in many other countries and races has not been defined.

SPECIES SPECIFICITY. Reflux commonly occurs in other animals. Rabbits, rats, and other rodents are almost uniformly affected yet never suffer any measurable loss of renal function (Gruber, 1929). A high incidence (80%) has been observed in puppies, though resolution by adulthood is the rule (Christie, 1971). Reflux is also found in other primates at variable rates that are both species- and age-specific. Interestingly, resolution occurs in rhesus monkeys, who are phylogenetically neighbors of humans, at rates that are similar to those noted in children with urinary infection (Roberts, 1974; Walker, 1991).

Inheritance

Like most genitourinary anomalies, vesicoureteral reflux appears to have a multifactorial origin, although a genetic component undoubtedly exists. **Siblings of patients with reflux have a much greater risk of having reflux than the normal population.** Up to 45% of siblings have been noted to have reflux (Van den Abbeele et al, 1987; Noe, 1992). **Notably, the large majority (75%) are asymptomatic.** Contrary to the findings in some earlier studies, there appears to be no relationship between the grade of reflux in index patients and that in their siblings. The presence of renal scars in the index case is probably also less important than was once supposed. There is a higher incidence in sisters of females with reflux.

The first large study to address this issue was performed by Dwoskin, who found reflux in 26% of siblings from 125 families of probands with reflux (Dwoskin, 1976). A subsequent report by Jerkins and Noe (1982) cited a 33% incidence in over 100 siblings of 78 index cases. Two follow-up studies by Noe have been revealing. The first noted a higher incidence of sibling reflux in probands without bladder dysfunction (38%) compared with those with bladder dysfunction (20%) (Noe, 1988). The second study placed a greater emphasis on **parent-to-child transmission** than on sibling-to-sibling transmission. In a select group of 23 parents with a known history of reflux, 24 of 36 (66%) progeny were also found to have the problem. In 69% of cases the mother was primarily affected, and reflux was discovered in 77% of female and 43% of male children (Noe, 1992b). **Although a polygenic mode of transmission is favored by some investigators** (Burger and Smith, 1971), **this type of data suggests a dominant inheritance pattern with variable penetrance.**

CLINICAL CORRELATE. The innocuous nature of sibling reflux amplifies the need for some form of screening. In Noe's study (1992) of 119 children with sibling reflux, 15 (13%) showed renal damage by excretory urography. In a smaller group of 16 children diagnosed with the condition who had never had urinary infections, renal scintigraphy (using dimercaptosuccinic acid [DMSA]) showed scarring in six (38%) (Buonomo et al, 1993). Voiding cystography is indicated as a screening test for reflux in babies and young children. In older children urinary ultrasonography should be performed. Although this study may not detect lower grades of reflux, families can be reassured that the kidneys are not grossly abnormal. Periodic checks of the blood pressure and urine are also appropriate. The appearance of one urinary infection or the presence of upper tract scarring or hydronephrosis also warrants further evaluation with standard or radionuclide cystography, which remain the only definitive tests for reflux (Van den Abbeele et al, 1987).

ETIOLOGY AND PATHOGENESIS

Anatomic Considerations

The normal ureter propels boluses of urine into the bladder in an antegrade fashion. To achieve this end certain criteria must be met. First, the three muscular layers (inner longitudinal, middle circular, and outer longitudinal) of the ureter must initiate effective peristalsis in response to a stretch reflex caused by the bolus. Second, the pressures in the recipient bladder must be low enough to allow the free egress of urine. Finally, the ureterovesical junction must occlude with the increases in pressure that inevitably occur with bladder filling or contraction. **To achieve this "flap-valve" effect, the intravesical ureter ideally has an oblique course as it enters the bladder, proper muscular attachments to provide fixation and posterior support to enable its occlusion, and adequate submucosal length** (Harrison, 1888; Johnson, 1962; King et al, 1974) (Fig. 61–1).

As the ureter approaches the bladder, its muscular layers disperse. The circular layer and the ureteral adventitia meld into the detrusor in the upper part of the hiatus to form Waldeyer's sheath, which attaches the ureter to the bladder. Distally, the longitudinal muscles continue alone with the submucosal intravesical ureter. Along this course the muscle fibers become decussated and interspersed with the detrusor musculature to form the borders of the superficial trigone. Some longitudinal fibers project beyond the ureteral orifice to meet those of the contralateral ureter, creating Bell's muscle of the posterior urethra. Others pass medially to form Mercier's bar and the intraureteric ridge (Mathisen, 1964).

Functional Correlates

The ureterovesical complex functions as a single unit that has both passive and active components. When a bolus of urine approaches the hiatus, the intravesical longitu-

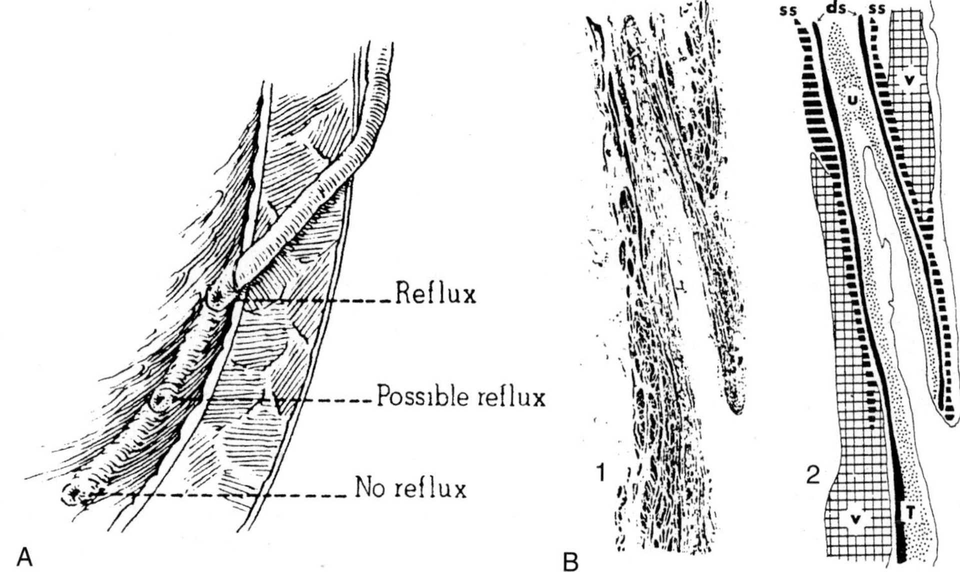

Figure 61–1. *A,* Refluxing ureterovesical junction has same anatomic features as nonrefluxing orifice, except for inadequate length of intravesical submucosal ureter. Some orifices with marginal submucosal tunnels may reflux intermittently. (From Glenn J, ed: Urologic Surgery, 2nd ed. New York, Harper & Row, 1975.) *B,* Ureterovesical junction in longitudinal section. 1, Photomicrograph. 2, Diagrammatic representation. Ureteral muscularis **(u)** is surrounded by superficial **(ss)** and deep **(ds)** periureteral sheaths, which extend in the roof of the submucosal segment and continue beyond the orifice into trigonal muscle **(T).** Relationship of superficial sheath to vesical muscularis **(v)** is clearly seen. Transverse fascicles in superior lip of ureteral orifice belong to superficial and deep sheaths. No true space seperates ureter from bladder. (From Elhadaiwi A: J Urol 1992; 107:224.)

dinal muscles contract. This action pulls the orifice toward the hiatus to shorten and widen the intravesical ureter, thus reducing resistance. The peristaltic pressures of the ureter (usually between 20 and 35 mm Hg) sufficiently propel the bolus into the bladder, which typically has low resting pressures (8 to 12 mm Hg). After the ureter relaxes it returns to its normal position beneath the bladder mucosa. Here a passive flap-valve mechanism prevents reflux during bladder filling. The intravesical ureter, a delicate and supple structure sandwiched between mucosa and the muscle, coapts with resting bladder pressure. During micturition, the longitudinal muscles of the ureterovesical junction close the meatus and submucosal tunnel to provide an "active" component during bladder contraction.

Primary Reflux

Primary reflux is a congenital anomaly of the ureterovesical junction in which a deficiency of the longitudinal muscle of the intravesical ureter results in an inadequate valvular mechanism. The factor most critical to a competent ureterovesical junction is the length of submucosal ureter relative to its diameter. Large-caliber ureters or those having short intravesical segments cannot be effectively shut by the junction's valvular mechanisms. **In one study a 5:1 ratio of tunnel length to ureteral diameter was found in normal children without reflux.** In contrast, children with reflux had a 1.4:1 ratio (Paquin, 1959). The relationship between intravesical (intramural and submucosal) ureteral length and ureteral diameter in normal children is shown in Table 61–2. Hutch estimated that the intravesical ureter averages 0.5 cm in neonates and 1.3 cm in adults (Hutch, 1961). Although the 5:1 ratio sets the standard for reimplantation surgery, it may not be absolutely necessary to achieve this ratio to obviate reflux.

Secondary Reflux

Anatomic and Functional Causes

Secondary reflux is that caused by bladder obstruction and its consequent elevated pressures. Such obstructions are ***anatomic*** or ***functional,*** although the outcomes can be the same. The chronicity and degree of obstruction undoubtedly influence the severity of secondary reflux. **The most common anatomic cause is posterior urethral valves, which are associated with reflux in approximately 50% of affected boys** (Henneberry and Stevens, 1980). Anatomic obstructions in females are extremely rare, although ureteroceles can block the bladder outlet and distort the anatomic relationships of the trigone in both sexes. Urethral stenosis remains commonly (and incorrectly) implicated by some urologists. **Instead, functional causes are far more com-**

Table 61–2. URETERAL TUNNEL LENGTHS AND DIAMETERS IN NORMAL CHILDREN (mean in mm)

Age (years)	Intravesical Ureteral Length	Submucosal Ureteral Length	Ureteral Diameter at Ureterovesical Junction
1–3	7	3	1.4
3–6	7	3	1.7
6–9	9	4	2.0
9–12	12	6	1.9

From Paquin AJ: J Urol 1959; 82:573.

mon in both sexes. These include ***neurogenic bladder, non-neurogenic neurogenic bladder,*** and ***bladder instability*** or dysfunction.

Any child with altered bladder dynamics is at risk for developing reflux. A poorly compliant bladder or abnormal interplay of the bladder with the urinary sphincter can result in increased intravesical pressure. This can gradually weaken and overcome the ureteral sphincter mechanism at the ureterovesical junction, causing reflux in patients with a previously normal response. **Patients with spina bifida and other types of neurogenic bladder are particularly prone to the development of reflux** (Bauer et al, 1982). Children with sacral agenesis or external signs of occult spinal dysraphism including a hair patch, sacral dimple, aberrant gluteal cleft, or decreased rectal tone or perineal sensation are also at risk.

In other cases, bladder dysfunction is apparently an acquired phenomenon resulting from abnormal voiding patterns in neurologically normal children. Young children commonly demonstrate a labile, infantile-type response to bladder filling in the form of uninhibited contractions. The child, who is typically in the early stages of toilet training and is attempting to maintain continence, responds to this instability by contracting the external sphincter (Allen, 1979). Variable degrees of incontinence result depending on the threshold volume for contractions and the effectiveness of the sphincter. Continence can be maintained but at the expense of abnormally elevated intravesical pressures. Complete emptying occurs, at least initially. On the far end of the spectrum are children with *non-neurogenic neurogenic bladders.* Here constriction of the urinary sphincter occurs during voiding in a voluntary form of detrusor-sphincter dyssynergia. Gradual bladder decompensation results in the presence of incomplete emptying and increasing amounts of residual urine. In addition, as many as 75% of children with this syndrome also have bladder instability (Hinman, 1986; Mayo and Burns, 1990).

The intravesical pressures seen with bladder dysfunction can be impressive, and vesicoureteral reflux is their common sequelae. Reflux is a common finding at presentation in children with non-neurogenic neurogenic bladders (Fig. 61–2). Koff and Murtaugh noted reflux in nearly 50% of children who were urodynamically evaluated for voiding dysfunction (Koff and Murtaugh, 1983). **Conversely, the most common urodynamic abnormality in patients with reflux is uninhibited bladder contractions** (Homsy et al, 1985). These were found in 75% of girls with reflux in one series (Taylor, 1982). Interestingly, both reflux and bladder dysfunction peak between the ages of 3 and 5 years. The normal ureterovesical junction is extremely resistant to reflux, even in the presence of the intermittently exceptional pressures that occur with normal voiding (greater than 100 cm of water in some young boys). Yet the sustained effects of chronically elevated intravesical pressures take a toll. **Decreases in bladder wall compliance, detrusor decompensation, and incomplete emptying gradually damage the complex anatomic relationships required of the ureterovesical junction.** The development of reflux further impairs bladder emptying and amplifies resting and filling pressures, thus initiating a self-perpetuating cycle of upper and lower urinary tract damage (Koff, 1992a). Immature bladders and ureters are especially prone to this sequence of events, though a similar scenario sometimes occurs in adults with bladder outlet obstruction.

Clinical Correlates

The identification and treatment of secondary causes of reflux often brings about its spontaneous resolution unless the ureterovesical junction has been irreparably damaged. In addition, failure to do so significantly jeopardizes any surgery that might inadvertently be done to correct the problem. The importance of identification is emphasized by the findings of the European arm of the International Reflux Study in Children (IRSC), which noted more frequent breakthrough urinary infections, greater variability in follow-up reflux grade, and increased persistence of reflux in patients with untreated bladder dysfunction (Van Gool et al, 1992). **The initial management of functional causes of reflux is medical. It is important for clinicians to inquire about and determine the voiding patterns of children with reflux.**

In addition to a careful physical examination, signs or symptoms of voiding dysfunction include dribbling, urgency, incontinence, and curtseying. Encopresis and constipation also suggest abnormal toilet behavior and altered dynamics of the external sphincter. Constipation is also associated with recurrent urinary infections (O'Regan et al, 1985). Incomplete evacuation, residual urine on voiding studies or ultrasonography, and a thick bladder wall or multiple diverticula are other suggestive findings.

Treatment of bladder dysfunction and instability, regardless of severity or cause, is directed at dampening uninhibited contractions and lowering intravesical pressures. Neurologically normal children with reflux and uninhibited bladder contractions who were treated with anticholinergics showed statistically different rates of resolution compared to normal children with a combination of reflux and bladder hyperreflexia and/or some degree of abnormal urinary sphincter activity. Oxybutynin contributed to the resolution or downgrading of reflux in 62% of ureters in 37 children in one report (Homsy et al, 1985). In another study in which diazepam, baclofen, or other muscle-relaxing agents were used in 53 children, reflux resolved in 92% of ureters and decreased in the remainder (Seruca, 1989).

There is a strong association between intravesical pressures of more than 40 cm of water and the presence of reflux in patients with myelodysplasia and neuropathic bladders. If pressures at typical capacity (average catheterization volume) or leak point are kept below this standard, reflux often resolves, even when it is significant (Flood et al, 1994). High-grade reflux (grades III to V) either ceased or lessened in 18 of 33 patients (55%) with myelodysplasia when intravesical pressures were lowered and emptying was facilitated. In a larger series of 200 myelodysplastic patients with neurogenic bladder, reflux lessened or resolved in 124 (62%) (Kaplan and Firlit, 1983). When medical management is unsuccessful in correcting abnormal bladder dynamics and resolving secondary reflux, enterocystoplasty, vesicostomy, or some other form of urinary diversion becomes a necessary option in management.

When residual urine is present, a finding that can be amplified by the yo-yo effect of high-grade reflux, treatment is directed at facilitating emptying. In normal children with-

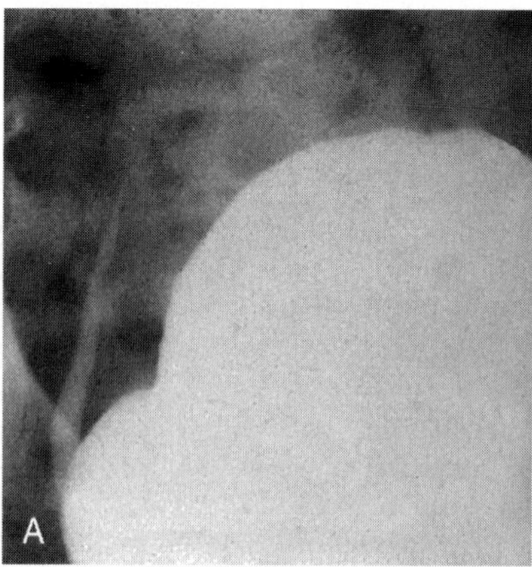
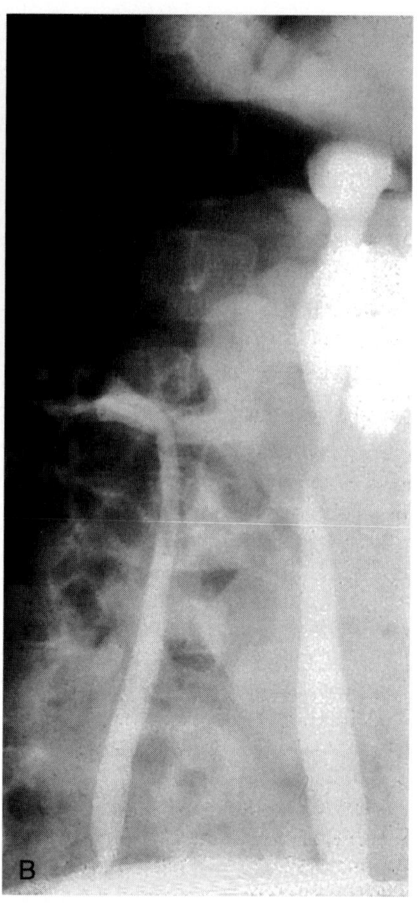

Figure 61–2. *A,* Voiding cystogram in a child having urinary accidents, encopresis, and recurrent urinary infections. Large bladder and incomplete emptying were not addressed. *B,* Two years later, reflux is now bilateral to level of kidneys. Variable reflux is common finding with voiding dysfunction.

out bladder dysfunction, this includes double voiding. Otherwise, relaxation techniques or biofeedback aimed at lessening constriction of the external sphincter is sometimes successful in patients with a non-neurogenic neurogenic picture (Hellstrom, 1987b). Occasionally, intermittent catheterization combined with medication becomes the key to management (Lapides et al, 1972).

Lower Urinary Tract Infection

Bladder infection (urinary tract infections [UTI]) and their accompanying inflammation can also cause reflux by lessening compliance, elevating intravesical pressures, and distorting and weakening the ureterovesical junction (Van Gool and Tanagho, 1977). The ureteral atony caused by gram-negative endotoxins can also be a contributing factor (Jeffs and Allen, 1962). For the same reasons, the spontaneous resolution of reflux normally expected of some ureters may be delayed (Roberts and Riopelle, 1978). In some patients transient reflux occurs only during episodes of acute cystitis that resolves with treatment and the dissipation of inflammation (Kaplan, 1980). The immature or damaged ureterovesical junction may be particularly prone to this phenomenon. The cystitis that results from the chemotherapeutic agent Cytoxan can have a similar effect.

Clinical Correlates

Because of the bladder changes that result from cystitis, the recommendation for the timing of voiding cystourography (VCUG) remains open to debate. Some clinicians defer the study for a few weeks to allow the inflammation to resolve and to avoid so-called false-positive studies. This approach, however, risks overlooking reflux that occurs only with infection, so others perform the study during its active phase. If parenteral antibiotics have been taken for a few days, the latter course seems reasonable because cystography itself poses little risk in the presence of reflux without bacteriuria. Finally, because residual urine is a fertile medium for bacteria and also potentially alters bladder dynamics, additional attention is given to complete bladder emptying in any patient who has recurrent urinary infections, whether reflux is present or not.

CLASSIFICATION AND GRADING

Several systems for grading vesicoureteral reflux have been proposed in the past three decades. In the early classifications reflux was graded in relation to the physiologic state of the bladder. The terms high pressure and low pressure were introduced to describe reflux that occurred during bladder emptying or bladder filling (Hinman and Hutch, 1962; Lattimer et al, 1963; Melick et al, 1962; Smellie and Normand, 1968). Later classifications relied on the degree of pelvicalyceal dilatation as well as ureteral diameter (Bridge and Roe, 1969; Heikel and Parkkulainen, 1966; Howerton and Lich, 1963; Dwoskin and Perlmutter, 1973; Rolleston et al, 1975). The Heikel and Parkkulainen system gained popularity in Europe a few years before the Dwoskin

Table 61–3. INTERNATIONAL CLASSIFICATION OF VESICOURETERAL REFLUX

Grade I	Into the nondilated ureter
Grade II	Into the pelvis and calyces without dilation
Grade III	Mild to moderate dilation of the ureter, renal pelvis, and calyces with minimal blunting of the fornices
Grade IV	Moderate ureteral tortuosity and dilation of the pelvis and calyces
Grade V	Gross dilation of the ureter, pelvis, and calyces, loss of papillary impressions, and ureteral tortuosity

and Perlmutter system became widely accepted in the United States. **The International Classification System** devised by the International Reflux Study represents a meld of the two systems and **provides the current standard for grading that is based on the appearance of contrast in the ureter and upper collecting system during voiding cystourethrography** (International Reflux Study Committee, 1981) (Table 61–3 and Fig. 61–3). Because reflux appears as a continuum on cystography, any grading system suffers from being somewhat arbitrary (Lebowitz, 1992). However, a classification system that is widely accepted allows for sequential comparisons in individual patients and comparisons of different patients or groups of patients despite this and other drawbacks.

One shortcoming of the International Classification System and other systems based primarily on calyceal appearance is that the degree of ureteral dilatation may not correlate with the degree of pyelocalyceal dilatation. Some lower ureteral segments are impressively dilated yet are associated with little if any proximal reflux. Whether the natural history of these segments is similar to that of ureters of the caliber typically found with similar grades of reflux remains unclear (Fig. 61–4). In addition, inconsistencies occur because the degree of ureteral dilatation can vary with bladder pressure and filling at the time of each film. Finally, accurate grading of reflux is impossible if coexisting ipsilateral obstruction is present. If obstruction is unrecognized, the grade of reflux will be falsely elevated. The permanent calyceal distortion associated with postinfection scarring or nonobstructive dilatation can also lead to overestimation of the severity of reflux. To be accurate, grading systems must reflect the degree of primary reflux unaltered by associated pathology (Lebowitz, 1992).

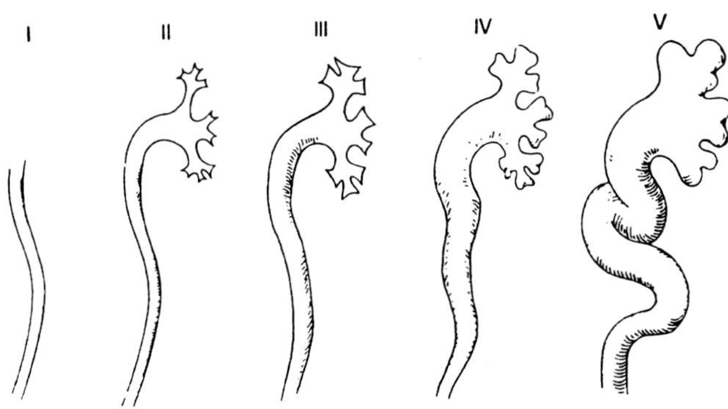

Figure 61–3. International classification of vesicoureteral reflux.

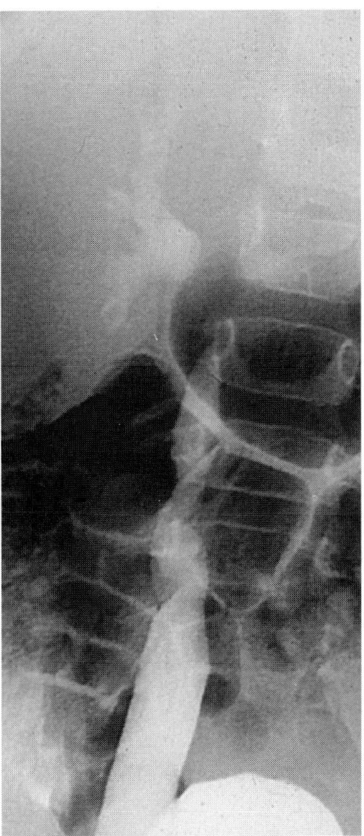

Figure 61–4. Refluxing ureter with significant dilatation of lower segment but no distortion of collecting system may be different from typical system with grade II reflux.

Other problems arise during comparisons of standard voiding cystourethrography and radionuclide cystography (RNC), which is commonly used for follow-up screening (see later discussion). **Classifying reflux with RNC is difficult because it is impossible to assess ureteral and pelvicalyceal anatomy accurately with radionuclide tracer.** In response to this dilemma, Willi and Treves (1985) devised a system for grading RNC that correlates closely with the International Classification System. The three degrees of reflux identified within this schema are shown in Figure 61–5. Nevertheless, **when management decisions depend on comparisons of grade and trends in the degree of reflux, it is preferrable to revert to standard cystography.**

DIAGNOSIS AND EVALUATION

Clinical Presentations

Most patients with reflux present initially with some symptoms that suggest a UTI, although newborns typi-

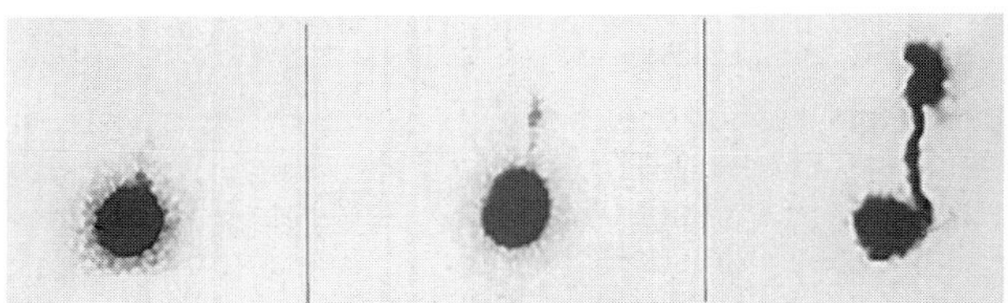

Figure 61–5. Nuclear voiding cystogram showing right-sided reflux. Radionuclide tracer can be quantitated as (from left to right) Grade 1, Grade I International Grading System; Grade 2, Grade II to III International Grading System; Grade 3, Grade IV to V International Grading System.

cally show nonspecific symptoms. Failure to thrive and lethargy are worrisome signs, whereas high fevers are uncommon. Infants and younger children arrive with fever, malodorous urine, dysuria and urinary frequency, lethargy, and gastrointestinal symptoms including nausea and vomiting. Pyelonephritis usually causes vague abdominal discomfort rather than localized flank pain. Even in the absence of an infection, children and adults with vesicoureteral reflux sometimes describe abdominal or flank discomfort, usually with a full bladder or immediately after voiding. When reflux has gone undetected and renal scarring has occurred, children of any age can present with renal insufficiency, hypertension, and impaired somatic growth.

To summarize, **a urine culture should be included in the evaluation of any infant or child who presents with fever or malaise.** Unfortunately, UTIs and reflux are often overlooked, and their ill-defined presentations are mistakenly attributed to otitis media, viral gastroenteritis, respiratory infections, or fever of unknown origin. Until a proper diagnosis is made, severe renal damage can be incurred. **The presence of fever may be an indicator of upper urinary tract involvement but is not always a reliable sign** (Farnsworth et al, 1991). However, if fever (and presumably pyelonephritis) is present, the likelihood of discovering vesicoureteral reflux is significantly increased (Govan and Palmer, 1969; Woodard and Holden, 1976; Smellie et al, 1981). A variety of laboratory tests have been used to localize infection including B_2-macroglobulin, lactic dehydrogenase, and antibody-coated bacteria, but these are of equivocal value (Neal, 1989). Elevated cytokines including interleukin-1β, interleukin-6, and interleukin-8 have also been observed in patients with acute urinary infections, and interleukin-8 may provide a marker of renal scarring (Haraoka et al, 1996).

Documenting Urinary Tract Infections

When a urinary tract infection is suspected from the clinical history, a urine culture is essential for making the diagnosis. Microscopy alone may not provide a valid assessment of the urine, although the use of dipsticks combined with microscopy increases sensitivity. Specimens should be immediately refrigerated at 4°C until they can be cultured. The method of collection also is extremely important. **In toilet-trained children, a *midstream-voided* specimen is adequate.** The first portion of the urine, which contains the bulk of the bacterial contaminant of the periurethral region, is omitted. Any growth of greater than 100,000 colonies per high-power field per milliliter of urine (CFU/ml) is considered significant from a midstream specimen. ***Catheterization* is also an excellent way of obtaining a urine sample with minimal contamination and is the preferred method in infants or older children. Contamination is suspected in specimens collected otherwise.** Catheterized specimens with bacterial counts of more than 1000 CFU/ml are considered significant. Finally, ***suprapubic aspiration* is the most sensitive but challenging means of assessing bacteriuria in children.** Many children void during the procedure because of anxiety or pain, making collection difficult. In addition, needle trauma can cause microscopic hematuria that clouds the diagnostic picture. When the bladder is not extremely full, ultrasonic needle guidance is helpful. Any growth from a suprapubic aspiration sample warrants further evaluation. **Collection of urine specimens with *adhesive bags* is the most widely used method, but the least reliable.** These specimens carry a high risk of contamination and should probably be condemned in the symptomatic patient. Approximately 10% of samples yield growths of greater than 50,000 CFU/ml that have no correlation whatsoever with actual urinary infection (Wettergren, 1985). Bagged specimens may also be unreliable despite yielding pure growths of more than 100,000 CFU/ml.

Evaluating Urinary Tract Infections

Vesicoureteral reflux is found in 29% to 50% of children with UTIs (International Reflux Study Committee, 1981). Approximately 30% of these already have some evidence of renal parenchymal scarring that is usually proportional to the severity of reflux (Bellinger and Duckett, 1984; Blickman et al, 1985). Baker and colleagues (1966) found that reflux was more commonly associated with UTIs in younger children. In contrast, Smellie and associates did not find any age-related differences in the incidence of reflux in children with urinary infections. In addition, there were thought to be no reliable clinical features that distinguished children with reflux from those without (Smellie et al, 1981; Johnson et al, 1985). **Renal scarring can occur after only a single UTI, even in the absence of fever** (Ransley and Risdon, 1981; Smellie et al, 1985; Rushton et al, 1992). These data amplify the need for a thorough evaluation of any child in whom a urinary infection is suspected.

The diagnostic work-up is tailored to the individual according to age, gender, and clinical history. **Complete evaluations that include voiding cystourethrography (VCUG) and ultrasonography are required in three groups of patients: any child under the age of 5 years with a valid documented UTI; children with a febrile UTI regardless of age; and any boy with a UTI unless he is sexually active or has a past urologic history** (Burbige et al, 1984). Children who have had one UTI are highly prone (80% to 85%) to have another. As many as half are asymptomatic. As a result, **work-ups are recommended after the first urinary infection to rule out anatomic risk factors.** If none are present, parents can be reassured that the urinary tract is normal and that further UTIs should generally remain confined to the lower urinary tract and do not pose a serious health threat. Therapeutic efforts are then directed at improving the child's toilet hygiene (timed voids, relaxation to facilitate emptying, treatment of constipation, and so on). Older children who present with asymptomatic bacteriuria or UTIs that manifest solely with lower tract symptoms can be initially screened with ultrasonography alone, reserving cystography for those with abnormal upper tracts or recalcitrant infections. Radiographic evaluations of black children are usually reserved for those with recurrent or febrile UTIs because of the low incidence of the anomaly in such children (Askari and Belman, 1982). Finally, detection of asymptomatic reflux is becoming increasingly common because the anomaly is the cause of many cases of antenatally diagnosed hydronephrosis (Fig. 61–6). **Newborns with a moderate to severe degree of upper tract dilatation should be fully evaluated with VCUG, as should any baby who had**

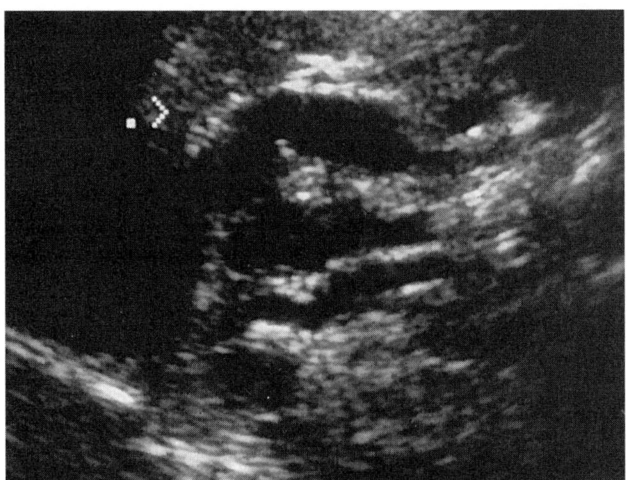

Figure 61–6. Antenatal ultrasound demonstrates bilateral ureteral and pelvic dilatation. Reflux is a common cause of such a finding.

intermittent hydronephrosis as a fetus, another common presentation of the problem. Postnatal ultrasound examination alone is a poor screening technique for reflux in the neonate; it was normal in 25% of patients with antenatal hydronephrosis who had reflux on voiding cystourethrography (Lebowitz, 1993).

Lower Urinary Tract Assessment—Cystography

The presence of vesicoureteral reflux can be established with either fluoroscopic or radionuclide voiding cystography, though certain factors affect the diagnostic yield. **Some reflux can only be appreciated during detrusor contractions and active voiding, making it easy to miss in the anxious or stubborn child who is unable to void** (Poznanski and Poznanski, 1969). **Cystograms performed with a Foley catheter or while the patient is anesthetized are static studies that inaccurately screen for reflux or sometimes exaggerate its degree because of bladder overfilling.** In addition, general anesthesia can also influence the severity of reflux by reducing glomerular filtration and urinary output (Mazze et al, 1963). As a result, studies performed under general anesthesia are of equivocal value. Conversely, excessive hydration may mask low grades of reflux because diuresis can blunt the retrograde flow of urine (Ekman et al, 1966). Finally, some reflux is demonstrated only during active infection when cystitis weakens the ureterovesical junction with edema or increases intravesical pressure (Van-Gool and Tanagho, 1977; Kaplan, 1980). In addition, cystograms obtained during active infections can overestimate the grade of reflux because the endotoxins produced by some gram-negative organisms can paralyze ureteral smooth muscle and exaggerate ureteral dilatation (Roberts, 1975; Boyarsky et al, 1978; Hellstrom et al, 1987). **Unless the detection of infection-related reflux will alter management or there is a social situation that warrants a prompt evaluation, most radiologists advise performing the voiding cystourethrogram after an infection-free period of a few weeks.**

Fluoroscopic VCUG is an outpatient procedure that should provide more information than mere anatomic detail. Children who are old enough are asked to void in the bathroom. After the perimeatal area is cleansed, a small-caliber lubricated feeding tube (No. 5 Fr in newborns, 8 Fr in others) is placed through the urethra into the bladder. The postvoid residual urine is measured, and a sample is sent for culture. Diluted contrast agent is then instilled via gravity (not to exceed 100 cm H_2O) under fluoroscopic control. Given the small catheter sizes used, the intravesical pressures generated during gravity filling are independent of the height of the bottle (Koff et al, 1979). Once the contrast agent ceases to drip, the bladder capacity can be calculated from the end-point of infusion. Intermittent fluoroscopic scans are used to assess the presence of reflux during filling and voiding. A complete VCUG also includes views of the ureterovesical junctions and urethra during voiding, and a film of the bladder after voiding is a useful way to assess emptying. When reflux is present, delayed films are obtained to assess upper tract drainage. Contrast material that is refluxed proximally should return readily to the bladder. Its hang up may implicate a coexisting obstruction in the renal moiety. Leibovic and Lebowitz (1980) showed that a comprehensive voiding study can be completed using a minimum (average 36 seconds) of fluoroscopic time. **The accuracy of cystography is improved by repeating the procedure during several cycles of filling and voiding.** In one study of cyclic cystography, a 12% increase in incidence of reflux or change in grade was seen when the procedure was repeated (Paltiel, 1992). Cyclic voiding cystourethrography is time intensive and requires more fluoroscopic exposure but is indicated in patients in whom reflux that is not appreciated on a single-sequence study is strongly suspected (Jequier and Jequier, 1989; Paltiel et al, 1992).

Nuclear cystography (RNC) is the scintigraphic equivalent of conventional cystography. **Although the technique does not provide the anatomic detail of fluoroscopic studies, it is an accurate method for detecting and following reflux.** Technetium-99m pertechnetate, instilled into the bladder in saline, provides doses of radiation that are 100-fold lower than those of a standard VCUG (Blaufox et al, 1971). **In addition to minimizing radiation exposure, the technique allows prolonged observation under the gamma camera, which enhances sensitivity** (Fig. 61–7). These advantages make nuclear cystography an effective means of screening for reflux, for following reflux after its initial grading and anatomic detail has been obtained by standard VCUG, and for making sure that the reflux has resolved after corrective surgery. When reflux is initially discovered by RNC, VCUG often becomes necessary to grade reflux more accurately and better delineate the lower urinary tract anatomy (Willi and Treves, 1983).

Indirect cystography uses intravenously injected technetium-99m diethyl-enetriamine-pentan-acetic acid (Pollet et al, 1981). This agent is cleared by glomerular filtration and excreted into the bladder within 20 minutes. The child can then be scanned for reflux, thus avoiding catheterization (Conway et al, 1975). Unfortunately, the method has a high percentage of false-negative studies and is particularly unreliable in patients with milder grades of reflux.

Ultrasonic cystography offers an ideal screening tool for reflux because there is no exposure to radiation. Sonicated

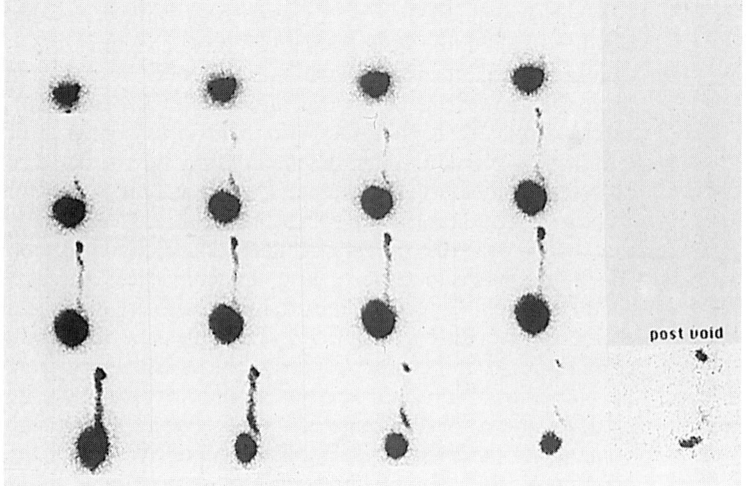

Figure 61–7. Radionuclide cystogram shows right-sided reflux that worsens with bladder filling. Upper collecting system drains with voiding.

human serum albumin, composed of three to five times 108 air-filled echogenic spheres per milliliter, can be detected by ultrasound and has been successfully used to detect reflux in animal models (Fig. 61–8) (Atala et al, 1993c) and in preliminary studies in humans (Atala et al, 1994c). Until the latter are completed, the modality must be considered a research tool.

Diagnostic Drawbacks

It is important to know whether reflux is present before upper tract functional studies are completed (excretory urogram, renal scintigraphy) **because reflux can cause both under- and overestimation of renal function** (Lebowitz and Avni, 1980; Blickman et al, 1985). For example, contrast material or radionuclide excreted from one kidney can reflux into a nonfunctioning contralateral partner to mimic function. Conversely, the reflux of nonopaque or unlabeled urine into the collecting system of a kidney with good function can dilute excreted material, causing underestimation of function. **To avoid such artifacts, catheter drainage of the bladder is required in any renal functional studies in known refluxers.** To avoid multiple manipulations, catheters are also placed before the performance of functional studies that precede the VCUG in patients undergoing initial evaluation.

Upper Tract Assessment

***Ultrasonography* has replaced the excretory urogram (intravenous pyelogram [IVP]) as the diagnostic study of choice in the initial evaluation of the upper urinary tract in patients with suspected or proven vesicoureteral reflux. Ultrasound alone cannot effectively rule out reflux, especially the lower grades of reflux that do not cause renal pelvic dilatation, and VCUG is required in children in whom reflux is suspected** (Scott et al, 1991; Blane et al, 1993). However, the information gleaned from the study can be invaluable. Urinary ultrasound includes views of the bladder as well as the kidneys and offers baseline assessments of overall renal size, parenchymal thickness, and the presence of scars, hydronephrosis, or other renal and ureteral anomalies (Fig. 61–9). Postvoid residual urine and bladder wall thickness are also useful information in children with suspected bladder dysfunction. A yearly ultrasound examination is recommended in patients with reflux who are being medically managed to follow interval renal growth and to detect grossly evident renal scarring, although the study does not provide the sensitivity of scintigraphy in defining subtleties of the latter (see later discussion). Some centers also advocate serial sonography for a few years after the resolution of reflux to monitor long-term renal development.

Doppler ultrasound allows visualization of the ureteric

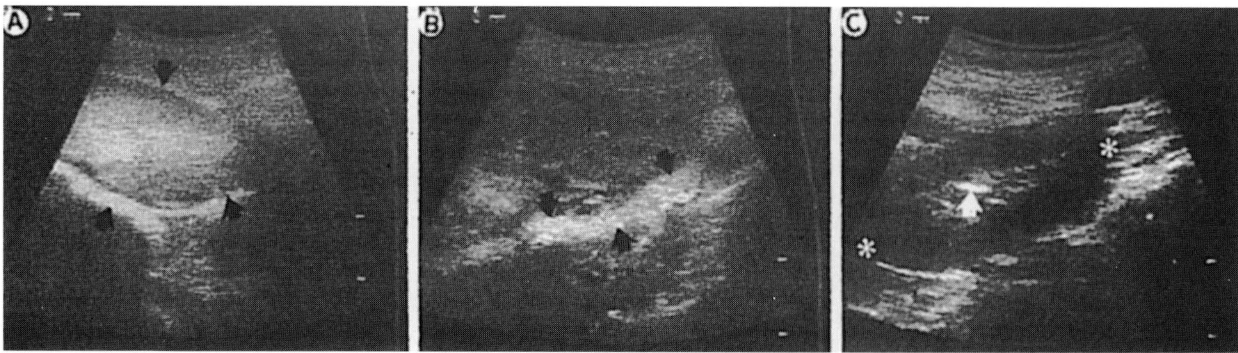

Figure 61–8. Sonographic visualization of sonicated albumin. *A,* diffuse echogenicity produced in bladder by filling it with albumin and saline *(arrows outline bladder). B,* Sonicated albumin that refluxes into ureter produces bright echogenic band *(arrows). C,* Echogenic area caused by albumin that has refluxed into renal pelvis.

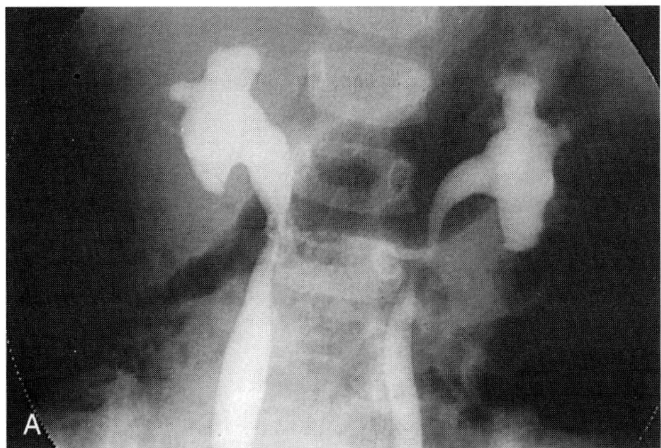

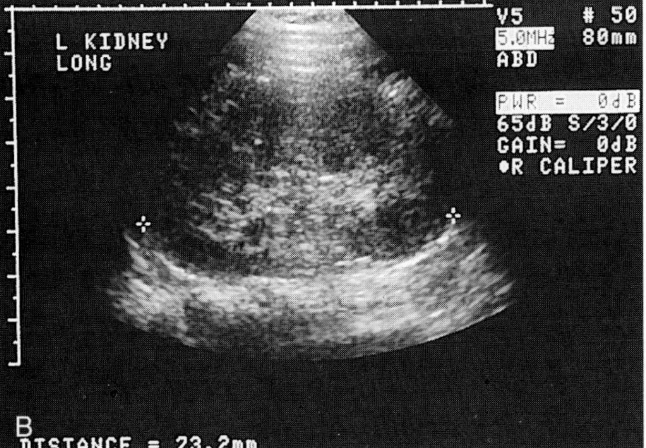

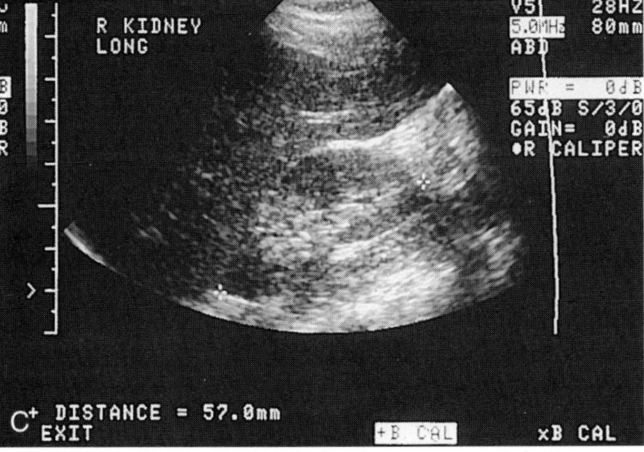

Figure 61–9. *A,* Bilateral reflux (R, V; L, IV). Ultrasound shows *B,* normal left kidney (73 mm length). *C,* Small, scarred right kidney (57 mm) with significant thinning of the upper pole.

jet created by the passage of a urine bolus through the ureterovesical junction. Usually, two to six peristaltic waves occur per minute (Elejalde and DeElejalde, 1983). Color Doppler facilitates visualization of the anteromedially directed jet in the bladder. Although severe renal parenchymal scarring reduces the frequency and amplitude of jets, Doppler analysis fails to allow the diagnosis or exclusion of reflux (Jequier et al, 1990; Marshall et al, 1990).

Functional studies are required in patients with severely scarred kidneys when the question of salvagability is raised. A baseline functional study is also usually obtained in anticipation of reimplantation surgery but is probably unnecessary with a normal renal ultrasound. Several findings on excretory urography suggest the presence of reflux. These include pyelonephritic scarring without obstruction (Claesson and Lindberg, 1977), renal growth retardation (Ginalski et al, 1985), and the presence of a retrograde ureteral jet on the bladder phase of an IVP (Kuhns et al, 1977). Any of these findings in a patient with or without suspected reflux prompt further evaluation with voiding cystography.

Excretory urography (IVP) once provided the gold standard for the imaging of kidneys associated with reflux. Rough measures of function and assessment of scars and parenchymal thinning are gradually being displaced by the more sophisticated information provided by scintigraphy (Fig. 61–10).

Renal scintigraphy **using technetium-99m (^{99m}Tc) labeled DMSA is the best study for detecting pyelonephritis and the cortical renal scarring that sometimes results.** Radionuclide uptake is directly proportional to functional proximal tubular mass and correlates well with glomerular filtration rates (Taylor, 1982). Pyelonephritis impairs tubular uptake and causes areas of photon deficiency in the cortical outline. Many cases completely resolve, especially with prompt medical treatment, but others persist as actual scars resulting from irreparable tubular damage (Rushton et al, 1988). A 98% specificity and a 92% sensitivity in detecting renal scars was noted in a study of 79 children who were followed for 1 to 4 years after a proven urinary infection (Merrick et al, 1980). The role of scintigraphy is changing with the altered understanding of upper urinary tract infections. Contrary to historical belief, **pyelonephritis does not usually result from infection that relies on reflux as its delivery system but from infection alone** (Bjorgvinsson et al, 1991). This was recently shown in a prospective study performed by Majd and colleagues, who found that 63% of children (mean age 3 years) with DMSA-proven pyelonephritis did not have vesicoureteral reflux, even when evaluated for it at the same admission (Majd et al, 1991). A similar prevalence of cortical defects in the absence of reflux was also noted by Ditchfield and his associates (Ditchfield et al, 1994).

High-resolution single-photon emission computerized tomography (SPECT), which involves 360-degree imaging and computer reconstruction, was proposed as another means of obtaining greater renal cortical detail (Joseph et al, 1990). This technology, which has the capacity to provide coronal, sagittal, and transaxial imaging, has been applied to DMSA scans in an effort to enhance the detection of acute pyelonephritis. Tarkington and colleagues (1990) compared the findings of SPECT and standard pinhole imaging in 33 children with various acute and chronic pathologic renal conditions. They found that SPECT imaging improved the ability to identify cortical defects compared to the more commonly used imaging techniques. Itoh and colleagues (1995) also reported that SPECT scintigraphy was more effective in demonstrating anatomic damage to the renal parenchyma than planar scintigraphy in patients with various urologic disorders (Fig. 61–11).

Because scan results do not alter treatment or the need for further work-up, its role in the evaluation of any child presenting clinically with acute pyelonephritis remains unclear. However, because of the nonspecific presentation of UTIs in many children, **the study is an invaluable aid to**

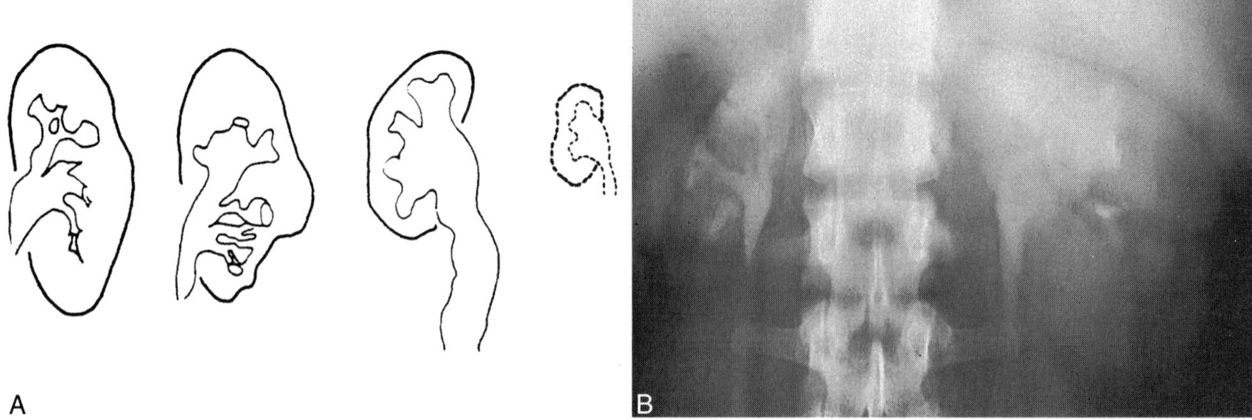

Figure 61–10. *A,* Classification of renal scarring based on alterations in renal size and contour seen on excretory urography. (From Smellie J, Edwards D, Hunter N, et al: Kidney Int, 1975; 8:S65.) *B,* Excretory urogram demonstrates bilateral renal scarring.

diagnosis when pyelonephritis is suspected but has not been proved (Verber et al, 1988). In addition, because of its sensitivity in detecting scars, DMSA scans are now being used by some clinicians for periodic screening (every 2 years) of patients with known reflux who are being medically managed.

***Cystoscopy* has a limited role in the diagnosis of reflux. There is little additional information to be gained in defining the anatomy of the ureters, urethra, and bladder neck that is not provided by voiding cystourethrography and ultrasonography.** The utility of cystoscopy was originally underscored by the study of Lyon and colleagues, who described four orifice configurations of increasing abnormality ranging from the normal or cone shape to the stadium, horseshoe, and golf-hole configurations. These assumed progressively lateral positions, had shorter intramural tunnel lengths, and were increasingly likely to be associated with reflux (Fig. 61–12) (Lyon et al, 1969). Although these descriptive terms linger in the literature, their implications have assumed less importance with time. A few years later, measurements of submucosal tunnel lengths using calibrated ureteral catheters were also emphasized by King and his coworkers as having important prognostic implications for the outcome of reflux (King et al, 1974). In actuality, it is now well known that progressive bladder filling gives an orifice a more abnormal appearance. In addition, the muscular hiatus slides along the extravesical ureter as the bladder fills, in effect shortening the length of the submucosal tunnel. This phenomenon helps to explain reflux that is seen only when the bladder is filled to extreme limits. **Orifice configuration was subsequently found to be of little value in**

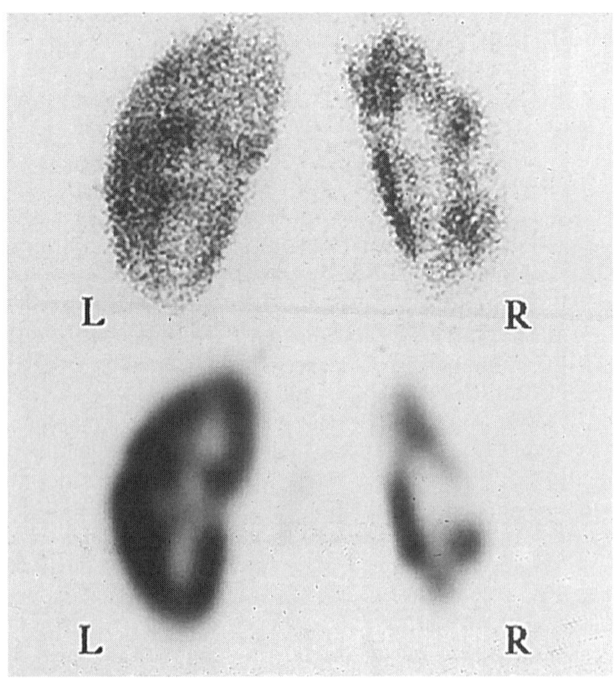

Figure 61–11. DMSA renal scintigraphy. Pinhole imaging shown above. Normal left kidney. Right kidney demonstrates multiple cortical defects. Single photon emission computerized tomography (SPECT) study shown below.

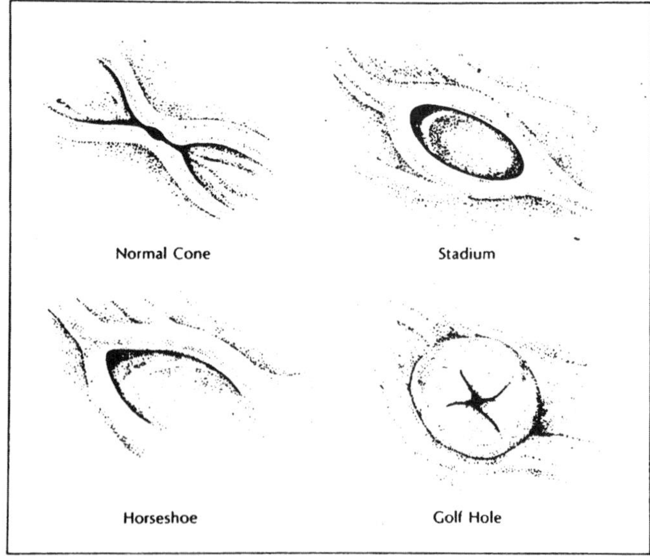

Figure 61–12. Configurations of ureteral orifice as classically taught. So-called stadium appearance suggests a short intravesical ureter. The horseshoe configuration signifies a significant loss of submucosal tunnel. The Golf hole configuration occurs with an extremely short or absent tunnel. Less significance is given to cystoscopic findings than in the past.

sion or the severity of scarring unless preexisting dysplasia was present (Wolfish et al, 1993).

The elimination or spontaneous resolution of reflux does not reverse the predisposition to hypertension if scarring is present. Wallace and colleagues, for example, reported hypertension despite successful ureteral reimplantation in 18.5% of children with bilateral scarring and in 11.3% with unilateral scarring after more than 10 years of follow-up (Wallace et al, 1978). **Removing the offending renal parenchyma by partial or total nephrectomy can improve or correct hypertension in some patients** (Dillon and Smellie, 1984). Patients with one small, scarred, poorly functioning kidney and a normal contralateral kidney may be reasonable candidates. Confirmation with selective renal vein renin determinations (ratio greater than 1.5) is instrumental to selection of patients but may still not ensure success with ablative surgery. Patients with diffuse bilateral scarring are less than ideal candidates because localization is difficult and sparing the renal parenchyma assumes primary importance.

Renal Growth

Factors that might contribute to the effects of reflux on renal growth include the congenital dysmorphism that is often associated with (30%) but is not caused by reflux; the number and type of urinary infections and the nephropathy resulting from them; the quality of the contralateral kidney and its implications for compensatory hypertrophy; and the grade of reflux in the affected kidney. Studies that might be used to evaluate renal growth are unreliable. In addition to the variability in interpretation that occurs with excretory urography or ultrasound (Redman et al, 1974; Hodson et al, 1975a), the response of the kidney to scarring, with its polar contracture and intermediate hypertrophy, makes interpretation of renal length alone unreliable. Other parameters used to measure growth have included parenchymal thickness, renal area and length, and bipolar thickness (Lyon, 1973; Klare et al, 1980; Hannerz et al, 1989). Claesson and colleagues (1981) used planimetry to measure urograms and formulate a nomogram that allows determination of renal mass in relation to somatic size (Fig. 61–18).

With the exception of kidneys that are developmentally arrested, most studies implicate infection as the cause of altered renal growth. Impaired growth was seen in kidneys with long-term reflux before the era of prophylactic antibiotics (Ibsen et al, 1977). It was subsequently shown that acceptable growth occurred if urinary infections could be controlled. In a study of 111 kidneys with reflux that were managed medically, Smellie and his associates (1981a) found slow growth in 11 kidneys, 10 of which had documented UTIs. **Successful antireflux surgery can accelerate renal growth but may not allow affected kidneys to regain their normal size** (McRae et al, 1974; Willscher et al, 1976). In one study of 22 kidneys with reflux nephropathy, significant growth after reimplantation occurred in 15 (68%), 7 of which grew proportionally to their mates (Carson et al, 1982). The potential for renal growth was less optimistically portrayed in the studies of Hagberg and colleagues (1984) and Shimada and associates (1988), who reported that 75% of kidneys with significant nephropathy remained stunted despite reimplantation. In contrast, kidneys without radiographic evidence of scarring usually show rebound growth when reflux is surgically corrected or resolves spontaneously. In addition, the results from the Birmingham Reflux Study Group (1987) and the International Reflux Study (Olbing et al, 1992; Weiss et al, 1992a and b) showed no significant difference in rates of growth or parenchymal scarring in patients who were managed medically and those managed with surgery.

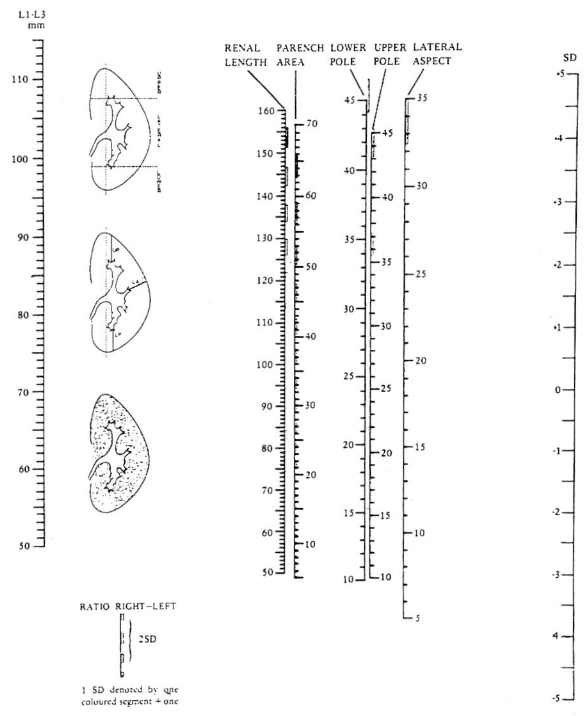

Figure 61–18. Nomogram for measuring renal parenchymal thickness and area measured by planimetry allows comparison of observed and expected renal mass. (From Winberg J, Claesson I, Jacobsson B, et al: Renal growth after acute pyelonephritis in childhood: An epidemiological approach. *In* Hodson CJ, Kincaid-Smith P, eds: Reflux Nephropathy. New York, Masson Publishing 1979, pp 309–322.)

Renal Failure and Function

Renal failure is an uncommon consequence of vesicoureteral reflux, with a risk estimated at less than 1% (Haycock, 1986). Nevertheless, the implications of recurrent bouts of pyelonephritis cannot be ignored, especially in young patients. Severe scarring and renal failure probably do not occur after isolated episodes of pyelonephritis in adults. However, in a study by Jacobson and colleagues (1989) every adult who had his or her first infection during infancy had decreased renal function, one third had hypertension, and 10% had end-stage renal disease. Chronic pyelonephritis was reported as the cause of end-stage renal disease in 15% to 25% of children and young adults in earlier studies (Scharer, 1971; Human Renal Transplant Registry, 1975; Smellie and Norman, 1985), although the presence of active reflux is probably less common, occurring in an estimated 10% (Salvatierra and Tanagho, 1977). Increased awareness and improved management should continue to exert positive effects on the incidence of this complication. For example, chronic pyelonephritis accounted for less than 2.2% of cases of end-stage renal disease in a recent report of the North American Pediatric Renal Transplant Cooperative Study (1994).

Lesser degrees of renal impairment can also occur with reflux in a progressive manner that has been likened to that seen with partial ureteral obstruction. The increased pressure of reflux presumably affects the distal nephron initially, although its effects are difficult to separate from those of associated infection. Defects in concentrating ability result that appear to be independent of infection and are inversely proportional to the grade of reflux. Improvement often occurs with the cessation of reflux (Walker et al, 1973). Other parameters of tubular function may also be affected including fractional excretion of magnesium and sodium (Walker, 1991). **Glomerular function is usually unaffected unless global parenchymal damage has occurred.** Proteinuria often accompanies significant renal insufficiency and scarring (Torres, 1983). Genetic markers, including HLA-B12 in females, HLA-B8 with A9 or BW15 in males, and HLA-BW15 in both sexes, have been found with end-stage reflux nephropathy and may represent a link to the genetic susceptibility to renal damage (Torres et al, 1980).

Somatic Growth

Children with vesicoureteral reflux tend to be small for their age (Dwoskin and Perlmutter, 1973), **especially those with a history of recurrent urinary infections.** Eliminating infections with prophylactic antibiotics maintained normal somatic growth in 51 girls with known reflux (Smellie et al, 1983). Surgically correcting reflux has also been shown to affect somatic growth positively (Merrell and Mowad, 1979). It remains unclear whether one form of treatment offers preferential benefit in this aspect of development because there are no comparative studies in a large series of children with extended follow-up (Sutton and Atwell, 1989).

ASSOCIATED ANOMALIES AND CONDITIONS

Ureteropelvic Junction Obstruction

The incidence of vesicoureteral reflux associated with ureteropelvic junction (UPJ) obstruction ranges from 5% to 25% (DeKlerk et al, 1979; Lebowitz and Blickman, 1983; Maizels et al, 1984; Hollowell et al, 1989). Most of the patients reported in these studies had incidental reflux that resolved spontaneously with time. Conversely, the incidence of UPJ obstruction in patients with reflux ranges from 0.8% to 14% (Lebowitz and Blickman, 1983; Hollowell et al, 1989; Leighton and Mayne, 1989). **UPJ obstructions associated with reflux can amplify its grade because of the collecting system dilatation that results. Therefore, the management of reflux in this setting cannot be made on the basis of cystography alone.** In addition, cases of high-grade reflux cause kinking of the ureter and pelvic junction that can result in obstruction. Impaired or absent filling of the pelvis by reflux that causes dilatation of the ureter below the UPJ is a suspicious radiologic sign (Fig. 61–19). Whether UPJ obstructions associated with reflux are similar to those that occur primarily is unclear, but the dual nature of the problem poses a management dilemma.

Therapy is directed at preserving renal function. **When scintigraphy with catheter drainage shows obstruction, pyeloplasty rather than reimplantation should be performed.** To correct the reflux initially risks amplifying obstruction because of the distal ureteral edema that results. In addition, improving urinary outflow is thought by some to increase the likelihood of cessation of reflux, although reimplantation is often necessary in patients in whom high-grade reflux persists after successful pyeloplasty. If, however, the pelvic dilatation associated with reflux is thought to be nonobstructive, ureteroneocystostomy is the procedure of choice. Three or four days of stent drainage is advisable during the early postoperative period to minimize any amplification of upper ureteral obstruction resulting from distal ureteral edema.

Ureteral Duplication

Vesicoureteral reflux is the most common abnormality associated with complete ureteral duplication. The anatomy of patients with ureteral duplication typically follows the Weigert-Meyer rule (Meyer, 1946; Weigert, 1887) wherein the upper pole ureter enters the bladder distally and medially and the lower pole ureter enters the bladder proximally and laterally. **The incidence of reflux is increased in patients with complete ureteral duplication.** Although urine may reflux into either ureter, **it more commonly involves the ureter from the lower pole** because of its lateral position and shorter submucosal tunnel (Fig. 61–20). Contrary to historical teaching, **the frequency of resolution of reflux appears to be the same whether the patient has a single ureter or double ureters,** although the duration of resolution may be somewhat increased in patients with ureteral duplication. A series of children with grades I, II, and III reflux into the lower pole of a duplicated collecting system showed no significant differences in resolution of reflux or incidence of new scars than a control group of children with single ureters (Ben-Ami et al, 1989). Although management must be individualized, a more aggressive approach is not warranted in patients with reflux into duplicated systems (Husman and Allen, 1991).

Bladder Diverticula

Bladder diverticula are mucosal herniations through areas of weakness in the muscular bladder wall. They were initially thought to occur only with bladder outlet obstruction and secondary detrusor hypertrophy and trabeculation. Hutch (1961) was the first to recognize that bladder diverticula were also congenital abnormalities that occurred primarily in smooth-walled normal bladders in children. **The most common location for diverticula is lateral and cephalad to the ureteral orifice** (Boechat and Lebowitz, 1978). These occasionally expand within Waldeyer's fascia to cause ure-

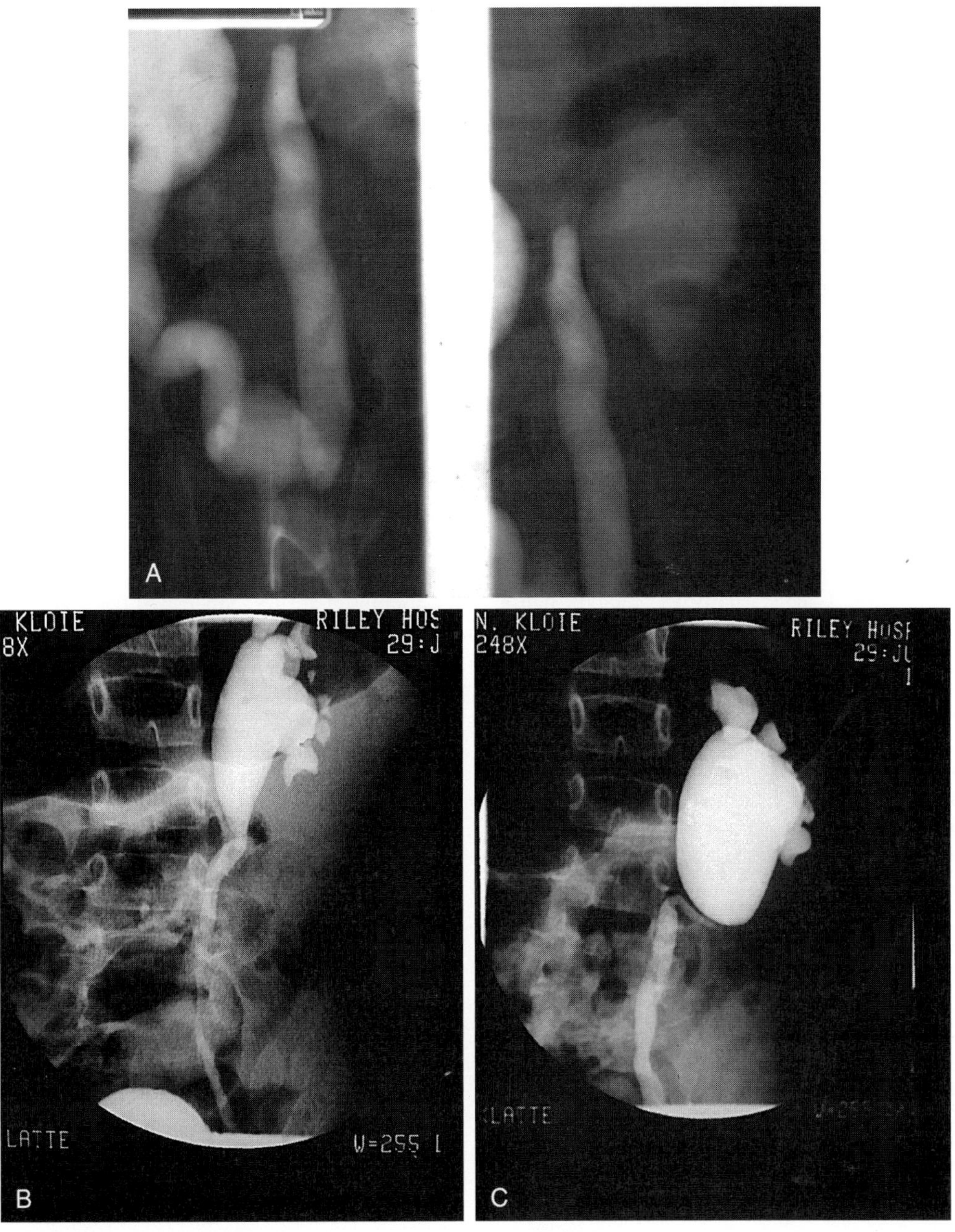

Figure 61–19. Reflux and ureteropelvic junction obstructions. *A,* Significant reflux fills the left ureter to the level of the ureteropelvic junction. Minimal filling of the pelvis can be a sign of obstruction at that level. *B,* In another patient, reflux is seen as bladder fills. *C,* Significant kinking of the ureteropelvic junction occurs with voiding.

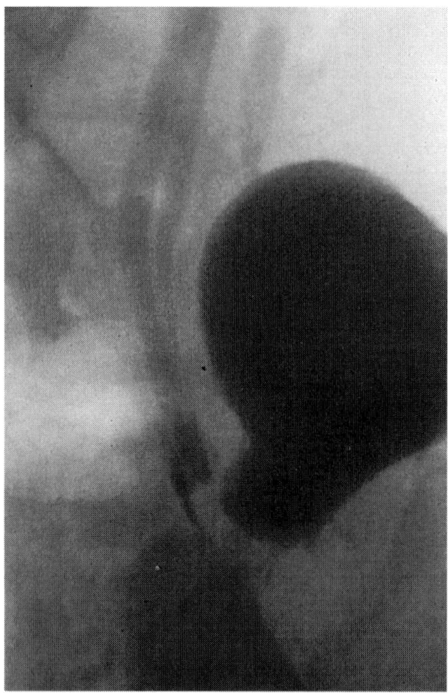

Figure 61–20. Reflux into both ureters of a complete duplication as shown is less common than reflux into the lower pole ureter alone.

teral obstruction or project intraluminally to obstruct the bladder neck or urethra. Usually, however, they prolapse outside the bladder at the expense of paraureteral mucosa. This alters the anatomy of the ureterovesical junction and allows either transient or permanent reflux (Fig. 61–21). The management of reflux associated with diverticula differs from that of primary reflux depending on the degree of anatomic distortion that results. **Reflux associated with small diverticula resolves at a rate similar to that of primary reflux and can be managed accordingly. In contrast, reflux with paraureteral large diverticula is less likely to resolve and usually requires surgical correction. In any case, surgery is recommended where the ureter enters the diverticulum, regardless of size** (Atala and Retik, 1993).

PREGNANCY AND VESICOURETERAL REFLUX

The morphology of the urinary tract is altered with the onset of pregnancy and increases throughout gestation (Beydoun, 1985). **Bladder tone decreases owing to edema and hyperemia, changes that predispose the patient to bacteriuria. In addition, urine volume increases in the upper collecting system as the physiologic dilatation of pregnancy evolves. The slower drainage that results can enhance the growth of organisms and increase the propensity to develop pyelonephritis.** It seems logical to assume that during pregnancy the presence of vesicoureteral reflux in a system already prone to bacteriuria would lead to increased morbidity. A number of studies have been conducted during the last four decades to examine this relationship.

The presence of active reflux appears to present a risk factor for the affected mother. In 1958, Hutch described a higher incidence of pyelonephritis during pregnancy in 23 women with a history of reflux and recurrent bacteriuria. Heidrick and associates (1967) evaluated 321 women with cystography during either the last trimester or within 30 hours of delivery. The incidence of pyelonephritis was 33% in women with reflux compared to less than 5% in women without reflux. Finally, cystograms performed 4 to 6 months postpartum in 100 women with a history of asymptomatic bacteriuria during pregnancy showed reflux in 21%. Bacteriuria was easier to clear in patients without reflux (67%) than in those with reflux (33%) (Williams et al, 1968).

Maternal history is also a factor if past reflux, renal scarring, or a tendency to urinary infections is present.

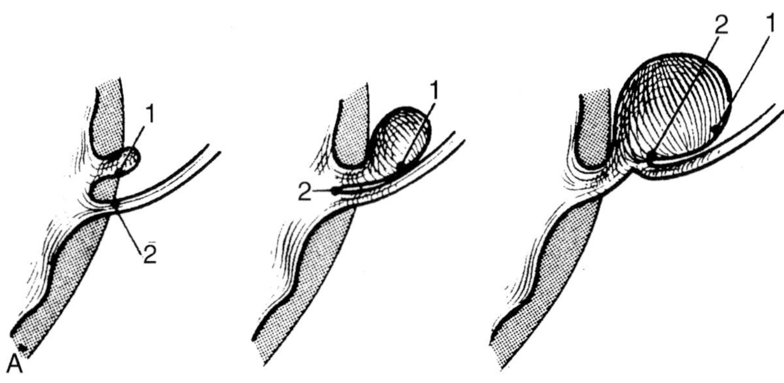

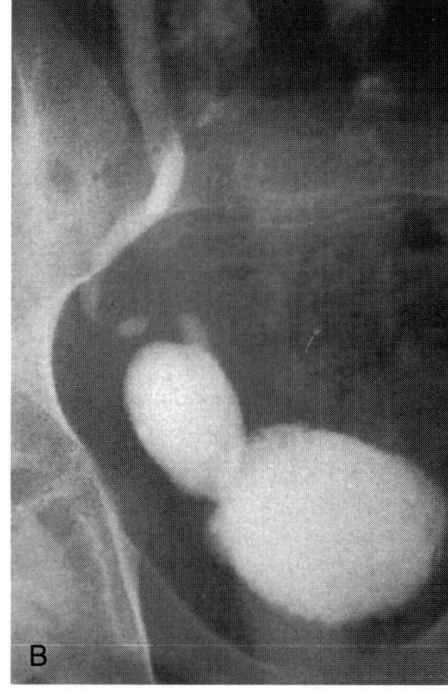

Figure 61–21. *A,* Schematic representation of bladder diverticulum. A small amount of mucosa initially herniates through a congenital defect in the bladder musculature. This enlarges with voiding. Finally, the ureteral orifice is incorporated into the diverticulum. (From Hernanz-Schulman M, Lebowitz RL: The elusiveness and importance of bladder diverticula in children. Pediatr Radiol 1985; 15:399–402. Copyright © Springer-Verlag.) *B,* Reflux into right-sided paraureteral diverticulum and ureter seen on voiding cystogram.

Martinell and colleagues (1990) compared the outcome of pregnancy in matched controls to that in 41 women with and without renal scarring after childhood urinary infections. They found that women with a history of prior infections had a high incidence of bacteriuria during pregnancy, whereas those with renal scarring and persistent reflux were prone to develop acute pyelonephritis. In a similar study, the outcome of pregnancy was assessed in 88 women with previous bacteriuria. Women with known renal scars had a 3.3-fold incidence of hypertension, a 7.6-fold risk of preeclampsia, and a higher rate of obstetric interventions. Women with normal kidneys and reflux had an increased risk of hypertension during the last trimester (McGladdery, 1992). Pregnant women with bilateral renal scars were also shown to have a higher incidence of preeclampsia than those with unilateral scarring (24% versus 7%) (El-Khatib, 1994), and those with elevated creatinine are also at risk (Jungers, 1987).

More recently, Austenfeld and Snow (1988) found an increased risk of urinary infections and fetal loss in 31 women who had undergone ureteral reimplantation as children despite correction of the anomaly. In a follow-up study of the same patients compared to a new cohort of historical controls, Mansfield and colleagues (1995) noted that women with urinary infections and reflux who had undergone reimplantation (suggesting an initially higher degree of reflux and increased renal scarring) were still at significant risk of urinary infection during pregnancy but had no higher risk of miscarriage than the general population.

In summary, the majority of studies that have examined the effects of vesicoureteral reflux on pregnancy suggest that **women with a history of *reflux and renal scarring* have increased morbidity** during pregnancy because of infection-related complications, ***whether or not the reflux has been corrected*. The morbidity during pregnancy of women with *persistent reflux without renal scarring* remains poorly defined, but a tendency toward urinary infection appears to be increased. Because of the difficulty of predicting an outcome for this subset of patients, most clinicians recommend surgical correction for girls with reflux that persists beyond puberty.**

NATURAL HISTORY AND MANAGEMENT

Spontaneous Resolution

Vesicoureteral reflux resolves spontaneously in many children, although **the rates of resolution depend on the initial grade of reflux and the age at presentation.** In theory, two mechanisms contribute to this phenomenon. The first is elongation of the submucosal tunnel that occurs with interval growth of the bladder and longitudinal muscles of the ureter (Stephens and Lenaghan, 1962). The second, especially in neonates and infants, is a beneficial change in bladder dynamics from a small-capacity, hyperreflexic voiding pattern to a more mature pattern with a larger capacity and a lower intravesical pressure. In addition, experimental studies in puppies have implicated changes in the autonomic nervous system and an increase in adrenergic innervation as factors that contribute in some way to the presence of reflux (Kiruluta et al, 1986). The clinical data in this regard are revealing.

Grade of Reflux

Most low grades (I to II) of reflux resolve spontaneously (King et al, 1974). Edwards and colleagues cited an 85% rate and Smellie and Normand cited an 80% rate of resolution in children with ureters of normal caliber (Edwards et al, 1977; Smellie and Normand, 1979). Similar results were reported by the Southwest Pediatric Nephrology (SPN) study group, which noted resolution in 82% of children with grade I and 80% of those with grade II reflux after 5 years of medical management, whereas Duckett reported resolution in 63% of those with grade II reflux (Arant, 1992; Duckett, 1983). Skoog and associates, using long-term medical management, noted resolution in 90% of children with grade I to III reflux after 5 years (Skoog et al, 1987). Intermediate grade (III) reflux will resolve in approximately 50% of patients (Arant, 1992; Duckett, 1983). A similar rate of resolution was reported after 5 years of medical management by McLorie and colleagues (1990).

High-grade (IV to V) reflux seldom resolves spontaneously. Historically, a more aggressive surgical stance has usually been taken with this degree of reflux, especially in the United States. The results of the International Reflux Study, which commenced in 1980 to evaluate children with grades III and IV reflux, appear to support this bias. In the European arm of the study, 82 patients with bilateral grade III or IV reflux were followed. Cessation of reflux occurred in only seven (9%). Similarly, reflux resolved in only 4 (11%) of 31 children with grade III or IV reflux on one side and low grade (I to II) reflux on the other. Children with unilateral reflux had a more optimistic prognosis with reflux abating in 23 of 38 (61%). The results from the 41 patients entered in the American arm of the study were similarly discouraging with reflux persisting in 75% of patients, although the outcome of unilateral versus bilateral involvement was not reported (Weiss et al, 1992a and b; Tamminen-Mobius et al, 1992). Resolution rates of 41% for grades III to V (Smellie and Normand, 1979), 30% for grade IV and 12% for grade V (McLorie et al, 1990), and as low as 9% for grade IV have been reported (Skoog et al, 1987).

Age at Diagnosis

The age of the patient is also important in any discussion of the spontaneous resolution of reflux. Grade III reflux in a 3-year-old child, for example, is probably different from that in a 3 month old and, in fact, may have been grade V reflux if a diagnosis had been made at an earlier age. **Younger children are more likely to have reflux, and reflux appears to be more likely to resolve spontaneously in such children regardless of grade.** In a study of perinatally diagnosed reflux, Burge and associates (1992) noted resolution in 54% of children with grades III and IV reflux within 3 years. The significance of the period of early development was also suggested by Skoog and colleagues (1987), who noted a significantly shorter duration of reflux in children in whom the problem was diagnosed before 1 year of age

(1.44 versus 1.85 years). In contrast, McLorie and associates (1990) found no difference in degree of resolution of high-grade (III and IV) reflux between children less than 1 year of age and those who were older.

Assuming that the theories of lower urinary tract development required to bring about the resolution of reflux are correct, intervals of significant growth and beneficial urodynamic change are most likely to effect change. This seems especially true in neonates and infants (Belman, 1995). During childhood, gradual growth brings about a more slowly cumulative constant change as suggested by the 15% to 20% overall yearly rate of resolution offered by Smellie and Normand (1979). **If resolution is to occur, it usually does so within the first few years after reflux has been diagnosed.** Skoog and colleagues noted resolution rates of 30% to 35% per year in their study of low- and moderate-grade reflux. Interestingly, the different grades had similar disappearance curves, although the higher grades took longer to disappear (grade II, 1.56 years; grade III, 1.97 years) (Skoog et al, 1987). **The absence of improvement in the degree of reflux on serial cystograms is a worrisome sign that resolution may not occur with interval growth.** The duration of observation that should be allowed for the maturation of reflux remains undefined. However, in one series, 92% of cases of grade III reflux that resolved did so within 4 years (McLorie et al, 1990). **Resolution of reflux sometimes occurs after 5 years but is especially uncommon if little improvement has occurred in the interim.** The onset of puberty does not initiate a period of accelerated resolution of reflux. Instead, **with the cessation of longitudinal growth the likelihood that reflux will resolve presumably ends,** although this has never been proved. In addition, the implications of reflux in adults need to be more clearly defined.

DECISIONS IN MANAGEMENT

The surgeries designed to correct vesicoureteral reflux have always set a high standard against which medical management is measured. Ninety-nine percent success rates are not uncommon (Duckett et al, 1992). Nevertheless, **it has become increasingly apparent that medical treatment will be effective for many children with reflux.** Both modalities bring attendant risks and benefits that must be weighed in light of the natural history of the anomaly and its implications for the patient, as discussed earlier. Walker summarized the premises that anchor decision making in management of reflux (Walker and Flack, 1994):

1. Spontaneous resolution of reflux occurs in many infants and children but is less likely to occur at puberty.
2. More severe grades of reflux are less likely to resolve spontaneously.
3. Sterile reflux does not appear to cause significant nephropathy.
4. Extended courses of prophylactic antibiotics are well tolerated by children.
5. Antireflux surgeries are highly successful in capable hands.

An outline of rigid algorithms in management would be unfair both to patients, for whom treatment should be individualized, and to clinicians, who must gauge parental compliance with medical management and periodic radiologic follow-up, factor in socioeconomic concerns, and also weigh their own personal experience with the anomaly. Nevertheless, some generalized recommendations can be made based on the likelihood of grade-related spontaneous resolution and the natural history of reflux as previously discussed.

Medical management is initially recommended for prepubertal children with grade I, II, or III reflux on the assumption that most cases will resolve. A period of observation and medical therapy also seems to be warranted for most patients with grade IV reflux, especially younger children and those with unilateral disease. Some trend toward improvement should become evident within 2 or 3 years. If not, surgery is recommended. Finally, grade V reflux is unlikely to resolve spontaneously. Surgery is recommended after infancy, although, again, a period of observation seems reasonable for children with perinatally diagnosed disease, especially because correcting megaureters in newborns can be challenging.

The onset of puberty and the cessation of longitudinal growth alter the recommendations for adolescents in whom reflux is being medically managed. **Surgery is recommended for most girls with reflux that persists to avoid the implications of active reflux for future pregnancies** (see earlier discussion). **This is especially true if they have nephropathy or have shown a tendency toward urinary infections in the past.** Some clinicians discontinue antibiotics in adolescent girls as puberty approaches (Belman, 1995). Girls with normal kidneys or those whose reflux is discovered serendipidously during sibling screening are particularly good candidates for this approach. Its risks must be fully understood by the family and treating physician, although episodes of pyelonephritis are uncommon, and the development of scarring decreases with age. Surgery is reserved for those who develop significant infections. **Because older boys are less prone to UTIs, prophylaxis can be discontinued and most reflux can be observed** unless infections or other symptoms arise. Reimplantation is recommended for adults in whom reflux is discovered because of urinary tract infections. It is noted, although rarely discussed, that reimplantation surgery in females is far more challenging after puberty. Maturation of the pelvic adnexa makes ureteral mobilization difficult and increases bleeding.

MEDICAL MANAGEMENT

There has been no clear-cut demonstration that nephropathy develops in children with reflux whose urine is kept free of infection. To achieve this end medical management consists of low-dose prophylactic antibiotics that are continued until reflux resolves as expected. A variety of different medications achieve high urinary concentrations and effectively control a broad range of uropathogens, but preferences do exist. Medications are usually given as suspensions once daily at half the standard therapeutic dose. Nighttime dosing in toilet-trained children is most effective because this dose precedes the longest period of urinary retention when infection is most likely to develop.

Amoxicillin or ampicillin is recommended for children up to 6 weeks of age. Although these medications favor the development of resistant fecal flora they have the fewest side effects in the newborn. **After 6 weeks the biliary system is mature enough to handle trimethoprim-sulfamethoxazole (Septra), which usually becomes the antibiotic of choice.** Side effects include gastrointestinal symptoms, allergies, Stevens-Johnson syndrome, and leukopenia, which resolves with discontinuance of the drug. A complete blood count is obtained before surgery in any child taking this medication, but periodic blood counts are probably unnecessary. **Nitrofurantoin (Macrodantin) is another acceptable option for prophylaxis and is the best medication for minimizing fecal resistance. Pulmonary fibrosis and interstitial pneumonia are rare but well-recognized complications of this medication.** Other side effects include nausea and vomiting, hemolytic anemia, peripheral neuropathies, and exfoliative dermatitis. Nitrofurantoin should not be used in children less than 2 months old. Alternating trimethoprim-sulfamethoxazole and nitrofurantoin every other day or taking one in the morning and the other at night has been effective in children who develop organisms that are resistant to single-agent therapy. Other options in prophylaxis for children who develop allergies include nalidixic acid, trimethoprim alone, or the cephalosporins.

Improving toilet hygiene and bladder emptying by timed voids, double voiding, proper perineal wiping, and elimination of constipation also help to achieve the goals of medical management. When present, bladder dysfunction should be treated with anticholinergics. Periodic urine cultures are obtained every 3 months to evaluate breakthrough infections. **Negative cultures are usually reliable regardless of collection technique. When questions of culture validity arise, confirmation with catheterization becomes necessary.**

Yearly radiologic studies are also necessary, although some clinicians maintain follow-up at 18-month intervals. The latter allows more time for interval growth, is cost-effective, and requires only two catheterizations for cystography in a 3-year period. The tradeoff is that 6 additional months of unnecessary medication may be given if reflux has resolved. **A combination of ultrasonography and nuclear cystography provide adequate follow-up of the urinary tract for directing the continuance or cessation of medical therapy.** Prophylaxis is discontinued whenever cystography documents resolution of reflux. A repeat confirmatory cystogram is unnecessary in the asymptomatic child. Families should be aware, however, that these children sometimes remain prone to urinary infections, and they are instructed to continue their efforts to maintain proper toilet hygiene. When infections do occur they generally become manifest with lower urinary tract symptoms. Complete re-evaluations are required in children who develop pyelonephritis.

The likelihood of resolution of reflux and the expectations of medical management should be frankly discussed with the parents. The requirements of periodic radiologic follow-up and, in some cases, long-term prophylaxis cannot be fulfilled by certain families. **Intermittent treatment of infections is ineffective. Data from patients who are treated only during symptomatic episodes demonstrate progressive nephropathy compared to those maintained on continuous prophylaxis.** For example, Lenaghan and colleagues (1976) noted a 21% incidence of new renal scarring when intermittent antibiotics were given, in contrast to the 1% incidence noted with continuous antibiotics (Smellie et al, 1975). **If compliance is an issue, some children are best served by correcting their reflux surgically rather than embarking on a futile course of medical management.**

Clinical Studies

Since Smellie and Normand's (1979) early work in following a large group of children with reflux on continuous low-dose chemotherapy, a number of clinical studies have been done to assess the efficacy of medical management of reflux and better define certain aspects of its natural history. These include the following:

THE INTERNATIONAL REFLUX STUDY IN CHILDREN. This study compared the medical and surgical management of high-grade (grades III and IV) reflux after randomization in children under 9 years of age in Europe and the United States (Table 61–6). **Surgery was more effective than medical therapy in preventing pyelonephritis** (10% versus 21%), **but the overall incidence of urinary infections between the two groups** (38% and 39%) **was the same.** Both modalities were equally effective in preventing new renal scarring, although scars did develop regardless of therapy, providing further proof of the importance of host defense and bacterial virulence factors. In this regard, the European arm of the study considered the effects of dysfunctional voiding on reflux. When this was present (18%) and untreated, patients had more infections, greater variability in reflux grade during follow-up, and an increased rate of persistent reflux. Reflux nephropathy was not increased (Weiss et al, 1992a; Tamminen-Mobius et al, 1992; Van Gool et al, 1992). Cessation of reflux was seen in 34 of 151 patients (23%) who were medically managed in the European arm, although bilateral reflux was less likely to resolve (10%).

THE BIRMINGHAM REFLUX STUDY. This study used a design similar to that used by the IRSC in treating 104 patients with severe reflux. Surgical and medical management was equally effective in preventing new renal scars. Between 50% and 80% of medically treated patients still had reflux after a 5-year period (Birmingham Reflux Study Group, 1987).

OTHER STUDIES. The Southwest Pediatric Nephrology Group Study prospectively evaluated the medical management of low- and moderate-grade reflux (grades I to III) in 84 ureters in 59 patients. Grade-dependent resolution was seen in 67% of ureters. Despite strict medical therapy and close surveillance, breakthrough urinary infections occurred in one-third of the patients, and grade-related renal scarring occurred in 16%. No comparisons with surgery were made (Arant, 1992). In another prospective randomized study by Scholtmeijer (1993) 135 ureters in 93 children with varying

Table 61–6. RENAL SCARRING—MEDICAL AND SURGICAL THERAPY

Registrant	Number	New Scars	Thinning
European—Medical	155	19 (12%)	11 (7%)
European—Surgical	151	20 (13%)	15 (10%)
USA—Medical	66	14 (20%)	9 (13%)
USA—Surgical	64	16 (25%)	2 (3%)

grades of reflux were studied. Spontaneous resolution occurred in 27 of 47 (57%) cases of grade III and IV reflux with 5 years of follow-up. Fifteen (32%) children required cross-over to reimplantation because of breakthrough infections. New scars developed in two patients with grade II or III reflux who were being medically managed and in six who were surgically treated. Other prospective studies of reflux have been done, although not in randomized fashion. Each emphasized the need to control breakthrough urinary infections (Edwards et al, 1977; King, 1977; Dunn et al, 1978).

SURGICAL MANAGEMENT

The treatment of vesicoureteral reflux should be individualized. Before recommending surgery, consideration is given to the severity of the reflux, the possible underlying risk factors including bladder dysfunction, the age at presentation and duration of the disorder, and the presence and quality of urinary infections that may have occurred while the patient was on medical management. Knowing that corrective surgery is usually successful does not allow a broadening of its indications. Errors in selection set the stage for postoperative complications. **Typical indications for antireflux surgery include:**

1. **Breakthrough urinary tract infections despite prophylactic antibiotics.**
2. **Noncompliance with medical management.**
3. **Severe reflux (grades IV or V), especially with pyelonephritic changes.**
4. **Failure of renal growth, the presence of new renal scars, or deterioration of renal function on serial ultrasound examinations or scans.**
5. **Reflux that persists in girls as full linear growth is approached at puberty.**
6. **Reflux associated with congenital abnormalities at the ureterovesical junction (e.g., bladder diverticula).**

The expectations for the results of surgery must be understood beforehand. **Successful ureteral reimplantation should decrease but will not eliminate** the incidence of pyelonephritis in children with reflux. A significant decrease (from 50% to 10%) was reported by Govan and Palmer (1969) after successful surgery. In the IRSC study the incidence of pyelonephritis in the surgical group (10%) was less than half that in the medically controlled group (21%) (Jodal et al, 1992). Unfortunately, however, UTIs persist despite surgery. Bacteriuria is reported in as many as 40% of patients postoperatively, although most do not develop pyelonephritis (Willscher et al, 1976; Wacksman et al, 1978; Weiss et al, 1992a). However, like medical management, surgery cannot completely protect the kidney. This is undoubtedly the consequence of host abnormalities such as dysfunctional voiding and bacterial virulence factors, especially because the incidence of bacteriuria is similar to that in children without reflux or those whose reflux is being treated medically.

A variety of techniques have been described to correct vesicoureteral reflux. These are categorized anatomically as *extravesical, intravesical,* or combined, depending on the approach to the ureter, and *suprahiatal* or *infrahiatal,* depending on the position of the new submucosal tunnel in relation to the original hiatus. **Common to each is the creation of a valvular mechanism that allows ureteral compression with bladder filling and contraction, replicating normal anatomy and function. A successful ureteroneocystostomy provides a submucosal tunnel for reimplantation that has sufficient length and adequate muscular backing. A tunnel length of five times the ureteral diameter is cited as necessary to eliminate reflux** (Paquin, 1959). Deviation from this basic principle is the most common cause of failure of reimplantation and explains the lack of success seen with many earlier reimplantation techniques that are no longer employed (Winter, 1969). The technical details of the more widely used repairs follow.

Politano-Leadbetter Technique

The Politano-Leadbetter technique has been a reliable method of correcting vesicoureteral reflux since it was described in 1958, although its popularity appears to be waning (Politano and Leadbetter, 1958). Any reluctance to use this suprahiatal, intravesical repair stems from the somewhat "blind" nature of the transfer of the ureter behind the bladder, especially compared with the relatively simple cross-trigonal reimplant. This drawback can be overcome by using the technique described here. Many surgeons still prefer the Politano-Leadbetter technique for unilateral reimplants because it avoids possible disruption of the valvular mechanism of the contralateral ureter. Success rates of between 97% and 99% are cited in the literature (Brannon et al, 1973), although some authors have noted a slightly higher complication rate compared to the cross-trigonal method (Carpentier et al, 1982).

Method (Fig. 61–22)

1. A transverse skin incision is made along a skin crease two finger breadths above the symphysis pubis (Fig. 61–22*A*).
2. After opening the anterior rectus fascia, flaps are developed superiorly and inferiorly above the muscles. The rectus and pyramidalis muscles are separated in the midline.
3. The transversalis fascia and peritoneum are swept from the dome of the bladder with the finger.
4. The bladder is opened in the midline with cautery to 2 cm above the bladder neck, and its inferior and lateral edges are sutured to the anterior rectus fascia. This elevates the bladder floor and aids in placement of the Denis-Brown retractor, whose lateral blades are positioned within the bladder.
5. Multiple moist 4 × 4 sponges are placed in the dome of the bladder behind the superior blade to further elevate the bladder floor. When the trigone is flattened and tense the exposure is sufficient to proceed. Manipulation of the bladder with sponges, suction, or forceps is minimized to prevent edema and bleeding.
6. Ureteral dissection is performed with minimal tissue handling. A 5-0 chromic suture is placed above and below the orifice within the future perimeatal cuff. Placement of a fine (No. 3.5 or 5 Fr) feeding tube aids in the initial dissection of the ureter (Fig. 61–22*B*).
7. A generous mucosal cuff is outlined around the meatus using a needle-tip cautery. This facilitates later suturing of the ureter and helps avoid compromise of its lumen (Fig. 61–22*C*).

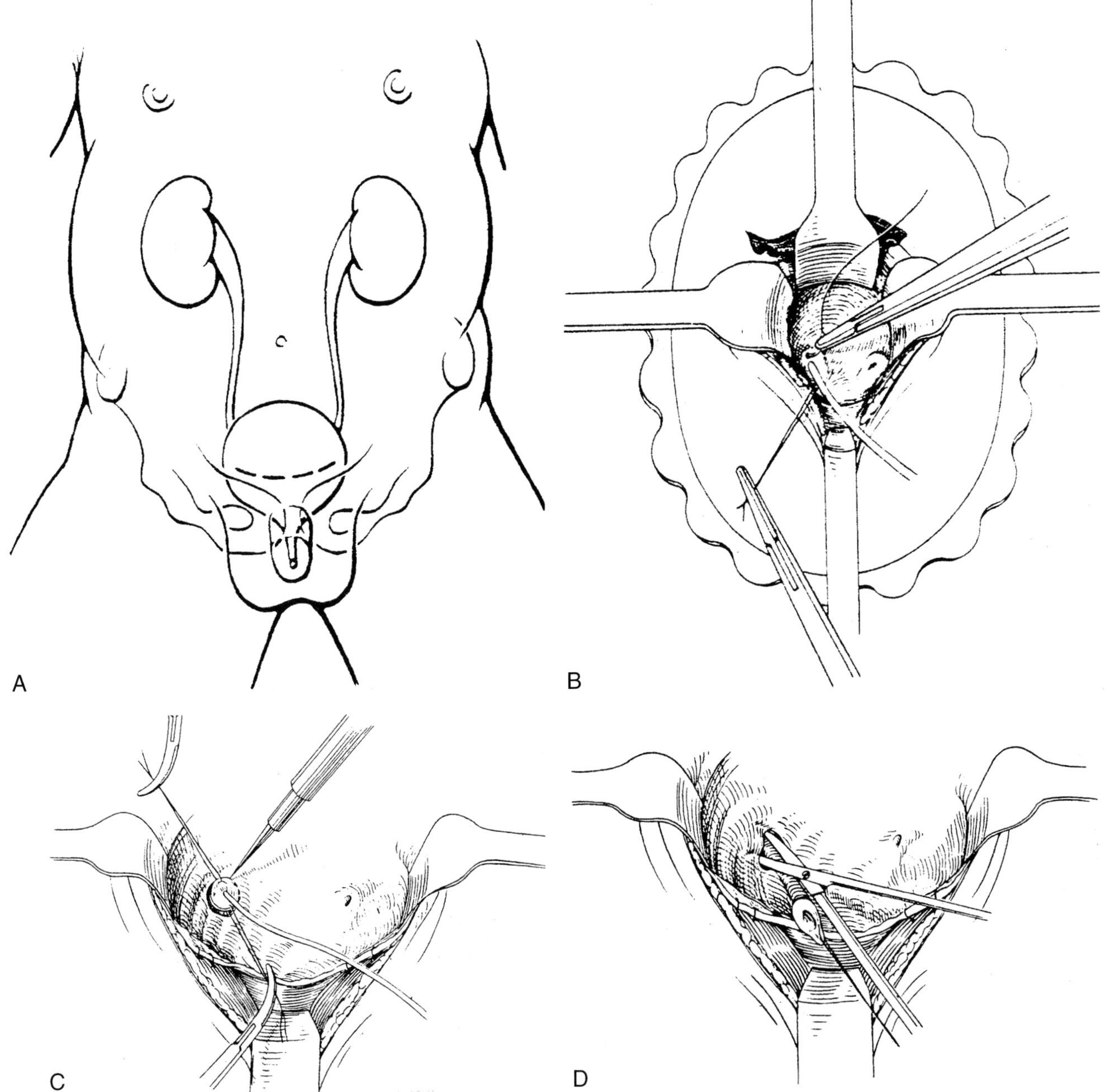

Figure 61–22. Politano-Leadbetter technique. *A,* Typical approach to the bladder for reimplantation. A transverse, lower abdominal incision is made along a skin crease one or two finger breadths above the symphysis pubis. *B,* Fine sutures are placed above and below the ureteral orifice for handling. A feeding tube in the ureter aids in the initial dissection. *C,* A needle-tip cautery outlines a circumferential incision around the orifice. *D,* Tenotomy scissors initially establish the plane of dissection inferiorly, where ureteral damage can be avoided. The plane is then carried around the ureter.

Illustration continued on following page

8. After incising the mucosa and taking down the superficial detrusor, the plane for ureteral dissection is found inferiorly by spreading a snap (Fig. 61–22*D*). Excessive dissection of the surrounding detrusor is unnecessary and causes annoying bleeding.

9. Sharp dissection parallel to the ureter with tenotomy scissors establishes the correct plane. It is important not to skeletonize the ureter and damage its adventitia. Hemostasis is accomplished with selective cautery using fine hemostats on the periureteral attachments. Kinks and angulations should be straightened. If the distal ureter is narrow or unhealthy after being mobilized, it is excised back to healthy viable tissue and spatulated to avoid stenosis.

10. Visualization of the perivesical region and site for the neohiatus is aided by spreading the musculature of the old hiatus with a blunt right-angle clamp.

11. A fine gauze dissector is used to sweep the peritoneum from the posterior bladder wall with the aid of a lighted suction tip and two Senn retractors (Fig. 61–22*E*). The peritoneum must be completely swept from the proposed new hiatus to avoid placing the ureter through the peritoneum or viscera. The vas in males is visualized and

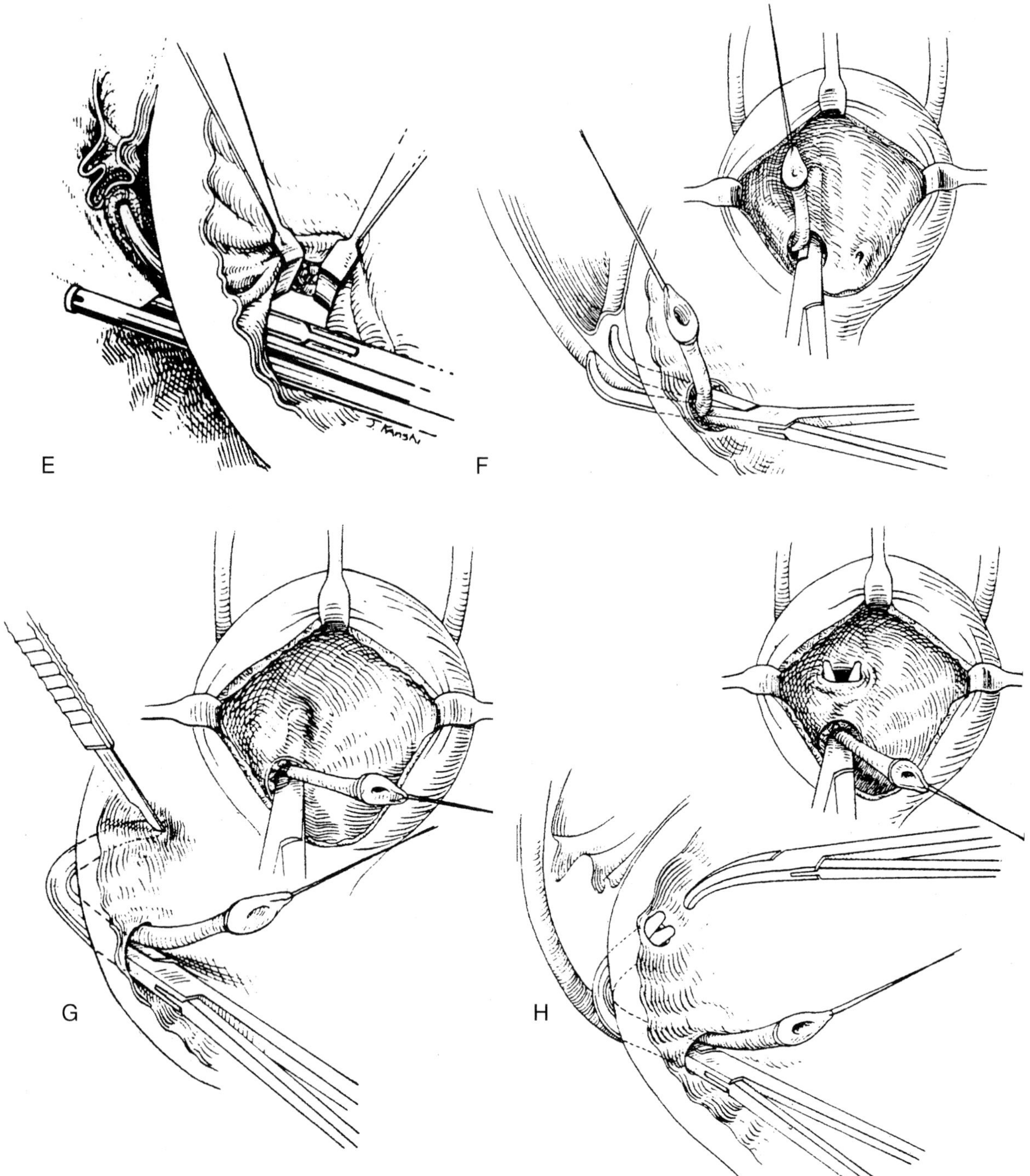

Figure 61–22 *Continued E,* With the aid of a lighted suction tip and two Senn retractors, a fine gauze dissector is used to sweep the peritoneum from the posterior bladder wall. *F,* After sweeping the peritoneum away, blunt right-angle clamp indents the bladder from behind at a new hiatus approximately 2.5 cm superior and somewhat medial to the original hiatus. *G,* The clamp is incised on from within and generously spread to make certain the new hiatus is wide enough. *H,* A second right angle follows the first from within the bladder to the original hiatus.

swept away as it crosses the peritoneum while the perivesical vessels are fulgurated.

12. Adequate mobilization and length are mandatory. Mobilization usually is possible with 6 to 8 cm of dissection, which leaves the ureter untethered on gentle traction. In some cases it is necessary to elevate the peritoneum from the ureter to gain adequate length.

13. The right-angle clamp hugs the posterior wall and indents the proposed new hiatus from without. This location is superior, medial, and, in most instances, 2 to 2.5 cm from the old hiatus (Fig. 61–22*F*). The site of the new hiatus must be carefully chosen. Excessive lateral placement can lead to ureteral obstruction as the bladder fills. Obstruction can also occur with an excessively superior position if the ureter has not been adequately mobilized.

14. The mucosa and muscle are then sharply incised, and the right-angle clamp is spread generously upon entering the bladder (Fig. 61–22*G*). Incomplete separation of the detrusor

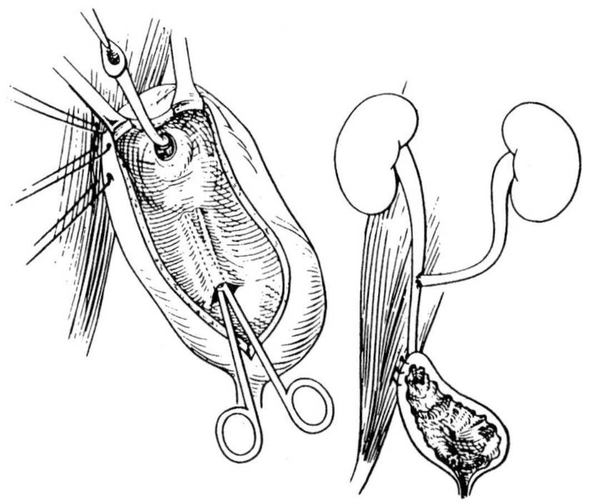

Figure 61–29. Psoas hitch can be used to effectively bridge significant ureteral defects. Combination with transureteroureterostomy is ideal when both ureters are addressed in the reoperative setting. (From Keating MA, Retik AB: Management of failures of ureteroneocystostomy. In McDougal WS, ed: Difficult Problems in Urologic Surgery. Chicago, Year Book, 1988, p 140.)

tiveness. Decision making in the management of reflux often depends on balancing the uncertainty of spontaneous resolution against surgical morbidity. A significant reduction in the latter would very likely shift management decisions in favor of surgery in selected patients (Atala and Casale, 1990).

Any endoscopic material used in the treatment of reflux should have two major characteristics. The first, "anatomic integrity," is the capability of the material for easy delivery and conservation of volume; the second, "material safety," refers to the material's biocompatibility, nonantigenicity, and nonmigratory qualities. A number of different nonautologous and autologous options have been offered to meet these criteria.

General Endoscopic Technique

All patients are given a broad-spectrum preoperative antibiotic. The patient is placed in the dorsal lithotomy position. Routine cystoscopy is performed, and the ureters are visualized. A 20-gauge needle is advanced through the working channel. The needle tip is inserted under direct vision at the 6 o'clock position into the subureteral space, approximately 4 to 6 mm distal to the ureteral orifice. Occasionally, proper placement of the needle may be facilitated by placing a 3 Fr catheter in the ureter. The needle is then advanced proximally. The bulking material is injected slowly until a bulge nearly obliterates the ureteral orifice. A precise single injection should be made because multiple puncture sites can allow extravasation of the material. The needle is kept in position for 2 to 3 minutes before it is withdrawn to minimize extravasation of the injected material through the needle track. Clinical studies have shown that such procedures can be performed in an outpatient setting and completed in less than 15 minutes; they have a low morbidity (Geiss et al, 1990).

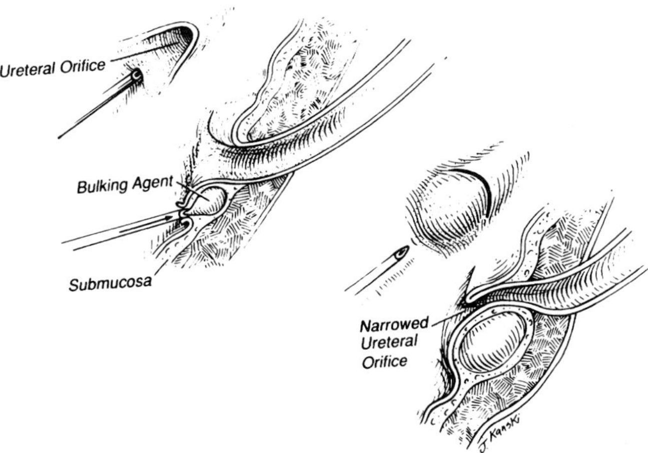

Figure 61–30. Principle of endoscopic treatment of reflux. Bulking agent is injected beneath ureteral orifice with needle. The buttress that is provided helps coapt the distal ureter.

Nonautologous Materials

Teflon

The endoscopic treatment of vesicoureteral reflux originated with otolaryngologists, who treated patients with vocal cord paralysis by injecting their cords with polytetrafluoroethylene (Teflon) paste (Arnold, 1962). Berg (1973) and Politano and colleagues (1974) realized the potential urologic applications of this bulking agent and applied the technology as a solution to urethral incontinence. The endoscopic treatment of reflux was first introduced by Matouschek (1981), who injected Teflon paste (Polytef) into the subureteral region of a patient. O'Donnell and Puri (1984) later popularized the technique as the Sting procedure. Success rates vary from 66% to 92% depending on the grade of reflux and the number of repeat treatments needed, which may be required in as many as a third of patients (Dewan and Guiney, 1992; Bhatti et al, 1993).

Teflon has not fared well in the urinary tract, however. **Teflon particles are phagocytized into the reticuloendothelial system and are able to migrate locally and to distant sites.** This was first documented in a 76-year-old man who was successfully treated for urinary incontinence following a radical prostatectomy but was noted to have pulmonary Teflon granulomas at autopsy 4 years later (Mittleman and Marraccini, 1983). Malizia and colleagues (1984) subsequently demonstrated Teflon particle migration and granuloma formation in the lung, brain, and lymph nodes of dogs and monkeys after periurethral injection. Additional descriptions of Teflon's migration in animals after periureteral injection followed these initial reports (Claes et al, 1989; Aaronson et al, 1993), although the particles are thought by some to be artifacts (Miyakita and Puri, 1994). Concerns of similar results in children have prevented the widespread use of this substance for the treatment of reflux in children (Ferro et al, 1988; Rames and Aaronson, 1991).

Collagen

Collagen has been used as an injectable soft tissue substitute for years, although its application as a cystoscopically delivered antireflux agent is a novel development. Zyderm, Zyplast, and Contigen (Collagen Corporation, Palo Alto, CA, and Bard Corporation, Covington, GA) are commercially available injectable cross-linked bovine corium collagen pastes composed almost solely of type I collagen (Frey et al, 1994). In vitro human and porcine cell culture studies demonstrate a simulatory effect on fibroblasts by collagen causing ingrowth of the material. In the largest clinical study to date, a success rate of 63% was reported after one injection of collagen in 204 ureters of children with variable grades of reflux (Frey et al, 1995). Retreatment with a second injection in initial failures increased the success rate to 79% 3 months after treatment. However, long-term results were not provided. Notably, patients who failed to respond to endoscopic treatment and required reimplantation were shown to have received improperly placed injections, a validation of the concept of endoscopic treatment. In another study of 92 ureters treated with collagen an overall success rate of 65% was achieved, although second (33%) and third (5%) injections were common (Leonard et al, 1991).

The major flaw of collagen is that its volume decreases with time. Biodegradation explains the high frequency of recurrent reflux and the need for retreatment reported in Frey's and other studies (Leonard et al, 1991; Frey et al, 1995). Similar long-term failure rates have been reported with collagen used for the treatment of urinary incontinence (Monga et al, 1995). As opposed to incontinence, reflux is largely a silent disease whose presence can be determined only with invasive radiologic testing. The major problem with any bulking agent that loses its volume is not knowing when reflux might reappear. "Successfully treated" patients may in fact redevelop recurrent reflux and its attendant health risks. For these reasons, collagen has not been approved for the treatment of vesicoureteral reflux by the Food and Drug Administration (FDA).

Silicone Microimplants

Textured silicone macroparticles suspended in hydrogel have been used for the endoscopic treatment of urethral incontinence and vesicoureteral reflux (Buckley et al, 1991; Henly et al, 1995). The substance is composed of fully vulcanized polydimethylsiloxane particles and water-soluble polyvinylpyrrolidone (PVP). The adverse publicity surrounding silicone gel-filled implants does not extend to these types of silicone elastomers. However, safety concerns do exist. In vivo experiments in animals have demonstrated particle migration to distant organs after their submucosal injection in the bladder (Buckley et al, 1991; Henly et al, 1995). Distant migration probably occurs more commonly when silicone particles less than 100 μ in size are included in the suspension. Nevertheless, these types of findings preclude the use of this material.

Polyvinyl Alcohol

Polyvinyl alcohol (Ivalon) has had a variety of medical usages since it was first introduced as a postpneumonectomy prosthesis in 1940. Since then it has also been used to reconstruct cardiac valves and close septal defects, cover burn victims and embolize vascular and neoplastic lesions in the head, neck, and spine. Because this inert material uniquely absorbs water and withstands the actions of most acids, alkalis, and detergents it retains mass over time (Tadavarthy et al, 1975). In fact, Ivalon has been shown to remain as long as 20 years after implantation in other organ systems. Its potential application in the treatment of vesicoureteral reflux was studied by Merguerian and associates (1990) in rabbits. They showed significant fibrotic reactions that gradually stabilize after bladder injections and submucosal retention for 3 months without migration. Combination therapy with collagen may increase the potential long-term success of the latter if polyvinyl alcohol ever becomes widely accepted by urologists, which seems unlikely. Fibroblastic proliferation and tumor development, including sarcoma, in animals are worrisome considerations for clinicians (Canning, 1991).

Injectable Bioglass

Bioglass is a ceramic composed of oxides of silicone, calcium, and sodium and calcium silicone that is biocompatible and bonds to animal soft tissues (Wilson et al, 1981). Fine particles of the material are suspended and delivered in sodium hyaluronate, a natural viscous polysaccharide that is also minimally reactive (Balasz and Denlinger, 1988). These properties are ideal for the treatment of reflux. Preliminary studies show no evidence of instability or migration in rabbits, although additional investigation is warranted (Walker et al, 1992; Walker and Flack, 1994). Difficulty has been experienced in delivering bioglass beads through small needles to treat reflux, and additional work with the substance is still in progress.

Deflux System

The Deflux system combines dextranomer microspheres with sodium hyaluranan, a common polysaccharide (Stenberg and Lackgren, 1995). The microspheres initially induce fibroblast and collagen deposition after their injection in the bladder. They disappear by 1 week, but endogenous tissue augmentation remains. Deflux has been used to treat grade III and IV reflux in 101 ureters of 75 patients. Satisfactory results were achieved in 88% of those with grade III reflux and 62% of those with grade IV, and treatment failed in 25 ureters. Follow-up was limited, however, and detracts somewhat from these impressive results, especially because this material is biodegradable. Concerns about long-term efficacy, as with collagen, will determine the role of this agent in the treatment of reflux.

Detachable Membranes

A detachable, self-sealing silicone balloon has also been developed for the endoscopic treatment of vesicoureteral reflux (Fig. 61–31) (Atala et al, 1992). The balloon is cystoscopically maneuvered into the submucosa beneath the ureter and filled with hydroxyethylmethyl acrylate (HEMA) through a catheter, which is then withdrawn, leaving the membrane intact. HEMA is a biocompatible, nondegradable polymer that is also used as a bonding agent with hip prostheses and as a component of contact lenses. Ferrous sulfate is added to HEMA just before it is injected into the membrane to initiate its polymerization and solidification within 1 to 2 hours. Experiments in a pig model have documented high rates of success with this novel system. HEMA-filled membranes cause minimal reaction, remain

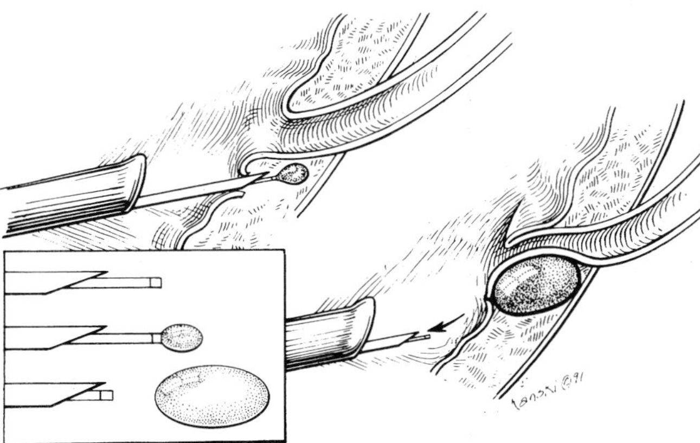

Figure 61–31. Detatchable balloon system. Balloon is delivered through a needle into the subureteral space to provide similar antirefluxing action as a bulking agent.

intact, and do not migrate. The system has been recently approved by the FDA to assess the performance of membranes in the treatment of incontinence.

Autologous Injectable Materials

Autologous Fat

Autologous fat has been used as a bulking agent by plastic surgeons to sculpt new body contours for years. **Its major drawback stems from its extremely unreliable volume conservation.** Peer (1956) described a 50% volume loss 1 year after open harvest and implantation. Autologous fat has been used for the treatment of urethral incontinence with equivocal success (Santiago et al, 1989). Animal studies also raise concerns about its stability when used as an antireflux agent. Matthews and his associates (1994) cites a 25% to 100% loss in 66% of rabbit bladders injected with fat, although no inflammatory response was present. Until these conservation characteristics are better defined, fat is unlikely to gain little acceptance as a treatment option for reflux.

Alginate and Chondrocytes

Alginate, a biodegradable polymer, can be seeded with chondrocytes to serve as a synthetic substrate for the injectable delivery and maintenance of cartilage in vivo. Alginate-bovine chondrocyte cell allografts contain viable cartilage cells for as long as 6 months after implantation in athymic mice. The new cartilage that is formed retains the approximate shape and volume of the injected template (Atala et al, 1993a). Relying on these characteristics, harvested chondrocytes effectively eliminated reflux in a mini-pig model (Atala et al, 1994b). The chondrocyte-alginate gel suspension meets all of the necessary criteria desired of an ideal substance. Because it is a biodegradable, injectable material that is nonmigratory and nonantigenic and conserves its volume, the alginate-chondrocyte mixture may be ideal for the treatment of reflux as well as urinary incontinence. FDA-approved clinical trials are now underway.

Alginate and Bladder Muscle

Using the same reasoning applied to chondrocyte technology, autologous muscle cells have been combined with synthetic alginate to treat reflux. Using a similar series of experiments, progressive alginate replacement and muscular differentiation were shown in athymic mice (Atala et al, 1994a). Again, reflux was obviated in a mini-pig model using harvested muscle cells (Cilento and Atala, 1995). Histologic examinations have shown that muscle cells survive after being harvested, expanded in culture, and injected in the subureteral mucosa. Muscle-alginate complex offers the same advantages as chondrocyte-alginate complex and may be applicable to any reconstructive procedure that requires a biocompatible and injectable bulking agent.

Summary

The endoscopic treatment of vesicoureteral reflux can be effective. The task remains to discover a material that is safe and provides long-term efficacy. The next several years will be instrumental in determining which autologous or nonautologous bulking agent is best for this innovative solution to reflux.

LAPAROSCOPIC MANAGEMENT

Major advances have been made in laparoscopic surgery during the past decade. The advantages of this approach over open surgery include smaller incisions, less discomfort, brief hospitalization, and quicker convalescence. The recent surge in laparoscopic urologic procedures and equipment (Winfield et al, 1991) has led several investigators to explore so-called noninvasive alternatives to open ureteroneocystostomy. The first successful correction of reflux in an animal was reported by Atala and his colleagues (1993b), who applied a laparoscopic modification of the Lich-Gregoir extravesical reimplant, described subsequently, to mini-pigs (Lich et al, 1961; Gregoir and Van Regermortar, 1964). Serial cystograms demonstrated resolution of reflux in every animal, and IVP showed no evidence of obstruction. Later reports confirmed that laparoscopic correction of reflux was technically feasible in other animal models (Schimberg et al, 1994; McDougall et al, 1995) and in humans (Atala, 1993; Ehrlich et al, 1994).

There is a learning curve to be broached with laparoscopy, and experience is essential to the success of this approach. As with any new technique, patients must be carefully selected. The procedure is initially limited to older children with unilateral reflux and nondilated ureters. Indications are broadened with further experience, although drawbacks remain. Laparoscopy requires a team with at least two surgeons; the repair is converted from an extraperitoneal to an intraperitoneal approach; many of the available instruments are less than ideal for use in children, operative time is greater than with open techniques, and cost is increased because of the lengthier surgery and the expense of disposable equipment. These considerations explain why, after an initial flurry of interest, laparoscopic reimplantation has not been used. It may be that improved instrumentation and more experience will allow better acceptance of the laparoscopic approach to reflux.

LAPAROSCOPIC TECHNIQUE (Fig. 61–32). A Verris needle is placed beneath the umbilicus, and pneumoperitoneum is obtained by insufflating CO_2 (at a rate of 2 L/min) up to a pressure of 15 mm Hg. After adequate insufflation has been achieved, two 10-mm trocars are placed, one at the side opposite the refluxing ureter at the midclavicular line 1 cm above the umbilicus (for various instruments), and one in the infraumbilical midline (camera). Two 10-mm trocars are then positioned in the left and right midclavicular line, 2 cm above the level of the anterior superior iliac spine (dissecting instruments, retractors). The table is then laterally rotated with the refluxing side up, allowing the bladder and viscera to fall away from the area of repair.

Ureteral mobilization is begun by identifying the obliterated umbilical artery along the pelvic sidewall. The bladder is then shifted away from the operative side by grasping and retracting its dome. This stretches the obliterated umbilical artery, which is traced deep into the pelvis until the ureter is seen passing beneath it. After dividing the artery, periureteral adventitial tissue is gently grasped to retract the ureter away from the bladder. Blunt dissection is used to mobilize 4 cm of the ureter proximal to the ureterovesical junction (UVJ) to permit its placement within a bladder trough. Small vessels are isolated and carefully fulgurated with cautery, and the UVJ is cleared of any bulky surrounding tissues. The bladder wall trough is created by incising the detrusor with electrocautery along a line from the UVJ superiorly for approximately 3 cm and inferiorly for 1 cm. Gentle spread-

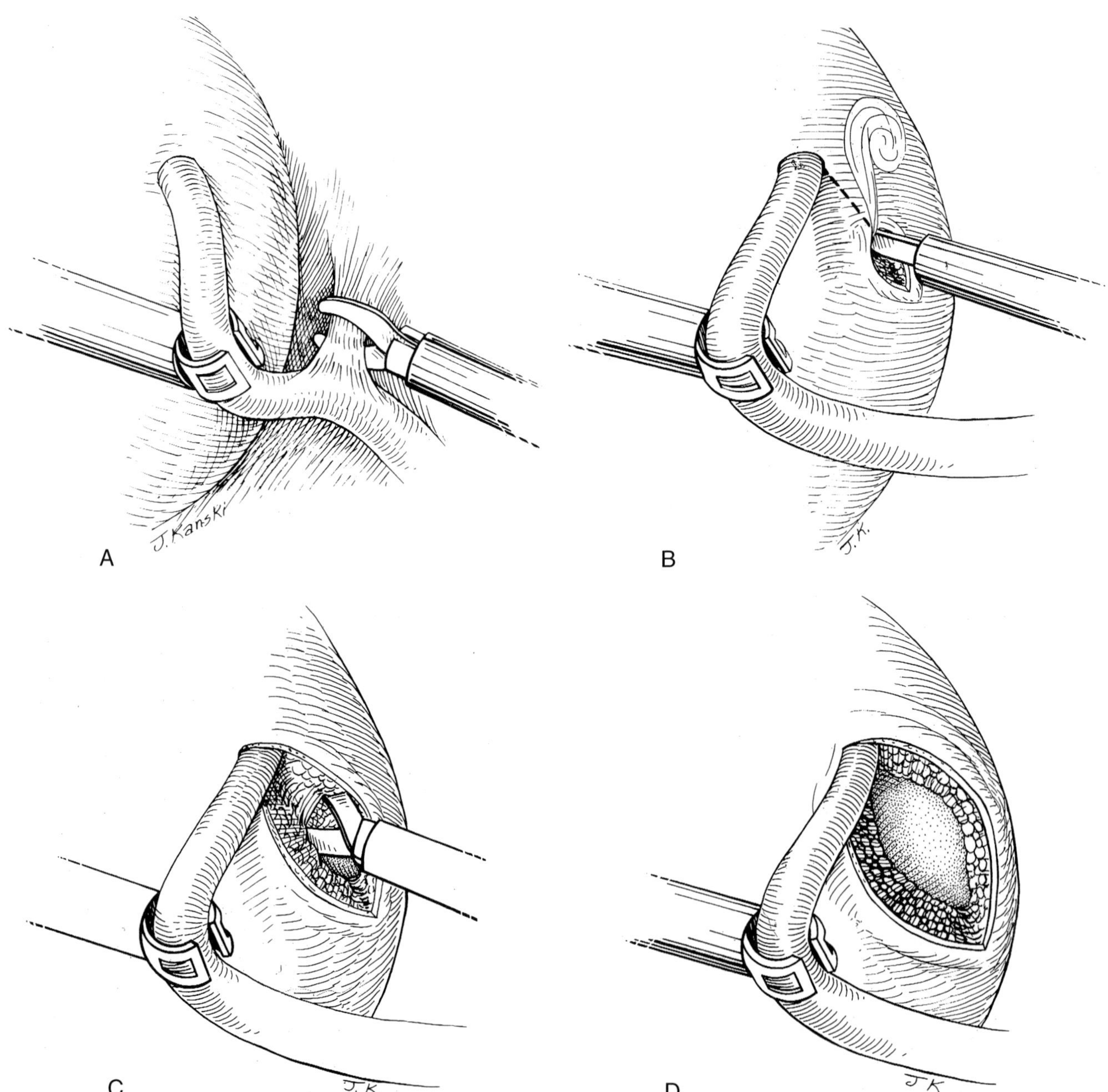

Figure 61–32. Laparoscopic reimplant. *A,* Ureteral mobilization. The ureter is grasped gently, and the periureteral tissue is dissected bluntly toward the ureterovesical junction. *B* to *D,* Creation of bladder wall trough. Bladder wall is incised with electrocautery 3 cm proximal to the ureterovesical junction. Muscle fibers are gently cut and spread. Dissection is complete when mucosal tissue bulges outward.

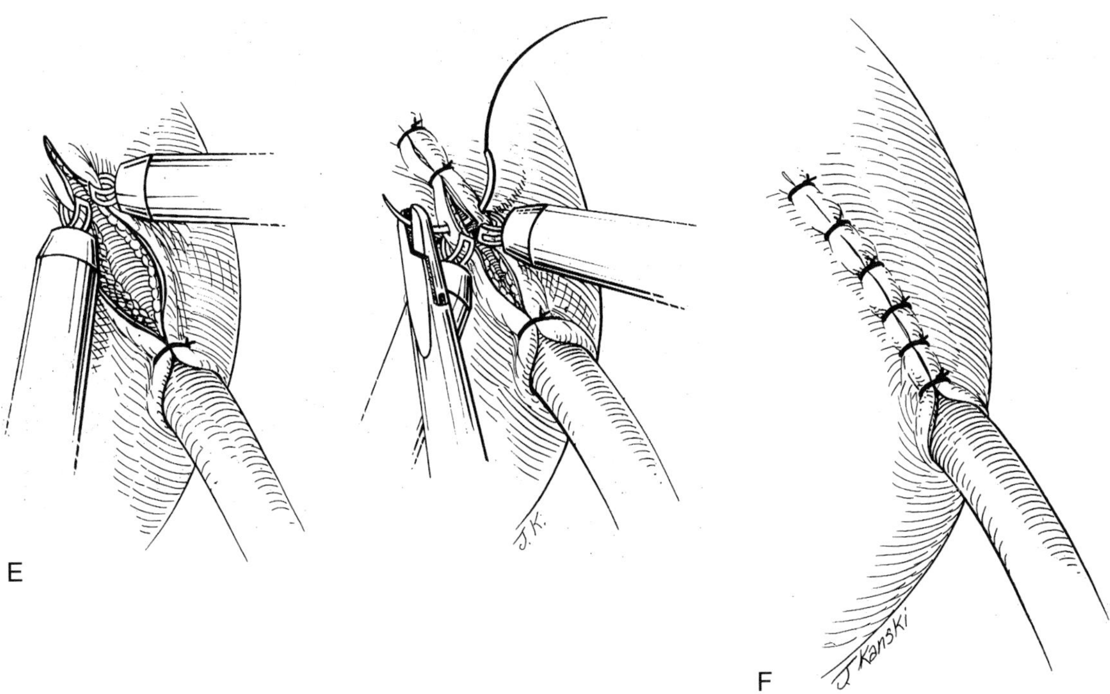

Figure 61–32 *Continued E,* After placing the ureter in the trough, grasping instruments wrap the superior aspect of the bladder wall around the ureter and a suture is placed proximally, immobilizing the ureter in the trough *(left).* Remaining sutures are placed throughout the length of the tunnel *(right). F,* Completed repair.

ing of the muscle fibers opens the trough until the mucosa bulges outward. This level of dissection is developed for the entire length of the tunnel. Muscle fibers around the UVJ are also spread slightly, but no attempt is made to perform extensive dissection of the UVJ free of the bladder wall.

The ureter is advanced by placing a pexing suture that approximates lateral muscle at the distal end of the trough and distal ureter and medial bladder muscle tissue at the end of the trough. Once the advancement is complete, detrusor is approximated over the ureter with a continuous long-lasting absorisxanone suture (PDS, Ethicon, Cincinnati, OH). A Lapra-Ty (Ethicon) is extremely useful for this portion of the procedure. This device laparoscopically applies absorbable anchors onto sutures. The anchor secures the suture and acts as a knot. Two grasping instruments are used to wrap the superior aspect of the bladder wall trough around the ureter, and a suture is placed at the distalmost point, bringing the edges of the bladder muscle together over the ureter. A Lapra-Ty anchor is placed at the end of the suture. This tie serves to maintain traction on the bladder wall trough as a running suture is initiated from the distalmost portion of the trough. Additional Lapra-Ty anchors are placed along the anastomosis to keep the suture under appropriate tension during the closure.

After the repair is complete, instruments and trocars are removed after checking for trocar site bleeding or visceral injury. The fascial defects and skin of each port are closed with absorbable sutures. A bladder catheter may be kept overnight.

MEGAURETER

The spectrum of anomalies known as megaureter (MGU) continues to challenge today's urologists and fuels one of the livelier debates in the field. Like reflux, the surgical solutions to the anomaly are reliable. Where controversy arises is in differentiating nonobstructive from obstructive variants and in better defining the indications for surgery. It is increasingly apparent that many urinary tract dilatations are distortions of the collecting system that, although at times quite severe, may not represent an obstructive threat to their associated renal moiety. Examples that have been recognized for some time include MGU found with prune-belly syndrome and the postobstructive upper tract dilatation associated with urethral valves (Glassberg et al, 1982).

More recently, perinatal ultrasonography has altered the understanding and management of other urologic anomalies and dilatations, and megaureters are no exception (Arger et al, 1986). In one series, MGU comprised 20% of antenatally diagnosed urologic anomalies, a percentage inordinately higher than that in historical series of urinary tract abnormalities, in which most abnormalities were discovered only after they became symptomatic (infection, calculi, and so on) (Preston and Lebowitz, 1989). Surgery usually was necessary. Today, with prenatal detection, the majority of children present with abnormalities that are totally asymptomatic. The denominator increased, and, for obvious reasons, its characteristics changed. If left undetected, many MGUs would never become symptomatic, an observation that raises serious questions about treatment. In the same manner, expectant treatment and serial ultrasonic follow-up have dramatically redefined the natural history of multicystic dysplastic kidneys (Wacksman and Phipps, 1993), ureteroceles, and variants of ureteropelvic junction (UPJ) obstruction (Homsy et al, 1986; Grignon et al, 1986, Johnson et al, 1987). The last are particularly significant because mechanisms that affect the ureter at its junction with the renal pelvis and bring about resolution of hydronephrosis may be similar to those that influence nonrefluxing MGUs.

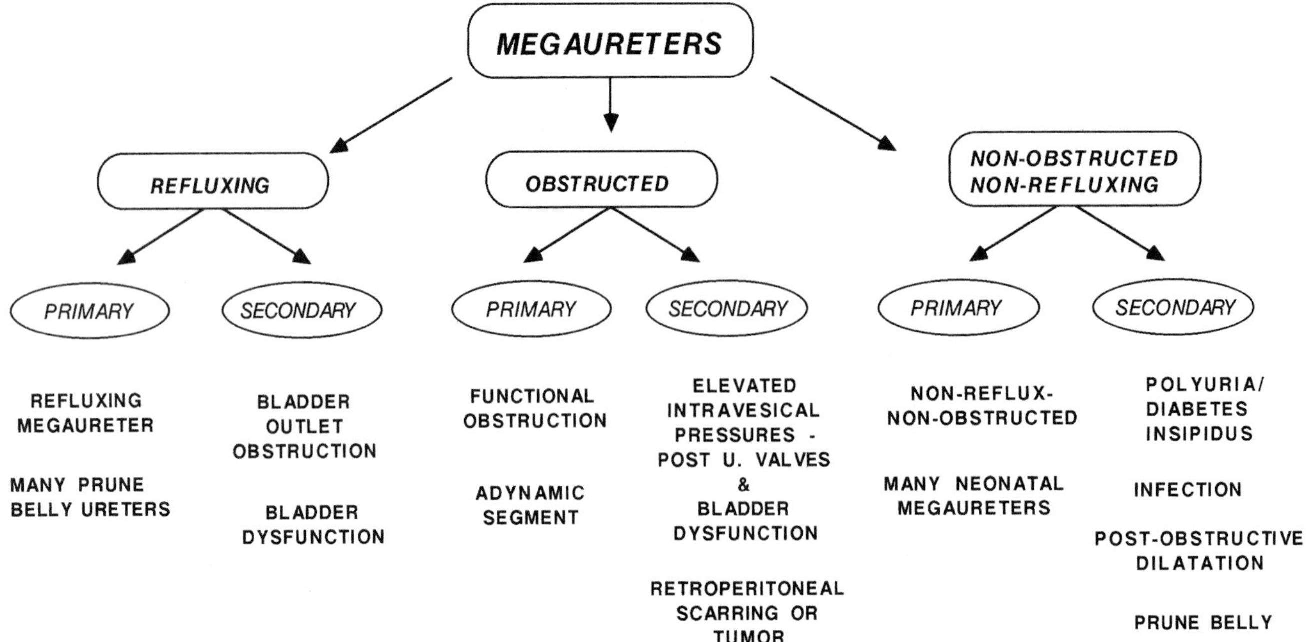

Figure 61–33. Three major classifications of megaureter based on primary and secondary etiologies. A combination of reflux and obstruction can also be seen with some megaureters.

Definitions

The term megaureter could be applied to any dilated or "big" (*mega*) ureter and has a generic connotation because it does not refer to any particular entity. This caused some confusion in the earlier literature until an international classification system was created (Smith et al, 1977) that forms the basis of today's designations and serves as a useful guide for management *when categorization is possible* (Fig. 61–33) (King, 1980). **The dilated ureter or MGU can be classified into one of four groups based on the cause of the dilatation. These include (1) refluxing, (2) obstructed, (3) both refluxing and obstructed, and (4) nonrefluxing and nonobstructed.** Further subdivisions into primary or secondary causes assume additional importance for obvious reasons. Therapeutic recommendations depend on proper categorization, and a thorough evaluation of the entire urinary tract is required in every case.

Pathophysiology

PRIMARY AND SECONDARY REFLUXING MEGAURETER. The cause of primary and secondary refluxing MGU was discussed earlier. **In addition, a small group of patients have an element of obstruction combined with reflux.** In one series of over 400 refluxing ureters, obstruction was present in approximately 2% of cases (Weiss and Lytton, 1974). A dysgenetic distal ureteral segment that not only fails to coapt within the intramural tunnel but also has ineffective peristalsis is implicated. Identification is important because the management of obstruction often differs from that of reflux alone.

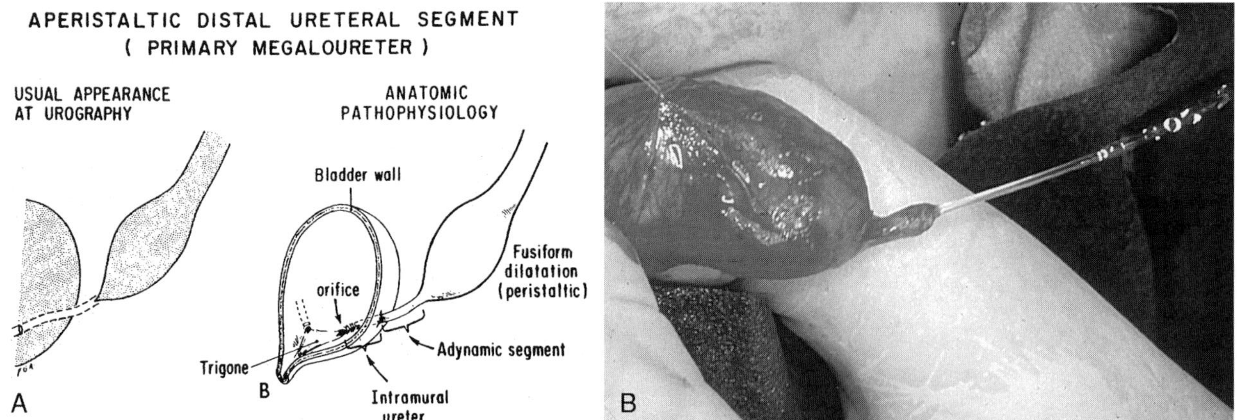

Figure 61–34. *A,* Artist's rendition of megaureter. Ureteral dilatation begins above the ureterovesical junction, usually a few millimeters or more above the bladder. (Courtesy of Dr. AP McLaughlin III.) *B,* Typical appearance of distal portion of megaureter at exploration.

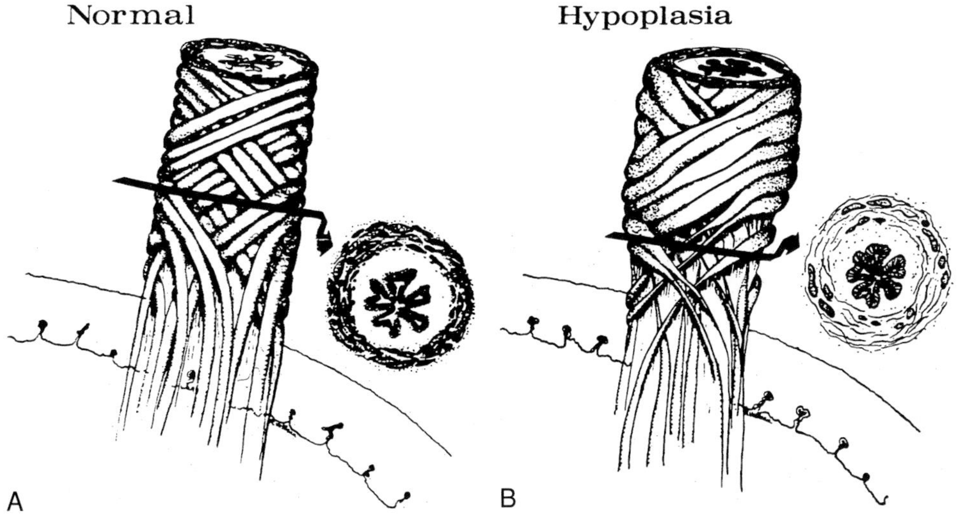

Figure 61–35. *A,* Normal ureteral muscular orientation sometimes seen with megaureters. *B,* Hypoplasia and atrophy of muscle is more common. (From McLaughlin AP III, Pfister RC, Leadbetter WF, et al: The pathophysiology of primary megaureter. J Urol, 1973; 109:805–811. Copyright © 1973 by The Williams & Wilkins Company.)

PRIMARY OBSTRUCTIVE MEGAURETER. It is generally agreed that the cause of primary obstructive MGU is an aperistaltic juxtavesical segment 3 to 4 cm long that is unable to propagate urine at acceptable flow rates. The cause of this segmental aberrancy remains unclear (Fig. 61–34). True stenosis is rarely found, but a variety of histologic and ultrastructural abnormalities have been described. These include disorientation of muscle (Tanagho, 1973; MacKinnon, 1977), muscular hypoplasia, muscular hypertrophy, and mural fibrosis (McLaughlin et al, 1973) (Fig. 61–35). Excess collagen deposition has been a common finding in light and electron microscopic studies (Gregoir and Debled, 1969; Hanna et al, 1976; Pagano and Passerini, 1977) (Figs. 61–36 and 61–37). In theory, increased matrix deposition alters cell-to-cell junctions and disrupts myoelectrical propagation and peristalsis. Why the distal ureter is usually involved is unclear but may be related to arrested development of its musculature, which is the last to develop (Tanagho, 1973). **Regardless of cause, altered peristalsis prevents the free outflow of urine, and func-**

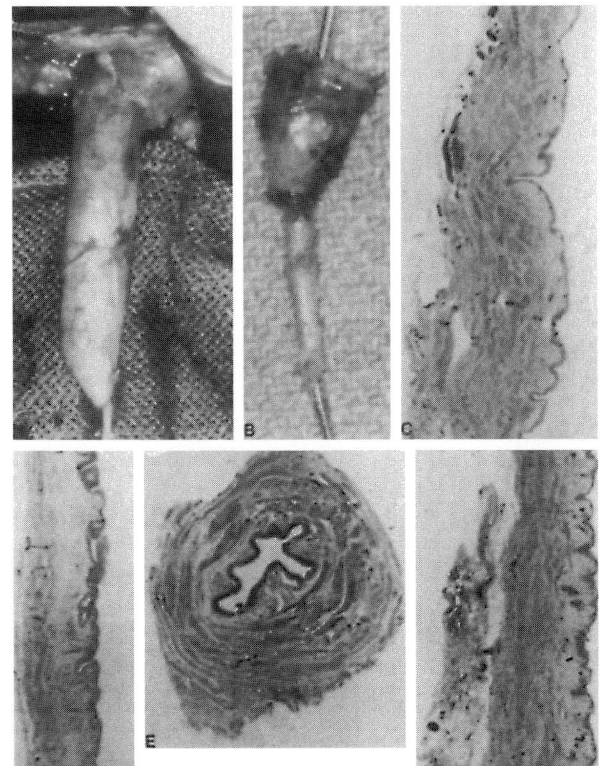

Figure 61–36. Primary obstructive megaureter. Light microscopic findings show various abnormalities. *A,* Operative exposure. *B,* Specimen. Obstructed segment admits probe. *C,* No abnormality seen on longitudinal section. *D,* Reduced muscle bulk seen in some megaureters. *E,* Preponderance of circular muscle. *F,* Thickened adventitia. (From Hanna MK, Jeffs RD, Sturgess JM, et al: Ureteral stricure and ultrastructure. J Urol 1978; 116:728. Copyright © 1978 by The Williams & Wilkins Company, Baltimore.)

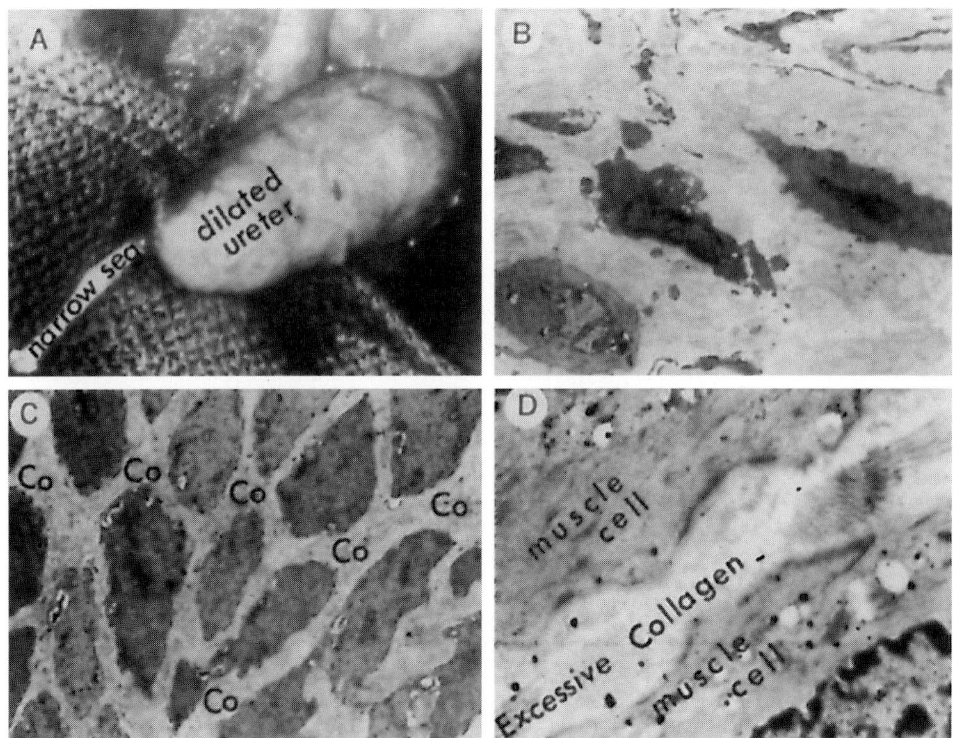

Figure 61–37. Primary obstructive megaureter. Electron microscopic findings. *A,* Operative specimen. *B,* Muscle cell atrophy, absent nexus, and excessive ground substance and collagen in intracellular space from dilated ureter. *C,* Abnormal collagen fibers between muscle cells (reduced × 4000). *D,* Abnormality from narrow ureter (reduced from 17,000). (From Hanna MK, Jeffs RD, Sturgess JM, et al: Ureteral stricure and ultrastructure, part II. J Urol 1978; 116:728. Copyright © 1978 by The Williams & Wilkins Company.)

tional obstruction results. Retrograde regurgitation occurs as successive boluses of urine are unable to traverse the aberrant distal segment fully. The degree of ureteral dilatation that results depends on the amount of urine forced to coalesce proximally owing to incomplete passage. This in turn is determined by the degree of distal obstruction and urinary output (Hutch and Tanagho, 1965). This disruption in ureteral dynamics has obvious implications for the renal parenchyma if the collecting system is unable to dampen the proximal pressures that can develop. Other rare causes of primary obstructive MGU include congenital ureteral strictures (Allen, 1970) and ureteral valves (Albertson and Talner, 1972).

SECONDARY OBSTRUCTIVE MEGAURETER. This form of MGU most commonly occurs with neurogenic and non-neurogenic voiding dysfunction or infravesical obstructions such as posterior urethral valves. The ureter experiences increasing difficulty with the propulsion of urine when an elevated pressure differential (greater than 40 cm of water) exists across the ureterovesical junction. Progressive ureteral dilatation, reflux, and renal damage can be expected if such pressures continue unchecked. The dilatation that occurs in most cases largely resolves once the cause of the elevated intravesical pressures has been addressed. Other ureters remain permanently dilated owing to what appears to be altered compliance or a permanent insult to the organ's peristaltic mechanisms. Transmural scarring due to chronic infection is implicated in some cases. Obstruction is not present within such ureters, but their ability to buffer the kidney is lessened as elevated intravesical pressures are projected proximally as a noncompliant column (Jones et al, 1988). Other causes of ureteral dilatation, the management of which is discussed in more detail elsewhere, include ureteroceles, bladder diverticula, periureteral postreimplant fibrosis, neurogenic bladder, and external compression by retroperitoneal tumors, masses, or aberrant vessels.

SECONDARY NONOBSTRUCTIVE, NONREFLUXING MEGAURETER. Nonobstructed, nonrefluxing MGUs are more common than was once recognized and often have an identifiable cause. **Significant ureteral dilatation can result from acute UTIs as a consequence of bacterial endotoxins that inhibit peristalsis.** Resolution is expected with appropriate antibiotic therapy (Retik et al, 1978). Nephropathies and other medical conditions that cause significant increases in urinary output can also lead to progressive ureteral dilatation as the collecting system complies to handle the output from above. These conditions include lithium toxicity, diabetes insipidus or mellitus, sickle cell nephropathy, and psychogenic polydipsia (Keating, 1990). The most extreme examples of nonobstructed ureteral dilatations occur with the prune-belly syndrome. A spectrum of severity exists, but it is common to have markedly dilated and tortuous MGUs that belie the presence of a well-preserved and normally functioning renal parenchyma (Berdon et al, 1977; Keating and Duckett, 1993).

PRIMARY NONOBSTRUCTIVE, NONREFLUXING MEGAURETER. Once reflux, obstruction, and secondary causes of dilatation are ruled out, the designation of primary nonrefluxing nonobstructed MGU is appropriate. Most MGUs in newborns fall into this category (Keating et al, 1989; Rickwood et al, 1992; Baskin et al, 1994b). In addition, many MGUs discovered in adults in which the distal ureteral spindle alone is dilated, are similarly categorized (Fig. 61–38). Explanations for the ureteral transformations that occur during development remain to be clarified. However, a multifactorial cause with a basis in transitional renal physiology and ureteral histoanatomy seems likely. The fetal kidney reportedly produces four to

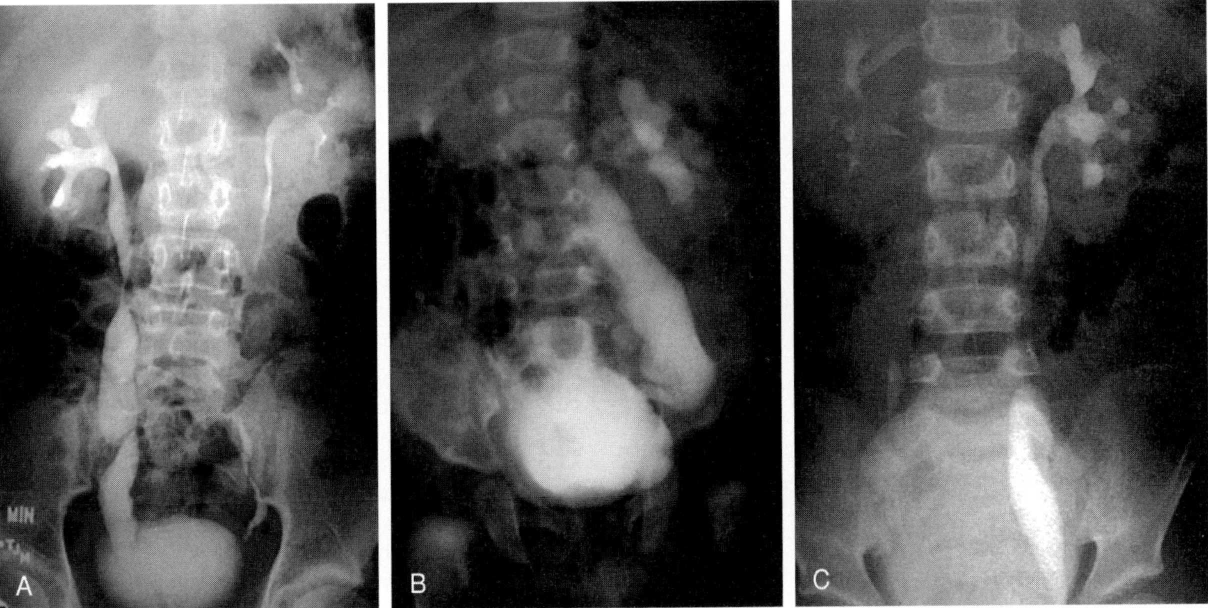

Figure 61–38. *A,* Megaureter in adult is usually discovered serendipitously. Most are asymptomatic. Distal ureteral spindle is typically involved. *B,* Megaureter discovered antenatally and evaluated in newborn period. Believed to be a nonobstructive variant. *C,* Same child 2 years later. Continued maturation leaves ureter with similar appearance to that of adult.

six times more urine before delivery than it does afterward owing to differences in glomerular filtration, renal vascular resistance, and concentrating ability (Campbell et al, 1973). This deluge from above might "imprint" dilatation on the fetal ureter in a manner similar to that described for the polyuric nephropathies, especially if a transient distal obstruction is present. Persistent fetal folds (Fig. 61–39) (Ostling, 1942), delays in the development of ureteral patency (Ruano-Gil et al, 1975), and immaturity of normal peristalsis are plausible causes of the obstruction. The less compliant, hyperreflexic bladder of infancy (Baskin et al, 1994a) or a transient urethral obstruction that causes altered bladder compliance may also be implicated. Developmental alterations in ureteral compliance and changes in configuration may also result from differences in the deposition and orientation of elastin, collagen, and other matrices at different stages of development (Escala et al, 1989). The newborn ureter is a more compliant conduit than that of the adult, an impression borne out by the tortuous dilatations seen with distal obstruction in the infant compared to the "pipe stem" response seen at older ages. As a result, the kidneys of affected newborns are probably better buffered from the pressures of any partial or transient obstruction that might occur early in development than kidneys obstructed at more proximal levels (UPJ) or at a later age.

Evaluation

Ultrasound is the initial study obtained in any child in whom a urinary abnormality is suspected. It provides useful anatomic detail of the renal parenchyma, collecting system, and bladder and also offers an invaluable baseline standard of the degree of hydroureteronephrosis that can be used in serial follow-up (Fig. 61–40). Once ureteral dilatation is detected, a voiding cystourethrogram is obtained in most cases to rule out reflux and assess the quality of the bladder and urethra, in which neurogenic dysfunction or outlet obstruction are common causes of secondary MGU. A study is also performed to judge renal function and the degree of obstruction, if any. *Excretory urography* (IVP) is rarely performed because its functional data must be inferred. Substandard quality of this study also presents a problem with neonates because of renal immaturity and bowel gas. The anatomic detail provided by an IVP is useful when the level of obstruction cannot be defined, but this information can also be provided by retrograde pyelography at surgery. Instead, a *diuretic renogram* is preferred because it offers objective reproducible parameters of function and obstruction. Technetium-99m diethylenetriamine pentaacetic acid (^{99m}Tc DTPA) and technetium-99m mertiatide (MAG3) are the radionuclides most commonly used to provide parameters of function and clearance in assessment of obstruction. The diuretic renogram, however, suffers from its own shortcomings. Tracer and diuretic dosing must be standardized to ensure valid comparison of test results. Subjective estimates must be made both of the area of interest, which should include the lower ureter (Koff et al, 1984), and of the degree of filling of the affected system. These make timing the administration of the diuretic largely empirical, especially in patients with MGU. In addition, the immature glomeruli of the newborn kidney have a blunted response to diuretics. Whenever possible, it is preferable to defer the study for approximately 3 months to allow glomerular maturation. Scans that evaluate drainage (T1/2) alone often yield values indicative of obstruction because of the dilatation of the collecting system. As evaluators of function, however, these represent false-positive studies. Useful information is provided when there is no evidence of obstruction (Fig. 61–41).

Radionuclide scans can also be used to estimate glomerular filtration rates and absolute renal function by measuring

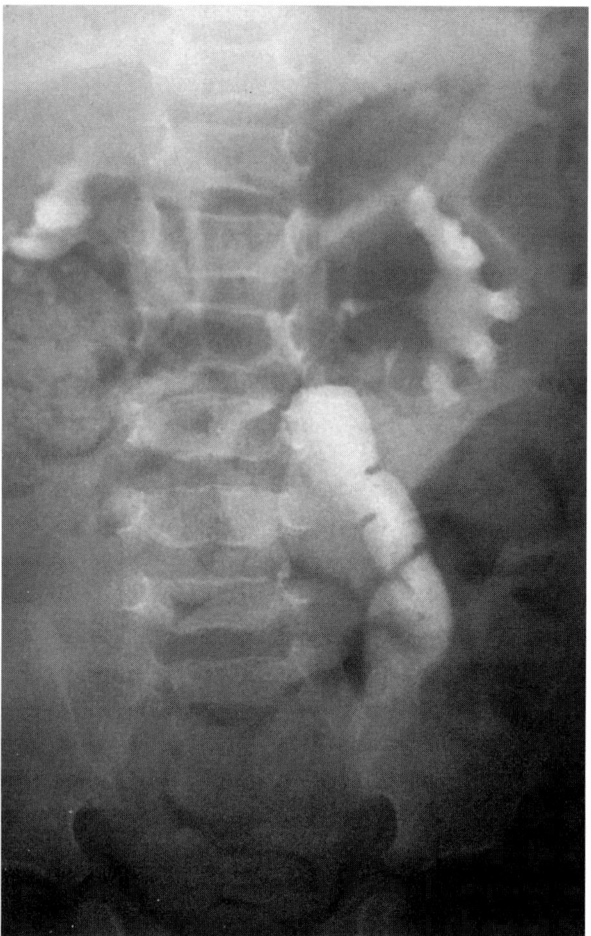

Figure 61–39. Ureteral folds perhaps implicated in early developmental obstructions. Lengthening with interval growth may bring about resolution.

the uptake of radionuclide (DPTA) early after its systemic administration. Correlation with glomerular filtration is high (Heyman and Duckett, 1988). The percentage of the total dose, the so-called extraction factor, filtered by the kidneys can then be calculated and has been adopted by some institutions as a means of providing a more objective parameter for gauging significant obstruction. **Ideally, these types of determinations offer functional correlates to hydroureteronephrosis by quantitating the effects of obstruction where it matters most, at the parenchymal level, rather than within the collecting system, where slow rates of washout are to be expected because of dilatation.** Nevertheless, differentiating truly obstructive dilatations of the urinary tract from those that appear to be no more than nonobstructive variants remains difficult (see Chapter 9).

Whitaker's perfusion test (Whitaker, 1973) can also be used to evaluate obstruction, although its invasiveness is a drawback in children. In addition, the rate of flow (10 ml/min) at which intrapelvic pressures are measured are excessive for younger children, and the parameters of obstruction are somewhat empirically defined. The correlation of pressure perfusion with diuretic renography is good, but the study provides little additional data than that offered by scintigraphy (Kass et al, 1985). Exceptions include renal moieties with extremely poor function or patients in whom the diuretic renogram is equivocal or difficult to interpret because of a capcious collecting system. Cystoscopy is done in concert with surgery if it becomes necessary. Retrograde imaging is rarely included in the initial evaluation of MGU, whose anatomy can usually be defined by other means.

Recommendations

The therapeutic recommendations for MGUs that are truly obstructed and those that reflux are fairly well agreed on. Where disagreement does arise is in the differentiation of primary obstructed MGU from the nonrefluxing nonobstructed variants, especially in the neonate. Unfortunately, given the constraints of the available diagnostic studies, classification is not always possible.

PRIMARY REFLUXING MEGAURETER. As discussed previously, the management of refluxing MGUs has changed with the advent of antenatal detection. **The rote recommendation for surgery in newborns and infants with grades IV and V reflux no longer applies. Instead, medical management is appropriate during infancy and is continued if a trend to resolution is noted.** Otherwise, surgery remains the recommendation for persistent high-

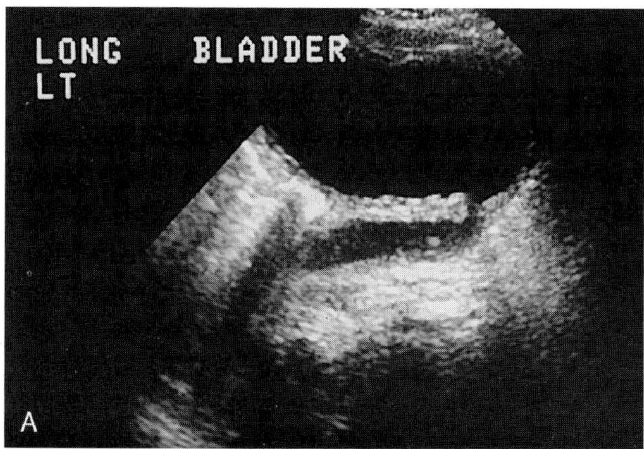

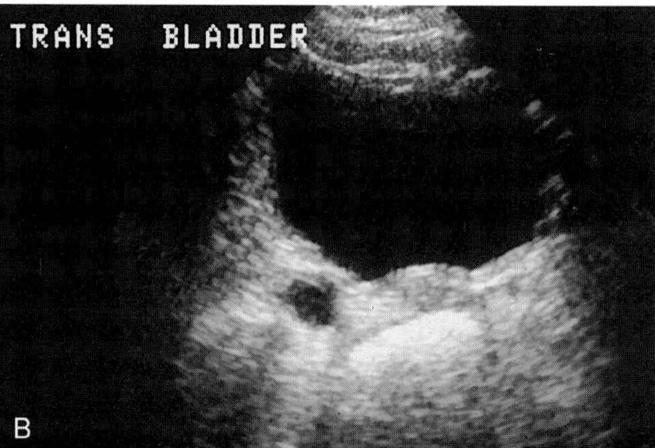

Figure 61–40. Urologic ultrasound includes evaluation of the upper urinary tract as well as the pelvis and the bladder. *A,* Longitudinal study shows ureteral dilatation. *B,* Transverse study shows same behind the bladder on the right.

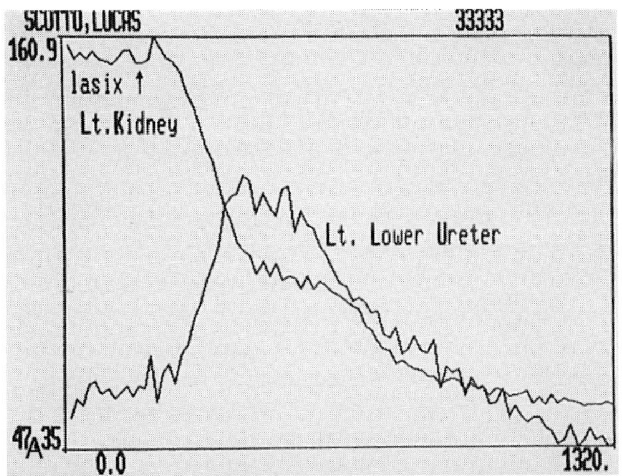

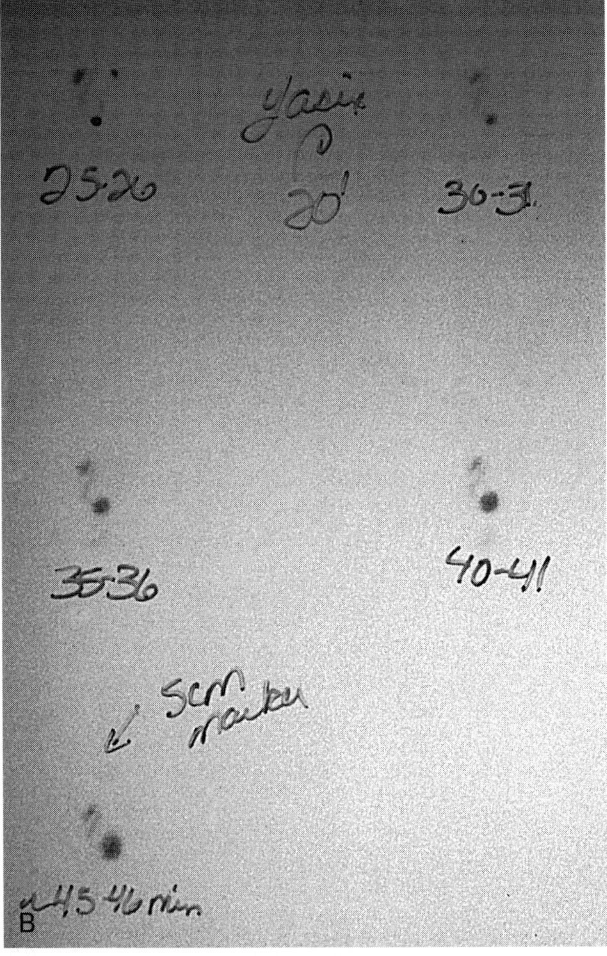

Figure 61–41. Diuretic renography (DTPA) of megaureter shown in 61–38*B*. *A*, Washout curve from area of interest shows no evidence of obstruction, although delayed washout is commonly seen with such variants. *B*, Equal function was present on early sequences. Drainage is slightly impaired on the left.

grade reflux in older children and adults. In the rare infant who fails medical management but is considered too small for reconstruction, distal ureterostomy for unilateral reflux or vesicostomy for bilateral disease provides an ideal temporizing solution.

SECONDARY REFLUXING OR OBSTRUCTIVE MGU. The management of secondary MGU is directed at its cause. For example, impressive degrees of reflux and dilatation often improve with the ablation of urethral valves or medical management of neurogenic bladder. Other diseases that lead to secondary MGU, including the prune-belly syndrome, **diabetes insipidus, or infection, require no more than observation alone.** Chronic congenital distention, regardless of its source, imprints permanent dilatation on many collecting systems. As a result, some degree of nonobstructed hydroureteronephrosis usually persists even after primary or secondary causes have been corrected. This dilation can be amplified with bladder filling, a finding that can pose a diagnostic dilemma because it mimics persistent or recurrent obstruction at the ureterovesical junction. Reevaluation is often necessary.

PRIMARY OBSTRUCTIVE OR NONOBSTRUCTIVE MEGAURETER. Deciding between surgery or expectant treatment sometimes becomes a function of clinical impression and experience. However, any haste in correcting MGU in the newborn is tempered by the realization that their repair represents a technical challenge in smaller infants. Even in experienced hands, the complication rate of surgery is higher than it is in older children. For example, repeat surgeries were required in 5 of 42 (12%) infants who were operated on before 8 months of age (Peters et al, 1989). **In the light of clinical observation, most clinicians now believe that as long as renal function is not significantly affected and urinary infections do not become a problem, expectant management is preferable. Antibiotic suppression and close radiologic surveillance are appropriate in most cases.** Periodic checks of the urine and ultrasound examinations every 3 to 6 months during the first year of life are appropriate. Renography is also sometimes repeated. The duration between studies is then extended if improvement in the degree of dilatation is seen. **If hydroureteronephrosis is severe and shows no signs of improvement or if the clinical status worsens, correction is undertaken when it is technically feasible, usually between the ages of 1 and 2 years.** In the occasional newborn who presents with massive ureteral dilatation and poor renal function (which is rare with MGU) or who develops recurrent infections, distal ureterostomy provides an effective panacea for poor drainage until the child is old enough to undergo reimplantation.

Clinical Correlates—Nonobstructive Megaureter

Past studies that have surgically addressed urinary tract obstructions or dilatations at both the UPJ and ureterovesical junction (UVJ) suffer from two weaknesses. They (1) lack a diagnostic modality that allows a uniform and reliable differentiation of nonobstructive from obstructive dilatations, and (2) are unable to predict the degree of renal recovery that might occur after the dilatation or obstruction has been corrected. In addition, data from surgical "correction" of urinary tract dilatation in the neonate are skewed by a paradox peculiar to therapy at this age. That is, although truly obstructed kidneys are helped by surgery, operations also appear to benefit kidneys with preoperative dilatation that are not obstructed because of the increases in glomerular and tubular function that occur with normal renal maturation. Obviously, the efficacy of surgery is difficult to judge in either instance (King et al, 1984; Peters et al, 1989; Koff and Campbell, 1992).

Antenatally diagnosed MGUs are different. Keating and colleagues evaluated 23 ureters in 17 newborns with observation alone (Keating et al, 1989). Renal scintigraphy (DTPA) and assessment of function rather than drainage defined the parameters of obstruction. Comparative IVPs were also obtained in most. Notably, 20 of the 23 ureters (87%) were deemed nonobstructive variants that showed no significant decrease in function and were followed medically (Fig. 61–42). None showed a decrease in renal function after an average of 7 years follow-up, and the improvement in dilatation that occurred in most was impressive (Baskin et al, 1994b). Others have since noted the same phenomenon, although functional deterioration or breakthrough urinary infections occurred in 13 of 82 neonatal MGUs (16%) in the combined series of Rickwood and colleagues (1992) and Liu and associates (1994). The rate of improvement that occurs with MGU is higher than the approximate 50% improvement seen in most series of ureteropelvic junction obstruction (Homsy et al, 1986; Johnson, 1987). Expectant treatment of this type of MGU is not novel, however. Nearly three decades ago, Williams and Hulme-Moir identified a subgroup of patients with obstructive ureters who had mild or negligible symptoms. Conservative management was recommended, although long-term follow-up of this series is unavailable (Williams and Hulme-Moir, 1970). Pitts and Muecke (1974) later followed a series of 80 patients with congenital MGU, 40% of whom required no therapy. The radiographic appearance of primary MGU coincidentally found in adults usually remains stable over many years (Heal, 1973; Pfister and Hendren, 1978). Fusiform dilatations of the distal ureteral spindle comprise the most common variants, although the entire ureter can be affected. Pyelocaliectasis is either absent or mild (Hanna and Wyatt, 1975). **It now appears that many perinatally diagnosed MGUs represent the anomaly at an earlier stage in its natural history and are precursors of the nonobstructive variants discovered serendipidously in adults in the past.**

Surgical Options

Once it has been determined that correction of a MGU is necessary regardless of its cause, the surgical objectives of ureteroneocystostomy are the same as those used with nondilated ureter. **Ureteral tailoring (excision or plication) is usually necessary to achieve the proper length-diameter ratio required for successful reimplants. Narrowing the ureter also theoretically allows its walls to coapt properly, leading to more effective peristalsis. Revising the distal segment intended for reimplantation is all that is usually required.** The proximal segments of most MGUs regain tone once they are unobstructed. Kinking is usually nonobstructive and resolves. Rarely, massively dilated and tortuous ureters require straightening with removal of excess length and proximal revision (Hanna, 1979). Instead, extended stent drainage after tapering such a ureter decompresses the system and allows peristaltic recovery.

Two methods can be used to remodel MGUs. Plication or infolding is useful for the moderately dilated ureter. Ureteral vascularity is preserved, and the revision can be taken down and redone if vascular compromise is suspected (Bakker et al, 1988) (Fig. 61–43). **Bulk poses a problem with an extremely large ureter, however. Excisional tapering is preferred for more severely dilatated ureters or those that are markedly thickened.** Plication of ureters greater than 1.75 cm in diameter resulted in more complications in one series (Parrott et al, 1990). Remodeled MGUs have generally been reimplanted using standard cross-trigonal or Leadbetter-type techniques, but extravesical repairs can also be done successfully (Perovich, 1994). Success with reimplantation of remodeled MGUs, regardless of technique, is not as high as with nondilated ureters, yet the 90% to 95% success rate approximated in most contemporary series is commendable (Hendren, 1969; Retik et al, 1978; Parrott et al, 1990).

Technique (Fig. 61–44)

1. The bladder is opened through a Pfannenstiel incision, and the ureter is dissected from its intravesical and extravesical attachments as previously described. In some instances it is possible to mobilize the dilated ureter adequately by staying within the bladder. When this is the case, the maneuvers for reimplantation using either the Cohen or Politano-Leadbetter method are repeated after ureteral tailoring. However, when very large ureters are being tapered, it is advisable to go outside the bladder if there is any difficulty with mobilization to better define the blood supply.
2. If the Politano-Leadbetter method of reimplantation is chosen, it is wise to create the new hiatus before moving outside the bladder. The hiatus is widened with a right-angle clamp, and the peritoneum is swept from the base of the bladder, again using the lighted suction and Senn retractors. The clamp is incised upon and spread at an appropriate superior-medial location for the new hiatus. A red rubber catheter, which helps to guide the ureter through its new hiatus, is engaged and carried extravesically and then back into the bladder, where it is snapped.
3. Dissection outside the bladder is begun by sweeping the lateral peritoneal attachments superiorly with a Kittner dissector. A right-angle clamp is used to pass the ureteral cuff stitch through the old hiatus to the pervesical space, and the ureter is then brought extravesically.
4. The adventitia and blood supply to the lower ureter, which usually emanates medially, are carefully preserved. When dissecting outside the bladder, it is helpful to divide the obliterated hypogastric artery to aid in the dissection and to eliminate it as a possible source of obstruction. Excessive mobilization and removal of proximal kinks are unnecessary.
5. After excision of any obstructive distal ureter or excessive length, ureteral tailoring is performed over a No. 10 Fr red rubber catheter (8 Fr in a baby). If the ureter is snug over the catheter, revisions are unnecessary. Otherwise, ureteral remodeling is recommended using one of the following methods:

TAPERING (Fig. 61–45). The technique used is similar to that originally described by Hendren (1969). Baby Allis clamps are placed laterally to define any redundant ureter while preserving the medial vascular blood supply. Atraumatic clamps are applied around the catheter, and any excessive portion of the ureter is excised. Narrowing of the lumen should be avoided. A running, locking (to avoid reefing) 6-0

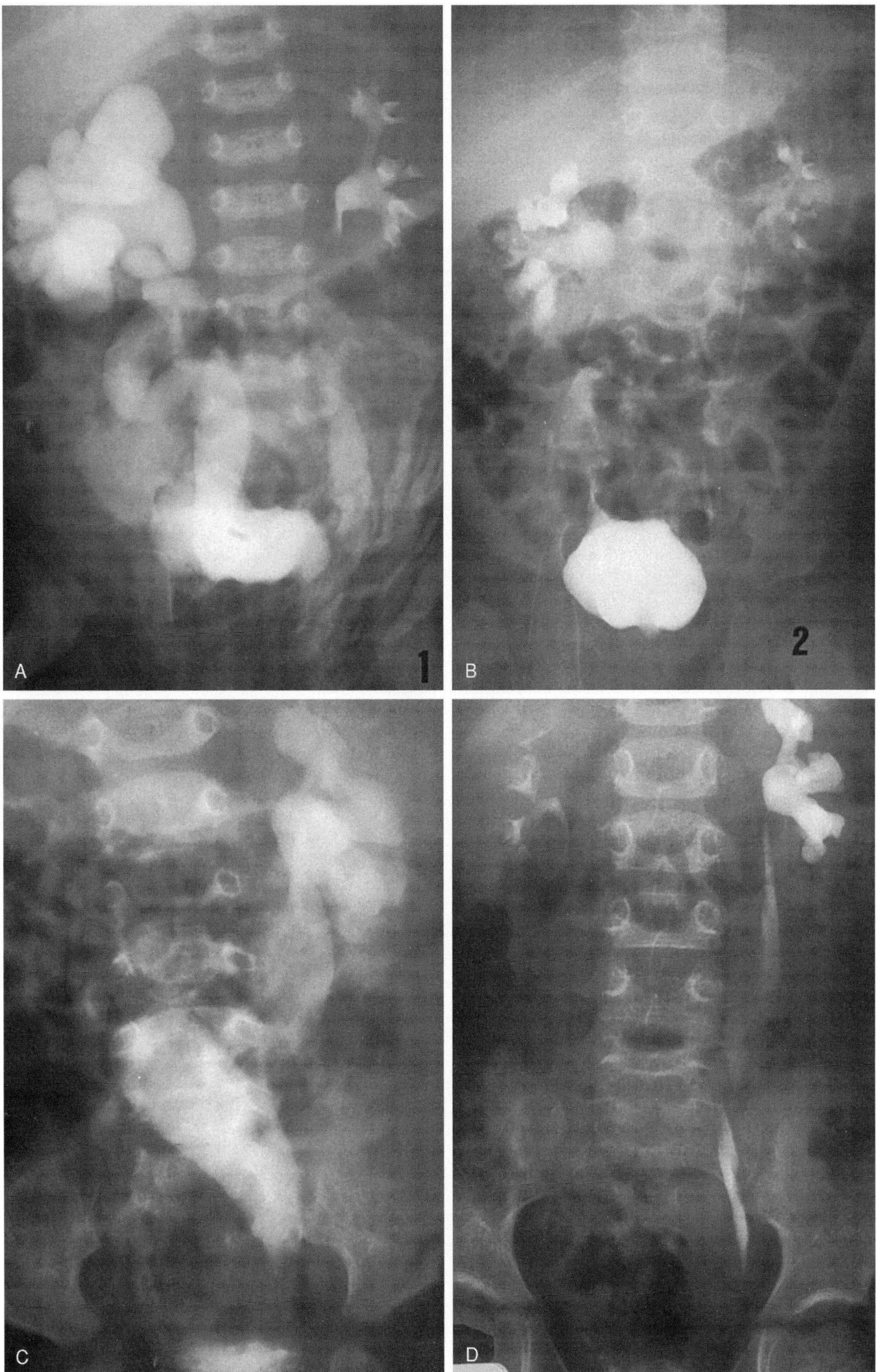

Figure 61–42. Neonatal megaureters are managed expectantly. *A,* Excretory urogram at 3 weeks of age shows impressive dilatation of right ureter. Renal scan documented good function but delayed drainage. *B,* Excretory urogram in same patient 2 years later. *C,* Excretory urogram demonstrates impressively dilated left megaureter in a 6-week-old child. *D,* Three years later appearance is nearly normal.

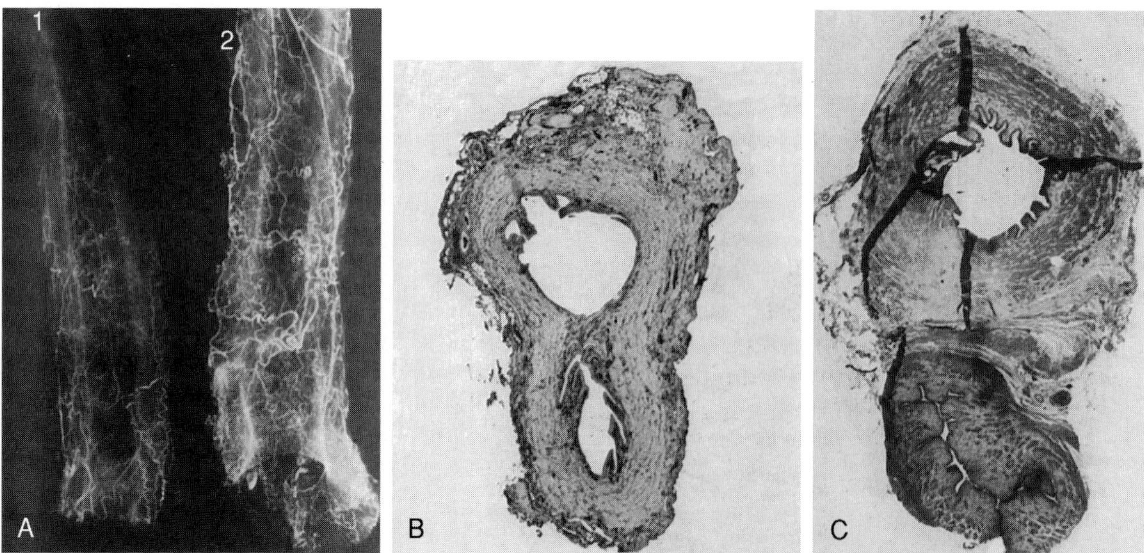

Figure 61–43. *A,* Comparison of microvasculature preservation in specimens obtained by excisional tapering *(1)* and folding techniques *(2)*. *B,* Histologic section of folded ureter 3 weeks postoperatively shows no obliteration of underfolded segment. *C,* Underfolded segment shows progressive obliteration at 3 months, although the lumen remains patent. (From Bakker HHR, Scholtaneijer RJ, Klopper PJ: Comparison of 2 different tapering techniques in megaureters. J Urol 1988; 140:1237.)

polydiaxanone suture is used to reapproximate the proximal two thirds of the tapered ureter. Interrupted sutures complete the repair to allow any shortening that may be necessary. The proximal portion of the revised ureter should remain just outside the bladder after reimplantation with either tapering or plications is completed.

STARR PLICATION (Fig. 61–46). Redundant ureter is again defined by briefly applying atraumatic clamps to mark the degree of necessary plication and preserve the best vascularized portion of ureter. Starting proximally, the ureter is plicated anteriorly using interrupted 6-0 polydioxanone sutures placed in Lembert fashion along the clamp impressions (Starr, 1979).

KALICINSKY PLICATION (Fig. 61–47). Two 6-0 polydioxanone sutures are placed along the clamp impressions, one at the proximal extent of the proposed revision and the other at the new meatus. The ureter is divided longitudinally by weaving one suture toward the other in running fashion, thus creating two lumens. The ureter is then reduced by folding its nonfunctional portion over the catheterized lumen (Kalicinsky et al, 1977)

6. The reimplantation is completed using either the cross-trigonal or Politano-Leadbetter technique. If the latter is used, a right-angle clamp brings the revised ureter back into the bladder through the new hiatus using the previously placed catheter as a guide. It is often helpful to combine the repair with a psoas hitch, especially in smaller children.

7. Tapered ureters are stented for 5 to 7 days. Stentograms are unnecessary because leaks rarely occur. Obstruction is also uncommon, although the stent itself often obstructs. Plicated ureters, in general, do not require stenting.

Results and Complications

Reimplantation of MGU is associated with the same complications, persistent reflux and obstruction, that accompany reimplantation of nondilated ureters but at increased rates. Some authors have noted better results with obstructive MGU and higher rates of unresolved reflux following the tailoring of refluxing variants (Johnson and Farkas, 1975). This finding has been attributed to a higher incidence of bladder dysfunction associated with the latter and to more dramatic abnormalities of the musculature. A histologic study by Lee and colleagues (1992) demonstrated increased collagen deposition in refluxing MGUs and altered smooth muscle ratios that might severely affect function. In contrast, obstructive MGUs were not statistically different from controls. On rare occasions, reflux persists despite adequate ureteral tunnels in both tapered and normal-sized ureters. This may be due to intrinsic ureteral dysfunction resulting from the transmural scarring of repeated infections or to the insult of prior surgeries. The rigid distal ureter is incapable of normal peristalsis or appropriate coaptation during bladder contractions. Transureteroureterostomy is ideal for patients with unilateral disease. Bilateral cases can be treated by excising the scarred distal ureter and creating exaggerated ureteral tunnels whose diameter-length ratios may exceed 10:1.

The Dilated Duplex Ureter

Duplications of the ureter are associated with anomalies commonly associated with reflux or obstruction that result in dilatation of one or both ureters. Examples include ureteroceles and ectopic ureters. In the presence of salvageable renal function, a number of surgical options can be tried depending on the cause, degree of dilatation, and whether one or both ureters are abnormal.

Ureteroureterostomy provides an ideal solution when only one ureter of a duplex ureter needs to be addressed. This can be done above the bladder through a lower abdominal extraperitoneal approach. Ureteropyelostomy is another option but leaves a segment of lower ureter unless a two-incision approach is used. When both ureters require correc-

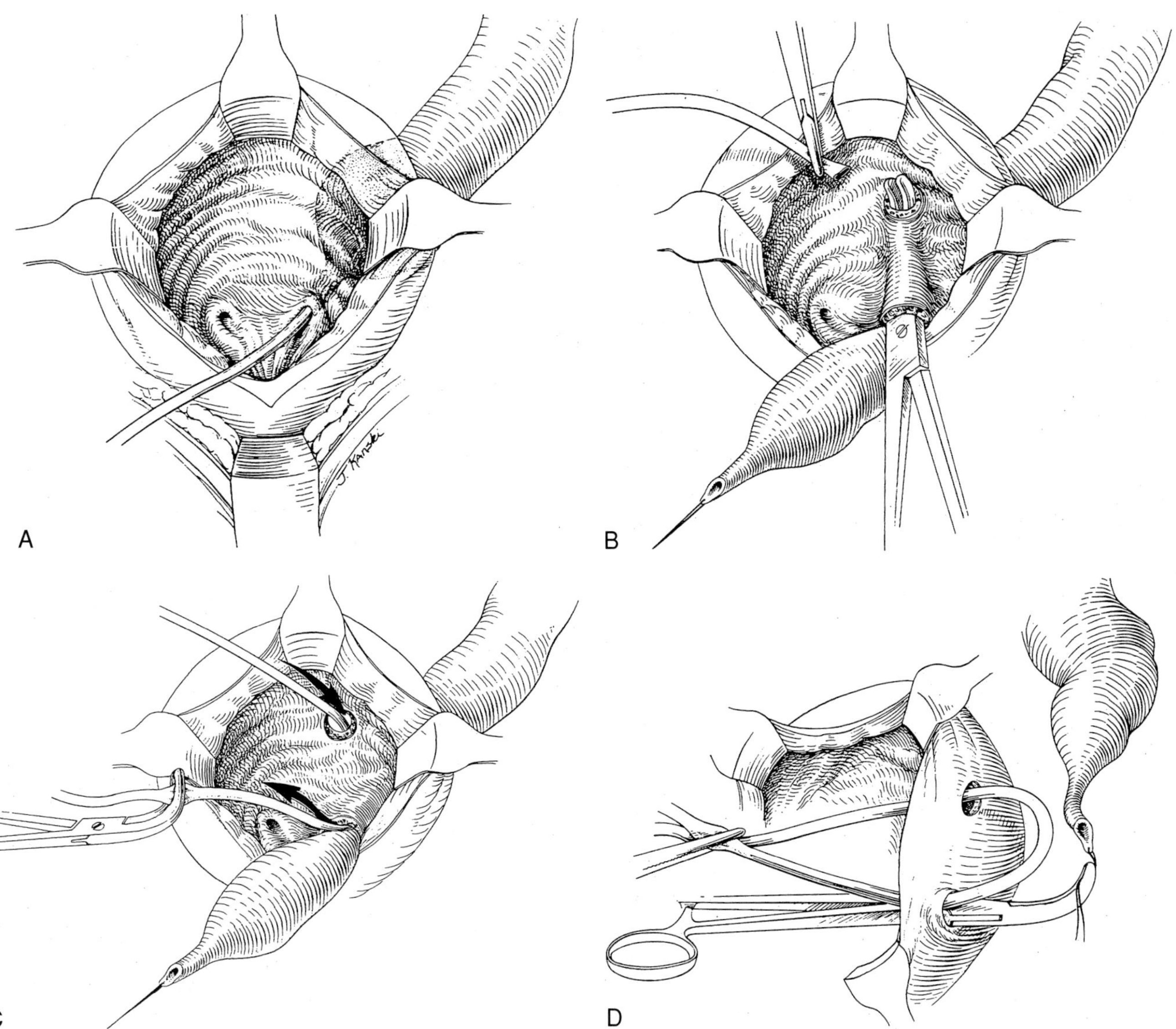

Figure 61–44. Technique for repair of megaureter. *A,* A No. 5 Fr feeding tube typically passes up a normal caliber intravesical segment of primary obstructive megaureter. *B,* After the megaureter is freed from its intravesical and extravesical attachments, a blunt right angle is used to clear the peritoneum from the posterior and base of the bladder. If an extravesical dissection is necessary, it is advisable to make the new hiatus prior to moving outside the bladder. A right-angle clamp is incised on and spread. *C,* A fine red rubber catheter marks the new hiatus by being pulled from within the bladder to the outside and then through the old hiatus. *D,* A right-angle clamp is guided from within the bladder to the perivesical space, where it is identified and incised upon. The ureter is brought extravesically by grasping the traction suture in the ureter.

Illustration continued on following page

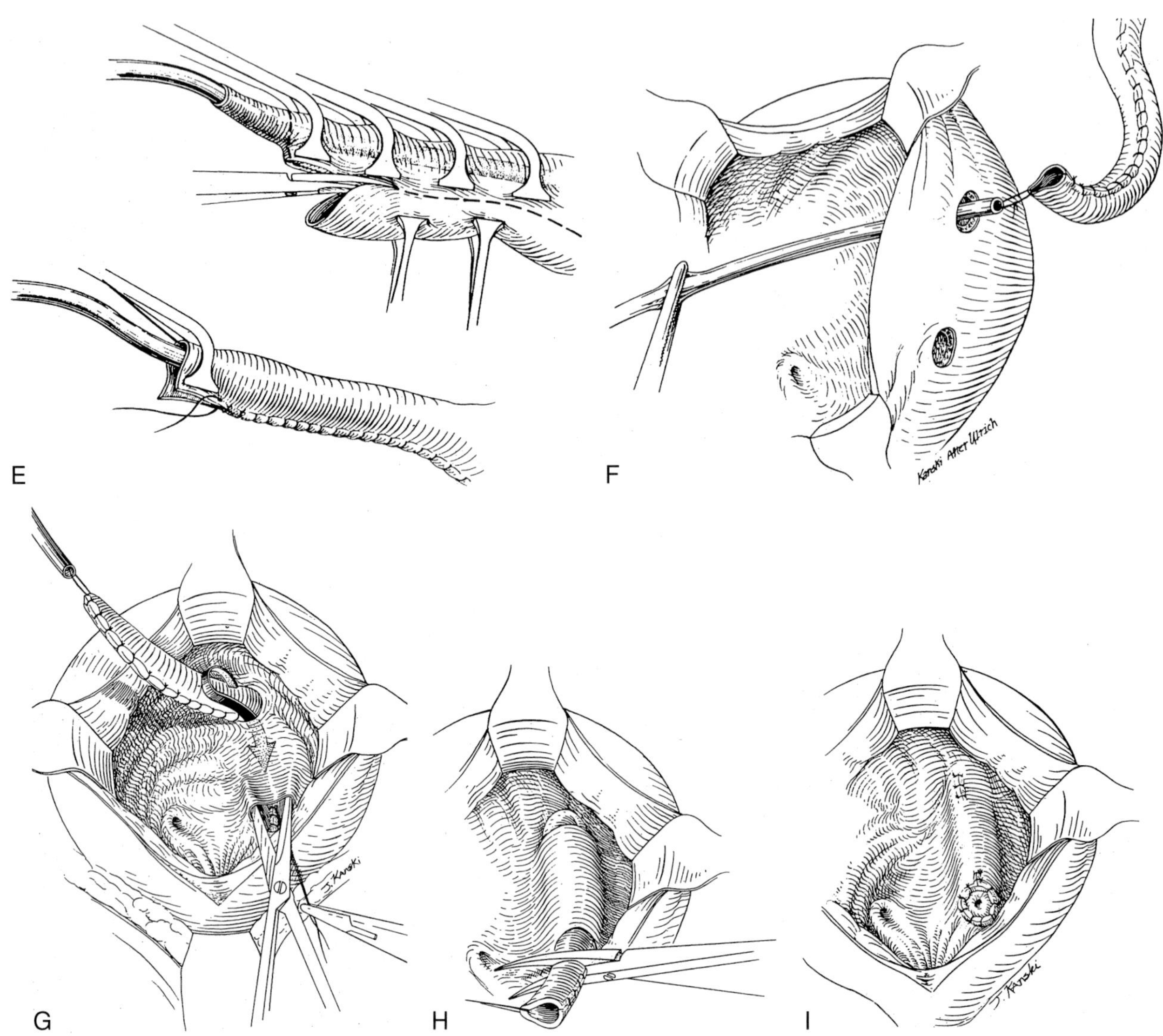

Figure 61–44 *Continued E,* Ureteral tailoring is completed. Tapering is done over a No. 8 Fr red rubber catheter in infants and No. 10 Fr catheter in older children and adults. After vascularity is defined, special atraumatic clamps are placed over the catheter. Baby Allis clamps help retract the portion of ureter to be resected, which is usually lateral. It is important not to resect too much ureter. A running 5-0 polydiaxanone or chromic suture is used to reapproximate the proximal two thirds of the ureter. Its distal third is closed with interrupted sutures to allow for shortening. *F,* The tailored ureter is brought back into the bladder through the new hiatus. *G,* After closing the original hiatus, a new submucosal tunnel is made to the new hiatus. *H,* The distal portion of ureter is resected to match the length of the tunnel. *I,* The revised ureter is anastomosed to the bladder with fine interrupted sutures. (From Retik AB, Colodny AH, Bauer SB: Pediatric urology. *In* Paulson DF, ed: Genitourinary Surgery, Vol 2. New York, Churchill Livingstone, 1984, pp 767–774.)

Jones BW, Headstream JW: Vesicoureteral reflux in children. J Urol 1958; 80:114.

Jones DA, Holden D, George NJR: Mechanisms of upper tract dilatation in patients with thick-walled bladders, chronic retention of urine and associated hydroureteronephrosis. J Urol 1988; 140:326.

Joseph DB, Young DW, Jordan SP: Renal cortical scintigraphy and single proton emission computerized tomography (SPECT) in the assessment of renal defects in children. J Urol 1990; 144:595.

Jungers T, Forget D, Houllier T, et al: Pregnancy in IgA nephropathy, reflux nephropathy, and focal glomerulosclerosis. Am J Kidney Dis 1987; 9:334.

Kaack MB, Roberts JA, Baskin G: Maternal immunization with P fimbriae for the prevention of neonatal pyelonephritis. Infect Immunol 1988; 56:1.

Kalicinsky ZH, Kansy J, Kotarbinska B, et al: Surgery of megaureters: Modification of Hendren's operation. J Pediatr Surg 1977; 12:183.

Kallenius G, Mollby R, Svenson SB, et al: Occurrence of P-fimbriated *Escherichia coli* in urinary tract infections. Lancet 1981; 2:1369.

Kaplan GW: Postinfection reflux. Soc Pediatr Urol Newslett April 9, 1980.

Kaplan WE, Firlit CF: Management of reflux in the myelodysplastic child. J Urol 1983; 129:1195.

Kass EJ, Majd M, Belman AB: Comparison of the diuretic renogram and pressure-perfusion study in children. J Urol 1985; 134:92.

Keating MA: A different perspective of the perinatal primary megaureter. *In* Kramer SA (ed): Problems in Urology. Philadelphia, 1990 J.B. Lippincott, p 583.

Keating MA, Duckett JW: Prune-belly syndrome. *In* Ashcraft KW, Holder TM (eds): Pediatric Surgery. Philadelphia, W. B. Saunders, 1993, p 721.

Keating MA, Escala J, Snyder HM, et al: Changing concepts in management of primary obstructive megaureter. J Urol 1989; 142:636.

Keating MA, Retik AB: Management of failures of ureteroneocystostomy. *In* McDougal WS (ed): Difficult Problems in Urologic Surgery. Chicago, Year Book Medical Publishers, 1989, pp 118–142.

King LR: Megaloureter: Definition, diagnosis and management. J Urol 1980; 123:222.

King LR, Coughlin PWF, Bloch EC, et al: The case for immediate pyeloplasty in the neonate with ureteropelvic junction obstruction. J Urol 1984; 132:725.

King LR, Kazmi SO, Belman AB: Natural history of vesicoureteral reflux: Outcome of a trial of nonoperative therapy. Urol Clin North Am 1974; 1:144.

Kiruluta HG, Fraser K, Owen L: The significance of the adrenergic nerves in the etiology of vesicoureteral reflux. J Urol 1986; 136:232.

Klare B, Geiselhardt B, Wesch H, et al: Radiological kidney size in childhood. Pediatr Radiol 1980; 9:153.

Koff SA: Relationship between dysfunctional voiding and reflux. J Urol 1992; 148:1703.

Koff SA, Campbell K: Nonoperative management of unilateral neonatal hydronephrosis. J Urol 1992; 148:525.

Koff SA, Fischer CP, Poznanski AK: The effect of reservoir height upon intravesical pressure. Pediatr Radiol 1979a; 8:21.

Koff SA, Lapides J, Piazza DH: Association of urinary tract infection and reflux with uninhibited bladder contractions and voluntary sphincter obstruction. J Urol 1979b; 122:373.

Koff SA, Murtaugh DS: The uninhibited bladder in children: Effect of treatment on recurrence of urinary infection and on vesicoureteral reflux resolution. J Urol 1983; 130:1138.

Koff SA, Shore RM, Hayden LJ, et al: Diuretic radionuclide localization of upper urinary tract obstruction. J Urol 1984; 132:513.

Kollerman VMW: Überbewertung der pathogenetischen Bedeutung des vesiko-ureteralen Refluxes im Kindesalter. Z Urol 1974; 67:573.

Kretschmer HL: Cystography, its value and limitations in surgery of the bladder. Surg Gynecol Obstet 1916; 23:709.

Kramer SA: Vesicoureteral reflux. *In* Kelalis P, King LR, Belman AB (eds): Clinical Pediatric Urology. Philadelphia, W. B. Saunders, 1992, pp 441–499.

Kuhns LD, Hernandez R, Koff S, et al: Absence of vesicoureteral reflux in children with ureteral jets. Radiology 1977; 124:185.

Lapides J, Diokno AC, Silber SJ, et al: Clean intermittent catheterization in the treatment of urinary tract disease. J Urol 1972; 107:458.

Lamesch AJ: Retrograde catheterization of the ureter after antireflux plasty by the Cohen technique of transverse advancement. J Urol 1981; 125:73.

Lattimer JK, Apperson JW, Gleason D, et al: The pressure at which reflux occurs: An important indicator of prognosis and treatment. J Urol 1963; 89:395.

Lebowitz RL, Avni F: Misleading appearances in pediatric uroradiology. Pediatr Radiol 1980; 10:15–31.

Lebowitz RL, Blickman JG: The coexistence of ureteropelvic junction obstruction and reflux. AJR 1983; 140:231.

Lebowitz RL: The detection and characterization of vesicoureteral reflux in the child. J Urol 1992; 148:1640.

Lebowitz RL: Neonatal vesicoureteral reflux: What do we know? Radiology 1993; 187:17.

Lee BR, Partin AW, Epstein JI, et al: A quantitative histologic analysis of the dilated ureter of childhood. J Urol 1992; 148:1482.

Leibovic SJ, Lebowitz RL: Reducing patient dose in voiding cystourethrography. Urol Radiol 1980; 2:103–107.

Leighton DM, Mayne V: Obstruction in the refluxing urinary tract—a common phenomenon. Clin Radiol 1989; 40:271.

Lenaghan D, Whitaker J, Jensen F, et al: The natural history of reflux and long term effects of reflux on the kidney. J Urol 1976; 115:728.

Leonard MP, Canning DA, Peters CA, et al: Endoscopic injection of glutaraldehyde cross-linked bovine dermal collagen for correction of vesicoureteral reflux. J Urol 1991; 145:115.

Lich R, Howerton LL, Davis LA: Recurrent urosepsis in children. J Urol 1961; 86:554.

Lich R, Howerton LW, Goode LS, et al: The ureterovesical junction of the newborn. J Urol 1964; 92:436.

Lichodziejewska M, Steadman R, Verrier Jones K: Variable expression of P fimbriae in *Escherichia coli* urinary tract infection. Lancet 1989; 1:1414.

Lines D: 15th century ureteric reflux. Lancet 1982; 2:1473.

Linn R, Ginesin Y, Bolkier M, et al: Lich-Gregoir antireflux operation: A surgical experience and 5–20 years of follow-up in 149 ureters. Eur Urol 1989; 16:200.

Liu HYA, Dhillon HK, Yeung CK, et al: Clinical outcome and management of prenatally diagnosed primary megaureters. J Urol 1994; 152:614.

Lombard H, Hanson LA, Jacobsson B, et al: Correlation of P blood group, vesicoureteral reflux and bacterial attachment in patients with recurrent pyelonephritis. N Engl J Med 1983; 308:1189.

Lomberg H, Cedergren B, Leffler H, et al: Influence of blood group on the availability of receptors for attachment of uropathogenic *Escherichia coli.* Infect Immunol 1986; 51:919.

Lomberg H, Hellstrom M, Jodal U, et al: Virulence-associated traits in *Escherichia coli* causing first and recurrent episodes of urinary tract infections in children with and without vesicoureteral reflux. J Infect Dis 1984; 150:561.

Lyon RP: Renal arrest. J Urol 1973; 109:707.

Lyon RP, Marshall S, Tanagho EA: The ureteral orifice: Its configuration and competency. J Urol 1969; 102:504.

MacKinnon KC: Primary megaureter. Birth Defects 1977; 13:15.

McCord JM, Fridovich I: The biology and pathology of oxygen radicals. Ann Intern Med 1978; 89:122.

McDougall EM, Urban DA, Kerbl K, et al: Laparoscopic repair of vesicoureteral reflux utilizing the Lich-Gregoir technique in the pig model. J Urol 1995; 153:497.

McGladdery SL, Aparicio S, Verrier-Jones K, et al: Outcome of pregnancy in an Oxford-Cardiff cohort of women with previous bacteriuria. Q J Med 1992; 83:533–539.

McLaughlin AP, Pfister RC, Leadbetter WF, et al: The pathophysiology of primary megaloureter. J Urol 1973; 109:805.

McLorie GA, McKenna PH, Jumper BM, et al: High grade vesicoureteral reflux: Analysis of observational therapy. J Urol 1990; 144:537.

McRae CU, Shannon FT, Utley WLF: Effect on renal growth of reimplantation of refluxing ureters. Lancet 1974; 1:1310.

Mackie GG, Stephens FD: Duplex kidneys: A correlation of renal dysplasia with position of the ureteral orifice. J Urol 1975; 114:274.

Maizels M, Smith CK, Firlit CF: The management of children with vesicoureteal reflux and ureteropelvic junction obstruction. J Urol 1984; 131:722.

Majd M, Rushton HG, Jantausch B, et al: Relationship among vesicoureteral reflux, P-fimbriated *E. coli,* and acute pyelonephritis in children with febrile urinary tract infection. J Pediatr 1991; 119:578.

Malizia AA, Reiman HM, Myers RP, et al: Migration and granulomatous reaction after periurethral injection of polytef (Teflon). JAMA 1984; 251:3277.

Manivel JC, Pettinata G, Reinberg Y, et al: Prune belly syndrome: Clincopathologic study of 29 cases. Pediatr Pathol 1989; 9:691.

Manley CB: Reflux in blond haired girls. Soc Pediatr Urol Newslett 1981; Oct 14.

Mansfield JT, Snow BW, Cartwright PC, Wadsworth K: Complications of pregnancy in women after childhood reimplantation for vesicoureteral reflux: An update with 25 years of follow-up. J Urol 1995; 154:787.

Marberger M, Altwein JE, Straub E, et al: The Lich-Gregoir antireflux plasty: Experiences with 371 children. J Urol 1978; 120:216.

Marshall JL, Johnson ND, DeCampo MP: Vesicoureteral reflux in children: Prediction with color Doppler imaging. Radiology 1990; 175:355.

Marra G, Barbieri G, Dell'Agnola CA, et al: Congenital renal damage associated with primary vesicoureteral reflux detected prenatally in male infants. J Pediatr 1994; 124:726.

Martinell J, Jodal U, Lidin-Janson G: Pregnancies in women with and without renal scarring after urinary infections in childhood. Br Med J 1990; 300:840.

Mathisen W: Vesicoureteral reflux and its surgical correction. Surg Gynecol Obstet 1964; 118:965.

Matouschek E: Die Behandlung des vesikorenalen Refluxes durch Transuretherale (Einspritzung von polytetrafluoroethylenepaste). Urologe 1981; 20:263.

Matthews RD, Christensen JP, Canning DA: Persistence of autologous free fat transplant in bladder mucosa of rats. J Urol 1994; 152:819–821.

Mayo ME, Burns MW: Urodynamic studies in children who wet. Br J Urol 1990; 65:641.

Mazze RI, Schwartz FD, Slocum HC, et al: Renal function during anesthesia and surgery: 1. Effects of halothane anesthesia. Anesthesiology 1963; 24:279.

Melick WF, Brodeur AE, Karellos DN: A suggested classification of ureteral reflux and suggested treatment based on cineradiographic findings and simultaneous pressure recordings by means of the strain gauge. J Urol 1962; 83:35.

Mendoza J, Roberts JA: Effects of sterile high pressure vesicoureteral reflux on the monkey. J Urol 1983; 148:1721.

Merguerian PA, McLorie GA, Khoury AE, et al: Submucosal injection of polyvinyl alcohol foam in rabbit bladder. J Urol 1990; 144:531–533.

Merrell RW, Mowad JJ: Increased physical growth after successful antireflux operation. J Urol 1979; 122:523.

Merrick M, Utley W, Wild S: The detection of pyelonephritic scarring in children by radioisotope imaging. Br J Radiol 1980; 53:544.

Meyer R: Normal and abnormal development of the ureter in the human embryo—a mechanistic consideration. Anat Rec 1946; 96:355.

Middleton RG: Routine use of the psoas hitch in ureteral reimplantation. J Urol 1980; 123:352.

Miller T, Phillips S: Pyelonephritis: The relationship between infection, renal scarring and antimicrobial therapy. Kidney Int 1981; 19:654.

Mittleman RE, Marraccini JV: Pulmonary Teflon granulomas following periurethral polytetrafluoroethylene injection for urinary incontinence. Arch Pathol Lab Med 1983; 107:611.

Miyakita H, Puri P: Particles found in lung and brain following subureteal injection of polytetrafluoroethylene paste are not Teflon particles. J Urol 1994; 152:636.

Monga AK, Robinson D, Stanton SL: Periurethral collagen injections for genuine stress incontinence: A 2 year follow-up. Br J Urol 1995; 76:156–160.

Najmaldin A, Burge DM, Atwell JD: Fetal vesicoureteral reflux. Br J Urol 1990; 65:403.

Neal DE: Localization of urinary tract infections. AUA Update Series 1989; 8:4.

Noe HN: The role of dysfunctional voiding in the failure or complication of ureteral reimplantation for primary reflux. J Urol 1985; 134:1172.

Noe HN: The relationship of sibling reflux to index patient dysfunctional voiding. J Urol 1988; 140:119.

Noe HN: The long-term result of prospective sibling reflux screening. J Urol 1992; 148:1739.

Noe HN, Wyatt RJ, Peeden JN Jr, et al: The transmission of vesicoureteral reflux from parent to child. J Urol 1992; 148:1869.

North American Pediatric Renal Transplant Cooperative Study: Annual Report, 1994.

O'Donnell B, Puri P: Treatment of vesicoureteric reflux by endoscopic injection of Teflon. Br Med J 1984; 289:5–9.

Olbing H, Claesson I, Ebel K, et al: Renal scars and parenchymal thinning in children with vesicoureteral reflux: The International Reflux Study in Children (European branch) J Urol 1992; 148:1653.

O'Regan S, Yerbeck S, Schick E: Constipation, bladder instability, urinary tract infection syndrome. Clin Nephrol 1985; 23:152.

Orskov I, Ferencz A, Orskov F: Tamm-Horsfall protein or uromucoid is the normal urinary slime that traps type I fimbriated *Escherichia coli.* Lancet 1980; 1:887.

Ostling K: The genesis of hydronephrosis. Particularly with regard to the changes at the ureteropelvic junction. Acta Chir Scand (Suppl) 1942; 86:72.

Pagano P, Passerini G: Primary obstructed megaureter. Br J Urol 1977; 49:469.

Paltiel JH, Rupich RC, Kiruluta HG: Enhanced detection of vesicoureteral reflux in infants and children with use of cylic voiding cystourethrography. Radiology 1992; 184:753.

Paquin AJ: Ureterovesical anastomosis. The description and evaluation of a technique. J Urol 1959; 82:573.

Parrott TS, Woodard JR, Wolpert JJ: Ureteral tailoring: A comparison of wedge resection with infolding. J Urol 1990; 144:328.

Parsons LC, Greenspan C, Mulholland GS: The primary antibacterial defense mechanism of the bladder. Invest Urol 1975; 13:72.

Peer LA: The neglected free fat graft. Plast Reconstr Surg 1956; 18:233.

Perovich S: Surgical treatment of megaureters using detrusor tunneling extravesical ureteroneocystostomy. J Urol 1994; 152:618.

Peters CA, Mandell J, Lebowitz RL, et al: Congenital obstructed megaureters in early infancy: Diagnosis and treatment. J Urol 1989; 142:641.

Peters PC, Johnson DE, Jackson JH Jr: The incidence of vesicoureteral reflux in the premature child. J Urol 1967; 97:259.

Pfister RC, Hendren WH: Primary megaureters in children and adults. Clinical and pathophysiologic features in 150 ureters. Urology 1978; 12:160.

Pitts WR, Muecke EC: Congenital megaureter. A review of 80 patients. J Urol 1974; 111:468.

Polk HC Jr: Notes on Galenic urology. Urol Survey 1965; 15:2.

Politano VA: Vesicoureteral reflux in children. JAMA 1960; 172:1252.

Politano VA: Periurethral polytetrafluoroethylene injection for urinary incontinence. J Urol 1982; 127:439.

Politano VA, Leadbetter WF: An operative technique for the correction of vesicoureteral reflux. J Urol 1958; 79:932.

Politano VA, Small MP, Harper JM, Lynne CM: Teflon injection for urinary incontinence. J Urol 1974; 111:180.

Pollet JE, Sharp PF, Smith RW, et al: Intravenous radionuclide cystography for the detection of vesicoureteral reflux. J Urol 1981; 125:75.

Poznanski E, Poznanski AK: Psychogenic influences on voiding: Observations from voiding cystourethrography. Psychosomatics 1969; 10:339.

Pozzi S: Ureteroverletzung bei Laparotomie. Zentrlbl Gyncol 1893; 17:97.

Press SM, Badlani GH: Injection therapy for urinary incontinence. AUA Update Series 1995; 14:14–20.

Preston A, Lebowitz RL: What's new in pediatric uroradiology. Urol Radiol 1989; 11:217.

Prout GR Jr, Koontz WW Jr: Partial vesical immobilization: An important adjunct to ureteroneocystostomy. J Urol 1970; 103:147.

Rames RA, Aaronson IA: Migration of Polytef paste to the lung and brain following intravesical injection for the correction of reflux. Pediatr Surg Int 1991; 6:239.

Ransley PG, Risdon RA: Renal papillary morphology and intrarenal reflux in the young pig. Urol Res 1975; 3:105.

Ransley PG, Risdon RA: Reflux and renal scarring. Br J Radiol Suppl 1978; 14:1.

Ransley PG, Risdon RA: Reflux nephrophathy: Effects of antimicrobial therapy on the evolution of the early pyelonephritic scar. Kidney Int 1981; 20:733.

Redman JF, Scriber LJ, Bissad NK: Apparent failure of renal growth secondary to vesicoureteral reflux. Urology 1974; 3:704.

Retik AB, McElvoy JP, Bauer SB: Megaureters in children. Urology 1978; 11:231–236.

Rickwood AMK, Jee LD, Williams MPL, et al: Natural history of obstructed and pseudoobstructed megaureters detected by prenatal ultrasonography. Br J Urol 1992; 70:322.

Ring E, Petritsch P, Riccabona M, et al: Primary vesicoureteral reflux in infants with a dilated fetal urinary tract. Eur J Pediatr 1993; 152:523.

Roberts JA: Vesicoureteral reflux in the primate. Invest Urol 1974; 12:88.

Roberts JA: Experimental pyelonephritis in the monkey. III. Pathophysiology of ureteral malfunction induced by bacteria. Invest Urol 1975; 13:117.

Roberts JA: Vesicoureteral reflux and pyelonephritis in the monkey: A review. J Urol 1992; 148:1721.

Roberts JA: Mechanisms of renal damage in chronic pyelonephritis (reflux nephropathy). Curr Top Pathol 1995; 88:265.

Roberts JA, Kaack MB, Baskin G: Treatment of experimental pyelonephritis in the monkey. J Urol 1990; 143:150.

Roberts JA, Kaack MB, Fussell EF, et al: Immunology of pyelonephritis VII: Effect of allopurinol. J Urol 1986; 136:960.

Roberts JA, Riopelle AJ: Vesicoureteral reflux in the primate: III. Effect of urinary tract infection on maturation of the ureterovesical junction. Pediatrics 1978; 61:853.

Rolleston GL, Maling TMJ, Hodson CJ: Intrarenal reflux and the scarred kidney. Arch Dis Child 1974; 49:531.

Rolleston GL, Shannon FT, Utley WLF: Follow-up of vesicoureteric reflux in the newborn. Kidney Int 1975; 8:59.

Rose JS, Glassberg KI, Waterhouse K: Intrarenal reflux and its relationship to scarring. J Urol 1975; 113:400.

Ruano-Gil D, Coca-Payeras A, Tejedo-Mateu A: Obstruction and normal recanalization of the ureter in the human embryo. Its relation to congenital ureteral obstruction. Eur Urol 1975; 1:293.

Rushton HG: Genitourinary infections: Nonspecific infections. *In* Kelalis PP, King LR, Belman AB (eds): Clinical Pediatric Urology. Philadelphia, W. B. Saunders, 1992, pp 286–331.

Rushton HG, Majd M, Chandra R, Yim D: Evaluation of 99m-technetium-dimercaptosuccinic acid renal scans in experimental acute pyelonephritis in piglets. J Urol 1988; 140:1169.

Rushton HG, Majd M, Jantausch B, et al: Renal scarring following reflux and nonreflux pyelonephritis: Evaluation with 99m-technetium-dimercaptosuccinic acid scintigraphy. J Urol 1992; 147:1327.

Salvatierra O Jr, Tanagho EA: Reflux as a cause of end stage kidney disease: Report of 32 cases. J Urol 1977; 117:441.

Sampson JA: Ascending renal infections: With special reference to the reflux of urine from the bladder into the ureters as an etiological factor in its causation and maintenance. J Hopkins Hosp Bull 1903; 14:334.

Santiago AM, Castro MJ, Castillo JM, et al: [Endoscopic injection of autologous adipose tissue in the treatment of female incontinence] [Spanish]. Arch Esp Urol 1989; 42:143.

Savage JM, Koh CT, Shah V, et al: Renin and blood pressure in children with renal scarring and vesicoureteral reflux. Lancet 1978; 8:441.

Savage JM, Koh CT, Shah V, et al: Five-year prospective study of plasma renin activity and blood pressure in patients with long-standing reflux nephropathy. Arch Dis Child 1987; 62:678.

Scharer K: Incidence and causes of chronic renal failure in childhood. *In* Cameron D, Fries D, Ogg CS (eds): Dialysis and Renal Transplantation. Berlin, Pitman Medical, 1971, pp 211–217.

Schimberg W, Wacksman J, Rudd R, et al: Laparoscopic correction of vesicoureteral reflux in the pig. J Urol 1994; 151:1664.

Scholtmeijer RJ: Treatment of vesicoureteric reflux: Results of a prospective study. Br J Urol 1993; 71:346.

Schulman CC: Macroplastique: A new uro-implant for the endoscopic correction of reflux (abstract). Second International Congress of Endoscopic Paediatric Urology, October 7–9, 1993.

Scott JES, Stansfeld JM: Ureteric reflux and kidney scarring in children. Arch Dis Child 1968; 43:468.

Scott JES, Lee REJ, Hunter EW, et al: Ultrasound screening of newborn urinary tract. Lancet 1991; 338:1571.

Semblinow VI: Zur Pathologie der duech Bacterien bewinkten ambsteifenden Nephritis (1883 dissertation). Cited by Alksne J: Folia Urol 1907; 1:338.

Seruca H: Vesicoureteral reflux and voiding dysfunction: A prospective study. J Urol 1989; 142:494.

Shannon A, Feldman W: Methodologic limitations in the literature on vesicoureteral reflux: A critical review. J Pediatr 1990; 117:171.

Shimada K, Matsui T, Ogino T, et al: Renal growth and progression of reflux nephropathy in children with reflux. J Urol 1988; 140:1097.

Shopfner CE: Vesicoureteral reflux: Five year re-evaluation. Radiology 1970; 95:637.

Skoog SJ, Belman AB: Primary vesicoureteral reflux in the black child. Pediatrics 1991; 87:538.

Skoog SJ, Belman AB, Majd M: A nonsurgical approach to the management of primary vesicoureteral reflux. J Urol 1987; 138:941.

Slotki IN, Asscher AW: Prevention of scarring in experimental pyelonephritis in the rat by early antibiotic therapy. Nephron 1982; 30:262.

Smellie JM, Edwards D, Hunter N, et al: Vesicoureteral reflux and renal scarring. Kidney Int 1975; (Suppl 4) 8:65.

Smellie JM, Edwards D, Normand ICS, et al: Effect of vesicoureteral reflux on renal growth in children with urinary tract infection. Arch Dis Child 1981a; 56:593.

Smellie JM, Normand ICS: The clinical features and significance of urinary infection in childhood. Proc R Soc Lond 1966; 59:415.

Smellie JM, Normand ICS: Experience of follow-up of children with urinary tract infection. *In* O'Grady F, Brumditte W (eds): Urinary Tract Infection. London, Oxford University Press, 1968, p 123.

Smellie JM, Normand C: Reflux nephropathy in childhood. *In* Hodson CJ, Kincaid-Smith P (eds): Reflux Nephropathy. New York, Masson Publishing USA, 1979, pp 14–20.

Smellie JM, Normand ICS: Urinary tract infections in children 1985. Postgrad Med 1985; 61:895.

Smellie JM, Normand ICS, Katz G: Children with urinary infection: A comparison of those with and those without vesicoureteral reflux. Kidney Int 1981b; 20:717.

Smellie JM, Preece MA, Paton AM: Normal somatic growth in children receiving low-dose prophylactic cotrimoxazole. Eur J Pediatr 1983; 140:301.

Smellie JM, Ransley PG, Normand ICS, et al: Development of new renal scars: A collaborative study. Br Med J 1985; 290:1957.

Smith ED, et al: Report of working party to establish an international nomenclature for the large ureter. *In* Bergsman D, Duckett JW (eds): Birth Defects Orginal Articles Series 1977; 13(5):3–8.

Solok V, Erozenci A, Kural A, et al: Correction of vesicoureteral reflux by the Gil-Vernet procedure. Eur Urol 1988; 14:214.

Sommer JT, Stephens FD: Morphogenesis of nephropathy with partial ureteral obstruction and vesicoureteral reflux. J Urol 1981; 125:67.

Starr A: Ureteral plication; A new concept in ureteral tapering for megaureter. Invest Urol 1979; 17:153.

Stecker JF, Rose JG, Gillenwater JY: Dysplastic kidneys associated with vesicoureteral reflux. J Urol 1973; 110:341.

Steinhardt GF: Reflux nephropathy. J Urol 1985; 134:855.

Stenberg A, Lackgren G: A new bioimplant for the endoscopic treatment of vesicoureteral reflux: Experimental and short-term clinical results. J Urol 1995; 154:800–803.

Stephens FD, Lenaghan D: The anatomical basis and dynamics of vesicoureteal reflux. J Urol 1962; 87:669.

Sutton R, Atwell JD: Physical growth velocity during conservative treatment and following subsequent surgical treatment for primary vesicoureteric reflux. Br J Urol 1989; 63:245.

Tadavarthy SM, Moller JH, Amplatz K: Polyvinyl alcohol (Ivalon)—a new embolic material. AJR 1975; 125:609.

Tamminen-Mobius, Brunier E, Ebel KD, et al: Cessation of vesicoureteral reflux for 5 years in infants and children allocated to medical treatment. The International Reflux Study in Children. J Urol 1992; 148:1662.

Tanagho EA: Intrauterine fetal ureteral obstruction. J Urol 1973; 109:196.

Tanagho EA, Hutch JA, Meyers FH, et al: Primary vesicoureteral reflux: Experimental studies of its etiology. J Urol 1965; 93:165.

Tarkington MA, Fildes RD, Levin K, et al: High-resolution single photon emission computerized tomography (SPECT) 99m-technetium-dimercaptosuccinic acid renal imaging: A state of the art technique. J Urol 1990; 144:598.

Taylor CM, Corkery JJ, White RHR: Micturition symptoms and unstable bladder activity in girls with primary vesicoureteric reflux. Br J Urol 1982; 54:494.

Taylor A Jr: Quantitation of renal function with static imaging agents. Semin Nucl Med 1982; 12:330.

Torres VE, Moore SB, Kurtz SB, et al: In search of a marker for genetic susceptibility to reflux nephropathy. Clin Nephrol 1980; 14:217.

Torres VE, Malek RS, Svensson JP: Vesicoureteral reflux in the adult: II. Nephropathy, hypertension and stones. J Urol 1983; 130:41.

Torres VE, Kramer SA, Holley KE, et al: Effect of bacterial immunization on experimental reflux nephropathy. J Urol 1984; 131:772.

Urrutia EJ, Lebowitz TL: Re-reflux in blonde haired girls. Soc Pediatr Urol Newslett Oct 14, 1983.

Vaisanen V, Tallgren L, Makela P, et al: Mannose-resistant hemagglutination and P-antigen recognition are characteristic of *Escherichia coli* causing primary pyelonephritis. Lancet 1981; 2:1366.

Van den Abbeele AD, Treves ST, et al: Vesicoureteral reflux in asymptomatic siblings of patients with known reflux: Radionuclide cystography. Pediatrics 1987; 79:147.

Van Gool J, Tanagho EA: External sphincter activity and recurrent urinary tract infection in girls. Urology 1977; 10:348.

Van Gool D, Hjalmas K, Tamminen-Mobius T, et al: Historical clues to the complex of dysfunctional voiding, urinary tract infection, and vesicoureteral reflux. The International Reflux Study in Children. J Urol 1992; 148:1699.

Verber IG, Strudley MR, Meller ST: 99mTc dimercaptosuccinic acid (DMSA) scan as the first investigation of urinary tract infection. Arch Dis Child 1988; 63:1320.

Wacksman J, Anderson EE, Glenn JF: Management of vesicoureteral reflux. J Urol 1978; 119:814.

Wacksman J: Initial results with the Cohen cross-trigonal ureteroneocystostomy. J Urol 1983; 129:1198.

Wacksman J, Gilbert A, Sheldon CA: Results of the renewed extravesical reimplant for surgical correction of vesicoureteral reflux. J Urol 1992; 148:359.

Wacksman J, Phipps L: Report of the multicystic kidney registry: Preliminary findings. J Urol 1993; 150:1870.

Walker RD: Vesicoureteral reflux. *In* Gillenwater JY, Grayhack JT, Howards SS, et al (eds): Adult and Pediatric Urology, Vol. 2. Chicago, Year Book Medical Publishers, 1991, pp 1889–1920.

Walker RD: Vesicoureteral reflux update: Effect of prospective studies on current management. Urology 1994; 43:279.

Walker RD, Duckett JW, Bartone F, et al: Screening school children for urologic disease. Pediatrics 1977; 60–239.

Walker RD, Flack C: Experimental use of injectable bioglass. Use of nonautologous substances in VUR and incontinence treatment. Dial Pediatr Urol 1994; 17:1–8.

Walker RD, Richard GA, Dobson D, et al: Maximum urinary concentration: Early means of identifying patients with reflux who may require surgery. Urology 1973; 1:343.

Walker RD, Wilson T, Clark AE: Injectable bioglass as a potential substitute for injectable polytetrafluoroethylene. J Urol 1992; 148:645.

Wallace DMA, Rothwell DL, Williams DI: The long term follow-up of surgically treated vesicoureteral reflux. Br J Urol 1978; 50:479.

Weigert C: Ueber einige Bildungsfehler der Ureteren. Virchows Arch (Pathol Anat) 1887; 70:490.

Weinstein AJ, Bauer SB, Retik AB, et al: The surgical management of megaureters in duplex system: The efficacy of ureteral tapering and common sheath reimplantation. J Urol 1988; 139:328.

Weiss RM, Lytton B: Vesicoureteral reflux and distal ureteral obstruction. J Urol 1974; 111:245.

Weiss R, Duckett J, Spitzer A, on behalf of the International Reflux Study in Children: Results of a randomized clinical trial of medical vs. surgical management of infants and children with grades III and IV primary vesicoureteral reflux (United States). J Urol 1992a; 148:1667.

Weiss R, Tamminen-Mobius T, Koskimies O, et al, on behalf of the International Reflux Study in Children: Characteristics of entry in children with severe primary vesicoureteral reflux recruited for a multicenter international therapeutic trial comparing medical and surgical management. J Urol 1992b; 148:1644.

Wettergren B, Jodal U, Jonasson G: Epidemiology of bacteriuria during the first year of life. Acta Paediatrica Scandinavica 1985; 74(6):925–933.

Whitaker RH: Methods of assessing obstruction in dilated ureter. Br J Urol 1973; 45:15.

Williams DI, Hulme-Moir I: Primary obstructive mega-ureter. Br J Urol 1970; 42:140.

Williams GL, Davies DKL, Evans KT, Williams JE: Vesicoureteral reflux in patients with bacteriuria in pregnancy. Lancet 1968; 2:1202.

Willscher MK, Bauer SB, Zammuto PJ, et al: Renal growth and urinary infection following antireflux surgery in infants and children. J Urol 1976; 115:722.

Wilson J, Pigott GH, Schoen FJ, Hench LL: Toxicology and biocompatibility of bioglass. J Biomed Mat Res 1981; 15:805.

Winberg J, Andersen HJ, Bergstrom T, et al: Epidemiology of symptomatic urinary tract infection in childhood. Acta Pathol Scand Suppl 1974; 252:1.

Winberg J: Commentary: Progressive renal damage from infection with or without reflux. J Urol 1992; 148:1733.

Winfield HN, Donovan JF, See WA, et al: Urological laparoscopic surgery. J Urol 1991; 146:941.

Winter AL, Hardy BE, Alton DJ, et al: Acquired renal scars in children. J Urol 1983; 129:1190.

Winter CC: Vesicoureteral Reflux and Its Treatment. New York, Appleton-Century-Crofts, 1969.

Wiswell TE, Roscelli JD: Corroborative evidence for the decreased incidence of urinary tract infections in circumcised male infants. Pediatrics 1986; 78:96.

Wiswell TE, Enzenauer RM, Holton ME, et al: Declining frequencies of circumcision: Implications for changes in the incidence of male to female sex ratio of upper tract infection in early infancy. Pediatrics 1987; 79:338.

Wolfish NM, Delbrouck NF, Shanon A: Prevalence of hypertension in children with primary vesicoureteral reflux. J Pediatr 1993; 123:559.

Woodard JR, Keats G: Ureteral reimplantation: Paquin's procedure after 12 years. J Urol 1973; 109:891.

Woodard JR, Holden S: The prognostic significance of fever in childhood urinary infections: Observations in 350 consecutive patients. Clin Pediatr (Phila) 1976; 15:1051.

Woodard JR, Borden TS: Determination of true intravesical filling pressure in patients with vesicoureteral reflux by Fogarty catheter occlusion of ureters. J Urol 1982; 127:1149.

Woodside JR, Borden TS: Determination of true intravesical filling pressure in patients withi vesicoureteral reflux by Fogarty occlusion of ureters. J Urol 1982; 127:1149.

Young HH: Johns Hopkins Hosp Bull 1898; 9:100.

Zaontz MR, Maizels M, Sugar EC, et al: Detrusorrhaphy: Extravesical ureteral advancement to correct vesicoureteral reflux in children. J Urol 1987; 138:947.

Zerin JM, Ritchey ML, Chang AC: Incidental vesicoureteral reflux in neonates with antenatally detected hydronephrosis and other renal abnormalities. Radiology 1993; 187(1):157.

62
PRUNE-BELLY SYNDROME

John R. Woodard, M.D.
Edwin A. Smith, M.D.

Prune-belly syndrome is the most common term for the congenital absence, deficiency, or hypoplasia of the abdominal musculature accompanied by a large hypotonic bladder, dilated and tortuous ureters, and bilateral cryptorchidism (Osler, 1901). Known since Frolich's description in 1839, it has been of interest to urologists since 1895 when Parker described the genitourinary involvement. Because of the involvement of the abdominal musculature, urinary tract, and testicles, the term triad syndrome is commonly used. It is also frequently referred to as the Eagle-Barrett syndrome (Eagle and Barrett, 1950). The syndrome occurs primarily in boys and is rare, with a **reported incidence of approximately 1 in 35,000 to 50,000 live births** (Garlinger and Ott, 1974).

Historically, infants born with the full-blown syndrome have had a poor prognosis for long-term survival, a high percentage dying from urinary sepsis, renal failure, or both (Lattimer, 1958; McGovern and Marshall, 1959; Burke et al, 1969; Barnhouse, 1972). Although the prognosis for these patients has certainly improved, controversy has arisen between those who believe a more aggressive approach toward surgical reconstruction of the urinary tract might improve the quality of life of these unfortunate infants (Hendren, 1972; Jeffs et al, 1977; Woodard and Parrott, 1978a; Randolph et al, 1981; Fallat et al, 1989) and those who advocate limited or no surgical intervention (Woodhouse et al, 1979; Duckett, 1980).

In rare instances, a girl is affected by absence of the abdominal muscles, but it is exceptional to find the characteristic urinary tract anomaly at the same time (Aaronson and Cremin, 1980). Virtually by definition, the fully developed syndrome occurs almost exclusively in boys. Infants with the prune-belly syndrome may be born of entirely normal pregnancies; however, oligohydramnios is more often the rule and is responsible for some of the associated and complicating conditions, especially the pulmonary and skeletal variety. With the increased use of diagnostic fetal ultrasound, it is no longer novel for a presumptive diagnosis of prune-belly syndrome to be made in utero. The clinical significance of such a fetal diagnosis is discussed further later in this chapter. The appearance of the neonate is now so well known to neonatologists and pediatricians that it is unlikely to be missed (Fig. 62–1). The abdominal wall is thin and lax and, because of the sparsity of subcutaneous tissue, tends to be creased and wrinkled like a wizened prune. The liver edge, spleen, intestines, and distended bladder are often quite evident on viewing the abdominal wall externally.

The cause of the prune-belly syndrome remains unknown. Some have suggested that both the abdominal wall defect and the intra-abdominal cryptorchidism are secondary to distention of the urinary tract during early fetal development. **Obstruction in the posterior urethra is a possible cause** of this distention and would explain the predominance of male patients (Pagon et al, 1979; Nakayama et al, 1984). This theory suggests that testicular descent is blocked by a distended bladder and that the abdominal wall defect is secondary to either urinary tract distention or fetal ascites. However, other types of severe obstruction in the posterior urethra, such as posterior urethral valves, do not result in either a similar abdominal wall defect or the same type of

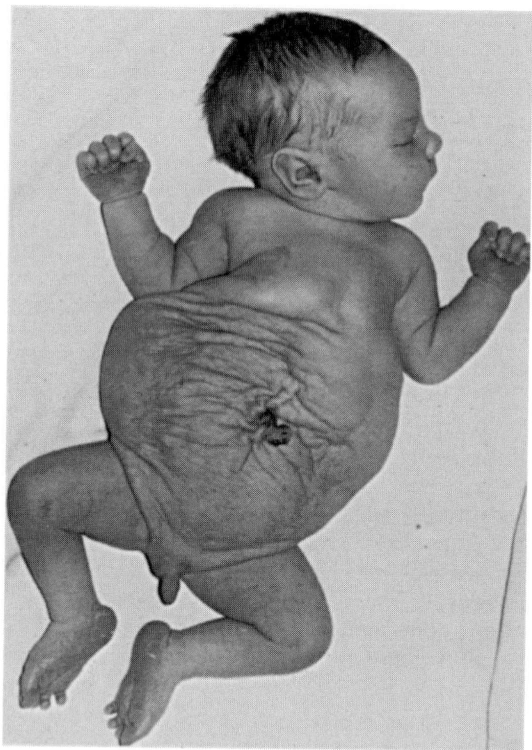

Figure 62–1. Newborn infant with the prune-belly syndrome, showing the characteristic appearance of the abdominal wall, the empty scrotum, and the talipes equinovarus.

upper urinary tract distortion. In addition, a similarly high incidence of cryptorchidism has not been observed in other obstructive uropathies.

Several investigators (Monie and Monie, 1979; Moerman et al, 1984) **have suggested that prostatic dysgenesis and fetal ascites are key factors in the causation of the syndrome,** with fetal ascites producing the abdominal wall defect. Although ascites is rarely present in patients with prune-belly syndrome (Smythe, 1981), it is speculated that ascites may be transient with absorption toward the end of gestation. Another commonly quoted and at one time more popular theory is that **a primary mesodermal error might account for both the abdominal wall defect and the genitourinary abnormalities because both arise from the paraxial intermediate and lateral plate mesoderm** (Smith, 1970). A genetic basis has been explored, but no clear inheritance pattern has emerged.

PATHOPHYSIOLOGY

Genitourinary Abnormalities

Kidney

Although the kidneys may be normal, **renal dysplasia and hydronephrosis are the two renal abnormalities typically associated with the syndrome.** Dysplasia may be present in more than 50% of cases, but involvement varies widely and is often asymmetric (Rogers and Ostrow, 1973). For example, a completely dysplastic multicystic kidney may be present on one side with the contralateral kidney demonstrating a completely normal histology. This feature, which is an important determinant of prognosis, seems to be more severe in patients who have urethral stenosis, megalourethra, or imperforate anus (Potter, 1972).

Most patients with prune-belly syndrome display some degree of hydronephrosis, which similarly follows a spectrum of severity and does not appear to be related to the severity of abdominal wall deficiency. Dilation of the calyces may be random or global, and the renal pelvis may be of normal caliber or grossly dilated (Berdon et al, 1977). The severity of the hydronephrosis is often less than that anticipated from the degree of dilation of the ureter. It is also common to find that the renal parenchyma is thicker and of better quality than might be expected from the amount of distortion in the drainage system. Although these findings have prognostic importance, they also suggest that the mechanism for the hydronephrosis might differ from that characteristic of other obstructive uropathies.

Occasional patients may also have ureteropelvic junction obstruction, and this possibility must not be overlooked in deciding on a plan of management. However, **recurrent infection rather than obstruction generally represents the greatest threat to renal parenchyma** that may already be compromised by an element of renal dysplasia.

Ureter

Ureteral abnormalities are detected at each level of pathologic observation. The gross features are tortuosity and segments of massive dilation alternating with segments of more normal caliber or even stenosis. **The proximal ureter usually displays a more normal appearance, an important feature when considering corrective surgery** (Fig. 62–2). Microscopically, the prune-belly ureter shows a reduced number of smooth muscle cells, which are replaced by fibrous connective tissue (Palmer and Tesluk, 1974). Although involvement may be patchy, there is no greater fibro-

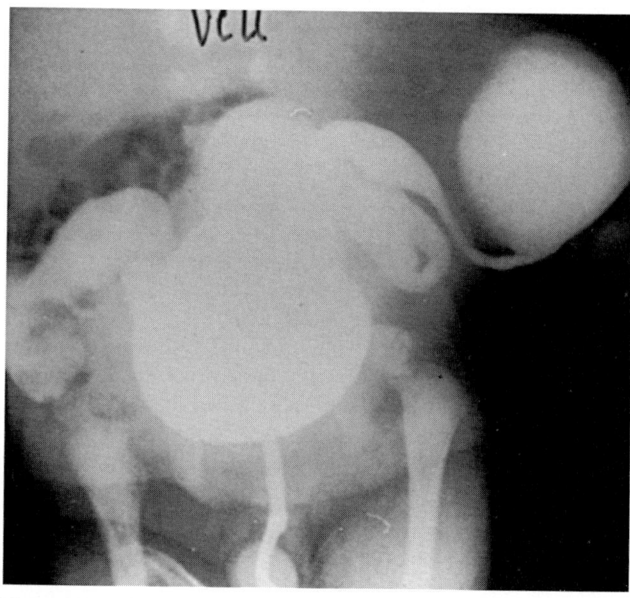

Figure 62–2. Cystogram showing massive bilateral vesicoureteral reflux. Note the marked difference in caliber of the left upper ureter as compared with the lower ureter.

sis in regions of dilation or narrowing (Nunn and Stephens, 1961). However, the smooth muscle cell population is best represented proximally, where it may be arranged into normal layers. Aberrations in innervation of the ureter may also be present. A decrease in the number of nerve plexuses and "obstruction of the nerve fibers by fibrous septae" has been reported (Ehrlich and Brown, 1977). Electron microscopy has demonstrated ultrastructural defects with both thick and thin myofilaments reduced in number and less distinct (Hanna et al, 1977).

The prune-belly ureter is disadvantaged mechanically by multiple factors. Severe ureteral dilation prohibits the luminal coaptation necessary for effective propulsion of urine. Also, the normal ureter allows a conduction wave to be propagated from smooth muscle cell to smooth muscle cell through intracellular junctions. In the prune-belly ureter the excitatory wave reaches a smooth muscle cell population that is reduced in number, separated by a collagen meshwork, and may be less capable of generating an effective contraction due to an abnormal myofilament content. Furthermore, the urine bolus that is moved forward reaches a progressively more severely affected segment of the ureter. Fluoroscopic observation confirms that these ureters may have markedly depressed peristaltic activity or may even be functionally inert (Nunn and Stephens, 1961; Williams and Burkholder, 1967). The resulting stasis within the upper tracts provides an opportunity for infection.

Bladder and Urachus

The ureters enter the bladder in a lateral and posterior position, and, if discernible, the interureteric ridge is elongated and often asymmetric (Barnhouse, 1972). Given the position and frequently patulous configuration of the ureteral orifices, **the high rate of vesicoureteral reflux** (Fig. 62–3), **which may approach 85%,** is not surprising (Goulding and Garret, 1978). As with the ureteral architecture, there is replacement of the bladder smooth muscle with connective tissue. The bladder wall may be severely thickened by this process, yet the gross appearance of hypertrophied interlacing muscle bundles and trabeculation consistent with obstruction is absent. No abnormality in innervation has been detected. The large-capacity bladder is often elongated with a wide urachal diverticulum that provides an hourglass configuration (Fig. 62–4). **Patency of the urachus occurs most commonly when urethral atresia is present but may occur without definite urethral obstruction.**

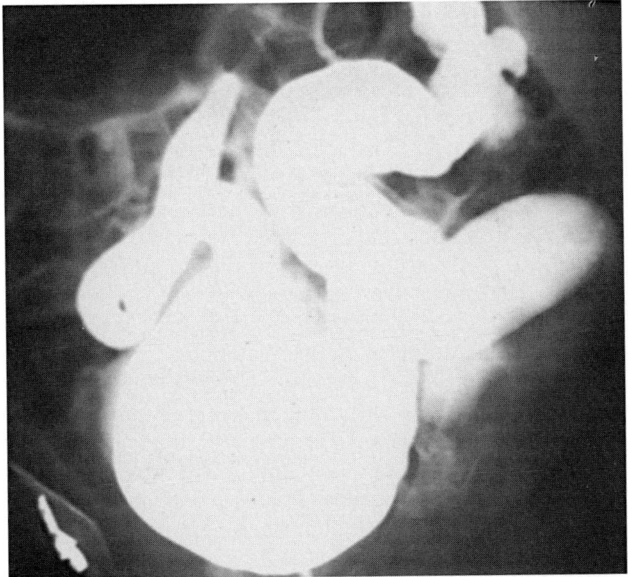

Figure 62–3. Cystogram in a boy with prune-belly syndrome, showing massive bilateral reflux. The upper ureter has an abrupt upper termination without any filling of the renal pelvis, an appearance that is characteristic of the multicystic kidney.

Usually the cystometrogram reveals **excellent detrusor compliance; the end filling pressure assumes a normal value, and the bladder functions well as a reservoir.** However, bladder sensation during filling is shifted to the right with a delayed first sensation to void, and bladder capacity may be more than double the normal volume (Snyder et al, 1976). Less consistent and less favorable results are seen with the voiding profile. The **compressor capabilities of the detrusor are diminished** by the frequent presence of vesicoureteral reflux and reduced detrusor contractility (Kinahan et al, 1992). Despite these disadvantages, nearly 50% of patients can void spontaneously, and a few may display normal voiding pressures and generate normal flow rates with minimal postvoid residuals (Nunn and Stephens, 1961; Snyder et al, 1976; Kinahan et al, 1992). Both **spontaneous improvement as well as deterioration in the efficiency of voiding have been observed,** however, underscoring the importance of regular urodynamic monitoring in those patients who can void spontaneously (Kinahan et al, 1992). In most cases in which a significant postvoid residual is present, there is no anatomic evidence of outflow obstruction, and the voiding pressure is not elevated (Williams and Burkholder, 1967; Snyder et al, 1976). The term unbalanced voiding has been used to describe the development of postvoid residuals as a consequence of the disproportion between detrusor contractility and the normal, although impeding, outflow resistance offered by the urethra. Internal urethrotomy has been employed to reduce urethral resistance and improve voiding efficiency (Snyder et al, 1976; Cukier, 1977).

Prostate and Accessory Sex Organs

The characteristically wide bladder neck merges with a grossly dilated prostatic urethra, so that the junction is nearly imperceptible both radiographically and by gross inspection (Fig. 62–5). The prostatic urethra does, however, taper to a relatively narrow membranous urethra at the urogenital diaphragm. This configuration produces an image on voiding cystourethrography that resembles that of posterior urethral valves. In fact, true anatomic obstruction of the posterior urethra by atresia, segmental stenosis, or posterior urethral valves is only rarely seen in the surviving infant (Rogers and Ostrow, 1973; Welch and Kearney, 1974; Aaronson, 1983). Significant lesions have been more frequently reported in necropsy series of fetuses and neonates (Popek et al, 1991; Stephens and Gupta, 1994). Cystourethrography may also reveal reflux of contrast material into the ejaculatory ducts, and a utricular diverticulum (see Fig. 62–5) is also often seen during the voiding phase (Kroovand et al, 1982).

Prostatic hypoplasia is responsible for the dilated ra-

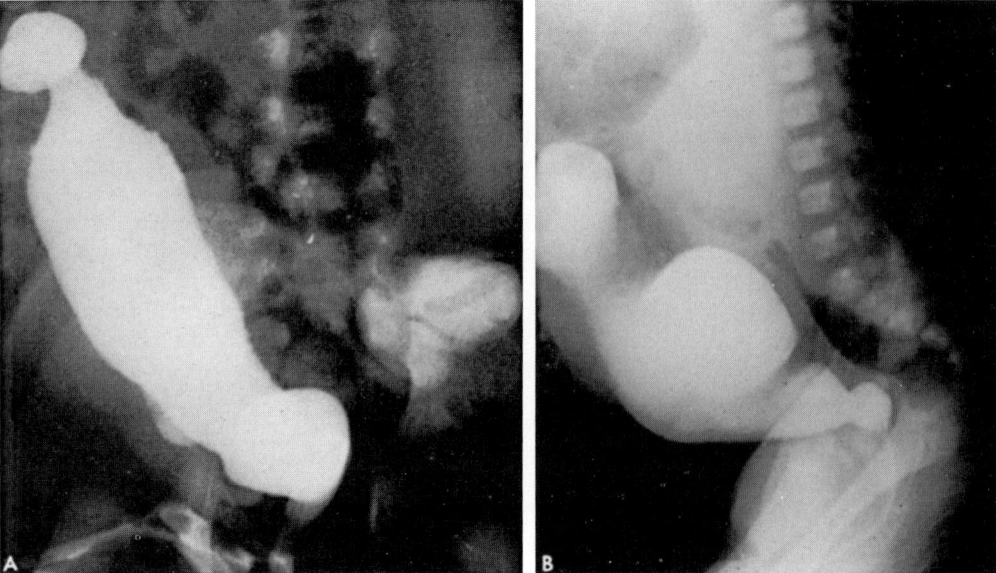

Figure 62–4. *A* and *B,* Voiding cystograms in two patients, showing the pseudodiverticulum configuration of the dome of the bladder. Note the wide, triangular prostatic urethra in both cystograms and the small utricular diverticulum in *B*.

diographic appearance of the prostatic urethra. This is a uniform feature of the syndrome that is represented pathologically by a marked reduction in epithelial elements, reduced smooth muscle fibers, and increased connective tissue content (Deklerk and Scott, 1978; Popek et al, 1991). The configuration of severe prostatic sacculation combined with an obliquely implanted urethra has also been proposed as a mechanism of functional outflow obstruction (Monie and Monie, 1979). Involvement of other accessory sex organs has also been reported. In an autopsy series of affected fetuses and neonates, the seminal vesicles were in some cases rudimentary or absent, the vas deferens segmentally atretic, and the epididymal attachment to the testis tenuous (Stephens and Gupta, 1994).

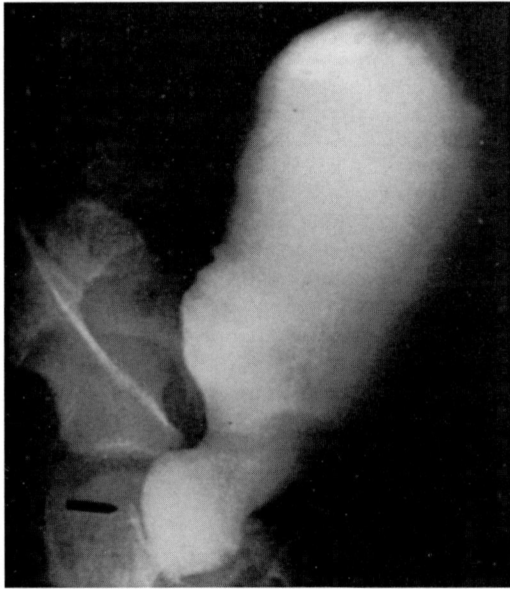

Figure 62–5. Voiding cystogram in a boy, showing the abrupt narrowing of urethra and apex of the wide, triangular prostatic portion. Note the utricular diverticulum *(arrow)*.

Urethra

The anterior urethra and the penis are normal in most prune-belly patients. However, it is well known that **congenital megalourethra** is occasionally associated with the syndrome. **Both the scaphoid variety, represented by maldevelopment of the spongiosum** (Fig. 62–6), **and the more severe fusiform megalourethra, with its absent corpora, have been reported** (Sellars et al, 1976). The scaphoid variety seems to occur with the greatest frequency (Shrom et al, 1981). In one patient series (Kroovand et al, 1982), the association of penile and urethral anomalies was rather prominent; cases of both ventral and dorsal chordee, and hypospadias were noted.

Testis

Bilateral cryptorchidism is a central feature of the syndrome, and in most patients both testes are intra-abdominal, overlying the ureters at the pelvic brim near the sacroiliac level. Obstructed descent by the dilated urinary system (Silverman and Huang, 1950), gubernacular insufficiency as a consequence of its defective precursor mesenchyme (Rajfer and Walsh, 1978), and an intrinsic abnormality of the testis have all been proposed as causes of cryptorchidism in the prune-belly patient. In support of the theory of an intrinsic testicular defect, some investigators have found an absence of spermatogonia in prune-belly testes (Uehling, 1984; Hadziselimovic, 1984). Spermatogonia were, however, observed in fetal seminiferous tubules by Orvis and his colleagues (Orvis et al, 1988). There are two important implications of this finding. First, early orchiopexy may preserve spermatogenesis, and second, these patients should not be considered immune to the development of germ cell tumors (Massad et al, 1991).

Little information is available on sexual function in men with prune-belly syndrome. **Erection and orgasm are apparently normal, but no cases of paternity have been reported.** The potential for fertility in these patients is com-

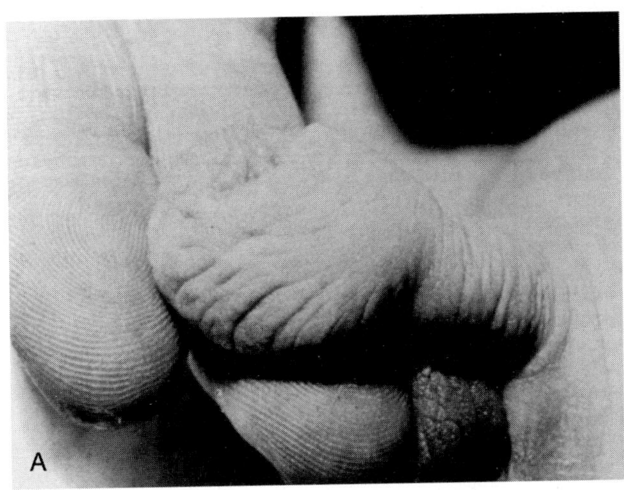

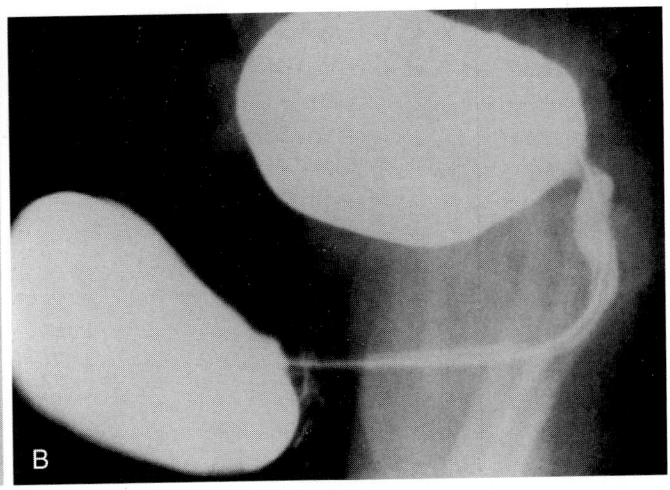

Figure 62–6. *A* and *B*, Elongated penis with ventral skin redundancy accompanying a scaphoid megalourethra demonstrated by cystourethrography. (Reprinted by permission of the publisher from Shrom SH, Cromie WJ, Duckett JW: Megalourethra. Urology 1981; 17:152. Copyright 1981 by Elsevier Science.)

promised not only by testicular abnormalities but also by multiple extratesticular factors. As mentioned, epididymal, vasal, and seminal vesical abnormalities may be present. The prostatic epithelium is hypoplastic, and the bladder neck is open. Therefore, retrograde ejaculation is common, and analysis of seminal fluid or postejaculation urine reveals azoospermia (Woodhouse and Snyder, 1985).

Extragenitourinary Abnormalities

Extragenitourinary abnormalities are frequently associated with prune-belly syndrome. Excluding the abdominal wall defect that is a consistent feature of the syndrome, as many as three quarters of the patients may have other clinically significant problems (Geary et al, 1986). The range of possible abnormalities is listed in Table 62–1.

Table 62–1. EXTRAGENITOURINARY ABNORMALITIES

Cardiac	Patent ductus arteriosus
	Ventricular septal defect
	Atrial septal defect
	Tetralogy of Fallot
Pulmonary	Lobar atelectasis
	Pulmonary hypoplasia
	Pneumothorax
	Pneumomediastinum
Gastrointestinal	Intestinal malrotation
	Intestinal atresias or stenoses
	Omphalocele
	Gastroschisis
	Hirschsprung's disease
	Imperforate anus
	Hepatobiliary anomalies
Orthopedic	Pectus excavatum, pectus carinatum
	Skin dimple at knee or elbow
	Varus deformity of feet
	Congenital hip dislocation
	Severe leg maldevelopment
Miscellaneous	Splenic torsion
	Adrenal cystic dysplasia

Abdominal Wall Defect

Although most affected infants have a similar appearance, the abdominal wall defect varies in severity and is often asymmetric and patchy in distribution. **Characteristically, the abdominal muscles are absent in the lower and medial parts of the abdominal wall, although the upper rectus muscles and outer oblique muscles are developed.** Some practitioners (Welch and Kearney, 1974) have observed that the muscles are present but hypoplastic, whereas others (Afifi et al, 1972) have found that the deficiency ranges from slight hypoplasia to complete absence of muscles. In addition, although the muscle layers may be thin, their normal arrangement is preserved, or they may be fused to form a single fibrotic layer (Afifi et al, 1972). Innervation by the anterior spinal nerves, however, is intact (Nunn and Stephens, 1961).

A definite but nonspecific myopathology has been observed both histologically and ultrastructurally. Variation in muscle fiber diameter with haphazard arrangement of both atrophic and hypertrophic fibers, an increase in fibrous tissue surrounding the muscle fibers, and fatty infiltration are present. Disorganization persists at the ultrastructural level with disarray of myofibrils, mitochondrial proliferation, and clumping of glycogen granules (Afifi et al, 1972; Mininberg et al, 1973). Unfortunately, the myopathologic findings are common to a number of neuromuscular disorders and provide little insight into the etiology of the prune-belly syndrome.

These features translate into a lax and redundant abdominal wall with bulging flanks and secondary flaring of the lower rib cage. The **poor support of the lower chest wall interferes with an effective cough mechanism and contributes to a greater vulnerability to respiratory infections.** These children also have difficulty in sitting up from the supine position. Although the wrinkled appearance is typical of the abdominal wall in the infant, it tends to take on a potbellied appearance in the older child (Fig. 62–7).

Surprisingly, the defective abdominal wall causes little difficulty for the surgeon. Wound healing proceeds satisfactorily despite the absence of layers for suturing. Wound dehiscence and other wound complications are rare.

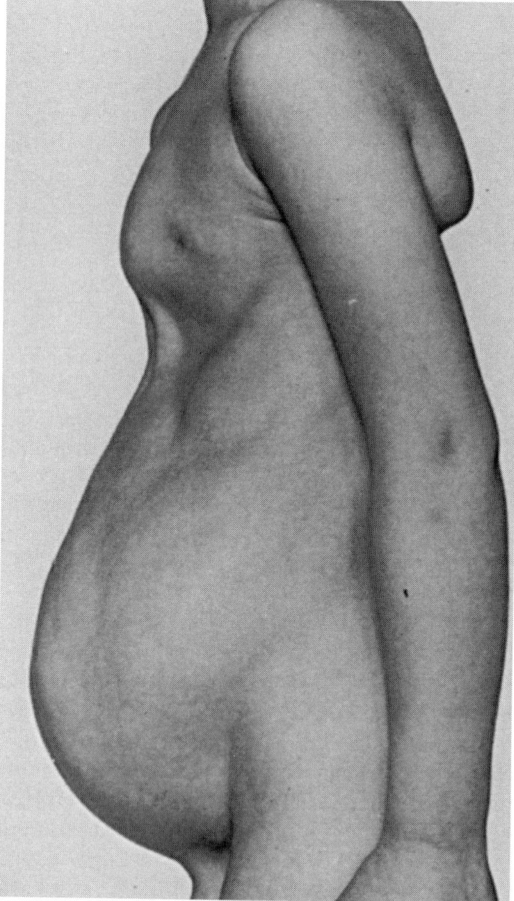

Figure 62–7. Older child with the prune-belly syndrome, showing the absence of wrinkling, the "potbelly" appearance, and the consequent deformity of the lower ribs.

Pulmonary Aspects

The pulmonary status of the infant with prune-belly syndrome is particularly critical, and survival may be threatened by a variety of pulmonary complications. **Pulmonary hypoplasia** (Fig. 62–8) **precipitated by oligohydramnios is particularly ominous.** Moreover, pneumomediastinum or pneumothorax is a common occurrence in patients with hypoplastic lungs. Neonates in this category commonly die from respiratory failure. If the patient does survive the neonatal period, the lungs grow and eventually attain adequate capacity (Alford et al, 1978). As the patient becomes older, however, he still may have respiratory problems secondary to the deficiency of accessory muscles in the abdominal wall.

The other major category of pulmonary complications includes a tendency toward lobar atelectasis and pneumonia. Because the abdominal walls are important structures in powerful expiration, patients with prune-belly syndrome have a decreased ability to generate an effective cough. Consequently, they are more vulnerable to complications during periods of excess mucus production. A number of anesthetic complications have been reported (Hannington-Kiff, 1970; Karamanian et al, 1974). Sedatives and analgesics must be used judiciously to avoid respiratiory depression. Apnea monitors play an important role in the neonatal surveillance of these patients.

Cardiac Anomalies

Ventricular septal defect, atrial septal defect, and tetralogy of Fallot occur with increased frequency in this patient population. The **incidence of cardiac abnormalities in prune-belly patients is approximately 10%** (Adebonojo, 1973).

Gastrointestinal Anomalies

Most individuals with this syndrome have **intestinal malrotation secondary to a universal mesentery with an unattached cecum** (Silverman and Huang, 1950). Much less frequent is an imperforate anus, which is more likely to occur in association with urethral atresia and renal dysplasia (Morgan et al, 1978). Gastroschisis and Hirschsprung's disease have also been reported in these patients (Willert et al, 1978; Cawthern et al, 1979). Constipation also appears to be a problem; it is secondary to deficiency of the abdominal musculature and may lead to acquired megacolon. Hepatobiliary anomalies including paucity of intralobar bile ducts (Aanpreung et al, 1993) and splenic torsion have also been reported (Heydenrych and DuToit, 1978).

Orthopedic Deformities

On a literature review of 188 cases of prune-belly syndrome, Loder and associates noted a 45% incidence of musculoskeletal involvement. Although the most frequent and benign finding is a dimple on the outer aspect of the knee (Fig. 62–9), **the club foot deformity occurs in 26%, hip dysplasia with dislocation in 5%, and spinal deformities in 5% of patients** (Loder et al, 1992). Pectus carinii and pectus excavatum deformities are also found relatively frequently. Fetal compression secondary to oligohydramnios is believed to be the cause of the various limb deformities. More severe malformations including lower extremity hypoplasias and even amelias rarely occur. Because the lower extremities only are involved, compression of the iliac vessels by a distended bladder has been suggested as the patho-

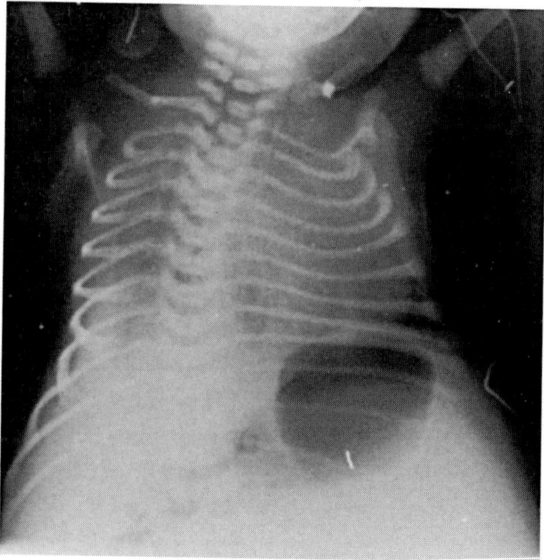

Figure 62–8. Chest radiograph of an infant who died shortly after birth from pulmonary hypoplasia.

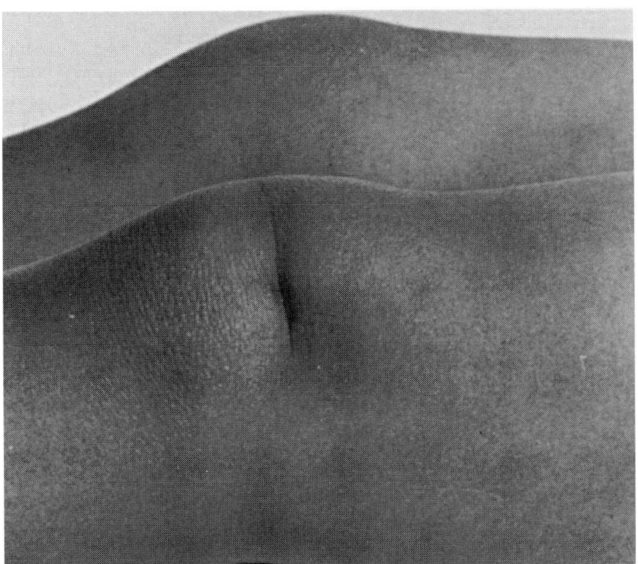

Figure 62–9. The dimple on the outer aspect of the knee characteristic of the prune-belly syndrome.

genic mechanism (Ralis and Forbes, 1971). The prevalence of orthopedic deformities and improving survival ensures a greater role for the orthopedic surgeon in the future.

CLINICAL PRESENTATION AND NATURAL HISTORY

Prenatal Diagnosis

Successful prenatal diagnosis of prune-belly syndrome by obstetric ultrasonography has been made as early as 20 weeks of gestation. However, the suggestive features of dilated ureters, bladder distention, and irregular dilation of the abdominal circumference (Bovicelli et al, 1980; Christopher et al, 1982; Shih et al, 1982) are more readily imaged at 30 weeks (Okulski, 1977). **In clinical practice it has proved difficult to distinguish the fetus with prune-belly syndrome from one with primary vesicoureteral reflux or posterior urethral valves** (Kramer, 1983). Misinterpretation of prenatal sonographic findings has resulted in application of in utero drainage procedures in 14 cases of prune-belly syndrome (Elder et al, 1987; Sholder et al, 1988). No evidence of benefit has been ascertained from this experience. Therefore, although the increasing use of maternal-fetal ultrasound has increased the frequency of fetal diagnosis of prune-belly syndrome, the incidence of the syndrome and its clinical management remain unchanged (Woodard, 1990).

Neonate

Although all cases should be recognized by the pediatrician or neonatalogist on routine postnatal examination, there is a considerable variability in the severity of the disorder and in the urgency with which urologic advice is sought. This is obviously a syndrome with a wide range of severity. Patients can be grouped according to severity. The classification shown in Table 62–2 is simple and clinically useful.

Category I includes neonates with severe pulmonary or marked renal dysplasia, either of which precludes survival beyond the first days of life. Some of these infants have a patent urachus and complete urethral obstruction. The more severely affected babies in this category may be stillborn. Because of severe oligohydramnios, others may have some of the features characteristic of renal agenesis, such as Potter's facies. The serum creatinine level is normal at birth but steadily rises thereafter. If these babies do not die quickly from pulmonary hypoplasia, they succumb only slightly later from renal failure. Drainage procedures result in a very scanty flow of dilute urine. In a few of these cases, in which there appears to be a chance for survival, a simple drainage procedure such as a vesicostomy may be justified.

Patients in category II have the potential to survive the neonatal period. They have the typical full-blown uropathy with diffuse dilatation of the urinary tract and hydronephrosis. Renal dysplasia may exist, but it is unilateral or less severe than that found in patients with category I disease. Most of these infants are able to void urine from the bladder and often do so with apparent ease. Others suffer a general failure to thrive with enormous abdominal distention. All such infants should be transferred to medical centers staffed by pediatric nephrologists, urologists, and other neonatal experts before any instrumentation is permitted.

Category III includes infants with definite but relatively mild or incomplete features of the syndrome. Some uropathy is present, but the renal parenchyma is apparently of high quality, renal function is normal, and urinary stasis is generally less marked. General agreement exists that patients in category III may require little if any urologic reconstructive surgery. However, they may later show signs of progressive upper tract deterioration, particularly if they are prone to urinary infection. They will also be candidates for treatment of cryptorchidism. All surviving patients require surveillance.

Childhood and Adolescence

Protection against further renal compromise is a challenge that continues through the individual's childhood and adolescence. **Chronic pyelonephritis and obstruction have been shown to play a significant role in the loss of renal**

Table 62–2. THE SPECTRUM OF THE PRUNE-BELLY SYNDROME

Distinguishing Characteristics	Category Classification
Oligohydramnios, pulmonary hypoplasia, or pneumothorax. May have urethral obstruction or patent urachus and club foot	I
Typical external features and uropathy of the full-blown syndrome but no immediate problem with survival. May have mild or unilateral renal dysplasia. May or may not develop urosepsis or gradual azotemia	II
External features may be mild or incomplete. Uropathy is less severe; renal function is stable	III

function, underscoring the need to maintain sterility of the urinary tract and the need for surgery for reflux and obstruction (Reinberg et al, 1991). Despite these efforts, as many as 30% of patients, generally those with impaired renal function at initial evaluation, may develop chronic renal failure during childhood or adolescence (Geary et al, 1986). Renal transplantation is necessary for these patients to ensure normal growth and development, and success with transplantation in prune-belly patients can be expected to equal that in other age-matched groups (Reinberg et al, 1989). Among patients with normal renal function, normal growth may be expected in the majority, although growth retardation in the absence of renal compromise was observed in one third of patients in one series (Geary et al, 1986). A normal pattern of secondary sexual development can be expected (Woodhouse and Snyder, 1985).

Adult Presentation

Although the diagnosis of prune-belly syndrome is usually made in the neonatal period or during early infancy, adult presentation still occasionally occurs. Symptoms of renal failure with associated hypertension most commonly bring these patients to medical attention (Lee, 1977; Wallner and Kramar, 1990; Kerbl and Pauer, 1993). In one case, a history of urinary tract infections was absent (Texter and Koontz, 1980). However, urinary stasis represents a persistent opportunity for infection, and patients have been reported who seem to do well for years with little treatment or no treatment only to succumb to urinary sepsis as adults (Culp and Flocks, 1954).

Female Syndrome

In the strictest sense, only a male patient may harbor the complete syndrome. Yet about 3% of reported cases occur in genetic females. When less strict criteria for diagnosis are applied, the percentage quoted is sometimes higher. Affected female patients appear to have no urethral abnormality. The defect involves the abdominal wall, bladder, and upper urinary tract (Rabinowitz and Schillinger, 1977). Actually, fewer than 20 cases have been reported, and the principles of management are essentially the same as those for males. Many of the female patients have had incomplete forms of the syndrome with normal upper urinary tracts.

Incomplete Syndrome

Although it is exceptionally rare to encounter a normal urinary tract in association with the characteristic abdominal wall defect in a male, the converse is not unusual. Some patients (with "pseudo-prune-belly syndrome") with a normal or relatively normal abdominal wall exhibit many or all of the internal urologic features, usually in a less severe form. These features may include dysplastic or dysmorphic kidneys or may include dilated and tortuous ureters.

Genetic Aspects

The possibility of a genetic basis for prune-belly syndrome is suggested by the curious male-to-female ratio, the occasional occurrence of affected male siblings or cousins, and the rare patient with a karyotypic abnormality. Mendelian inheritance patterns that have been considered include autosomal chromosome abnormalities, X chromosome abnormalities, and polygenic transmission (Garlinger and Ott, 1974; Adenyokunna et al, 1975; Riccardi and Grum, 1977; Lockhart et al, 1979). The possibility of genetic heterogeneity also exists, further confounding the delineation of a genetic basis. One of the most powerful arguments against a genetic etiology rests with the observation of 100% discordance among all twins in which monozygosity has been proved (Fig. 62–10) (Ives, 1974). Environmental factors, teratogens, and maternal factors have not been clearly implicated. The fact that the syndrome has rarely occurred in siblings, however, is important in counseling parents of affected infants.

Although the karyotypic analysis is nearly always normal in these patients, a few cases of chromosomal abnormalities have been reported. These include the association of prune-belly syndrome with a minute additional chromosome in one case (Halbrecht et al, 1972); one case of mosaic monosomy 16 (Harley et al, 1972); two cases each of trisomy 13 (Frydman et al, 1983) and trisomy 18 (Beckman et al, 1984); and four cases of Turner's syndrome (Lubinsky et al, 1980; Adenyokunna and Familusi, 1982). Although no clear pattern has emerged, the variable chromosome abnormalities may suggest the involvement of multiple loci on different chromosomes.

MANAGEMENT

Initial Diagnostic Evaluation

The syndrome is now well known and, because of the typical external features, the diagnosis of prune-belly syn-

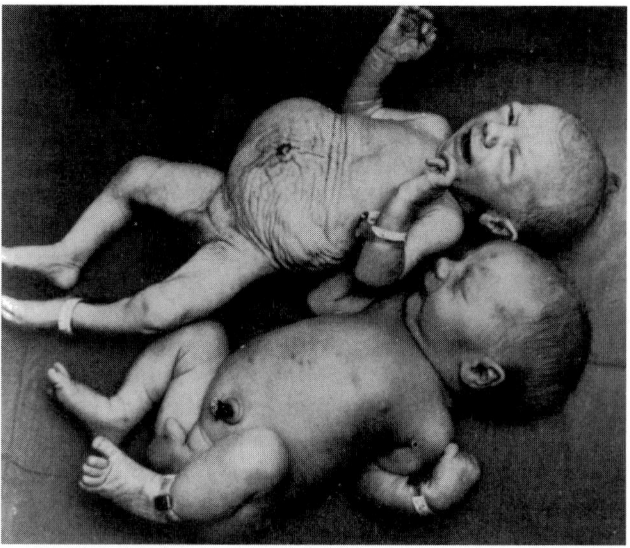

Figure 62–10. Infant with prune-belly syndrome and his unaffected identical twin brother at age 3 days. (From Ives EJ: The abdominal muscle deficiency triad syndrome—experience with ten cases. Birth Defects 1974, 10:127.)

drome and the presence of prune-belly uropathy are seldom in doubt. Although the urologist is usually notified immediately, the affected neonate rarely represents a true urologic emergency. **The most urgent matters are actually those concerned with cardiopulmonary function.** Pulmonary complications including pulmonary hypoplasia, pneumomediastinum, pneumothorax, and cardiac abnormalities must be excluded. Following stabilization, urologic evaluation proceeds with physical examination and ultrasonography. Renal volume as well as the presence of dilated upper tracts may be palpated through the thin abdominal wall, and the infant is observed for its voiding pattern and for the presence of a patent urachus. Further parenchymal assessment and definition of the collecting system, ureter, and bladder are provided by an ultrasound examination (Fig. 62–11). Serial electrolytes and routine urine culture complete an early urologic profile. An orthopedic examination should also be done initially.

If the baby is in stable condition and the serum creatinine level remains normal, one may wait for several days before obtaining a radioisotopic renal scan or an excretory urogram. However, these studies should be done, and the remainder of the diagnostic evaluation must then be tailored in accordance with one's attitude toward definitive management (Fig. 62–12). **Studies that require instrumentation and therefore risk infection are avoided unless they influence immediate management decisions.** Vesicoureteral reflux may be assumed to be present, and prophylactic antibiotics are routinely provided.

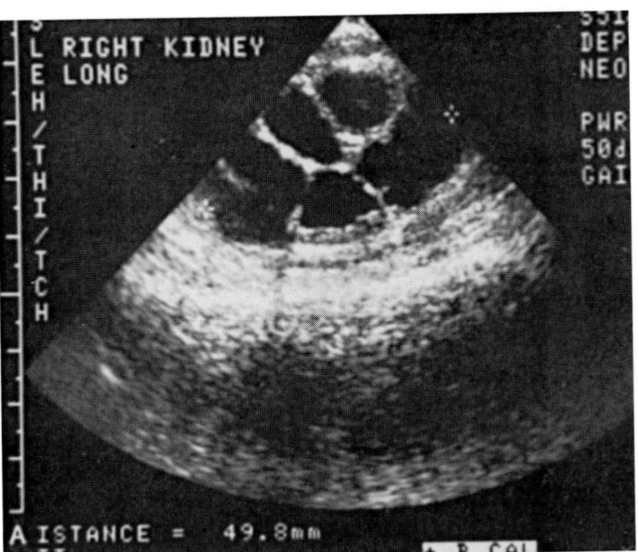

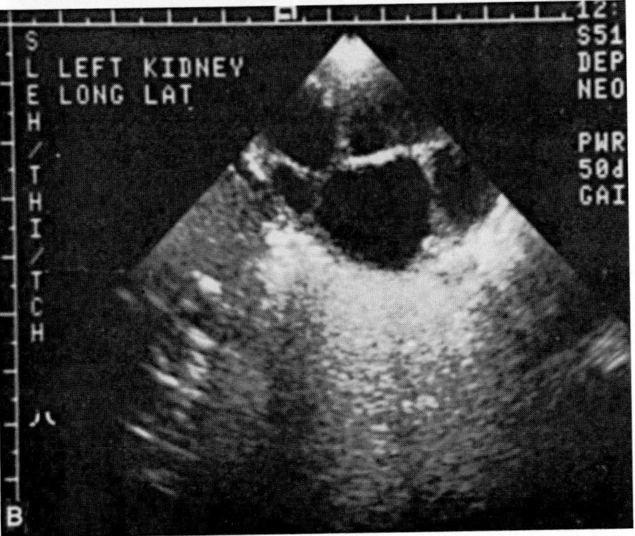

Figure 62–11. Right *(A)* and left *(B)* kidneys in a 1-day-old infant with typical prune-belly syndrome. The infant was seen at birth, placed on antibiotics, and followed closely with urine cultures, serum creatinine determinations, and renal ultrasound imaging. (From Woodard JR, and Zucker I: Current management of the dilated urinary tract in prune-belly syndrome. Urol Clin North Am 1990; 17[2]:413.)

By following the serum creatinine levels, urine bacteriology, and pyelographic and sonographic findings, it is possible to formulate a reasonable plan of clinical management. Evidence of infection or deteriorating renal function is usually an indication for surgical intervention. In the absence of such complications, one should monitor the respiratory function closely for 2 to 3 months, at which time a more thorough urologic evaluation may be appropriate. Many different approaches have been advocated for the management of prune-belly uropathy, each with its rationale and each with its own proponents. All methods have the same ultimate aim of maintaining renal function and preventing urinary infection.

Controversies in Management of the Category II Patient

The motivation for aggressive surgical intervention was initially derived from observation of the poor prognosis for category II infants as a group. Because 20% were either stillborn or died in the neonatal period and an additional 30% died during the first 2 years of life, the outlook was dismal (Lattimer, 1958). Compilation of the reported cases in the literature between 1950 and 1970 by Waldbaum and Marshall revealed that 86% of the 56 accurately traceable patients had died, with or without surgical intervention (Waldbaum and Marshall, 1970). The obvious implication was that a more aggressive approach was necessary to improve the fate of the infant with prune-belly syndrome. With the recognition that infection and progressive renal insufficiency are the factors that most often pose the greatest threat to quality of life and survival, surgical reconstruction to normalize the anatomy and function of the genitourinary tract was advocated. Early retailoring of the urinary system to reduce stasis and eliminate reflux or obstruction has included ureteral shortening, tapering and vesicoureteral reimplantation, and reduction cystoplasty. Reconstruction is best delayed until the child is approximately 3 months of age to allow for pulmonary maturation. This approach has been successful in achieving anatomic and functional improvement based on stable radiographic studies, stable creatinine values, and a reduced occurrence of infection (Waldbaum and Marshall, 1970; Jeffs et al, 1977; Woodard and Parrott, 1978a; Randolph et al, 1981). Review of the author's experience with 17 category II patients followed from the neonatal period who underwent early reconstruction has shown that 15 patients have maintained a normal creatinine level and only two have demonstrated moderate renal insufficiency; follow-up has ranged from 2 to 27 years (Smith et al, 1995).

An alternative approach of limited surgical intervention has also been applied. Proponents advocate close surveil-

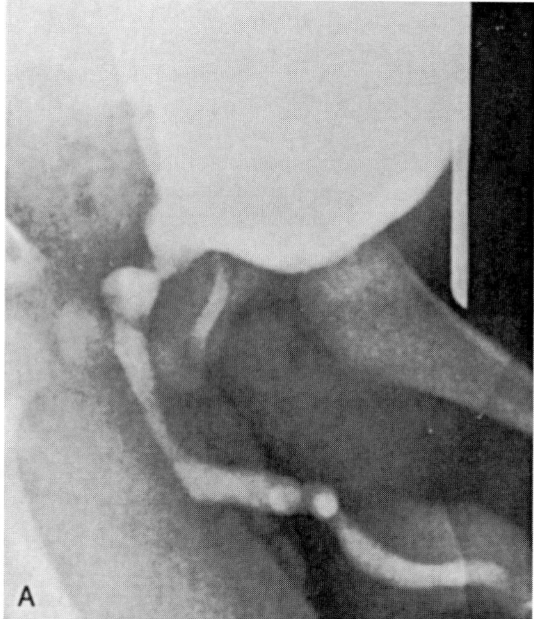

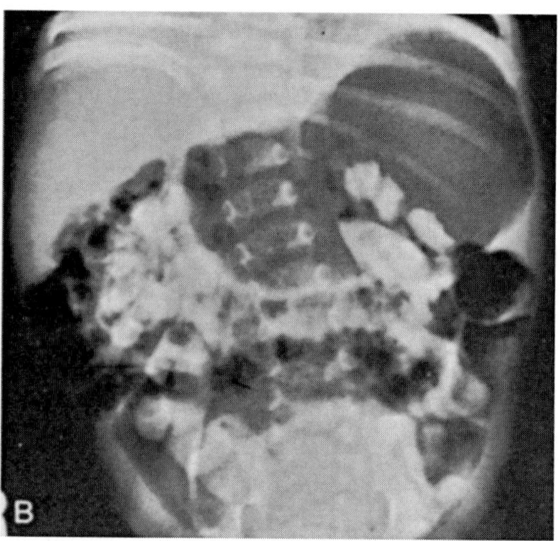

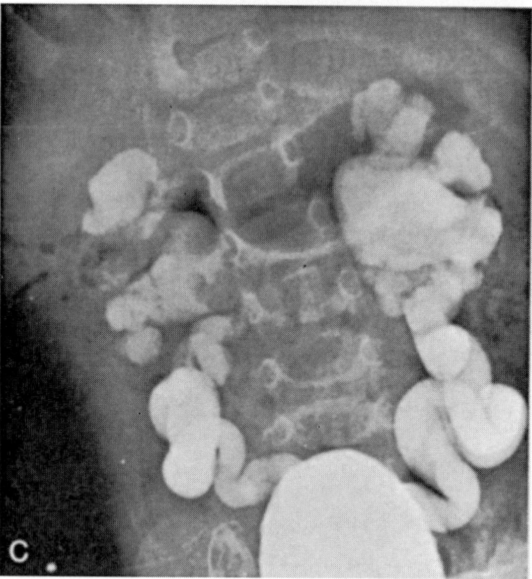

Figure 62–12. Same infant as shown in Figure 62–11 when he was re-evaluated at the age of 1 month with voiding cytourethrogram *(A)*. Note reflux posterior to bladder and typical wide bladder neck with long triangular prostatic urethra. *B,* Film from intravenous urogram, also at 1 month of age. *C,* Film from voiding cystogram made as part of his re-evaluation 7 months later. Note grade V bilateral vesicoureteral reflux with marked ureteral tortuosity. Patient underwent major reconstructive surgery following this study. (From Woodard JR, and Zucker I: Current management of the dilated urinary tract in prune-belly syndrome. Urol Clin North Am 1990; 17[2]:413.)

lance with medical management of bacteriuria and surgical intervention only in patients with proven obstruction or intractable infection. Opinions vary about the management of vesicoureteral reflux in the prune-belly population, although there is no reason to believe that reflux in this population is any less important, and correction of high-grade reflux seems prudent. Success with minimal surgical intervention has been reported (Woodhouse et al, 1979; Duckett, 1980; Tank and McCoy, 1983; McMullin et al, 1988). Woodhouse and his associates (1979) reviewed a series of prune-belly patients who had been managed conservatively. Nine of eleven of these patients, who were followed from infancy, remained well except for a few urinary tract infections for periods of up to 24 years. They were said to have normal voiding patterns and normal renal function. Certainly, patients in category III are candidates for this type of management (Fig. 62–13).

The paucity of long-term data for category II patients, the probable variation in assignment of disease severity in treatment groups, and the variable natural history of the disease make comparison of these retrospective studies difficult. Spontaneous improvement in ureteral appearance and function may occur with normal growth and elongation of the ureters (Duckett, 1980). Also, some patients with gross abnormalities of the urinary collecting system have survived decades without medical attention (Asplund and Laska, 1975; Lee, 1977; Texter and Koontz, 1980). Yet progressive uropathy is also well known to occur, and many patients with prune-belly syndrome ultimately require renal transplantation (Reinberg et al, 1989). Controversy will persist over category II patients until accurate application of a medical or surgical approach is possible based on distinct clinical features.

Nonoperative Management

When obstruction and vesicoureteral reflux have been excluded, a nonoperative stance may be taken toward pa-

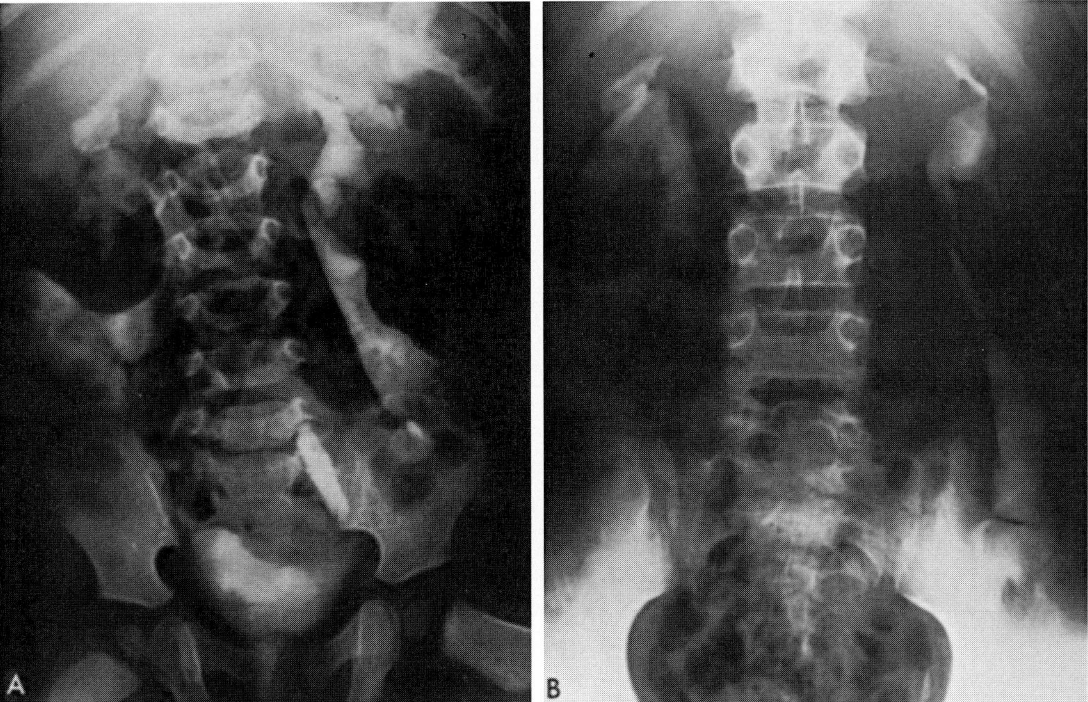

Figure 62–13. Intravenous urogram in a boy with prune-belly syndrome. *A,* At age 2 years, showing classic appearance of tortuous, dilated ureters with relatively well-preserved kidneys. *B,* At age 19 years, showing improvement in ureteric dilation without surgical treatment and no deterioration in renal function.

tients with normal renal function despite gross dilation of the upper and lower urinary tracts. This position demands close surveillance for the development of urinary tract infections, continuous monitoring of renal function, and routine radiographic imaging. Generally, antibiotic prophylaxis is provided, and urinalysis is performed each month with cultures performed as indicated. The upper tracts are monitored for increasing dilation and for evidence of obstruction by functional studies (radionuclide imaging). Suspicion of obstruction that cannot be fully defined with more routine studies should be further evaluated with a Whitaker's test.

Surgical Management of Prune-Belly Syndrome

Surgical management of prune-belly syndrome uropathy is directed toward both correction of vesicoureteral dysfunction including vesicoureteral reflux, upper tract obstruction, and severe upper tract stasis, and correction of vesicourethral dysfunction including improvement of bladder emptying. As discussed, the timing of surgical intervention may be early in an attempt to protect a threatened system from further compromise, or it may be delayed until obstruction or infection mandate intervention. Orchiopexy is necessary in all patients. Abdominal reconstruction depends on the severity of the abdominal defect, but when indicated it should be performed early to allow development of a normal physique as the child progresses through the formative years.

Vesicoureteral Dysfunction

Temporary Diversion

Earlier efforts to improve the prognosis of the infant with prune-belly syndrome employed routine high supravesical urinary diversion followed by extensive reconstruction in infants with stable renal function (Carter et al, 1974; Burbige et al, 1987). Although enthusiasm for routine proximal diversion in the neonatal period has justifiably diminished, there remain situations in which urinary diversion is indicated. **In the presence of intractable infection or deterioration in renal function a temporizing drainage procedure must be considered. Cutaneous vesicostomy should be considered first in this situation.** Vesicostomy is relatively simple to perform and generally effective and will not compromise a more extensive reconstructive effort if such is indicated at a later date (Fig. 62–14). The procedure is performed through a small transverse incision midway between the umbilicus and the symphysis pubis. A small ellipse of skin and rectus fascia is excised. The dome of the bladder is mobilized and delivered into the incision, at which point it is sutured to the rectus fascia and skin, and a small bladder stoma is fashioned (Duckett, 1974). The urine is allowed to drain freely into a diaper, using no collection device or tubes. Vesicostomy is useful as a preliminary drainage procedure prior to a more extensive reconstructive operation at a later date.

More proximal drainage in the form of a cutaneous pyelostomy remains useful in the unusual case of ureteropelvic junction or ureterovesical junction obstruction, or in patients with unremitting infection. Although not as simple as a vesicostomy, it is still an expedient procedure and has the advantage of providing good proximal drainage to each kidney while permitting inspection and biopsy of the kidney at the time of operation. By allowing subsequent evaluation of differential kidney function, it may also aid in the planning of subsequent reconstructive operations. **Proximal ureterostomy should be avoided because it jeopardizes the segment of the ureter that is most useful in subsequent reconstruction.**

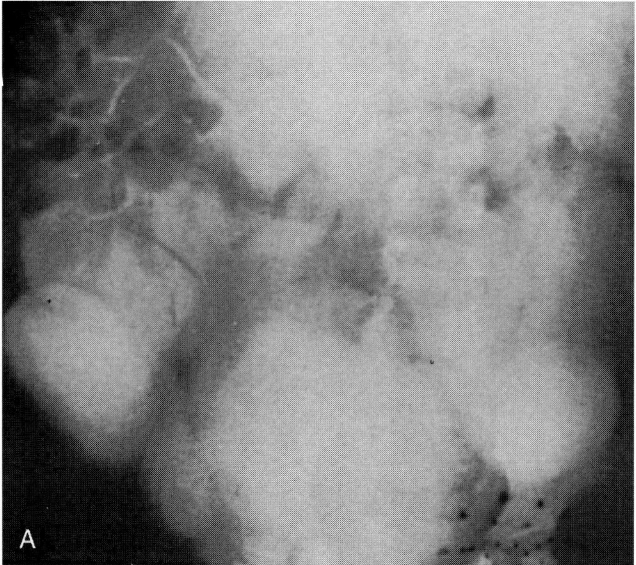

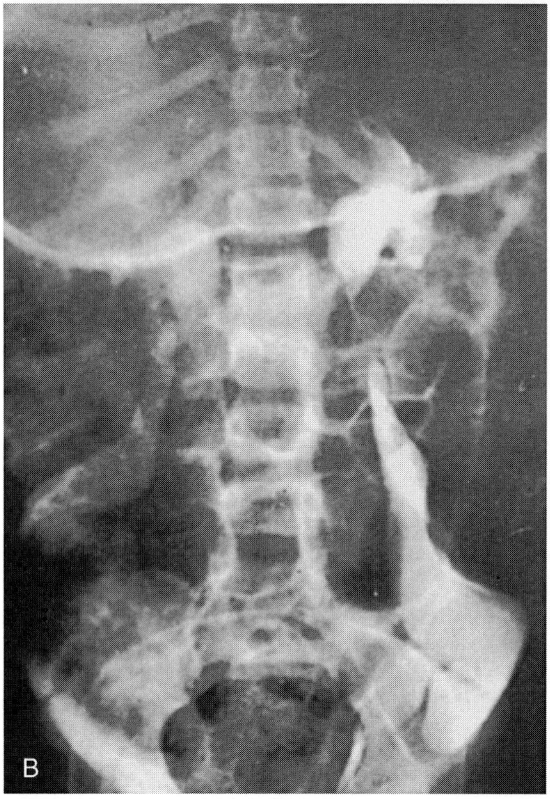

Figure 62–14. Vesicostomy drainage. *A,* Intravenous pyelogram in an 18-month-old boy with prune-belly syndrome. *B,* Intravenous pyelogram 10 years later with cutaneous vesicostomy alone.

Ureteral Reconstruction

The role of extensive surgical remodeling of the urinary tract in patients with prune-belly syndrome is understandably controversial because some patients appear to do well without major reconstruction and others seem to have been harmed by unsuccessful surgical attempts. There is little question, however, that the urinary tract in patients with prune-belly syndrome is characterized by stasis and that this stasis predisposes to bacteriuria, which may lead to deterioration of renal function as well as to troublesome clinical symptoms. Therefore, it is likely that many surgeons will continue their efforts to remodel these distorted urinary tracts.

Success in these surgical reconstructions depends to a great extent on the use of the upper few centimeters of ureter, which are usually less dilated, less tortuous, and morphologically better than the distal ureter. Meticulous surgical technique with adherence to established principles of ureteral tailoring and reimplantation surgery is required (Fig. 62–15*E–G*). Unfortunately, both the bladder and the ureter, by the very nature of this bizarre uropathy, are difficult structures with which to work. Despite these inherent difficulties, in experienced hands a reasonably high degree of success is possible with this extensive reconstructive surgery, both in the neonate as a primary procedure (Figs. 62–16 and 62–17) and in the older infant or child (Fig. 62–18) as a primary or staged procedure (Woodard and Parrott, 1978a; Woodard, 1990a).

Vesicourethral Dysfunction

Reduction Cystoplasty

Through reconfiguration of the bladder, the goal of reduction cystoplasty is to maximize the efforts of the poorly contractile detrusor. The most aggressive description of the procedure entails not only removal of the wide urachal diverticulum but also reshaping of the bladder into a more spherical form, either by further excision of the bladder dome or by overlapping the redundant detrusor muscle (Perlmutter, 1976; Hanna, 1982). Benefit was believed to follow from removal of the tubelike dome, which often emptied poorly, and from alleviation of the acentric detrusor contraction caused by urachal tethering. The more spherical shape should also maximize the intravesical pressure generated by a detrusor contraction as described by Laplace's law (Perlmutter, 1976). Some initial improvement in voiding dynamics may be achieved by aggressive bladder remodeling. However, with long-term follow-up, there has been no evidence that this improvement is maintained, and excessive bladder volumes tend to recur with time (Bukowski and Perlmutter, 1994). Current use of reduction cystoplasty should be limited to simple excision of the large urachal diverticulum when it exists (see Fig. 62–15*F*).

Internal Urethrotomy

Internal urethrotomy is indicated in the rare patient with true anatomic urethral obstruction or in patients with urodynamic evidence of urethral obstruction by pressure flow studies. Application has been extended, however, to include those children who develop large postvoid residuals as a consequence of "unbalanced" vesicourethral function. Proponents suggest that improved flow rates and improved bladder emptying may be achieved by lowering urethral resistance (Snyder et al, 1976; Cukier, 1977). The procedure usually is considered in a child with increasing postvoid residuals, vesicoureteral reflux, or worsening ureteral dilation. Lower resting urethral pressures, improved flow rates, and a reduction in postvoid residuals with lowered infection rates have been reported (Snyder et al, 1976;

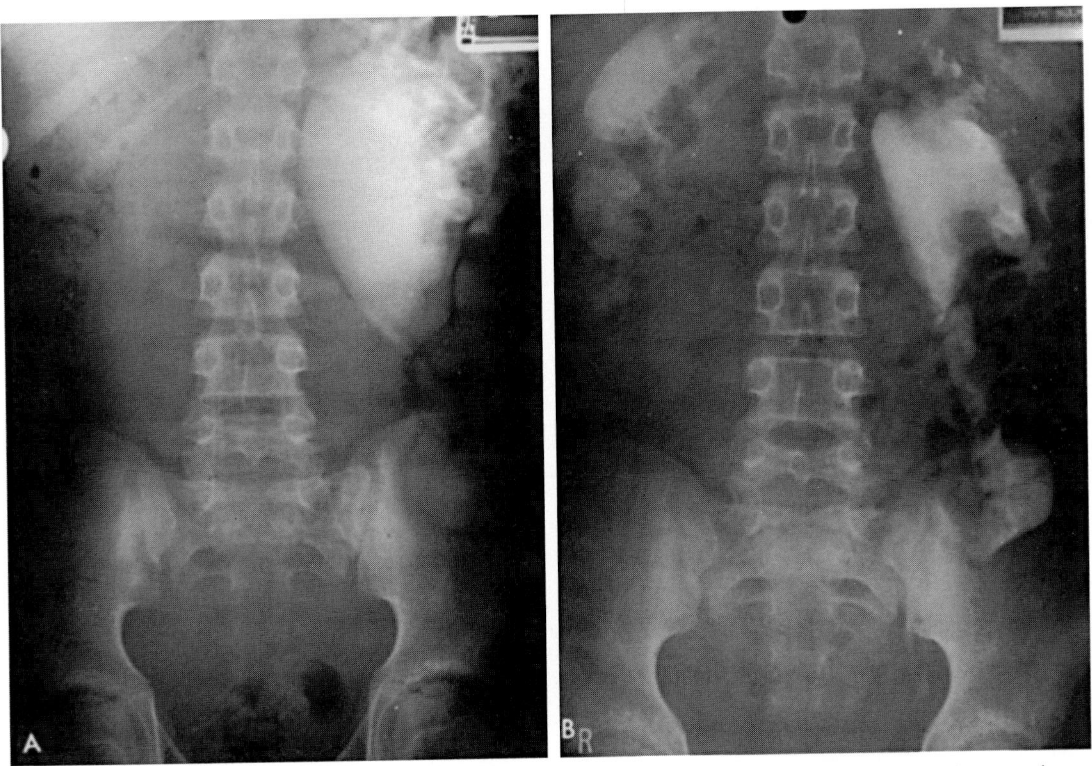

Figure 62–19. Intravenous urograms in a 12-year-old boy with prune-belly syndrome. *A*, At presentation with residual urine volume of 2 liters. *B*, Following Otis urethrotomy.

and the urethra, basing the reconstruction on the principles of hypospadias repair.

Management of Cryptorchidism

The potential for fertility in patients with prune-belly syndrome is doubtful. However, germ cells are known to be present in the testes of affected infants, and testicular hormonal function will allow normal puberty. Therefore, orchiopexy is attempted in most patients. However, because the standard surgical techniques of orchiopexy are rarely successful, one of three alternatives is usually employed.

EARLY TRANSABDOMINAL ORCHIOPEXY. In the neonate and in patients up to at least 6 months of age, transabdominal complete mobilization of the spermatic cord almost always allows the testis to be positioned in the dependent portion of the scrotum without dividing the vascular portion of the spermatic cord (Fig. 62–20) (Woodard and Parrott, 1978b). This procedure was found to be particularly applicable to infants undergoing extensive ureteral reconstructive procedures during the neonatal period because it could be done simultaneously. In patients who do not require reconstructive surgery, one may wait 3 or 4 months to ensure stability of the upper urinary tract as well as that of the cardiopulmonary system before performing the operation.

FOWLER-STEPHENS (LONG LOOP VAS) TECHNIQUE. The Fowler-Stephens technique for performing orchiopexy in patients with intra-abdominal testes has become part of the standard urologic armamentarium (Fowler and Stephens, 1963). The operation relies on the presence of vascular anastomoses between the vessels of the vas deferens and the distal spermatic artery and on the redundancy of the looping vas deferens, which extends down beyond the testis and then returns superiorly to the epididymis. Preservation of the peritoneum over the vas deferens is important for protection of the collateral vessels. The spermatic vessel is divided above the level of the internal ring before its convergence with the vas. The vas and accompanying vasculature then allow placement of the testis in a scrotal position.

In patients with prune-belly syndrome the operation is done transperitoneally with a wider-than-usual exposure; the success rate has been reported as approximately 75% (Gibbons et al, 1979). This procedure, therefore, represents a reasonable approach to the intra-abdominal testis in the patient with prune-belly syndrome and may allow greater flexibility in the timing of the procedure. Enthusiasm has been generated for the so-called staged Fowler-Stephens operation, in which the spermatic vessels are ligated several months prior to the orchiopexy operation itself. The rationale for this modification is to allow the development of increased collateral circulation between the vasal and distal testicular arteries, which may improve the success rate of the Fowler-Stephens procedure in these patients.

MICROVASCULAR AUTOTRANSPLANTATION. It is technically feasible to perform autotransplantation of the abdominal testis to the scrotum using microvascular anastomoses of the spermatic vessels to the inferior epigastric vessels. Although enthusiasm for this procedure is limited, the technique has been applied successfully in patients of various ages with prune-belly syndrome (McMahon et al, 1976; Wacksman et al, 1980). Despite the improbability of fertility in a patient with prune-belly syndrome, advances in the treatment of infertility may reduce the importance of

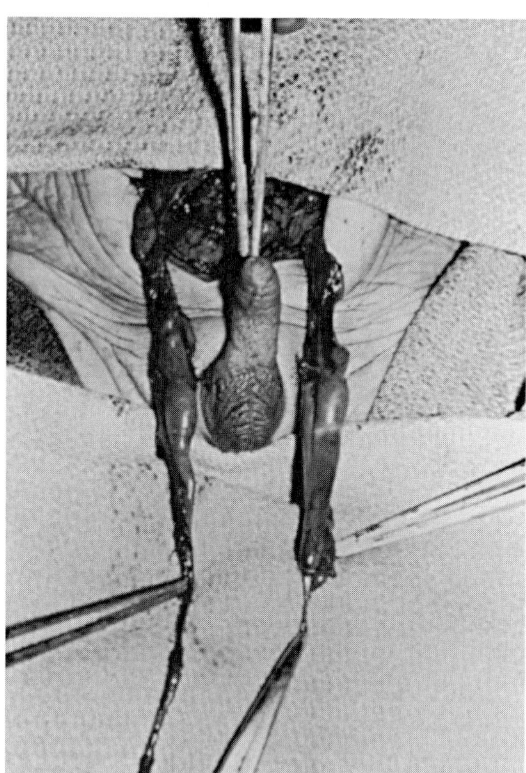

Figure 62–20. Operative photograph showing the ease with which the testes reach the scrotum following neonatal transabdominal mobilization of the spermatic cords.

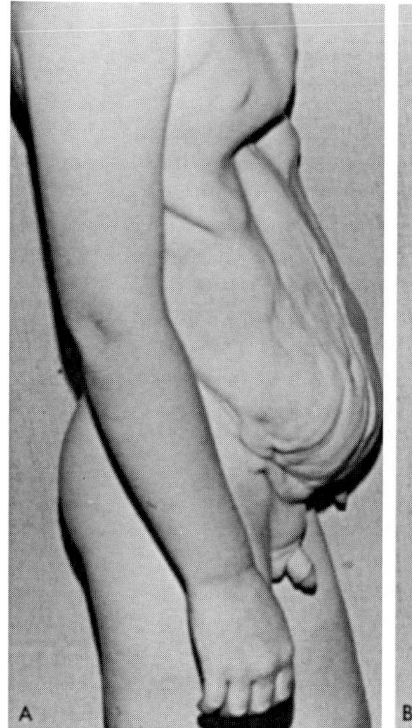

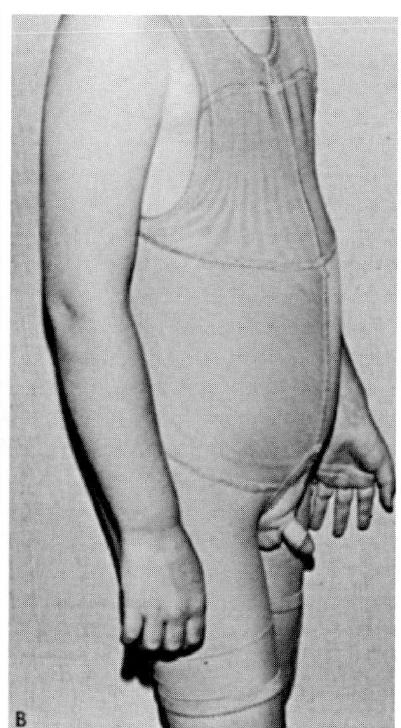

Figure 62–21. Photograph of a 4-year-old boy without *(A)* and with *(B)* his elasticized corset.

extratesticular factors in these patients. Early orchiopexy may then assume even greater importance in preserving spermatogonia.

ABDOMINAL WALL RECONSTRUCTION

Correction of the abdominal wall defect should be recognized as an important part of the management of patients with prune-belly syndrome. Not only does such a reconstruction produce a significant improvement in cosmesis and psychological well-being, it also may improve bladder, bowel, and pulmonary function (Woodard et al, 1995). External support devices remain useful as a noninvasive means of managing abdominal wall support (Fig. 62–21). However, most parents and patients desire more definitive correction of the defect. Randolph and his colleagues carefully delineated the abdominal wall muscular defect by both electromyographic mapping and anatomic description. The lateral and upper parts of the abdominal wall are clearly the most normal and the suprapubic region is the most affected (Randolph et al, 1981; Fallat et al, 1989). This information forms the basis for each of the three procedures suggested for abdominal wall reconstruction.

RANDOLPH TECHNIQUE. The procedure developed by Randolph and colleagues (1981) **involves full-thickness removal of the abnormal region** using a transverse incision extending from the tip of the 12th rib down to the symphysis pubis and back to the tip of the contralateral 12th rib. The redundant skin and deficient fascia are marked and excised, and the more healthy fascia is reapproximated to the anterior iliac spines, pubic tubercle, and fascia below. This procedure does succeed in reducing the protuberance of the abdomen, and the incision is carried out so that innervation to the anterior abdominal muscles is preserved. However, it does

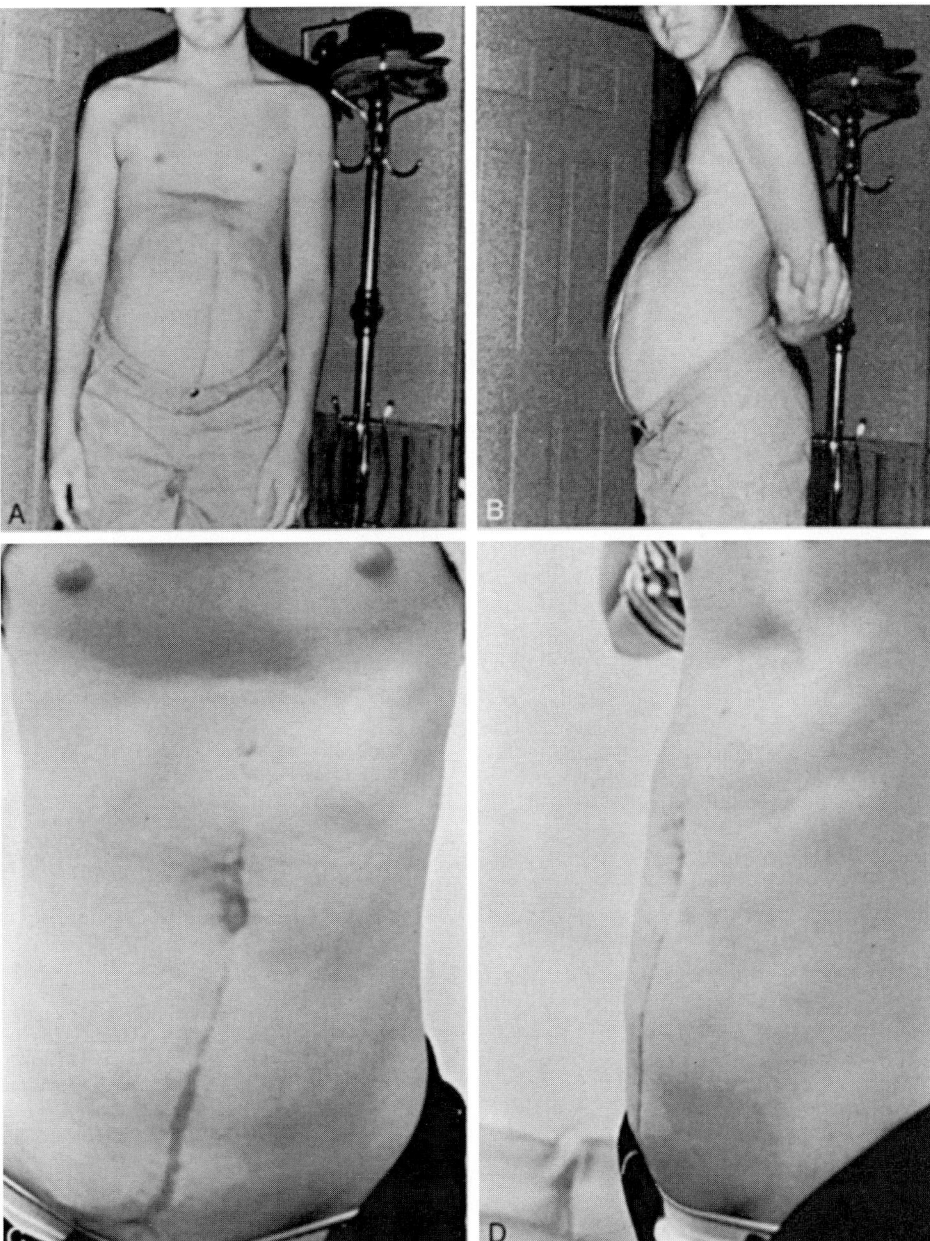

Figure 62–22. *A* and *B,* Anterior and lateral views of the abdomen of a 14-year-old boy who underwent major surgical remodeling of the urinary tract during early infancy with good results. Note typical abdominal configuration. *C* and *D,* Anterior and lateral views of the same boy 1 month after undergoing abdominoplasty using the technique described by Monfort.

not improve abdominal wall thickness, and lateral bulging tends to remain uncorrected.

EHRLICH TECHNIQUE. Both the Ehrlich technique and the Monfort technique employ vertical overlapping of the abdominal fascia to eliminate redundancy, improve abdominal wall thickness, and generate a more normal physique (Fig. 62–22). Ehrlich's technique uses a midline incision followed by elevation of the skin and subcutaneous tissue from the attenuated muscular and fascial layers. A double-breasted overlapping advancement of each side toward the contralateral flank is then performed (Ehrlich et al, 1986). Preservation of the umbilicus requires mobilization on a vascular pedicle using the inferior epigastric vessels and appropriate repositioning during skin closure (Ehrlich and Lesavoy, 1993).

MONFORT ABDOMINOPLASTY. The Monfort abdominoplasty (see Fig. 62–15*A–D* and *H–J*) uses a vertically oriented elliptical incision to isolate the redundant skin, which is then elevated from the underlying fascia and excised. The umbilicus is circumscribed with a second incision and is left undisturbed. The abdominal cavity is then entered lateral to the rectus fascia, taking care to avoid interrupting the epigastric vessels at the superior and inferior aspects of the incision. Advancement of the lateral fascia over the central plate eliminates redundancy and provides increased thickness to the abdominal wall. Excellent results with a high degree of patient satisfaction have been reported with both the Erhlich and Monfort techniques. Both procedures also provide adequate exposure for performance of concomitant genitourinary reconstruction (Ehrlich et al, 1986; Monfort et al, 1991).

OUTLOOK

The considerable improvements achieved in the medical, surgical, and urodynamic management of patients born with the prune-belly syndrome will certainly result in a prognosis far better than that previously reported, both for survival and for quality of life. The syndrome is clearly a disorder with a wide spectrum of severity. Some patients may benefit from major urologic reconstruction, but others require little if any such surgery. All patients need careful evaluation and individualized management and, because urodynamics may change with age, long-term surveillance and periodic reappraisal are necessary.

REFERENCES

Aanpreung P, Beckwith B, Gelansky SH, et al: Association of paucity of interlobular bile ducts with prune belly syndrome. J Pediatr Gastroenterol Nutr 1993; 16(1):81.

Aaronson IA: Posterior urethral valve masquerading as the prune belly syndrome. Br J Urol 1983; 55:508.

Aaronson IA, Cremin BJ: Prune-belly syndrome in young females. Urol Radiol 1980; 1:151.

Adebonojo FO: Dysplasia of the abdominal musculature with multiple congenital anomalies: prune belly or triad syndrome. J Natl Med Assoc 1973; 65:327.

Adenyokunna AA, Adenyi TM, Kolewole TM, et al: Prune-belly syndrome: A study of ten cases in Nigerian children with common and uncommon manifestations. East Afr Med J 1975; 52:438.

Adenyokunna AA, Familusi JB: Prune belly syndrome in two siblings and a first cousin. Am J Dis Child 1982; 136:23.

Affifi AK, Rebiez JM, Andonian SJ, et al: The myopathology of the prune belly syndrome. J Neurol Sci 1972; 15:153.

Alford BA, Peoples WM, Resnick JS, et al: Pulmonary complications associated with the prune-belly syndrome. Pediatr Radiol 1978; 129:401.

Asplund J, Laska J: Prune belly syndrome at the age of 37. Scand J Urol Nephrol 1975; 9:297.

Barnhouse DH: Prune belly syndrome. Br J Urol 1972; 44:356.

Beckman H, Rehder H, Rauskolb R: Letter to the editor: Prune belly sequence associated with trisomy 13. Am J Med Genet 1984; 19:603.

Berdon WE, Baker DH, Wigger HJ, et al: The radiologic and pathologic spectrum of the prune belly syndrome—The importance of urethral obstruction in prognosis. Radiol Clin North Am 1977; 15:83.

Bovicelli L, Rizzo N, Orsini LF, et al: Prenatal diagnosis of the prune belly syndrome. Clin Genet 1980; 18:79.

Bukowski TP, Perlmutter AD: Reduction cystoplasty in the prune belly syndrome: A long-term followup. J Urol 1994; 152:2113.

Burbige KA, Amodio J, Berdon WE, et al: Prune belly syndrome: 35 years of experience. J Urol 1987; 137:86.

Burke EC, Shin MH, Kelalis PP: Prune-belly syndrome. Am J Dis Child 1969; 117:668.

Carter TC, Tomskey GC, Ozog LS: Prune-belly syndrome—Review of ten cases. Urology 1974; 3:279.

Cawthern TH, Bottene CA, Grant D: Prune-belly syndrome associated with Hirschsprung's disease. Am J Dis Child 1979; 133:652.

Christopher CR, Spinelli A, Severt D: Ultrasonic diagnosis of prune-belly syndrome. Obstet Gynecol 1982; 59:391.

Cukier J: Resection of the urethra in prune-belly syndrome. Birth Defects 1977; 13:95.

Culp DA, Flocks RH: Congenital absence of abdominal musculature. J Iowa State Med Soc 1954; 44:155.

Deklerk DP, Scott WW: Prostatic maldevelopment in the prune belly syndrome: A defect in prostatic stromal-epithelial interaction. J Urol 1978; 120:341.

Duckett JW Jr: Cutaneous vesicostomy in childhood: The Blocksom technique. Urol Clin North Am 1974; 1:485.

Duckett JW Jr: The prune-belly syndrome. *In* Holder TM, Ashcroft KW, eds: The Surgery of Infants and Children. Philadelphia, W. B. Saunders, 1980, pp 802.

Eagle JF, Barrett GS: Congenital deficiency of abdominal musculature with associated genitourinary anomalies: A syndrome: Reports of 9 cases. Pediatrics 1950; 6:721.

Ehrlich RM, Brown WJ: Ultrastructural anatomic observations of the ureter in the prune-belly syndrome. Birth Defects 1977; 8:101.

Ehrlich RM, Lesavoy MA: Umbilicus preservation with total abdominal wall reconstruction in prune-belly syndrome. Urology 1993; 41:3.

Ehrlich RM, Lesavoy MA, Fine RN: Total abdominal wall reconstruction in the prune-belly syndrome. J Urol 1986; 136:282.

Elder JS, Duckett JW, Snyder HM: Intervention for fetal obstructive uropathy: Has it been effective? Lancet 1987; 10:1007.

Fallat ME, Skoog SJ, Belman AB, et al: The prune-belly syndrome: A comprehensive approach to management. J Urol 1989; 142:802.

Fowler R Jr, Stephens FD: The role of testicular vascular anatomy in the salvage of high undescended testes. *In* Stephens FD, ed: Congenital Malformations of the Rectum, Anus, and Genitourinary Tract. Baltimore, Williams & Wilkins, 1963.

Frydman M, Magenis RE, Mohandas TK, et al: Chromosome abnormalities in infants with prune belly anomaly: Association with trisomy 18. Am J Med Genet 1983;15:145.

Garlinger P, Ott J: Prune-belly syndrome—possible genetic implications. Birth Defects 1974; 10:173.

Geary DF, MacLusky IB, Churchill BM, et al: A broader spectrum of abnormalities in the prune belly syndrome. J Urol 1986; 135:324.

Gibbons MD, Cromie WJ, Duckett JW: Management of the abdominal undescended testis. J Urol 1979; 122:76.

Goulding FJ, Garrett RA: Twenty-five year experience with prune belly syndrome. Urology 1978; 7:329.

Hadziselimovic F: Personal communication, July, 1984.

Halbrecht I, Komlos L, Shabtal F: Prune-belly syndrome with chromosomal fragment. Am J Dis Child 1972; 123:518.

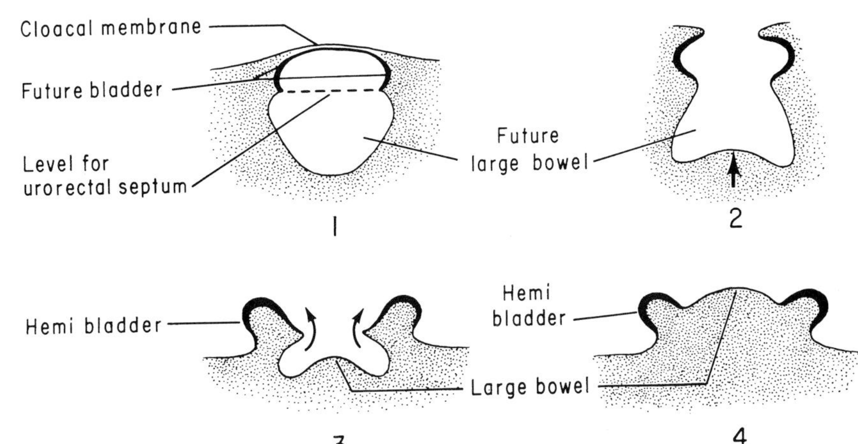

Figure 63–4. Diagram of eventration of cloaca to form cloacal exstrophy.

Duplicate Exstrophy

Duplicate exstrophy occurs when a superior vesical fissure opens, but there is later fusion of the abdominal wall and a portion of the bladder elements (mucosa) remains outside. In a case report by Muecke (1986), the patient had exstrophy of the mucosa but a normal bladder inside (Fig. 63–7). The patient had a very widened symphysis and a stubby, upward-pointing penis. Three additional cases have been reported by Arap and Giron (1986) in which the patients had classic musculoskeletal defects and two of the three were continent. In the two male patients, one had an associated complete epispadias, whereas the other had a completely normal penis. Thus, the external genital manifestations of duplicate exstrophy can be variable.

Covered Exstrophy

Besides pseudoexstrophy, superior vesical fissure, and duplicate exstrophy, isolated occurrences of a fourth entity—covered exstrophy—have been reported (Narasimharao et al, 1985; Cerniglia et al, 1989). These anomalies have also been referred to as split symphysis variants. A common factor present in these patients is the musculoskeletal defect associated with classic exstrophy with no significant defect of the urinary tract. However, in most cases reported as covered exstrophy (Narasimharao et al, 1985; Cerniglia et al, 1989), an isolated ectopic bowel segment has been present on the inferior abdominal wall near the genital area. This can be either colon or ileum and has no connection with the underlying gastrointestinal tract or epispadias in male patients (Fig. 63–8).

Anatomic Considerations

In bladder exstrophy, most anomalies are related to defects of the abdominal wall, bladder, genitalia, rectum, and anus (Fig. 63–9). Children presenting with bladder exstrophy are frequently robust, full-term babies, with the anomalous development confined to structures adjacent to the cloacal membrane.

Musculoskeletal Defects

All cases of exstrophy have the characteristic widening of the symphysis pubis caused by the outward rotation of the innominate bones. **New data from Sponseller and associ-**

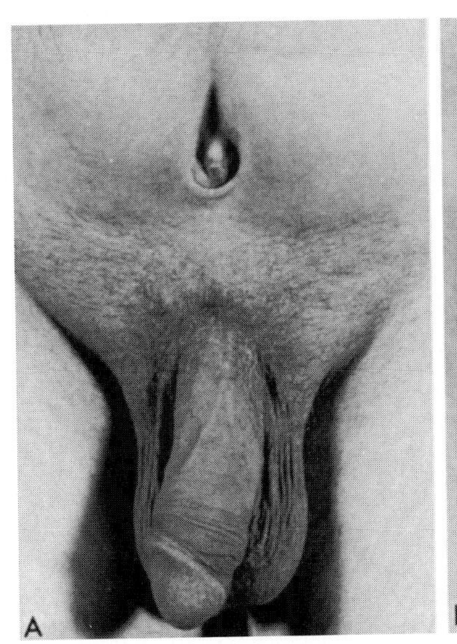

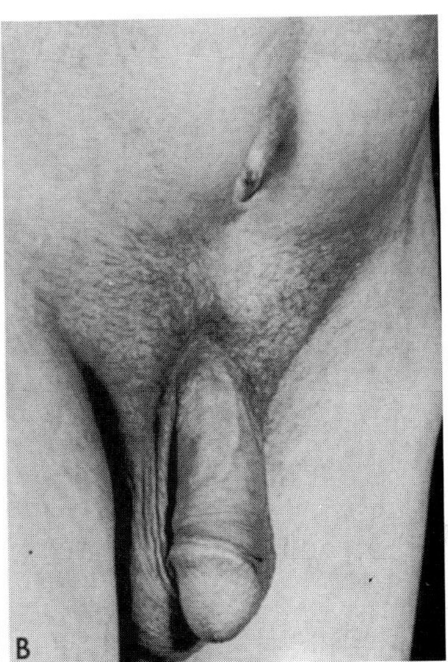

Figure 63–5. Pseudoexstrophy in an adult male patient. Musculoskeletal deformity characteristic of exstrophy is present, but the urinary tract is intact.

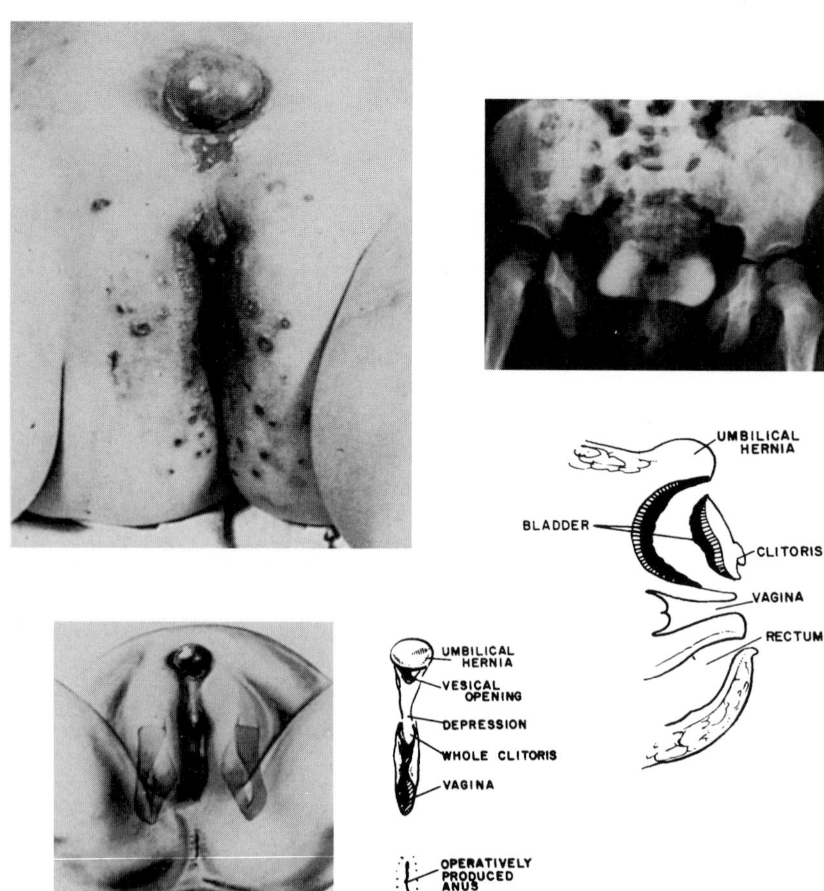

Figure 63–6. Superior vesical fissure in a girl. Musculoskeletal deformities are those typical of exstrophy of the bladder.

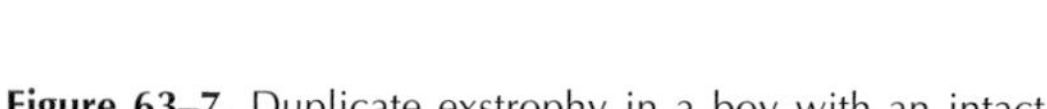

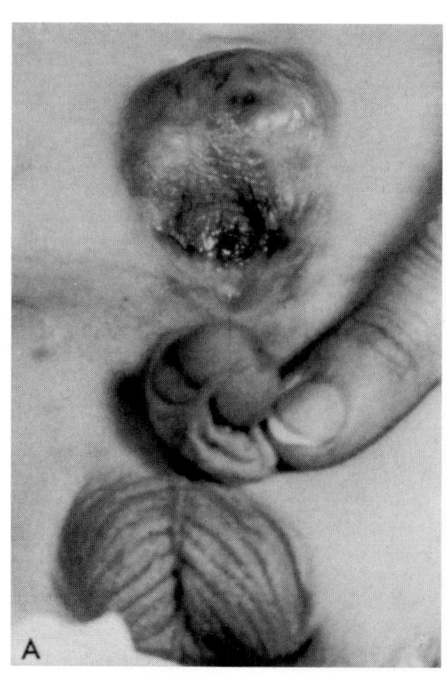

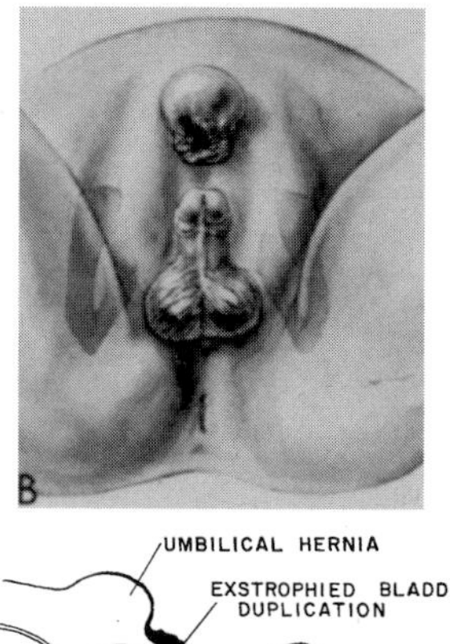

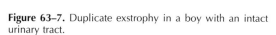

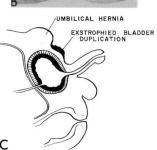

Figure 63–7. Duplicate exstrophy in a boy with an intact urinary tract.

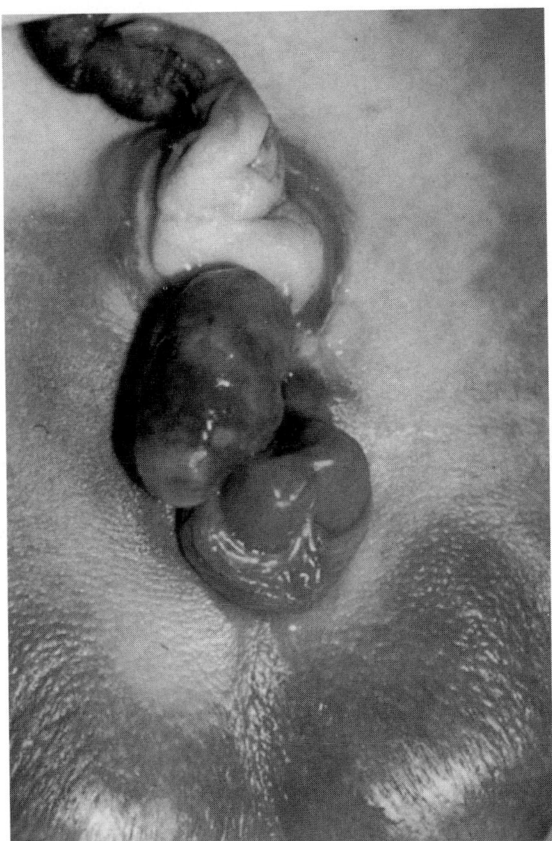

Figure 63–8. Covered exstrophy with isolated ectopic bowel segment present on the inferior abdominal wall, just above the penis. (Courtesy of Dr. Frank Cerniglia.)

ates (1995) using pelvic computed tomography scans of 24 patients with bladder exstrophy have accurately described the bony pelvic deformity for the first time. This study reveals a 12-degree outward rotation of the posterior pelvis on each side, retroversion of the acetabuli, 15-degree external rotation and 30% shortening of the pubic rami, and progressive diastasis of the symphysis pubis (Fig. 63–10). These rotational deformities of the pelvic skeletal structures may contribute to a short, pendular penis. The outward rotation and lateral displacement of the innominate bones accounts for the increased distance between the hips and the outward rotation of lower limbs in these children, which causes little disability.

A waddling gait develops secondary to the external rotation of the lower extremities, resulting from the posterolateral position of the acetabulum (Cracchiolo and Hall, 1970). Foot progression angle is 20 to 30 degrees externally rotated above normal limits in early childhood, but the anomaly soon corrects itself with age and leaves no orthopedic problems (Sponseller et al, 1995).

Abdominal Defects

The triangular defect caused by the premature rupture of the abnormal cloacal membrane is occupied by the open bladder. The fascial defect is limited inferiorly by the intersymphyseal band, which represents the divergent urogenital diaphragm. The anterior sheath of the rectus muscles, seeking midline attachment, has a fanlike extension behind the urethra and bladder neck, which inserts into the intersymphyseal band.

At the upper end of the triangular defect and bladder is the umbilicus. In bladder exstrophy, the distance between the umbilicus and the anus is always foreshortened. Because the umbilicus is situated well below the horizontal line of the iliac crest, there is an unusual expanse of uninterrupted abdominal skin. Although an umbilical hernia is always present, it is usually of insignificant size. The umbilical hernia should be repaired at the time of the abdominal wall closure. Omphaloceles, although rarely associated with the exstrophy-epispadias complex, are usually small and can be closed with the bladder. If a large omphalocele is associated with bladder exstrophy, this defect is treated initially and treatment of the exstrophy defect is postponed until circumstances allow bladder closure.

Anorectal Defects

The perineum is short and broad. **The anus, situated directly behind the urogenital diaphragm, is displaced anteriorly and corresponds to the posterior limit of the triangular fascial defect.** The anal sphincter mechanism is also anteriorly displaced, and it should be preserved intact in case internal urinary diversion is required in the future.

The divergent levator ani and puborectalis muscles, and the distorted anatomy of the external sphincter contribute to varying degrees of anal incontinence and rectal prolapse. (Gearhart et al, 1993). Anal continence is usually imperfect at an early age. In some patients, the rectal sphincter mechanism may never be adequate to control liquid content of the bowel. Rectal prolapse frequently occurs in untreated exstrophy patients with a widely separated symphysis. It is usually transient and reduced without difficulty. The prolapse is frequently exacerbated by the child's straining and crying, which causes spasm of the irritated, exposed bladder. Prolapse virtually always disappears after bladder closure or cystectomy and urinary diversion. The appearance of prolapse is an indication to proceed with definitive management of the exstrophied bladder.

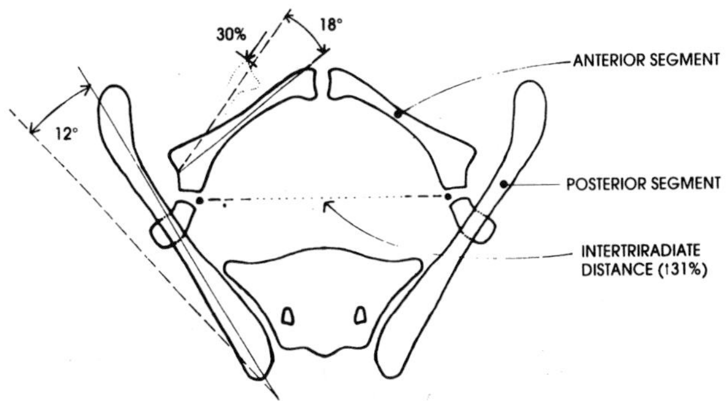

Figure 63–9. Abnormal anatomy seen in classic bladder exstrophy. The posterior segment is externally rotated a mean of 12 degrees on each side, but the length is not different. The anterior segment is externally rotated 18 degrees (6 degrees more than the posterior segment) and is shortened by a mean of 30%. The distance between the triradiate cartilage is increased by 31%.

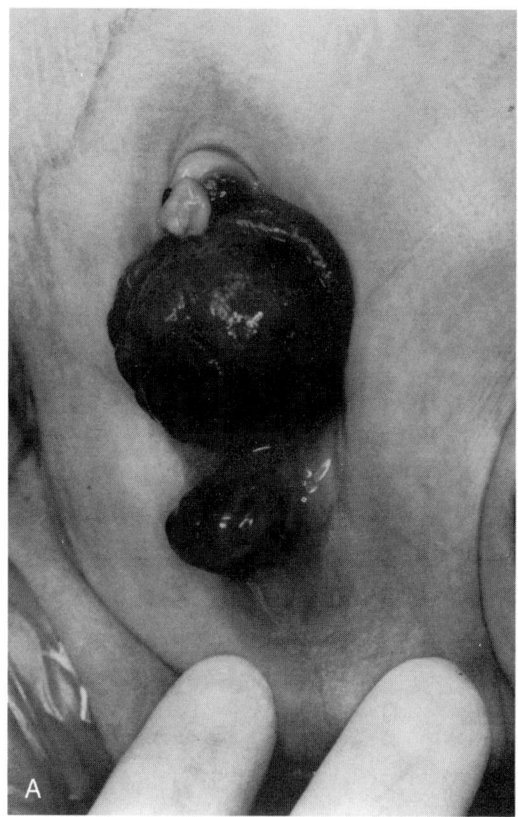

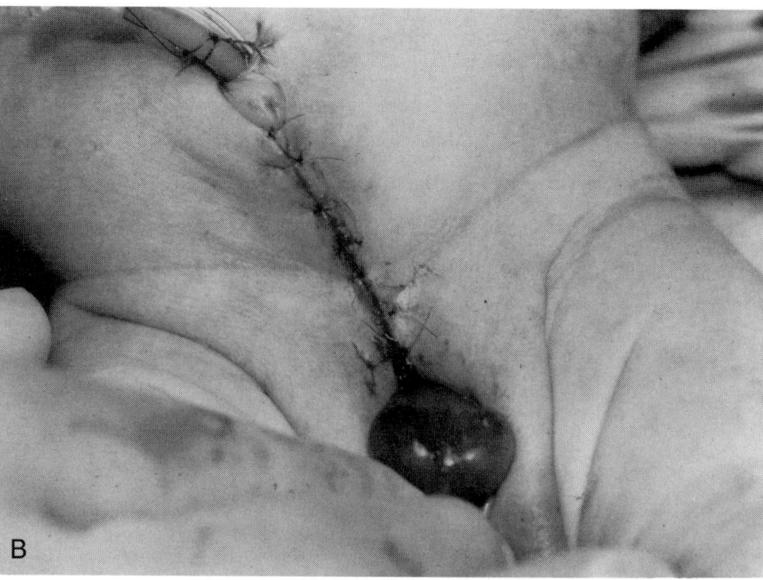

Figure 63–10. *A,* Newborn male exstrophy with nice-sized bladder template but short urethral groove. *B,* Same patient at end of surgical procedure. Note exit of suprapubic tubes and ureteral stents from neoumbilicus.

Male Genital Defects

The male genital defect is severe and may be the most troublesome aspect of the surgical reconstruction, independent of the decision to treat by staged closure or by urinary diversion (Fig. 63–11). Formerly, the individual corpus cavernosa in bladder exstrophy were thought to be of normal caliber and length and the penis foreshortened because of the wide separation of the crural attachments, prominent dorsal chordee, and the shortened urethral groove. However, by using MRI measurements of the corpora in exstrophy in adults and normal controls, Silver and associates (1996) found that the total corpora length is shorter on the anterior segment, which is not attached to the pubic ramus, but is of normal length on the posterior part, which is attached to the ramus. Also, the diameter of the posterior corporal segment is greater than that in normal males. The urethral groove may be so short and the dorsal chordee so severe that the glans becomes located adjacent to the verumontanum. A functional and cosmetically acceptable penis can be achieved

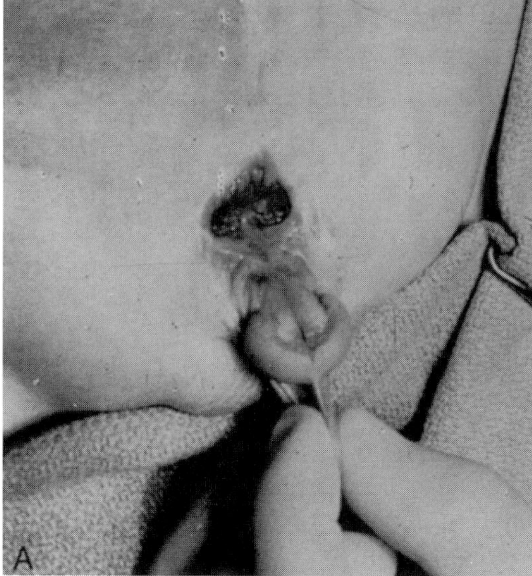

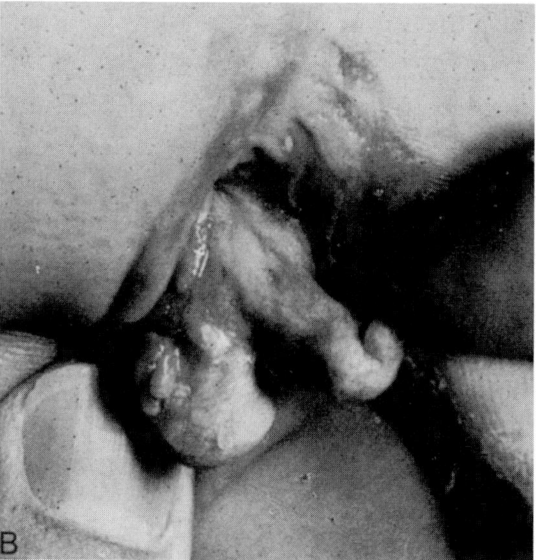

Figure 63–11. Difficult genital reconstruction. *A,* Short penis and very small bladder. *B,* Duplex penis.

plete epispadias with incontinence while preserving renal function. Secondarily, the best management for the incontinence and epispadias will be determined in a later stage or stages. (Table 63–1).

OSTEOTOMY

When patients are seen within the first 48 hours of life, the bladder and pelvic ring closure can usually be carried out without osteotomy because of the malleability of the pelvic ring (Ansell, 1983). However, when the separation is unduly wide or when delay in referral occurs, osteotomy will be required to achieve anterior closure of the pelvic ring. Osteotomy should be carried out at the same time as bladder closure. A well-coordinated surgical and anesthesia team can carry out osteotomy and proceed to bladder closure without undue loss of blood or risk of prolonged anesthesia. However, osteotomy along with bladder closure is a 5- to 7-hour procedure in these patients.

At present, two separate approaches are being used for osteotomy in the exstrophy group: posterior bilateral iliac osteotomy or anterior bilateral transverse innominate osteotomy combined with a vertical iliac osteotomy performed through the same anterior incision. Both of these approaches

Table 63–1. INITIAL PRESENTATION AND MANAGEMENT OF PATIENTS WITH EXSTROPHY OF BLADDER

Age	Problem	Possible Solution
Initial Presentation		
0–72 hours	Classic exstrophy with reasonable capacity and moderate symphyseal separation; long urethral groove; mild dorsal chordee	I: Midline closure of bladder, fascia, and symphysis to level of posterior urethra; no osteotomy
0–72 hours	Above-mentioned findings with short urethra and severe dorsal chordee	II: Close as in I, adding lengthening of dorsal urethral groove by paraexstrophy skin (cautiously)
0–72 hours or late presentation	Above-mentioned findings with very wide separation of symphysis or late presentation of patient (beyond 72 hours up to 1–3 years) for initial treatment	Osteotomy (combined anterior and vertical iliac) and closure as in I or II
0–2 weeks	Male, penis duplex or extremely short	Consider female sex of rearing and closure as in I or II
0–2 weeks	Very small, nondistensible bladder patch	Prove by examination under anesthesia, then nonoperative expectant treatment awaiting internal or external diversion
Incontinent Period After Initial Closure		
1 month–4 years	Infection with residual resulting from outlet stenosis	Urethral dilatation, occasional meatotomy or bladder neck revision
	Infection, grade III reflux, with pliable outlet resistance	Continuous antibiotic suppression with plan for early ureteroneocystostomy
	Partial dehiscence at bladder neck or partial prolapse of bladder (both prevent bladder capacity increase)	Reclosure of bladder neck with osteotomy (with epispadias repair if older than 1 year of life)
Epispadias Repair and Continence		
2 years	Closed bladder with incontinence, normal intravenous pyelogram, and good penile size and length of urethral groove	Epispadias repair after preparation with testosterone
	Epispadiac penis, short with severe chordee, before bladder neck reconstruction	Correction of chordee, lengthening of urethral groove, and epispadias repair; prepare with testosterone; consider osteotomy to aid in achieving increased penile length
4–5 years	Epispadias repaired, capacity greater than 60 ml	Proceed to bladder neck plasty and ureteroneocystostomy
4 years and older	Completed repair of bladder, bladder neck, and epispadias with dry interval but wet pants	Patience, biofeedback, oxybutynin chloride (Ditropan), imipramine, and time (up to 2 years)
	Above-mentioned problems with marked stress incontinence and good bladder capacity	Wait—may require bladder neck revision or endoscopic injection or possible artificial sphincter
	Small capacity bladder unchanged by time, epispadias repair or attempted bladder neck reconstruction	Consider augmentation cystoplasty and bladder neck reconstruction; acceptance of intermittent catheterization with abdominal or urethral access may be necessary
4–7 years	Late presentation of untreated exstrophy, unsuitable for closure	Consider temporary diversion by colon conduit with plan to undivert to bladder using bladder to form urethra and conduit for augmentation; in patients older than 7 years, artificial sphincter or continent diversion can be considered
4–7 years	Small closed exstrophy unsuitable for bladder neck reconstruction or augmentation	Consider permanent external or internal diversion; internal diversion direct by ureterosigmoidostomy or indirect by colocolostomy; evaluate day continence of anal sphincter and nighttime seepage before surgery or continent neobladder
5–15 years	Closed exstrophy with epispadias repaired with uncontrolled stress or dribbling incontinence	Consider (1) revision of bladder neck reconstruction, (2) endoscopic injection, (3) augmentation and bladder neck revision, (4) artificial sphincter with omental wrap, and (5) continent diversion
10–20 years	Closed penis with inadequate penis	Consider penile lengthening, urethral reconstruction using free graft, pedicle grafts, and tissue transfer
10–20 years	Diverted exstrophy with inadequate penis	As above-mentioned recommendations or penile lengthening without urethral reconstruction (prostatic fistula at base)

can improve symphyseal approximation in the exstrophy patient. With appropriate approximation, tension on the midline abdominal closure is lessened. Also, in our experience, the dehiscence rate is lower if osteotomies are performed (Gearhart et al, 1993a). **In addition, pubic closure allows approximation of the levator and puborectal sling, inclusion of the bladder neck and urethra within the pelvic ring, and improved eventual continence rate (Oesterling and Jeffs, 1987; Gearhart and Jeffs, 1992).**

Several reports have demonstrated experience with an anterior approach through the innominate bone just above the acetabulum (Montagnani, 1988; Gokcora et al, 1989; Sponseller et al, 1990). Although our experience with posterior iliac osteotomy reveals no failure of initial closures, the authors were disappointed with the poor mobility of the pubis, the occasional delayed union or malunion of the ilium, and most importantly the need to turn the patient from the prone to the supine position. Initially, our interest in anterior osteotomy was in those patients who had failed an initial exstrophy closure with or without prior posterior iliac osteotomy (Sponseller et al, 1996). The results with that approach were so satisfactory that a new combination of anterior innominate in conjunction with vertical posterior iliac osteotomy (Gearhart et al, 1996) is now being used for both primary and secondary closures of bladder exstrophy (Fig. 63–17). The anterior iliofemoral approach to the pelvis was performed in a similar manner to that of a Salter osteotomy. Both sides were exposed simultaneously and a horizontal innominate anterior osteotomy was performed using a Gigli saw. If the patient is younger than 6 months, an oscillating saw was used instead of a Gigli saw (Sponseller et al, 1990). The level of the osteotomy is from 5 mm above the anterior-inferior iliac spine to the most cranial part of the sciatic notch in order to leave a sizeable inferior segment for fixation. A secondary osteotomy incision is then made in a ventral direction just medial to the S-I joint bilaterally. An external fixator is commonly used, and the pins are inserted before wound closure (Fig. 63–18). A horizontal mattress suture of No. 2 nylon is placed between the fibrous cartilage of the pubic rami and tied anterior to the pubic closure at the time of bladder closure. If the suture works loose or cuts through the tissues during subsequent healing, the anterior placement of the knot in the horizontal mattress suture ensures that it will not erode into the urethra and interfere with the bladder or urethral lumen.

Posterior iliac osteotomy is still used in some institutions and is performed through bilateral incisions over the sacroiliac region. The posterior iliac osteotomy is performed vertically and close to the midline to allow the two wings of the pelvis to hinge and come together without anterior-to-posterior flattening of the true pelvic ring. Success of the posterior osteotomy is demonstrated in the review by Andalen and coworkers (1980). Among 100 patients who underwent posterior iliac osteotomy, for those who achieved symphyseal approximation of less than 2 cm, there was a higher continence rate than for those who achieved pubic diastasis greater than 2 cm. In addition, Frey and Cohen (1989) and Schmidt and coworkers (1993) have used a superior pubic ramotomy to facilitate pubic closure and report satisfactory results.

Bladder and Prostatic Urethra Closure

The various steps in primary bladder closure are illustrated in Figure 63–19. A strip of mucosa, 2 cm wide, extending from the distal trigone to below the verumontanum in the male and to the vaginal orifice in the female, outlines prostatic and posterior urethral reconstruction. The male urethral groove length may be adequate, and no transverse incision of the urethral plate need be made for urethral length. **However, when the length of the urethral groove from the verumontanum to the glans is so short that it interferes with eventual penile length, the urethral groove is elongated after the manner of Johnston (1974) or Duckett (1977).** However, great care must be used in designing and applying these flaps in the exstrophy patient because they can be associated with a significantly high complication rate (Gearhart et al, 1993c).

The diagrams indicate that an incision is made outlining the bladder mucosa and the prostatic plate (Fig. 63–19*C, D*). If possible, the urethral groove is left intact and continuity is maintained between the thin, mucosa-like, non–hair-bearing skin adjacent to the posterior urethra and bladder neck and the skin and mucosa of the penile shaft and glans.

Penile lengthening is achieved by exposing the corpora cavernosum bilaterally and freeing the corpora from their attachments to the suspensory ligaments and the anterior part of the inferior pubic rami. If the mucosal plate has been transected, the bare corpora are covered with flaps of the thin paraexstrophy skin, which are rotated medially to be attached to the distal mucosa of the posterior plate (Fig. 63–19*C*1 through *C*3). These flaps are inward rotation flaps and not long paraexstrophy skin flaps running along the lateral aspect of the exstrophied bladder. The urethra in the female patient does not require lengthening at the time of closure.

Bladder closure proceeds by excision of the umbilical area. The redundant skin adjacent to the superior aspect of the bladder mucosa is discarded, and the bladder muscle is freed from the fused rectus sheaths on each side. This dissection is facilitated by exposing the peritoneum above the umbilicus and carefully dissecting extraperitoneally, to enter the retropubic space on each side from above (Fig. 63–19*E, F*). The wide band of fibers and muscular tissue representing the urogenital diaphragm is detached subperiosteally from the pubis bilaterally (Fig. 63–19*G, H*). The dissection must be extended onto the inferior ramus of the pubis to allow the bladder neck and posterior urethra to fall back and achieve a position deep within the pelvic ring. Reluctance to free the bladder neck, urethra, and urogenital diaphragm fibers from the inferior ramus of the pubis will certainly move the neobladder opening cephalad away from the penile base should separation of the pubis occur during healing. The mucosa and muscle of the bladder and posterior urethra are closed in the midline anteriorly. This orifice should accommodate a No. 14 Fr sound comfortably (Fig. 63–19*I, J*). The size of the opening should allow enough resistance to aid in bladder adaptation and to prevent prolapse but not enough outlet resistance to cause upper tract changes. The posterior urethra and bladder neck are buttressed with a second layer of local tissue, if possible (see Fig. 63–19*J*).

The bladder is drained by a suprapubic Malecot catheter for a period of 4 weeks (Fig. 63–19*K*). The urethra is not stented in order to avoid pressure necrosis or the accumulation of infected secretions in the neourethra. Ureteral stents provide drainage during the first 10 to 14 days, when swelling or the pressure of closure of a small bladder may obstruct

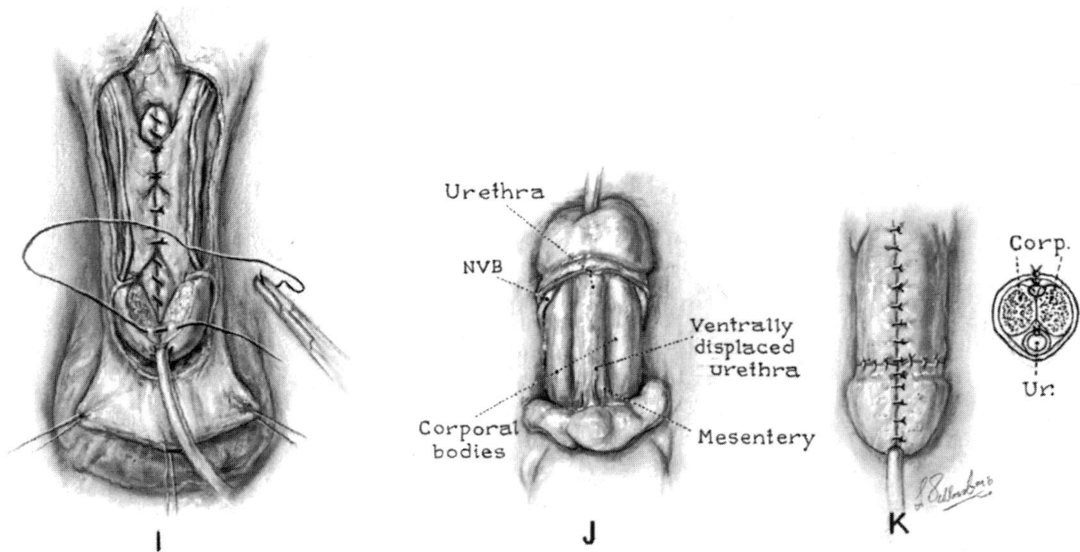

Figure 63–21 *Continued I*, Further sutures placed distally to further bury urethra under corporal bodies at glandular junction with initial coaptation of glandular tissue. *J* and *K*, Completed repair with urethra below corporal bodies and skin closure of the penis. (Drawings by Leon Schlossberg.)

the dissection is extended proximally along the corpora to dissect the urethral plate free from the corporal bodies (see Fig. 63–21*F*). Initially, the authors believed that difficulties would be encountered dissecting proximally where the paraexstrophy skin flaps had been sutured to the urethral plate but this has not been encountered when one keeps the dissection just on the corporal body while proceeding proximally. The urethral plate is also dissected distally past the level of the junction of the glans with the corporal bodies. Unless adequate mobilization is obtained, it will be difficult to bring the corporal bodies over the urethra (see Fig. 63–21*G*). The neurovascular bundles, situated between Buck's fascia and the corporeal wall, are then dissected free from the corporeal bodies, with vessel loops being placed around these structures (see Fig. 63–21*G*). This method ensures that the neurovascular bundles will not be compromised when incisions are made in the corpora and the corpora are rotated medially over the neourethra.

The urethral strip is closed in a linear manner from the prostatic opening to the glans over a No. 8 silicone stent with 6-0 polydioxanone sutures (see Fig. 63–21*H*). After this is accomplished, transverse incisions are made in the corporal bodies at the point of maximum dorsal curvature of the corporal bodies, opening a diamond-shaped defect in the erectile tissue (see Fig. 63–21) The corpora are then closed over the neourethra with two running sutures of 5-0 polydioxanone acid, and the diamond-shaped defects in adjacent areas of the corpora are sutured to each other. This procedure displaces the urethra ventrally. Not only does this cause a downward deflection of the penis but it also allows for additional length with dorsal rotation and approximation of the corporal bodies over the neourethra. After the urethra has been transferred to the ventrum, further sutures of 5-0 polyglycolic acid are placed between the corporal bodies to bury the urethra further, especially at the level of the junction of the glans and corporal bodies.

The glans wings are closed over the glandular urethra using subcuticular sutures of 5-0 polyglycolic acid (see Fig. 63–21*I*). The glans epithelium is then closed with 6-0 polyglycolic acid sutures. The ventral skin is then brought up and sutured to the ventral edge of the corona, and flaps are fashioned to provide adequate coverage of the dorsum of the penis. The skin is reapproximated with interrupted 5-0 polyglycolic acid sutures (see Fig. 63–21*J, K*). The Z plasty at the base of the penis is closed with interrupted 5-0 polyglycolic acid sutures. The silicone stent is left indwelling in the neourethra to provide drainage.

Incontinence and Antireflux Procedures

The bladder capacity is measured yearly under general anesthesia, after the child reaches the second year of life. **When the bladder capacity is 60 ml or greater, bladder neck reconstruction can be planned if the child is old enough to be interested in a postoperative voiding program and wants to be dry. This usually occurs around 4 to 5 years of age.** The incontinence and antireflux procedures are illustrated in Figure 63–22*A* through *I*. The bladder is originally opened through a transverse incision at the bladder neck, but a vertical extension is used (see Fig. 63–22*A, B*). The midline closure of this incision narrows the width of the bladder neck area and enlarges the vertical dimension of the bladder, which in exstrophy is often short. The illustrator depicts a Cohen (1975) type of transtrigonal advancement procedure for correcting reflux in which a new hiatus lateral to the original orifice is selected prior to advancing the ureter across the bladder above the trigone. Also, the ureter can be taken in a more cephalad direction, the cephalotrigonal reimplant (see Fig. 63–22*C*)(Canning et al, 1989). In addition, if the ureters are low on the trigone and there is a need to move the ureteral hiatus higher on the trigone, the hiatus is simply cut in a cephalad direction and cross-trigonal reimplants are performed on the upper aspect of the trigone (see Fig. 63–22*C*).

The procedure for incontinence is begun by selecting a posterior strip of mucosa 15 to 18 mm wide and 30 mm long that extends distally from the midtrigone to the prostate

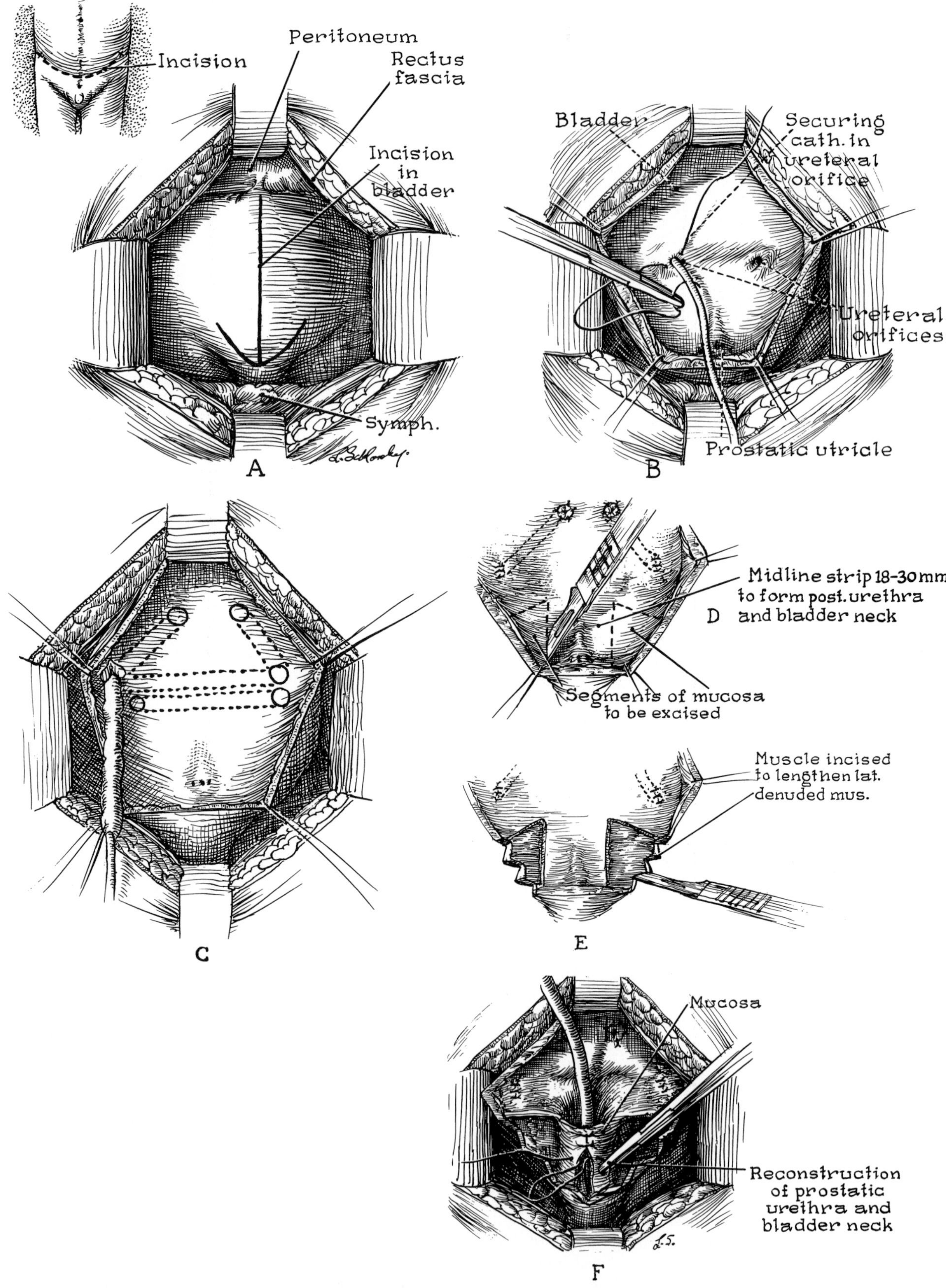

Figure 63–22. *A* to *I*, Steps in the Cohen transtrigonal or cephalotrigonal reimplantation of ureters in bladder neck reconstruction for continence. *A*, Transverse bladder incision with vertical extension subsequently closed in the midline to narrow bladder near the bladder neck. *B* to *F*, Ureteral mobilization with either transtrigonal or cephalotrigonal course for reimplantation. Mucosal strip of trigone to form bladder neck and prostatic urethra. Lateral denuded muscle triangles are lengthened by several small incisions to allow tailoring and funneling of the bladder neck reconstruction area.

were severe stricture of the posterior urethra (6), bladder prolapse (6), dehiscence (9), failure to gain capacity after initial closure (9), and failure to gain capacity after bladder neck reconstruction (5). Multiple reconstructive techniques were used to create the continent stoma, including Indiana pouch in 1, Mitrofanoff in 19, Benchekroun in 12, tapered revision in 2, and Mainz type stoma in 7. Series by Kramer (1989) and Mitchell and Piser (1987) also show the applicability of bladder augmentation or continent urinary diversion to the child with a small bladder associated with the exstrophy condition.

Bladder Neck Reconstruction

Urinary continence, defined as a 3-hour dry interval, is usually achieved within 1 year following bladder neck reconstruction. Delayed achievement of urinary continence has been associated with puberty in the male patient (Kramer and Kelalis, 1982a). The increasing urethral length associated with prostatic enlargement may provide additional resistance to urinary outflow. **In our experience, patients who do not achieve a 3-hour dry interval within 1 to 2 years following bladder neck reconstruction seldom develop a sufficient continence mechanism.** These incontinent individuals may be treated by the following means: (1) repeat Young-Dees-Leadbetter bladder neck reconstruction with or without simultaneous bladder augmentation; (2) tubularization of the remaining bladder into a neourethra and bladder augmentation by colocystoplasty (Arap et al, 1976); (3) insertion of an artificial urinary sphincter device (Decter et al, 1988); (4) transurethral injection to enhance outlet resistance; (5) transection of the bladder neck, bladder augmentation, and creation of a catheterizable abdominal stoma; and (6) as a last resort, urinary diversion (see Table 63–1).

A patulous bladder neck with adequate bladder capacity is best managed by repeating the Young-Dees-Leadbetter procedure (Gearhart et al, 1991; Gearhart et al, 1993a). In the first series, six of seven patients who underwent repeat Young-Dees-Leadbetter procedures without augmentation are dry for greater than 3 hours and are voiding by way of the urethra. However, the majority of patients who fail initial Young-Dees-Leadbetter procedures typically need bladder augmentation along with a continence procedure (Gearhart et al, 1991).

In a recent series, Ben-Chaim and associates (1995a) used bovine collagen following Young-Dees-Leadbetter bladder neck reconstruction in 15 patients. Repeated injections were performed in 10 patients after a mean interval of 12 months. After a mean follow-up of 26 months (range 9–84 months), improvement of continence was noted in 53% of patients and four patients had a significant improvement in their continence rate. Nine of the ten patients who underwent repeated collagen injections showed added improvement with the additional injections. Collagen injection into the bladder neck after Young-Dees-Leadbetter bladder neck reconstruction is safe and simple, and has a reasonable success rate. Unfortunately, this procedure is not enough to create continence by itself and should be used only as an adjunct to bladder neck reconstruction.

Although others have reported good results with the artificial urinary sphincter in the exstrophy patient and report an excellent continence rate in those in whom the sphincter is working, the authors have not enjoyed the same success (Decter et al, 1988). Similar experiences have been reported with anti-incontinence devices in complete epispadias (Hanna, 1981; Kramer and Kelalis, 1982a). The artificial sphincter may be useful in older children who have well-vascularized bladder neck tissues or in those who have a mature omentum that can be interposed between the cuff and the reconstructed bladder neck.

The authors have recently treated over 35 patients with multiple failures of exstrophy reconstruction including prior bladder neck reconstructions. The ultimate choices in this very difficult group of patients are (1) placement of an artificial urinary sphincter and bladder augmentation; (2) reoperative bladder neck reconstruction, bladder augmentation, and a continent urinary stoma; or (3) a continent urinary stoma along with bladder augmentation or replacement (Gearhart et al, 1995b).

Although bladder augmentation and bladder neck reconstruction alone can certainly render the child continent, two problems exist that may make this option less attractive: (1) the bladder may be so small that once a bladder neck reconstruction is performed, little bladder is left for ureteral reimplantation and bladder augmentation, and (2) reliable intermittent catheterization through a reconstructed urethra and bladder neck area often is difficult or impossible. Because methods of bladder augmentation and continent urinary diversions were presented in other chapters, the authors' comments are limited to the approach to a small bladder with a prior failed bladder neck reconstruction. Whether bladder augmentation and a continent stoma or complete bladder replacement with continent stoma is chosen depends on several factors. These include (1) the size of the template after opening the bladder, (2) competence of the bladder neck, and (3) the type of continence mechanism that will be employed.

The size of the bladder at the time of surgery dictates whether an additional outlet procedure along with bladder augmentation and continent stoma can be accomplished or if the bladder neck will need to be transected and augmentation and a continent stoma required. If the bladder is so small that it is of no use to the reconstructive effort, then it can be removed and a urinary reservoir and continent stoma constructed.

The method of dealing with the incompetent bladder neck is of prime importance. Some authors have recommended trying to tighten the bladder neck so that a so-called high-pressure pop-off valve would exist so that the reservoir would not be isolated and the risk of spontaneous perforation would be lessened. However, patients who have undergone multiple failed repairs have extensive scarring and poor tissue quality in the region. This situation obviates further bladder neck reconstruction or tightening. Transection of the bladder neck should be a last resort. When transection is performed, it is done above the verumontanum so that any fertility function will be preserved.

Genital-Urethral Reconstruction

The most common complication in exstrophy patients after urethral reconstruction is a urethrocutaneous fistula

occurring in 12% in our current experience. Modern techniques of hypospadias surgery, including optical magnification, de-epithelialized skin flaps, testosterone stimulation, and so forth can make most of these fistulas straightforward to repair. However, the three most common problems observed in these boys are as follows: (1) need for additional penile length, (2) correction of residual chordee, and (3) unsightly scars of old suture lines.

Certainly, in the young patient, extensive mobilization of the penile skin with or without further dissection of the corpora from the pubic ramus will add some length (see Table 63–1). However, in the adolescent and older patient, this technique alone may not be adequate to gain additional length (Woodhouse, 1989). Through this approach, the corpora can be mobilized more completely from the pubis, and any tethering scar tissue can be excised. The authors like to use rhomboid flaps (Kramer and Jackson, 1986), because this technique allows good access to the base of the phallus.

The need for additional correction of chordee varies. Mesrobian and associates (1986) found little need for additional correction of chordee in older patients because the majority of patients, even those with a curved penis, could have satisfactory intercourse. This improved experience may simply be due to better penile lengthening at the time of initial closure and at the time of epispadias repair (Gearhart and Jeffs, 1989a). However, patients are seen who need further corrective procedures. Certainly, even several intraoperative erections may be needed to assess the true curvature of the penis. Cavernosography may also be required preoperatively in the most severe cases (Woodhouse, 1989).

In many cases, the urethra is too short and may have to be transected and replaced with a free graft (Devine and Horton, 1980). If the amount of curvature is not significant after immobilization of all the scar tissue and the corporal bodies, then a Nesbit procedure may correct any remaining upward chordee (Frank et al, 1981; Brzezinski et al, 1986). Also, one may use the ventrum of the phallus and perform a Koff corporal rotation procedure to direct the phallus in a more downward manner (Koff and Eakins, 1984). If the amount of remaining chordee is significant, a transverse incision must be made on the dorsum of the penis at the point of greatest curvature. When this procedure needs to be performed, the urethra typically has to be transected. This incision, when properly performed, will leave an elliptic defect in the tunica albuginea, which must be closed with a graft. The authors' experience has been only with full-thickness skin grafts or dermal grafts to cover the defect (Brzezinski et al, 1986).

Some older adolescents and adults simply dislike the unsightly scars from suture lines on the phallus. The technique chosen for urethroplasty and penile elongation dictates to a large extent the type of skin coverage remaining on the penis. If there is adequate penile skin, the authors have simply excised the area and effected a plastic type closure. However, if there is a paucity of skin, enough usually remains to cover most of the shaft. Rhomboid skin flaps (Kramer, 1986) can be used to cover the proximal shaft and corpora. Also, full-thickness skin grafts can be used for penile coverage after scar excision.

OTHER TECHNIQUES

Not all children born with bladder exstrophy are candidates for staged functional closure, usually because of small bladder plates or significant hydronephrosis. Additional reasons for seeking other methods of treatment include failure of initial closure with a small remaining bladder and failure of incontinence surgery (see previous section). Therefore, excluding those patients with failure in initial treatment (see preceding section), this discussion deals with options available if staged functional closure is not suitable or is not chosen by the surgeon for other reasons.

Whichever diversion option is chosen, the upper tracts and renal function initially are usually normal. This occurrence allows the reimplantation of normal-sized ureters in a reliable nonrefluxing manner into the colon or other suitable urinary reservoir. Historically, ureterosigmoidostomy was the first form of diversion to be popularized in the exstrophy patient group. Although the initial series had multiple metabolic problems, when newer techniques of reimplantation of the ureter into the colon were introduced, the results improved markedly (Leadbetter, 1955; Zarbo and Kay, 1986). Ureterosigmoidostomy is favored by some because of the lack of an abdominal stoma. However, this form of diversion should not be offered until one is certain that anal continence is normal and after the family has been made aware of the potential for serious complications, including pyelonephritis, hyperchloremic acidosis, rectal incontinence, ureteral obstruction, and late development of malignancy (Spence et al, 1979; Duckett and Gazak, 1983; Stockel et al, 1990).

Because of the many complications associated with ureterosigmoidostomy, several alternative techniques of urinary diversion for bladder exstrophy have been described. Maydl (1894) described a method of trigonosigmoidostomy, and patients were followed for a mean interval of 10 years. Renal function, assessed by excretory urography, was normal in 21 patients (91%); stones formed in two (9%); and hypokalemic acidosis developed in approximately 50%. However, only a few individuals required chronic alkalinization, and reoperation was performed in only two patients (9%).

All of the children achieved daytime continence; overall, 18 cases (78%) were considered to have good results. Kroovand's (1988) update of Boyce's 37-year experience (Boyce and Vest, 1952) with this procedure shows that the majority of patients had stable upper urinary tracts, minimal leakage, and no electrolyte imbalances or malignant change in the vesicorectal reservoir. The Heitz-Boyer-Hovelaque (1912) procedure included diverting the ureters into an isolated rectal segment and pulling the sigmoid colon through the anal sphincter muscle just posterior to the rectum. Taccinoli and co-workers (1977) reviewed 21 staged Heitz-Boyer-Hovelaque procedures for bladder exstrophy, which were followed between 1 and 16 years. They reported 95% fecal and urinary continence, no cases of urinary calculi, electrolyte abnormalities, or postoperative mortality. Three patients (14%) developed urethrorectal strictures requiring surgical revision. Isolated cases in North America treated with this approach have been subject to multiple and severe complications.

The early results following ileal conduit urinary diversions suggested that this technique might be ideal for urinary drainage in patients with bladder exstrophy because fecal contamination and acidosis due to reabsorption were avoided. Unfortunately, significant long-term complications developed in children 10 to 15 years following ileal conduit diversion mostly due to infection, stomal stenosis, and ureteral obstruction (Jeffs and Schwartz, 1975; Shapiro et al,

1975). Ileal conduit diversion is not acceptable for children with exstrophy, who may have a normal life expectancy (MacFarlane et al, 1979).

As an alternative method of treatment, Hendren (1976) first established an antirefluxing colonic conduit and later undiverted this conduit into the sigmoid colon. The nonrefluxing ureterointestinal anastomosis represents the primary advantage of colon conduits. The colon conduit is constructed at 1 year of age. When anal continence is achieved and there is no reflux or upper tract deterioration, the conduit is undiverted into the colon at age 4 to 5 years. Sixteen colon conduits and 11 subsequent colocoloplasties were reported by Hendren (1976); the only reported postoperative complications were intestinal obstruction in three patients (19%) and ureteral obstruction in one patient (6%). No cases of stomal complications, persistent reflux, pyelonephritis, or upper tract deterioration have been reported in the Hendren series. The long-term assessment of renal function and continence following colon conduit diversion and subsequent colocoloplasty requires further investigation. Despite the authors' preference for primary functional bladder closure for bladder exstrophy, colon conduit urinary diversion represents the most attractive alternative because a nonrefluxing anastomosis is achieved and undiversion can be performed when clinically indicated.

An additional innovative approach by Rink and Retik (1987) was the creation of a nonrefluxing ileocecal segment that can be rejoined to the sigmoid colon. The proximity of the fecal and urinary streams may predispose the child to later risk of malignancy. In a recent series reported by Gearhart and colleagues (1995a) success was obtained in these multiple failed exstrophy reconstructions by the use of multiple reconstructive techniques, including the Mitrofanoff and Benchekroun principles, along with the continent urinary diversion.

Arap and colleagues (1976) managed bladder exstrophy by initially constructing a colon urinary conduit. The entire bladder was subsequently tubularized into a 5- to 6-cm neourethra, and the colon conduit was anastomosed to the urethrovesical tube. This technique may be useful for the patient with a failed Young-Dees-Leadbetter bladder neck procedure and a small contracted bladder or for the initial treatment of a bladder exstrophy when the bladder capacity is less than 3 ml.

The best method for urinary diversion in children is the nonrefluxing colon conduit, which requires an external stoma and appliance. However, techniques of continent urinary diversion are rapidly improving, as are the results in the treatment of the bladder exstrophy patient, especially those with an initial failure. However, the authors believe that the accepted form of treating bladder exstrophy today is the staged functional reconstructive approach. Those patients with small bladders unsuitable for closure, late closures, or multiple closures who do not develop an adequate bladder capacity after the first-stage reconstruction are problematic. These patients are best treated with any of the multiple reconstructive procedures mentioned previously.

ASSOCIATED CONCERNS

Growth of Secondary Sex Organs

In the past, it was thought that prostatic growth at puberty would lead to eventual continence in patients with exstrophy. Ritchey and associates (1988) found that this was true in those patients with complete epispadias who gained continence at puberty. However, this was not true in the exstrophy group. **Gearhart and co-workers (1993d) reviewed magnetic resonance imaging scans of the prostate gland in 14 adult patients with classic bladder exstrophy. The volume and cross-sectional area of the prostate gland was the same in patients with exstrophy as in normal, age-matched controls.** However, the configuration of the prostate gland in exstrophy patients was very unusual and did not surround the urethra in any patient voiding through the urethra. The seminal vesicle length was normal in all exstrophy patients when compared with normal controls. Whether the prostate gland and its unusual configuration aid eventual continence is unknown, but the data of Ritchey and colleagues (1988) suggest that it does not in patients with exstrophy. Personal experience has shown that some patients with incomplete continence become dry at night as puberty advances.

Malignancy

In the 1920s, it was estimated that 50% of individuals with bladder exstrophy died by 10 years of age (Mayo and Hendricks, 1926). The development of operative techniques that preserve renal function, the availability of broad-spectrum antibiotics, and an understanding of the metabolic disorders associated with urinary diversion have resulted in 91% of patients with this disorder surviving to the age of 30 years (Lattimer et al, 1978). This extended survival has uncovered two latent malignant processes that are associated with bladder exstrophy. Of carcinomas identified in exstrophied bladders, 80% are adenocarcinomas (Kandzari et al, 1974). The prevalence of adenocarcinoma in exstrophied bladders is approximately 400-fold greater than that in normal bladders (Engel and Wilkerson, 1970). According to Mostofi (1954), chronic irritation, infection, and obstruction can induce a metaplastic transformation of the urothelium to cystitis glandularis, a premalignant lesion. Adenocarcinoma may also develop from the malignant degeneration of embryonic rests of gastrointestinal tissue that is incorporated into the exstrophied bladder (Engel and Wilkinson, 1970). The inherent malignant potential of the closed exstrophy bladder has not been determined because long-term follow-up of a large number of patients with bladder exstrophy without urinary tract infection, obstruction, and chronic irritation has not been performed.

Bladder abnormalities, including squamous metaplasia, acute inflammation, fibrosis, and epithelial submucosal inclusions, were observed in exstrophy bladders of patients at 2 weeks of age (Culp, 1964). This observation suggests that exstrophied bladders are inherently abnormal. In comparison, consider the case of the 17-year-old boy who underwent primary exstrophy closure at 1 year of age and developed normal urinary control with preservation of the upper urinary tracts. He was killed in an automobile accident, and serial section of the bladder revealed no evidence of malignant or premalignant changes* (Fig. 63–23). Until the malignant potential of the exstrophied bladder is determined, a high

*Jeffs RD: Personal communication, 1979.

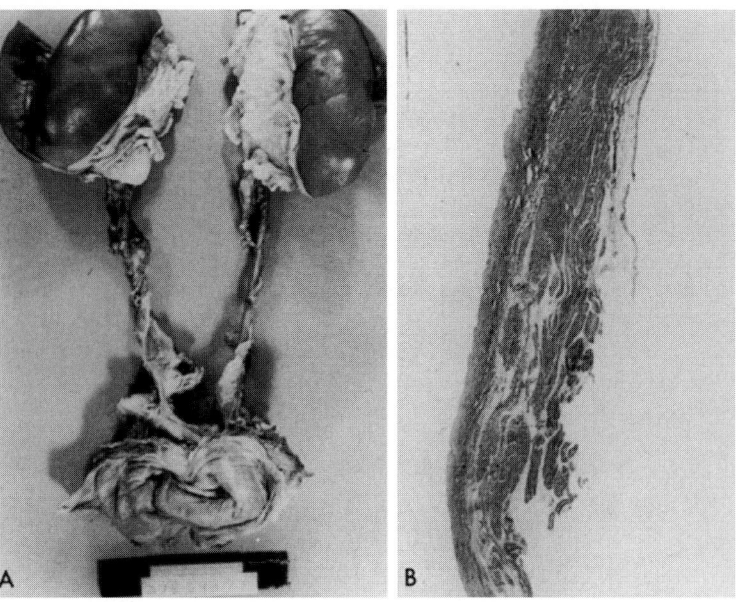

Figure 63-23. Gross *(A)* and microscopic *(B)* views of bladder of exstrophy patient who died accidentally after 17 years of normal bladder function.

suspicion should be maintained for potential malignant degeneration. Only two epithelial malignancies have been reported in patients closed at birth. Both bladder tumors were squamous in nature.

In untreated exstrophied bladders that are left everted, the patient is predisposed to develop adenocarcinoma secondary to repeated trauma. Squamous cell carcinoma accounted for only four of 57 (7%) of the carcinomas reported in exstrophied bladders (Kandzari et al, 1974). Rhabdomyosarcoma has been observed in three individuals with bladder exstrophy (Semerdjian et al, 1972; Engel, 1973).* **Krishnansetty and co-workers (1988) found 104 cases of malignancy in untreated bladder exstrophy patients and, as previously reported, the majority are adenocarcinomas with occasional squamous cell carcinomas and rhabdomyosarcomas.** In a review by Hartmann and colleagues (1984), adenocarcinoma was found in 93%, squamous cell carcinoma in 3%, undifferentiated carcinoma in 2%, and rhabdomyosarcoma in 1% of 97 patients with untreated bladder exstrophy.

Adenocarcinoma of the colon adjacent to the ureterointestinal anastomosis in an exstrophy patient was initially described by Dixon and Weisman (1948). The risk of adenocarcinoma of the colon in exstrophy patients following ureterosigmoidostomy is 7000 times that of the general population 25 years of age or younger (Krishnansetty et al, 1988). Spence and associates (1979) surveyed the literature to identify patients with bladder exstrophy who developed tumors following ureterosigmoid diversion. The mean latency interval from the time of ureterointestinal anastomosis to the diagnosis of intestinal tumor in these cases was 10 years, and the longest interval was 46 years. Of 35 compiled tumors, 28 were malignant and 24 were adenocarcinomas. Approximately half of the adenocarcinomas had metastasized at the time of diagnosis. In a large series of cancers associated with ureterosigmoidostomy in exstrophy patients, Krishnansetty and co-workers (1988) reported a review of the world's literature and discovered 90 cases.

*Jeffs RD: Personal communication, 1979.

Fertility and Pregnancy

Reconstruction of the male genitalia and preservation of fertility were not primary objectives of the early surgical management of bladder exstrophy. **Sporadic accounts of pregnancy or the initiation of pregnancy by men with bladder exstrophy had been reported.** In two prior exstrophy series, male fertility was rarely reported. Only three of 68 men (Bennett, 1973) and four of 72 men (Woodhouse et al, 1983) had successfully fathered children. In a more recent series by Ben-Chaim and associates (1996), 16 adult males were reviewed. Of four married males, two have fathered children (two and three children respectively). One unmarried male patient also fathered a child. Ten of 16 males (63%) ejaculate a few milliliters in volume, whereas a clear history of retrograde ejaculation was reported in six patients. Semen analysis was obtained in four patients with an average volume of 0.4 ml (range 0.1–1 ml), three of whom had azoospermia and one had oligospermia.

Hanna and Williams (1976) compared semen analyses between men who had undergone primary bladder closure and ureterosigmoidostomy. A normal sperm count was found in only one of eight men following functional bladder closure and in four of eight men with urinary diversions. The difference in fertility potential was attributed to iatrogenic injury of the verumontanum during functional closure. Retrograde ejaculation may also account for the low sperm counts observed following functional closure.

Six of 26 and 7 of 27 women with bladder exstrophy in these respective series successfully delivered offspring. A survey of 2500 exstrophy and epispadias patients conducted by Shapiro and colleagues (1984) identified 38 men who had fathered children and 131 women who had borne offspring.

Clementson (1958) successfully reviewed 45 women with bladder exstrophy who delivered 49 normal offspring. **The main complication following pregnancy was cervical and uterine prolapse, which occurred in six of seven women (Krisiloff et al, 1978).** A large review of 40 women ranging from 19 to 36 years of age who were treated in infancy for bladder exstrophy was performed by Burbige and co-workers

(1986). There were 14 pregnancies in 11 women, which resulted in nine normal deliveries, three spontaneous abortions, and two elective abortions. Uterine prolapse occurred in seven of 11 patients, all of whom underwent previous diversions during pregnancy. The patient must be informed of the likelihood of uterine prolapse following pregnancy. Spontaneous vaginal deliveries were experienced by women who had undergone functional bladder closure to eliminate stress on the pelvic floor and to avoid traumatic injury to the delicate urinary sphincter mechanism (Krisiloff et al, 1978; Lattimer et al, 1978).

Psychosocial and Sexual Function

Formerly, little was known or published about the psychosocial effect of bladder exstrophy on both the child and the family. **Reiner and associates (1996) performed a pilot study of 40 patients of various ages with bladder exstrophy and their parents. Both groups were assessed with standardized psychiatric diagnosis questionnaires and interviews. It was found that 70% of the adolescents and 33% of school-age children had behavioral, social, and school competency problems. Both externalizing and depressive problems were present with avoidance of social contacts. These behaviors tended to deteriorate with age. Also, concern about the children's sexual function or sexual disfigurement was present in nearly 70% of the participants and their parents. Initiation of sexual activity tended to be delayed in both girls and boys until early adulthood. The mechanics of sexual intercourse as well as anxiety about the appearance and adequacy of their genitalia were seen as a barrier to relationships by both adults and all of the older adolescents (Reiner et al, 1996).**

Sexual function remains an interesting part of the exstrophy patient's life. Ben-Chaim and co-workers (1996) recently reviewed 20 adult (16 male, 4 female) exstrophy patients who answered an anonymous questionnaire and had their charts reviewed. All males experienced normal erections, which were described as unsatisfactory in seven because of a small penis, and 12 (75%) experienced satisfactory orgasms. Ten patients had sexual intercourse, with full partner satisfaction in 9 of them. Libido, as in the series conducted by Woodhouse and associates (1983), was very high. Of the four female patients who engage in sexual intercourse, three experienced orgasms, which were described as satisfactory by two.

Half of the males and all of the females describe their intimate relationship as serious and long term. Ten patients are in college, five study in the university, three have graduated from high school, and one each finished 5th grade and 8th grade, respectively.

Feitz and colleagues (1994) looked specifically at the psychosexual and socioeconomic development in 22 patients, most of whom were diverted. Although most had a positive attitude toward life, only one of the ten males describe his erections as satisfactory and four complain of retrograde ejaculation. Also, penile length and chordee were a most embarrassing issue for these young men. **The studies by Ben-Chaim and co-workers (1996), Feitz and associates (1994) and Woodhouse and colleagues (1983) all suggest that (1) education, employment and family life have not been substantially affected; (2) that erection, sexuality, and sexual function are well preserved, although patients are bothered by their small penile length and dorsal chordee; and (3) females have normal fertility, sexuality, and sexual function.**

CLOACAL EXSTROPHY

Cloacal exstrophy, also known as vesicointestinal fissure or exstrophia splanchnia, is the most severe defect that can occur in the formation of the ventral abdominal wall. Fortunately, this entity is extremely rare, occurring in one in 200,000 to 400,000 live births. Formerly, the incidence between sexes was thought to be similar; current reports indicate a 2:1 male-to-female ratio (Gearhart and Jeffs, 1992). With newer techniques of prenatal ultrasound, this condition can reliably be diagnosed by the presence of sacral myelomeningocele (usually present in 50%), rocker-bottom feet, splaying of the pubic rami, and a large cystic mass protruding from the infraumbilical anterior abdominal wall. The mode of inheritance of this condition is unknown because offspring have never been produced from individuals with this disorder. With reliable prenatal diagnosis, prenatal counseling can be undertaken and perinatal management enhanced (Gearhart et al, 1995a).

Anatomy and Embryology

Anatomically, there is exstrophy of the foreshortened hindgut or cecum, which displays its bulging mucosa between the two hemibladders (Fig. 63–24). The orifices of the terminal ileum, the rudimentary tailgut, and a single or paired appendix are apparent on the surface of the everted cecum. The tailgut is blind ending, and the ileum is usually prolapsed (Fig. 63–25). The anatomy of the bony pelvis in cloacal exstrophy has generally been described in the past

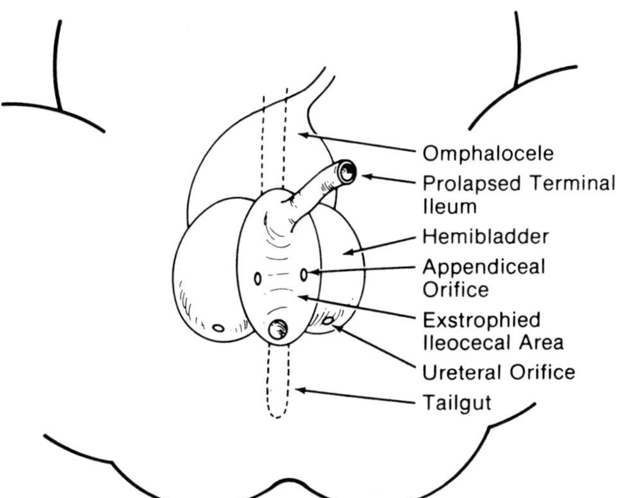

Figure 63–24. Schematic drawing showing gastrointestinal and urinary defects in children of either sex born with cloacal exstrophy. (Courtesy of Dr. Richard Hurwitz.)

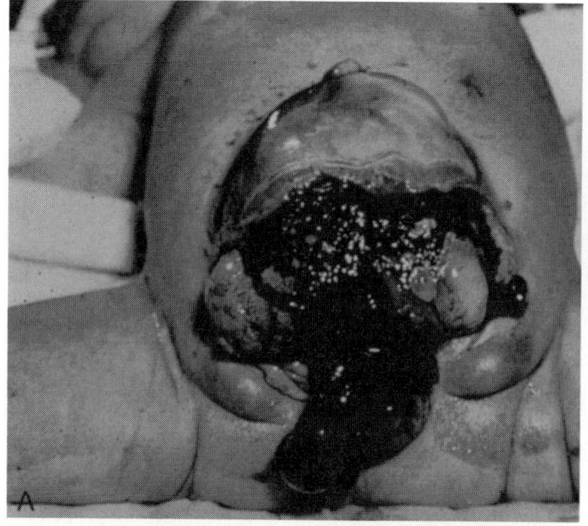

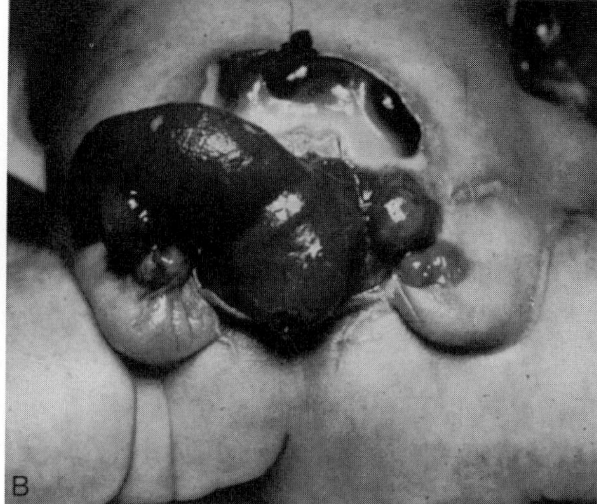

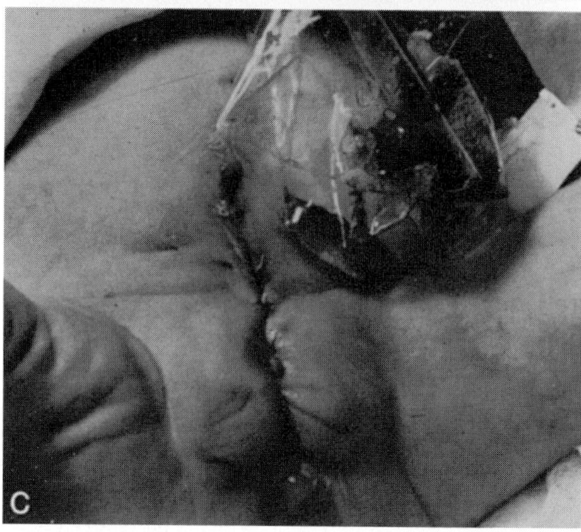

Figure 63–25. Cloacal exstrophy. *A,* Newborn female showing omphalocele, prolapsed ileum, and symmetric bladder halves. *B,* Male patient with similar appearance but also demonstrating orifice of small hindgut and bifid penis. *C,* Closure (patient shown in *B*) to conform to female sex of rearing; left-sided ileostomy.

as a widened symphysis pubis with hips that are externally rotated and abducted (Gearhart and Jeffs, 1992).

Bony and Genitourinary Abnormalities

Sponseller and associates (1995) have described the markedly severe abnormalities of the bony pelvis associated with cloacal exstrophy. Using computed tomography scans of the pelvis in controls and patients with cloacal exstrophy, the interpubic diastasis was found to have a mean of 0.5 cm in controls and 8.0 cm in patients with cloacal exstrophy. The anterior segment length (distance from the triradiate cartilage to the pubis) was 37% shorter in patients with cloacal exstrophy versus controls. Also, the angle of the iliac wing was markedly increased at 45 degrees, showing the amount of external rotation. Likewise, the ischiopubic angle was markedly increased in patients with cloacal exstrophy. **Overall, patients with cloacal exstrophy have extreme abnormalities of the pelvis as well as asymmetry between the sides, sacroiliac joint malformations, and occasional hip malformations (Sponseller et al, 1995).**

Müllerian and Testis Anomalies

Duplication anomalies of the uterus and vagina are the most commonly found müllerian anomalies. Hurwitz found duplication of the vagina in 43%, whereas Tank found this anomaly in 65% of patients (Tank and Lindenaver, 1970; Hurwitz et al, 1987). In addition, vaginal agenesis is common, occurring in 25% to 43% of patients (Hurwitz et al, 1987). Partial or complete duplication of the uterus has been described in up to 95% of patients (Hurwitz et al, 1987). Normal ovarian tissue was found in six of seven female patients in Hurwitz's series (1987). In both the series by Hurwitz and colleagues (1987) and Ricketts and co-workers (1991), the testis position was undescended in the majority of patients. Because almost all males with cloacal exstrophy need gender reassignment along with bilateral orchiectomy, the need for orchiopexy is rare. However, most müllerian structures should be preserved because these can be used in lower urinary tract reconstructive efforts later in life. Skeletal system anomalies of both the vertebral bodies and lower limb are commonly seen in the cloacal exstrophy patient. **Vertebral anomalies have been reported in up to 80% of patients (Diamond, 1990). Lower limb abnormalities are seen in 12% to 65% of patients.** These include clubfoot, congenital hip dislocation, agenesis, and severe deformity of both the foot and leg (Hurwitz et al, 1987; Diamond, 1990).

The phallus is usually separated into right and left halves with adjacent scrotum or labia. Occasionally, the penis is together in the midline but the structure is diminutive and the corporal bodies small so that the female sex of rearing

(Gearhart and Jeffs, 1990). The choice between a catheterizable urethra or an abdominal stoma depends on the adequacy of the urethra and bladder outlet, the intellect and dexterity of the child, and the child's orthopedic status regarding the spine, hip joints, braces, and ambulation.

The time to initiate management of urinary incontinence is determined by the age at which the child can understand and manage the type of bladder emptying that will be required. Social factors, intelligence, school support, and mobility are important considerations for this group.

Occasionally, hindgut is available for bladder enhancement but ileum is the bowel segment that has traditionally been used. In an effort to avoid further loss of absorptive surface by preserving both hindgut and ileum, Mitchell has used gastrocystoplasty with good success (Adams et al, 1988). Regardless of which bowel segment is chosen, bladder augmentation should be delayed until bowel function is mature and nutrition and acidosis are no longer a problem (Gearhart and Jeffs, 1990).

Some patients are found to have a functioning bladder and can void through a reconstructed bladder outlet. However, innovative methods may be needed to construct a continent outlet in those patients without substantial native urethral tissues (Gearhart and Jeffs, 1995). Some of these techniques include use of the vagina to form a urethra, with reimplantation of the vagina into the bladder for continence, or an ileal nipple, as described by Hendren (1992).

Continence Results in the Patient with Cloacal Exstrophy

The authors are following 23 patients with cloacal exstrophy, of whom 14 have undergone continence procedures. Four patients underwent Young-Dees bladder neck plasty only, one underwent patient bladder neck suspension, three underwent Young-Dees-Leadbetter bladder neck plasty and augmentation, and four underwent Young-Dees-Leadbetter plasty, augmentation, and creation of a continent abdominal stoma. The upper tracts remained normal in 21 of 21 patients. Two patients required revision of their continent stomas due to catheterization difficulties. One patient required injection of collagen into the reconstructed bladder neck, and one patient who had both bladder neck reconstruction and bladder augmentation underwent reoperation with bladder neck closure and ileal Mitrofanoff continent diversion for failure to achieve continence (Longaker, 1989). Overall, 12 patients (86%) experience diurnal continence, whereas 79% are dry at night. Twelve are on a continuous intermittent catheterization regimen, and two are voiding spontaneously (Ben-Chaim et al, 1995b).

Despite the complexity of this anomaly, a staged approach to lower tract reconstruction can produce urinary continence. An individualized approach is required to find the most suitable solution for each patient's bladder and bowel anatomy and function, according to their intellectual, neurologic, and orthopedic capabilities. Ricketts and associates (1991) have developed a scoring system to analyze both bladder and bowel continence. In the absence of multiple cases due to the rarity of this condition, use of this scoring system may allow a collective experience to be analyzed and thus to optimize future management of this most complex disorder.

An innovative approach is required to find the most suitable solution for each individual patient concerning bladder size and function, and mental, neurologic, and orthopedic status. With the advent of modern pediatric anesthesia and intensive care, the survival rate is high. This high survival rate makes reconstructive techniques applicable to a large percentage of infants born with this condition. The type II variants demand variation and innovation in the aforementioned schema of treatment.

EPISPADIAS

Epispadias varies from a glandular defect in a covered penis, to the penopubic type with complete incontinence, to the complete variety associated with exstrophy of the bladder.

Male Epispadias

Epispadias in males is classified according to the position of the dorsally displaced urethral meatus. The degree of penile deformity and the occurrence of urinary incontinence are related to the extent of the dorsally displaced urethral meatus. The displaced meatus may be found in the glans, penile shaft, or penopubic region. All types of epispadias are associated with varying degrees of dorsal chordee. In penopubic or subsymphyseal epispadias, the entire penile urethra is open and the bladder outlet may be large enough to admit the examining finger, indicating obvious gross incontinence. The pubis symphysis is divergent and contributes to the deficiency of the external urinary sphincter mechanism. The divergence of the pubis symphysis and the shortened urethral plate results in prominent dorsal chordee and a penis that appears short. **The penile deformity is virtually identical to that observed in bladder exstrophy. In a combined study, Dees (1949) reported the incidence of complete epispadias to be one in 117,000 males and one in 484,000 females.** The reported male-to-female ratio of epispadias varies between 3:1 (Dees, 1949) and 5:1 (Kramer and Kelalis, 1982).

Kramer and Kelalis (1982) reviewed their surgical experience of 82 males with epispadias. Penopubic epispadias occurred in 49 cases, penile epispadias in 21, and glandular epispadias in 12. Urinary incontinence was observed in 46 of 49 patients with penopubic epispadias, in 15 of 21 patients with penile epispadias, and in no patients with glandular epispadias.

Associated Anomalies

The anomalies associated with complete epispadias are usually confined to deformities of the external genitalia, diastasis of the pubic symphysis, and deficiency of the urinary continence mechanism. The only renal anomaly observed in 11 cases of complete epispadias was agenesis of the left kidney (Campbell, 1952). In a review by Arap and colleagues (1988), one case of unilateral renal agenesis and one ectopic pelvic kidney occurred in 38 patients. **The ureterovesical junction is inherently deficient in complete epispadias, and reflux has been reported in a number of**

series to be around 30% to 40% (Kramer and Kelalis, 1982a; Arap et al, 1988).

Surgical Management

The objectives for the repair of penopubic epispadias include achievement of urinary continence with preservation of the upper urinary tract and reconstruction of functional and cosmetically acceptable genitalia. The surgical management of incontinence in penopubic epispadias is virtually identical to that of a closed bladder exstrophy.

Young (1922) reported the first cure of incontinence in a male patient with complete epispadias. Since Young reported his approach to obtain continence, results have progressively improved (Burkholder and Williams, 1965; Kramer and Kelalis, 1982a; Arap et al, 1988; Peters et al, 1988). In patients with complete epispadias and good bladder capacity, epispadias and bladder neck reconstruction can be performed in a single stage. Urethroplasty formerly was performed after bladder neck reconstruction (Kramer and Kelalis, 1982a; Arap et al, 1988). However, our results with the small bladder associated with exstrophy (Gearhart and Jeffs, 1989a) and the small bladder associated with epispadias (Peters et al, 1988) have led us to perform urethroplasty and penile elongation prior to bladder neck reconstruction. A small incontinent bladder with reflux is hardly an ideal situation for bladder neck reconstruction and ureteral reimplantation. With urethroplasty prior to bladder neck reconstruction, there was an average increase in bladder capacity of 95 ml within 18 months in those patients with a small bladder capacity initially associated with epispadias and a continence rate overall of 87% after the continence procedure (Peters et al, 1988). In a recent series exclusively composed of patients with complete male epispadias, bladder capacity increased by an average of 42 ml within 18 months following urethroplasty. Nine of 11 patients (82%) were dry day and night after an average of 9 months.

In the epispadias group, much as in the exstrophy group, bladder capacity is the most predominant indicator of eventual continence (Ritchey et al, 1988). Also, in a current series, Arap and co-workers (1988) obtained a much higher continence rate in those with adequate bladder capacity (71%) prior to bladder neck reconstruction than in those with inadequate capacity (20%). In addition, in Arap's group of complete epispadias patients, most attained continence within 2 years, much like those patients with classic bladder exstrophy.

A firm intersymphyseal band bridges the divergent symphysis, and an osteotomy is not usually performed. The Young-Dees-Leadbetter bladder neck plasty, Marshall-Marchetti-Krantz bladder neck suspension, and ureteral reimplantation are performed when the bladder capacity reaches approximately 60 ml, which usually occurs between 3 and 4 years of age.

The genital reconstruction and urethroplasty in epispadias and exstrophy are similar. The following must take place: release of dorsal chordee and vision of suspensory ligaments; dissection of the corpora from their attachment to the inferior pubic ramus; lengthening of the urethral groove; and lengthening of the corpora, if needed, by incision and anastomosis or grafting, or by medial rotation of the ventral corpora in a more downward direction.

Urethral reconstruction in complete epispadias can be as simple as a modified Young urethroplasty to even a two-stage repair (Kramer and Kelalis, 1982a). All modern techniques of hypospadias repair have been used to aid in the treatment of epispadias, including the use of the prepuce to the bladder mucosa and even full-thickness skin grafts. A transverse ventral island flap has been performed by Monfort (1987). The urethra, once reconstructed, can be positioned between and below the corpora (Cantwell, 1895; Ransley et al, 1989). The glandular and skin closure is performed in a manner similar to the reconstruction of the penis in patients with bladder exstrophy (see the previous section).

The achievement of urinary continence following bladder neck reconstruction in patients with epispadias is summarized in Table 63–8 (Dees, 1989; Burkholder and Williams, 1965; Arap et al, 1988; Kramer and Kelalis, 1982a; Peters et al, 1988; Ben-Chaim et al, 1995c). The majority of these patients underwent reconstruction by means of a Young-Dees-Leadbetter bladder neck plasty. Urinary continence was achieved in 82% of males (Ben-Chaim et al, 1995c). Urinary diversion should seldom be considered in the initial management of complete epispadias. Delayed achievement of urinary continence occurred in more than half the males with complete epispadias who eventually became continent following the continence procedures (Kramer and Kelalis, 1982a). The effect that urethral lengthening and prostatic enlargement have on increasing bladder outlet resistance is emphasized by these observations in the epispadias group. However, in a series by Arap and colleagues (1988), establishment of continence had no relationship to puberty and usually occurred within 2 years; in a majority of patients, continence preceded puberty by several years.

The results of urethroplasty for epispadias have been reviewed by Kramer and Kelalis (1982a). A Thiersch-Duplay procedure (modified Young urethroplasty) was selected in 49 of 67 cases (73%), and various other reconstructive techniques were selected in the remaining 18 cases. Urethral fistulas requiring surgical repair occurred in 21% of these urethroplasties. In Ben-Chaim's series, 13 patients underwent a Young urethroplasty and 2 patients a Cantwell-Ransley repair. Urethrocutaneous fistulae occurred in 20% of patients. Because more patients are undergoing Cantwell-Ransley repair, this incidence should decrease appreciably.

Kramer and associates (1986) reported the success of genital reconstruction in epispadias with a straight penis angled downward in almost 70% of patients with normal erectile function. Of this group, 80% had satisfactory intercourse, and of 29 married patients, 19 have fathered children. The carefully constructed and well-planned approach to the management of urinary incontinence and genital deformities associated with complete epispadias should provide a satisfactory cosmetic appearance, normal genital function, and preservation of fertility potential in most patients.

Female Epispadias

Female epispadias is a rare congenital anomaly, occurring in one in 484,000 female patients (Gearhart and Jeffs, 1992). Three degrees of epispadias occur in female patients, and we use the classification of Davis for female epispadias (Davis, 1928). In the lesser degree of epispadias,

Table 63–8. URINARY CONTINENCE FOLLOWING BLADDER NECK RECONSTRUCTION IN PATIENTS WITH COMPLETE EPISPADIAS

	Ben-Chaim et al (1995c)	Gearhart and Jeffs (1993)	Kramer and Kelalis (1982a)	Arap et al (1988)	Burkholder and Williams (1965)
Total number of patients with complete epispadias	15	11	53	38	27
Number of males with complete epispadias treated with BNR	11	—	32*	21	17
Number of males with surgically corrected incontinence	9	—	22	15	8
Percentage of males with surgically corrected incontinence	82	—	69	71	47
Number of females with complete epispadias treated with BNR	0	9	8	9	10
Number of females with surgically corrected incontinence	0	8	8	7	7
Percentage of females with surgically corrected incontinence	0	87	88	77	70

*Male patients with penopubic epispadias and total incontinence included.
BNR, bladder neck reconstruction

the urethral orifice appears patulous. In intermediate epispadias, the urethra is dorsally split along most of the urethra. In the most severe degree of epispadias, the urethral cleft involves the entire length of the urethra and the sphincteric mechanism is rendered incompetent (Fig. 63–28).

The genital defect is characterized by a bifid clitoris. The mons is depressed in shape and covered by a smooth, glabrous area of skin. Beneath this area, there may be a moderated amount of subcutaneous tissue and fat or the skin may be closely applied to the anterior and inferior surfaces of the symphysis pubis. The labia minora are usually poorly developed and terminate anteriorly at the corresponding half of the bifid clitoris, where there may be a rudiment of the preputial fold. Although these external appearances are most characteristic, on separation of the labia, one sees the urethra, which may vary considerably as mentioned previously. The symphysis pubis is usually closed but may be represented by a narrow fibrous band. The vagina and internal genitalia are usually normal.

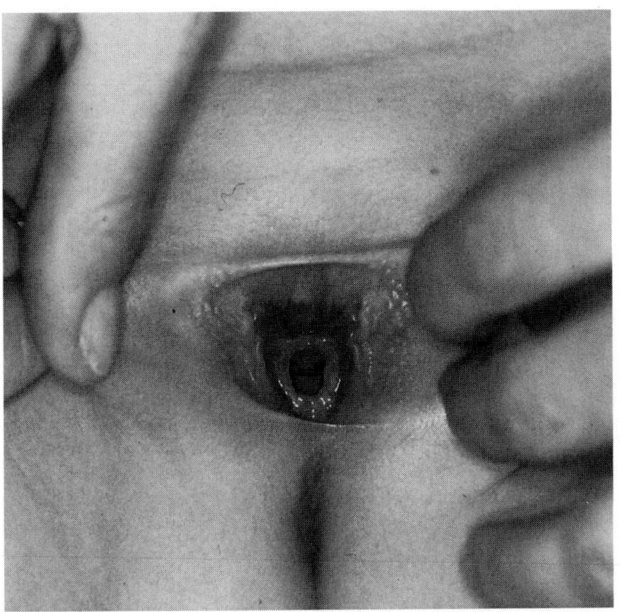

Figure 63–28. Gravity cystogram showing complete duplication of the bladder and urethra.

Associated Anomalies

The ureterovesical junction is inherently deficient in cases of epispadias, and the ureters are often laterally placed and enter the bladder with a straight course so that reflux occurs. **The incidence of reflux in epispadias is reported to be 30% to 75% (Kramer and Kelalis, 1982b; Gearhart and Jeffs, 1992).** Because there is no outlet resistance, the bladder is small and the wall is thin. However, after urethral reconstruction, the mild urethral resistance created allows the bladder to develop an acceptable capacity so that in the future the child can undergo bladder neck reconstruction.

Surgical Anomalies

The objectives for the repair of female epispadias parallel those devised in the male: (1) achievement of urinary continence, (2) preservation of the upper urinary tract, and (3) reconstruction of functional and cosmetically acceptable external genitalia.

Operative Technique

With the patient in the lithotomy position, the defect of female epispadias with incontinence is apparent (Fig. 63–29*A*). The two halves of the clitoris are widely apart, and the roof of the urethra is cleft from the 9 o'clock to the 3 o'clock positions. The smooth mucosa of the urethra tends to blend in cephalad with the thin hairless skin over the mons. The urethral incision is begun at the cephalad end of the vertical incision at the base of the mons and brought inferiorly through the full thickness of the urethral wall at the 9 o'clock and 3 o'clock positions (Fig. 63–29*B, C*). Sutures can be placed in the urethra at this juncture and used to retract the cephalad extent of the urethra downward so that the roof of the urethra is excised up a level near the bladder neck. Often, one will find that the dissection is under the symphysis at this junction (Fig. 63–29*D*). An inverting closure of the urethra is then performed over a No. 12 Fr

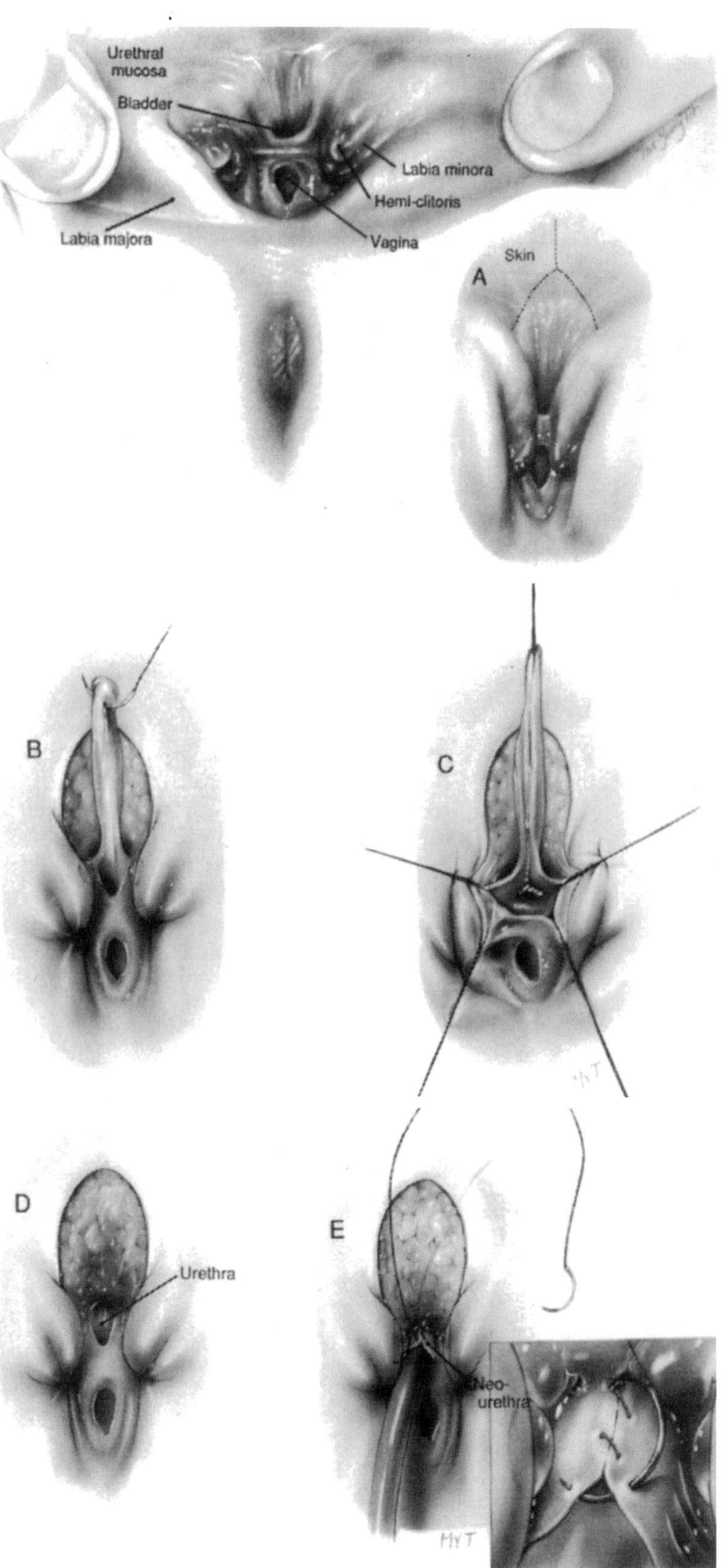

Figure 63–29. *A,* Typical appearance of female epispadias. Inset shows initial incision for surgical repair. *B* and *C,* Excision of glabrous skin of mons and parallel urethral incisions taken cephalad toward bladder neck. *D* and *E,* Urethral reconstruction begun over catheter with running suture of 5-0 polyglycolic acid.

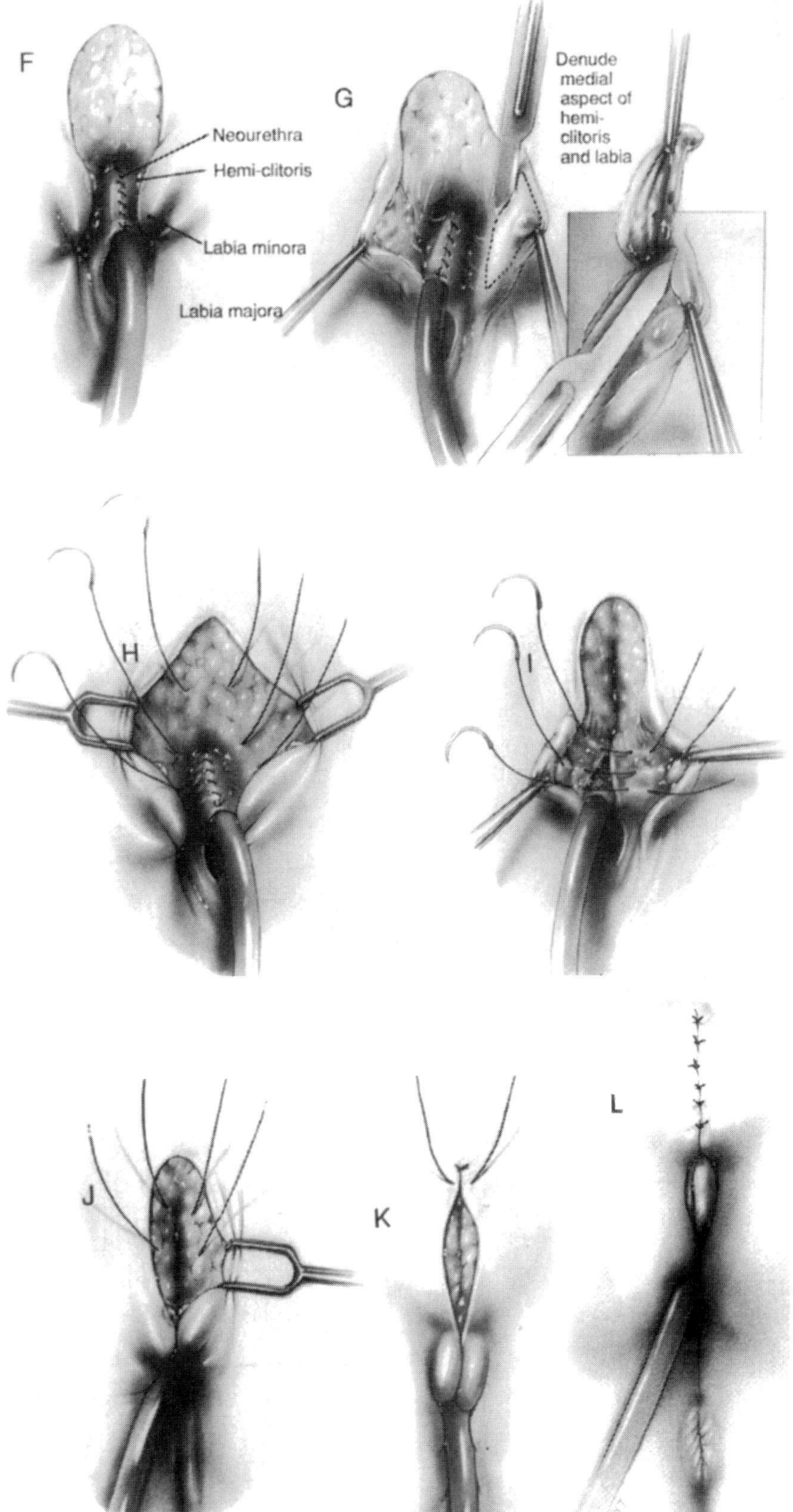

Figure 63–29 *Continued F* and *G,* Completed urethral reconstruction with denuding medial aspect of labia minora and clitoris. *H* and *I,* Closure of periurethral tissues over neourethra with coaptation of labia and clitoral halves. *J* and *K,* Closure of subcutaneous area to build up mons area and skin closure. *L,* Completed urethral and genital reconstruction.

Foley catheter. The suture is begun near the bladder neck and progresses from above downward until narrowing of the neourethra is accomplished (Fig. 63–29*E*, *F*).

Attention is then given to denuding the medial half of the bifid clitoris and labia minora so that proper genital coaptation can be obtained (Fig. 63–29*G*). After this is done, fat from the mons and subcutaneous tissue can be used to cover the suture line and obliterate the space in front of the pubic symphysis (Fig. 63–29*H*). The two halves of the clitoris and labia minora are brought together using interrupted sutures of 6-0 polyglycolic acid. The corpora may be partially detached from the anterior ramus of the pubis to aid in urethral closure. Also, bringing these tissues together may contribute added distal resistance to the urethra. Mons closure is further aided by mobilizing subcutaneous tissue laterally and bringing it medially to fill any prior depression that remains. The subcutaneous layer is closed with 4-0 polyglactin in an interrupted fashion (see Fig. 63–29*I*). The skin is closed with interrupted sutures of 6-0 polypropylene (Fig. 63–29*J* through *L*). A No. 12 Fr Foley catheter is left indwelling for 5 to 7 days. Should the patient undergo simultaneous bladder neck reconstruction, a Foley catheter is not left in the urethra and the patient is then placed in the supine position for the abdominal part of the procedure.

Achievement of a satisfactory cosmetic appearance of the external genitalia and of satisfactory urinary continence in the female child with epispadias represents a formidable surgical challenge. Many operations have been reported to control incontinence in the epispadias group but the results were disappointing. These procedures included transvaginal plication of the urethra and bladder neck, reefing procedures of the urethra, muscle transplantations, urethral twisting, cauterization of the urethra, interposition of the uterus, bladder flap and Marshall-Marchetti vesicourethral suspension (Stiles, 1911; Davis, 1926; Marshall et al, 1949; Gross and Cresson, 1952). Certainly, these procedures may increase urethral resistance, but they do not correct incontinence or the malformed anatomy of the urethra, bladder neck, and genitalia.

The challenge of the small bladder in female patients with epispadias and incontinence is comparable to a situation often seen with closed bladder exstrophy. The small incontinent bladder with or without reflux is hardly an ideal setting for successful bladder neck reconstruction and ureteral reimplantation. A third of all incontinent epispadias patients have a small bladder capacity (less than 60 ml) in the authors' series and that of Kramer and Kelalis (1982b). Bladder augmentation or polytetrafluoroethylene (Teflon) injection in the bladder neck area and/or simultaneous bladder neck reconstruction and bladder augmentation have been offered as a solution to this challenge. However, primary closure of the epispadiac urethra in children with closed exstrophy was found to increase bladder capacity without causing hydronephrosis, and this approach has been applied to male and female patients with epispadias (Peters et al, 1988; Gearhart and Jeffs, 1989a).

Although we typically perform urethral and genital reconstruction between 18 months and 2 years of age, we advocate delaying bladder neck reconstruction until the child is 4 to 5 years old. Not only does this delay allow the bladder to adapt and increase the capacity after urethral and genital reconstruction but deferring an operation until this age allows the child to accept essential instruction in toilet training. This factor is critical in achievement of satisfactory continence.

Surgical Results

The continence rate of 87.5% in our female patients is comparable to that of Klauber and Williams (1974), who found a 67% continence rate in female patients with a good bladder capacity, and those of Kramer and Kelalis (1982b), who found an 83% continence rate in patients with adequate bladder capacity (defined as 50 ml capacity). All of the authors' patients seen for primary treatment have achieved a capacity in excess of 80 ml.

Hendren (1981) and Kramer and Kelalis (1982b) have shown that genital, urethral, and bladder neck reconstruction can all be accomplished in one procedure with satisfactory results. The authors' patients who underwent prior urethral and genital reconstruction had a mean bladder capacity at bladder neck reconstruction of 121 ml, making the bladder suitable for bladder neck reconstruction and eventual continence without the use of augmentation cystoplasty and its attendant need for intermittent catheterization.

The time interval to achieve total continence was a mean of 18 months in patients who underwent genital, urethral, and bladder neck reconstruction in one procedure versus 23 months in patients who underwent preliminary urethroplasty and genital reconstruction before bladder neck reconstruction. In a series by Klauber and Williams (1974), the mean interval to acceptable continence was 2.25 years. Also, in a series by Kramer and Kelalis (1982b), some patients became continent within a short period, while complete continence was delayed for several years in others. The time delay for achieving continence may represent increased pelvic musculature development, as suggested by Kramer and Kelalis. When assessing the interval to continence, no advantage appears to be gained by preliminary urethroplasty. However, the authors believe that the advantage gained by increased bladder capacity at the time of bladder neck reconstruction outweighs any advantage gained by a combined approach.

OTHER BLADDER ANOMALIES

Agenesis and Hypoplasia

Agenesis of the bladder is an extremely rare congenital anomaly, with only 44 cases reported in the English literature up to 1988. Campbell (1952) reported seven cases in 19,046 autopsies (two were anocephalic monsters, and in all seven, other severe anomalies coexisted). Glenn (1959) found only one case in 600,000 patients seen at Duke University Hospital in 28 years. Agenesis of the bladder is seldom compatible with life, and only 15 live births have been reported, all except one being females (Akdas et al, 1988; Aragona et al, 1988; Krull et al, 1988).

The cause of agenesis of the bladder is uncertain. Because the hindgut is normal in these infants, it may be assumed that embryologic division of the cloaca into the urogenital sinus and anorectum has proceeded normally. Bladder agenesis may be the result of secondary atrophy of the anterior division of the cloaca, perhaps because of a lack of distention advocate conservative treatment initially, while reserving radical surgical excision of the urachus for persistent cases or recurrences. Similarly, simple drainage of a urachal cyst is associated with recurrent infections in 30% of cases, and late occurrence of adenocarcinoma has been reported (Nix et al, 1958; Blichert-Toft and Nielson, 1971b). However, a recent large series from Cilento and colleagues (1994) recommends both excision of the anomaly and a cuff of bladder routinely.

In the treatment of benign urachal lesions in children, it is rarely necessary to remove the umbilicus; whenever possible, cosmetic considerations should prevail. In infants, a small, curved, subumbilical incision is usually ample, because at this age, the bladder dome is still high and readily accessible through this exposure.

A transverse midhypogastric incision is adequate exposure in older children and adults, and allows for both superior and inferior dissection. Surgical management of umbilical anomalies is depicted in Figure 63–34. The urachal stalk or fibrous urachal remnant should be detached from the dermis posterior to the umbilicus. A buttonhole in the umbilical area is of no consequence. Application of a small gauze pledget under the dressing obliterates dead space, maintains umbilical configuration, and allows the skin to close secondarily.

When peritoneum and umbilical ligaments are adherent to the inflammatory mass, these structures should be excised in continuity with the lesion. A vertical midline incision is the best approach for removal of an extensive inflammatory mass. Elliptic excision of the umbilicus may be necessary if it is involved in the inflammatory process, especially with an external urachal sinus or alternating sinus. A suppurative infection within a cyst or external sinus may require initial incision and drainage and treatment as for an abscess. After healing is complete, an internal excision of urachal tissue should be performed.

REFERENCES

Abramson J: Double bladder and related anomalies: Clinical and embryological aspects in a case report. Br J Urol 1965; 33:195.

Adams MC, Mitchell ME, Rink RC, et al: Gastrocystoplasty: An alternate solution to the problem of urological reconstruction in severely compromised patients. J Urol 1988; 140:1152.

Akdas A, Iseri C, Ozgur S, Kirkali Z: Bladder agenesis. Int Urol Nephrol 1988; 20:261.

Allen NH, Atwell JD: The paraureteric diverticulum in children. Br J Urol 1980; 52:264.

Ambrose SS, O'Brien DP: Surgical embryology of the exstrophy-epispadias complex. Surg Clin North Am 1974; 54:1379.

Andalen RM, O'Phelan EH, Chisholm JC, et al: Exstrophy of the bladder. Long-term results of bilateral posterior iliac osteotomies and two-stage anatomic repair. J Clin Orthop 1970; 68:156.

Ansell JE: Exstrophy and epispadias. *In* Glenn JF, ed: Urologic Surgery. Philadelphia, J. B. Lippincott Company, 1983, p 647.

Aragona F, Passerini G, Zarembella P, Zorzi C, et al: Agenesis of the bladder: A case report and review of the literature. Urol Radiol 1988; 10:207.

Arap S, Giron AM: Duplicated exstrophy: Report of three cases. Eur Urol 1986; 12:451.

Arap S, Giron A, Degoes GM: Complete reconstruction of bladder exstrophy. Urology 1976; 7:413.

Arap S, Nahas WC, Giron AM, et al: Incontinent epispadias: Surgical treatment of 38 cases. J Urol 1988; 140:577.

Avni EF, Matos C, Diard F, Schuman CC: Midline omphalovesical anomalies in children. Contribution of ultrasound imaging. Urol Radiol 1988; 2:189.

Bandler CG, Milbed AH, Alley JL: Urachal calculus. N Y State J Med 1942; 42:2203.

Barrett DM, Malek RS, Kelalis PP: Observation of vesical diverticulum in children. J Urol 1976; 116:234.

Begg RC: The urachus and umbilical fistulae. J Anat 1927; 64:170.

Ben-Chaim J, Jeffs RD, Reiner WG, Gearhart JP: The outcome of patients with classic bladder exstrophy in adult life. J Urol 1996; 155:1251.

Ben-Chaim J, Jeffs RD, Peppas DS, Gearhart JP: Submucosal bladder neck injections of glutaraldehyde cross-linked bovine collagen for treatment of urinary incontinence in patients with exstrophy/epispadias complex. J Urol 1995a; 154:862.

Ben-Chaim J, Peppas DS, Sponseller PD, et al: Applications of osteotomy in the cloacal exstrophy patient. J Urol 1995b; 154:865.

Ben-Chaim J, Peppas DS, Jeffs RD, Gearhart JP: Complete male epispadias: Genital reconstruction and achieving continence. J Urol 1995c; 153:1665.

Bennett AH: Exstrophy of the bladder treated by ureterosigmoidostomies. Urology 1973; 2:165.

Berman SM, Tolia BM, Laor E, et al: Urachal remnants in adults. Urology 1988; 31:17.

Blichert-Toft M, Nielson OV: Diseases of the urachus simulating intraabdominal disorders. Am J Surg 1971a; 122:123.

Blichert-Toft M, Nielson OV: Congenital patient urachus and acquired variants. Acta Chir Scand 1971b; 137:807.

Boyce WH, Vest SA: A new concept concerning treatment of exstrophy of the bladder. J Urol 1952; 677–503.

Brzezinski AE, Homsy YL, Leberg I: Orthoplasty in epispadias. J Urol 1986; 136:259.

Burbige KA, Hensle TW, Chambers WJ, et al: Pregnancy and sexual function in women with exstrophy. Urology 1986; 28:12.

Burkholder GV, Williams DI: Epispadias and incontinence: Surgical treatment of 27 children. J Urol 1965; 94:674.

Burns JE: A new operation for exstrophy of the bladder. JAMA 1924; 82:1587.

Campbell M: Epispadias: A report of fifteen cases. J Urol 1952; 67:988.

Canning DA, Gearhart JP, Peppas DS, Jeffs RD: The cephalotrigonal reimplant in bladder neck reconstruction for patients with exstrophy or epispadias. J Urol 1992; 150:156.

Cantwell FV: Operative technique of epispadias by transplantation of the urethra. Ann Surg 1895; 22:689.

Cendron J: La reconstruction vesicale. Ann Chir Infant 1971; 12:371.

Cerniglia FR, Roth DA, Gonzalez ET: Covered exstrophy and visceral sequestration in a male newborn: Case report. J Urol 1989; 141–903.

Chisholm TC: Pediatric Surgery, Vol 2. Chicago, Year Book Medical Publishers, 1962, p 933.

Chisholm TC: Exstrophy of the urinary bladder. *In* Kiesewetter WB, ed: Long-term Follow-up in Congenital Anomalies, Vol 6. Pittsburgh, Pediatric Surgical Symposium, Pittsburgh Children's Hospital, 1979, p 31.

Cilento BG, Retik AB, Peters CA, et al: Urachal abnormalities: Experience with 45 cases over 25 years. Abstract #93. American Academy of Pediatrics, Urology Section, Dallas, Texas, October 23, 1994.

Clark M, O'Connell KJ: Scanning and transmission electron microscopic studies of an exstrophic human bladder. J Urol 1973; 110:481.

Clemetson CAB: Ectopia vesicae and split pelvis. J Obstet Gynaecol Br Monnw 1958; 65–973.

Coffey RC: Transplantation of the ureter into the large intestine in the absence of a functioning bladder. Surg Gynecol Obstet 1921; 32:383.

Cohen SJ: Ureterozstoneostomie eine neve antirefluxtechnik. Aktuel Urol 1975; 6:24.

Conner JP, Lattimer JK, Hensle TW, Burbige KA: Primary bladder closure of bladder exstrophy: Long-term functional results in 137 patients. J Pediatr Surg 1988; 23:1102.

Connolly JA, Peppas DS, Jeffs RD, Gearheart JP: Prevalence and repair of inguinal hernias in children with bladder exstrophy. J Urol 1995; 154:1901.

Cracchiolo A III, Hall CB: Bilateral iliac osteotomy. Clin Orthop 1970; 68:156.

Culp DA: The histology of the exstrophied bladder. J Urol 1964; 91:538.

Davis DM: Epispadias in females and its surgical treatment. Surg Gynec Obstet 1928; 47:600.

Davis HH, Nilhaus FW: Persistent omphalomesenteric duct and urachus in the same case. JAMA 1926; 86:685.

Decter RM, Roth DR, Fishman IJ, et al: Use of the AS 800 device in exstrophy and epispadias. J Urol 1988; 140:1202.

Dees JE: Congenital epispadias with incontinence. J Urol 1949; 62:513.

Devine CJ Jr, Horton CE, Scarff JE Jr: Epispadias: Symposium of pediatric urology. Urol Clin North Am 1980; 7:465.

Dixon CF, Weisman RE: Polyps of the sigmoid occurring 30 years after bilateral ureterosigmoidostomies for exstrophy of the bladder. Surgery 1948; 24:6.

Duckett JW: Use of paraexstrophy skin pedicle grafts for correction of exstrophy and epispadias repair. Birth Defects 1977; 13:171.

Duckett JW, Gazak JM: Complications of ureterosigmoidostomy. Urol Clin North Am 1983; 10:473.

Engel RM, Wilkinson HA: Bladder exstrophy. J Urol 1970; 104:699.

Engel RM: Bladder exstrophy: Vesicoplasty or urinary diversion. Urology 1973; 2:29.

Ezwell WW, Carlson HE: A realistic look at exstrophy of the bladder. Br J Urol 1970; 42–197.

Feitz WF, Van Gruns-Venn EJ, Froeling FM, de Vries JD: Outcome analysis of psychosexual and socioeconomic development of adult patients born with bladder exstrophy. J Urol 1994; 152:1417.

Frank JD, Mor SB, Pryor JP: The surgical correction of erectile deformities of the penis of 100 men. Br J Urol 1981; 53:645.

Frey P, Cohen SJ: Anterior pelvic osteotomy. A new operative technique facilitating primary bladder exstrophy closure. Br J Urol 1989; 64:641.

Gearhart JP, Ben-Chaim J, Jeffs RD, Sanders R: Accurate prenatal diagnosis of classic bladder exstrophy. Am J Obstet Gynecol, 1995a; 85:961

Gearhart JP, Canning DA, Jeffs RD: Failed bladder neck reconstruction: Options for management. J Urol 1991; 146:1082.

Gearhart JP, Canning DA, Peppas DS, Jeffs RD: Techniques to create continence in the failed bladder exstrophy patient. J Urol 1993a; 150:441.

Gearhart JP, Forschner DC, Jeffs RD, et al: A combined vertical and horizontal pelvic osteotomy approach for primary and secondary repair of bladder exstrophy. J Urol 1996; 155:689.

Gearhart JP, Jeffs RD: The use of parenteral testosterone therapy in central reconstructive surgery. J Urol 1987; 138:1077.

Gearhart JP, Jeffs RD: Augmentation cystoplasty in the failed exstrophy reconstruction. J Urol 1988; 139:790.

Gearhart JP, Jeffs RD: Bladder exstrophy: Increase in capacity following epispadias repair. J Urol 1989a; 142:525.

Gearhart JP, Jeffs RD: Reconstruction of the lower urinary tract in cloacal exstrophy. Dial Pediatr Urol 1990; 13:4.

Gearhart JP, Jeffs RD: State of the art reconstructive surgery for bladder exstrophy at the Johns Hopkins Hospital. Am J Dis Child 1989b; 143:1475.

Gearhart JP, Jeffs RD: Techniques to create urinary continence in cloacal exstrophy. J Urol 1991; 146:616.

Gearhart JP, Jeffs RD: Exstrophy of the bladder, epispadias and other bladder anomalies. *In* Walsh PC, Retik AB, Stamey TA, Vaughn ED, eds: Campbell's Urology, Vol 2, 6th ed. Philadelphia, W. B. Saunders Company, 1992, p 1772.

Gearhart JP, Jeffs RD: Techniques for continence in the cloacal exstrophy patient. J Urol 1991; 146:616.

Gearhart JP, Lee BR, Perlman E, Partin AW: An analysis of collagen subtypes in the newborn exstrophy bladder. J Urol 1996; in press.

Gearhart JP, Leonard MP, Bingers JK, Jeffs RD: The Cantwell-Ransley technique for repair of epispadias. J Urol 1992; 148:851.

Gearhart JP, Peppas DS, Jeffs RD: The failed exstrophy closure: strategy for management. Br J Urol 1993a; 71:217.

Gearhart JP, Peppas DS, Jeffs RD: Complete genitourinary reconstruction in female epispadias. J Urol 1993b; 149:1110.

Gearhart JP, Peppas DS, Jeffs RD: Complications of paraexstrophy skin flaps in the reconstruction of classical bladder exstrophy. J Urol 1993c; 150:627.

Gearhart JP, Peppas DS, Jeffs RD: The application of continent urinary stomas to bladder augmentation or replacement in the failed exstrophy reconstruction. Br J Urol 1995b; 75:87.

Gearhart JP, Sciortino CM, Ben-Chaim J, et al: The Cantwell-Ransley epispadias repair in exstrophy/epispadias: Lessons learned. Urology 1995c; 46:92

Gearhart JP, Williams KA, Jeffs RD: Intraoperative urethral pressure profilometry as an adjunct to bladder neck reconstruction. J Urol 1986; 136:1055.

Gearhart JP, Yang A, Leonard MP, et al: prostate size and configuration in adults with bladder exstrophy. J Urol 1993d; 149:308.

Geist D: Patent urachus. Am J Surg 1952; 84:118.

Glenn JR: Agenesis of the bladder. JAMA 1959; 169:2016.

Gokcora IH, Yazar T: Bilateral transverse iliac osteotomy in the correction of neonatal bladder exstrophy. Int Surg 1989; 74:123.

Gross RE, Cresson SL: Exstrophy of the bladder: Observations from eighty cases. JAMA 1952; 149:1640.

Hammond G, Yglesias L, David JE: The urachus, its anatomy and associated fasciae. Anat Rec 1941; 80:271.

Hanna MK, Williams DJ: Genital function in males with vesical exstrophy and epispadias. Br J Urol 1972; 44:1969.

Hanna MK: Artificial urinary sphincter for incontinent children. Urology 1981; 18:370.

Hartmann R, Schuberg LGE, Bichler KH: Bladder exstrophy and cancer. Aktuel Urol 1984; 15:116.

Harvard BM, Thompson GJ: Congenital exstrophy of the urinary bladder: Late results of treatment by the Coffey-Mayo method of ureterointestinal anastomosis. J Urol 1951; 65:223.

Hector A: Les vestiges de l'ouraque et leur pathologie. J Chir (Paris) 1961; 81:449.

Heitz-Boyer M, Hovelaque A: Creation d'une nouvelle vessie et d'une nouvelle uretre. J Urol 1912; 1:237.

Hendren WH: Exstrophy of the bladder: An alternative method of management. J Urol 1976; 115:195.

Hendren WH: Penile lengthening after previous repair of epispadias. J Urol 1979; 12:527.

Hendren WH: Congenital female epispadias with incontinence. J Urol 1981; 125:58.

Hendren WH: Ileal nipple for continence in cloacal exstrophy. J Urol 1992; 148;372.

Herbst WP: Patent urachus. South Med J 1937; 30:711.

Higgins CC: Exstrophy of the bladder: Report of 158 cases. Am Surg 1962; 28:99.

Hinman F Jr: Surgical disorders of the bladder and umbilicus of urachal origin. Surg Gynecol Obstet 1961; 113:605.

Howell C, Caldamone A, Snyder H, et al: Optimal management of cloacal exstrophy. J Pediatr Surg 1983; 18:365.

Hurwitz RS, Manzoni GA, Ransley PG, Stephens FD: Cloacal exstrophy: A report of 34 cases. J Urol 1987; 138:1060.

Husmann DA, McLorie GA, Churchill BM: A comparison of renal function in the exstrophy patient treated with staged reconstruction vs. urinary diversion. J Urol 1988; 140:1204.

Husmann DA, McLorie GA, Churchill BM: Closure of the exstrophic bladder: An evaluation of the factors leading to its success and its importance on urinary continence. J Urol 1989a; 142:522.

Husmann DA, McLorie GA, Churchill BM: Phallic reconstruction in cloacal exstrophy. J Urol 1989b; 142:563.

Ives E, Coffey R, Carter CO: A family study of bladder exstrophy. J Med Genet 1980; 17:139.

Janssen P: Die operation der blasnektopic ohne inanspruchnahme des intestinums. Zentralbl Chir 1933; 60:2657.

Jeffs RD, Charrios R, Many M, Juransz AR: Primary closure of the exstrophied bladder. *In* Scott R, ed: Current Controversies in Urologic Management. Philadelphia, W. B. Saunders Company, 1972, p 235.

Jeffs RD, Guice SL, Oesch I: The factors in successful exstophy closure. J Urol 1982; 127:974.

Jeffs RD, Schwartz GR: Ileal conduit urinary diversion in children: Computer analysis follow-up from 2 to 16 years. J Urol 1975; 114:285.

Johnston JH: Vesical diverticula without urinary obstruction in childhood. J Urol 1960; 84:535.

Johnston JH: Lengthening of the congenital or acquired short penis. Br J Urol 1974; 46:685.

Kandzari SJ, Majid A, Ortega AM, Milam DF: Exstrophy of the urinary bladder complicated by adenocarcinoma. Urology 1974; 3:496.

Kapoor R, Saha MM: Complete duplication of the bladder, common urethra and external genitalia in the neonate: A case report. J Urol 1987; 137:1243.

Kenigsberg K: Infection of umbilical artery simulating patient urachus. J Pediatr 1975; 86:151.

Klauber GT, Williams DI: Epispadias with incontinence. J Urol 1974; 111:110.

Koff SA, Eakins M: The treatment of penile chordee using corporeal rotation. J Urol 1984; 131:931.

Kossow JH, Morales PA: Dupication of bladder and urethra and associated anomalies. Urology 1973; 1:71.

Kramer SA: Augmentation cystoplasty in patients with exstrophy-epispadias. J Pediatr Surg 1989; 24:1293.

Kramer SA, Jackson IT: Bilateral rhomboid flaps for reconstruction of the external genitalia in epispadias-exstrophy. Plast Reconstr Surg 1986; 77:621.

Kramer SA, Kelalis PP: Assessment of urinary continence in epispadias: A review of 94 patients. J Urol 1982a; 128:290.

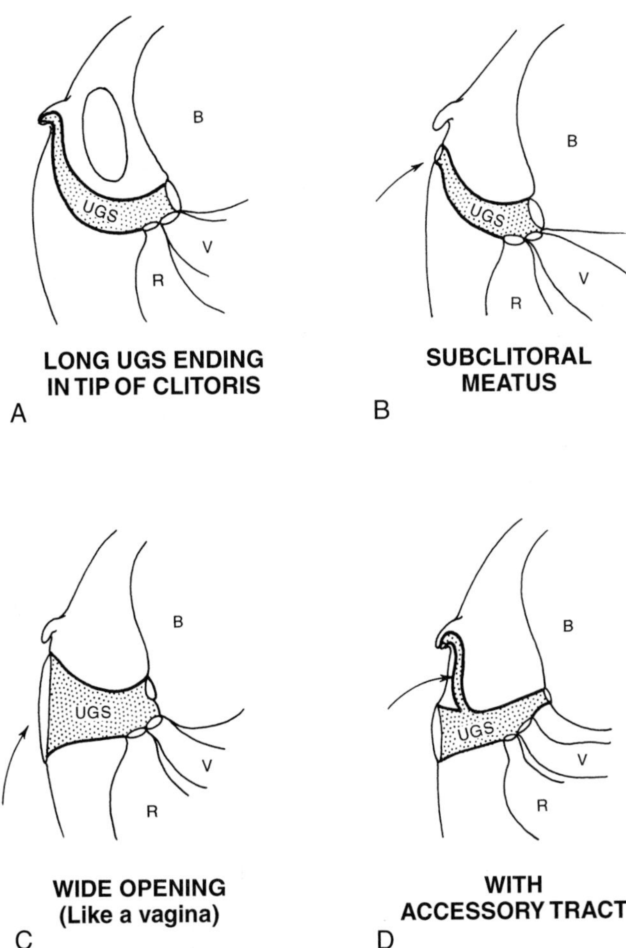

Figure 64–2. Urogenital sinus (UGS) variations, which can differ widely. *A,* A long urogenital sinus, which ends in a small aperture at the tip of the phallic structure. This finding is usually associated with a severe cloacal malformation. Cutting the UGS back a few millimeters at birth facilitates endoscopy and intermittent catheterization to decompress the lower urinary tract. *B,* Subclitoral meatus. *C,* A wide opening of the UGS. This opening will need to be tapered to construct a urethra from it. *D,* A rare variant showing a nonfunctional accessory tract leading forward from the UGS to the tip of the phallus. It should be marsupialized at the time of a definitive reconstruction.

the urogenital sinus. In others, there is a high confluence, so that all three systems—bladder, vagina, and rectum—converge at the same high level. Similarly, these structures may converge in the trigone of the bladder, so that there is no bladder neck, which poses an even greater task for the reconstructive surgeon.

Vagina

Great variability is found in the vaginal anatomy (Fig. 64–4). It is important to define this anatomy preoperatively. In 60 cases, a single vagina with a single uterine cervix was found. However, in 55 cases, two vaginas were discovered, and these vaginas can vary greatly in their anatomy. Most commonly, the two vaginas lie side by side with a midline septum between them. They can be easily converted into a single vaginal passage by incising the center of the septum with a cutting electrode, from its lower end up to the level of the two cervices, which lie on each side of the septum at the apex of the two vaginas. In some cases, the lower vaginas are adjacent but soon diverge, one to each side of the pelvis. Rarely, two separate ostia are present, each entering separately into the side walls of the urogenital sinus.

Other variations include the absence of a vagina but the presence of its uterus, and the absence of both the vagina and the uterus. There was no vagina in 20 of the author's cases. When there are two separate vaginas, they can sometimes be joined into one. In other cases, it may be better to retain one and remove the other. Sometimes the vagina is very large. In other cases, however, it can be small, offering no chance for bringing it to the perineum except by using an extension of bowel.

The technique of creating a bowel extension for a vagina has been described previously (Hendren, 1986). The segment of bowel to be used is brought down to the perineum between the opening for the urethra and the anus, employing a combined abdominal-perineal access. When the bowel segment has been joined to the perineum, the short vagina is anastomosed to it in end-to-end or end-to-side fashion, depending on the length of the bowel segment and the size of the vagina. If colon is used for this, it may be the part that was the previously dilated terminal rectal segment, and the next higher level of bowel is used for the pull-through procedure. Conversely, if the lower colon is well suited as rectum, a piece of sigmoid colon may be brought down as the extension for the vagina. Alternatively, an isolated segment of small bowel can be used to extend the vagina if the colon is not adaptable for that purpose. The caliber of small bowel is too narrow and should be tailored to double its width, a process that has been described previously (Hendren and Atala, 1994).

Lower Rectum

The most common location for entry of the rectum into a cloaca is at the posterior margin of the vaginal orifice, as shown in Figure 64–5, or at the base of the vaginal septum, when one exists. Usually, the dilated terminal colon is located just above the entry site. Occasionally, the fistula is a long tract running the full length of the vagina, so that the dilated lower colon is high in the pelvis and enters just behind the uterus. The relationship of the rectal fistula and the vaginas can be transposed, so that the rectal opening lies anterior to the single or duplicated vaginal openings. Obviously, it is very important for the surgeon to work out such anatomic vagaries preoperatively to guide the operative repair of the anomaly.

Urinary Tract

Vesicoureteral reflux is common in these patients. The ureter often enters laterally without a suitable tunnel, as seen routinely in patients with exstrophy of the bladder after primary bladder closure. In other cases, the ureters may be located ectopically too close to the bladder neck. A wide variety of other associated problems has been encountered, including ureterocele, megaureter, ureteropelvic junction ob-

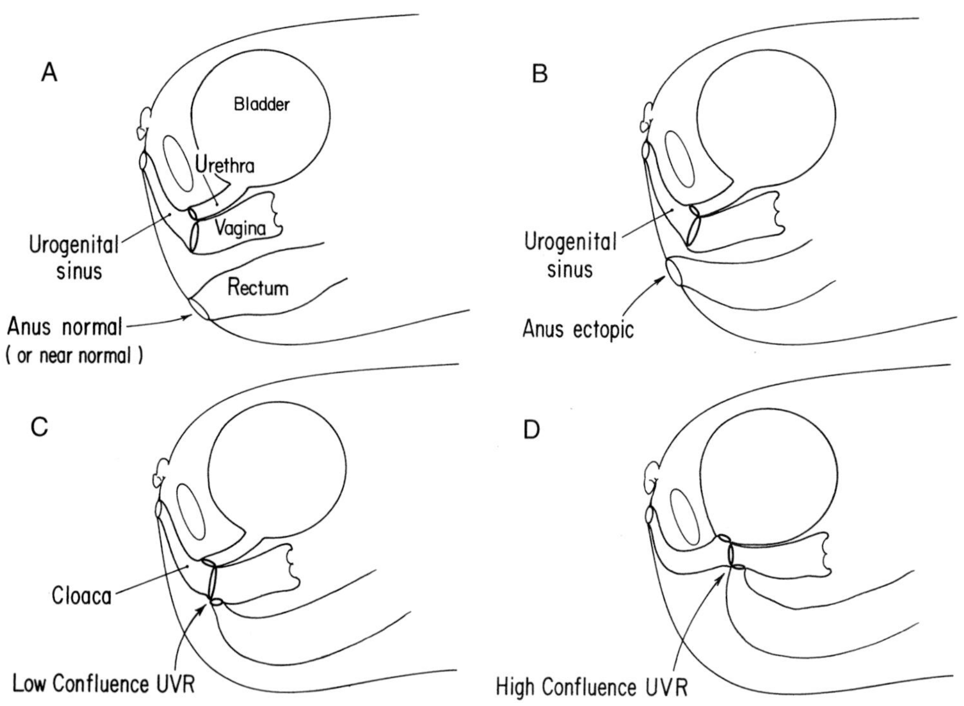

Figure 64–3. The spectrum of anatomy seen in urogenital sinus and cloacal malformations. *A,* The rectum in normal position. *B,* The anorectal canal clearly farther forward than normal but not actually joining the urogenital sinus. *C,* Low cloacal malformation, which can usually be repaired through a posterior sagittal approach. *D,* High confluence of the three organ systems, which may require an abdominal approach as well.

struction, and so forth. The urologic aspects of cloacal malformations are life threatening if not properly managed.

In the past, many of these children underwent abdominal-perineal pull-through procedures of the rectum to allow them to have bowel movements from below; correction of the genitourinary problems was deferred. This practice led to disastrous consequences with the upper urinary tracts when there was massive reflux with infection. It is the author's firm conviction that in some of these patients the first requirement is a urologic procedure early in life, such as correction of reflux; the genital and gastrointestinal tracts can be dealt with later. Occasionally, when the urologic aspects of a case have been mild, the author and his associates have elected to deal with the major cloacal reconstruction first (i.e., the urogenital sinus, vagina, and colon) and with the urologic problem later. However, this writer is

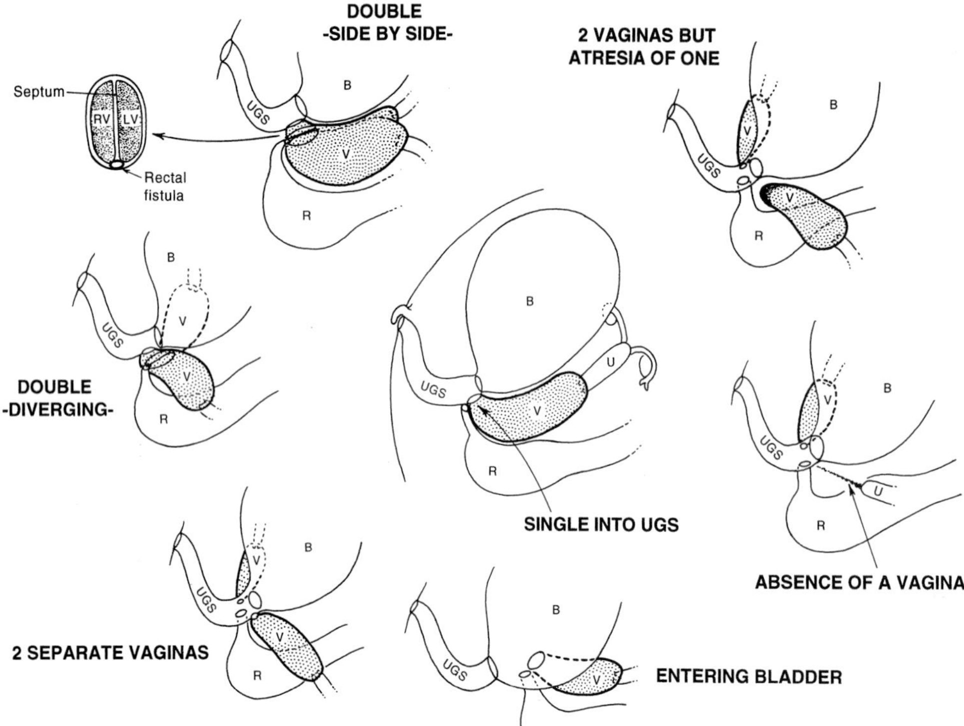

Figure 64–4. Variations in vaginal anatomy in cloacal malformations. Most commonly, there is a single vagina entering the urogenital sinus (UGS), with the rectal fistula entering at 6 o'clock adjacent to it or just inside the vaginal opening. As shown, there can be two vaginas side by side; two vaginas that diverge laterally; two separate vaginas, each with its own opening into the UGS; atresia of a vagina; absence of a vagina, but presence of a uterus on that side; and entry of the vagina, or two vaginas, directly into the bladder. (B, bladder; V, vagina; R, rectum.)

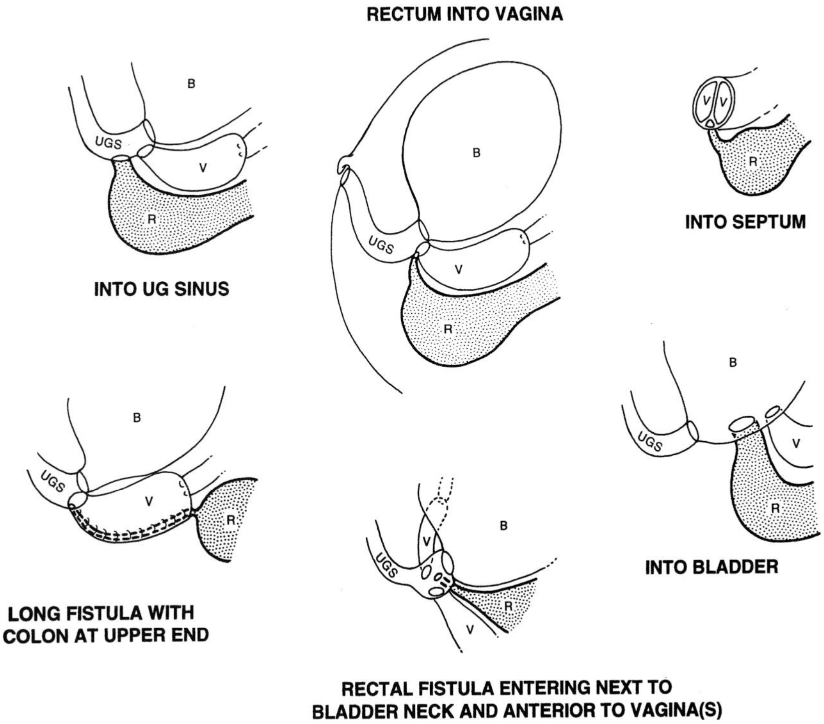

Figure 64–5. Variations in the rectal anatomy in cloacal malformations. Most commonly, the rectum enters at 6 o'clock in the vaginal orifice. When there are two vaginas, it usually enters at the base of the intervaginal septum. Rarely, the rectum opens into the urogenital sinus distal to the opening of the vagina. Occasionally, there is a long fistula, which opens in the usual location, but the actual rectal segment to be mobilized and pulled through is much higher. The rectal fistula can lie adjacent to the bladder neck, anterior to the vaginal opening(s). The bowel may enter the bladder itself, usually seen in cases with severely deranged anatomy. (B, bladder; R, rectum; UGS, urogenital sinus; V, vagina.)

firmly convinced that there is absolutely no place today for an isolated rectal pull-through reconstruction early in life, deferring the more difficult aspects of the anomaly until later, "when the child grows up."

MANAGEMENT OF THE NEWBORN WITH CLOACAL MALFORMATION

At birth, or soon thereafter, the female infant with a severe cloacal malformation usually presents with abdominal distention and is noted to have an abnormal perineum characterized by imperforate anus and variable development of an external opening and labia. In the most severe cases, the phallus is similar to the primitive genital tubercle of the early embryo. At first, some of these infants are thought to be sexually ambiguous. However, an infant with this appearance is a genetic female with a cloacal malformation.

Plain radiographs of the abdomen often show a large, fluid-filled structure in the lower abdomen, as seen in Figure 64–6. In some patients, this structure is the bladder, but more often it is a very distended vagina (or vaginas) filled with urine. If diagnosis is delayed for a day or two, air may enter this structure, confusing the picture further if the clinician is not aware of the cloacal malformation.

Decompressive colostomy should be performed immediately. The location of the colostomy, in the author's opinion, should be in the right upper quadrant to maintain intact the blood supply of the left colon, sigmoid colon, and rectum. This approach will provide greater flexibility during a definitive reconstructive operation later. The colostomy should be divided to prevent continuing spillover of fecal material into the distal colon, which communicates with the urogenital sinus. It is tempting to perform an exploratory laparotomy simultaneously to view the pelvic organs; however, the author thinks this procedure should be avoided to minimize the extent of the laparotomy for the distended infant and to avoid creating more postoperative bowel adhesions, which can cause intestinal obstruction.

Decompression of the Urinary Tract

In some patients with cloacal anatomy, the urogenital sinus is not obstructed, the infant empties the bladder easily, and the vagina is not dilated. In many of these cases, however, decompression of the urinary tract is needed urgently. Typically, the vagina is distended, pushing the bladder forward and causing severe hydronephrosis, as shown in Figure 64–7.

Intermittent catheterization is begun immediately to see if it will decompress the lower urinary tract. This procedure can be done with a small plastic catheter or a small metal catheterizing sound. It may be necessary to cut back the urogenital sinus a few millimeters to facilitate catheterization. Almost invariably the catheter enters the distended vagina, not the bladder, because the passage into the bladder is angulated forward sharply, allowing the catheter to pass more easily into the vagina.

In some neonates, the author and his colleagues have performed endoscopy immediately after the colostomy, introducing a No. 5 Fr plastic feeding catheter into the vagina and another into the bladder to decompress both structures. This procedure can be accomplished by passing a No. 8 Fr endoscope through the urogenital sinus into the vagina, removing the telescope, and passing the No. 5 Fr plastic catheter through it. The wide end of the catheter is cut off so that the endoscopic sheath can be withdrawn, leaving the catheter in place.

After the distended vagina is decompressed, the same

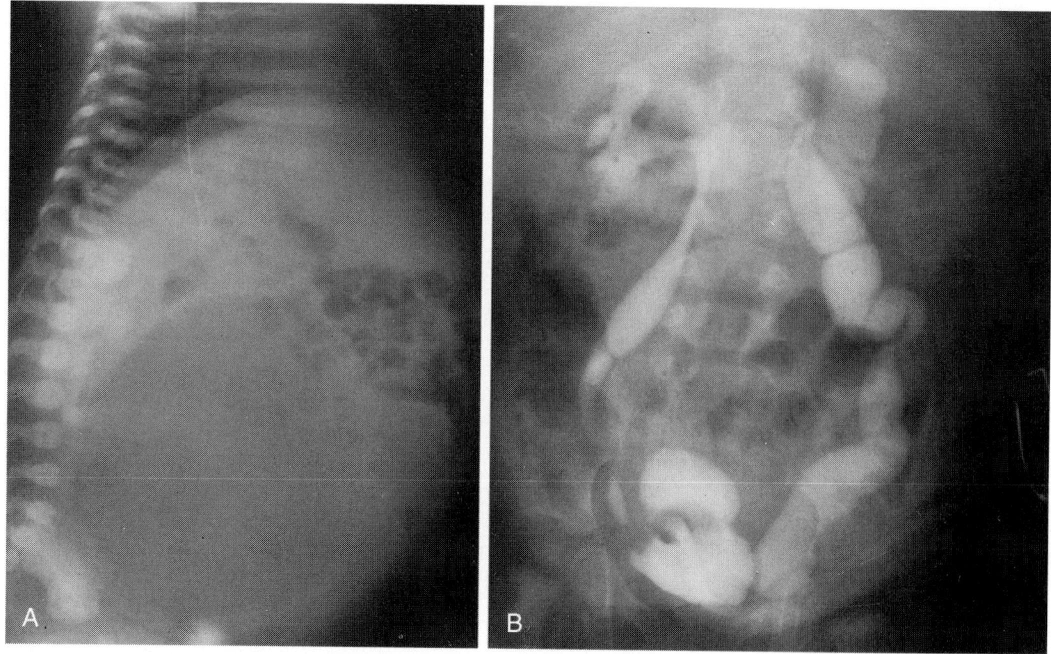

Figure 64–6. Roentgenograms from a typical cloacal case. *A,* Plain film showing large, rounded structure in lower abdomen. This structure was the vagina. *B,* Subsequent intravenous pyelogram after colostomy and decompression of the urinary tract, showing bilateral hydroureteronephrosis.

maneuver can be repeated for the bladder. The two tubes are fastened in place, thereby securing good drainage for several days until the infant's course is stabilized and the colostomy begins to function. These tubes also allow introduction of contrast medium into the bladder and vagina to delineate the anatomy. The rectal anatomy can be demonstrated by introducing contrast medium into the distal limb of the colostomy.

If intermittent catheterization of the distended vagina fails to decompress the lower urinary tract, vesicostomy and/or tube vaginostomy can be considered. However, the author and his group believe that these measures have been used more than needed. The author treated two infants for whom vesicostomy had been performed at birth. In these infants there was obstruction of the urogenital sinus because it was tethered across the pubic symphysis by the vesicostomy, which had been performed high to avert prolapse of the bladder—a known complication of vesicostomy. The author

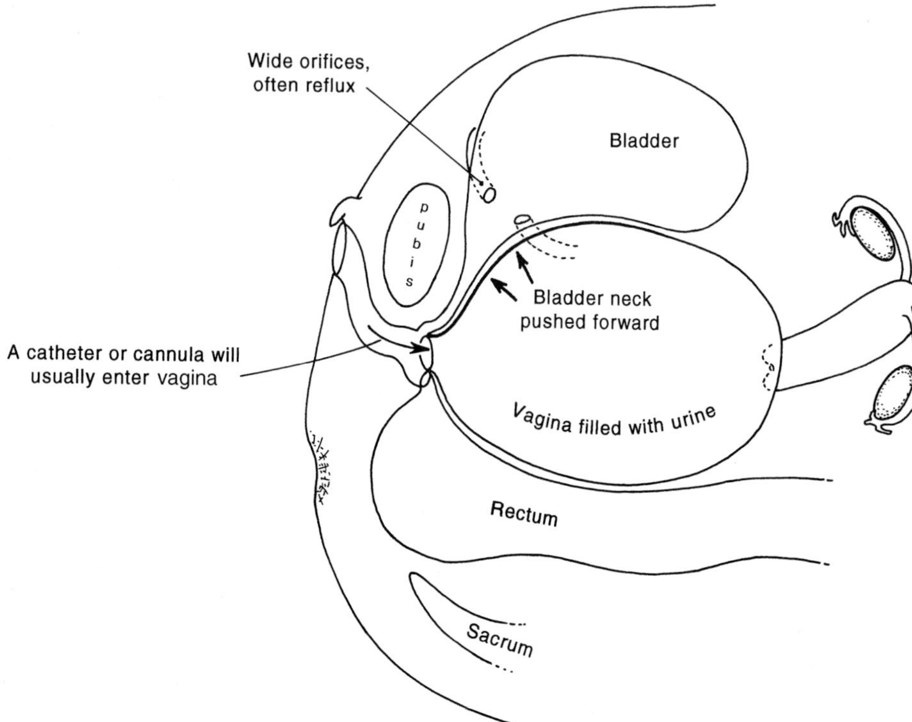

Figure 64–7. Obstruction of the lower urinary tract by compression from vagina, which fills with urine in some cloacal malformations. At endoscopy, it may prove impossible to visualize the urethra or bladder neck until passing the endoscope into the vagina to drain it. During cystoscopy, the anterior displacement of the bladder is readily apparent. Ureteral orifices are often laterally placed and wide in caliber, consistent with reflux. Alternatively, they can be normal in appearance and location, or they can be ectopic near the bladder neck.

also treated an infant in whom the distended vagina had been exteriorized in the anterior midline under the mistaken impression that it was the bladder. This procedure deformed the right side of the bladder and its ureter, causing right hydronephrosis. Vesicostomy had been performed later in that patient, resulting in an unusual situation in which there was a vaginostomy in the lower anterior midline and a vesicostomy superior to it.

Diagnostic Imaging

Radiologic findings and imaging recommendations in cloacal patients have been described (Jaramillo et al, 1990). The upper urinary tract can be studied by ultrasound examination or intravenous pyelogram if necessary. Contrast medium introduced into the urogenital sinus should disclose its anatomy and its relationship to the bladder neck, vagina(s), and rectal fistula. Contrast medium can be introduced into the distal limb of the colostomy to study the point of entry of the gastrointestinal tract into the cloaca. In a secondary case in which vesicostomy or vaginostomy has been performed, those openings can also be used for introduction of contrast medium.

These examinations are time consuming. The greater the experience of the radiologist, the higher the yield of information. Since the advent of magnetic resonance imaging (MRI) of the lumbosacral spine, this examination has become routine to exclude the presence of tethering of the spinal cord. Normally, the spinal cord ends at the level of the first lumbar vertebra. If it is tethered to a lower level, sometimes with an associated lipoma of the spinal canal, it can produce a neurologic deficit. Neurosurgical release of the spinal cord may prove helpful in preventing such a deficit. Once a deficit is established, it is unlikely to be improved if the cord is detethered (Warf et al, 1993). One third of cases have spinal cord tethering, but all patients with the related anomaly, cloacal exstrophy, have tethering. The experience of the author and his associates with that group of malformations was reported recently (Lund and Hendren, 1993).

Endoscopic Evaluation

An unhurried endoscopic examination is mandatory before the physician embarks on the definitive correction of a cloacal malformation. If the vagina fills when the endoscope is introduced into the urogenital sinus, it can displace the bladder neck so far forward that visualization of the bladder entry is impossible. In this instance, the bladder and vagina should be emptied, and the endoscope should be passed again along the anterior wall of the urogenital sinus, looking for the opening to the bladder just anterior to the opening of the vagina. When the rectal fistula is identified, it is convenient to pass a ureteral catheter through it, turning the endoscope 180 degrees so that its beak points backward. This technique usually allows it to enter the rectal fistula, permitting visualization of the interior of the colon.

If there is old fecal material or impacted mucus in the distal colon, it should be cleaned out to prevent contamination of the operative field during subsequent reconstructive surgery. Impacted fecal material can be washed out from above, through the distal limb of the colostomy, or from below, by directing the endoscope up through the rectal fistula, washing from below upward and irrigating the material out through the colostomy. It is important to use a physiologic salt solution for such prolonged irrigation of the colon, not water, which can be absorbed and may cause water intoxication.

If the patient has undergone a simple loop colostomy, there may be an enormous amount of fecal impaction in the distal colon segment. Thorough cleansing can take several hours and a very large volume of irrigating fluid. It is better to spend this time cleaning the bowel properly than to proceed with stool in the bowel. Forceful to and fro irrigation using an Ellik evacuator can break up and wash out inspissated fecal material. By adhering rigidly to this principle, wound contamination and pelvic sepsis can be avoided in cloacal reconstructions.

This type of prolonged endoscopy should precede a definitive operation by several days to give the child ample time to recover fully from the anesthetic. In some particularly complex malformations, it has been helpful to invite the radiologist into the operating room to study the patient with a C-arm fluoroscopy device. As each orifice entering the urogenital sinus is visualized endoscopically, a catheter is introduced and contrast medium is instilled. The events are recorded radiographically, and the information is correlated with the endoscopy findings.

DEFINITIVE REPAIR OF CLOACAL MALFORMATIONS

Reconstructions of cloacal malformations are usually long and difficult and should be deferred until the child is about 1 year of age, so that she will be better able to withstand major surgery. In addition to the preliminary washout of the defunctioned distal colon, the proximal bowel is prepared by giving the infant clear liquids by mouth the day before surgery and administering GoLytely gastrointestinal lavage solution (Braintree Laboratories, Braintree, MA). Expert anesthesiology is mandatory and includes monitoring blood gases, acid-base balance, arterial pressure, serial hematocrit determinations, and urine output. Latex allergy is being encountered and recognized today in some children who undergo multiple operations. Therefore, the author's group now avoids exposing these patients to latex. They are routinely placed on "latex alert," and latex gloves, tubes, drains, and so on are avoided (Holzman, 1993). Latex allergy can precipitate life-threatening bronchospasm intraoperatively.

No muscle relaxants are used in these patients because they inhibit electrical stimulation of the muscle sphincters, which is important in the proper placement of the rectum. This prohibition includes even short-acting agents because if there is a lack of response after use of such drugs the surgeon has no way to judge whether the agent is not reversed or whether the muscle reflex is simply deficient. Nitrous oxide anesthesia is also avoided, even for induction of anesthesia, because it causes distention of the bowel, which can be very troublesome if it becomes necessary to enter the abdomen.

As shown in Figure 64–8, the patient is prepared and draped circumferentially, with the legs sterilely wrapped.

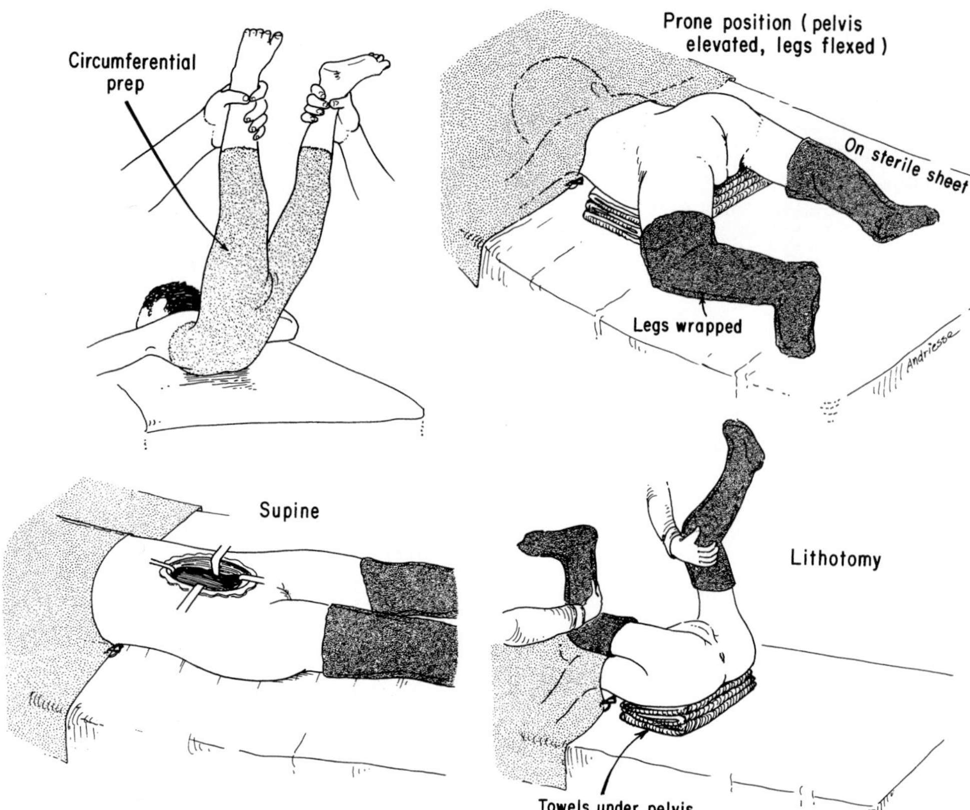

Figure 64–8. Preparation of patient to allow prone, supine, and lithotomy positions during operation. Note that the entire patient is circumferentially prepared, and the legs are sterilely wrapped. The patient is on a double thickness of sterile sheets. Beneath the sterile sheets are lamb's wool padding and a heating blanket. The upper sterile drape is clipped loosely enough so that the patient can be turned intraoperatively. After each turning, the exposed side is swabbed once again with povidone-iodine (Betadine) solution. A stack of sterile towels is placed beneath the patient when he or she is in prone or lithotomy positions.

The uppermost drapes in the surgical field are fastened loosely to allow the patient to be turned intraoperatively. This arrangement permits the surgeon to work on the patient in the supine position (through the abdomen); in the prone, jackknifed position (for posterior sagittal access); or in the lithotomy position. Frequently, all three positions are used in a given case. When the patient is turned, the arms and all attached monitoring lines and tubes are brought straight up above the head to allow turning without dislodging them. Two anesthesiologists remain at the head of the table during turning.

In the author's initial experience with cloacal reconstructive surgery, these operations were performed using a combined abdominal-perineal exposure, holding the patient's legs upward to work in the lithotomy position, and dropping them to gain access to the belly. Since 1982, after deVries and Peña (1982) emphasized the usefulness of the posterior sagittal position in correcting anorectal malformations, the author has used that approach in these cases (Peña, 1990). In a straightforward case in which there is a low confluence of all structures, the entire repair can be performed through a posterior sagittal approach, separating the rectum, vagina, and urogenital sinus and bringing each to the perineum. However, in some cases it is better to start in the abdomen if there has been a vesicostomy or vaginostomy, which tethers those structures upward, or if there is a very high entry of the rectum into the vagina or back wall of the bladder. Separation of the rectum in these circumstances may be more easily accomplished from above, later turning the patient and using the posterior sagittal approach for performing the actual reconstruction. In several patients with cloacal malformations the author and colleagues have encountered major anomalies of the abdominal aorta and its branches (Dykes et al, 1993). In two the abdominal aorta ran up to the navel and then branched into the iliac arteries. In two the iliac artery crossed the pelvis behind the bladder to supply the contralateral leg. It could be a disaster to divide such a vessel owing to failure to recognize this entity.

When commencing work in the posterior sagittal position, as shown in Figure 64–9, the perineum is electrically stimulated to mark the point of maximum contraction of the sphincter muscles at which the anus will be located. This point is marked boldly, using brilliant green dye and a toothpick or wooden applicator. Similarly, the locations for the perineal body, the vagina, and the urethra are marked.

A vertical midline incision is made in the gluteal cleft, progressing in the midline down to the underlying structures. The author finds it easier to stay in the exact midline by holding the buttocks apart with the thumb and third finger of the left hand. If two surgeons each hold a buttock apart with unequal tension, it is easy to stray from the midline. It is vital to place a metal sound in the urogenital sinus, holding it upward and dissecting down in the midline to the metal sound to approach the urogenital sinus, urethra or bladder neck, vagina, and rectum.

If the urogenital sinus is wide and needs to be tapered to construct a urethra of the proper size, the incision into it should start at the skin, proceeding upward from there until the openings of the other structures are identified. However, if the urogenital sinus is of the normal caliber for a urethra, it is preserved, incising it at a higher level where the converging structures will be found.

The rectal fistula usually enters the back wall of the vagina at 6 o'clock, but this is not always the case. If it

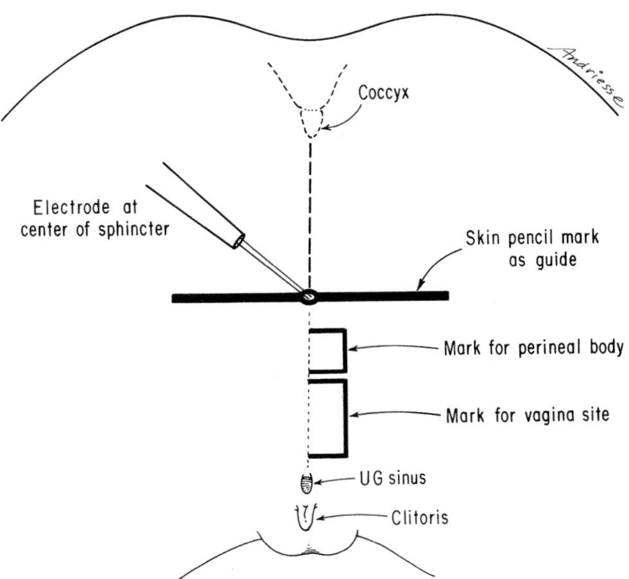

Figure 64–9. Identifying landmarks by electrical stimulation. It is helpful to mark heavily the line where anal sphincter contraction is maximal, renewing this marking intraoperatively as needed. Marks are placed also for the anticipated location of the perineal body and the vagina. These marks, together with visualization and stimulation of the muscle mass intraoperatively, are helpful in placing the three openings accurately. UG, urogenital.

enters very high, well above the level of the coccyx into the apex of the vagina, it may be impossible to reach it through the posterior sagittal approach. Also, the rectal fistula can enter adjacent to the bladder neck and anterior to the entry of the vagina, especially if there are two diverging vaginas. It is for this reason that it is so important to determine the anatomy preoperatively by appropriate imaging and endoscopy.

The author has encountered 11 cases in which no vagina was seen on preoperative imaging, including ultrasound examination, or on endoscopic study. A vagina was indeed present, but it did not communicate with the urogenital sinus. The surgeon must maintain a high degree of suspicion that such an occult vagina may be present. In one complex urogenital sinus case, a sigmoid vaginoplasty was performed, during which the presence of a small vagina was not appreciated. At menarche, a large midline blood-filled mass appeared, which was subsequently anastomosed to the previously reconstructed sigmoid vagina! Others have also noted genital tract complications at puberty in females with imperforate anus (Mollitt et al, 1981; Hall et al, 1985; Fleming et al, 1986).

The rectum can be freed in one of two ways. The first is to incise the back wall of the rectum, visualizing the fistula from its interior, circumscribing it, and then dissecting the rectum away from the vagina with the lower rectum open. The rectal wall should never be grasped with tooth forceps, which will cause damage during its mobilization. Instead, many fine silk sutures are placed along the cut edge to exert gentle traction. The author routinely employs this approach in ordinary imperforate anus cases, in which the rectum is being mobilized from the urethra or bladder neck in the male, or from the posterior vaginal fourchette in the female.

A second way to mobilize the rectum is to place a Foley catheter in its ostium, partially filling its balloon and securing it with purse-string sutures around the fistulous opening. The balloon catheter provides a convenient means of exerting traction on the rectal pouch while dissecting it from the surrounding tissues. Occasionally, it is helpful to inflate the rectum with air through the Foley catheter as an aid in identifying the plane of dissection. In patients undergoing reoperation, usually older patients, in whom the rectum is surrounded by scar tissue, it is very helpful to put an index finger into the rectal lumen as a guide in this dissection.

As a further precaution against contamination of the operative field, a povidone-iodine–soaked gauze sponge is placed in the rectal lumen to prevent possible soiling of the operative field despite thorough bowel preparation. In reoperative anorectal procedures employing these general principles, the author's group has been able to complete the procedure without performing a complementary colostomy. Virtually all previously unoperated cloacal patients have the original colostomy in place during the definitive reconstruction.

One of the most tedious parts of cloacal surgery is separating the vagina(s) from the bladder neck and posterior bladder wall. The vagina usually wraps halfway around the urogenital sinus and is closely related to the bladder neck. Partially opening the lower vagina and placing traction sutures on its edges is a great help in initiating this separation. It is useful to fill the bladder with saline solution or air to distend its wall to help identify this plane of cleavage. It is important not to inadvertently enter the back wall of the bladder or bladder neck because doing so will predispose the patient to development of a urinary tract fistula postoperatively. Thus, if either structure is to be violated during this dissection, it is better to make holes in the vagina, not the bladder.

The lateral attachments of the vagina must be dissected quite high to gain adequate length to bring it to the perineum. Surprisingly, the author has found that some vaginas, although large in size, do not come down easily to the perineum. Formerly, flaps of vaginal wall were used to reach the perineum, but these passages usually require enlarging at a later time. A short discrepancy in vaginal length can be overcome by making flaps from skin of the perineum. When there is a great gap, however, it is better to consider the use of a bowel segment to bridge the distance between the vagina and the perineum. The bowel segment can be taken from the lower rectum, the sigmoid colon, or even the terminal ileum.

The author performed a secondary reconstruction in a patient whose vagina had sloughed during a reconstruction elsewhere. Interposing a bowel segment between the pulled-through colon and the repaired urogenital sinus was difficult. When the vagina has been mobilized, its lateral walls are usually intact. Rotating the vagina so that an intact wall of vagina overlies the closure of the bladder neck and urogenital sinus will offer protection against the development of a fistula, which can occur with adjacent suture lines.

Some surgeons use cautery to separate these converging structures. Although it makes a bloodless dissection, the author prefers not to use cautery in order to avoid thermal burn of the tissues, which must heal per primum if fistulization is to be avoided. Therefore, he uses a sharp knife or fine scissors and optical magnification to perform these dissections, which have been accomplished to date without occurrence of a postoperative fistula.

Closure of the bladder neck and urogenital sinus is performed in two layers. The first layer is a running, inverted continuous suture of 4-0 or 5-0 polydioxanone suture (PDS). A second layer of adjacent muscle is closed over this using interrupted horizontal mattress sutures of the same material. In some cases, the urogenital sinus is of satisfactory caliber to be used as a urethra. In that case, it is opened only at its upper end, to accomplish separation of the rectum and vagina, and then is closed as described previously. However, if the urogenital sinus is a large, funnel-shaped passageway, it is opened fully. Later, its caliber is reduced by trimming the mucosa on each side and fashioning it into a urethra of appropriate size. The posterior sagittal approach not only allows very accurate division of the three organ systems but also ensures accurate placement of the structures within the pelvic muscles.

A segment of bowel can be used to extend the vagina in two ways. First, one can insert a large, stuffed drain of the appropriate size at the site where the bowel extension will be placed after the urogenital sinus is closed and the bowel is placed in its ideal position in the anorectal sphincter muscle. Turning the patient and using the abdominal approach, the bowel segment can be pulled through into the space temporarily occupied by the stuffed drain. The bowel segment is sewn to the perineum with the patient in the lithotomy position. Its upper end is anastomosed to the vagina in need of extension.

Alternatively, the bowel can be pulled down. The patient is turned once more to the prone position, and the bowel segment is sutured in place, completing the rectal pull-through. Then the patient is turned back to the supine position to finish the procedure in the abdomen. When the rectal pull-through is performed, dilated bowel is tapered to the appropriate size. If a higher segment of bowel that is not so dilated is used, the author sometimes simply imbricates its wall, in the manner described by Kalicinski and co-workers (1977) for the imbrication of the wall of a megaureter.

At the end of a cloacal reconstruction, the child's face is usually edematous from having been positioned in the prone jackknifed position. This problem is accentuated by the large fluid requirements needed to maintain satisfactory urinary output during these long procedures, particularly if abdominal surgery is required. Thus, it is routine for these children to spend the next day or two postoperatively in the intensive care unit, often with ventilatory support. For several days postoperatively they are kept flat, not partially upright, a position that can increase venous pressure in the pelvis and cause edema of the pelvic organs.

Postoperatively, the urinary tract is drained by a small straight plastic catheter placed in the urogenital sinus. The author does not use a Foley catheter for this drainage because he prefers to avoid having an inflated balloon adjacent to a repaired bladder neck and urogenital sinus. Relying on a balloon to hold the catheter in place can be risky because it may deflate. Similarly, inadvertent pulling of an inflated balloon through a repaired urogenital sinus could prove disastrous.

A straight catheter that is adequately secured is safer. If the abdomen was entered during the repair, a suprapubic tube is placed in the bladder as an additional means of drainage. Twelve days postoperatively, the urethral catheter is removed, and a "pull-out urethrogram" is obtained. This study confirms that the repair is intact. The child is then allowed to void, and the suprapubic tube is opened every 3 to 4 hours to estimate the amount of residual urine. If voiding is uneventful, the suprapubic tube is soon removed. Sometimes, however, these children are unable to void temporarily, or for a longer period of time.

The parents are instructed in the process of catheterization. When that is accomplished, the suprapubic catheter can be removed. If catheterization is not easy, parental instruction is delayed for at least another week to allow further healing of the repair. If catheterization continues to be difficult, endoscopy is performed gently to ascertain why catheterization is difficult. Sometimes a mucosal fold is blocking the passage of the catheter; this can be remedied by making an incision endoscopically. In some cases, the parent is brought to the operating room to observe the endoscopy on a television monitor. The parent passes the catheter while the child is asleep to become acquainted with the technique.

Cloacal surgery is long and difficult and must be performed meticulously if satisfactory results are to be achieved. It is important for the procedure to be performed by either a team of surgeons, who together have expertise in all of the organ systems involved and can work in a coordinated fashion, or by a single surgeon who is thoroughly conversant with surgery of the urinary tract, the genital tract, and the gastrointestinal tract.

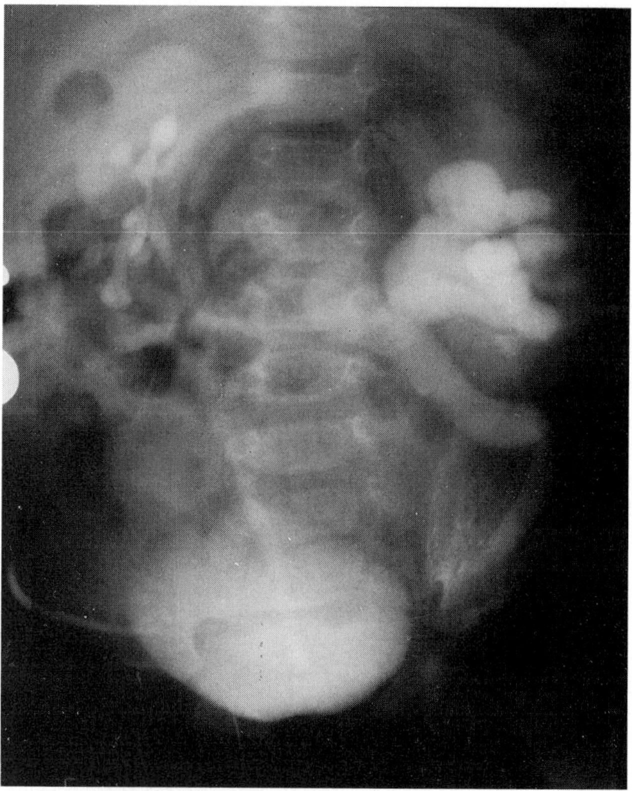

Figure 64–10. *(Case 1)* Intravenous pyelogram of patient as an infant, showing hydronephrosis. This condition disappeared after cutback of the urogenital sinus and intermittent catheterization of the vagina by the mother.

CASE STUDIES

The following cases illustrate most of the cardinal points required in cloacal reconstruction. It is important to realize that each case of cloacal malformation differs in some aspects from every other case. Nevertheless, the same general principles apply in dealing with all of them. These general principles include precise delineation of anatomy, separation of the three organ systems, and the need to bring each to the perineum without tension while avoiding adjacent suture lines, which can cause fistulization from one structure to another.

Case 1

An Uncomplicated Case Repaired Solely Through the Posterior Sagittal Approach. An infant was referred at age 16 months in 1986. Colostomy had been performed at birth. Urologic investigation showed severe hydronephrosis (Fig. 64–10), but this disappeared after intermittent catheterization of the vagina was begun. The anatomy, as shown in Figure 64–11, included two side-by-side vaginas and a rectal fistula opening at the base of the vaginal septum.

At operation, the intervaginal septum was incised endoscopically,

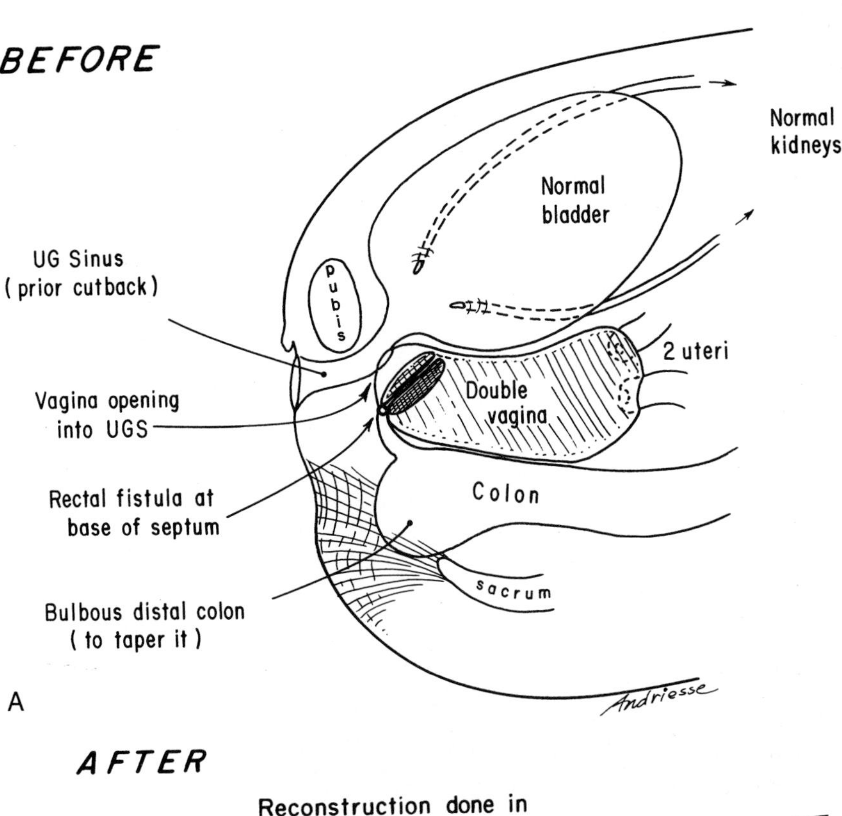

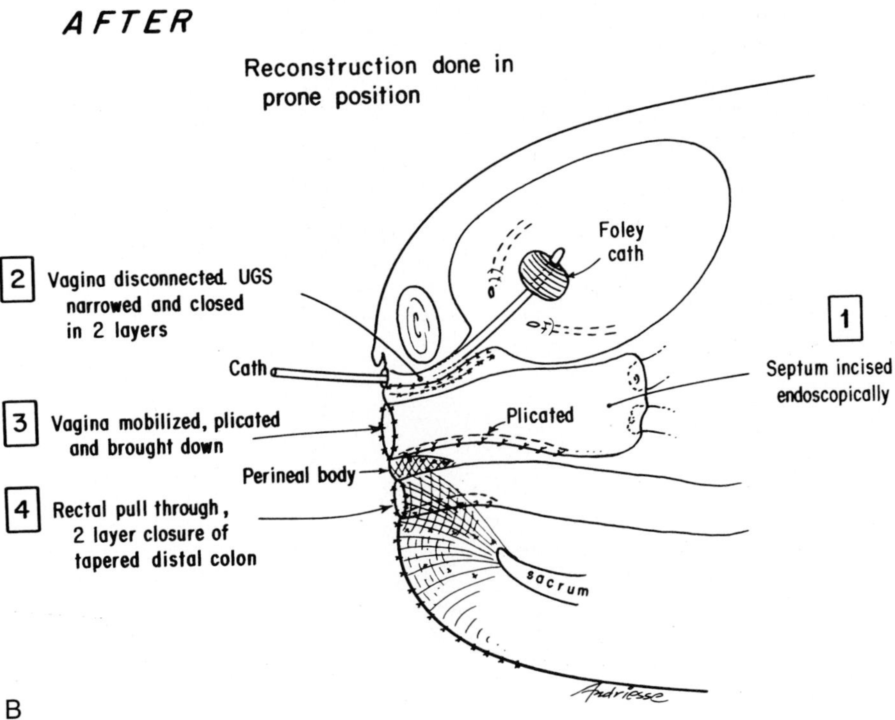

Figure 64–11. *(Case 1) A,* Preoperative anatomy showing moderately high confluence of the vaginas into urogenital sinus (UGS). *B,* After reconstruction, which was possible from a posterior sagittal approach with pull through of vagina and rectum, without need to enter abdomen.

converting it to a single passage. The vagina was disconnected from the urogenital sinus, which was narrowed and closed. After mobilization, the vagina was brought to the perineum, a perineal body was constructed, and the tapered rectum was pulled through to the perineum, closing the levators and sphincter muscles appropriately around it.

The patient was discharged from the hospital 12 days postoperatively. Her mother passed a 9- to 10- Hegar dilator into the vagina and rectum every day to prevent postoperative contracture. The colostomy was closed 3 months later. The patient is now 10 years old. She has normal urinary control and a normal upper urinary tract on intravenous pyelography. She required periodic soapsuds enemas initially to move her bowels but later established completely normal bowel control. Barium study showed a normal appearing rectum, as seen in Figure 64–12. MRI studies of the lumbosacral spine showed normal findings.

Comment. The anatomy in this child was very favorable for repair because she had no other serious problems and the hydronephrosis resolved on intermittent catheterization of the vagina. Preoperative and postoperative views of the perineum are shown in Figure 64–13.

Case 2

Cloaca with Diverging Vaginas and Rectal Fistula Anterior to Them. A 3-year-old girl was referred in 1988. Colostomy had been performed at birth. No urinary decompression was required because there was no obstructive uropathy; the patient was completely incontinent.

Evaluation showed a solitary, normal left kidney with compensatory hypertrophy. Cystogram showed a small-capacity bladder with an incompetent bladder neck and grade 3 reflux. MRI of the lumbosacral spine showed normal findings. Inspection revealed a large perineal opening that had the appearance of a normal vaginal introitus. Urine flowed freely from it. Endoscopically, two vaginal orifices were visible with a septum between them. The rectal opening was not immediately apparent but could be seen by injecting saline and air into the distal colostomy limb. It lay near the bladder neck and anterior to the two vaginas.

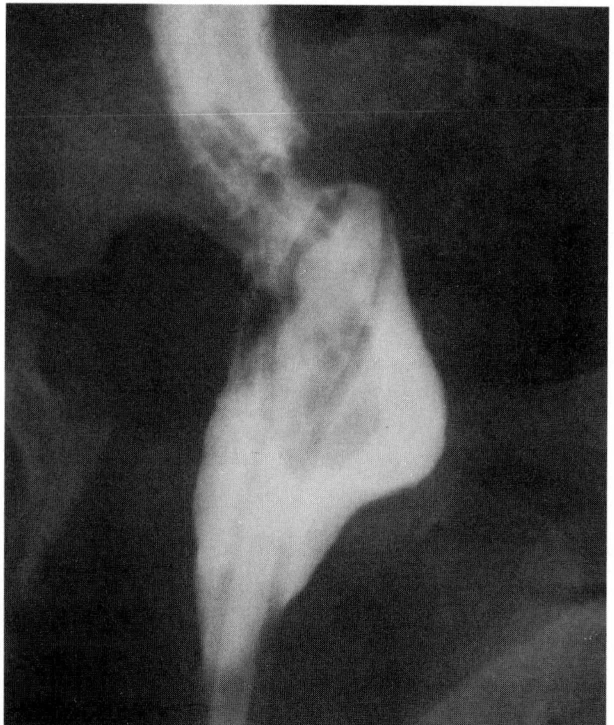

Figure 64–12. *(Case 1)* Postoperative barium enema showing normal rectum, with slight tapering of the back wall.

One week later, reconstructive surgery was performed, as seen in Figure 64–14. It was accomplished with the patient in the prone jackknifed position using a posterior sagittal approach. The two vaginas, colon, and bladder neck were separated. The coccyx and a cyst adjacent to it were removed. A urethra was constructed from the roof of the wide urogenital sinus. The two vaginas were opened, sewn together, and brought to the perineum. They were rotated 90 degrees to cover the urethra with an intact vaginal wall, thereby avoiding the presence of adjacent suture lines, which might fistulize. The perineal body was constructed. The dilated lower rectum was tapered, and the rectum was placed within the sphincter and levator muscles.

The urethral catheter was removed 2 weeks postoperatively. No difficulty with urinary retention occurred. The patient was discharged 3 weeks postoperatively on a program of daily dilatation of the anorectal canal and vaginal opening using a 10-Hegar dilator. When evaluated 9 months later, the patient had developed some continence from her new urethra, but grade 3 reflux into the ectopic ureter was present in the bladder neck. Nine months later a second operation was performed to close the colostomy. There was a 4:1 discrepancy in the size of the two limbs of the colostomy. The ectopic ureter was reimplanted diagonally across the back wall of the bladder, and a Young-Dees bladder neck lengthening and narrowing procedure was performed to gain more outlet resistance. The belly was a mass of intra-abdominal adhesions resulting from the original exploratory laparotomy in the neonatal period. An incidental cecal duplication was resected.

When the suprapubic tube was clamped intermittently 2 weeks later, the patient was able to void only small amounts. The mother was taught how to perform clean intermittent catheterization, and the suprapubic tube was removed. The patient was discharged 4 weeks postoperatively. She was soon able to void, and intermittent catheterization was discontinued. The mother reported normal urinary and bowel control 3 months later.

Comment. This child's cloacal malformation presented an entirely different technical problem from that described in Case 1. The vaginas could not be made into one by simply incising a vaginal septum. The author has encountered a case similar to this, in which the vaginas were too short to reach the perineum; thus, they were joined together and extended using a segment of bowel. Note also that this patient had essentially no effective urethra; the bladder neck emptied directly into the large urogenital sinus. The anterior position of the rectal opening was unusual but not rare. This case underscores the importance of defining the specific anatomy in each cloaca before embarking on its repair. The patient is now 10 years old, is dry, and has normal bowel control.

Case 3

Cloaca and Large Pelvic Tumor; Tube Diversion Since Birth. A 15-month-old girl was referred in 1987 with the unusual problem of a large sacrococcygeal teratoma and a cloacal malformation, as seen in Figure 64–15*A*. At birth, suprapubic cystostomy and left upper quadrant loop colostomy had been performed.

An aortogram showed displacement of the iliac vessels by the intrapelvic component of the tumor (Fig. 64–16*A*). Preoperative roentgenographic evaluation (Fig. 64–16*B*) showed high confluence of bladder, vagina, and rectum and a wide urogenital sinus. Reconstruction was performed as shown in Figure 64–15*B*.

Beginning with the patient in the prone jackknifed position, an elliptical incision was made around the teratoma, leaving the involved skin with it, and extending the incision forward to allow posterior sagittal exposure access. The coccyx was transected with

65
NEUROGENIC DYSFUNCTION OF THE LOWER URINARY TRACT IN CHILDREN

Stuart B. Bauer, M.D.

At least 25% of the clinical problems seen in pediatric urology are the result of neurologic lesions that affect lower urinary tract function. In the 1960s, urinary diversion was the mainstay of treatment for these children with either intractable incontinence or normal or abnormal upper urinary tracts (Smith, 1972). The advent of clean intermittent catheterization (CIC) in the early 1970s by Lapides (Lapides et al, 1972) and refinements in techniques of urodynamic studies in children (Gierup and Ericcson, 1970; Blaivas, et al, 1977; Blaivas, 1979) dramatically changed the way this pediatric population was traditionally managed. Along with this change came a greater understanding of the pathophysiology of the many diseases that affect children primarily. With the increased reliability of data collection, the applicability of urodynamic testing has expanded to the point where most pediatric urologic centers now believe that functional assessment of the lower urinary tract is an essential element in the evaluation process and is as important as x-ray visualization in characterizing and managing these abnormal conditions (McGuire et al, 1981; Bauer et al, 1984). The natural outcome of early functional investigation has been the advocacy of proactive or early aggressive management of children who are now considered at risk of urinary tract deterioration based on specific hostile urodynamic parameters (Perez et al, 1992; Edelstein et al, 1995; Kaufman et al, 1995). Because urodynamic testing has become such an integral part of any discussion of the subject, this chapter first defines the testing process as it applies to children, outlines its pitfalls and advantages, and then elaborates on the various neurourologic abnormalities that are prevalent in children.

URODYNAMIC EVALUATION

Before a urodynamic study is performed, it is important for the child and his family to have full knowledge of the procedure. Therefore, an explanation of the test and a questionnaire are sent to each family prior to the appointment. A booklet is provided so that parents will know what to expect and can explain the test to their child. If the child is old enough, he can read about it himself. Attempts are made to minimize the anxiety level in children who are able to understand what will happen by providing reasons for specific portions of the test and explaining exactly what the child will experience. The questionnaire tries to elicit information about the mother's pregnancy history, the child's birth and development, his or her current bladder and bowel habits, and any other information that might be pertinent at the time of the procedure.

Sometimes in very anxious children over 1 year of age, meperidine, 1 mg/kg of body weight, is administered intramuscularly to reduce the discomfort and anxiety level; this does not alter the child's level of cooperation or responsiveness (Ericsson et al, 1971). If at all feasible, however, no medication is given, but the child is conscientiously attended to in order to minimize his or her fears. Since 1993, EMLA cream, a topical anesthetic, has been applied to the perineum about 45 minutes before the electromyographic needle is inserted to record sphincter activity. If possible, the child is instructed to come to the urodynamic suite with a full bladder to obtain an initial representative uroflow. The time of the child's previous urination is noted to calculate an average rate of urine production per unit of time. In addition, this information allows the nurse to record a reliable residual urine volume when catheterizing the child after voiding. The flowmeter is located in a private bathroom that contains a one-way mirror so that voiding can be viewed unobtrusively. This allows the investigator to see if a Credé or Valsalva maneuver is employed by the individual to help empty the bladder.

Next, the nurse reviews the test and shows the child all the equipment in an attempt to make him or her feel as comfortable as possible. The child is catheterized with either a No. 7 or 11 Fr triple-lumen urodynamic catheter (Cook Urological Inc, Spencer, IN) after a small amount of liquid Xylocaine (1%) has been injected into the urethra and held in place for a moment or two. Then the residual urine is carefully measured. Sometimes it is necessary to aspirate the catheter to get accurate information on the volume of residual urine, especially if the bladder is hypotonic (particularly if the child is taking anticholinergic medication) or has been previously augmented and secretes mucus because it may not drain completely following insertion of a catheter.

A small balloon catheter is passed into the rectum at this time to measure intra-abdominal pressure during the cystometrogram to identify artifacts of motion and monitor increases in abdominal pressure during the filling and emptying phases of the study (Bates et al, 1970; Bauer, 1979). Uninhibited contractions and straining to empty can be clearly differentiated by this maneuver.

Prior to filling the bladder, a urethral pressure profile is sometimes obtained by infusing saline through the side-hole channel at a rate of 2 ml/minute as the catheter is withdrawn at a rate of 2 mm/second (Yalla et al, 1980). Some urodynamicists advocate using a balloon or microtipped transducer catheter to measure urethral resistance instead of a saline infusion (Tanagho, 1979). When the maximum resistance is known, the catheter is positioned so that the urethral pressure port is located at that or any other point of interest. This area can then be monitored throughout the urodynamic study.

Urethral pressure profilometry (UPP) measures the passive resistance of a particular point within the urethra to stretch (Gleason et al, 1974). Many factors contribute to this resistance, including the elastic properties of the tissues surrounding the lumen and the tension generated by the smooth and skeletal muscles of the urethra, which are constantly changing during the micturition cycle (Fig. 65–1) (Abrams, 1979; Evans et al, 1979). Thus, the static urethral pressure profile is a measure of resistance in a specific set of circumstances (Yalla et al, 1979). It is difficult to extrapolate data obtained when the bladder is empty and apply it to periods

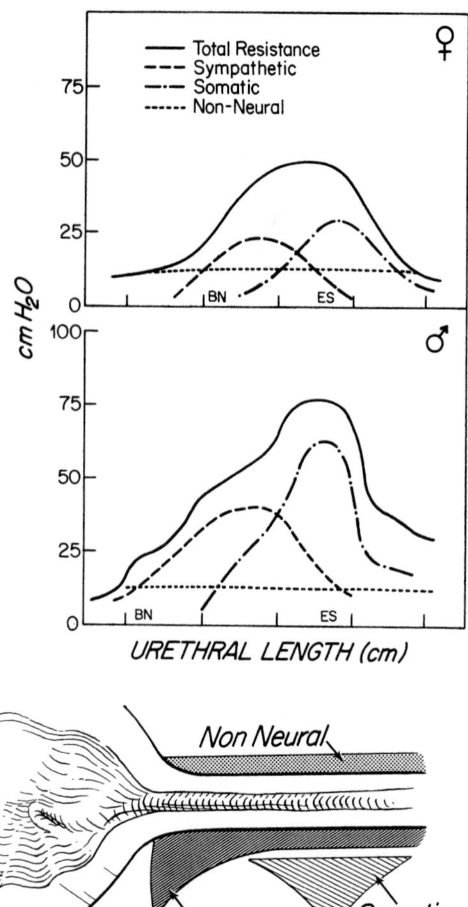

Figure 65–1. Components of urethral wall tension according to their geographic distribution and effect along the urethra in males and females (BN, bladder neck; ES, external sphincter). (From Bauer SB: Urodynamic evaluation and neuromuscular dysfunction. *In* Kelalis PP, King LR, Belman AB, eds: Clinical Pediatric Urology, 2nd ed, Vol I. Philadelphia, W. B. Saunders Company, 1985, pp 283–310.)

when the bladder is full, is responding to increases in abdominal pressure, or is in the process of emptying (Fig. 65–2). Failure to recognize this fact will lead to false assumptions and improper treatment.

External urethral sphincter electromyography (EMG) is performed using a 24-gauge concentric needle electrode (Diokno et al, 1974; Blaivas et al, 1977b) inserted perineally in males or paraurethrally in females and advanced into the skeletal muscle component of the sphincter until individual motor unit action potentials are seen or heard on a standard electromyographic recorder. Alternatively, perineal (Maizels and Firlit, 1979) or abdominal patch electrodes (Koff and Kass, 1982), or anal plugs (Bradley et al, 1974) have been used to record the bioelectric activity in the sphincter muscle. Disagreements exist between the accuracy of these surface electrode measurements versus needle electrodes, particularly during voiding. The intactness of sacral cord function is easily measured with needle electrodes by (1) looking at the characteristic wave form of individual motor unit action potentials when the patient is relaxed and the bladder empty, (2) performing and recording the responses to bulbocavernosus and anal stimulation and Credé and Valsalva maneuvers,

Table 65–5. TYPES OF OCCULT SPINAL DYSRAPHISMS

Lipomeningocele
Intradural lipoma
Diastematomyelia
Tight filum terminale
Dermoid cyst/sinus
Aberrant nerve roots
Anterior sacral meningocele
Cauda equina tumor

hammer or claw digits, a discrepancy in muscle size and strength from one leg to the other with weakness at the ankle and/or a gait abnormality, especially in older children, due to shortness of one leg (Dubrowitz et al, 1965; Weissert et al, 1989). Absent perineal sensation and back pain are not uncommon symptoms in older children or young adults (Linder et al, 1982; Yip et al, 1985; Weissert et al, 1989). Lower urinary tract function is abnormal in 40% of affected individuals (Mandell et al, 1980). The child may experience difficulty with toilet training, urinary incontinence after an initial period of dryness following toilet training (especially during the pubertal growth spurt), recurrent urinary infections, and/or fecal soiling. Occasionally, some patients without an obvious back lesion escape detection until they develop urinary symptoms after puberty owing to delayed traction on the spinal cord (Satar et al, 1995).

Findings

When these children are evaluated in the newborn period or early infancy, the majority are perfectly normal on neurologic examination (Atala et al, 1992). Urodynamic testing, however, reveals abnormal lower urinary tract function in about one third of babies under the age of 1½ years (Fig. 65–16) (Keating et al, 1988). In fact, these studies may provide the only evidence of a neurologic injury involving the lower spinal cord (Keating et al, 1988; Foster et al, 1990; Atala et al, 1992). When present, the most likely abnormality is an upper motor neuron lesion characterized by detrusor hyperreflexia and/or hyperactive sacral reflexes; mild forms of detrusor sphincter dyssynergy are rarely noted. Lower motor neuron signs with denervation potentials in the sphincter or detrusor areflexia occur in only 10% of young children.

In contrast, practically all individuals over 3 years of age who have not been operated on or in whom an occult dysraphism has been belatedly diagnosed have either an upper motor neuron or lower motor neuron lesion on urodynamic testing (92%) (see Fig. 65–16) or neurologic signs of lower extremity dysfunction (Yip et al, 1985; Kondo et al, 1986; Keating et al, 1988; Atala et al, 1992; Satar et al, 1995). There does not seem to be a preponderance of one type of lesion over the other (upper versus lower motor neuron); each occurs with equal frequency, and often the child shows signs of both (Kondo et al, 1986; Hellstrom et al, 1986; Satar et al, 1995).

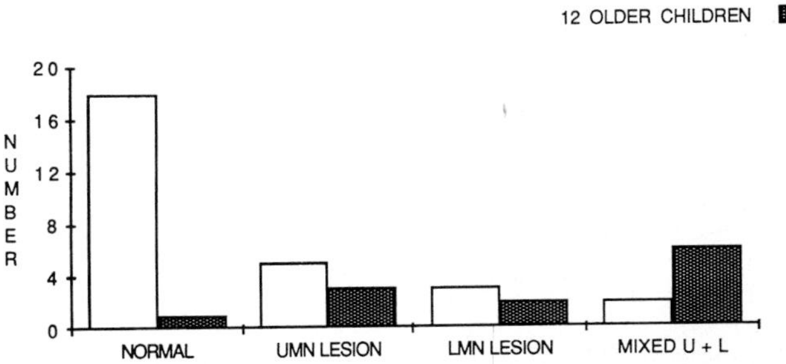

Figure 65–16. Most newborns with a covered spinal dysraphism have normal lower urinary tract function, whereas older children tend to have both upper (UMN) and lower motor neuron (LMN) lesions.

Pathogenesis

The reason for this difference in neurologic findings may be related to (1) compression on the cauda equina or sacral nerve roots by an expanding lipoma or lipomeningocele (Yamada et al, 1983) or (2) tension on the cord from tethering secondary to different growth rates in the bony vertebrae and neural elements (Dubrowitz et al, 1965). Under normal circumstances, the conus medullaris ends just below the L2 vertebra at birth and recedes upward to T12 by adulthood (Barson, 1970). When the cord does not "rise" because of one of these lesions, ischemic injury may ensue (Yamada et al, 1981). Correction of the lesion in infancy has resulted not only in stabilization but also in improvement in the neurologic picture in some instances (Fig. 65–17). Sixty percent of babies with abnormal urodynamic findings preoperatively revert to normal postoperatively, with improvement noted in 30%; 10% become worse with time. In older children there is a less dramatic change following surgery, with only 27% becoming normal, 27% improving, 27% stabilizing, but 19% actually becoming worse with time (see Fig. 65–17) (Keating et al, 1988; Satar et al, 1995). Older children with hyperreflexia tend to improve, whereas those with

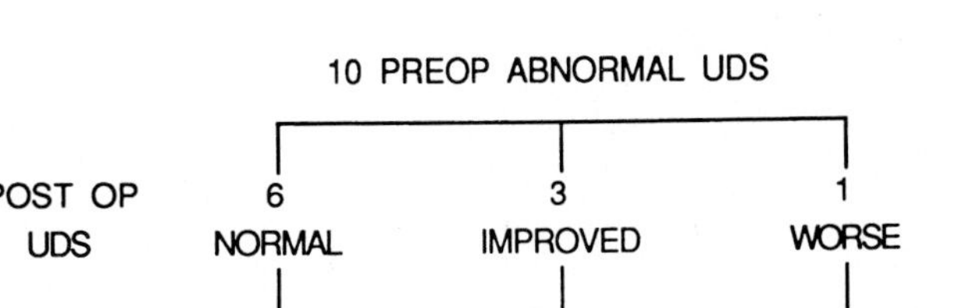

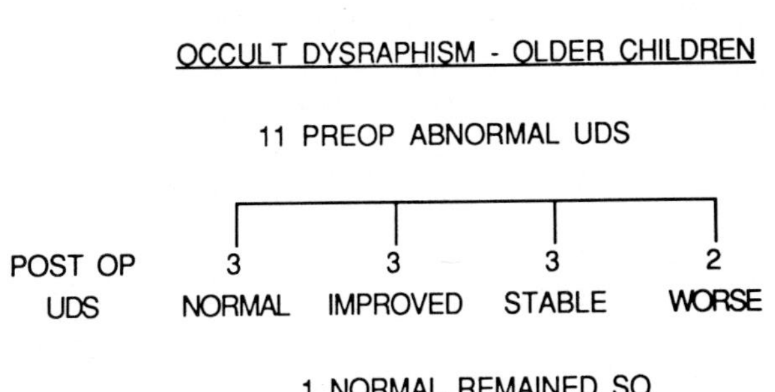

Figure 65–17. The potential for recoverable function is greatest in infants (6 of 10, 60%) and less so in older children (3 of 11, 27%). The risk of damage to neural tissue at the time of exploration to those with normal function is small (2 of 19, 11%). (UDS, urodynamic study.)

areflexic bladders do not (Kondo et al, 1986; Hellstrom et al, 1986; Flanigan et al, 1989). Finally, 20% of children operated on in early childhood develop secondary tethering when followed for several years, suggesting that early surgery has both beneficial and sustaining effects in patients with this condition (Satar et al, 1995a).

As a result of these findings, it is apparent that urodynamic testing may be the only way to document that an occult spinal dysraphism is actually affecting lower spinal cord function (Keating et al, 1988; Khoury et al, 1990). Some investigators have shown that posterior tibial somatosensory evoked potentials are an even more sensitive indicator of tethering and should be an integral part of the urodynamic evaluation (Roy et al, 1986). The implication of this lies in the fact that early detection and intervention can both reverse the progress of the lesion, which does not happen in the older child (Yamada et al, 1983; Tami et al, 1987; Kaplan et al, 1988) and offer a degree of protection from subsequent tethering, which seems to be a frequent occurrence when the lesion is not dealt with expeditiously in infancy (Chapman, 1982; Seeds and Jones, 1986).

Recommendations

Consequently, in addition to magnetic resonance imaging (MRI) (Tracey and Hanigan, 1990), urodynamic testing should be performed in everyone who has a questionable cutaneous or bony abnormality of the lower spine (Packer et al, 1986; Hall et al, 1988; Campobasso et al, 1988). If the child is less than 4 to 6 months of age, ultrasound may be useful to visualize the spinal canal before the vertebral bones have had a chance to ossify (Fig. 65–18) (Raghavendra et al, 1983; Scheible et al, 1983). In the past, these conditions were usually treated by removing only the superficial skin lesions without delving further into the spinal canal to remove or repair the entire abnormality. Today, most neurosurgeons advocate laminectomy and removal of the intraspinal process as completely as possible without injuring the nerve roots or cord to release the tether and prevent further injury with subsequent growth (Linder et al, 1982; Kondo et al, 1986; Kaplan et al, 1988; Foster et al, 1990; Atala et al, 1992).

Sacral Agenesis

Sacral agenesis has been defined as the absence of part or all of two or more lower vertebral bodies. The cause of this condition is still uncertain, but teratogenic factors may play a role because insulin-dependent mothers have a 1% chance of giving birth to a child with this disorder. Conversely, 16% of children with sacral agenesis have an affected mother (Passarge and Lenz, 1966; Guzman et al, 1983). Often the mothers may have only gestational insulin-dependent diabetes. The disease has been reproduced in chicks when their embryos were exposed to insulin (Landauer, 1945; White and Klauber, 1976). Recently, maternal insulin–antibody complexes have been noted to cross the placenta, and their concentration in the fetal circulation is directly correlated with macrosomia (Menon et al, 1990). It is possible that a similar cause-and-effect phenomenon occurs in sacral agenesis.

Diagnosis

The diagnosis is often delayed until failed attempts at toilet training bring the child to the attention of a physician. Sensation, including sensation in the perianal dermatomes,

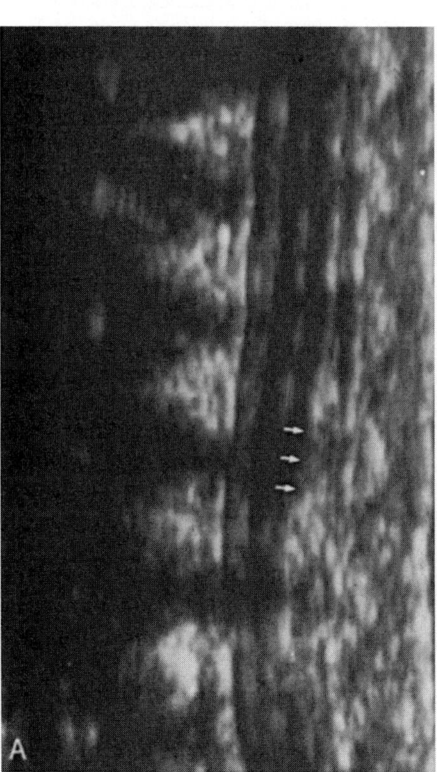

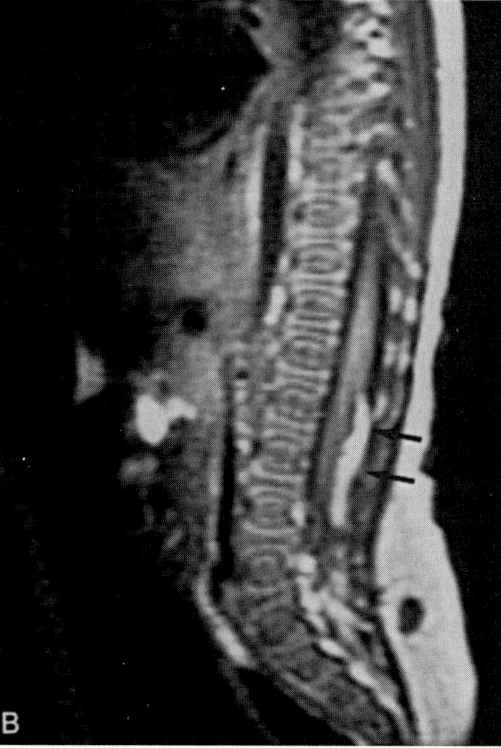

Figure 65–18. *A,* During the first few months of life, ultrasound can clearly demonstrate intravertebral anatomy because the posterior arches have not completely ossified. Note that the spinal cord along with its central canal is displaced anteriorly *(white arrows)* beginning at L-3 because of an intradural lipoma. *B,* The MRI is juxtaposed to confirm the ultrasound findings. The longitudinal white intraspinal mass is the lipoma; the longitudinal gray mass is the spinal cord.

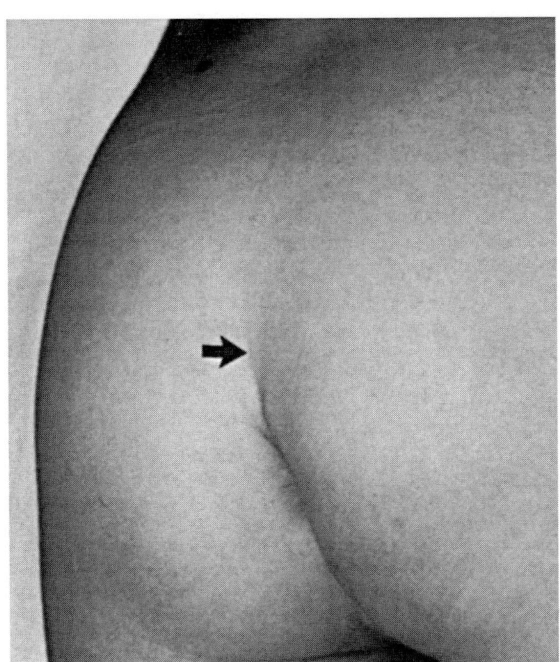

Figure 65–19. Characteristically, the gluteal crease is short and seen only inferiorly *(below arrow)* because of the flattened buttocks in sacral agenesis.

is usually intact, and lower extremity function is normal (Koff and DeRidder, 1977; Jakobson et al, 1985). Because these children have normal sensation and little or no orthopedic deformity in the lower extremities (although high arched feet or claw or hammer toes may be present), the underlying lesion is often overlooked. In fact, 20% of these children escape detection until the age of 3 or 4 (Guzman et al, 1983). The only clue, besides a high index of suspicion, is flattened buttocks and a low short gluteal cleft (Fig. 65–19) (Bauer, 1990). Palpation of the coccyx is used to detect the absent vertebrae (White and Klauber, 1977). The diagnosis is most easily confirmed with a lateral film of the lower spine because this area is often obscured by the overlying gas pattern on an anteroposterior projection (Fig. 65–20) (White and Klauber, 1976; Guzman et al, 1983). Recently, MRI has been used to visualize the spinal cord in these cases, and a sharp cut-off level of the conus seems to be a consistent finding (Fig. 65–21) (Pang, 1993).

Findings

On urodynamic studies an almost equal number of individuals manifest either upper or lower motor neuron lesions (35% versus 40%, respectively), whereas 25% have no signs of denervation at all (Guzman et al, 1983; Boemers et al, 1994). Upper motor neuron lesions are characterized by detrusor hyperreflexia, exaggerated sacral reflexes, absence of voluntary control over sphincter function, detrusor-sphincter dyssynergy, and no EMG evidence of denervation potentials in the sphincter (White and Klauber, 1976; Koff and DeRidder, 1977; Guzman et al, 1983). A lower motor neuron lesion is noted when detrusor areflexia and partial or complete denervation of the external urethral sphincter with diminished or absent sacral reflexes are seen. The presence or absence of the bulbocavernosus reflex is an indicator (but

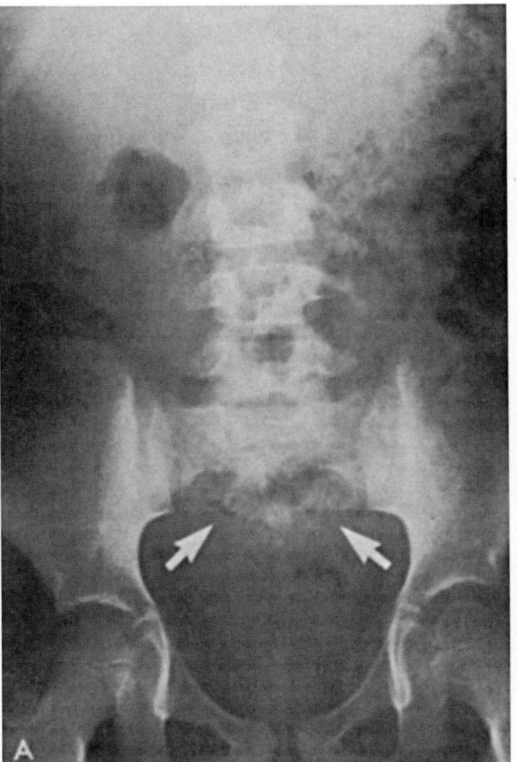

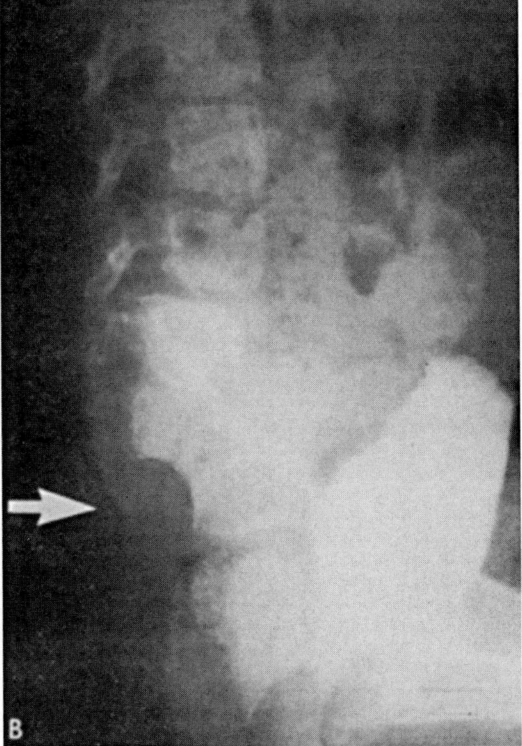

Figure 65–20. The diagnosis of partial or complete sacral agenesis is easily confirmed on an anteroposterior *(A)* or lateral *(B)* film of the spine (if bowel gas obscures the sacral area). (From Bauer SB: Urodynamic evaluation and neuromuscular dysfunction. *In* Kelalis PP, King LR, Belman AB, eds: Clinical Pediatric Urology, 2nd ed, Vol I. Philadelphia, W. B. Saunders Company, 1985, pp 283–310.)

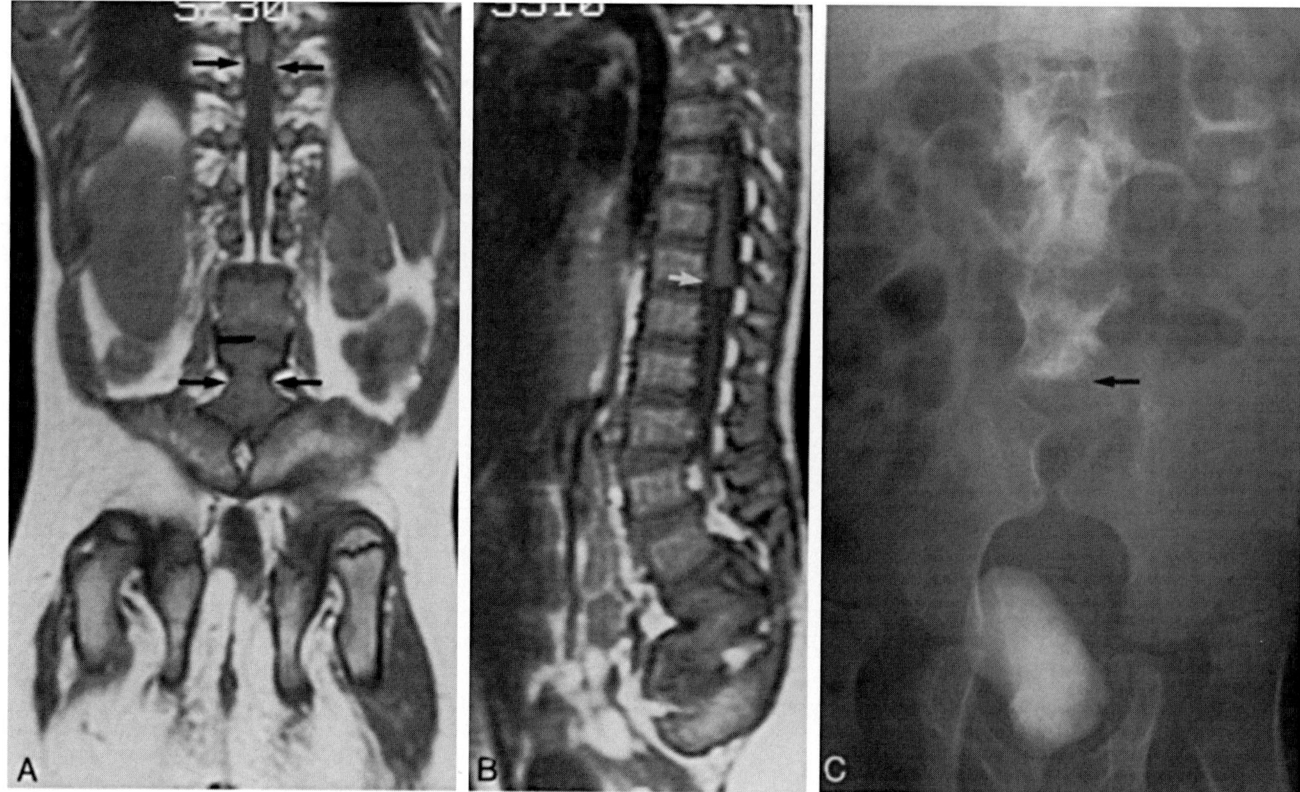

Figure 65–21. Coronal *(A)* and sagittal *(B)* MR images in a 10-year-old boy with sacral agenesis beginning at L-5. Note the squared lower limit of the cord adjacent to T-11 *(upper arrows* in *A* and *white arrow* in *B)* and the two sacroiliac joints *(lower arrows* in *A),* which are in the midline because of absence of the sacrum. *C,* An anteroposterior radiograph from an excretory urogram shows no vertebral bodies below L-4 *(arrow).*

not a foolproof one) of an upper or lower motor neuron lesion, respectively (Schlussel et al, 1994). The number of affected vertebrae does not seem to correlate with the type of motor neuron lesion present (Fig. 65–22) (Boemers et al, 1994). The injury appears to be stable and shows no signs of progressive denervation as the child ages. Interestingly, sacral sensation is relatively spared, even in the presence of extensive sacral motor defects (Boemers et al, 1994; Schlussel et al, 1994).

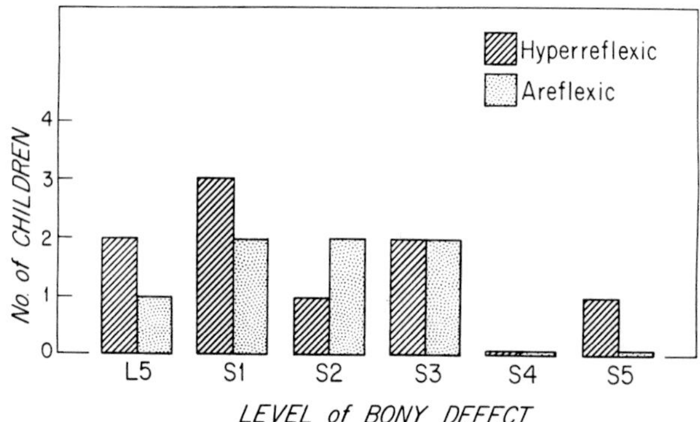

Figure 65–22. Bladder contractility is unrelated to the number of absent vertebrae. (From Bauer SB: Urodynamic evaluation and neuromuscular dysfunction. *In* Kelalis PP, King LR, Belman AB, eds: Clinical Pediatric Urology, 2nd ed, Vol I. Philadelphia, W. B. Saunders Company, 1985, pp 283–310.)

Recommendations

Management depends on the specific type of neurourologic dysfunction seen on urodynamic testing. Anticholinergic agents should be given to children with upper motor neuron findings of uninhibited contractions, whereas intermittent catheterization and alpha-sympathomimetic medications may have to be given to individuals with lower motor neuron deficits who cannot empty their bladders or stay dry between catheterizations. The bowels manifest a similar picture of dysfunction and need as much characterization and treatment as the lower urinary tract. It is important to identify these individuals as early as possible so that they can become continent and toilet trained at an appropriate age, thus avoiding the social stigma of fecal or urinary incontinence.

Associated Conditions

Imperforate Anus

Imperforate anus is a condition that can occur alone or as part of a constellation of anomalies that has been called the VATER or VACTERL syndrome (Barry and Auldist, 1974). This mnemonic stands for all the organs that can possibly be affected (V, vertebral; A, anal; C, cardiac; TE, tracheo-esophageal fistula; R, renal; L, limb). Urinary incontinence is not common unless the spinal cord is involved or the pelvic floor muscles or nerves are injured during imperforate anus repair. A plain film of the abdomen and an ultrasound

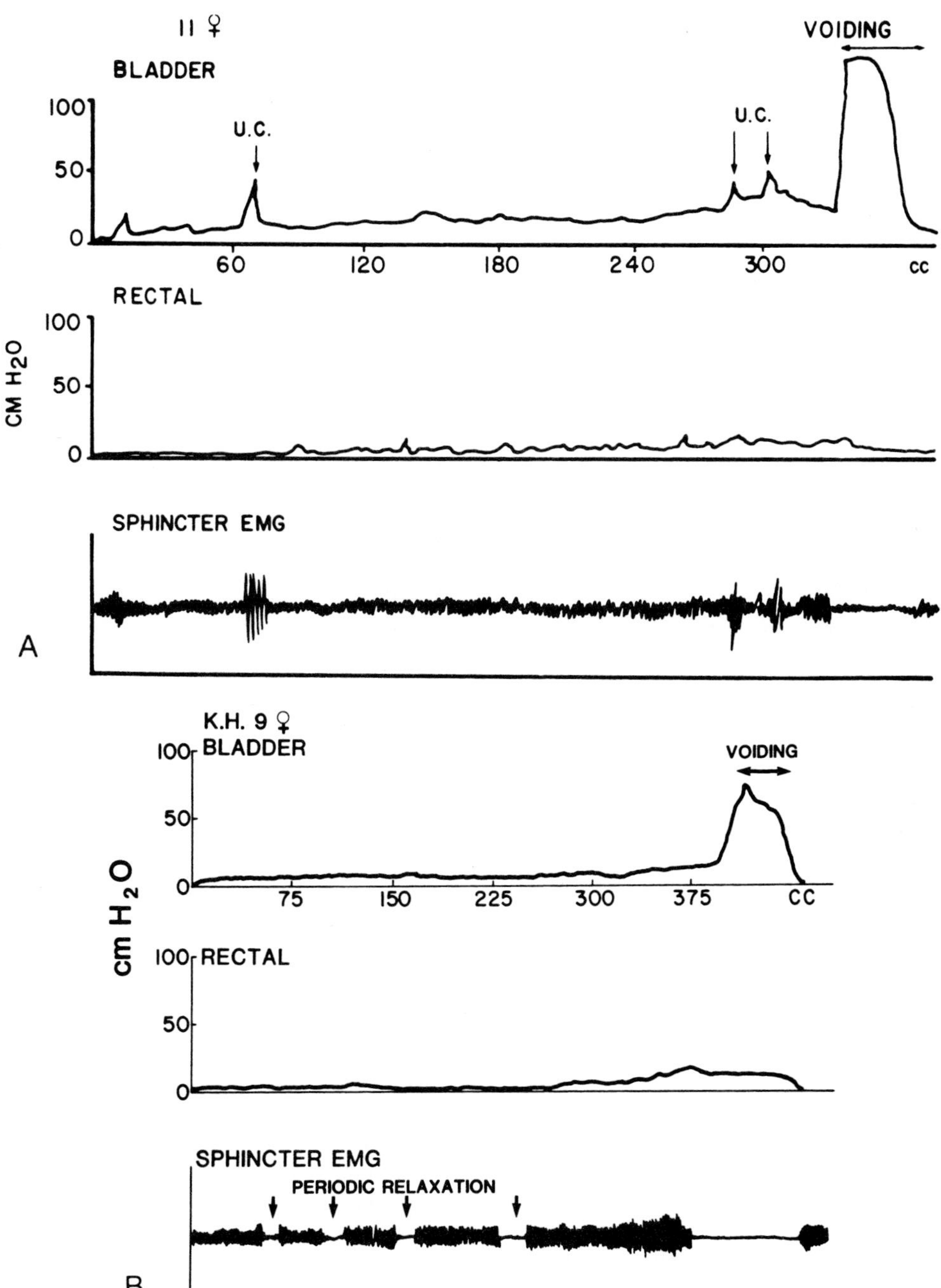

Figure 65–30. *A,* Uninhibited contractions (U.C.) of the bladder are associated with a rise in electromyographic (EMG) activity. During voluntary voiding, a coordinated vesicourethral unit exists. (From Bauer SB: Urodynamic evaluation and neuromuscular dysfunction. *In* Kelalis PP, King LR, Belman AB, eds: Clinical Pediatric Urology, 2nd ed, Vol I. Philadelphia, W. B. Saunders Company, 1985, pp 283–310.) *B,* Some children manifest only periodic relaxation of the sphincter without a rise in detrusor pressure as an early phase of a hyperreflexic bladder, producing urgency and incontinence.

et al, 1983). The uninhibited contractions are thought to be responsible for the symptoms (McGuire and Savastano, 1984).

These findings may be the result of a cerebral insult, however mild, in the perinatal period, but more commonly they are linked to delayed maturation of the reticulospinal pathways and the inhibitory centers in the midbrain and cerebral cortex. Thus, total control over vesicourethral function may be lacking (Mueller, 1960; MacKeith et al, 1973; Yeats, 1973). Several investigators have found a similar urodynamic picture in a significant number of adults with nocturnal enuresis and/or daytime symptoms (Torrens and Collins, 1975). Parents who exhibit the same behavior pattern as their children may have a genetically determined delayed rate of central nervous system maturation.

On occasion, children with profound constipation develop uninhibited contractions of the bladder and urinary incontinence secondary to them (O'Regan et al, 1985). The cause of this is unclear, but treatment of the bowel distention has resulted in dramatic improvement in the bladder dysfunction (O'Regan et al, 1986).

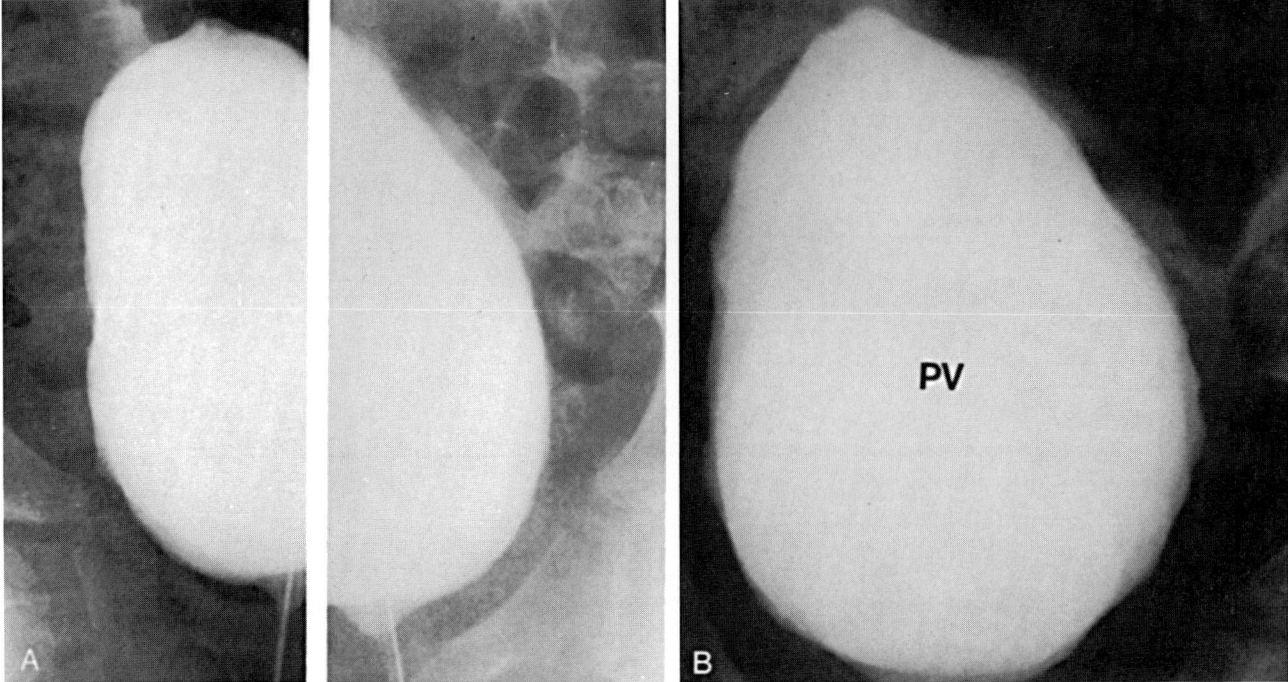

Figure 65–31. *A,* A large-capacity bladder with no reflux is noted in a 10-year-old girl with an infrequent voiding pattern. *B,* The postvoid (PV) residual volume is large.

Sometimes repeated urinary infection may produce an identical urodynamic picture. Detrusor hyperreflexia occurs as a result of the inflammatory response in the bladder wall that irritates the receptors located in the submucosa or detrusor muscle layers (Koff and Murtagh, 1983). Therefore, all children with these findings should be screened for infection. It has been postulated that a hyperactive detrusor may lead to inappropriate voiding. When the child realizes what is happening, he or she tightens the sphincter to reverse this process, which shuts the distal urethra first and the bladder neck second, causing the column of urine to be "milked back" into the bladder (Webster et al, 1984). This has the effect of carrying bacteria from the meatal opening up into the bladder, creating the potential for infection in the residual volume of urine, especially if the child does not immediately make an attempt to empty the bladder (Koff and Murtagh, 1983).

Anticholinergic medications (oxybutynin, propantheline, glycopyrrolate, and imipramine), alone or in combination, have been used successfully to manage this condition (Kondo et al, 1983). If infection is present it should be treated simultaneously (Buttarazzi, 1977; Firlit et al, 1978; Kass et al, 1979; Bauer et al, 1980; Mayo and Burns, 1990).

The Infrequent Voider—Lazy Bladder Syndrome

Most children urinate four to five times per day and defecate daily or at most every other day (Bloom et al, 1993; Weaver and Steiner, 1984). Some children, primarily girls, may void only twice a day, once in the morning (either at home or after they are in school) and again at night (DeLuca et al, 1962). It is not unusual for these children to shun bathrooms completely while in school. These children had normal voiding patterns as infants, but after toilet training they learned to withhold micturition for extended periods of time. Their parents may have instilled in them, however unintentionally, the idea that it is bad to wet or soil themselves. As a result, a few develop a fear of strange bathrooms or mimic their mother's pattern of infrequent urination and defecation (Bauer et al, 1980). Others may have experienced an aversive event or an infection associated with dysuria around the time of training that led to the infrequent pattern of micturition. Some children are excessively neat or have a fetish for cleanliness that causes them to avoid bathrooms. Often they void only enough to relieve the pressure to urinate and fail to empty the bladder completely.

The infrequent voiding and incomplete emptying produce an ever-increasing bladder capacity and a diminished stimulus to urinate (Webster et al, 1984). The chronically distended bladder is prone to urinary infection or overflow or stress incontinence. Sometimes these signs are the first manifestations of the abnormal voiding pattern. When the child is carefully questioned, the aberrant micturition pattern is easily detected. More often, the problem is diagnosed following a voiding cystourethrogram when a larger than normal capacity (for age) is noted and the residual urine volume on initial catheterization is measured; the child is questioned afterward about his or her voiding habits (see Fig. 65–31*A* and *B*) (Webster et al, 1984). In addition, the cystogram usually reveals a smooth-walled bladder without reflux.

Urodynamic studies demonstrate a very large capacity, highly compliant bladder with either normal, unsustained, or absent detrusor contractions (Fig. 65–32*A*) (Bauer et al, 1980). Straining to void is a common form of emptying. Sphincter EMG reveals normal motor unit potentials at rest

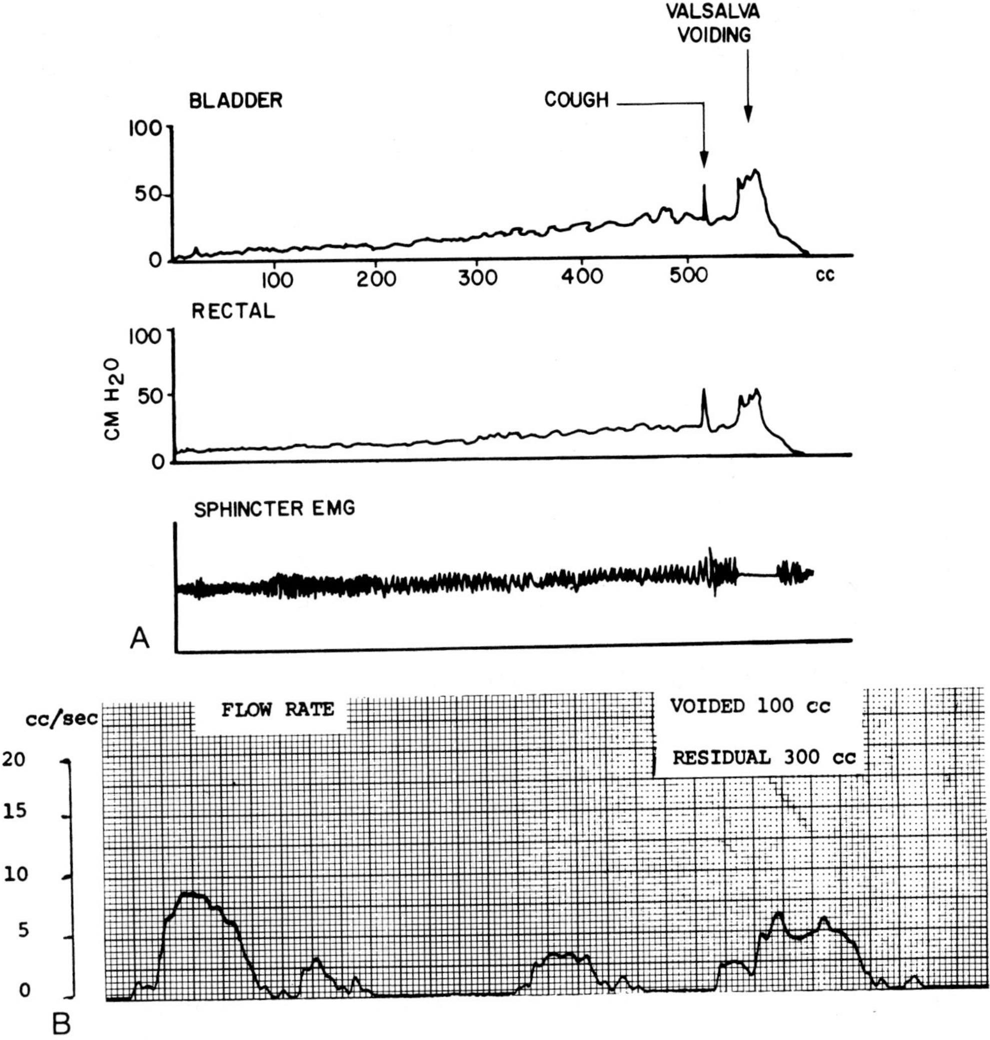

Figure 65–32. *A,* Urodynamic evaluation reveals a very large capacity bladder with no voiding contraction. The child empties by straining after relaxing the sphincter. *B,* The flow rate is characteristic of this effort to empty and leads to a considerable volume of residual urine. (From Bauer SB: Urodynamic evaluation and neuromuscular dysfunction. *In* Kelalis PP, King LR, Belman AB, eds: Clinical Pediatric Urology, 2nd ed, Vol I. Philadelphia, W. B. Saunders Company, 1985, pp 283–310.)

and normal responses to various sacral reflexes, bladder filling, and attempts at emptying. The urinary flow rate may be intermittent with sudden peaks coinciding with straining, or it may be normal but short-lived secondary to an unsustained detrusor contraction (Webster et al, 1984). Unless strongly encouraged, the child will not completely empty his or her bladder during voiding (Fig. 65–32*B*) (Bauer et al, 1980). This picture is consistent with myogenic failure resulting from chronic distention (Koefoot et al, 1981).

Changing the child's voiding habits is of paramount importance. Keeping to a rigid schedule of toiletting and encouraging the child to empty each time he or she voids is mandatory (Masek, 1985). Behavioral therapy techniques to get the child to comply are helpful. Occasionally, bethanechol chloride is administered to increase the sensitivity to regular voiding. Rarely, intermittent catheterization may be necessary to allow the detrusor muscle to regain its contractility and ability to empty. Antibiotics are needed when urinary infection is present; they are continued until the voiding pattern improves.

Psychologic Non-Neuropathic Bladder (Hinman's Syndrome)

There is a group of children with an apparent "syndrome" of voiding dysfunction that mimics neuropathic bladder disease but may be a learned disorder. At first this condition was believed to be an isolated neurologic lesion (Johnston and Farkas, 1975; Williams et al, 1975; Mix, 1977), but now it is thought to be an acquired abnormality (Hinman, 1974; Allen, 1977; Allen and Bright, 1978; Bauer et al, 1980). It is produced by an active contraction of the sphincter during voiding that creates a degree of outflow obstruction. Some investigators think this may be a result of persistence of the transitional phase of gaining control whereby the child learns to prevent voiding by voluntarily contracting the external sphincter (Allen, 1977; Rudy and Woodside, 1991), whereas others think this pattern results from the child's normal response to uninhibited contractions (McGuire and Savastano, 1984). This behavior becomes habitual because the child has difficulty in distinguishing between involuntary

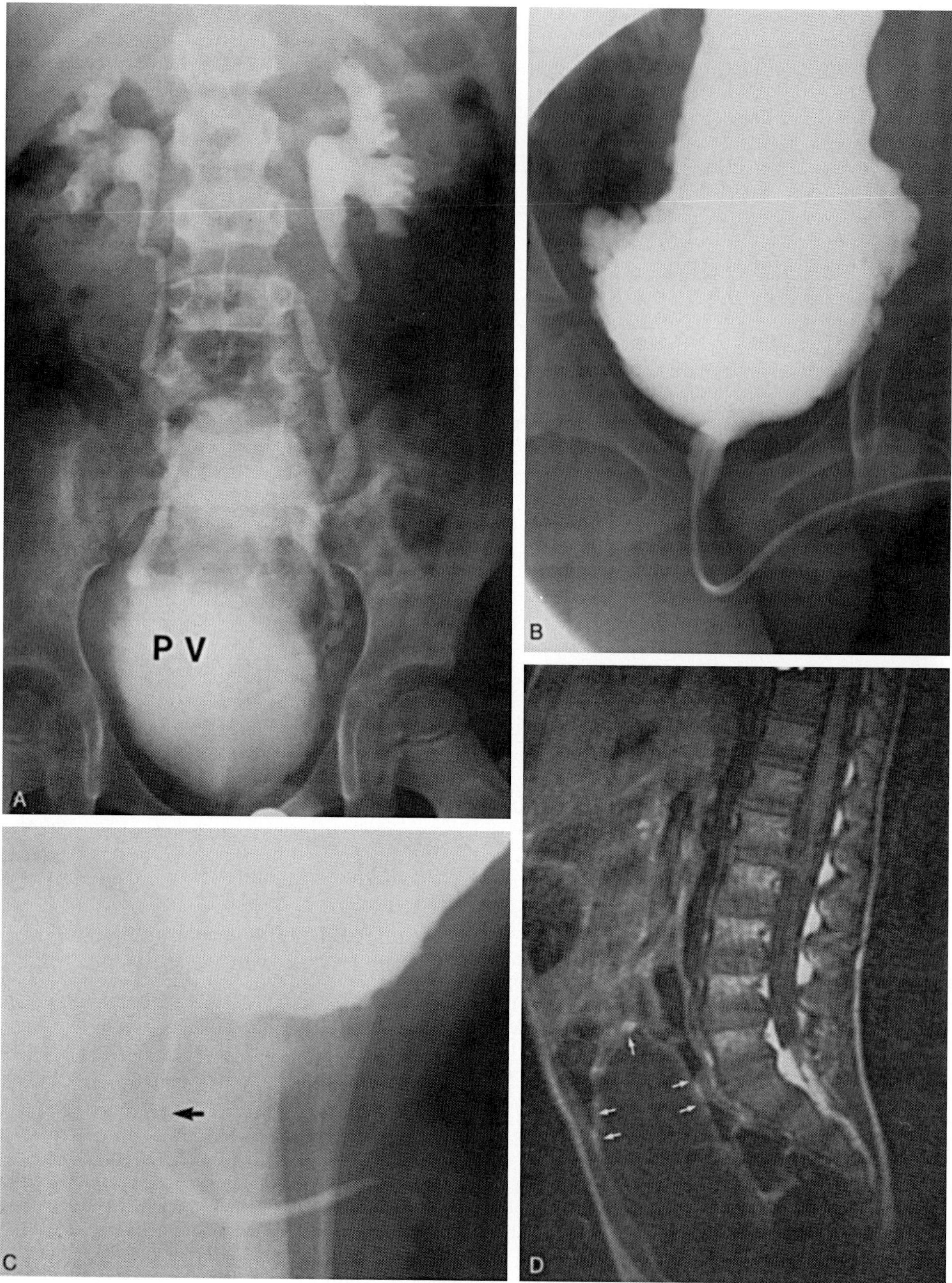

Figure 65–33. *A,* An excretory urogram in a 7-year-old boy with day and nighttime wetting and fecal soiling demonstrates bilateral hydronephrosis and a large bladder with incomplete emptying. *B* and *C,* Voiding cystogram reveals no reflux but severe trabeculation and a weak, narrow urine stream. *D,* An MRI scan of the spine is normal but note the large bladder *(arrows).* (PV, postvoid.)

and voluntary voiding; as a consequence, the inappropriate sphincter activity occurs all the time (Bauer et al, 1980).

The condition is characterized by urgency, urge or stress incontinence, infrequent voluntary voiding, intermittent urination associated with straining, recurrent urinary infections, and irregular bowel movements with fecal soiling between times (Bauer et al, 1980). The most striking factor is the similarity of the pattern of family dynamics, which is disclosed on careful observation and questioning of family members (Table 65–10) (Allen and Bright, 1978). The parents, especially the father, tend to be domineering, exacting, unyielding, and intolerant of weakness or failure. Delayed training or continued wetting is viewed as such a characteristic. Divorce and alcoholism are common threads that only exacerbate the situation. Wetting is perceived as immature, defiant, and purposeful behavior that the parents feel must be counteracted with stern reprimands. The children are often punished, both mentally and physically, for their ineptness. Confusion, depression, and withdrawal for fear of wetting with its added punitive response becomes the child's prevalent attitude because he does not know how to nor can he prevent this provocative behavior. The child tries to withhold urination and defecation further by keeping the sphincter muscle tight, aggravating the situation. Thus, wetting becomes more commonplace and abdominal pain from chronic constipation is not unusual.

X-ray evaluation reveals profound changes in the urinary tract. Hydroureteronephrosis with or without pyelonephritic scarring from recurrent infection occurs in two thirds of the children (Fig. 65–33*A*) (Bauer et al, 1980). Fifty percent have severe vesicoureteral reflux. Nearly every child has a grossly trabeculated, large-capacity bladder with a considerable postvoid residual urine volume (Fig. 65–33*B*). Voiding films show either persistent or intermittent narrowing in the region of the external sphincter in almost half the children (see Fig. 65–33*B*). Finally, the scout film from the excretory urogram displays considerable fecal material in the colon consistent with chronic constipation.

Urodynamic studies demonstrate a large-capacity bladder with poor compliance, uninhibited contractions and either high-pressure or ineffective detrusor contractions during voiding (Fig. 65–34*A*) (Kass et al, 1979; Bauer et al, 1980). Sometimes Valsalva voiding is needed to empty the bladder. The urinary flow rate is often intermittent because of failure of the external sphincter to relax (Fig. 65–34*B*). The bethanechol supersensitivity test may be positive; in the past, it was this response that led to the belief that these children had neuropathic bladder dysfunction (William et al, 1975). EMG recordings, however, reveal normal sphincter innervation and exclude the possibility of a sacral spinal cord lesion.

Table 65–10. FEATURES OF PSYCHOLOGIC NON-NEUROPATHIC BLADDER

Daytime and nighttime wetting
Encopresis, constipation, fecal impaction
Recurrent urinary tract infection
Parental characteristics
Domineering, exacting
Divorce
Alcoholism
Punishments (mental and physical) inflicted for wetting

Table 65–11. TREATMENT OF PSYCHOLOGIC NON-NEUROPATHIC BLADDER

Psychotherapy
Behavioral modification
Biofeedback
Drugs
Oxybutynin
Flavoxate
Bethanechol
Diazepam
Antibiotics
Intermittent catheterization
Bowel re-regulation program
Stool softeners
Bulking agents
Laxatives, enemas

The sphincter fails to relax completely and may actually tighten episodically once voiding commences (Rudy and Woodside, 1991); this finding, along with the uninhibited contractions, suggests an upper motor neuron lesion, but usually no other signs are present to confirm this urodynamic hypothesis. Recently, spinal canal imaging with MRI has failed to reveal any intraspinal process as a cause of the voiding dysfunction in these children (see Fig. 65–32*C*) (Hinman, 1986).

The dyssynergy created by the incoordination between the bladder and the sphincter muscles leads to high voiding pressures initially and later to ineffective detrusor contractions (Rudy and Woodside, 1991). Depending on which phase of the micturition cycle the child is at, a low or intermittent flow rate and either a significant or minimal postvoid residual urine volume is noted.

Before this "syndrome" was recognized and the pathophysiology elucidated, many children underwent multiple operations to improve bladder emptying and correct vesicoureteral reflux. The lack of success of these procedures led to urinary diversion in a number of instances. Reversal of diversion was eventually possible in some of these individuals at an older age after they outgrew the conditions that caused the dysfunction in the first place. Today, an entirely different approach is taken. Treatment is focused on improving the child's ability to empty and alleviating the psychosocial pressures that contribute to the aggravation of the voiding dysfunction (Table 65–11) (Masek, 1985; Hinman, 1986). A frequent emptying schedule accompanied by biofeedback techniques to relax the sphincter during voiding, anticholinergic drugs to abolish uninhibited contractions, and improved bowel emptying regimes are instituted (Bauer et al, 1980). Bethanechol chloride and prazosin (an alpha-blocking agent) may be added if the detrusor exhibits poor contractility. Despite these measures, intermittent catheterization may be needed in children who fail to respond and in those who require immediate decompression of the upper urinary tract (Snyder et al, 1982). In some cases, the outflow obstruction may have produced severe renal damage and even chronic kidney failure, which must be managed accordingly.

Psychotherapy is an integral part of the rehabilitative process to re-educate both the child and his parents in appropriate voiding habits. Punishments are stopped and a reward system initiated to improve the child's self-image and confidence (Masek, 1985).

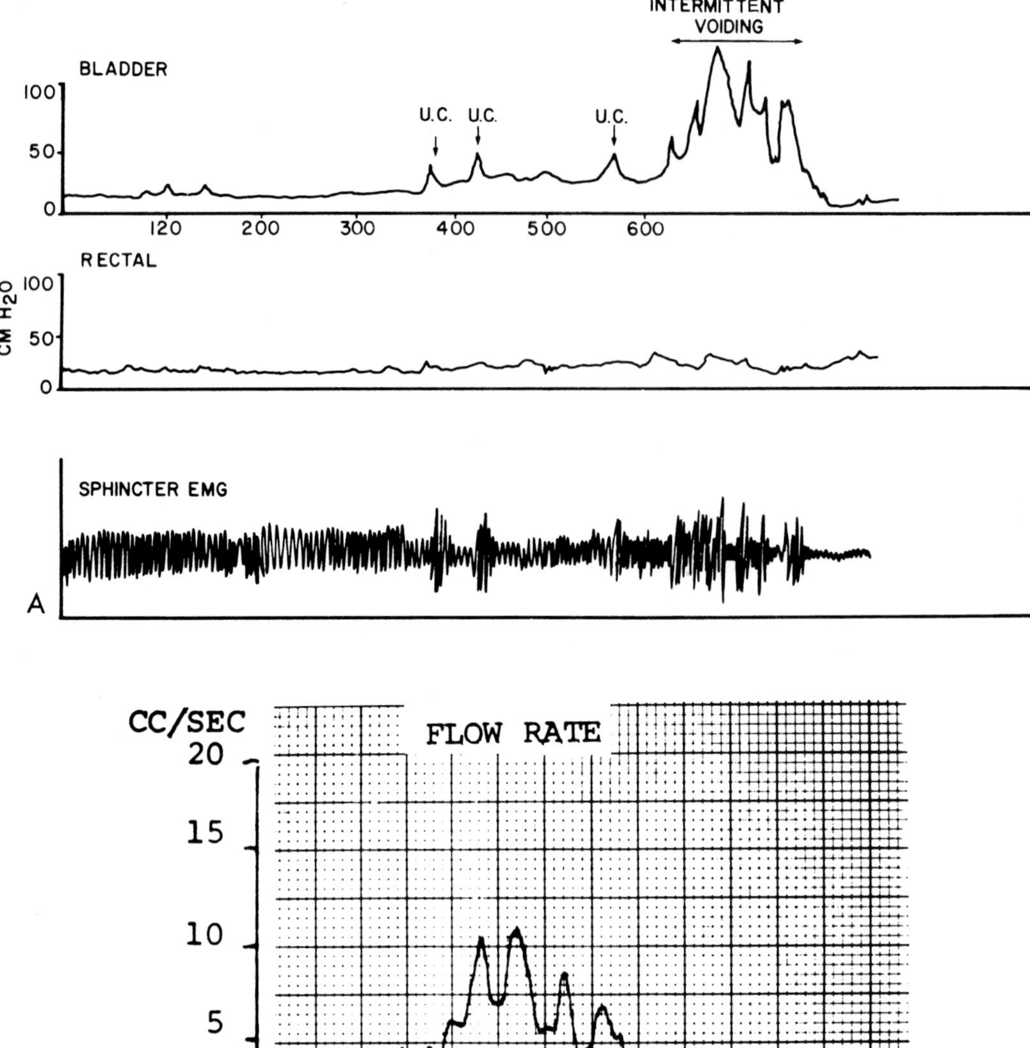

Figure 65–34. *A,* The urodynamic picture reveals both uninhibited contractions (U.C.) and high voiding pressures with a nonrelaxing sphincter. *B,* The urinary flow rate reflects the voiding pattern seen on urodynamic evaluation. (From Bauer SB: Urodynamic evaluation and neuromuscular dysfunction. *In* Kelalis PP, King LR, Belman AB, eds: Clinical Pediatric Urology, 2nd ed, Vol I. Philadelphia, W. B. Saunders Company, 1985, pp 283–310.)

REFERENCES

Introduction

Bauer SB, Hallet M, Khoshbin S, et al: The predictive value of urodynamic evaluation in the newborn with myelodysplasia. JAMA 1984; 152:650.

Blaivas JG, Labib KB, Bauer SB, Retik AB: Changing concepts in the urodynamic evaluation of children. J Urol 1977; 117:777.

Blaivas JG: A critical appraisal of specific diagnostic techniques. *In* Krane RJ, Siroky MB, eds. Clinical Neurourology. Boston, Little, Brown, 1979, pp 69–110.

Edelstein RA, Bauer SB, Kelly MD, et al: The long-term urologic response of neonates with myelodysplasia treated proactively with intermittent catheterization and anticholinergic therapy. J Urol 1995; 154:1500.

Gierup J, Ericsson NO: Micturition studies in infants and children: Intravesical pressure, urinary flow and urethral resistance in boys with intravesical obstruction. Scand J Urol Nephrol 1970; 4:217.

Kaufman AM, Roberts AC, Rudy DC, et al: Decreased bladder compliance in myelomeningocele patients managed by radiologic observation (Abstract 199). Presented at the Annual Meeting of the American Urological Association, Las Vegas, April 24, 1995.

Lapides J, Diokno AC, Silber SJ, Lowe BS: Clean intermittent self-catheterization in the treatment of urinary tract disease. J Urol 1972; 107:458.

McGuire EJ, Woodside JR, Borden TA, Weiss RM: The prognostic value of urodynamic testing in myelodysplastic patients. J Urol 1981; 126:205.

Perez LM, Khoury J, Webster GD: The value of urodynamic studies in infants less than one year old with congenital spinal dysraphism. J Urol 1992; 148:584.

Smith ED: Urinary prognosis in spina bifida. J Urol 1972; 108:115.

Urodynamic Evaluation

Abrams PH: Perfusion urethral profilometry. Urol Clin North Am 1979; 6:103.

Bates CP, Whiteside CG, Turner-Warwick RT: Synchronous cine/pressure/flow/cysto-urethrography with special reference to stress and urge incontinence. Br J Urol 1970; 42:714.

Bauer SB: Pediatric Neurourology. *In* Krane RJ, Siroky MB, eds: Clinical Neurourology. Boston, Little, Brown, 1979, pp 275–294.

Bauer SB: Urodynamics in children: indications and methods. *In* Barrett DM, Wein AJ, eds: Controversies in Neuro-urology. New York, Churchill-Livingstone, 1983, pp 193–202.
Blaivas JG: A critical appraisal of specific diagnostic techniques. *In* Krane RJ, Siroky MB, eds: Clinical Neurourology. Boston, Little, Brown, 1979a; pp 69–110.
Blaivas JG: EMG: Other uses. *In* Barrett DM, Wein AJ, eds: Controversies in Neuro-urology. New York, Churchill Livingstone, 1979b; pp 103–116.
Blaivas JG, Labib KB, Bauer SB, Retik AB: A new approach to electromyography of the external urethral sphincter. J Urol 1977a; 117:773.
Blaivas JG, Labib KB, Bauer SB, Retik AB: Changing concepts in the urodynamic evaluation of children. J Urol 1977b; 117:777.
Bradley WE, Timm GW, Scott FB: Sphincter electromyography. Urol Clin North Am 1974; 1:69.
Diokno AC, Koff SA, Bender LF: Periurethral striated muscle activity in neurogenic bladder dysfunction. J Urol 1974; 112:743.
Ericsson NO, Hellstrom B, Negardth A, Rudhe U: Micturition urethrocystography in children with myelomeningocele. Acta Radiol Diagn 1971; 11:321.
Evans AT, Felker JR, Shank RA, Sugarman SR: Pitfalls of urodynamics. J Urol 1979; 122:220.
Fairhurst JJ, Rubin CME, Hyde I, et al: Bladder capacity in infants. J Pediatr Surg 1991; 26:55.
Gierup J, Ericsson NO, Okmain L: Micturition studies in infants and children. Scand J Urol Nephrol 1969; 3:1.
Gleason DM, Reilly RJ, Bottacini MR, Pierce MJ: The urethral continence zone and its relation to stress incontinence. J Urol 1974; 112:81.
Joseph DB: The effect of medium-fill and slow-fill cystometry on bladder pressure in infants and children with myelodysplasia. J Urol 1992; 147:444.
Kerr LA, Bauer SB, Staskin DR: Abnormal detrusor function precipitating hydronephrosis identified by extended voiding cystometry. J Urol 1994; 152:89.
Koff SA: Estimating bladder capacity in children. Urology 1983, 21:248.
Koff SA, Kass EJ: Abdominal wall electromyography: A noninvasive technique to improve pediatric urodynamic accuracy. J Urol 1982; 127:736.
Maizels M, Firlit CF: Pediatric urodynamics. Clinical comparison of surface vs. needle pelvic floor/external sphincter electromyography. J Urol 1979; 122:518.
Mandell J, Bauer SB, Hallett M, et al: Occult spinal dysraphism: A rare but detectable cause of voiding dysfunction. Urol Clin North Am 1980; 7:349.
Mayo ME: Detrusor hyperreflexia: The effect of posture and pelvic floor activity. J Urol 1978; 119:635.
Scott FB, Quesada EM, Cardus D: Studies on the dynamics of micturition. J Urol 1964; 92:455.
Tanagho EA: Membrane and microtransducer catheters. Their effectiveness for profilometry of the lower urinary tract. Urol Clin North Am 1979; 6:110.
Turner-Warwick RT: Some clinical aspects of detrusor dysfunction. J Urol 1975; 113:539.
Yalla SV, Rossier AB, Fam B: Vesico-urethral pressure recordings in the assessment of neurogenic bladder functions in spinal cord injury patients. Urol Int 1979; 32:161.
Yalla SV, Sharma GURK, Barsamian EM: Micturitional static urethral pressure profile method of recording urethral pressure profiles during voiding and implications. J Urol 1980; 124:649.

Myelodysplasia

Adams MC, Mitchell ME, Rink RC: Gastrocystoplasty: An alternative solution to the problem of urological reconstruction in the severely compromised patient. J Urol 1988; 140:1152.
Atala A, Bauer SB, Hendren WH, Retik AB: Effect of gastric augmentation on bladder function. J Urol 1993; 149:1099–1102.
Barbalias GA, Klauber GT, Blaivas JG: Critical evaluation of the Credé maneuver: A urodynamic study of 207 patients. J Urol 1983; 130:720.
Barrett DM, Furlow WL: The management of severe urinary incontinence in patients with myelodysplasia by implantation of the AS791/792 urinary sphincter device. J Urol 1982; 128:44.
Bauer SB: Vesico-ureteral reflux in children with neurogenic bladder dysfunction. *In* Johnston JH, ed: International Perspectives in Urology, Vol. 10. Baltimore, Williams & Wilkins, 1984a; pp 159–177.
Bauer SB: Myelodysplasia: Newborn evaluation and management. *In* McLaurin RL, Ed. Spina Bifida: A Multidisciplinary Approach. New York, Praeger, 1984b, pp 262–267.
Bauer SB: The management of spina bifida from birth onwards. *In* Whitaker RH, Woodard JR, eds: Paediatric Urology. London, Butterworths, 1985, pp 87–112.
Bauer SB: Early evaluation and management of children with spina bifida. *In* King LR, ed: Urologic Surgery in Neonates and Young Infants. Philadelphia, WB Saunders, 1988, pp 252–264.
Bauer SB: Bladder neck reconstruction. *In* Glenn JF, Graham SD, eds: Urologic Surgery. Philadelphia, JB Lippincott, 1990, pp 509–522.
Bauer SB: Evaluation and management of the newborn with myelomeningocele. *In* Gonzales ET, Roth DR, eds: Common Problems in Urology. St. Louis, Mosby–Year Book, 1991, pp 169–180.
Bauer SB, Colodny AH, Retik AB: The management of vesico-ureteral reflux in children with myelodysplasia. J Urol 1982; 128:102.
Bauer SB, Hallet M, Khoshbin S, et al: The predictive value of urodynamic evaluation in the newborn with myelodysplasia. JAMA 1984; 152:650.
Bauer SB, Kelly MD, Darbey M, Atala A: Late onset detrusor instability in patients with the artificial urinary sphincter (Abstract 597). Presented at the Annual Meeting of the American Urologic Association, San Antonio, May 18, 1993.
Bauer SB, Labib KB, Dieppa RA, et al: Urodynamic evaluation in a boy with myelodysplasia and incontinence. Urology 1977; 10:354.
Bauer SB, Reda EF, Colodny AH, Retik AB: Detrusor instability: A delayed complication in association with the artificial sphincter. J Urol 1986; 135:1212.
Begger JH, Meihuizen de Regt MJ, Hogen Esch I, et al: Progressive neurologic deficit in children with spina bifida aperta. Z Kinderchir 1986; 41(Suppl 1):13.
Ben-Chiam J, Jeffs RD, Peppas DS, Gearhart JP: Submucosal bladder neck injections of glutanaldehyde cross-linked bovine collagen for treatment of urinary incontinence in patients with exstrophy/epispadias complex (Abstract 123). Presented at the Annual Meeting of the Section on Urology of the American Academy of Pediatrics, Dallas, October 24, 1994.
Bihrle R, Klee LW, Adams MC, et al: Transverse colon-gastric tube composite reservoir. Urology 1991; 37:36–40.
Blaivas JG, Sinka HP, Zayed AH, et al: Detrusor-sphincter dyssynergia: A detailed electromyographic study. J Urol 1986; 125:545.
Bloom DA, Knechtel JM, McGuire EJ: Urethral dilation improves bladder compliance in children with myelomeningocele and high leak point pressures. J Urol 1990; 144:430.
Bomalaski MD, Bloom DA, McGuire EJ, Panz LA: Glutaraldehyde cross-linked collagen in the treatment of urinary incontinence in children. J Urol 1996; 155:699.
Bomalaski MD, Teague JL, Brooks B: The long-term impact of urologic management on the quality of life in children with spina bifida. J Urol 1995; 156:778.
Bosco PJ, Bauer SB, Colodny AH, et al: The long-term follow-up of artificial urinary sphincters in children. J Urol 1991; 146:396.
Cartwright PC, Snow BW: Bladder autoaugmentation: Early clinical experience. J Urol 1989a; 142:505.
Cartwright PC, Snow BW: Bladder autoaugmentation: Partial detrusor excision to augment bladder without use of bowel. J Urol 1989b; 142:1050.
Cass AS: Urinary tract complications of myelomeningocele patients. J Urol 1976; 115:102.
Cass AS, Bloom BA, Luxenberg M: Sexual function in adults with myelomeningocele. J Urol 1986; 136:425.
Chiaramonte RM, Horowitz EM, Kaplan GA, et al: Implications of hydronephrosis in newborns with myelodysplasia. J Urol 1986; 136:427.
Cohen RA, Rushton HG, Belman AB, et al: Renal scarring and vesicoureteral reflux in children with myelodysplasia. J Urol 1990; 144:541.
Cromer BA, Enrile B, McCoy K, et al: Knowledge, attitudes and behavior related to sexuality in adolescents with chronic disability. Dev Med Child Neurol 1990; 32:602.
Czeizel AE, Dudas I: Prevention of the first occurrence of neural-tube defects by preconceptional vitamin supplementation. N Engl J Med 1992; 321:1832.
Dator DP, Hatchett L, Dyro EM, et al: Urodynamic dysfunction in walking myelodysplastic children. J Urol 1992; 148:362–365.
Dees JE: Congenital epispadias with incontinence. J Urol 1949; 62:513.
Duckett JW: Cutaneous vesicostomy in childhood. Urol Clin North Am 1974; 1:485.
Duckett JW, Snyder HM III: Continent urinary diversion: Variations of the Mitrofanoff principle. J Urol 1986; 136:58.

Edelstein RA, Bauer SB, Kelly MD, et al: The long-term urologic response of neonates with myelodysplasia treated proactively with intermittent catheterization and anticholinergic therapy. J Urol 1995; 154:1500.

Elder JS: Periurethral and pubovaginal sling repair for incontinence in patients with myelodysplasia. J Urol 1990; 144:434.

Epstein F: Meningocele: Pitfalls in early and late management. Clin Neurosurg 1982; 30:366.

Flood HD, Ritchey ML, Bloom DA, et al: Outcome of reflux in children with myelodysplasia managed by bladder pressure monitoring. J Urol 1994; 152:1574.

Geranoitis E, Koff SA, Enrile B: Prophylactic use of clean intermittent catheterization in treatment of infants and young children with myelomeningocele and neurogenic bladder dysfunction. J Urol 1988; 139:85.

Ghoniem GM, Bloom DA, McGuire EJ, Stewart KL: Bladder compliance in meningocele children. J Urol 1989; 141:1404.

Goldwasser B, Barrett DM, Webster GD, Kramer SA: Cystometric properties of ileum and right colon after bladder augmentation, substitution and replacement. J Urol 1987; 138:1007.

Gonzalez R, Reid C, Remberg Y, Buson H: Seromuscular enterocystoplasty lined with urothelium (SEIU). Experience with 12 patients. J Urol 1994; 151:235.

Gosalbez R Jr, Woodard JR, Broecker BH, Warshaw B: Metabolic complications of the use of stomach for urinary reconstruction. J Urol 1993; 150:710.

Greenfield SP, Fera M: The use of intravesical oxybutynin chloride in children with neurogenic bladder. J Urol 1991; 146:532.

Griffiths DM, Malone PS: The Malone antegrade continence enema. J Pediatr Surg 1995; 30:68–71.

Hayden P: Adolescents with meningomyelocele. Pediatr Rev 1985; 6:245.

Hendren WH: Reconstruction of the previously diverted urinary tracts in children. J Pediatr Surg 1973; 8:135.

Hendren WH: Urinary tract refunctionalization after long-term diversion. Am Surg 1990; 212:478.

Hernandez RD, Hurwitz RS, Foote JE, et al: Nonsurgical management of threatened upper urinary tracts and incontinence in children with myelomeningocele. J Urol 1994; 152:1582.

Hinman F Jr: Selection of intestinal segments for bladder substitution: Physical and physiological characteristics. J Urol 1988; 139:519.

Hinman F Jr: Functional classification of conduits for continent diversion. J Urol 1990; 144:27.

Jeffs RD, Jones P, Schillinger JF: Surgical correction of vesico-ureteral reflux in children with neurogenic bladder. J Urol 1976; 115:449.

Joseph DB, Bauer SB, Colodny AH, et al: Clean intermittent catheterization in infants with neurogenic bladder. Pediatrics 1989; 84:78.

Just M, Schwarz M, Ludwig B, et al: Cerebral and spinal MR findings in patients with post repair myelomeningocele. Pediatr Radiol 1990; 20:262.

Kaplan WE, Firlit CF: Management of reflux in myelodysplasic children. J Urol 1983; 129:1195.

Kasabian NG, Bauer SB, Dyro FM, et al: The prophylactic value of clean intermittent catheterization and anticholinergic medication in newborns and infants with myelodysplasia at risk of developing urinary tract deterioration. Am J Dis Child 1992; 146:840.

Kasabian NG, Vlachiotis JD, Lais A, et al: The use of intravesical oxybutynin chloride in patients with detrusor hypertonicity and detrusor hyperreflexia. J Urol 1994; 151:944.

Kass EJ, Koff SA, Lapides J: Fate of vesico-ureteral reflux in children with neuropathic bladders managed by intermittent catheterization. J Urol 1981; 125:63.

Khoury AE, Hendrick EB, McLorie GA, et al: Occult spinal dysraphism: Clinical and urodynamic outcome after division of the filum terminale. J Urol 1990; 144:426.

Kock NG: Ileostomy without external appliances: A survey of 25 patients provided with intra-abdominal intestinal reservoir. Ann Surg 1971; 173:545.

Kroovand RL, Bell W, Hart LJ, Benfeld KY: The effect of back closure on detrusor function in neonates with myelodysplasia. J Urol 1990; 144:423.

Kropp KA, Angwafo FF: Urethral lengthening and reimplantation for neurogenic incontinence in children. J Urol 1986; 135:533.

Lais A, Kasabian NG, Dyro FM, et al: Neurosurgical implications of continuous neuro-urological surveillance of children with myelodysplasia. J Urol 1993; 150:1879–1883.

Landau EH, Churchill BM, Jayanthi VR, et al: The sensitivity of pressure specific bladder volume versus total bladder capacity as a measure of bladder storage dysfunction. J Urol 1994; 152:1578.

Lapides J, Diokno AC, Silber SJ, Lowe BS: Clean intermittent self-catheterization in the treatment of urinary tract disease. J Urol 1972; 107:458.

Laurence KM: A declining incidence of neural tube defects in UK. Z Kinderchir 1989; 44:(Suppl 1) 51.

Laurence KM, Beresford A: Continence, friends, marriage and children in 51 adults with spina bifida. Dev Med Child Neurol 1975: 17(Suppl 35):128.

Laurence KM, James M, Miller MH, et al: Double-blind randomized controlled trial of folate treatment before conception to prevent recurrence of neural tube defects. Br Med J 1981; 282:1509.

Leadbetter GW Jr: Surgical correction for total urinary incontinence. J Urol 1964; 91:261.

Levesque PE, Bauer SB, Atala A, et al: Ten-year experience with artificial urinary sphincter in children. J Urol 1996; 156:625.

Light JK, Hawila M, Scott FB: Treatment of urinary incontinence in children: The artificial sphincter vs. other methods. J Urol 1983; 130:518.

Light JK, Scott FB: Use of the artificial urinary sphincter in spinal cord injury patients. J Urol 1983; 130:1127.

Loening-Baucke V, Desch L, Wolraich M: Biofeedback training for patients with myelomeningocele and fecal incontinence. Dev Med Child Neurol 1988; 30:781.

Mandell J, Bauer SB, Colodny AH, Retik AB: Cutaneous vesicostomy in infancy. J Urol 1981; 126:92.

Massad CA, Kogan BA, Trigo-Rocha FE: The pharmacokinetics of intravesical and oral oxybutynin chloride. J Urol 1992; 148:548.

McGuire EJ, Wang CC, Usitalo H, Savastano J: Modified pubovaginal sling in girls with myelodysplasia. J Urol 1986; 135:94.

McGuire EJ, Woodside JR, Borden TA, Weiss RM: The prognostic value of urodynamic testing in myelodysplastic patients. J Urol 1981; 126:205.

McLorie GA, Perez-Morero R, Csima AL, Churchill BM: Determinants of hydronephrosis and renal injury in patients with myelomeningocele. J Urol 1986; 140:1289.

Mitchell ME, Piser JA: Intestinocystoplasty and total bladder replacement in children and young adults: Follow-up of 129 cases. J Urol 1987; 138:1140.

Mitrofanoff P: Cystometrie continente trans-appendiculaire dans le traitement de vessies neurologiques. Chir Pediatr 1980; 21:297.

MRC Vitamin Study Research Group: Prevention of neural tube defects: Results of the Medical Research Council Vitamin Study. Lancet 1991; 338:131.

Myers GJ: Myelomeningocele: The medical aspect. Pediatr Clin North Am 1984; 31:165.

Nasrallah PF, Aliabadi HA: Bladder augmentation in patients with neurogenic bladder and vesicoureteral reflux. J Urol 1991; 146:563.

Nguyen DH, Bain MA, Salmonson KL, et al: The syndrome of dysuria and hematuria in pediatric urinary reconstruction with stomach. J Urol 1993; 150:707.

Nguyen DH, Carr MF, Bagli DJ, Mitchell ME: Demucosalized gastrocystoplasty with auto-augmentation: A clinical experience (Abstract 204). Presented at the Annual Meeting of the American Urological Association, Las Vegas, April 24, 1995.

Oi S, Yamada H, Matsumoto S: Tethered cord syndrome versus low-placed conus medullaris in an over-distended cord following initial repair for myelodysplasia. Child Nerv Syst 1990; 6:264.

Perez LM, Khoury J, Webster GD: The value of urodynamic studies in infants less than one year old with congenital spinal dysraphism. J Urol 1992; 148:584.

Peters CA, Bauer SB, Colodny AH, et al: The use of rectus fascia to manage urinary incontinence. J Urol 1989; 142:516.

Pontari MA, Keating M, Kelly MD, et al: Retained sacral function in children with high level myelodysplasia. J Urol 1995; 154:775.

Raghavendra BN, Epstein FJ, Pinto RS, et al: The tethered spinal cord: Diagnosis by high-resolution real-time ultrasound. Radiology 1983; 149:123.

Raz S, Ehrlich RM, Ziedman EJ, et al: Surgical treatment of the incontinent female patient with myelomeningocele. J Urol 1988; 139:524.

Riedmiller H, Burger R, Muller S, et al: Continent appendix stoma: A modification of the Mainz pouch technique. J Urol 1990; 143:1115.

Reigel DH: Tethered spinal cord. Concepts Pediatr Neurosurg 1983; 4:142.

Rinck C, Berg J, Hafeman C: The adolescent with myelomeningocele: A review of parent experiences and expectations. Adolescence 1989; 24:699.

Roth DR, Vyas PR, Kroovand RL, Perlmutter AD: Urinary tract deterioration associated with the artificial urinary sphincter. J Urol 1986; 135:528.

Rowland RG, Mitchell ME, Birhle R, et al: Indiana continent urinary reservoir. J Urol 1987; 137:1136.

Salle JLP, Amarante FA, Silveira ML, et al: Urethral lengthening with anterior bladder wall flap for urinary incontinence: A new approach. J Urol 1994; 152:803.

Scarff TB, Fronczak S: Myelomeningocele: A review and update. Rehab Lit 1981; 42:143.

Schwarz GR, Jeffs RD: Ileal conduit urinary diversion in children: Computer analysis of follow-up from 2 to 16 years. J Urol 1975; 114:285.

Shapiro SR, Lebowitz RL, Colodny AH: Fate of 90 children with ileal conduit urinary diversion a decade later: Analysis of complications, pyeloplasty, renal function and bacteriology. J Urol 1975; 114:289.

Sidi AA, Aliabadi H, Gonzalez R: Enterocystoplasty in the management and reconstruction of the pediatric neurogenic bladder. J Pediatr Surg 1987; 22:153.

Sidi AA, Dykstra DD, Gonzalez R: The value of urodynamic testing in the management of neonates with myelodysplasia: A prospective study. J Urol 1986; 135:90.

Skinner DG, Lieskovsky G, Boyd SD: Construction of a continent ileal reservoir (Kock pouch) as an alternative to cutaneous urinary diversion: An update after 250 cases. J Urol 1987; 137:1140.

Smith ED: Urinary prognosis in spina bifida. J Urol 1972; 108:115.

Spindel MR, Bauer SB, Dyro FM, et al: The changing neuro-urologic lesion in myelodysplasia. JAMA 1987; 258:1630.

Squire R, Kiely EM, Carr B, et al: The clinical application of the Malone antegrade colonic enema. J Pediatr Surg 1993; 28:1012–1015.

Stark GD: Spina Bifida: Problems and Management. Oxford, Blackwell Scientific Publications, 1977.

Stein SC, Feldman JG, Freidlander M, et al: Is myelomeningocele a disappearing disease? Pediatrics 1982; 69:511.

Steinhardt GF, Goodgold HM, Samuels LD: The effect of intravesical pressure on glomerular filtration rates in patients with myelomeningocele. J Urol 1986; 140:1293.

Teichman JMH, Scherz HC, Kim KD, et al: An alternative approach to myelodysplasia management: Aggressive observation and prompt intervention. J Urol 1994; 152:807.

Torrens M, Abrams P: Cystometry. Urol Clin North Am 1979; 6:79.

VanGool JD, Kuijten RH, Donckerwolcke RA, Kramer PP: Detrusor-sphincter dyssynergia in children with myelomeningocele: A prospective study. Z Kinderchir 1982; 37:148.

Venes JL, Stevens SA: Surgical pathology in tethered cord secondary to meningomyelocele repair. Concepts Pediatr Neurosurg 1983; 4:165.

Watson HS, Bauer SB, Peters CA, et al: Comparative urodynamics of appendiceal and ureteral Mitrofanoff conduits in children. J Urol 1995; 154:878.

Woodard JR, Anderson AM, Parrott TS: Ureteral reimplantation in myelodysplastic children. J Urol 1981; 126:387.

Woodhouse CRJ: The sexual and reproductive consequences of congential genitourinary anomalies. J Urol 1994; 152:645.

Woodhouse CRJ, Malone PR, Cumming J, Reilly TM: The Mitrofanoff principle for continent urinary diversion. Br J Urol 1989; 63:53.

Woodside JR, McGuire EJ: Techniques for detection of detrusor hypertonia in the presence of urethral sphincter incompetence. J Urol 1982; 127:740.

Young HH: An operation for the cure of incontinence of urine. Surg Gynecol Obstet 1919; 28:84.

Lipomeningocele and Other Spinal Dysraphisms

Anderson FM: Occult spinal dysraphism: A series of 73 cases. Pediatrics 1975; 55:826.

Atala A, Bauer SB, Dyro FM, et al: Bladder functional changes resulting from lipomeningocele repair. J Urol 1992; 148:592.

Barson AJ: The vertebral level of termination of the spinal cord during normal and abnormal development. J Anat 1970; 106:489.

Bruce DA, Schut L: Spinal lipomas in infancy and childhood. Brain 1979; 5:192.

Campobasso P, Galiani E, Verzerio A, et al: A rare cause of occult neuropathic bladder in children: The tethered cord syndrome. Pediatr Med Chir 1988; 10:641.

Chapman PH: Congenital intraspinal lipomas: Anatomic considerations and surgical treatment. Child's Brain 1982; 9:37.

Dubrowitz V, Lorber J, Zachary RB: Lipoma of the cauda equina. Arch Dis Child 1965; 40:207.

Flanigan RF, Russell DP, Walsh JW: Urologic aspects of tethered cord. Urology 1989; 33:80.

Foster LS, Kogan BA, Cogan PH, Edwards MSB: Bladder function in patients with lipomyelomeningocele. J Urol 1990; 143:984.

Hall WA, Albright AL, Brunberg JA: Diagnosis of tethered cord by magnetic resonance imaging. Surg Neurol 1988; 30 (Suppl 1):60.

Hellstrom WJ, Edwards MS, Kogan BA: Urologic aspects of the tethered cord syndrome. J Urol 1986; 135:317.

James CM, Lassman LP: Spinal Dysraphism: Spina Bifida Occulta. New York, Appleton-Century-Crofts 1972.

Kaplan WE, McLone DG, Richards I: The urologic manifestations of the tethered spinal cord. J Urol 1988; 140:1285.

Keating MA, Rink RC, Bauer SB, et al: Neuro-urologic implications of changing approach in management of occult spinal lesions. J Urol 1988; 140:1299.

Khoury AE, Hendrick EB, McLorie GA, et al: Occult spinal dysraphism: Clinical and urodynamic outcome after diversion of the filum terminale. J Urol 1990; 144:426.

Kondo A, Kato K, Kanai S, Sakakibara T: Bladder dysfunction secondary to tethered cord syndrome in adults: Is it curable? J Urol 1986; 135:313.

Linder M, Rosenstein J, Sklar FH: Functional improvement after spinal surgery for the dysraphic malformations. Neurosurgery 1982; 11:622.

Mandell J, Bauer SB, Hallett M, et al: Occult spinal dysraphism: A rare but detectable cause of voiding dysfunction. Urol Clin North Am 1980; 7:349.

Packer RJ, Zimmerman RA, Sutton LN, et al: Magnetic resonance imaging of spinal cord diseases of childhood. Pediatrics 1986; 78:251.

Raghavendra BN, Epstein FJ, Pinto RS, et al: The tethered spinal cord: Diagnosis by high-resolution real-time ultrasound. Radiology 1983; 149:123.

Roy MW, Gilmore R, Walsh JW: Evaluation of children and young adults with tethered spinal cord syndrome. Utility of spinal and scalp recorded somatosensory evoked potentials. Surg Neurol 1986; 26:241.

Satar N, Bauer SB, Shefner J, et al: The effects of delayed diagnosis and treatment in patients with an occult spinal dysraphism. J Urol 1995; 154:754.

Satar N, Bauer SB, Scott RM, et al: Late effects of early surgery on lipoma and lipomeningocele in children under 1 year of age. J Urol. In press.

Scheible W, James HE, Leopold GR, Hilton SW: Occult spinal dysraphism in infants: Screening with high-resolution real-time ultrasound. Radiology 1983; 146:743.

Seeds JW, Jones FD: Lipomyelomeningocele: Prenatal diagnosis and management. Obstet Gynecol 1986; 67 (Suppl):34.

Tami S, Yamada S, Knighton RS: Extensibility of the lumbar and sacral cord. Pathophysiology of the tethered cord in cats. J Neurosurg 1987; 66:116.

Tracey PT, Hanigan WC: Spinal dysraphism: Use of magnetic resonance imaging in evaluation. Clin Pediatr 1990; 29:228.

Weissert M, Gysler R, Sorensen N: The clinical problem of the tethered cord syndrome—A report of three personal cases. Z Kinderchir 1989; 44:275.

Yamada S, Knierim D, Yonekura M, et al: Tethered cord syndrome. J Am Paraplegic Soc 1983; 6 (Suppl 3): 58.

Yamada S, Zincke DE, Sanders D: Pathophysiology of "tethered cord syndrome" J Neurosurg 1981; 54:494.

Yip CM, Leach GE, Rosenfeld DS, et al: Delayed diagnosis of voiding dysfunction: Occult spinal dysraphism. J Urol 1985; 124:694.

Sacral Agenesis

Bauer SB: Urodynamics in children. *In* Ashcraft KW, ed: Pediatric Urology. Orlando, Grune & Stratton, 1990, pp 49–76.

Boemers TM, VanGool JD, deJong TPVM, Bax KMA: Urodynamic evaluation of children with caudal regression syndrome (caudal dysplasia sequence). J Urol 1994; 151:1038.

Guzman L, Bauer SB, Hallet M, et al: The evaluation and management of children with sacral agenesis. Urology 1983; 23:506.

Jakobson H, Holm-Bentzen M, Hald T: Neurogenic bladder dysfunction in sacral agenesis and dysgenesis. Neurourol Urodynam 1985; 4:99.

Koff SA, DeRidder PA: Patterns of neurogenic bladder dysfunction in sacral agenesis. J Urol 1977; 118:87.

Landauer W: Rumplessness of chicken embryos produced by the injection of insulin and other chemicals. J Exp Zool 1945; 98:65.

Menon RK, Cohen RM, Sperling MA, et al: Transplacental passage of insulin in pregnant women with insulin-dependent diabetes mellitus. N Engl J Med 1990; 323:309.

Pang D: Sacral agenesis and caudal spinal cord malformations. Neurosurgery 1993; 32:755.

Passarge E, Lenz K: Syndrome of caudal regression in infants of diabetic mothers: Observations of further cases. Pediatrics 1966; 37:672.

Schlussel RN, Bauer SB, Kelly MD, et al: The clinical and urodynamic findings in 35 patients with sacral agenesis (Abstract 412). Presented at the Annual Meeting of the American Urological Association, San Francisco, May 16, 1994.

White RI, Klauber GT: Sacral agenesis. Analysis of twenty-two cases. Urology 1976; 8:521.

Imperforate Anus

Barnes PD, Lester PD, Yamanashi WS, Prince JR: MRI in infants and children with spinal dysraphism. Am J Radiol 1986; 147:339.

Barry JE, Auldist AW: The Vater syndrome. Am J Dis Child 1974; 128:769.

Boemers TM, VanGool JD, deJong TPVM, Bax KMA: Urodynamic evaluation of children with the caudal regression syndrome (caudal dysplasia sequence). J Urol 1994; 151:1038.

Carson JA, Barnes PD, Tunell WP, et al: Imperforate anus: The neurologic implication of sacral abnormalities. J Pediatr Surg 1984; 19:838.

Greenfield SP, Fera M: Urodynamic evaluation of the patient with imperforate anus. A prospective study. J Urol 1991; 146:539.

Kakizaki H, Nonomura K, Asano Y, et al: Preexisting neurogenic voiding dysfunction in children with imperforate anus: Problems in management. J Urol 1994; 151:1041.

Karrer FM, Flannery AM, Nelson MD Jr, et al: Anal rectal malformations: Evaluation of associated spinal dysraphic syndromes. J Pediatr Surg 1988; 23:45.

Parrott T, Woodard J: Importance of cystourethrography in neonates with imperforate anus. Urology 1979; 13:607.

Peña A: Posterior sagittal approach for the correction of anal rectal malformations. Adv Surg 1986; 19:69.

Rivosecchi M, Lucchetti MC, Zaccara A, et al: Spinal dysraphism detected by magnetic resonance imaging in patients with anorectal anomalies: Incidence and clinical significance. J Pediatr Surg 1995; 30:488.

Scott JES: The anatomy of the pelvic autonomic nervous system in cases of high imperforate anus. Surgery 1959; 45:1013.

Sheldon C, Cormier M, Crone K, Wacksman J: Occult neurovesical dysfunction in children with imperforate anus and its variants. J Pediatr Surg 1991; 26:49.

Tunnell WP, Austin JC, Barnes TP, Reynolds A: Neuroradiologic evaluation of sacral abnormalities in imperforate anus complex. J Pediatr Surg 1987; 22:58.

Uehling DT, Gilbert E, Chesney R: Urologic implications of the VATER syndrome. J Urol 1983; 129:352.

Williams DI, Grant J: Urologic complications of imperforate anus. Br J Urol 1969; 41:660.

Cerebral Palsy

Brodak PP, Sherz HC, Packer MG, Kaplan GW: Is urinary screening necessary for patients with cerebral palsy? U Urol 1994; 152:1586.

Decter RM, Bauer SB, Khoshbin S, et al: Urodynamic assessment of children with cerebral palsy. J Urol 1987; 138:1110.

Kuban KCK, Leviton A: Cerebral palsy. N Engl J Med 1994; 330:188.

Kyllerman M, Bogen B, Bensch J, et al: Dyskinetic cerebral palsy. I. Clinical categories associated neurological abnormalities and incidences. Acta Pediatr Scand 1982; 71:543.

Mayo ME: Lower urinary tract dysfunction in cerebral palsy. J Urol 1992; 147:419.

McNeal DM, Hawtrey CE, Wolraich ML, Mapel JR: Symptomatic neurogenic bladder in a cerebral-palsied population. Dev Med Child Neurol 1983; 25:612.

Naeye RL, Peters EC, Bartholomew M, Landis R: Origins of cerebral palsy. Am J Dis Child 1989; 143:1154.

Nelson KB, Ellenberg JH: Antecedents of cerebral palsy. N Engl J Med 1986; 315:81.

Reid CJD, Borzyskowski M: Lower urinary tract dysfunction in cerebral palsy. Arch Dis Child 1993; 68:739.

Traumatic Injuries to the Spine

Adams C, Babyn PS, Logan WJ: Spinal cord birth injury: Value of computed tomographic myelography. Pediatr Neurol 1988; 4:109.

Anderson JM, Schutt AH: Spinal injury in children: A review of 156 cases seen from 1950 through 1978. Mayo Clin Proc 1980; 55:499.

Barkin M, Dolfin D, Herschorn S, et al: The urologic care of the spinal cord injury patient. J Urol 1983; 129:335.

Cass AS, Luxenberg M, Johnson CF, Gleich P: Management of the neurogenic bladder in 413 children. J Urol 1984; 132:521.

Decter RM, Bauer SB: Urologic management of spinal cord injury in children. Urol Clin North Am 1993; 20:475.

Donnelly J, Hackler RH, Bunts RC: Present urologic status of the World War II paraplegic: 25-year follow-up comparison with status of the 20-year Korean War paraplegic and 5-year Vietnam paraplegic. J Urol 1972; 108:558.

Fanciullacci F, Zanollo A, Sandri S, Cantanzaro F: The neuropathic bladder in children with spinal cord injury. Paraplegia 1988; 26:83.

Guttmann L, Frankel H: The value of intermittent catheterization in the early management of traumatic paraplegia and tetraplegia. Paraplegia 1966; 4:63.

Hadley MN, Zabramski JM, Browner CM, et al: Pediatric spinal trauma: Review of 122 cases of spinal cord and vertebral column injuries. J Neurosurg 1988; 68:18.

Iwatsubo E, Iwakawa A, Koga H, et al: Functional recovery of the bladder in patients with spinal cord injury—prognosticating programs of an aseptic intermittent catheterization. Acta Urol Japon 1985; 31:775.

Lanska MJ, Roessmann U, Wiznitzer M: Magnetic resonance imaging in cervical cord birth injury. Pediatrics 1990; 85:760.

Ogawa T, Yoshida T, Fujinaga T: Bladder deformity in traumatic spinal cord injury patients. Acta Urol Japon 1988; 34:1173.

Pang D, Pollack IF: Spinal cord injury without radiographic abnormalities in children. The SCIWORA syndrome. J Trauma 1989; 29:654.

Pang D, Wilberger JE Jr.: Spinal cord injury without radiographic abnormalities in children. J Neurosurg 1982; 57:114.

Pearman JW: Urologic follow-up of 99 spinal cord injury patients initially managed by intermittent catheterization. Br J Urol 1976; 48:297.

Pollack IF, Pang D, Sclabassi R: Recurrent spinal cord injury without radiographic abnormalities in children. J Neurosurg 1988; 69:177.

Ruge JR, Sinson GP, McLone DG, et al: Pediatric spinal injury: The very young. J Neurosurg 1988; 68:25.

Functional Voiding Disorders

Bauer SB: Overview: My approach to neurogenic bladder. *In* Gonzales ET, Paulson DF, eds: Problems in Urology, Vol 8. Philadelphia, J. B. Lippincott, 1994, pp 441–459.

Bauer SB, Retik AB, Colodny AH, et al: The unstable bladder of childhood. Urol Clin North Am 1980; 7:321.

Bellman N: Encopresis. Acta Paediatr Scand 1966; (Suppl 1) 70:1.

Fergusson DM, Hons BA, Horwood LJ, Shannon FT: Factors related to the age of attainment of nocturnal bladder control: An eight year longitudinal study. Pediatrics 1986; 78:884.

MacKeith RL, Meadow SR, Turner RK: How children become dry. *In* Kolvin I, MacKeith RL, Meadow SR, eds: Bladder Control and Enuresis. Philadelphia, J. B. Lippincott, 1973, pp. 3–15.

Yeats WK: Bladder function in normal micturition. *In* Kolvin I, MacKeith RC, Meadow SR, eds: Bladder Control and Enuresis. Philadelphia, J. B. Lippincott, 1973, pp 28–41.

Small Capacity Hypertonic Bladder

Bauer SB, Retik AB, Colodny AH, et al: The unstable bladder of childhood. Urol Clin North Am 1980; 7:321.

Dyro FM, Bauer SB, Hallett M, Khoshbin S: Complex repetitive discharges in the external urethral sphincter in a pediatric population. Neurourol Urodynam 1983; 2:39.

Hansson S, Hjalmas K, Jodal U, Sixt R: Lower urinary tract dysfunction in girls with untreated asymptomatic or covert bacteriuria. J Urol 1990; 143:333.

Lebowitz RL, Mandell J: Urinary tract infection in children: Putting radiology in its place. Radiology 1987; 165:1.

Masek BJ: Behavioral management of voiding dysfunction in neurologically normal children. Dial Pediatr Urol 1985; 8:7.

Mayo ME, Burns MW: Urodynamic studies in children who wet. Br J Urol 1990; 65:641.

Rudy DC, Woodside JR: Non-neurogenic neurogenic bladder: The relationship between intravesical pressure and the external sphincter EMG. Neurourol Urodynam 1991; 10:169.

Saxton HM, Borzyskowski M, Mundy AR, Vivian GC: Spinning top deformity: Not a normal variant. Radiology 1988; 168:147.

Tanagho EA, Miller EA, Lyon RP: Spastic striated external sphincter and urinary tract infection in girls. Br J Urol 1971; 43:69.

VanGool JD, Tanagho EA: External sphincter activity and recurrent urinary tract infection in girls. Urology 1977; 10:348.

to be an important factor in explaining this variability. Studies that use a urethral catheter and high filling rates have higher incidences of instability than those using a suprapubic tube inserted in advance of the study and low flow rates. Likewise, when provocative testing aimed at eliciting instability is used such as positional alterations (sitting and standing cystometry) or micturition stop testing, a very high incidence of instability (78% to 84%) can be elicited (Giles et al, 1978; Mahoney et al, 1981). In detailed awake urodynamic studies performed by Norgaard and colleagues (Norgaard 1989a, 1989b; Norgaard et al, 1985a, 1989a, 1989c), children with monosymptomatic nocturnal enuresis demonstrated bladder instability in only 16% of bladder fillings, a rate that is similar to normal (Hjälmåas, 1976).

Urodynamic studies that monitor natural bladder filling during sleep have helped clarify the pathophysiology of sleep wetting. Gastaut and Broughton (1965) and Broughton (1968) were the first to characterize the features of a typical enuretic episode as a series of high-pressure bladder contractions that culminated in micturition. Enuretics who happened not to wet during the study still displayed the same degree of bladder hyperactivity, but pressures were lower and the frequency of contractions were less than those preceding an enuretic event. In contrast, normal nonenuretic individuals displayed few, if any, low-pressure bladder contractions during sleep monitoring. More recently, studies by Norgaard and co-workers (1989b) have found that an enuretic wetting episode is nearly identical to voluntary daytime voiding, with a single contraction producing the discharge of urine. The differences between wetting at night and voiding in the daytime were slight: At night, the bladder was usually full when it contracted, the contraction time was longer, and the maximum bladder pressure was higher. In addition, simultaneous pelvic floor activity usually indicated that arousal would occur and led to voluntary voiding, whereas a silent pelvic floor was associated with sleep wetting (Norgaard, 1989b, 1989c). They also confirmed that in enuretics, bladder instability occurred much more commonly at nighttime (49%) than in the daytime (16%). Also, although instability would not necessarily lead to sleep wetting, it was just as likely to lead to awakening.

Urodynamic studies that actively fill the bladder during sleep at faster filling rates (30 ml/minute) give additional insight into the relationship between instability and enuresis and demonstrate that bladder instability (contractions) can be provoked in nearly 100% of patients, but that the patients' responses to the contractions were just as likely to be an enuretic event as an awakening to voluntarily void (Norgaard, 1989c).

In summary, daytime bladder instability does not occur in children with monosymptomatic nocturnal enuresis at a rate higher than normal. Bladder instability during sleep, however, normally occurs in about 50% of enuretics and can be provoked in nearly all simply by actively filling the bladder. Although nocturnal enuresis cannot occur without a bladder contraction, these contractions per se are not sufficient to produce incontinence because, in most children, the contraction is just as likely to lead to awakening to void as to wetting. Therefore, cures for monosymptomatic nocturnal enuresis that aim to eliminate bladder instability (such as anticholinergic medication) are predictably ineffective.

Sleep Factors

The fact that wetting occurs during sleep suggests that enuretics might have a disturbance of sleep that causes them to either sleep too deeply or to fail to awaken from sleep. Objective evaluation of the relationship between sleep and wetting during sleep requires careful monitoring throughout the night of multiple physiologic variables including electroencephalography (EEG), eye movement, urodynamic parameters, and pulse and blood pressure. Such studies have demonstrated that sleep is not simply the progressive and passive slowing of body and brain processes, and that the relationships between sleep, arousal, and sleep wetting are neither simple nor intuitive.

Normal sleep begins with so-called nonrapid eye movement (NREM) sleep, which is divisible into four progressively deeper stages of sleep (stages 1–4), each characterized by specific EEG changes. In addition, a particularly light stage of sleep is recognized and characterized by bursts of conjugate rapid eye movements (REM sleep). REM sleep is associated with increased autonomic activity, generalized muscle atonia, and dreaming.

Normal sleep structure is composed of cycles of NREM sleep, REM sleep, and occasional awakenings. In older children and adults, these cycles last about 1 to 1.5 hours, and the percentage of time spent in REM sleep increases as the cycles progress through the night (Rechtschaffen and Kales, 1968).

Recognizing that enuretics often appear to be very deep sleepers, enuresis was originally considered to be the result of sleeping too soundly or awakening with difficulty (Broughton, 1968; Lowy, 1970; Anders and Weinstein, 1972; Kales and Kales, 1974). Early sleep studies supported these views by demonstrating that enuresis often occurred during deep sleep and that older enuretics were often very deep sleepers whose wetting could be improved by amphetamines used to lighten their sleep (Strom-Olsen, 1950). Clearly, when children are aroused from deep sleep, they are often hard to awaken and appear to be confused and disoriented, and stumble when they walk to the toilet. Although it has been suggested, unconvincingly, that this so-called sleep drunkenness is more exaggerated in enuretics, the observation that enuretics are especially deep sleepers is biased by the fact that parents do not usually attempt to awaken their nonenuretic children. When they do attempt to awaken nonwetting siblings, they are usually surprised to find them sleeping equally soundly (Hallgren, 1957; Boyd, 1960; McKendry et al, 1968; Lowy, 1970; Graham, 1973). Controlled sleep studies have shown that children with enuresis sleep no more soundly than do normals and that a number of enuretics actually wet during very light sleep or even while temporarily awake (Ritvo et al, 1969). They have also demonstrated that neither hypothesis, deep sleep or an arousal disorder, is an accurate description of enuretic sleep or a cause for wetting. Enuretics are observed to sleep no more deeply than age-matched controls, and enuretic events were associated neither with deep sleep nor with any specific transition between sleep stages or signs of awakening. Instead, enuretic episodes were noted to occur throughout the night on a random basis with a tendency toward the first two sleep cycles and wetting occurred in each sleep stage in proportion to the time actually spent in that stage (Kales et al, 1977; Mikkelson et al, 1980; Inoue et al, 1987; Norgaard et al, 1989a, 1989b; Reimao, 1993). **These findings convincingly indicate that enuretic sleep patterns are not appreciably different from the sleep patterns of normal children, and that most enuretics do not wet as a consequence of sleeping too deeply or having a disorder of awakening.**

Recent nocturnal sleep and bladder monitoring studies by Robert and others (1993) have been able to distinguish three different types of enuretic episodes. The first pattern is similar to the classic description by Gastaut and Broughton (1965), in which gradually undulating elevations in bladder pressures culminate in wetting and are associated with prominent somatic and visceral reactions, including tachycardia, prominent body movements, increasing respirations, and a progressive awakening reaction. It appears as if the awakening reaction is very strong and the child is struggling to keep from wetting. The second pattern is a very quick micturition associated with minimal body movement and visceral signs; the awakening reaction is very brief, and the struggle not to wet very limited. The third pattern involves complete parasomnia, a total lack of central nervous system (CNS) reaction and response to bladder stimuli. Neither bladder filling nor bladder contraction is registered on the EEG; as a result, involuntary voiding occurs without any modification of sleep.

Watanabe and Azuma (1989) have defined three discrete types of enuresis based on cystometric and EEG observations (Table 66–2) Follow-up analysis of patients with these three types of patterns indicates that of patients with type IIb enuresis 20% will change to IIa and 60% to I, whereas 78% of patients with type IIa will change to type I (Watanabe et al, 1994; Watanabe, 1995). The evolution of these distinct patterns of EEG and urodynamic responses suggests that, with time, developmental changes are taking place, which include increasing CNS recognition of bladder fullness and contraction and increasing CNS control over the micturition reflex. **Rather than indicating disordered sleep as a cause for enuresis, these observations suggest alternatively that, in many cases, enuresis may indeed be caused by a developmental delay, actually a dual delay, in the development of the perception and inhibition of bladder filling and contraction by the CNS (Koff, 1995).**

Alterations in Vasopressin Secretion and Nocturnal Polyuria

It has been recognized for at least 100 years that less urine is normally excreted during the night than during the day. In 1975, George and associates demonstrated that a circadian rhythm of plasma arginine vasopressin (AVP), which increased during the night, was responsible for this change in urinary output. However, some children with enuresis appear to have stable levels of AVP during both the day and night, which causes them to produce larger amounts of dilute urine at night (Puri, 1980; Norgaard, 1985b; Rittig, 1989a). This can result in nocturnal urine production that equals or exceeds diurnal output and, in some children, may exceed functional bladder capacity (Norgaard et al, 1985b; Rittig, 1989a; Norgaard, 1989a). Although these authors found a close relationship between nocturnal polyuria due to a lack of AVP excretion and enuresis, and suggest that AVP deficiency may be etiologic in nocturnal enuresis, other opinions have been contradictory. In studies by Vulliamy (1956), no difference between day and night urine output was observed when enuretic and nonenuretic children were compared on standardized diets and fluid intakes, whereas Steffens and colleagues (1993) found that only 14 of 55 (25%) children with nocturnal enuresis had a significant decrease in nocturnal AVP compared with controls. Likewise, in large population studies Kawauchi and Watanabe (1993) found no significant difference in nocturnal urine osmolality between enuretic and nonenuretic children at any age. Although failure of AVP to increase during the night and its effect on urinary output appear to be factors in some children with enuresis, the frequency, mechanism, and pathophysiologic significance of altered AVP excretion in enuresis requires further clarification.

Table 66–2. TYPES OF ENURESIS BASED ON CYSTOMETRIC AND EEG OBSERVATIONS

Type I:	A stable bladder with an EEG response during an enuretic episode
Type IIa:	A stable bladder with no EEG response during an enuretic episode
Type IIb:	An unstable bladder with no EEG response during an enuretic episode

From Watanabe H, Azuma Y: A proposal for a classification system of enuresis based on overnight simultaneous monitoring of electroencephalography and cystometry. Sleep 1989; 12:257–264.
EEG, Electroencephalographic.

AVP is stored in the posterior pituitary and is released into the blood stream in response to action potentials in nerve fibers that synthesize the hormone (Ohne 1995). In addition to well-recognized factors, such as changes in serum osmotic pressure and extracellular fluid volume, a variety of other stimuli can alter vasopressin secretion, such as pain, emotion, exercise, and medication. Moreover, established patterns of AVP secretion can be modified by sleep and light. Sleep is known to affect pituitary hormone secretion, and this effect can be seen in individuals who nap after lunch and have increases in AVP secretion. Likewise, alterations in sleep produce changes in established AVP circadian rhythms, a phenomenon that is well recognized in night-shift workers who display a reversal of their AVP circadian rhythm (Aschoff, 1965; Moore-Ede, 1986).

Recent evidence suggests that AVP secretion may also be influenced by bladder fullness. In clinical studies, Kawauchi and associates (1993) observed that (1) following supravesical urinary diversion, the normal difference between day and night levels of AVP disappeared; and (2) during cystometry, AVP levels were higher when the bladder was full than when it was empty. Experimental studies by Ohne (1995) examined the effect of urinary retention on AVP production and found that within 2 hours of urethral obstruction, there occurred increased activity in hypothalamic cells that produce AVP. It was hypothesized that bladder wall fullness and wall stretching induced by urinary retention affects, via neuronal stimulation, the regulation of AVP secretion from the hypothalamus. **These observations suggest that bedwetting, by emptying the bladder during the night, may actually be the cause for enuretics to have low levels of nocturnal AVP secretion because the empty bladder removes a stimulus for the secretion of AVP.**

Evidence also suggests that the absence of an AVP circadian rhythm in some enuretics may be more aptly considered a delay in development rather than a true pathophysiologic process (Koff, 1995). Measurement of urinary osmolality in first morning urine specimens from enuretic and nonenuretic children demonstrated that children under age 4 years have significantly lower osmolality than children older than age 5 years, yet there was no difference in osmolality between enuretic and nonenuretic children (Kawauchi and Watanabe, 1993). This immaturity in nighttime urine concentration does not appear to be due to renal concentrating ability, which reaches adult levels by 18 months of age; nor does it appear to be due to serum AVP levels, which reach adult levels by 12 months of age (Winberg, 1959; Rascher et al, 1986). It suggests alternatively that it may be due to immaturity in the circadian rhythmicity of AVP. Observations by Knudsen and co-workers (1991) that 25% of enuretics who initially lacked AVP rhythmicity ultimately developed a circadian rhythm of AVP support the concept that the circadian rhythm of AVP may be delayed developmentally and improve with time. Interestingly, after developing an increase in nocturnal AVP secretion, these patients were improved but were not cured of their enuresis.

Developmental Delay

The aforementioned alterations in urodynamic function, sleep, AVP secretion, and urinary osmolality that include bladder instability in the day, uncontrolled bladder contractions at night, failure to respond or awaken to bladder fullness or contraction, and altered AVP excretion with low urinary concentration at night all occur normally in infants and young children. Nocturnal enuresis, therefore, appears to represent a true arrest in development, and each one of these associated physiologic alterations tends to improve with time and to resolve spontaneously in most children. Children displaying these abnormalities do not manifest any obvious evidence of neuropathy, and neurologic disease is rarely identified in patients with monosymptomatic nocturnal enuresis. It is likely that these phenomena are simply diverse expressions of neurophysiologic immaturity.

The hypothesis that enuresis represents a delay in CNS control or development is attractive and well supported by a number of eclectic clinical observations. These include the fact that nonorganic disturbances, such as social pressures and stress, can delay the development of urinary control and influence the duration of enuresis. Bedwetting is more common in lower socioeconomic groups and occurs twice as often among unskilled workers as compared with professionals (Essen and Peckham, 1976).

In families undergoing stressful circumstances, the likelihood of enuresis increases threefold (Miller et al, 1960). MacKeith (1968) has pointed out that the second to the fourth year is a particularly sensitive period in the development of nocturnal urinary control; children with a significant anxiety-producing episode during this period have an increased chance for developing enuresis. Young and Morgan (1973) have suggested further that the difference between primary and secondary enuresis is simply related to the timing of stressful events: Primary enuresis results from stress during this sensitive period, whereas stress after this period contributes to secondary enuresis.

Despite the fact that neuroanatomic pathways are usually intact in nocturnal enuretics, population control studies have shown a wide variety of developmental delays in these patients that do not occur in nonwetting controls (Stein and Susser, 1967; Mimouni et al, 1985; Jarvelin, 1989). These delays, which reflect immaturity in CNS regulatory function, include fine and gross motor clumsiness, perceptual dysfunction, and delays in speech. A significant number of children with enuresis display retardation in skeletal maturation (bone age) and many have been small-for-gestational-age infants. Delay in development is also reflected in the tendency for encopresis to occur more commonly in enuretics (10% to 25%) and supports the generally accepted clinical observation that children who are retarded in one aspect of sphincter control tend to be retarded in another.

In summary, these findings suggest that achieving urinary control at night is an integral and normal part of a child's general development that can be delayed or retarded by nonorganic internal and external factors. In most cases, nocturnal enuresis simply represents an arrest of development that, to the casual observer, may appear to be an isolated event. However, careful study of these children has shown that this delay is not isolated, that it is associated with other lags in development, and that in almost all cases, it will improve with time.

Genetic Factors

It is an old but valid observation that enuresis tends to run in families. In multiple series, over a third of fathers and a fifth of mothers of enuretics have an enuretic history themselves (Frary, 1935; Hallgren, 1957). Bakwin (1971, 1973) showed that when both parents had enuresis, 77% of children were enuretic, whereas when one parent was enuretic, 44% of children developed wetting. These figures contrast with a 15% incidence of enuresis in children of nonenuretic parents. Also, studies in twins indicate that when one twin has enuresis, the other is also predisposed to develop wetting (Bakwin, 1971). Response to desmopressin (DDAVP) also appears to have a genetic predisposition; Hogg and Husmann (1993) noted that whereas an overall response rate to DDAVP could be achieved in 75% of patients, the response by patients with a positive history of enuresis was 91%.

Organic Urinary Tract Disease

Children with enuresis, particularly girls, are predisposed to develop urinary tract infections (Dodge et al, 1970). Many of these children do not have monosymptomatic nocturnal enuresis but do have diurnal symptoms due to bladder instability. Boys with enuresis are less prone to develop urinary tract infections, even if they have diurnal symptoms associated with bladder instability (Koff and Murtagh, 1983).

Excluding bladder instability, most children with monosymptomatic nocturnal enuresis do not have an organic urinary tract cause for their wetting; the incidence of organic disease is less than 10% and probably closer to 1% (Hallgren, 1957; Forsythe and Redmond, 1974; McKendry and Stewart, 1974). Historically, however, diseases that nowadays would be classified as normal variants or minor abnormalities were regularly invoked as common causes for enuresis, and many children underwent some type of surgical procedure (Fisher and Forsythe, 1954; Mahony, 1971; Arnold and Ginsberg, 1973). It is now generally appreciated that these minor disorders, such as meatal stenosis, do not cause enuresis, and that cure of enuresis is unlikely to occur following an operation, such as meatotomy (Kunin et al, 1970). In contrast to pure nocturnal enuresis, Cutler and colleagues (1978) found an increased incidence of organic abnormalities in children with diurnal symptoms, although not all series have substantiated this finding (Redman and Seibert, 1979). This finding does suggest that **children with nocturnal enuresis and associated daytime symptoms, especially boys, should have their urinary tracts screened with at least an ultrasonogram to exclude obstruction: bladder wall thickening, hydronephrosis, or incomplete emptying.**

Psychologic Factors

The occurrence of emotional disturbances in enuretic children is probably slightly higher than in the general population, but most enuretics do not suffer from significant psychologic disease (Werry, 1967; Fergusson et al, 1986). From a psychodynamic viewpoint, if enuresis were the sole somatic expression of an emotional disorder, its elimination might produce unwanted results either by worsening the psychopathology or by causing substitute symptoms to develop (Young and Morgan, 1973). Most therapists find that precisely the opposite occurs after enuresis is cured—childhood adjustment tends to improve rather than worsen (Baker, 1969). Bindelglas and Dee (1978) and Stromgren and Thomsen (1990) reported the fate of enuretics who had been successfully treated with imipramine or conditioning years earlier. These and other studies convincingly put to rest the notion that enuresis is a symptom of severe psychopathologic disturbance and demonstrate that treatment of enuresis not only does not produce any negative effect on adolescent health, growth, or development but is beneficial (Moffatt, 1989).

In some instances, enuresis and a psychopathologic disorder may coexist, although disturbed children are not particularly prone to enuresis. Occasionally, an emotional disturbance may actually be caused by or made worse by enuresis when wetting places an additional burden on an already compromised child suffering from multiple difficulties (Young and Morgan, 1973).

Miscellaneous Factors

Although there is no objective evidence relating allergy to enuresis for most patients, in small subsets of selected individuals, such an association may exist and be treatable (Egger, 1992). Zaleski and associates (1972) have shown that food allergy may cause bladder hyperactivity and a reduced functional bladder capacity. These problems were observed to improve after elimination of the dietary allergen. However, in enuresis caused by food allergy, no differences were observed in the level of immunoglobulins often associated with allergenic phenomena (immunoglobulin [IgE]) in enuretics as compared with controls (Kaplan, 1973).

Enuretics have a higher incidence of EEG abnormalities compared with normal children, although many of these described abnormalities are nonspecific and minor (Campbell and Young, 1966; Kajtor et al, 1967; Fermaglich, 1969). This finding may reflect mild degrees of cerebral dysfunction, or more likely, it provides corroborating evidence for delayed maturation of the CNS.

Sudden-onset enuresis and urinary frequency in young girls may be due to *Enterobius vermicularis* (pinworm) infestation, even in the absence of perineal itching. Diagnosis is made by the recovery of characteristic eggs in feces, from perianal skin, or from under fingernails. Immediate and dramatic relief of symptoms follow appropriate antihelminthic therapy (Sachdev and Howards, 1975).

EVALUATION

The family of a child with enuresis seeks medical attention for a variety of reasons and at different times. Families with a history of bedwetting tend to be more tolerant of wetting and more likely to await spontaneous cure. They often bring an older child for evaluation of persisting wetting specifically to exclude organic disease. In families in which no others have been bedwetters, the enuretic may be blamed and punished for wetting and be brought for evaluation at a very young age; this can place great pressure on the physician to perform tests to identify a cause and to produce a cure. However, urologic tests are rarely indicated for monosymptomatic bedwetters, yet out of frustration, the physician may be tempted to perform radiographic testing or cystoscopy and to attach pathologic significance to minor anatomic variations and treat them aggressively. Such an approach is inappropriate and unwarranted.

Most children with enuresis do not have an organic lesion, and those who do are readily detected by routine evaluation. A careful screening evaluation that includes a history, physical examination, and urinalysis and culture is needed for all children with monosymptomatic bedwetting, and when the results are normal, these procedures are all that is needed. Radiographic studies, such as intravenous pyelography or voiding cystourethrography and invasive urologic testing with cystoscopy, are not required or indicated when the screening evaluation is negative (Table 66–3)

The goal of screening is to identify and separate the small number of children with possible urologic disease who need further investigation from the majority who need no further

Table 66–3. CHARACTERISTICS OF A NEGATIVE SCREENING EVALUATION FOR ENURESIS

Age: prepubertal
Enuresis has been lifelong
Wetting occurs only at night
No daytime symptoms of wetting, urgency, or polyuria
No history of urinary infection
Negative urinalysis and culture
Normal physical examination, including lumbosacral spine

evaluation. Specific features that can help distinguish these patients and guide treatment include urinary tract infection or a history of urinary tract infection, pattern of incontinence (day symptoms?), presence of constipation, positive family history (when did they stop wetting?), apparent deep sleeping, age and success of toilet training, and prior therapeutic trials. As part of the routine physical examination, a pertinent neurologic examination is required and should include careful inspection and palpation of the lumbosacral spine to look for hairy patches, lipomata, tracts, or bony irregularities that suggest spinal dysraphism.

This noninvasive approach usually separates children into three groups: (1) children with monosymptomatic nocturnal enuresis who require no further evaluation, (2) children with urinary infection or overt neuropathy who require full urologic investigation, and (3) children without infection or apparent neuropathy who have day and night incontinence or other symptoms of dysfunctional voiding. Although many children in the third group are often ultimately found to have urodynamic disturbances, such as bladder instability, it is necessary first to exclude anatomic urinary tract abnormalities. This can be accomplished noninvasively with an ultrasound examination that includes the kidneys, ureters, and bladder before and after voiding. This approach excludes hydroureteronephrosis and bladder wall thickening as well as assesses completeness of bladder emptying. When the ultrasonogram is normal, an empirical therapeutic trial of pharmacologic agents may be instituted as an alternative to performing urodynamic studies if symptoms are not severe. If voiding dysfunction is severe or persists, urodynamic studies are indicated to exclude neuropathy and to guide further treatment.

TREATMENT

Throughout history, enuresis has been viewed as more of a social bane than a medical problem, and a variety of different programs have been used to treat it (Glicklich, 1951). These programs range from home remedies and nonspecific measures, such as decreasing fluids and awakenings during the night, to sophisticated behavioral and medication regimens. Because children spontaneously improve and eventually outgrow enuresis, it has been genuinely difficult to objectively evaluate the effectiveness of even seemingly well-controlled treatment programs. This difficulty reflects a spontaneous remission rate of approximately 15% per year and a placebo improvement effect as high as 68% (Forsythe and Redmond, 1974; Mishra et al, 1980). Despite this analytic handicap, reproducibly effective therapy does exist for many children with enuresis and has evolved along two main lines: drug therapy and behavior modification.

Before beginning therapy, the physician must realize that once organic causes are excluded, not all families actually desire medical treatment because of risks, inconvenience, or responsibility, and some lack the motivation, intelligence, or commitment needed. Also, parents have been shown to have very different attitudes and expectations about bedwetting and its cure than do physicians. About 60% of surveyed parents believe that bedwetting is a significant problem, severe enough in 35% to punish the child. Also, most parents generally believe that their child should be dry at a much younger age than does their physician; yet only 63% of parents believe that enuresis should actually be treated as compared with nearly 90% of physicians. Likewise, the vast majority of parents (93%) have communicated that medication is not a good form of treatment for bedwetting (Haque et al, 1981). Although therapy for enuresis has been well shown to be advantageous by providing psychologic benefits to the patient, especially in improved self-image and behavior and reduced anxiety, the best time to start treatment is less well defined. In most families, pure nocturnal wetting is not perceived to be a problem before age 4 to 5, because at age 5, about 15% of the population still are wetting. Because of patient and family motivation and the relative lack of social pressures, I generally discourage treatment before age 7 years and have not witnessed many treatment successes prior to this age. This is the age when children, their peers, and parents generally begin to expect dryness and when bedwetting starts to interfere with social activities such as sleep-overs (Moffatt,1994).

Drug Therapy

Autonomic Agents

Effective drug therapy exists for enuresis but not in the form of sedatives, stimulants, or sympathomimetic agents (Blackwell and Currah, 1973). Overall, anticholinergic drug therapy has been disappointing. Its effectiveness has been in the range of 5% to 40%, and in some series, therapy was not at all different from placebo effect (Harrison and Albino, 1970; Kunin et al, 1970). Although anticholinergic drugs have been shown to increase the functional capacity of the bladder, elimination of enuresis does not occur in about half of cases (Johnstone, 1972). However, because these agents are very useful in eliminating bladder instability, they are definitely effective for treating enuretics with instability who typically do not have monosymptomatic nocturnal enuresis. Indeed, Kass and co-workers (1979) found anticholinergic therapy to be very effective (87.5%) in treating enuretic patients who had symptoms of bladder instability, such as urgency, frequency, and day and night incontinence, and even more effective (91%) in those with urodynamically proven instability. The success rate was much less (50%) in patients with purely nocturnal enuresis and was only 11% in those with normal urodynamic findings. Anticholinergic drugs appear to be of little value for children with monosymptomatic enuresis and normal urodynamic findings (Person-Junemann et al, 1993).

Agents Affecting Urinary Output

Reduction of urine output at night is theoretically attractive for treating bedwetting. However, simply limiting fluids or using diuretics during the daytime to produce relative dehydration at night has not been particularly effective (Scott and Morrison, 1980). In contrast, manipulation of antidiuretic hormone levels appears useful because of observations that some enuretics demonstrate reduced nocturnal vasopressin levels and have nocturnal polyuria (see the section above entitled Alterations in Vasopressin Secretion and Nocturnal Polyuria).

Until recently, however, any preparation containing natural vasopressin was not useful for enuresis control because the drug effect was too short and was associated with unpleasant smooth muscle side effects. With the development of DDAVP, an analogue of vasopressin, a potential application for treating enuresis became available. This drug can be given intranasally or orally, has no pressor or smooth muscle activity in the therapeutic dose range, and its effect lasts 7 to 12 hours.

In double-blind studies, DDAVP has been shown to be more effective than placebo in treating enuresis. Its mechanism of action is believed to be due to its antidiuretic effect. The usual clinical dose ranges between 20 and 40 μg per night for the nasal spray and between 200 and 400 μg per night for the tablet; response may be dose dependent. In Moffatt's 1993 review of the extant literature on randomized clinical studies using DDAVP therapy, all but one study demonstrated a statistically significant reduction in wet nights, yet only 25% of patients actually became dry for 14 or more consecutive days on therapy (Table 66–4). DDAVP thus appears to be much more effective at reducing the number of wet nights per week than at curing bedwetting. This finding has been confirmed by others (Harris, 1989; Klauber, 1989; Miller et al, 1989; Rew and Rundle, 1989; Bloom, 1993). The therapeutic effect of DDAVP is temporary, and after treatment, most children resume wetting. Oral DDAVP appears to be about as effective as the nasal preparation (Fjellestad-Paulsen et al, 1987; Matthiesen et al, 1994).

Short-term studies with follow-up of less than 1 year have generally shown ease of administration and a rapid initial effect; longer term studies show that after treatment is stopped, no adverse effects are observed on vasopressin secretion, diurnal urinary output, and urine osmolality (Knudsen et al, 1991). However, DDAVP is capable of producing side effects. Nonserious side effects are infrequent, the most common being nasal irritation associated with the nasal spray. Potentially serious side effects relate to the fact that DDAVP is a potent antidiuretic. The possibility of water intoxication leading to hyponatremic seizures exists and has been reported in 21 separate cases between 1974 and June 1992 (Hjälmåas and Bengtsson, 1993), with additional cases reported since then (Beach et al 1992). This potentially serious side effect requires caution whenever DDAVP is used; parents should be instructed to limit fluids prior to administering DDAVP and for the duration of its therapeutic effect (12 hours) (Beach et al, 1992). It is not yet clear what type of evaluation or monitoring, if any, is required when DDAVP is used for the long term, but long-term use should probably be reserved for older patients who understand the potential seriousness of water intoxication and can be expected to comply with fluid restrictions.

In summary, although DDAVP is effective in decreasing the number of wet nights per week, it cures less than 1/3 of patients and its effect is temporary. Because it is relatively expensive, is less effective than the body worn urinary alarm, and may occasionally be associated with serious side effects, it should not be used as a first line of therapy in treating nocturnal enuresis.

Table 66–4. DDAVP CURE RATE IN NOCTURNAL ENURESIS

Author	Number of Patients	Mean Wet Nights: *Placebo*	Mean Wet Nights: *DDAVP*	Percent Totally Dry
Aladjem et al, 1982	32	8.8	3	35
Birkasova et al, 1978	22	11	4.2	23
Dimson, 1977	17	9.9	6.9	12
Ferrie, 1984	22	8.8	7.9	N/S
Fjellestad-Paulsen, 1987	30	9.0	5.6	10
Janknegt and Smans, 1990	22	10.6	6.8	N/S
Pedersen et al, 1985	37	7.7	5.0	16
Post et al, 1983	52	10	7.8	12
Ramsden et al, 1982	24	8	4.3	38
Rittig, 1989b	28	6.7	1.8	86
Sukhai et al, 1989	28	5.8	3.8	58
Terho, 1991	52	9.4	5.0	29
Tuvemo, 1978	18	8.0	3.2	44
Wille, 1986	50	9.8	13.8	N/S

Number Totally Dry/Total Number Subjects = 24.5%

From Moffatt MEK, Harlos S, Kirshen AJ, Burd L: Desmopressin acetate and nocturnal enuresis: How much do we know? Pediatrics 1993; 92:420–425. Reproduced by permission of Pediatrics, vol 92, pp 420–425, copyright 1993.

N/S, Not stated.

Imipramine

Imipramine typifies a class of tricyclic antidepressants and before the introduction of DDAVP was one of the most widely studied and widely used of all antienuretic medications. Since its effect on enuresis was first observed by MacLean in 1960, it has proved to be significantly effective compared with placebo in large numbers of well-controlled clinical studies. Results range widely, but enuresis has reportedly been cured in more than 50% of children and improved in up to 80%. However, discontinuation of medication causes up to 60% of patients to relapse (Hägglund and Parkkulainen, 1965; Poussaint et al, 1966; Kardash et al, 1968; Miller et al, 1968; Milner and Hills, 1968; Shaffer et al, 1968; Esperanca and Gerrard, 1969b; Liederman et al, 1969; Harrison and Albino, 1970; Kunin et al, 1970; Martin, 1971; Blackwell and Currah, 1973; Furlanut et al, 1989; Fritz et al, 1994). Although imipramine (Tofranil) is the most widely used tricyclic agent, other drugs in this class, such as nortriptyline (Aventyl), amitriptyline (Elavil), and desipramine (Pertofrane), have similar effects.

Imipramine has several different pharmacologic actions on both the peripheral nervous system and CNS that could account for its antienuretic effects, yet its precise mechanism of action remains unknown. Its peripheral effects include (1) weak anticholinergic activity that is 1/160 as active as atropine on bladder smooth muscle (Sigg, 1959) but that is ineffective in abolishing uninhibited detrusor contractions (Diokno et al, 1972); (2) direct in vitro antispasmodic activity on bladder smooth muscle that is inapparent at clinically effective antienuretic doses (Labay and Boyarsky, 1973; Stephenson, 1979); and (3) a complex effect on sympathetic input to the bladder, which interferes with norepinephrine action on alpha receptors and enhances its effect on beta receptors by inhibiting norepinephrine reuptake (Labay and Boyarsky, 1973; Stephenson, 1979). Combined, these peripheral actions of imipramine tend to increase bladder capacity, the development of which has been reported to exert beneficial effects on enuresis (Hägglund, 1965).

Imipramine's influence on the CNS includes antidepressant activity and effects on sleep. It is unlikely that its antienuretic effect is related to antidepressant activity because the time course of action in enuresis is immediate, whereas the effect on depression is often delayed and usually requires a much higher dosage (Rapoport et al, 1980). Imipramine alters sleep by decreasing the amount of time spent in REM sleep and increasing the time spent in light NREM sleep. This REM sleep suppression occurs primarily during the first two thirds of the night. As a result, enuretic events become less common during these early sleep periods and more common during the last third. In sleep studies, imipramine reduces the total number of wetting episodes but does not alter the sleep stage at which wetting occurs. Just as in normals, incontinence occurs in each sleep stage roughly in proportion to the time spent in that stage (Ritvo et al, 1969; Kales et al, 1977; Rapoport et al, 1980). Imipramine works by eliminating night wetting not by converting enuresis to nocturia and treatment with imipramine does not lead to more frequent night awakenings than does placebo. This suggests that its effect on sleep and on sleep stages is relatively independent of its effect on enuresis (Kales et al, 1977; Rapoport et al, 1980).

In some studies, the clinical response to imipramine has been shown to correlate with plasma levels; this has provided a better understanding of drug action and potentially a more rational approach to therapy (Jorgensen et al, 1980; Rapoport et al, 1980; De Gatta et al, 1984). Although high serum levels tend to be associated with better responses, serum levels can vary by sevenfold at standard dosage levels, and not all patients with high serum levels respond to the drug (Fritz et al, 1994). This limits the clinical usefulness of serum level monitoring.

Imipramine is generally prescribed at a dose of 25 mg for children between 5 and 8 years of age and 50 mg for older children. On a weight basis, the usual recommended dosage is 0.9 to 1.5 mg/kg/day (Maxwell and Seldrup, 1971). Although dosage of up to 2.5 mg/kg/day can be well tolerated without significant side effects, disproportionate increases in plasma levels are observed as doses begin to rise above 2.0 mg/kg (Fritz et al, 1994). Unfortunately, the recommended dosage results in an optimal therapeutic plasma concentration in only 30% of patients (Jorgensen et al, 1980), a finding that may explain the variability in clinical effect noted in some early reports. An increase in the dose of three- to fivefold would be required to achieve a therapeutic level in all patients, but this cannot be justified because nearly toxic levels would result for certain patients (Stephenson, 1979). However, even high plasma levels will not ensure a response in all instances because true nonresponders do exist (up to 25%), as do patients who develop a tolerance to the drug. Likewise, clinical response does not always correlate directly with serum concentration; some patients respond well when serum levels are low. Therefore, routine measurement of the serum concentration of imipramine or its metabolites is not useful or recommended (DeVane et al, 1984).

Imipramine is generally given once per day, usually shortly before bedtime. The exact time of administration does not appear critical, although some children who wet very early at night may benefit from late afternoon administration (Alderton, 1970). A 2-week trial is generally adequate to assess drug responsiveness. Thereafter, adjustments in the dosage and timing can be made, if necessary. It is not entirely clear how long a satisfactorily responding child can safely be kept on medication. Because the long-term effects of tricyclic therapy in children are unknown, long-term use is difficult to justify except in exceptional instances. When the decision is made to stop medication, it may be advisable to wean the drug rather than stopping it abruptly in order to reduce the rate of relapse (Martin, 1971).

Imipramine drug therapy has two potentially problematic consequences. The first is drug toxicity, and although side effects are usually infrequent, personality changes, adverse effects on sleep and appetite, gastrointestinal symptoms, and nervousness have been reported (Kardash et al, 1968; Shaffer et al, 1968). Because of the low ratio between beneficial effect and toxic effect, toxic overdose is a potential hazard. At greatest risk are the younger siblings of enuretics who unwarily ingest the medication in large amounts. Poisoning is characterized by severe myocardial depression and electrocardiographic changes that are not observed at therapeutic levels (Fouron and Chicoine, 1971; Koehl and Wenzel, 1971; Martin, 1973; Rohner and Sanford, 1975). Should a toxic reaction occur, careful attention must be given to specific therapeutic protocols aimed at reversal of the drug effect (Green and Cromie, 1981).

The second potentially problematic effect of imipramine is its ability to improve wetting symptoms not only in cases of enuresis but also when incontinence is due to an organic abnormality, such as neuropathy (Cole and Fried, 1972; Epstein and DeQuevedo, 1964). As a result, the use of imipramine as a therapeutic test to distinguish organic from nonorganic incontinence is not advisable.

Behavior Modification

Modification of behavior to control enuresis has met with varying success. Although generalized supportive measures designed to improve self-confidence and provide encouragement are unpredictably effective, certain specific approaches, when determinedly applied to a motivated child, produce the most effective rate of sustained cure and **should be considered as the first-line approach to the management of enuresis.**

Techniques that have been used include bladder training, responsibility reinforcement, and classical conditioning therapy that incorporates a urinary alarm. Often, a successful treatment program combines several behavioral techniques that may be used in conjunction with drug therapy.

Bladder Training

Bladder training, specifically retention control training (Kimmel and Kimmel, 1970), was developed to counteract the reduced functional bladder capacity that characterizes many enuretics. Because an increase in the functional capacity of the bladder correlates positively with reduced bedwetting, the rationale for this treatment appears well founded and the initial results were promising.

The goal of therapy is to progressively increase the time interval between voidings so that the functional bladder capacity is enlarged. Parents typically encourage their child to retain urine for as long as possible after first feeling an urge to void. Positive reinforcement is provided as the child retains urine for longer intervals and demonstrates larger recorded urine volumes. With retention control therapy, mean bladder capacity can be increased sizably in enuretic subjects compared with controls (approximately 35%). Unfortunately, this increase does not generally translate into an improvement in bedwetting for most children (Doleys, 1977; Harris and Purohit, 1977). However, when retention control is combined with conditioning therapy using the urinary alarm (see later), results can be highly successful (Geffken et al, 1986; Scott et al, 1992).

Responsibility Reinforcement

Behavior modification techniques are successful in treating enuresis, but they require a motivated child, conscientious parents, and rapport between the physician and family. The components of a successful responsibility reinforcement program include motivation, reward, response shaping, and reinforcement. The program aims to motivate the child to assume both the responsibility for wetting and the credit for dryness. The child keeps a progress record or gold star chart, and tries to determine what factors are responsible for wetting, attempts to reduce enuresis, and tries to keep totally dry. Progressively longer dry intervals and dry nights are rewarded by stars or an equivalent. The consequence of these stepwise rewards for changes in behavior results in a generalized molding of responses and progressive attainment of continence.

The results of a responsibility reinforcement program are difficult to evaluate on a controlled basis because better results are observed when the child takes an active role in therapy compared with a passive role. For selected children, improvement may be more rapid and the relapse rate lower than with other types of programs (Marshall et al, 1973). Responsibility reinforcement is particularly useful as part of a multicomponent behavioral program (Scott et al, 1992).

Conditioning Therapy

Randomized controlled trials and clinical studies have both shown that conditioning therapy using a urinary alarm is the most effective means of eliminating bedwetting (Werry and Cohrsen, 1965; DeLeon et al, 1966; McKendry et al, 1975; Moffatt et al, 1987; Butler et al, 1990; Devlin et al, 1990; Van Londen et al, 1993). Conditioning therapy using a urinary alarm has evolved from the bell and pad popularized by Mowrer and Mowrer in 1938. It originally consisted of a battery-operated detector pad on which the child slept. The detector is activated by urine, and ideally, the child is awakened by a bell, turns off the alarm, and then gets up and completes voiding into the toilet. The success of the urinary alarm method depends on awakening to the alarm and getting up to complete micturition, and has been explained by classical conditioning theory. If the alarm that awakens the child and initiates inhibition of micturition is repeatedly followed by the onset of normal voiding, then ultimately those factors present and associated with micturition during sleep, such as the sensation of a full bladder, would be conditioned to produce the same inhibition response as the alarm and awaken the child before wetting is completed (Doleys, 1977). Although not all investigators agree with the theoretical basis of success (Lovibond, 1963), **conditioning therapy using a urinary alarm appears to be the most effective therapy available for nocturnal enuresis.**

In its modern form, a small transistorized battery-powered device is attached either to the collar or worn as a wristband and is connected by a fine wire to underclothes, where only a few drops of urine is required for alarm activation. It has been determined that the body-worn urinary alarm is well accepted, safe, and relatively inexpensive.

The single most important cause for failure is a lack of parental understanding and cooperation. This can be minimized by proper instruction and supervision. However, before embarking on this program, parents and child must be motivated and well selected, and must recognize that the period of therapy can be lengthy, possibly lasting several months. Once enuresis has been cured completely (for at least 14 days) or converted to nocturia, relapse can be prevented by using overlearning techniques (Young and Morgan, 1972). These techniques involve forcing fluids prior to bedtime to promote bladder overdistention in order to provide a stronger conditioning stimulus. The likelihood for relapse can also be reduced by having the alarm sound intermittently on some nights but not others.

In controlled studies, the urinary alarm is superior to drug therapy, imipramine or DDAVP, with a cure rate of 60% to 100% (80% in my experience). When compared directly with DDAVP, the alarm cure rate is significantly better, and after therapy, the relapse rate with DDAVP is ten times greater (Wagner et al, 1982; Wille, 1986). Although as many as 25% of patients may relapse with the alarm, in many instances, this is preventable with overlearning techniques. In addition, retreatment usually produces a secondary cure in a significant proportion (Forsythe and Redmond, 1970; Young and Morgan, 1973; Doleys, 1977; Forsythe et al, 1989; Butler et al 1990; Scott et al, 1992). Conditioning therapy is effective under a variety of circumstances; age and intelligence are not factors in achieving dryness, nor is the degree or frequency of wetting.

Conditioning therapy using the urinary alarm may be combined with pharmacotherapy or behavior modification to create individually tailored treatment. With this strategy, the prospect for success is excellent (Geffken et al, 1986; Sukhai et al, 1989). Along these lines, Houts and Liebert (1984) developed full spectrum home training, a multicomponent behavioral treatment program aimed at improving the results of basic urinary alarm treatment while reducing the length of therapy and minimizing relapse. It includes four components: (1) the basic urinary alarm treatment, (2) overlearning, (3) cleanliness training, and (4) retention control training. About 80% of children so treated are cured (dry for 14 consecutive days), whereas only 24% relapse (Houts et al, 1986)

Miscellaneous Therapy

In addition to the aforementioned programs, numerous other treatments have been used for enuresis. Hypnotherapy and psychotherapy are highly effective for selected patients who have a stressful emotional cause for their wetting or in whom enuresis accompanies psychologic disturbance. However, for most enuretics, these modalities are inappropriate and inefficient (Fraser, 1972).

Certain children show a marked improvement in wetting following elimination of specific foods, drink, or dietary ingredients. The approach to diagnosis is similar to that used to identify food allergies. It involves serial elimination of foods such as chocolate, dairy products, and red-dye–containing substances (Esperanca and Gerrard, 1969b; Miller, 1993). Of course, foods and drinks that contain caffeine may worsen enuresis by producing diuresis that may overwhelm the functional capacity of the bladder, and therefore, these foods and drinks should be avoided.

ADULT ENURESIS

Enuresis occurring in adults is seen in two contexts: (1) persistent primary enuresis, which occurs in more than 1% of the population (Levine, 1943; Miller et al, 1973); **and (2) secondary or adult-onset enuresis.** In contrast to children with primary enuresis, a higher proportion of adults with persisting primary enuresis display overt urodynamic abnormalities (ranging from 28% to 70%). This is generally in the form of bladder instability (Torrens and Collins, 1975; Whiteside and Arnold, 1975; Karaman et al, 1992). These abnormalities are generally not due to any readily identifiable neuropathic or anatomic obstructive process, and may persist for many years as fixed urodynamic disturbances. Some of these adults may display subtle diurnal symptoms that are useful in suspecting bladder instability as a cause and may help guide empiric pharmacologic therapy (Hindmarsh and Byrne, 1980).

In the absence of overt neuropathy, urinary infection, or obstructive symptoms, **the incidence of organic disease does not appear to be appreciably greater for adults with persistent primary nocturnal enuresis than for children** (Torrens and Collins, 1975; Karaman et al, 1992). Even though the presence of diurnal symptoms may increase the likelihood of urodynamic findings of instability in these patients, it has not been demonstrated that diurnal symptoms increase the likelihood of organic disease. Consequently, clinical judgment must be individualized in each case to determine the need for any urologic investigation in excess of the evaluation ordinarily required for childhood enuresis. Once a diagnosis of primary enuresis has been established, treatment may follow the general guidelines described for children. It is noteworthy, however, that elimination of caffeine significantly reduces bedwetting in adult enuretics, suggesting that caffeine intake should first be reduced before other forms of treatment are initiated (Karacan et al, 1976; Edelstein, 1984).

In contrast, acquired or adult-onset enuresis is not generally a solitary symptom but occurs more commonly in association with generalized bladder spasticity or with other disturbances of micturition and continence. Even in the absence of urinary infection, patients usually require a thorough anatomic evaluation as well as a careful neurologic and urodynamic study, recognizing that occult neurologic dysfunction or anatomic disease can masquerade as a disturbance of genitourinary tract function and present as adult-onset enuresis.

Urologists must also be aware that obstructive sleep apnea can present as or be associated with nocturnal enuresis in adults as well as children and that removal of upper airway obstruction by surgical intervention has resulted in elimination of the enuresis. The mechanism is related to the increased diuresis during sleep that occurs in these patients as a result of elevated intrathoracic pressures from diaphragmatic contraction against a closed upper airway that causes release of atrial natriuretic peptide and activation of the renin-angiotensin system but does not cause an increase in vasopressin secretion (Krieger et al, 1991; Yokoyama et al, 1995).

SUMMARY

The physician who cares for patients with enuresis must keep in mind certain principles and develop an orderly, practical, and effective approach to the large number of children who present with this complaint:

1. Medically serious conditions such as urinary infection, neuropathy, and obstruction must be excluded; for most enuretics, a systematic history, physical examination, and urinalysis are sufficient.
2. Parents and child should be reassured that bedwetting is medically harmless, is not their child's fault, may have been inherited from the parents, is subject to a high (15% per year) spontaneous cure rate, and usually disappears by puberty.
3. Recognize that not all parents want and not all children are ready for a treatment program.
4. Determine if the child is sufficiently mature and motivated (usually by age 7) and the family is sufficiently supportive to begin a treatment program that might be lengthy and may not be successful initially.
5. Recommend the body-worn urinary alarm as the initial treatment. Statistically, it is the most effective means of achieving complete dryness and has no known side effects.
6. Avoid use of drugs as the initial therapy because most children do not achieve complete dryness during or after drug therapy and side effects can occur.
7. Reassure the family that relapses following successful therapy are often transient and respond well to retreatment.

REFERENCES

Aladjem M, Wohl R, Boichis H, et al: Desmopressin in nocturnal enuresis. Arch Dis Child 1982; 57:137.

Alderton HR: Imipramine in childhood enuresis: Further studies on the relationship of time of administration to effect. Can Med Assoc J 1970; 102:1179.

Anders TF, Weinstein P: Sleep and its disorders in infants; A review. Pediatrics 1972; 50:312.

Arnold SJ, Ginsberg A: Enuresis, incidence and pertinence of genitourinary disease in healthy enuretic children. Urology 1973; 2:437.

Aschoff J: Circadian rhythms in man: A self-sustained oscillator with an inherent frequency underlies 24-hour periodicity. Science 1965; 148:1427–1432.

Baker BL: Symptom treatment and symptom substitution in enuresis. J Abnorm Psychol 1969; 74:42.

Bakwin H: Enuresis in twins. Am J Dis Child 1971; 121:222.

Bakwin H: The genetics of enuresis. *In* Kolvin I, MacKeith RC, Meadow SR, eds: Bladder Control and Enuresis. London, W. Heinemann Medical Books Ltd., 1973, pp 73–77.

Beach PS, Beach RE, Smith LR: Hyponatremic seizures in a child treated with desmopressin to control enuresis. Clin Pediatr 1992; 31:566–569.

Bindelglas PM, Dee G: Enuresis treatment with imipramine hydrochloride: A 10-year follow-up study. Am J Psychiatry 1978; 135:12.

Birkasova M, Birkas O, Flynn MJ, et al: Desmopressin in the management of nocturnal enuresis in children: A double blind study. Pediatrics 1978; 62:970.

Blackwell B, Currah J: The psychopharmacology of nocturnal enuresis. *In* Kolvin I, MacKeith RC, Meadow SR, eds: Bladder Control and Enuresis. London, W. Heinemann Medical Books Ltd., 1973, pp 231–257.

Bloom D: The American experience with desmopressin. Clin Pediatr 1993; Special No: 28–31.

Booth CM, Gosling JA: Histologic and urodynamic study of the bladder in enuretic children. Br J Urol 1983; 55:367–370.

Boyd MM: The depth of sleep in enuretic school children and nonenuretic controls. J Psychosom Res 1960; 4:274.

Broughton RJ: Sleep disorders: Disorders of arousal? Science 1968; 159:1070.

Butler RJ, Forsythe WI, Robertson J: The body worn alarm in the treatment of childhood enuresis. Br J Clin Pract 1990; 44:237.

Campbell EW Jr, Young JD Jr: Enuresis and its relationship to electroencephalographic disturbances. J Urol 1966; 96:947.

Cole AT, Fried FA: Favorable experiences with imipramine in the treatment of neurogenic bladder. J Urol 1972; 107:44.

Cutler C, Middleton AW, Nixon GW: Radiographic findings in children surveyed for enuresis. Urology 1978; 11:480.

De Gatta MF, Garcia MJ, Acosta A: Monitoring of serum levels of imipramine and desipramine and individualization of dose in enuretic children. J Ther Drug Monit 1984; 6:438–443.

DeLeon G, Mandell AJ: A comparison of conditioning and psychotherapy and the treatment of functional enuresis. J Clin Psychol 1966; 22:326–330.

DeVane CL, Walker RD, Sawyer WP, Wilson JA: Concentrations of imipramine and its metabolites during enuresis therapy. Pediatr Pharmacol 1984; 4:245–251.

Devlin JB, O'Cathain C: Predicting treatment outcome in nocturnal enuresis. Arch Dis Child 1990; 65:1158–1161.

Dimson SB: Desmopressin as treatment for enuresis. Lancet 1977; 1:1260.

Diokno AC, Hyndman CW, Hardy DA, Lapides J: Comparison of action of imipramine (Tofranil) and propantheline (ProBanthine) on detrusor contractions. J Urol 1972; 107:42.

Diokno AC, Koff SA, Bender L: Periurethral striated muscle activity in neurogenic bladder dysfunction. J Urol 1974; 112:743.

Dodge WF, West EF, Bridgforth EB, Travis LB: Nocturnal enuresis in 6 to 10 year old children: Correlation with bacteriuria, proteinuria and dysuria. Am J Dis Child 1970; 120:32.

Doleys DM: Behavioral treatments for nocturnal enuresis in children: A review of the recent literature. Psychol Bull 1977; 1:30.

Edelstein BA, Keaton-Brasted C, Burd MM: Effects of caffeine withdrawal on nocturnal enuresis, insomnia, and behavioral restraints. J Consult Clin Psychol 1984; 52:857–862.

Egger J, Carter CH, Soothill JF, Wilson J: Effect of diet treatment on enuresis in children with migraine or hyperkinetic behavior. Clin Pediatr 1992; 31:302–307.

Epstein SJ, DeQuevedo A: The control of enuresis with imipramine in the presence of organic bladder disease. Am J Psychiatry 1964; 120:908.

Esperanca M, Gerrard JW: Nocturnal enuresis: Studies in bladder function in normal children and enuretics. Can Med Assoc J 1969a; 101:324.

Esperanca M, Gerrard JW: Nocturnal enuresis. Comparison of the effect of imipramine and dietary restriction on bladder capacity. Can Med Assoc J 1969b; 101:721.

Essen J, Peckham C: Nocturnal enuresis in childhood. Dev Med Child Neurol 1976; 18:577.

Fergusson DM, Horwood LJ, Shannon FT: Factors related to the age of attainment of nocturnal bladder control: An eight-year longitudinal study. Pediatrics 1986; 78:884–890.

Fermaglich JL: Electroencephalographic study of enuretics. Am J Dis Child 1969; 118:473.

Ferrie BC, MacFarlane J, Glen S: DDAVP in young enuretic patients: A double-blind trial. Br J Urol 1984; 56:376.

Fisher OD, Forsythe WI: Micturating cystourethrography in the investigation of enuresis. Arch Dis Child 1954; 29:460.

Fjellestad-Paulsen A, Wille S, Harris AS: Comparison of intranasal and oral desmopressin for nocturnal enuresis. Arch Dis Child 1987; 62:674–677.

Forsythe WI, Butler RJ: Fifty years of enuretic alarms. Arch Dis Child 1989; 64:879–885.

Forsythe WI, Redmond A: Enuresis and the electric alarm: Study of 200 cases. Br Med J 1970; 1:211.

Forsythe WI, Redmond A: Enuresis and spontaneous cure rate: Study of 1129 enuretics. Arch Dis Child 1974; 49:259.

Fouron J, Chicoine R: ECG changes in fatal imipramine (Tofranil) intoxication. Pediatrics 1971; 48:777.

Frary LG: Enuresis: A genetic study. Am J Dis Child 1935; 49:553.

Fraser MS: Nocturnal enuresis. Practitioner 1972; 208:203.

Fritz GK, Rockney RM, Yeung A: Plasma levels and efficacy of imipramine treatment for enuresis. J Am Acad Child Adolesc Psych 1994; 33:1.

Furlanut M, Montanari P, Benetello P, et al: Steadystate serum concentrations of imipramine, its main metabolites and clinical response in primary enuresis. Pharm Rev 1989; 21:561.

Gastaut H, Broughton R: A clinical and polygraphic study of episodic phenomena during sleep. *In* Wortis J, ed: Recent Advances in Biological Psychiatry. New York, Plenum Press, 1965, pp 197–221.

Geffken G, Johnson SB, Walker D: Behavioral interventions for childhood nocturnal enuresis: The differential effect of bladder capacity on treatment, progress and outcome. Health Psychol 1986; 5:261–272.

George CPL, Messeril FH, Gennest J, et al: Diurnal variation of plasma vasopressin in man. J Endocrinol Metab 1975; 41:332.

Giles GR, Light K, Van Blerk PJP: Cystometrogram studies in enuretic children. S Afr J Surg 1978; 16:33.

Glicklich LB: An historical account of enuresis. Pediatrics 1951; 8:859.

Goellner MH, Ziegler EE, Fomon SJ: Urination during the first three years of life. Nephron 1981; 28:174.

Graham P: Depth of sleep and enuresis: A critical review. *In* Kolvin I, MacKeith RC, Meadow, SR, eds: Bladder Control and Enuresis. London, W. Heinemann Medical Books Ltd., 1973, pp 78–83.

Green AS, Cromie WJ: Treatment of imipramine overdose in children. Urology 1981; 18:314.

Hägglund TB: Enuretic children treated with fluid restriction or forced drinking: A clinical and cystometric study. Ann Paediatr Fenn 1965; 11:84.

Hägglund TB, Parkkulainen KV: Enuretic children treated with imipramine (Tofranil). Ann Paediatr Fenn 1965; 11:53.

Hallgren B: Enuresis: A clinical and genetic study. Acta Psychiatr Neurol Scand (Suppl) 1957; 114:1.

Hallman N: On the ability of enuretic children to hold urine. Acta Paediatr 1950; 39:87.

Haque M, Ellerstein NS, Gundy JH, et al: Parental perceptions in enuresis, a collaborative study. Am J Dis Child 1981; 135:809.

Harris AS: Clinical experience with desmopressin: Efficacy and safety in central diabetes insipidus and other conditions. J Pediatr 1989; 114:711–718.

Harris LS, Purohit AP: Bladder training and enuresis: A controlled trial. Behav Res Ther 1977; 15:485.

Harrison JS, Albino VJ: An investigation into the effects of imipramine hydrochloride on the incidence of enuresis in institutionalized children. S Afr Med J 1970; 44:253.

Hindmarsh JR, Byrne PO: Adult enuresis—a symptomatic and urodynamic assessment. Br J Urol 1980; 52:88.

Hjälmåas K: Micturition in infants and children with normal lower urinary tract. Scand J Urol Nephrol (Suppl) 1976; 37:1–150.

Hjälmåas K, Bengtsson B: Efficacy, safety, and dosing of desmopressin for nocturnal enuresis in Europe. Clin Pediatr 1993; Special No: 19–24.

Hogg RJ, Husmann D: The role of family history in predicting response to desmopressin in nocturnal enuresis. J Urol 1993; 150:444–445.

Houts AC, Liebert RM: Bedwetting: A Guide for Parents and Children. Springfield, IL, Charles C. Thomas, 1984.

Houts AC, Peterson JK, Whelan JP: Prevention of relapse in full-spectrum home training for primary enuresis: A component analysis. Behavior Therapy 1986; 17:462–469.

Inoue M, Shimojima H, Shiba H, et al: Rhythmic slow wave observed on nocturnal sleep encephalogram in children with idiopathic nocturnal enuresis. J Sleep 1987; 10:570–579.

Janknegt RA, Smans AJ: Treatment with desmopressin in severe nocturnal enuresis in childhood. Br J Urol 1990; 66:535–537.

Jarvelin MR: Developmental history and neurological findings in enuretic children. Dev Med Child Neurol 1989; 31:728–736.

Johnstone JMS: Cystometry and evaluation of anticholinergic drugs in enuretic children. J Pediatr Surg 1972; 7:18.

Jorgensen OS, Lober M, Christiansen J, et al: Plasma concentration and clinical effect in imipramine treatment of childhood enuresis. Clin Pharmacokinet 1980; 5:386.

Kajtor F, Ovary I, Zsadanyi O: Nocturnal enuresis: Electroencephalographic and cystometric examinations. Acta Med Acad Sci Hung 1967; 23:153.

Kales A, Kales JD: Sleep disorders: Recent findings in the diagnosis and treatment of disturbed sleep. N Engl J Med 1974; 290:487.

Kales A, Kales JD, Jacobson A, et al: Effect of imipramine on enuretic frequency and sleep stages. Pediatrics 1977; 60:431.

Kaplan G: Serum IgE and allergy in enuresis. Presented at Section on Urology, American Academy of Pediatrics, Chicago, Illinois, Oct. 22, 1973.

Karacan I, Thornby JI, Anch AM, et al: Dose-related sleep disturbances induced by coffee and caffeine. Clin Pharmacol Ther 1976; 20:682–689.

Karaman MI, Esen T, Kocak T, et al: Rationale of urodynamic assessment in adult enuresis. Eur Urol 1992; 21:138–140.

Kardash S, Hillman ES, Werry J: Efficacy of imipramine in childhood enuresis: A double blind control study with placebo. Can Med Assoc J 1968; 99:263.

Kass EJ, Diokno AC, Montealegre A: Enuresis: Principles of management and result of treatment. J Urol 1979; 121:794.

Kawauchi A, Watanabe H: Development of bladder capacity, nocturnal urinary volume and urinary behavior in non-enuretic and enuretic children. Nippon Hinyokika Gakkai Zasshi 1993; 84:1811–1820.

Kawauchi A, Watanabe H, Kitamori T, et al: The possibility of centripetal stimulation from the urinary bladder for vasopressin excretion. J Kyoto Pref Univ Med 1993; 102:747–752.

Kimmel HD, Kimmel EC: An instrumental conditioning method for the treatment of enuresis. J Behav Ther Exp Psychiatry 1970; 1:121.

Klauber GT: Clinical efficacy and safety of desmopressin in the treatment of nocturnal enuresis. J Pediatr 1989; 114:719–722.

Knudsen UB, Rittig S, Norgaard JP, et al: Long term treatment of nocturnal enuresis with desmopressin. Urol Res 1991; 19:237–240.

Koehl GW, Wenzel JE: Severe postural hypotension due to imipramine therapy. Pediatrics 1971; 47:71.

Koff SA: Why is desmopressin sometimes ineffective at curing bedwetting? Scand J Urol Nephrol 1995; 29(Suppl 173):103–108.

Koff SA, Murtagh DS: The uninhibited bladder in children: Effect of treatment on recurrence of urinary infection and on vesicoureteral reflux resolution. J Urol 1983; 130:1138.

Krieger J, Follenius M, Sforza E, et al: Effects of treatment with nasal continuous positive airway pressure on atrial natriuretic peptide and arginine vasopressin release during sleep in patients with obstructive sleep apnea. Clin Sci 1991; 80:443–449.

Kunin SA, Limbert DJ, Platzker ACG, McGinley J: The efficacy of imipramine in the management of enuresis. J Urol 1970; 104:612.

Labay P, Boyarsky S: The action of imipramine on the bladder musculature. J Urol 1973; 109:385.

Lapides J, Sweet RB, Lewis LW: Role of striated muscle in urination. J Urol 1957; 77:247.

Levine A: Enuresis in the Navy. Am J Psychiatry 1943; 100:320.

Liederman PC, Wasserman DH, Liederman VR: Desipramine in the treatment of enuresis. J Urol 1969; 101:314.

Linderholm BE: The cystometric findings in enuresis. J Urol 1966; 96:718.

Lovibond SH: The mechanism of conditioning treatment of enuresis. Behav Res Ther 1963; 1:17.

Lowy FH: Recent sleep and dream research: Clinical implications. Can Med Assoc J 1970; 102:1069.

MacKeith RC: A frequent factor in the origins of primary nocturnal enuresis: Anxiety in the third year of life. Dev Med Child Neurol 1968; 10:465.

MacLean REG: Imipramine hydrochloride (Tofranil) and enuresis. Am J Psychiatry 1960; 117:551.

Mahony DT: Studies of enuresis: I. Incidence of obstructive lesions and pathophysiology of enuresis. J Urol 1971; 106:951.

Mahony DT, Laferte RO, Blais DJ: Studies on enuresis: IX. Evidence of a mild form of compensated detrusor hyperreflexia in enuretic children. J Urol 1981; 126:520.

Marshall S, Marshal HH, Lyon RP: Enuresis: An analysis of various therapeutic approaches. Pediatrics 1973; 52:813.

Martin GI: ECG monitoring of enuretic children given imipramine. JAMA 1973; 244:902.

Martin GI: Imipramine pamoate in the treatment of childhood enuresis: A double-blind study. Am J Dis Child 1971; 122:42.

Matthiesen TB, Rittig S, Djurhuus JC, Norgaard, JP: A dose titration, and an open 6-week efficacy and safety study of desmopressin tablets in the management of nocturnal enuresis. J Urol 1994; 151:460–463.

Maxwell C, Seldrup J: Imipramine in the treatment of childhood enuresis. Practitioner 1971; 207:809.

McGuire EJ, Savastanes JA: Urodynamic studies in enuresis and the non-neurogenic bladder. J Urol 1984; 132:229–302.

McKendry JBJ, Stewart DA: Enuresis. Pediatr Clin North Am 1974; 21:1019.

McKendry JBJ, Stewart DA, Kahnna F, Netley C: Primary enuresis: Relative success of three methods of treatment. Can Med Assoc J 1975; 113:953–955.

McKendry JBJ, Williams HAL, Broughton C: Enuresis—a study of untreated patients. Appl Ther 1968; 10:815.

Mikkelsen EJ, Rapoport JL, Nee L, et al: Childhood enuresis: I. Sleep patterns and psychopathology. Arch Gen Psychiatry 1980; 37:1139.

Miller FJW, Court SDM, Walton NG, Knox EG: Growing up in Newcastle upon Tyne. London, Oxford University Press, 1960.

Miller FJW, Knox EG, Brandon S: Children who wet the bed. *In* Kolvin I, MacKeith RC, Meadow, SR, eds: Bladder Control and Enuresis. London, W. Heinemann Medical Books Ltd., 1973, pp 47–52.

Miller K: Concomitant nonpharmacologic therapy in the treatment of primary nocturnal enuresis. Clin Pediatrics 1993; July:32–37.

Miller K, Goldberg S, Atkin B: Nocturnal enuresis: Experience with long-term use of intranasally administered desmopressin. J Pediatr 1989; 114:723–726.

Miller PR, Champelli JW, Dinello FA: Imipramine in the treatment of enuretic school children. Am J Dis Child 1968; 115:17.

Milner G, Hills NF: A double-blind assessment of antidepressants in the treatment of 212 enuretic patients. Med J Aust 1968; 1:943.

Mimouni M, Schuper A, Mimouni F, et al: Retarded skeletal maturation in children with primary enuresis. J Pediatr 1985; 144:234–235.

Mishra PC, Agarwal VK, Rahman H: Therapeutic trial of amitriptyline in the treatment of nocturnal enuresis—a controlled study. Indian Pediatr 1980; 17:279.

Moffatt MEK: Nocturnal enuresis—is there a rationale for treatment? Scand J Urol Nephrol Suppl 1994; 163:55–67.

Moffatt MEK: Nocturnal enuresis: Psychologic implications of treatment and nontreatment. J Pediatr 1989; 114:697–704.

Moffatt MEK, Harlos S, Kirshen AJ, Burd L: Desmopressin acetate and nocturnal enuresis: How much do we know? Pediatrics 1993; 92:420–425.

Moffatt MEK, Kato C, Pless IB: Improvements in self-concept after treatment of nocturnal enuresis: Randomized controlled trial. J Pediatr 1987; 110:647–652.

Moore-Ede MC: Physiology of the circadian timing system: Predictive vs reactive homeostasis. Am J Physiol 1986; 250:737–752.

Mowrer OH, Mowrer WM: Enuresis—a method for its study and treatment. Am J Orthopsychiatry 1938; 8:436.

Muellner SR: Development of urinary control in children. JAMA 1960; 172:1256.

Nash DFE: The development of micturition control with special reference to enuresis. Ann R Coll Surg Engl 1949; 5:318.

Norgaard JP: Urodynamics in enuretics. I. Reservoir function. Neurourol Urodyn 1989a; 8:199–211.

Norgaard JP: Urodynamics in enuretics. II. A pressure-flow study. Neurourol Urodyn 1989b; 8:213–217.

Norgaard JP, Hansen JH, Nielsen JB, et al: Simultaneous registration of sleep stages and bladder activity in enuresis. Urology 1985a; 26:316–319.

Norgaard JP, Hansen JH, Nielsen JB, et al: Sleep patterns in enuretics. A polygraphic study of EEG and bladder activity. Scand J Urol Nephrol 1989a; 125:73–78.

Norgaard JP, Hansen JH, Wildschiotz G: Cystometries in children with nocturnal enuresis. J Urol 1989b; 141:1156.

Norgaard JP, Pederson EB, Djurhuus JC: Diurnal antidiuretic hormone levels in enuretics. J Urol 1985b; 134:1029.

Norgaard JP, Ritting S, Djurhuus J.: Nocturnal enuresis: An approach to treatment based on pathogenesis. J Pediatr 1989c; 114:705–710.

Ohne T: The increase in c-Fos expression in vasopressin- and oxytocin-immunoreactive neurons in paraventricular and supraoptic nucleus of the hypothalamus following urinary retention. J Kyoto Pref Univ Med 1995; 104:393–403.

Oppel WC, Harper PA, Rider RV: The age of attaining bladder control. Pediatrics 1968; 42:614.

Pedersen PS, Hejl M, Kjoller SS: Desamino-D-arginine vasopressin in childhood nocturnal enuresis. J Urol 1985; 133:65–66.

Person-Junemann C, Seemann O, Kohrmann KU, et al: Comparison of urodynamic findings and response to oxybutynin in nocturnal enuresis. Eur Urol 1993; 24:92–96.

Pompeius R: Cystometry in pediatric enuresis. Scand J Urol 1971; 5:222.

Post EM, Richman RM, Blackett PR, et al: Desmopressin response in enuretic children. Effects of age and frequency of enuresis. Am J Dis Child 1983; 137:962–963.

Poussaint AF, Ditman KS, Greenfield R: Amitriptyline in childhood enuresis. Clin Pharmacol Ther 1966; 7:21.
Puri VN: Urinary levels of antidiuretic hormone in nocturnal enuresis. Indian Pediatr 1980; 17:675.
Ramsden PD, Hindmarch DA, Price DA, et al: DDAVP for adult enuresis: A preliminary report. Br J Urol 1982; 54:256–258.
Rapoport JL, Mikkelsen EJ, Zavodil A, et al: Childhood enuresis. II. Arch Gen Psychiatry 1980; 37:1146.
Rascher W, Rauh W, Brandeis WE, et al: Determinants of plasma arginine-vasopressin in children. Acta Paediatr Scand 1986; 75:111–117.
Rechtschaffen A, Kales A, eds: A Manual of Standardized Terminology, Techniques and Scoring System for Sleep Stages of Human Subjects. Los Angeles, Brain Information Service/Brain Research Institute, UCLA, 1968, pp 1–12.
Redman JF, Seibert JJ: The uroradiographic evaluation of the enuretic child. J Urol 1979; 122:799.
Reimao R, Pachelli LC, Carneiro R, Faiwichow G: Primary sleep enuresis in childhood. Polysomnographic evidences of sleep stage and time modulation. Arq Neuropsiquiatr 1993; 51:41–45.
Rew DA, Rundle JSH: Assessment of the safety of regular DDAVP therapy in primary nocturnal enuresis. Br J Urol 1989; 63:352–353.
Rittig S, Knudsen UB, Norgaard JP, et al: Abnormal diurnal rhythm of plasma vasopressin and urinary output in patients with enuresis. Am J Physiol 1989a; 256:664.
Rittig S, Knudsen UB, Sorensen S, et al: Long-term double-blind cross-over study of desmopressin intranasal spray in the management of nocturnal enuresis. *In* Meadow SR, ed: Desmopressin in Nocturnal Enuresis. Horus Medical Publication, 1989b, pp 43–54.
Ritvo ER, Ornitz EM, Gottlieb F, et al: Arousal and non-arousal enuretic events. Am J Psychiatry 1969; 126:115.
Robert M, Averous M, Besset A, et al: Sleep polygraphic studies using sleep cystomanometry in twenty patients with enuresis. Eur Urol 1993; 24:97–102.
Rohner TJ, Sanford EJ: Imipramine toxicity. J Urol 1975; 114:402.
Sachdev YV, Howards SS: *Enterobius vermicularis* infestation and secondary enuresis. J Urol 1975; 113:143.
Scott MA, Barclay DR, Houts AC: Childhood enuresis: etiology, assessment, and current behavioral treatment. Prog Behav Modif 1992; 28:83–117.
Scott R, Morrison LH: Diuretic treatment of enuresis: Preliminary communication. J R Coll Surg Edinb 1980; 25:470.
Shaffer D, Costello AJ, Hill ID: Control of enuresis with imipramine. Arch Dis Child 1968; 43:665.
Sigg EB: Pharmacological studies with Tofranil. Can Psychiatr Assoc J 1959; 4:75.
Starfield B: Functional bladder capacity in enuretic and non-enuretic children. J Pediatr 1967; 55:777.
Steffens J, Netzer M, Isenberg E, et al: Vasopressin deficiency in primary nocturnal enuresis. Results of a controlled prospective study. Eur Urol 1993; 24:366–370.
Stein ZM, Susser MW: Social factors in the development of sphincter control. Dev Med Child Neurol 1967; 9:692.
Stephenson JD: Physiological and pharmacological basis for the chemotherapy of imipramine. Psychol Med 1979; 9:249.
Stromgen A, Thomsen PH: Personality traits in young adults with a history of conditioning-treated childhood enuresis. Acta Psychiatr Scand 1990; 81:538–541.
Strom-Olsen R: Enuresis in adults and abnormality of sleep. Lancet 1950; 2:133.
Sukhai RN, Mol J, Harris AS: Combined therapy of enuresis alarm and desmopressin in the treatment of nocturnal enuresis. Eur J Pediatr 1989; 148:465–467.
Terho P: Desmopressin in nocturnal enuresis. J Urol 1991; 145:818–820.
Torrens MJ, Collins CD: The urodynamic assessment of adult enuresis. Br J Urol 1975; 47:433.
Troup CW, Hodgson NB: Nocturnal functional bladder capacity in enuretic children. J Urol 1971; 129:132.
Tuvemo T: DDAVP in childhood nocturnal enuresis. Acta Pediatr Scand 1978; 67:753.
Van Londen A, Van Londen-Barensten MWM, Van Son MJM, Mulder GALA: Arousal training for children suffering from nocturnal enuresis: A 2½-year follow-up. Behav Res Ther 1993; 31:613–615.
Vulliamy D: The day and night output of urine in enuresis. Arch Dis Child 1956; 31:439–443.
Wagner W, Johnsson SS, Walker D, et al: A controlled comparison of two treatments for nocturnal enuresis. J Pediatr 1982; 101:302–307.
Watanabe H, Kawauchi A, Kitamori T, Azuma Y: Treatment system for nocturnal enuresis according to an original classification system. Eur Urol 1994; 25:43–50.
Watanabe H, Azuma Y: A proposal for a classification system of enuresis based on overnight simultaneous monitoring of electroencephalography and cystometry. Sleep 1989; 12:257–264.
Watanabe H, Kawauchi A, Kitamori T, Azuma Y: Treatment system for nocturnal enuresis according to an original classification system. Eur J Urol 1994; 25:43–50.
Werry JS: Enuresis—a psychosomatic entity? Can Med Assoc J 1967; 97:319.
Werry JS, Cohrsen J: Enuresis: An etiologic and therapeutic study. J Pediatr 1965; 67:423–431.
Whiteside CG, Arnold EP: Persistent primary enuresis: A urodynamic assessment. Br Med J 1975; 1:364.
Wille S: Comparison of desmopressin and enuresis alarm for nocturnal enuresis. Arch Dis Child 1986; 61:30–33.
Winberg J: Determination of renal concentration capacity in infants and children without renal disease. Acta Paediatr Scand 1959; 48:318.
Wu HHH, Chen M-T, Lee Y-H: Urodynamics studies and primary nocturnal enuresis. Chin Med J (Taipei) 1988; 41:227–232.
Yeates WK: Bladder function in normal micturition. *In* Kolvin I, MacKeith RC, Meadow SR, eds: Bladder Control and Enuresis. London, W. Heinemann Medical Books Ltd., 1973, pp 28–36.
Yokoyama O, Lee S-W, Ohkawa M, et al: Enuresis in an adult female with obstructive sleep apnea. Urology 1995; 45:150.
Young GC, Morgan RTT: Overlearning in the conditioning treatment of enuresis. Behav Res Ther 1972; 10:147–151.
Young GC, Morgan RTT: Conditioning technics and enuresis. Med J Aust 1973; 2:329.
Zaleski A, Shokeir MK, Gerrad JW: Enuresis: Familial incidence and relationship to allergic disorders. Can Med Assoc J 1972; 106:30.

67 POSTERIOR URETHRAL VALVES AND OTHER URETHRAL ANOMALIES

Edmond T. Gonzales, Jr., M.D.

The embryology of the male urethra is complex and is not completely understood. Development of the urethra can be considered in two separate phases: differentiation of the urogenital sinus portion, the posterior urethra; and tubularization of the urethral plate, the anterior urethra. The mature male urethra is generally divided into four segments: (1) the prostatic urethra—from the bladder neck to the proximal margin of the urogenital diaphragm; (2) the membranous urethra—the segment that traverses the urogenital diaphragm (the striated sphincter); (3) the bulbous urethra—the portion from the distal margin of the membranous urethra to the penoscrotal angle; and (4) the penile urethra—the segment that traverses the length of the penile shaft, including the glans.

The prostatic and membranous portions of the urethra are not entirely androgen dependent because these segments of the urethra also develop in the female. However, it is obvious that androgen action on the tissues of the prostate gland and the mesonephric ducts (the embryologic anlage of the male genital ducts) has a significant impact on the final differentiation of these segments of the male urethra.

The bulbous and penile segments of the urethra are uniquely male and are entirely dependent on androgen action for differentiation. The presence of inadequate androgenization in peripheral tissues due to abnormal androgen receptor number or function, 5α-reductase deficiency, or inadequate androgenic steroid production by the testes will result in incomplete tubularization of the anterior segments of the male urethra. These multiple disorders represent the various syndromes of incomplete virilization that can be seen in genotypic (XY) males and span the anatomic spectrum from mild degrees of hypospadias to complete phenotypic females (testicular feminization syndrome) (Griffin and Wilson, 1989).

This chapter, however, is concerned with anomalies of the male urethra not known or believed to result from androgen deficiency and includes the following topics:

1. Posterior urethral valves
2. Anterior urethral valves
3. Syringoceles
4. Megalourethra
5. Urethral duplications
6. Prostatic urethral polyps

Normal urethral embryology is described elsewhere. This chapter emphasizes the abnormal embryology, as generally understood, to explain the individual anomalies discussed here.

POSTERIOR URETHRAL VALVES

Young is generally given credit for the first clear description and classification of posterior urethral valves. He recognized three distinct varieties of congenital proximal urethral obstructions and classified these as types I, II, and III urethral valves (Fig. 67–1) (Young et al, 1919).

A type I urethral valve is an obstructing membrane that radiates in a distal direction from the posterior edge of the verumontanum toward the membranous urethra, inserting anteriorly near the proximal margin of the membranous urethra. Although type I valves are usually represented in

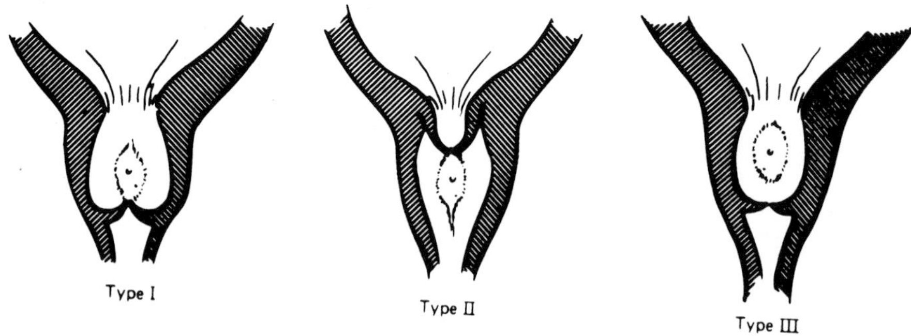

Figure 67–1. The original classification and diagrammatic depiction of urethral valves as presented by Young and co-workers. (Adapted from Young HH, et al: J Urol 1919;3:289.)

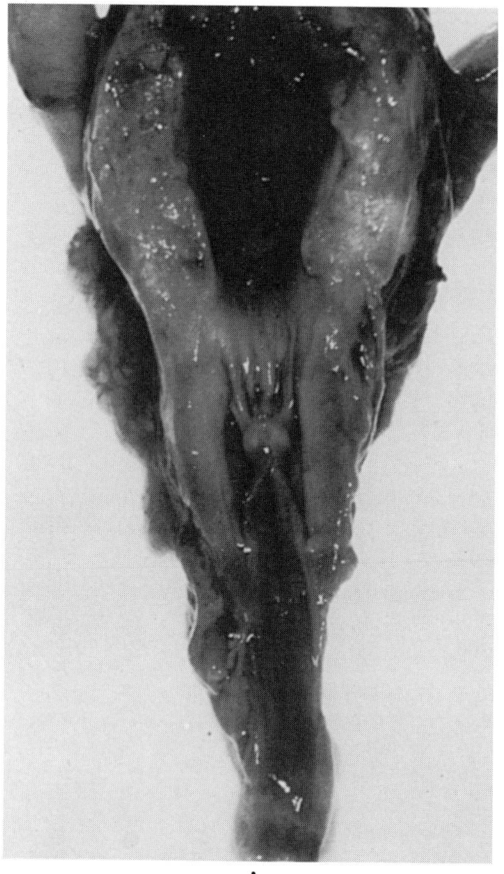

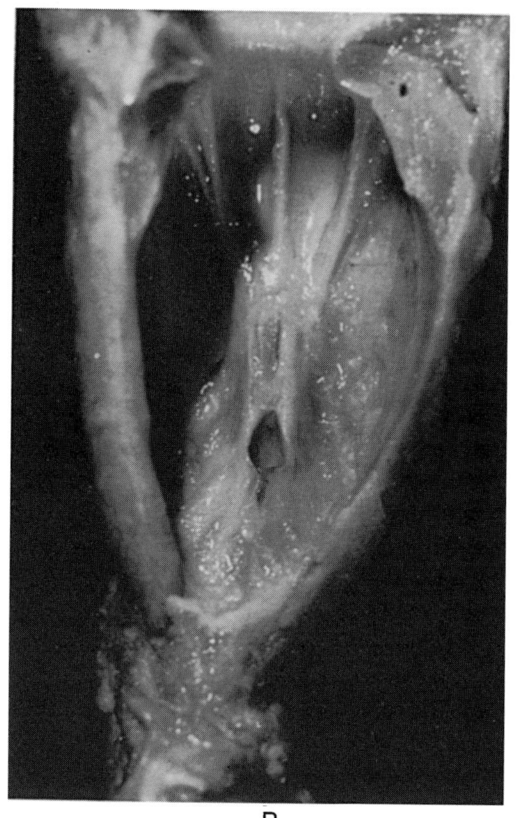

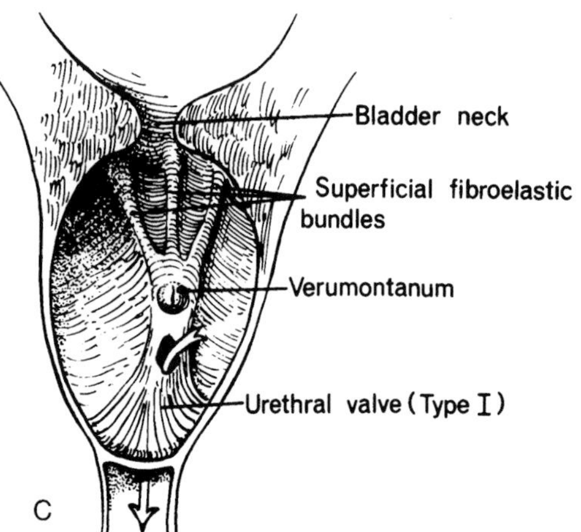

Figure 67–2. *A,* A posterior urethral valve specimen unfolded after an anterior urethra midline incision gives the impression of two folds coapting in the midline. *B,* Another specimen opened by unrooting rather than incising anterior urethral wall shows the folds to be an oblique diaphragm fused anteriorly. Note also the proximal folds, which could be confused with type II valves. (From Robertson WB, Hayes JA: Br J Urol 1969;41:592.) *C,* Drawing of typical appearance of type I urethral valve.

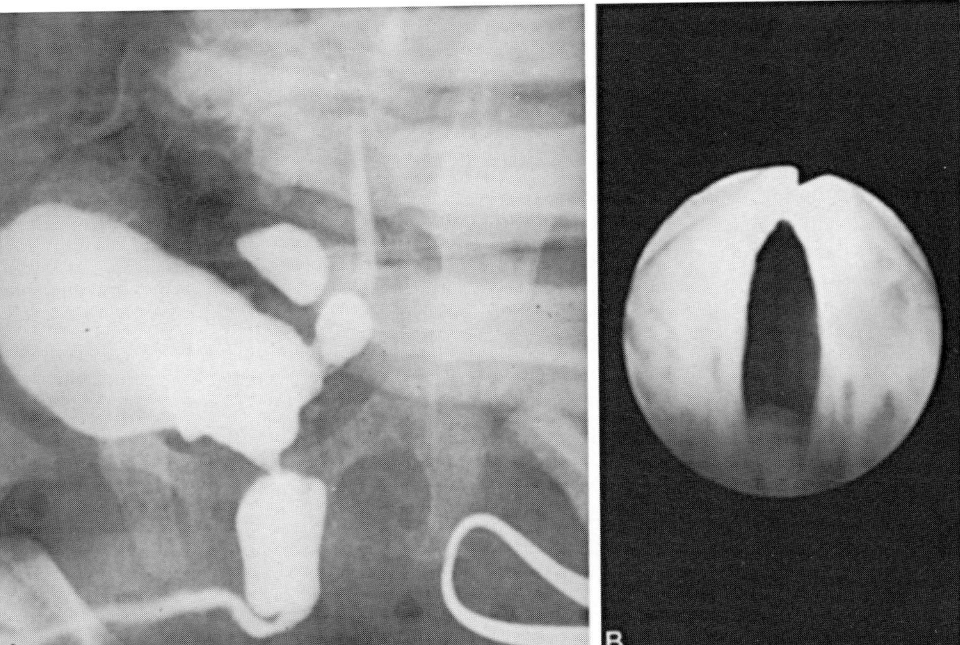

Figure 67–3. *A,* Radiologic appearance of type I urethral valve. Note the bulging anterior membrane, the posteriorly positioned perforation in the valve, the dilated prostatic urethra, and the narrowed and thickened bladder neck. These findings are typical of type I valves when the urethra is viewed in an oblique position. *B,* Cystoscopic picture of type I valve. The verumontanum is the small nodule at the 6 o'clock position.

line sketches as two coapting folds, they actually are a single membranous structure with the opening in the membrane positioned posteriorly near the verumontanum (Fig. 67–2) (Robertson and Hayes, 1969). During voiding, the fused anterior portion of the membrane bulges into the membranous urethra and possibly into the bulbous urethra, leaving only a narrow opening along the posterior wall of the urethra. This predictable anatomy gives type I urethral valves a characteristic radiologic appearance (Fig. 67–3).

The embryology of type I valves is not completely understood, but it is generally believed that these valves are the end result of anomalous insertion of the mesonephric ducts into the primitive fetal cloaca. Normally, the mesonephric ducts insert laterally on the cloaca. As the cloaca folds inward in its midportion to separate the anorectal canal from the urogenital sinus, the ostium of each mesonephric duct migrates posteromedially and cranially to assume a final position at the verumontanum. In the normal male urethra, this pathway of migration persists as the plicae colliculi—delicate mucosal folds that emanate from the verumontanum in a distal and slightly lateral direction along the posterior (dorsal) floor of the urethra. Type I posterior urethral valves are thought to develop when the mesonephric ducts enter the cloaca in a more anterior position than normal. During infolding and separation of the cloaca, their migration is impeded and they may fuse in the midline anteriorly (Stephens, 1983). Children with classic type I valves do not have plicae colliculi (Fig. 67–4).

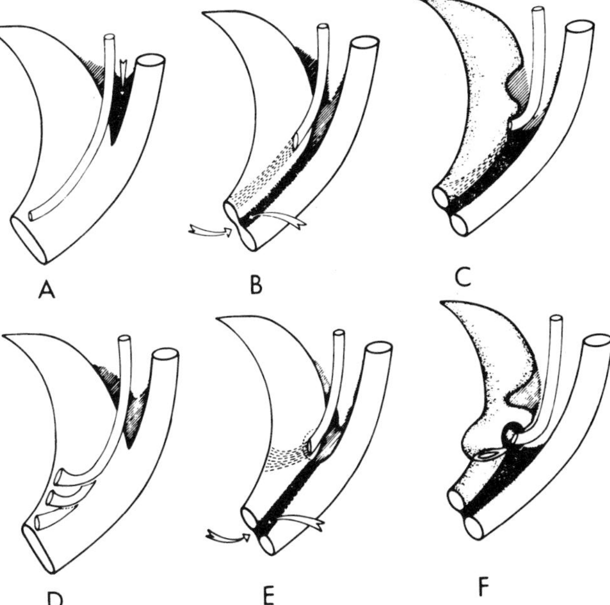

Figure 67–4. Development of type I valves.

A to *C,* Development of the normal urethral crest. Migration of the orifice of the wolffian duct from its anterolateral position in the cloaca to the site of the Müller tubercle on the posterior wall of the anorectal septum occurs synchronously with cloacal division. (Dots denote pathway of migration.) This wolffian remnant is more lateral and posterior and remains as the normal inferior crest and the plicae colliculi.

D, Abnormal anterior positions of the wolffian duct orifices.

E, Abnormal migration of the terminal ends of the ducts.

F, Circumferential obliquely oriented ridges that compose the valve.

(From Kelalis PP, King LR, eds.: Clinical Pediatric Urology. Philadelphia, W. B. Saunders Company, 1976.)

Type II urethral valves were initially described as folds radiating in a cranial direction from the verumontanum to the posterolateral aspect of the bladder neck. It is now generally accepted that these folds are not obstructive and, in fact, that type II valves as a clinical entity do not exist. These folds represent hypertrophy of the strip of superficial muscle that runs from the ureteral orifice to the verumontanum (muscle derived from the tissue of the mesonephric ducts that forms the layer of bladder muscle known as the superficial trigone). In response to increased resistance to voiding, hypertrophy of these muscle bands occurs. Such hypertrophy is found in the presence of true mechanical obstruction as well as in cases of functional obstruction (neuropathic bladder, detrusor-sphincter dyssynergy).

Type III valves are believed to represent incomplete dissolution of the urogenital membrane. The obstructing membranes are situated distal to the verumontanum, at the level of the membranous urethra (Fig. 67–5). Classically described as discrete ringlike membranes with a central aperture, these lesions can assume bizarre configurations, depending on the elasticity of the membrane and the location of the perforation in the membrane (Fig. 67–6). Long, willowy folds may prolapse well down into the urethra during voiding, suggesting rather a bulbar urethral obstruction—the classic wind-sock valve described by Field and Stephens (1974) (Fig. 67–7).

Although it is generally accepted that type II valves do not exist, the traditional classification scheme is so ingrained in the urologic vernacular that the usual congenital obstructions of the proximal urethra continue to be described as type I and type III. This accepted classification is continued in this chapter.

Overall, type I urethral valves make up more than 95% of the lesions in large series; type III valves make up the remainder. However, despite their different embryology, there is no clear difference in the clinical presentation, pathophysiology, or management of children with either anomaly, and the following discussion applies to both anomalies. Although the number of children with type III valves is small, as a group they seem to have a worse prognosis than children with type I valves (Rosenfeld et al, 1994).

The incidence of congenital valvular obstruction is not clearly known, in part because the presentation is variable and different series include patients of many different ages and degrees of obstruction. The incidence is generally accepted to be somewhere between 1 in 5000 and 1 in 8000 male births, although large screening studies of fetuses with hydronephrosis place the likely incidence slightly higher (in one study [Gunn et al, 1995], the incidence was one case of urethral valves in 1250 fetal ultrasound studies).

Stephens (1983) suggested the existence of an additional type of proximal urethral obstruction, which he dubbed a type IV valve. Seen most often in children with the prune-belly syndrome, these obstructions occur when a flabby, poorly supported prostate folds on itself and causes relative outlet obstruction. This phenomenon is not discussed in this chapter.

Clinical Presentation

Children with congenital posterior urethral obstruction present in a variety of ways, depending primarily on the degree of obstruction. Classically, presenting symptoms are age dependent. In the newborn, the presence of palpable abdominal masses (distended bladder, hydronephrosis), asci-

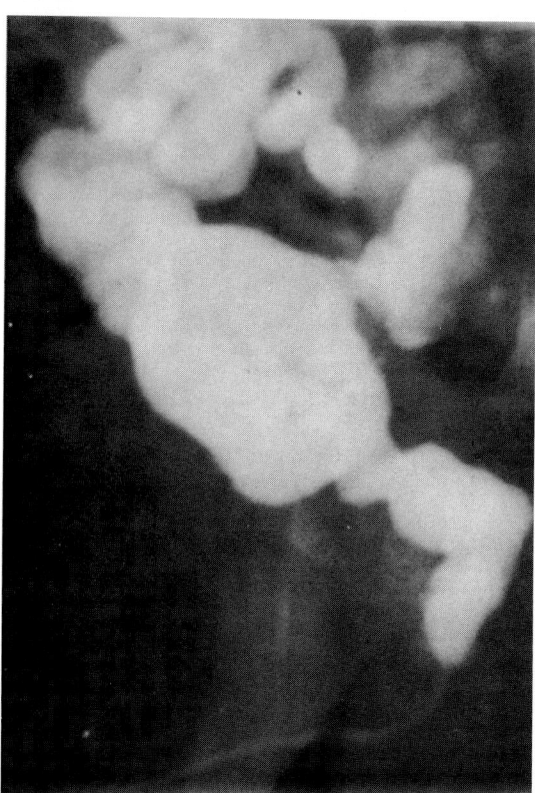

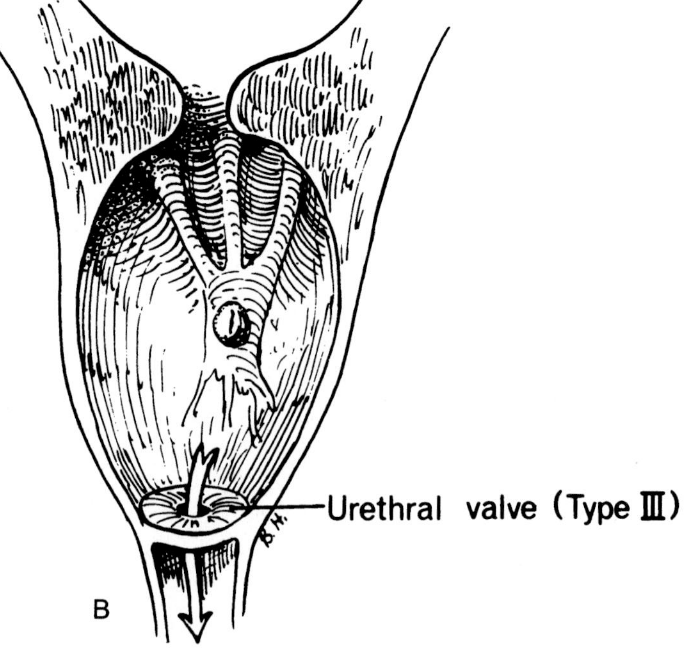

Figure 67–5. *A*, Congenital urethral membrane (Young's type III urethral valve) causing severe obstruction with bilateral renal dysplasia; a retrograde catheter could not be passed. *B*, Drawing of typical appearance of type III urethral valve.

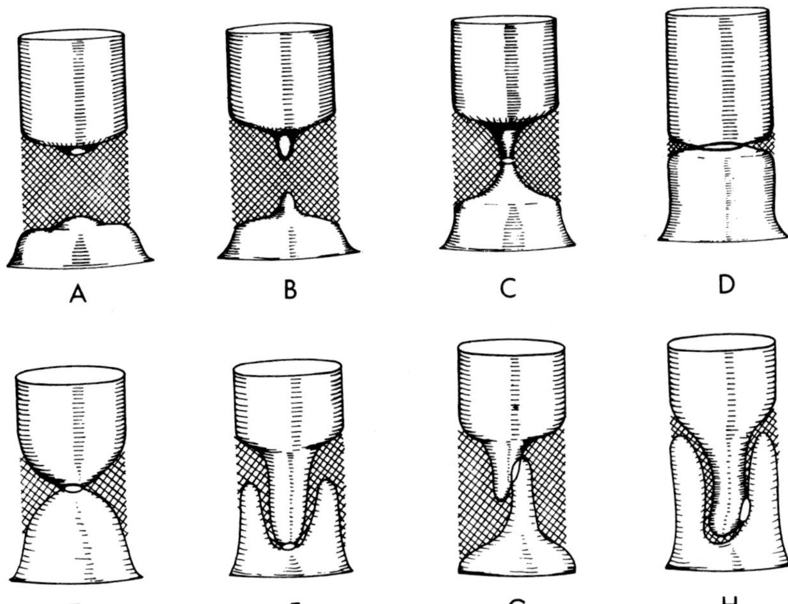

Figure 67–6. Development of congenital urethral membranes (type III valves).

A to *D*, Normal canalization of the urogenital membrane. *D* shows normal slight constriction at the level of the perineal membrane.

E, Stricture formation.

F, Canalization by central downgrowth and circumferential ingrowth resulting in bulging membrane with a central stenotic orifice.

G and *H*, Side openings creating valvular wind-sock membranes. (Drawings and descriptions supplied through the courtesy of Dr. FD Stephens. From Kelalis PP, King LR, eds: Clinical Pediatric Urology. Philadelphia, W. B. Saunders Company, 1976.)

tes, or respiratory distress resulting from pulmonary hypoplasia suggests the possibility of severe bladder outlet obstruction. Other features may include an obstetric history of oligohydramnios (the bulk of the amniotic fluid is composed of fetal urine) and findings in the neonate consistent with Potter's syndrome (dysmorphic facial features, fetal growth retardation, positional limb deformations, pulmonary hypoplasia). The neonate with severely obstructing valves has a very thick-walled bladder that is easily palpable through the flaccid abdomen of infants of this age group, even when the bladder empties completely. The dilated renal pelves and large, tortuous, tense ureters are often readily felt on abdominal examination.

Neonatal ascites results from many diverse causes, but in nearly 40% of the cases, urinary ascites is secondary to obstructive uropathy, most often infravesical in location (Fig. 67–8) (Adzick et al, 1985). The ascites actually represents a transudation of retroperitoneal urine across the thin and permeable peritoneum of the neonate. Extravasation may develop at any number of sites but is seen most often at the renal fornix (Fig. 67–9). Although newborns with urinary ascites may develop severe electrolyte abnormalities and life-threatening abnormal fluid shifts shortly after birth, the presence of ascites actually indicates a more favorable prognosis regarding ultimate renal function than the absence of ascites in a similar group of children (Rittenberg et al, 1988).

Pulmonary hypoplasia is frequently associated with severe obstructive uropathy, especially when oligohydramnios is present also. Although several theories have been proposed to explain the cause of pulmonary hypoplasia, the most accepted one suggests that oligohydramnios prevents normal chest mobility and lung expansion in utero (Landers and Hanson, 1990). At birth, these infants are cyanotic and have low Apgar scores. They require immediate pulmonary resuscitation with endotracheal intubation and positive-pressure ventilation, and they may develop pneumothorax or

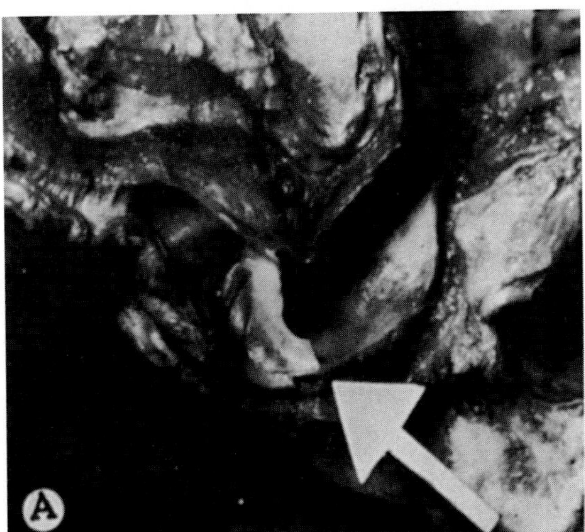

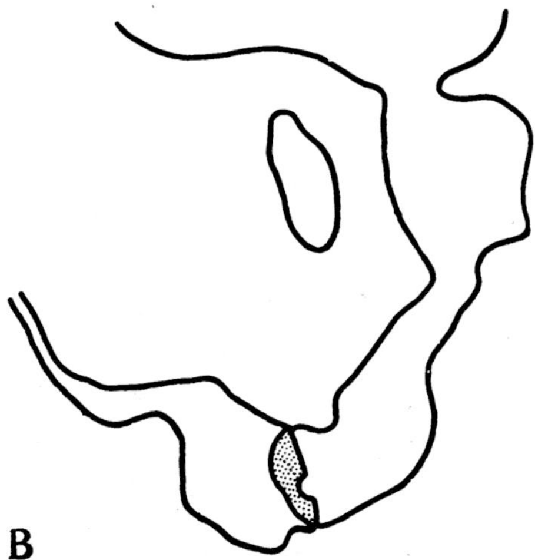

Figure 67–7. Wind-sock membrane. *A*, Obstructing membrane attached in membranous urethra and ballooned like wind sock into expanded bulbous urethra (autopsy specimen). *B*, Diagram of the anatomic findings. (From Field PL, Stephens FD: J Urol 1974;111:250.)

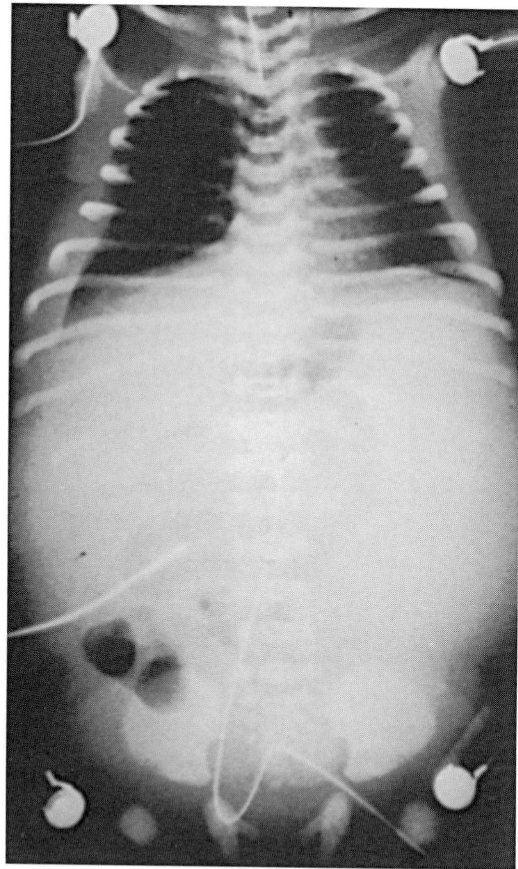

Figure 67–8. Typical radiographic findings with urinary ascites in a neonate, showing the centrally positioned bowel loops, ground glass appearance of the abdomen, and bulging flanks.

pneumomediastinum, which necessitates placement of chest tubes. Some centers are employing the technique of extracorporeal membrane oxygenation (ECMO) to assist the severely affected infant during the early postpartum period (Detjer and Gibbons, 1990; Gibbons et al, 1993). Today, most neonates who die as a result of posterior urethral valves die from respiratory causes—not from renal or infectious causes. Indeed, newborns with urethral valves and significant pulmonary hypoplasia still have a mortality rate as high as 50% (Nakayama et al, 1986).

Severely affected neonates who are not recognized at birth most commonly present within a few weeks with urosepsis, dehydration, and electrolyte abnormalities. Some infants may have only failure to thrive from renal insufficiency. Less commonly, a dribbling urinary stream may call attention to the problem.

Patients presenting during the toddler years are more likely to have somewhat better renal function and generally present because of urinary infection or voiding dysfunction. School-aged boys—the least common age of children at presentation—more often have voiding dysfunction as their primary complaint, which is generally recognized as urinary incontinence (Pieretti, 1993).

Today, the majority of infants with bladder outlet obstruction are recognized on prenatal ultrasound examination and are promptly evaluated and managed before continuing obstruction or infection does further renal parenchymal damage (Fig. 67–10). Our current ability to diagnose this problem before birth also raises the possibility that intervention before birth (by percutaneous placement of vesicoamniotic shunts or primary fetal surgery) may better preserve renal and pulmonary function in some babies than if we wait to initiate treatment electively at birth. A more detailed discussion of prenatal diagnosis and the issues surrounding fetal intervention follows the later section on clinical management of urethral valves.

Pathophysiology

Congenital urethral obstruction causes a broad array of abnormalities in the urinary tract, including damage to the renal parenchyma as well as to the smooth muscle function of the ureter and bladder. These changes may persist despite successful relief of the primary obstruction. Because urethral valves are present during the earliest phase of fetal development, primitive tissues mature in an abnormal environment of high intraluminal pressures and organ distention. Increasingly, studies are demonstrating that this situation results in permanent maldevelopment and long-lasting functional abnormalities (McConnell, 1989; Keating, 1994). The pathophysiology of the urinary tract associated with congenital urethral obstruction is discussed under five categories: reduced glomerular filtration, abnormal renal tubular function, hydronephrosis (luminal dilatation), vesicoureteral reflux, and detrusor dysfunction.

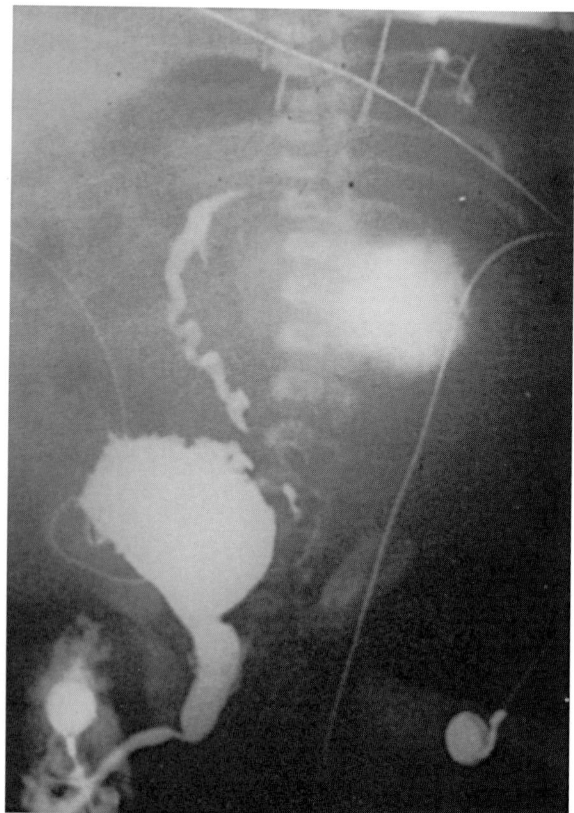

Figure 67–9. Voiding cystourethrogram in the patient with ascites shown in Figure 67–8. In this study, reflux occurred on the left, demonstrating the site of urinary extravasation to be at the renal fornix.

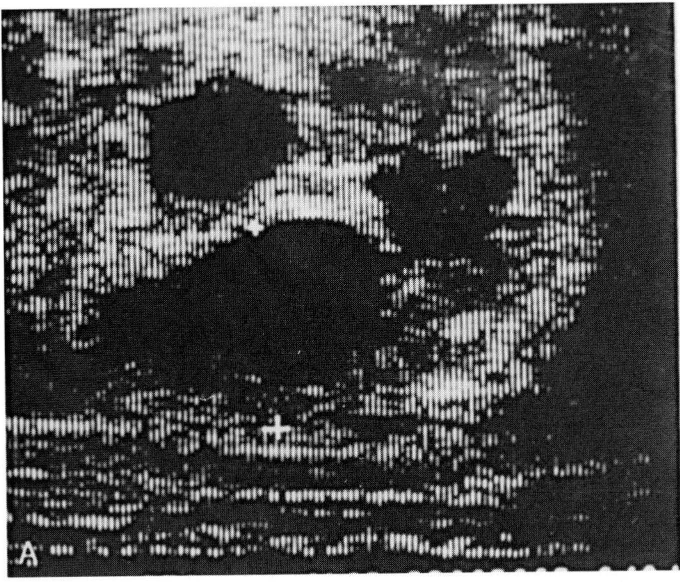

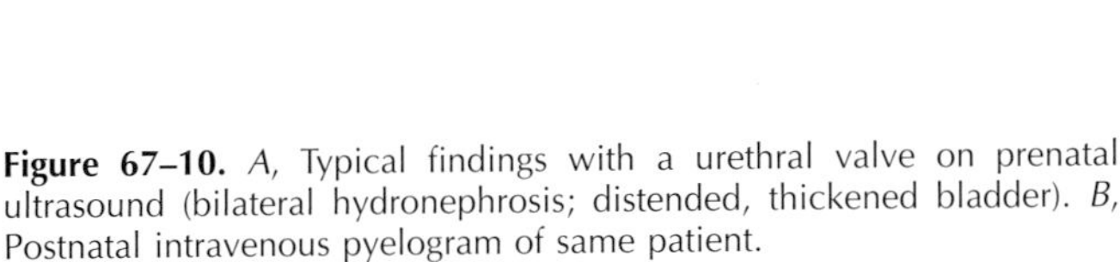

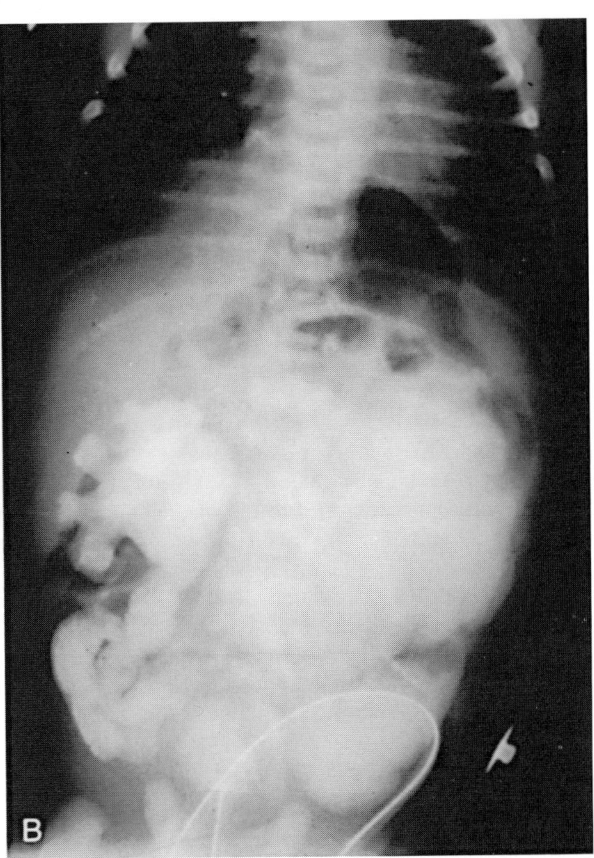

Figure 67–10. *A*, Typical findings with a urethral valve on prenatal ultrasound (bilateral hydronephrosis; distended, thickened bladder). *B*, Postnatal intravenous pyelogram of same patient.

Glomerular Filtration

The ultimate goal of management of posterior urethral valves is to maximize and preserve glomerular filtration. Although this issue has always been the area of primary concern, it is especially acute now because of our ability to make the diagnosis of urethral valves with substantial accuracy in the fetus. Today, our decisions regarding management of the unborn, related to both timing and technique, may have a significant impact on the ultimate renal function of the child. The data relative to patient survival as well as the anticipated levels of renal function are gradually being rewritten.

Two decades ago, 25% of children with urethral valves died within the first year of life, 25% died later in childhood, and the remaining half survived into the young adult years with varying degrees of renal insufficiency (Churchill et al, 1983). Today, neonatal deaths from renal insufficiency or sepsis are rare. Dialysis and, ultimately, renal transplantation are available to the youngest babies. Neonatologic and nephrologic support is universally available, and the overall outlook is greatly improved. Children who die within the neonatal period generally die from respiratory insufficiency resulting from pulmonary hypoplasia (Churchill et al, 1990). Nonetheless, children with urethral valves may have severe renal insufficiency at birth, are at risk of infection even after relief of the obstruction because of stasis of urine or reflux, may develop hypertension with its deleterious effects on renal function, and, in some cases, demonstrate a tendency toward gradually deteriorating renal function over time, the cause of which often remains elusive (Burbige and Hensle, 1987). Decreasing renal function may be a result of renal parenchymal dysplasia, hydronephrotic damage, infectious atrophy, and, perhaps, progressive glomerulosclerosis due to hyperfiltration.

Renal parenchymal dysplasia is commonly associated with urethral valves. The renal dysplasia seen in association with urethral valves tends to be microcystic in nature and develops most severely in the peripheral cortical zone. It has long been suspected that this dysplasia is a result of maturation of the primitive metanephric blastema in the presence of high intraluminal pressures. Experimental data suggest that this probably does play a role. Beck first reported the development of cystic, dysplastic changes in the kidneys of fetal sheep that underwent ureteral obstruction created in the midtrimester (Beck, 1971). Subsequent experimental studies by Glick and co-workers (1984) and by Gonzalez and associates (1990) in lambs and by McVary and Maizels (1989) in the chick embryo have also demonstrated the development of dysplastic changes in normal fetal kidneys after creation of fetal ureteral and urethral obstruction.

Henneberry and Stephens (1980), however, have argued that the dysplasia seen with urethral valves may also be a primary embryologic abnormality resulting from an abnormal position of the primitive ureteral bud along the mesonephric duct. In a careful anatomic dissection of the trigone in 11 cases of urethral valves (22 renal units), they noted that, in 11 instances, the ureters were very laterally ectopic (D position) and that these kidneys were more dysplastic than those associated with more normally positioned ureters. Hoover and Duckett (1982) have observed that a relationship exists between nonfunction of a kidney (severe dysplasia) and the presence of ipsilateral massive vesicoureteral reflux in patients with urethral valves. Commonly known as the VURD syndrome (*v*alves, *u*nilateral *r*eflux, *d*ysplasia), this finding is thought to be another clinical manifestation of abnormal ureteral budding in this anomaly.

Regardless of the mechanism that initiates the abnormal parenchymal histology, it is clear that the development of dysplasia is an early embryologic event. The presence of renal dysplasia is the single most significant abnormality that will determine ultimate renal function, and it is perhaps the only aspect of this congenital disorder over which the clinician has no influence.

On the other hand, satisfactory relief of the high intravesical and intraureteral pressures associated with urethral obstruction should prevent progressive renal parenchymal damage resulting from the obstruction. What is not clearly known is which therapeutic approach to the management of valves (primary ablation, temporary diversion, and so forth) is most likely to prevent further damage as well as possibly allow some recovery of renal function. In the newborn and very young infant, in particular, data suggest that satisfactory relief of obstruction allows growth of new renal tissue as well as an absolute measurable increase in glomerular filtration (Mayor et al, 1975). This item is discussed later in greater detail under the specifics of management, but controversy exists about the optimal approach to therapy in relation to ultimate renal function.

Other causes for progressive renal failure are recurring urinary tract infection and perhaps glomerulosclerosis associated with hyperfiltration. Although the child who has had a urethral valve is at risk of recurring urinary infection because of the presence of vesicoureteral reflux, ureteral stasis, or incomplete bladder emptying, careful selected surgical intervention and the use of long-term chemoprophylaxis, when necessary, should prevent significant, progressive damage from infection. The importance of hyperfiltration remains very controversial (Brenner et al, 1982). When experimental animals with a significant reduction in renal mass are fed diets that result in a high renal solute load, thereby requiring considerable renal work to excrete the metabolic by-products, progressive deterioration of renal function occurs much faster than it does in a similar group of animals fed a diet with a low renal solute load. Whether this phenomenon might play a role in the child who has had valves and who now has moderate renal insufficiency remains unclear. Of the major food groups, protein provides a higher renal solute load by weight than either fats or carbohydrates. Experimentally, diets high in protein are most often associated with progressive renal functional deterioration. At this time, however, it is not entirely clear what effect severely limiting protein intake in children would have on somatic and central nervous system growth, and there is still no great enthusiasm for embracing a severely protein-restricted diet in an infant with significant renal insufficiency (Klahr, 1989).

Several anatomic conditions associated with urethral valves appear to be associated also with generally improved renal function, presumably by allowing lower intraluminal pressures during fetal development (Conner et al, 1988; Rittenberg et al, 1988). These conditions include the following: (1) massive unilateral vesicoureteral reflux, (2) large bladder diverticula, and (3) urinary ascites. In each situation, there is a pop-off valve, which potentially absorbs high intraluminal pressures, thereby allowing the fetal renal parenchyma to develop in a more normal environment.

Renal Tubular Function

Because high ureteral pressures always affect the most distal aspect of the nephron first, some patients with urinary obstruction encounter more difficulty with urinary concentrating ability than with reduction in glomerular filtration (Dinneen et al, 1995). This abnormality (an acquired form of nephrogenic diabetes insipidus) results in persistently high urinary flow rates regardless of fluid intake or the state of hydration. This phenomenon has two important consequences.

The newborn or infant with fixed high urinary flow rates is particularly prone to severe episodes of dehydration and electrolyte imbalances whenever there is increased fluid loss elsewhere, such as with excessive gastrointestinal losses (vomiting, diarrhea), high fever, or third space fluid sequestration. As long as adequate fluid and electrolytes are taken orally, the high urinary output is of limited significance. If the infant is unable to maintain adequate oral intake, he or she will rapidly become dehydrated because of the persistently high urinary output despite significant total body water depletion.

The second major consequence of high urinary flows involves ureteral and vesical dysfunction. Significantly high ureteral flow rates may cause persistent ureteral dilation that would be less significant with a lower urinary flow rate. In addition, high urinary flow rates rapidly fill the bladder. When poor bladder compliance is present, higher resting bladder pressures are achieved much more quickly. High urinary flow rates can be controlled to some extent with the use of diets that provide a low renal solute load. Hormonal therapy with antidiuretic hormone is generally not successful because this renal diabetes insipidus results from damage to the collecting ducts.

Hydronephrosis

In the presence of significant urethral obstruction, ureteral dilatation of variable but usually considerable degree is expected. After satisfactory relief of the obstruction, either by endoscopic destruction of the valve or by vesicostomy, a gradual but substantial reduction in the degree of hydronephrosis generally occurs (Fig. 67–11). When this does not happen, several specific diagnostic possibilities must be investigated to elucidate the cause of the problem. Is the persistent dilatation a result of true ureterovesical junction obstruction? Is the ureteral musculature faulty and unable to generate effective peristalsis (Gearhart et al, 1995)? In this situation, the dilatation of the ureters may be a permanent facet of the child's disorder. Are these changes the result of high intravesical pressures, or are they secondary to high urinary flow rates? Each of these factors may play a role in an individual case.

Johnston and Kulatilake (1971) demonstrated many years ago that it may take years after primary valve ablation for final improvement in ureteral caliber to occur. They suggested that the responsible physician should not be anxious to proceed with further surgical therapy on the ureter in young infants as long as renal function is stable and urinary

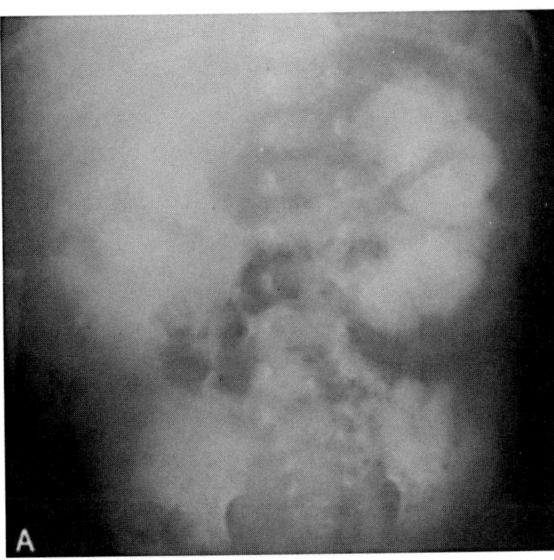

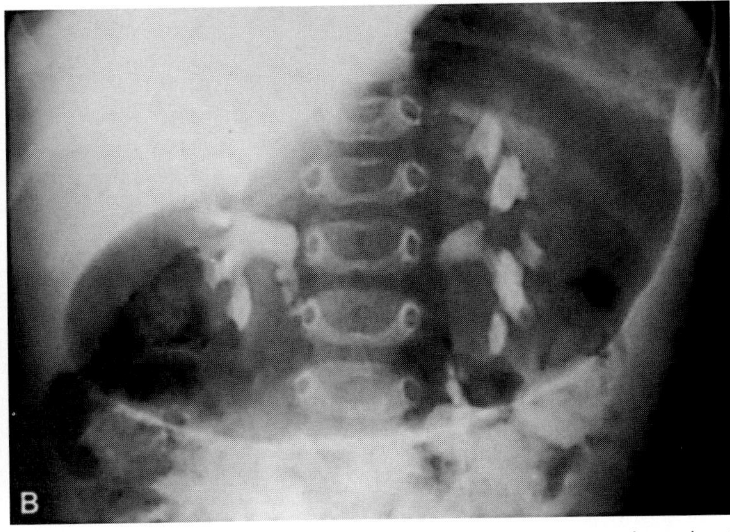

Figure 67–11. *A,* Initial intravenous pyelogram (IVP) at the time of diagnosis of urethral valves. *B,* IVP 3 months after valve ablation alone, showing marked reduction in the degree of hydronephrosis.

infection is controlled. When it becomes evident that substantial recovery is not going to occur, it is then necessary to address the role of each of the issues noted previously (Fig. 67–12).

Properly performed vesical urodynamic studies are essential. If the child has a noncompliant bladder associated with high intravesical pressures, this condition must be corrected before any attempt at surgical remodeling of the ureter is considered. Correction of the bladder dysfunction may be sufficient to allow the hydronephrosis to resolve. Dynamic flow studies of the upper urinary tract may be necessary to determine whether true ureterovesical junction obstruction is present (Whitaker, 1973). Percutaneous pressure-flow studies of the upper urinary tract (Whitaker test) are often necessary to differentiate nonobstructive ureteral dilatation from true ureterovesical junction obstruction. Diuretic-enhanced renograms are less invasive but difficult to interpret in the presence of relatively poor renal function, dilute urine with high-volume flow, and dilated ureters.

When investigators looked critically at this issue, they discovered that true ureterovesical obstruction is rare. In Whitaker's series, only 4 of 17 ureters in children with urethral valves and suspected secondary ureterovesical junction obstruction were actually found to have signs consistent with obstruction when both pressures and flow were considered. In the Whitaker test, flow is constant and pressure varies. Woodbury (1989) described an upper tract urodynamic test in which pressure is stable but flow may vary. Whether this additional diagnostic tool will offer a reassessment of older data remains unknown at this time.

An accurate assessment of a timed sample of urine volume is also an important factor in this evaluation. As noted previously, many children who have urethral valves have significant hyposthenuria and excrete a very large volume of urine. As in children with primary diabetes insipidus, this excessive, high-flow state may also contribute to persistent ureteral dilatation.

Vesicoureteral Reflux

Vesicoureteral reflux is commonly found in association with posterior urethral valves. Between one third and one half of children with valves have reflux at the time of initial diagnosis. Most often, this probably represents secondary vesicoureteral reflux resulting from high intravesical pressures, development of paraureteral diverticula, and loss of ureterovesical valvular competence. In some instances, however, the reflux may be primary and may be due to a ureteral bud anomaly. As noted previously, Henneberry and Stephens (1980), in their study of fetuses and newborn infants with severe posterior urethral valves, reported a significant incidence of lateral ectopia of the ureteral orifice.

The presence of vesicoureteral reflux should not in itself influence the initial management of children with posterior urethral valves (Johnston, 1979). In about a third of cases, the reflux resolves spontaneously after the obstruction has been eliminated. In another third of cases, the reflux may persist but causes no problem so long as the child is maintained on chemoprophylaxis. Decisions about reimplantation should then be made after a period of observation following the initial valve ablation so long as urinary infection is controlled with maintenance chemoprophylaxis. Even if reflux persists, the dilated ureters generally decrease in caliber over time. If reimplantation is ultimately necessary, it probably can be accomplished without extensive tailoring or remodeling of the ureter. About one third of patients have problems associated with reflux during follow-up and are best managed by earlier reimplantation.

Vesical Dysfunction

It has been recognized for many years that some children with urethral valves (as many as 25%) have varying degrees of abnormal bladder function. Most often, this abnormality presents as urinary incontinence. Many years ago investigators assumed that this incontinence was due primarily to incompetent sphincter function as a result of either primary maldevelopment of the membranous urethra and bladder neck (because of the anatomic location of the valve at the level of the voluntary sphincter, which caused distention and dilatation of that region of the urethra during embryogenesis) or direct injury to the sphincter at the time of endoscopic valve ablation. However, with the application of modern

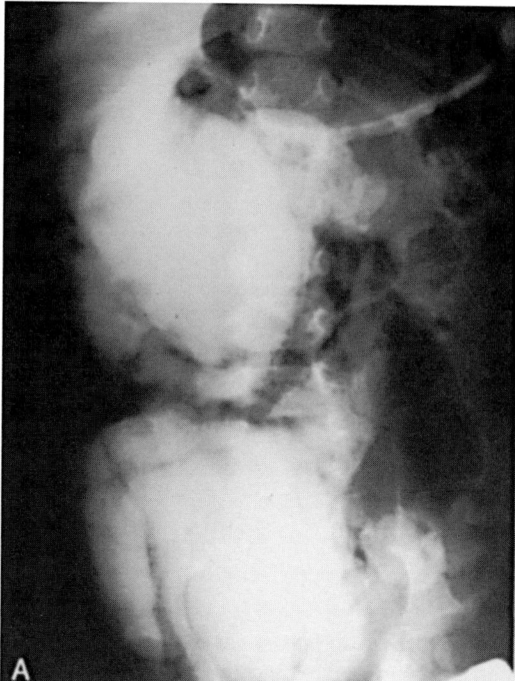

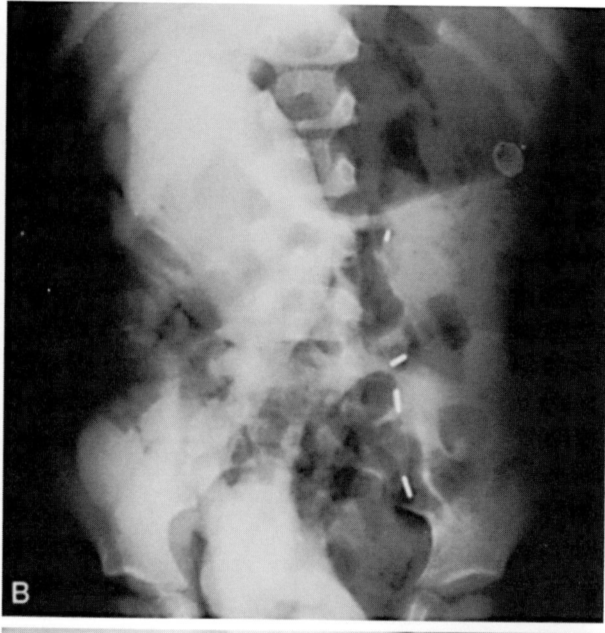

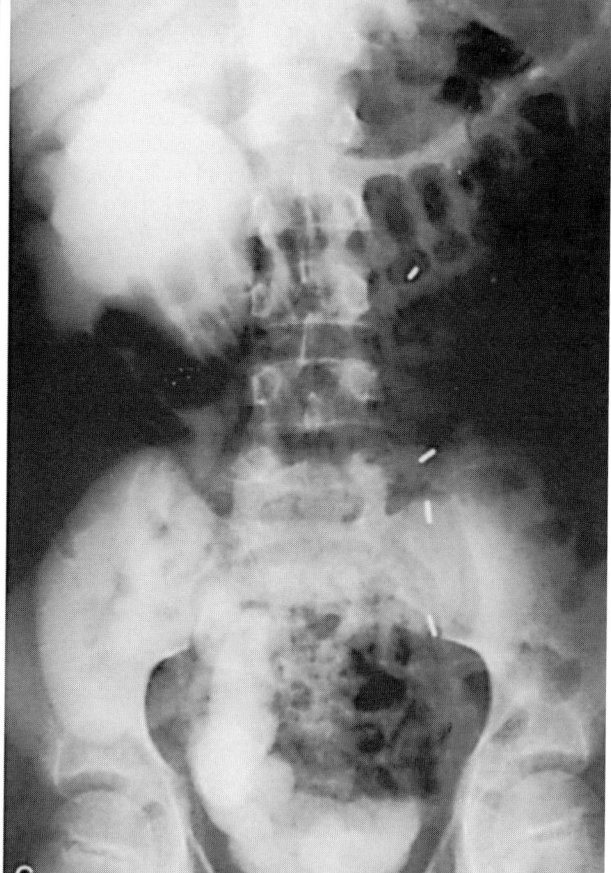

Figure 67–12. Series of intravenous pyelogram (IVP) films in a child with urethral valves, a functioning right kidney, and a nonfunctioning left kidney.

A, IVP at diagnosis.

B, IVP 1 year after valve ablation and left nephroureterectomy. The voiding urethrogram appeared normal, and no vesicoureteral reflux was present. Little or no improvement in the degree of hydronephrosis is apparent.

C, IVP 4 years later. The degree of hydronephrosis remains essentially unchanged. Urodynamic studies revealed a compliant bladder, which emptied satisfactorily, and a Whitaker study was thought to be normal. Renal function has remained stable at a serum creatinine level of 0.6 mg/dl.

urodynamic techniques to pediatric urology, it has become increasingly obvious that primary vesical dysfunction is commonly associated with urethral valves and that this vesical dysfunction does not necessarily abate after relief of the obstruction and ultimately has a significant impact on prognosis as well.

Tanagho (1974) and Lome and associates (1972) first brought to our attention the difficulties encountered in establishing adequate bladder volume after a period of bladder dysfunction in some children with urethral valves (usually after high loop urinary diversion). Review of these data from the 1960s and 1970s shows that many children included in these series had also had previous bladder surgery or placement of indwelling suprapubic tubes for initial management of the urethral valves. The extent of the impact of this previous bladder surgery on final bladder function was not clearly defined. Several groups of investigators, including Glassberg and colleagues (1982), Bauer and associates (1979), and Campaiola and co-workers (1985), studied a series of children who had urethral valves and reported several abnormalities of detrusor function, including primary myogenic failure, uninhibited bladder activity, and findings consistent with poor compliance of the detrusor muscle. In a more recent study, Holmdahl and associates (1995) demonstrated that urodynamic patterns can change when bladder function is evaluated over time in infants with urethral valves. In this study of 16 infants, all underwent urodynamic testing prior to valve ablation, and all were followed with serial urodynamic studies postoperatively. Preoperatively, in all boys the bladder was small in capacity and hypercontractile. After destruction of the valves, bladder capacity increased, although the bladder continued to show some instability, and some boys demonstrated incomplete emptying. The cause of detrusor dysfunction remains unclear, although experimental evidence suggests that fetal urethral obstruction results in irreversible changes in the organization and function of the smooth muscle cells of the bladder (Karim et al, 1992, 1993) and may also result in deposition of abnormal quantities of intercellular collagen (Keating, 1994; Peters, 1994).

Vesical dysfunction not only contributes to problems of urinary incontinence but also may be a primary factor in maintaining persistent ureterectasis and high intravesical and intraureteral pressures that ultimately may cause deterioration of renal function. Parkhouse and associates (1988) reported on a series of children with urethral valves who were surveyed repeatedly from childhood into adolescence. They observed that children who were incontinent during childhood developed more severe degrees of renal insufficiency in adolescence than did those who had normal urinary control. They proposed that children who were incontinent had more severe bladder dysfunction than those who had normal urinary control. Presumably, at puberty the development of the prostate increases outlet resistance, improving continence but raising intravesical pressure and producing unfavorable effects on renal function. Unfortunately, routine urodynamic studies were not performed consistently in all of these children to support these observations and conclusions beyond question.

Depending on the extent and nature of bladder dysfunction and the ability of the bladder to empty, management may consist of anticholinergic therapy to reduce uninhibited detrusor contractions, clean, intermittent catheterization to afford satisfactory bladder emptying, or bladder augmentation to improve bladder volume and compliance (Glassberg, 1985). In older, cooperative boys, a program of planned, timed voidings might keep bladder volumes sufficiently low to maintain intravesical pressures at an acceptable level.

Management

Management of the child with posterior urethral valves depends on the degree of renal insufficiency and the age of the child. Older children who have voiding dysfunction or urinary tract infection but satisfactory renal function are easily and effectively treated initially by endoscopic destruction of the urethral valves alone. Decisions about selective surgery for persistent vesicoureteral reflux, lingering ureterovesical junction obstruction (uncommon), or detrusor dysfunction are made on an individual basis.

The main issues in treatment of urethral valves involve very young infants. In these patients, the potential for recovering renal function is believed to be significant. In addition, the increasing recognition of urethral valves in the fetus raises ongoing questions about the timing of intervention and offers the responsible physician an opportunity to perform procedures that will decompress the urinary tract, allowing maximum recovery of renal function during a period when growth of new renal tissue is ongoing.

In the past, most infants with urethral valves came to medical attention because of urosepsis or failure to thrive. These infants were often dehydrated and had renal insufficiency, severe acidosis, and electrolyte abnormalities. In either case, management was usually begun by placing a small transurethral catheter to provide unobstructed vesical drainage and initiating appropriate antibiotics and parenteral fluid rehydration. Initiation of these measures allowed immediate improvement of renal function in most cases. In general, 5 to 7 days of catheter drainage should allow the physician to assess adequately the existing level of glomerular filtration. Currently, more patients with posterior urethral valves are being recognized by the observation of hydronephrosis on prenatal ultrasound than by the more traditional signs described earlier. At birth, these children have renal function parameters equivalent to those of maternal renal function. The placement of a urethral catheter and initiation of prophylactic antibiotic management allow assessment of the baseline level of renal function during the first few days after birth. In each of these situations, further management is dictated by the level of renal function.

In the presence of normal or satisfactory renal function (most often described as a serum creatinine of less than 1.0 mg/dl in the newborn after several days of catheter drainage, although a healthy neonate at 4 weeks of age may have a serum creatinine of 0.2 to 0.4 mg/dl), endoscopic destruction of the valves is considered. Today, endoscopes with excellent optics and sufficiently small caliber are available for even the tiniest newborn. Most endoscopic systems today accept small operating cauterizing electrodes that are sufficient to destroy the valve. For the child whose urethra is too small to accept the available endoscopes, antegrade destruction of the valve by percutaneous access to the bladder has been described by Zaontz and Firlit (1985). MacAninch (personal communication) has suggested that this technique is made easier by using the rigid ureteroscope. The longer instrument allows the endoscopist increased maneuverability, which is one of the limiting factors of this technique when the short pediatric cystoscope is used. Other techniques employed for primary destruction of urethral valves include use of the neodymium-yttrium-aluminum-garnet laser (Ehrlich and Shanberg, 1988; Biewald and Schier, 1992) or of the cautery hook as originally described by Williams and improved by Deane and co-workers (1988), antegrade extraction of a balloon catheter (Kolicinski, 1988), and use of the valvulotome (Cromie et al, 1994).

Valve ablation must be done carefully. Only a single wire (not a loop) or a small electrode should be used. The current on the electrosurgical unit should be set just high enough to incise the valve but not high enough to diffuse thermal injury to surrounding urethral tissues. I prefer to incise the valve at the 4:00, 8:00, and 12:00 o'clock positions, but I believe that the 12:00 o'clock incision is most important because it is the one that separates the anteriorly fused membrane. The cautery wire or electrode is advanced in an antegrade fashion from the proximal margin of the membranous urethra into the dilated prostatic urethra (Fig. 67–13). If the bladder is distended during valvulotomy, the increased luminal pressure balloons the valve, making antegrade incision easy and safe. This approach significantly minimizes the risk of injury to the urethral sphincter that might occur if the valve were pulled down in a retrograde fashion by the resectoscope wire. A small transurethral catheter may be left in place for 1 or 2 days, but this is generally not necessary.

After satisfactory destruction of the valve has been accomplished, one should follow the child expectantly with regular estimates of renal function as well as imaging studies that assess improvement in the degree of hydronephrosis or the presence of vesicoureteral reflux. A follow-up voiding cystourethrogram is generally done 2 months after valve destruction to be sure that the obstruction was satisfactorily relieved. If renal function remains stable and infection is avoided (chemoprophylaxis is generally recommended), improvement in the anatomy of the urinary tract and continued stable renal function can be expected. The improvement in ureteral dilation can be gradual and may take months or occasionally years.

Careful endoscopic destruction of valves, even in the newborn, has not been associated with a significant incidence of urethral stricture. In the unusual situation in which the newborn urethra seems too small to accommodate the available endoscopes, an elective vesicostomy is appropriate and safe. Indeed, Walker and Padron prefer vesicostomy to endoscopic ablation in the neonate, believing that this technique may be safer and may reduce the incidence of urethral stricture. However, a review of their approach did not suggest any overall improvement of renal function compared with endoscopic management of valves only (Walker and Padron, 1990).

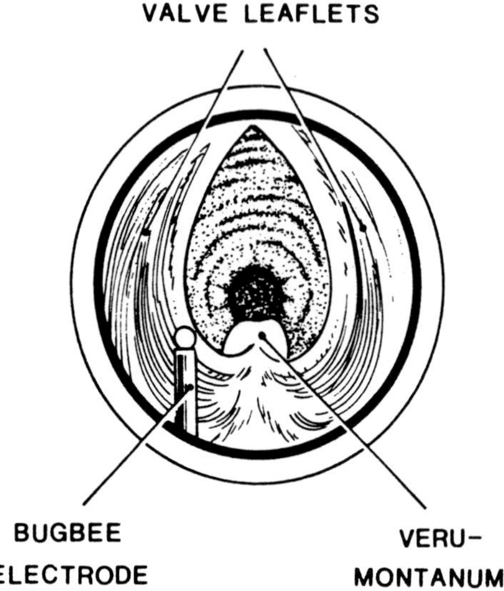

Figure 67–13. Endoscopic visualization of type I posterior urethral valve for electrosurgical ablation. Note that the electrode is positioned distal to the valve and will be advanced toward the prostatic urethra. (From Kaplan GW, Scherz HC: Infravesical obstruction. *In* Kelalis PP, King LR, Belman AB, eds: Clinical Pediatric Urology, 3rd ed. Philadelphia, W. B. Saunders Company, 1992, p 846.)

The major area of continuing controversy involves the most appropriate therapeutic approach to infants in whom significant renal insufficiency persists after a satisfactory period of transurethral drainage. The options for managing this group of children include endoscopic destruction of urethral valves only, elective vesicostomy, and high-loop temporizing ureteral diversion. The issue of concern is which therapeutic approach maximizes recovery of renal function and restores the urodynamics of the upper urinary tract most nearly to normal (Gonzales, 1990).

During the 1960s, high-loop ureterostomy was a commonly performed, generally accepted approach to the initial management of infants with urethral valves (Johnston, 1963). After ureterostomy, renal function often improved initially and then remained stable, ureteral diameter decreased, and the infant often exhibited surprisingly good health. Reconstruction of the ureters and valve ablation were then done electively within 1 to 2 years in a larger, more robust child.

During the same period, a few investigators experimented with different techniques designed to destroy the valves transurethrally. Johnston (1966) demonstrated that many infants treated in this manner also showed stabilized or improved renal function and a gradual but progressive reduction in the degree of hydronephrosis. When better endoscopes became available in the 1970s, most pediatric urologists switched to primary endoscopic destruction of valves as their preferred form of management.

Krueger and associates (1980a) published a provocative article in 1980 that compared two series of children with posterior urethral valves; one group was treated by high-loop ureterostomy and a second group was treated by endoscopic ablation only. Their data suggested that children who presented with renal insufficiency and were managed by high-loop cutaneous ureterostomy ultimately showed an improved glomerular filtration rate and somatic growth potential compared with children presenting with similar renal function degree who were managed by endoscopic destruction of valves only. They proposed that high-loop diversion probably lowered ureteral luminal pressures more, thereby allowing the renal parenchyma to recover in an environment more nearly normal than that achieved by valve ablation only. This report has been challenged by Duckett and Norris (1989) and Reinberg and associates (1992a, 1992b) on the basis that it is not a controlled study and that similar data of their own do not support this conclusion; they maintain that comparable groups treated by valve ablation or temporizing diversion show no difference in outcome. This area remains controversial, although the author believes it is honest to say that even fewer temporizing diversions are being done now than in the recent past.

The decision to proceed with a high-loop ureterostomy is a significant one because it commits the child to a major reconstructive procedure later with all its attendant complications; therefore, the indications for high-loop ureteral diversion are limited. Severe urosepsis that does not respond to

(Reinberg et al, 1992a; Jee et al, 1993). In one other study, patients who were recognized early in gestation (less than 24 weeks) fared much worse in regard to renal function than those who were first recognized later in pregnancy or at birth after a normal earlier fetal ultrasound examination (Hutton et al, 1994).

Prognosis

The prognosis for children with urethral valves is improving, and current management is gradually rewriting the historical data. In most modern large series, neonatal deaths occur in only 2% to 3% of the patients (Churchill et al, 1990). Early (prenatal) recognition, control of infection, appropriate and selective surgery, recognition of harmful urodynamic abnormalities, modern nephrologic management methods, and eventual dialysis and transplantation all combine to increase survival now to an extent unheard of in the recent past. The original series reported total mortality as high as 50% by the end of the adolescent period (Johnston and Kulatilake, 1972). Certainly those statistics no longer hold true today. In all series, prognosis relates closely to the nadir serum creatinine level. Warshaw and associates (1985) noted that infants with a serum creatinine of less than 1.0 mg/dl at 1 year of age generally fared well, although a serum creatinine at this level does not ensure long-term satisfactory renal function. The fact remains that many children with urethral valves have significant degrees of parenchymal dysplasia and demonstrate gradual but progressive loss of renal function during their lifetime (Tejani et al, 1986; Burbige and Hensle, 1987; Parkhouse et al, 1988; Reinberg et al, 1992a). It is important that parents be aware that the diagnosis of urethral valves means a long-term commitment to surveillance and care and that even today the eventual outcome is unclear in many instances.

One bright spot is the success of renal transplantation in the management of patients with urethral valves. Despite the recognized bladder dysfunction in many patients, overall graft survival approaches that in patients who require transplants but have no uropathy whatsoever (Bryant et al, 1991; Groenewegen et al, 1993). Careful urodynamic evaluation and selective vesical reconstruction (including enterocystoplasty and clean intermittent catheterization) ensure the best chance for successful management of renal failure (Zaragoza et al, 1993). Even when the patient has a supravesical diversion, transplantation into the native bladder has generally been successful (Ross et al, 1994). One study has shown an increased risk of urinary infection after transplantation in boys who had urethral valves compared to that in a similar matched group who had normal bladders, although the long-term significance of the observation in regard to graft survival remains unknown (Mochon et al, 1992).

As the outlook for boys with urethral valves improves, it is becoming increasingly evident that a significant number of these patients will have problems with fertility. The cause of this is not always clear and may be multifaceted. Injury to the ejaculatory ducts at the time of valve ablation and retrograde ejaculation are two possible sequelae of the treatment itself (Parkhouse and Woodhouse, 1990). About 10% of boys with valves also have cryptorchidism (Krueger, 1980b). Again, the reasons are unclear, but this observation suggests that there may be a primary mesonephric anomaly that is responsible for both the valve and the cryptorchidism. But overall, the majority of men with urethral valves demonstrate normal erectile function and ejaculation, and many, if not all, are able to father children (Parkhouse and Woodhouse, 1990).

ANTERIOR URETHRAL OBSTRUCTION

Congenital obstruction of the more distal urethra is much less common than obstruction of the proximal urethra. Forms of congenital obstruction of the anterior urethra are varied and can include anterior urethral valves (congenital diverticulum of the urethra), valvular obstruction of the fossa navicularis, and cystic dilation of the ducts of Cowper's glands (syringoceles). Of these, the most common abnormality is anterior urethral valves.

An anterior urethral valve in nearly all cases is actually a congenital urethral diverticulum (Fig. 67–16) (Tank, 1987). During voiding, the diverticulum expands, ballooning ventrally and distally beneath the thinned corpus spongiosum. The flap-like dorsal margin of the diverticulum then extends into the urethral lumen, occluding urinary flow (an obstructing valve). Anterior urethral valves have been described in every portion of the anterior urethra with nearly equal rates of occurrence. They may be small, minimally obstructive, and of limited clinical concern (Fig. 67–17). Often, though, they are severely obstructive and result in all of the findings seen with posterior urethral valves.

The diagnosis of anterior urethral valves is confirmed by voiding cystourethrography. At times, difficulty with catheterization may be encountered because the catheter preferentially slips into the diverticulum. However, this occurs less often than one might suspect because the proximal wall of the diverticulum is often not hollowed out nearly as extensively as the distal wall. Because the diverticula are nearly always placed in the midline ventrally, a dorsally oriented coudé-tipped catheter can usually be negotiated with less difficulty into the more proximal urethra. To establish the diagnosis, the entire penile urethra must be included in the voiding phase of the cystourethrogram; otherwise, more distally located lesions will be missed.

The cause of these anomalies is not entirely clear, but they seem to represent incomplete fusion of a segment of the urethral plate. Another possible cause may be focally incomplete development of the corpus spongiosum with ballooning of the urethral mucosa due to inadequate support. Small, nonobstructive diverticula often appear to remain stable for many years and do not show continuous enlargement and progressively worsening obstruction.

Initial management of the child with a congenital anterior urethral valve parallels that of the child with the more common posterior urethral valve. Initial imaging studies assess the extent of hydronephrosis, the thickness and quality of the renal parenchyma (echogenicity on renal ultrasound, uptake on renal scan), and the presence or absence of vesicoureteral reflux. Infants presenting with urosepsis or severe renal insufficiency require a period of transurethral or suprapubic (by the percutaneous route) catheter drainage for stabilization, a course of antibiotics, management of electro-

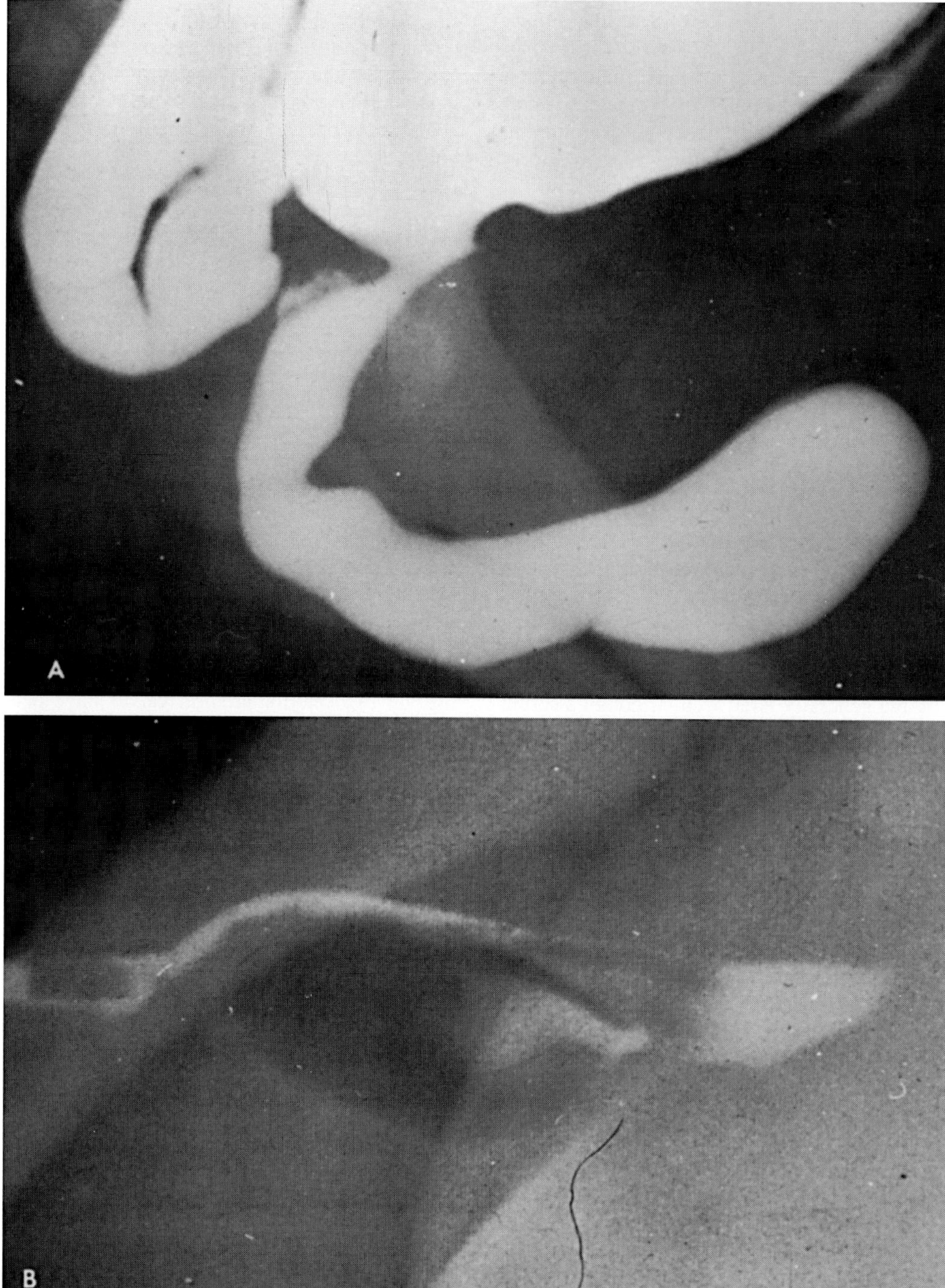

Figure 67–16. *A*, Anterior urethral diverticulum (valve). This voiding cystourethrogram in a newborn boy shows severe obstruction associated with reflux into a dysplastic left kidney and compromised right renal function. *B*, Demonstration of anterior diverticulum, using air injected retrograde with compression of urethra in perineum, followed by contrast injection, showing neck of diverticulum and mechanism of obstruction.

lytes, and assessment of renal functional improvement. As with infants with posterior urethral valves, a temporizing tubeless diversion (vesicostomy, loop ureterostomy) may be performed in individual cases (Rushton et al, 1987).

Management of the urethral anomaly may be done by endoscopic or open surgical methods. A hooked, single-wire electrocautery knife can engage the distal margin of the diverticulum and incise it in the midline. When performing this procedure, the surgeon must be very careful not to place the tip of the wire too close to the floor of the diverticulum. At this location, the wall of the urethra can be very thin, and thermal injury may result in the development of a urethrocutaneous fistula. Even after satisfactory destruction of the leaflet, postoperative urethrography is often disappointing because the appearance of the diverticulum may be unchanged. One must carefully assess the quality of urine flow (using a flow rate study if the child is old enough) and the extent of filling of the urethra distal to the anomaly to evaluate the results of the procedure.

Some surgeons have advocated open resection and recon-

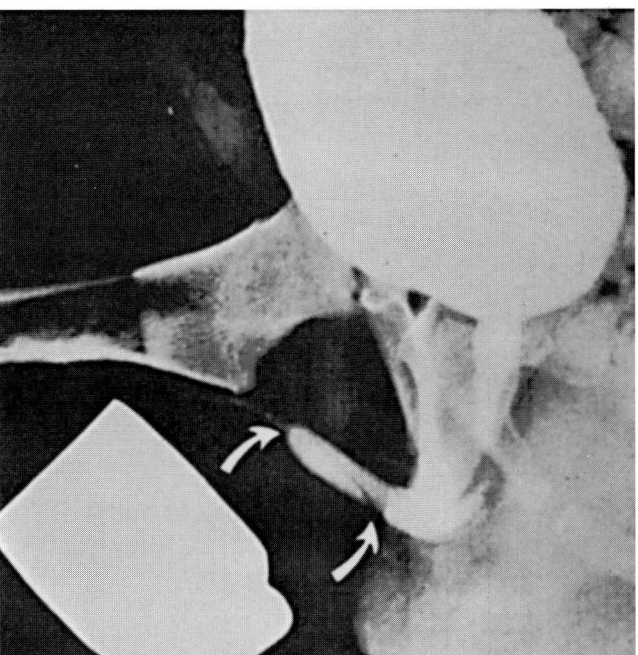

Figure 67–17. Anterior urethral diverticulum (valve) demonstrated by voiding cystourethrogram in 4-year-old boy with symptoms of straining to void and a fine stream.

struction of the diverticulum (Tank, 1987). This technique allows one to excise the distal lip completely and provide a more homogeneous caliber to the urethra. In most cases, a patch graft urethroplasty is the preferred procedure. If the diverticulum is on the penile shaft, a sleeve dissection of the penile shaft skin from the corona to the penoscrotal angle allows completion of the urethroplasty without ending up with overlapping suture lines.

Some anterior urethral valves may not be associated with a urethral diverticulum. DeCastro and colleagues (1987) described three children who had anterior urethral membranes without an associated diverticulum. Scherz and associates (1987) described valvular obstruction in the region of the fossa navicularis in three children. Whether these isolated variations represent a portion of the spectrum of abnormality described previously is unclear.

Syringoceles are cystic dilatations of the duct of Cowper's gland within the bulbous urethra (Maizels et al, 1983). They are generally small, inconsequential lesions but, rarely, are sufficiently large to cause varying degrees of outlet obstruction. Management, when necessary, is generally accomplished by endoscopic unroofing. After unroofing, a diverticulum-like defect may result on the posterolateral wall of the bulbous urethra. However, these defects are rarely obstructive and do not need further management.

MEGALOURETHRA

Nonobstructive urethral dilatation (megalourethra) is a rare entity that is associated with abnormal development of the corpus spongiosum and occasionally with abnormal development of the corpora cavernosa. Traditionally, megalourethra has been divided into two varieties: scaphoid megalourethra and fusiform megalourethra. In the scaphoid variety, the corpus spongiosum is generally thought to be the only abnormal segment, whereas the fusiform variety is associated with defects of the corpora cavernosa also. However, this distinction is arbitrary and is not based on any recognized embryologic difference between the two entities (Appel et al, 1986). Although megalourethra may be an isolated entity, it is often associated with upper tract abnormalities. Appropriate imaging of the urinary tract is indicated in every case. Megalourethra is especially common in association with the prune-belly syndrome and may represent a defect in development of the mesoderm, one of the proposed causes of the prune-belly anomaly (Mortensen et al, 1985).

Management of the megalourethra itself is primarily cosmetic if the upper tracts are satisfactorily normal (Fig. 67–18). The large bulbous urethra can be trimmed and tailored to achieve a more homogeneous and normal urethral caliber. If the corpora cavernosa are severely deficient, consideration of a change in the sex of rearing in the newborn is appropriate.

An interesting subset of boys with megalourethra is often classified as having a variant of hypospadias. These anomalies have been described by Duckett and Keating (1989) as the "megameatus, intact prepuce." The patient presents with a coronally positioned, wide-mouthed meatus and a fully formed foreskin. For a centimeter or so the urethra is often very large, and the corpus spongiosum is very thin. Ventral chordee is not present. This anomaly contrasts with the more usual variety of hypospadias, thought to represent a fetal androgen deficiency, in which the meatus is often small, the distal urethra is narrowed and inelastic, the foreskin is unfused ventrally, and ventral chordee is expected.

URETHRAL DUPLICATION

Duplication of the urethra is an uncommon anomaly. Urethral duplications are complex anomalies, and different embryologic abnormalities are thought to be responsible for the many variations seen. A universally accepted classification has not yet been described (Ortolano and Nasaralloh, 1986). Urethral duplications are conveniently divided into dorsal duplications and ventral duplications. Most duplications occur in the same sagittal plane—that is, they occur one on top of the other (Fig. 67–19). Less commonly, duplex urethras lie side by side. This is the usual finding in children with a completely duplicated phallus, but occasionally it can occur when the phallus is fused but widened. This anatomic appearance is also more common when the bladder is completely duplicated.

In the dorsal variety, in which a meatus is positioned above a glandular meatus, the normal urethra is the ventrally positioned channel that generally ends in a normal meatus on the glans. The accessory (abnormal) channel opens on the shaft in an epispadiac position anywhere from the glans to the base of the penis. Often dorsal penile chordee is present, and the foreskin may be unfused dorsally. The abnormal dorsal segment extends proximally beneath the symphysis pubis for a variable length. Many urethras end blindly before reaching the bladder. If these abnormal urethras do reach the bladder, the patient is usually incontinent. Widening of the symphysis pubis may also be found. These

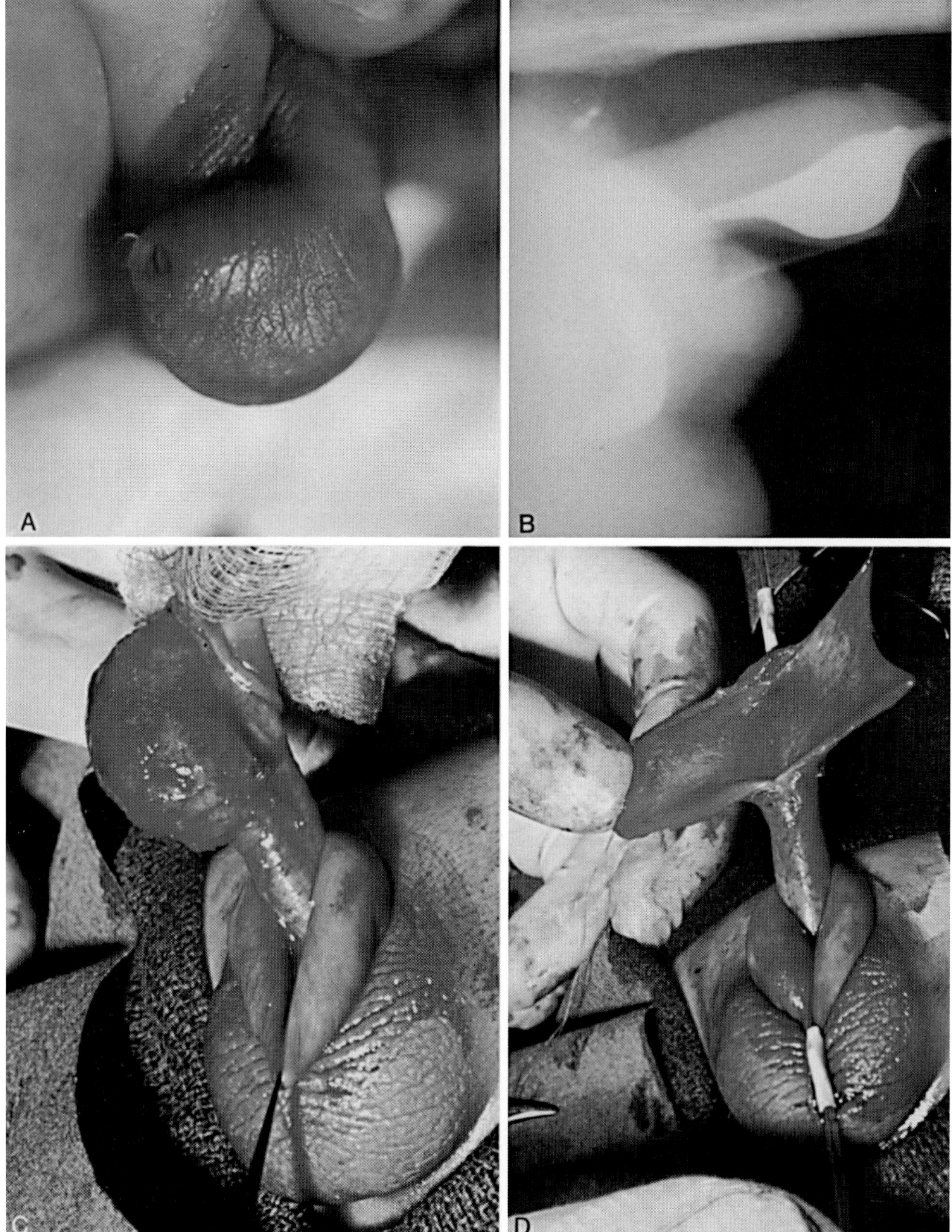

Figure 67–18. *A*, Photograph with megalourethra of a newborn male. This photograph was taken during the act of micturition.
B, Voiding urethrogram of same patient.
C, Appearance of the urethra after degloving of the penis.
D, The dilated segment of the urethra has been opened. Excess urethral tissue is excised, leaving just enough to reconstruct a urethra of normal caliber.

68 HYPOSPADIAS

John W. Duckett, M.D.

The surgical goal in patients with hypospadias is to construct a straight penis with the meatus as close as possible to the normal site to allow a forward-directed stream and normal coitus. Culp and McRoberts (1968) stated, "It is the inalienable right of every boy to be a pointer instead of a sitter by the time he starts school and to write his name legibly in the snow."

Hypospadiology is liberally sprinkled with eponyms, each representing a symbol for a technique or principle. It seems appropriate to continue this descriptive method that is so entrenched in surgery today. There have probably been over 200 reported original methods of urethral reconstruction, and they continue today as modifications of modifications. Although certain surgeons have arrived at perfection, their success has not been accepted or at least transferable to colleagues. David M. Davis wrote in 1951, "I would like to say that I believe the time has arrived to state that the surgical repair of hypospadias is no longer dubious, unreliable, or extremely difficult. If tried and proven methods are scrupulously followed, a good result should be obtained in every case. Anything less than this suggests that the surgeon is not temperamentally fitted for this kind of surgery." Much depends on experience, but even more necessary is a familiarity with all the options available. Indeed, with this familiarity as a prerequisite, **hypospadiology** would be an appropriate term for this discipline (Duckett, 1981a).

CLASSIFICATION

The abnormal urethral opening in a boy with hypospadias may be anywhere along the shaft of the penis or into the perineum. The more proximal the meatus, the more likely it is that ventral curvature (chordee) will occur (Fig. 68–1).

The most commonly used classification of hypospadias (Browne, 1936) is based on the location of the meatus (glanular, distal penile, proximal penile, penoscrotal junction, and perineal). However, the severity of hypospadias cannot always be defined by the original site of the meatus. The meatus may be close to the tip of the glans yet have significant curvature. The author, therefore, prefers a classification based not on the original site but on the new location after correction of the associated curvature (orthoplasty), as proposed by Barcat (1973).

Welch (1979) estimated that 62% of the openings were subcoronal or penile, 22% were at the penoscrotal angle, and 16% were in the scrotum or perineum. Using the Barcat classification, Juskiewenski and colleagues (1983) reported that of 536 patients with hypospadias 71% of openings were anterior, 16% were in the middle, and 13% were posterior. Of the anterior group (383 patients), 13% were classified as balantic, 43% as subcoronal, and 38% as distal shaft; the prepuce was intact in 6% (megameatus intact prepuce).

The author's own experience at The Children's Hospital of Philadelphia corresponds to these reports: 50% of openings were anterior, 30% were in the middle or midpenile, and 20% were posterior (Duckett and Snyder, 1992) (see

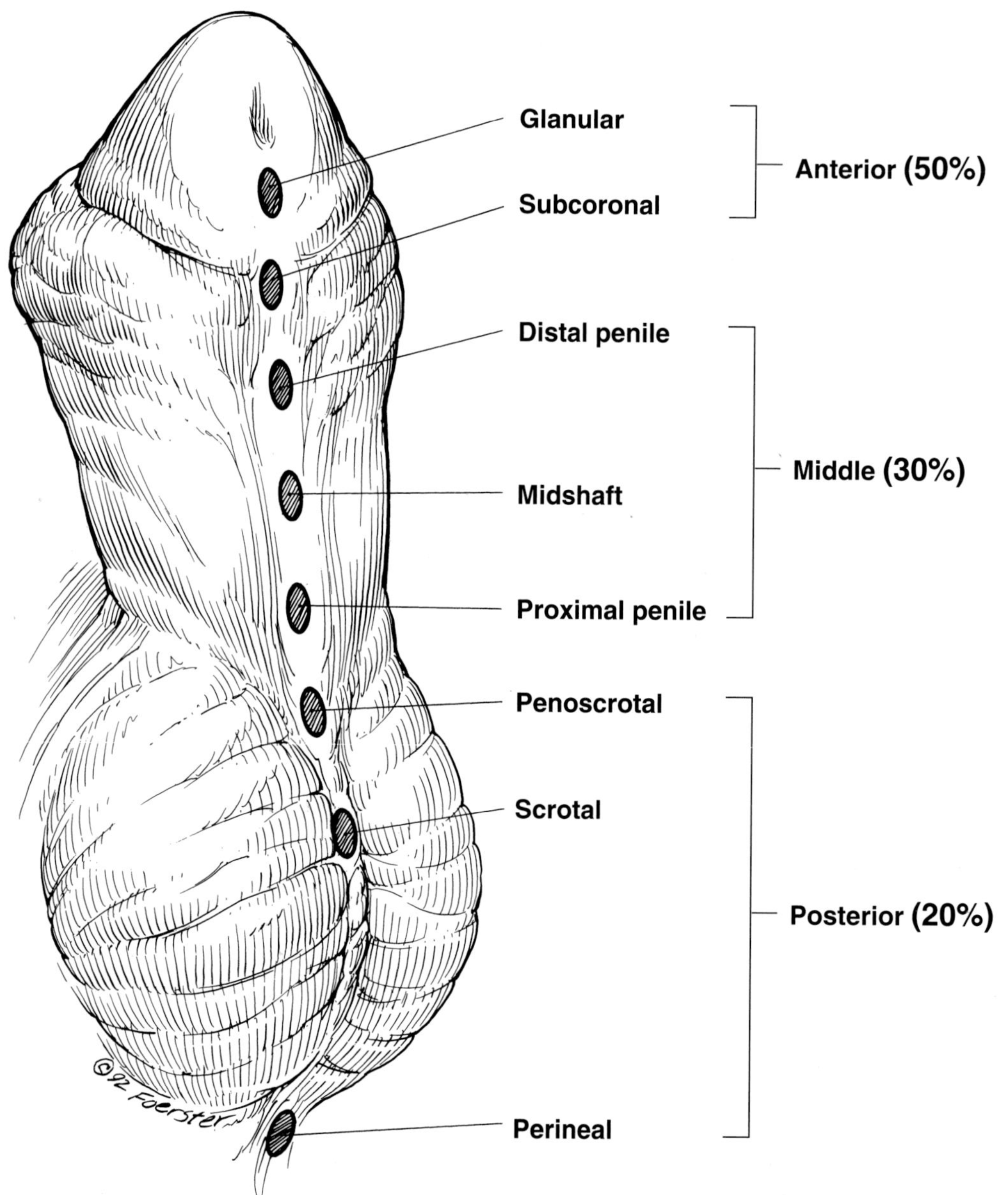

Figure 68–1. Classifying hypospadias. The location of the meatus after correction of curvature provides the most practical classification of hypospadias. The glanular and coronal types constitute anterior hypospadias, which accounts for 50% of all cases. The distal penile midshaft and proximal penile types account for 30% of cases. Penoscrotal, scrotal, and perineal types make up the 20% that are classified as posterior. (From Duckett JW: Successful hypospadias repair. Contemporary Urology 1992, 4:42–55. Copyright Medical Economics Company.)

Fig. 68–1). The anterior group was further classified as 19% glanular, 47% coronal, and 34% distal shaft.

EMBRYOLOGY

The midline *genital tubercle* fuses by the sixth week while the lateral mesoderm heaps up to form the urethral and *genital folds*. These mesodermal components retain the capacity to convert testosterone to dihydrotestosterone, thus heralding the first signs of sexual differentiation. From the indifferent state, the external genital structures develop a typically male configuration under the influence of testosterone. As the phallus elongates, the urethral groove extends to the level of the corona. Gradually, the urethral folds coalesce in the midline, closing the urethra and forming the median raphe of the scrotum and penis.

The distal glans channel is most likely induced by hormonal and local factors, forming a solid core that tunnels to join the proximal urethra (Glenister, 1954). This core later undergoes canalization, forming a complete urethra. Because this is the last step in the formation of the normal urethra, there is a higher incidence of hypospadias in which the meatal opening is in the subcoronal region (Sommer and Stephens, 1980) (Fig. 68–2).

The prepuce forms as a ridge of skin from the corona that gradually grows to enclose the glans circumferentially, fusing with the glans epithelium. The preputial defect associated with hypospadias consists of a deficient ventral segment and resultant dorsal hood. In hypospadias the normal scrotal and penile raphe divides into a Y shape running onto the dorsal preputial hood around the glans in varying configurations. Even with the severe scrotal meatus, this defect of the raphe is apparent, fusing the penis into a vulviform appearance; even a penoscrotal transformation may occur. A glanular cleft may exist with a normal intact foreskin (Kumar, 1986). The author has designated this variant the *megameatus intact prepuce* (MIP) (Duckett and Keating, 1989).

The abnormal ventral curvature of the penis (chordee) is a poorly understood entity. It has been accepted for over 150 years that the deficient mesenchyme that would normally form the corpus spongiosum and fascial layers distal to the hypospadiac meatus in the normal urethra persists as fibrous tissue that causes downward curvature by a "bowstring" effect (Mettauer, 1842). It is more likely, however, that during penile development a growth differential between the normally formed dorsal tissue of the corporal bodies and the deficient ventral tissue and urethra results in the curvature (Kaplan and Lamm, 1975; Bellinger, 1981; Kaplan and Brock, 1981). In the experience of the author, fibrous chordee tethering the penis to the meatus in a bowstring manner occurs in less than 15% of cases with curvature.

INCIDENCE AND GENETICS

The incidence of hypospadias has been calculated as 1 in 300 live male births (Sorenson, 1953; Sweet et al, 1974; Avellan, 1975). In the United States, about 6000 boys with hypospadias are born each year (Duckett, 1991).

Familial tendencies indicate some polygenic factors. Fathers of 8% of patients have hypospadias; 14% of male siblings are affected (Bauer et al, 1981). The condition is more common in whites than in blacks, and in Italians and Jews than in other groups (Welch, 1979). The higher incidence (8.5 times higher) in monozygotic twins (Roberts and Lloyd, 1973) may be explained by the demand of two fetuses on the placental production of human chorionic gonadotropin (hCG) in the first trimester.

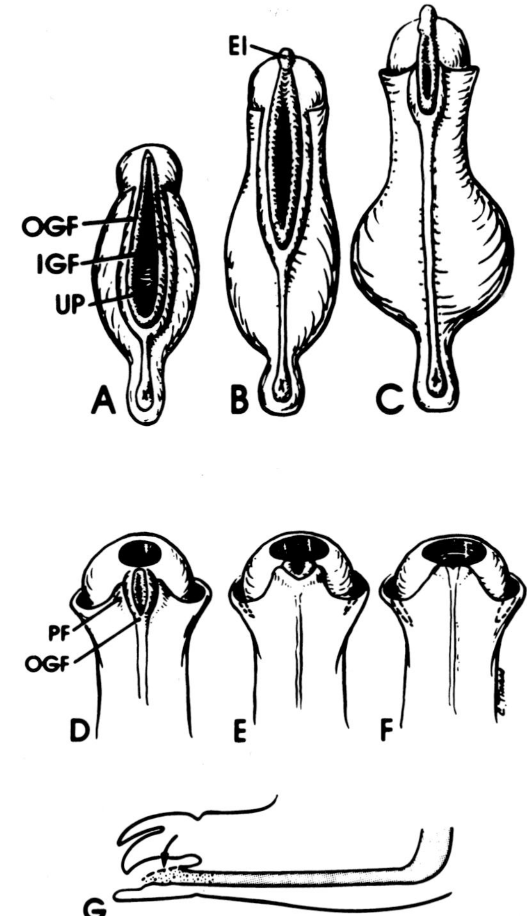

Figure 68–2. Embryology of penile and glanular urethra. *A* through *C*, The inner and outer genital folds cover the urethral plate (UP) and form the raphe. The glanular urethra is a compound of ectodermal pit at tip of glans and open end of the urethral groove. *D* through *F*, Further closure of the groove by outer genital and preputial folds, and orifice of the intervening septum to create one orifice, the fossa navicularis and the lacuna magna. *G*, Arrow indicates site of anastomosis between the ectodermal pit and the urethral groove. (OGF, outer genital folds; IGF, inner genital folds; PF, preputial folds; UP, urethral plate; EI, ectodermal tag marking site of ectodermal ingrowth.) (From Sommer JT, Stephens FD: Dorsal urethral diverticulum of the fossa navicularis: Symptoms, diagnosis and treatment. J Urol 1980; 124:94.)

ASSOCIATED ANOMALIES

The most common anomalies associated with hypospadias are undescended testes and inguinal hernia. Khuri and coworkers (1981) found a 9% incidence of undescended testes in patients with hypospadias. Third-degree hypospadias was associated with a 32% incidence of undescended testes; second-degree hypospadias, 6%; and first-degree hypospadias, 5%. They also found that the incidence of inguinal hernia was 9% in the total group, 17% in third-degree hypospadias; 8% in second-degree hypospadias; and 7% in first-degree hypospadias. Ross and colleagues (1959) reported a similar incidence of either cryptorchidism or hernia in 16% of these patients, whereas Cerasaro and co-workers (1986) found an incidence of 18%.

Significant anomalies of the upper urinary tract associated with isolated hypospadias are rare (1% to 3%) (Avellan, 1975; McArdle and Lebowitz, 1975; Shelton and Noe, 1985; Cerasaro et al, 1986). Khuri and co-workers (1981) found that hypospadias associated with other systemic anomalies increased the incidence of upper tract anomalies to 12% to 50%. With imperforate anus, the incidence of such anomalies was 46%; with myelomeningocele, it was 33%. They concluded that the urinary tract should be screened in all patients with hypospadias of any degree who had associated anomalies, whereas screening was not indicated in those with hypospadias alone with or without undescended testes or hernia.

Utricles

Utriculus masculinus (utricle) is a residual prostatic urethral outgrowth that may persist in patients with severe forms of hypospadias. The incidence of utricles may be as high as 10% to 15% in those with perineal or penoscrotal hypospadias (Shima et al, 1979; Devine et al, 1980). These represent either incomplete müllerian duct regression or incomplete masculinization of the urogenital sinus. There are no uterine elements. The vasa course in the lateral walls and must be divided if the utricle is removed, but there are few situations in which removal is required. Stone formation and infection may result from obstruction (Ritchey et al, 1988).

Intersex

The presence of hypospadias is thought by some to be a form of intersex. Certainly, the diagnosis of intersex must be ruled out in the more severe forms of hypospadias, especially in those with cryptorchidism (Rajfer and Walsh, 1976), but this decision is made when the child is a newborn. Intersex states that must be ruled out in a child with hypospadias presenting later include the following:

1. *Adrenogenital syndrome (AGS).* Clearly, if a baby has undescended testes, she is a girl until proved otherwise, no matter how masculinized.
2. *Mixed gonadal dysgenesis (MGD).* This is the second most frequent cause of ambiguous genitalia in the neonate. With a testis on one side and a streak gonad on the other, the most frequent karyotype is 45,XO/46,XY (Davidoff and Federman, 1973). Many of these MGD patients (60%) are severely undervirilized and have a micropenis at birth (phallus less than 2.5 cm). After inadequate response to testosterone stimulation, gender conversion may be appropriate.
3. *Incomplete male pseudohermaphroditism, type I; Reifenstein syndrome.* These boys have perineal scrotal hypospadias with azoospermia, infertility, incomplete virilization at puberty, and gynecomastia that develops at or after puberty. Severe manifestations may involve a vagina with small testes, which are cryptorchid. The etiology of this syndrome can be demonstrated by fibroblast culture to be a defect in androgen binding to a varying degree. In severe cases that are detected early the child should be gender converted to female, whereas in the milder forms the majority of children are phenotypic and physiologic males, and the hypospadias can be repaired. Supplemental testosterone, unfortunately, is not effective. A point mutation in the DNA-binding domain of the androgen receptor has recently been identified (Klocker et al, 1992).
4. *Incomplete male pseudohermaphroditism, type II; pseudovaginal-perineal-scrotal hypospadias–5α-reductase deficiency.* These very rare patients have a blind vaginal pouch of variable size opening either into the urogenital sinus or, more frequently, into the urethra immediately behind the urethral orifice (Opitz et al, 1972; Walsh et al, 1974). Unlike type I patients, they have well-developed and histologically normal testes as well as normal epididymides, vasa, and seminal vesicles, which terminate in the blind-ending vagina. Most patients are raised as females. Because of an enlarged clitoris, they are diagnosed early, and castration is performed early. If the condition is allowed to take its natural course, these children will develop profound masculinization at puberty with muscle development, phallomegaly, ejaculation, and erections. In some, the sperm count has even been normal. Such a population has been studied in the Dominican Republic (Peterson et al, 1977).
5. *True hermaphroditism.* In these rare cases, both an ovary and a testis or an ovotestis is present. The external genitalia display all gradations from male to female, but most children are masculinized to some degree. For this reason, 75% of patients have been reared as males. Twenty-five percent of patients have bilateral ovotestes; 35%, a unilateral ovotestis; 25%, a testis on one side and an ovary on the other; and 10%, indeterminate (Butler et al, 1969). Fifty percent have a 46,XX karyotype, 20% have an XY karyotype, and 30% are mosaics. Abdominal exploration with biopsy of both gonads is appropriate in these cases, and, in those sufficiently virilized to warrant male gender assignment, inappropriate ovarian tissue and müllerian structures should be removed. Repair of the hypospadias is indicated.
6. *Micropenis.* Micropenis is a miniature penis unaffected with hypospadias. Most often, it is due to a central defect of gonadotropin deficiency, but some are idiopathic.

Allen and Griffin (1984) presented evidence supporting the concept that hypospadias is not just a local dysmorphic problem but rather a local manifestation of a systemic endocrinopathy. They examined a variety of endocrine abnormalities but failed to confirm the impression that the principal defect lies in the inability of the target tissues to respond to androgen, either because of the numbers of androgen receptors or because of an inability to convert testosterone to dihydrotestosterone (Gearhart et al, 1988, 1989).

HISTORY OF SURGICAL PROCEDURES

The first account of hypospadias surgery was written by Heliodorus and Antyllus (100 to 200 A.D.). The repair consisted of amputation of the shaft distal to the existing meatus. Dieffenbach (1838) pierced the glans to the normal urethral meatus, allowing a cannula to remain in position until the channel became lined with epithelium—an unsuccessful procedure. Mettauer (1842) suggested that the "organ be liberated by multiple subcutaneous incisions," whereas Bouisson (1861) was the first to suggest a transverse incision at the point of greatest curvature. He also reported the use of scrotal tissue to reconstruct the urethra. Thiersch (1869) described local tissue flaps to repair epispadias, a technique he later used in hypospadias. Thiersch suggested performing perineal urinary diversion to divert the urine temporarily away from the urethral reconstruction. He also performed the first buttonhole flap in the prepuce to allow resurfacing of the ventrum of the penis with the prepuce.

Duplay (1874) used Bouisson's technique to release chordee and, as a later stage, formed a central flap, which was tubed and then covered with lateral penile flaps. He also stated that it did not matter if the central tube was incompletely formed because epithelialization would form a channel if the tube were buried under lateral flaps; this technique was later popularized by Denis Browne (1950). Wood (1875) created a meatus-based flap to form the urethral channel and combined this with the Thiersch-type buttonhole flap to cover the raw surface—a technique similar to that of Ombredanne (1932) and of Mathieu (1932).

Rosenberger (1891), Landerer (1891), Bidder (1892), and Bucknall (1907) all used scrotal tissue for urethroplasty and buried the penis in the scrotum to obtain skin coverage, as in the later similar techniques of Leveuf (1936) and Cecil-Culp (1951).

Hook (1896) described a vascularized preputial flap for urethroplasty that was similar to that used in the Davis procedure (1951). Hook further suggested using a lateral oblique flap from the side of the penis, later popularized by Broadbent (1951).

Beck and Hacker (1897) undermined and advanced the urethra onto the glans in subcoronal cases, as in the later technique of Waterhouse and Glassberg (1981). Beck (1897) and White and Martin (1917) employed adjacent rotation flaps from the scrotum for resurfacing after performing a Duplay-type urethroplasty; these flaps were similar to those of Marberger and Pauer (1981) and Turner-Warwick (1979). Nove-Josserand (1897 and 1914) reported attempts to repair hypospadias with split-thickness grafts, as in the technique of McIndoe (1937). Rochet (1899) chose a large, distally based scrotal flap for urethroplasty and buried this in a tunnel on the ventral surface of the penis. Edmunds (1913) was the first to transfer the skin of the prepuce to the ventral surface of the penis at the time of release of chordee. This abundant ventral skin was then used in a Duplay-type urethroplasty at a later stage, as in the techniques of Blair (1933) and, later, of Byars (1955). Bevan (1917) used a urethral meatus-based flap channeled through the glans for distal repair, similar to the procedure of Mustarde (1965). References for the aforementioned review are found in Horton and colleagues (1973).

Multistaged Repairs

In the standard two-stage repair, the chordee release (orthoplasty) was accomplished by dividing the urethral plate distal to the meatus, straightening the penis, and allowing the meatus to retract to a more proximal position. Skin cover of the ventrum was achieved by mobilizing the dorsal preputial and penile skin around to the ventrum so that it would be available in a later urethroplasty. Because the modern technique of artificial erection (Gittes and McLaughlin, 1974) was not used, residual chordee was not an unusual result of this type of urethroplasty. Secondary chordee releases were required before the surgeon could form the urethra.

Denis Browne (1953) was very influential in promoting the so-called buried strip principle for hypospadias repair. A ventral strip of skin was covered by generous mobilized skin flaps brought together in the midline with "beads and stops." The channel under the skin flaps epithelialized around a stenting catheter left in place for 3 to 6 weeks. Results were never very satisfactory until Van der Meulen (1964) demonstrated that a rotated skin cover from the dorsum closed with an eccentric suture line offered more successful healing. In fact, he avoided stenting and diversion of urine and had the patient void through the repair, leaving only subcutaneous drains for several days. The lifetime results have been dramatic—no fistulas (Van der Muelen, 1982)!

Byars (1955) further developed the two-stage method by extending the foreskin onto the glans in the first stage and rolling a complete tube in the second. Durham Smith (1973, 1990) refined the Byars approach by denuding the epithelium on one skin edge to allow "double-breasting" of raw surfaces. Smith's review (1990) of 503 repairs showing only 1.8% fistulas, 7.6% meatal stenoses, and 1% incomplete chordee correction is commendable.

In 1955, Elmer Belt devised a technique that he never published but that gained acclaim after Fuqua (1971) published his series. Hendren (1981) had the largest series, with excellent results.

Numerous other methods for repair of hypospadias have been introduced. Creevy (1958) and Backus and DeFelice (1960) have provided excellent reviews of the multistaged procedures performed up to 1960. A complete review of procedures up to 1970 has been published by Horton and his associates (1973). All of these methods must be studied to understand the pitfalls of this difficult surgery. However, emphasis in this chapter is placed on the one-stage methods that are currently popular.

One-Stage Repairs

In the late 1950s, when surgeons were more confident of their ability to remove chordee tissue in its entirety, one-stage hypospadias procedures became popular. In 1900, Russell had described a procedure for a one-stage repair of hypospadias using a urethral tube constructed from a flap developed on the ventral surface of the penis. This flap extended around the entire circumference of the corona to include a cuff of the prepuce. This new urethra was placed through a tunnel in the glans and secured to the tip of the glans. Broadbent and co-workers (1961) created a urethral tube from the skin of the penis and prepuce and laid this tube in the split glans. Des Prez and his colleagues (1961) developed a one-stage procedure similar to that of Broadbent and associates (1961). In 1954, McCormack reported a two-stage procedure in which a full-thickness tube graft urethroplasty was placed during the first procedure, but the proximal anastomosis closure was delayed. In 1955, Devine and Horton developed this technique further by using a free graft of preputial skin to replace the urethra after release of chordee; they then completed this McCormack procedure in one stage (Devine and Horton, 1961). In 1970 and 1972, Hodgson described three different procedures that used vascularized flaps from the dorsal prepuce as well as penile skin. This urethral flap was brought onto the ventral aspect using a buttonhole transposition (Hodgson, 1975).

One-stage hypospadias repair has withstood the test of time, supporting the feasibility of this type of surgery. Besides the desirability of completing the reconstruction in one operation, a one-stage procedure has the additional advantage of using skin that is unscarred from previous surgical procedures, the normal blood supply of which has not been disrupted. The main impediment to the success of this procedure, inadequate chordee release, has been nearly eliminated since the introduction of the artificial erection technique (Gittes and McLaughlin, 1974).

TREATMENT OF HYPOSPADIAS

The phases of surgical repair include (1) meatoplasty and glanuloplasty, (2) orthoplasty (straightening), (3) urethroplasty, (4) skin cover, and (5) scrotoplasty. These various elements of surgical technique can be applied sequentially or in various combinations to achieve surgical success.

Meatoplasty and Glanuloplasty

For many years, the two-stage techniques (e.g., Byars, 1955; Denis Browne, 1953) left the meatus just beneath the glans. We now make every effort to move the meatus to the tip, particularly in the more extensive one-stage repairs (e.g., Devine and Horton, 1961; Duckett, 1980a). Even in those with distal hypospadias, the trend is to achieve the same goal in patients with relatively minor defects. The meatal advancement and glanuloplasty (MAGPI) procedure (Duckett, 1981b) has come under considerable scrutiny in this regard. Using electronic video photography, MacMillan and co-workers (1985) recorded high-speed pictures of urinary streams after the MAGPI repair and concluded that the excellent cosmetic results are achieved with preservation of normal voiding.

Several different techniques can be used to achieve an apical meatus, depending on the variation of the proximal meatus (Gibbons and Gonzales, 1983). The **triangularized glans** (Devine and Horton, 1961) achieves a flap meatoplasty and avoids a circumferential meatal closure. Glans wings are developed, which wrap around the neourethra on the ventrum. Although this maneuver avoids meatal stenosis, the glans is flattened and its normal configuration is distorted. *Extension of the meatus onto the ventral glans* can be done using either a meatal-based flap (Mathieu) or an onlay vascularized flap as described later in this chapter. In this case, a strip of urethral plate remains between the glans wings, onto which a roof of urethra is placed with a glans wrap closure. The **glans split** (Barcat, 1973; Redman, 1987) permits deeper placement of the urethral extension in the glans tissue. The *glans fillet* described by Turner-Warwick (1979) and Cronin and Guthrie (1973) is a two-stage procedure in which preputial skin is laid onto the ventrum of the spatulated glans. The meatus can later be tubularized and the glans closed over it to achieve a normal-appearing glans with an apical meatus. This technique is more applicable to the adult penis that requires revision.

The **glans channel** technique that delivers the urethra to the apex is another method. Bevan (1917) devised a technique that created a proximal penile flap, which was converted into a urethral tube and pulled through a tunnel in the glans. Mays (1951) employed a staged technique that straightened the penis, bringing the prepuce over the glans to cover the ventral defect and constructing a preputial flap for a glanular urethra that was carried through a tunnel to the tip of the glans. Davis (1940, 1951) developed a similar procedure. Both Ricketson (1958) and Hendren (1981) channeled a full-thickness skin tube through the glans. Hinderer (1971) used a trocar to create the tunnel, entering the glans at the tip and emerging a few millimeters below the coronal sulcus through a "trap-door" flap of albuginea. Duckett (1980a, b, c) combined the glans channel with a transverse preputial island flap.

In more distal hypospadias, the configuration of the glans may dictate the type of meatoplasty used. If the glans furrow is deep, a Mathieu procedure (1932) may be preferred. In contrast, if the glans is broad and flat, an onlay island flap technique will allow rolling of the glans around the glanular vascularized urethral extension.

Orthoplasty

Curvature (Chordee)

The curvature of the penis is caused by a deficiency of the normal structures on the ventrum of the penis. Contributing factors include skin deficiency, dartos fascia fibrosis, and true fibrous chordee with tethering of the ventral shaft or corpora cavernosa disproportion.

The role played by skin deficiency is especially striking in manipulation of the penis without artificial erection, which creates an apparent curvature of the tip. The skin and fibrous dartos fascia beneath it together contribute to curvature with artificial erection, which is relieved after the skin drops back (Allen and Spence, 1968).

Fibrous Chordee

When associated with hypospadias, chordee has commonly been attributed to hypoplasia of the corpus spongiosum distal to the hypospadiac meatus (Mettauer, 1842). This situation results in a midline fibrous band or fan-shaped area of fibrosis, which tethers the penis ventrally. When this tissue is excised *(orthoplasty)*, the penis straightens. This simplified explanation is not altogether applicable to the variety of possible expressions of hypospadias or pure chordee without hypospadias. Certainly the concept of a "bowstring" tether that requires a simple incision is not true.

Kaplan and Lamm (1975) argued convincingly that chordee may indeed be an arrest of normal embryologic development analogous to failure of the testicles to descend. Thus, fibrosis is conspicuously absent in some clinical cases of chordee. Chordee may also result from differential growth of the dorsal and ventral aspects of the corpora (Bellinger, 1981), which is best corrected by shortening the dorsal tunica albuginea.

Devine and Horton (1973) divided chordee into three types, but this classification has not been widely accepted.

Artificial Erection

Introduced in 1974 by Gittes and McLaughlin, the technique of artificial erection has contributed significantly to the success of orthoplasty. By placing a tourniquet at the base of the penis and injecting the corpus cavernosum with saline, both corporal bodies fill, and it is possible to determine the extent of chordee and the success of chordee correction. The assurance of complete correction is essential before proceeding with a one-stage repair with urethroplasty. So far there has been no report of damage to the cavernous tissue with this technique. This technique has also been used extensively in adults with no untoward effects. Care must be taken to ensure that normal saline is used. Penile necrosis occurred when 50% saline was injected inadvertently. Injecting through the glans rather than on the side of the shaft avoids hematoma formation.

Technique of Orthoplasty

Orthoplasty, (from the Greek, *orthus,* straighten) is a term used in Europe to refer to excision of chordee and straightening of the penis. In true **fibrous chordee**, the penis is curved ventrally and there is only a short distance between the location of the meatus and the glans. An incision is made around the corona and is carried well below the glans cap just distal to the urethral meatus and down to the tunica albuginea of the corpora cavernosa. Proximal dissection is then performed, freeing the fibrous plaque of tissue closely adherent to the tunica albuginea using sharp dissection and moving from side to side as the ventral curvature is released. The urethra is elevated from the corpora in this en bloc dissection. In most cases, the chordee tissue surrounds the urethral meatus and extends proximally along the urethra for some distance. This tissue should all be freed well down to the penoscrotal junction and often into the scrotoperineal area as well. Once this urethral mobilization has been accomplished, the shaft of the penis, extending as far as the lateral shaft of the penis and distally below the glans, should be stripped of any fibrous tissue. Artificial erection is used to test the success of this excision.

Several further maneuvers have been devised to release the last bit of bend. A midline incision along the septum between the two corpora cavernosa has been effective in some cases (Devine, 1983). Lateral incisions in a stepwise manner may be effective in the groove between the dorsal corpora and the ventral aspect.

If, after adequate excision of all abnormal fibrous tissue, artificial erection continues to demonstrate curvature, corporal disproportion is present. This should be corrected by performing **tunica albugenia plication (TAP)** (Baskin and Duckett, 1994) (Fig. 68–3). Buck's fascia is elevated on either side of the midline (10 o'clock and 2 o'clock) to avoid the neurovascular bundle. Parallel incisions about 8 mm long and 5 to 8 mm apart are made through the tunica albuginea. The outer edges of the incisions are sutured together with permanent interrupted sutures (5-0 Prolene). This symmetrically tucks the dorsum to correct the ventral bend.

In rare cases, there is so much deficiency of the tunica albuginea on the ventrum that the tunica albuginea must be excised and replaced by dermal graft or tunica vaginalis (Hendren and Keating, 1988). Tunica vaginalis is obtained by exposing the testis and removing a patch of the tunica from around the testis.

Once the chordee has been released, a urethroplasty may proceed in the one-stage repair if a vascularized neourethra has been used. If a dermal graft has been placed on the ventrum, a neourethra composed of a free full-thickness skin graft will probably not succeed.

Congenital Curvature of the Penis (Chordee Without Hypospadias)

Congenital curvature of the penis without hypospadias is rare. Much more common in adults are the secondary curvatures associated with Peyronie's disease or periurethral sclerosis associated with urethral stricture. There are two kinds of primary curvature: those associated with a normal urethral spongiosum and those associated with a hypoplastic urethra.

Primary curvature with a normal corpus spongiosum comprises two thirds of penises with congenital curvature. The penis when flaccid looks normal and has a circular prepuce. During erection, the penis is usually curved downward but may have a lateral curvature of as much as 90 degrees. An upward curvature (without epispadias) is exceptional (Udall, 1980). This deformity becomes noticeable to the adolescent or young adult. However, many experience little difficulty with intercourse with this condition. The lateral deviations seen in about one third of cases are almost always to the left. With erection, disproportion of the corpora cavernosa is usually apparent.

Physiologic ventral curvature of the penis has been noted in the fetus at different stages of development (Kaplan and Lamm, 1975; Kaplan and Brock, 1981). It usually disappears by birth yet may be found in premature infants. This curvature slowly disappears in the first several years of life (Cendron and Melin, 1981).

In patients in whom the urethra is normal, treatment varies with the direction of the deviation and whether one believes that true chordee tissue is responsible for the ventral bend (Devine and Horton, 1975). Good results have been reported by Devine and Horton with resection of the fibrous dartos fascia beneath and beside the mobilized normal urethra. However, this rather extensive dissection does not offer consistent results (Kramer et al, 1982).

The procedure described by Nesbit in 1965 of taking tucks or plicating the disproportionally large tunica albuginea has been more accepted. This technique was first described by Philip Syng Physick, the "father of American surgery," in the early 19th century. He treated chordee by shortening the dorsal tunica albuginea (Pancoast, 1844). When the arc of maximum curvature is located with artificial erection, wedges of tunica albuginea can be excised in a stepwise fashion. These diamond-shaped wedges are closed transversely with permanent sutures until the penis is straight. It

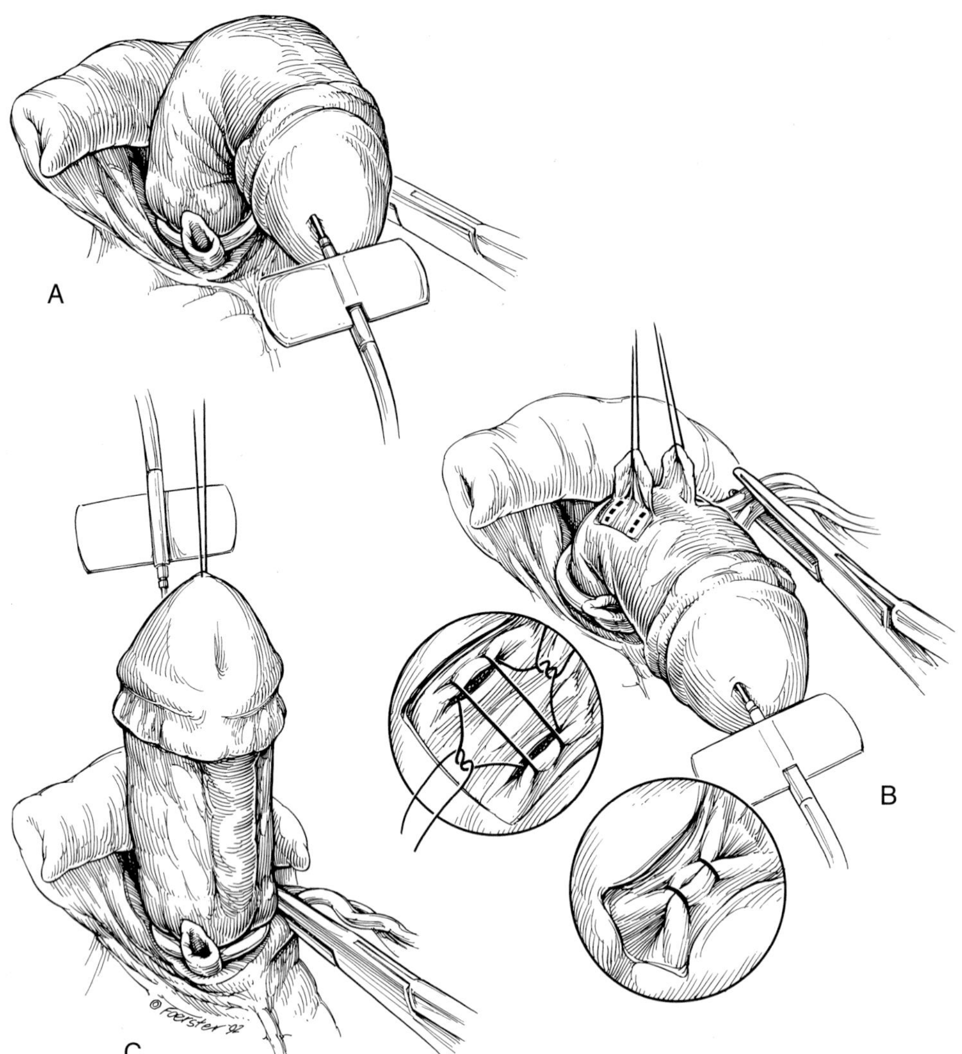

Figure 68–3. Tunica albugenia plication (TAP). *A,* After removing ventral fibrous tissue, either with the urethral plate intact or having divided the urethral plate, there is occasionally residual curvature noted with artificial erection. *B,* Buck's fascia flaps are elevated at 10 and 2 o'clock over the apex of the curvature in order to avoid the neurovascular bundle. Parallel incisions *(insert)* are made about 8 mm apart and about 8 mm long down to cavernous tissue. The outer edges of the parallel strips are approximated with two permanent 5–0 Prolene sutures. *C,* These tucks on each side usually achieve straightening. (From Duckett JW: Successful hypospadias repair. Contemporary Urology 1992; 4:42–55. Copyright Medical Economics Company.)

is possible to plicate the fascia without cutting the tunica by placing several rows of sutures at the maximum convex side. Nesbit (1966), however, reported long-term follow-up with this method as disappointing. Exposure for the surgical approach is achieved by retracting the penile skin toward the base as a sleeve.

The age at which this defect should be corrected is important. Cendron believes it should not be done too early for two reasons: The curvature may improve spontaneously with age, and there is risk of disturbing the growth of the phallus by altering the tunica of the corpora. For both of these reasons, it is better to perform the repair after puberty.

Primary curvature with a hypoplastic urethra is found in about one third of these congenital curvature cases (Cendron and Melin, 1981). In this type of curvature, the urethral meatus is well situated on the glans, but the foreskin is incomplete, and the ventral penis is not normal. The skin covering the urethra is very thin, and spongiosal tissue is absent on a large portion of the penis. Chordee is present with erection. Lengthening the frenulum and eliminating the penoscrotal web does not alter the curvature. Because the segment of urethra is hypoplastic, it may be considered a "concealed" hypospadias. Congenitally short urethra is another term for this condition.

Skin Cover

Once the urethroplasty has been accomplished, the ventral surface of the penis must be resurfaced with skin. Because of the abundant dorsal foreskin, coverage may be achieved by mobilizing the penile and preputial skin to the ventrum in most cases. The skin may be transferred by one of several techniques.

THE BUTTONHOLE. Transposition of skin is credited first to Thiersch (1869). However, Ombredanne (1932), Nesbit (1941), and Mustarde (1965) also selected this method. The major drawback is the lateral edges, which are difficult to fashion without leaving bulky wedges of skin. One must be cautious not to trim these lateral pedicles too much at this stage because to do so risks devascularizing the flap. The author has abandoned this technique.

BYARS' FLAPS. The prepuce may be split vertically and the bipedicled preputial skin brought around to the ventrum for resurfacing (see Fig. 68–4). If this is done in a symmetric fashion in the first stage of a two-stage procedure (as in the Blair-Byars technique), redundant preputial skin is relocated on the distal shaft and glans (Smith, 1981, 1990). If this technique is used to cover a urethroplasty in a one-stage

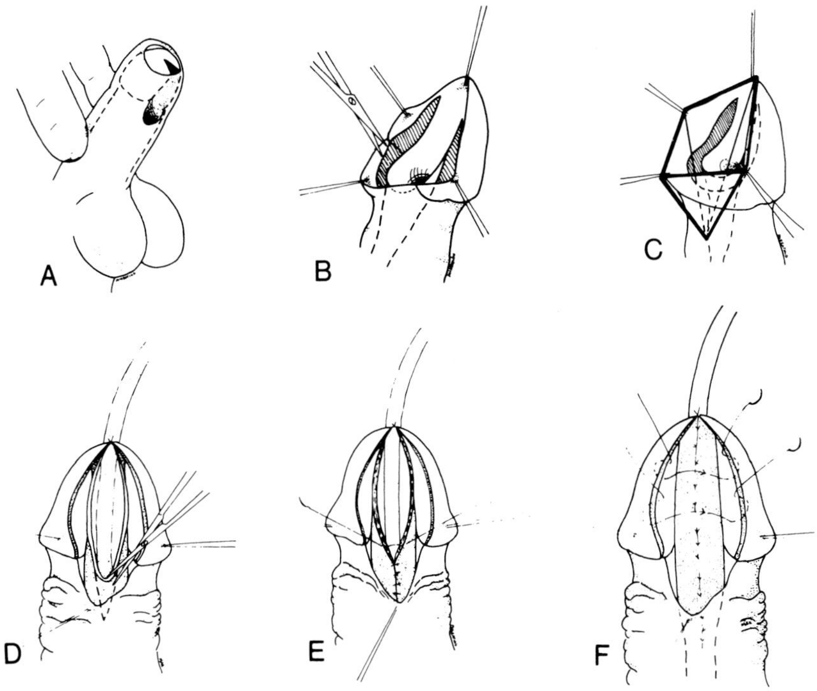

Figure 68–7. Pyramid procedure. *A,* Megameatus intact prepuce (MIP) variant. Intact prepuce conceals an often impressive anomaly. *B* and *C,* Traction sutures define the megameatus and pyramid base. *D,* Sharp dissection to the apex of the pyramid mobilizes urethra and glans wings. Widened distal urethra is tapered. *E,* Neourethra created by tubularizing the urethral plate. *F,* Repair completed by two-layer glans reapproximation. (From Duckett JW, Keating MA: Technical challenge of the megameatus intact prepuce hypospadias (MIP) variant: The pyramid procedure. J Urol 1989; 141:1407–1409.)

ventrum if the proximal urethra is deficient (Hollowell et al, 1990; Baskin et al, 1994). Even though the proximal meatus may be located near the corona, the urethra should be opened back to good spongiosum tissue, discarding the thin ventral urethra. Current results with this onlay flap technique have been satisfactory, with a secondary surgical rate of 5% to 6%. In most of these cases, the urethral meatus is in the middle third of the shaft (Elder et al, 1987; Hollowell et al, 1990; Baskin et al, 1994).

Other Techniques for the Anterior Meatus

The Thiersch-Duplay (1869) tubularization of the distal urethral plate has been used more recently by Nesbit (1966), King (1970, 1981), Perlmutter and Vatz (1975), and Belman and King (1979). The author does not favor this method as a routine procedure. Occasionally, it may have a place in repair of unique configurations such as the MIP.

The **tubularized incised plate urethroplasty** recently proposed by Snodgrass (1994) is a further extension of "hinging the urethral plate" that was described earlier (Rich et al, 1989). The urethral plate is incised deeply in the sagittal plane down to the corporal bodies so that a Thiersch-Duplay tubularization is accomplished.

The technique of the **Devine-Horton "flip flap"** with triangularization of the glans was popular in the past, but it has not been used even by its originators (Devine, 1983). It is now of historic interest only.

Likewise, the **Mustarde procedure** has not held up. This technique is a more extensive Mathieu procedure involving tubularization of the proximal parameatal-based flap. The main criticism of the technique relates to the viability of the pedicle flap, which is likely to be compromised as it goes through the glans channel. The author has found that the Mustarde technique is appropriate for some secondary cases that combine resection of residual chordee with a retrusive meatus.

TECHNIQUES FOR MIDDLE AND POSTERIOR HYPOSPADIAS

Middle and posterior hypospadias represent approximately 50% of all cases of hypospadias, which are certainly the most challenging to repair. Vascularized flaps of the preputial and penile skin may be mobilized to the ventrum for urethroplasty as island flaps, our preference being to use either onlay or tubularized flaps.

Asopa and colleagues (1971, 1984) employed a vascularized flap attached to the outer prepuce (Fig. 68–9). The ventral preputial skin is used for the new urethra but is left attached to the penile skin and is spiraled around to the ventrum. The result was asymmetric and bulky. The author made modifications in the form of a *double-faced island flap,* which improved the cosmetic result (Duckett, 1991). However, the fistula rate was not satisfactory, and this author has now abandoned the double-faced repair. Perhaps the extra tissue supplied by the pedicle was too much.

Transverse Preputial Island Flap and Glans Channel (Fig. 68–10)

This technique has been developed during the last 20 years as a modification of the Hodgson III and Asopa procedures. The author firmly believes that a vascularized urethral tube is preferable to a free graft. The blood supply to the inner preputial transverse island flap is abundant, with the vessels oriented in longitudinally (Quartey, 1983). This flap is dissected free from the penile and outer preputial skin,

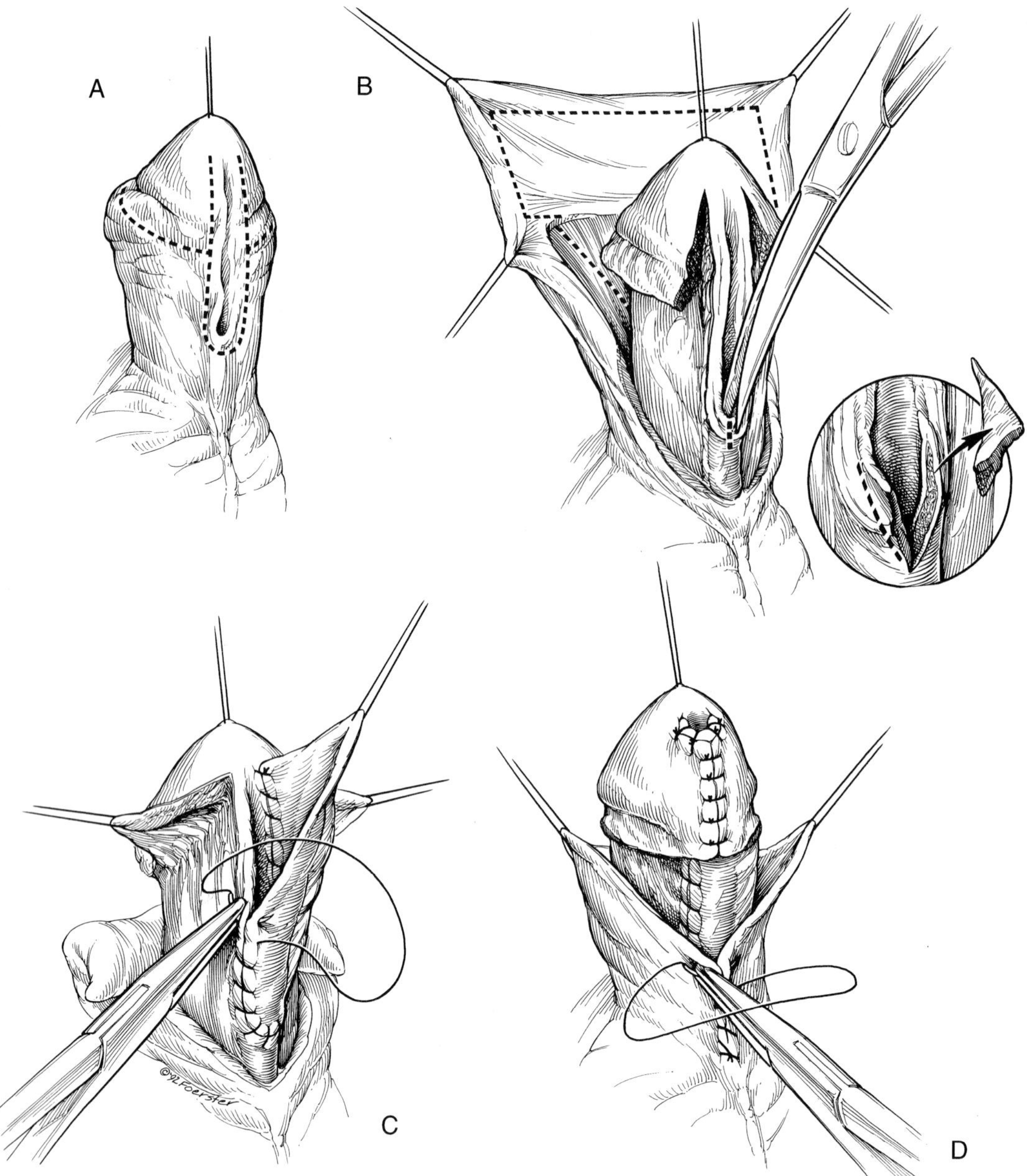

Figure 68–8. Onlay island flap. *A,* The urethral plate is left intact in all cases and the procedure starts with this outlined incision. *B,* Fibrous tissue on the ventrum is excised adjacent to the urethral plate to remove all dartos fascia tethering. Artificial erection often demonstrates a straight penis. The urethral plate is then left intact for the onlay. If curvature persists, a TAP procedure is done (see Fig. 68–3). Insert: The skin edges of the meatus are excised, and the urethra is cut back to good spongiosal tissue. *C,* A transverse preputial island flap is outlined and brought around to the ventrum. A lateral edge is sewn, and the flap is fashioned to make a No. 12-Fr–sized urethra. The urethral plate is about 4 to 6 mm wide, whereas the onlay is 6 to 8 mm wide. *D,* Glans wings are developed and brought around to the ventrum with a two-layer glans closure. Skin is then reapproximated with Byars' flaps. (From Duckett JW: Successful hypospadias repair. Contemporary Urology 1992; 4:42–55. Copyright Medical Economics Company.)

leaving the major vasculature on the island flap. Devascularization of the penile and preputial outer skin is in practice not as severe a problem as theoretically predicted (Hinman, 1991). Certainly, the outer extent of the preputial skin is not well vascularized and may slough if used in the ventral cover. This excess skin is excised during the skin cover phase (Byars' flaps).

In the past the *fully tubularized transverse preputial island flap* (TPIF) was used for shorter urethral replacements than it is today. Now we prefer the onlay island flap (OIF) whenever the urethral plate can be preserved. The TPIF is reserved for longer urethroplasties in more severe cases. When the glans is tethered to a scrotal or perineal meatus, the preputial skin is configured in a **horseshoe fashion.** When the TPIF is designed in these cases, the extent of the preputial skin can be broadly extended to form a long 5- to 6-cm vascularized island flap. The pedicle is wider and often can be deployed to the ventrum by using a midline buttonhole (Fig. 68–11).

The fully tubularized TPIF must be carefully calibrated using a No. 10 to 12 Fr bougie-à-boule. Otherwise, the distensible skin will form a fusiform diverticulum

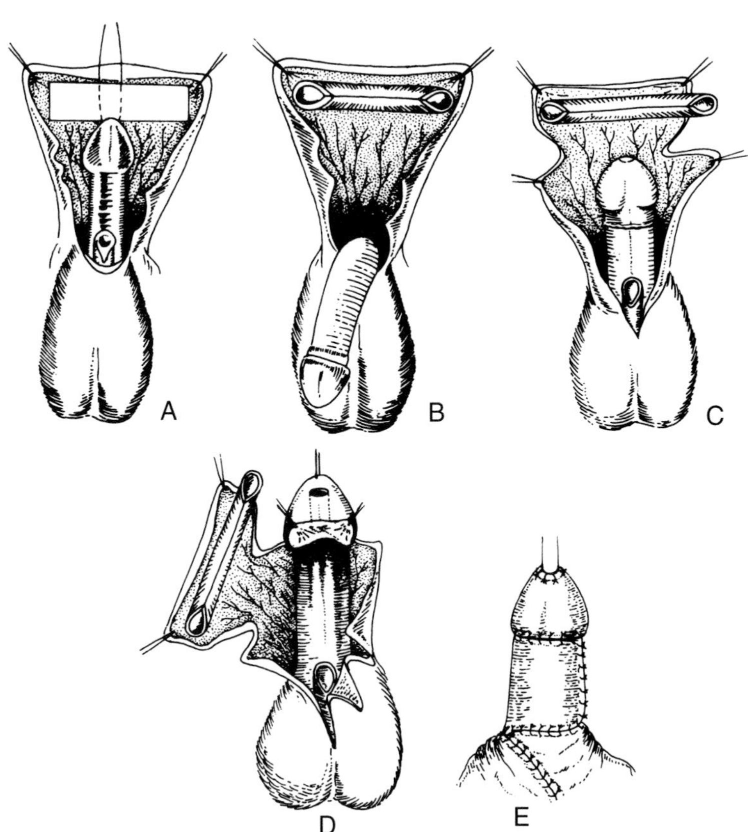

Figure 68–9. Asopa procedure. *A,* After chordee correction, the inner layer of the prepuce is arranged as a rectangle placed transversely and measured to the size of the urethral gap. *B,* The neourethral tube is formed with interrupted 6–0 polyglycolic suture. *C,* The outer preputial skin is cut on both sides obliquely, leaving the central part of the skin intact. *D,* A glans tunnel is created with scissors, and the flap is rotated around the right side. An oblique incision is made at the penoscrotal junction on the left side. *E,* The end of the neourethra is anastomosed to the spatulated native urethra, and the distal end is brought through the glans channel and anastomosed to the opening in the glans. A Z-plasty at the penoscrotal junction results in a transverse suture line at the penoscrotal area. The outer preputial skin is covering the ventral penis. Using this technique, Asopa reports a reoperation rate of 10% to 12%. (Courtesy of Hari Asopa, M.D.)

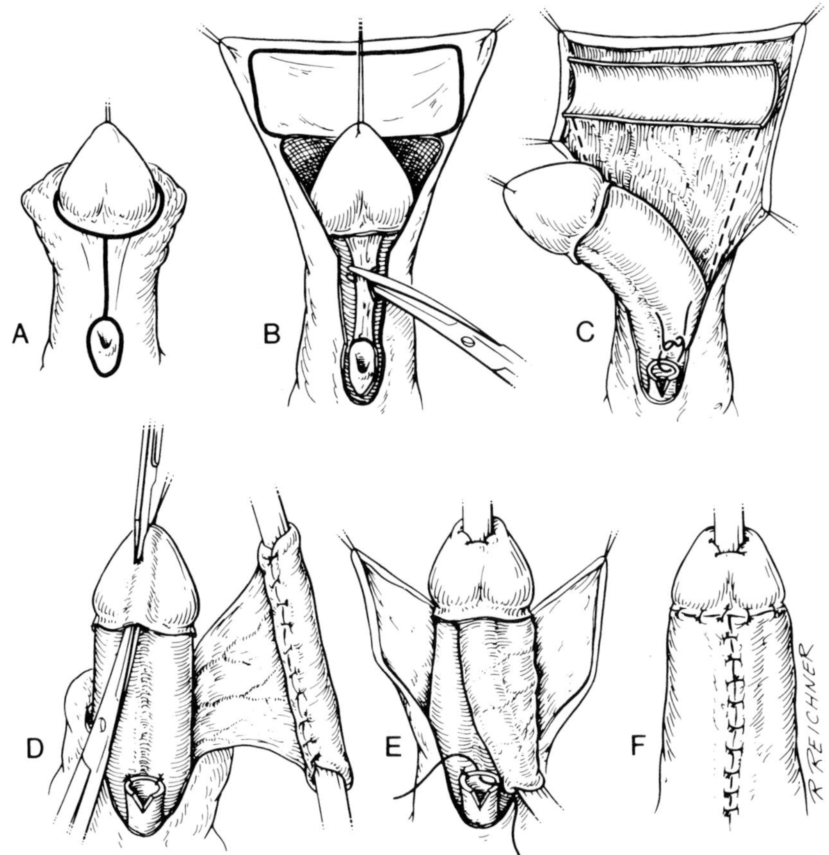

Figure 68–10. Transverse preputial island flap (TPIF) (Duckett). *A,* Circumferential incision is made around the corona. Marked chordee exists, and the urethral plate is not preserved. *B,* The fibrous chordee tissue is excised, and the penis straightened. If residual chordee persists, the TAP procedure is made on the dorsum. An outline of the inner preputial skin is designed. *C,* The inner preputial island flap is mobilized away from the dorsal preputial and penile skin to make a rectangle of shiny skin approximately 4 cm in length and 12 to 15 mm wide. *D,* The pedicle is mobilized down to the base of the penis so it may be rotated around to the ventrum without creating torsion to the penis. The proximal urethra after freeing of the curvature is fixed to the ventral corporal tissue and spatulated. *E,* A glans channel is made underneath the glans cap out to the tip of the penis and circumferential chromic sutures fix the meatus in place. The proximal neourethra is brought to the proximal native meatus, and redundant tissue is excised. The suture line lays against the corporal body. An oblique anastomosis is made proximally, and the pedicle covers the anastomosis. *F,* Byars' flaps resurface the penis. A urethral stent is left. (From Kodama RT, Winslow BH: Hypospadias. *In* Marshall FF, ed: Operative Urology, Philadelphia, W.B. Saunders Company, 1991, p. 519.)

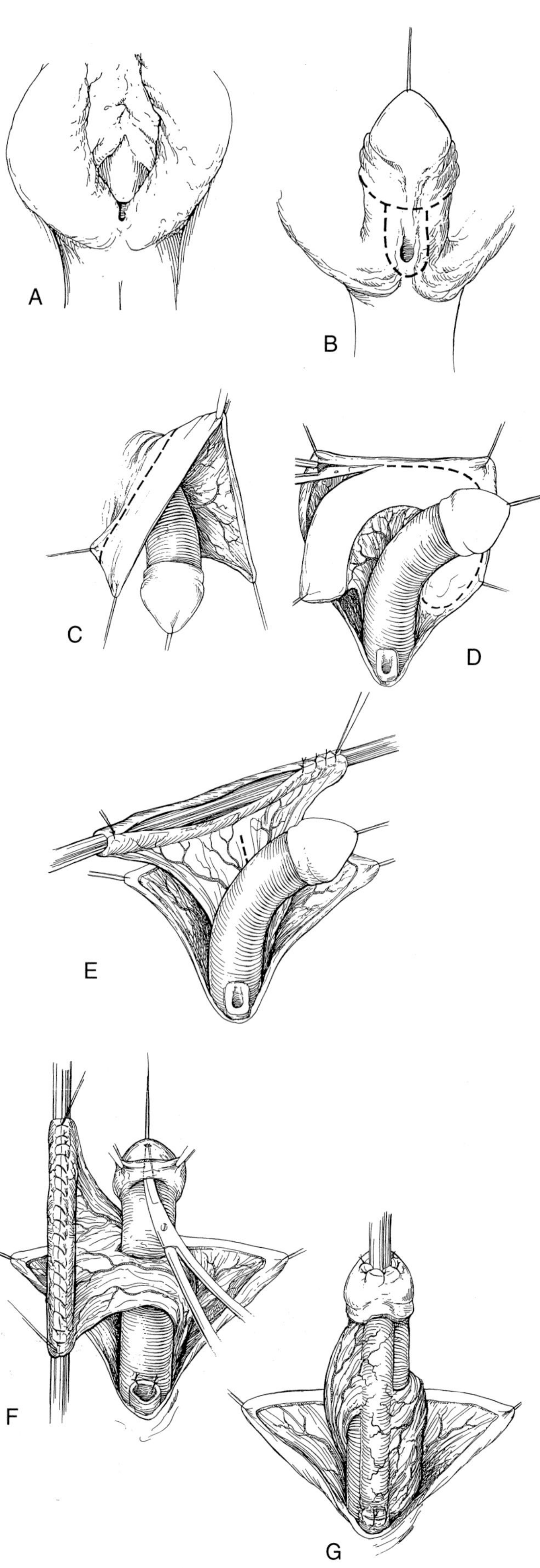

Figure 68–11. Scrotal hypospadias. *A,* In severe cases in which the glans is tethered with a short urethral plate to a scrotal or perineal meatus, a more extended preputial tubed urethroplasty is preferred over a two-stage procedure. *B,* Lines of incision dividing the short urethral plate tethered to the scrotal meatus. *C,* Mobilization of the penile and preputial skin; note the elongated preputial area in the form of a horseshoe. *D,* Consider the deployment of the preputial skin as a horseshoe permitting a 5- to 7-cm vascularized inner preputial flap. *E,* Tubularization of the lengthy flap maintaining vascularity to each end. Interrupted sutures on the ends of the tube permit excisions to tailor length. *F,* A buttonhole of the pedicle in the midline permits transposition to the ventrum with a bipedicle flap. The urethra should be stretched so that no redundancy exists. Both ends should be trimmed to fit perfectly. A glans channel is depicted. *G,* Note bipedicled flap for long urethroplasty. It is important to calibrate the width of the tubed urethra to no more than No. 10 to 12 Fr so that a diverticulum due to redundancy is avoided. Skin closure is done by rotating dorsal penile skin around to the ventrum (Byars' flaps). A urethral drip stent is used for 2 weeks.

("urethrocele"), which is a major complication requiring a reduction urethroplasty later (Aigen et al, 1987). As the tubed TPIF is stretched to fit the urethral defect, the ends are excised to reduce redundancy.

For a long tube, the meatus is attached first and the tube is stretched down into the perineum for the appropriate distance. Very rarely, a proximal extension of the urethra may be required for a perineal meatus (Duckett, 1987). An oblique anastomosis is made, fixing the native urethra to the tunica albuginea. The skin edges of the native urethra are excised, making good spongiosum available. Fixation of the neourethra to the tunica albuginea also prevents overlapping and kinking of the proximal anastomosis.

Once the neourethra is in place, bougienage to No. 10 to 12 Fr is done routinely to make sure there are no bumps, kinks, or lips. The urethra is filled with saline using an indwelling No. 8 Fr catheter to check for leaks after the repair is intact. Such leaks are oversewn.

The **glans channel** is made by performing sharp dissection against the corporal bodies out to the tip of the glanular groove. A button of glans epithelium is removed, and dissection is carried down into the glanular tissue, removing enough to create a broad channel through the glans. The neourethra and its vasculature must traverse this area without compression. A common error is making the glans channel too small, which will compress the pedicle. Interrupted fine chromic sutures are placed circumferentially to the glans meatus.

The **skin cover** for the TPIF is made by splitting the dorsal outer prepuce and stretching the lateral wings around to the ventrum. A midline closure is made using horizontal mattress 7–0 chromic sutures up to the glans. These preputial flaps are *not* rotated in a "huggy-bear" transposition. Excess skin is excised, leaving good viable penile and preputial skin for cover.

A No. 6 Fr Kendall **catheter** is placed in the bladder approximately 2 cm from the bladder neck and sutured to the glans and meatus with a 5–0 Prolene suture. The stent drips urine into the diaper. The patient does not void through the tube.

A sandwich-like **dressing** is applied using benzoin on the skin, a 4 × 4 gauze on the ventral repair, folded four times to apply pressure on the abdomen, and a bioocclusive dressing (Tagaderm), which compresses the penis against the abdomen. This dressing is removed in 72 hours, and no further dressing is used.

Although the tubed TPIF is used less now than it was in the past and only for the more severe cases, the **results** remain satisfactory, with a 10% to 15% secondary surgery rate. Fistulas require closure in half of these cases. Urethroceles remain the most serious complication and require reduction by excision; imbrication does not give satisfactory long-term correction.

Onlay Island Flap Technique

(see Fig. 68–8)

The onlay island flap **procedure** has become the technique most used by the author for correction of middle and posterior hypospadias during the past 10 years. The author attempts to maintain the urethral strip as he makes the initial incisions. The circumferential incision is made around the corona and up to the urethral plate, where parallel markings are made out to the glans tip. The incision is then brought proximally around the meatus, and the skin and dartos fascia are dissected, freeing the fibrous tethering. Once this skin drop-back has been made, an artificial erection is performed to see the extent of curvature. Often very little curvature is apparent after this skin drop-back. If mild to moderate curvature exists (25% to 30% in the author's experience), a **dorsal plication** (TAP) is used (see Fig. 68–3).

With the **urethral plate** outlined with parallel incisions about 4 to 6 mm wide, a strip is made to the tip of the glanular groove to develop the glanular wings, very similar to the procedure in a Mathieu-type repair. The proximal urethra is cut back to good spongiosum, and the skin edge is excised, making the urethral plate uniform.

Once this maneuver has been accomplished, a ventral preputial island flap is developed, making no attempt to measure the appropriate size. This flap is mobilized to the ventrum and placed alongside the urethral plate. A running 7–0 Vicryl suture closes one side of the onlay.

A marking pen outlines the size of the **onlay flap**. With a 4- to 6-mm urethral strip, the onlay need be no more than 6 to 8 mm wide for a neourethra with a No. 12 Fr caliber. The excess epithelium is excised from the onlay, and the pedicle is kept intact, supplying this strip of epithelium. The onlay is rolled over the urethral plate, and interrupted sutures are made around the horseshoe shape of the proximal urethra. A running suture closes the lateral side, completing the repair out to the tip of the glans. Throughout this onlay process, bougie-à-boules are used to calibrate the urethra to make sure it is not too wide. A diverticulum may form if there is too much redundant tissue. The urethra is distended with saline to check for leaks.

The lateral **glans wings** are brought around the ventrum of the urethral onlay to perform the meatoplasty. The glanular wings are brought over the onlay using deep Vicryl stitches and a superficial running chromic stitch. This completes the glanuloplasty and the meatoplasty.

The **pedicle** is splayed over the anastomosis and tacked to the tunica albuginea so that it is flattened out. Excess tissue is excised from the flap to avoid any bulkiness, taking care to avoid the axial blood supply.

Skin cover is achieved in the usual manner by dividing the dorsal preputial skin and stretching it around to the ventrum to attain a midline closure up to the glans. Horizontal chromic suture is used for this part of the procedure. A urethral stent, described previously, is placed to allow urine to drip into the diaper.

In a review of 5 years' experience with 1022 primary cases (Baskin and Duckett, 1994), 33% of patients underwent OIF procedures, whereas only 9% had a tubed TPIF. MAGPI or Mathieu procedures were performed in the remaining 58%. Although 62 patients (of 1022) required division of the urethral plate, 90% of these still required extra dorsal tucks (TAP) to straighten the penis completely. The **secondary surgery rate** (5% fistulas) for the 356 patients with the OIF is much better than the 10% to 15% achieved with the tubed TPIF; thus the author and his group prefer the onlay flap.

COMPLEX HYPOSPADIAS

Patients with multiple repairs that have failed have in the past been branded "hypospadias cripples," an unfortunate designation that should be abandoned. In these patients it is usually necessary to discard the problem-plagued urethra created previously and start anew. Problems occur in the free grafts of preputial skin but more commonly in the free full-thickness grafts of extragenital skin (inner arm or inguinal skin donor sites) years later. There appears to be a delay of many years before the appearance of a chronic inflammation similar to balanitis xerotica obliterans, which affects the entire graft (Hendren and Crooks, 1980; Akporiaye et al, 1995). Bladder mucosal grafts are not currently in vogue for the reconstruction of these urethral replacements. Buccal mucosal grafts are, however, encouraging (Duckett and Coplen, 1995).

Bladder mucosal grafts (BlMG) were used enthusiastically for a while both in primary cases (Li et al, 1981; Mollard et al, 1989) and in secondary cases (Ransley et al, 1987). However, a review of the published reports showed that the overall results were disappointing in the long view, especially the meatal eversion problem that appeared in 24% of patients (Keating et al, 1990). Fistulas, strictures, and graft failures were also prevalent, also in 24%. The morbidity associated with the elaborate harvesting effort for BlMG was a also negative factor.

Buccal mucosal grafts (BuMG) (Fig. 68–12*A* to *C*) were first used by the author as a substitute urethral graft in 1986 in a patient with epispadias (Duckett, 1986). The graft may be easily harvested from the cheek. No previous preparation is necessary in the mouth, but one must identify and avoid Stenson's duct. In an adult, the cheek will provide a 6-cm long graft with a tubularized caliber of No. 24 to 28 Fr. In a child, a length of 4 to 5 cm with a width of 1.5 to 2 cm is usually available. Compared with skin and bladder mucosa, immunohistochemical stains of buccal grafts demonstrate an abundant layer of vasculature just under the basement membrane of the epithelium in the outer layer of lamina propria (Duckett et al, 1995). The **lamina propria** must be thinned by excising the fat beneath the epidermis, a step that is most important in achieving success. The author has written in the past that the buccal graft is very thick, meaning that microscopically the epithelial layer has four times the depth of skin or bladder mucosal grafts. This does *not* mean that the graft itself should be thick. It is most important to thin it of subcutaneous tissue.

Meatal stenosis has caused trouble for the author if a circular meatus is made in the glans. A dart of glans tissue or an oblique anastomosis may be preferred from the outset to avoid meatal stenosis. The proximal anastomosis to the native urethra should be made in an oblique direction to avoid stricture. Immobilization of the graft should be maintained for 3 to 4 days to avoid shearing of the tissues. A suction drain should be placed for 24 hours to avoid any immediate postoperative hematoma formation.

BuMG for **onlay repairs** is now preferred to full tubularized grafts when a urethral plate can be left intact. The author has used buccal grafts for urethral strictures. They are especially effective for onlay repairs, leaving a dorsal strip of urethral mucosa intact. The well-vascularized bulbar cavernosus muscle will revascularize the graft sufficiently. The author has had success with BuMG onlays in performing glanular urethral repairs (Duckett et al, 1995).

The inner lip has been harvested for an onlay graft in several cases but is not wide enough to form a tubularized replacement for the urethra (Dessanti et al, 1992). The author has found that this harvest unroofs a number of submaxillary glands and that the inner lip is not as sturdy a urethral replacement as the cheek. A cheek harvest can be closed primarily so that there is very little discomfort, whereas the lip is left open, and resurfacing takes longer to complete.

Recently, Schonwetter (1995) has discovered that an antibacterial peptide (TAP) is abundant in the bovine tongue and probably enhances the healing process as well.

CURRENT CONTROVERSIES AND NEW CONCEPTS

Congenital Penile Curvature Versus Chordee

The concept of chordee as a bowstring tethering the hypospadiac penis ventrally has been so ingrained in the hypospadias literature that challenging the concept is treasonous. In 1842 Mettauer identified ventral penile curvature or chordee as a fibrous remnant of corpus spongiosum. Since then, the concept of dividing the urethral plate to release this bowstring or cord has become well established in hypospadiology.

After many years' experience, we now recognize that congenital curvature is not necessarily enhanced by division of a healthy urethral plate. This radical change in concept has led to an increase in preservation of the urethral plate and an increased number of OIF repairs of hypospadias (33% in the last 5 years versus 10% in the 5 previous years) (Hollowell et al, 1990; Baskin et al, 1994).

Congenital penile curvature (chordee) is often due to abnormal fixation of skin or dartos fascia (Daskalopoulos et al, 1993). Corporal disproportion is explained as the result of abnormal differential growth of the tunica albuginea of the corpora cavernosa, usually on the ventral aspects of the corpora. Dissection of the urethral plate from such an anomaly often does not straighten the curvature sufficiently. The author has, therefore, left the urethral plate intact and elected to use dorsal tunica albuginea plications (TAP) to repair both curvature due to primary hypospadias and curvature without hypospadias. This procedure is a modification of Nesbit's original tunica albuginea excision and plication technique (Baskin and Duckett, 1994). The author does not think this shortens the penis in a measurable way.

An alternative to dorsal plication is excision of ventral tissue and replacement of it with an elastic graft. Dermal graft is the most prevalent (Devine et al, 1991). Others have used tunica vaginalis, and recently vein grafting of the tunical incisions has been successful. The author believes that this is an unnecessarily elaborate option, although he has used it successfully in selected cases (see Fig. 68–3*A* to *C*).

The TAP is performed with the penis in the erect state to determine the point of maximum bend dorsally. Buck's fascia is elevated on either side of the midline at the 10- and 2-o'clock positions to lift the neurovascular bundle above the tunica albuginea. Parallel incisions about 8 mm long and approximately 6 to 8 mm apart are made through the tunica albuginea. The outer edges of the incisions are approximated with permanent sutures (5–0 polypropylene in infants) to bury the knot. A straight penis is confirmed by repeated

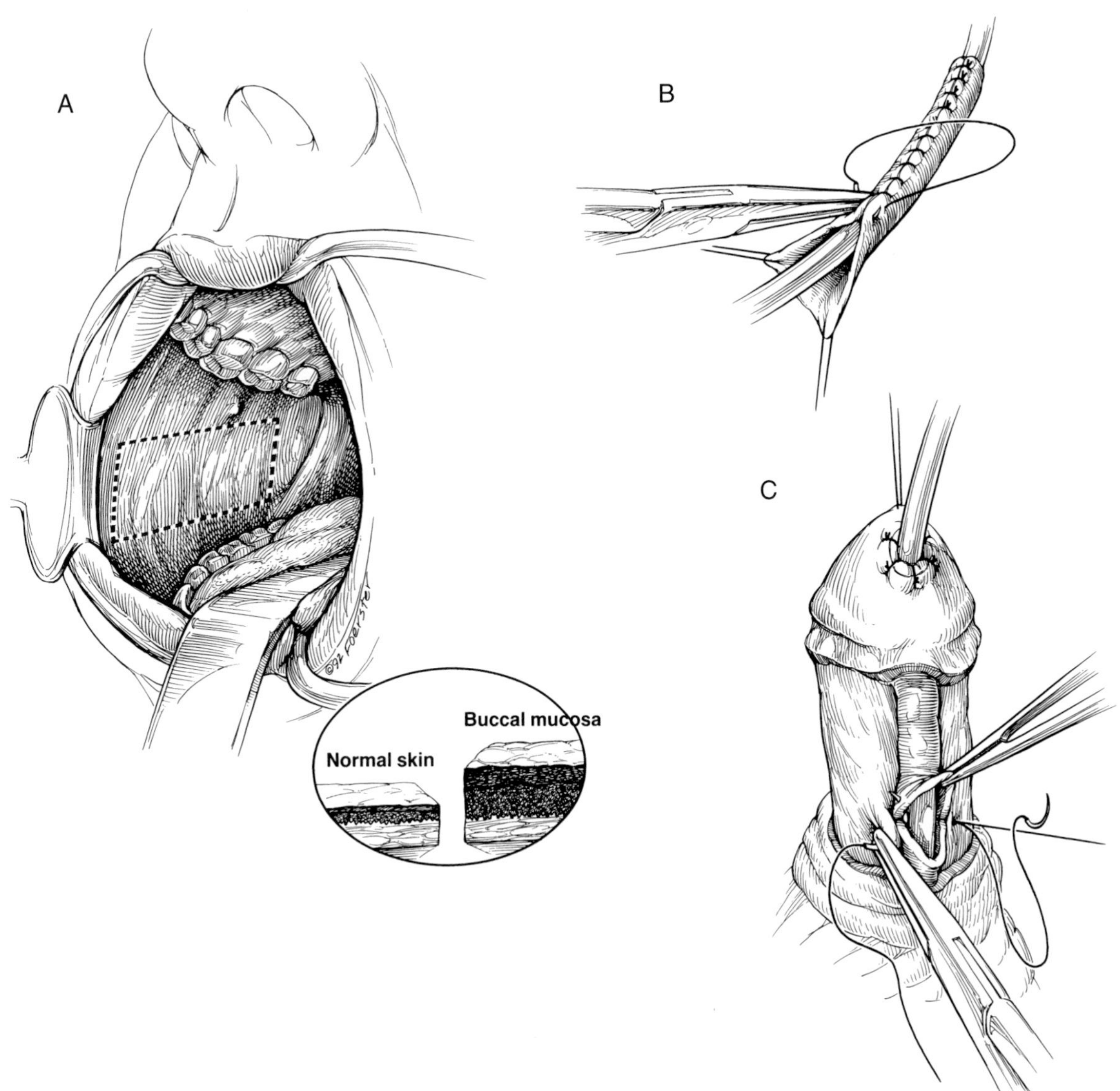

Figure 68–12. Buccal mucosal graft. The inner cheek is harvested for its thick mucosal lining using a mouth retractor. Stenson's duct is noted opposite the second molar. The graft is thinned to remove all fat and buccinator muscles. Insert: The epithelium of buccal mucosa is four times thicker than normal skin or bladder mucosa. The graft is either tubularized for urethral replacement or used as an onlay graft. (From Duckett JW: Successful hypospadias repair. Contemporary Urology 1992; 4:42–55. Copyright Medical Economics Company.)

performance of artificial erection. In rare cases, two separate plications are performed if the penis is long. However, if a bend of more than 20% to 30% is present, it may be preferable to incise the ventrum and replace the tissue with tunica vaginalis (Stewart et al, 1995).

Dissecting Beneath the Urethral Plate

One current controversy relates to the need to dissect underneath the urethral plate and lift it off the shaft. Some practitioners have tried the onlay technique and find it successful. Others, however, still find the Mettauer concept of fibrous tissue under the urethral plate difficult to jettison and insist on lifting the skin flap and removing the spongiotic tissue beneath the urethral plate (Mollard et al, 1991; Perovic and Vukadinovic, 1994; Mouriquand, 1995). This author refutes this concept (Duckett, 1995), whereas Mollard and Perovic both believe that this step is important. Time will tell only after more experience has been accumulated. This author believes that the spongiosum under the plate helps in supplying blood and reduces fistulas (5% versus 13% in Mollard's experience). But more important, the author has not seen photographic confirmation that penile curvature that was present with the plate intact was relieved by dissection under the plate alone, a challenge his detractors cannot meet.

Two-Stage Repairs for Severe Forms of Hypospadias

Others have been disappointed by the results of repairs for the severe forms of hypospadias and have turned back to the two-stage Byars' or Durham-Smith technique (Retik et al, 1994) or the Belt-Fuqua procedure (Greenfield et al, 1994). In the 39 cases reviewed by Greenfield and his colleagues (1994), 62% of the patients required Nesbit dorsal tucks. Fistulas occurred in only one patient (2.5%); however, 21% developed neourethral diverticulas, and 20% developed strictures. Retik and his colleagues (1994), on the other hand, using the Byars' technique, reported only 5% fistulas and no strictures or other complications. These reports concern patients with "very severe hypospadias."

It has been the experience of the author and his colleagues that even with a very proximal meatus in the perineum or deep scrotum (Fig. 68–13), it has always been possible to achieve a long transverse preputial tube urethroplasty stretching from the native urethra to the tip of the penis. The concept that only a rectangle of skin may be taken from the inner prepuce is not true. If one thinks of the foreskin deployment as a **horseshoe** extending from the scrotum around the top of the penis and back to the scrotum, the inner skin margin may be taken as a flap as long as 6 to 7 cm (see Fig. 68–11). The cosmetic and functional results achieved with these long flaps have been very satisfactory. The author believes that today there is no need to return to two-stage procedures. However, the technique used is critical to a good outcome.

Double-Faced Island Flap

In the past the author has left the outer preputial skin attached to the inner tubularized flap and transferred the double-faced island flap around to the ventrum (Duckett, 1986). Hinman (1991) has noted the theoretical advantage of leaving both layers attached. However, this led to a significantly higher fistula rate, probably due to an excessive tissue transfer that had to be supported by the pedicle. The procedure is similar to the Hodgson (1986) tangential tube and the Asopa (Asopa and Asopa, 1984) rotational flap (see Fig. 68–9), both of which are more secure than the double-faced procedure (Duckett, 1991). Chen and colleagues (1993) recently developed a modification of the Hodgson III procedure, a two-faced flap variation that may be an advantage.

Recent Procedures with Promise

Snodgrass (1994) has described a longitudinal incision made in the middle of the urethral plate, folding together the lateral edges as in a Thiersch-Duplay procedure.

The *Koyanagi ("manta-wing") repair* is a meatal-based flap that can be extended circumferentially to form a foreskin flap and has been developed during the past several years. The results in 120 patients were 91% successful (Koyanagi et al, 1994). Although this technique is innovative, this author has been opposed to leaving the native meatus attached to the skin because it is likely to develop diverticula and there may be difficulty in passing catheters. Nevertheless, these results are very interesting.

The *tunica vaginalis blanket wrap* (TVBW) interposition proposed by Snow (1986) is an adjunctive technique that was

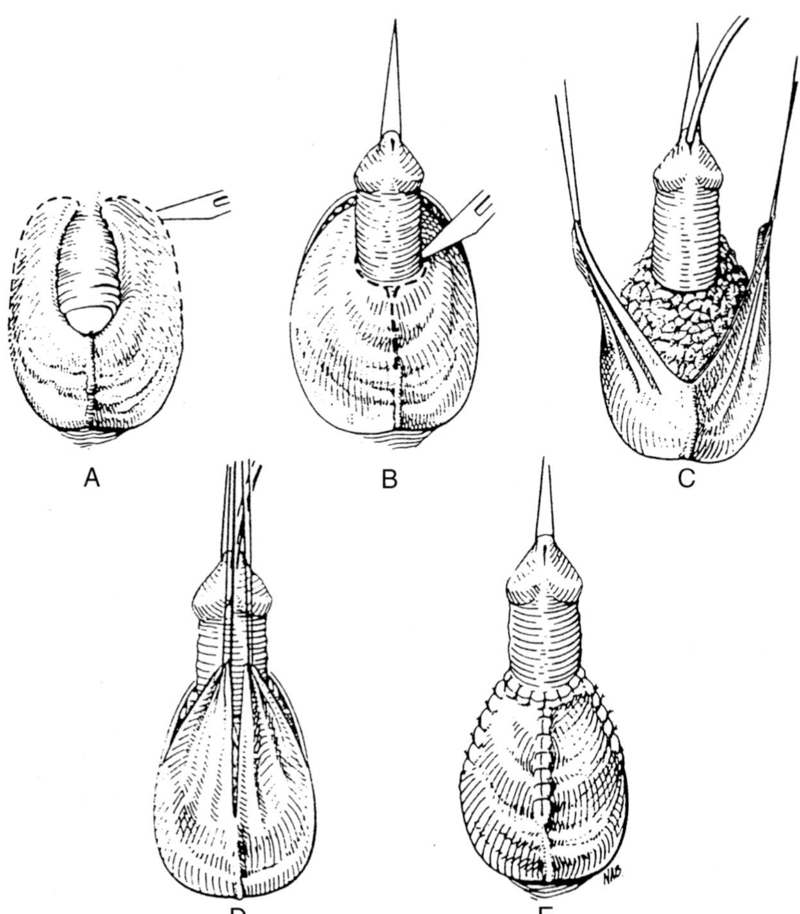

Figure 68–13. Scrotoplasty This procedure is performed 6 months after the urethroplasty to avoid compromising the penile skin vasculature after an island flap repair. *A* and *B,* Outline of incisions. *C,* Generous mobilization of scrotal skin flaps with correction of bifid scrotum in midline. *D,* Transpose skin to midline excising excess tissue; close base of penis to lateral abdominal skin. *E,* Final appearance.

Bellinger MF: Embryology of the male external genitalia. Urol Clin North Am 1981; 8:375–382.

Belman AB: Urethroplasty. Soc Pediatr Urol Newsletter, December 1977.

Belman AB: The Broadbent hypospadias repair. Urol Clin North Am 1981; 8:483.

Belman AB: The modified Mustarde hypospadias repair. J Urol 1982; 127:88–90.

Belman AB, Kass EJ: Hypospadias repair in children less than one year old. J Urol 1982; 128:1273–1274.

Belman AB, King LR: The urethra. *In* Kelalis PP, King LR, eds: Clinical Pediatric Urology. Philadelphia, W.B. Saunders, 1979, pp 576–594.

Berg R, Berg G: Penile malformation, gender identity and sexual orientation. Acta Psychiatr Scand 1983; 68:154–166.

Berg R, Svensson J, Astrom G: Social and sexual adjustment of men operated on for hypospadias during childhood: A controlled study. J Urol 1981; 125:313–317.

Bevan AD: A new operation for hypospadias. JAMA 1917; 68:1032–1033.

Brannen GE: Meatal reconstruction. J Urol 1976; 116:319–321.

Broadbent TR, Woolf RM, Toksu E: Hypospadias: One-stage repair. Plast Reconstr Surg 1961; 27:154–157.

Browne D: An operation for hypospadias. Lancet 1936; 1:141.

Browne D: A comparison of the Duplay and Denis Browne techniques for hypospadias operation. Surgery 1953; 34:787–793.

Brueziere J: How I perform the Mathieu technic in the treatment of anterior penile hypospadias. Ann Urol (Paris) 1987; 21:277–280.

Butler LJ, Snodgrass GJA, France NE, et al: True hermaphroditism or gonadal intersexuality. Arch Dis Child 1969; 44:666.

Byars LT: Technique of consistently satisfactory repair of hypospadias. Surg Gynecol Obstet 1955; 100:184–190.

Carmignani G, Belgrande E, Gabardi F, et al: Microsurgical one-stage repair of hypospadias with a rectangular transverse dorsal preputial vascularized skin flap. J Microsurg 1982; 3:222–227.

Cendron J, Melin Y: Congenital curvature of the penis without hypospadias. Urol Clin North Am 1981; 8:389–395.

Cerasaro TS, Brock WA, Kaplan GW: Upper urinary tract anomalies associated with congenital hypospadias: Is screening necessary? J Urol 1986; 135:537–542.

Chen S, Wang G, Wang M: Modified longitudinal preputial island flap urethroplasty for repair of hypospadias: Results in 60 patients. J Urol 1993; 149:814-816.

Coleman JW, McGovern JH, Marshall VF: The bladder mucosal graft technique for hypospadias repair. Urol Clin North Am 1981; 8:457–462.

Creevy CD: The correction of hypospadias: A review. Urol Surv 1958; 8:2–68.

Cromie WJ, Bellinger MF: Hypospadias dressing and diversions. Urol Clin North Am 1981; 8:545–558.

Cronin TD, Guthrie TH: Method of Cronin and Guthrie for hypospadias repair. *In* Horton CE, ed: Plastic and Reconstructive Surgery of the Genital Area. Boston, Little, Brown, 1973, pp 302–314.

Culp OS: Experiences with 200 hypospadiacs: Evolution of a therapeutic plan. Surg Clin North Am 1959; 39:1007–1023.

Culp OS, McRoberts JW: Hypospadias. *In* Alken CE, Dix V, Goodwin WE, et al, eds: Encyclopedia of Urology. New York, Springer-Verlag, 1968, pp 11307–11344.

Daskalopoulos EL, Baskin L, Duckett JW, Snyder HM: Congenital penile curvature (chordee without hypospadias). Urology 1993; 42:708–712.

Davidoff F, Federman DD: Mixed gonadal dysgenesis. Pediatrics 1973; 52:727–747.

Davis DM: Pedicle tube graft in surgical management of hypospadias, male, with new method of closing small urethral fistulas. Surg Gynecol Obstet 1940; 71:790–796.

Davis DM: Surgical treatment of hypospadias, especially scrotal and perineal. J Urol 1951; 65:595–602.

Des Prez JD, Persky L, Kiehn CL: A one-stage repair of hypospadias by island flap technique. Plast Reconstr Surg 1961; 28:405–410.

Dessanti A, Rigamonti W, Merulla V, et al: Autologous buccal mucosa graft for hypospadias repair: An initial report. J Urol 1992; 147:1081–1084.

DeSy WA: Aesthetic repair of meatal stricture. J Urol 1984; 132:678–679.

DeSy WA, Oosterlinck W: Urethral Advancement of Hypospadias Repair. Film presented at the International Congress of Urology, Vienna, 1985.

Devine CJ Jr: Chordee and hypospadias. *In* Glenn JF, Boyce WH, eds: Urologic Surgery, 3rd ed. Philadelphia, J. B. Lippincott, 1983, pp 775–797.

Devine CJ, Gonzales-Serva L, Stecker JF Jr, et al: Utricular configuration in hypospadias and intersex. J Urol 1980; 123:407–411.

Devine CJ Jr, Horton CE: A one-stage hypospadias repair. J Urol 1961; 85:166–172.

Devine CJ Jr, Horton CE: Chordee without hypospadias. J Urol 1973; 110:264–267.

Devine CJ Jr, Horton CE: Use of dermal graft to correct chordee. J Urol 1975; 113:56–58.

Devine CJ Jr, Blackley SK, Horton CE, Gilbert DA: The surgical treatment of chordee without hypospadias in men. J Urol 1991; 146:325–329.

Duckett JW: Transverse preputial island flap technique for repair of severe hypospadias. Urol Clin North Am 1980a; 7:423–431.

Duckett JW: Hypospadias. Clin Plast Surg 1980b; 7:149–160.

Duckett JW: Repair of hypospadias. *In* Hendry WF, ed: Recent Advances in Urology/Andrology. Vol. 3. New York, Churchill-Livingstone, 1980c, pp 279–290.

Duckett JW: Foreword: Symposium on Hypospadias. Urol Clin North Am 1981a; 8:371–373.

Duckett JW: MAGPI (meatal advancement and glanuloplasty): A procedure for subcoronal hypospadias. Urol Clin North Am 1981b; 8:513–520.

Duckett JW: The island flap technique for hypospadias repair. Urol Clin North Am 1981c; 8:503–511.

Duckett JW: Hypospadias. *In* Walsh PC, Gittes RF, Perlmutter AD, Stamey TA, eds: Campbell's Urology, 5th ed. Philadelphia, W.B. Saunders, 1986, pp 1969–1999.

Duckett JW: Use of buccal mucosa urethroplasty in epispadias. Meeting of Society of Paediatric Urologists, Southampton, England, 1986.

Duckett JW: Hypospadias. *In* Gillenwater JY, Grayhack JT, Howards SS, Duckett JW, eds: Adult and Pediatric Urology. Vol. 2. Chicago, Year Book Medical Publishers, 1987, pp 1880–1915.

Duckett JW: Advances in hypospadias repair. Festschrift honoring Sir David I. Williams. Postgrad Med J (London) 1990; 66:S62–S71.

Duckett JW: Hypospadias. *In* Gillenwater JY, Grayhack JT, Howards SS, Duckett JW, eds: Adult and Pediatric Urology, 2nd ed. Chicago, Mosby–Year Book, 1991, pp 2103–2110.

Duckett JW: Successful hypospadias repair. Contemp Urol 1992; 4:42–55.

Duckett JW: The current 'hype' in hypospadiology. Br J Urol 1995; 76(Suppl 3):1–7.

Duckett JW, Coplen D, Ewalt D, Baskin LS: Buccal mucosal urethral replacement. J Urol 1995; 153:1660–1663.

Duckett JW, Kaplan GW, Woodard JR, et al: Panel: Complications of hypospadias repair. Urol Clin North Am 1980; 7:443–452.

Duckett JW, Keating MA: Technical challenge of the megameatus intact prepuce hypospadias (MIP) variant: The pyramid procedure. J Urol 1989; 141:1407–1408

Duckett JW, Snyder HM: Hypospadias "pearls." Soc Pediatr Urol Newsletter 1985; 7:4.

Duckett JW, Snyder HM: The MAGPI hypospadias repair after 1,000 cases: Avoidance of meatal stenosis and regression. J Urol 1992; 147:665–669.

Duckett JW, Ueoka K, Seibold J, Snyder HM: Megameatus intact prepuce (MIP) variant in hypospadias. J Urol 1995; 153:340-A.

Ehrlich RM, Scardino PT: Surgical correction of scrotal transposition and perineal hypospadias. J Pediatr Surg 1982; 17:175–177.

Elder JS, Duckett JW, Snyder HM: Onlay island flap in the repair of mid and distal penile hypospadias without chordee. J Urol 1987; 138:376–379.

Filmer RB, Duckett JW, Sowden R: One-stage correction of hypospadias/chordee. Birth Defects 1977; 13:267–270.

Fuqua F: Renaissance of a urethroplasty: The Belt technique of hypospadias repair. J Urol 1971; 106:782.

Gearhart JP, Donohou PA, Brown TR, et al: Long-term endocrine follow-up of patients with hypospadias [Abstract 10]. J Urol 1989; 141:45-A.

Gearhart JP, Jeffs RD: The use of parenteral testosterone therapy in genital reconstructive surgery. J Urol 1987; 138:1077–1078.

Gearhart JP, Linhard HR, Berkovitz GD, et al: Androgen receptor levels and 5-alpha-reductase activities in preputial skin and chordee tissue of boys with isolated hypospadias. J Urol 1988; 140:1243–1246.

Gibbons AD, Gonzales ET Jr: The subcoronal meatus. J Urol 1983; 130:739–742.

Gittes RF, McLaughlin AP III: Injection technique to induce penile erection. Urology 1974; 4:473–475.

Glenister JW: The origin and fate of the urethral plate in man. J Anat 1954; 288:413–418.

Gonzales ET Jr, Veeraraghavan KA, Delaune J: The management of distal hypospadias with meatal-based, vascularized flaps. J Urol 1983; 129:119–120.

Greenfield SP, Sadler BT, Wan J: Two stage repair for severe hypospadias. J Urol 1994; 152:498-501.

Gunter JB, Forestner JE, Manley CB: Caudal epidural anesthesia reduces blood loss during hypospadias repair. J Urol 1990; 144:517–519.
Hendren WH: The Belt-Fuqua technique for repair of hypospadias. Urol Clin North Am 1981; 8:431–450.
Hendren WH, Crooks KK: Tubed free skin graft for construction of male urethra. J Urol 1980; 123:858–862.
Hendren WH, Horton CE Jr: Experience with one-stage repair of hypospadias and chordee using free graft of prepuce. J Urol 1988; 140:1259–1264.
Hendren WH, Keating MA: Use of dermal graft and free urethral graft in penile reconstruction. J Urol 1988; 140:1265–1269.
Hendren WH, Reda EF: Bladder mucosa graft for construction of male urethra. J Pediatr Surg 1986; 21:189–192.
Higgins CC: Hypospadias. Cleve Clin Q 1947; 14:176.
Hinderer U: New one-stage repair of hypospadias (technique of penis tunnelization). *In* Hueston JT, ed: Transactions of the 5th International Congress of Plastic and Reconstructive Surgery. Stoneham, MA, Butterworth Co., 1971, pp 283–305.
Hinman F Jr: The blood supply to preputial island flaps. J Urol 1991; 145:1232.
Hodgson NB: A one-stage hypospadias repair. J Urol 1970; 104:281–284.
Hodgson NB: In defense of the one-stage hypospadias repair. *In* Scott R Jr, Gordon HL, Scott FB, et al, eds: Current Controversies in Urologic Management. Philadelphia, W.B. Saunders, 1972, pp 263–271.
Hodgson NB: Hypospadias. *In* Glenn JF, Boyce WH, eds: Urologic Surgery, 2nd ed. New York, Harper & Row, 1975, pp 656–667.
Hodgson NB: Hypospadias and urethral duplication. *In* Harrison JH, ed: Campbell's Urology, 4th ed. Philadelphia, W.B. Saunders, 1978, pp 1566–1595.
Hodgson NB: Use of vascularized flaps in hypospadias repair. Urol Clin North Am 1981; 8:471–482.
Hodgson NB: Personal communication, 1986.
Hoffman WW, Hall WV: A modification of Spence's hood for one-stage surgical correction of distal shaft penile hypospadias. J Urol 1973; 109:1017–1018.
Hollowell JG, Keating MA, Snyder HM, et al: Preservation of urethral plate in hypospadias repair: Extended applications and further experience with the onlay island flap urethroplasty. J Urol 1990; 143:98–101.
Horton CE, Devine CJ, Baran N: Pictorial history of hypospadias repair techniques. *In* Horton CE, ed: Plastic and Reconstructive Surgery of the Genital Area. Boston, Little, Brown, 1973, pp 237–248.
Horton CE, Devine CJ, Graham JK: Fistulas of the penile urethra. Plast Reconstr Surg 1980; 66:407–418.
Humby G: A one-stage operation for hypospadias. Br J Surg 1941; 29:84–92.
Jensen BH: Caudal block for postoperative pain relief in children after genital operations: A comparison between bupivacaine and morphine. Acta Anesthesiol Scand 1981; 25:373–375.
Juskiewenski S, Vaysse P, Guitard J, et al: Traitement des hypospadias anterieurs. Chir Pediatr 1983; 24:75–79.
Juskiewenski S, Vaysse P, Moscovici J, et al: A study of the arterial blood supply to the penis. Anat Clin 1982; 4:101–107.
Kaplan GW: Repair of proximal hypospadias using a preputial free graft for neourethral construction and a preputial pedicle flap for ventral skin coverage. J Urol 1988; 140:1270–1272.
Kaplan GW, Brock WA: The etiology of chordee. Urol Clin North Am 1981; 8:383–387.
Kaplan SD, Hensle TW, Burbige KA, et al: Hypospadias: Associated behavior problems and male gender role development [Abstract 11]. J Urol 1989; 141:45A.
Kaplan GW, Lamm DL: Embryogenesis of chordee. J Urol 1975; 114:769–773.
Karl GW, Swedlon DB, Lee KW, et al: Epinephrine-halothane interaction in children. Anesthesiology 1983; 58:142–145.
Kass EJ, Bolong D: Single-stage hypospadias reconstruction without fistula. J Urol 1990; 144:520–522.
Keating MA, Duckett JW: Bladder mucosa in urethral reconstructions. J Urol 1990; 144:827–834.
Kenawi MM: Sexual function in hypospadias. Br J Urol 1975; 47:883–890.
Khuri FJ, Hardy BE, Churchill BM: Urologic anomalies associated with hypospadias. Urol Clin North Am 1981; 8:565–571.
Kim SH, Hendren WH: Repair of mild hypospadias. J Pediatr Surg 1981; 16:806–811.
King LR: One-stage repair without skin graft based on a new principle: Chordee is sometimes produced by skin alone. J Urol 1970; 103:660–662.
King LR: Cutaneous chordee and its implications in hypospadias repair. Urol Clin North Am 1981; 8:397–403.
Kirsch AJ, Miller MI, Hensle TW, et al: Results of a clinical trial using diode laser tissue welding in urinary tract reconstruction. J Urol 1995; 153:280-A.
Klocker H, Kaspar F, Eberle J, et al: Point mutation in the DNA binding domain of the androgen receptor in two families with Reifenstein Syndrome. Am J Hum Genet 1992; 50:1318–1327.
Koff SA: Mobilization of the urethra in the surgical treatment of hypospadias. J Urol 1981; 125:394–397.
Koff SA, Brinkman J, Ulrich J, Deighton D: Extensive mobilization of the urethral plate and urethra for repair of hypospadias: The modified Barcat technique. J Urol 1994; 151:466–469.
Koyanagi T, Nonomura K, Gotoh T, et al: One-stage repair of perineal hypospadias and scrotal transposition. Eur Urol 1984; 10:364–367.
Koyanagi T, Nonomura K, Yamashita T, et al: One-stage repair of hypospadias: Is there no simple method universally applicable to all types of hypospadias? J Urol 1994; 152:1232–1237.
Koyle MA, Ehrlich RM: The bladder mucosal graft for urethral reconstruction. J Urol 1987; 138:1093–1095.
Kramer SA, Aydin G, Kelalis PP: Chordee without hypospadias in children. J Urol 1982; 128:559–561.
Kumar S: Hypospadias with normal prepuce. J Urol 1986; 136:1056–1057.
Li ZC, Zheng ZH, Shen YX, et al: One-stage urethroplasty for hypospadias using a tube constructed with bladder mucosa—a new procedure. Urol Clin North Am 1981; 8:463–470.
MacMillan RDH, Churchill BM, Gilmore RF: Assessment of urinary stream after repair of anterior hypospadias by meatoplasty and glanuloplasty. J Urol 1985; 134:100–102.
Manley CB, Epstein ES: Early hypospadias repair. J Urol 1981; 125:698–700.
Marberger H, Pauer W: Experience in hypospadias repair. Urol Clin North Am 1981; 8:403–419.
Marshall M, Johnson SH, Price SE, et al: Cecil urethroplasty with concurrent scrotoplasty for repair of hypospadias. J Urol 1979; 121:335–339.
Marshall VF, Spellman RM: Construction of urethra in hypospadias using vesical mucosal graft. J Urol 1955; 73:335–342.
Mathieu P: Traitement en un temps de l'hypospadias balanique et juxtabalanique. J Chir (Paris) 1932; 39:481–484.
Mays HB: Hypospadias: A concept of treatment. J Urol 1951; 65:279–287.
McArdle F, Lebowitz R: Uncomplicated hypospadias and anomalies of upper urinary tract: Need for screening? Urology 1975; 5:712–716.
McCormack RM: Simultaneous chordee repair and urethral reconstruction for hypospadias. Plast Reconstr Surg 1954; 13:257.
Memmelaar J: Use of bladder mucosa in a one-stage repair of hypospadias. J Urol 1947; 58:68–73.
Mettauer JP: Practical observations on those malformations of the male urethra and penis, termed hypospadias and epispadias, with an anomalous case. Am J Med Sci 1842; 4:43.
Mollard P, Mouriquand P, Bringeon G, Bugmann P: Repair of hypospadias using a bladder mucosal graft in 76 patients. J Urol 1989; 142:1548–1551.
Mollard P, Mouriquand P, Felfela T: Appication of onlay island flap urethroplasty in penile hypospadias with severe chordee. Br J Urol 1991; 68:317–319.
Monfort G, Jean P, Lacoste M: One-stage correction of posterior hypospadias using a transverse pedicle flap (Duckett's operation). Chir Pediatr 1983; 24:71–74.
Monfort G, Lucas C: Dihydrotestosterone penile stimulation in hypospadias surgery. Eur Urol 1982; 8:201–203.
Montagnino BA, Gonzales ET Jr, Roth DR: Open catheter drainage after urethral surgery. J Urol 1988; 140:1250–1252.
Mouriquand PDE, Persad R, Sharma S: Hypospadias repair: Current principles and procedures. Br J Urol 1995; 76(Suppl 3):3–22.
Mustarde JC: One-stage correction of distal hypospadias and other people's fistulae. Br J Plast Surg 1965; 18:413–420.
Nasrallah PF, Minott HB: Distal hypospadias repair. J Urol 1984; 131:928–930.
Nesbit RM: Plastic procedure for correction of hypospadias. J Urol 1941; 45:699–702.
Nesbit RM: Congenital curvature of the phallus: Report of three cases with description of corrective operation. J Urol 1965; 93:230–232.
Nesbit RM: Operation for correction of distal penile ventral curvature with and without hypospadias. Trans Am Assoc Genitourin Surg 1966; 58:12–14.
Nonomura K, Koyanagi T, Imanaka K, et al: One-stage total repair of

severe hypospadias with scrotal transposition: Experience in 18 cases. J Pediatr Surg 1988; 23:177–180.

Ombredanne L: Precis Clinique et Operation de Chirurgie Infantile. Paris, Masson, 1932, p 851.

Opitz JM, Simpson JL, Sarto GE, et al: Pseudovaginal perineoscrotal hypospadias. Clin Genet 1972; 3:1.

Ossandon F, Ransley PG: Lasso tourniquet for artificial erection in hypospadias. Urology 1982; 19:656–657.

Pancoast JA: Treatise on Operative Surgery. Philadelphia, Carrey and Hart, 1844, pp 317–318.

Perlmutter AD, Vatz AD: Meatal advancement for distal hypospadias without chordee. J Urol 1975; 113:850–852.

Perovic S, Vukadinovic V: Onlay island flap urethroplasty for severe hypospadias: A variant of the technique. J Urol 1994; 151:711–714.

Peterson RE, Imperato-McGinley J, Gautier T, Sturla E: Male pseudohermaphroditism due to steroid 5-alpha-reductase deficiency. Am J Med 1977; 62:170.

Polus J, Lotte S: Chirurgie des hypospades: Une nouvelle technique esthetique et fonctionnelle. Ann Chir Plast 1965; 10:3–9.

Quartey JKM: One-stage penile/preputial cutaneous island flap urethroplasty for urethral stricture: A preliminary report. J Urol 1983; 129:284–287.

Rabinowitz R: Outpatient catheterless modified Mathieu hypospadias repair. J Urol 1987; 138:1074–1076.

Rajfer J, Walsh PC: The incidence of intersexuality in patients with hypospadias and cryptorchidism. J Urol 1976; 116:769–770.

Ransley PG. Duffy PG, Oesch IL, et al: The use of bladder mucosa and combined bladder mucosa/preputial skin grafts for urethral reconstruction. J Urol 1987; 138:1096–1098.

Redman JF: Experience with 60 consecutive hypospadias repairs using the Horton-Devine techniques. J Urol 1983; 129:115–118.

Redman JF: The balanic groove technique of Barcat. J Urol 1987; 137:83–85.

Retik AB, Keating MA, Mandel J: Complications of hypospadias repair. Urol Clin North Am 1988; 15:223–236.

Retik AB, Bauer SB, Mandell J, et al: Management of severe hypospadias with 2-stage repair. J Urol 1994; 152:749–751.

Rich MA, Keating MA, Snyder HM, et al: "Hinging" the urethral plate in hypospadias meatoplasty. J Urol 1989; 142:1551–1553.

Ricketson G: A method of repair for hypospadias. Am J Surg 1958; 95:279–283.

Ritchey ML, Benson RC Jr, Kramer SA, et al: Management of mullerian duct remnants in the male patient. J Urol 1988; 140:795–799.

Rober PE, Perlmutter AD, Reitelman C: Experience with 81 one-stage hypospadias/chordee repairs using free graft urethroplasties. J Urol 1990; 144:526–529.

Roberts CJ, Lloyd S: Observations on the epidemiology of simple hypospadias. Br Med J [Clin Res] 1973; 1:768–770.

Ross F, Farmer AW, Lindsay WK: Hypospadias—a review of 230 cases. Plast Reconstr Surg 1959; 24:357–368.

Russell RH: Operation for severe hypospadias. Br J Med [Clin Res] 1900; 2:1432.

Sauvage P, Rougeron G, Bientz J, et al: Use of the pedicled transverse preputial flap in the surgery of hypospadias: Apropos of 100 cases. Chir Pediatr 1987; 28:220–223.

Scherz HC, Kaplan GW, Packer MG, et al: Post-hypospadias repair of urethral strictures: A review of 30 cases. J Urol 1988; 140:1253–1255.

Schonwetter BS, Stolzenberg ED, Zasloff MA: Epithelial antibiotics induced at sites of inflammation. Science 1995; 267:1645–1648.

Schultz JR, Klykylo WM, Wacksman J: Timing of elective hypospadias repair in children. Pediatrics 1983; 71:342–351.

Secrest CL, Jordan GH, Winslow BH, et al: Repair of the complications of hypospadias surgery. J Urol 1993; 150:1415–1418.

Shelton TB, Noe HN: The role of excretory urography in patients with hypospadias. J Urol 1985; 135:97–100.

Shima H, Ikoma F, Terakawa T, et al: Developmental anomalies associated with hypospadias. J Urol 1979; 122:619–621.

Smith ED: A de-epithelialized overlap flap technique in the repair of hypospadias. Br J Plast Surg 1973; 26:106–109.

Smith ED: Durham-Smith repair of hypospadias. Urol Clin North Am 1981; 8:451–455.

Smith ED: Hypospadias. *In* Ashcraft K, ed: Pediatric Urology. Philadelphia, W.B. Saunders, 1990.

Snodgrass W: Tubularized, incised plate urethroplasty for distal hypospadias. J Urol 1994; 151:464–465.

Snow BW: Use of tunica vaginalis to prevent fistulas in hypospadias surgery. J Urol 1986; 136:861–863.

Snow BW, Cartwright PC, Unger K: Tunica vaginalis blanket wrap to prevent urethrocutaneous fistula: An 8 year experience. J Urol 1995; 153:472–473.

Snyder HM, Duckett JW: Hypospadias "pearls." Soc Pediatr Urol Newsletter, May 1984.

Sommer JT, Stephens FD: Dorsal ureteral diverticulum of the fossa navicularis: Symptoms, diagnosis and treatment. J Urol 1980; 124:94–98.

Song R, Wang X, Zuo Z: Hypospadias repair. Clin Plast Surg 1982; 9:91–95.

Sorenson R: Hypospadias with special reference to etiology. Op Dom Biol Hered Hum 1953; 31:1.

Spencer JR, Perlmutter AD: Sleeve advancement distal hypospadias repair. J Urol 1990; 144:523–525.

Standoli L: Correzione dell'ipospadias con tempo ad isola prepuziale. Rass Italia Chir Pediatr 1979; 21:82–91.

Standoli L: One-stage repair of hypospadias: Preputial island flap technique. Ann Plast Surg 1982; 9:81–88.

Stecker JF, Horton CE, Devine CJ, et al: Hypospadias cripples. Urol Clin North Am 1981; 8:538–544.

Stewart TS, Bartkowski DP, Perlmutter AD: Tunica vaginalis patch graft for treatment of severe chordee (Abstract 446). J Urol 1995; 153:340-A.

Sugar EC, Firlit CF: Urinary prophylaxis and postoperative care of children at home with an indwelling catheter after hypospadias repair. Urology 1989; 32:418–420.

Svensson J, Berg R: Micturition studies and sexual function in operated hypospadias. Br J Urol 1983; 55:422–426.

Sweet RA, Schrott HG, Kurland R, et al: Study of the incidence of hypospadias in Rochester, Minnesota, 1940–1970, and a case-control comparison of possible etiologic factors. Mayo Clin Proc 1974; 49:52–59.

Thiersch C: Ueber die Entstehungsweise und operative Behandlung der Epispadie. Arch Heitkunde 1869; 10:20.

Turner-Warwick R: The use of pedicle grafts in the repair of urinary tract fistulae. Br J Urol 1972; 44:644–656.

Turner-Warwick R: Observations upon techniques for reconstruction of the urethral meatus, the hypospadiac glans deformity and the penile urethra. Urol Clin North Am 1979; 6:643–655.

Udall DA: A correction of three types of congenital curvatures of the penis including the first reported case of dorsal curvature. J Urol 1980; 124:50–54.

Van der Meulen JC: Hypospadias Monograph. Leiden, The Netherlands, A.G. Stenfert, Kroese NV, 1964.

Van der Meulen JC: Hypospadias and cryptospadias. Br J Plast Surg 1971; 24:101–108.

Van der Meulen JC: Correction of hypospadias: Types I and II. Ann Plast Surg 1982; 8:403–411.

Wacksman J: Modification of the one-stage flip-flap procedure to repair distal penile hypospadias. Urol Clin North Am 1981; 8:527–530.

Wacksman J: Repair of hypospadias using new mouth-controlled microscope. Urology 1987; 29:276–278.

Walker RD: Outpatient repair of urethral fistulae. Urol Clin North Am 1981; 8:582–583.

Walsh PC, Madden JD, Harrod MJ, et al: Familial incomplete male pseudohermaphroditism, type 2. Decreased dihydrotestosterone formation in pseudovaginal perineoscrotal hypospadias. N Engl J Med 1974; 291:189–194.

Waterhouse K, Glassberg KI: Mobilization of the anterior urethra as an aid in the one-stage repair of hypospadias. Urol Clin North Am 1981; 8:521–525.

Welch KJ: Hypospadias. *In* Ravitch MM, Welch KJ, Benson CD, et al, eds: Pediatric Surgery, 3rd ed. Chicago, Year Book Medical Publishers, 1979, pp 1353–1376.

Wilson JD: Familial incomplete male pseudohermaphroditism, type 1. Evidence for androgen resistance and variable clinical manifestations in a family with Reifenstein syndrome. N Engl J Med 1974; 290:1097–1103.

Woodard JR, Cleveland R: Application of Horton-Devine principles to the repair of hypospadias. J Urol 1982;127:1155–1158.

Yeoman DM, Cooke R, Hain WR: Penile block for circumcision? A comparison with caudal block. Anesthesia 1983; 38:862–866.

69
CONGENITAL ANOMALIES OF THE GENITALIA

Jack S. Elder, M.D.

Neonatal genital anomalies are common and may result from a disorder of sexual differentiation, genital differentiation, or genital growth. Many genital anomalies are associated with developmental abnormalities of other organ systems. Although most genital deformities are recognized at birth, occasionally they may be detected in utero (Mandell et al, 1995).

Recognition of normal embryology is essential to understanding the pathogenesis of genital anomalies. **In the male embryo, differentiation of the external genitalia occurs between weeks 9 and 13 of gestation and requires production of testosterone by the testes as well as conversion of testosterone into dihydrotestosterone (DHT) under the enzymatic influence of 5α-reductase in the genital anlagen. Under the influence of DHT, the genital tubercle differentiates into the glans penis; the genital folds become the shaft of the penis, and the genital swellings migrate inferomedially, fusing in the midline to become the scrotum. In the female, because of the absence of testosterone and DHT, the genital tubercle develops passively into the clitoris, the genital folds become the labia minora, and the genital swellings become the labia majora.** The same changes may also occur in males with an abnormality in fetal testosterone production, a 5α-reductase deficiency, or an androgen receptor defect.

NORMAL GENITALIA

In a normal term male neonate, the penis is 3.5 ± 0.7 cm in stretched length and 1.1 ± 0.2 cm in diameter (Table 69–1). At birth, the inhibitory effect of maternal estrogens on the fetal pituitary is no longer present; this change in the hormonal milieu causes a rebound surge in gonadotropins that results in an **early transient surge in testosterone production by the Leydig cells, stimulating penile growth during the first 3 months of life.** During the remainder of childhood, the penis grows much more slowly. Normally, the penis has a fully developed foreskin and a median raphe on the shaft. However, **in 10% of males, the raphe deviates, usually to the left side** (Ben-Ari et al, 1985). Although deviation of the raphe may be associated with penile torsion or chordee without hypospadias, it is usually an insignificant finding. However, in the newborn

Table 69–1. STRETCHED PENILE LENGTH (CM) IN NORMAL MALE SUBJECTS

Age	Mean ± SD	Mean − 2.5 SD
Newborn 30 wk	2.5 ± 0.4	1.5
Newborn 34 wk	3.0 ± 0.4	2.0
0–5 mo	3.9 ± 0.8	1.9
6–12 mo	4.3 ± 0.8	2.3
1–2 yr	4.7 ± 0.8	2.6
2–3 yr	5.1 ± 0.9	2.9
3–4 yr	5.5 ± 0.9	3.3
4–5 yr	5.7 ± 0.9	3.5
5–6 yr	6.0 ± 0.9	3.8
6–7 yr	6.1 ± 0.9	3.9
7–8 yr	6.2 ± 1.0	3.7
8–9 yr	6.3 ± 1.0	3.8
9–10 yr	6.3 ± 1.0	3.8
10–11 yr	6.4 ± 1.1	3.7
Adult	13.3 ± 1.6	9.3

From Feldman KW, Smith DW: Fetal phallic growth and penile standards for newborn male infants. J Pediatr 1975; 86:895; and Schonfeld WA, Beebe GW: Normal growth and variation in the male genitalia from birth to maturity. J Urol 1987; 30:554.

male with deviation of the raphe, careful inspection of the glans is important. Congenital ventral or lateral curvature of the penis affects approximately 0.6% of male neonates (Yachia et al, 1993). A urethral deformity such as hypospadias or epispadias occurs in approximately 1 in 250 males.

The appearance of the normal female genitalia is much less variable. The clitoris, urethral meatus, and hymen may be visualized when the labia minora are separated. Between 3% and 13% of females have hymenal variants, such as tags or transverse bands (Jenny et al, 1987; Berenson, 1995). In the neonate, the vulva may be hyperpigmented and enlarged as a consequence of circulating maternal estrogens. The breadth of the newborn clitoris ranges from 2 to 6 mm, with a mean of 3.7 to 3.9 mm (Riley and Rosenbloom, 1980). Huffman (1976) reported a "clitoral index" obtained by multiplying the breadth of the glans by its length, an index of 4.35 being the upper limit of normal. Generally, infants with a clitoral breadth of greater than 6 mm or a clitoral index of more than 10 should be evaluated. The clitoris does not change in size during the first year of life.

GENITAL ANOMALIES AND ASSOCIATION WITH OTHER ABNORMALITIES

Congenital anomalies of the genitalia are often associated with abnormalities of other organ systems or are part of recognized syndromes (Table 69–2). **As many as 50% of children with congenital anorectal malformations also have an associated urologic malformation** (Hoekstra et al, 1983), and frequently the external genitalia are involved. For example, **in a series of boys with high imperforate anus, 29% had an abnormality of the external genitalia,** including hypospadias, penile duplication, micropenis, or scrotal deformity, whereas hypospadias was the primary genital abnormality in those with low imperforate anus (Hoekstra et al, 1983). **Among girls with imperforate anus, genital anomalies occur in 35%,** including bicornuate uterus, uterus didelphys, hypoplastic uterus, vaginal septum, vaginal agenesis, phallic urethra, imperforate hymen, and absence of the lower third of the vagina (Bellinger and Duckett, 1982; Hoekstra et al, 1983; Fleming et al, 1986). Among boys with esophageal atresia or tracheoesophageal fistula, genital deformities also are common, including hypospadias (6%), penile agenesis, penoscrotal transposition, scrotal malformation, and scrotal agenesis (1.5% each) (Berkhoff et al, 1989). Consequently, involvement of the urologist in the initial evaluation and long-term management of these patients is important.

Table 69–2. GENITAL ANOMALIES COMMONLY OCCURRING IN VARIOUS SYNDROMES

Male	Female
Microphallus/Ambiguous Genitalia/ Bifid Scrotum	**Hypoplastic Labia Majora**
Anencephaly	Escobar's syndrome
Aniridia-Wilms' tumor association	Popliteal pterygium syndrome
Bladder exstrophy	Robinow's syndrome
Borjeson-Forssman-Lehman syndrome	Trisomy 18
Carpenter's syndrome	9p−, 18q−
CHARGE association	**Double Vagina and/or Bicornuate Uterus**
Cloacal exstrophy	Cloacal exstrophy
Fraser's syndrome	Fraser's syndrome
Johanson-Blizzard syndrome	Johanson-Blizzard syndrome
Meckel-Gruber syndrome	Rokitansky's sequence
Noonan's syndrome	Trisomy 13
Opitz's syndrome	**Vaginal Atresia**
Pallister-Hall syndrome	Cloacal exstrophy
Popliteal pterygium syndrome	MURCS association
Prader-Willi syndrome	Rokitansky's sequence
Rapp-Hodgkin ectodermal dysplasia syndrome	Sirenomelia sequence
Rieger's syndrome	Turner's syndrome
Robinow's syndrome	Caudal regression
Schinzel-Giedian syndrome	
Short rib–polydactyly	
Smith-Lemin-Opitz syndrome	
Triploidy syndrome	
Trisomy 4p, 9p, 18, 20p, 21, 22	
9p, 10q, 11p, 15q deficiency	
XXY, XXXXY	

Adapted from Jones KL: Smith's Recognizable Patterns of Human Malformation, 4th ed. Philadelphia, W. B. Saunders, 1988.

MALE GENITAL ANOMALIES

Penile Anomalies

Phimosis

At birth, there is a physiologic phimosis or inability to retract the foreskin in the majority of neonates because natural adhesions exist between the prepuce and the glans. During the first 3 to 4 years of life, as the penis grows, epithelial debris (smegma) accumulates under the prepuce, gradually separating the foreskin from the glans. Intermittent penile erections aid in allowing the foreskin eventually to become retractable. **By 3 years of age, 90% of foreskins are retractable,** and less than 1% of males have phimosis by 17 years of age (Oster, 1968).

Early forceful retraction of the foreskin generally is not recommended because recurrent adhesions between the de-epithelialized glans may occur, and a cicatricial preputial ring may form, causing secondary phimosis. However, in some boys with phimosis who develop balanitis or balanoposthitis, manual retraction of the foreskin with lysis of adhesions should be considered. This may be done during an office visit. It may be helpful to apply Eutectic mixture of local anesthetics (EMLA) cream topically prior to the procedure (MacKinley, 1988). In uncircumcised boys in whom the tip of the foreskin remains tight after the age of 4 to 5 years as well as in young boys with phimosis that causes ballooning of the foreskin or recurrent balanitis, strong consideration should be given to performing a circumcision or dorsal slit.

Circumcision

In pediatrics, few topics generate as much controversy as whether the newborn male should undergo circumcision, perhaps because it is the most common surgical procedure in the United States and because it is usually performed for social reasons. In 1975, the American Academy of Pediatrics declared, "There is no absolute medical indication for routine circumcision of the newborn" (Thompson et al, 1975). This stance was supported by the American College of Obstetricians and Gynecologists.

Reasons given in support of circumcision include prevention of penile cancer, sexually transmitted diseases, and phimosis and lessening of the risk of balanitis. Although carcinoma of the penis develops primarily in uncircumcised men, in Scandinavian countries, where few men are circumcised and genital hygiene is excellent, the incidence of penile cancer is exceedingly low.

It has become apparent that **uncircumcised newborns are predisposed to urinary tract infections (UTIs)** in the neonatal period. For example, in a study of 100 neonates with UTIs, Ginsburg and McCracken (1982) found that only 3 of the 62 males (5%) who developed a UTI were circumcised. Subsequently, Wiswell and colleagues (1985) studied more than 2500 male infants and found that 41 had symptomatic UTIs; of these 88% were uncircumcised. In that study, uncircumcised males were nearly 20 times more likely to develop UTIs than circumcised neonates. Other studies of larger groups of infants have corroborated these reports (Wiswell, 1992). **The increased risk seems to affect males at least through 5 years of age** (Craig et al, 1996). Presumably, UTIs result from colonization of the prepuce by urinary pathogens (Fussell et al, 1988; Wiswell et al, 1988). In view of these findings, the American Academy of Pediatrics reviewed its policy and published an updated scholarly report on neonatal circumcision (AAP Task Force on Circumcision, 1989). The report reviews penile hygiene, cancer of the penis, UTIs, sexually transmitted diseases, cervical carcinoma, pain, local anesthesia, contraindications, and complication and concludes, **"Newborn circumcision has potential medical benefits and advantages as well as disadvantages and risks. When circumcision is being considered, the benefits and risks should be explained to the parents and informed consent obtained."** The report is very readable and should be given to families who are undecided about the issue. In general, **neonatal circumcision is safe, although there is a complication rate of 0.2% to 3%** (Ross, 1995). Dorsal penile nerve block with either lidocaine or bupivacaine significantly reduces the pain associated with the procedure (Ryan et al, 1994).

Circumcision should not be performed in neonates with hypospadias, chordee without hypospadias, a dorsal hood deformity, or webbed penis or in those with a small penis. In addition, many neonates with a large hydrocele or hernia are more likely to develop secondary phimosis and a buried penis if circumcision is performed.

Some newborn males are not circumcised owing to either illness (prematurity, sepsis) or parental choice, and when the child is older the family requests that a circumcision be performed under anesthesia. The most common indications for "delayed" circumcision include balanoposthitis (23% to 36%), social reasons (23% to 39%), improved hygiene (13%), urinary tract infection (7%), coincident with other surgery (27%), and phimosis (3%) (Larsen and Williams, 1990; Wiswell et al, 1993). An alternative to circumcision for phimosis is "preputial plasty," which is essentially a minimal dorsal slit through the phimotic ring (Cuckow et al, 1994).

Penile Cysts

The most common cystic lesion of the penis is accumulation of epithelial debris, or smegma, under the unretractable foreskin. In young boys the foreskin should not be retracted unless infection or inflammation is associated because eventually it will retract by itself.

Congenital epidermal cysts occasionally form along the median penile raphe. Epidermal inclusion cysts may form following circumcision, hypospadias repair, or other forms of penile surgery, and result when islands of epithelium are left behind in the subcutaneous tissue. These cystic lesions should be treated with simple excision.

Inconspicuous Penis

The term **inconspicuous penis** refers to a penis that appears to be small (Bergeson et al, 1993). **Several entities are included in this term including webbed penis, concealed penis, and trapped penis, in which the penis is normal in size, and micropenis, in which the penis is abnormally small.** When an infant is found to have an inconspicuous penis, prompt evaluation is necessary for proper treatment, and the family must be informed that the penis is or is not normal.

Webbed Penis

Webbed penis is a condition in which the scrotal skin extends onto the ventrum of the penis (Fig. 69–1). When this condition is congenital, the penis, urethra, and the remainder of the scrotum typically are normal, and the **deformity represents an abnormality of the attachment between the penis and the scrotum.** This condition also may be iatrogenic following circumcision or other penile surgery, in which case it results from excessive removal of ventral penile skin.

Although the webbed penis is usually asymptomatic, the cosmetic appearance is often unacceptable. Occasionally this condition may be corrected by incising the web transversely, separating the penis from the scrotum, and closing the skin vertically (Perlmutter and Chamberlain, 1972; Kenawi, 1973). In other cases a circumferential incision is made 1.5 cm proximal to the coronal sulcus, Byars' preputial skin flaps are transferred to the ventral surface of the penis, and the redundant foreskin is excised. The scrotum may be anchored to the base of the penis to prevent recurrence of the webbed appearance. **In rare cases the distal urethra is hypoplastic, necessitating urethral reconstruction.**

Concealed (Buried or Hidden) Penis

A concealed penis is a normally developed penis that is camouflaged by the suprapubic fat pad; this anomaly may be congenital or iatrogenic following circumcision (Fig. 69–2). In infants and young children the congenital condition has been thought to result from the inelasticity of the dartos fascia (which normally allows the penile skin to slide freely on the deep layers of the shaft), thus restricting extension of the penis (Devine, 1989), and because the penile skin is not anchored to the deep fascia. In older children and obese adolescents, the abundant fat on the abdominal wall may hide the penile shaft.

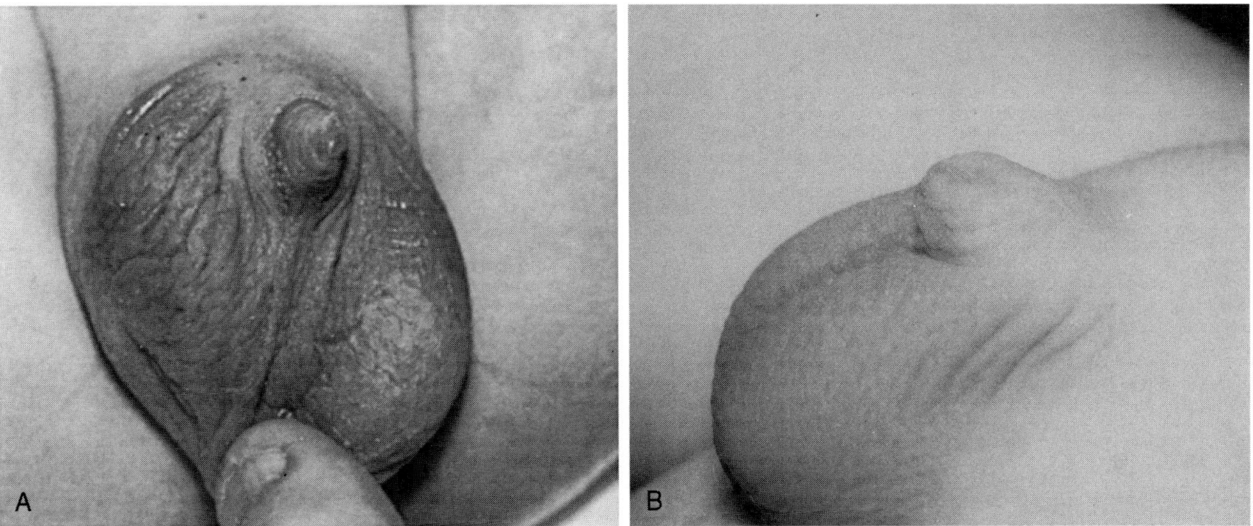

Figure 69–1. *A* and *B*, Examples of webbed penis. Penile shaft is normal in length. In *A*, there is also scrotal engulfment of the penile shaft.

On inspection, the contour of the penile shaft and the glans cannot be seen. However, careful palpation allows one to determine that the penile shaft actually is concealed and normal in size and not a microphallus or a penis that has undergone circumcision injury. It is important to determine whether the glans can be exposed simply by retracting the skin covering the glans. If so, it remains the surgeon's judgment whether or not correction is warranted.

Several techniques have been described to correct the concealed penis (Redman, 1985; Donahoe and Keating, 1986; Maizels et al, 1986; Shapiro, 1987; Lim et al, 1995). The indications for this type of surgery as well as the timing of reconstruction are controversial. In moderately severe cases, the dysgenic bands of tissue, which are located primarily on the dorsal surface of the shaft of the penis, must be removed. In addition, the subcutaneous tissue on the dorsal aspect of the penis should be fixed to the pubic fascia, and the subcutaneous tissue of the scrotum should be fixed to the ventral aspect of the base of the penile shaft with nonabsorbable suture. In the most severe cases, the suspensory ligament of the penis must be divided, suprapubic fat must be excised, and the spermatic cords must be protected. Liposuction has been reported to be helpful in severe cases (Maizels et al, 1986). In some cases, an island pedicle of ventral preputial skin may be used to cover the penis and aid in reconstruction.

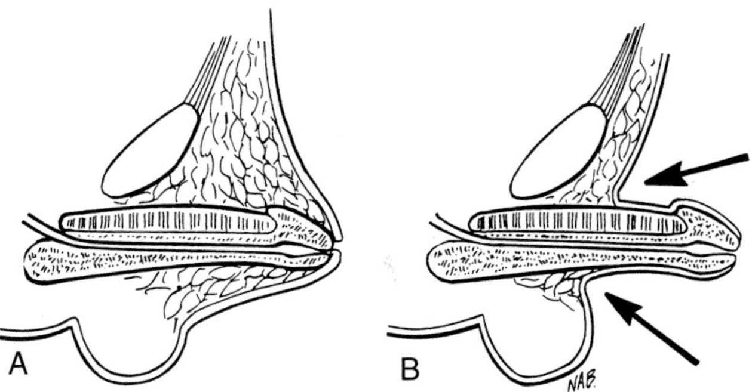

Figure 69–2. Concealed penis *(A)*, which may be visualized by retracting skin lateral to penile shaft *(B)*.

Trapped Penis

Trapped penis is an acquired form of inconspicuous penis and refers to a phallus that becomes embedded in the suprapubic fat pad following circumcision. This deformity may occur after neonatal circumcision in a baby who has significant scrotal swelling due to a hydrocele or hernia or after routine circumcision in a baby with a webbed penis. In some neonates, the penile shaft seems to retract naturally into the scrotum, and if circumcision is performed in this situation, the skin at the base of the penis may form a cicatrix over the retracted phallus (Fig. 69–3). In its most severe form, **this complication can cause a predisposition to UTIs and may cause urinary retention.** Elective repair of the trapped penis is recommended. The surgical technique is similar to that for concealed penis.

Micropenis

Micropenis is defined as a normally formed penis that is at least 2.5 standard deviations below the mean in size (Aaronson, 1994) (Fig. 69–4*A*). **Typically, the ratio of the length of the penile shaft to its circumference is normal.** In a few cases, the corpora cavernosa are severely hypoplastic. The scrotum usually is fused but often is diminutive. The testes usually are small and frequently are undescended.

Assessment of length is made by measuring the penis from its attachment to the pubic symphisis to the tip of the glans (Fig. 69–4*B*). In an obese infant or child, one must be careful to depress the suprapubic fat pad completely to obtain an accurate measurement. Stretched penile length is used because it correlates more closely with erectile length than the relaxed length of the penis. The measurements should be compared with standards for penile length (see Table 69–1). **In general, the penis of a term newborn should be at least 1.9 cm long.** A webbed or concealed penis often resembles micropenis, but examination shows a normal penile shaft.

Knowledge of the endocrinologic regulation of penile development fosters an understanding of how micropenis occurs. Differentiation of the male external genitalia is com-

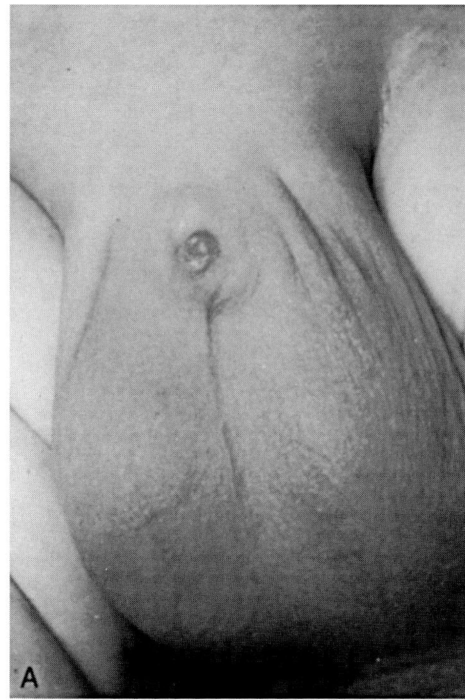

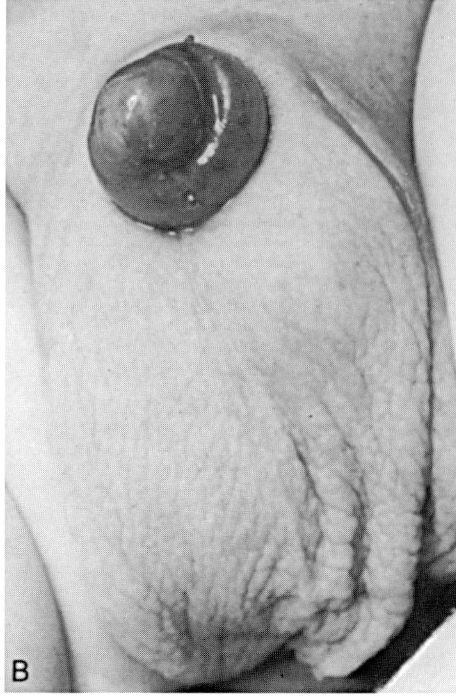

Figure 69–3. *A,* Concealed penis resulting from circumcision. *B,* Same patient following revision of circumcision.

plete by the 12th week of gestation and requires a normal testis producing testosterone, stimulated by maternal chorionic gonadotropin. During the second and third trimesters, growth of the penis occurs under the direction of fetal androgen, which is controlled by the secretion of fetal luteinizing hormone (LH). An abnormality in the production or use of testosterone results not only in a small penis but usually in hypospadias also, whereas a true micropenis often seems to be a consequence of a deficiency of gonadotropic hormones. Thus, **micropenis results from a hormonal abnormality that occurs after 14 weeks of gestation.**

There are numerous causes of micropenis, including isolated gonadotropin defects without involvement of other organ systems and generalized endocrinopathies that may be associated with central nervous system defects. **The most common causes of micropenis include (1) hypogonadotropic hypogonadism, (2) hypergonadotropic hypogonadism (primary testicular failure), and (3) idiopathic** (Lee et al, 1980b; Gonzales, 1983). In addition, micropenis is often associated with major chromosomal defects including Klinefelter's syndrome (47,XXY), other X polysomy syndromes, and translocations, deletions, and trisomy involving chromosomes 8, 13, and 18 (Aaronson, 1994).

The most common cause of micropenis is failure of the hypothalamus to produce an adequate amount of gonoadotropin-releasing hormone. This condition, termed

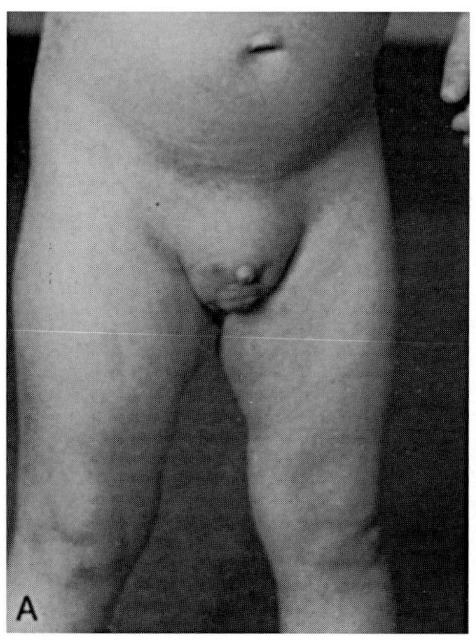

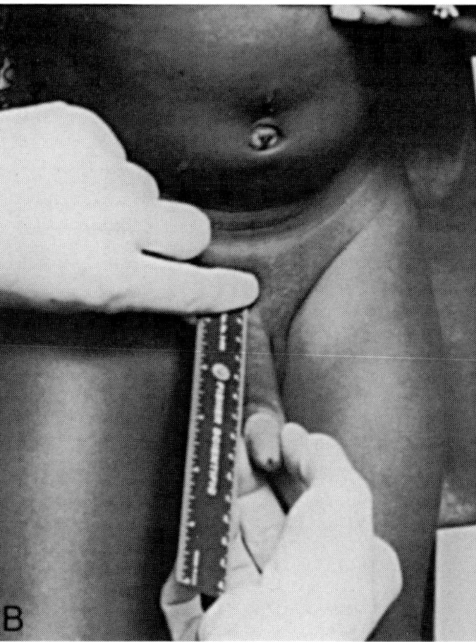

Figure 69–4. *A,* Microphallus. *B,* Technique of measuring stretched penile length.

hypogonadotropic hypogonadism, may result from hypothalamic dysfunction, such as **Kallmann's syndrome** (genito-olfactory dysplasia), **Prader-Willi syndrome,** and Lawrence-Moon-Biedl syndrome (Walsh et al, 1978; Danish et al, 1980). In other cases, there is an associated **growth hormone deficiency** (Burstein et al, 1979) or neonatal hypoglycemia secondary to congenital hypopituitarism (Lovinger et al, 1975). Other major causes include congenital pituitary aplasia and midline brain defects such as agenesis of the corpus callosum and occipital encephalocele.

Another cause of micropenis is primary testicular failure. Micropenis secondary to **hypergonadotropic hypogonadism** may result from **gonadal dysgenesis or rudimentary testes** syndrome, and also occurs in **Robinow's syndrome** (Lee et al, 1980b). Failure of serum testosterone to rise appropriately following human chorionic gonadotropin (hCG) stimulation has been the test most frequently used to identify this subgroup. However, in patients with Kallmann's syndrome and undescended testes, the serum testosterone level may not increase following hCG administration. Rarely, a patient with partial androgen insensitivity syndrome has micropenis; more commonly, however, the patient has sexual ambiguity.

Some patients may have an idiopathic form of micropenis, and endocrine studies demonstrate a normal hypothalamic-pituitary-testicular axis. In these cases, micropenis may result from improper timing or delayed onset of gonadotropin stimulation in the fetus (Lee et al, 1980a).

A karyotype should be performed in all patients with micropenis. Consultation generally is obtained from the pediatric endocrinology service to help determine the cause of the micropenis and to assess whether other abnormalities are present as well. Several issues need to be addressed, the most important of which is the growth potential of the penis. In addition, the endocrine abnormality needs to be defined. **Testicular function may be assessed by measuring serum testosterone levels before and after hCG stimulation.** Primary testicular failure would show an absent response and elevated basal LH and follicle-stimulating hormone (FSH) levels. In some cases, a gonadotropin-releasing hormone stimulation test is done also. **Anterior pituitary screening tests include serial measurements of serum glucose, sodium and potassium concentrations, serum cortisol levels, and thyroid function tests.** The endocrine evaluation of patients with micropenis is not standardized. **Magnetic resonance imaging (MRI) should be done to determine the anatomic integrity of the hypothalamus and the anterior pituitary gland as well as the midline structures of the midbrain.**

Before extensive evaluation of the hypothalamic-pituitary-testicular axis, **androgen therapy should be administered to determine the end-organ response. In general, testosterone enanthate, 25 mg monthly for 3 months, is given.** Although prolonged treatment might advance skeletal maturation, short courses of treatment do not affect height (Burstein et al, 1979). If the penis does not respond to testosterone, gender reassignment probably should be performed. Transdermal testosterone also has been utilized in these patients (Choi et al, 1993).

If androgen treatment in a neonate with a micropenis increases the size of the penis so that it falls within the normal range, what will happen at puberty? This is an unanswered question, but most think that the response of the penis to the increase in serum testosterone levels at puberty probably will not be striking. Indeed, in the hypogonadotropic hypogonadal penis there is experimental evidence that significant prepubertal exposure of the penis to androgens may significantly reduce the ultimate growth response to androgens (Husmann and Cain, 1994; McMahon et al, 1995). Preliminary clinical observations in children with hypogonadotropic hypogonadism also suggest that use of extensive androgen therapy before puberty may significantly reduce eventual penile size (Cain et al, 1994).

In an important long-term retrospective study, Reilly and Woodhouse (1989) reported on 20 patients with a primary diagnosis of micropenis in infancy. Of these, 8 patients were prepubertal and 12 were postpubertal; nearly all had received androgen therapy during childhood. Only one child in the prepubertal group had a stretched penile length above the tenth percentile. None of the adults had a penis in the satisfactory range. In the prepubertal group, all parents considered their children normal boys and thought that the penile appearance was satisfactory but expressed concern about the size of the penis and wondered whether sexual function in adulthood would be a problem. All boys stood to urinate. In the adult group, 9 of the 12 patients had a normal male appearance; three appeared eunuchoid despite regular testosterone therapy. All of the patients had a strong male identity, although half had experienced teasing because of the genital appearance. Nine of the twelve patients were sexually active. This study demonstrated that, **although the ultimate penile size in these patients may not fall within what is considered a normal range, the majority can still function satisfactorily.** Another option that may be beneficial for some of these patients is insertion of a penile prosthesis (Burkholder and Newell, 1983).

Penile Torsion

Penile torsion is a rotational defect of the penile shaft (Fig. 69–5). **Almost always it occurs in a counterclockwise direction, that is, to the left side.** In most cases, penile development is normal, and the condition is unrecognized until circumcision is performed or until the foreskin is retracted. Penile torsion may also be associated with hypospadias or a dorsal hood deformity without a urethral abnormality. In most cases of penile torsion, the median raphe spirals obliquely around the shaft. In general, the defect has primarily cosmetic significance, and **correction is unnecessary if the rotation is less than 60 to 90 degrees from the midline.**

Although the glans may be directed more than 90 degrees from the midline, the orientation of the corporeal bodies and the corpus spongiosum at the base of the penis is normal. In the milder forms of penile torsion, the penile skin may be degloved and simply reoriented so that the median raphe is restored to its normal position (Pomerantz et al, 1978). However, in boys with penile torsion greater than or equal to 90 degrees, simply rearranging the skin on the shaft of the penis is insufficient. In these more severe forms of the disorder, the base of the penis must be mobilized so that dysgenic bands of tissue can be identified and incised. If the penis still remains rotated, correction may be accomplished by placing a nonabsorbable suture through the lateral aspect of the base of the corpora cavernosa on the side opposite

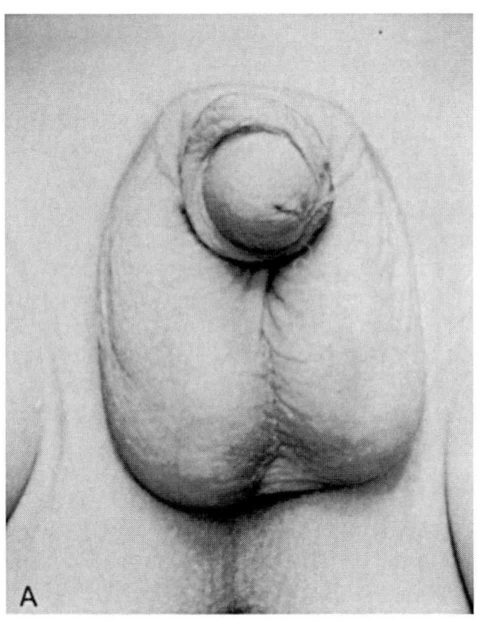

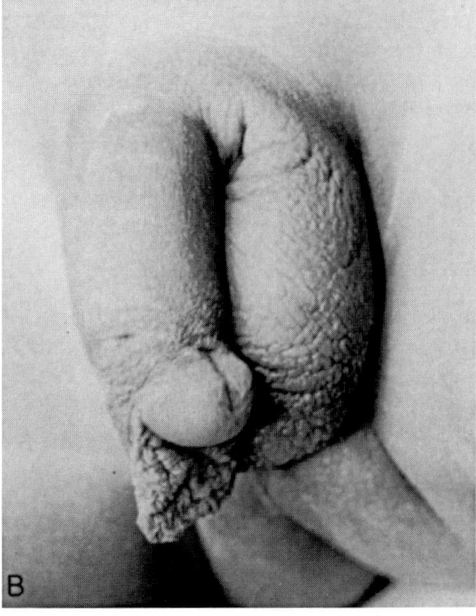

Figure 69–5. Penile torsion in a 1-year-old infant *(A)* and a 9-year-old child *(B)*.

the direction of the abnormal rotation (i.e., on the right corporeal body) and fixing it to the pubic symphysis dorsal to the penile shaft.

Lateral Curvature of the Penis

Lateral penile curvature usually is caused by overgrowth or hypoplasia of one corporeal body (Fitzpatrick, 1976). **Lateral penile curvature usually is congenital;** however, it is often unrecognized until later in childhood because the penis is normal when flaccid, and the disparity in corporeal size becomes apparent only during an erection. Surgical repair of this lesion involves degloving the penis and performing a modified Nesbit procedure, in which ellipses of tunica albuginea are excised from the site of maximum curvature to allow straightening of the penis (Gavrell, 1974). The intraoperative technique of artificial erection is critical to the procedure's success (Gittes and McLaughlin, 1974). During correction, one must be careful to avoid injury to the neurovascular bundles.

Aphallia

Penile agenesis results from failure of development of the genital tubercle. The disorder is rare and has an estimated incidence of 1 in 10,000,000 births; approximately 70 cases have been reported. In these cases, **the karyotype almost always is 46,XY, and the usual appearance is that of a well-developed scrotum with descended testes and an absent penile shaft** (Fig. 69–6). The anus generally is displaced anteriorly. The urethra often opens at the anal verge adjacent to a small skin tag; in other cases it opens into the rectum.

Associated malformations are common, including cryp-

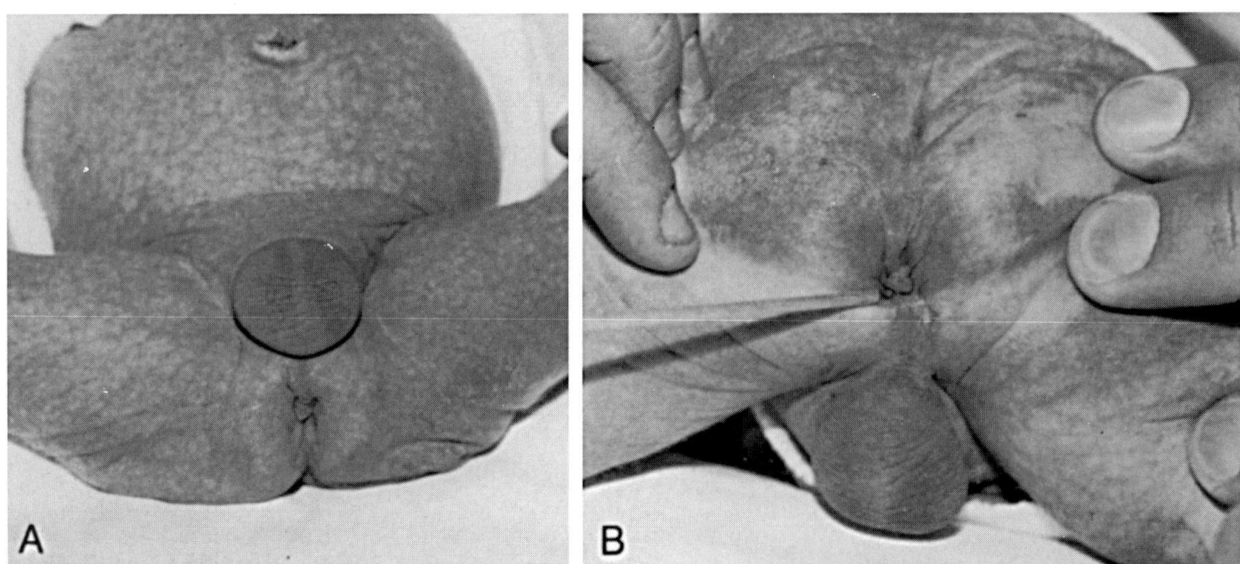

Figure 69–6. *A,* Neonate with aphallia. *B,* Urethral meatus at skin tag on anal verge.

torchidism, vesicoureteral reflux, horseshoe kidney, renal agenesis, imperforate anus, and musculoskeletal and cardiopulmonary abnormalities (Oesch et al, 1987; Skoog and Belman, 1989). **The connection between the genitourinary and gastrointestinal tract is variable** (Gilbert et al, 1990). Skoog and Belman (1989) reviewed 60 reports of aphallia and found that the more proximal the urethral meatus, the higher the incidence of other anomalies and the greater the likelihood of neonatal death. At least 60% of patients had a postsphincteric meatus located on a peculiar appendage at the anal verge (Fig. 69–6*B*). There were an average of 1.2 associated anomalies, and mortality was 13%. Among the 28% of patients who had a presphincteric urethral communication (prostatorectal fistula), mortality was 36%. In the 12% with a vesicorectal fistula and urethral atresia, there were an average of four anomalies per patient, and mortality was 100%.

Children with this lesion should be evaluated immediately with a karyotype and other appropriate studies to determine whether there are associated malformations of the urinary tract or other organ systems. **Gender reassignment is recommended in the newborn,** with orchiectomy and feminizing genitoplasty. At a later age, construction of a neovagina is necessary. Because of the proximity of the urethra to the rectum, this reconstruction can be a formidable procedure. Construction of an intestinal neovagina through a posterior sagittal and abdominal approach in two patients with penile agenesis has been described (Stolar et al, 1987).

Diphallia

Duplication of the penis is a rare anomaly and has a range of appearances from a small accessory penis (Fig. 69–7) **to complete duplication** (Hollowell et al, 1977). In some cases, each phallus has only one corporeal body and urethra, whereas others seem to be a variant of twinning, with each phallus having two corpora cavernosa and a urethra. The penes usually are unequal in size and lie side by side. Associated anomalies are common, including hypospadias, bifid scrotum, duplication of the bladder, renal agenesis or ectopia, and diastasis of the pubic symphysis (Rao and Chandrasekharam, 1980; Kapoor and Saha, 1987). Anal and cardiac anomalies also are common. Evaluation should include imaging of the entire urinary tract. Sonography has been reported to aid in assessment of the extent of phallic development (Marti-Bonmati et al, 1989). Treatment must be individualized to attain a satisfactory functional and cosmetic result.

Meatal Stenosis

Meatal stenosis is a condition that almost always is acquired and occurs following neonatal circumcision. One theory is that following disruption of the normal adhesions between the prepuce and glans and removal of the foreskin, a significant inflammatory reaction occurs, causing severe meatal inflammation and cicatrix formation and resulting in an extremely narrow meatus, a membranous web across the ventral aspect of the meatus, or an eccentric healing process that results in a prominent lip of ventral meatal tissue. Symptoms of meatal stenosis vary with the appearance. Another theory is that the abnormality results from meatal devascularization due to cutting the frenular artery during circumcision (Persad et al, 1995).

In most cases meatal stenosis does not become apparent until after the child is toilet trained. **If the meatus is pinpoint, boys void with a forceful, fine stream that has a great casting distance. Some boys have a dorsally deflected stream and prolonged voiding times.** Dysuria, frequency, terminal hematuria, and incontinence are symptoms that may lead to discovery of meatal stenosis but generally are not attributable to this abnormality. In other boys with meatal stenosis deflection of the urinary stream is the only sign. These concepts of meatal stenosis reflect the philosophy espoused by the Urology Section of the American Academy of Pediatrics (Committee from the Urology Section, 1978).

In a boy with suspected meatal stenosis, the meatus should be calibrated with a bougie à boule (Table 69–3) or assessed with infant sounds. Not infrequently, an asymptomatic boy with suspected meatal stenosis actually has a compliant meatus of normal caliber. If the meatus is diminished in size

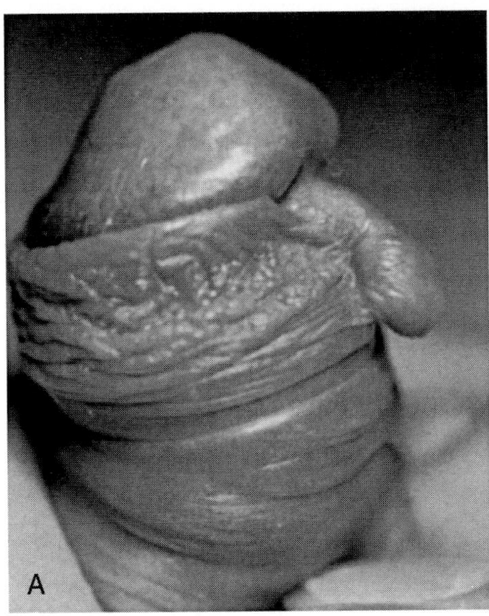

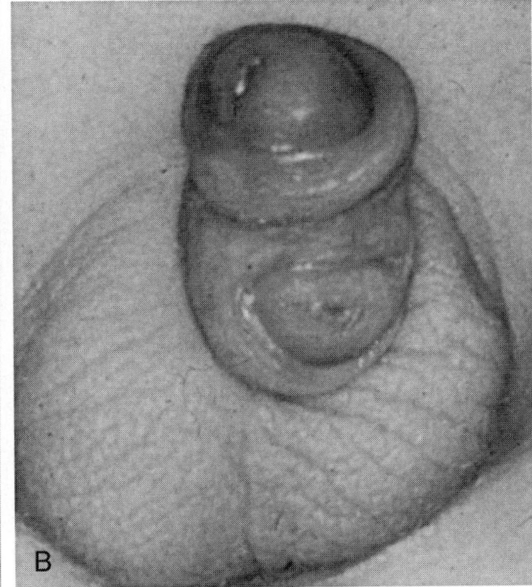

Figure 69–7. *A,* Diphallia. (Courtesy of Dr. Richard Hurwitz.) Urethra in diminutive phallic structure. *B,* Second example of diphallia.

Table 69–3. NORMAL MEATAL SIZE IN BOYS

Age	Size (Fr)	Number (%)	Size (Fr)	Number (%)
6 weeks–3 years	<8	62/425 (15)	10	363/425 (85)
4–10 years	tight 8	41/508 (8)	12	384/508 (76)
11–12 years	<10	4/85 (5)	14	64/85 (75)

Adapted from Litvak AS, Morris JA Jr, McRoberts JW: Normal size of the urethral meatus in boys. J Urol 1976; 115:736; and Morton HG: Meatus size in 1,000 circumcised children from two weeks to sixteen years of age. J Fla Med Assoc 1986; 50:137.

or if the child has abnormal voiding symptoms, a renal and bladder ultrasound examination is indicated. Furthermore, if the child has a history of UTIs, a voiding cystourethrogram should be done also. However, **meatal stenosis rarely causes obstructive changes in the urinary tract.** In boys with UTIs, it is often uncertain whether the infection is the result of meatal stenosis. In a series of 280 children with meatal stenosis, 5% of the patients had surgically significant lesions on voiding cystourethrograms (VCUG), and only 1% had upper tract abnormalities (Noe and Dale, 1975). All of the patients with radiologic findings had experienced UTIs.

In most cases, meatoplasty can be accomplished in the physician's office using EMLA cream for local anesthesia (Cartwright and Snow, 1996). In addition, 1% lidocaine with 1:100,000 epinephrine may be infiltrated into the ventral web with a 26-gauge needle for local anesthesia and vasoconstriction. A ventral incision is made toward the frenulum long enough to provide a meatus of normal caliber, which can be checked with the bougie. The urethral mucosa is sutured to the skin with fine chromic catgut sutures. If the procedure is performed under general anesthesia, the bladder may be filled with saline and compressed manually to be certain that the stream is straight. **Cystoscopy is unnecessary unless the child has obstructive symptoms and has not had a VCUG.**

When meatal stenosis is congenital, it occurs primarily in neonates with coronal or subcoronal hypospadias. Obstruction in these cases is unusual, but occasionally UTI occurs or catheterization is necessary during hospitalization and meatoplasty is necessary.

In rare cases a boy with suspected meatal stenosis and obstructive symptoms may have an anterior urethral valve in the fossa navicularis (Scherz et al, 1987). Another form of meatal stenosis that can result in urinary retention is balanitis xerotica obliterans. In these cases, application of steroid cream may be effective in reducing the risk of recurrent meatal stenosis.

Congenital Urethral Fistula

A rare anomaly is the congenital urethral fistula, in which the urethra and meatus are normal and a urethrocutaneous fistula is present, usually coronal or subcoronal (Fig. 69–8).

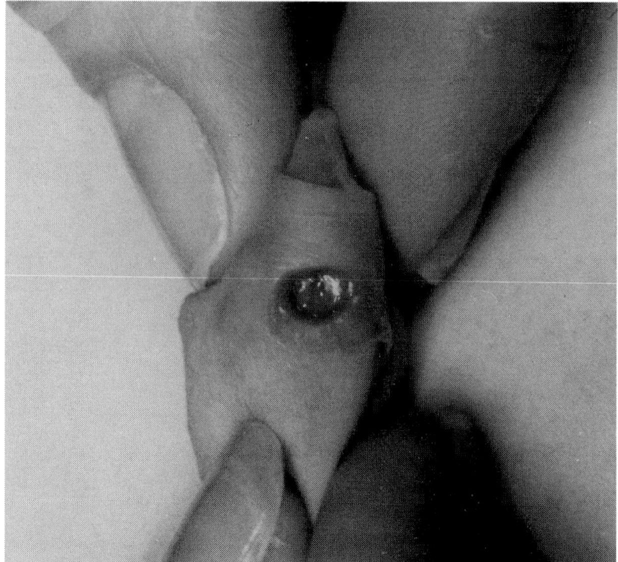

Figure 69–8. Infant with subcoronal congenital urethral fistula.

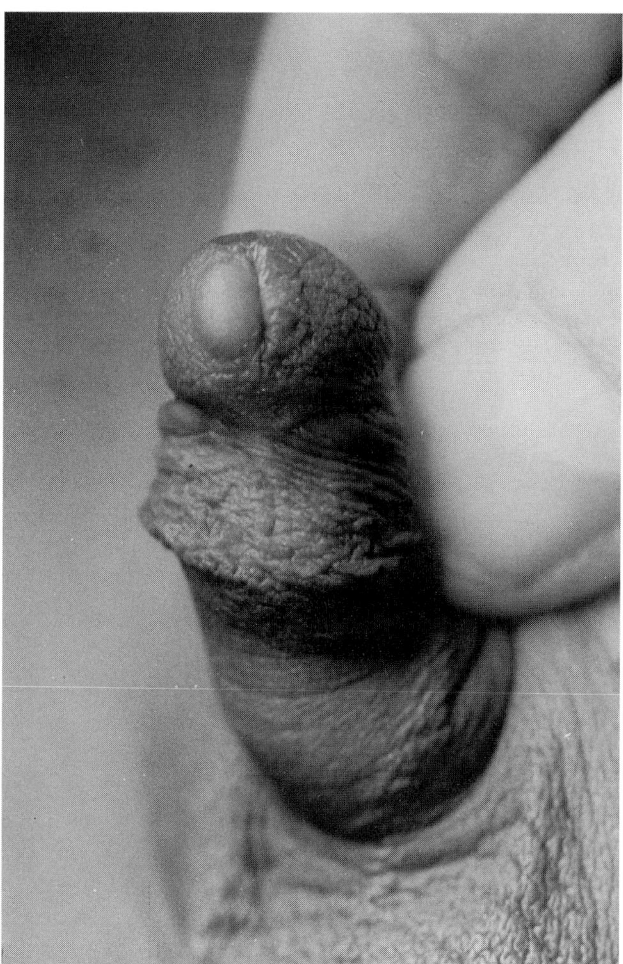

Figure 69–9. Example of parameatal urethral cyst.

This abnormality usually is an isolated deformity, but it may be associated with imperforate anus or ventral chordee (Ritchey et al, 1994). In the patient portrayed in Figure 69–8, at birth there was a small ventral penile cyst, resembling an epithelial inclusion cyst, that ruptured at 1 to 2 weeks of age and became a small fistula. The cause of congenital urethral fistula is unknown but probably involves a focal defect in the urethral plate that prevents fusion of the urethral folds. Some reported patients have undergone circumcision before diagnosis (Tennenbaum and Palmer, 1994), raising the possibility that in some of these cases the fistula may have been iatrogenic rather than congenital. Treatment usually consists of one of two techniques: (1) the fistula can be circumscribed and then closed in multiple layers, similar to a urethrocutaneous fistula after hypospadias repair, or (2) if the glans bridge is thin, the ventral glans can be opened through the distal urethra, and then the distal urethra is closed using a Thiersch-Duplay technique.

Parameatal Urethral Cysts

The parameatal urethral cyst is another rare anomaly (Fig. 69–9). Shiraki (1975) suggested that these cysts may result from occlusion of paraurethral ducts, whereas in other cases they may result from faulty preputial separation from the glans along the coronal sulcus. The cyst wall has been reported to consist of transitional and squamous as well as columnar epithelium (Hill and Ashken, 1977).

Scrotal Anomalies

Penoscrotal Transposition (Scrotal Engulfment)

Penoscrotal transposition may be complete or partial (Figs. 69–10 and 69–11). **Its less severe forms have been termed bifid scrotum, doughnut scrotum, prepenile scrotum, and shawl scrotum.** Frequently, the condition occurs in conjunction with perineal, scrotal, or penoscrotal hypospadias with chordee. The condition also has been associated with caudal regression (Lage et al, 1987), Aarskog syndrome (Shinkawa et al, 1983), and sex chromosome abnormalities (Cohen-Addad et al, 1985; Yamaguchi et al, 1989). Presumably, this anomaly results from incomplete or failed inferomedial migration of the labioscrotal swellings.

When the abnormality is associated with severe hypospadias, hypospadias repair is generally accomplished using a transverse preputial island flap in conjunction with Thiersch-Duplay tubularization of the proximal urethra. To minimize the possibility of devascularizing the preputial flap, correction of the scrotal engulfment generally is done as a second-stage procedure 6 months later (Elder and Duckett, 1990). If the penis is normal, scrotoplasty can be accomplished when the child is 6 to 12 months of age.

Scrotoplasty is begun by circumscribing the superior aspects of each half of the vertical aspect of the scrotum and extending these incisions laterally to include at least half of the scrotum (see Fig. 69–11). The medial aspects of the incision are joined on the ventral aspect of the penis, and the incision is carried down the midline along the median raphe for 4 or 5 cm. Prior to making the incision, it is helpful to infiltrate the skin with 1% lidocaine with 1:100,000 epinephrine to diminish bleeding. Traction sutures are placed on the superior aspect of the scrotal flaps, and these are dissected out in the areolar layer (Fig. 69–12). Deeper dissection may result in cutting the tunica vaginalis, which is unnecessary and may injure the spermatic cord. The scrotal wings are rotated medially under the penis and are sutured together in the midline in an everted manner. During this dissection, moderate oozing from the areolar tissue frequently occurs, and it may be necessary to leave a small dependent drain in place for 24 to 48 hours. In many

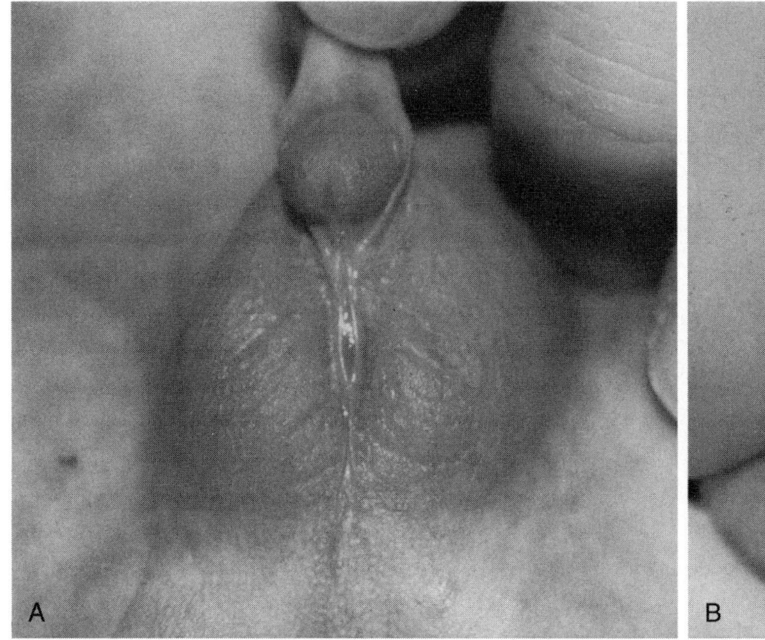

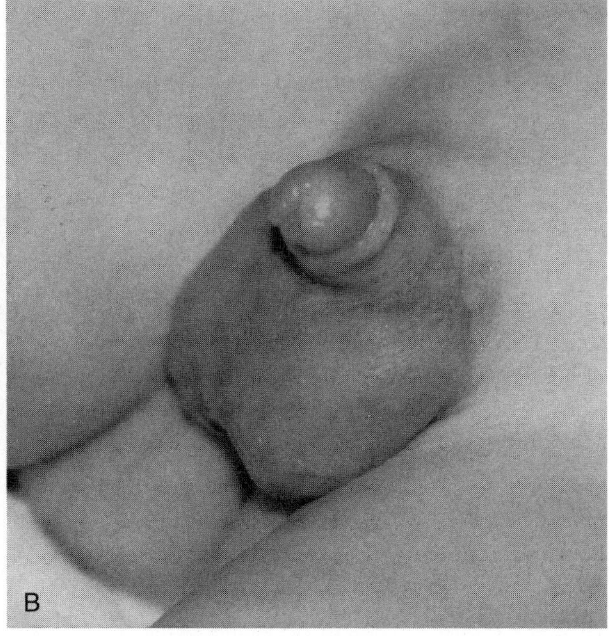

Figure 69–10. *A,* Scrotal engulfment in child with penoscrotal hypospadias. *B,* Same patient following transverse preputial island flap hypospadias repair and scrotoplasty.

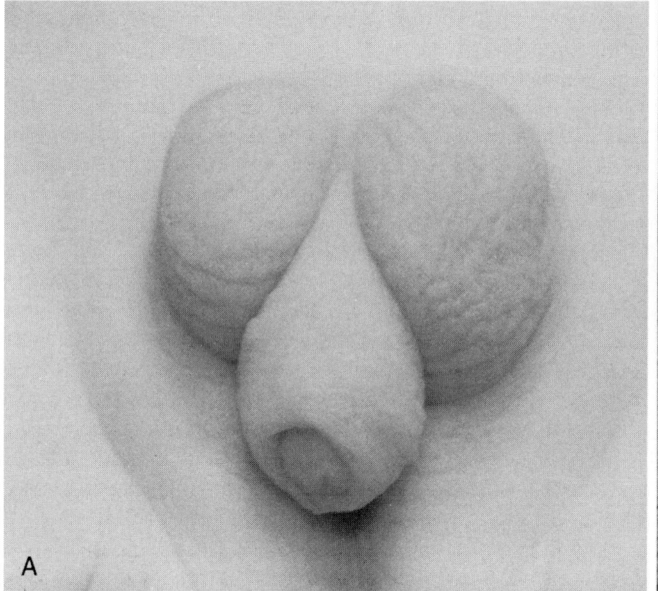

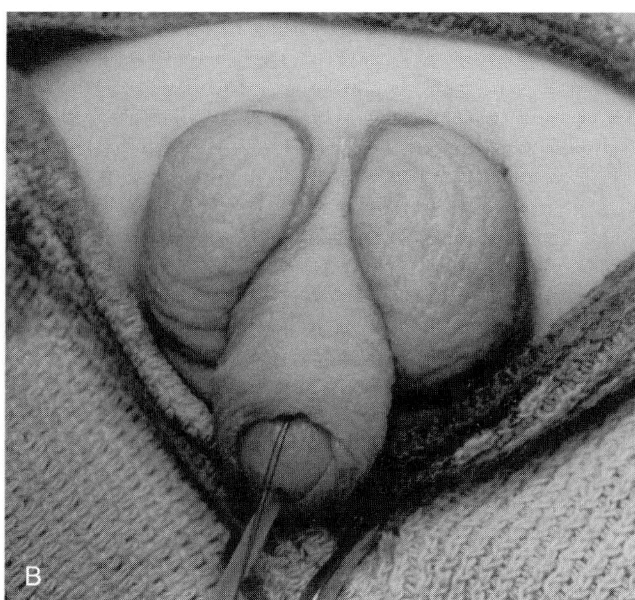

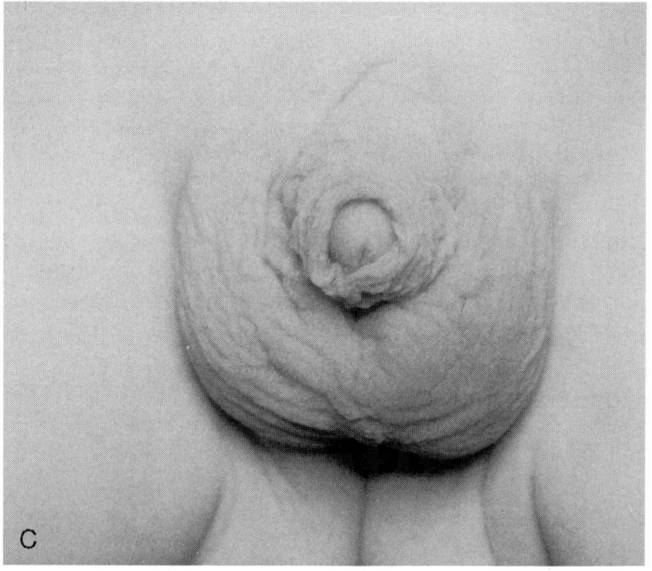

Figure 69–11. *A,* Complete penoscrotal transposition. The urethral meatus is at the tip of the glans, but the urethra is short. *B,* Skin flaps for scrotoplasty. *C,* Completed two-stage repair; first stage, scrotoplasty; second stage, urethroplasty.

cases, the bare area on either side of the penis can be closed. However, in more severe cases of penoscrotal transposition, dorsal interposition flaps may be necessary, allowing caudal advancement of the skin of the abdominal wall (Dresner, 1982). Usually, scrotoplasty can be accomplished as an outpatient procedure.

Ectopic Scrotum

Ectopic scrotum is rare and refers to the anomalous position of one hemiscrotum along the inguinal canal. Most commonly, it is suprainguinal (Fig. 69–13), although it may also be infrainguinal or perineal (Lamm and Kaplan, 1977; Elder and Jeffs, 1982). This anomaly has been associated with cryptorchidism, inguinal hernia, and exstrophy as well as the popliteal pterygium syndrome (Cunningham et al, 1989). In one review, 70% of patients with a suprainguinal ectopic scrotum exhibited ipsilateral upper urinary tract anomalies, including renal agenesis, renal dysplasia, and ectopic ureter (Elder and Jeffs, 1982). Another study indicated that an associated perineal lipoma was found in 83% of these children; 68% of those with a lipoma had no associated anomalies, whereas 100% of those without a lipoma had associated genital or renal malformations. Consequently, children with this anomaly should undergo upper urinary tract imaging. Because the embryology of the gubernaculum and scrotum is intimately related chronologically and anatomically, it seems likely that the ectopic scrotum results from a defect in distal gubernacular formation that prevents migration of the labioscrotal swellings. Scrotoplasty and orchiopexy may be performed at 6 to 12 months of age, or earlier if other surgical procedures are necessary.

Bifid Scrotum

Bifid scrotum refers to the deformity in which the labioscrotal folds are completely separated, and nearly always this anomaly is associated with proximal hypospadias (Fig. 69–14).

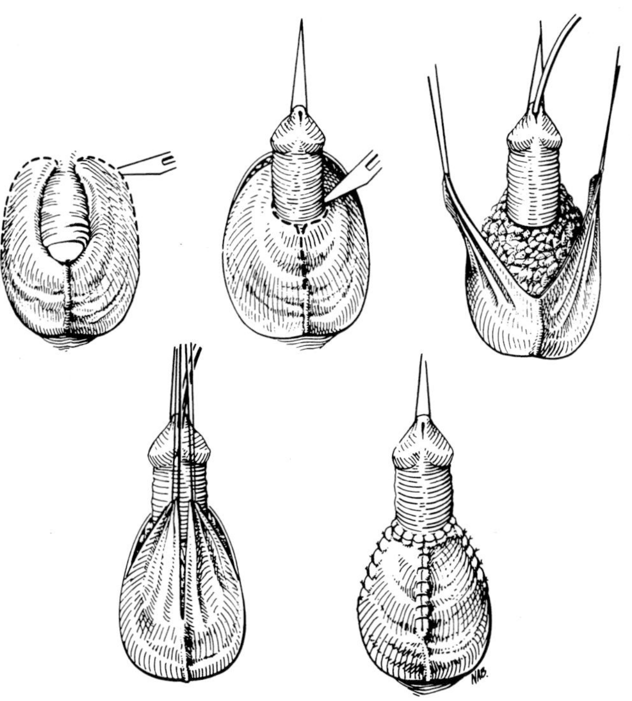

Figure 69–12. Repair of penoscrotal transposition. (See discussion in text.)

Scrotal Hypoplasia

Scrotal hypoplasia is the underdevelopment of one or both sides of the scrotum. This anomaly **occurs most commonly in boys with an undescended testis** (Fig. 69–15) **and frequently is noted in infants with genital ambiguity.** The deformity probably results from lack of gubernacular swelling of the labioscrotal folds.

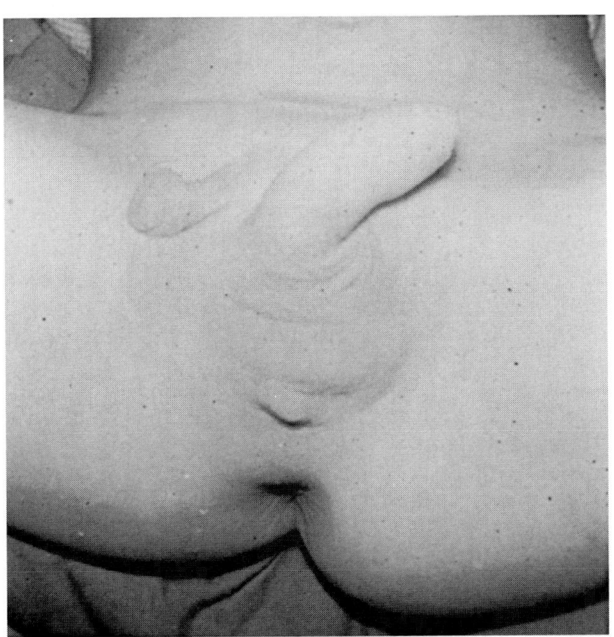

Figure 69–13. Child with ectopic scrotum.

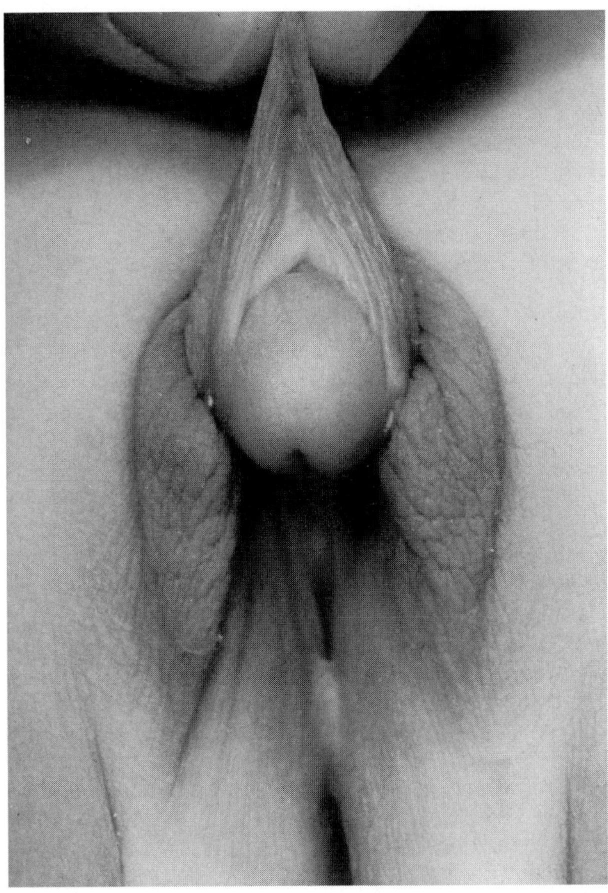

Figure 69–14. Child with bifid scrotum and perineal hypospadias.

Scrotal Hemangioma

Congenital hemangiomas are common and affect the genitalia in approximately 1% of cases (Alter et al, 1993).

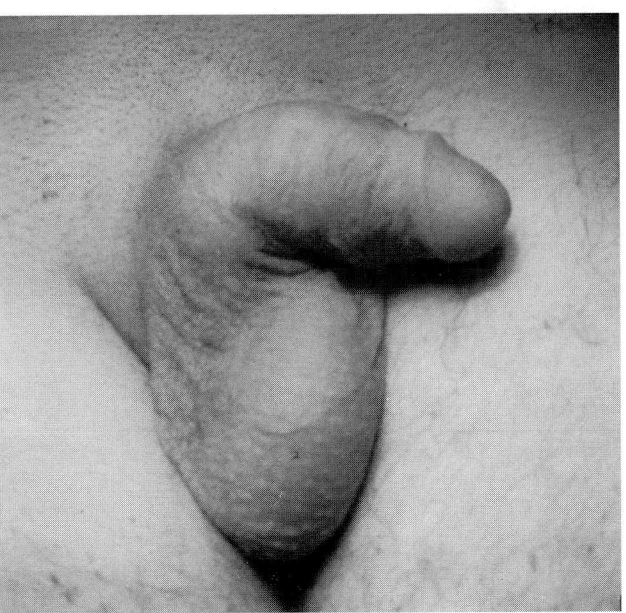

Figure 69–15. Boy with hypoplastic right hemiscrotum and right undescended testis.

Strawberry hemangiomas, the most common type, result from proliferation of immature capillary vessels. These are also categorized as cutaneous hemangiomas because they occur on the skin. Although the lesions may undergo a period of rapid growth lasting 3 to 6 months, **gradual involution is common, and most lesions require no treatment** (Casale and Menashe, 1989). If ulceration develops, intervention is necessary to prevent complications from bleeding. The most popular form of therapy is short-term oral steroid therapy. In some cases, surgical excision is necessary.

Recently, there has been interest in the use of the laser in managing these lesions. In 1990 Smith reported using an argon laser to treat a bladder hemangioma because the pigments melanin and hemoglobin absorb the argon laser, which emits a wave length of 488 to 524 nm. Then, because of limited tissue penetration, he abandoned the argon laser in favor of the neodymium:YAG laser. However, the high degree of scatter with resultant tissue injury and the twofold increase in depth of penetration makes use of this laser potentially dangerous in the treatment of cutaneous hemangiomas of the genitalia in the pediatric population. **The potassium thiophosphate (KTP) laser** is a frequency-doubled neodymium:YAG laser. The 1060-nm wave length of the neodymium:YAG laser is passed through a potassium thiophosphate crystal in this laser, producing a **wave length of 532 nm, which is highly absorbed in hemoglobin and produces less tissue scatter.** Preliminary work with the potassium thiophosphate laser in children with cutaneous and urethral hemangiomas has been encouraging (Kennedy et al, 1993).

Subcutaneous hemangiomas, also referred to as **cavernous hemangiomas,** are much less common than the cutaneous variety (Ferrer and McKenna, 1995). They may be detected at birth or later in life. In contrast to cutaneous hemangiomas, which tend to involute, cavernous hemangiomas tend to enlarge gradually. Physical examination reveals a "bag of worms" sensation similar to that of a varicocele, although the lesions tend to be firm and do not decompress when the patient is recumbent. Because examination does not disclose the extent of the lesion, ultrasound is advised to delineate the size of the hemangioma. Definitive treatment by en bloc resection is advised.

A related condition is the **scrotal arteriovenous malformation** (Sule et al, 1993). Although this lesion is thought to be congenital, it usually is not diagnosed until the teenage years or young adulthood. Examination discloses a loud bruit over the lesion. Treatment consists of surgical excision, and preoperative angioembolization may be helpful to reduce the size of the mass and the risk of bleeding.

Miscellaneous Genital Anomalies

Cysts of the median raphe can occur on the perineum, scrotum, or shaft of the penis (Little et al, 1992). The lesions probably result from epithelial rests that become buried during the urethral infolding process. Excision is recommended unless the cysts are small and asymptomatic.

Juvenile xanthogranulomas appear as one or more lesions of rapid onset; they measure 2 to 20 mm in diameter and are orange, gold, or brown in color. These lesions can affect the penis (Hautmann and Bachor, 1993) or scrotum (Goulding and Traylor, 1983). As many as 20% are present at birth. The lesion often is self-limited, and a period of 1 year of expectant waiting is advised to avoid potentially unnecessary ablative genital surgery.

Meconium peritonitis may cause genital manifestations on occasion, among them meconium hydrocele (Ring et al, 1989) and congenital rupture of the scrotum (Pippi Salle et al, 1992). When an unusual inflammatory condition of the scrotum is detected, one should suspect meconium peritonitis and proceed with the appropriate evaluation.

FEMALE GENITAL ANOMALIES

Although minor variations in the appearance of the female genitalia are common, significant abnormalities are uncommon and may represent a disorder in sexual differentiation. The female reproductive system is derived primarily from the müllerian ducts. **In the absence of androgen production by the fetal ovary, the wolffian ducts regress, and in the absence of müllerian-inhibiting factor, the paired müllerian ducts, lateral to the wolffian ducts, move medially and fuse in the midline. The fused müllerian ducts join the urogenital sinus at the müllerian tubercle, and, following fusion of their distal portions and absorption of the septum, the single uterovaginal canal is formed. The fused portion of the müllerian ducts forms the uterus and upper two thirds of the vagina,** whereas the proximal nonfused portions form the fallopian tubes.

The presence of a normal wolffian duct contiguous with the müllerian system is important for the latter's development (Gruenwald, 1941). An abnormality in the wolffian duct may result in anomalous differentiation of the internal female genitalia. In the absence of androgen, the primitive external genital anlagen develop into female external genitalia. The genital tubercle forms the clitoris, the genital swellings fuse posteriorly to form the posterior fourchette and enlarge laterally to form the labia majora, and the genital folds develop into the labia minora.

Labial/Clitoral Anomalies

Labial Adhesion

Labial adhesion usually results from chronic inflammation of the vulva and rarely is present at birth. It also has been associated with sexual abuse. Labioscrotal fusion is a different entity from labial adhesion and refers to virilization of the female external genitalia. In many girls, labial adhesions are asymptomatic (Fig. 69–16). However, in some cases, the introitus is nearly completely sealed, which can lead to **vaginal voiding and classically results in urinary dribbling when the child stands after voiding.** In addition, **urinary stasis predisposes the child to UTIs** (Leung and Robson, 1993). At times, the condition is not recognized until the child is to be catheterized for a VCUG.

Treatment of labial adhesions traditionally consists of application of estrogen cream to the labia three times daily for 7 to 10 days. However, the cream rarely is effective, **and in most cases, the adhesion must be lysed manu-**

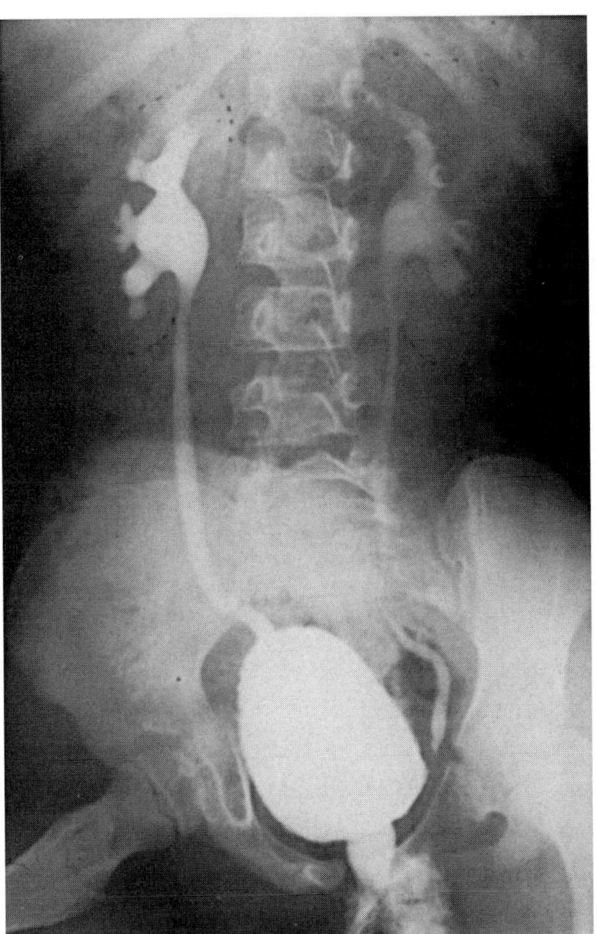

Figure 69–24. Voiding cystourethrogram (VCUG) demonstrating spinning top urethra and bilateral vesicoureteral reflux.

the distal third of the urethra and that in all cases the bougie à boule passed easily through the bladder neck. Furthermore, vigorous overdilation of the urethra (No. 28 to 32 Fr) reportedly often resulted in restoration of a normal voiding pattern and elimination of recurrent UTIs (Lyon and Smith, 1963). The site of distal urethral narrowing came to be known as Lyon's ring.

At birth there is no apparent evidence of the distal urethral ring (Fisher et al, 1969). However, during the first few months, the ring reportedly develops as a normal anatomic structure that calibrates at No. 14 Fr at 2 years of age and at 16 Fr between the ages of 4 and 10 (Lyon and Tanagho, 1965). At puberty, the ring disappears. Thus, it has been speculated that absence of estrogens leads to the development of the lesion.

Tanagho and Smith (1966) reported that the inner longitudinal detrusor muscle fibers continue as the inner longitudinal fibers of the urethra, the outer longitudinal detrusor fibers continue into the urethra as the outer circular coat of fibers, and the middle circular fibers of the detrusor do not enter the urethra. The striated external sphincter surrounds the two layers of urethral musculature, and the inner and outer layers of urethral musculature appear to insert into a dense collagenous tissue ring situated in the distal urethra. The overabundance of collagen was thought to encroach upon and indent the lumen of the distal urethral segment, which was the anatomic basis of the ring (Lyon, 1974). It was thought that rupture of the ring was accomplished by urethral dilation. Lyon (1974) noted that adequate urethral dilation should result in urethral bleeding and that a large catheter should be placed for 30 to 60 minutes as a tamponade. Lyon and Marshall (1971) reported that in the 15% to 20% of children who continued to experience chronic bacilluria, repeat calibration disclosed a persistent "ring" of between 26 and 30 Fr that did not require dilation. Subsequently, internal urethrotomy also became a popular method of dealing with the obstructing ring, and several modifications of this procedure were developed (Halverstadt and Leadbetter, 1968).

At that time, however, Immergut and co-workers (1967) reported the mean size of the urethral meatus and distal urethra in 136 girls undergoing tonsillectomy (Table 69–4), and it became apparent that these measurements were not dissimilar from those previously reported by Lyon in girls with recurrent UTIs. Subsequently, Immergut and Wahman (1968) demonstrated that the urethral caliber in 77 girls with recurrent UTIs was larger than the urethral size in normal uninfected girls. Graham and colleagues (1967) reported that dilation of a urethra that calibrated at No. 14 Fr or less was most likely to result in improvement in symptoms; however, they also noted that the narrow caliber was often probably coincidental and actually normal in the majority of girls in whom it was found. Later, Kaplan and co-workers (1974) compared urethral dilation, internal urethrotomy, and antimicrobial therapy in girls with UTIs and found no differences in treatment results.

What, then, accounts for the abnormal urethral appearance? Many of these girls have interrupted, staccato streams that are consistent with obstruction. Johnston and associates (1978) speculated that this finding is more likely due to different degrees of distensibility of various parts of the urethra and that the spinning top is normal in girls with high voiding rates. **The spinning top urethra probably is related more to detrusor instability or detrusor-sphincter dyssynergia** (Saxton et al, 1988). Hausegger and colleagues (1991) studied 102 girls referred for VCUG and found that 28 (27%) had a spinning top urethra. Of the 28, 16 (57%) had bladder instability on urodynamic investigation. Conversely, of the 29 girls with bladder instability, 13 (45%) had a normal urethra. Consequently, **the spinning top urethra should be interpreted as a sign of possible bladder instability, and urge incontinence and squatting to prevent loss of urine are common symptoms of this.** Many of these girls also have recurrent UTIs, for which combined therapy with anticholinergic medications and antimicrobial suppression is indicated.

Currently, most girls with UTIs or incontinence, or both, respond to medical management and do not require cysto-

Table 69–4. CALIBER OF NORMAL FEMALE URETHRA

Age (years)	Median (Fr)
2–4	14
6–10	16
12	20
≥14	24

Adapted from Immergut M, Culp D, Flocks RH: The urethral caliber in normal female children. J Urol 1967; 97:693.

scopic evaluation. Consequently, urethral calibration and dilation is performed infrequently at present. However, if a girl is undergoing endoscopic evaluation for these problems and the urethra is found to be less than No. 14 to 16 Fr, dilation to these sizes often is performed. Internal urethrotomy should be avoided because overvigorous incision of the bladder neck in these girls can result in incontinence (Kessler and Constantinou, 1986).

Hypospadias

Hypospadias in an otherwise normal girl is a rare condition and when present is usually not symptomatic. Generally, it becomes significant only as a result of difficulty with urethral catheterization. Although it might be thought to result in symptoms of vaginal voiding (i.e., postmicturition incontinence), girls who experience vaginal voiding almost always have normal external genital anatomy. A form of hypospadias may occur in girls with urogenital sinus abnormalities.

Vaginal Anomalies

Hydrocolpos refers to the accumulation of secretions in the vagina caused by excessive intrauterine stimulation of the infant's cervical mucous glands by maternal estrogen in association with obstruction of the genital tract by an intact hymen, vaginal membrane, or vaginal atresia. Hydrometrocolpos refers to the accumulation of secretions in the vagina and uterus. These two conditions generally result in a lower midline abdominal or bulging perineal mass in the newborn or infant. Hematometrocolpos refers to the accumulation of menstrual products caused by an imperforate hymen or other obstruction at menarche. These terms do not define the cause of the obstruction.

Vaginal anomalies may be classifed by their etiology (Table 69–5). **Disorders of vertical fusion result either from an abnormality in caudal development of the müllerian duct and/or canalization of the vaginal plate, whereas disorders of medial fusion result from failure of medial fusion of the two müllerian ducts.** Internal genital anomalies occur in one third of girls with anorectal anomalies (Fleming et al, 1986) and are common in girls with urogenital sinus and cloacal anomalies also. **Because differentiation of the müllerian duct is intimately associated with development of the wolffian duct, females with vaginal agenesis or disorders of medial fusion often have associated congenital upper urinary tract anomalies. In contrast, obstructive disorders of vertical fusion often cause secondary obstructive effects on the urinary tract that resolve following treatment, but congenital urinary tract anomalies are uncommon. The *Mayer-Rokitansky syndrome* generally refers to vaginal agenesis.** However,

Table 69–5. CONGENITAL VAGINAL ANOMALIES

Disorders of Vertical Fusion
Obstructive
Vaginal agenesis
Transverse vaginal septum
Imperforate hymen
Nonobstructive
Incomplete transverse vaginal septum
Disorders of Medial Fusion
Obstructive
Unilateral obstructing vaginal septum
Nonobstructive
Longitudinal vaginal septum
Vaginal duplication

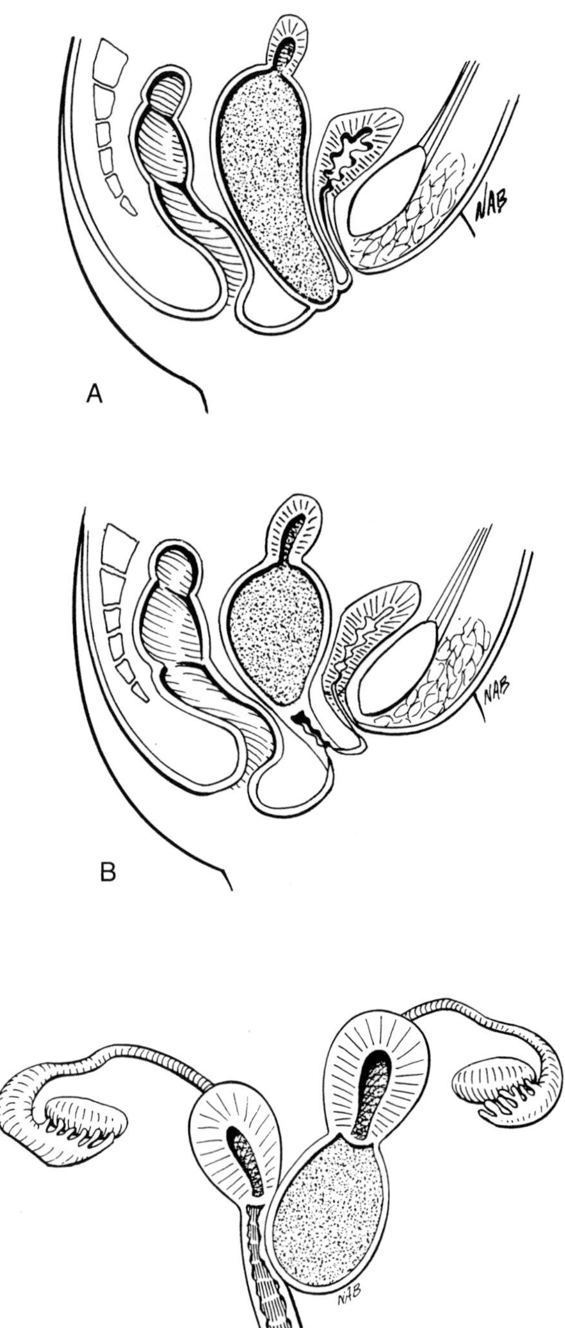

Figure 69–25. *A,* Hydrocolpos secondary to imperforate hymen. *B,* Hydrocolpos secondary to high transverse vaginal septum. *C,* Obstructed hemivagina in patient with uterus didelphys.

it has been proposed that the name be applied to the entire spectrum of müllerian anomalies, with or without renal anomalies, in genotypic and phenotypic females with normal endocrine status, specifically excluding those with associated anorectal or cloacal malformations (Tarry et al, 1986).

Disorders of Vertical Fusion

***Vaginal agenesis* occurs in 1 of every 4000 to 5000 females and is the second most common cause of primary infertility in women after gonadal dysgenesis** (Rock and Azziz, 1987). **Vaginal agenesis probably results from incomplete or absent canalization of the vaginal plate,** which begins at the 11th week of gestation and is completed by the 20th week. **Characteristically, the uterus in these patients is rudimentary without a lumen, although normal fallopian tubes are present, and ovarian function is normal** (Fraser et al, 1973). Approximately one third of these women have renal anomalies (Griffin et al, 1976), most commonly renal agenesis or ectopia. In addition, **renal fusion anomalies, such as horseshoe kidney, are common.** Furthermore, skeletal anomalies have been reported in 12% of these patients (Griffin et al, 1976; Chitayat et al, 1987), two thirds of whom have anomalies of the spine, ribs, or limbs, including polydactyly. The MURCS association of anomalies refers to *mü*llerian duct aplasia, *r*enal agenesis, and *c*ervicothoracic *s*omite abnormalities (Duncan et al, 1979).

Vaginal agenesis usually is diagnosed at puberty in girls with amenorrhea. The external genitalia are normal in appearance, and the vagina is either absent or may consist of a shallow pouch of 2 to 3 cm deep. However, the diagnosis should also be suspected in any female child with an absent or blind vagina.

Timing of vaginoplasty is variable. Traditionally, it has been performed late in the teenage years, but recently interest has been shown in performing vaginoplasty early in childhood (Sheldon et al, 1994). It is generally accomplished with either a full-thickness skin graft or an isolated segment of ileum or sigmoid colon (Hensle and Dean, 1992). In girls with an associated cloacal anomaly, a posterior sagittal approach often provides optimal exposure to the vagina (Hendren, 1992).

Another disorder of vertical fusion is the *transverse vaginal septum*, which can be high, in the middle third of the vagina, or in the lower third of the vagina (Fig. 69–25); it affects 1 in 80,000 females. **High transverse septa are the most common, occurring in 46% of cases, whereas obstruction in the middle or lower third of the vagina is found in 35% and 19% of cases, respectively** (Rock et al, 1982). **These anomalies result from abnormal canalization of the vaginal plate.** Septa in the upper part of the vagina frequently are incomplete, whereas in the lower third of the vagina, the septa are usually obstructive (Rock and Azziz, 1987).

The diagnosis of transverse vaginal septum generally is made following the development of hydrocolpos, which is detectable on bimanual examination. At times, the mass may be large enough to obstruct venous return from the lower extremities, resulting in lymphedema (Tran et al,

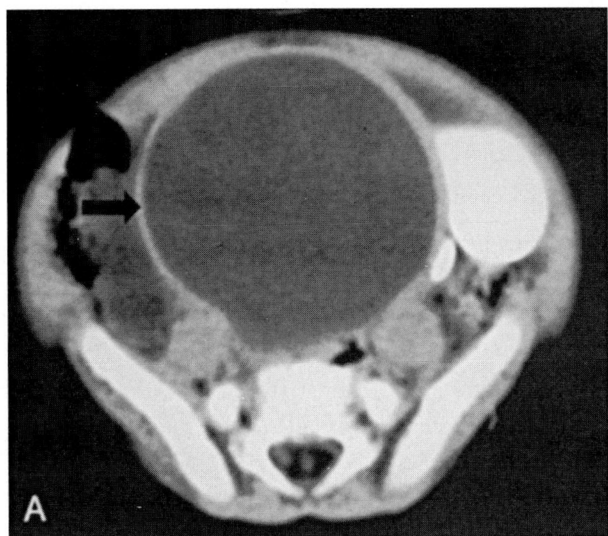

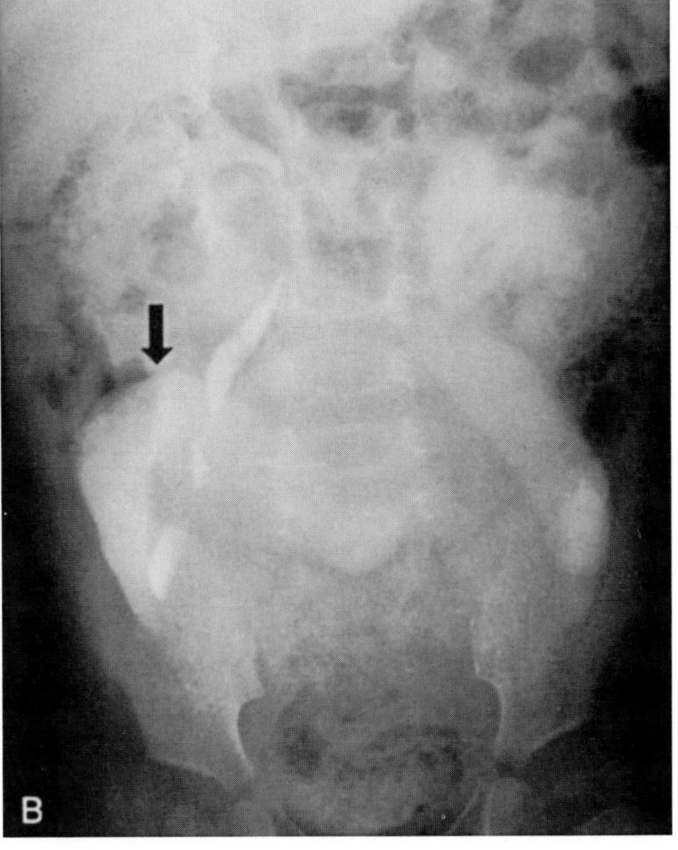

Figure 69–26. *A,* Computed tomography scan in an infant with hydrocolpos *(arrow)* secondary to transverse vaginal septum. *B,* Intravenous pyelogram (IVP) showing left hydroureteronephrosis and bilateral ureteral deviation. (Arrow points to displaced bladder.)

1987). Abdominal ultrasonography demonstrates a large midline sonolucent mass with debris. **Upper urinary tract obstruction is common,** and an IVP or CT scan may demonstrate hydronephrosis, whereas a VCUG may show anterior displacement of the bladder (Fig. 69–26). At times, **percutaneous needle aspiration and injection of contrast material may aid in the diagnosis.** In the infant who does not develop an abdominal mass, the transverse septum is not detected until adolescence, when the patient develops amenorrhea, cyclic abdominal pain, and an abdominal mass secondary to hematocolpos.

Treatment of an obstructing transverse vaginal septum varies, depending on the anatomy, and often an exploratory laparotomy is necessary (Rock and Azziz, 1987). Prompt therapy of an obstructing transverse vaginal septum is important because otherwise ultimate fertility may be decreased, apparently because of a high incidence of endometriosis resulting from prolonged obstruction of menses (Rock et al, 1982). In a female with a high transverse vaginal septum or vaginal obstruction associated with a urogenital sinus abnormality, the Ramenofsky-Raffensperger abdominoperineal pull-through vaginoplasty (Ramenofsky and Raffensperger, 1971; Fig. 69–27) may be indicated.

In the neonate, hydrocolpos secondary to an *imperforate hymen* usually appears as a bulging cystic interlabial mass (see Fig. 69–21). In addition, a suprapubic abdominal mass may be evident. An imperforate hymen usually is not associated with other congenital anomalies. Preoperatively, sonographic assessment of the urinary tract should be done; if hydronephrosis is present, it should be monitored until it resolves following definitive therapy. Treatment of an imperforate hymen is hymenotomy, using a cruciate incision and oversewing the cut edges with absorbable sutures. A small drain should be inserted through the introitus to prevent adhesion of the raw edges, and antibiotics are administered to prevent infection.

Disorders of Medial Fusion

The process of fusion of the paired müllerian structures can be arrested at any stage of development. If there is partial fusion of these structures, a *bicornuate uterus* with a single vagina results (Sayer and O'Reilly, 1986). If they are completely separated, *uterus didelphys* with *vaginal duplication* results. Often, one side of the duplex vagina is obstructed (see Fig. 69–25*C*; Burbige and Hensle, 1984), whereas in other cases there is a nonobstructing longitudinal septum. **An obstructed hemivagina and bicornuate uterus are almost always associated with ipsilateral renal agenesis** (Woolf and Allen, 1953; Gilsanz and Cleveland, 1982). Consequently, **women with unilateral renal agenesis should be evaluated radiologically for an anomaly of the female genital system.** Rarely, the vaginal duplication may extend through the lower third of the vagina

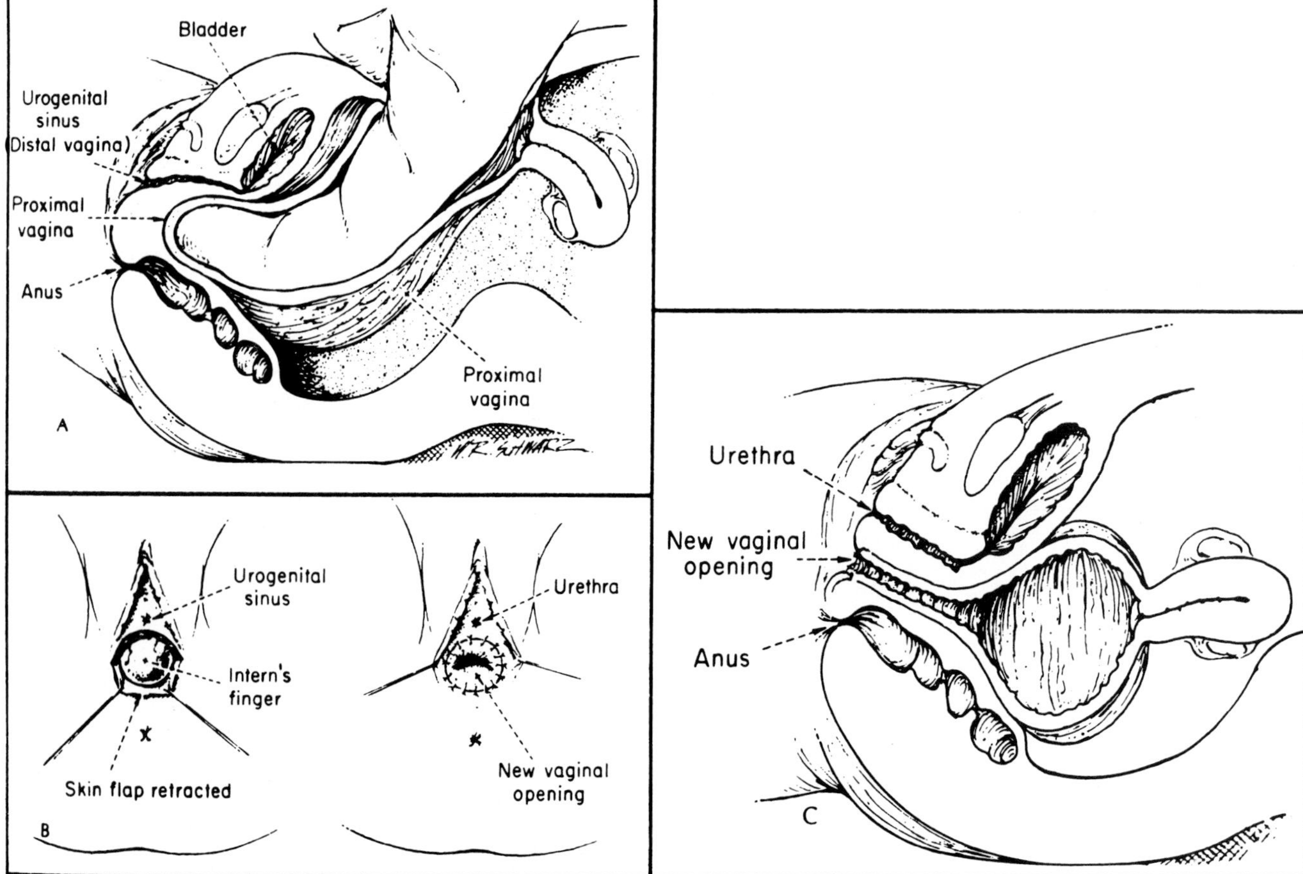

Figure 69–27. Ramenofsky-Raffensperger abdominoperineal pull-through vaginoplasty. (From Ramenofsky ML, Raffensperger JG: An abdominoperineal-vaginal pull-through for definitive treatment of hydrometrocolpos. J Pediatr Surg 1971; 6:381.)

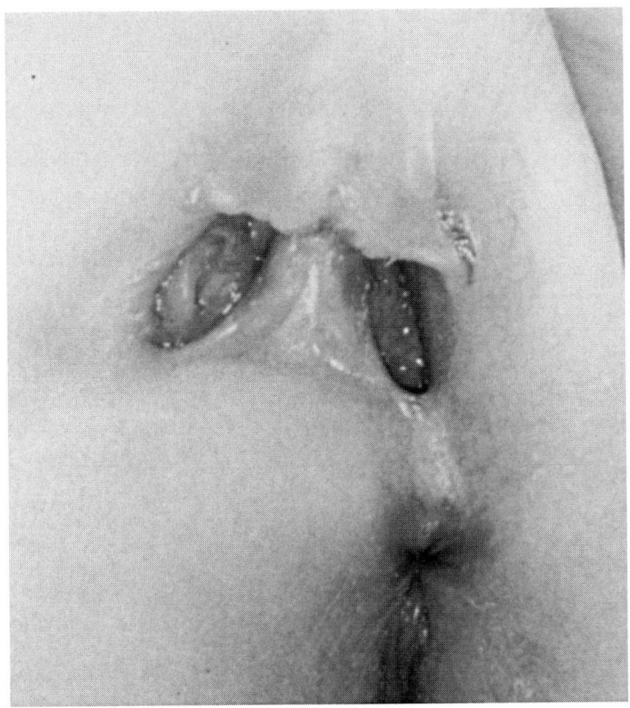

Figure 69–28. Infant with vaginal duplication.

and hymen (Fig. 69–28), probably secondary to incomplete caudal twinning.

The obstructed hemivagina may be detected in the neonate following detection of an abdominal mass on physical examination or ultrasound. However, it may not be detected until puberty in girls who experience cyclic abdominal pain and develop an abdominal mass. In these patients, one horn of the uterus functions normally, and thus menstrual flow is not affected (Foglia et al, 1987; Tolete-Velcek et al, 1989). The internal genital anatomy as well as the urinary tract must be evaluated carefully prior to definitive treatment. Often, the finding of unilateral agenesis helps to provide the diagnosis. In some cases, the distended chamber may be incised by a vaginal approach, whereas in others a pull-through vaginoplasty may be necessary. If one of the duplex uterine chambers is infected, it may have to be excised.

REFERENCES

Anomalies of the Male Genitalia

AAP Task Force on Circumcision: Report of the Task Force on Circumcision. Pediatrics 1989; 84:388.

Aaronson IA: Micropenis: Medical and surgical implications. J Urol 1994; 152:4.

Alter GJ, Trengove-Jones G, Horton CE Jr: Hemangioma of penis and scrotum. Urology 1993; 42:205.

Ben-Ari J, Merlob P, Mimouni F, Reisner SH: Characteristics of the male genitalia in the newborn: Penis. J Urol 1985; 134:521.

Bergeson PS, Hopkin RJ, Bailey RB Jr, et al: The inconspicuous penis. Pediatrics 1993; 92:794.

Berkhoff WBC, Scholtmeyer RJ, Tibboel D, Molenaar JC: Urogenital tract abnormalities associated with esophageal atresia and tracheoesophageal fistula. J Urol 1989; 141:362.

Burkholder GV, Newell ME: New surgical treatment for micropenis. J Urol 1983; 129:832.

Burstein S, Grumbach MM, Kaplan SL: Early determination of androgen-responsiveness is important in the management of microphallus. Lancet 1979; 2:193.

Cain MP, Levy J, Zimmerman D, Husmann DA: Micropenis secondary to hypogonadotropic hypogonadism: A clinical evaluation of early versus delayed hormonal therapy. Presented at the meeting of the Urology Section, American Academy of Pediatrics, Dallas, Texas, October 1994.

Cartwright PL, Snow BW: Urethral meatotomy in the office using EMLA anesthetic cream. J Urol 1996. In press.

Casale AJ, Menashe DS: Massive strawberry hemangioma of the male genitalia. J Urol 1989; 141:593.

Choi SK, Han SW, Kim DH, de Lignieres B: Transdermal dihydrohydrotestosterone therapy and its effects on patients with microphallus. J Urol 1993; 150:657.

Cohen-Addad N, Zarafu IW, Hanna MK: Complete penoscrotal transposition. Urology 1985; 26:149.

Committee from the Urology Section, American Academy of Pediatrics: Urethral meatal stenosis in males. Pediatrics 1978; 61:778.

Craig JC, Knight JF, Suresh Kumar P, et al: Effect of circumcision on incidence of urinary tract infection in preschool boys. J Pediatr 1996; 128:23.

Cuckow PM, Rix G, Mouriquand PDE: Preputial plasty: A good alternative to circumcision. J Pediatr Surg 1994; 29:561.

Cunningham LN, Keating MA, Snyder HM, Duckett JW: Urological manifestations of the popliteal pterygium syndrome. J Urol 1989; 141:910.

Danish RK, Lee PA, Mazur T, et al: Micropenis: II. Hypogonadotropic hypogonadism. Johns Hopkins Med J 1980; 146:177.

Devine CJ Jr: Comment. *In* Hinman F, Jr: Atlas of Urologic Surgery. Philadelphia, W. B. Saunders, 1989, p 67.

Donahoe PJ, Keating MA: Preputial unfurling to correct the buried penis. J Pediatr Surg 1986; 21:1055.

Dresner ML: Surgical revision of scrotal engulfment. Urol Clin North Am 1982; 9:305.

Elder JS, Duckett JW: Complications of hypospadias surgery. *In* Smith RB, Ehrlich RM, eds: Complications of Urologic Surgery. Philadelphia, W. B. Saunders, 1990, p 549.

Elder JS, Jeffs RD: Suprainguinal ectopic scrotum and associated anomalies. J Urol 1982; 127:336.

Feldman KW, Smith DW: Fetal phallic growth and penile standards for newborn male infants. J Pediatr 1975; 86:395.

Ferrer FA, McKenna PH: Cavernous hemangioma of the scrotum: A rare benign genital tumor of childhood. J Urol 1995; 153:1262.

Fitzpatrick TJ: Hemihypertrophy of the human corpus cavernosum. J Urol 1976; 115:560.

Fussell EN, Kaack MB, Cherry R, Roberts JA: Adherence of bacteria to human foreskins. J Urol 1988; 140:997.

Gavrell GJ: Congenital curvature of the penis. J Urol 1974; 112:489.

Gilbert J, Clark RD, Koyle MA: Penile agenesis: A fatal variation of an uncommon lesion. J Urol 1990; 143:338.

Ginsburg CM, McCracken GH Jr: Urinary tract infections in young infants. Pediatrics 1982; 69:409.

Gittes RF, McLaughlin AP III: Injection technique to induce penile erection. Urology 1974; 4:473.

Gonzales JR: Micropenis. AUA Update Series 1983; 2(39):1.

Goulding FJ, Traylor RA: Juvenile xanthogranuloma of the scrotum. J Urol 1983; 129:841.

Hautmann RE, Bachor R: Juvenile xanthogranuloma of the penis. J Urol 1993; 150:456.

Hill JT, Ashken MH: Parameatal urethral cysts: A review of 6 cases. Br J Urol 1977; 49:323.

Hoekstra WJ, Scholtmeijer RJ, Molenaar JC, et al: Urogenital tract abnormalities associated with congenital anorectal anomalies. J Urol 1983; 130:962.

Hollowell JG Jr, Witherington R, Ballagas AJ, Burt JN: Embryologic consideration of diphallus and associated anomalies. J Urol 1977; 117:728.

Husmann DA, Cain MP: Microphallus: Eventual phallic size is dependent on the timing of androgen administration. J Urol 1994; 152:734.

Kapoor R, Saha MM: Complete duplication of the bladder, urethra and external genitalia in a neonate—a case report. J Urol 1987; 137:1243.

Kenawi MM: Webbed penis. Br J Urol 1973; 45:569.

Kennedy WA II, Hensle TW, Giella J, et al: Potassium thiophosphate laser treatment of genitourinary hemangioma in the pediatric population. J Urol 1993; 150:950.

Lage JM, Driscoll SG, Bieber FR: Transposition of the external genitalia associated with caudal regression. J Urol 1987; 138:387.

Lamm DL, Kaplan GW: Accessory and ectopic scrota. Urology 1977; 9:149.
Larsen GL, Williams SD: Postneonatal circumcision: Population profile. Pediatrics 1990; 85:808.
Lee PA, Danish RK, Mazur T, Migeon CJ: Micropenis: III. Primary hypogonadism, partial androgen insensitivity syndrome, and idiopathic disorders. Johns Hopkins Med J 1980a; 147:175.
Lee PA, Mazur T, Danish R, et al: Micropenis: I. Criteria, etiologies and classification. Johns Hopkins Med J 1980b; 146:156.
Lim DJ, Barraza MA, Stevens PS: Correction of retractile concealed penis. J Urol 1995; 153:1668.
Little JS Jr, Keating MA, Rink RC: Median raphe cysts of the genitalia. J Urol 1992; 148:1872.
Litvak AS, Morris JA Jr, McRoberts JW: Normal size of the urethral meatus in boys. J Urol 1976; 115:736.
Lovinger RD, Kaplan SL, Grumbach MM: Congenital hypopituitarism associated with neonatal hypoglycemia and microphallus: Four cases secondary to hypothalamic hormone deficiencies. J Pediatr 1975; 87:1171.
MacKinley GA: Save the prepuce: Painless separation of preputial adhesions in the outpatient clinic. Br Med J 1988; 297:590.
McMahon DR, Kramer SA, Husmann DA: Micropenis: Does early treatment with testosterone do more harm than good? J Urol 1995; 154:825.
Maizels M, Zaontz M, Donovan J, et al: Surgical correction of the buried penis: Description of a classification system and a technique to correct the disorder. J Urol 1986; 136:268.
Mandell J, Bromley B, Peters CA, Benacerraf BR: Prenatal sonographic detection of genital malformations. J Urol 1995; 153:1994.
Marti-Bonmati L, Menor F, Gomez J, et al: Value of sonography in true complete diphallia. J Urol 1989; 142:356.
Morton HG: Meatus size in 1,000 circumcised children from two weeks to sixteen years of age. J Fla Med Assoc 1986; 50:137.
Noe HN, Dale GA: Evaluation of children with meatal stenosis. J Urol 1975; 114:455.
Oesch IL, Pinter A, Ransley PG: Penile agenesis: A report of six cases. J Pediatr Surg 1987; 22:172.
Oster J: Further fate of the foreskin: Incidence of preputial adhesions, phimosis, and smegma among Danish schoolboys. Arch Dis Child 1968; 43:200.
Perlmutter AD, Chamberlain JW: Webbed penis without chordee. J Urol 1972; 107:320.
Persad R, Sharma S, McTavish J, et al: Clinical presentation and pathophysiology of meatal stenosis following circumcision. Br J Urol 1995; 75:91.
Pippi Salle JL, de Fraga JCS, Wojciechowski M, Antunes CRH: Congenital rupture of the scrotum: An unusual complication of meconium peritonitis. J Urol 1992; 148:1242.
Pomerantz P, Hanna M, Levitt S, Kogan S: Isolated torsion of penis: Report of 6 cases. Urology 1978; 11:37.
Rao TV, Chandrasekharam V: Diphallus with duplication of cloacal derivatives: Report of a rare case. J Urol 1980; 124:555.
Redman JF: A technique for the correction of penoscrotal fusion. J Urol 1985; 133:432.
Reilly JM, Woodhouse CRJ: Small penis and the male sexual role. J Urol 1989; 142:569.
Ring KS, Axelrod SL, Burbige KA, Hensle TW: Meconium hydrocele: An unusual etiology of a scrotal mass in the newborn. J Urol 1989; 141:1172.
Ritchey ML, Sinha A, Argueso L: Congenital fistula of the penile urethra. J Urol 1994; 151:1061.
Ross JH: Circumcision: Pro and con. *In* Elder JS, ed: Pediatric Urology for the General Urologist. New York; Igaku-Shoin, 1996, p 49.
Ryan CA, Finer NN: Changing attitudes and practices regarding local analgesia for newborn circumcision. Pediatrics 1994; 94:230.
Scherz HC, Kaplan GW, Packer MG: Anterior urethral valves in the fossa navicularis in children. J Urol 1987; 138:1211.
Schonfeld WA, Beebe GW: Normal growth and variation in the male genitalia from birth to maturity. J Urol 1942; 48:759.
Shapiro SR: Surgical treatment of the "buried" penis. Urology 1987; 30:554.
Shinkawa T, Yamauchi Y, Osada Y, Ishisawa N: Aarskog syndrome. Urology 1983; 22:624.
Shiraki IW: Parameatal cysts of the glans penis: A report of 9 cases. J Urol 1975; 114:544.
Skoog SJ, Belman AB: Aphallia: Its classification and management. J Urol 1989; 141:589.
Smith JA Jr: Laser treatment of bladder hemangioma. J Urol 1990; 143:282.
Stolar CJH, Wiener ES, Hensle TW, et al: Reconstruction of penile agenesis by a posterior sagittal approach. J Pediatr Surg 1987; 22:1076.
Sule JD, Lemmers MJ, Barry JM: Scrotal arteriovenous malformation: Case report and literature review. J Urol 1993; 150:1917.
Sule JD, Skoog SJ, Tank ES: Perineal lipoma and the accessory labioscrotal fold: An etiological relationship. J Urol 1994; 151:475.
Tennenbaum SY, Palmer LS: Congenital urethrocutaneous fistula. Urology 1994; 43:98.
Thompson HC, King LR, Knox E, Keanes SB: Report of the ad hoc task force on circumcision. Pediatrics 1975; 56:610.
Walsh PC, Wilson JD, Allen TD, et al: Clinical and endocrinological evaluation of patients with congenital microphallus. J Urol 1978; 120:90.
Wiswell TE: Prepuce presence portends prevalence of potentially perilous periurethral pathogens. J Urol 1992; 148:739.
Wiswell TE, Miller GM, Gelston HM Jr, et al: Effect of circumcision status on periurethral bacterial flora during the first year of life. J Pediatr 1988; 113:442.
Wiswell TE, Smith FR, Bass JW: Decreased incidence of urinary tract infections in circumcised male infants. Pediatrics 1985; 75:90l.
Wiswell TE, Tencer HL, Welch CA, Chamberlain JL: Circumcision in children beyond the neonatal period. Pediatrics 1992; 92:791.
Yachia D, Beyar M, Aridogan IA, Dascalu S: The incidence of congenital penile curvature. J Urol 1993; 150:1478.
Yamaguchi T, Hamasuna R, Hasui Y, et al: 47,XXY/48,XXY, +21 chromosomal mosaicism presenting as hypospadias with scrotal transposition. J Urol 1989; 142:797.

Anomalies of the Female Genitalia

Anveden-Hertzberg L, Gauderer MWL, Elder JS: Urethral prolapse: An often misdiagnosed cause of urogenital bleeding in girls. Pediatr Emerg Med 1995; 11:212.
Belis JA, Hrabovsky EE: Idiopathic female intersex with clitoromegaly and urethral duplication. J Urol 1979; 122:805.
Bellinger MF, Duckett JW: Accessory phallic urethra in the female patient. J Urol 1982; 127:1159.
Berenson AB: A longitudinal study of hymenal morphology in the first 3 years of life. Pediatrics 1995; 95:490.
Brock JW III, Morgan W, Anderson TL: Congenital hemangiopericytoma of the clitoris. J Urol 1995; 153:468.
Burbige KA, Hensle TW: Uterus didelphys and vaginal duplication with unilateral obstruction presenting as a newborn abdominal mass. J Urol 1984; 132:1195.
Caldamone AA, Snyder H III, Duckett JW: Ureteroceles in children: Follow-up of management with upper tract approach. J Urol 1984; 131:1130.
Carpenter SE, Rock JA: Procidentia in the newborn. Int J Obstet Gynecol 1987; 25:151.
Chitayat D, Hahm SYE, Marion RW, et al: Further delineation of the McKusick-Kaufman hydrometrocolpos-polydactyly syndrome. Am J Dis Child 1987; 141:1133.
Dershwitz RA, Levitsky LL, Feingold M: Vulvovaginitis: A cause of clitoromegaly. Am J Dis Child 1984; 138:887.
Duncan PA, Shapiro LR, Stangel JJ, et al: The MURCS association: Mullerian duct aplasia, renal aplasia, and cervicothoracic somite dysplasia. J Pediatr 1979; 95:399.
Fisher RE, Tanagho EA, Lyon RP, Tooley WH: Urethral calibration in newborn girls. J Urol 1969; 102:67.
Fleming SE, Hall R, Gysler M, McLorie GA: Imperforate anus in females: Frequency of genital tract involvement, incidence of associated anomalies, and functional outcome. J Pediatr Surg 1986; 21:146.
Foglia RP, Kim SH, Cleveland RH, Donahoe PK: Complications of vaginal atresia in association with a duplicated müllerian duct. J Pediatr Surg 1987; 22:653.
Fraser IS, Baird DT, Hobson BM, et al: Cyclical ovarian function in women with congenital absence of the uterus and vagina. J Clin Endocrinol Metab 1973; 36:634.
Gilsanz V, Cleveland RH: Duplication of the müllerian ducts and genitourinary malformation, parts I and II. Radiology 1982; 144:793.
Graham JB, King LR, Kropp KA, Uehling DT: The significance of distal urethral narrowing in young girls. J Urol 1967; 97:1045.
Greenfield SP, Rutigliano E, Steinhardt G, Elder JS: Genitourinary tract malformations and cocaine abuse. Urology 1991; 37:455.
Greer DM Jr, Pederson WC: Pseudo-masculinization of the phallus. Plast Reconstr Surg 1981; 68:787.
Griffin JE, Edwards C, Madden JD, Harrod MJ, Wilson JD: Congenital

absence of the vagina: The Mayer-Rokitansky-Kuster-Hauser syndrome. Ann Intern Med 1976; 85:224.
Gruenwald P: The relation of the growing müllerian duct to the wolffian duct and its importance for the genesis of malformations. Anat Rec 1941; 81:1.
Halverstadt DB, Leadbetter GW, Jr: Internal urethrotomy and recurrent urinary tract infection in female children: I. Results in the management of infection. J Urol 1968; 100:297.
Hausegger KA, Fotter R, Sorantin E, Schmidt P: Urethral morphology and bladder instability. Pediatr Radiol 1991; 21:278.
Hendren WH: Cloacal malformations: Experience with 105 cases. J Pediatr Surg 1992; 27:890.
Hensle TW, Dean GE: Vaginal replacement in children. J Urol 1992; 148:677.
Huffman JW: Some facts about the clitoris. Postgrad Med 1976; 60:245.
Immergut M, Culp D, Flocks RH: The urethral caliber in normal female children. J Urol 1967; 97:693.
Immergut MA, Wahman GE: The urethral caliber of female children with recurrent urinary tract infections. J Urol 1968; 99:189.
Jenny C, Kuhns MLD, Arakawa F: Hymens in normal female infants. Pediatrics 1987; 80:399.
Johnson CF: Prolapse of the urethra: Confusion of clinical and anatomic characteristics with sexual abuse. Pediatrics 1991; 87:722.
Johnston JH, Koff SA, Glassberg KL: The pseudo-obstructed bladder in enuretic children. Br J Urol 1978; 50:505.
Kaplan GW, Sammons TA, King LR: A blind comparison of dilatation, urethrotomy and medication alone in the treatment of urinary tract infection in girls. J Urol 1973; 109:917.
Karlin G, Brock W, Rich M, Pena A: Persistent cloaca and phallic urethra. J Urol 1989; 142:1056.
Kessler R, Constantinou CE: Internal urethrotomy in girls and its impact on the intrinsic and extrinsic continence mechanisms. J Urol 1968; 136:1248.
Kizer JR, Bellah RD, Schnaufer L, Canning DA: Meconium hydrocele in a female newborn: An unusual cause of a labial mass. J Urol 1995; 153:188.
Klee LW, Rink RC, Gleason PE, Ganesan GS: Urethral polyp presenting as interlabial mass in young girls. Urology 1993; 41:132.
Klein FA, Vick CW III, Broecker BH: Neonatal vaginal cysts: Diagnosis and management. J Urol 1986; 135:371.
Leung AKC, Robson WLM: Labial fusion and asymptomatic bacteriuria. Eur J Pediatr 1993; 152:250.
Lowe FC, Hill GS, Jeffs RD, Brendler CB: Urethral prolapse in children: Insights into etiology and management. J Urol 1986; 135:100.
Lyon RP: Distal urethral stenosis. *In* Johnston JH, Goodwin WE, eds: Reviews in Paediatric Urology. Amsterdam, Excerpta Medica, 1974, p 1.
Lyon RP, Marshall S: Urinary tract infections and difficult urination in girls: Long-term follow-up. J Urol 1971; 105:314.
Lyon RP, Smith DR: Distal urethral stenosis. J Urol 1963: 89:414.
Lyon RP, Tanagho EA: Distal urethral stenosis in little girls. J Urol 1965; 93:379.
McHenry CR, Reynolds M, Raffensperger JG: Vaginal neoplasms in infancy: The combined role of chemotherapy and conservative surgical resection. J Pediatr Surg 1988; 23:842.
Nussbaum AR, Lebowitz RL: Interlabial masses in little girls: Review and imaging considerations. AJR 1983; 141:65.
Ramenofsky ML, Raffensperger JG: An abdomino-perineal-vaginal pull-through for definitive treatment of hydrometrocolpos. J Pediatr Surg 1971; 6:381.
Richardson DA, Hajj SN, Herbst AJ: Medical treatment of urethral prolapse in children. Obstet Gynecol 1982; 59:69.
Riley WJ, Rosenbloom AL: Clitoral size in infancy. J Pediatr 1980; 96:918.
Rock JA, Azziz R: Genital anomalies in childhood. Clin Obstet Gynecol 1987; 30:682.
Rock JA, Zacur HA, Dlugi AM, et al: Pregnancy success following surgical correction of imperforate hymen and complete transverse vaginal septum. Obstet Gynecol 1982; 59:448.
Saxton HM, Borzyskowski M, Mundy AR, Vivian GC: Spinning top urethra: Not a normal variant. Radiology 1988; 168:147.
Sayer T, O'Reilly PH: Bicornuate and unicornuate uterus associated with unilateral renal aplasia and abnormal solitary kidneys: Report of 3 cases. J Urol 1986; 135:110.
Sheldon CA, Gilbert A, Lewis AG: Vaginal reconstruction: Critical technical principles. J Urol 1994; 152:190.
So EP, Brock W, Kaplan GW: Ectopic labium and VATER association in a newborn. J Urol 1980; 124:156.
Sule JD, Skoog SJ, Tank ES: Perineal lipoma and the accessory labioscrotal fold: An etiological relationship. J Urol 1994; 151:475.
Tanagho EA, Smith DR: The anatomy and function of the bladder neck. Br J Urol 1966; 38:54.
Tarry WF, Duckett JW, Stephens FD: The Mayer-Rokitansky syndrome: Pathogenesis, classification and management. J Urol 1986; 136:648.
Tolete-Velcek F, Hansbrough F, Kugaczewski J, et al: Uterovaginal malformations: A trap for the unsuspecting surgeon. J Pediatr Surg 1989; 24:736.
Tran ATB, Arensman RM, Falterman KW: Diagnosis and management of hydrohematometrocolpos syndromes. Am J Dis Child 1987; 141:632.
Williams DI: Urology in Childhood. Berlin, Springer-Verlag, 1958, p 73.
Wilson DA, Stacy TM, Smith EI: Ultrasound diagnosis of hydrocolpos and hydrometrocolpos. Radiology 1978; 128:451.
Woolf RB, Allen WM: Concomitant malformations. Obstet Gynecol 1953; 2:236.

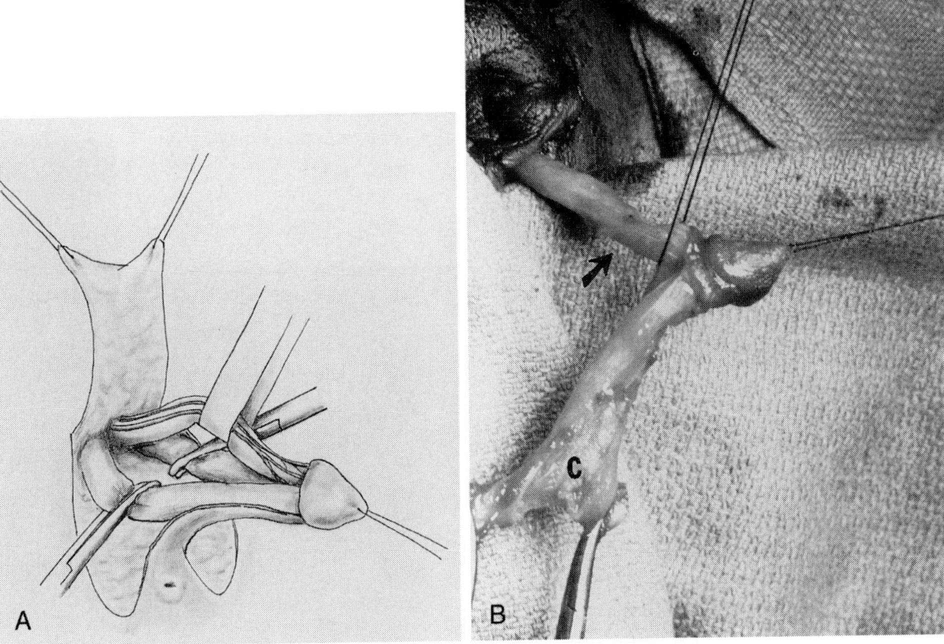

Figure 71–3. *A*, Line drawing of separation of neurovascular bundle from corporal bodies. *B*, Clinical photo of detached corporal bodies (C) and intact neurovascular bundle (*arrow*).

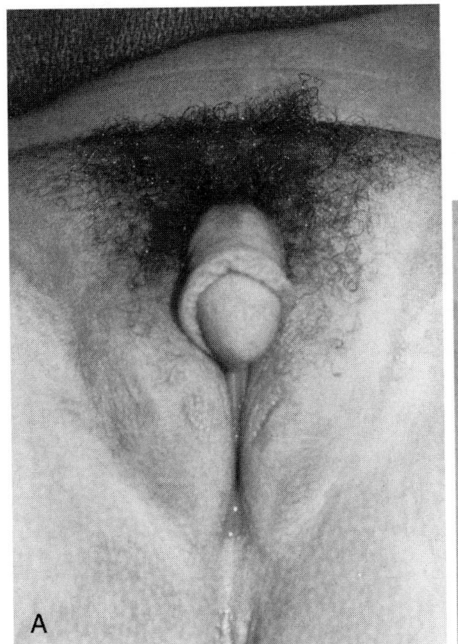

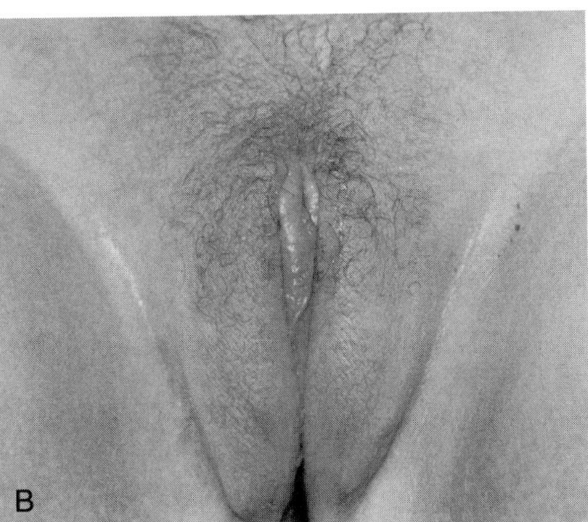

Figure 71–4. *A*, Preoperative photo of a 12-year-old patient with clitoromegaly secondary to CAH. *B*, Postoperative photo of the same patient 6 months after reduction clitoroplasty.

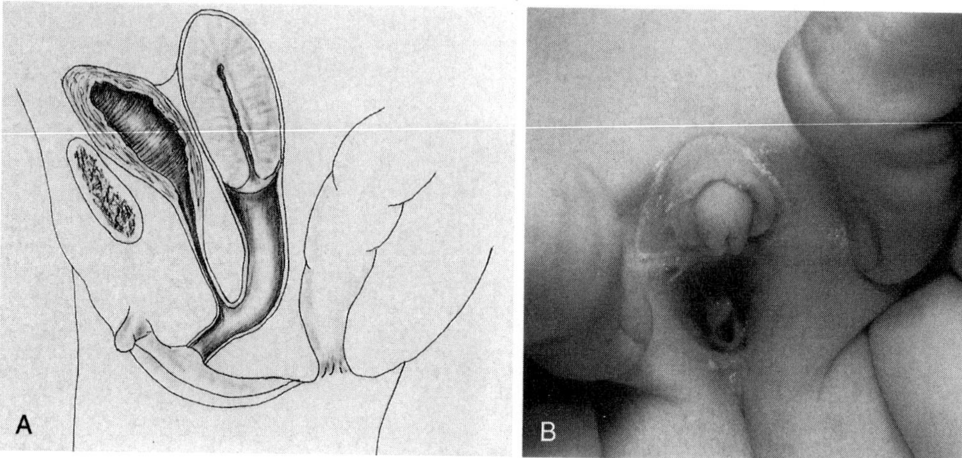

Figure 71–5. *A*, Line drawing of urogenital sinus with a low confluence. *B*, Clinical photo of an infant with CAH and a very low urogenital sinus defect.

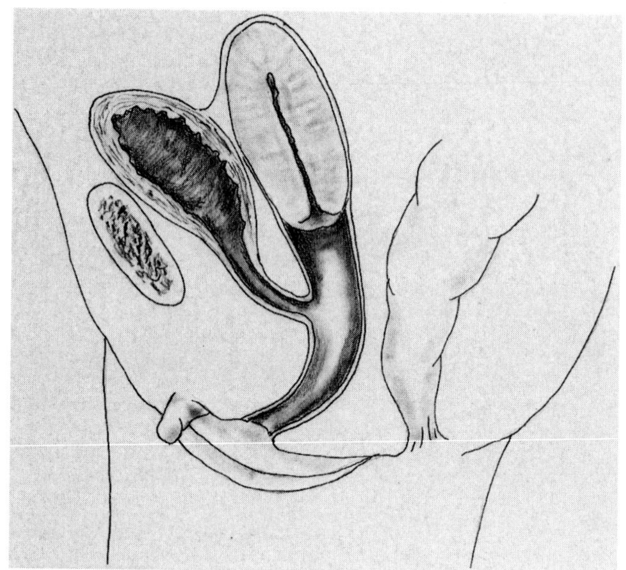

Figure 71–6. Entry of vagina in the midportion of the urogenital sinus.

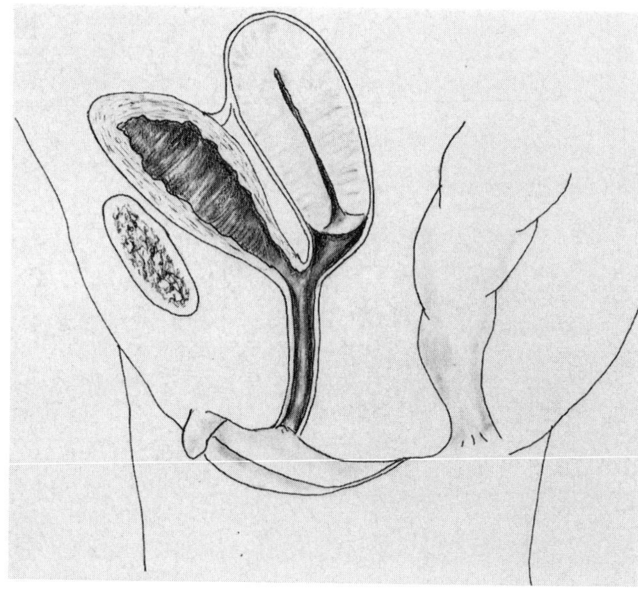

Figure 71–7. High confluence of the vagina and urogenital sinus at the area of the urinary sphincter.

repair can be performed, and if the junction is just at or proximal to the sphincter (Fig. 71–7), a high vaginal repair should be planned.

Low vaginoplasty is best performed using a flap of perineal skin. The procedure is performed with the patient in the lithotomy position, and the endoscope is used at that time in order to fully understand the anatomy and define the surgical landmarks. A catheter is placed into the bladder anteriorly, and an inverted U-flap of perineal skin is outlined and developed using electrocautery (Fig. 71–8*A* and *B*). The perineal skin flap is held with traction sutures, and the length of the flap should roughly correspond to the length of urogenital sinus to be opened. Once the perineal U-flap has been developed, the urogenital sinus is opened in the midline posteriorly until the vagina is identified and entered (Fig. 71–9*A*). The vagina can then be gently separated from the rectum posteriorly. It is often helpful to have placed a rectal tube preoperatively or the nondominant index finger intraoperatively to help identify the anterior rectal wall. The inverted U-flap of perineal skin is then turned in to join the apex of the posterior vagina and sutured in place using interrupted long acting absorbable sutures (see Fig. 71–9*B* and *C*). The dorsal shaft skin of the phallus, which is mobilized during the clitoral recession, is then divided in the midline and brought inferiorly to join the newly exposed urogenital sinus, thereby creating labia minora (Fig. 71–10*A* and *B*). The labioscrotal folds can then be mobilized, reduced in size and bulk, and sutured inferiorly to create labia majora. Postoperatively, the vaginoplasty is stented for 3 days using either antibiotic impregnated gauze packing or a vaginal stent of appropriate caliber (Fig. 71–11). A Foley catheter is left in place for as long as the vaginal stent remains.

High Vaginal Repair

In a small number of individuals with female pseudohermaphroditism, the virilization is severe and the vagina enters the urogenital sinus just at or proximal to the urinary sphincter. In those instances, vaginoplasty becomes much more complex and the risk of injury to both rectum and to the urinary continence mechanism becomes far greater. In 1969, Hendren and Crawford originally described extensive introital reconstruction using a vaginal pull-down technique in combination with both perineal and laterally based skin flaps. In that procedure, after a small balloon (Fogarty) catheter is placed into the vaginal introitus with the aid of an endoscope (Fig. 71–12), the urogenital sinus is approached perineally (Hendren and Atala, 1995), just as one would do in a low-flap vaginoplasty. In dissecting anteriorly, it is often helpful to use a nerve stimulator to avoid injury to the urinary sphincter. The dissection is carried out superiorly between the rectum and the urogenital sinus until the catheter is encountered (Fig. 71–13). The vagina is then divided just where it joins the urethra. The proximal portion of the urogenital sinus can then be tubularized for a short distance and closed in two layers in order to create a longer functional urethra and avoid the problem of female hypospadias.

At this point, the vagina is mobilized anteriorly from the bladder and posteriorly from the rectum. Traction sutures on the lateral vaginal wall help maintain the landmarks in this very tight perineal space. Because there is very little anterior vaginal tissue to bring to the perineum, both lateral skin flaps and perineal skin U-flap have to be mobilized (Fig. 71–14) to bring up into the high vagina (Fig. 71–15). It is not unusual for patients to require multiple vaginal dilations following this kind of procedure, and often, home dilation is necessary.

More recently, Passerini-Glazel (1989) has described a transvesical approach to the high vagina (Fig. 71–16), in which the vagina is separated from the urogenital sinus anteriorly through the posterior wall of the bladder. In this procedure, the phallus is degloved and reduced in a fashion similar to that already described. The corporal bodies are freed and resected, and the urogenital sinus is mobilized

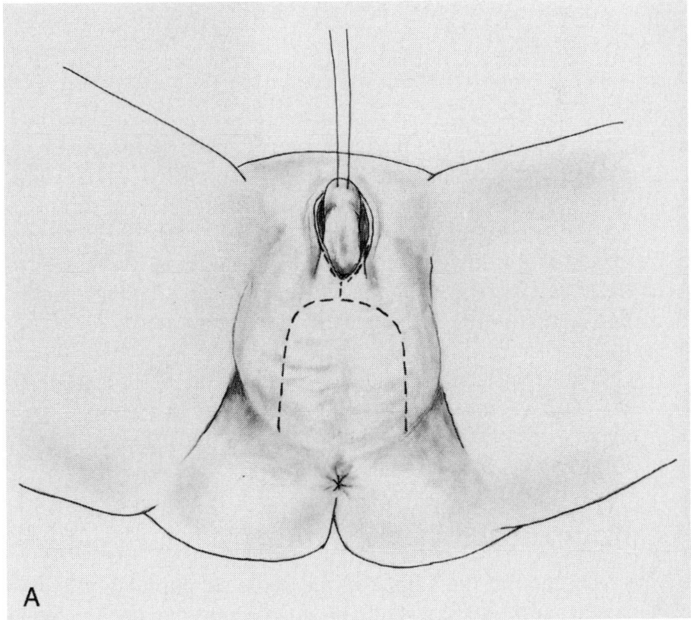

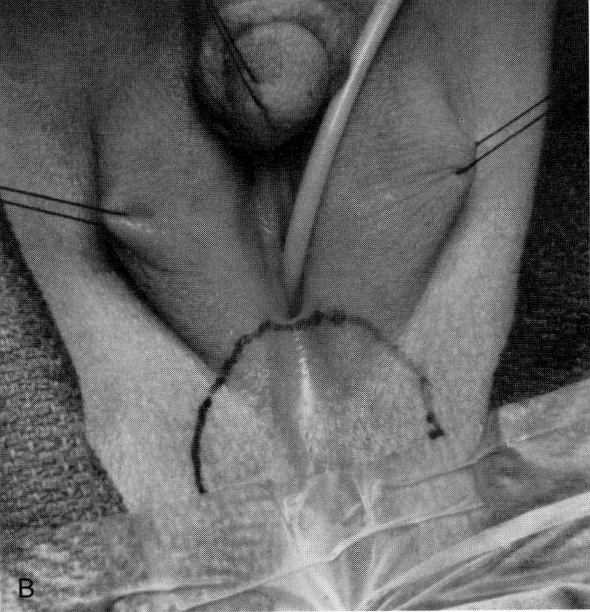

Figure 71–8. *A*, Inverted perineal U-flap is outlined. *B*, U-flap outlined with traction sutures in the labioscrotal folds, and catheter in the urethra.

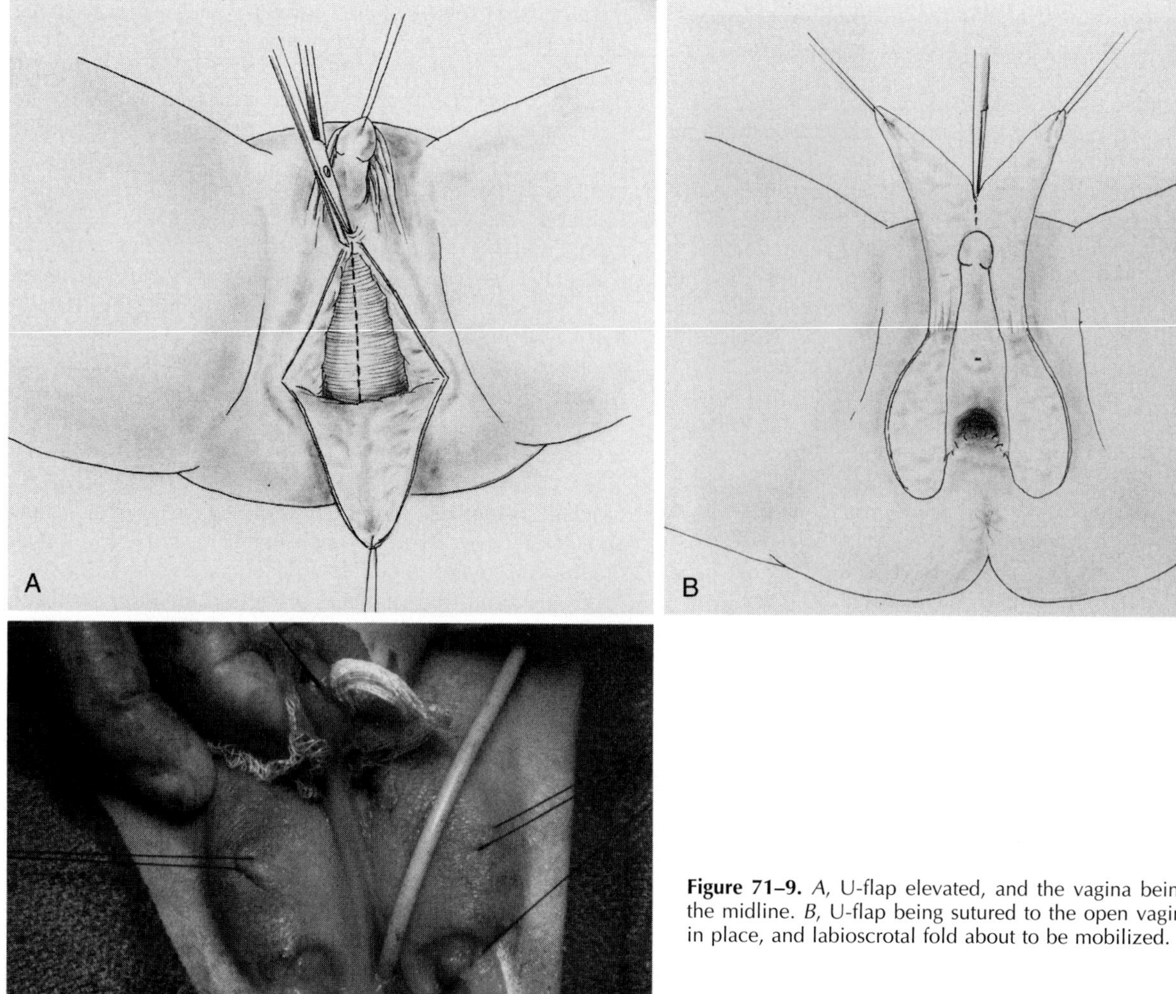

Figure 71–9. *A*, U-flap elevated, and the vagina being opened in the midline. *B*, U-flap being sutured to the open vagina. *C*, U-flap in place, and labioscrotal fold about to be mobilized.

inferiorly. Once this has been accomplished, the anterior phallic shaft skin is mobilized both anteriorly and inferiorly, and divided in the midline (Fig. 71–17). The urogenital sinus is then opened anteriorly with a Y incision, and the previously mobilized anterior phallic skin flaps are brought inferiorly and sutured to the open urogenital sinus (Fig. 71–18) and tubularized (Fig. 71–19). This procedure allows the urethral meatus to be in the normal subclitoral position and allows the mobilized, tubularized skin flaps to be free and redundant enough to move up into the perineum for anastomosis to the divided vagina.

The bladder can then be opened, and the posterior wall of the bladder can be split in the midline. This dissection is carried to the junction of the urogenital sinus and the vagina, with much of the mobilization carried out under the bladder neck, and it can be very difficult. It is often helpful to place a Fogarty catheter in the vaginal opening preoperatively to allow better identification of the junction of the urogenital sinus and vagina. Once the area has been identified and divided, the urogenital sinus can be closed under direct vision to avoid postoperative fistulization. The mobilized phallic skin tube is then carried through the perineal opening and brought upward subtrigonally for an anastomosis to the high vagina (Fig. 71–20). Postoperatively, vaginal packing and a urethral catheter usually remain in place for 4 to 5 days (Fig. 71–21).

The significant advantage of this kind of procedure for the high vagina is that it can be performed in one stage, it avoids postoperative vaginal stenosis, and it leaves the urethral meatus in a normal position.

Construction of the Neovagina

Absence of the vagina in the pediatric population is associated with intersex states in which there has been a female gender assignment in a chromosomal male, such as male

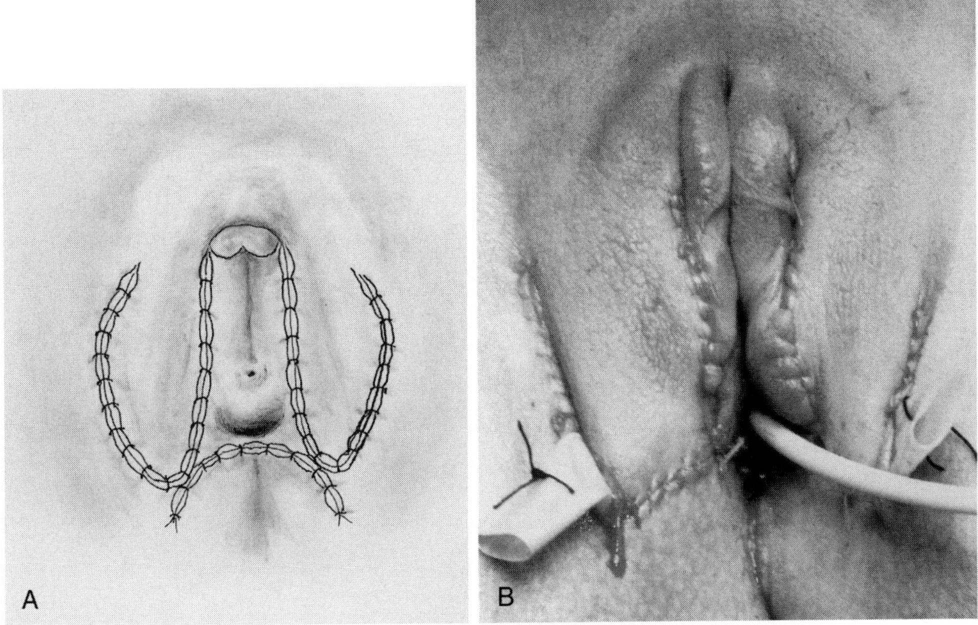

Figure 71–10. *A*, Suture line completed with labioscrotal folds creating labia majora and shaft skin creating labia minora. *B*, Completed low vaginoplasty and genitoplasty.

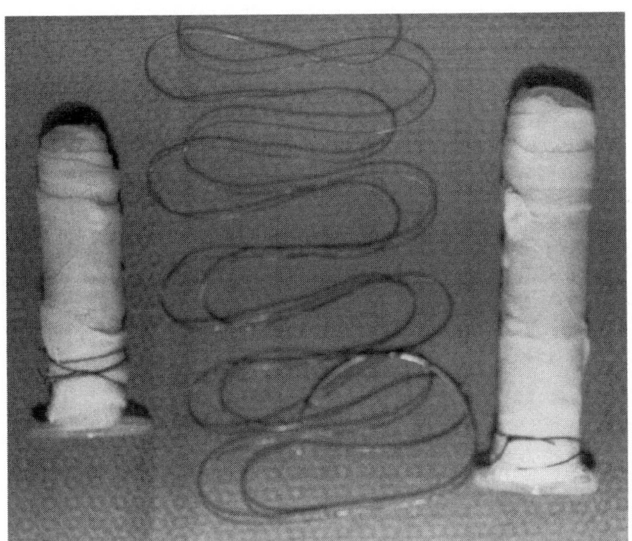

Figure 71–11. Vaginal stents using barrel of 3-, 5-, or 10-ml syringe covered with xeroform gauze.

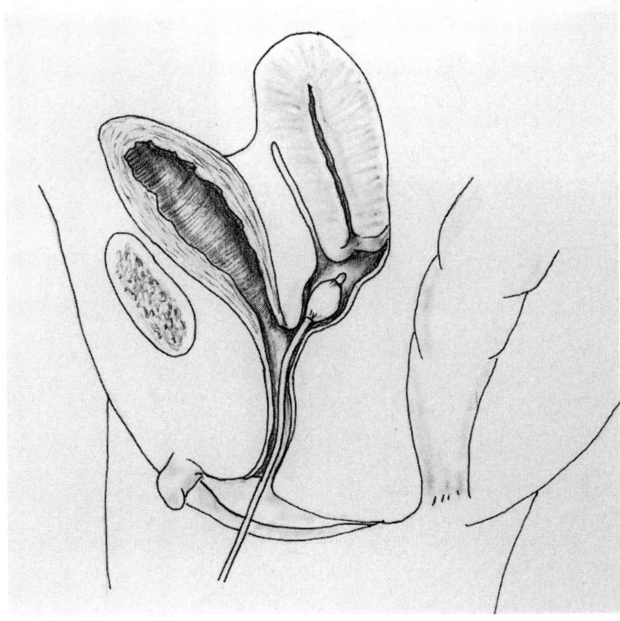

Figure 71–12. Lateral view of high confluence of vagina and urogenital sinus with Fogarty catheter in vagina as a guide.

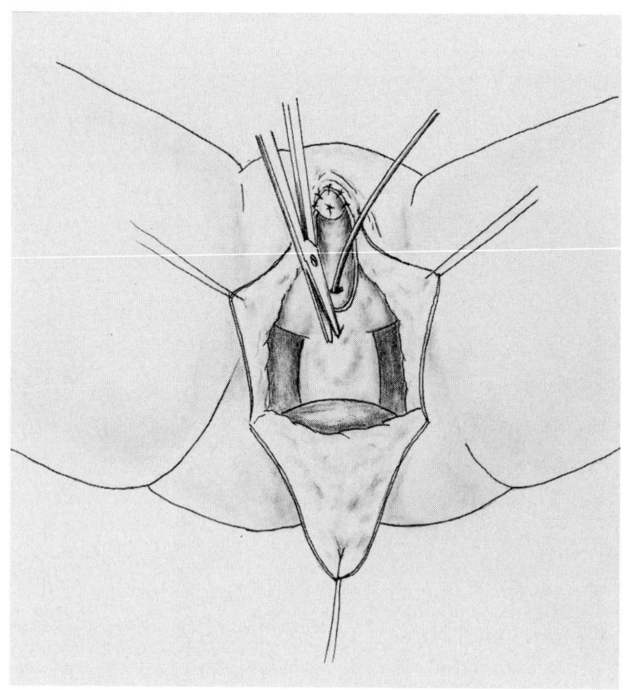

Figure 71–13. Perineal U-flap is raised, and vaginal cut back is begun.

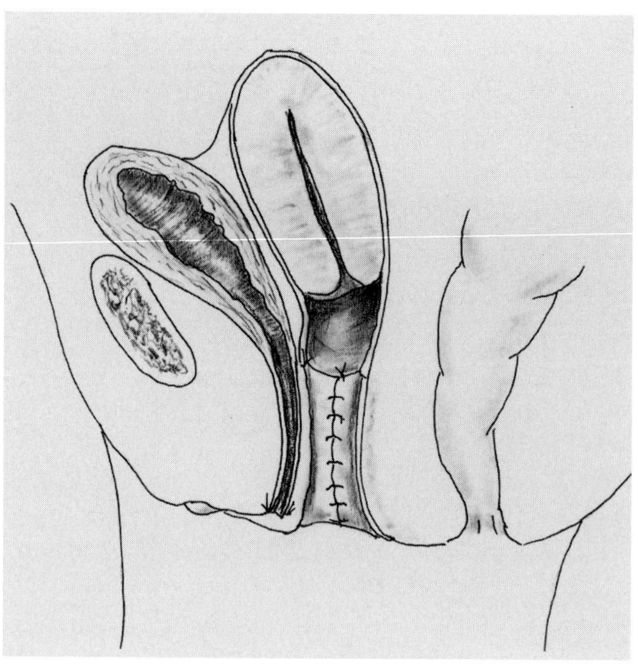

Figure 71–15. Lateral view of flaps extended up to meet the high vagina.

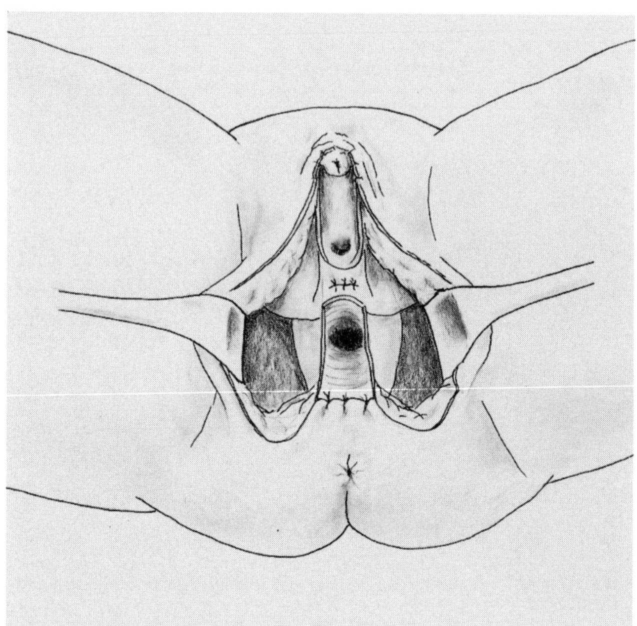

Figure 71–14. Perineal skin flap in place and lateral flap being mobilized.

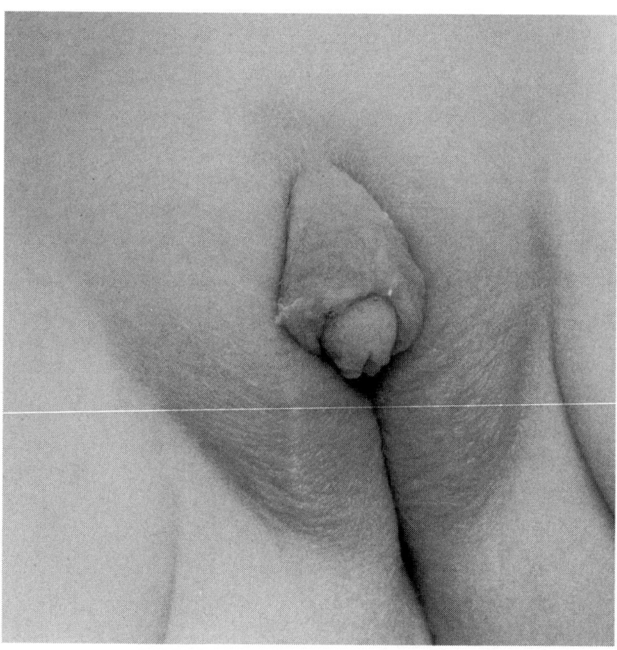

Figure 71–16. Preoperative photo of a virilized child with CAH and a very high confluence of vagina and urogenital sinus, as pictured in Figure 71–7.

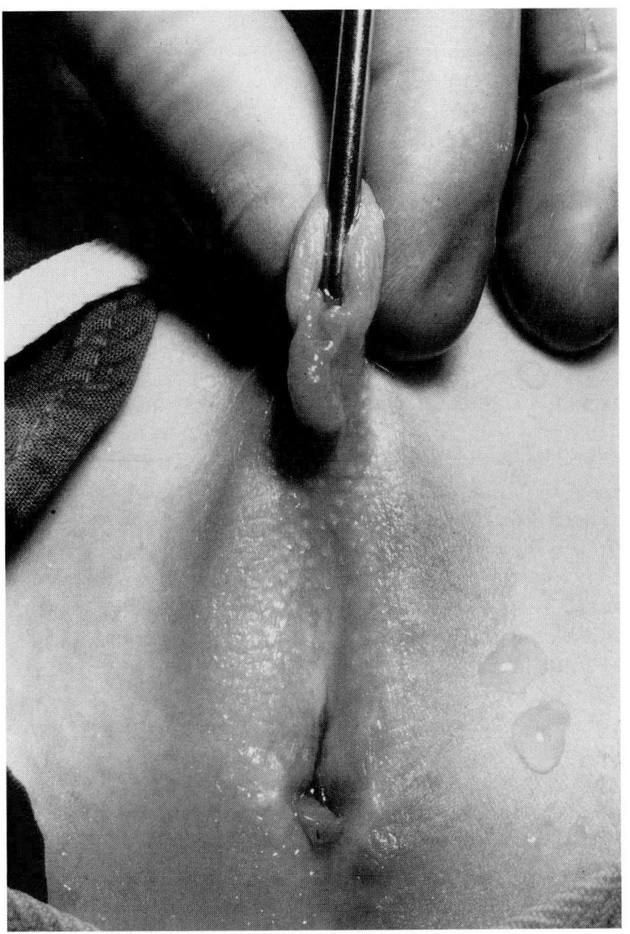

Figure 71–30. 46XY neonate with microphallus, nonpalpable gonads, and a fused perineum.

the male gender assignment would be complete androgen insensitivity syndrome.

The reconstruction of these individuals often requires surgical staging. The first stage consists of straightening the severe chordee, and the second stage involves construction of a neourethra. Often, additional surgeries are needed to repair penoscrotal transposition and to perform orchiopexies (Fig. 71–32).

First-Stage Hypospadias Repair

The size of the phallus dictates the timing of the first stage of the repair, with a sizable phallus repaired at 6 months of age and a small phallus repaired only after 1 year of age. For hypospadias repairs of this magnitude, it is often advisable to divert the urine with a cystotomy. During the first stage of the hypospadias repair, the shaft skin is circumscribed distal to the corona of the glans and the chordee is straightened by resecting the atretic and fibrotic copora spongiosa tissue. The foreskin is then transferred to cover the ventral surface of the shaft. Excess skin may be used later to construct a neourethra. A series of multiple Z-plasty closures may be performed to ensure that the penis is straight, and a Nesbitt procedure may be necessary.

Second-Stage Hypospadias Repair

The second stage of the hypospadias repair with a composite graft is performed 6 months after the initial surgery. The composite graft that forms the neourethra consists of a portion of midscrotal tubularized tissue and foreskin that was previously transposed to a ventral position. If sufficient tissue is not available on the ventrum of the shaft, a bladder graft or buccal mucosa may be used. Closure of the scrotum over the proximal portion of the composite graft can correct a bifid scrotum.

Correction of Penoscrotal Transposition

The penoscrotal hypospadias associated with intersexuality is frequently associated with a prepenile dislocation of the scrotum. Correction is delayed until 6 months after construction of the neourethra to await complete healing of the urethral graft and ventral shaft skin closure. In this repair, the base of the penis is advanced cephalad, while abdominal flaps are rotated posteriorly. The rotated abdominal flaps are joined on the ventral midline to the base of the penis. Midline and lateral closure of the scrotum completes the repair.

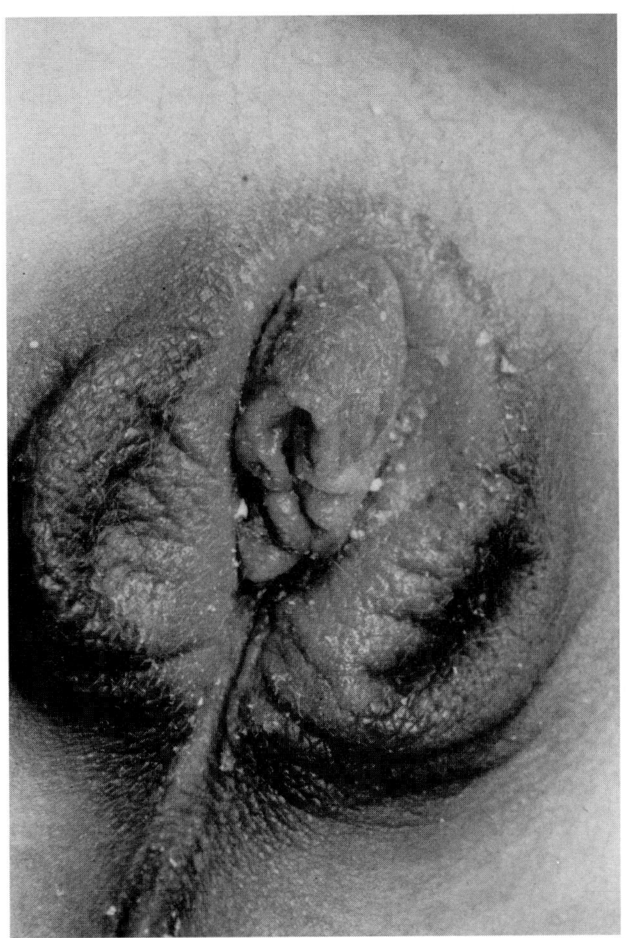

Figure 71–31. 46XY neonate with microphallus and poorly virilized genitalia.

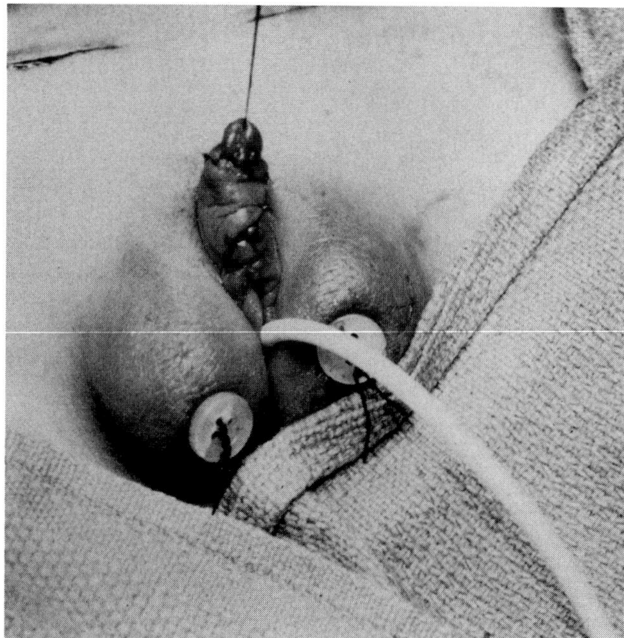

Figure 71–32. Same patient following orchiopexy, first-stage hypospadias repair, and androgen stimulation.

Surgical Management of the Retained Abnormal Gonadal Tissue

The retained gonad in an intersex patient requires careful evaluation. In patients with an undescended testis without obvious intersex abnormalities, the risk of malignancy is 20 to 46 times greater than that of the normal population (Batata et al, 1982). The risk is related to the abnormal testis itself and not to its position, because correction of cryptorchidism alone does not prevent carcinogenesis. Scrotal positioning, however, does permit more accurate follow-up. Frequent examinations, prompt diagnosis of changes, and expeditious treatment are mandatory.

One third of patients with mixed gonadal dysgenesis develop gonadoblastomas, and an additional one third develop highly malignant germ cell tumors (Robboy et al, 1982). Early removal of these gonads is recommended in this select group of patients.

Resection of Tissue Inappropriate to Sexual Assignment

Patients with true hermaphroditism, rare variants of mixed gonadal dysgenesis, and persistent müllerian duct syndrome have retained müllerian ducts that join the urethra at the prostatic utricle. The consequences of reflux of urine into the retained müllerian structure can lead to recurrent urinary tract infections, epididymitis, and retrograde ejaculation. Removal of the müllerian structures may appear simple, but the vas often conjoins either the uterine or the vaginal wall, where it can be severed. Preservation of the vas should be attempted during surgery to protect the future potential for fertility (Donahoe, 1988). The uterus, and often the dilated vagina, are mobilized distally to the point where the vagina takes off from the posterior urethra. The vas usually implants into the side wall of the dilated vagina. A broad strip of vaginal wall, on the side of the vas, is left behind after the vagina, uterus, and fallopian tube have been resected. This strip may then be tubularized and used to create a neoseminal vesicle.

CONCLUSION

Adequate long-term results for multiple large series of children undergoing genital reconstruction for management of intersexuality by current surgical techniques are not yet available. Details concerning adult sexual function are still scant; however, preliminary reports appear favorable with a feminizing genitoplasty and neovaginal construction (Azziz et al, 1986; Turner-Warwick and Kirby, 1990; Hensle and Dean, 1992; Wesley and Coran, 1992). Experience with adults with an inadequate phallus who try to function in the male gender role supports reconstructive efforts toward a female gender assignment in infancy when phallic adequacy is questioned. The sex of assignment and rearing are often the most important factors in attaining a satisfactory sexual identity.

Ultimately, our goals should be directed toward better detection of carriers of genetic intersex states and early in utero detection in pregnancies of families at risk. These efforts, coupled with our expanded understanding of the molecular genetics and pathophysiology of these intersex abnormalities may soon lead to gene replacement therapies. Until such a time comes, it is our responsibility as physicians and surgeons to diagnose and gender assign these infants rapidly, through the use of reconstructive surgery, so that they may achieve an adequate functional role in society.

REFERENCES

Ansell JS, Rajfer J: A new and simplified method for concealing the hypertrophied clitoris. J Pediatr Surg 1981; 16:681–684.

Azziz R, Mulaikas RM, Migeon CJ, et al: Congenital adrenal hyperplasia: Long-term results following vagina reconstruction. Fertil Steril 1986; 46:1011–1014.

Baldwin JF: The formation of an artificial vagina by intestinal transplantation. Ann Surg 1904; 40:398–403.

Baldwin JF: Formation of an intestinal transplantation. American Journal of Obstetrical Diseases of Women and Children 1907; 56:636–640.

Batata MA, Chu FCH, Hilaris BS, et al: Testicular cancer in cryptorchids. Cancer 1982; 49:1023–1030.

Beemer W, Hopkins MP, Morley GW: Vaginal reconstruction in gynecologic oncology. Obstet Gynecol 1988; 72:911–914.

Berkovitz GD, Rock JA, Urban MD, Migeon CJ: True hermaphroditism. Johns Hopkins Med J 1982; 151:290–297.

Burger RA, Riedmiller H, Knapstein PG, et al: Ileocecal vaginal construction. Am J Obstet Gynecol 1989; 161:162–167.

Buss JG, Lee RA: McIndoe procedure for vaginal agenesis: Results and complications. Mayo Clin Proc 1989; 64:758–761.

de Souza AZ, Mariangela M, Perin PM, et al: Surgical treatment of congenital uterovaginal agenesis: Mayer-Rokitansky-Kuster-Hauser syndrome. Int Surg 1987; 72:45–47.

Dean GE, Hensle TW: Intestinal vaginoplasty. Current Surgical Techniques in Urology 1994; 7:1–8.

Donahoe PK: Neoseminal vesicle created from retained müllerian duct to preserve the vas in male infants. J Pediatr Surg 1988; 23:272–274.

Fall FH: A simple method for making an artificial vagina. Am J Obstet Gynecol 1940; 40:906–917.

Federman DD: Abnormal Sexual Development: A Genetic and Endocrine

Approach to Differential Diagnosis. Philadelphia, W. B. Saunders Company, 1967.

Glassberg KI, Laungani G: Reduction clitoroplasty. Urology 1981; 17:604–605.

Hendren WH, Atala A: Repair of the high vagina in girls with severely masculinized anatomy from the adrenogenital syndrome. J Pediatr Surg 1995; 30:91–94.

Hendren WH, Crawford JD: Adrenogenital syndrome: The anatomy of the anomaly and its repair. Some new concepts. J Pediatr Surg 1969; 4:49–58.

Hendren WH, Crawford JD: The child with ambiguous genitalia. Curr Probl Surg 1972; Nov:1–64.

Hensle TW, Dean GE: Vaginal replacement in children. J Urol 1992; 148:677–679.

Imperato-McGinley J, Peterson RE, Gautier T, Sturla E: Androgens and the evolution of male-gender identity among male pseudohermaphrodites with 5-alpha reductase deficiency. N Engl J Med 1974; 300:1233–1237.

Kogan SJ, Smey P, Levitt SB: Subtunical total reduction clitoroplasty: A safe modification of existing techniques. J Urol 1983; 130:746–748.

Kumar H, Kiefer JH, Rosenthal IE, Clark SS: Clitoroplasty: Experience during a 19 year period. J Urol 1974; 111:81–84.

McIndoe AH: Treatment of congenital absence and obliterative conditions of vagina. Br J Plast Surg 1950; 2:254–267.

Passerini-Glazel G: A new one-stage procedure for clitorovaginoplasty in severely masculinized female pseudohermaphrodites. J Urol 1989; 142:565–568.

Permutter AD: Management of intersexuality. *In* Harrison JH, Gittes RF, Perlmutter AD, et al, eds: Cambell's Urology. Philadelphia, W. B. Saunders Company, 1979, p 1535.

Radhakrishnan J: Colon interposition vaginoplasty: A modification of the Wagner-Baldwin technique. J Pediatr Surg 1987; 22:1175–1176.

Randolph JG, Hung W: Reduction clitoroplasty in females with hypertophied clitoris. J Pediatr Surg 1970; 5:224–231.

Robboy SJ, Miller T, Donahoe P, et al: Dysgenesis of testicular and streak gonads in the syndrome of mixed gonadal dysgenesis. Hum Pathol 1982; 13:700–716.

Snyder HM, Retik AB, Bauer SB, Colodny AH: Feminizing genitoplasty: A synthesis. J Urol 1983; 129:1024–1026.

Spence HM, Allen TD: Genital reconstruction in the female with adrenogenital syndrome. Br J Urol 1973; 45:126–130.

Stefan H: Surgical reconstruction of the external genitalia in female pseudohermaphrodites. Br J Urol 1967; 39:347–352.

Turner-Warwick R, Kirby RS: The construction and reconstruction of the vagina with the colocecum. Surg Gyn Obstet 1990; 170:132–136.

Wesley JR, Coran AG: Intestinal vaginoplasty for congenital absence of the vagina. J Pediatr Surg 1992; 27:885–889.

72 CONGENITAL ANOMALIES OF THE TESTIS AND SCROTUM

Jacob Rajfer, M.D.

CRYPTORCHIDISM

Cryptorchidism means a hidden testis. In humans, this anomaly occurs when the testis fails to descend into its normal postnatal anatomic location, the scrotum. Because the testis develops originally in the abdominal region, its descent may be inhibited anywhere along its normal pathway. Alternatively, the testis may be diverted from this route into an ectopic location.

Cryptorchidism represents one of the most common disorders of childhood. All races are affected, and there does not seem to be any geographic propensity for the disorder. Although cryptorchidism may be associated with a number of chromosomal and hereditary disorders in which a specific defect can be identified, at the present time the majority of cases appear to be isolated, probably because relatively little is known about what actually causes the human testis to migrate from the abdomen into the scrotum. As technologic and scientific advances continue to be made in the fields of genetics, molecular biology, and reproductive endocrinology, it is hoped that the actual mechanisms involved in the migration of the fetal testis will be ascertained. More clinical cases of cryptorchidism may therefore be identified as the phenotypic expression of a more generalized systemic disorder.

Why the Testis Descends

For the testis to produce viable and mature spermatozoa, in most mammalian species it must descend from the warmer intra-abdominal environment into the cooler scrotum (Felizet and Branca, 1902; Moore and Quick, 1924; Cooper, 1929; Wangensteen, 1935; Pace and Cabot, 1936). The slight temperature difference of 1.5 to 2.0°C between these two locations is sufficient to inhibit spermatogenesis (Mieusset et al, 1993).

If the timing of testicular descent in various animal species is compared, interesting observations can be made about the thermoregulation of spermatogenesis. The primate is the only species in which the testis completely descends at or near the time of birth (Wislocki, 1933). In the monkey, the testes retract from the scrotum to the inguinal canal at about the fifth postnatal day only to return permanently to the scrotum between the third and fifth years of life, which is the normal time of puberty in this species. In certain hibernating animals, the testes, which are intra-abdominal during the winter months, descend into the scrotum only during the breeding season (Bishop, 1945). In other animals, the testes remain intra-abdominal except during copulation, when they descend into the scrotum (Deming, 1936). In the whale, the testes are located intra-abdominally and are probably cooled by the animal's constant contact with cool water (Huberman and Israeloff, 1935). The testes of birds are located in the lumbar region and presumably are cooled by the air stream that constantly flows over them during flight. Therefore, cooling of the testes via migration into the scrotum appears to be a phylogenetic mechanism that humans have retained in order to propagate the species.

Embryology of Testicular Descent

To comprehend how the testis migrates into the scrotum, a knowledge of the related embryology is essential (Hamilton et al, 1957; Arey, 1965). **In the human, by the sixth week of gestation the primordial germ cells have migrated from the wall of the embryonic yolk sac along the dorsal mesentery of the hindgut to invade the genital ridges** (Witschi, 1948). At this stage of development in the male, the gubernaculum first appears as a ridge of mesenchymal tissue that extends from the genital ridge through a gap in the anterior abdominal wall musculature to the genital swellings, which are the site of the future scrotum (Backhouse, 1964). This gap in the anterior abdominal wall is the future inguinal canal.

By 7 weeks of gestation, under the influence of the SRY protein whose secretion is under the regulation of a gene located on the short arm of the Y chromosome (Page et al, 1987), **the indifferent gonad differentiates into the fetal testis. During the eighth week of gestation in the male embryo, the fetal testis begins to secrete two hormones, testosterone and müllerian-inhibiting factor** (Jost, 1953a; Jost, 1953b). **Testosterone, which is synthesized and secreted by the fetal Leydig cells** (Siiteri and Wilson, 1974; Payne and Jaffe, 1975), **is under the regulation of maternal human chorionic gonadotropin (hCG)** at this stage of development (Clements et al, 1976) **and induces the ipsilateral wolffian duct to form the epididymis and vas deferens.**

Müllerian-inhibiting factor, which is secreted by the fetal Sertoli cells (Josso, 1972, 1973; Guerrier et al, 1989), **causes regression of the müllerian ducts,** leaving only the appendix testis, a remnant of the müllerian ductal system. At this time, the processus vaginalis, an outpouching of peritoneum, is ventral to the gubernaculum (Wyndham, 1943; Lemeh, 1960). The future muscle fibers of **the cremaster, an embryologic derivative of the internal oblique muscle,** may also appear at this time along the developing processus vaginalis. The processus vaginalis forms as a hernia in the weak triangle that consists of peritoneum backed only by the jelly of the gubernaculum (Gier and Marion, 1970). The margins of the triangle are formed dorsally by the internal iliac artery and vein and ventrolaterally by the most posterior bands of the transversus abdominis muscle.

Between the 8th and 16th weeks of gestation, the external genitalia develop (Jirasek et al, 1968). **In the male embryo, testosterone, which is also secreted systemically by the fetal testis, is picked up by the tissues of the external genitalia and converted to dihydrotestosterone (DHT) by the 5α-reductase enzyme within the tissues of the external genitalia** (Siiteri and Wilson, 1974). **DHT is the active androgen that induces differentiation of the external genitalia in the male embryo** (Siiteri and Wilson, 1974). After the development of the testis, ductal system, and external genitalia, the testis lies on top of the conically shaped gubernaculum, awaiting descent (Backhouse, 1981). The gubernaculum can be seen from the cauda epididymis distally through the inguinal canal toward the genital swellings. The growth of the gubernaculum is believed to be regulated by substances secreted by the fetal testis (Wensing, 1968, 1973; Fentener Van Vlissingen et al, 1988). Under continued androgenic stimulation, the genital swellings are transformed into the scrotum. The testis has now assumed an intra-abdominal position right behind the internal inguinal ring. In reality, the testis is never more than 1.3 mm from the internal inguinal ring at any time during its development (Wyndham, 1943; Hutson, 1986).

The process of testicular descent remains relatively dormant between the 12th week and the 7th month of gestation. During this time, the processus vaginalis slowly extends into the scrotum (Wyndham, 1943). At about the seventh month of gestation, just prior to actual descent of the testis, rapid alterations occur simultaneously in the gubernaculum, processus vaginalis, and other surrounding structures. The size of the vas deferens and testicular vessels increases, the gubernaculum begins to swell, and the processus vaginalis extends rapidly into the scrotum (Backhouse, 1964; Backhouse and Butler, 1960; Heyns et al, 1986). A separation now occurs between the gubernaculum and the scrotal wall. As the scrotum and inguinal canal are stretched by the developing gubernaculum, the gonad, which sits on top of the gubernaculum, slips very rapidly into the scrotum (Wyndham, 1943; Schechter, 1963; Backhouse, 1981; Heyns, 1987). During descent, the epididymis precedes the testis in its journey into the scrotum. After descent, the scrotal part of the processus vaginalis persists as the tunica vaginalis, and the upper part is obliterated. The gubernaculum subsequently atrophies. **If the processus vaginalis fails to obliterate, a hernia or hydrocele may form.**

Incidence of Testicular Descent

Cryptorchidism represents one of the most common disorders in humans. The genitourinary system is well represented by the cryptorchid state in a multitude of congenital and hereditary abnormalities (Frey et al, 1981). In some premature babies, birth may occur prior to the onset of normal testicular descent during the last trimester of gestation. Scorer and Farrington (1971) found that **of 1500 full-term** (birth weight greater than 2500 g) **infants examined at birth, 3.4% had true undescended testes,** whereas 30.3%

of 142 premature infants had undescended testes (Table 72–1). This differential in the incidence of testicular descent between full-term and premature infants has also been reported by other investigators (Buemann et al, 1961), and there is some preliminary evidence that these estimates of two decades ago may need to be revised upward in the years to come (Cryptorchidism Study Group, 1992). Nevertheless, the smaller the birth weight of the infant, the greater the incidence of cryptorchidism. However, once these babies, particularly the premature ones, begin to gain weight and advance in age, the testes begin to descend.

By 1 year of age, the incidence of testicular maldescent is between 0.8% and 1.5%, a marked decrease during this short time period (Villumsen and Zachau-Christiansen, 1966; Scorer and Farrington, 1971; Berkowitz et al, 1993; Cryptorchidism Study Group, 1992). These data show that approximately 75% of full-term cryptorchid testes and up to 95% of premature cryptorchid testes spontaneously descend by 1 year of age. **Most of the testes that descend during the first year of life actually do so within the first 3 months after birth.** If descent has not occurred by this time, descent of the testis is never completed, and this testis remains relatively smaller than the contralaterally descended testis.

It is assumed, although it has not been proved, that the reason the testis may descend within the first year is the elevated level of androgens in the plasma during the first 3 months of life (Table 72–2) (Scorer, 1964; Forest et al, 1974). The rise in plasma testosterone level that occurs during the first 3 months in the male gradually falls to prepubertal levels (Forest et al, 1974; Winter et al, 1976). The Leydig cells, the source of the testosterone, become inactive and remain so until puberty. Despite the fact that the Leydig cells are inactive during the prepubertal years, they nevertheless retain the potential to respond to human chorionic gonadotropin (hCG) stimulation. This response to exogenous gonadotropin has been amply demonstrated in both prepubertal normal testes and prepubertal cryptorchid testes (Winter et al, 1972; Grant et al, 1976; Merksz et al, 1992).

The cryptorchid state is most easily determined at birth, when the scrotum is relatively large, minimal subcutaneous fat exists, and the cremasteric reflex is absent (Scorer and Farrington, 1971). However, **the cremasteric reflex is most active between the second and seventh years of age, and, as a result, a falsely high incidence of cryptorchidism may be obtained during childhood** (McCutcheon, 1938; Ward and Hunter, 1960). In fact, in a number of studies, the incidence of cryptorchidism at or about the fifth year of age was estimated at about 10% (Farrington, 1968). This high percentage was probably due to the inclusion of unrecognized cases of retractile testes. For example, if the incidence of cryptorchidism is the same at 1 year and at adulthood (approximately 1.0%), this incidence cannot change at any time between these ages because human testes do not ascend permanently in the postnatal period. This ascent is what Farrington and the author term a true retractile testis (Rajfer et al, 1986). Consequently, if there appears to be an increase in the incidence of cryptorchidism to more than 1% at other ages, it must be due to testes that retract and then descend at a later date. Indeed, the author would term the gliding testis, one that glides between the external ring and the top of the scrotum, not a retractile testis but a true undescended testis (Lais et al, 1993). When Cour-Palais (1966) reexamined those cases of undescended testes of various age groups, the majority were indeed found to be retractile testes. In Cour-Palais's series, the true incidence of cryptorchidism was 0.76% at age 5 years, 0.95% at age 8 years, and 0.64% at age 11 or thereafter.

Table 72–1. INCIDENCE OF CRYPTORCHIDISM

Age	Incidence (%)
Pre-term infant	30.3
Full-term infant	3.4
One year	0.8
Adulthood	0.8

Adapted from Scorer CG, Farrington GH: Congenital Deformities of the Testis and Epididymis. New York, Appleton-Century-Crofts, 1971.

Table 72–2. PLASMA TESTOSTERONE (mg/dl) IN HUMANS

	1–15 days	1–3 months	1 Year	Prepuberty	Adulthood
Male	68 ± 60	208 ± 68	7 ± 5	7 ± 3	572 ± 135
Female	12 ± 6	9 ± 4	6 ± 3	7 ± 3	37 ± 10

Adapted from Forest MG, et al: J Clin Invest 1974; 53:819. Reproduced from the Journal of Clinical Investigation, 1974, 53, 819, by copyright permission of the Journal of Clinical Investigation.

In adults, Cour-Palais found that the incidence of cryptorchidism was slightly less than 1% of the male population. In addition to this careful study, other studies attest to the fact that the incidence of cryptorchidism at adulthood is less than 1%. Baumrucker (1946) determined that the incidence of cryptorchidism in 10,000 consecutive United States Army inductees was 0.8%. Others have noted similar incidences: 0.5% in 10,000 Scottish recruits (Southam and Cooper, 1927), 0.7% in male autopsies, and 0.55% in almost 3 million United States Selective Service registrants between 1940 and 1944 (Campbell, 1959). **The true incidence of cryptorchidism remains relatively constant from 1 year of age until adulthood,** without any geographic distinction. The recent findings by some investigators (Chilvers et al, 1984; Cryptorchidism Study Group, 1992) that the incidence of cryptorchidism appears to be increasing has not been corroborated by others (Berkowitz et al, 1993).

In surgical explorations for cryptorchidism, **absence of one or both testes may be encountered in 3% to 5% of cases** (Goldberg et al, 1974). **In 10% of patients with cryptorchidism, the defect is bilateral; in 3%, one or both testes are absent** (Scorer and Farrington, 1971). A familial incidence is apparent in certain patients with cryptorchidism. Approximately 14% of boys with undescended testes have family members with the same condition (Bishop, 1945; Brimblecomb, 1946; Wiles, 1934).

Mechanisms of Testicular Descent

Since Hunter's (1841) treatise, various mechanisms have been proposed to be responsible for the final placement of the testes into the scrotum (Table 72–3). Foremost are certain physical factors, which include (1) traction of the testis by the gubernaculum or cremaster muscle, or both; (2) differen-

Table 72–3. MECHANISMS OF TESTICULAR DESCENT

Traction
Differential growth
Intra-abdominal pressure
Epididymal maturation
Genitofemoral nerve
Hormonal

tial growth of the body wall in relation to a relatively immobile gubernaculum; (3) intra-abdominal pressure pushing the testis through an inguinal canal that is engorged by the swollen gubernaculum; (4) development and maturation of the epididymis being responsible for testicular migration, and (5) the effect of the genitofemoral nerve.

The traction theory adheres to the concept that the gubernaculum or the cremaster muscle, or both, pulls the testis into the scrotum (Curling, 1840; Sonneland, 1925). Support for this concept comes from the observation that severance of the genitofemoral nerve, which innervates the gubernaculum, prevents testicular descent in rodents (Tayakkononta, 1963). However, severance of the gubernaculum in a variety of animal species did not prevent the testis from descending into the scrotum (Wells, 1944; Bergh et al, 1978). In addition, in the human fetus there is only a weak attachment between the gubernaculum and the scrotum, and this is probably insufficient to support any traction on the testis (Wyndham, 1943; Tayakkononta, 1963, Bergh et al, 1978). Regarding the cremaster, it is well established that the sole function of this muscle is to retract the testis. Consequently, traction of the testis into the scrotum by the cremaster muscle is unlikely.

The differential growth theory adheres to the concept that as the body wall grows, the testis is kept in proximity to the internal inguinal ring. It is then pulled into the scrotum by the relatively immobile gubernaculum as a result of rapid growth of the body wall during the last trimester of pregnancy (McMurrich, 1923; Hunter, 1927). However, it has been demonstrated that the gubernaculum actually increases in size prior to descent and that it actually grows faster than the body as a whole (Hunter, 1927; Lemeh, 1960), thereby casting doubt on the validity of this theory.

The intra-abdominal pressure theory states that an increase in intra-abdominal pressure is the primary force causing the testis to leave the abdomen and enter the inguinal ring (Schechter, 1963; Bergin et al, 1970; Gier and Marion, 1970). A number of investigators have provided theoretical and experimental evidence that appears to support the concept of intra-abdominal pressure as a promoter of testicular descent (Elder et al, 1982; Frey et al, 1983; Frey and Rajfer, 1984; Attah and Hutson, 1993).

The epididymal theory of testicular descent (Hadziselimovic, 1981), which is based on the assumption that differentiation and maturation of the epididymis induce testicular descent, has been investigated in depth and may not be as important as initially thought (Frey and Rajfer, 1982; Elder, 1992).

Although it is difficult to refute unequivocally the aforementioned mechanical theories of testicular descent, and indeed all may play some role, it is generally accepted that **endocrine factors somehow play the major role in promoting the descent of the testis into the scrotum.** The endocrine regulation of testicular descent was initially inferred by Engle (1932), who induced premature testicular descent in the monkey by the use of gonadotropins. Thereafter, testosterone was found to be as efficacious as gonadotropins in inducing testicular descent in humans (Goldman et al, 1926; Thompson et al, 1937; Arnheim 1938; Bigler et al, 1938; Hamilton and Hubert, 1938; Hamilton, 1938). Although it has been demonstrated that dihydrotestosterone, the 5α-reduced product of testosterone, appears to be the active androgen involved in testicular descent in at least two animal species (Rajfer and Walsh, 1977; Rajfer, 1982), inhibition of the 5α-reductase enzyme and the androgen receptor to male rodents postnatally failed to retard descent (Ngyuen et al, 1991; Bluestein et al, 1991). If, however, drugs that block the 5α-reductase enzyme or androgen receptor are given to pregnant rats during the period of sexual differentiation of the male offspring, cryptorchidism may be induced in these newborn animals (Spencer et al, 1991; Husmann and McPhaul, 1991).

The theory that the genitofemoral nerve is involved in modulating the gubernaculum to induce testicular descent (Tayakkononta, 1963; Beasley and Hutson, 1987) has regained some adherents after it was shown in animal experiments that androgens exert an effect on the nuclei of the genitofemoral nerve. After exposure to androgens, the nuclei of this nerve, which are located in the spinal cord, stimulate the release or production of factors, possibly calcitonin gene-related peptide (CGRP), by the nerve terminals to modulate gubernacular development or function (Larkins and Hutson, 1991; Larkins et al, 1991; Yamanaka et al, 1992, 1993). Clinical evidence to support this theory comes from the observation that **boys with spinal cord defects at and below the level of the nuclei of the genitofemoral nerve have a higher incidence of undescended testes** (Hutson et al, 1988). However, Houle and Gagne (1995) recently showed in animals that hCG but not CGRP had a positive effect on promoting testis descent.

Endocrine Aspects of Cryptorchidism

If gonadotropins and androgens are necessary for testicular descent to occur, it follows that abnormalities in the hypothalamic-pituitary-testicular axis may result in cryptorchidism. Indeed, **in a variety of clinical syndromes characterized by defects in gonadotropin production, androgen synthesis, or androgen action, cryptorchidism may be observed** (Fig. 72–1). In Kallmann's syndrome, an inherited disorder in which there is a deficiency of gonadotropin-releasing hormone (GnRH) secretion from the hypothalamus, cryptorchidism may be a presenting feature (Bardin et al, 1969; Santen and Paulsen, 1972). In anencephaly or developmental abnormalities of the pituitary gland, such as hypoplasia or aplasia, undescended testes are very common (Ch'in, 1938; Steiner and Boogs, 1965; Sadeghi-Nejad and Senior, 1974). In disorders of androgen synthesis or androgen action, cryptorchidism may also be a presenting feature (Grumbach and Van Wyk, 1974). In patients with defects of the 5α-reductase enzyme that converts testosterone into dihydrotestosterone, cryptorchidism is frequent (Opitz et al, 1972; Walsh et al, 1974).

Although hormonal involvement in testicular descent ap-

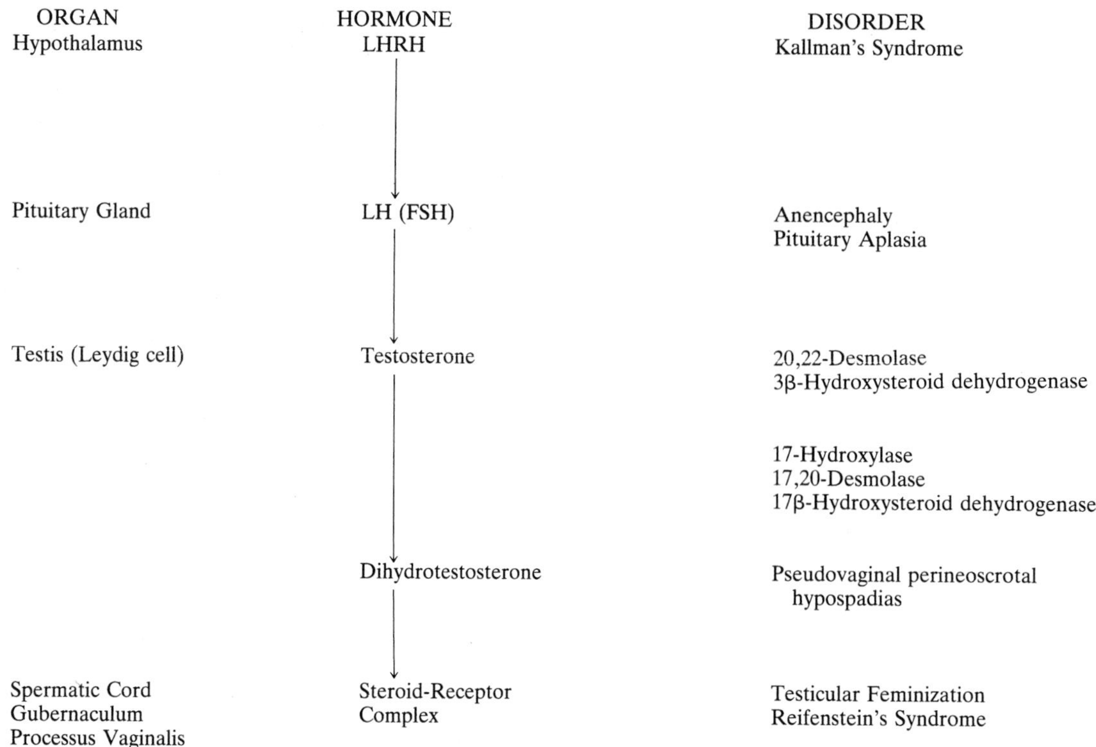

Figure 72–1. Disorders of the hypothalamic-pituitary-testicular axis in the presence of cryptorchidism. (From Rajfer J, Walsh PC: Hormonal regulation of testicular descent: Experimental and clinical observations. J Urol 1977; 118:985. © Williams & Wilkins.)

pears to be clear-cut, there is nevertheless some discrepancy in the literature as to whether patients with cryptorchidism have discernible abnormalities in the hypothalamic-pituitary-testicular axis. Walsh and associates (1976) found no difference in plasma testosterone levels following hCG stimulation between children with cryptorchidism and normal children. In contrast, Cacciari and colleagues (1976) found a subnormal testosterone response to gonadotropin in children with cryptorchidism. When these workers used GnRH to stimulate the hypothalamic-pituitary axis, they found no difference in pituitary luteinizing hormone (LH) and follicle-stimulating hormone (FSH) secretion between the children with cryptorchidism and normal children. This finding was confirmed by Sizonenko and associates (1978), Van Vliet and associates (1980), and deMuinck Keizer-Schrama and associates (1986). However, the data of Hadziselimovic (1983) and Job and Gendrel (Gendrel et al, 1977, 1978, 1980a and b; Job et al, 1977) suggest that infants and children with cryptorchidism do indeed have abnormalities in the hypothalamic-pituitary-testicular axis, as evidenced by a decrease in basal LH and testosterone levels and a blunted response of LH and testosterone to GnRH stimulation (Fig. 72–2). This deficiency in secretion of LH and testosterone in infants with cryptorchidism persists through early puberty but disappears at midpuberty. No significant abnormality in the FSH levels of these patients was seen, although an occasional patient did demonstrate elevated basal FSH levels indicative of seminiferous tubular damage.

Despite these data, the exact mechanism by which androgens act to promote testicular descent is still unknown. It is apparent, based on embryologic observations and some experimental data, that the gubernaculum is intimately involved with this important physiologic event. George and Peterson (1988) demonstrated some DHT binding within the gubernaculum of the postnatal rat, suggesting that the gubernaculum may be the androgen target tissue involved in testicular descent. The finding that the nuclei of the genitofemoral nerve, which innervates the gubernacular tissue, is androgen responsive adds credence to this theory (Hutson et al, 1988).

Classification of Undescended Testes

Undescended testes can be classified as (1) abdominal—located inside the internal inguinal ring; (2) canalicular—located between the internal and external inguinal rings; (3) ectopic—located away from the normal pathway of descent between the abdominal cavity and the bottom of the scrotum, and (4) retractile—the fully descended testis moves freely between the bottom of the scrotum and the groin, where it enters the superficial inguinal pouch (Browne, 1949). This pouch is actually a subcutaneous pocket lined by thin fibrous tissue situated in front of and lateral to the external inguinal ring.

The intra-abdominal testis, by definition, is impalpable. Very commonly, the testis is located just at the internal inguinal ring, and at the time of surgical exploration slight abdominal pressure usually causes the testis to pop into the inguinal canal. The canalicular testis is farther along the pathway of descent than the intra-abdominal testis. It may be located within the canal, or it may become emergent from within the canal to lie at the top of the scrotum. When it is located in the inguinal canal, the tension of the aponeurosis

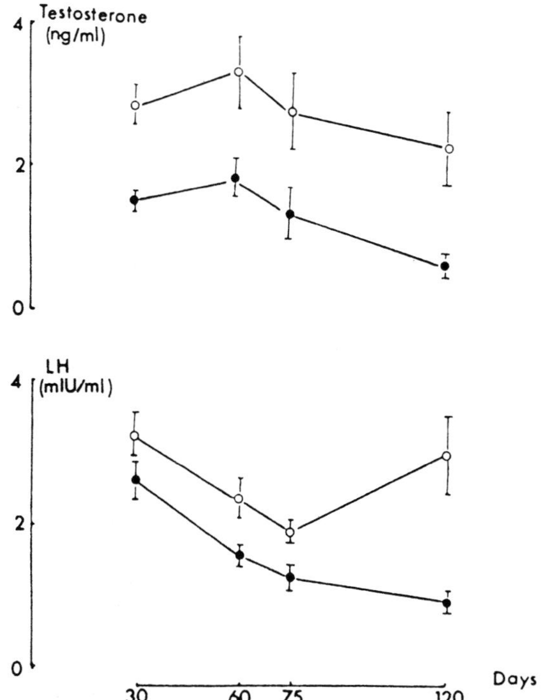

Figure 72–2. Age-dependent plasma testosterone and LH (mean ± SEM) values in newborn infants who presented at birth with undescended testes. One group (○) had spontaneous descent by 4 months, whereas the other group (●) had no testicular descent. (From Gendrel D, et al: J Pediatr 1980; 97:217.)

of the external oblique muscle may be too firm a barrier to allow the testis to become palpable (Scorer and Farrington, 1971).

On rare occasions, the testis may migrate from its normal pathway of movement between the abdominal cavity and the bottom of the scrotum and become located in an ectopic position. **The five major sites of testicular ectopia are the perineum, the femoral canal, the superficial inguinal pouch, the suprapubic area, and the opposite scrotal compartment** (Fig. 72–3). Testicular ectopia is believed to be directly related to the development of the gubernaculum. The gubernaculum is known to be divided into five branches, one each going to the aforementioned areas (Lockwood, 1888; Schechter, 1963). The scrotal area normally contains the bulk of the gubernaculum, and the testis normally follows this path during its descent. It has been suggested that when one of the other four branches contains the bulk of the gubernaculum, the testis is misdirected from its normal pathway of descent into the ectopic location. Clinically, **the most common ectopic location is the superficial inguinal pouch,** which is a subcutaneous pocket lined by thin fibrous tissue situated in front of and lateral to the external ring (Browne, 1949). Transverse testicular ectopia is the rarest of all ectopic conditions but should be considered in any patient with an empty hemiscrotum and an additional mass in the contralateral hemiscrotum (Davis, 1957; Mukerjee and Amesur, 1965; Dajani, 1969).

The single most common factor that leads to an inaccurate diagnosis of an undescended testis is the presence of testicular retraction. Testicular retraction results from spontaneous or provoked activity of the cremaster muscle. **It is most apparent in boys 5 to 6 years of age.** In a survey of some 600 normal boys, Farrington (1968) found that in those under the age of 12 years, up to 20% of the testes were in the superficial inguinal pouch at initial inspection. In boys between 6 months and 11 years of age, deliberate stimulation of the cremasteric reflex resulted in withdrawal of up to 80% of fully descended testes from their scrotal positions, leaving a seemingly empty hemiscrotum. Some 25% of these testes retract fully into the superficial inguinal pouch, and the remainder retract into the neck of the scrotum. From the fifth to sixth year of age until puberty, a gradual decline occurs in the number of testes that fully retract out of the scrotum. At 11 years of age, in half of the boys who were showing evidence of the onset of puberty, only half of the testes retracted upon stimulation of the cremasteric reflex. At 13 years of age, the testis was usually found to be no longer retractile.

This retraction of the normal testis into the upper part of the scrotum or the superficial inguinal pouch during boyhood seems to be a protective reflex. Why this reflex appears to dissipate at the time of puberty is unknown. Therefore, **it is of paramount importance to determine and record in an infant's chart whether the testes are palpable in the scrotum at birth or within the first year of life.** During the physical examination, manual traction is gently placed on the testis to try to bring it down to the bottom of the scrotum (Wylie, 1984). If it reaches the bottom of the scrotum, this is considered a retractile testis. If it does not, the patient returns on another visit for a second attempt at "milking the testis down." If it fails a second time, consideration is given to hormonal therapy (Rajfer et al, 1986b).

Although there are reports in the literature of ascending testes, the author has been unable to confirm or document unequivocally such a finding at his institution and is unable to explain its occurrence scientifically (Belman, 1988; Robertson et al, 1988). Testes with such a diagnosis that have been sent to us for evaluation turn out to be either true ectopic testes or retractile testes. Nevertheless, it has been reported that such testes may show histologic abnormalities (Saito and Kumamoto, 1989) and orchiopexy of such as-

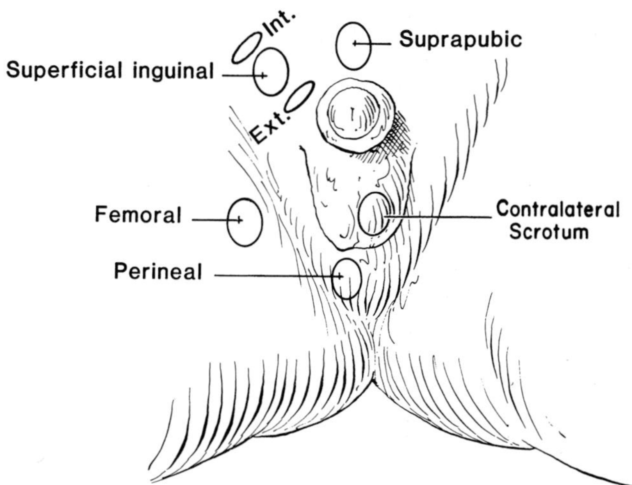

Figure 72–3. Schematic representation of sites of ectopic testes (int, internal inguinal ring; ext, external inguinal ring). (From Rajfer J: Urol Clin North Am 1982; 9:422.)

cended testes may result in improvement in sperm counts (Nistal and Paniagua, 1984).

If a testis is not palpable, it is intracanalicular, intra-abdominal, or absent (Scorer and Farrington, 1971). The diagnosis of bilateral anorchia should always be considered in the presence of bilateral nonpalpable testes (Goldberg et al, 1974). **If the basal gonadotropin levels (FSH in particular) are elevated in a boy less than 9 years of age, further work-up is not necessary to diagnose bilateral anorchia** (Jarow et al, 1986). **If the FSH levels are not elevated in a boy with bilateral nonpalpable testes, hCG stimulation tests are applied to help determine the presence or absence of testicular tissue,** in particular, the presence of Leydig cells (Winter et al, 1972; Grant et al, 1976). A short course of hCG (2000 IU daily for 3 days) may be used to distinguish bilateral anorchia from bilateral cryptorchidism. In bilateral anorchia, there is no testosterone response to exogenous hCG.

Recently, Whitaker (1992) and Kaplan (1993) have proposed an improved and simplified classification of the undescended testis based on the determination of whether the testis is palpable or not (Table 72–4).

Imaging of Undescended Testes

The unilateral impalpable testis itself poses a unique diagnostic problem. Its presence must be verified and appropriate therapy taken either to make it palpable or to remove it. A variety of tests are employed in clinical practice to search for the impalpable testis. These include herniography, ultrasonography, computed tomography (CT) scanning, testicular arteriography or venography, and magnetic resonance imaging (MRI).

Herniography (White et al, 1970, 1973) is the oldest of these tests and has an unacceptably high incidence of false-positive and false-negative results. For these reasons, it is used rarely in routine clinical practice today. Ultrasound scanning has been helpful in locating the testis only if the testes is located in the superficial inguinal pouch or within the inguinal canal (Madrazo et al, 1979). If the testis is located underneath the aponeurosis of the external oblique muscle or is intra-abdominal, ultrasound may not be very reliable (Maghnie et al, 1994). CT scanning may be useful in documenting the location of bilateral impalpable testes, but the test is expensive, emits radiation, and sometimes is difficult to perform in the young child (Lee et al, 1980; Pak et al, 1981; Rajfer et al, 1983; Wolverson et al, 1983). MRI may be helpful in locating the impalpable testis (Fritzsche et al, 1987; Landa et al, 1987), but, like CT scanning, it may be difficult to perform in the young child. It is, however, the least invasive of all current procedures (Maghnie et al, 1994).

Table 72–4. CLASSIFICATION OF CRYPTORCHIDISM

1. Palpable
   A. Normal
   B. Retractile
   C. Ectopic
   D. Undescended
2. Nonpalpable
   A. Canalicular
   B. Intra-abdominal
   C. Emergent
   D. Absent
      (1) Agenesis
      (2) Atrophy

Adapted from Kaplan GW: Eur J Pediatr 1993; 152:S17.

Angiography of the testicular vessels is technically difficult, and its complications (e.g., femoral thrombosis) may have disastrous consequences (Ben-Menachem et al, 1974; Vitale et al, 1974). Testicular venography has less morbidity than arteriography but is still an invasive procedure. Venography relies on the fact that when the pampiniform plexus of veins is present, the testis presumably is always present (Amin and Wheeler, 1976; Weiss et al, 1979). However, if the plexus is not visualized or if the testicular vein is blind-ending, one cannot state unequivocally that the testis is absent on that side (Weiss et al, 1979). For this reason, the test has its drawbacks.

Recently, Hrebinko and Bellinger (1993) reported on the usefulness of all the different imaging techniques in the management of children with cryptorchidism and concluded that these techniques rarely helped the physician. They found that **the overall accuracy of radiologic testing was 44%.** Physical examination was 53% accurate when performed by the referring physician and 84% accurate when done by the attending pediatric urologist. In no case did radiographic assessment influence the decision to operate, the surgical approach, or the viability or salvageability of the involved testes.

Pediatric laparoscopy has evolved as an important tool in the search for the impalpable testis (Silber and Cohen, 1980). **If the testicular vessels are seen to end blindly, this signifies that the testis is absent on that side and that no surgical exploration is necessary. If the vessels are seen to enter the internal inguinal ring, an inguinal exploration or laparoscopic assisted orchiectomy or orchiopexy is all that is required** (Froeling et al, 1994). When the testis is seen in the abdomen, a decision may be made either to perform an intra-abdominal exploration and attempt to place the testis in the scrotum (Naslund et al, 1989) or to clip the testicular vessels and perform an orchiopexy at a later date (Ransley et al, 1984; Bloom et al, 1988; Jordan and Winslow, 1994; Holcomb et al, 1994).

Histology

In 1929, Cooper published her classic paper on the histology of the cryptorchid testis. She noted that **the longer a testis remained cryptorchid, the more likely it was to be histologically abnormal.** The higher the testis lay from the bottom of the scrotum, the more pronounced the histologic abnormality. **These histologic alterations in the cryptorchid testis appear by 1½ years of age and include smaller seminiferous tubules, fewer spermatogonia, and more peritubular tissue.** Since Cooper's work, a multitude of papers have appeared confirming these histologic alterations in the cryptorchid testis. (Sohval, 1954; Mack et al, 1961; Scorer and Farrington, 1971; Mengel et al, 1974). Although the seminiferous tubules are definitely altered by the cryptorchid state, there is conflicting histologic evidence about whether the Leydig cells are affected.

The electron microscope has been used to document certain ultrastructural changes in the seminiferous tubules as early as the second year of life (Hadziselimovic and Seguchi, 1973; Hadziselimovic, 1977; Zarzycki et al, 1977; Mengel et al, 1981). These changes include (1) degeneration of the mitochondria, (2) loss of ribosomes in both the cytoplasm and the smooth endoplasmic reticulum, and (3) an increase in the collagen fibers in the spermatogonia and Sertoli cells. Ultrastructural data about changes in the Leydig cells are conflicting. It is still uncertain whether the known changes in the cryptorchid testis represent a primary defect or only an alteration secondary to the cryptorchid state. Support for the idea that the testis itself is defective lies in the observation that **some of these histologic changes may also occur in the contralateral scrotal testis of the unilateral cryptorchid male** (Mengel et al, 1974).

Complications

Neoplasia

A strong association exists between neoplasia and cryptorchidism. **Approximately 10% of testicular tumors arise from an undescended testis** (Gilbert, 1941; Gordon-Taylor and Wyndham, 1947; Campbell, 1959; Abratt et al, 1992). Statistically, **the undescended testis is reported to be 35 to 48 times more likely to undergo malignant degeneration than the normal testis** (Johnson et al, 1968; Jones and Scott, 1971; Martin and Menck, 1975).

The fact that neoplastic degeneration of an undescended testis is in itself a rare entity allows some surgeons to state that orchiectomy may not be the only choice of therapy in the postpubertal patient with cryptorchid testis (Welvaart and Tijssen, 1981). In 1985, Farrer and associates addressed this issue and, using data available at that time, concluded that **the true annual incidence of germ cell testis tumors in patients with cryptorchidism is one tumor per 2550 cases.** Employing the same statistical data, these investigators also concluded that **after age 32, the patient with cryptorchidism is at greater risk of death from orchiectomy than from testicular malignancy** (Fig. 72–4). Therefore, the author and his associates have modified their policy so that **all impalpable testes are either removed or placed in a position to allow palpation.** If a testis is undescended but palpable, they observe patients who are 32 years of age or older. For patients with palpable undescended testes less than 32 years of age, observation or orchiopexy is recommended depending on the patient's wishes.

With regard to location, an abdominal testis is four times more likely to undergo malignant degeneration than an inguinal testis (Campbell, 1959). **Tumors in undescended testes occur mainly at the time of puberty or after,** although some neoplasms have occurred in children and infants (Gordon-Taylor and Wyndham, 1947). For this reason, if surgical correction of the cryptorchid testis is to be performed, it should be carried out before puberty.

In 1972, Skakkebaek reported finding carcinoma in situ in the testis of an infertile man with an undescended testis who developed a germ cell tumor 16 months later. Since then, **the prevalence of carcinoma in situ has been determined to be 1.7% in patients with cryptorchidism.** As a result, these European investigators recommend that all patients between 18 and 20 years of age with a history of cryptorchidism, treated or untreated, should be offered an open testis biopsy (Giwercman et al, 1987, 1989). If carcinoma in situ is not found on the biopsy, the risk of developing future testicular cancer in that gonad is extremely low. If carcinoma in situ is discovered, the gonad is removed.

Because testicular tumors have occurred in patients who have undergone orchiopexy as early as 5 years of age (Alt-

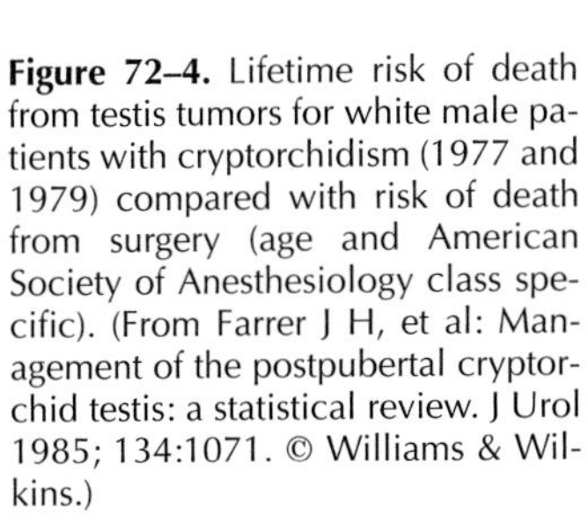

Figure 72–4. Lifetime risk of death from testis tumors for white male patients with cryptorchidism (1977 and 1979) compared with risk of death from surgery (age and American Society of Anesthesiology class specific). (From Farrer J H, et al: Management of the postpubertal cryptorchid testis: a statistical review. J Urol 1985; 134:1071. © Williams & Wilkins.)

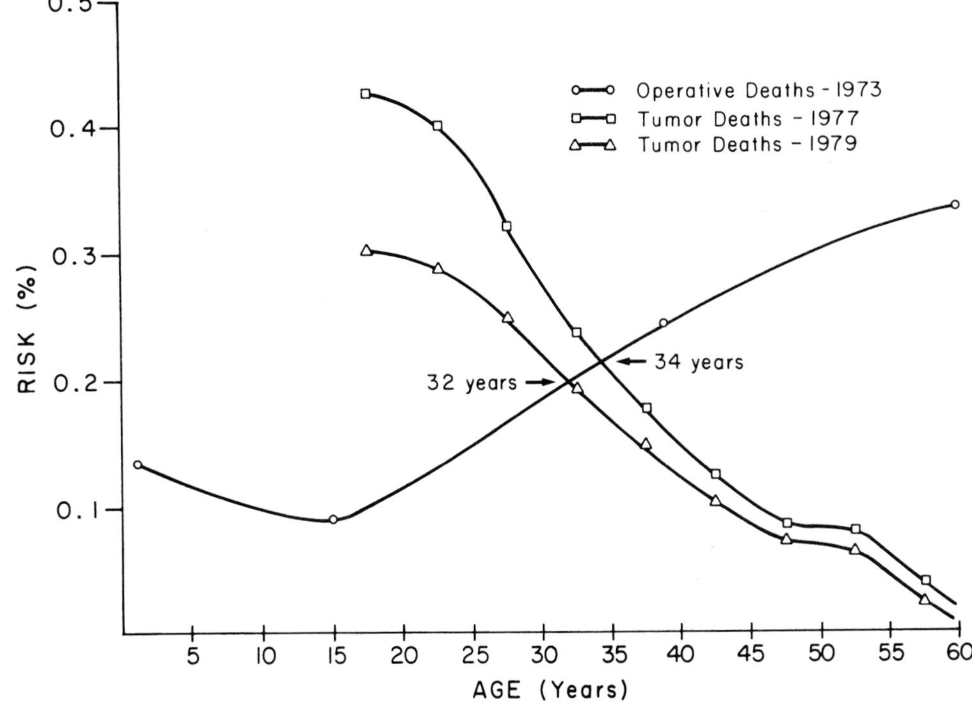

man and Malament, 1967), **most workers currently recommend surgical correction between 1 and 1½ years of age,** especially in light of the fact that ultrastructural changes begin to occur in the undescended testis at this early age (Mengel et al, 1974, 1981; Hadziselimovic, 1977). Whether this earlier surgical correction will deter the subsequent development of neoplasia in the undescended testis remains to be seen (United Kingdom Testicular Cancer Study Group, 1994). Further support for the concept that there is an underlying pathologic process that affects both testes in the patient with unilateral cryptorchidism comes from the data of Johnson and associates (1968). They showed that **one in five testicular tumors occurring in patients with cryptorchidism develop in the contralateral, supposedly normal, scrotal testis.**

In patients with bilateral cryptorchidism, there is a 15% chance of developing a tumor in the opposite testis if one of the testes becomes involved with a tumor (Gilbert and Hamilton, 1970). If both testes are intra-abdominal and one testis becomes malignant, there is a 30% chance of the other testis becoming malignant. Seminoma followed by embryonal cell carcinoma are the two most frequent neoplasms encountered in cryptorchid testes (Gilbert and Hamilton, 1970; Martin, 1979; Batata et al, 1980).

In patients with certain intersex disorders in which cryptorchidism is a presenting feature, gonadoblastoma is the most common tumor (Scully, 1970). **Although gonadoblastomas themselves are nonmalignant tumors, they often coexist with germ cell tumors in the same gonad** (Fig. 72–5). Evidence exists that gonadoblastomas develop because of a deletion of part of the long arm of the Y chromosome (Page, 1987).

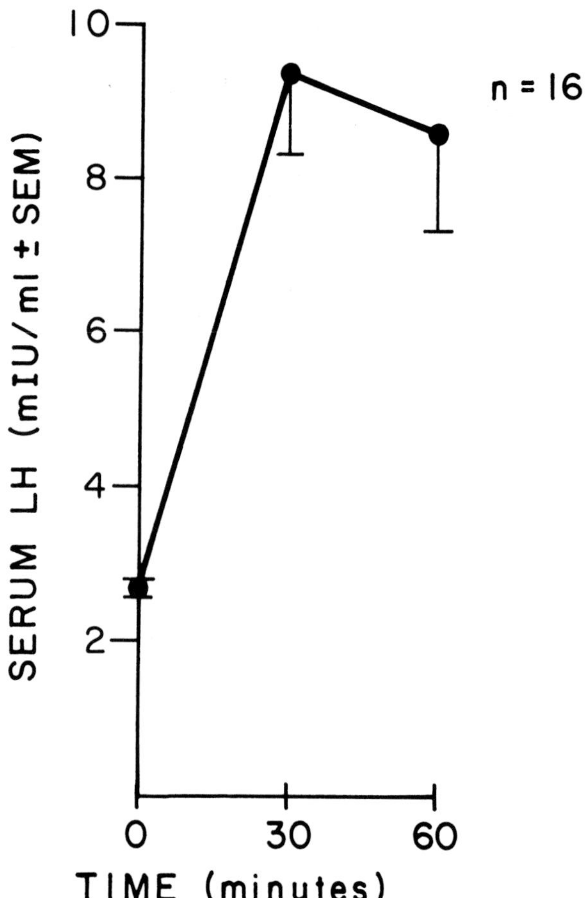

Figure 72–5. Mean serum LH levels among boys with cryptorchidism treated with intranasal GnRH. (From Rajfer J, et al: N Engl J Med 1986; 314:466. Used by permission.)

Torsion

The increased susceptibility of the testis to undergo torsion is due to a developmental anatomic abnormality between the testis and its mesentery. If the testis is broader than its mesentery, it is more likely to twist on its stalk (Scorer and Farrington, 1971). Therefore, **the incidence of torsion is greatest in the postpubertal period when the testis usually increases in size.** Similarly, **the undescended testis is more susceptible to torsion by any mechanism that causes an increase in testicular size, e.g., a tumor.** In a review of the literature, Rigler (1972) found that 64% of adults with torsion in an undescended testis had an associated germ cell tumor. **The presentation of a patient with abdominal pain and an ipsilateral empty hemiscrotum should alert the physician to the possibility of torsion of a cryptorchid testis** (Cilento et al, 1993).

Hernia

As stated in the previous section on embryology, the processus vaginalis is intimately associated with the structures involved in testicular descent. Following descent, which occurs at or about the seventh month of fetal life, **the processus vaginalis, which connects the peritoneal cavity to the tunica vaginalis, closes between the eighth month of fetal life and the first month after birth. However, when the testis fails to descend, the processus vaginalis remains patent.** This may permit some of the intra-abdominal contents to enter the tunica vaginalis through the processus vaginalis and appear clinically as a hernia or a hydrocele. Although the true incidence is unclear, **hernia sacs may be found in more than 90% of patients with cryptorchidism** (Scorer and Farrington, 1971; Elder, 1992).

Infertility

Testicular maldescent retards the production of spermatozoa. Therefore, the fertility of patients with bilaterally retained testes is generally very poor (Hansen, 1949; Mack, 1953; Scott, 1962; Scorer, 1967; Albescu et al, 1971; Wolloch et al, 1980). **The higher and longer the testis resides away from the bottom of the scrotum, the greater the likelihood of damage to the seminiferous tubules.** The earlier the testis is brought down into the scrotum, the greater the potential for recovering spermatogenic activity, although recent data suggest that this may not be the case (McAleer et al, 1995). Consequently, it seems prudent to perform orchiopexy before degeneration of the seminiferous tubules occurs (Ludwig and Potempa, 1975).

A defect may be present in the spermatogenic activity of the contralateral scrotal testis in the patient with unilateral cryptorchidism (Hecker and Heinz, 1967; Scorer, 1967; Woodhead et al, 1973). By comparing the sperm density of normal adults with that of adults who had undergone successful unilateral orchiopexy during childhood, Lipschultz and associates (1976) discovered that **men with unilateral cryptorchidism had much lower than expected sperm counts.** This observation further supports the hypothesis that there may be an inherent defect in both testes of the patient with unilateral cryptorchidism.

In addition to the defect in spermatogenesis, clinical and experimental evidence suggests that cryptorchidism may also affect the interstitial compartment of the testis. In cryptorchid animals, sex accessory tissue weight has been shown to be retarded, and the testicular enzymes necessary for testosterone synthesis may be inhibited (Korenchevsy, 1931; Clegg, 1960). It has also been demonstrated that the testosterone response of prepubertal children with cryptorchidism to exogenous hCG stimulation is retarded (Job et al, 1977; Gendrel et al, 1977, 1978, 1980a and b). Postpubertally, however, there appears to be no difference in the hCG response between children with cryptorchidism and normal children. If, indeed, cryptorchidism does have an adverse effect on testosterone synthesis, the defect is probably not clinically significant because **most patients with bilateral cryptorchidism are normally androgenized both at birth and at adulthood.**

Associated Anomalies

Some question exists in the literature about the incidence of chromosomal abnormalities in patients with uncomplicated unilateral cryptorchidism (Mininberg and Bragol, 1973; Dewald et al, 1977). Genetic syndromes associated with the undescended testis are extremely rare and are associated with poor survival. Of these, the best known are Klinefelter's, Noonan's, and Prader-Willi syndromes. Most patients with Klinefelter's syndrome are sterile, and the disease therefore cannot be passed to offspring. However, an occasional patient has a mosaic chromosomal constitution and may be potentially fertile. Noonan's syndrome, or male Turner's syndrome, is an endocrine disorder in which cryptorchidism is common (Redman, 1973; Sasagawa et al, 1994). As in Klinefelter's syndrome, a patient with Noonan's syndrome may occasionally be fertile, but the disorder is usually not passed to the offspring. Patients with Prader-Willi syndrome, which is believed to be secondary to a hypothalamic defect, are usually obese, mentally retarded, hypotonic, and short in stature (Laurence, 1967). Treatment is currently directed at replacement of the deficient hypothalamic hormones.

Vasal and epididymal abnormalities have long been associated with the undescended testis (Marshall, 1982). The epididymis may be extended in length, may undergo partial or total atresia, or may be totally disassociated from the testis (Scorer and Farrington, 1971). The same abnormalities may be seen with the vas deferens. **In cystic fibrosis, in which there is a very high incidence of congenital absence of the vasa deferentia, cryptorchidism is frequent** (Landing et al, 1969; Holschaw et al, 1971; Toussig et al, 1972; Shwachman et al, 1977; Goshen et al, 1992). Experimental evidence that epidermal growth factor is important in the development of the wolffian duct in utero suggests a possible cause of the vasal and epididymal abnormalities seen in these patients (Cain et al, 1994).

Epididymal defects have also been described in the male offspring of women exposed to diethylstilbestrol during pregnancy (Bibbo et al, 1975; McLachlan et al, 1975; Cosgrove et al, 1977). The most common abnormalities in these patients are cryptorchidism and cystic dilatations of the epididymis. Although this finding may suggest that some cases of cryptorchidism may be due to elevated in utero levels of estrogen, which may act either through the hypothalamic-pituitary-testicular axis or through a direct effect on the tissues themselves, all fetuses are normally bathed in estrogen during the entire gestational period, yet the incidence of these disorders is relatively infrequent in the normal population.

Treatment

The reasons for correcting the undescended testis are (1) to permanently correct a defect that is obvious and visible to both parents and patient; (2) to prevent or alleviate certain psychopathologic tendencies that surface initially around the fifth year of age, when the child enters school (Cytryn et al, 1967); (3) to place the testis in a site where it can be easily palpated because the undescended testis has an increased susceptibility to malignant degeneration; and (4) to enhance the possibility of future fertility.

Because the prognosis for fertility in patients with bilateral cryptorchidism is extremely poor, every conceivable effort should be made to salvage at least one, or preferably both, of the testes and place them in the scrotum. Placement of the testis should be accomplished as early as 12 to 18 months of age. In the unilateral cryptorchid male, a determined effort should be made to deliver the retained testis into the scrotum in light of reports that suggest that fertility may otherwise be impaired. It is the author's policy at the present time to salvage all testes if at all possible and position them in a site where they are readily palpable. Otherwise, an orchiectomy is performed. Orchiectomy is also reserved for the older postpubertal male patient (Farrer et al, 1985), if the patient so desires, and for the patient with certain intersex disorders in which the testis is dysgenetic and prone to malignant degeneration (Scully, 1970).

Two avenues of therapy are available for placing the cryptorchid testis in the scrotum: hormonal and surgical. The optimal time for attempting to place the retained testis in the scrotum is debatable. It appears, from the data on the changes occurring in the seminiferous tubules by the second year of age and from the observation that a testis not descended by 1 year of age will probably remain undescended, that **treatment probably should be rendered as early as possible, preferably during or prior to the second year of life.**

Hormonal Therapy

Hormonal therapy is the only medical therapy available for the undescended testis. At present, there are two types of hormonal therapy: hCG and GnRH (gonadotropin or luteinizing hormone–releasing factor, or LHRH). The hormone **hCG is given on the premise that stimulation of the Leydig cells will result in an increase in plasma testosterone, which will promote testicular descent.** GnRH is used on the premise that children with cryptorchidism have an abnormality in the secretion of GnRH (LHRH) from the hypothalamus, as evidenced by a decrease in basal LH levels in certain cryptorchid patients. Replacement therapy with exogenous GnRH should reverse this defect or deficiency.

A number of studies have been done in which hCG has been given parenterally to induce testicular descent in children with cryptorchidism, and the success rate has varied from 14% to 50% (Bigler et al, 1938; Ehrlich et al, 1969; Job et al, 1982). The total dose of hCG has varied from 3000 IU to more than 40,000 IU. The frequency of injection has ranged from daily to weekly, and the duration of treatment has ranged from a few days to several months.

Job and associates (1982) demonstrated that **in order to obtain maximal stimulation of the Leydig cells from hCG, a total dose of at least 10,000 IU is needed;** however, with a dose of over 15,000 IU side effects may occur. With a dose of 15,000 IU of hCG or under, testicular histology does not change and bone age is not affected. Rarely, there is a transient increase in the size of the penis, which regresses following cessation of therapy.

The less than ideal results achieved with exogenous hCG and the fact that it has to be given parenterally, along with the data of Job and colleagues (1977) that gonadotropin levels are deficient in infants with cryptorchidism, led to studies using exogenous GnRH as a form of therapy. The dose of native GnRH that has been found to be effective in stimulating LH is 1.2 mg/day as a perinasal spray for 4 weeks (Rajfer et al, 1986a). The efficacy of this form of hormonal therapy in patients with cryptorchidism has been reported to be successful in up to 70% of patients treated (Bartsch and Frick, 1974; Job et al, 1974; Happ et al, 1975, 1978a; Illig et al, 1977, 1980; Pirazzoli et al, 1978; Spona et al, 1979; Zabransky, 1981; Hadziselimovic, 1982). However, in other clinics (deMuinck Keizer-Schrama et al, 1986; Rajfer et al, 1986b, Olsen et al, 1992), the success rate in inducing descent with GnRH is, at best, 6% to 18%.

This low success rate with GnRH is not due to defective LH and testosterone secretion (Figs. 72–5 and 72–6) by the hypothalamus and testis, respectively (Rajfer et al, 1986b). Synthetic, long-lasting analogues of GnRH, which may have a paradoxical effect on serum LH concentration, have also been used, but results are reported to be less effective in inducing descent than those of native GnRH (Happ et al, 1978b; Frick et al, 1980), and there are no long-term follow-up data from these investigators reporting short-term improvement in testicular histology following GnRH analogue therapy (Hadziselimovic, 1987). No side effects, such as precocious growth, have been reported with native GnRH, although the relapse rate after 6 months of therapy approximates 10%. In addition, there does not appear to be a difference in the success rate between unilateral and bilateral cryptorchidism. Some evidence suggests that hCG injections subsequent to GnRH therapy may have an additional effect in promoting descent in the testes (Hadziselimovic, 1982; Lala et al, 1993), but this method of hormonal therapy has never been fully embraced. Indeed, the serum testosterone levels during therapy for cryptorchidism in prepubertal boys are much higher with hCG than those with GnRH (see Fig. 72–6).

One explanation for the markedly different success rates with GnRH among various investigators may be due to the fact that retractile testes were not carefully excluded. Of the 56 patients who were referred to the author and his associates for treatment of undescended testes with either hCG or GnRH, 13 (23%) were found to have retractile testes rather than true cryptorchid testes (Rajfer et al, 1986b). The author believes that this may explain the high success rate of GnRH therapy in earlier studies compared with later data from a variety of investigators.

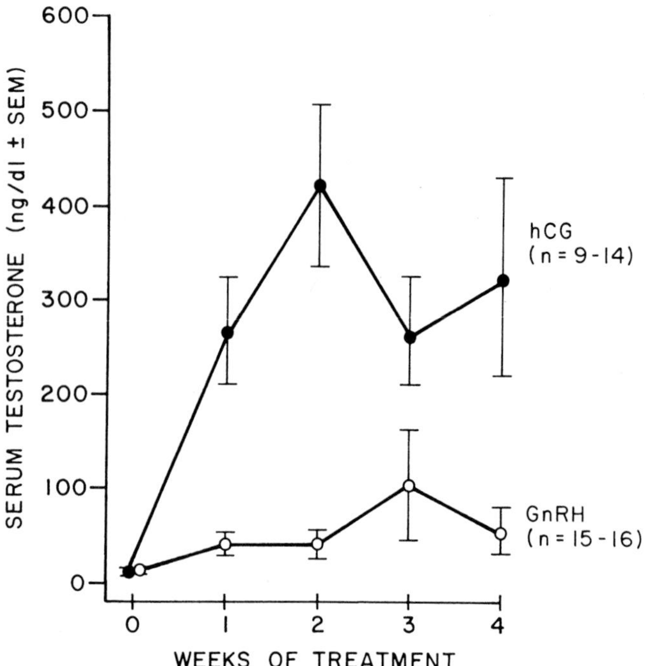

Figure 72–6. Mean serum testosterone levels among boys with cryptorchidism treated with weekly parenteral human chorionic gonadotropin or daily intranasal gonadotropin-releasing hormone. (From Rajfer J, et al: N Engl J Med 1986; 314:466–470.)

The term **retractile testes** refers to those testes that migrate freely between the bottom and upper parts of the scrotum or superficial inguinal pouch. They **are most common between 5 and 7 years of age** (Farrington, 1968). In 1949, Browne observed that of every five patients referred to him for surgery, four actually had **retractile testes** and were misdiagnosed by the referring physician. Puri and Nixon (1977) later demonstrated that children with **retractile testes do not require any interventional therapy such as surgery because at adulthood these testes are of normal volume and fertility.** Wylie (1984) recommended that if a testis on physical examination can be milked down to the bottom of the scrotum, it is a retractile testis and does not require therapy. However, when the testis can be milked down only to the upper scrotum, this testis at adulthood will have a smaller volume that a normal descended testis and therefore should be treated as a true undescended testis.

It has been proposed that a significant number of retractile testes are still being misdiagnosed as true undescended testes and are being treated surgically. As an example, Chilvers and colleagues (1984) reported that between 1962 and 1981 the diagnosis of cryptorchidism and the rate of orchiopexy increased tenfold during a time when the incidence of cryptorchidism in the general population remained stable at 0.8% of all boys. Cooper and Little (1985) reported that in Nottingham, England, where the population and incidence of cryptorchidism have remained stable for decades, approximately five times the expected number of orchiopexies per year are performed. Approximately 14,070 orchiopexies were actually performed annually instead of the expected 3150. These data tend to suggest that the inclusion of retractile testes in population groups of true cryptorchid testes is very common among both primary physicians and specialists.

Therefore, if a simple diagnostic test could be made available to these primary physicians and specialists to allow them to make an accurate distinction between retractile testes and true undescended testes, a huge number of children could be spared the trauma, morbidity, and expense of orchiopexy. Some data in the literature suggest that retractile testes treated with hCG almost always descend (Deming, 1936; Cooper and Little, 1985; Rajfer et al, 1986b). Intranasal GnRH has never been used to help in this differentiation of retractile from true undescended testes. As a result, it has been proposed that **hCG should be given to all children with palpable but undescended testes to help differentiate retractile testes (those that descend) from true undescended testes** (those that do not descend). However, hCG requires a series of injections, and this itself is traumatic to both parent and child. If intranasal GnRH were found to be as effective as hCG in promoting descent of retractile testis, this would provide a simple and nontraumatic means of differentiating a retractile from a true cryptorchid testis. In turn, such a result would encourage its use by all primary physicians, urologists, and surgeons as the preliminary step in the diagnosis and work-up of a patient with a testis outside the scrotum (Hazebroek et al, 1987). Until this occurs, we recommend hCG to help in this differentiation (Rajfer et al, 1986b).

INGUINAL HERNIA IN INFANCY AND CHILDHOOD

In clinical practice, **the majority of infantile inguinal hernias appear in the first year,** the diagnosis being made most commonly in the first month after birth. New cases are less frequent in older children. The overall incidence in the pediatric population has been variously reported as 1.0% to 4.4%. In immature infants, those weighing less than 2000 g at birth, the incidence rises to over 13%. **The condition affects boys nine times more frequently than girls** (Venugopal, 1993).

The cause of the hernia is believed to be strictly anatomic—a patent processus vaginalis. However, some experimental evidence suggests that patients susceptible to hernias may have an abnormality in collagen synthesis in the inguinal area (Friedman et al, 1993). **Once the hernia is identified, it is advisable not to postpone surgery, particularly in infants, because the rate of incarceration is high in those less than 12 months of age** (Stylianos et al, 1993).

Bilateral Inguinal Hernias

Controversy has arisen about the desirability of routine bilateral exploration in cases of apparent unilateral inguinal hernia. For instance, Gunnlaugsson and colleagues (1967) reported that on surgical exploration 60% of such patients were found to have in addition a clinically undiagnosed hernial sac on the contralateral side. Although accepting that these and other workers have shown it to be likely that a patent sac is present on the opposite side in early childhood, it seems pertinent to inquire whether this is of practical significance, as long as the sac does not accept abdominal viscera. **It is estimated that between 6% and 10% of patients with unilateral hernias subsequently develop a clinical hernia on the contralateral unexplored side** (Hamrick and Williams, 1962; Surana and Puri, 1993). Hence, it may reasonably be argued that routine operation on the second side of a younger child may be unnecessary in up to 90% of cases (Othersen, 1993).

When additional consideration is given to the close association of the spermatic vessels and vas deferens to the patent processus vaginalis, it is apparent that routine exploration cannot be done without risk to the testicular apparatus. Indeed, there is an incidence of testicular atrophy of approximately 0.5% following infantile hernia repair. **Occasionally, a vas deferens is seen by the pathologist in the resected hernia sac. The author recommends that no attempt be made in this case to reconstruct or reconnect the vas,** but the patient's family should be made aware of the situation should a problem with infertility arise later during adulthood. However, if laparoscopy ever becomes the accepted method of treating the infantile hernia, both sides may then be repaired with very little risk to the spermatic structures (Easter, 1992; Lobe and Schropp, 1992).

Diagnosis

The majority of patients with infantile inguinal hernias present to the physician within the first 3 months of life. The parent describes the sudden appearance of a bulge in the child's groin, often after a period of crying, coughing, or straining at stool. The swelling is generally absent in the morning and becomes more noticeable later in the day.

The diagnosis is sometimes simple to make—a fullness is visible in one groin compared with the other, and a cough or cry makes the swelling briefly more obvious. Gentle pressure on the abdomen may provoke the child to grunt and cause the swelling to reappear. Palpation reveals an indistinct swelling in the area, accompanied by an impulse of coughing or crying. On occasion, there is no immediately visible abnormality, but the child's parents are convinced that they have seen a swelling, that the child was distressed at the time, but that the swelling has since disappeared. Careful synchronous palpation, in which both spermatic cords are rolled gently over the pubic tubercles, may reveal that the cord on the suspected side is more bulky and more tangible than the more delicate structure on the other side. The presence of a patent processus does seem to impart a palpable thickness and substance to the spermatic cord. Such a finding gives reliable confirmation to the parent's account. To complete the examination, it is important to inspect the scrotum, ensuring that both testes are fully descended, because **up to 6% of congenital inguinal hernias are associated with incomplete descent.**

Inguinal Hernia in Girls

Some 1.6% of girls with inguinal hernias prove to have a 46,XY genotype with intra-abdominal testes but with female external genitalia and female endocrine function (i.e., the testicular feminization syndrome). **Karyotypes should routinely be performed in all female infants presenting with inguinal hernias, particularly if these are bilateral.** The importance lies in the realization that the hernial sac may contain not an ovary (as is commonly the case with girls with inguinal hernias) but a testis. **If a testis is found, it does not have to be excised during childhood** and may be placed back into the abdomen until the postpubertal period. **After the patient has passed puberty and growth and feminization are complete, the testis can be excised because it is liable to undergo malignant changes like any other undescended testis.**

Support for leaving the testis in situ until the postpubertal period lies in the endocrine alterations that ensue during puberty (Griffin and Wilson, 1980). Because gonadotropins are secreted at puberty, the testes begin to secrete testosterone and some estrogen. Because the androgen receptor is absent or defective in these patients, the serum testosterone cannot inhibit gonadotropin secretion from the pituitary gland, thereby allowing the serum LH level to remain remarkably elevated, along with the serum testosterone level. The high circulating testosterone is converted to 17β-estradiol by the aromatase enzyme found in the peripheral fatty tissues. The high serum 17β-estradiol level coupled with a totally ineffective serum testosterone level provides the feminization that these individuals undergo at puberty. In adult life, these patients become phenotypically normal women. Anatomically normal female external genitalia develop, although the vagina tends to be hypoplastic. They have normal breast development and female social behavior. Because the uterus and ovaries are absent, there is primary amenorrhea, which may be the presenting feature that brings some of these patients to clinical recognition.

INFANT HYDROCELE

A hydrocele is a collection of fluid between the parietal and visceral layers of the tunica vaginalis. Hydroceles usually occur during infancy or at adulthood. **During infancy, it is believed that a patent processus vaginalis contributes to the collection of peritoneal fluid in the tunica vaginalis.** In adulthood, some theoretical evidence exists that an imbalance in the secretory and absorptive capacities of the parietal and visceral layers of the tunica vaginalis is responsible for the collection of fluid within the tunic (Rinker and Allen, 1951; Ozdilek, 1957).

Clinical Presentation

Hydroceles are very common after birth, occurring in about 6% of full-term boys (Scorer and Farrington, 1977). The abnormality appears as a transilluminating, painless, oval, scrotal swelling that may extend along the spermatic cord. Because a hydrocele at birth is almost universally secondary to a patent processus vaginalis, **therapy should be delayed until after the processus closes, which may occur spontaneously within the first year of life.** The patent processus vaginalis also explains why the size of the infant hydrocele may vary daily. Although this fact suggests that the hydrocele fluid can be manually reduced back into the peritoneal cavity, this is usually not the case. The presence of mesenteric adenitis may also accentuate the size of a hydrocele. Occasionally, an inguinal hernia or a torsion (if a testis cannot be palpated) may be suspected in a patient with a hydrocele. A history of no previous scrotal pain or swelling and an adequate physical examination usually rule out torsion or an inguinal hernia.

Therapy involves observation during the first year of life, but thereafter surgical intervention is necessary. In the pediatric age group, surgery involves ligation of the patent processus vaginalis either via an inguinal incision or laparoscopically (McKay et al, 1958; Lobe and Schropp, 1992). **Sclerosing agents are not used in children because the patent processus vaginalis allows the agent to pass freely into the peritoneal cavity, producing chemical peritonitis.** Aspiration of the hydrocele fluid from the tunic is usually unsuccessful because the fluid re-collects owing to the patency between the peritoneum and the tunic. Occasionally, aspiration is necessary to allow careful palpation of the testis. However, aspiration poses a risk of introducing infection and possible peritonitis.

TESTICULAR TORSION

Torsion or twisting of the testis is considered a surgical emergency because the gonad may be lost. When torsion occurs, obstruction of the venous blood supply, with secondary edema and hemorrhage and subsequent arterial obstruction, results. This ultimately leads to necrosis of the entire gonad. **Although testicular torsion is possible at any age, it is most common during adolescence (between the ages of 12 and 18 years),** after which the incidence slowly decreases (Scorer and Farrington, 1971). The incidence is estimated to be approximately 1 in 4000 male patients less than 25 years of age (Barada et al, 1989). **Testicular torsion may also appear during the neonatal period** (Scorer and Farrington, 1971).

Although a variety of predisposing factors for testicular torsion have been mentioned, Scorer and Farrington believe that **torsion occurs because of a narrow mesenteric attachment from the cord onto the testis and epididymis** (Fig. 72–7). This narrow mesenteric attachment allows the testis to fall forward. Within the vaginal cavity, the testis is free to rotate like a clapper in a bell (Caesar and Kaplan, 1994). When the mesenteric attachment to the testis and epididymis is broad, the testis does not fall forward but attains a more upright position, thereby making it less likely to rotate on its axis. This characteristic explains why **the pubertal testis has a higher propensity for undergoing torsion than its prepubertal counterpart because at puberty the testis increases in volume approximately fivefold to sixfold** (Marshall and Tanner, 1980). This ability also explains why the onset of **torsion in an undescended testis may signal the development of a tumor because tumors also increase the size of the testis in relation to its mesentery** (Rigler, 1972). This anatomic abnormality is

Frey HL, Rajfer J: The role of the gubernaculum and intraabdominal pressure in the process of testicular descent. J Urol 1984; 131:574.

Frey HL, Peng S, Rajfer J: Synergy of androgens and abdominal pressure in testicular descent. Biol Reprod 1983; 29:1233.

Frick J, Danner C, Kunit G, et al: The effect of chronic administration of a synthetic LH-RH analogue intranasally in cryptorchid boys. Int J Androl 1980; 3:469.

Fritzsche PJ, Hricak H, Kogan BA, et al: Undescended testis value of MR imaging. Radiology 1987; 164:169.

Froeling FM, Sorber MJ, et al. The nonpalpable testis and the changing role of laparoscopy. Urology 1994; 43:222.

Gendrel D, Chaussain JL, Roger M, Job JC: Simultaneous postnasal rise of plasma LH and testosterone in male infants. J Pediatr 1980a; 97:600.

Gendrel D, Job JC, Roger M: Reduced postnatal rise of testosterone in plasma of cryptorchid children. Acta Endocrinol 1978; 89:372.

Gendrel D, Roger M, Chaussain JL, et al: Correlation of pituitary and testicular responses to stimulation tests in cryptorchid children. Acta Endocrinol 1977; 86:641.

Gendrel D, Roger M, Job JC: Plasma gonadotropin and testosterone values in infants with cryptorchidism. J Pediatr 1980b; 97:217.

George FW, Peterson KG: Partial characterization of the androgen receptor of the newborn rat gubernaculum. Biol Reprod 1988; 39:536.

Gier HT, Marion GB: Development of the mammalian testis. *In* Johnson AD, Gomes WR (eds): The Testis. New York, Academic Press, 1970, pp 1–45.

Gilbert JB: Studies in malignant testis tumors. V. Tumors developing after orchiopexy. J Urol 1941; 46:740.

Gilbert JB, Hamilton JB: Incidence and nature of tumors in ectopic testes. Surg Gynecol Obstet 1970; 71:731.

Giwercman A, Bruun E, Frimodt-Mollerf C, Skakkebaek N: Prevalence of carcinoma in situ and other histopathological abnormalities in testes of men with a history of cryptorchidism. J Urol 1989; 142:998.

Giwercman A, Grinsted J, Hansfen B, et al: Testicular cancer risk in boys with maldescended testis: A cohort study. J Urol 1987; 138:1214.

Goldberg LM, Skaist LB, Morrow JW: Congenital absence of testis: Anorchia and monorchism. J Urol 1974; 111:840.

Goldman A, Stein L, Lapin J: The treatment of undescended testes by the anterior pituitary-like principle. NY State J Med 1926; 36:15.

Gordon-Taylor G, Wyndham NR: On malignant tumors of the testis. Br J Surg 1947; 35:6.

Goshen R, Kerem E, Shoshani T: Cystic fibrosis manifested as undescended testis and absence of vas deferens. Pediatrics 1992; 90:982.

Grant DB, Laurence BM, Atherden SM, Ryness J: hCG stimulation test in children with abnormal sexual development. Arch Dis Child 1976; 51:596.

Grumbach MM, Van Wyk JJ: Disorders of sex differentiation. *In* Williams RH (ed): Textbook of Endocrinology, 4th ed. Philadelphia, W. B. Saunders, 1974, p 481.

Guerrier DT, et al: The persistent mullerian duct syndrome: A molecular approach. J Clin Endocrinol Metab 1989; 68:46.

Hadziselimovic F: Cryptorchidism: Ultrastructure of cryptorchid testes development. Adv Anat Embryol Cell Biol 1977; 53:3.

Hadziselimovic F: Pathogenesis of cryptorchidism. Clin Androl 1981; 7:147.

Hadziselimovic F: Treatment of cryptorchidism with GnRH. Urol Clin North Am 1982; 9:413.

Hadziselimovic F: Cryptorchidism. Management and Implications. Heidelberg, Springer-Verlag, 1983.

Hadziselimovic F, Seguchi H: Electron microscope investigations in cryptorchidism (Elektronen Mikroskopische Untersuchungen beim Kryptorchismus). Z Kinderchir 1973; 12:376.

Hadziselimovic F, Snyder H, Duckett J, Howards S: Testicular histology in children with unilateral testicular torsion. J Urol 1986; 136:208.

Hamilton JB: The effect of male hormone upon the descent of the testes. Anat Rec 1938; 70:533.

Hamilton JB, Hubert G: Effect of synthetic male hormone substance on descent of testicles in human cryptorchidism. Proc Soc Exp Biol Med 1938; 39:4.

Hamilton WJ, Boyd JD, Mossman JD: Human Embryology. Cambridge, W. Heffer and Sons, 1957, pp 255–256.

Hansen TS: Fertility in operatively treated and untreated cryptorchidism. Proc R Soc Med 1949; 42:645.

Happ J, Kollmann F, Krawehl C, et al: Intranasal GnRH therapy of maldescended testes. Horm Metab Res 1975; 7:440.

Happ J, Kollmann F, Krawehl C, et al: Treatment of cryptorchidism with perinasal gonadotropin-releasing hormone therapy. Fertil Steril 1978a; 29:546.

Happ J, Weber T, Callnesee W, et al: Treatment of cryptorchidism with a potent analog of gonadotropin-releasing hormone. Fertil Steril 1978b; 29:552.

Hazebroek FWJ, deMuinck Keizer-Schrama SMPF, van Maarschalkerweerd M, et al: Why luteinizing hormone-releasing-hormone nasal spray will not replace orchiopexy in the treatment of boys with undescended testes. J Pediatr Surg 1987; 22:1177–1182.

Hecker WC, Heinz HA: Cryptorchidism and fertility. J Pediatr Surg 1967; 2:513.

Heyns CF, Human HJ, deKlerk DP: Hyperplasia and hypertrophy of the gubernaculum during testicular descent in the fetus. J Urol 1986; 135:1043.

Heyns CF: The gubernaculum during testicular descent in the human fetus. J Anat 1987; 153:93.

Holcomb G, Brock J, Neblett W, et al: Laparoscopy for the nonpalpable testis. Am Surg 1994; 60:143.

Holschaw DS, Perlmutter AD, Joclin H, Shwachman H: Genital abnormalities in male patients with cystic fibrosis. J Urol 1971; 106:568.

Houle A-M, Gagne D: Human chorionic gonadotropin but not the calcitonin gene-related peptide induces postnatal testicular descent in mice. J Androl 1995; 16:143.

Hrebinko RL, Bellinger MF: The limited role of imaging techniques in managing children with undescended testes. J Urol 1993; 150:458.

Huberman J, Israeloff H: The application of recent theories in the treatment of undescended testes. J Pediatr 1935; 7:759.

Hunt JB, Witherington R, Smith AD: The midline approach to orchiopexy. Am Surg 1981; 47:184.

Hunter JA: A description of the situation of the testis in fetus with its descent into the scrotum. *In* Observations on Certain Parts of the Animal Oeconomy. New Orleans, John J. Haswell and Co., 1841, pp 42–50.

Hunter PA: The etiology of congenital inguinal hernia and abnormally placed testes. Br J Surg 1927; 14:125.

Husmann DA, MacPhaul MJ: Time specific androgen blockade with flutamide inhibits testicular descent in the rat. Endocrinology 1991; 129:1409.

Hutson JM: Testicular feminization: A model for testicular descent in mice and men. J Pediatr Surg 1986; 21:195.

Hutson JM, Beasley SW, Bryan AD: Cryptorchidism in spina bifida and spinal cord transection: A clue to the mechanism of transinguinal descent of the testis. J Pediatr Surg 1988; 23:275.

Illig R, Bucher H Prader A: Success, relapse and failure after intranasal LH-RH treatment of cryptorchidism in 55 prepubertal boys. Eur J Pediatr 1980; 133:147.

Illig R, Kollman F, Borkenstein M, K et al: Treatment of cryptorchidism by intranasal synthetic luteinizing-hormone releasing hormone. Lancet 1977; 2:518.

Imperato-McGinley J, Binienda Z, Gendey J, Vaughn E D Jr: Nipple differentiation in fetal male rats treated with an inhibitor of the enzyme 5-reductase: Definition of a selective role for dihydrotestosterone. Endocrinology 1986; 118:132.

Jarow JP, Berkovitz GD, Migeon CJ, et al: Elevation of serum gonadotropins establishes the diagnosis of anorchism in prepubertal boys with belated cryptorchidism. J Urol 1986; 136:277.

Jirasek JE, Raboch J, Uher J: The relationship between the development of the gonads and external genitals in human fetuses. Am J Obstet Gynecol 1968; 101:803.

Job JC, Canlorbe P, Garagorri JM, Toublanc JE: Hormonal therapy of cryptorchidism with human chorionic gonadotropin (hCG). Urol Clin North Am 1982; 9:405.

Job JC, Garnier PE, Chaussain JL, et al: Effect of synthetic luteinizing hormone-releasing hormone on the release of gonadotropins in hypophyseal disorders of children and adolescents. IV. Undescended testes. J Pediatr 1974; 84:371.

Job JC, Gendrel D, Safar A, R et al: Pituitary LH and FSH and testosterone secretion in infants with undescended testes. Acta Endocrinol 1977; 85:644.

Johnson DE, Woodhead DM, Pohl DR, Robinson JR: Cryptorchidism and testicular tumorigenesis. Surgery 1968; 63:919.

Jones HW, Scott WW: Cryptorchidism. *In* Jones HW, Scott WW (eds): Hermaphroditism, Genital Anomalies and Related Endocrine Disorders, 2nd ed. Baltimore, Williams & Wilkins, 1971, p 363.

Jordon GH, Winslow BH: Laparoscopic single stage and staged orchiopexy. J Urol 1994; 152:1249.

Josso N: Evolution of the müllerian-inhibiting activity of the human testis. Biol Neonate 1972; 20:368.

Josso N: In vitro synthesis of müllerian-inhibiting hormone by seminiferous tubules isolated from the calf fetal testis. Endocrinology 1973; 93:829.

Jost A: A new look at the mechanisms controlling sex differentiation in mammals. Johns Hopkins Med J 1953a; 130:8.

Jost A: Problems of fetal endocrinology: The gonadal and hypophyseal hormones. Rec Prog Horm Res 1953b; 8:379.

Kaplan GW: Nomenclature of cryptorchidism. Eur J Pediatr 1993; 152:S17.

Kaplan LM, Koyle MA, Kaplan GW, et al: Association between abdominal wall defects and cryptorchidism. J Urol 1986; 136:645.

Korenchevsy V: The influence of cryptorchidism and of castration on body-weight, fat deposition, the sexual and endocrine organs of male rats. J Pathol Bacteriol 1931; 33:607.

Lais A, Caterino S, Talamo M, et al: The gliding testis: Minor degree of true undescended testis? Eur J Pediatr 1993; 152: S20.

LaQuaglia MP, Bauer SB, Eraklis A, et al: Bilateral neonatal torsion. J Urol 1987; 138:1051.

Lala R, Matarazzo P, Chiabotto P, et al: Combined therapy with LHRH and hCG in cryptorchid infants. Eur J Pediatr 1993; 152:S31.

Landa HM, Gylys-Morin V, Mattrey RF, et al: Magnetic resonance imaging of the cryptorchid testis. Eur J Pediatr 1987; 146 (Suppl 2):S16.

Landing BH, Wells TR, Wong CI: Abnormality of the epididymis and vas deferens in cystic fibrosis. Arch Pathol 1969; 88:569.

Larkins SL, Williams MPL, Hutson JM: Localization of calcitonin gene-related peptide within the spinal nucleus of the genitofemoral nerve. Pediatr Surg Int 1991; 6:176.

Larkins SL, Hutson JM: Fluorescent antegrade labelling of the genitofemoral nerve shows that it supplies the scrotal region before migration of the gubernaculum. Pediatr Surg Int 1991; 6:167.

Laurence BM: Hypotonia, mental retardation, obesity, cryptorchidism associated with dwarfism and diabetes in children. Arch Dis Child 1967; 42:126.

Lee JK, McClennan BL, Stanley RJ, Sagel SS: Utility of computed tomography in the localization of the undescended testis. Radiology 1980; 135:121.

Lemeh CN: A study of the development and structural relationships of the testis and gubernaculum. Surg Gynecol Obstet 1960; 110:164.

Levitt SB, Kogan SJ, Engel RM, et al: The impalpable testis: A rational approach to management. J Urol 1978; 120:515.

Lipschultz LI, Caminos-Torres R, Greenspan CS, Snyder PJ: Testicular function after orchiopexy for unilaterally undescended testis. N Engl J Med 1976; 195:15.

Lockwood CG: Development and transition of the testis, normal and abnormal. J Anat Physiol 1888; 22:505.

Ludwig G, Potempa J: Der optimale Zeitpunkt der Behandlung des Kryptorchismus. Dtsch Med Wochenschr 1975; 100:680.

Mack WSL: Discussion on male fertility. Proc R Soc Med 1953; 46:840.

Mack WS, Scott, LS, Ferguson-Smith MA, Lennox B: Ectopic testis and true undescended testis: A histological comparison. J Pathol Bacteriol 1961; 82:439.

Madrazo BL, Klugo RC, Parks JA, DiLoreto R: Ultrasonographic demonstration of undescended testes. Radiology 1979; 123:181.

Maghnie M, Vanzulli A, Paesano P, et al: The accuracy of magnetic resonance imaging and ultrasonography compared with surgical findings in the localization of the undescended testis. Arch Pediatr Adolesc Med 1994; 148:699.

Marshall FF: Anomalies associated with cryptorchidism. Urol Clin North Am 1982; 9:339.

Martin DC: Germinal cell tumors of the testis after orchiopexy. J Urol 1979; 121:422.

Martin DC, Menck HR: The undescended testis: Management after puberty. J Urol 1975; 114:77.

McAleer IM., Packer MG, Kaplan GW, et al: Fertility index analysis in cryptorchidism. J Urol 1995; 153:1255.

McCutcheon AB: Further observations on delayed testis. Med J Aust 1938; 1:654.

McLachlan JA, Newbold RR, Bullock B: Reproductive tract lesions in male mice exposed prenatally to diethylstilbestrol. Science 1975; 90:991.

McMurrich JP: The Development of the Human Body. A Manual of Human Embryology, 7th ed. Philadelphia, P. Blakiston's Son and Co., 1923, pp 374–376.

Mengel W, Heinz HA, Sippe WG, Hecker WCH: Studies on cryptorchidism: A comparison of histological findings in the germinal epithelium before and after the second year of life. J Pediatr Surg 1974; 9:445.

Mengel W, Wronecki K, Zimmerman FA: Comparison of the morphology of normal cryptorchid testes. *In* Fonkaslrud EW, Mengal W (eds): The Undescended Testis. Chicago, Year Book Medical Publishers, 1981, p 72.

Merksz M, Toth J, Pirot L: Testosterone secretion in children with undescended testis. Int Urol Nephrol 1992; 24:429.

Mieusset R, Fouda PJ, Vaysse P, et al: Increase in testicular temperature in case of cryptorchidism in boys. Fertil Steril 1993; 59:1319.

Mininberg DT, Bragol N: Chromosomal abnormalities in undescended testis. Urology 1973; 1:98.

Moore CR, Quick WJ: The scrotum as a temperature regulator for the testes. Am J Physiol 1924; 68:70.

Mukerjee S, Amesur NR: Transverse testicular ectopia with unilateral blood supply. Ind J Surg 1965; 27:547.

Naslund MJ, Gearhart JP, Jeffs RD: Laparoscopy: Its selected use in patients with unilateral nonpalpable testis after human chorionic gonadotropin stimulation. J Urol 1989; 142:108.

Nistal M, Paniagua R: Infertility in adult males with retractile testes. Fertil Steril 1984; 41:395.

Ngyuen MM, Lemmi CAE, Rajfer J: Effect of 5-alpha reductase inhibitor, 4-MAPC, on testicular descent in male rat. J Urol 1991; 145:1096–1098.

Olsen LH, Genster HG, Mosegaard A, et al: Management of the non-descended testis: Doubtful value of luteinizing-hormone-releasing-hormone (LHRH). A double-blind, placebo-controlled multicentre study. Int J Androl 1992; 15:135.

Optitz JM, Simpson JL, Sarto GE, et al. Pseudovaginal perineoscrotal hypospadias. Clin Genet 1972; 3:1026.

Pace JM, Cabot M: A histological study in 24 cases of retained testes in the adult. Surg Gynecol Obstet 1936; 63:16.

Page DC: Hypothesis: A Y-chromosomal gene causes gonadoblastoma in dysgenetic gonads. Development 1987; 101(Suppl):157.

Page DC, Mosher R, Simpson EM, et al: The sex determining region of the human Y chromosome encodes a finger protein. Cell 1987; 51:1091–1104.

Pak K, Sakaguchi N, Takeuchi H, Tomoyoshi T: Computed tomography of carcinoma of the intra-abdominal testis: A case report. J Urol 1981; 125:253.

Payne AH, Jaffe RB: Androgen formation from pregnenolone sulfate by fetal neonatal adult human testes. J Clin Endocrinol Metab 1975; 40:102.

Pirazzoli P, Zappulla F, Bernardi F, et al: Luteinizing hormone-releasing hormone nasal sprays as therapy for undescended testicle. Arch Dis Child 1978; 53:235.

Puri P, Nixon MH: Bilateral retractile testes—subsequent effects on fertility. J Pediatr Surg 1977; 12:563–566.

Rajfer J: An endocrinological study of testicular descent in the rabbit. J Surg Res 1982; 33:158.

Rajfer J, Handelsman DJ, Swerdloff RS, et al: Luteinizing hormone follicle-stimulating hormone responses to intranasal gonadotropin-releasing hormone. Fertil Steril 1986a; 45:794–799.

Rajfer J, Handelsman DJ, Swerdloff RS, et al: Hormonal therapy of cryptorchidism. N Engl J Med 1986b; 312:466.

Rajfer J, Tauber A, Zinner N, et al: The use of computerized tomography scanning to localize the impalpable testis. J Urol 129:978, 1983.

Rajfer J, Walsh PC: Hormonal regulation of testicular descent: Experimental and clinical observations. J Urol 1977; 118:985.

Ransley PG, Vordermark JS, Caldamone AA, Bellinger MF: Preliminary ligation of the gonadal vessels prior to orchiopexy for the intra-abdominal testicle: A staged Fowler-Stephens procedure. World J Urol 1984; 2:266.

Redman J: Noonan's syndrome and cryptorchidism. J Urol 1973; 109:909.

Rigler HC: Torsion of intra-abdominal testes. Surg Clin North Am 1972; 52:371.

Robertson JFR, Azmy A, Cochran W: Assent to ascent of the testis. Br J Urol 1988; 61:146.

Sadeghi-Nejad A, Senior B: A familial syndrome of isolated aplasia of the anterior pituitary. J Pediatr 1974; 84:79.

Saito S, Kumamoto Y: The number of spermatogonia in various congenital testicular disorders. J Urol 1989; 141:1166.

Santen RJ, Paulsen CA: Hypogonadotropic eunuchoidism. Gonadal responsiveness to exogenous gonadotropins. J Clin Endocrinol Metab 1972; 36:47.

Sasagawa I, Nakada T, Kubota Y, et al: Gonadal function and testicular histology in Noonan's syndrome with bilateral cryptorchidism. Arch Androl 1994; 32:135.

Schechter J: An investigation of the anatomical mechanisms of testicular descent (thesis for Master of Arts degree). Baltimore, Johns Hopkins University, 1963.

Scorer CG: The descent of the testis. Arch Dis Child 1964; 39:605.
Scorer CG: Early operation for the undescended testis. Br J Surg 1967; 54:694.
Scorer CG, Farrington GH: Congenital Deformities of the Testis and Epididymis. New York, Appleton-Century-Crofts, 1971.
Scott LS: Unilateral cryptorchidism; Subsequent effects on fertility. J Reprod Fertil 1961; 2:54.
Scott LS: Fertility in cryptorchidism. Proc R Soc Med 1962; 55:1047.
Scully RE: Gonadoblastoma. A review of 74 cases. Cancer, 1970; 25:1340.
Shwachman H, Kowlski M, Khaw K: Cystic fibrosis: A new outlook. Medicine 1977; 56:129.
Siiteri PK, Wilson JD: Testosterone formation and metabolism during male sexual differentiation in the human embryo. J Clin Endocrinol Metab 1974; 38:113.
Silber SJ, Cohen R: Laparoscopy for cryptorchidism. J Urol 1980; 124:928.
Sizonenko PC, Schindler RA, Roland W, et al: Evidence for a possible prepubertal regulation of its secretion by the seminiferous tubules in cryptorchid boys. J Clin Endocrinol Metab 1978; 46:301.
Skakkebaek NE: Possible carcinoma in situ of the testis. Lancet 1972; 1:516.
Sohval AR: Histopathology of cryptorchidism. Am J Med 1954; 16:346.
Sonneland CG: Undescended testicle. Surg Gynecol Obstet 1925; 40:535.
Southam AH, Cooper ERA: Hunterian lecture on the pathology and treatment of the retained testis in childhood. Lancet 1927; 1:805.
Spencer JR, Torrado T, Sanchez RS, et al: Effects of flutamide and finasteride on rat testicular descent. Endocrinology 1991; 129:741.
Spona J, Gleispach H, Happ J, et al: Changes of serum testosterone and of LH-RH test after treatment of cryptorchidism by intranasal LH-RH. Endocrinol Exp 1979; 13:204.
Steiner MD, Boggs JD: Absence of the pituitary gland, hypothyroidism, hypoadrenalism and hypogonadism in a 17-year-old dwarf. J Clin Endocrinol Metab 1965; 25:1591.
Tayakkononta K: The gubernaculum testis and its nerve supply. Aust N Z J Surg 1963; 33:61.
Toussig LM, Lobeck LC, DiSant'Aznese PA, et al: Fertility in males with cystic fibrosis. N Engl J Med 1972; 287:586.
United Kingdom Testicular Cancer Study Group: Aetiology of testicular cancer: Association with congenital abnormalities, age at puberty, infertility, and exercise. Br Med J 1994; 308:1393.
Van Vliet G, Caufriez A, Robyn C, Wolter R: Plasma gonadotropin values in prepubertal cryptorchid boys: Similar increase of FSH in unilateral and bilateral cases. J Pediatr 1980; 97:253.
Villumsen AL, Zachau-Christiansen B: Spontaneous alterations in position of the testis. Arch Dis Child 1966; 41:198.
Vitale PJ, Khademi M, Seebode JH: Selective gonadal angiography for testicular localization in patients with cryptorchidism. Surg Forum 1974; 25:538.
Walsh PC, Curry N, Mills RC, Siiteri PK: Plasma androgen response to hCG stimulation in prepubertal boys with hypospadias and cryptorchidism. J Clin Endocrinol Metab 1976; 42:52.
Walsh PC, Madden JD, Harrod MJ, et al: Familial incomplete male pseudohermaphroditism, type 2. Decreased dihydrotestosterone formation in pseudovaginal perineoscrotal hypospadias. N Engl J Med 1974; 291:944.
Wangensteen OH: The undescended testis. Ann Surg 1935; 102:875.
Ward B, Hunter WM: The absent testicle, a report on a survey carried out among schoolboys in Nottingham. Br Med J 1960; 1:1110.
Weiss RM, Glickman MG, Lytton B: Clinical implications of gonadal venography in the management of the non-palpable undescended testis. J Urol 1979; 121:745.
Wells LJ: Descent of the testis. Anatomical and hormonal considerations. Surgery 1943; 14:436.
Wells LJ: Descensus testiculorum: Descent after severance of the gubernaculum. Anat Rec 1944; 88:465.
Wensing CJG: Testicular descent in some domestic mammals. I. Anatomical aspect of testicular descent. Proc Kon Akad Wetensch 1968; C71:423.
Wensing CJG: Testicular descent in some domestic animals. II. The nature of the gubernacular change during the process of testicular descent in the pig. Proc Kon Akad Wetensch 1973; C76:190.
Welvaart K, Tijssen JPG: Management of the undescended testis in relation to the development of cancer. J Surg Oncol 1981; 17:218.
Whitaker RH: Undescended testis — the need for a standard classification. Br J Urol 1992; 70:1.
White JJ, Haller JA Jr, Dorst JP: Congenital inguinal hernia and inguinal herniography. Surg Clin North Am 1970; 50:823.
White JJ, Shaker IJ, Oh KS: Herniography: A diagnostic refinement in the management of cryptorchidism. Ann Surg 1973; 39:624.
Wiles P: Family tree showing hereditary undescended right testis and associated deformities. Proc R Soc Med 1934; 28:157.
Winter JSD, Hughes IA, Reyes FI, Faiman C: Pituitary-gonadal relations in infancy: 2. Patterns of serum gonadal steroidal concentrations in man from birth to two years of age. J Clin Endocrinol Metab 1976; 42:679.
Winter JSD, Teraska S, Faiman C: The hormonal response to hCG stimulation in male children and adolescents. J Clin Endocrinol Metab 1972; 34:348.
Wislocki GB: Observation on the descent of the testes in the macaque and in the chimpanzee. Anat Rec 1933; 57:133.
Witschi E: Migration of the germ cells of human embryos from the yolk sac to the primitive gonadal folds. Contrib Embryol Carnegie Inst 1948; 32:67.
Wollach Y, Shaher E, Schachter A, Dintsman M: Fertility and sexual development after bilateral orchiopexy for cryptorchidism. Isr J Med Sci 1980; 16:707.
Wolverson MK, Jagannadharao B, Sundaram M, et al: CT localization of impalpable cryptorchid testes. Am J Roentgenol 1980; 134:725.
Woodhead DM, Pohl DR, Johnson DE: Fertility of patients with solitary testes. J Urol 1973; 100:66.
Wylie GC: The retractile testis. Med J Aust 1984; 140:403–405.
Wyndham NR: A morphological study of testicular descent. J Anat 1943; 77:179.
Yamanaka J, Metcalfe SA, Hutson JM: Demonstration of calcitonin gene-related peptide receptors in the gubernaculum by computerized densitometry. J Pediatr Surg 1992; 27:876.
Yamanaka J, Metcalfe SA, Hutson JM, Mendelsohn FAO: Testicular descent, II. Ontogeny and response to denervation of calcitonin gene-related peptide receptors in neonatal rat gubernaculum. Endocrinology 1993; 132:280.
Zabransky S: LH-RH Nasal spray (Kryptocur), ein neuer Aspekt in der hormonellen Behandlung des Hodenhoch-Standes. Klin Paediatr 1981; 193:382.
Zarzycki J, Szroeder J, Michaelowski WL: Ultrastructure of seminiferous tubule cells and interstitial cells in cryptorchid human testicles. Acta Med Pol 1977; 18:38.

Inguinal Hernia in Infancy and Childhood

Easter DW: Inguinal hernia in pediatrics: Initial experience with laparoscopic inguinal exploration of the asymptomatic contralateral side. J Laparoendosc Surg 1992; 2:361.
Friedman DW, Boyd CD, Norton P, et al: Increases in type III collagen gene expression and protein synthesis in patients with inguinal hernias. Ann Surg 1993; 218:754.
Griffin JE, Wilson JD: The syndromes of androgen resistance. N Engl J Med 1980; 302:198.
Gunnlaugsson GH, Dawson B, Lynn HB: Treatment of inguinal hernia in infants and children: Experience with contralateral exploration. Mayo Clin Proc 1967; 42:129.
Hamrick LC, Williams JO: Is contralateral exploration indicated in children with unilateral inguinal hernias? Am J Surg 1962; 104:52.
Lobe TE, Schropp KP: Inguinal hernias in pediatrics: Initial experience with laparoscopic inguinal exploration of the asymptomatic contralateral side. J Laparoendosc Surg 1992; 2:135.
Othersen HB: The pediatric inguinal hernia. Surg Clin North Am 1993; 73:853.
Stylianos S, Jacer NN, Harres BH: Incarceration of inguinal hernia in infants prior to elective repair. J Pediatr Surg 1993; 28:582–583.
Surana R, Puri P: Is contralateral exploration necessary in infants with unilateral inguinal hernia? J Pediatr Surg 1993; 28:1026.
Venugopal S: Inguinal hernia in children. West Indian Med J 1993; 42:24.

Infant Hydrocele

McKay DG, Fowler R, Barnett JS: The pathogenesis and treatment of primary hydroceles in infancy and childhood. Aust N Z Surg 1958; 28:2.
Ozdilek S: The pathogenesis of idiopathic hydrocele and a simple operative technique. J Urol 1957; 77:282.
Rinker JR, Allen L: Lymphatic defect in hydrocele. Am Surg 1951; 17:681.
Scorer GC, Farrington GH: Congenital anomalies of the testis. *In* Harrison JH, Gittes R, Perlmutter A, et al (eds): Campbell's Urology, 4th ed. Vol. 2. Philadelphia, W. B. Saunders, 1977, p 1564.

Testicular Torsion

Akgur FM, Kilinc K, Tanyel FC, et al: Ipsilateral and contralateral testicular biochemical acute changes after unilateral testicular torsion and detorsion. Urology 1994; 44:413.

Atkinson GO Jr, Patrick LE, Ball TI Jr, et al: The normal and abnormal scrotum in children: Evaluation with color Doppler sonography. Am J Roentgenol 1992; 138:613.

Backhouse KM: Embryology of testicular descent and maldescent. Urol Clin North Am 1982; 9:315.

Barada IH, Weingarten JL, Cromie WJ: Testicular salvage and age-related delay in the presentation of testicular torsion. J Urol 1989; 142:746.

Bartsch G, Frank S, Marberger H, Mikuz G: Testicular torsion: late results with special regard to fertility and endocrine function. J Urol 1980; 124:375.

Burton JA: Atrophy following testicular torsion. Br J Surg 1972; 59:422.

Caesar RE, Kaplan GW: Incidence of bell-clapper deformity in an autopsy series. Urology 1994; 44:114.

Campobasso P, Donadio P, Spata E, et al: Acute scrotum in children: Analysis of 265 consecutive cases. Pediatr Med Chir 1994; 16:521.

Chapman RH, Walton AJ: Torsion of the testis and its appendages. Br Med J 1972; 1:164.

Datta NS, Mishkin F: Radionuclide imaging and intrascrotal lesions. JAMA 1975; 231:1060.

Dominguez C, Martinez Verduch M, Estornell F, et al: Histological study in contralateral testis of prepubertal children following unilateral testicular torsion. Eur Urol 1994; 26:160.

Dresner M: Torsed appendage: Blue dot sign. Urology 1973; 1:63.

Holder LE, Martine JR, Holmes ER, Wagner HN: Testicular radionuclide angiography and static imaging: Anatomy, scintigraphic interpretation, and clinical indications. Radiology 1977; 125:739.

Ingram S, Hollman AS: Colour Doppler sonography of the normal paediatric testis. Clin Radiol 1994; 49:266.

Jarow JP: Intratesticular arterial anatomy. J Androl 1990; 11:255.

Korbel EI: Torsion of the testis. J Urol 1974; 111:521.

Krarup T: The testes after torsion. Br J Urol 1978; 50:43.

Levy BJ: The diagnosis of torsion of the testicle using the Doppler ultrasonic stethoscope. J Urol 1975; 113:63.

Macnicol MF: Torsion of the testis in childhood. Br J Surg 1974; 61:905.

Marshall JC, Tanner JM: Variations in pattern of pubertal changes in boys. Arch Dis Child 1980; 45:13.

Rigler HC: Torsion of intra-abdominal testes. Surg Clin North Am 1972; 52:371.

Scorer CG, Farrington GH: Congenital Deformities of the Testis and Epididymis. London, Butterworth and Co, 1971.

Sparks JP: Torsion of the testis in adolescents and young adults. Clin Pediatr 1972; 11:484.

Stone KT, Kass EJ, Cacciarelli AA, Gibson DP: Management of suspected antenatal torsion: What is the best strategy? J Urol 1995; 153:782.

Thompson IM, Latourette H, Chadwick S, et al: Diagnosis of testicular torsion using Doppler ultrasonic flowmeter. Urology 1975; 6:706.

Tryfonas G, Violaki A, Tsikopoulos G, et al: Late postoperative results in males treated for testicular torsion during childhood. J Pediatr Surg 1994; 29:553.

Yazbeck S, Patriquin HB: Accuracy of Doppler sonography in the evaluation of acute conditions of the scrotum in children. J Pediatr Surg 1994; 29:1270.

Varicocele

Atassi O, Kass EJ, Steinert BW: Testicular growth afer successful varicocele correction in adolescents: Comparison of artery sparing techniques with the Palomo procedure. J Urol 1995; 153:482.

Belloli G, D'Agostino S, Pesce C, Fantuz E: Varicocele in childhood and adolescence and other testicular anomalies: An epidemiological study. Pediatr Med Chir 15:159, 1993.

Belman AB: The dilemma of the adolescent varicocele. Cont Urol 1991; 3:21.

Berger OG: Varicocele in adolescence. Clin Pediatr 1980; 19:810.

Braedel HU, Steffens J, Ziegler M, Polsky MS: Out-patient sclerotherapy of idiopathic left-sided varicocele in children and adults. Br J Urol 1990; 65:536.

Buch JR, Cromie WJ: Evaluation and treatment of the preadolescent varicocele. Urol Clin North Am 1985; 12:3.

Clarke BG: Incidence of varicocele in normal men and among men of different ages. JAMA 1966; 198:1121.

Dubin L, Amelar RD: Etiologic factors in 1294 consecutive cases of male infertility. Fertil Steril 1971; 22:469–474.

El-Gohary MA: Boyhood varicocele: An overlooked disorder. Ann R Coll Surg Engl 1984; 66:36.

Fussell EN, Lewis RW, Roberts JH, Harrison RM: Early ultrastructural findings in experimentally produced varicocele in the monkey testis. J Androl 1981; 2:111.

Gorenstein A, Katz S, Schiller M: Varicocele in children: "To treat or not to treat" — venographic and manometric studies. J Pediatr Surg 1986; 21:1046.

Haans LCF, Laven JSE, Male WPTM, et al: Testis volumes, semen quality, and hormonal patterns in adolescents with and without a varicocele. Fertil Steril 1991; 56:731.

Heinz HA, Voggenthaler J, Weissbach L: Histological findings in testes with varicocele during childhood and their therapeutic consequences. Eur J Pediatr 1980; 133:139.

Holschneider AM, Butenandt O, Schuster L, et al: Operative therapy of varicocele in childhood. Z Kinderchir 1978; 24:252.

Hudson RW: The endocrinology of varicoceles. Fertil Steril 1988; 49:199.

Johnsen SG, Agger P: Quantitative evaluation of testicular biopsies before and after operation for varicocele. Fertil Steril 1978; 29:58–63.

Kass EJ, Belman AB: Reversal of testicular growth failure by varicocele ligation. J Urol 1987; 137:475.

Kass EJ, Chandra RS, Belman AB: Testicular histology in the adolescent with a varicocele. Pediatrics 1987; 79:996.

Kass EJ, Freitas JE, Bour JB: Pituitary-gonadal function in adolescence with a varicocele. J Urol 1988; 139:207.

Kass EJ, Reitelman C: Adolescent varicocele. Urol Clin North Am 1995; 22:151.

Levitt S, Gil B, Katlowitz N, et al: Routine intraoperative post-ligation venography in the treatment of the pediatric varicocele. J Urol 1987; 137:716.

Lyon RP, Marshall S, Scott MP: Varicocele in childhood and adolescence: Implication in adulthood infertility? Urology 1982; 19:641.

Lyon RP, Marshall S, Scott MP: Varicocele in youth. West J Med 1983; 138:832.

McFadden MR, Mehan DJ: Testicular biopsies in 101 cases of varicocele. J Urol 1978; 119:372.

Okuyama A, Nakamura M, Namiki M, et al: Surgical repair of varicocele at puberty: Preventive treatment for fertility improvement. J Urol 1988; 139:562.

Oster J: Varicocele in children and adolescents. An investigation of the incidence among Danish school children. Scand J Urol Nephrol 1971; 5:27.

Parrott TS, Hewatt L: Ligation of the testicular artery and vein in adolescent varicocele. J Urol 1994; 152:791.

Rajfer J, Turner TT, Rivera F, et al: Inhibition of testicular testosterone biosynthesis following experimental varicocele in rats. Biol Reprod 1987; 36:933.

Rajfer J, Pickett S, Klein SA: Laparoscopic occlusion of testicular veins for clinical varicocele. Urology 1992; 40:113–116.

Reidl P, Lunglmayr G, Stackl W: A new method of transfemoral testicular vein obliteration for varicocele using a balloon catheter. Radiology 1981; 139:323.

Reyes BL, Trerotola SO, Venbrux AC, et al: Percutaneous embolotherapy of adolescent varicocele: Results and long-term follow-up. J Vasc Interv Radiol 1994; 5:131.

Risser WL, Lipschultz LI: Frequency of varicocele in black adolescents. J Adolesc Health Care 1984; 5:28.

Rodriguez-Rigau LJ, Weiss DB, Zuckerman Z, et al: A possible mechanism for the detrimental effect of varicocele on testicular function in man. Fertil Steril 1978; 30:577.

Saypol DC, Turner TT, Howards SS, Miller ED: Influence of surgically induced varicocele on testicular blood flow, temperature and histology in adult rats and dogs. J Clin Invest 1981; 68:39.

Steeno O, Knops J, Declerck L, et al: Prevention of fertility disorders by detection and treatment of varicocele at school and college age. Andrologia 1976; 8:47.

Vermuelen A, Bandeweghe M, Deslypere JP: Prognosis of subfertility in men with corrected or uncorrected varicocele. J Androl 1986; 7:147.

Wylie GG: Varicocele and puberty — the critical factor? Br J Urol 1985; 57:194.

Zorgniotti AW, MacLeod J: Studies in temperature, human semen quality and varicocele. Fertil Steril 1973; 24:854.

73 SURGERY OF THE SCROTUM AND TESTIS IN CHILDREN

Thomas Rozanski, MD
David A. Bloom, MD
Arnold Colodny, MD

Surgical procedures for scrotal disorders were prominent among the earliest operative interventions. Two factors accounted for this: scrotal disorders were common, and the site was easily accessible. Peter Lowe, founder of the Royal College of Physicians and Surgeons in Glasgow and author of the first complete surgical text in English, wrote about scrotal surgery in 1597. He called the scrotum and testes the codde and stones:

> ***In the Coddes, are situated the stones, which are ordained by nature for the generation of man, which are subject to divers tumors and inflammations so that sometime the stones doe swell, to the greatness of a goose egg, accompanied with dolor and hardness, so that the heart, liver, & brains feel the grief.***
>
> LOWE, 1597

Today, just as Lowe wrote four centuries ago, the causes of scrotal grief are external and internal. Cryptorchidism, hernia, hydrocele, trauma, torsion, tumors, and varicocele remain the usual reasons for which surgeons are called on to bring relief.

SURGERY FOR CRYPTORCHID TESTES

Cryptorchidism means hidden or obscure testis and is generally synonymous with undescended testis (UDT). The incidence of UDT at birth is around 3%, and 15% of these are bilateral. Spontaneous descent may occur up to 1 year of age, when the incidence of UDT falls to 0.8%. The three main reasons for relocating the testis to a scrotal position are (1) the environment, which favors normal organ maturation and function, (2) the accessibility of the gonad for self-examination later in life, and (3) the psychologic disadvantage of an empty scrotum. Infertility is more common in men with a history of UDT, and fertility potential may be improved by early orchiopexy. Histologic studies support the benefit of surgical intervention at around 1 year of age. Orchiopexy is safe and effective in boys even younger than 1 year of age (Kogan, 1990). Testis biopsies during orchiopexy demonstrate a higher number of spermatogonia per tubule (Canavese et al, 1993) and a larger diameter of the seminiferous tubule in boys under 1 year of age compared to older boys (Kogan, 1990). In a review of over 750 boys with UDT, Cendron and associates noted a relative decrease in the volume of the ipsilateral testis by 6 months of age (Cendron et al, 1993). Recently, Lugg and colleagues presented work indicating that early orchiopexy may reverse histologic changes in cryptorchid testes in an animal model (Lugg et al, 1995). These findings suggest that damage to the germinal epithelium is acquired and progressive.

The basic principles of orchiopexy include testis localization, mobilization, cord dissection, isolation of the patent processus vaginalis, and relocation to the scrotum without tension. A cryptorchid testis may be substantively intra-abdominal (at least 1 cm above the internal ring), high annular (living at the internal ring and peeping into the abdominal cavity), canalicular, in the superficial inguinal pouch of Denis Browne, distantly ectopic (perineal, femoral, penopubic), or high scrotal (Fig. 73–1).

Some locations suggest migration arrest during the normal course of testicular descent, whereas ectopic testes are found outside the usual anatomic path of descent. Maneuvers during physical examination that facilitate identification of an elusive testis include lubricating jelly on the skin to decrease tactile friction and a crossed leg position to relax the cremasteric muscles. It is important to distinguish a retractile from a true undescended testis. The catcher or squat position may help in older boys who can stand. If a testis has to be manipulated into the scrotum and if it drifts or pops back into the inguinal area, it is most likely cryptorchid and not merely retractile. Some UDTs in superficial inguinal pouches that extend down toward the scrotal inlet may appear properly descended but with age and growth become more obviously truly undescended. Most UDTs are palpable and are amenable to standard orchiopexy. Nonpalpability is a special circumstance of cryptorchidism, which occurs in approximately 20% of UDT. Assessment of nonpalpable testes (NPT) reveals that 45% of the gonads are absent, 30% are in a truly abdominal position, and 25% are lower testes missed on palpation (Bloom and Semm, 1991). Success rates for orchiopexy are directly related to anatomic position. Docimo's analysis of 8425 undescended testes revealed that orchiopexy was successful in 92% of testes below the external ring, 89% of inguinal testes, 84% of microvascular orchiopexies, 81% of standard abdominal orchiopexies, 77% of staged Fowler-Stephens orchiopexies, and 67% of standard Fowler-Stephens orchiopexies (Docimo, 1995).

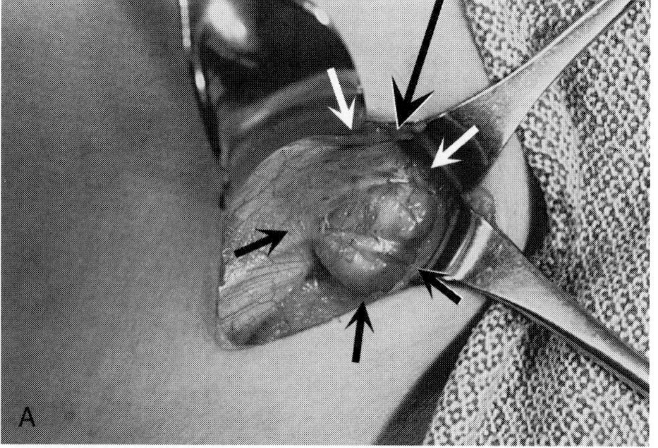

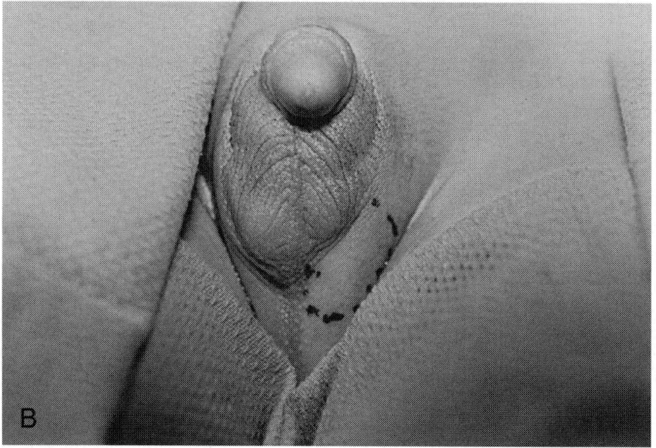

Figure 73–1. Cryptorchid variants. *A*, Testis in superficial inguinal pouch *(large arrow)*. *B*, Femoral testis.

Standard Orchiopexy

Make a transverse skin incision over the midinguinal canal and cut with cautery through the dermis. Watch for a testis in the superficial inguinal pouch that may bulge into the wound as Scarpa's fascia is opened. Identify the testis, which is usually still lying within its tunics, and divide the gubernacular attachments. Open the tunics, measure the testis, and describe the epididymal configuration (Fig. 73–2). Incise the external oblique fascia in the direction of its fibers and preserve the ilioinguinal nerve. The testis with the spermatic cord must be completely mobilized to allow tension-free placement in the scrotum. Key steps needed to achieve adequate cord length are (1) complete transsection of the fused fibers between the cremasteric muscle and the internal oblique muscle, (2) separation of cord structures from the patent processus vaginalis and from the peritoneum above the internal ring, and (3) division of the lateral spermatic fascia to bring the cord medially. If these maneuvers do not result in adequate cord length, further retroperitoneal dissection is necessary. An army-navy retractor in the internal ring helps with retroperitoneal exposure, which additionally can be enhanced by incising the superior lateral margin of the internal ring 1 to 2 cm.

Experimental evidence suggests that transparenchymal suture fixation may cause testicular damage by inducing an inflammatory reaction (Bellinger et al, 1989; Dixon et al, 1993). Because cryptorchid patients are at risk for fertility problems, it seems logical to avoid any transparenchymal sutures. The testis can be adequately secured in the scrotum using a dartos pouch alone (Redman, 1990) or by closing the dartos fascia around the spermatic cord with circumferential sutures in the dartos window (Ritchey and Bloom, 1995). The dartos pouch orchiopexy has a long and proven record of success. The most critical factor for retention in the pouch is adequate cord mobilization. Eversion of the tunica vaginalis, allowing contact of the tunica albuginea with the scrotal wall, is also important. Suture fixation may be necessary for 12 to 15 days while collagen is deposited to produce long-term fixation (Rodriguez and Kaplan, 1988).

After mobilizing the testis and cord, finger dissection defines and enlarges the scrotal cavity. The finger must seek

by incising the muscle medially or using a Prentiss-type maneuver to bring the testis and pedicle medial to the epigastric vessels. The peritoneum is closed on either side of the vasal peritoneal pedicle. One does not want to compromise the delicate vascularity of the vasal pedicle, yet the peritoneal cuff must be small enough to prevent visceral descent through it. On the right side, the appendix is prone to follow the vasal peritoneal pedicle downward, and occasionally an inversion appendectomy must be performed (Garcia and Bloom, 1986). Muscle is reapproximated to regain the integrity of the inguinal floor. This operation can be performed as an outpatient procedure. Jordan and Bloom have developed laparoscopic techniques to perform the Fowler-Stephens orchiopexy in one or two completely laparoscopic steps (Jordan and Bloom, 1994).

Follow-up After Orchiopexy

Children are evaluated 1 year after surgery to assess the testis location, size, and viability. Parents must be cognizant of potential infertility and tumorigenesis. At puberty, boys are re-examined and are instructed to perform monthly testicular self-examination. Son and father may be given the self-examination pamphlet of the American Cancer Society. The diagnosis of cryptorchidism early in a boy's life has far-reaching ramifications, and the education and long-term follow-up of these patients is just as important as the operative procedure.

TESTIS BIOPSY

Testis biopsies are sometimes performed at the time of orchiopexy in younger boys to assess testis potential but usually are reserved for adolescents and adults to answer questions relating to fertility or malignancy. A fertility index based on a biopsy taken at the time of childhood orchiopexy correlates with subsequent fertility (Cendron et al, 1989). Gonadal biopsies also may be performed during abdominal or laparoscopic exploration for disorders of sexual differentiation. Testicular biopsies were once routine in boys with acute lymphocytic leukemia (ALL). The testis has been suggested to be a potential sanctuary for leukemic cells because the blood-testis barrier may prevent effective levels of chemotherapeutic agents from reaching the tumor. Testicular relapse, however, may occur primarily in the interstitium and not necessarily in the tubules where the supposed barrier would favor recurrence. Occult testicular leukemia occurs in 10% to 20% of boys who are otherwise in remission following treatment for ALL. Ultrasonography and magnetic resonance imaging are not helpful in detecting occult ALL in boys with a normal scrotal examination (Klein et al., 1986). In the last several years, pediatric oncologists have abandoned routine testis biopsies in ALL patients for two reasons. New multidrug chemotherapy regimens including methotrexate are more effective in preventing testicular relapse, and survival has been shown to be similar whether a boy is treated for occult testicular ALL or gross recurrence elsewhere. Currently, testis biopsies are performed for ALL only when a scrotal examination suggests a mass or tumor within the testis. Prepubertal testicular tumors are uncommon and normally present obviously enough to schedule an inguinal orchiectomy. If, however, malignancy is suspected but is less obvious, a biopsy is performed after inguinal exposure and cord occlusion.

An open testis biopsy is performed with the testis delivered through a short transverse scrotal incision or through a small window with the testis remaining inside the scrotum. A No. 11 blade creates a small transverse opening in the tunica albuginea. The exposed testis tubules are excised with the belly of the knife placed against the extruded wedge of parenchyma stabilized by the tunical edge. The specimen is placed in Bouin's solution in preference to formalin. One or two 6–0 absorbable sutures close the tunica albuginea, and the scrotum is then reapproximated.

Percutaneous testis biopsy under local anesthesia with a spring-loaded needle device is safe, rapid, and effective in adults (Morey et al, 1994), although there is little experience with this method in children. Flow cytometric analysis of testicular aspirates in cryptorchid testes has demonstrated excellent correlation with standard histologic sections in postpubertal boys (Ring et al, 1990). The testis is well suited to DNA flow cytometric analysis because there are a number of cell populations with different DNA content (haploid spermatozoa and spermatids, diploid germ cells and stromal cells, tetraploid spermatocytes). Three distinct DNA ploidy patterns correspond to normal spermatogenesis, maturation arrest, and Sertoli-cell-only syndrome. In the postpubertal male, fine needle aspiration biopsy with DNA flow analysis to predict fertility potential is safe and effective and has a lower potential for injury than open testis biopsy.

TESTICULAR PROSTHESES

The silicone gel prosthesis, with a consistency similar to that of the testis, has a long and successful history of clinical use. Anecdotal reports of autoimmune disease in patients with silicone breast implants have caused suppliers to retreat from the market, although no substantive scientific data support a causal relationship between silicone and autoimmune disorders. The American Urological Association issued a policy statement on testicular implants in May, 1992. The statement has been revised twice and was reaffirmed in January, 1995 as follows:

> The silicone gel testicular implant is made of a liquid material and can possibly leak through the prosthesis shell. Silicone gel testicular prostheses have been voluntarily withdrawn from the market and are no longer available in the United States. It is prudent at this time not to use this prosthesis. There is a silicone elastomer testicular prosthesis currently on the market. The placement of a silicone elastomer testicular prosthesis may be considered, if the benefits, such as psychological benefit to the patient, outweigh any potential risk. A potential risk could be leachables from the silicone elastomer testicular prosthesis. Such information should be included in an informed consent. If a silicone gel-filled prosthesis is already in place, in the absence of apparent rupture or local complications, the risk of removal may be greater than the risk of allowing the prosthesis to remain in place.

In most boys with monorchia, a solitary testis creates enough mass effect to produce a satisfactory locker room appearance. In contrast, bilateral absent testes, anorchia, result in a flat, small, empty scrotum that is visually very

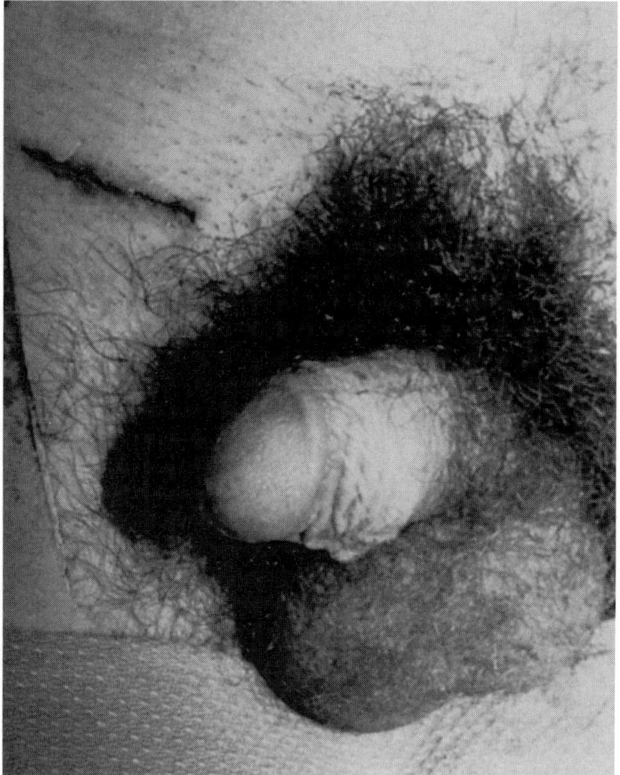

Figure 73–6. Subinguinal incision for right testicular prosthesis.

abnormal. Prostheses offer two primary benefits to boys with anorchia. The child and parents benefit psychologically; furthermore, the prostheses expand the scrotum to permit placement of a larger prosthesis after puberty. Prostheses are advantageous at an early age in boys with anorchia to avoid the emotional and physical disadvantage of a flat hypoplastic scrotum throughout childhood.

Testicular prostheses are implanted through an inguinal or subinguinal incision because the device may erode a scrotal incision (Fig. 73–6). Perioperative broad-spectrum antibiotics are administered. The scrotal space is developed with blunt dissection. The prosthesis can be anchored to the dependent dartos muscle; however, if an anchoring suture is not placed in a perfectly dependent position, the prosthesis may assume an abnormal lie and look odd. It is preferable to close the scrotal inlet securely and leave the implant free to move within the hemiscrotum. Oral cephalosporins are given for 1 week postoperatively. Elder and colleagues reported on 41 boys under age 5 who underwent insertion of a testicular prosthesis. There were no significant complications, and long-term results were excellent, with over 90% of families reporting a good cosmetic appearance and satisfaction with their decision to place a prosthesis (Elder et al, 1989).

TORSIONS

Testicular Torsion

Failure to diagnose torsion of the testis is one of the more litigious issues in urologic practice. Any child with acute pain in the scrotum should be presumed to have torsion until proved otherwise, although torsion is the cause in only 25% to 35% of all pediatric patients with acute scrotal pain. The majority of testicular torsions occur between the ages of 12 and 18, and adolescents with acute scrotal pain have a 50% to 60% chance of having torsion (Melekos et al, 1988). Symptoms include acute pain, nausea, and abdominal discomfort. Patients have difficulty in walking and often describe previous similar transient episodes (torsion-detorsion) that resolved spontaneously. Physical examination reveals a tender scrotum with landmarks that are difficult to differentiate owing to edema and inflammation. A reactive hydrocele may develop, and the cremasteric reflex is usually but not always absent. The differential diagnosis of an acute scrotum in children includes torsion of an appendage, epididymitis, orchitis, hernia, varicocele, tumor, trauma, idiopathic scrotal edema, fat necrosis, viral inflammation, and Henoch-Schönlein purpura. Reduction of the spermatic cord twist within 6 hours affords a good chance of salvaging the testis.

Some boys are anatomically predisposed to torsion of the spermatic cord. Normally, the parietal tunica vaginalis surrounds the entire testis and most of the epididymis. A small bare area posterior to the epididymis and the entire spermatic cord lie outside of the parietal and visceral tunica vaginalis. This anatomic situation does not allow twisting of the spermatic cord within the tunics. The bell clapper deformity occurs when the testis, epididymis, and part of the spermatic cord lie entirely within the tunica vaginalis, permitting the structures to hang freely within the sac and allowing complete rotation around the vascular axis. The testis may have a horizontal lie (Fig 73–7). Caesar and Kaplan reported finding the bell clapper deformity in 12% of males in an autopsy series (Caesar and Kaplan, 1994). This may occur bilaterally.

When the history and examination suggest torsion, immediate surgical exploration should be performed. If an operating room is not immediately available, manual detorsion may be attempted with sedation or spermatic cord block. The testis usually torses in an inward or medial direction. Turn the testis two or three rotations in a lateral-outward direction (when viewing the scrotum from the feet). Release

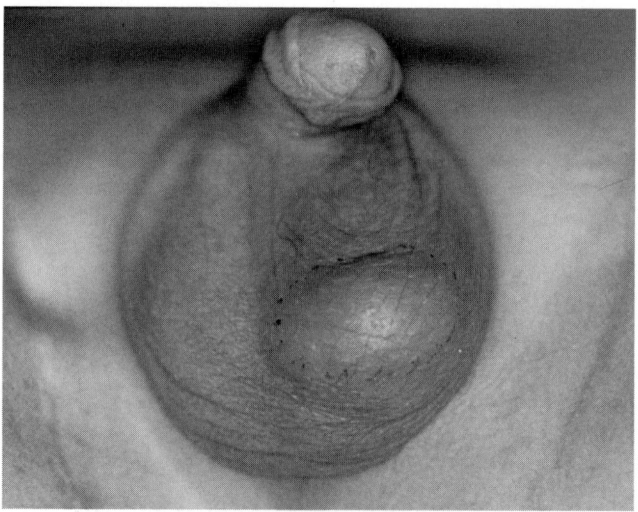

Figure 73–7. Horizontal lie of left testis.

and elongation of the cord and rapid relief of symptoms occur when detorsion is complete. Manual detorsion is not a definitive solution, and surgical fixation must still be performed, although perhaps not as an emergency procedure. A pitfall of manual detorsion is partial reduction of the twisted spermatic cord, which produces symptomatic relief but does not resolve the ischemia. Alternatively, the testis can be cooled with an ice pack on the way to the operating room.

All boys with acute scrotal pain do not require immediate exploration, and if the presentation is not classic for torsion further evaluation is indicated. Nuclear imaging to assess testicular blood flow occasionally may be helpful but is not always readily available; also, it delays intervention and is expensive. Color Doppler ultrasound is rapid and noninvasive and is more readily available. This technique can be used to assess blood flow and has the added benefit of displaying scrotal anatomy to reveal a hematoma, torsed appendage, or hydrocele. Kass and associates found that differentiation of torsion from other conditions was reliable with color Doppler ultrasound. Seventy-one percent of boys thus evaluated for acute scrotal pain did not require immediate exploration (Kass et al, 1993). False-positive and false-negative findings occur with color Doppler ultrasound as well as with nuclear imaging (Bomalaski et al, 1995).

Younger boys are explored under a general anesthetic, whereas spinal or epidural techniques can be used in adolescents. The scrotum is incised, the tunica vaginalis is opened, and hydrocele fluid is evacuated. The testis is delivered and the color noted, and the spermatic cord is inspected for twisting. The cord may be rotated in multiples of 360 degrees. The testis is detorsed and observed for return of its normal color. If it remains dark and the hydrocele fluid is bloody, the testis is probably nonviable. The testis is wrapped in a warm saline gauze while contralateral orchiopexy is performed. After the contralateral testis has been fixed, the torsed testis is re-examined for viability. The tunica albuginea may be incised to assess for bleeding. Tunical bleeding is not equivalent to parenchymal viability, so the testicular tissue should be examined specifically. If there is no hope for survival of the testis, orchiectomy is performed. If the testis appears viable, the entire tunica albuginea is exposed, and the paratesticular tissue is secured to the dartos in three places. There is debate about the site of suture fixation of the testis. Jarrow has shown that the medial aspect of the upper pole is the safest site for a suture in terms of vascularity. Adequate gonadal fixation, however, can be accomplished in children by placing paratesticular sutures that do not contact the testicular parenchyma or the gonadal vessels (Jarrow, 1990). The dartos and skin are reapproximated with absorbable sutures. Contralateral orchiopexy is recommended, but the testis and its vasculotubular structures must not be compromised. An alternative to suture fixation of the tunica albuginea to the scrotal wall is placement of the testis in a modified dartos pouch as used for undescended testes. The pouch is developed before the tunica vaginalis is opened, and fixation sutures are placed through the dartos and paratesticular tunics.

Complications of orchiopexy include hematoma formation and retorsion. Orchiopexy does not guarantee against future torsion, and therefore patients and parents must be aware of that possibility. The child must be evaluated immediately for subsequent episodes of pain or swelling. The most important factor in promoting adhesions between the testis and the scrotal wall is exposure of the tunica albuginea by excision or eversion of the tunica vaginalis.

Torsion of Appendages

The appendix testis is a müllerian duct remnant, whereas epididymal appendages are vestigial remnants of the wolffian duct system. The etiology for appendiceal torsion is not known; however, the clinical scenario may mimic that of testicular torsion. The onset of pain usually occurs gradually over a day or two, although it can be acute and severe. A reactive hydrocele often confounds the examination, and nausea and abdominal discomfort may occur. The classic blue dot sign, wherein the infarcted appendage can be visualized through thin scrotal skin or palpated as the point of isolated tenderness at the upper pole of the testis, is pathognomonic (Dresner, 1973). Certainty of diagnosis precludes exploration, and the symptoms resolve with scrotal support, bed rest, and nonsteroidal anti-inflammatory agents given over several days to a week or more. If there is any doubt about the diagnosis, spermatic cord torsion must be ruled out, usually by surgical exploration. A torsed gonadal appendage results in a fibrinous exudate around the entire gonad, so that the blue dot sign may not be evident later in the natural history of the process.

Perinatal Torsion

Newborn boys with gonadal torsion have a firm, hard scrotal mass. Most torsions are extravaginal, occurring above or outside the reflection of the tunica vaginalis on the spermatic cord. The weak attachments of the testicular tunics to the scrotal wall early in the neonatal period seem to predispose to extravaginal torsion. Das and Singer noted that 92% of cases of perinatal torsion were extravaginal, and up to 21% were bilateral (Das and Singer, 1990). Perinatal torsion can occur in utero (prenatal torsion) or within 30 days of birth (neonatal torsion). Prenatal torsion presents at birth as an asymptomatic, dusky, edematous, swollen scrotum that cannot be transilluminated. Neonatal torsion occurs in an infant who had a normal scrotum on examination at birth but subsequently develops scrotal swelling, ecchymosis, or a mass; this condition constitutes a surgical emergency. Exploration is warranted in these infants to establish the diagnosis and remove the testis. Contralateral orchiopexy is controversial but in the opinion of the authors is indicated because 8% of perinatal torsions are intravaginal, and delayed contralateral torsions have occurred. Furthermore, even if contralateral torsion is not *more* likely than average in this population, loss of a solitary testis is such a catastrophe that it seems hard to argue against the modest additional operative time needed for prophylactic fixation orchiopexy. The principles of atraumatic fixation orchiopexy are especially important in this group of patients, the key being to avoid transparenchymal sutures. The differential diagnosis of an infant with a hard scrotal mass includes hydrocele, hematocele, inguinal hernia, infection, infarction, ectopic splenic or adrenal rests, meconium peritonitis, and tumor. Exploration should therefore be performed through an inguinal incision because intrascrotal malignancy is a possibility, the spermatic cord torsion may occur high in the canal, and concomitant hernia may exist.

ORCHIECTOMY

Orchiectomy can be performed through a scrotal incision or higher on the cord through an inguinal incision. In pediatrics the primary reason for scrotal orchiectomy is a nonviable testis due to spermatic cord torsion. Inguinal orchiectomy is indicated for testicular tumors to control spermatic vessels early during the dissection. A painless scrotal mass is the most common manifestation of a prepubertal testicular tumor. These rare lesions are sometimes misdiagnosed as hydroceles, delaying treatment. Yolk sac tumor is the most common testicular tumor in childhood. Alpha-fetoprotein (AFP) is elevated in 90% of patients with yolk sac tumors, and tumor markers should be checked prior to orchiectomy. AFP, however, is markedly high in the normal neonate and does not fall to normal levels until after 6 months of age (Brewer and Tank, 1993). Teratoma is the second most frequent prepubertal testicular tumor. Physical examination should include assessment of sexual development and gynecomastia because some gonadal-stromal tumors are hormonally active. In contrast to adult teratomas, the pediatric variant does not tend to metastasize. Testicular swelling in patients with a history of ALL mandates testicular biopsy. Up to 10% of prepubertal intrascrotal tumors are paratesticular rhabdomyosarcomas. These lesions are treated by high inguinal orchiectomy. If the scrotum has been violated by an incision, biopsy, or previous scrotal surgery, a hemiscrotectomy is performed.

Scrotal orchiectomy is accomplished through a short transverse scrotal incision. The dartos and cremasteric layers are incised to expose the tunica vaginalis. Blunt dissection will free the tunica vaginalis from the scrotal wall, and the testis within the tunica vaginalis can be delivered through the incision. The distal cord and the vas deferens are identified and ligated. The cord can be divided into two or three segments and each ligated with a free tie and suture-ligature. When a testis is removed for torsion, contralateral orchiopexy is performed. The most likely postoperative complication is hematoma formation, so good hemostasis should be ensured.

Inguinal orchiectomy is performed through a skin crease over the midinguinal canal. Scarpa's fascia is divided to expose the external ring and external oblique aponeurosis. The external oblique fascia is opened carefully to avoid the underlying ilioinguinal nerve. The edges of the fascia are grasped and elevated, and the cord is mobilized at the level of the pubic tubercle. The cord is freed to the level of the internal inguinal ring. A noncrushing clamp occludes the proximal spermatic cord. Blunt dissection frees the testis from the scrotal wall, and division of the gubernaculum allows delivery of the testis into the inguinal area. The field is draped and the tunica vaginalis opened to inspect the testis. If a tumor is present, the cord is divided above the occluding clamp. The vas deferens is separated and ligated, and the cord is then divided into several segments. Each cord segment should be securely ligated with nonabsorbable suture, leaving tags long enough to allow identification if subsequent retroperitoneal lymphadenectomy and excision of the spermatic cord stump are necessary. The external oblique fascia and Scarpa's fascia are reapproximated and the skin is then closed in subcuticular fashion.

HYDROCELES AND HERNIAS

A hydrocele is a fluid collection within the tunica vaginalis of the testis or along the spermatic cord. Hydroceles are common in newborn boys and are due to persistence of a patent processus vaginalis (PPV) from the peritoneum or to residual peritoneal fluid that has yet to be reabsorbed after processus closure. A PPV accompanies the testis during normal descent and normally fuses spontaneously after the testis reaches the scrotum. Incomplete obliteration of the PPV can result in simple hydrocele, hydrocele of the cord, communicating hydrocele through a narrow PPV, or a widely patent processus with complete inguinal hernia. Most simple hydroceles resolve by 1 year of age and require no intervention. Physical examination reveals a transilluminating mass that may or may not reduce with pressure or in the supine position. The ipsilateral testis must be palpated to avoid missing an undescended testis with associated PPV. Premature and low-birth-weight infants have a higher incidence of hydroceles and bilateral lesions.

Fluctuating hydrocele size and persistent scrotal swelling after the age of 1 year suggest a communicating hydrocele, which is, in fact, an indirect inguinal hernia. This is repaired through an inguinal approach. Surgeons must be prepared for unexpected findings within the hernia sac (Bloom, Wan, Key, 1992). Failure to recognize bladder or bowel can be disastrous. Hernia precautions should be explained to parents of all children with scrotal swelling. Incarceration and strangulation of abdominal structures is a risk when hydroceles/hernias are followed expectantly. Less often a hydrocele can become acutely symptomatic when the PPV itself obstructs by intussusception (Bloom et al, 1993).

High Ligation of Communicating Hydroceles

A short transverse skin incision is made midway between the internal and external inguinal rings. Cauterize through the dermis to Scarpa's fascia, which is a distinct layer in children and can be confused with the external oblique fascia. Open Scarpa's fascia and expose the external oblique fascia and the external ring. Open the external oblique fascia by elevating the external ring with scissors and incising in the direction of the fibers, preserving the ilioinguinal nerve. Alternatively, incise the aponeurosis with a knife above the external ring and divide it proximally and distally with scissors. Separate the cremaster fibers to reveal the internal spermatic fascia and cord. The hernia sac is located on the anteromedial aspect of the cord and may appear as a widely patent, well-defined structure, or it may be a barely visible thin fibrous stalk. Place hemostats on the sac edges and use careful blunt dissection to separate the posterior sac wall from the anterior cord (Fig. 73–8*A*). If it is difficult to identify the sac, deliver the testis into the field without dividing the gubernaculum and open the tunic over the testis.

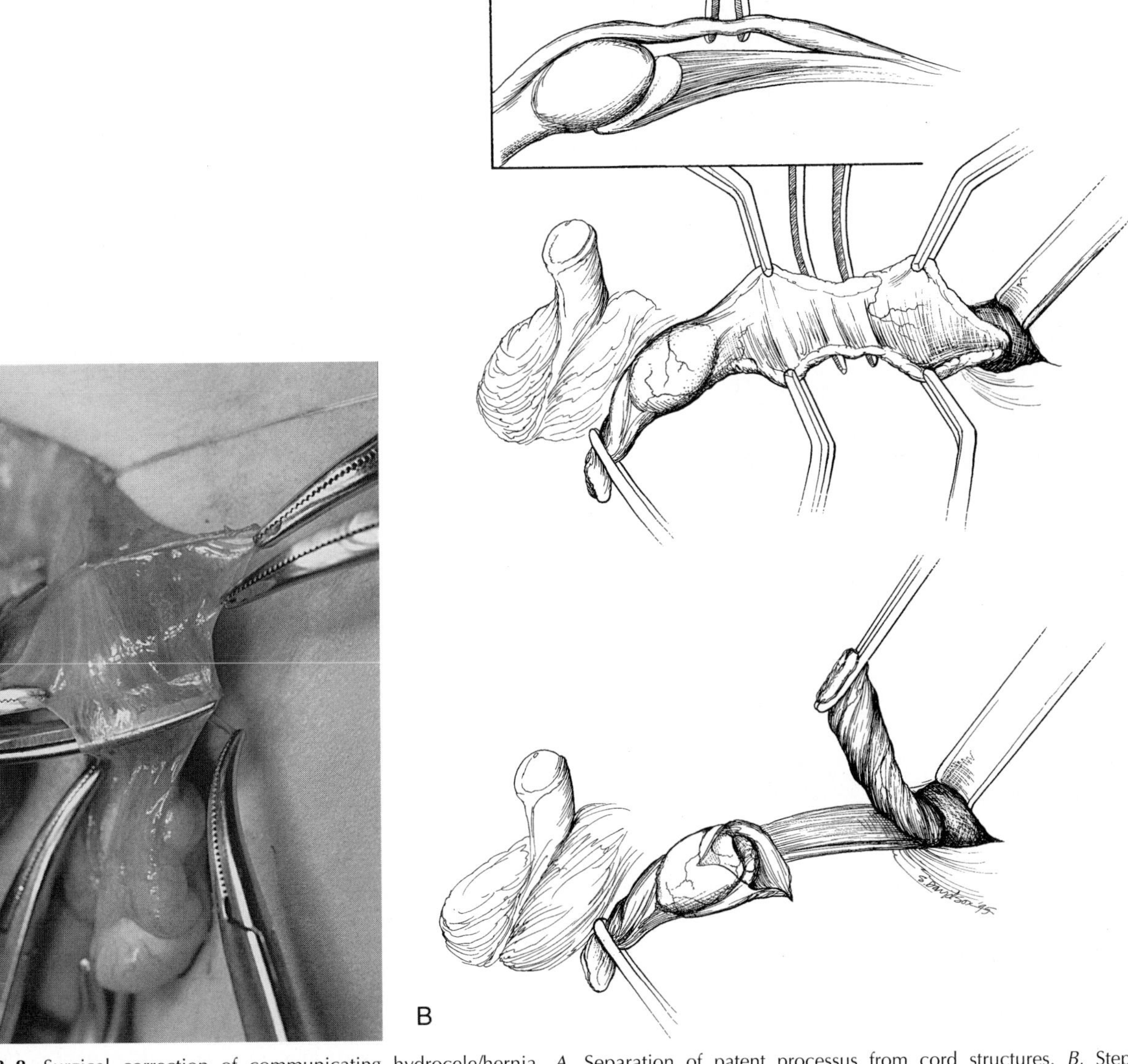

Figure 73–8. Surgical correction of communicating hydrocele/hernia. *A*, Separation of patent processus from cord structures. *B*, Steps of herniorrhaphy.

The sac can be traced from its distal termination up into the proximal cord. Once the sac has been separated from the cord, gather it in a single clamp, divide it distally, and free it proximally to the internal ring. Twist the sac to reduce any contents and ligate it at the internal ring (Fig. 73–8*B*). Excise excess sac distal to the suture, and the stump of peritoneum will retract into the internal ring. If the hydrocele extends into the scrotum, open the distal extent of the sac carefully without taking down the gubernaculum. There is no need to remove the distal sac. If the internal ring is patulous, reapproximate the transversalis fascia, taking care not to create too narrow a ring leading to possible cord ischemia.

Routine contralateral inguinal exploration is controversial. Up to 20% of patients undergoing unilateral repair have a subsequent contralateral hernia; however, the chances of finding an occult PPV are greatest in the first few months of life, particularly in premature infants (Skoog and Conlin, 1995). Given and Rubin evaluated 904 children and found that subsequent clinical contralateral hernias developed in only 5.7% of boys, and none were complicated by incarceration or strangulation (Given and Rubin, 1989). In older children, routine contralateral exploration is probably not warranted and must be weighed against the risks of injury to the vas deferens and spermatic vessels. Routine contralateral exploration is best reserved for premature infants and children with a potential for elevated intra-abdominal pressures (i.e., peritoneal dialysis, ascites, and ventriculoperitoneal shunts). An alternative to open contralateral exploration is endoscopic inspection of the contralateral internal ring through the ipsilateral PPV (Horgan and Brock, 1994) (Fig. 73–9). The ipsilateral PPV is isolated and divided but not ligated. A 5-mm trocar is passed into the sac, which is then tied around the sheath. Modest insufflation usually permits enough visualization to allow endoscopic inspection of the contralateral internal ring. If a hernia is present, it is repaired.

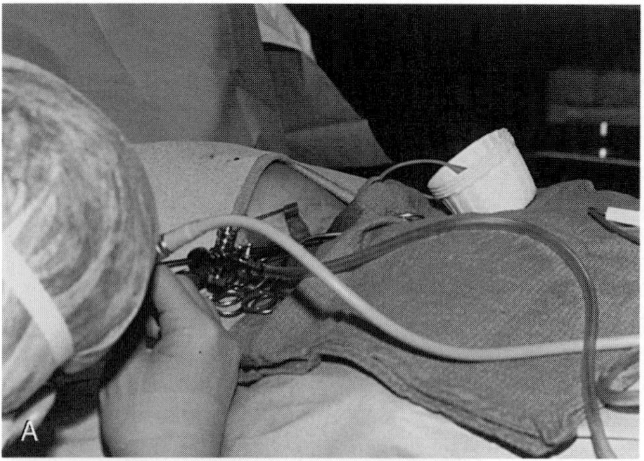

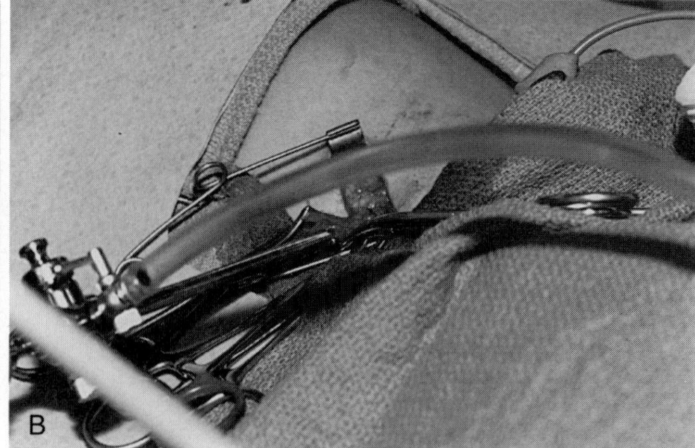

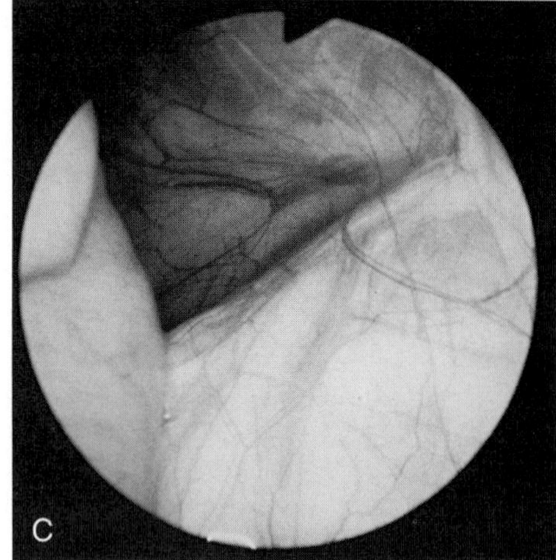

Figure 73–9. Hernioscopy. *A,* Small-caliber endoscope is passed into patent processus vaginalis. *B,* Processus is tied around the scope. *C,* Endoscopic view—no contralateral patent processus; normal wishbone at closed left internal ring.

Complications of hernia repair include wound infection, recurrence, atrophy of the testis, and injury to the vas deferens. If the vas deferens is inadvertently divided or resected, the ends are marked with permanent suture, and vasovasostomy is delayed until after puberty.

Acute simple hydroceles can develop in boys owing to trauma, torsion, tumor, inflammation, or infection, or they may be idiopathic. If acquired hydroceles persist in older boys and the history is not suggestive of communication, a scrotal approach may be used, although this usually is not our preference. Because the vast majority of pediatric hydroceles are due to a PPV, the surgeon must carefully consider the risks of scrotal exploration and the need for extension of the incision and high ligation of a hernia sac.

Simple Hydrocele Repair (Lord and Bottle Procedures)

Push the hydrocele against the anterior scrotum and make a short transverse incision between the skin vessels. Incise through the dartos to the tunica vaginalis, which appears as a blue cyst. Bluntly dissect and separate the dartos fascia from the hydrocele sac circumferentially to deliver the hydrocele and testis into the operative field. Large lesions can be aspirated to allow delivery through a small incision. Open the tunica vaginalis, inspect the testis and epididymis, and confirm that the sac does not communicate proximally. Plicate the tunica vaginalis with 4–0 absorbable suture by lifting the free edge and taking small bites of the peritoneal surface every centimeter until the junction with the testis is reached. Place six to eight sutures circumferentially, which can be tied sequentially as placed or following placement of all plicating sutures. Close the dartos and skin with absorbable suture. A disadvantage of this method, the Lord plication, is the presence of excess tissue bulk within the scrotum. Alternatively, the excess sac can be excised, leaving a 1 cm rim of sac adjacent to the testis and epididymis. Sac edges are cauterized or run with a chromic suture for hemostasis. If a larger margin of sac is left around the testis (2 cm), the edges can be brought behind the testis and epididymis, reapproximated, and run with chromic suture in bottle neck fashion. Do not close the bottle neck so tight that the cord is compromised (Fig. 73–10).

Complications of simple hydrocele repair include infection, hematoma, injury to the vas deferens, and recurrence. The most likely reason for recurrence is a missed patent processus vaginalis. A ventriculoperitoneal shunt that slips down through a ligated patent processus is a rare cause of recurrent hydrocele.

VARICOCELE

Varicocele is an abnormal dilation of the spermatic veins within the scrotum. The lesion occurs in approximately 15%

Redman JF: Simplified technique for scrotal pouch orchiopexy. Urol Clin North Am 1990; 17:9–12.

Ring KS, Burbige KA, Benson MC, et al: The flow cytometric analysis of undescended testes in children. J Urol 1990; 144:494–498.

Ritchey ML, Bloom DA: Modified dartos pouch orchiopexy. Urology 1995; 45:136–138.

Rodriguez LE, Kaplan GW: An experimental study of methods to produce intrascrotal testicular fixation. J Urol 1988; 139:565–567.

Rozanski TA, Bloom DA: The undescended testis: Theory and management. Urol Clin North Am 1995; 22:107–118.

Rozanski TA, Wojno K, Bloom DA: The remnant orchiectomy. J Urol 1996; 155:712.

Sayfan J, Soffer Y, Orda R: Varicocele treatment. Prospective randomized trial of three methods. J Urol 1992; 148:1447.

Silber SJ, Kelly J: Successful autotransplantation of an intraabdominal testis. J Urol 1976; 115:452.

Silicone Testicular Implants. American Urological Association Board of Director's Minutes. Baltimore, Maryland, January, 1995.

Skoog SJ, Conlin MJ: Pediatric hernias and hydroceles: The urologist's perspective. Urol Clin North Am 1995; 22:119–130.

Snyder H III: Editorial: Testicular autotransplantation. J Urol 1995; 154:562.

Steinhardt GF, Kroovand RL, Perlmutter AD: Orchidopexy: Planned 2-stage techniques. J Urol 1985; 133:434.

Szabo R, Kessler R: Hydrocele following internal spermatic vein ligation: A retrospective study and review of the literature. J Urol 1984; 132:924–925.

Turek PJ, Lipshultz LI: The varicocele controversies. II. Diagnosis and management. AUA Update Series 1995; 14:114–119.

Upton J, Schuster SR, Colodny AH, Murray JE: Testicular auto-transplantation in children. Am J Surg 1983; 145:514.

Wacksman J, Dinner M, Straffon RA: Technique of testicular auto-transplantation of the intra-abdominal testis using a microvascular anastomosis. Surg Gynecol Obstet 1980; 150:399.

Zaontz MR, Firlit CF: Use of venography as an aid in varicocelectomy. J Urol 1987; 138:1041–1042.

74
PEDIATRIC ONCOLOGY

Howard M. Snyder III, M.D.
Giulio J. D'Angio, M.D.
Audrey E. Evans, M.D.
R. Beverly Raney, M.D.

WILMS' TUMOR AND OTHER RENAL TUMORS OF CHILDHOOD

History

Rance, in 1814, apparently was the first to describe the tumor; Max Wilms, in 1899, better characterized the tumor that has become associated with his name. Other more descriptive terms commonly used include mixed tumor of the kidney, embryoma of the kidney, and nephroblastoma.

These neoplasms often are massive in size before they become clinically evident; thus, only rare efforts were made to excise them, and most children died. By the 1930s, better surgical techniques, especially improvements in anesthesia, and better understanding of pediatric surgical care led to a lowering of operative mortality rates, and survival rates of 25% had been achieved by the 1940s (Gross and Neuhauser, 1950).

The multimodal approach to the management of pediatric solid tumors originated with the treatment of Wilms' tumor because it was learned that this tumor was responsive to **radiation therapy.** With this addition to the treatment options, survivals rose to the 50% range, where they remained until the advent of chemotherapy.

The introduction of aminopterin in the 1940s for the treatment of leukemia opened the era of chemotherapy for pediatric cancers. Sidney Farber and co-workers at the Boston Children's Hospital reported that actinomycin D was an effective treatment for Wilms' tumor in 1956. This marked the first successful treatment of a pediatric solid neoplasm by chemotherapy. By 1966, Farber reported a survival rate of 81% for children with Wilms' tumor treated by surgery, radiotherapy, and chemotherapy with **actinomycin D** at the Boston Children's Hospital compared with a 40% survival rate for children treated by surgery and radiotherapy only. Wolff and associates (1968) reported that multiple courses of chemotherapy were more effective than a single course.

At about the same time, the *b Vinca* alkaloids were found to be effective oncolytic agents. Sutow and Sullivan reported in 1965 the successful use of vincristine as a single agent in the treatment of Wilms' tumor. **Vincristine** was also shown to be effective in patients who had previously been treated with actinomycin D (Sutow et al, 1963). Subsequently, high-dose cyclophosphamide (Finkelstein et al, 1969) and doxorubicin (Adriamycin [Adria, Columbus, OH]) (Wang et al, 1971) were demonstrated to be helpful in the treatment of Wilms' tumor.

The evolution of modern treatment of Wilms' tumor owes much to the cooperative studies carried out in many medical centers to compare different modes of treatment. The intergroup National Wilms' Tumor Study (NWTS) in the United States and trials conducted by the International Society of Pediatric Oncology (SIOP) and the United Kingdom Medical Research Council helped guide the development of current treatment.

Incidence

Wilms' tumor is the **most common malignant neoplasm of the urinary tract in children** and is responsible for 8% of all solid tumors in children. It comprises more than 80% of genitourinary cancers in children younger than 15 years (Young et al, 1978). Approximately 7 new cases occur per million children per year in the United States, resulting in about 350 new cases per year. In about 75% of cases the diagnosis is made in children between 1 and 5 years of age. Of all patients, 90% are seen before age 7, and the peak incidence occurs between ages 3 and 4 years. The male-to-female ratio is almost equal (0.97:1.0). Occasionally, the tumor occurs in adults (Olsen and Bischoff, 1970). Familial cases are rare (1%).

Etiology and Embryology

Wilms' tumor is thought to be the result of an abnormal proliferation of **metanephric blastema without normal differentiation into tubules and glomeruli.** The median age incidence of 3½ years makes it unlikely that Wilms' tumor is a truly congenital neoplasm, although there clearly is a hereditary component. Evidence (Bove and McAdams, 1976; Machin, 1980*a* and *b*) suggests that lesions of the nephroblastomatosis complex may function as a carrier state, bringing blastemal tissue to a point at which subsequent change leads to the development of clinical Wilms' tumor. The two-stage mutational model of Knudson and Strong (1972) suggests separation of Wilms' tumors into two classes: hereditary and nonhereditary, depending on whether or not the initial tumor mutational event occurred in a germ cell. Patients with familial or bilateral tumors and tumors associated with aniridia or genitourinary anomalies present at a younger age and appear to represent hereditary cases.

In the **etiology** of Wilms' tumor, the loss of allelic heterozygosity on the distal portion of chromosome 11p (seen in a third of sporadic cases) suggests that the **loss of function of a recessive tumor suppressor gene in the 11p13 (WT1) region** is important (Hoffman, 1989; Koufos et al, 1984). Mutational events at other gene loci are also involved. In some cases, the allelic heterozygosity is **distal to 11p13 in the distal portion of 11p15 (WT2),** seen with Wilms' tumor in the Beckwith-Wiedemann syndrome (Manners et al, 1988; Reeve et al, 1989). Thus it appears that during tumor formation, maternal chromosome 11 alleles are preferentially lost (Schroeder et al, 1987; Williams et al, 1989). Of additional particular interest is the demonstration that WT1 is important in normal kidney embryogenesis. Kreidberg and colleagues (1993) found that deletion of the WT1 alleles in mice led to major genitourinary maldevelopments. These issues have been reviewed recently by Coppes and associates (1994).

The **association of pseudohermaphroditism, nephron disorders, and Wilms' tumor** raises the question of whether an embryologic event might occur before the differentiation of renal and genital structures, thereby affecting both (Drash et al, 1970). Teratogens in animal models have also produced Wilms' tumor as well as other neoplasms. Expression of a transforming gene on the maternal chromosome may be muted by genomic imprinting (Wilkins, 1989), raising the possibility of paternal occupational exposure as a possible risk factor. Children of machinists have been identified as being at higher risk of Wilms' tumor (Bunin et al, 1989; Olshan et al, 1990), although the exact nature of the exposure remains to be identified.

Associated Anomalies

About 15% of children with Wilms' tumor have **other congenital abnormalities** (Miller, 1968; Miller et al, 1964; Pendergrass, 1976). ***Aniridia*** was found in 1.1% of the children in the first NWTS. Whereas the occurrence of aniridia in the general population is 1 in 50,000 persons, it is present in about 1 in 70 patients with Wilms' tumor. The sporadic form of aniridia rather than the familial form is associated with Wilms' tumor. In children with sporadic aniridia, especially when it is associated with the 11p deletion, there is an approximate 33% risk of Wilms' tumor. The full syndrome, in addition to the tumor and congenital eye lesions, includes presentation generally before 3 years of age, genitourinary anomalies, deformities of the external ear, mental retardation, and, less frequently, facial or skull dysmorphism, inguinal and umbilical hernias, and hypotonia (Haicken and Miller, 1971). This combination has become known as the WAGR syndrome—Wilms' tumor, aniridia, genitourinary anomalies, and retardation (Narahara et al, 1984).

Hemihypertrophy, characterized by an asymmetry of the body, has been found in 2.9% of patients with Wilms' tumor, not necessarily lateralized to the side of the tumor. It may even become evident after the Wilms' tumor has appeared (Janik and Seeler, 1976). The incidence of hemihypertrophy in the general population is 1 in 14,300 persons, whereas in those with Wilms' tumor, it is found in 1 of 32 cases. An increased incidence of other cancers is associated with hemihypertrophy, e.g., embryonal carcinomas, especially adrenal cortical carcinomas and hepatoblastomas. These patients often manifest multiple pigmented nevi, hemangiomas, and genitourinary anomalies (Meadows and Jarrett, 1978).

The ***Beckwith-Wiedemann syndrome*** (Fig. 74–1) consists of visceromegaly involving the adrenal cortex, kidney, liver, pancreas, and gonads. Additionally, omphalocele, hemihypertrophy, microcephaly, mental retardation, and macroglossia

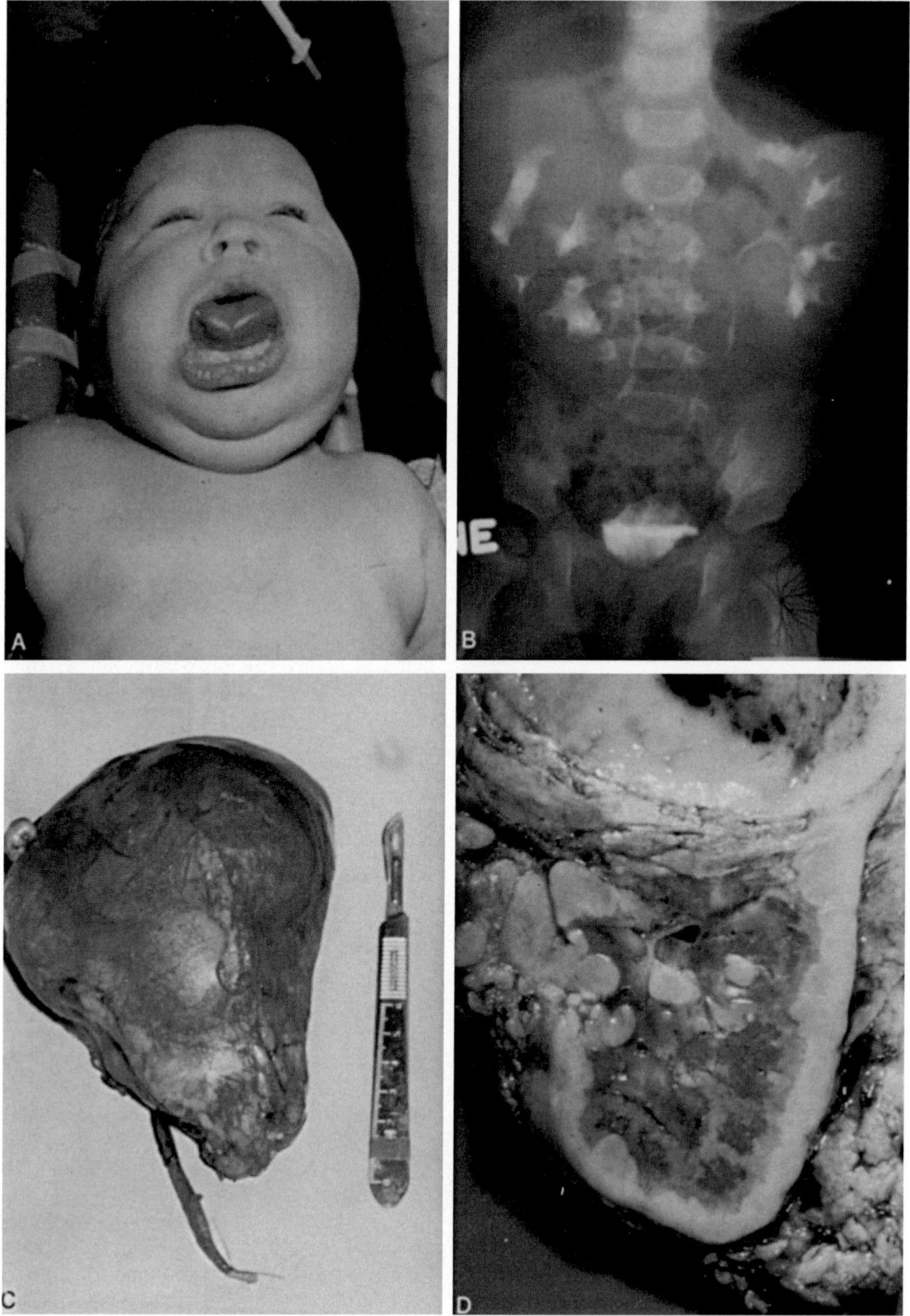

Figure 74–1. Bilateral Wilms' tumor and Beckwith-Wiedemann syndrome. *A*, Associated macroglossia. *B*, Intravenous pyelogram showing calyceal distortion in both kidneys. *C*, Right kidney with large upper pole Wilms' tumor. *D*, Cut specimen showing Wilms' tumor and inferior rim of nephroblastomatosis and Wilms' tumorlets.

may be found. Approximately one in ten children with this syndrome develops a neoplasm (Sotelo-Avila et al, 1980). The malignancies affect the liver, adrenal cortex, and kidney; the same organs are at risk in children with hemihypertrophy. Many cases listed as hemihypertrophy may represent incomplete forms of the Beckwith-Wiedemann syndrome.

Musculoskeletal anomalies have been found in 2.9% of patients with Wilms' tumor, who demonstrate a 7.9% incidence of hamartomas, including hemangiomas, multiple nevi, and café-au-lait spots. A 30-fold increase in the incidence of ***neurofibromatosis*** has been reported in patients with Wilms' tumor (Stay and Vawter, 1977), but the association remains tenuous (Clericuzio, 1993).

Genitourinary anomalies are found in 4.4% of cases. Most often seen are renal hypoplasia, ectopia, fusions, duplications, cystic disease, hypospadias, cryptorchidism, and pseudohermaphroditism. As mentioned earlier, this finding suggests that the primary event in the genesis of this tumor occurs before the differentiation of renal and genital structures has taken place and accordingly affects both.

A number of associated ***second malignant neoplasms*** have been reported in long-term survivors of Wilms' tumor. The incidence of these neoplasms is up to 15%, and the tumors include sarcomas, adenocarcinomas, and leukemias. Most of the sarcomas, generally osteogenic, and carcinomas have been found in previous fields of radiation therapy. Such tumors may be induced by previous treatment or may result from a genetic predisposition to the second tumor. Perhaps others are a result of a combination of these factors.

A recent review by the NWTS reports a cumulative incidence of 2% in children who survive 15 years after the diagnosis. The risk was increased in patients who received radiation therapy, especially when combined with doxorubicin (Breslow et al, in press).

Pathology

Gross Features

Classic Wilms' tumor is a sharply demarcated and usually **encapsulated solitary tumor** occurring in any part of the kidney (Fig. 74–2). The cut tumor bulges with a fleshy tan surface. Necrosis is frequent. It may lead to hemorrhage or the appearance of cyst formation. True cysts are seen occasionally. The tumor distorts the calyceal anatomy, accounting for the typical radiographic picture. Uncommonly, the tumor grows into the renal pelvis, where it may lead to hematuria or obstruction. Renal venous invasion occurs in 20% of cases (Fig. 74–3). Although lymph node metastases often appear to be present at surgery, histologic examination frequently proves this impression to be false, making gross assessment of nodal involvement unreliable (Martin et al, 1979).

It may be possible from gross examination to distinguish Wilms' tumor from some other renal tumors. Congenital mesoblastic nephroma on examination of the cut surface has a typical interlacing pattern, which is similar to a uterine fibroid (Fig. 74–4). If multiple small lesions are present, they suggest the diagnosis of nephroblastomatosis with or without Wilms' tumor.

Rarely, extrarenal Wilms' tumors have been found (Aterman et al, 1979) in the retroperitoneum and inguinal regions or as part of complex teratomas. Other sites include the posterior mediastinum, retroperitoneum, posterior pelvis, inguinal canal, and sacrococcygeal area (Coppes et al, 1991; McCauley et al, 1979).

Microscopic Features

It is difficult to describe a "typical" Wilms' tumor because the neoplasm can exhibit a wide variety of the structures of the metanephros and mesoderm from which it takes its origin. The tumor is **triphasic.** The most diagnostic feature is a **swirl of "nephrogenic" cells that have a tubuloglomerular pattern against a background of "stromagenic" cells** (Fig. 74–5). These cells are undifferentiated and generally compact, but they may have a mixoid appearance. The stromal component may occasionally differentiate into striated muscle (frequent), cartilage or fat (rare), or bone (very rare). The epithelial component of Wilms' tumor can be well differentiated, with characteristic mature tubules, or it may be very primitive.

Experience with the pathologic features of large numbers of specimens has suggested histologic characteristics that tend to be associated with a favorable or an ominous prognosis. Chatten (1976) recognized that epithelial predominance may indicate a better prognosis (Lawler et al, 1977). Although data from the Medical Research Council Nephroblastoma Trial supported this concept, data from the NWTS did not (Beckwith and Palmer, 1978). The reason for this difference may be that overall survival for Wilms' tumor is now so high (approaching 90%) that it may be impossible to distinguish histologic features that confer a particularly favorable prognosis. Although the poor outlook predicted for those with tumors having unfavorable histologic features may be confirmed by the clinical course, it may be that especially favorable histologic variants cannot be recognized because the overall success of treatment prevents singling out these cases.

Unfavorable Histologic Types

One of the first important pathologic correlations to come from the NWTS was the recognition of three particularly unfavorable histologic types. Although these three categories made up only about 10% of the cases studied, they accounted for at least 60% of the deaths.

Anaplasia is strictly defined as a threefold variation in nuclear size with hyperchromatism and abnormal mitotic figures. These features may be found in any of the various elements of a Wilms' tumor. When anaplasia is diffuse rather than focal, the prognosis is more unfavorable. This type of tumor has a greater incidence in older children.

The definitions of focal and diffuse anaplasia have recently been revised (Faria and Beckwith, 1993). The term focal now indicates circumscribed clusters of anaplastic cells, whereas diffuse connotes such cells distributed throughout the lesion. The prognosis is worse with the latter (Green et al, in press).

The second unfavorable category, which is no longer believed to be a form of Wilms' tumor, is the **rhabdoid tumor,** which, although comprising only 2% of the renal tumors entered in the NWTS, is and continues to be the **most lethal**

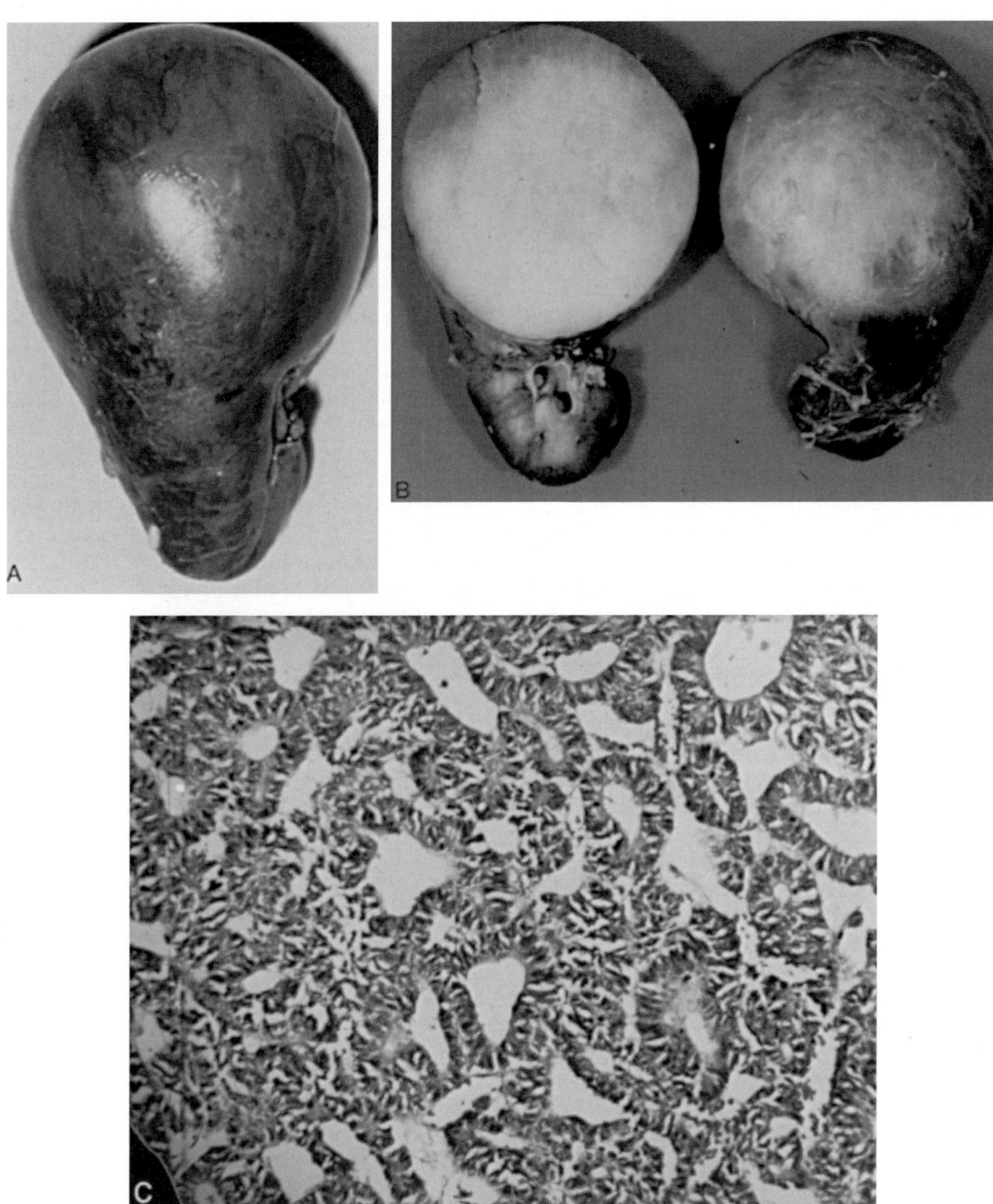

Figure 74–2. Wilms' tumor with epithelial differentiation. *A*, Kidney with large upper pole tumor. *B*, Cut specimen showing well-encapsulated tumor. *C*, Well-differentiated Wilms' tumor with epithelial component forming tubules (favorable histology) (× 320).

(82% died from tumor) (Fig. 74–6) (Sotelo-Avila et al, 1986; Weeks et al, 1987). Histologically, the cells are uniform and large with large nuclei and very prominent nucleoli. The cytoplasm contains eosinophilic inclusions, which can be shown to be fibrils on electron microscopy. These large cells are suggestive of rhabdomyoblasts and give the tumor its name, but neither light nor electron microscopy actually confirms the presence of muscle. Indeed, if striated muscle can be identified, as in conventional Wilms' tumors, it excludes the diagnosis of a rhabdoid tumor, and the outlook is not bad. In fact, these neoplasms may not be a form of Wilms' tumor at all. They are now considered by many to be a distinct sarcoma of childhood that is not of metanephric origin. They tend to **metastasize to the brain** and have a high association with independent primary central nervous system tumors (Palmer and Beckwith, 1981).

The third unfavorable variant has been referred to as ***clear cell sarcoma*** **of the kidney** and seems to be the same tumor as the "bone metastasizing renal tumor of childhood" described by Marsden and Lawler (1980). In NWTS-III, this tumor formed 3% of entered renal tumors and was equal in frequency to anaplastic Wilms' tumor. It also is now identified as separate from Wilms' tumor. Histologically, the tumors are characterized by a spindle cell pattern with a vasocentric arrangement. The nucleoli are not prominent, and the cytoplasm is scanty and has variably eosinophilic characteristics. Because tubules can be seen in the primary tumor but not in metastatic sites, it is possible that they are

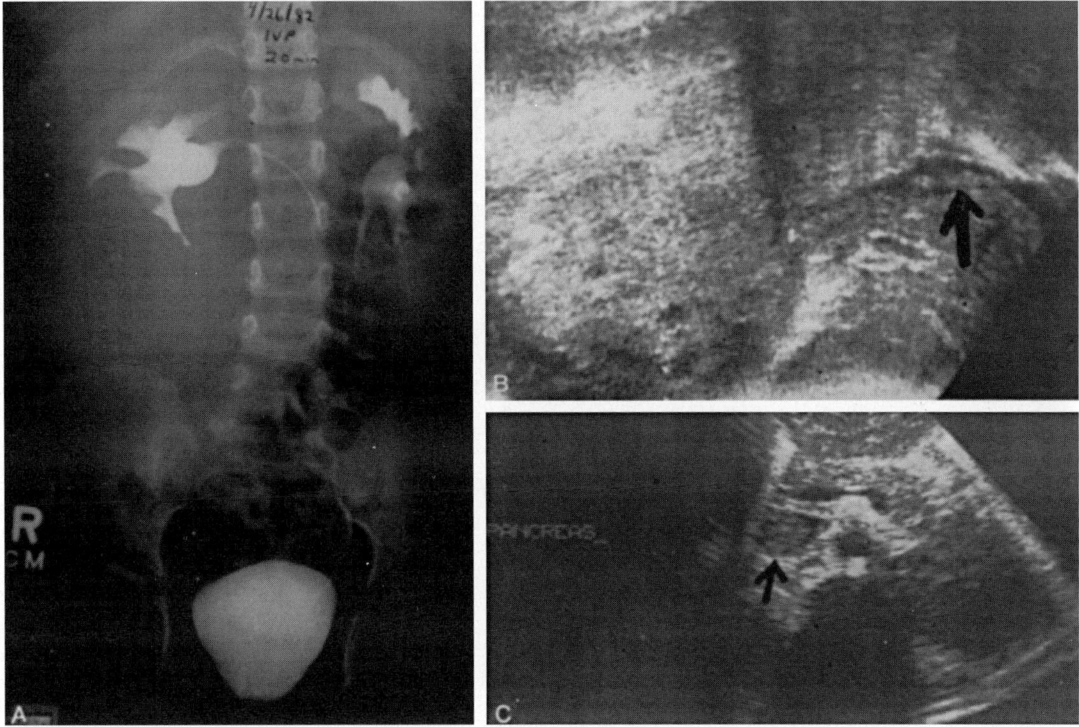

Figure 74–3. Wilms' tumor with caval invasion. *A,* Intravenous pyelogram showing a large right lower pole intrarenal tumor displacing the collecting system upward. Note course of ureter coursing over tumor. Abdominal ultrasound study showing tumor *(arrow)* in inferior cava on sagittal *(B)* and transverse *(C)* views.

merely being trapped by the tumor. The tumor characteristically **metastasizes to bone** (Morgan and Kidd, 1978) and is frequent in males.

Opinion is building to classify this tumor as a distinct entity rather than as a variant of Wilms' tumor (Carcassonne et al, 1981). Some ultrastructural studies have suggested that the tumor may be derived from blastemal cells (Novak et al, 1980). Clear cell sarcoma may reflect a malignant phase of the normally benign congenital mesoblastic nephroma. In NWTS-III, a better prognosis was achieved for patients with clear cell sarcoma when doxorubicin (Adriamycin) was added to treatment protocols (D'Angio et al, 1989).

Favorable Histologic Types

Several other renal lesions found in children have a characteristic morphology and tend to have a relatively benign course. Their exact relationship to classic Wilms' tumor continues to be debated, but perhaps they are best considered variants rather than distinct pathologic entities (Ganick et al, 1981).

MULTILOCULAR CYST. The characteristic aspect of a multilocular cyst (MLC) is its gross appearance. Typically, the lesion is round and smooth on its external border. It consists of a localized cluster of cysts within the kidney and is almost always unilateral. There are two peaks in the age incidence of MLC (Coleman, 1980; Banner et al, 1981). The first occurs in the pediatric age group and is characterized by the presence of blastema in the septa of the cyst. Although this lesion may have the potential to develop eventually into a classic Wilms' tumor (Fig. 74–7), the MLC itself has a benign course. Local excision constitutes adequate treatment.

The second peak in incidence occurs in the adult and more commonly in females than in males. Histologically, more mature fibrous tissue is found in the wall. Again, this is a benign tumor. Unfortunately, not all cystic localized lesions of the kidney can be divided into such a straightforward classification (Cho et al, 1979). Joshi (1979) and Joshi and Beckwith (1989) defined another entity in the spectrum of these cyst tumors—the cystic, partially differentiated nephroblastoma (CPDN), in which typical elements of Wilms' tumor are seen in the septae. Here, a simple nephrectomy but not a partial one appears to be curative. Because of such cases, it is wise to perform a frozen-section analysis before deciding to carry out a partial nephrectomy.

CONGENITAL MESOBLASTIC NEPHROMA. The patient with this renal tumor typically presents in early infancy before the age peak for classic Wilms' tumor (Howell et al, 1982). A frequent association with polyhydramnios has been reported (Blank et al, 1978). A male predominance has been noted. Grossly, this is a massive, firm tumor, which on cut surface demonstrates interlacing bundles of whitish tissue grossly resembling a leiomyoma (see Fig. 74–4). Microscopically, the tumor consists of sheets of spindle-shaped uniform cells (Bolande, 1973, 1974), and ultramicroscopically, the cells appear to be fibroblasts or myofibroblasts (Wockel et al, 1979). The margin of the tumor tends to show local infiltration rather than the pseudocapsule of classic Wilms' tumor. Cartilaginous tissue may appear at the tumor margin, a characteristic suggesting dysplasia.

When completely excised, classic congenital mesoblastic nephroma (CMN) has a uniformly **benign** course (Snyder et al, 1981). Greater morbidity has arisen from the treatment of small infants with radiation therapy and chemotherapy

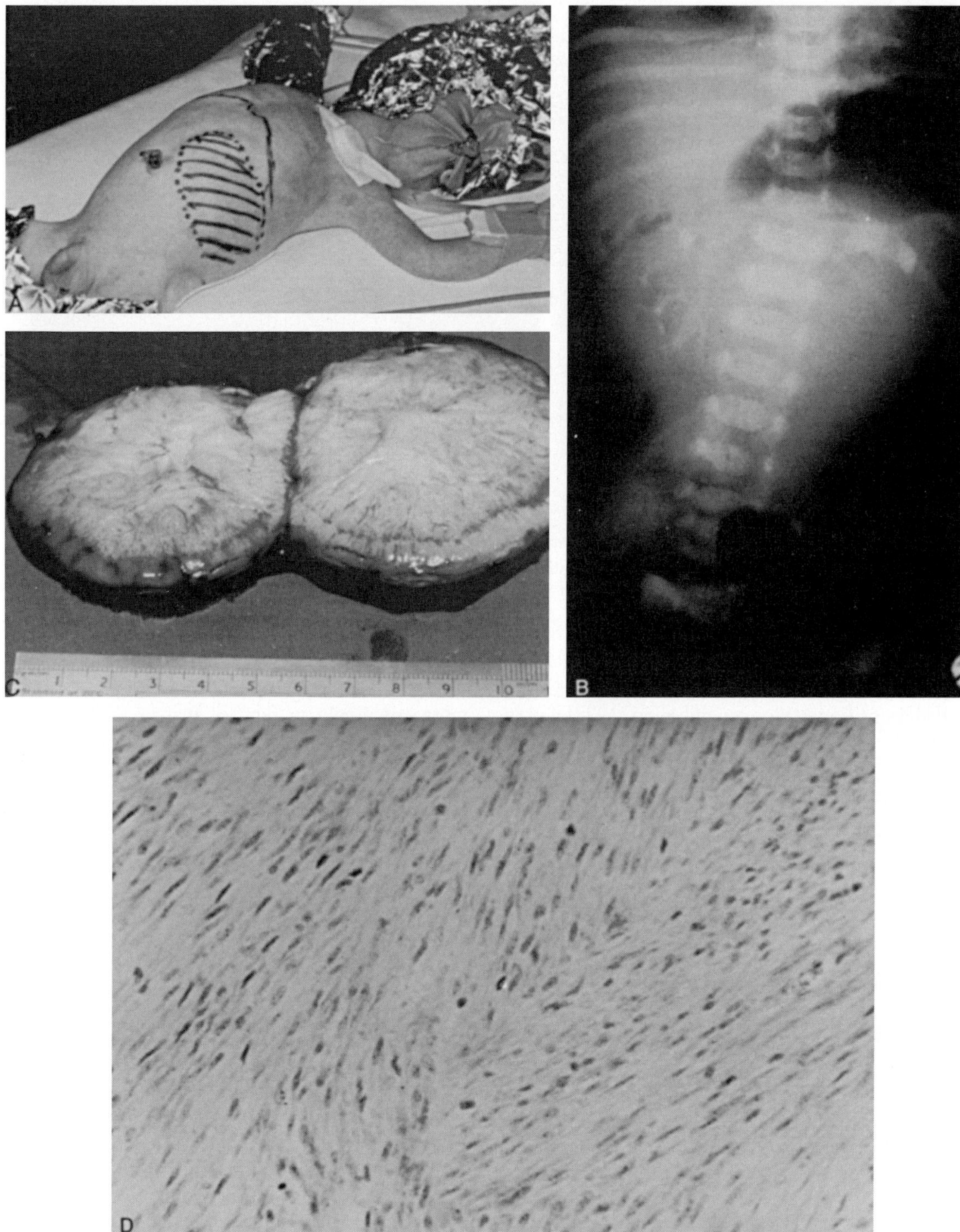

Figure 74–4. Congenital mesoblastic nephroma. *A,* Newborn infant who presented with a left flank mass (outlined). *B,* Intravenous pyelogram showing large left lower pole renal tumor displacing collecting system superiorly. *C,* Gross specimen shows characteristic dense, pale tumor composed of interlacing bundles grossly resembling a leiomyoma. *D,* Histology is tumor composed of sheets of uniform spindle-shaped cells with no capsule.

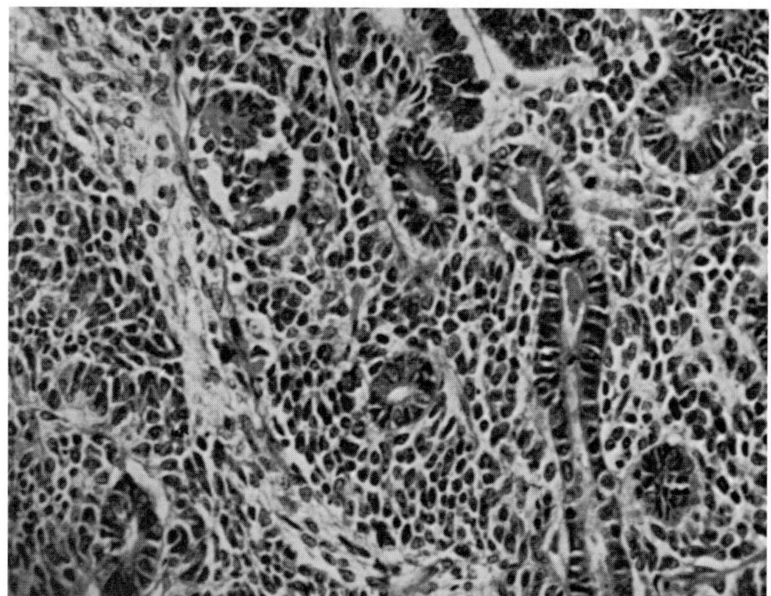

Figure 74–5. Wilms' tumor pathology: Classic triphasic histology showing swirls of primitive renal blastema and tubules against a background of undifferentiated stroma.

than from the tumor itself in the belief that CMN was a true Wilms' tumor. Wigger (1969) argued that this tumor is a hamartoma and not a form of Wilms' tumor.

Occasionally, a **"cellular variant" of CMN** is seen. This tumor has a higher mitotic index and a more sarcomatous appearance. The distinction between this variant and clear cell sarcoma of the kidney may be difficult. Indeed, the age and sex incidence, spindle morphology, prominent vascularity, and trapping of mature renal elements may suggest that the clear cell sarcoma is the malignant counterpart of the normally benign classic CMN (Hartman, 1981).

RHABDOMYOSARCOMA TUMOR. This is a rare Wilms' tumor variant with a favorable outcome, characterized by the presence of fetal striated muscle. It should not be confused with the unfavorable rhabdoid tumor, which does not contain muscle (Harms et al, 1980).

Any high grade of differentiation in pediatric renal tumors tends to impart a better prognosis in the various lesions grouped under the term nephroblastoma.

Nephrogenic Rests, Nephroblastomatosis, and Relation to Wilms' Tumor

In the 1970s our understanding of the pathogenesis of Wilms' tumor improved considerably with the description of what was then called the nephroblastomatosis complex of lesions (Bove and McAdams, 1976; Machin, 1980*a* and *b*). This complex of pathologic entities has been re-examined by Beckwith and co-workers (1993). A new classification and terminology have been suggested, which have the poten-

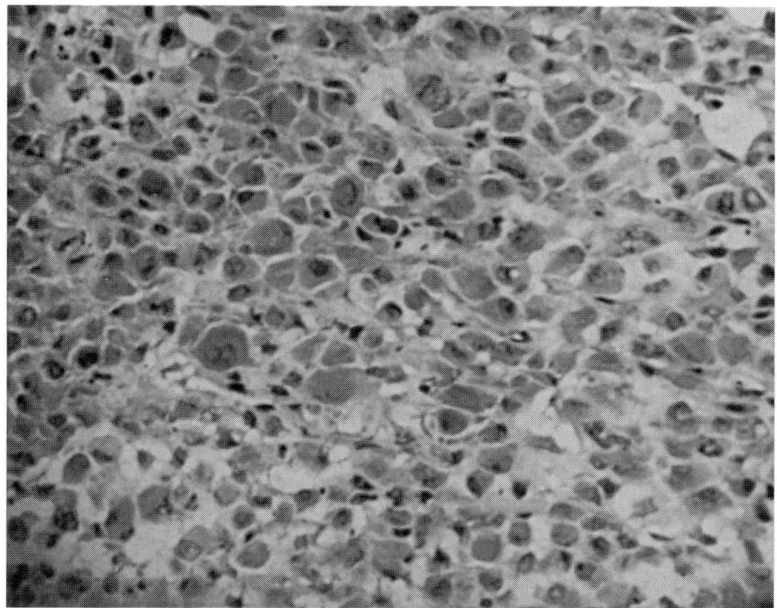

Figure 74–6. Rhabdoid Wilms' tumor: Unfavorable histology. Uniform cells with large nuclei and prominent nucleoli. The cytoplasm contains eosinophilic inclusions, which by electron microscopy can be shown to be fibrils.

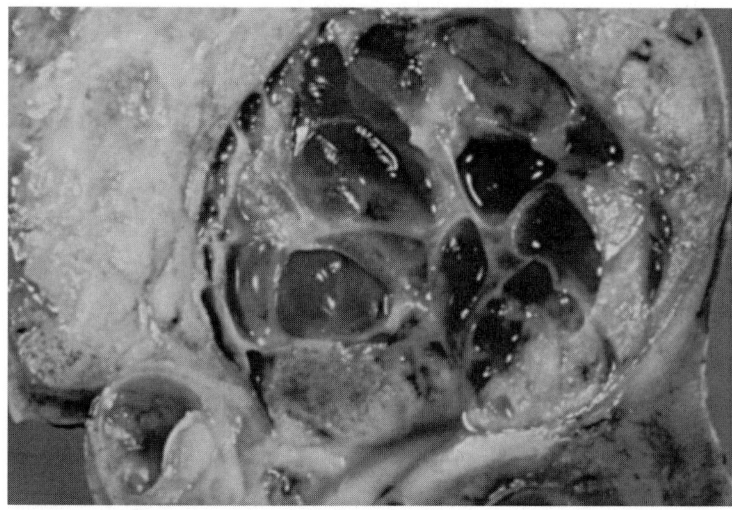

Figure 74–7. Wilms' tumor containing a multilocular cyst that demonstrates a typical characteristic series of adjacent cysts with an overall round configuration.

tial to simplify what was previously a very confusing topic. As an embryonic tumor, Wilms' tumor has a rather late presentation at 3 years, suggesting that it is not a truly congenital tumor. It has been speculated that lesions that are precursors of Wilms' tumor are present and may undergo a second "hit" in the two-step process of oncologic induction (Knudson and Strong, 1972). It was postulated that these previously noted pathologic entities, representing the persistence of nephrogenic elements beyond the end of nephrogenesis at 36 weeks, might be such a carrier state, permitting the persistence into childhood of embryologic tissue capable of completing evolution into Wilms' tumor.

Such potential embryologic precursors for Wilms' tumor have been found in approximately 1% of infant postmortem examinations (Bennington and Beckwith, 1975). Such lesions have been found in 30% to 44% of kidneys removed for Wilms' tumor (Bove and McAdams, 1976).

Beckwith's (1993) recommendation is to define a ***nephrogenic rest*** as a **focus of abnormally persistent nephrogenic cells** that retains cells that can be induced to form a Wilms' tumor. ***Nephroblastomatosis* is defined as the diffuse or multifocal presence of nephrogenic rests or their recognized derivatives.** The term also is applied to cases in which the prior presence of rests can be inferred (i.e., multicentric or bilateral cases of Wilms' tumor). The main categories of nephrogenic rests are ***intralobar*** (ILNR) and ***perilobar*** nephrogenic rests (PLNR). This categorization stresses the relationship between renal lobar topography and the chronology of renal development.

The medullary pyramid is the earliest portion of the renal lobe to form. The juxtamedullary nephrons are thus the oldest, and the ones nearest the lobar surface are the youngest. Theoretically, the location of a nephrogenic rest might provide an important clue to the timing of the teratogenic event that led to its formation. Events occurring late in fetal life would be located at the lobar periphery. This would include lesions along the columns of Bertin, which are at the periphery. Earlier events would be manifest deeper in the cortex or medullary areas. A very early disturbance could produce a total disruption of lobar organization.

The intralobar position of ILNRs implies that an earlier developmental event led to their creation than would be postulated for PLNRs. The two categories are not absolute, and overlapping cases are probable. A number of morphologic differences are found between PLNRs and ILNRs (Table 74–1).

The patterns of **nephrogenic rest distribution** are **unifocal, multifocal, and diffuse.** Diffuse patterns are those that have been previously referred to as nephroblastomatosis. In an effort to help clarify the fate of nephrogenic rests, Beckwith and associates (1990) suggested a subclassification of PLNRs and ILNRs (Table 74–2).

Most commonly, rests undergo retrogressive changes with time **(sclerosing, regressing, and obsolescent nephrogenic rests).** Rests that do not involute may show progressive changes in two patterns: (1) growth of the rest as a whole **(hyperplastic nephrogenic rests)** and (2) localized cell proliferation within the rest **(neoplastic nephrogenic rests)** (Fig. 74–8). This last category of neoplastic nephrogenic rests may be either benign appearing (adenomatous) or early

Table 74–1. MORPHOLOGICAL FEATURES DISTINGUISHING PLNR FROM ILNR

	PLNR	ILNR
Position in lobe	Periphery	Random, including cortex, medulla, sinus, and caliceal wall
Number	Usually numerous	Often single, usually sparse
Relation to adjacent nephrons	Demarcated, no nephrons inside rest	Interstitial, nephrons mingled with rest cells
Structure	Blastemal or epithelial Stroma sparse or sclerotic	Stroma usually prominent Blastema forms cuffs around tubules

From Beckwith JB: Precursor lesions of Wilms' tumor: Clinical and biological implications. Med Pediatr Oncol 1993; 21:158.

Table 74–2. SUBCLASSIFICATION OF NEPHROGENIC RESTS*

Rest Subtype	Description
I. Nascent or dormant rests	Microscopic size; composed of blastemal or other embryonal cell types
II. Maturing, sclerosing, and obsolescent rests	Few or no blastemal cells; differentiating epithelial or stromal cells in maturing rests; stromal hyalinization in sclerosing and obsolescent rests
III. Hyperplastic rests	Grossly visible lesions of same shape as original dormant rests; blastemal or embryonal cells during growth phase, but sclerosing hyperplastic rests are often observed
IV. Neoplastic rests	Any of the above three rest types containing one or more spherical, expanding nodular lesions; compressed remnants or rest around the nodules
A. Adenomatous rests	Neoplastic nodules contain only well-differentiated cells, with few to absent mitoses
B. Nephroblastomatous rests	Neoplatic nodules of any size are composed of crowded embryonal cells identical to Wilms' tumors; mitoses numerous

*Appies to perilobar and intralobar nephrogenic rests.
Data from Beckwith JB, Kiviat NB, Bonadio JF: Nephrogenic rests, nephroblastomatosis, and the pathogenesis of Wilms' tumor. Pediatr Pathol 1990; 10(1–2):1–36.

Wilms' tumors, and both types may coexist. Several of these different subclassifications may occur in the same rest.

Because the incidence of nephrogenic rests on routine autopsies is about 100 times the incidence of clinical Wilms' tumor, it is evident that **most rests do involute without tumor formation.** In Beckwith's reviews, most of the rests were PLNRs; ILNRs are rare. Interestingly, Wilms' tumors associated with ILNRs appear in a younger age group (Breslow et al, 1988). The Wilms' tumors associated with PLNRs have purely blastemal or epithelial cells with scanty stroma and only rare heterogeneous elements, such as muscle. In contrast, Wilms' tumors arising in association with ILNRs have more variation and more stroma. They may replicate early nephrogenesis. More heterogenic cell types, such as muscle, are seen.

Beckwith and co-workers (1990) report a 22% incidence of ILNRs with Wilms' tumor, a 17% incidence of PLNRs, and a 3% incidence of both types of nephrogenic rests, giving a total incidence of 41% of Wilms' tumors associated with nephrogenic rests. Table 74–3 summarizes the prevalence of nephrogenic rests (Beckwith, 1993).

In bilateral synchronous Wilms' tumors, there is almost a 100% incidence of nephrogenic rests, with PLNRs being twice as common as ILNRs. Both types coexist in 6% of cases. When an ILNR is seen in association with a unilateral Wilms' tumor, there appears to be an increased risk of a later metachronous contralateral Wilms' tumor. The implications are that ILNRs are less often multifocal, but, as stated earlier, such rests are more likely than PLNRs to undergo transformation into Wilms' tumors.

The association of nephrogenic rests with Wilms' tumor syndromes is interesting. In the WAGR syndrome, aniridia and the 11p13 deletion are associated with a high incidence of ILNRs. A younger age at presentation is characteristic. In the Drash syndrome, again, ILNRs are commonly seen. In contrast, in hemihypertrophy and in the Beckwith-Wiedemann syndrome, PLNRs are prevalent; however, there is a moderate frequency of ILNRs, which may coexist, producing combined nephroblastomatosis. The mean age at presentation of patients with this group of Wilms' tumors is similar to that for the overall incidence of the tumor.

A number of important clinical inferences can be drawn from experience with nephrogenic rests. One of the most important is that the microscopic appearances of Wilms' tumor and nephrogenic rests can be indistinguishable. Accordingly, the growth characteristics of the lesion as manifested on serially repeated imaging studies may be more important in revealing the biologic nature of the lesion than its histology. Indeed, repeated imaging with computed tomographic (CT) scans, ultrasound, or perhaps magnetic resonance imaging (MRI) may provide more clinically useful information than a second-look procedure and biopsy.

Absence of the long arm of chromosome 16 has been identified in 20% of Wilms' tumor specimens (Maw et

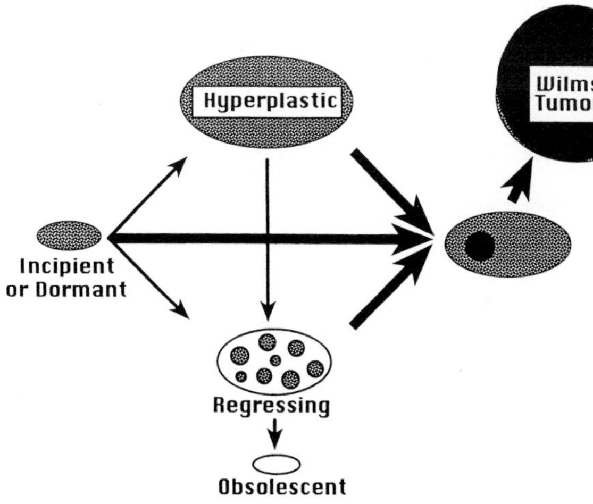

Figure 74–8. Nephrogenic rest classification. Heavy arrows indicate tumor induction. (From Beckwith JB: Precursor lesions of Wilms' tumor: Clinical and biological implications. Med Pediatr Oncol 1993; 21:158. Copyright © (1993) John Wiley & Sons, Inc. Reprinted by permission of Wiley-Liss, Inc., a subsidiary of John Wiley & Sons, Inc.)

Table 74–3. APPROXIMATE PREVALENCE OF NR

Population (ref.)	PLNR (%)	ILNR (%)
Infant autopsies [3]	1	0.01*
Renal dysplasia [6]	3.5	Unknown
Unilateral WT [1]	25	15
Bilateral WT (synchronous) [1]	74–79	34–41
Bilateral WT (metachronous) [1]	42	63–75
BWS/HH/WT† [1]	70–77	47–56
Aniridia/WB [1]	12–20	84–100
Drash/WT [1]	11	78

*Author's unpublished observation (2 cases with ILNR in 2000 infant autopsies).
†BSW/HH, Beckwith–Wiedemann syndrome/hemihypertrophy.
From Beckwith JB: Precursor lesions of Wilms' tumor: Clinical and biological implications. Med Pediatr Oncol 1993; 21:158. Copyright © (1993) John Wiley & Sons, Inc. Reprinted by permission of Wiley-Liss, Inc., a subsidiary of John Wiley & Sons, Inc.

al, 1992). Subsequent studies have suggested a correlation between 16 q and 1 p loss of heterozygosity and a worse prognosis (Grundy et al, 1994). These observations form the basis for the major hypothesis being tested in the Fifth National Wilms' Tumor Study Clinical Trial. Thus, the NWTS, launched in 1969, has advanced beyond tests of competing therapies and morphometric definitions. It has now reached the stage of attempting to link features at the molecular level within the tumors and their subsets that remain resistant to conventional treatment.

Further underlining the importance of imaging is the fact that ILNRs can occur deep in the parenchyma, as can PLNRs in association with the column of Bertin. Because most of these precursor nephrogenic rests do not seem to be headed for the development of a frank Wilms' tumor, their routine removal need not be advocated. However, careful imaging to detect growth of a tumor, which might indicate the need for early intervention, is required for this approach. When nephrogenic rests are bilateral or multiple, the key is to preserve nephrons. Because chemotherapy tends to obliterate only proliferating cells, nephrogenic rests with a malignant potential may well be the ones most likely to be affected. The more benign ones, such as sclerosing rests and those with extensively differentiated elements, may not disappear after chemotherapy. Accordingly, serial imaging is important in planning appropriate intervention and in avoiding unnecessary removal of benign rests.

Wilms' Tumor Presentation

Discovery of an **abdominal mass** and **increasing abdominal girth** are the most frequent presenting signs leading to the diagnosis of Wilms' tumor. These signs are seen in more than three quarters of cases. Usually the child is well and has no history of worrisome symptoms. About one third of patients present with **abdominal pain.** This pain may range from vague, poorly localized discomfort to acute flank pain reflecting hemorrhage into the tumor. A history of acute onset of pain with fever, abdominal mass, anemia, and hypertension suggests Wilms' tumor with sudden subcapsular hemorrhage (Ramsey et al, 1977). Rarely, a child may present with signs of an **acute abdomen secondary to intraperitoneal rupture** of the tumor (Thompson et al, 1973). Although gross **hematuria** is uncommon, microscopic blood may be found in up to 25% of cases. A history of minor renal trauma is often elicited.

On **physical examination** a **firm, nontender, smooth, unilateral abdominal mass** is most common. Very large tumors may cross the midline, but most do not. This finding is in contrast to neuroblastoma, which often appears with a more nodular irregular tumor growing across the midline. The child with neuroblastoma also usually looks sick.

Hypertension may be found in Wilms' tumor patients if the blood pressure is carefully checked—a practice not common in the past. The incidence of hypertension has been reported to range from 25% to as high as 63%. Hypertension may result from compression of normal renal tissue (renal ischemia) or from direct production of renin by the tumor itself (Marosvari et al, 1972; Ganguly et al, 1973).

Rare cases of Wilms' tumor associated with polycythemia secondary to erythropoietin production by the tumor have been reported (Shalet et al, 1967). Occasionally, a patient with Wilms' tumor is found to have an associated nephrotic syndrome, leading to the term Wilms' nephritis. This may be a chance association because neither problem is rare; however, it has been proposed that both conditions may result from a common embryologic renal misadventure, and, thus, the relationship may not be due to chance alone (Drash et al, 1970).

Even more rare presentations of Wilms' tumor have included varicocele, hernia, enlarged testis, congestive heart failure due to propagation of tumor into the heart or intrarenal arteriovenous fistula, hypoglycemia, Cushing's syndrome, hydrocephalus resulting from a brain metastasis, and acute renal failure (Sanyal et al, 1976). Occasionally, pulmonary metastases may lead to an initial presentation with cough, pleural effusion, or pleural pain.

Differential Diagnosis

The differential diagnosis for Wilms' tumor is the same as that for any abdominal mass (Table 74–4). Renal tumors can usually be distinguished from nonrenal ones by a combination of intravenous pyelography and ultrasonography. Neuroblastoma may cause diagnostic problems even after these two tests, particularly if the tumor arises intrarenally (Shende et al, 1979), but a bone marrow aspiration with positive results for neuroblastoma cells or elevation of the urinary catecholamine levels is conclusive. The diagnosis of other malignant tumors is usually not difficult once the origin of the abdominal mass has been identified correctly. Most benign abdominal masses can be distinguished from Wilms' tumor by intravenous pyelography or ultrasonography. An intrarenal abscess may be confusing if signs of sepsis are not prominent (Simonowitz and Reyes, 1976). Splenomegaly is occasionally confused with a left-sided Wilms' tumor.

Age is important in the differential diagnosis; in the newborn period, a renal mass is most likely to be a ureteropelvic junction obstruction or a multicystic dysplastic kidney. Infantile polycystic disease usually appears with bilateral nephromegaly. The rare congenital mesoblastic nephroma, found early in life, requires histopathologic examination for accurate diagnosis. In the first NWTS, 5% of patients were misdiagnosed preoperatively (Ehrlich et al, 1979). The most

Table 74–4. DIFFERENTIAL DIAGNOSIS FOR WILMS' TUMOR

Malignant Tumors
Renal: renal cell carcinoma
Neuroblastoma
Rhabdomyosarcoma
Hepatoblastoma
Lymphoma, lymphosarcoma
Benign Abdominal Masses
Renal: renal abscess, multicystic dysplastic kidney, hydronephrosis, polycystic kidney, congenital mesoblastic nephroma
Mesenteric cysts
Choledochal cysts
Intestinal duplication cysts
Splenomegaly

common errors were a diagnosis of neuroblastoma or renal cystic disease.

Diagnostic Imaging

Ultrasound, CT, and MRI have assumed dominant roles in the imaging of Wilms' tumor. The conventional **intravenous pyelogram (IVP),** however, usually suffices for the diagnosis of this tumor and for initial management (D'Angio et al, 1993). It is readily available in most institutions and is less costly than CT or MRI. The characteristic radiographic appearance on **IVP is deformation and distortion of the calyceal morphology by an intrarenal mass** (see Figs. 74–1*B* and 74–3*A*). Radiolucent areas may be produced by hemorrhage or necrosis in the tumor. The initial plain film of the abdomen should be examined carefully. Calcification is rarely present but, when found, has a characteristic peripheral "egg-shell" pattern resulting from old hemorrhage. If a stippled pattern is found, the diagnosis of neuroblastoma is probable. The IVP also permits assessment of the kidney opposite the side of the clinical mass. It is important to make certain that a contralateral renal anomaly is not present before removing the tumor. About 10% of Wilms' tumors are bilateral.

Nonvisualization of the affected kidney on IVP occurs in about 10% of cases (Nakayama et al, 1988). This finding may suggest complete blockage of the urinary outflow tracts (pelvis and/or ureter) or, less commonly, severe obstruction of the renal vein or massive parenchymal replacement by tumor. **Ultrasound is particularly valuable in the evaluation of a nonvisualizing kidney.**

Modern real-time **ultrasonography** has eliminated much of the diagnostic doubt that occasionally surrounded renal masses in the past. Renal agenesis, hydronephrosis, and multicystic kidneys can be rapidly distinguished from Wilms' tumor, which has a characteristic echogenic pattern distinct from that of a number of other infiltrative renal diseases (Hunig and Kinser, 1973). Although Wilms' tumor may be completely solid or predominantly cystic, the tumor **characteristically exhibits a heterogeneous echo pattern,** reflecting necrosis and hemorrhage in the tumor as well as the varied tissues that may be present (Jaffe et al, 1981). Another benefit of ultrasound is that, when used to follow a Wilms' tumor in a patient receiving chemotherapy, the appearance of new anechoic areas may indicate a response even when the overall size of the tumor has not changed (Shimizu et al, 1987).

Ultrasound also permits an **assessment of the renal vein** and inferior vena cava for intraluminal tumor (see Fig. 74–3*B, C*) (Green et al, 1979). When a tumor thrombus is identified in the cava, extension into the right atrium can be determined. Given the increased morbidity associated with resecting a tumor of this extent through a thorocoabdominal approach, preoperative chemotherapy is increasingly being elected. Retroperitoneal nodes and possible liver metastases may be ascertained. By observing movement of the tumor in relation to the liver during breathing, it may be possible to determine whether there is direct involvement of the liver. Assessment of the contralateral kidney may detect small tumors missed by IVP and may show a pattern suggestive of nephroblastomatosis. This is important in directing attention toward specific areas of the opposite kidney for biopsy. In the majority of cases, ultrasonography and IVP establish the diagnosis and extent of disease accurately and obviate the need for other time-consuming and costly examinations.

MRI has assumed an increasingly important role in the evaluation of abdominal masses in children and is becoming more important in the imaging of Wilms' tumor (Belt et al, 1986; Hricak et al, 1988). The extent and size of tumor are accurately assessed by MRI. The signal intensity of the tumor is variable in most cases. On T1-weighted pulse sequences, areas of hemorrhage show increased signal intensity, whereas areas of necrosis show a decreased signal. Both areas show increased signal intensity on T2-weighted pulse sequences. Unfortunately, MRI is not able to differentiate Wilms' tumor from other renal tumors by relaxation times. On postoperative follow-up, MRI studies may be the most cost-effective single imaging technique.

Arteriography, which carries significant morbidity in childhood, is recommended by the NWTS only in cases for which (1) the mass is not clearly intrarenal; (2) the mass is so small that it cannot be assessed by other modalities; (3) the tumors are suspected to be bilateral, especially if heminephrectomy is being considered; and (4) the kidney cannot be visualized and cannot be adequately assessed by other means. In practice, **angiography is rarely needed.** Inferior vena cavography to evaluate renal vein or caval involvement is subject to false-positive studies caused by blood shunting from the Valsalva effect during crying. The opaque column is forced into the paravertebral plexus of veins, suggesting inferior vena caval obstruction. Ultrasound is more reliable.

CT provides precise anatomic delineation of renal and retroperitoneal anatomy but requires a general anesthetic in the small child and is usually not necessary in Wilms' tumor patients. This study may have a greater role in the evaluation of neuroblastoma. Renal scans are usually needed only for the evaluation of a possible renal pseudotumor. In this situation a ^{99m}Tc-dimercaptosuccinic acid (DMSA) or glucoheptonate renal scan is useful (Katz and Landau, 1979). A renal pseudotumor shows normal function, whereas a Wilms' tumor is cold.

A **retrograde ureteropyelogram is rarely needed** today. It is indicated in the presence of hematuria, especially when the kidney is not visualized by IVP. Ureteral metastases due to calyceal invasion (Stevens and Eckstein, 1976) and direct ureteral invasion by Wilms' tumor have occasionally been reported, and diagnosis of these is important to permit an en bloc resection.

Evaluation for metastatic disease in children with Wilms' tumor routinely involves careful imaging of the chest because the lungs are the most frequent sites of metastases. Chest radiographs in frontal, lateral, and both oblique views are advocated by some (D'Angio et al, 1993) and appear to be effective for clinical purposes. Others stress the need for initial CT scans (Cohen, 1994). It remains to be seen whether the indubitably more sensitive but more ambiguous and costly CT results in a better outcome (D'Angio et al, 1993).

Other imaging studies are generally not carried out until pathologic studies have been done. If a rhabdoid tumor is found, imaging of the brain by radionuclear scan or CT is indicated because of the high incidence of central nervous system (CNS) involvement with either metastases or second independent brain tumors. The finding of a clear cell sarcoma should lead to a skeletal survey or radionuclide bone scan because of the high incidence of bone metastases with this tumor. These studies are complementary (Feusner et al, 1990).

Laboratory Studies

Standard laboratory evaluations of a child with a retroperitoneal mass include a complete blood count and urinalysis. To help rule out neuroblastoma in questionable cases, the LaBrosse spot test for urinary catecholamines is helpful (Evans et al, 1971). Bone marrow aspiration and biopsy usually are not carried out unless the diagnosis of neuroblastoma is suspected. Wilms' tumor rarely infiltrates the marrow in the absence of bone metastases, if then. A blood urea nitrogen (BUN) and serum creatinine level as well as liver enzyme determinations are usually performed to provide baseline comparisons. Although formal creatinine clearances are seldom needed before surgery, they may be useful for assessing renal function following treatment. Glomerular filtration rate calculations by nuclear medicine techniques can provide similar follow-up information.

Surgical Treatment

Until the introduction of radiotherapy, increased survival in patients with Wilms' tumor experienced in this century correlated with improved surgical and anesthetic techniques. The hallmark of success with Wilms' tumor continues to be the complete removal of the tumor. Although surgery is no longer regarded as the emergency it once was, exploration of the abdomen should be undertaken as soon as the child can be completely evaluated diagnostically and his or her condition has been stabilized appropriately.

The authors usually position the child with rolls beneath the back to hyperextend the back with the involved side elevated approximately 30 degrees. A very generous incision is made from below the tip of the 12th rib on the involved side to the lateral margin of the opposite rectus muscle. This incision generally affords excellent exposure, and, today, the authors rarely find a need to resort to the thoracoabdominal approach. The extent of the tumor is evaluated first. The liver should be inspected and palpated as well as the paraaortic and hilar lymph nodes and cava. Although node assessment can be frustratingly inaccurate at surgery, the presence of large node masses should certainly lead to biopsy (Othersen et al, 1990).

Exploration of the contralateral kidney should be carried out before efforts are begun to remove the tumor. The colon is reflected and Gerotas's capsule is entered with enough mobilization of the uninvolved kidney to permit careful palpation and visual study of its entire surface. The presence of nephrogenic rests may be suggested by an abnormal-looking cleft or discoloration on the surface of the kidney. Some authorities believe that MRI is sufficiently sensitive that inspection of the opposite kidney is no longer warranted (Koo et al, 1992). False-negative MRI examinations have been recorded (Ritchey et al, 1995). **It continues to be the responsibility of the surgeon to visualize both surfaces of the contralateral kidney adequately.** Biopsy should be performed for any suspicious-looking lesion.

The resectability of the tumor must then be determined. It is not unusual for Wilms' tumor to invade through the renal capsule and adhere to or invade adjacent organs such as the adrenal gland, duodenum, liver, pancreas, spleen, diaphragm, colon, or muscles of the abdominal wall. Although it may be appropriate to perform limited resection of these involved organs to permit primary extirpation of the tumor, a heroic initial undertaking is not justified. Pretreatment with chemotherapy with or without radiation therapy will shrink the size of a tumor and allow its removal.

The approach to the tumor begins with reflection of the colon on the involved side. If the mesocolon appears to be adherent, it may be left with the tumor because the bowel is generally adequately vascularized through the marginal vessel (Williams and Martin, 1982). When approaching a large left-sided tumor, it may be helpful to reflect the cecum and the base of the mesentery to permit exposure of the infrarenal vena cava. This maneuver quickly permits exposure of the left renal vein and artery, which can thus be ligated using a right-sided approach (Todani et al, 1976). The authors usually begin the tumor mobilization by establishing a plane of dissection against the posterior abdominal wall inferiorly and along the great vessels medially. The ureter is divided early, below the level of the iliac vessels and along with the gonadal vessels. The advantage of establishing these planes of dissection is that they are as far away from the tumor as possible, thus helping to avoid rupture of the tumor. Dissection along the great vessels leads to early identification of the renal vessels.

It is consistent with the basic principles of cancer surgery to try always to ligate the renal artery and vein before mobilizing the tumor to avoid hematogenous spread. With renal tumors, division of the renal artery before the renal vein has been advocated to avoid venous engorgement of the tumor. Although the authors do try to adhere to this principle, they do not hesitate to divide the renal vein first when exposure of the artery is difficult. They have not noted that this approach has materially affected the tumor or the difficulty of the operation.

Great effort should be made to avoid tumor rupture and spillage of viable cells into the peritoneal cavity. This event has been shown to be associated with an increased incidence of relapse in the abdomen (Cassady et al, 1973; Breslow et al, 1985). Occasionally limited rupture occurs, but this can be contained by judicious application of surgical sponges or suction. Preventing diffuse spillage will avoid the need for total abdominal irradiation.

The adrenal gland is removed with the tumor if the tumor involves the upper pole. However, the adrenal gland may be spared when the upper pole of a kidney is normal.

It is important to establish by careful palpation whether the renal vein and inferior vena cava contain tumor because renal vein ligation when a tumor thrombus is present may lead to separation of a tumor embolus (Shurin et al, 1982). Engorged retroperitoneal venous collaterals indicate obstruction of the renal vein. Surgical management requires cross-clamping of the cava above the neoplastic plug and opening of the renal vein and cava, if necessary, to extract the thrombus. The tumor is usually free and may be extracted with surprising ease. If a right-sided mass has grown into the wall of the cava, the vessel can be resected up to the level of the hepatic veins. The left kidney has adequate venous collaterals through gonadal and adrenal veins to survive caval resection (Duckett et al, 1973). Preliminary chemotherapy is advocated for major caval involvement, especially if the tumor extends to the atrium, to avoid the morbidity of a major vascular procedure or cardiopulmonary bypass (Nakayama et al, 1986; Ritchey et al, 1988). The preoperative embolization of Wilms' tumor to facilitate removal has been reported (Danis et al, 1979); however, the authors have not found this procedure necessary.

Although some authors have advocated a formal radical lymph node dissection for Wilms' tumor (Martin and Reyes, 1969), no improvement in survival was achieved by radical dissection when the nodes were positive (Jereb et al, 1980). In patients with Wilms' tumor, there are often enlarged hilar or para-aortic nodes, which are reactive and do not contain tumor. Nonetheless, **biopsies of these nodes should always be performed** and the site of large masses of matted nodes marked with metal clips. The presence of **positive nodes has important prognostic implications.** When tumor excision has been incomplete, it is advisable to use a limited number of metal clips to mark the extent of tumor. This approach assists the radiation specialist in designing the treatment. Many clips are inadvisable because they interfere with CT scanning of the area postoperatively if it becomes necessary.

When a tumor seems **unresectable,** consideration should be given to pretreatment with chemotherapy, radiation therapy, or both, with a subsequent surgical attempt at tumor removal. This approach to pretreatment has become popular in Europe and is being considered more often in the United States, primarily to lower intraoperative morbidity (Keating and D'Angio, 1988). Radiation therapy, as well as actinomycin D and vincristine, has been shown to produce good preoperative shrinkage of tumors (Waggert and Koop, 1970; Lemerle et al, 1976, 1983; Bracken et al, 1982). The NWTS has shown that, in the United States, preoperative diagnostic error is about 5%. Because of this rate of error and concerns that treatment might change the pathologic findings, making it more difficult to ascertain the need for subsequent treatment, pretreatment before surgical exploration of a tumor has not been popular (D'Angio, 1983). No evidence indicates that pretreatment with radiotherapy (Lemerle et al, 1976) or chemotherapy (D'Angio et al, 1976; Lemerle et al, 1983) influences long-term survival. However, the incidence of surgical rupture of the tumor has been shown by SIOP to be decreased by preoperative radiation or chemotherapy (Lemerle et al, 1976, 1983). SIOP data have also shown that preoperative actinomycin D and vincristine produce results at least as good as those achieved with preoperative radiotherapy (Lemerle et al, 1983).

Staging

A number of different staging systems have been advocated for Wilms' tumor, notably that of Garcia as modified by others (Cassady et al, 1973). The clinical-pathologic staging system created by the NWTS has been the one most widely adopted (Table 74–5).

One problem that emerged from NWTS-I and NWTS-II was that there was no adequate discrimination between groups II and III. In NWTS-II, the 2-year relapse-free survival rates for patients in groups II and III were 80% and 72%, with survival rates of 86% and 84%, respectively. **Lymph node involvement was associated with a poor prognosis** (Jereb and Eklund, 1973). The previous NWTS grouping system was therefore changed to the current staging system. All patients with positive lymph nodes were assigned to stage III. Analyses based on NWTS-II experience showed relapse-free survival rates for NWTS-II patients of 85% and 69% for stages II and III, and survival rates of 94% and 79%, respectively. Better discrimination between these two forms of localized but extensive disease promises to be useful.

Results and Conclusions from National Wilms' Tumor Studies I to III

NWTS-I, which ran from 1969 to 1974, began to open new vistas for the treatment of this common tumor. The adverse prognostic effect of anaplasia was clear. It was shown that routine radiotherapy conferred no advantage for stage I tumors in patients younger than 2 years if actinomycin D were given for 15 months. Vincristine and actinomycin D together were better than either drug alone. Treatment of stage IV tumors with preoperative vincristine showed no advantage in those treated postoperatively with radiation therapy, actinomycin D, and vincristine.

Delays of more than 10 days in starting radiation therapy had a deleterious effect on outcome. In patients who underwent tumor biopsy or in whom local spillage occurred, whole abdomen irradiation was demonstrated to confer no advantage over localized flank irradiation. Thus, it was realized that a confined spill of tumor cells or tumor biopsy was not an indication to upstage the tumor. When the tumor was completely excised, the extension of Wilms' tumor into the renal vein or local direct extension beyond the kidney itself had no adverse effect on outcome (D'Angio et al, 1976, 1978, 1980).

NWTS-II was conducted from 1974 to 1979 and was more revealing. For patients with stage I tumors, 6 months of actinomycin D and vincristine were shown to be as effective as 15 months of therapy with these drugs (D'Angio et al, 1981). Stage II, III, and IV tumors did better when doxorubicin was added to actinomycin D and vincristine. With the improvements in chemotherapy, neither patient age over 2 years or tumor size of more than 250 g appeared to be important prognostic variables. An adverse effect was shown to result from the presence of local nodal disease in the abdomen (Thomas et al, 1984; Breslow et al, 1985).

NWTS-III ran from 1979 to 1985 and provided further important information. In patients with stage II tumors, radiotherapy conferred no additional benefit. In patients with stage III tumors, a radiation dose of 1000 cGy provided as good an outcome as 2000 cGy. In patients with stage II and III tumors, no benefit was obtained from adding doxorubicin to vincristine and actinomycin D. Patients with stage I tumors with a favorable histology appeared to do as well with vincristine and actinomycin D for 10 weeks as for 6 months. However, subset analysis showed a possible benefit for the

Table 74–5. NATIONAL WILMS' TUMOR STAGING SYSTEM*

Stage I:	Tumor limited to kidney and completely excised. The surface of the renal capsule is intact. Tumor was not ruptured before or during removal. There is no residual tumor apparent beyond the margins of resection.
Stage II:	Tumor extends beyond the kidney but is completely removed. There is regional extension of the tumor, i.e., penetration through the outer surface of the renal capsule into perirenal soft tissues. Vessels outside the kidney substance are infiltrated or contain tumor thrombus. The tumor may have undergone biopsy or there has been local spillage of tumor confined to the flank. There is no residual tumor apparent at or beyond the margins of excision.
Stage III:	Residual nonhematogenous tumor confined to the abdomen. Any one or more of the following occur: a. Lymph nodes on biopsy are found to be involved in the himus, the periaortic chains, or beyond. b. There has been diffuse peritoneal contamination by tumor, such as by spillage of tumor beyond the flank before or during surgery, or by tumor growth that has penetrated through the peritoneal surface. c. Implants are found on the peritoneal surfaces. d. The tumor extends beyond the surgical margins either microscopically or grossly. e. The tumor is not completely resectable because of local infiltration into vital structures.
Stage IV:	Hematogenous metastases. Deposits beyond stage III, e.g., lung, liver, bone, and brain.
Stage V:	Bilateral renal involvement at diagnosis. An attempt should be made to stage each side according to the above criteria on the basis of extent of disease before biopsy.

*Staging, which is on the basis of gross and microscopic tumor distribution, is the same for tumors with favorable and with unfavorable histologic features. The patient should be characterized, however, by a statement of both criteria, e.g., stage II, favorable histologic features or stage III, unfavorable histologic features. Tumors of unfavorable type are those with focal or diffuse anaplasia, or those with sarcomatous histology (D'Angio et al., 1989).

Data from D'Angio GJ, Breslow W, Beckwith JB, et al: Treatment of Wilms' tumor: Results of the Third National Wilms' Tumor Study. Cancer 1989; 64:349–360.

6-month course, providing the rationale for using this standard in NWTS-IV.

It was recognized that patients with stage I anaplastic tumors did as well as their counterparts with stage I favorable histology and thus did not require more intensive treatment. The same favorable outlook is associated with tumors showing focal anaplasia (Green et al, 1994). Cyclophosphamide added to dactinomycin, vincristine, and doxorubicin led to a better outlook for children with diffusely anaplastic tumors, but the prognosis is guarded even so (Green et al, 1994). Clear cell sarcoma was recognized to be responsive to doxorubicin, and patients with three-drug therapy responded almost as well at 2 years as those with comparative stages of favorable histology Wilms' tumor. Four-year rates were not as good, however. Rhabdoid sarcoma continued to be an enigma, and no therapeutic regimens were found that improved its dismal outcome. The current survival data for NWTS-III are given in Table 74–6 (D'Angio et al, 1989).

Prognostic Factors

From all the knowledge gained from the first three NWTS, **four important prognostic aspects** of the tumor have emerged. Most important has been ***histology.*** Anaplasia is characterized by the presence of mitotic figures, a threefold enlargement in the nuclei, and a hyperchromatic pattern. Flow cytometry may now enable us to identify these cases more simply (Rainwater et al, 1987). The incidence of anaplasia increases with age (Bonadio et al, 1985). Patients with anaplasia make up approximately 5% of all patients with Wilms' tumor. In this group, the relapse rate is four times higher and the death rate nine times higher than in those in whom anaplasia is absent (Zuppan et al, 1988).

Table 74–6. RESULTS OF THE NATIONAL WILMS' TUMOR STUDY III

Stage	Histology	4-Year Postnephrectomy Survival (%)
I	Favorable	97
II	Favorable	92
III	Favorable	84
IV	Favorable	83
I–III	Unfavorable	68
IV	Unfavorable	55
All patients	Unfavorable	89
Clear cell sarcoma		75
Rhabdoid sarcoma		26

Adapted from D'Angio GJ, et al: Cancer 1989; 64:349–360.

The second unfavorable prognostic determinant is the presence of ***hematogenous metastases,*** whether they involve the lung (most common) or the liver, bone, or brain. Aggressive chemotherapy has dramatically improved the prognosis in this group.

The third prognostic factor is the presence of ***lymph node involvement.*** In NWTS-III, patients with positive involvement of lymph nodes were placed in stage III because it was recognized from NWTS-II that there was an 82% overall survival for those with negative nodes versus a 54% survival for those with positive nodes. This fact emphasizes the importance of careful node sampling to stage Wilms' tumor accurately.

The fourth prognostic area relates to ***tumor extension at the site of the primary tumor*** (Weeks et al, 1987). The presence of an inflammatory pseudocapsule or invasion of the tumor into the capsule or the intrarenal veins was associated with an increased risk of local relapse. The tumor tends to spread into the renal sinus initially, and tumor in this area has also been associated with an increased rate of local relapse. One or more of these features was seen in 100% of relapsed stage I Wilms' tumors with favorable histology.

Careful study of NWTS-II and NWTS-III results revealed a subgroup of patients with relapsed tumors in which the postrelapse survival rate for 3 years exceeded 40%, thus constituting a favorable group (Grundy et al, 1989). The five favorable characteristics in this patient group were as follows: (1) tumors with favorable histology that recurred only in the lung, (2) local relapse in the abdomen when radiation therapy had not been previously given, (3) tumors that were

Malignant neoplasms include soft tissue sarcomas, bone tumors, especially osteosarcomas (Tucker et al, 1987), hepatomas, thyroid carcinomas, and leukemias (Li et al, 1975b). Colon cancer has also been reported (Opitz, 1980). Most of these secondary malignancies have developed in fields of prior radiation therapy.

The cumulative probability of a second cancer in long-term survivors of Wilms' tumor who were treated with radiotherapy has been calculated as 17% over 5 to 25 years, the peak incidence occurring 15 to 19 years after the initial diagnosis (Li et al, 1975b). Mike and colleagues (1982) found a lower incidence of secondary neoplasms (3%) among 20-year survivors of Wilms' tumor, a figure more consistent with recent data compiled by Breslow and associates (1996). Lifelong surveillance is nonetheless important for those cured of Wilms' tumor.

Bilateral Wilms' Tumor

In the NWTS, the incidence of **synchronous bilateral Wilms' tumor** was reported to be approximately 4.2% (Breslow and Beckwith, 1982). Bilateral Wilms' tumors have a number of features distinct from those of unilateral tumors (Table 74–12) (Bond, 1975a; Blute et al, 1987).

Mothers of children with bilateral Wilms' tumor tend to be older, and the children tend to present at a younger age. A positive family history for cancer was found in 42% of patients with a 21% incidence of genitourinary malignancy. Associated anomalies are more frequent in patients with bilateral Wilms' tumor. The incidence of genitourinary anomalies is four times that seen in patients with unilateral Wilms' tumor, and hemihypertrophy is twice as common. The incidence of aniridia and hypertension is similar in patients with unilateral and bilateral Wilms' tumor.

A pathologic examination showed multicentric involvement and nephrogenic rests in 61% of cases. Beckwith and co-workers (1990) believe that this figure may be underreported because samplings from the tumor were restricted in many cases at the initial biopsy. The fact that many of these children have very large tumors and do very well despite that may be related to the fact that these tumors are often compound neoplasms composed of a number of low-stage tumors. Unfavorable histology was seen in 10% (15 patients), an incidence similar to that for unilateral tumors. Of the 15 children, 12 were females, indicating a dominance of anaplasia in girls. Discordant histology between the tumors in opposite kidneys was seen in 6 of the 145 bilateral cases presented by Blute and associates (1987). This figure represented 4% of the series as a whole but 40% of the subset with unfavorable histology. Of the 15, 11 had stage III or IV disease in the more advanced neoplasm, and 10 died during follow-up.

Table 74–12. FEATURES OF UNILATERAL AND BILATERAL WILMS' TUMOR

	Unilateral	Bilateral
Distribution	Unifocal (usual)	Multifocal (nephroblastomatosis)
Patient age (average)	42 mo	15 mo
Mother's age (average)	28 yr	34 yr
Associated anomalies	4%	45%
Inheritance	sporadic	?dominant

Adapted from Bond JV: Lancet 1975; 2:721; and Blute ML, et al: J Urol. 1987; 138:968–973.

Beckwith and colleagues (1990) believe that **bilateral Wilms' tumors exhibit nephrogenic rests in 100% of cases.** In their review, they reported a prevalence of PLNRs in synchronous Wilms' tumors. This figure contrasts with the approximately equal prevalence of the two types of rests in unilateral Wilm's tumor cases. Beckwith postulates that PLNRs are more likely to be seen in both kidneys, accounting for this finding. ILNRs are seen less frequently in bilateral cases. When a metachronous bilateral Wilms' tumor is seen, it is more characteristically associated with an ILNR. Beckwith and his associates attribute this to the fact that ILNRs tend to be multifocal less often; however, when this type of rest is present, it has a probability of eventually developing into a Wilms' tumor. Metachronous bilateral Wilms' tumors were reported in only 0.6% of NWTS patients (Jones, 1982). However, the prognosis for these patients is poor, with only 39% free of disease 2 or more years after developing the second Wilms' tumor.

The overall survival of patients with synchronous bilateral Wilms' tumor is excellent (76% 3-year survival). Bilateral Wilms' tumors clearly respond as well to chemotherapy as unilateral tumors. In the review by Blute and co-workers (1987), several interesting characteristics of this tumor were revealed. Outcome did not appear to be influenced by whether the initial tumor underwent a resection or merely a biopsy. The presence of residual disease did not influence outcome, and, indeed, in only 38% of the patients was all tumor resected at one or more operations. Outcome was not influenced by the presence or absence of nephrectomy nor of salvage radiotherapy. This last finding suggests that residual disease after more intensive initial chemotherapy does not tend to respond to radiation therapy. **Aggressive chemotherapy appears to be the mainstay of therapy in the care of patients with synchronous bilateral Wilms' tumor.**

From analysis of the experience of Blute and associates (1987) and Asch and colleagues (1985), a number of prognostic variables appear to be important. The age at diagnosis is important in children younger than 3 years of age with tumors of favorable histology, who have an 86% survival rate, compared with a 57% survival in those older than 3 years. The majority of young patients presented with stage I disease; older children more commonly presented with advanced stage tumors. Anaplasia was observed infrequently in children younger than 2 years old, also helping to explain this age-related variable. Histology was also pivotal as in unilateral Wilms' tumor. In the NWTS series, 16% of patients with tumors of unfavorable histology survived compared with 84% of those with favorable histology. **The stage of the most advanced lesion and histology thus were the most important prognostic variables.**

Additionally, **positive lymph nodes were important.** If lymph node biopsy showed positive results, survival was only 56% compared with 85% when node biopsies showed negative results. Overall, the survival of more than 75% of NWTS patients with synchronous bilateral Wilms' tumor indicates the favorable prognosis for patients with this tumor. The results in this series are similar to those reported by

Bishop and co-workers (1977) (87%) and Wikstrom and co-workers (1982) (83%).

In surgical management, **the importance of initial exploration of the contralateral kidney when disease appears to be unilateral** is emphasized by the fact that the preoperative diagnosis of bilateral Wilms' tumor in Blute's series (1987) was only 64%. Thus, more than one third of bilateral cases were detected by careful inspection of both surfaces of the contralateral kidney. This failure of diagnostic imaging to detect contralateral disease is supported by the radiologic review of Kirks and associates (1981).

In the past, the traditional initial surgical approach to bilateral Wilms' tumor was to perform a nephrectomy for the larger tumor and a biopsy for the smaller one. This approach has changed because the NWTS (Kelalis, 1985) now recommends a renal-sparing approach. The official NWTS surgical recommendation is for an initial transabdominal transperitoneal staging laparotomy without nephrectomy. Careful tumor biopsy and sampling of the nodes are performed, and an excisional biopsy is carried out only if two thirds of the total renal parenchyma can be spared.

Chemotherapy is undertaken for a period of 6 weeks to a maximum of 6 months following standard Wilms' tumor chemotherapy protocols based on the stage of the more advanced tumor. At second-look surgery, a partial nephrectomy or excisional biopsy is carried out only if all tumor can be removed. If this appears to be impossible, then the recommendation is to close the incision and continue with more chemotherapy with the addition of focal radiotherapy.

A third-look operation is then carried out in less than 6 months. Surgery at this time continues to focus on maximal preservation of the renal parenchyma. In patients with stage II or III tumors with unfavorable histology at initial biopsy, a more aggressive surgical approach is appropriate. Because of the poor prognosis for these patients, renal-preserving approaches are of secondary importance. After the initial biopsy, three-drug chemotherapy and radiation therapy are instituted, followed by a more radical second surgical look. Unfortunately, to date survival in this group has been poor.

Special techniques such as bench surgery have been used in bilateral cases (Altman et al, 1977), and it is important to keep such techniques in mind while making efforts to spare the renal parenchyma. Bilateral nephrectomy and renal transplantation may be required rarely in patients with bilateral tumors but may be more appropriate for those in whom anaplasia is encountered (deLorimier et al, 1971). If transplantation is contemplated, some investigators advocate a waiting period of 2 years to be certain that no metastatic disease is present (Penn, 1979).

Future Considerations

The history of the treatment of Wilms' tumor has been one of the success stories of pediatric oncology, and the future offers hope for further advances. Experience with bilateral Wilms' tumor suggests that, in the future, surgery focused on the preservation of renal parenchyma may become an important consideration even in children with unilateral disease. The goal of NWTS-V is to continue the effort to minimize the morbidity of chemotherapy and radiation therapy for patients with a favorable prognosis. Conversely, patients with poor prognostic characteristics continue to be treated more intensively with new therapeutic regimens in an effort to salvage more of them. Epidemiologic studies are underway to seek possible environmental and genetic causes of Wilms' tumor. The long-term effects of successful therapy on the gonads, lungs, and other treated organs are also being studied with the goal of preventing some of these problems in the future.

Other Renal Tumors of Childhood

Primary renal neoplasms of childhood other than Wilms' tumor are rare; **renal cell carcinoma** is the most common of them. Although it is the most frequent malignant tumor of the kidney in adults, it accounts for less than 7% of all renal tumors in those younger than 21 years. Most children with renal cell carcinoma are 5 years old or older at the time of diagnosis, but cases have been reported of patients in the first year of life (Castellanos et al, 1974). The signs and symptoms are the same as those seen in adults: hematuria, abdominal or flank pain, an abdominal mass, or nonspecific symptoms such as weight loss, anorexia, and fever. IVP reveals calyceal deformation resembling that seen in Wilms' tumor, but calcifications are more common. Metastatic renal cell carcinoma spreads to the regional lymph nodes, bones, lungs, and liver. Renal vascular invasion or the absence of a pseudocapsule around the tumor are ominous anatomic features (Dehner et al, 1970).

Most renal cell carcinomas in children appear sporadically, as in adults, but some families with an increased incidence have been reported. The tumor in one family with 10 involved members appeared to be passed on as an autosomal dominant trait with a characteristic chromosomal translocation (Cohen et al, 1979). An increased incidence of renal cell carcinoma has also been reported in patients with von Hippel-Lindau disease and polycystic kidney disease (Kantor, 1977).

Reviews of renal cell carcinoma in childhood by Raney and co-workers (1983), Castellanos and co-workers (1974), and Dehner and co-workers (1970) reveal an overall survival rate of about 50%. The outlook seems best in children under 11 years of age and in those with stage I lesions. All six children under age 11 and all five with stage I lesions survived in the series reported by Raney and colleagues (1983). Radiation therapy, chemotherapy, and hormonal therapy did little if anything to improve survival over that produced by nephrectomy alone. At present, the most effective **treatment continues to be radical nephrectomy** with regional lymph node dissection.

In 1980 Chatten and associates reported two male infants who had what was termed **ossifying tumor of the infantile kidney.** The infants presented with hematuria and were found to have small calcified renal masses, which appeared to be calculi. On histologic examination, dense cores of bone were found surrounded by a periphery of undifferentiated cells that were firmly adherent to the renal parenchyma. These investigators postulated that these tumors were derived from urothelium rather than from metanephric blastema. They also postulated that the tumors were separate **benign** pediatric renal tumors that were distinct from Wilms' tumors.

Additional very rare primary intrarenal tumors are found in children including the following: **neuroblastoma, rhabdomyosarcoma, leiomyosarcoma, fibroma, hemangiopericytoma, cholesteatoma, lymphangioma, and hamartoma.** The diagnosis of these tumors is rarely made before histologic examination. The renal *angiomyolipoma* is a form of hamartoma usually seen in adults but rarely observed in children (Bennington and Beckwith, 1975). This tumor is very common in patients with tuberous sclerosis and may be bilateral. Diagnostic and therapeutic measures are similar to those used in adults. Although more commonly found in the pararenal retroperitoneal space, *teratomas* may rarely occur as intrarenal tumors.

By far the most common **secondary tumor** seen in the kidney is that produced by non-Hodgkin's **lymphoma or leukemia.** Tumor involvement is generally diffuse. Unlike the other non-Wilms' renal tumors discussed previously, therapy consists of radiation therapy, chemotherapy, or both.

Although rare, both **benign and malignant tumors of the renal pelvis and ureter** have also been reported. Ureteral lesions are most commonly benign fibrous polyps located in the upper third of the ureter. Symptoms usually consist of intermittent pain resulting from obstruction. Treatment consists of local excision with a ureteroureterostomy or ureteral pyelostomy (Colgan et al, 1973). Rarely, a transitional epithelial cancer of the renal pelvis may be seen in infancy or childhood (Koyanagi et al, 1975).

NEUROBLASTOMA

History

Virchow was the first, in 1864, to characterize neuroblastoma, which he labeled glioma. Marchand, in 1891, commented on the histologic similarities between neuroblastoma and developing sympathetic ganglia. Herxheimer (1914), using a specific neural silver stain, showed that fibrils of neuroblastoma shared staining characteristics with nervous tissue. This finding contributed to the establishment of the tissue of origin of this tumor.

The biochemical aspects of neuroblastoma began to be understood as Mason and co-workers, in 1957, reported the presence of pressor amines in the urine of a child with neuroblastoma. Subsequently, elevated levels of norepinephrine, its precursors, and metabolites in the urine of patients with this tumor have been recognized.

Another early landmark in our understanding of neuroblastoma came in 1927 when Cushing and Wolbach reported for the first time a transformation of neuroblastoma into benign ganglioneuroma. Everson and Cole (1966) noted that this event generally occurred in infants under the age of 6 months. That spontaneous regression of neuroblastoma may be more common than is clinically evident was suggested by Beckwith and Perrin (1963), who noted microscopic clusters of neuroblastoma cells in the adrenal glands in a number of infants under 3 months of age who had died of other causes. They called these foci of tumor cells **"neuroblastoma in situ".** They estimated that neuroblastoma in situ occurs about 40 times more often than the number of cases of neuroblastoma that are clinically diagnosed. Under normal circumstances, recession usually appears to be complete after 3 months of age.

Etiology

For many years the actual incidence of neuroblastoma was thought to be higher than that diagnosed, based on the work by Beckwith and Perrin (1963), who detected small tumors in the adrenals of infants dying from other causes (they were studying sudden infant death syndrome). The massive screening effort mounted in the past 10 years, first in Japan and more recently in other countries, has shown that the actual incidence is indeed twice that originally reported (Takeda et al, 1989). The increase is due to detection of infants with low-stage "favorable" tumors, which presumably regressed spontaneously before they became clinically evident.

Although the cause of neuroblastoma, like most other carcinomas, is unknown, it **arises from cells of the neural crest that form the sympathetic ganglia and adrenal medulla**. Bolande (1979) has termed this tumor a type of **"neurocristopathy."** Other neurocristopathies include pheochromocytoma, paraganglioma, medullary carcinoma of the thyroid, carcinoid melanoma, neurocutaneous melanosis, neurofibromatosis, and multiple endocrine neoplasia. Sympathetic nervous system tumors can apparently differentiate along two lines: the pheochromocytoma line and the sympathoblastoma line. The sympathoblastoma line includes the neuroblastoma, ganglioneuroblastoma, and ganglioneuroma forms.

A genetic influence is apparent in this tumor. Knudson and Strong (1972) suggested that approximately 20% of cases arise in children who have a predisposition to the tumor through a dominant transmittable mutation. Knudson and Meadows (1976) suggested that familial cases result from a prezygotic mutation and that nonfamilial ones result from a postzygotic somatic mutation. Rare families have been described in which more than one member is affected with this tumor (Chatten and Voorhees, 1967; Arenson et al, 1976).

Incidence

Neuroblastoma is the **most common malignant tumor of infancy** and, after brain tumors, the most common malignant solid tumor of childhood (Young and Miller, 1975). Neuroblastoma accounts for 6% to 8% of all childhood malignancies. In the United States, the incidence is 9.6 per million in white children and 7.0 per million in black children per year. There is a slight male predominance of 1.1 to 1 (Miller et al, 1968). The actual incidence is much higher than the reported incidence because of the proclivity for spontaneous regression of neuroblastoma in situ.

Although neuroblastoma may occur throughout childhood and occasionally in adulthood, the tumor predominantly develops early in life. Of all cases, 50% occur in children under the age of 2, and more than 75% of cases have been encountered by the fourth year of life (Fortner et al, 1968; Peterson et al, 1969). This is a younger age of presentation than that for Wilms' tumor. Unlike Wilms' tumor, there is a low incidence of associated congenital anomalies. One exception is an increased incidence of brain and skull defects approaching 2% in children with neuroblastoma (Miller et al, 1968). An association with neurofibromatosis and Hirschsprung's disease has been noted (Hope et al, 1965; Knudson and Amromin, 1966).

Pathology

Neuroblastoma

On gross examination, small tumors usually are well encapsulated and firm. The cut surface of the tumor is fairly soft and lobulated with a grayish-to-pink color. The tumor has a tendency to break through its pseudocapsule and infiltrate surrounding tissues. When it does, it is found to be friable and soft with hemorrhage and necrosis. Cystic areas may be present.

Histologically, neuroblastoma is **one of the small round cell tumors of childhood.** Light microscopy shows a similarity between neuroblasts, lymphocytes, and the cells of lymphomas, embryonal myosarcomas, and Ewing's sarcomas. When the tumor cells are seen to form themselves into rosettes and neurofibrils are evident, the degree of differentiation is good, and the tumor is recognizable as a neuroblastoma. Unfortunately, these signs are often absent. Ewing's sarcoma and rhabdomyosarcoma usually contain glycogen, which can be seen by periodic acid—Schiff (PAS) staining.

Marrow is a frequent site of metastasis, and if the cells clump and form **rosettes,** they can be considered diagnostic. If they are more primitive, neuroblastoma-specific monoclonal antibodies can differentiate them from leukemia or other small round cell tumors of childhood (Kleihues et al, 1987).

Neuroblastoma lacks glycogen. Neuroblastoma cells can be recognized by using a rapid fluorescence assay for intracellular catecholamines or a tissue culture assay for neurite outgrowth (Reynolds et al, 1981). Neuron-specific enolase staining of tumor has also been reported to be fairly specific for neuroblastoma (Odelstad et al, 1982). This test is useful for distinguishing neuroblastoma from poorly differentiated Wilms' tumor. The importance of this distinction lies in the different responses to chemotherapy of these neoplasms.

The **ultrastructure of neuroblastoma** is distinctive and reflects the neural crest derivation of neuroblasts. Characteristic peripheral dendritic processes that contain longitudinally oriented microtubules are seen. Small, spherical, membrane-coated granules with electron-dense cores representing cytoplasmic accumulations of catecholamines are seen. The larger number of granules seen in some tumors reflects a higher degree of differentiation and has been reported by Romansky and colleagues (1978) to be a favorable prognostic factor. Conventional microscopy, occasionally supplemented by electron microscopy, usually allows identification and then diagnosis of a bone marrow aspirate as neuroblastoma, avoiding the need for an open biopsy in a child with disseminated disease.

For a number of years efforts have been made to correlate the histologic characteristics of neuroblastoma with the biologic behavior of this tumor. A grading system devised by Shimada and associates (1984) analyzes the number of mitotic cells per high-power field, the tumor stroma, the distribution of immature cells, and the age of the patient to identify patients with a favorable versus an unfavorable prognosis. This histologic grading system is now recognized as a pivotal factor in selecting patients for a more or less intensive therapeutic approach (Silber et al, 1991).

Ganglioneuroma

At the other end of the spectrum of neuroblastoma lies the **benign** counterpart—the ganglioneuroma. By definition, these tumors do not metastasize, but they can recur following resection. They can become rather large and have projections that envelop adjacent structures and occasionally extend through the intervertebral foramina, producing neurologic symptoms by way of cord compression. On cut surface they tend to be more firm and better encapsulated than neuroblastoma. Histologically, they are composed of large, mature ganglion cells with abundant cytoplasm and a large nucleus. They are scattered throughout a collagen-rich background with bundles of neurofibrils.

Ganglioneuroblastoma

This tumor is **intermediate** between neuroblastoma and ganglioneuroma. Histologically, there are grades of ganglioneuroblastoma that cover the full spectrum from benign ganglioneuroma to malignant neuroblastoma. The **outcome is varied.**

Location, Presentation, and Differential Diagnosis

Because neuroblastomas and their more benign variants may occur **anywhere along the sympathetic chain** from the head to the pelvis, their presentation and differential diagnosis vary with the site of tumor origin (Fig. 74–9). More than half of neuroblastomas originate in the **abdomen,** and two thirds of these arise in the *adrenal gland.* When a tumor originates in the **adrenal gland,** there is less likelihood of metastasis than there is from nonadrenal abdominal paravertebral sites. A mass is the most common presenting symptom. This is characteristically an irregular, firm, nontender, fixed mass that often extends beyond the midline. In comparison, Wilms' tumor usually occurs with a smooth flank mass that does not cross the midline.

Neuroblastomas have been separated as retroperitoneal, adrenal, and celiac. It has been found that retroperitoneal and adrenal tumors did as well as those at all other sites. Tumors in the region of the **celiac axis do very poorly.** Abdominal tumors do less well than those in other sites, but this negative effect arises solely from celiac axis tumors.

Neuroblastoma that arises from an **abdominal paravertebral sympathetic ganglion** has a greater likelihood of growing through an intervertebral foramen to form a dumbbell-shaped tumor that compresses the spinal cord (Traggis et al, 1977; Akwari et al, 1978). In about 40% of these cases, the intraspinal component is asymptomatic. **Paravertebral tumors always warrant evaluation for possible intraspinal extension.** There is no uniform agreement on the best

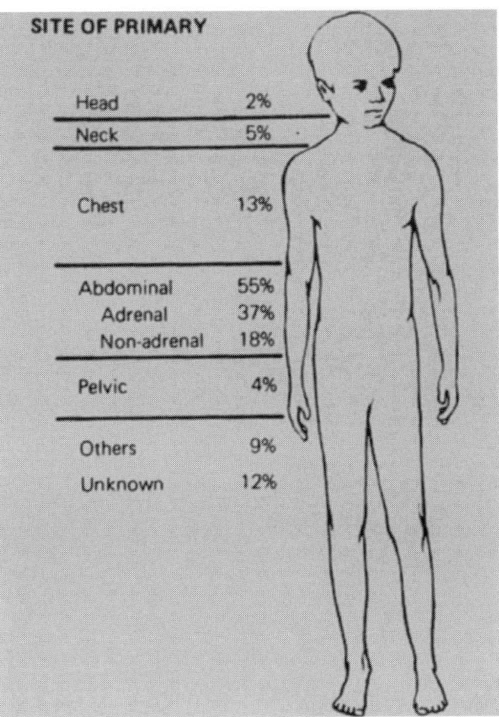

Figure 74–9. Neuroblastoma: Site of primary tumor. Composite data from the literature. (From Williams TE, Donaldson MH: Neuroblastoma. *In* Sutow WW, Vietti TJ, Fernback DJ, eds: Clinical Pediatric Oncology. St. Louis, C. V. Mosby Co., 1973, p 388.)

treatment for intraspinal extensions that cause cord signs. Low-dose irradiation is usually effective, although concern has been expressed that initial swelling may cause a transient increase in paralysis. Chemotherapy avoids the surgical complications, but the effect is not always sufficiently rapid. Surgical decompression is the most rapidly effective measure, but unless the spine is reconstructed (a procedure some neurosurgeons are not willing to do as part of the primary surgery), scoliosis frequently results. If the paralysis is only partial, chemotherapy should be tried first. The most striking aspect of this complication is the regenerative powers of the infant nervous system. Children with complete paralysis of some days or weeks' duration may have an excellent recovery with few sequelae. The exception to this rule is the neonate who is born paralyzed and may have been paralyzed for many weeks in utero. Early intervention may be warranted because patients with these dumbbell-shaped neuroblastomas generally have an excellent prognosis. These tumors may be more mature or even completely benign within the spinal canal and less mature in the abdominal extension. They must be differentiated from primary intraspinal tumors.

Neuroblastoma may also arise in the **presacral** region, presumably from the organ impar or along the aorta from the organs of Zuckerkandl. In the pelvis, the tumor may lead to urinary frequency or retention due to extrinsic pressure on the bladder (Hepler, 1976). Constipation may also result. These tumors are rare, constituting only 4% of neuroblastomas. The differential diagnosis of abdominal and pelvic neuroblastomas includes other abdominal and retroperitoneal tumors, such as Wilms' tumors, teratomas, and rarer primary neoplasms in the pancreas or liver.

One of the rarest primary sites for a neuroblastoma is the **olfactory bulb (esthesioneuroblastoma).** This tumor usually presents with unilateral nasal obstruction and epistaxis. It tends to occur later in life than the typical neuroblastoma arising in other sites (Homzie and Elkin, 1980) and is now considered a peripheral neuroectodermal tumor rather than a true neuroblastoma.

Neuroblastomas originating in the **cervical sympathetic ganglion** account for approximately 5% of these tumors. Horner's syndrome may result with inward sinking of the eyeball, ptosis of the upper eyelid, elevation of the lower eyelid, pupillary constriction, narrowing of the palpebral fissure, and anhidrosis. Because the sympathetic nervous system is involved in the development of pigmentation in the iris, neuroblastoma affecting the ophthalmic sympathetic nerves can lead to heterochromia iridis, an unequal color between the two irises. Both syndromes may occur together (Jaffe et al, 1975). Hoarseness may indicate compression of the recurrent laryngeal nerve by tumor. Cervical neuroblastoma may appear as a neck mass and must be differentiated from branchial cleft cysts, benign adenopathy, lymphoma, and leukemia, and other malignant tumors found in the neck.

Thoracic neuroblastoma, accounting for 13% of tumors, may become massive before becoming clinically evident. More often, these lesions are discovered by radiographs taken for the diagnosis of an unrelated disease. The patient may have cough, dyspnea, or pulmonary infection resulting from tracheal or bronchial compression. The superior vena cava may be compressed. Weakness of an upper extremity may indicate brachial plexus involvement. Pain in the neck, back, abdomen, or pelvis may be caused by a dumbbell extension of the tumor producing spinal cord compression. In the posterior mediastinum, neuroblastoma must be differentiated from teratomas, esophageal duplications, and bronchogenic cysts.

In its early stages, neuroblastoma is usually a silent tumor. **Metastatic dissemination** of the tumor may occur early and does not appear to be related to the size of the primary tumor. **Up to 70% of patients have metastatic disease at the time of diagnosis** (Gross et al, 1959). In the young, metastases tend to go to the liver; in older children, bony metastases are more common. Unexplained fever, general malaise, anorexia, weight loss, irritability, bone pain, and pallor secondary to anemia are all common manifestations of widespread disease. Occasionally, such symptoms may be noted without evidence of dissemination. The high incidence of disseminated disease in patients with neuroblastoma accounts for the more frequent presentation of a child who is generally unwell in contrast to that of a child with Wilms' tumor, who usually seems well and robust.

The **liver** suffers the brunt of metastatic dissemination, especially in the infant (Fig. 74–10*A*). The tumor may appear as a rapidly growing hepatic neoplasm, which may embarrass respiration (Bond, 1976). Primary hepatoblastoma must be differentiated.

Often, the first symptoms of neuroblastoma reflect *bony* involvement. The skull and long bones are most commonly involved. Metastatic disease usually occurs in the diaphysis and may be bilaterally symmetric. On radiographs, metastases appear as lytic defects with an irregular margin and some periosteal reaction. Symptoms may include local bone pain or a limp. Metastatic bone lesions must be differentiated

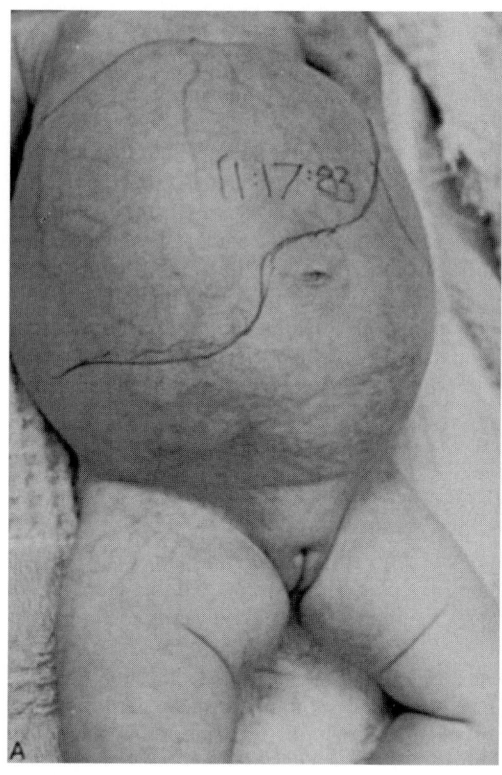

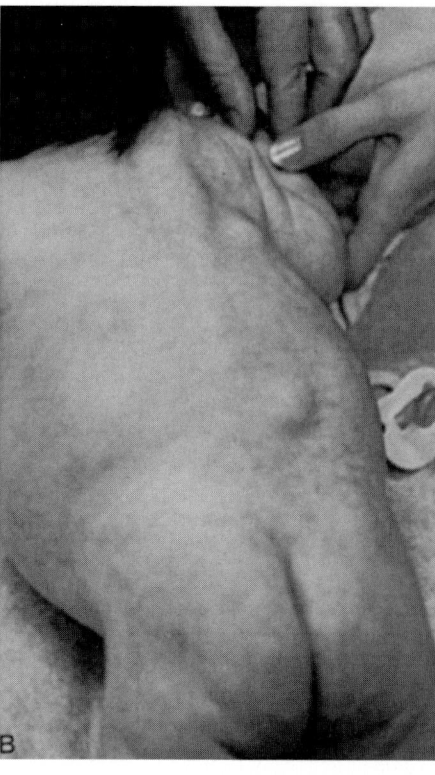

Figure 74–10. Neuroblastoma: Stage IV-S. *A*, Liver metastases causing abdominal distention. *B*, Skin metastases on back.

from primary bone tumors, lymphorecticular malignancies, or infectious processes.

More than 50% of children with neuroblastoma have **bone marrow** involvement, even in the absence of radiographic evidence of change in the bone (Finklestein et al, 1970). Bone marrow replacement with depletion of one or more cell lines in the peripheral blood may lead to an incorrect diagnosis of aplastic anemia or other diseases that may cause thrombocytopenia or anemia (Quinn and Altman, 1979). Neuroblastoma cells in the bone marrow can usually be distinguished from leukemic infiltration because neuroblastoma cells appear in small clusters and may have rosette shapes and neurofibrils. Electron microscopy, as mentioned earlier, may occasionally be useful in distinguishing neuroblastoma from other malignancies that invade the bone marrow. The recognition of neuroblastoma may also be assisted by appropriate monoclonal antibodies and fluorescence microscopy (Kemshed and Coakham, 1983; Cheung et al, 1985; Horne et al, 1985).

Subcutaneous nodules (Fig. 74–10*B*) are also a common metastatic pattern for neuroblastoma in infants. A not uncommon presentation in infants is hepatomegaly, sometimes accompanied by skin nodules and occasional tumor cells in the bone marrow. When these patients have small primary tumors and do not have bone lesions, they fit the classification of IV-S disease with a strong likelihood of spontaneous regression (see later). The skin nodules often have a bluish color, and the babies have been termed "blueberry muffin" babies. Such subcutaneous nodules have been reported in up to one third of neonates with neuroblastoma (Schneider et al, 1965). These skin lesions may become erythematous for several minutes after palpation and then blanch, presumably as a result of vasoconstriction attributable to catecholamine release from the tumor cells. When present, this reaction may be a diagnostic sign of neuroblastoma (Hawthorne et al, 1970). These nodules must be differentiated from leukemic infiltrates of the skin.

Periorbital metastatic disease is also common in children with neuroblastoma (Fig. 74–11). Retrobulbar soft tissue involvement may cause periorbital edema and proptosis. Periorbital ecchymoses may produce a "raccoon-like" appearance. Ecchymosis typically occurs in the upper eyelid,

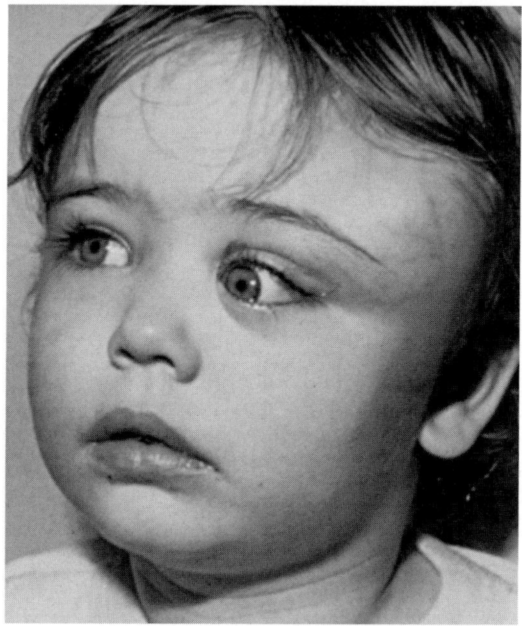

Figure 74–11. Neuroblastoma. Retrobulbar metastases producing proptosis.

whereas ecchymosis of the lower eyelid more commonly occurs with trauma.

Some organs are rarely the site of metastases; these include the heart, lungs, brain, and spinal cord. Pulmonary metastases are occasionally seen in children with very advanced disease secondary to extensive lymphatic spread or direct growth through the diaphragm.

Occasionally, symptoms are produced by the biochemical activity of the tumor. As neural crest tumors, neuroblastomas usually **secrete catecholamines**. Occasional children are seen with paroxysmal attacks of sweating, pallor, headaches, hypertension, palpitations, and flushing. Voute and co-workers (1970) reported six mothers who had these symptoms in the eighth and ninth months of pregnancy and subsequently delivered infants in whom neuroblastoma was diagnosed during the first few months of life. The mothers' symptoms presumably were caused by fetal catecholamines entering the maternal circulation. When symptoms of catecholamine release are prominent, neuroblastoma may simulate pheochromocytoma.

Children have also presented with intractable watery diarrhea and hypokalemia. This presentation is due to tumor secretion of an enterohormone known as **vasoactive intestinal peptide (VIP)** (Mitchell et al, 1976; El Shafie et al, 1983). A variety of other tumors besides neuroblastoma, including pancreatic tumors and bronchiogenic carcinoma, have been shown to secrete VIP. Pearse (1978) suggested that these tumors share a common ancestor cell in the neural crest. The tumors have similar cytochemical characteristics, the most important of which is the ability to absorb amines from the environment and convert them into hormones or hormone-like products. This ability is referred to as amine precursor uptake and decarboxylation (APUD), and these tumors are thus termed APUDomas.

One of the most interesting systemic manifestations of neuroblastoma is **acute myoclonic encephalopathy.** This condition is seen in approximately 2% of children with neuroblastoma. The syndrome consists of rapid multidirectional eye movements (opsoclonus), myoclonus, and truncal ataxia in the absence of increased intracranial pressure (Senelick et al, 1973). Although it was initially thought that the encephalopathy was caused by a toxic neurologic effect of circulating catecholamine catabolites, at least one child has been reported who developed this neurologic symptom 7 months after a primary tumor was removed and previously elevated levels of urinary catecholamines had returned to normal (Delalieux et al, 1975). An alternative explanation may be the existence of an autoimmune factor, perhaps an antibody directed against a neuroblastoma antigen, which is cross-reacting with a common antigen in the cells of the cerebellum, resulting in damage (Bray et al, 1969). Tumors associated with this syndrome are often well differentiated and located in the thorax, and are associated with a good prognosis (Altman and Baehner, 1976).

On rare occasions, a neonate presents with a syndrome that may mimic **erythroblastosis.** Massive metastasis to the liver and bone marrow may produce jaundice, anemia, and hepatosplenomegaly. This syndrome may mimic hemolytic disease in the newborn. Two cases of congenital neuroblastoma were reported by Anders and colleagues (1973); these patients had congenital neuroblastoma that was metastatic to the liver and placenta, and they were thought to have hydrops fetalis.

From these descriptions of the multiple possible sites and presentations for neuroblastoma, it should be evident why this **tumor has been referred to as the "great mimicker."** A prepared mind is required to make a proper diagnosis in many of these enigmatic cases (Jaffe, 1976).

Diagnostic Evaluation

The work-up of a patient with neuroblastoma depends in part on the presenting symptoms and signs. The tumor tends to fall into **two categories, "favorable" and "unfavorable," the first arising in infants and remaining localized, and the second appearing in older children with metastasis.** A good history and physical examination will go a long way toward suggesting which type of neuroblastoma is present. A healthy looking infant with an asymptomatic mass is likely to have a localized favorable tumor, whereas an anemic, febrile, anorectic child who complains of aches and pains probably has metastatic disease. The early suspicions help to direct the flow of the work-up.

Hematologic Studies

The complete blood count (CBC) is usually normal in a child with neuroblastoma until the disease becomes disseminated. With dissemination, anemia may be present because of bone marrow involvement by tumor or hemorrhage into the tumor. Rarely, thrombocytopenia may be present because of bone marrow involvement or platelet trapping in the tumor. Liver involvement may cause a bleeding diathesis through disseminated intravascular coagulopathy. The erythrocyte sedimentation rate is usually elevated in the child with systemic disease.

Bone marrow aspiration is indicated in all cases of neuroblastoma, and usually bilateral iliac crest procedures are performed. The timing depends on the suspected outcome. In patients with "favorable" disease who are proceeding to primary surgery, it can be postponed until the patient is under general anesthesia. In "unfavorable" cases it should be done early, if possible, and may obviate the need for a tissue biopsy. These cells form clusters and occasionally pseudorosettes with pink neurofibrillary processes that mark the "core" of the rosette. Rarely, cells are so undifferentiated that it is not possible to distinguish them from other small round cell tumors of childhood or acute leukemia. At such times, neuron-specific enolase (Odelstad et al, 1982) or neuroblastoma-specific monoclonal antibodies (Kleihues et al, 1987) can be employed to differentiate one from another. It is important to obtain adequate samples of positive bone marrow aspirates because this is likely to be the only tissue available for the cytogenetic studies such as the *N-myc* amplification factors used in determining the prognosis.

As many as 70% of bone marrow aspirates in patients with neuroblastoma have been reported to be positive (Finklestein et al, 1970). Although it is not unusual to find tumor cells in the bone marrow aspirate that show no evidence of skeletal metastases, occasionally a patient may demonstrate widespread bony metastases with no cells in the marrow. As discussed previously, neuroblastoma frequently forms pseudorosettes in the bone marrow. This feature helps to distinguish neuroblastoma in the marrow from leukemia and metastatic carcinomas, such as lymphosarcoma, retinoblastoma, Ewing's sarcoma, and other small round cell tumors that have a proclivity to metastasize to bone. In the child with disseminated disease, careful evaluation of the bone marrow may obviate the need for an open biopsy of the tumor.

Catecholamine Excretion

Since the first report of urinary catecholamine excretion in neuroblastoma was made by Mason and associates in 1957, much attention has been paid to the biochemical products of this tumor. The two major metabolites of catecholamine production by neuroblastoma are vanillylmandelic acid (VMA) and homovanillic acid (HVA). Williams and Greer (1963) reported that 95% of patients with neuroblastoma have elevated levels of urinary VMA, HVA, or both. Occasional patients are seen with no elevation of catecholamine excretion (Voorhees, 1971). These tumors are most commonly found in the thorax and probably arise from the dorsal spinal nerve roots and ganglia, which are nonsecretors of catecholamines. No correlation has been found between the pattern of catecholamine excretion and the age of the patient, symptomatology, or histologic pattern.

Because hypertension is not common in patients with neuroblastoma, it is interesting to speculate on why elevated catecholamine production does not lead to clinical symptoms in most cases. It may be that norepinephrine is catabolized within the tumor and thus does not become systemically active (LaBrosse and Karon, 1962). Also, it is possible that the initial enzyme in catecholamine synthesis, tyrosine hydrolase, is subject to normal feedback inhibition by norephinephrine, dopamine, and dopa (Imashuku et al, 1971). These factors may help to explain why high levels of serum norepinephrine and hypertension are uncommon with neuroblastoma; in comparison, in patients with pheochromocytoma, excessive amounts of tyrosine hydrolase are present because feedback inhibition is absent.

Although quantitative determination of all catecholamines and their metabolites in a 24-hour urine specimen is clearly the most accurate method of obtaining a biochemical diagnosis of neuroblastoma, the collection of 24-hour urine specimens in infants and small children is difficult. This problem led Gitlow and co-workers (1970) to propose performing a simultaneous assay of VMA, HVA, and creatinine in a single spot urine specimen. The upper limits of normal have been found to be 20 μg/mg of creatinine for VMA and 40 μg/mg of creatinine for HVA. Although this test provides an accurate diagnostic approach, it is rather cumbersome.

In 1968, LaBrosse developed a **filter paper spot test for VMA in the urine.** This test has approximately a 75% accuracy when used in the diagnosis and follow-up of patients with neuroblastoma (Evans et al, 1971a). It is, however, generally agreed that VMA screening tests, although useful, lack total reliability and that confirmation by specific quantitative assays is important (Johnsonbaugh and Cahill, 1975).

Elevation of cystathionine and carcinoembryonic antigen levels has also been reported in patients with neuroblastomas. The lack of specificity of these products for neuroblastoma, however, has limited the clinical usefulness of urinary assays.

Imaging

Appropriate roentgenographic and nuclear medicine diagnostic studies can localize the site of primary disease and define the presence and extent of metastatic spread. Plain films of the chest and abdomen can be done on admission and frequently offer valuable information. Chest films, including oblique views, can be examined for posterior mediastinal or supraclavicular masses, extension into the posterior mediastinum from an abdominal mass, and pulmonary metastases (more consistent with a Wilms' tumor), and the bony skeleton can be scrutinized for the presence of metastases. Examination of the ribs may show splaying and thinning of a rib adjacent to a tumor, suggesting long-standing pressure, and examination of the spine may show enlargement of the intraspinal foramina, suggesting extradural extension. Abdominal films may show a mass with "stippled" calcification, organs displaced by the mass, or hepatomegaly, and again the bones can be examined for evidence of metastatic spread. As the initial work-up proceeds and the radiographs identify the tumor origin, more definitive studies can be ordered, usually **CT scans.** Such scans are likely to show the mass, its consistency and extent, the presence of enlarged lymph nodes, and the placement of major vessels. Tumors arising in the adrenal area frequently cause displacement or dysfunction of the kidney (Figs. 74–12 and 74–13) and can be distinguished from a Wilms' tumor, which tends to cause more distortion of the kidney. Very rarely, intrarenal neuro-

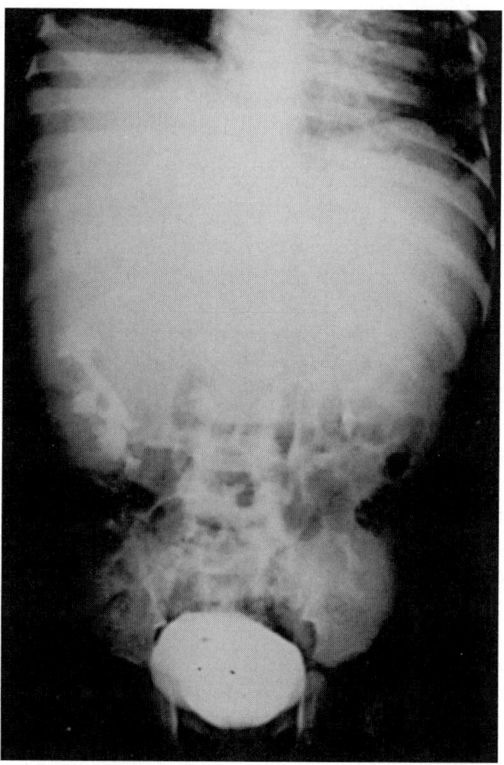

Figure 74–12. Neuroblastoma: Intravenous pyelogram showing inferior and lateral displacement of right kidney by adrenal neuroblastoma.

MacKenzie AR, Whitmore WF, Melamed MR: Myosarcomas of the bladder and prostate. Cancer 1968; 22:833.

Mahour GH, Soule EH, Mills SD, Lynn HB: Rhabdomyosarcoma in infants and children: A clinicopathologic study of 75 cases. J Pediatr Surg 1967; 2:402.

Mann JR, Pearson D, Barrett A: Results of the United Kingdom Children's Cancer Study Groups' malignant germ cell tumor studies. Cancer 1989; 63:1657.

Maurer HM: The Intergroup Rhabdomyosarcoma Study II: Objectives and study design. J Pediatr Surg 1980; 15:371.

Maurer HM, Donaldson M, Gehan EA, et al: The Intergroup Rhabdomyosarcoma Study: Update, November 1978. NCI Monogr 1981; 56:61.

Maurer HM, Moon T, Donaldson M, et al: The Intergroup Rhabdomyosarcoma Study: A preliminary report. Cancer 1977; 40:2015.

McKeen EA, Bodurtha J, Meadows AT, et al: Rhabdomyosarcoma complicating multiple neurofibromatosis. J Pediatr 1978; 93:992.

Mierau GW, Favara BE: Rhabdomyosarcoma in children: Ultrastructural study of 31 cases. Cancer 1980; 46:2035.

Norris HJ, Bagley GP, Taylor HB: Carcinoma of the infant vagina: A distinctive tumor. Arch Pathol 1970; 90:473.

Ortega JA: A therapeutic approach to childhood pelvic rhabdomyosarcoma without pelvic exenteration. J Pediatr 1979; 94:205.

Patton RB, Horn RC Jr: Rhabdomyosarcoma: Clinical and pathological features and comparison with human fetal and embryonal skeletal muscle. Surgery 1962; 52:572.

Pinkel D, Pickren J: Rhabdomyosarcoma in children. JAMA 1961; 175:293.

Pollack RS, Taylor HC: Carcinoma of the cervix during the first two decades of life. Am J Obstet Gynecol 1979; 53:135.

Ramani P, Yeung CK, Habeebu SS: Testicular intratubular germ cell neoplasia in children and adolescents with intersex. Am J Surg Pathol 1993; 17:1124.

Raney B Jr, Carey A, Snyder HM, et al: Primary site as a prognostic variable for children with pelvic soft tissue sarcomas. J Urol 1986; 136:874–878.

Raney RB Jr, Donaldson MH, Sutow WW, et al: Special considerations related to primary site in rhabdomyosarcoma: Experience of the Intergroup Rhabdomyosarcoma Study, 1972–1976. NCI Monogr 1981; 56:69–74.

Raney RB Jr, Gehan EA, Hays DM, et al: Primary chemotherapy with or without radiation therapy and/or surgery for children with localized sarcoma of the bladder, prostate, vagina, uterus and cervix. Cancer 1990; 66:2072–2081.

Ray B, Grabstald H, Exelby PR, Whitmore WW Jr: Bladder tumors in children. Urology 1973; 11:426.

Rivard G, Ortega J, Hittle R, et al: Intensive chemotherapy as primary treatment for rhabdomyosarcoma of the pelvis. Cancer 1975; 36:1593.

Rodary C, Flamant F, Maurer H, et al: Initial lymphadenectomy is not necessary in localized and completely resected paratesticular rhabdomyosarcoma. Med Pediatr Oncol (Abstract) 1992; 20:430.

Ruymann FB, Gaiger AM, Newton W: Congenital anomalies in rhabdomyosarcoma. *In* Programs and Abstracts of the Conference on Congenital Birth Defects, Memphis, June 9–11, 1977.

Ruymann RB, Maddux HR, Ragab A, et al: Congenital Anomalies Associated with Rhabdomyosarcoma: An Autopsy Study of 115 Cases. A report from the Intergroup Rhabdomyosarcoma Study Committee (representing the Children's Cancer Study Group, the Pediatric Oncology Group, the United Kingdom Children's Cancer Study Group, and the Pediatric Intergroup Statistical Center). Med Pediatr Oncol 1988; 16:33.

Sagerman RH, Tretter P, Ellsworth RM: The treatment of orbital rhabdomyosarcoma of children with primary radiation therapy. Am J Roentgenol 1972; 114:31.

Schoenberg HS, Murphy JJ: Neurofibroma of the bladder. J Urol 1961; 85:899.

Sheng V, Soukup S, Ballard E, et al: Chromosomal analysis of sixteen human rhabdomyosarcomas. Cancer Res 1988; 48:983–987.

Stevens MJ, Norman AR, Dearnaley DP: Prognostic significance of early serum tumor marker half-life in metastatic testicular teratoma. J Clin Oncol 1995; 13:87.

Stobbe GC, Dargeon HW: Embryonal rhabdomyosarcoma of the head and neck in children and adolescents. Cancer 1950; 3:826.

Sutow WW, Sullivan MP, Ried HL, et al: Prognosis in childhood rhabdomyosarcoma. Cancer 1970; 25:1384.

Tefft M: Radiation of rhabdomyosarcoma in children: Local control in patients enrolled into the Intergroup Rhabdomyosarcoma Study. NCI Monogr 1981; 56:75.

Uehling DT, Phillips E: Residual retroperitoneal mass following chemotherapy for infantile yolk sac tumor. J Urol 1994; 152:185.

Ulfelder H: The stilbestrol-adenosis-carcinoma syndrome. Cancer 1976; 38:426.

Visfeldt J, Jorgensen N, Müller J: Testicular germ cell tumours of childhood in Denmark, 1943–1989: Incidence and evaluation of histology using immunohistochemical techniques. J Pathol 1994; 174:39.

Voute PA, Vos A: Combination chemotherapy as primary treatment of children with rhabdomyosarcoma to avoid mutilating surgery or radiotherapy Procceedings of the American Association for Cancer Research 1977; 18:327.

Voute PA, Vos A, deKraker J: Chemotherapy at initial treatment in rhabdomyosarcoma (Abstract C-341). Proc Am Soc Clin Oncol 1984; 3:87.

Weiner ES, Lawrence S, Hays D, et al: Retroperitoneal node biopsy in childhood paratesticular rhabdomyosarcoma. J Pediatr Surg 1994; 29:171.

Wilbur JR: Combination chemotherapy of embryonal rhabdomyosarcoma. Cancer Chemother Rep 1974; 58:281.

Yeung CK, Ward HS, Ransley PG: Bladder and kidney function after cure of pelvic rhabdomyosarcoma in childhood. Br J Cancer 1994; 70:1000.

Young JL, Miller RW: Incidence of malignant tumors in U.S. children. J Pediatr 1975; 86:254.

Testicular Tumors

Banowsky LH, Shultz GN: Sarcoma of the spermatic cord and tunics: Review of the literature, case report and discussion of the role of retroperitoneal lymph node dissection. J Urol 1970; 103:628.

Batata MS, Whitmore WF Jr, Chu FCH, et al: Cryptorchidism and testicular cancer. J Urol 1980; 124:382.

Bracken RB, Johnson DE: Sexual function and fecundity after treatment for testicular tumors. Urology 1976; 7:35.

Brosman SA: Testicular tumors in prepubertal children. Urology 1979; 18:581.

Brown NJ: Teratomas and yolk-sac tumors. J Clin Pathol 1976; 29:1021.

Byrd RL: Testicular leukemia: Incidence and management results. Med Pediatr Oncol 1981; 9:493–500.

Campbell HE: Incidence of malignant growth of the undescended testicle: A critical and statistical study. Arch Surg 1942; 44:353.

Campbell HE: The incidence of malignant growth of the undescended testicle: A reply and re-evaluation. J Urol 1959; 81:663.

Carney JA, Kelalis PP, Lynn HB: Bilateral teratoma of testis in an infant. J Pediatr Surg 1973; 8:49.

Colodny A, Hopkins TB: Testicular tumors in infants and children. Urol Clin North Am 1977; 4:347.

DeCamargo B, Pinus J, Lederman H, Saba L: Intrascrotal metastasis from Wilms' tumor. Med Pediatr Oncol 1988; 16:381–383.

Drago JR, Nelson RP, Palmer JM: Childhood embryonal carcinoma of testes. Urology 1978; 12:499.

Einhorn LH, Donohue JP: Combination chemotherapy in disseminated testicular cancer: The Indiana University experience. Semin Oncol 1979; 6:87.

Exelby PR: Testis cancer in children. Semin Oncol 1979; 6:116.

Fonkalsrud EW: Current concepts in the management of the undescended testis. Surg Clin North Am 1970; 50:847.

Gallager HS: Pathology of testicular and paratesticular neoplasms. *In* Johnson DE, ed. Testicular Tumors, 2nd ed. Flushing, NY, Medical Examination Publishing, 1976.

Giguere JK, Stablein DM, Spaulding JT, et al: The clinical significance of unconventional orchiectomy approaches in testicular cancer: A report from the Testicular Cancer Intergroup Study. J Urol 1988; 139:1225.

Grabstald H: Germinal tumors of the testis. CA Cancer J Clin 1975; 25:82.

Griffin GC, Raney RB, Tefft M, et al: Soft tissue sarcomas arising in the retroperitoneal space in children: A report from the Intergroup Rhabdomyosarcoma Study (IRS) Committee. Cancer 1985; 56:2125–2132.

Hinman F Jr: Unilateral abdominal cryptorchidism. J Urol 1979; 122:71.

Hopkins GB, Jaffe N, Colodny A, et al: The management of testicular tumors in children. J Urol 1978; 120:96.

Houser R, Izant RJ, Persky L: Testicular tumors in children. Am J Surg 1965; 110:876.

Hu LM, Phillipson J, Barsky SH: Intratubular germ cell neoplasia in infantile yolk sac tumor. Verification by tandem repeat sequence in situ hybridization. Diagnostic Molecular Pathology 1992; 1(2):118.

Ilondo MM, Van der Mooter F, Marchal G, et al: A boy with Leydig cell tumor and precocious puberty: Ultrasonography as a diagnostic aid. Eur J Pediatr 1981; 137:221.

Ise T, Ohtsuki H, Matsumoto K, Sano R: Management of malignant testicular tumors in children. Cancer 1976; 37:1539.

Jeffs RD: Management of embryonal adenocarcinoma of the testis in childhood: An analysis of 164 cases. *In* Gooden JA, ed: Cancer in Childhood. Toronto, The Ontario Cancer Treatment and Research Foundation, 1972.

Johnstone G: Prepubertal gynecomastia in association with an interstitial cell tumor of the testis. Br J Urol 1967; 39:211.

Karamehmedovic O, Woodtli W, Pluss HJ: Testicular tumors in childhood. J Pediatr Surg 1975; 10:109.

Kramer SA: Embryonal cell carcinoma in children. Pediatr Urol Letter Club, October 21, 1981.

Kurman RJ, Scardino PT, McIntire KR, et al: Cellular localization of alpha-feto-protein and human chorionic gonadotrophin in germ cell tumors of the testis using an indirect immunoperoxidase technique: A new approach to classification utilizing tumor markers. Cancer 1977; 40:2136.

Lamm DL, Kaplan GW: Urological manifestation of Burkitt's lymphoma. J Urol 1974; 112:402.

Leopold GR, Woo VL, Scheible FW, et al: High-resolution ultrasonography of scrotal pathology. Radiology 1979; 131:719.

Li FP, Fraumeni JF Jr: Testicular cancers in children: Epidemiologic characteristics. J Natl Cancer Inst 1972; 48:1575.

Manger D: Pathology of tumors of the testis in children. *In* Gooden JO, ed: Cancer in Childhood. New York, Plenum Press, 1973, p 60.

Manuel M, Katayama KP, Jones HW Jr: The age of occurrence of gonadal tumors in intersex patients with a Y chromosome. Am J Obstet Gynecol 1976; 124:293.

Martin DC: Germinal cell tumors of the testis after orchiopexy. J Urol 1979; 121:422.

Mostofi FK, Price EB: Tumors of the male genital system. Armed Forces Institute of Pathology, Fascicle 8, 2nd series. Washington, D.C., Armed Forces Institute of Pathology, 1973, p 99.

Mulvihill JJ, Wade WM, Miller RM: Gonadoblastoma in dysgenetic gonads with a Y chromosome. Lancet 1975; 1:863.

Oakhill A, Mainwaring D, Hill FGH, et al: Management of leukemic infiltration of the testis. Arch Dis Child 1980; 55:564.

Olive D, Flamant F, Zucker JM, et al: Para-aortic lymphadenectomy is not necessary in the treatment of localized paratesticular rhabdomyosarcoma. Cancer 1984; 54:1283–1287.

Olive-Sommelet D: Paratesticular rhabdomyosarcoma. Dialog Pediatr Urol 1989; 12(11):1–8.

Olney LE, Narayana A, Leoning S, Culp DA: Intrascrotal rhabdomyosarcoma. Urology 1979; 14:113.

Pierce GB, Bullock WK, Huntington RW Jr: Yolk-sac tumors of the testis. Cancer 1970; 25:644.

Pomer FA, Stiles RE, Graham JH: Interstitial cell tumors of the testis in children: Report of a case and review of the literature. N Engl J Med 1954; 250:233.

Price EB: Epidermoid cysts of the testis: A clinical and pathologic analysis of 69 cases from the testicular tumor registry. Urology 1969; 102:708.

Raney RB Jr, Hays DM, Lawrence W Jr, et al: Paratesticular rhabdomyosarcoma in childhood. Cancer 1978; 42:729.

Raney RB Jr, Tefft M, Lawrence W Jr, et al: Paratesticular sarcoma in childhood and adolescence: A report from the Intergroup Rhabdomyosarcoma Studies I and II, 1973–1983. Cancer 1987; 60:2337–2343.

Rosvoll RV, Woodard JR: Malignant Sertoli cell tumor of the testis. Cancer 1968; 22:8.

Scully RE: Gonadoblastoma: A review of 74 cases. Cancer 1970; 25:1340.

Staubitz WJ, Jewett TC Jr, Magoss IV, et al: Management of testicular tumors in children. J Urol 1965; 94:683.

Tefft M, Lattin PB, Jereb B, et al: Acute and late effects on normal tissues following combined chemo- and radiotherapy for childhood rhabdomyosarcoma and Ewing's sarcoma. Cancer 1976; 37:1201.

Teilum G: Endodermal sinus tumors of ovary and testis: Comparative morphogenesis of the so-called mesonephroma ovarii (Schiller) and extra-embryonic (yolk sac-allantoic) structures of the rat's placenta. Cancer 1959; 23:1092.

Urban MD, Lee PA, Plotnick LP, Migeon CJ: The diagnosis of Leydig cell tumors in childhood. Am J Dis Child 1978; 132:494.

Viprakasit D, Navarro G, Guarin UK, Garnes H: Seminoma in children. Urology 1977; 9:568.

Weissbach L, Altwein JE, Stiens R: Germinal testicular tumors in childhood. Eur Urol 1984; 10:73.

Wong KY, Ballard ET, Strayer FH, et al: Clinical and occult testicular leukemia in long-term survivors of acute lymphoblastic leukemia. J Pediatr 1980; 96:569.

INDEX

Note: Page numbers in *italics* refer to illustrations; page numbers followed by t refer to tables.

ISBN 0-7216-4463-5

18